DIAGNOSIS AND TREATMENT IN INTERNAL MEDICINE

T0177928

DIAGNOSIS AND TREATMENT IN INTERNAL MEDICINE

Edited by

Patrick Davey

Consultant Cardiologist, Northampton General Hospital NHS Trust, Northampton, UK

David Sprigings

Formerly Consultant Physician, Northampton General Hospital NHS Trust, Northampton, UK

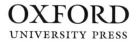

OXFORD
UNIVERSITY PRESS

OXFORD
UNIVERSITY PRESS

Great Clarendon Street, Oxford, OX2 6DP,
United Kingdom

Oxford University Press is a department of the University of Oxford.
It furthers the University's objective of excellence in research, scholarship,
and education by publishing worldwide. Oxford is a registered trade mark of
Oxford University Press in the UK and in certain other countries

© Oxford University Press 2018

The moral rights of the authors have been asserted

First Edition published in 2018

Impression: 1

All rights reserved. No part of this publication may be reproduced, stored in
a retrieval system, or transmitted, in any form or by any means, without the
prior permission in writing of Oxford University Press, or as expressly permitted
by law, by licence or under terms agreed with the appropriate reprographics
rights organization. Enquiries concerning reproduction outside the scope of the
above should be sent to the Rights Department, Oxford University Press, at the
address above

You must not circulate this work in any other form
and you must impose this same condition on any acquirer

Published in the United States of America by Oxford University Press
198 Madison Avenue, New York, NY 10016, United States of America

British Library Cataloguing in Publication Data

Data available

Library of Congress Control Number: 2018941300

ISBN 978–0–19–956874–1

Printed and bound in China by
C&C Offset Printing Co., Ltd.

Oxford University Press makes no representation, express or implied, that the
drug dosages in this book are correct. Readers must therefore always check
the product information and clinical procedures with the most up-to-date
published product information and data sheets provided by the manufacturers
and the most recent codes of conduct and safety regulations. The authors and
the publishers do not accept responsibility or legal liability for any errors in the
text or for the misuse or misapplication of material in this work. Except where
otherwise stated, drug dosages and recommendations are for the non-pregnant
adult who is not breast-feeding

Links to third party websites are provided by Oxford in good faith and
for information only. Oxford disclaims any responsibility for the materials
contained in any third party website referenced in this work.

Preface

Diagnosis and Treatment in Internal Medicine came about through our experience on the acute medical take. Here, sick patients present in large numbers with a vast range of problems. What all patients need, as the bedrock of management, is a differential diagnosis, and the central aim of our book is to help doctors formulate this. We asked experts in their field to provide succinct and authoritative guidance across the breadth of internal medicine. The assessment of symptoms or presenting problems is a major element of the book, but there is also comprehensive coverage of disorders of the body systems, including psychological aspects and palliative care. Chapters are structured so that key information can rapidly be found. Doctors need a broad perspective on health and its promotion, and there are sections addressing nutrition, lifestyle, and prevention of disease.

This book approaches medicine from the patient's perspective, through the stories that patients tell us about their illness, and provides the knowledge that turns these narratives into diagnoses, treatment, health, and longevity. Throughout, our focus has been on meeting the needs of doctors in the clinic, in the emergency department, or on the ward.

Our eternal thanks go out to our contributors. Some 200 outstanding doctors have produced admirably compact and lucid chapters. Throughout the lengthy gestation of the book, we have been ably supported by the staff at Oxford University Press, who have encouraged us and orchestrated the project. All praise should be directed to the authors, and any mistakes are ours. Please do let us have your suggestions for improvements (you can contact us at david.sprigings@gmail.com and pftame@gmail.com).

Patrick Davey
David Sprigings

Contents

PART 1 THE APPROACH TO THE PATIENT

PART 2 ASSESSMENT OF SYMPTOMS AND PRESENTING PROBLEMS

PART 3 CARDIOVASCULAR DISORDERS

PART 4 RESPIRATORY DISORDERS

PART 5 INTENSIVE CARE MEDICINE

PART 6 DISORDERS OF THE KIDNEY AND URINARY TRACT, AND ELECTROLYTE AND METABOLIC DISORDERS

PART 7 DIABETES MELLITUS AND ENDOCRINE DISORDERS

PART 8 GASTROINTESTINAL DISORDERS

CONTENTS

PART 9 DISORDERS OF THE LIVER

PART 10 NEUROLOGICAL DISORDERS

PART 11 DISORDERS OF THE SKIN

CONTENTS

Normal values

Common haematology values	
Haemoglobin	men: 130–180 g/l
	women: 115–160 g/l
Mean cell volume, MCV	76–96 fl
Platelets	150–400 × 10⁹/l
White cells (total)	4–11 × 10⁹/l
• neutrophils	40%–75%
• lymphocytes	20%–45%
• eosinophils	1%–6%
Blood gases	
pH	7.35–7.45
PaO₂	>10.6 kPa (75–100 mm Hg)
PaCO₂	4.7–6 kPa (35–45 mm Hg)
Base excess	±2 mmol/l
U&ES (urea and electrolytes)	
Sodium	135–145 mmol/l
Potassium	3.5–5 mmol/l
Creatinine	70–120 µmol/l
Urea	2.5–6.7 mmol/l
eGFR	>90
LFTs (liver function tests)	
Bilirubin	3–17 µmol/l
Alanine aminotransferase, ALT	5–35 IU/l
Aspartate transaminase, AST	5–35 IU/l
Alkaline phosphatase, ALP	30–150 IU/l (non-pregnant adults)
Albumin	35–50 g/l
Protein (total)	60–80 g/l
Cardiac enzymes	
Troponin T	<0.1 µg/l
Creatine kinase	25–195 IU/l
Lactate dehydrogenase, LDH	70–250 IU/l
Lipids and other biochemical values	
Cholesterol	<5 mmol/l desired
Triglycerides	0.5–1.9 mmol/l
Amylase	0–180 Somogyi U/dl
C-reactive protein, CRP	<10 mg/l
Calcium (total)	2.12–2.65 mmol/l
Glucose, fasting	3.5–5.5 mmol/l
Prostate-specific antigen, PSA	0–4 ng/ml
T4 (total thyroxine)	70–140 mmol/l
Thyroid-stimulating hormone, TSH	0.5–5.7 mU/l

Abbreviations: eGFR, estimated glomerular filtration rate; PaCO₂, partial pressure of carbon dioxide in arterial blood; PaO₂, partial pressure of oxygen in arterial blood.

Reproduced from M Longmore and IB Wilkinson et al., *Oxford Handbook of Clinical Medicine, Ninth Edition*, 2014, with permission from Oxford University Press

Abbreviations

γGT	gamma-glutamyl transferase	ALL	acute lymphocytic leukaemia
5-ASA	5-aminosalicylic acid	ALP	alkaline phosphatase
6MP	6-mercaptopurine	ALS	amyotrophic lateral sclerosis
AA	AA protein-related renal amyloidosis	ALT	alanine aminotransferase
AAA	abdominal aortic aneurysm	AMA	anti-mitochondrial antibody
AAFB	acid- and alcohol-fast bacteria	AMD	age-related macular degeneration
AASV	antineutrophil cytoplasmic antibody-associated systemic vasculitis	AMI	acute myocardial infarction
		AML	acute myeloid leukaemia
Ab	antibody	AMP	adenosine monophosphate
ABC	Airway, Breathing, and Circulation	ANA	antinuclear antibody
ABCDE	Airway, Breathing, Circulation, Disability, and Exposure	ANC	absolute neutrophil count
		ANCA	antineutrophil cytoplasmic antibody
ABG	arterial blood gas	ANS	alcohol nurse specialist
ABP	arterial blood pressure	anti-dsDNA	anti-double-stranded DNA antibody
ABPA	allergic bronchopulmonary aspergillosis	anti-HBc	antibody to the hepatitis B core antigen
ABPI	ankle–brachial pressure index	anti-HBe	antibody to the hepatitis B e antigen
ABPM	ambulatory blood-pressure monitoring	anti-HBs	antibody to the hepatitis B surface antigen
AC	air conduction	anti-LKM	anti-liver kidney microsomal type 1 antibody
ACD	anaemia of chronic disorders	anti-LPA	anti-liver–pancreas antigen antibody
ACE	angiotensin-converting enzyme	anti-SLA	anti-soluble liver antigen antibody
ACE-I	angiotensin converting-enzyme inhibitor	anti-SMA	smooth muscle antibody
ACPA	anti-citrullinated protein/peptide antibody	anti-TNF	anti-tumour necrosis factor
ACR	albumin–creatinine ratio	ANZDATA	Australia and New Zealand Dialysis and Transplant Registry
ACS	acute coronary syndrome		
ACT	activated clotting time	APACHE	Acute Physiology and Chronic Health Evaluation
ACTH	adrenocorticotropic hormone	APC	activated protein C
AD	autosomal dominant	APKD	adult polycystic kidney disease
ADA	adenosine deaminase	APS	antiphospholipid syndrome
ADC	apparent diffusion coefficient	APTT	activated partial thromboplastin time
ADH	antidiuretic hormone	APTTr	activated partial thromboplastin time ratio
ADP	adenosine diphosphate	AR	autosomal recessive
ADT	androgen deprivation therapy	ARB	angiotensin II receptor blocker
AEIPF	acute exacerbation of idiopathic pulmonary fibrosis	ARDS	acute respiratory distress syndrome
AF	atrial fibrillation	ARF	acute renal failure
AFB	acid-fast bacilli	ARPKD	autosomal recessive polycystic kidney disease
AH	atrium–His	ARR	aldosterone:renin activity ratio
AHF	acute heart failure	ARSAC	Administration of Radioactive Substances Advisory Committee
AHI	apnoea hypopnoea index		
AI	adrenal insufficiency	ART	antiretroviral therapy
AIDS	acquired immune deficiency syndrome	ARVC	arrhythmogenic right ventricular cardiomyopathy
AIH	autoimmune hepatitis	ARVC/D	arrhythmogenic right ventricular cardiomyopathy/dysplasia
AIN	anal intra-epithelial neoplasia		
AION	anterior ischaemic optic neuropathy	AS	ankylosing spondylitis
AIP	autoimmune pancreatitis	ASAS	Assessment of SpondyloArthritis International Society
AIVR	accelerated idioventricular rhythm		
AJCC	American Joint Committee on Cancer	ASD	atrial septal defect
AKI	acute kidney injury	AST	aspartate aminotransferase
AL	amyloid light chain	AT	antithrombin
ALA	amoebic liver abscess	ATG	antithymocyte globulin
ALD	alcoholic liver disease	ATL	adult T-cell leukaemia
ALERT	Acute Life-threatening Events Recognition and Treatment	ATN	acute tubulointerstitial nephritis
		ATP	adenosine triphosphate
ALF	acute liver failure	AUDIT	Alcohol Use Disorders Identification Test

AV	atrioventricular		CCF	congestive cardiac failure
aVF	augmented voltage unipolar left foot lead		CCP	cyclic citrullinated peptide
AVIR	accelerated idioventricular rhythm		CCS	Canadian Cardiovascular Society
aVL	augmented voltage unipolar left arm lead		CD	Crohn's disease
AVN	atrioventricular node		CDC	Centers for Disease Control
AVNRT	atrioventricular nodal re-entrant tachycardia		CDI	cranial diabetes insipidus
AVP	arginine vasopressin		CF	counting fingers
AVPU	Alert, Voice, Pain, or Unresponsive		CGD	chronic granulomatous disease
AVRT	atrioventricular re-entrant tachycardia		CHD	coronary heart disease
AVSD	atrioventricular septal defect		CHF	congestive heart failure
AZA	azathioprine		CI	confidence interval
BAE	bronchial artery angiography and embolization		CIDP	chronic inflammatory demyelinating polyradiculoneuropathy
BAL	bronchoalveolar lavage		CIPO	chronic idiopathic pseudo-obstruction
BC	bone conduction		CIS	carcinoma in situ
BCC	basal cell carcinoma		CJD	Creutzfeldt–Jakob disease
BCLC	Barcelona Clinic Liver Cancer		CK	creatine kinase
BCNIE	blood culture-negative infective endocarditis		CKD	chronic kidney disease
BCP	basic calcium phosphates		CLL	chronic lymphoid leukaemia
BCR	B-cell receptor		CMAP	compound muscle action potential
BCT	broad-complex tachycardia		CMC	carpometacarpal
BD	brain death		CML	chronic myeloid leukaemia
BDD	body dysmorphic disorder		CMRI	cardiac magnetic resonance imaging
BI	bacterial index		CMT	Charcot–Marie–Tooth disease
BIMA	bilateral internal mammary artery		CMV	cytomegalovirus
BIPAP	bi-level positive airway pressure		CNS	central nervous system
BIPSS	bilateral inferior petrosal sinus sampling		COCP	combined oral contraceptive pill
BMD	bone mineral density		COP	cryptogenic organizing pneumonia
BMI	body mass index		COPD	chronic obstructive pulmonary disease
BMRC	British Medical Research Council		CPAP	continuous positive airways pressure
BMT	bone marrow transplantation		CPB	cardiopulmonary bypass
BNP	brain natriuretic peptide		CPEX	cardiopulmonary exercise testing
BO	Barrett's oesophagus		CPP	combined physical and psychological programme
BP	blood pressure		CPPD	calcium pyrophosphate dihydrate deposition
BPH	benign prostatic hypertrophy		CrAG	cryptococcal antigen
bpm	beats per minute		CRAO	central retinal artery occlusion
BPPV	benign paroxysmal positional vertigo		CRF	clinical risk factor for parental hip fracture
BRAO	branch retinal artery occlusion		CRH	corticotrophin-releasing hormone
BRF	bone risk factor		CRP	C-reactive protein
BrS	Brugada syndrome		CRT	cardiac resynchronization therapy
BRVO	branch retinal vein occlusion		CRVO	central retinal vein occlusion
BSA	body surface area		CS	corticosteroid
BSD	brainstem death		CSF	cerebrospinal fluid
BSE	bovine spongiform encephalopathy		CSH	carotid sinus hypersensitivity
BSG	British Society of Gastroenterology		CSM	carotid sinus massage
BTS	British Thoracic Society		CT	computed tomography
CABG	coronary artery bypass graft surgery		CTA	computed tomography angiography
CAD	coronary artery disease		CTD	connective tissues disease
CADASIL	cerebral autosomal dominant arteriopathy with subcortical infarcts and leucoencephalopathy		CTEPH	chronic thromboembolic pulmonary hypertension
CAH	congenital adrenal hyperplasia		CTPA	computed tomography pulmonary angiography
CAM	Confusion Assessment Method		CVA	cerebral vascular accident
cANCA	cytoplasmic antineutrophil cytoplasmic antibody		CVD	cardiovascular disease
CAP	community-acquired pneumonia		CVID	common variable immunodeficiency
CaSR	calcium-sensing receptor		CVP	central venous pressure
CBCD	chronic bullous disease of childhood		CVPT	catecholaminergic polymorphic ventricular tachycardia
CBD	common bile duct		CWS	cotton-wool spot
CBG	cortisol-binding globulin		CXR	chest X-ray
CBT	cognitive behavioural therapy		CYC	cyclophosphamide
CBZ	carbimazole		DA	dermatitis artefacta
CCB	calcium-channel blocker			

DADS	distal acquired demyelinating symmetrical
DAH	diffuse alveolar haemorrhage
DAS	Disease Activity Score
DAT	drug action team
DBS	deep brain stimulation
DCM	dilated cardiomyopathy
DEXA	dual-energy X-ray absorptiometry
DF	Maddrey discriminant function
DHEA	dehydroepiandrosterone
DHEAS	dehydroepiandrosterone sulphate
DI	diabetes incipidus
DIC	disseminated intravascular coagulopathy
DILD	drug-induced lung disease
DILS	diffuse infiltrative lymphocytosis syndrome
DIP	distal interphalangeal
DIS	dissemination in space
DIT	dissemination in time;
DLCO	diffusing capacity of the lung for carbon monoxide
DLE	discoid lupus erythematosus
DM	diabetes mellitus
DMARD	disease-modifying anti-rheumatic drug
DOT	directly observed therapy
DPP-4	dipeptidyl peptidase-4
DRE	digital rectal examination
dsDNA	double-stranded DNA
DSE	dobutamine stress echocardiography
DST	dexamethasone suppression test
DU	duodenal ulcer
DVLA	Driver and Vehicle Licensing Agency
DVP	diastolic blood pressure
DVT	deep-vein thrombosis
DWI	diffusion-weighted imaging
EBUS-TBNA	endobronchial ultrasound-guided transbronchial needle aspiration
EBV	Epstein–Barr virus
ECG	electrocardiogram
Echo	echocardiography
ECOG	Eastern Cooperative Oncology Group
EDTA	ethylenediamine tetra-acetic acid
EEG	electroencephalogram
EGDT	early goal-directed therapy
eGFR	estimated glomerular function rate
EHEC	enterohaemorrhagic *Escherichia coli*
EIA	enzyme immunoassay
ELISA	enzyme-linked immunosorbent assay
EMG	electromyography
ENA	extractable nuclear antigen antibody
ENT	ear, nose, and throat
EOTR	end-of-treatment response
EPAP	expiratory positive airway pressure
EPO	erythropoietin
EPP	erythropoietic protoporphyria
ePPi	extracellular pyrophosphate
EPR	electronic patient record
EPS	electrophysiological study
ERCP	endoscopic retrograde cholangiopancreatography
EROA	effective regurgitant orifice area
ESC	European Society of Cardiology
ESR	erythrocyte sedimentation rate
ESRD	end-stage renal disease

ET	essential tremor
EUA	examination under anaesthesia
EUS	endoscopic ultrasound
FAP	familial amyloid polyneuropathy
FAST	Face Arm Speech Test
FBC	full blood count
FDA	Food and Drug Administration
FDG	fluorodeoxyglucose
FDP	fibrinogen degradation products
FEV_1	forced expiratory volume in 1 second
FFA	free fatty acid
FFR	fractional flow reserve
FFS	five-factor score
FHH	familial hypocalciuric hypercalcaemia
FI	faecal incontinence
FiO_2	inspired fraction of oxygen
FISH	fluorescent in situ hybridization
FLAIR	fluid attenuated inversion recovery
FLI	fatty liver index
FNAC	fine-needle aspiration cytology
FOB	faecal occult blood
FSGS	focal segmental glomerulosclerosis
FSH	follicle-stimulating hormone
FTD	frontotemporal dementia
FUO	fever of unknown origin
FVC	forced vital capacity
FVL	factor V Leiden
FXTAS	fragile X-associated tremor/ataxia syndrome
G1	Genotype 1
G2	Genotype 2
G3	Genotype 3
G6PD	glucose-6-phosphate dehydrogenase
GA	general anaesthesia
GABA	gamma-aminobutyric acid
GAD	glutamic acid decarboxylase
GAD65	glutamic acid decarboxylase autoantibody
GALT	gut-associated lymphoid tissue
GAS	Group A streptococcus
GBM	glomerular basement membrane
GBS	Guillain–Barré syndrome
GCA	giant cell arteritis
GCS	Glasgow Coma Scale
GFR	glomerular filtration rate
GGO	ground-glass opacity
GH	growth hormone
GI	gastrointestinal
GIST	gastrointestinal stromal tumour
GMC	General Medical Council
GN	glomerulonephritis
GnRH	gonadotropin-releasing hormone
GOLD	Global Initiative for Chronic Obstructive Lung Disease
GORD	gastro-oesophageal reflux disease
GOS	Glasgow Outcome Score
GP	general practitioner
GPA	granulomatosis with polyangiitis
GPI	glycosyl-phosphatidylinositol
GRA	glucocorticoid-responsive aldosteronism
GU	gastric ulcer
GUM	genito-urinary medicine

GvHD	graft-vs-host disease
HAART	highly active antiretroviral therapy
HAP	hospital-acquired pneumonia
HAS	human albumin solution
HAV	hepatitis A virus
Hb A	adult haemoglobin
Hb A1c	haemoglobin A1c (glycosylated haemoglobin)
Hb F	fetal haemoglobin
Hb	haemoglobin
HBc	hepatitis B core protein
HBeAg	hepatitis B e antigen
HBPM	home blood-pressure monitoring
HBsAg	hepatitis B surface antigen
HBV	hepatitis B virus
HCC	hepatocellular carcinoma
HCM	hypertrophic cardiomyopathy
HCV	hepatitis C virus
HD	Huntington's disease
HDL	high-density lipoprotein
HDU	high-dependency units
HDV	hepatitis D virus
HER2	human epidermal growth factor receptor 2
HEV	hepatitis E virus
HF	heart failure
HFmrEF	heart failure with mid-range ejection fraction
HFpEF	heart failure with preserved ejection fraction
HFrEF	heart failure with reduced ejection fraction
HHT	hereditary haemorrhagic telangiectasia
HHV6	human herpes virus 6
HHV7	human herpes virus 7
HHV8	human herpes virus 8
HIFU	high-intensity focused ultrasound
HIGM	hyperimmunoglobulin M
HIT	heparin-induced thrombocytopenia
HIV	human immunodeficiency virus
HLA	human leukocyte antigen
HM	hand movements
HMW	high molecular weight
HNPCC	hereditary non-polyposis colorectal cancer
HNPP	hereditary neuropathy with liability to pressure palsies
HPA	hypothalamic–pituitary–adrenal
HPIV	human parainfluenza virus
HPV	human papilloma virus
HRA	Human Rights Act 1998
HRCT	high-resolution computed tomography
HRS	hepatorenal syndrome
HS	hereditary spherocytosis
HSCT	haemopoietic stem cell transplantation
HSP	Henoch–Schönlein purpura
HSV	herpes simplex virus
HTLV1	human T-lymphotrophic virus 1
HUS	haemolytic–uraemic syndrome
HUV	hypocomplementaemic urticarial vasculitis
HV	His–ventricle
IA2	islet antigen 2 autoantibody
IAA	insulin autoantibody
IABP	intra-aortic balloon pump
IAH	intra-abdominal hypertension
IAP	intra-abdominal pressure
IBA	identification and brief advice

IBD	inflammatory bowel disease
IBS	irritable bowel syndrome
IC	intermittent claudication
ICA	islet cell autoantibody
$I_{Ca,L}$	L-type calcium current
ICD	implantable cardioverter defibrillator
ICH	intracranial haemorrhage
ICP	intracranial pressure
ICU	intensive care unit
ID	infectious disease
IDL	intermediate-density lipoprotein
IDU	intravenous drug users
IE	infective endocarditis
IFD	invasive fungal disease
IFN	interferon
IFN-alpha	interferon alpha
IgA	immunoglobulin A
IgE	immunoglobulin E
IgG	immunoglobulin G
IgM	immunoglobulin M
IGRA	interferon gamma release assays
IHD	ischaemic heart disease
I_{K1}	inward rectifier potassium current
I_{Kr}	rapidly activating component of the delayed rectifier potassium current
I_{Ks}	slowly activating component of the delayed rectifier potassium channel
IL	interleukin
IL-6	interleukin 6
ILD	interstitial lung disease
IM	intramuscular
IMD	inherited metabolic disease
IMIg	intramuscular immunoglobulin
IMPACT	Ill Medical Patients' Acute Care and Treatment
I_{Na}	sodium current
$I_{Na,K}$	sodium–potassium pump current
I_{NCX}	sodium-calcium exchanger current
INR	international normalized ratio
IPAP	inspiratory positive airway pressure
IPD	idiopathic Parkinson's disease
IPF	idiopathic pulmonary fibrosis
IPG	implantable pulse generator
IPI	International Prognostic Index
IPJ	interphalangeal joint
IRIS	immune reconstitution inflammatory syndrome
IRRT	intermittent renal replacement therapy
IRT	immunoreactive trypsinogen
ISS	International Staging System
IST	inappropriate sinus tachycardia
ITP	immune thrombocytopenia
ITT	insulin tolerance test
ITU	intensive therapy unit
IUD	intrauterine device
IV	intravenous
IVC	inferior vena cava
IVDU	intravenous drug use
IVF	in vitro fertilization
IVIg	intravenous immunoglobulin
IVUS	intravascular ultrasound
JVP	jugular venous pulse

KCO	carbon monoxide transfer coefficient	MDS	myelodysplasia
KDIGO	Kidney Disease: Improving Global Outcomes	MDT	multidisciplinary team
KEEP	Kidney Early Evaluation Program	MELAS	mitochondrial encephalomyopathy with lactic acidosis and stroke-like episodes
KS	Kaposi's sarcoma	MELD	Model for End-Stage Liver Disease
KSHV	Kaposi's sarcoma-associated herpesvirus	MEN	multiple endocrine neoplasia
LACS	lacunar stroke	MERRF	myoclonic epilepsy with ragged red fibres
LAD	left anterior descending	MG	myasthenia gravis
LAE	left atrial enlargement	MGUS	monoclonal gammopathy of unknown significance
LAVAT	local anaesthetic video-assisted thoracoscopy	MHC	major histocompatibility complex
LBBB	left bundle branch block	MHRA	Medicines and Healthcare Products Regulatory Agency
LBC	liquid-based cytology	MI	myocardial infarction
LBD	Lewy body dementia	MIC	minimum inhibitory concentration
LBP	low back pain	MM	malignant melanoma
LCIS	lobular carcinoma in situ	MMA	methylmalonic acidaemia
LCSD	left cervicothoracic sympathetic denervation	MMR	measles, mumps, rubella
LCX	left circumflex artery	MMSE	Mini-Mental State Examination
LDCT	low-dose computed tomography	MND	motor neuron disease
LDH	lactate dehydrogenase	MOAI	monoamine oxidase inhibitor
LDL	low-density lipoprotein	MODY	maturity-onset diabetes of the young
LEMS	Lambert–Eaton myasthenia syndrome	MOF	multi-organ failure
LET	linear-energy transfer	MPO	myeloperoxidase
LFT	liver function test	MPS	myocardial perfusion scan
LH	luteinizing hormone	MR	mitral regurgitation
LIMA	left internal mammary artery	MRA	magnetic resonance angiography
LMN	lower motor neuron	MRA	magnetic resonance angiography
LMWH	low-molecular-weight heparin	MRC	Medical Research Council
LN	lymph node	MRCP	magnetic resonance cholangiopancreatography
LOS	lower oesophageal sphincter	MRI	magnetic resonance imaging
LP	lumbar puncture	MRSA	meticillin-resistant *Staphylococcus aureus*
LPA	Lasting Power of Attorney	MRV	magnetic resonance venography
LPP	lichen planopilaris	MS	multiple sclerosis
LQTS	long-QT syndrome	MSE	mental state examination
LR	likelihood ratio	MSF	Mediterranean spotted fever
LSMDT	local skin cancer multidisciplinary team	MSM	men who have sex with men
LT	leukotriene	MSU	monosodium urate
LTBI	latent infection with *Mycobacterium tuberculosis*	MSUD	maple syrup urine disease
LTNP	long-term non-progressor	MTP	metatarsophalangeal
LV	left ventricular	MTX	methotrexate
LVAD	left ventricular assist device	MUP	minimum unit price
LVEF	left ventricular ejection fraction	MuSK	muscle-specific kinase
LVESD	left ventricular end-systolic diameter	MUST	Malnutrition Universal Screening Tool
LVH	left ventricular hypertrophy	NAAT	nucleic acid amplification test
LVNC	left ventricular non-compaction	NAC	N-acetylcysteine
LVOT	left ventricular outflow tract	NAD	nicotinamide adenine dinucleotide
LVRS	lung volume reduction surgery	NADPH	nicotinamide adenine dinucleotide phosphate
MAC	*Mycobacterium avium* complex	NAFLD	non-alcoholic fatty liver disease
MALT	mucosa-associated lymphoid tissue	NAPQI	N-acetyl-p-benzoquinone imine
MAP	mean arterial pressure	NASH	non-alcoholic steatohepatitis
MAT	multifocal atrial tachycardia	NCRN	National Cancer Research Network
MBL	mannan-binding-lectin	NCS	nerve conduction study
MCA	middle cerebral artery	NEWS	National Early Warning Score
MCandS	microscopy, culture, and sensitivities	NFD	nephrogenic fibrosing dermopathy
MCBT	mindfulness-based cognitive therapy	NGT	nasogastric tube
MCH	mean cell haemoglobin	NHL	non-Hodgkin's lymphoma
MCHC	mean cell haemoglobin concentration	NICE	National Institute for Health and Care Excellence
MCI	mild cognitive impairment	NIHL	noise-induced hearing loss
MCP	metacarpophalangeal	NIHSS	National Institutes of Health Stroke Scale
MCV	mean corpuscular volume	NIPPV	nasal intermittent positive pressure ventilation
MDM	multidisciplinary meeting		
MDR	multidrug-resistant		

NIV	non-invasive ventilation	PET	positron emission tomography
NK	natural killer	PEX	plasma exchange
NMO	neuromyelitis optica	PFT	pulmonary function testing
NMS	neuroleptic malignant syndrome	PG	prostaglandin
NP	nosocomial pneumonia	PH	pulmonary hypertension
NPL	no perception of light	PHT	pressure half-time
NRH	nodular regenerative hyperplasia	PI	pancreatic insufficiency
NRT	nicotine replacement therapy	PIP	proximal interphalangeal
NS	nephrotic syndrome	PISA	proximal isovelocity surface area
NSAID	non-steroidal anti-inflammatory drug	PJP	*Pneumocystis jiroveci* pneumonia
NSCLC	non-small cell lung carcinoma	PJRT	persistent junctional reciprocating tachycardia
NSLBP	non-specific low back pain	PK	pyruvate kinase
NSTEMI	non-ST-elevation myocardial infarction	PKU	phenylketonuria
NSVT	non-sustained ventricular tachycardia	PL	perception of light
NTA	National Treatment Authority	PLAX	parasternal long-axis view
NTG	glyceryl trinitrate (nitroglycerin)	PLE	polymorphic light eruption
NTM	non-tuberculous mycobacteria	PLMS	periodic leg movements during sleep
NT-pro-BNP	N-terminal brain natriuretic peptide	PLS	primary lateral sclerosis
NYHA	New York Heart Association	PML	progressive multifocal leucoencephalopathy
OA	osteoarthritis	PML	progressive multifocal leukoencephalopathy
OAC	oral anticoagulation	PMN	polymorphonuclear
OCP	oral contraceptive pill	PMT	pacemaker-mediated tachycardia
OCSP	Oxfordshire Community Stroke Project	PNH	paroxysmal nocturnal haemoglobinuria
ODI	oxygen desaturation index	PNS	peripheral nervous system
OGD	oesophagogastroduodenoscopy	POF	premature ovarian failure
OHS	obesity hypoventilation syndrome	POI	premature ovarian insufficiency
OLM	ocular larva migrans	POTS	postural tachycardia syndrome
ONJ	osteonecrosis of the jaw	PPH	primary pulmonary hypertension
OPSI	overwhelming post-splenectomy infection	PPI	proton-pump inhibitor
OSA	obstructive sleep apnoea	PPM	permanent pacemaker
PABA	para-aminobenzoic acid	PPMS	primary progressive multiple sclerosis
PACNS	primary angiitis of the central nervous system	PPV	polysaccharide pneumococcal vaccine
$PaCO_2$	partial pressure of carbon dioxide in arterial blood	pred.	predicted
PAH	pulmonary arterial hypertension	PRES	posterior reversible encephalopathy syndrome
PAI	primary adrenal insufficiency	PRR	pattern recognition receptors
PAMP	pathogen-associated molecular patterns	PS	performance status
pANCA	perinuclear antineutrophil cytoplasmic antibody	PSA	prostate-specific antigen
PAO_2	partial pressure of alveolar oxygen	PsA	psoriatic arthritis
PaO_2	partial pressure of oxygen in arterial blood	PSAX	parasternal short-axis view
PAT	Paddington Alcohol Test	PSC	primary sclerosing cholangitis
PBC	primary biliary cholangitis	PSP	primary spontaneous pneumothorax
PC_{20}	the provocative concentration required to cause a 20% fall in the forced expiratory volume in 1 second	PT	prothrombin time
		PTA	pure tone audiogram
PCI	percutaneous coronary intervention	PTCA	percutaneous transluminal coronary angioplasty
PCO_2	partial pressure of carbon dioxide	PTH	parathyroid hormone
PCOS	polycystic ovary syndrome	PTU	propylthiouracil
PCP	pneumocystis pneumonia	PUD	peptic ulcer disease
PCR	polymerase chain reaction	PUJ	pelvic–ureteric junction
PCT	porphyria cutanea tarda	PUO	pyrexia of unknown origin
PCV	pneumococcal conjugate vaccine	PUVA	psoralen plus ultraviolet light A
PD	Parkinson's disease	PVC	premature ventricular complex
PDA	patent ductus arteriosus	PVE	prosthetic valve endocarditis
PE	pulmonary embolus	PVL	Panton–Valentine leukocidin
PEA	pulseless electrical activity	PVT	portal vein thrombosis
PEEP	positive end-expiratory pressure	RA	rheumatoid arthritis
PEFR	peak expiratory flow rate	RAPD	relative afferent pupillary defect
PEG	percutaneous endoscopic gastrostomy	RAS	reticular activating system
PEG-IFNα	pegylated interferon alpha	RAST	radioallergosorbent testing
PEI	percutaneous ethanol injection	RBBB	right bundle branch block
PEM	protein-energy malnutrition	RBC	red blood cell

RBV	ribavirin	SPECT	single-photon emission computed tomography
RCC	red-cell count	SQTS	short-QT syndrome
RCM	restrictive cardiomyopathy	SRH	stigmata of recent haemorrhage
RCT	randomized control trial	SSP	secondary spontaneous pneumothorax
RDT	rapid diagnostic test	SSRI	selective serotonin reuptake inhibitor
REM	rapid-eye-movement	ssRNA	single-stranded RNA
RF	rheumatoid factor	SSSS	staphylococcal scalded skin syndrome
RFA	radiofrequency ablation	STD	sexually transmitted disease
RIP	Riyadh Intensive Care Programme	STEMI	ST-elevation myocardial infarction
RIPA	ristocetin-induced platelet aggregation	STI	sexually transmitted infection
RNP	ribonucleoprotein	STIR	short T1 inversion recovery
RNS	repetitive nerve stimulation	SUA	serum uric acid
ROSIER	Recognition of Stroke In the Emergency Room	SUDEP	sudden unexpected death in epilepsy
RPGN	rapidly progressive glomerulonephritis	SUNCT	short-lasting neuralgiform headache with conjunctival injection and tearing
RR	relative risk	SV40	simian virus 40
RRT	renal replacement therapy	SVC	superior vena cava
RS	reactive site	SVR	sustained virologic response
RSV	respiratory syncytial virus	SVT	supraventricular tachycardia
RTA	road traffic accident	SWEDD	subjects without evidence of dopaminergic deficits
RUQ	right upper quadrant	T3	triiodothyronine
RV	right ventricular	T4	thyroxine
RVAD	right ventricular assist device	TAA	thoracic aortic aneurysm
RVOT	right ventricular outflow tract	TACE	trans-arterial chemo-embolization
RVOTO	right ventricular outflow tract obstruction	TB	tuberculosis
SAA	serum amyloid A protein	TBG	thyroxine-binding globulin
SAAG	serum–ascites albumin gradient	TBNA	transbronchial needle aspiration
SAB	*Staphylococcus aureus* bacteraemia	TCA	tricyclic antidepressant
SAECG	signal-averaged electrocardiogram	TCR	T-cell receptor
SAH	subarachnoid haemorrhage	TdP	torsades de pointes
SAI	secondary adrenal insufficiency	TE	thromboembolism
SALT	speech and language therapists	TFPI	tissue factor pathway inhibitor
SaO$_2$	arterial oxygen saturation	TFT	thyroid function test
SAPS	Simplified Acute Physiology Score	TGA	transposition of the great arteries
SARS	severe acute respiratory syndrome	Th	T helper
SBP	systolic blood pressure	Th2	T-helper type 2
SCA	sudden cardiac arrest	TIA	transient ischaemic attack
SCC	squamous cell carcinoma	TIN	tubulointerstitial nephritis
SCD	sudden cardiac death	TINU	tubulointerstitial disease with uveitis
SCID	severe combined immune deficiency	TIPS	transjugular intra-hepatic portosystemic shunt
SCLC	small cell lung carcinoma	TK	tyrosine kinase
SCLE	subacute cutaneous lupus erythematosus	TKI	tyrosine kinase inhibitor
ScvO$_2$	central venous oxygen saturation	TLC	total lung capacity
SD	standard deviation	TLCO	transfer factor for carbon monoxide
SF	synovial fluid	TLoC	transient loss of consciousness
SHBG	sex hormone-binding globulin	TLR	Toll-like receptor
SIADH	syndrome of inappropriate antidiuretic hormone excretion	TLS	tumour lysis syndrome
SIRS	systemic inflammatory response syndrome	TM	tympanic membrane
SIV	simian immunodeficiency virus	TNFα	tumour necrosis factor alpha
SLE	systemic lupus erythematosus	TNM	tumour, node, and metastases
SLNB	sentinel lymph node biopsy	TOE	transoesophageal echocardiography
SMA	smooth muscle antibody	TPMT	thiopurine methyltransferase
SMART	Specific, Measurable, Achievable, Realistic, and Timed	TPO	thyroid peroxidase
		TPR	total peripheral resistance
SMR	standard mortality ratio	TRH	thyrotropin-releasing hormone
SNHL	sensorineural hearing loss	TRUS	trans-rectal ultrasound
SNRT	sinus node re-entrant tachycardia	TSE	transmissible spongiform encephalopathy
SOD	sphincter of Oddi dysfunction	TSH	thyroid-stimulating hormone
SOFA	Sequential Organ Failure Assessment	TT	thrombin time
SOV	single-organ vasculitis	TTE	transthoracic echocardiography

TTP	thrombotic thrombocytopenic purpura		VC	vital capacity
TURBT	trans-urethral resection of bladder tumour		VCD	vocal cord dysfunction
TURP	trans-urethral resection of the prostate		VCLAD	very long-chain acyl-coenzyme A dehydrogenase deficiency
TWI	T-wave inversion		VDRL	Venereal Disease Research Laboratory
UA	undifferentiated arthritis		VEGF	vascular endothelial growth factor
U&E	urea and electrolytes		VF	ventricular fibrillation
UC	ulcerative colitis		VGCC	voltage-gated calcium channel
UCD	urea cycle disorder		VGKC	voltage-gated potassium channel complex
UDCA	ursodeoxycholic acid		VKA	vitamin K antagonist
UGIH	upper gastrointestinal haemorrhage		VLDL	very-low-density lipoprotein
UKPDS	UK Prospective Diabetes Study		VLM	visceral larva migrans
UKRR	UK Research Reserve		VOC	volatile organic compound
ULN	upper limit of normal		VPC	premature ventricular complex
ULT	urate-lowering therapy		VQ	ventilation–perfusion
UMN	upper motor neuron		VSD	ventricular septal defect
UNSCEAR	United Nations Scientific Committee on the Effects of Atomic Radiation		VT	ventricular tachycardia
URTI	upper respiratory tract infection		VTE	venous thromboembolism
USRDS	United States Renal Data System		VUJ	vesicoureteric junction
USS	ultrasound scan		VZV	varicella zoster virus
UTI	urinary tract infection		WBC	white blood cell
UUN	urinary urea nitrogen		WCC	white-cell count
UV	ultraviolet		WG	Wegener's granulomatosis (granulomatosis with polyangiitis)
UVA	ultraviolet light A		WG–MPA	Wegener's granulomatosis–microscopic polyangiitis
UVB	ultraviolet light B		WHO	World Health Organization
V_A	effective alveolar volume		WPW	Wolff–Parkinson–White syndrome
VaD	vascular dementia		XO	xanthine oxidase
VAD	ventricular assist devices		XP	xeroderma pigmentosum
VAP	ventilator-associated pneumonia			
VATS	video-assisted thoracoscopic surgery			

Contributors

Richard Abbott
Consultant Neurologist, Leicester Royal Infirmary, Leicester, UK

Yasir Abu-Omar
Consultant Cardiothoracic and Transplant Surgeon, Papworth Hospital, Papworth Everard, UK

Bhavyang Acharya
Consultant in Palliative Medicine, Cynthia Spencer Hospice, Northamptonshire Healthcare NHS Foundation Trust, Northampton, UK

David Adlam
Senior Lecturer in Acute and Interventional Cardiology and Honorary Consultant Cardiologist, University of Leicester, Leicester, UK

Joshua Agbetile
Consultant Respiratory Physician, Homerton University Hospital, London, UK

Daniel Ajzensztejn
Consultant Clinical Oncologist, Oxford University Hospitals NHS Foundation Trust, Oxford, UK

Raza Alikhan
Consultant Haematologist, University Hospital of Wales, Cardiff, UK

Rob Andrews
Associate Professor of Diabetes University of Exeter, Exeter, UK

Tim Anstiss
Member, British Psychological Society, and Fellow, Royal Society of Arts

Charles M. G. Archer
Specialist Registrar in Dermatology, Churchill Hospital Oxford, UK

Clive B. Archer
Consultant Dermatologist, Guy's and St Thomas' NHS Foundation Trust, London, UK

Richard Armstrong
Consultant Neurologist, Royal Berkshire NHS Foundation Trust, Reading, UK, and Oxford University Hospitals NHS Foundation Trust, Oxford, UK

Kaleab Asrress
St Thomas' Hospital, London, King's College London; Royal North Shore Hospital, University of Sydney, Australia

Stephen Aston
National Institute for Health Research Academic Clinical Lecturer in Infectious Diseases, University of Liverpool, Liverpool, UK

Mona Bafadhel
Consultant Respiratory Physician, Oxford University Hospitals NHS Foundation Trust, and Senior Clinical Researcher, University of Oxford, Oxford, UK

Fahd Baig
Clinical Research Fellow, University of Oxford, Oxford, UK

Peter G. Bain
Reader and Honorary Consultant in Clinical Neurology, Charing Cross Hospital, London, UK

Amitava Banerjee
Senior Clinical Lecturer in Clinical Data Science and Honorary Consultant Cardiologist, University College London, London, UK

Phil Barber
Consultant Respiratory Physician, University Hospital of South Manchester, Manchester, UK

Simon Barry
Consultant in Respiratory Medicine, University Hospital Llandough, Penarth, UK

Dirk Bäumer
Consultant Neurologist, Peterborough and Stamford Hospitals NHS Foundation Trust, Peterborough, UK

Mike Beadsworth
Consultant in Infectious Diseases and General Medicine, Royal Liverpool University Hospital, Liverpool, UK

Nick Beeching
Senior Lecturer and Honorary Consultant in Infectious Diseases, Liverpool School of Tropical Medicine and Royal Liverpool University Hospital, Liverpool, UK

Tony Bentley
Consultant Microbiologist, Northampton General Hospital NHS Trust, Northampton, UK

Anthony Bewley
Consultant Dermatologist, Barts Health NHS Trust, London, UK, and Honorary Senior Lecturer, University of London, London, UK

Kailash P. Bhatia
Professor of Clinical Neurology, University College London, London, UK, and Honorary Consultant Neurologist, National Hospital for Neurology and Neurosurgery, London, UK

Malini Bhole
Consultant Immunologist, The Dudley Group NHS Foundation Trust, Dudley, UK

Benjamin Bloch
Consultant Orthopaedic Surgeon, Nottingham University Hospitals NHS Trust, Nottingham, UK

James Bonnington
Consultant Intensivist, Nottingham University Hospital NHS Trust, Nottingham, UK

Ian Bowler
Consultant and Deputy Clinical Lead in Microbiology, John Radcliffe Hospital, Oxford, UK

Marilyn Bradley
Consultant Physician in Genitourinary Medicine, Royal Liverpool and Broadgreen University Hospitals NHS Trust, Liverpool, UK

Rowland J. Bright-Thomas
Consultant Respiratory Physician, University Hospital of South Manchester, Manchester, UK

Elaine Buchanan
Consultant Physiotherapist, Oxford University Hospitals NHS Foundation Trust, Oxford, UK

Chris Bunch
Consultant Physician and Clinical Haematologist, John Radcliffe Hospital, Oxford, UK

Sarah Cader
Consultant Neurologist, Basingstoke and North Hampshire Hospital, Basingstoke, UK

Caroline Cardy
Consultant Rheumatologist, Worcestershire Royal Hospital, Worcester, UK

Alan Carson
Consultant Neuropsychiatrist, NHS Lothian, Edinburgh, UK, and Reader, University of Edinburgh, Edinburgh, UK

Matteo Cella
Lecturer in Clinical Psychology, King's College London, London, UK

Aron Chakera
Consultant Nephrologist, Sir Charles Gairdner Hospital, Perth, Australia

Trudie Chalder
Professor of Cognitive Behavioural Psychotherapy, King's College London, London, UK

John Chambers
Professor of Clinical Cardiology and Consultant Cardiologist, Guy's and St Thomas' NHS Foundation Trust, London UK

Hannah Chapman
Specialist Registrar in Clinical Oncology, Mount Vernon Cancer Centre, Northwood, UK

Mas Chaponda
Consultant in Infectious Diseases and General Medicine, Royal Liverpool University Hospital, Liverpool, UK

Mimi Chen
Consultant Endocrinologist, St.George's University Hospitals Foundation NHS Trust, London, UK

Nigel Clayton
Senior Chief Clinical Physiologist, Wythenshawe Hospital, Manchester, UK

Sian Coggle
Consultant in Infectious Diseases and Acute Internal Medicine, Cambridge University Hospitals NHS Foundation Trust, Cambridge, UK

Graham Collins
Clinician Scientist, Imperial College, London, UK

Cris S. Constantinescu
Professor of Neurology and Consultant Neurologist, Nottingham University Hospital NHS Trust, Nottingham, UK

Graham Cooke
Reader Infectious Diseases, Imperial College, London, UK

Susan Cooper
Consultant Dermatologist and Honorary Senior Clinical Lecturer, Oxford University Hospitals NHS Foundation Trust, Oxford, UK

Lucy Cottle
Consultant Physician in Infectious Diseases, Leeds Teaching Hospitals NHS Trust, Leeds, UK

Anthony Cox
Senior Lecturer in Clinical Pharmacy and Drug Safety, University of Birmingham, Birmingham, UK

Sonya Craig
Consultant Respiratory and Sleep Physician, Aintree University Hospital, Liverpool, UK

Anjali Crawshaw
Consultant Respiratory Physician, Queen Elizabeth Hospital, University Hospitals Birmingham NHS Foundation Trust, Birmingham, UK

Paul Cullinan
Professor of Occupational and Environmental Respiratory Disease, National Heart and Lung Institute, Imperial College, London, UK

Nicola Curry
Consultant Haematologist, Churchill Hospital, Oxford, UK

David Cutter
Consultant Clinical Oncologist, Oxford University Hospitals NHS Foundation Trust, Oxford, UK

Adam Darowski
Consultant Physician, John Radcliffe Hospital, Oxford, UK, and Honorary Senior Lecturer, Oxford University, Oxford, UK

Parthajit Das
Consultant Rheumatologist, Kettering General Hospital NHS Foundation Trust, Kettering, UK

Patrick Davey
Consultant Cardiologist, Northampton General Hospital NHS Trust, Northampton, UK

Emily Davies
Consultant Dermatologist, Gloucestershire Royal Hospital, Gloucester, UK

Geraint Davies
Reader in Infection Pharmacology and Consultant in Infectious Diseases, University of Liverpool, Liverpool, UK

Paul Davies
Consultant Neurologist, Northampton General Hospital NHS Trust, Northampton, UK

Sam Dawkins
Specialist Registrar in Cardiology, John Radcliffe Hospital, Oxford, UK

David de Berker
Consultant Dermatologist and Honorary Senior Lecturer, University Hospitals Bristol NHS Foundation Trust, Bristol, UK

Aminda De Silva
Consultant Gastroenterologist, Royal Berkshire NHS Foundation Trust, Reading UK

Sarah Deacon
Consultant Respiratory Physician, Worcestershire Royal Hospital, Worcester, UK

Miguel Debono
Consultant Endocrinologist and Honorary Senior Lecturer, Royal Hallamshire Hospital, Sheffield, UK

Patrick Deegan
Metabolic Physician, Addenbrooke's Hospital, Cambridge, UK

Alastair Denniston
Consultant Ophthalmologist, University Hospitals Birmingham NHSFT & Hon Professor, University of Birmingham, Birmingham, UK

Dhananjay Desai
Consultant Respiratory Physician, University Hospital Coventry, Coventry, UK

Michael Doherty
Professor of Rheumatology and Head of Division of Academic Rheumatology, School of Medicine, University of Nottingham, Nottingham, UK

Moutaz El-Kadri
Consultant Cardiologist and Electrophysiologist, Sheikh Khalifa Medical City, Abu Dhabi, UAE

Michelle Ellinson
Freelance Dietitian, London, UK

Christine Elwell
Consultant Oncologist, Northampton General Hospital NHS Trust, Northampton, UK

Clare England
Senior Research Associate, University of Bristol, Bristol, UK

Ben Esdaile
Consultant Dermatologist, Whittington Hospital, London, UK

Robin Ferner
Honorary Professor of Clinical Pharmacology, University of Birmingham, Birmingham, UK

Tom Fletcher
Wellcome Trust/Ministry of Defence Research Training Fellow and Speciality Registrar in Infectious Diseases, Liverpool School of Tropical Medicine, and Royal Liverpool University Hospital, Liverpool, UK

Colin Forfar
Consultant Cardiologist, Oxford University Hospitals NHS Foundation Trust, Oxford, UK

Martin Fotherby
Consultant Stroke Physician, Leicester Royal Infirmary Leicester, UK

Anthony Frew
Professor of Allergy and Respiratory Medicine, Royal Sussex County Hospital, Brighton, UK

Paul Frost
Consultant in Intensive Care Medicine, University Hospital of Wales, Cardiff, UK

Hill Gaston
Emeritus Professor of Rheumatology, University of Cambridge, Cambridge, UK

David J. Gawkrodger
Professor Emeritus in Dermatology, University of Sheffield, Sheffield, UK

Sir Ian Gilmore
Honorary Consultant, Royal Liverpool University Hospital, and Honorary Professor, University of Liverpool, Liverpool, UK

William Gilmore
Research Fellow, National Drug Research Institute, Curtin University, Perth, Australia

Sherif Gonem
National Institute for Health Research Clinical Lecturer in Respiratory Medicine, University of Leicester, Leicester, UK

Lynsey Goodwin
Specialist Trainee in Infectious Diseases and General Medicine, Royal Liverpool University Hospital, Liverpool and North Manchester General Hospital, Manchester, UK

Warren Grant
Consultant Clinical Oncologist, Cheltenham General Hospital, Cheltenham, UK

Tracey Graves
Consultant Neurologist, Addenbrooke's Hospital, Cambridge, UK, and Hinchingbrooke Hospital, Huntingdon, UK

Alexander L. Green
Spalding Associate Professor and Consultant Neurosurgeon, John Radcliffe Hospital, Oxford, UK

Seamus Grundy
Consultant Respiratory Physician, Aintree University Hospital, Liverpool, UK

Pranabashis Haldar
Senior Clinical Lecturer in Respiratory Medicine, University of Leicester, Leicester, UK

George Hart
Honorary Research Professor, University of Manchester, Manchester, UK

Yvonne Hart
Consultant Neurologist, Newcastle Upon Tyne NHS Foundation Trust, Newcastle, UK

Catherine Harwood
Professor in Dermatology and Honorary Consultant Dermatologist, Queen Mary University of London, London, UK

Victoria Haunton
Consultant and Honorary Senior Lecturer in Geriatric Medicine, University Hospitals of Leicester NHS Trust, Leicester, UK

Neil Herring
Associate Professor of Cardiovascular Physiology, University of Oxford, Oxford, UK, and Consultant Cardiologist, Oxford University Hospitals NHS Trust, Oxford, UK

William G. Herrington
Honorary Consultant Nephrologist, Churchill Hospital, Oxford, UK

Melvyn Hillsdon
Associate Professor of Exercise and Health Behaviour, University of Exeter, Exeter, UK

Stephan Hinze
Consultant Neurologist, Great Western Hospital, Swindon, UK

Sandeep Hothi
Bye Fellow, University of Cambridge, Cambridge, UK, and Specialist Registrar in Cardiology and General Internal Medicine, Glenfield Hospital, Leicester, UK

Jonathan A. Hyam
Consultant Brain and Comprehensive Spinal Neurosurgeon, National Hospital for Neurology and Neurosurgery, London, UK, and Honorary Senior Lecturer in Neurosurgery, University College London, London, UK

CONTRIBUTORS

Sarosh Irani
Honorary Consultant Neurologist and Senior Clinical Fellow, John Radcliffe Hospital, Oxford, UK

Simon Jackson
Consultant Urogynaecologist, Oxford University Hospitals NHS Foundation Trust, Oxford, UK

Kassim Javaid
Honorary Consultant Rheumatologist, University of Oxford, Oxford, UK

Rachel Jeffery
Consultant Rheumatologist, Northampton General Hospital NHS Trust, Northampton, UK

Andrew A. Jeffrey
Consultant Respiratory Physician and Director of Medical Education, Northampton General Hospital NHS Trust, Northampton, UK, and Honorary Senior Lecturer, University of Oxford, Oxford, UK

Liberty Jenkins
Fellow in Neuromuscular Medicine, Stanford University Hospital, Palo Alto, CA, USA

Andrew M. Jones
Consultant Respiratory Physician, University Hospital of South Manchester, Manchester, UK

Michael Jones
Clinical Fellow in Cardiology, Oxford University Hospitals NHS Foundation Trust, Oxford, UK

Nerissa Jordan
Consultant Neurologist, Fiona Stanley Hospital, Perth, Australia

Elizabeth Justice
Consultant Rheumatologist, Queen Elizabeth Hospital Birmingham, Birmingham, UK

Manish Kalla
Lecturer in Medicine and Clinical Research Fellow, University of Oxford, Oxford, UK

Alexandra Kent
Research Fellow, John Radcliffe Hospital, Oxford, UK

Satish Keshav
Gastroenterologist and Honorary Senior Lecturer, John Radcliffe Hospital, Oxford, UK

Saifudin Khalid
Consultant Respiratory Physician, Royal Blackburn Hospital, Blackburn, UK

Richard Knight
Professor of Clinical Neurology, National CJD Research And Surveillance Unit, Edinburgh, UK

Robin Lachmann
Consultant in Metabolic Medicine, National Hospital for Neurology and Neurosurgery, London, UK

Ajit Lalvani
Chair of Infectious Diseases, Director of the National Institute of Health Research Health Protection Research Unit, Director of the Tuberculosis Research Centre, and Head of Respiratory Infections, National Heart and Lung Institute, Imperial College London, London, UK

Chris Lavy
Professor of Orthopaedic and Tropical Surgery, and Consultant Orthopaedic and Spine Surgeon, University of Oxford, Oxford, UK

Richard Lessells
Senior Infectious Diseases Specialist, University of KwaZulu-Natal, Durban, South Africa

Andrew Lever
Professor of Infectious Diseases, University of Cambridge, Cambridge, UK, and Honorary Consultant Physician, Addenbrooke's Hospital, Cambridge, UK

Keir Lewis
Professor of Respiratory Medicine, University of Swansea, Swansea, UK

Su-Yin Lim
Specialist Registrar in Neurology, Leicester General Hospital, Leicester, UK

Mark P. Little
Senior Investigator, National Cancer Institute, Bethesda, MD, USA

Yoon Loke
Professor of Medicine and Pharmacology, University of East Anglia, Norwich, UK

Melanie Lord
Speech and Language Therapist, Fen House, Ely, UK

Raashid Luqmani
Professor of Rheumatology, University of Oxford, Oxford, UK

Linda Luxon
Professor Emeritus of Audiovestibular Medicine and Honorary Consultant Physician in Neuro-otology, University College London and University College Hospitals NHS Trust, London, UK

Graz Luzzi
Consultant in Genitourinary Medicine, Wycombe General Hospital, High Wycombe, UK, and Honorary Senior Clinical Lecturer, University of Oxford, Oxford, UK

Robert MacKenzie-Ross
Respiratory Consultant, Royal United Hospital, Bath, UK

Rubeta Matin
Consultant Dermatologist, Churchill Hospital, Oxford, UK

Jane McGregor
Consultant Dermatologist, Barts Health NHS Trust, London, UK

Tess McPherson
Consultant Dermatologist, Churchill Hospital, Oxford, UK

Benedict Michael
National Institute for Health Research Senior Clinician Scientist Fellow University of Liverpool, Liverpool, UK, and Post-Doctoral Researcher/Lecturer, Massachusetts General Hospital/Harvard Medical School Boston, MA, USA

Siraj Misbah
Consultant Clinical Immunologist, John Radcliffe Hospital, Oxford, UK, and Honorary Senior Clinical Lecturer, Oxford University, Oxford, UK

Amit Mistri
Consultant in Stroke Medicine, Leicester Royal Infirmary, Leicester, UK

Sajjan Mittal
Consultant Haematologist, Northampton General Hospital NHS Trust, Northampton, UK

Susan Mollan
Consultant Ophthalmologist, University Hospitals Birmingham NHSFT & Clinical Fellow, University of Birmingham, Birmingham, UK

Rhiain Morris
Clinical Psychologist, Oxfordshire Counselling and Psychology Practice, Oxford, UK

Karen Morrison
Associate Dean for Education and Student Experience, Director of Medical Education, and Professor of Neurology, University of Southampton, Southampton, UK, and Honorary Consultant Neurologist, University Hospital Southampton, Southampton, UK

Alia Munir
Consultant Endocrinologist, Royal Hallamshire Hospital, Sheffield, UK

Louisa Murdin
Consultant Audiovestibular Physician, Guy's and St Thomas' NHS Foundation Trust, London, UK

Elaine Murphy
Consultant in Inherited Metabolic Disease, National Hospital for Neurology and Neurosurgery, London, UK

Chandramouli Nagarajan
Consultant Haematologist and Adj. Assistant Professor, DUKE-NUS Medical School, Singapore General Hospital, Singapore

Pradip Nandi
Consultant Rheumatologist, Northampton General Hospital NHS Trust, Northampton, UK

Abdul Nasimudeen
Consultant Chest Physician, Northampton General Hospital NHS Trust, Northampton, UK

Pavithra Natarajan
Consultant in Infectious Diseases, North Manchester General Hospital, Manchester, UK

John Newell-Price
Professor of Endocrinology and Consultant Endocrinologist, University of Sheffield, Sheffield, UK

Jim Newton
Consultant Cardiologist, Oxford University Hospitals NHS Foundation Trust, Oxford, UK

Pippa Newton
Consultant in Infectious Diseases, Manchester University NHS Foundation Trust, Manchester, UK

Kannan Nithi
Consultant Neurologist and Neurophysiologist, Northampton General Hospital NHS Trust, Northampton, UK

Christopher A. O'Callaghan
Professor of Medicine and Honorary Consultant Physician and Nephrologist, University of Oxford, Oxford, UK

Liz Orchard
Consultant Cardiologist, John Radcliffe Hospital, Oxford, UK

Rakesh Panchal
Consultant Respiratory Physician, Glenfield Hospital, Leicester, UK

Manish Pareek
Senior Clinical Lecturer in Infectious Diseases, University of Leicester, Leicester, UK, and Honorary Consultant in Infectious Diseases, Leicester Royal Infirmary, Leicester, UK

Joanna Pepke-Zaba
Consultant Respiratory Physician, Papworth Hospital, Papworth Everard, UK

Erlick A. C. Pereira
Senior Lecturer in Neurosurgery, St George's, University of London, London, UK, and Consultant Neurosurgeon, St George's Hospital, London, UK

Jeremy Perkins
Consultant Vascular Surgeon, John Radcliffe Hospital, Oxford, UK

Joanna Peters
Locum Consultant in Infectious Diseases and Medical Microbiology, Royal Sussex County Hospital, Brighton, Sussex, UK

Katrina Pollock
National Institute for Health Research Clinical Lecturer in Genitourinary Medicine, Imperial College London, London, UK

Jenny Powell
Consultant Dermatologist, Basingstoke and North Hampshire Hospital, Basingstoke, UK

Jonathan Price
Clinical Tutor in Psychiatry, University of Oxford, Oxford, UK

Natalia Price
Consultant Urogynaecologist, John Radcliffe Hospital, Oxford, UK

Susan Price
Consultant in Clinical Genetics, Oxford Regional Genetics Service, Oxford, UK

Norman Qureshi
Consultant Cardiologist and Electrophysiologist, Imperial College Healthcare NHS Trust, London, UK

Kazem Rahimi
Professor of Medicine, University of Oxford, Oxford, UK

Kim Rajappan
Consultant Cardiologist, John Radcliffe Hospital, Oxford, UK

Tommy Rampling
Academic Clinical Fellow, University College London, London, UK

James Ramsden
Consultant ENT Surgeon, John Radcliffe Hospital, Oxford, UK

Anna Rathmell
Medical Manager, Takeda UK Ltd, Wooburn Green, UK, and Lay Member, South Central–Oxford C Research Ethics Committee, Bristol, UK

David Ratliff
Consultant Vascular Surgeon, Northampton General Hospital NHS Trust, Northampton, UK

Karim Raza
Professor of Clinical Rheumatology, University of Birmingham, Birmingham, UK

Dave Riley
Palliative Medicine Consultant and Clinical Director, Northamptonshire Healthcare NHS Foundation Trust, Northampton, UK

Simon Rinaldi
MRC Clinician Scientist and Honorary Consultant Neurologist, University of Oxford, Oxford, UK

Joanna Robson
Consultant Senior Lecturer in Rheumatology, University of the West of England, Bristol, UK

Kufre Sampson
Consultant Clinical Oncologist, Leicester Royal Infirmary, Leicester, UK

John Saunders
Consultant Gastroenterologist, Royal United Hospital, Bath, UK

Alys Scadding
Consultant in Respiratory Medicine, Glenfield Hospital, Leicester, UK

Matthew Scarborough
Consultant in Clinical Infection, John Radcliffe Hospital, Oxford, UK

Alexander Schmidt
Director, Professor of Musicians' Medicine, and Consultant Neurologist, Kurt Singer Institute for Music Physiology and Musicians' Health, Berlin, Germany

Susanne Schneider
Consultant Neurologist, Ludwig-Maximilians-Universität München, München, Germany

Martin Scott-Brown
Consultant Oncologist, University Hospital Coventry, Coventry, UK

Aung Sett
Consultant Stroke Physician, Fairfield General Hospital, Bury, UK

Shireen Shaffu
Consultant Rheumatologist, Leicester Royal Infirmary, Leicester, UK

Karen K. K. Sheares
Respiratory Consultant, Papworth Hospital, Papworth Everard, Cambridge

Jackie Sherrard
Consultant Physician, Department of Sexual Health, Churchill Hospital, Oxford, UK

Cheerag Shirodaria
Honorary Consultant Cardiologist, John Radcliffe Hospital, Oxford, UK

Ehoud Shmueli
Consultant Gastroenterologist, Northampton General Hospital, NHS Trust, Northampton, UK

Kevin Shotliff
Consultant Diabetologist, Chelsea and Westminster Hospital, London, UK

Salman Siddiqui
Clinical Senior Lecturer , Glenfield Hospital, Leicester, UK

Muthu Sivaramakrishnan
Consultant Dermatologist, Ninewells Hospital and Medical School, Dundee, UK

Jacky Smith
Professor of Respiratory Medicine, University of Manchester, Manchester, UK, and Honorary Consultant, University Hospital of South Manchester, Manchester, UK

Roger Smyth
Consultant Psychiatrist, Royal Infirmary of Edinburgh, Edinburgh, UK

Tom Solomon
Professor of Neurology, University of Liverpool, Liverpool, UK

Christine Soon
Consultant Dermatologist, Northampton General Hospital NHS Trust, Northampton, UK

David Sprigings
Formerly Consultant Physician, Northampton General Hospital NHS Trust, Northampton, UK

Robert Stevens
Consultant Rheumatologist, Doncaster Royal Infirmary, Doncaster, UK

Jon Stone
Consultant Neurologist and Honorary Reader in Neurology, University of Edinburgh, Edinburgh, UK

Sarah Stoneley
Consultant Geriatrician, Leicester Royal Infirmary, Leicester, UK

Michael Stroud
Consultant Gastroenterologist and Professor of Clinical Nutrition, Southampton University Hospital, Southampton, UK

Kenny Sunmboye
Consultant Rheumatologist and UKNIHR CRN East Midlands Musculoskeletal Disorders Specialty Lead, University Hospitals of Leicester, Leicester, UK

Ravi Suppiah,
Consultant Rheumatologist, Auckland District Health Board, Auckland, New Zealand

Joanna Szram
Consultant Respiratory Physician, Royal Brompton and Harefield NHS Foundation Trust, London, UK

David Taggart
Professor of Cardiovascular Surgery, John Radcliffe Hospital, Oxford, UK

Kathy Taghipour
Consultant Dermatologist, Whittington Health NHS Trust, London, UK

James Taylor
Consultant Rheumatologist, Northampton General Hospital NHS Trust, Northampton, UK

Sherine Thomas
Consultant in Infectious Diseases and General Medicine, Barts Health NHS Trust, London, UK

Bryan Timmins
Consultant Neuropsychiatrist, Northamptonshire Healthcare NHS Trust, Northampton, UK

Jonathan Timperley
Consultant Cardiologist, Northampton General Hospital NHS Trust, Northampton, UK

Stacy Todd
Consultant in Infectious Diseases and General Medicine, Royal Liverpool University Hospital, Liverpool, UK

Palak Trivedi
Academic Clinical Lecturer and Specialist Registrar in Hepatology and Gastroenterology, University of Birmingham, Birmingham, UK

Martin R. Turner
Professor of Clinical Neurology and Neuroscience, John Radcliffe Hospital, Oxford, UK

Jaime Vera,
Clinical Senior Lecturer, Brighton and Sussex Medical School, Brighton, UK

Raman Verma
Specialist Registrar in Respiratory Medicine and Honorary National Institute for Health Research Lecturer, Glenfield Hospital University, Leicester, UK

Sarah Wakelin
Consultant Dermatologist and Honorary Senior Lecturer, Imperial College Healthcare NHS Trust, London, UK

Ben Wakerley
Consultant Neurologist, Gloucestershire Royal Hospital, Gloucester, UK

Emma Wall
Academic Clinical Lecturer, University College London, London, UK

Pippa Watson
Consultant Rheumatologist, University Hospital of South Manchester, Manchester, UK

Andrew Weir
Consultant Neurologist, Royal Berkshire Hospital, Reading, UK, and John Radcliffe Hospital, Oxford, UK

Sophie West
Consultant Physician, Freeman Hospital, Newcastle, UK

Matt Wise
Physician, University Hospital of Wales, Cardiff, UK

Martyn Wood
Consultant in Sexual Health and HIV Medicine, Royal Liverpool and Broadgreen University Hospitals NHS Trust, Liverpool, UK

Chee-Seng Yee
Consultant Rheumatologist, Doncaster Royal Infirmary, Doncaster, UK

PART 1

The approach to the patient

1 Diagnostic reasoning

David Sprigings

Introduction

It was an ordinary medical outpatient clinic. I was seeing a ward follow-up, a 25-year-old woman who had been admitted a couple of months earlier with a non-specific febrile illness, anaemia, and raised inflammatory markers. She was now feeling well. I began the examination by taking her blood pressure. But for some reason I couldn't feel her brachial pulse. What was going on?

Diagnostic reasoning is the mental process by which we turn such information about the patient into the name of a disease. In the patient above, this proved to be Takayasu arteritis. To do this we must gather and evaluate evidence relevant to the clinical problem, and then choose a diagnosis or make a decision about management. Like detective work, with which it has many similarities, we have to reason from observed effects to their possible causes. In this chapter we will explore the thinking behind diagnostic reasoning, drawing on insights from cognitive psychology, philosophy, and the design of computer programs. If we have a deeper understanding of the reasoning that underpins making a diagnosis, we may be more astute diagnosticians, and better able to teach the skill to novices. And, however we arrive at a diagnosis, we need to be able to articulate our reasoning to the patient and our colleagues. But first, let's clarify what we mean by a diagnosis.

Patients with diseases exist in the real world. A diagnosis, however, is a mental construct with which we reason about disease. In essence, it is an explanation for what is happening to the patient.

It resembles a scientific hypothesis, but differs in that there are agreed criteria for its confirmation or exclusion. It is often the name of a disease, but can be much broader than this: for example, it could be a syndrome—a cluster of clinical features—such as heart failure or malabsorption, or a category of disease like cancer or sepsis. A diagnosis summarizes our thoughts about what is happening to the patient, guides our actions, and helps us foretell the future. It need only be as precise as is required by the circumstances and the next step to be taken. This may be at the level of investigation (if we diagnose heart failure, we order an echocardiogram), or treatment (if we diagnose cardiac arrest, we start life support).

Like other human reasoning, diagnostic reasoning is fallible. Ten per cent or more of diagnoses are wrong, and for certain diseases (such as rare diseases) the rate of misdiagnosis (failure or delay in diagnosis) is often higher. Because so much of our management hinges on the diagnosis, errors in diagnosis typically lead to poor outcomes. Perhaps unfairly, patients regard misdiagnosis as more negligent than technical errors or complications. Many factors contribute to misdiagnosis (Table 1.1), amongst which errors in diagnostic reasoning are prominent. The single most common failing we need to guard against is 'premature closure', that is too readily accepting a diagnosis which seems to fit the facts, without considering better alternatives. Formulating a **differential diagnosis** (asking yourself 'What else could this be?') helps avoid this trap.

Table 1.1 Factors contributing to diagnostic error	
Factor	**Comment**
Doctor related	
Lack of knowledge of specific diseases	Diseases such as subdural empyema, cerebral venous sinus thrombosis, oesophageal rupture, and mesenteric ischaemia are sufficiently rare to mean that we may not have encountered them in our training, and so do not consider them in the relevant setting.
Failure to appreciate the spectrum of clinical presentations of diseases we know	Many diseases have a broad range of clinical manifestations. Examples include pulmonary embolism, aortic dissection, infective endocarditis, and phaeochromocytoma, as well as multisystem diseases such as vasculitis or amyloidosis.
Inadequate data collection	Failure to take an adequate history, perform an appropriate examination, or order relevant investigations inevitably increases the risk of misdiagnosis.
Errors in diagnostic reasoning	We may ignore, misunderstand, or misinterpret relevant clinical data. We may put too much store by 'normal' results in ruling out disease (e.g. we may wrongly believe that a normal ECG excludes acute coronary syndrome). We may accept a working diagnosis without subjecting it to proper scrutiny, or considering better alternatives.
Other human factors	Biases, fatigue, distraction, and lapses of memory may lead us astray.
Patient/setting related	
Older patients	Older patients are more likely to have more than one disease. The presentation of diseases may be modified with age.
Patients with psychiatric symptoms or disease	Diagnostic error is more common in patients with both physical and psychiatric symptoms. Psychiatric symptoms may in fact be due to physical disease. Psychiatric disease and its treatment may affect the response to physical disease (e.g. reduced pain perception in schizophrenia).
Patients in intensive care	Information from the history is reduced, and physical examination may be more difficult. The spectrum of disease is different, and patients often have multiple, interrelated diseases.
System related	
Management of healthcare records	Access to previous paper and electronic healthcare records may be difficult; as a consequence, key facts about the patient may not be known when diagnoses are being made.
Management of test results	Doctors may not be alerted to abnormal test results (e.g. of patients who have been discharged from hospital or who are outpatients) and so these results go unrecognized.
Communication across healthcare interfaces	Diagnostic information may not be passed between primary and secondary care, or between hospitals.

Table 1.2 Diagnostic features of Ehlers–Danlos syndrome type IV		
Defining characteristics (present in all patients)	**Consistent features (present in >75% of patients)**	**Variable features (present in <75% of patients)**
Cultured dermal fibroblasts synthesize abnormal type III procollagen molecules Identification of a mutation in the gene for type III procollagen (*COL3A1*)	Autosomal dominant inheritance Easy bruising Thin skin with visible veins Characteristic facial features	Hypermobility of large joints Hyperextensibility of skin Arterial rupture, dissection, or aneurysm formation Uterine rupture Gastrointestinal perforation

Diagnosis, disease, and clinical features

The exact number of diseases is uncertain, but likely to be in excess of 30 000 (the current International Classification of Diseases (ICD-10) has 12 420 codes; online *Mendelian Inheritance in Man* (OMIM™), which focuses primarily on inherited genetic disorders, has just under 20 000 entries). We recognize diseases by their clinical features—the symptoms, signs, imaging, and other data they are associated with. For a given disease, there are **defining characteristics**—those abnormalities which confirm the presence of the disease and distinguish it from other diseases; **consistent features**, seen (arbitrarily) in >75% of patients with the disease; and **variable features**, seen in <75% of patients. Defining characteristics may change over time, with advances in understanding of the genetic and molecular mechanisms of the disease. There is of course substantial overlap between diseases as regards their consistent and variable features but, by definition, the defining characteristics are unique to a single disease. Table 1.2 illustrates this for the collagen disorder, Ehlers–Danlos syndrome type IV (EDS IV).

In EDS IV, as in many other diseases, the defining characteristics relate to the results of laboratory investigations. The **clinical diagnosis** is the diagnosis based on the presence of clinical features most consistently associated with the disease. A patient presenting with easy bruising and who has typical facial features and thin skin could be given the clinical diagnosis of EDS IV. The **working diagnosis**—which we will return to in 'Making a diagnosis'—is the diagnosis about which we are sufficiently certain to use as the basis for action. If the patient with easy bruising had joint hypermobility but no other abnormal signs (and no other cause for easy bruising apparent), EDS IV might be our working diagnosis, leading us to request collagen and DNA studies. If these tests were both positive, EDS IV would be the **final (or confirmed) diagnosis**. A comprehensive final diagnosis should provide answers to three questions: which tissue, organ, region, or system of the body is diseased; what is the pathophysiological process causing the disease; and why has this process happened in this patient?

Making a diagnosis

The knowledge base of medicine is largely structured by disease, as reflected in the contents list of this book, but patients come to us with problems. A schematic description of the process through which we transform a clinical problem into a final diagnosis is shown in Figure 1.1.

Clinical problem

Actions	**Diagnostic process**
Initial data gathering	Clarification of the problem and context
Further data gathering by focused history, physical examination and bedside testing	Generation of a provisional diagnosis or differential diagnosis by pattern recognition, hypothetico-deductive reasoning or algorithm
Diagnostic testing	Diagnoses confirmed, refined or rejected
Review and integration of data Diagnosis and diagnostic reasoning discussed with patient and colleagues	Management of diagnostic uncertainty and avoidance of diagnostic error Formulation of working diagnosis

Working diagnosis

Plan of management

Actions	**Diagnostic process**
Observation of progress over time and response to treatment	Working diagnosis confirmed, refined or rejected
Definitive diagnostic testing	Formulation of final diagnosis

Final diagnosis

Figure 1.1 Diagnostic reasoning.

Table 1.3 Common causes of thrombocytopenia by clinical context, illustrating the powerful influence of context on the differential diagnosis

Context	Common causes (after exclusion of pseudothrombocytopenia due to platelet clumping)
Acute hospital admission	Sepsis
	Acute alcohol toxicity
	Disseminated intravascular coagulation
	Drug-induced thrombocytopenia
	Immune thrombocytopenic purpura
	Thrombotic thrombocytopenic purpura
Inpatient	Sepsis
	Disseminated intravascular coagulation
	Drug-induced thrombocytopenia
	Dilutional thrombocytopenia from transfusion of plasma-reduced red cells
	Post-transfusion purpura
Pregnancy and peripartum	Gestational thrombocytopenia
	Immune thrombocytopenic purpura
	HELLP syndrome (haemolysis, elevated liver enzymes, low platelet count)
	Disseminated intravascular coagulation
	Thrombotic thrombocytopenic purpura
Outpatient	Myelodysplasia
	Hypersplenism
	Immune thrombocytopenic purpura
	Antiphospholipid-antibody syndrome

Clarification of the problem and context

Over the first minute or two of the clinical encounter, we gather data to clarify the nature of the problem and its context. The opening remarks or appearance of the patient, the physiological observations, the contents of the referral letter, or the comments of the nurse—all may help define the problem. The context—which will include the age and sex of the patient, and the clinical setting (e.g. primary/secondary care)—exercises a powerful constraint on diagnostic possibilities. This influence of context is particularly important when dealing with clinical problems with a wide differential diagnosis. Thrombocytopenia, for example, has over 30 causes, when considered by mechanism. However, classification by context yields groups of 4–6 causes (Table 1.3), allowing us to focus on a much more manageable shortlist. We may need to cast our net wider if the shortlist does not contain a diagnosis which meets the standards of a good working diagnosis, but narrowing the field in this way makes the diagnostic process more efficient.

Generation of a provisional diagnosis or differential diagnosis

Our initial data gathering is followed by a more systematic process of focused history taking, physical examination, and bedside testing. By focused we mean that our thoughts about what might be the diagnosis drive our search for further information. We use three distinct methods to generate a provisional diagnosis or differential diagnosis: pattern recognition, hypothetico-deductive reasoning, and the use of algorithms. Broadly speaking, we solve easy cases by pattern recognition, and difficult cases by hypothetico-deductive reasoning. What counts as easy or difficult depends on our knowledge and experience: experts playing on their home ground will tend to use pattern recognition but, when faced with an unusual problem which does not yield to this, switch to hypothetico-deductive reasoning. Algorithms are helpful when the clinical picture is dominated by one feature with a relatively narrow differential diagnosis.

Pattern recognition

Consider the case of a 52-year-old woman who presented to the Emergency Department with headache. This is her account:

I was towel-drying my hair yesterday evening when I got a blinding headache. I think I blacked out for a few seconds.

I went to bed. The headache was still there. It was worse when I moved my head around and when I coughed. I could sometimes find a comfortable position. I've still got the headache now. I took a painkiller this morning which helped a bit. It's worse if I bend my head down.

Pattern recognition transforms clusters of clinical features—patterns—into diagnoses, based on their match with previously classified patterns in memory. In this case, the characteristics of the headache (its abrupt onset, association with syncope, and exacerbation by head movement and coughing) and the ensuing neck stiffness allow a pattern-recognition diagnosis of subarachnoid haemorrhage. The case is typical: all the features are consistent with subarachnoid haemorrhage, and none is discordant. The diagnosis can be made in a minute or two.

Of course, we soon learn that not all cases are typical. As we gain experience, we become familiar with unusual presentations—also called disease polymorphisms—such as the presentation of subarachnoid haemorrhage with pulmonary oedema or confusional state. These patterns can be thought of as 'illness scripts'—narratives of the features of the case. The more patients we see (or hear or read about), the more illness scripts we have in our memory and the better we become at recognizing patients with the same disease, even when the clinical features don't match those of the typical case. Pattern recognition is a fast and economical method of making a diagnosis, but has an Achilles heel: we have a tendency to assess less critically the diagnoses we make by pattern recognition.

Hypothetico-deductive reasoning

Hypothetico-deductive reasoning means thinking of possible explanations for the problem and testing them. We use hypothetico-deductive reasoning when we don't have all the relevant clinical information immediately to hand, and diagnosis by pattern recognition is not possible. Typically, we start with a tentative initial diagnosis ('Has he had a pulmonary embolism?', 'Could this be meningitis?'). As we progress with the case, seeking and organizing further information, we mentally adjust the probabilities of the diagnoses we are actively considering. We are particularly interested in those clinical features that are **defining characteristics** of a disease or syndrome (e.g. regional ST elevation in a patient with acute chest pain) or allow discrimination between different diseases. **Discriminatory features** are those whose presence or absence significantly increases or decreases the probability of a given diagnosis. In a patient presenting with exertional syncope, hair colour is of no discriminatory value, but the presence of a loud mid-systolic murmur is highly relevant, given its association with aortic stenosis and hypertrophic obstructive cardiomyopathy. Discriminatory features may be a combination of several signs. For example, the presence of an elevated jugular venous pressure together with pulsus paradoxus of >10 mm Hg and a large cardiac silhouette on the chest X-ray make cardiac tamponade the likely diagnosis in the breathless patient. Conversely, the absence of fever, or neck stiffness, or altered mental state—one or more of which are present in 99% of patients with meningitis—effectively excludes this diagnosis in the patient with headache. In general, the **presence** of features (single or composite) with a **low false-positive rate** rules **in** a diagnosis, and the **absence** of features with a **low false-negative rate** rules **out** a diagnosis. False-positive and false-negative rates are discussed further in 'Diagnostic testing'.

Red flags and worst-case scenarios

Many symptoms have a broad differential diagnosis ranging from self-limiting diseases such as minor viral infection to life-threatening disorders. When considering the cause of a patient's problem, we need to be mindful of the consequences of failure to diagnose rare but potentially lethal diseases. Various strategies have been proposed to force consideration of diagnoses which carry a high penalty if missed. 'Red flags' are the name given to symptoms or signs whose presence mandates further testing to exclude serious disease. The limitation of this focus on 'red flags' is that many patients with serious disorders do not have red-flag symptoms (in other words, these symptoms have a high false-negative rate), so their absence does not allow you to rule out the diagnosis. For example, subarachnoid haemorrhage may not cause abrupt-onset or severe headache. Nevertheless, it is a strategy that is helpful, especially when the prevalence of life-threatening disease is low.

A related strategy is to force consideration of life-threatening diseases in a given situation—a 'rule out worst-case scenario' strategy. In patients with acute chest pain, for example, it is useful always to consider acute coronary syndrome, pulmonary embolism, aortic dissection, and oesophageal rupture, and test the features of the case against these diagnoses. Many clinical aphorisms are of this sort ('In patients with abdominal pain, always consider acute appendicitis in the very young, the very old, and the pregnant.', 'Positive blood cultures are due to infective endocarditis until proven otherwise.').

The use of pivots

Often, the sheer volume of clinical features—most of which are not going to be relevant to the diagnosis—can make it difficult to know where to start with hypothetico-deductive reasoning. When faced with this situation, one fruitful approach is to focus on pivotal features. Pivotal clinical features are features which have to be explained—that is, they are rarely if ever seen in the absence of disease and, importantly, have a manageable differential diagnosis. Examples include pleuritic chest pain, finger clubbing, splenomegaly, extensor plantar response, and heavy proteinuria.

The use of a pivot can be illustrated by analysis of this case from the *British Medical Journal*:

A 70-year-old man presented with a 30-minute history of throbbing left-sided headache that woke him from sleep. He had no history of headache or recent head injury. He also described a four-day history of breathlessness when climbing one flight of stairs. He was taking tablets for type 2 diabetes mellitus, hypertension, and congestive cardiac failure. He did not smoke and drank seven units of alcohol a week. The patient was alert and oriented, with a heart rate of 100 beats/minute and a blood pressure of 150/90 mm Hg. Respiratory rate was 16 breaths per minute, oxygen saturation was 98% on air, and his lungs were clear to auscultation. An early diastolic murmur was heard at the base of the heart. He had no temporal artery tenderness or neck stiffness. Haemoglobin was 13.2 g/L; white blood cell count was 7×10^9/L; urea and electrolytes, liver function, and renal function were normal, and the erythrocyte sedimentation rate was 30 mm/hour (normal <20 mm/hour in men over 50). Electrocardiography showed sinus tachycardia. The results of chest radiography and computed tomography of the brain were normal.

Where to start? Well, amongst all the clinical features mentioned, only two stand out as clearly abnormal: the unilateral throbbing headache and the early diastolic murmur. An early diastolic murmur is usually due to aortic regurgitation, the causes of which can be divided into acute or chronic (see Table 1.4).

If we presume that aortic regurgitation started suddenly, which would account for the patient's breathlessness, then there are really only two diagnoses we need to consider: infective endocarditis and aortic dissection. Use of this pivot has simplified the problem—for the moment—to making a judgement as to which of these two diagnoses could explain the clinical features and, if both could, which is the more likely.

Both disorders are famous for their varied clinical presentation. Against a diagnosis of aortic dissection is the absence of chest pain, and the normal chest X-ray. However, in patients with proven aortic dissection, chest pain is absent in 15%, and the chest X-ray normal in a similar percentage. Against a diagnosis of infective endocarditis

Table 1.4 Causes of aortic regurgitation	
Acute aortic regurgitation	**Chronic aortic regurgitation**
Infective endocarditis	Bicuspid aortic valve
Aortic dissection	Calcification of a morphologically normal aortic valve
	Aortic root dilatation

is the absence of fever, the normal full blood count and only mildly raised ESR.

So both are possible. Aortic dissection is perhaps the more likely. But how to account for the headache? A unilateral throbbing headache suggests a local vascular cause, rather than a systemic cause related to infection. But can aortic dissection and headache be linked? At this point, most of us would need help. Fortunately, Google is usually to hand, and googling 'headache' and 'aortic dissection' returns several case reports of aortic dissection extending into the carotid artery and thus causing headache.

So we can now adopt a **working diagnosis** of painless proximal aortic dissection complicated by acute aortic regurgitation (resulting in breathlessness) and extension into the left carotid artery (causing unilateral headache). We don't yet have a **final or confirmed diagnosis**: this requires imaging to demonstrate an aortic dissection flap, the defining characteristic of aortic dissection. CT with contrast was done and this was found.

Pivots are useful because they reduce the diagnostic possibilities to a number we can hold in short-term memory (around five at a time), and take advantage of the fact that, although we are generally poor at estimating absolute probabilities of diseases, we are much better at comparing and ranking the relative probabilities of diseases.

Use of algorithms

An algorithm is defined as a set of rules designed to solve a specific problem by proceeding through a sequence of logical steps. Diagnostic algorithms are typically written by experts for non-experts, with reference to the evidence base, and follow an approach considered the most expeditious in the analysis of a clinical problem. They prompt us to seek specific information which discriminates between the choices at the branch points of the flowchart. For example, in relation to hypokalaemia (Figure 1.2), whether the urinary potassium-to-creatinine excretion is low or high and, if high, whether there is a metabolic alkalosis or acidosis. The diagnostic process of an algorithm is explicit, but its output still needs to be validated, as we would any provisional diagnosis.

Diagnostic support systems

We often find ourselves needing help with diagnoses, which usually comes from colleagues or a review of the relevant medical literature. Web-based diagnostic support (Table 1.5) is increasingly available where we see patients, and is underused. Google, as previously demonstrated, is a powerful tool, particularly when we have a cluster of definite abnormalities (i.e. findings that are unquestionably pathological) for which we are seeking a unifying diagnosis. For example, a middle-aged woman presented with breathlessness and was found to have hypoxia and a 9 cm diameter aortic root aneurysm, without significant aortic regurgitation. Extensive respiratory investigation drew a blank as to the cause of hypoxia. However, googling these two features gives the answer: distortion of the right atrium by the aortic root aneurysm allowing a right-to-left shunt across a patent foramen ovale (confirmed as the diagnosis by bubble-contrast echocardiography). With further development of the electronic patient record (EPR), automatic diagnostic support may be possible, using information taken directly from the EPR.

Diagnostic testing

We do diagnostic testing to confirm, refine, or reject possible diagnoses. A diagnosis is confirmed if its defining characteristics are found, and rejected if these are absent. Some tests are used to determine if a particular disease is present (e.g. measurement of urinary copper excretion for Wilson's disease), while others provide information relevant to a range of diseases (e.g. chest X-ray in acute breathlessness). Testing may also enable us refine a diagnosis (e.g. echocardiography in cardiac valve disease, or staging CT in carcinoma of the bronchus).

A perfect diagnostic test is abnormal or positive in every patient with the disease, and normal or negative in every patient without the disease. Most tests are less than perfect, and gold-standard tests of high accuracy may be invasive or costly. Bayes' theorem tells us explicitly how much we should adjust our assessment of the probability of disease in the light of a positive or negative result on a test that is not 100% accurate. There are several introductions to Bayes' theorem available on the web (e.g. http://yudkowsky.net/rational/bayes).

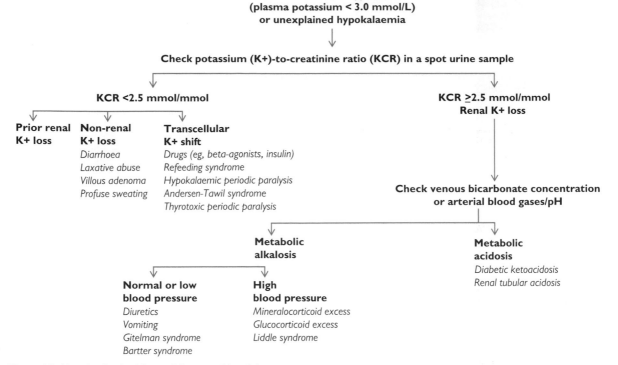

**Moderate to severe hypokalaemia
(plasma potassium < 3.0 mmol/L)
or unexplained hypokalaemia**

↓

Check potassium (K+)-to-creatinine ratio (KCR) in a spot urine sample

KCR <2.5 mmol/mmol   **KCR ≥2.5 mmol/mmol
Renal K+ loss**

**Prior renal
K+ loss**

**Non-renal
K+ loss**
Diarrhoea
Laxative abuse
Villous adenoma
Profuse sweating

**Transcellular
K+ shift**
Drugs (eg, beta-agonists, insulin)
Refeeding syndrome
Hypokalaemic periodic paralysis
Andersen-Tawil syndrome
Thyrotoxic periodic paralysis

**Check venous bicarbonate concentration
or arterial blood gases/pH**

**Metabolic
alkalosis**

**Metabolic
acidosis**
Diabetic ketoacidosis
Renal tubular acidosis

**Normal or low
blood pressure**
Diuretics
Vomiting
Gitelman syndrome
Bartter syndrome

**High
blood pressure**
Mineralocorticoid excess
Glucocorticoid excess
Liddle syndrome

Figure 1.2 Algorithm for the differential diagnosis of hypokalaemia.

A key insight from the theorem is that we must consider the probability of disease before we did the test (the pretest probability) when interpreting a test result.

To illustrate the practical application of Bayes' theorem, consider two patients you've seen in clinic: one is a 30-year-old woman, the other a 57-year-old man. Both have been referred because of a 6-month history of episodic retrosternal chest discomfort which may come on at rest (with no relation to meals) but sometimes occurs when they run up two flights of stairs at work. Both are smokers of ten cigarettes daily, with no other coronary risk factors. There is no other relevant past or family history. Examination and resting ECG are normal. You wonder about the possibility of coronary disease and arrange an exercise ECG. The test is positive in both patients, that is, exercise provokes ST depression of 2 mm (but no symptoms). Does this mean that both have coronary disease?

To answer this question, we need two pieces of information: first, how likely was coronary disease before we had the test result; and, second, how good is exercise ECG as a test for coronary disease?

We can estimate the probability of coronary disease from the age, sex, symptoms, and coronary risk factor profile of a patient. For a 30-year-old female smoker with atypical angina, the probability of coronary disease is <10%. It is substantially higher in a 57-year-old male smoker with atypical angina, at around 60%.

The relation between disease and test result can be depicted in a 2 × 2 table. Data on coronary disease and ST depression on exercise

ECG are shown in Table 1.6. This table tells us how likely a positive test result is in patients with coronary disease (70%, the true-positive rate (or sensitivity)). But we want to know the obverse: how likely is coronary disease in a patient with a positive test result?

From the data in the 2 × 2 table, we can calculate this likelihood. The likelihood ratio is the percentage of patients **with** coronary disease who show ST depression on exercise ECG (70%), divided by the percentage **without** coronary disease who also have a positive test (20%), that is, 3.5. So, a positive exercise test increases the likelihood of coronary disease by a factor of 3.5. The negative likelihood ratio is the percentage of patients **with** coronary disease who have a **negative** test (30%), divided by the percentage **without** coronary disease who have a negative test (80%), that is, 0.4. Likelihood ratios for positive and negative tests can be translated into approximate changes in the probability of disease (Table 1.7): a positive exercise test increases the probability of coronary disease by 20%–25%, while a negative test decreases it by a similar amount.

Table 1.5 Some web-based diagnostic support services

Website	Web address	Access
Google	http://www.google.co.uk	Open
DXplain	http://www.lcs.mgh.harvard.edu/projects/dxplain.html	Subscription
Isabel	http://www.isabelhealthcare.com	Subscription
DiagnosisPro	http://en.diagnosispro.com/	Open

Table 1.6 A 2 × 2 table showing the frequency of ST depression ≥1 mm on exercise ECG in patients with and without coronary artery disease (defined by angiography)

		Coronary artery disease	
		Present	Absent
ST depression ≥1 mm on exercise ECG	Present	70%	20%
		True positive	False positive
	Absent	30%	80%
		False negative	True negative
	Total	100%	100%

Note: True-positive rate (sensitivity) = 70%; true-negative rate (specificity) = 80%; positive likelihood ratio = true-positive rate/false-positive rate = 70%/20% = 3.5; negative likelihood ratio = false-negative rate/true-negative rate = 30%/80% = 0.4.

Data from Gianrossi R, Detrano R, Mulvihill D, et al. Exercise-induced ST depression in the diagnosis of coronary artery disease: A Meta-Analysis. *Circulation.* Volume 80 pp87-98 (1989).

Data averaged from several sources.

Table 1.7 Likelihood ratios and estimates of probability of disease. Likelihood ratios >1 increase the probability of the disease in question. Likelihood ratios between 1 and 0 decrease the probability of that disease

Likelihood ratio	Increase in probability of disease (%)	Likelihood ratio	Decrease in probability of disease (%)
2	+15	0.5	−15
5	+30	0.2	−30
10	+45	0.1	−45

Reproduced from *Journal of General Internal Medicine*, Volume 17, Issue 8, 2002, 'Simplifying likelihood ratios', McGee S., Copyright © 2002, Society of General Internal Medicine. With permission of Springer.

Returning to our patients, the positive exercise test therefore increases the likelihood of coronary disease to around 30% in the woman, and around 80% in the man. The same test result is associated with very different probabilities of disease, driven by the different pretest probabilities. We would now need to make a clinical judgement as to how to manage these patients, in the light of their individual probabilities of coronary disease. The limited diagnostic accuracy of exercise testing, as revealed in the relatively modest positive and negative likelihood ratios, is the principal reason why its use as a diagnostic test is declining in favour of other, more accurate tests such as CT coronary angiography and myocardial perfusion imaging.

The likelihood ratios of some commonly used diagnostic tests in acute medicine are given in Table 1.8. A positive finding on a test with a positive likelihood ratio >10 effectively rules in the disease in question, while a negative finding on a test with a negative likelihood ratio <0.1 effectively rules it out. Likelihood ratios have some important advantages over other measures of test performance, such as sensitivity and specificity (from which they can be calculated): they incorporate all the information in the 2×2 table of the test, and can be applied to individual patients, across the full range of pretest probabilities of disease. If we regard elements in the history and clinical examination as biomarkers of disease (e.g. abrupt-onset chest pain, pulse deficit, and aortic regurgitation in aortic dissection), we can use the likelihood ratios of these features to adjust our estimate of the probability of the disease as we assess the patient: we deal with this in more detail in the chapters on history taking (Chapter 3) and physical examination (Chapter 4).

Table 1.8 Likelihood ratios of selected diagnostic tests

Disease	Test	Positive LR	Negative LR
Coronary artery disease	Exercise electrocardiography	3.5	0.4
Coronary artery disease	CT coronary angiography	9.0	0.03
Pulmonary embolism	CT pulmonary angiography	5.9	0.18
Aortic dissection	Plasma D-dimer	2.6	0.06
Heart failure as the cause of acute dyspnoea	Plasma brain natriuretic peptide	3.8	0.14
Subarachnoid haemorrhage	Cranial CT and examination of CSF	3.0	0

Abbreviations: LR, likelihood ratio.
Data from several sources.

Box 1.1 Questions to ask yourself before you accept a working diagnosis

- Can I trust my working diagnosis? Are there discordant features which it doesn't explain?
- Let's assume my working diagnosis is wrong: what would be the next most likely diagnosis?
- Have I considered and excluded the most serious causes of this clinical problem?
- Am I relying on a normal test result to rule out a serious diagnosis? Do I know how much I can trust this test to do so?

Formulation of a working diagnosis

Formulation of a working diagnosis is a crucial step in diagnostic reasoning and misdiagnosis often stems from too readily accepting a diagnosis which seems to fit the facts, without considering better alternatives. Always starting with a differential diagnosis (e.g. the obvious cause, the less obvious cause and the cause we don't want to miss) defends against this. When considering the causes in our differential diagnosis, we need to subject these to intellectual as well as diagnostic testing. How well does each explain the significant positive and negative findings? Does it provide a plausible anatomical or physiological mechanism to link them, and account for the time course of events? Are there any significant findings not explained by the diagnosis (or another confirmed diagnosis)? Are any expected findings absent? Some questions we should ask ourselves before accepting a working diagnosis are given in Box 1.1.

Deciding between competing diagnoses may be difficult. In essence, one diagnosis is better than another if it explains more, that is, provides a more plausible mechanism and more convincing narrative, and unifies more findings, with fewer loose ends. Although we should prefer the more probable over the less probable diagnosis, other things being equal, the fine detail of the individual case may make a rare diagnosis more likely than a common one. As the cause of acute chest pain with minor ST/T-wave abnormalities, acute coronary syndrome is more common than oesophageal rupture (by a factor of >100); however, if the patient was weightlifting before the onset of pain, and has evidence of pneumomediastinum on chest X-ray, oesophageal rupture will be our diagnosis.

We may not be able to make a definite diagnosis after our first encounter with the patient. Often, this uncertainty can be resolved by further diagnostic testing. Alternatives are the use of tests of time and treatment. For example, in a young patient with non-specific chest pain and whose clinical features make serious disease unlikely, we may decide to observe progress over an appropriate period, without intervention. Or we may opt for a test of treatment, such as a course of proton-pump inhibitor, as an alternative to diagnostic testing. Whichever course we take, the progress of the patient is a crucial test of the correctness of our diagnosis. Each time we review patients, in clinic or on the ward, we should ask ourselves how well their progress matches what would be expected from our working diagnosis.

Diagnostic reasoning is a serious business, but also absorbing, satisfying, and often exhilarating. We can enjoy learning from our colleagues when a stunning diagnosis is made which transforms the care of a patient, and we should also learn from our mistakes. However good we are, we can always be better diagnosticians.

Further Reading

Brush JE. *The Science of the Art of Medicine: A Guide to Medical Reasoning*. Manakin-Sabot, VA: Dementi Milestone Publishing, Inc; 2015.
National Academies of Sciences, Engineering, and Medicine. *Improving Diagnosis in Health Care*. Washington, DC: National Academies Press; 2015.

2 Dealing with uncertainty

David Sprigings

Introduction

Uncertainty is a frequent and often uncomfortable element in our professional lives. Its many overlapping sources range from biological variation in patients and diseases, to the inherent unpredictability of the future (Table 2.1). In this chapter, we focus on dealing with uncertainty in diagnosis, prognosis, and management. How can we make better judgements and take wiser decisions, even though the information on which they are based is incomplete?

Dealing with diagnostic uncertainty

We can mismanage a patient even when we've got the right diagnosis but, given the central importance of the diagnosis to our choice of actions, if our diagnosis is wrong, our management will almost certainly be wrong as well. The strategies that may help us deal with diagnostic uncertainty can be illustrated by an analysis of this case:

A 58-year-old man, with a background of type 2 diabetes and hypertension, comes to the Emergency Department following an episode of central chest pain, without radiation, which came on abruptly while he was in a stressful meeting at work. He graded the pain 9/10 in severity. It was associated with sweating and faintness, was not affected by breathing or posture, and lasted for over an hour, settling after he was given morphine. When you see him, 2 hours following the onset of symptoms, he is free of pain, with normal findings on cardiovascular and general examination. His pulse is 80 beats per minute, and blood pressure 150/90 mm Hg. Oxygen saturation breathing air is 95%. ECG on admission showed sinus rhythm with no ST/T-wave abnormalities. His chest X-ray is normal.

Rule out worst-case scenario

The diagnostic process is a journey with certainty as its sometimes unattainable goal: from a problem which may have a dozen possible causes to the exact cause in our patient. For many presenting symptoms, the range of diagnoses extends from benign disorders to life-threatening diseases. Its many overlapping sources range from a useful approach which reminds us to consider life-threatening diseases (Table 2.2) before we accept a diagnosis of a benign disorder as the cause of acute chest pain. Does the patient have major risk factors for or typical clinical features of one of these diseases? Coronary disease is common in a middle-aged man with type 2 diabetes and hypertension, but of course this doesn't necessarily make acute coronary syndrome the diagnosis. The abrupt onset of non-pleuritic chest pain raises the question of aortic dissection, particularly given the normal ECG. There's nothing pointing strongly to pulmonary embolism or oesophageal rupture, but neither are there features allowing a positive diagnosis of an alternative benign disorder.

The clinical features of aortic dissection are notoriously diverse, but 'aortic pain'—defined as acute chest or back pain of onset within less than 2 minutes, tearing or ripping in quality—is the most common. Other features independently predictive of aortic dissection are pulse or blood pressure differences between the limbs, and mediastinal or aortic widening on chest X-ray. In a study of 250 patients with suspicion of aortic dissection, the absence of all three features made the probability of dissection low (<10%). However, 1 in 25 of patients who proved to have aortic dissection were in this group, making the point that low risk does not mean no risk of the disease. Conversely, any combination of the three features or isolated pulse/blood pressure differences indicated a high likelihood of dissection (>80%).

With one of the three features, abrupt-onset chest pain, this patient is at intermediate risk of dissection (around 30%). We must bear in mind, of course, that abrupt-onset chest pain is not exclusive to aortic dissection: it may be a feature of other aortic diseases (e.g. intramural haematoma), as well as acute coronary syndrome and oesophageal diseases (such as oesophageal rupture).

Table 2.1 Sources of uncertainty in medicine	
Source	**Comment**
Biological variation in patients and diseases	Patients with the same disease may have very different clinical manifestations, prognoses, and responses to treatment. Our understanding of the genetic and molecular differences which underlie this variation—the promise of personalized medicine—is still rudimentary.
Stochastic mechanisms of disease	The same initial conditions may result in a range of outcomes which can only be described by probability distributions and cannot be predicted with certainty for the individual patient (e.g. acute myocardial ischaemia may or may not result in ventricular fibrillation).
Limits of clinical data	We work with data which may be incomplete, inaccurate, unreliable, or missing. Elements in the history may be forgotten by the patient, or not elicited by the doctor. Examination findings may be overlooked or misinterpreted. Many diagnostic tests have limited accuracy.
Limits of the medical literature	The medical literature is vast, but of varying quality, with gaps, inaccuracies, and bias. Many clinical questions are not specifically addressed. It is often difficult to consult the literature at the point of care.
Limits of diagnostic and prognostic models	Models are imperfect: they may predict what proportion of patients have a diagnosis or will suffer an event, but cannot specify the outcome of individuals.
Limits of personal knowledge	Because of limited or faulty knowledge, our differential diagnosis may be too narrow and not contain the true diagnosis; even if it does contain the true diagnosis, we may wrongly reject this. Distinguishing between the limits of personal knowledge and the limits of medical knowledge may be difficult, especially early in one's career.
Limits of our ability to assess and interpret data	Experience generally improves our ability to interpret data; factors such as fatigue and distraction can reduce it. Heuristics (rules of thumb) and biases may lead us to make wrong judgements. We may respond to missing data with assumptions which prove to be unfounded.
The inherent unpredictability of the future	Predictions are necessarily provisional. The unexpected may happen. We cannot quantify unknown risks.

Table 2.2 Life-threatening causes of acute chest pain

	Acute coronary syndrome	Pulmonary embolism	Aortic dissection	Oesophageal rupture
Approximate incidence per 10^5 population per year	~300	~30	~3	~1

Data averaged from several sources.

Using clinical decision rules

Pulmonary embolism seems unlikely, but how confidently can we exclude it? We can sometimes extend (and calibrate) our analysis of the clinical features by use of a decision rule. A clinical decision rule gives an assessment of the probability of a disease, based on findings from the history, examination, and readily available investigations. Clinical decision rules are useful in situations where diagnosis is difficult, the consequences of misdiagnosis are serious, or there are opportunities to achieve savings (e.g. by reducing the use of costly investigations) without loss of quality. Clinical decision rules (like likelihood ratios) enable us to benefit from the collective medical experience of thousands of patients, far more than we will personally meet.

Perhaps surprisingly, there are no well-validated clinical decision rules for acute coronary syndrome or aortic dissection. However, for pulmonary embolism, the Wells score (see NICE Clinical Guideline 144 (2012)) is validated and easy to use. The Wells score includes uses readily available clinical information to yield a score between 0 and 12.5; the clinical probability of pulmonary embolism is dichotomized as 'unlikely' (probability <5%) if the score is ≤4, and 'likely' if >4. It may seem counter-intuitive that data on oxygen saturation, blood gases, or chest X-ray findings are not included in the score: the explanation is that while these data are relevant to the diagnosis, they lack discriminatory power. Our patient has a Wells score of 0, indicating that pulmonary embolism is very unlikely: pretty much what we thought.

Probability and consequences

Risk can be defined as a state of uncertainty in which some of the potential outcomes (present or future) are associated with harm or death. Risk has two dimensions: probability and consequences. As we reason about the case, we weigh up both of these dimensions of potential diagnoses (Table 2.3). Phrases like 'always consider diagnosis X' and 'have a high index of suspicion for diagnosis Y' are often used to remind us of diagnoses which may be unlikely in a given setting (low probability) but carry a high penalty if missed (serious consequences). The strategy of 'rule out worst-case scenario' shares the same philosophy. Given that the mortality rate of untreated aortic dissection is up to 1% per hour, definitive imaging by contrast CT is warranted to rule out the diagnosis. As the probability of pulmonary embolism is low, based on our clinical impression and supported by

the decision rule, a normal level of plasma D-dimer will be sufficient to exclude it.

Probability in the context of diagnostic reasoning is largely an expression of the strength of our belief in a diagnosis. There is an interplay between the strength of this belief—a 'subjective' probability—and the 'objective' probability, as found in descriptive studies of the epidemiology of acute chest pain. We may use the 'objective' probability (e.g. that 10% of adult patients presenting to the emergency department with acute severe chest pain have aortic dissection) as the starting point in our diagnostic assessment, adjusting the probability up or down as we incorporate additional findings about the patient in front of us. The logic underpinning our reasoning is that the presence of a recognized feature of the disease makes it more likely, and its absence, less likely. By how much more or less likely depends on the strength of the association between feature and disease (which can be summarized in its likelihood ratio). The absence of a feature characteristic of the disease (i.e. seen in >95% of patients), or the absence of two or three features each found in >80% of patients, is strong evidence against that disease being present. Making a positive diagnosis of one disease (by demonstrating its defining characteristics) also reduces the likelihood of other competing diagnoses, unless they can be linked pathophysiologically (e.g. proximal aortic dissection with involvement of a coronary ostium causing simultaneous acute coronary syndrome) or are comorbidities. So, for example, while oesophageal rupture should cross our mind in all patients with acute severe chest pain, we don't need to take the diagnosis further if none of the typical clinical features is present, and we can make a confident alternative diagnosis.

Diagnostic testing

Testing often helps us reduce diagnostic uncertainty. Likelihood ratios (see Chapter 1) are a useful summary measure of test performance, and can be applied to individual patients, across the full range of pretest probabilities of disease. A positive finding on a test with a positive likelihood ratio >10 effectively rules in the disease in question, while a negative finding on a test with a negative likelihood ratio <0.1 effectively rules it out. However, not many tests are this accurate.

Diagnostic testing is not without its problems. It may increase rather than reduce our uncertainty, if the test poorly discriminates between patients with and without the disease in question. We need

Table 2.3 Causes of acute chest pain under consideration in this case

	Comment	Probability of diagnosis	Consequences if untreated
Benign musculoskeletal disease	Onset and severity argue against benign musculoskeletal disease	<1% Very unlikely	Nil
Benign oesophageal disease (reflux/dysmotility)	No antecedent oesophageal symptoms	?10% Unlikely	Nil
Biliary colic	Location of pain (exclusively in the chest) and absence of associated nausea atypical for biliary colic	?10% Unlikely	Low
Acute coronary syndrome (ACS)	Several risk factors for coronary artery disease present; the normal ECG at presentation does not exclude ACS	?35% Possible	Moderate
Pulmonary embolism	Both intuitively and by the use of the clinical decision rule, pulmonary embolism is unlikely	?10% Unlikely	Moderate
Aortic dissection	Abrupt-onset pain, but this is not exclusive to aortic dissection, and its complete resolution within 2 hours would be unusual	?35% Possible	High
Oesophageal rupture	No clinical or radiological features in favour of this diagnosis; however, it is a diagnosis notoriously easy to miss	<1% Very unlikely	High

to integrate the test result with our assessment of the pretest probability of disease: when the pretest probability of disease is very high, a negative test result is more likely to be a false negative. Imaging tests are open to errors of technique and interpretation: a 'normal' chest X-ray or CT scan may not be normal when viewed by a more experienced eye. Testing also has costs and may have hazards (if the test is invasive or involves radiation or contrast media). Tests may reveal incidental findings which trigger further investigation, increasing costs without necessarily improving outcomes (e.g. the detection of pulmonary nodules on CT coronary angiography). And testing may delay appropriate management: for example, waiting for the result of contrast CT in a patient with a high clinical probability of aortic dissection rather than focusing on medical stabilization and transfer to a cardiothoracic surgical unit.

Combining diagnostic assessment with safe care

Patients understand that we can't always get the diagnosis right the first time, but they do expect us to minimize their exposure to harm. The evolution of diseases over time means that many diagnoses become apparent after the initial encounter, and we often need to observe and reassess the patient to come to the correct diagnosis. As a general rule, the sicker the patient, the more often should the assessment (particularly the examination) be repeated.

In many patients presenting after an episode of chest pain, we may not be able to make a confident diagnosis, despite observation (the evidence is that this should be for at least 6 hours), reassessment, and testing. Such patients usually have benign disease; we may accept the diagnostic uncertainty implicit in a label of non-specific chest pain, provided we have confirmed their low-risk status, as reflected in normal findings on examination, serial ECGs, chest X-ray, and measurement of biomarkers, as a minimum. How far to take testing for coronary artery disease (or other serious disease) beyond this is a common judgement call.

Safe care also involves giving information to discharged patients as to what symptoms should prompt them to seek further help, making appropriate provision for their follow-up, and ensuring that clinical information is promptly sent from secondary to primary care. These actions can reduce the risk to which the patient is exposed should we have got the diagnosis wrong.

Outcome of the case

Contrast CT was normal, with no evidence of aortic dissection. Serial ECGs showed minor anterolateral T-wave changes only. However, serum troponin I was raised at 8 ng/ml. Treatment was therefore started for non-ST elevation acute coronary syndrome. Coronary angiography the following day showed a severe stenosis in a large left circumflex artery marginal branch, which was treated by percutaneous intervention. The case illustrates the point that diagnostic ECG changes are not always seen in acute coronary syndrome: acute coronary syndromes in the left circumflex artery territory are less likely to result in diagnostic ECG changes than those involving other territories.

Prognostic and management uncertainty

Getting the diagnosis right is important, but we often have patients whose prognosis or management is uncertain, even though their

diagnosis is clear. For example, should a 75-year-old woman admitted with hypercapnic respiratory failure due to an acute exacerbation of severe chronic obstructive pulmonary disease have mechanical ventilation if non-invasive ventilation fails? Is anticoagulation necessary for a 68-year-old woman found to be in atrial fibrillation and who has hypertension but no other medical problems? Can we safely manage as an outpatient a 59-year-old man with pulmonary embolism confirmed on CT pulmonary angiography?

In each case, what we do will be strongly influenced by what we think the outcome (or range of possible outcomes) will be for the patient in question. In pulmonary embolism, for example, the risk of death extends from >50% to <1%, depending on the clinical features. How can we accurately predict the outcome for the patient before us, and so make the right decision?

Clinical acumen and experience are useful guides, but don't always get us to the right answer: we naturally give undue weight to the cases we remember which went particularly well or badly. And, if our experience is limited, what else can we rely on? Which features are the ones to which we should pay most attention when considering prognosis?

There is good evidence that our intuitive risk assessments are often wrong. As regards estimates of survival, doctors veer between the overly optimistic (e.g. overestimating survival in patients under their care with cancer) and overly pessimistic (e.g. underestimating the benefits of intensive care for patients admitted on-take with acute exacerbations of COPD). Prognostic and risk-assessment models are therefore useful to check and calibrate our clinical assessments. A valid model shows good discrimination (its ability to correctly separate patients into different groups (e.g. survivors/non-survivors) and calibration (the degree of correspondence between the estimated probability derived from the model and the actual observed probability in different patient groups). To gain acceptance, the model also needs to be based on readily available clinical or laboratory data, be easily remembered, and to have been validated in more than one patient population. Examples of risk-assessment models that have become part of standard clinical practice are given in Table 2.4.

Even though the use of validated risk-assessment models can improve our assessment of prognosis, we need to bear in mind that these models cannot specify the outcome of individuals: some 'high-risk' patients will inevitably fare better than some 'low-risk' ones. The longer the interval between the prediction and the event (e.g. predicting 1-year as compared to 30-day survival), the less accurate the prediction.

Decision-making in the face of uncertainty

In medicine, we often have to act (or choose not to act) despite uncertainty, and our style of decision-making is largely determined by the demands of the situation (Table 2.5). The approach adopted in relation to the case in the previous section can be characterized as analytical: we had the time to collect the information we wanted, consider it carefully, and, if necessary, ask a colleague for advice. When dealing with emergencies, however, we have to act under time pressure and with high stakes. Studies of doctors and of those in other professions with similar responsibilities (e.g. those in the armed forces, firefighters) reveal that, in emergencies, intuitive decision-making—triggered by situation recognition—usually

Table 2.4 Use of risk-assessment models in clinical practice		
Reasons for using the model	Examples	Model
The treatment is of low overall benefit: to identify patients most likely to benefit	Primary prevention with statin therapy	Joint British Societies model
The treatment is of moderate or large benefit but carries significant risk of harm: to identify patients for whom benefit exceeds risk	Anticoagulation in non-valvular atrial fibrillation	CHADS$_2$ and CHADS-Vasc score for risk of stroke HAS-BLED score for risk of bleeding with anticoagulation
The treatment is of limited availability	Liver transplantation for liver failure	Model for End-Stage Liver Disease (MELD) score
To identify patients who can safely be managed with only a brief or no inpatient stay	Community-acquired pneumonia	CURB65 score
	Upper gastrointestinal haemorrhage	Rockall score, Blatchford score
	Transient ischaemic attack	ABCD^2 score

Table 2.5 Approaches to medical decision-making

	Analytical	Intuitive
Setting	Used when time pressure is low and the situation is well defined	Used when urgency is high and immediate action needed
Example	Clinic: how should I manage this 78-year-old man with symptomatic severe aortic stenosis who has multiple comorbidities?	Emergency Dept: how should I manage this 78-year-old man admitted following a syncopal episode whose blood pressure is falling?
Concept of decision-making	A choice between alternative strategies, guided by calculation of utility: do A rather than B because A is predicted to have a superior outcome	A choice between actions, guided by the match between situation and appropriate action: do A rather than B because A is a better match to the situation
Drivers of decision-making	Information and analysis	Situation recognition and experience
Principal feature of uncertainty	Limited or ambiguous information	Doubt that hinders action
Response to uncertainty	Focused gathering of information Use of clinical decision rules, prognostic models, and risk-assessment models Use of formal decision analysis Second opinion Multidisciplinary team discussion	Not sure what's going on: rapidly gather the information needed to allow situation recognition Missing information: make assumptions based on the working diagnosis to fill gaps Not sure which course of action to take: weigh the pros and cons before acting; have a back-up plan to use if the first plan is unsuccessful

takes precedence over the analytical approach used when time is less critical. Because experience is of such importance in intuitive decision-making, experts usually perform better than novices in managing emergencies. Experts are generally more astute at recognizing what type of emergency they're dealing with (and when it differs from a typical pattern), more confident in matching their action to the situation, and better able to judge the time available for assessment before action. They are also more willing to change tack when unfolding events show that their initial approach was wrong, and can switch between intuitive and analytical decision-making as the circumstances require.

So, how can we accelerate our progress from novice to expert? Simulation exercises can supplement our clinical experience. Formal debriefing may help us learn more from the cases we have dealt with. And checklists can support our responses to common emergencies, providing us with an expert guide to action (and ensuring that we don't forget crucial information in the heat of the moment). At its simplest, a checklist can be a list of all the diagnoses to be considered in a given situation (e.g. the causes of cardiac arrest with pulseless electrical activity), but will typically specify a sequence of actions to be taken. The use of checklists to structure the management of medical emergencies is in its infancy but, given its success in improving the outcome of aviation emergencies, holds great promise.

Further Reading

http://understandinguncertainty.org/ This site, produced by the Winton Programme for the Public Understanding of Risk based in the Statistical Laboratory in the University of Cambridge, provides an excellent introduction to risk and related concepts.

Schwarze ML and Taylor LJ. Managing uncertainty—harnessing the power of scenario planning. *N Engl J Med* 2017; 377: 206–08.

Woodward M, Tunstall-Pedoe H, and Peters SAE. Graphics and statistics for cardiology: clinical prediction rules. *Heart* 2017; 103: 483–90.

3 Taking the history

David Sprigings

Introduction

Our aim as doctors is to understand the patient and the disease. Taking the history is key to both of these objectives. Only through talking to patients can we can get to know them as people, their personal experience of illness, and their concerns. And the history remains the richest source of information about their diseases. Most diagnoses are suggested by the history, with examination and investigation providing supporting and confirmatory evidence. By the same token, if we reach the end of the history without some idea as to the cause of the patient's problem, we need to go back and retake it, because our chances of arriving at the correct diagnosis without this map to guide us are slim.

History taking is a conversation with a purpose, not a cross-examination. In this chapter, we look at some aspects of history taking that are of particular relevance to diagnosis in internal medicine. Let's begin with what the patient tells us.

The patient's account

We need to give patients enough time to tell their story in their own words, without interruption, before we start asking questions. Sometimes the patient's account is so comprehensive that further questioning is superfluous (Box 3.1), but we will usually want to explore the detail of the symptoms, as this detail enables us to distinguish between diagnostic possibilities. For example, chest pain may arise from a broad range of thoracic and upper abdominal diseases, as well as being a sensation transiently experienced by healthy people. However, recurrent retrosternal chest pain, provoked by exertion and relieved promptly by rest, as described by this patient, has a much narrower differential diagnosis.

With experience, we become familiar with the range of diseases that can give rise to a given symptom. We also learn the varied ways patients express the symptoms of a given disease. The patient whose account is given in the box (who proved to have three-vessel coronary disease) was unusual in saying he experienced 'pain': most patients use words such as discomfort, heaviness, pressure, tightness, or 'like indigestion' to describe what myocardial ischaemia feels like. And some symptoms prove on closer questioning to be composites

Box 3.1 The typed account of his symptoms brought by a 63-year-old man to his first cardiology clinic appointment

'Sometimes (but rarely) the pain does not appear at all, especially if I walk slowly. But in the majority of cases it starts after about ¼ of a mile, or even sooner, especially if I walk fast. The pain stops completely and almost immediately (about 10 seconds) if I stop. If I start again the pain comes back after 50 yards or so. As I keep stopping and starting, the pain becomes milder, and frequently may disappear completely and not come back—provided I do not accelerate the pace. The pain seems to rise from the stomach and usually concentrates in the central-upper part of my chest. It takes the form of a hard lump, very much like food sticking in the oesophagus. When it disappears, it often seems to be sinking back. I often feel if I could expel air, I would be all right. Very often this happens and I do feel better afterwards. The pain seems to be worse on wet or humid days. By worse I mean that it starts sooner and does not get better as I keep stopping. Agitation or emotion seems to make matters worse.'

Table 3.1 Diagnostic questions to determine whether transient loss of consciousness is due to seizure or syncope

Question	Points (if yes)
At times do you wake with a cut tongue after your spells?	2
At times do you have a sense of déjà vu or jamais vu before your spells?	1
At times is emotional stress associated with losing consciousness?	1
Has anyone ever noted your head turning during a spell?	1
Has anyone ever noted that you are unresponsive, have unusual posturing, or have jerking limbs during your spells, or have no memory of your spells afterwards? *(Score as 'yes' for any positive response)*	1
Has anyone ever noted that you are confused after a spell?	1
Have you ever had lightheaded spells?	−2
At times do you sweat before your spells?	−2
Is prolonged sitting or standing associated with your spells?	−2

The patient has seizures if the point score is ≥1, and syncope if the point score is <1.

Reprinted from *Journal of the American College of Cardiology*, Volume 40, Issue 1, Sheldon R, et al., 'Historical criteria that distinguish syncope from seizures', pp. 142-148, Copyright © 2002 American College of Cardiology Foundation, with permission from Elsevier.

of several abnormal sensations. Exertional breathlessness in patients with chronic obstructive pulmonary disease, for example, often spans 'shallow breathing', 'can't get enough air in', and 'chest tightness', likely to reflect different pathophysiological mechanisms.

Interpreting the patient's symptoms—in this case, moving from the patient's account of around 200 words to a two-word summary, exertional angina—is a necessary step towards formulating a differential diagnosis, but one that introduces the possibility of error. And error at this point can have a profound influence on clinical outcome, as our formulation of the problem based on the history often determines the diagnostic pathway we take. To avoid misinterpretation, we need time to make sure we have grasped correctly the detail of the symptoms. Careful questioning can also help us distinguish between diagnoses. For example, the answers to nine questions can, in aggregate, determine (with >90% accuracy) whether transient loss of consciousness is due to seizure or syncope (Table 3.1).

The focused history

We must adapt our history taking to the clinical circumstances. When dealing with a patient who may have critical illness, initial history taking has to be abbreviated, and usually combined with an assessment of the physiological status. The focused history—the focus being diagnosis—is based on defining the problem, establishing its context, and then asking those questions which best discriminate between the diagnostic possibilities (Table 3.2).

We usually come to a view as to the nature of the clinical problem within a minute or two of meeting the patient. It's rarely the case that the patient's major symptom (the 'presenting complaint' in UK terminology, and 'chief complaint' in US terminology) is not central to the diagnosis, and overlooking or sidelining this carries a serious risk of diagnostic error. A 66-year-old woman with rheumatoid arthritis presented with erythema and swelling of her right arm following a fall. However, her main complaint was of diffuse severe

Table 3.2 The focused and the complete history

Focused history	Complete history*
Presenting problem and its context (age/sex of the patient; clinical setting; chronology of events)	History of each presenting complaint
Active medical problems (including comorbidities or long-term conditions) and major events in the past history	Past medical, surgical, and mental health history
Current medication	Medication record
Allergies	Relevant legal information
Concise social history: to include as a minimum usual functional status, home circumstances, tobacco and alcohol use	Allergies and adverse reactions
	Risk and warnings
	Social history
	Family history
	Systematic enquiry
	Patient's concerns, expectations, and wishes

* Recommended database for patients admitted to hospital.

Data from Health and Social Care Information Centre, Academy of Medical Royal Colleges (2013): Standards for the clinical structure and content of patient records.

pain in the arm. The importance of this was not recognized, and the correct diagnosis of necrotizing fasciitis was delayed.

The context of a problem has a powerful effect on the differential diagnosis. Context includes the age and sex of the patient, the clinical setting (e.g. primary/secondary care; inpatient/outpatient), and the patient's comorbidities. Grouping causes by context is an effective way of keeping the differential diagnosis manageable. For example, if we are seeing a young adult with delirium in the emergency department, our differential diagnosis will focus on meningoencephalitis, or alcohol or substance use; if called to the oncology ward because of delirium in an older patient receiving chemotherapy for lung cancer, we will be considering electrolyte disorders, metastatic disease, and opioid toxicity. When taking a focused history, we select those questions relevant to the problem and its context, aiming to narrow the differential diagnosis to a few possibilities at which examination and investigation can be directed.

The focused history must establish a clear chronology of events, because this is key to understanding causal relationships. In addition, the mode of onset, the time course, and the duration of symptoms are major clues to the underlying disease or pathophysiology. In neurological disorders, for example, the onset of symptoms over seconds or minutes suggests vascular disorders or epilepsy; over hours or days, infection or demyelination; and over weeks or months, neoplastic or degenerative diseases.

Comorbidities or 'long-term conditions' affect one in three of the UK adult population (one in two of those over 60) and are therefore frequently part of the clinical picture. Defining the patient's comorbidities is important, as these shape the differential diagnosis and often influence the choice of treatment. In suspected sepsis, for example, the range of infections to be considered is very different if there is a background of HIV–AIDS or of chronic liver disease. Establishing the patient's current (and recent) medication is also a central element of the focused history. A list of the patient's medication alerts you to comorbidities the patient may not have mentioned; and the presenting problem may be related to medication. You also need to ask specifically about allergies (and check for these in the patient's records). An abbreviated social history should be taken. As a minimum, you need to know the patient's usual functional status, home circumstances, and tobacco and alcohol use. The occupational, travel, and sexual history may all be relevant to a given problem.

A complete history (Table 3.2) remains central to the holistic care of the patient. In patients admitted to hospital, a complete history should be taken once their condition has been stabilized: this ensures that key diagnostic information has not been overlooked or misinterpreted, addresses psychosocial issues not covered in the focused history, and provides data relevant to longer-term care.

Getting the story straight

'Getting the story straight' is a crucial part of history taking: it is the process of summarizing the information we have gathered and

Box 3.2 A 36-year-old man with acute chest pain and breathlessness

Patient's story: 'I've not felt well for a few days. I thought I was going down with the flu. For the past day or so I've had this pain in the middle of my chest. If I lean right forward, it's a bit easier. The pain makes my breathing difficult.'

Novice trainee: 'The patient is a 36-year-old man with short history of pleuritic chest pain and breathlessness. He was previously well. He has a temperature of 38.0°C. There is a loud systolic murmur. His lungs are clear. His calves are soft and non-tender.'

Expert trainee: 'The patient is a 36-year-old man with central pleuritic chest pain which has developed in the context of a flu-like illness. He has had no previous episodes. There is no past history of connective tissue disease or other major illness. Examination shows him to be mildly unwell with a temperature of 38.0°C. A pericardial friction rub can be heard, with systolic and diastolic components. His jugular venous pressure is not raised and the lungs are clear. The rest of the examination is normal.'

Consultant: 'What do you think is the diagnosis?'

Novice trainee: 'He could have had a pulmonary embolism, which can happen even if you don't have risk factors for DVT. It could be pneumonia, although he hasn't had a productive cough and his lungs are clear. I can't explain the murmur. Infective endocarditis seems unlikely.'

Expert trainee: 'The patient has the features of acute pericarditis, with a diagnostic friction rub. This is likely to be viral in origin. There are no signs of myocarditis or cardiac tamponade. Pneumonia with pericarditis needs to be considered, but there are no clinical signs of pneumonia and he looks too well for purulent pericarditis.'

shaping it into a narrative or story that provides a coherent account of what has happened to the patient. This act of organization may lead us to the diagnosis. When it doesn't, it will usually narrow the differential diagnosis to a manageable number of possibilities, and direct our next steps. Box 3.2 illustrates how our ability to get the story straight is improved by experience, and also demonstrates the interplay between history taking and examination. The novice trainee has taken an adequate history but has failed to see the relevance of some of the answers, has misinterpreted a key physical sign, and cannot pull the information together into a working diagnosis. By contrast, the expert trainee has recognized the pericardial friction rub and deftly summarizes the features which make acute viral pericarditis the likely diagnosis.

So, how can we transform ourselves from novices into experts? Central to this transformation is the acquisition of a broad and deep knowledge of diseases and their clinical presentations. If it takes 10 000 hours practice to become an expert in other fields, it may well take experience of 10 000 patients to achieve this as a doctor. But as well as these clinical encounters, to become experts we have to practice presenting cases to colleagues, articulating the differential diagnosis, and defending our choice of working diagnosis.

Getting the story straight refers to the entirety of information in the history: as well as what we learn from the patient, this will often include the accounts of doctors, nurses, paramedics, and others and, depending on the problem, those of family members or carers. Memory is, of course, fallible, and we need to confirm and supplement these accounts with evidence from relevant documents. In a patient with a complex problem on a background of several major comorbidities, we can be dealing with a mass of information, often contained in multiple volumes of hospital notes. To manage this information effectively, we have to give it structure: we need a problem list.

Handling complexity: The use of problem lists

A problem list is a summary of all of the patient's medical problems, including psychiatric, social, and other factors that may be relevant to care. The problem list of a 66-year-old woman admitted on-take with acute kidney injury is shown in Table 3.3. Problems are stated at the

Table 3.3 The problem list of a 66-year-old woman admitted with acute kidney injury

Active problems	Inactive problems
Acute kidney injury? cause Dec 2014, normal renal function Nov 2014	Ulcerative colitis 2004
Acute coronary syndrome Nov 2014, single-vessel coronary disease, PCI of proximal LCX stenosis (bare-metal stent), normal LV systolic function on echocardiography	Right hip replacement 2008
	Left hip replacement 2009
Psoriasis with arthritis 2002	
Primary hypothyroidism 1990	

level of current understanding; unexplained clinical features or laboratory results should be included (e.g. Thrombocytopenia? cause). In the case of diseases such as diabetes or ischaemic heart diseases, which have a wide clinical spectrum, it is helpful to add relevant information in summary form, with dates. Inactive problems are those medical problems the patient has had in the past but do not currently need treatment.

A concise, up-to-date summary of all clinical problems benefits the patient in several ways. It helps offset the detrimental effects of care fragmented between medical shifts and between specialists. Discerning the potential interrelationships between problems is made easier by listing them. For example, in the case shown in the box, the onset of acute kidney injury shortly after percutaneous coronary intervention suggested cholesterol embolism, contrast nephropathy, or statin-induced rhabdomyolysis as possible mechanisms (it proved to be the last). The problem list also reminds us of those pieces of information (e.g. anaphylaxis from meropenem, renovascular disease), which might be buried in Volume 3 of the notes but are of great importance to safe prescribing.

The future

In most hospitals, we still write the history in the notes. But, as UK secondary care moves from paper to electronic records, history taking faces challenges and opportunities. A major challenge is to get hardware and software suited to the way we work. We don't want to be using desktop computers with keyboard entry of data into systems built around tick boxes: this will slow down the assessment of patients and degrade the quality of the information recorded. Rather, we need portable wireless devices with hand-writing, sketch, and voice-recognition software, so that we can easily gather complete information whether we are seeing the patient in the emergency department, on the ward, or in clinic. And the way in which the data are stored must preserve the richness of language.

With electronic recording comes the opportunity to use real-time diagnostic software, which could suggest a differential diagnosis as the history evolves, remind us of the relevant questions we haven't yet asked, and prompt us as to what information should be sought from the examination and investigation. Problem lists could be automatically generated from both primary and secondary care records, with links to source documents, imaging, and laboratory results. The diagnostic usefulness of the history, as well as its other functions, would be enhanced by these changes.

Whether written on paper or recorded electronically, the history—the narrative of the patient's illness—will remain the foundation of care. In the craft of bedside clinical assessment, history taking is closely linked to examination: examining the patient enables us to test immediately diagnoses suggested by the history, and the physical signs often evoke new diagnostic possibilities which can be explored by further questioning. In Chapter 4, we look critically at the place of physical examination in twenty-first-century medicine.

Further Reading

Charon R. Narrative medicine: A model for empathy, reflection, profession and trust. *JAMA* 2001; 286: 1897–902.

Haidet P and Paterniti DA. "Building" a history rather than "taking" one. A perspective on information sharing during the medical interview. *Arch Intern Med* 2003; 163: 1134–40.

Health and Social Care Information Centre, Academy of Medical Royal Colleges. *Standards for the clinical structure and content of patient records*. London: HSCIC, 2013. Available at https://www.aomrc.org.uk/wp-content/uploads/2016/05/Standards_for_the_Clinical_Structure_and_Content_of_Patient_Records_0713.pdf

Walsh SH. The clinician's perspective on electronic health records and how they can affect patient care. *BMJ* 2004; 328: 1184–7.

4 The physical examination

David Sprigings

Introduction

A 37-year-old man is admitted on the medical take with right hemiparesis. Examination shows Horner's syndrome contralateral to the weakness. Within a few moments, we have a working diagnosis of ischaemic stroke due to left carotid artery dissection. Although often focused on diagnosis, as powerfully demonstrated in this patient, the physical examination has broader purposes (Box 4.1). It has been traditionally defined as the evaluation of the body and its functions by the methods of inspection, palpation, percussion, and auscultation, but is more than this. Instruments such as the thermometer, stethoscope, tendon hammer, and ophthalmoscope increase the range and precision of our findings. And some tests which can be readily done at the bedside (such as measurement of oxygen saturation or blood glucose) have become incorporated into the examination, as they too provide immediately available data for integration into diagnostic thinking and patient management.

Notwithstanding the advances of the past 40 years in imaging—which is in effect an extension of the examination—the physical signs remain central to our assessment of patients, especially those with acute illness. And failure to detect these signs contributes to misdiagnosis. A study from a US hospital found that one-quarter of acute medical patients when re-examined had signs which had been overlooked on admission and which changed the diagnosis and management. To be effective clinicians, we must have a competent examination technique, but also need a clear understanding of what the signs can and can't tell us in a given clinical situation (Box 4.2).

Box 4.1 Purposes of the physical examination

- In acute illness, to define the physiological status of the patient and need for immediate organ support
- To test diagnostic hypotheses suggested by the history by the presence or absence of signs of disease
- To evoke diagnostic hypotheses
- To assess the severity of a known disease
- To contribute information (e.g. height and weight) to the database of the patient
- To check for asymptomatic abnormalities of diagnostic or prognostic importance (e.g. breast lump, enlarged prostate, hypertension)
- To meet the expectations of the patient, and strengthen the doctor–patient relationship
- To maintain clinical skills at examination

Box 4.2 Facts we need to know about physical signs

Significance

How likely is a patient with this sign to have disease?
Which diseases may give rise to this sign?
How often is this sign seen in a given disease?
How is this sign influenced by age and comorbidities?
How much does the presence or absence of this sign change the probability of a given disease?

Accuracy

How closely does this sign agree with an objective standard?

Reliability

How well do doctors agree with each other or with themselves on the presence or absence of this sign?

Let's begin by considering how we use examination findings in diagnostic reasoning.

Physical signs and diagnostic reasoning

There is two-way traffic between our thoughts about diagnosis and the physical signs. Diagnostic hypotheses suggested by the history can be tested by examination: if the signs of the disease in question are present, that disease becomes more likely, and if absent, less likely. And the examination may yield signs which suggest diagnoses we hadn't previously considered. As diagnosticians, we therefore need ready access to two categories of information: the diseases associated with a given sign, and the signs associated with a given disease.

Consider a 68-year-old man, an inpatient receiving chemotherapy for lung cancer, who has become breathless. As the medical registrar leading the night team, you are called to see him on the oncology ward. The differential diagnosis is wide and includes cardiac tamponade, superior vena caval (SVC) obstruction, and pleural effusion. You were told over the phone that he has an oxygen saturation of 90% breathing air, a pulse rate of 110, a blood pressure of 135/80, and a temperature of 38°C. Your first thought is that he has pneumonia. However, the chest examination is unremarkable, and the sign that strikes you is an elevated jugular venous pressure.

Cardiac tamponade now seems more likely than pneumonia. Pulmonary embolism and SVC obstruction also cross your mind. You also wonder about whether his chemotherapy could have resulted in heart failure. Indeed, a number of diagnoses are possible (Table 4.1). As you continue the examination, you weigh up the significance of the other findings and how they affect the likelihood of the diseases under consideration.

The logic driving your assessment is that the absence of a sign which is characteristic of a disease (seen in >95% of patients), or the absence of two or three signs each found in >80% of patients, is strong evidence against that disease being present. If this were cardiac tamponade causing breathlessness, you would expect a low blood pressure with pulsus paradoxus (Table 4.2), and your patient does not show these signs.

So, tamponade is not the leading diagnosis, but hasn't been definitively ruled out. How likely is pulmonary embolism? Here a clinical decision rule can sometimes help. The Wells score (see Chapter 101), which provides a guide to the likelihood of

Table 4.1 Possible causes of an elevated jugular venous pressure in a breathless 68-year-old man receiving chemotherapy for lung cancer

Pathophysiology	Mechanisms
Fluid overload	Acute kidney injury due to chemotherapy
	Excessive intravenous fluid administration
Superior vena caval obstruction	Extrinsic compression by the primary tumour or mediastinal lymphadenopathy
	Thrombosis around a central venous catheter
Mediastinal shift	Massive pleural effusion causing mediastinal compression
Raised intra-pericardial pressure	Metastatic pericardial disease with effusion
Raised right atrial pressure	Pulmonary embolism with right ventricular dysfunction
	Cardiomyopathy due to chemotherapy
	Acute inferior myocardial infarction with right ventricular infarction

Table 4.2 Frequency of physical signs in cardiac tamponade

Sign	Pooled frequency (95% confidence interval)
Pulsus paradoxus >10 mm Hg	82 (72–92)
Elevated jugular venous pressure	76 (62–90)
Tachycardia	77 (69–85)
Hypotension	26 (16–36)

Data from Roy CL, et al. Does this patient with a pericardial effusion have cardiac tamponade? *JAMA* volume 297: 1810-8, 2007.

Table 4.3 A 2 × 2 table showing the frequency of dullness to percussion in patients with and without pleural effusion

		Pleural effusion (by radiography)	
		Present	Absent
Dullness to conventional percussion	Present	89%	19%
	Absent	11%	81%

Reprinted from *Evidence Based Physical Diagnosis*, Steven McGee, p 288-290, Copyright 2012, with permission from Elsevier.

pulmonary embolism, is 4 (heart rate >100/min, immobilization, malignancy), indicating that the probability of pulmonary embolism is unlikely. As his breathlessness came on abruptly, you feel the likelihood of pulmonary embolism is higher than predicted by the score; however, he has been receiving prophylaxis against venous thromboembolism.

By examining the patient, and applying a knowledge of the significance of signs, within a few minutes you have been able to assemble a differential diagnosis in a complex clinical situation, and come to a rational decision about immediate management. No technology can rival this. Imaging will, of course, be part of your management, and we next consider the relation between examination and imaging.

Examination and imaging

The fact that examination may be an unreliable guide to the presence of disease leads some doctors to maintain it is better to get the relevant scan than to spend time examining the patient. This extreme view is clearly wrong (although has some attraction when one is faced with a complex neurological problem on a particularly heavy take), not least because the scan you want may not be immediately available and, in the setting of acute illness, can't do what the examination can, that is, define the physiological status of the patient and the need for immediate organ support. The information provided by the history and examination is crucial to our choice of imaging, our judgement as to how urgently it is needed, and the interpretation of the findings. Deciding if a patient has had an ischaemic stroke and should receive thrombolysis requires integration of clinical and CT data. Identical right upper lobe shadowing on the chest X-rays of two patients with cough and weight loss has a different significance for the 22-year-old student back from India and the 58-year-old smoker who has never travelled abroad. And if the scan result is discordant with the clinical findings, we will need to reassess the patient (and the scan).

Of course, doctors (and patients) may not be satisfied by a normal examination. There are many clinical situations in which the examination findings are of limited use in ruling in or ruling out serious disease. This is notoriously the case in relation to coronary artery disease. In the diagnosis of stable coronary disease, the examination is of little help (although may point to an alternative cause for angina, such as aortic stenosis or hypertrophic cardiomyopathy). Nor can the signs accurately identify patients with acute coronary syndrome. And the examination is a very poor guide to left ventricular systolic function, a key prognostic variable in coronary disease.

So we need to know the limitations of the examination in specific situations, and when imaging or laboratory testing is required in addition to clinical assessment. Imaging is often costly, may not improve outcomes, and if radiation based contributes to the risk of cancer: the challenge for healthcare systems is to define the appropriateness of imaging in a given clinical setting, and in which order tests should be done. The definition of appropriateness will necessarily be based on clinical assessment, and this brings us back to the value of physical signs.

How good is that sign?

As well as knowing its associations with diseases, to fully understand the significance of a sign, we need to have a feeling for its accuracy and reliability.

Accuracy

Accuracy is a measure of the extent to which the sign agrees with an objective standard. For example, consider dullness to percussion as a sign of pleural effusion. Table 4.3 shows the frequency of this sign in patients with pleural effusion defined by radiography. Dullness to percussion is not invariably present in patients with pleural effusion (as small effusions are not detected), nor invariably absent in patients without pleural effusion (as it may be found in other pleural, pulmonary, and diaphragmatic disorders). Nevertheless, we can see from the data in Table 4.3 that its presence makes the diagnosis of pleural effusion more likely, and its absence less likely. But by how much? Likelihood ratios (LRs) can help answer this question.

We met LRs in Chapter 1. Applied to the sign of dullness to percussion, the positive LR is the percentage of patients with pleural effusion who show the sign, divided by the percentage of patients without pleural effusion who also have the sign, that is, 89% divided by 81%, which gives an LR of 4.7. We can also calculate the negative LR, that is, the percentage of patients with pleural effusion who don't show dullness to percussion, divided by the percentage of patients without pleural effusion and who also lack the sign. The negative LR is 11% divided by 81%, which is 0.1. These LRs can be translated into approximate changes in the probability of disease (see Chapter 1). So, the presence of dullness to percussion means that the probability of pleural effusion is increased by around 30%; the absence of the sign equates to a decrease in probability of around 45%.

Accurate signs are therefore signs with high positive or low negative LRs. Signs with high positive LRs help rule in specific diseases, while signs with low negative LRs help rule these out. As can be seen from Table 4.4, few signs in isolation have the power definitively to rule in or rule out diseases (i.e. positive LR >10 or negative LR <0.1). Combinations of signs are more powerful in diagnosis. For example, the presence or absence of lung crackles, on its own, makes little difference to the likelihood of pneumonia. But the combination of fever >37.8°C, tachycardia, lung crackles, and reduced breath sounds has a positive LR of 8, increasing the likelihood of pneumonia (from whatever value is indicated by the clinical setting and the patient's symptoms) by around 40%.

Table 4.4 Accuracy of some physical signs

Sign	Positive LR	Negative LR
Conjunctival pallor as a sign of anaemia	4.7	0.6
Neck stiffness as a sign of subarachnoid haemorrhage	5.4	0.7
Lung crackles as a sign of pneumonia	1.8	0.8
Splenomegaly as a sign of cirrhosis in a patient with chronic liver disease	2.5	0.8
Presence of ascites as a sign of hepatocellular disease in the patient with jaundice	4.4	0.6
Palpable bladder, for detecting >400 ml urine in bladder	1.9	0.3
Extensor plantar response as a sign of unilateral cerebral hemispheric disease	8.5	Not significant

Abbreviations: LR, likelihood ratio.
Data from McGee S. *Evidence-Based Physical Diagnosis.* 3rd edition, 2012. Elsevier Saunders.

Reliability

Reliability usually refers to the extent to which two or more doctors agree on the presence or absence of the sign (inter-observer reliability). Doctors may disagree about examination findings for several reasons. The definition of the sign (e.g. an increased or decreased carotid pulse volume) may be imprecise. The sign may change with time or treatment (e.g. pericardial rub in acute pericarditis, or the jugular venous pressure in heart failure). The examination technique of one doctor may be flawed (e.g. failing to position the patient appropriately to hear the murmur of mitral stenosis or aortic regurgitation). The environment (e.g. a noisy emergency department) or factors such as fatigue and distraction may interfere with the examination. And, finally, a doctor's view as to the likely diagnosis may bias his or her interpretation of borderline abnormalities.

Reliability can be measured in several ways. The kappa statistic, which takes account of agreement by chance, is often used: this ranges from −1.0 (complete disagreement) through 0 (chance agreement) to +1.0 (perfect agreement). A kappa statistic of <0.4 indicates poor agreement, and one of >0.8, excellent agreement between doctors. When put to the test, the reliability of many signs is surprisingly limited. For example, one study of patients with respiratory diseases found that almost all signs (reduced chest movements, cyanosis, prolonged expiration, impalpable apex beat, cricosternal distance, tachypnoea, increased or decreased tactile fremitus, and displaced trachea) had kappa values of <0.4. Only finger clubbing had a kappa value over 0.4 (just—at 0.45). Other studies have shown similar results, although with better agreement as regards pleural rub and wheeze.

A low kappa value doesn't mean the sign has no value: provided the accuracy of the sign is high, and its intra-observer reliability is good (i.e. a doctor agrees with him- or herself about the presence or absence of the sign on repeated examinations), it may still be a very useful sign. The sign of spontaneous retinal vein pulsation exemplifies this. It's a difficult sign, but once you have learnt to see it, you will be confident as to its presence or absence. And its presence effectively establishes that intracranial pressure is normal (although the converse is not the case, as 10% of normal subjects don't show the sign).

Of course, issues of accuracy and reliability also apply to imaging tests: interpreting a scan requires the examination of the images. And we soon learn that a normal scan doesn't necessarily mean the absence of disease: as with physical examination, subtle findings can be missed, or the disease in question cannot be detected by that particular scan.

Other factors

The accuracy and reliability of the examination are strongly influenced by experience and training. Some signs, such as jaundice or hemiplegia, are readily apparent, whereas others (e.g. fixed splitting of the second sound) are harder to detect, and will often be missed by non-specialists. Specialists become better at the examination of their system as they do the examination more often, see more patients with abnormal signs, are highly motivated to interpret the signs correctly, and have their findings repeatedly compared with imaging and laboratory results. Of course, whether you are a novice or a specialist, physical signs will be missed if the patient is not examined systematically and thoroughly.

Aging and comorbidities also affect the accuracy and reliability of physical signs. A patient with end-stage kidney disease due to diabetes, treated by haemodialysis via an arteriovenous fistula, has many abnormal signs that may make distinguishing new from established disease difficult. The standard 70 kg man has been left behind in the twentieth century, and we must take account of the effects of obesity on the physical signs, particularly in relation to cardiovascular, respiratory, or intra-abdominal disease.

The future

The physical examination has changed over time and will continue to change. We no longer estimate cardiac size by percussion. Pulse oximetry is a much better guide to oxygen saturation than the presence or absence of cyanosis. Imaging with a portable ultrasound machine and immediate point-of-care measurement of biomarkers will be of increasing importance to our assessment of patients in the emergency department, on the ward, or in clinic. The information provided by these tests will require us to question which elements of the examination add value, and which are now redundant. But given the diagnostic and prognostic information yielded by physical examination, and the fact it can be done anywhere, repeated at any time, and needs no power source, it is safe to say the ability to examine a patient and make sense of the findings will remain a defining characteristic of a doctor.

Further Reading

The *Rational Clinical Examination* series in the *Journal of the American Medical Association* is highly recommended as a source of informative and thought-provoking reviews of the value of clinical assessment (http://jamaevidence.com/resource/523).

McGee S. *Evidence-Based Physical Diagnosis* (3rd edition), 2012. Elsevier Saunders. This remarkable single-author book contains a huge amount of information about examination technique and the value of physical signs.

5 The psychological examination

Jonathan Price

Approach to psychological diagnosis

Have broad aims

The aims of psychological assessment are broad:

1. to rule in/rule out common and important psychiatric diagnoses, including dementia, delirium, alcohol and substance use (harmful use, intoxication, dependence, withdrawal), depression, and health anxiety
2. to rule in/rule out possible risks of psychiatric illness, including their nature, degree, and timeline
3. to consider the influence on prognosis of the patient's beliefs about their illness
4. to rule in/rule out possible treatments, through patient's attitudes to treatments

Use an integrated, biopsychosocial approach

In medicine, psychological factors are often regarded as separate to physical factors, and psychological illness as distinct from physical illness. Yet health and illness states reflect multiple, interrelated physical, psychological, and social factors. In the weeks after myocardial infarction, the beliefs that a person has about their heart and damage to it will influence their willingness to take medicines and to engage in physical rehabilitation. Their mood will also be influential, as will social factors such as availability of a supportive partner, and opportunity for gainful employment.

Diagnose positively

Many doctors diagnose psychological illness through a process of exclusion of multiple physical causes. This is potentially harmful for two reasons: first, it means that psychological illness is diagnosed and treated late; and, second, it means that psychological factors, which contribute to the outcome of almost all patients, may not be considered at all.

Consider the risks

Assessing the nature, severity, and timeline of risks of psychiatric illness is a core component of the psychiatric assessment. When doctors think of the risks of psychiatric illness, they often think only of risk of harm to self (such as overdosing, jumping, or hanging) and risk of harm to others (such as assault or killing). However, there are several other important risks to consider (Table 5.1).

Stray outwith your comfort zone

Many doctors consider psychological assessment and management to be outwith their expertise or remit. They may refer on for formal psychiatric assessment, refer back to primary care, or simply ignore the issue. Doctors in any setting must be able to identify patients with core psychiatric problems and conduct a basic assessment.

Stay safe

The safety of the assessing doctor is paramount, and is often taken for granted in general hospital settings, whereas psychiatrists and doctors working in the community are acutely aware of their vulnerability.

Integrate information through time

Integrate information across background history, history of presenting complaints, and mental state examination (MSE). In the background, has the person harmed themselves before and, if so, how often, and how? In the recent history, has the person suffered from low mood, hopelessness about the future, or suicidal thoughts or impulses and, if so, have they acted on them? In the MSE, are they currently depressed, with hopeless thoughts, suicidal thoughts, or suicidal plans? If so, how detailed are their plans and how likely are they to act?

Key points in the history

Interview a corroborant

A corroborant is a person who knows the person's recent situation. Usually, this will simply confirm the patient's account, but sometimes it will refute the patient's account or give important new information. For example, an elderly woman asks her GP for help with rehousing, as her neighbours are threatening her through the walls. Is this real, or is she suffering from auditory hallucinations and persecutory delusions? Various corroborants can be helpful—most usual is a husband, wife, partner, or carer. Take care to obtain the patient's permission, or to be sure that this is not required (such as through focused history taking with a close relative of a patient with a confusional state).

Background history

Is there a family history of mental illness?

If so, which illness, and in which relative(s)? Draw a genogram. Is there a family history of suicide?

What is the nature of the person's social situation?

With whom do they live, and are those people supportive and reliable or unsupportive and chaotic? Is the person currently employed and, if so, does their job provide a clear structure for their day/week? Do they have dependents, such as children or ageing relatives?

Take a careful alcohol and illicit drug history

Be systematic: alcohol and illicit drugs are common contributors to mental illness. Harmful use may not be mentioned by the person because they are using alcohol or illicit substances such as cannabis as 'self-medication'.

Take a careful medicines history

Ask about prescribed medicines and non-prescribed medicines such as those available from chemists. Don't forget herbal remedies, vitamins, and minerals—these help our understanding of attitudes to health, illness, and treatment.

Don't forget the person's medical history

People with psychiatric disorder such as schizophrenia are at high risk of physical disorder, due to poor self-care, poor access to physical health care, and the metabolic side effects of some antipsychotics. People with physical disorder such as stroke are at high risk of psychiatric disorders such as depression, due to resulting disability, direct effects on brain function, and indirect effects on brain function via stroke-related medicines such as antihypertensives.

What is the person's past psychiatric history?

The past is a key predictor of the future. Have they had a mental illness before, and, if so, which? How were they treated? Have they been hospitalized? What risks were evident during these episodes? (See Table 5.1.)

Table 5.1 Risk assessment in the psychological examination

Risk	Example(s)
Suicide/risk of harm to self	Depression
Homicide/risk of harm to others	Schizophrenia
Deterioration in mental state	Any major mental illness
Wandering	Dementia
Abuse/exploitation (sexual, physical, financial)	Dementia
Driving/operating machinery	Drowsiness due to medication; poor concentration due to depression
Care of dependents, such as children and elderly	Moderate-severe depression;
Fire (due to fire-setting or inattention)	Mania, schizophrenia, cognitive impairment
Sexual disinhibition, leading to STIs/pregnancy/relationship breakdown	Mania
Overspending	Mania

History of presenting complaints

First, ascertain the main symptom(s), their duration, precipitants, and impacts.

Second, enquire specifically about symptoms and behaviours associated with the main symptoms. Table 5.2 outlines, within a biopsychosocial framework, the symptoms commonly associated with depression. Don't forget to enquire about risks, such as suicidal thoughts, suicidal impulses, and suicidal acts. Distinguish between **subjective** and **objective lethality**. As doctors, we may dismiss an overdose of ten amoxycillin tablets as trivial (objective lethality), and yet it might have high subjective lethality—the patient may report that they thought they would die because it is many times the standard dose.

Finally, what treatments have been tried, and how acceptable and effective have they been?

The psychological examination

The psychological examination is usually called the MSE. It aims to determine both current **symptoms** (what the patient reports about current psychological symptoms, such as mood, thoughts, beliefs, abnormal perceptions) and current **signs** (what you observe about the patient's current mood, thoughts, beliefs, abnormal perceptions). A symptom which has resolved, such as a belief held last week but not reported or evident today, is part of the history but not of the MSE. The MSE should not be used in isolation; rather, the background history, history of presenting complaint, corroborative history, MSE, and physical examination will all contribute to diagnostic decision-making.

Several aspects of the MSE involve complicated symptoms and signs of mental illness, some of which are rare. Therefore, any

Table 5.2 Features of depression

Risk	Example(s)
Biological	Low energy; poor sleep (including early morning waking); poor appetite; weight loss; constipation; amenorrhoea; low libido
Psychological	Poor motivation; self-neglect (e.g. eating, washing, medicating); poor enjoyment of usually pleasurable activities; diurnal mood variation (usually feeling worse in the morning); hopelessness (negative about the future); guilt (negative about the past); low self-esteem (negative about the present self); suicidal thoughts, impulses, and acts; homicidal thoughts, impulses, and acts; helplessness (negative about prospect of being helped by others or by treatment)
Social	Social withdrawal; absence from work; poor performance at work; relationship difficulties

observations made during an individual MSE should be used with caution, and only in their clinical context. It is also important to consider the diagnostic implications of any MSE abnormalities recorded, taking care not to document findings which have a high diagnostic specificity unless their presence is certain. For example, if someone laughs while describing a death, is this because they are uncomfortable (common, and normal) or is it 'incongruity of affect' (uncommon, abnormal, and seen specifically in schizophrenia alongside other symptoms and signs of the disease)?

A Bayesian approach to psychiatric diagnosis is desirable. Pretest probability (from the presenting complaints) informs an initial differential diagnosis, allowing the appropriate use of further specific questions during the history and MSE to rule in or rule out those diagnoses. For example, if a patient has a history of bipolar disorder and now presents with recent elevated mood, his pretest probability of a manic episode is high. In this case, it would be very appropriate to ask questions to further 'rule in' the diagnosis such as 'Have you been buying any interesting things recently?'—a question which would be much less useful if the pretest probability of bipolar disorder were low. In the same way, it is important to use general screening questions during the MSE to identify patients who may require further, more detailed questioning.

Preparation for the MSE

Preparation involves consideration of the needs of the patient (comfort, privacy) and the needs of the interviewer (safety). It is helpful to consider the questions 'Who?', 'Where?', 'With whom?', and 'With alarm?'.

Who is the patient?

How much risk does the patient pose to the interviewer? If this is unknown, assume a high risk. What risks are there for the patient? These include the risk of absconding with intent to self-harm, and the risk of being unforthcoming about their problems unless they are relaxed in a private, quiet setting.

Where is the patient to be seen?

The setting should be conducive to confidential discussion, but should never compromise the interviewer's safety. If there is a designated interview room, is this close to other staff, and is there an alarm button? Is the risk too high for such a room to be used? Seating should be arranged to ensure that the exit is easily accessible for the interviewer, and that any alarm button is within reach.

With whom is the patient to be seen?

It may be necessary to interview a patient with another member of staff. This is especially important if the patient is unknown to you or your team, may behave threateningly, or is sexually disinhibited, manipulative, or litigious. Should hospital security staff be called to supervise?

With alarm?

If an alarm system is in use, make sure you are familiar with its operation, and that you can activate it if needed. Know how to summon help, such as via the emergency number for your hospital's security service.

The components of the MSE

The MSE typically comprises seven areas of assessment: (1) appearance and behaviour, (2) speech, (3) mood, (4) thoughts, (5) perceptions, (6) cognition, and (7) insight. The interview begins with a brief explanation of the duration and purpose of the interview, followed by data gathering to illuminate the history. This allows the examiner to gain a general impression of the patient, while assessing (1) appearance and behaviour, and (2) speech, which require no direct questioning. These observations need to be recorded descriptively, rather than interpretatively, to allow other health professionals to reach their own conclusions from the 'raw' observations. Subsequent sections of the MSE are assessed both subjectively (by asking the patient) and objectively (by recording the observations of the interviewer).

Appearance and behaviour

Relevant aspects of the patient's appearance include apparent body mass index, posture, clothing (e.g. appropriateness and cleanliness), hygiene and grooming (e.g. hair, make-up), and evidence of self-harm or IV drug use. Relevant behavioural features include eye contact, facial expression, the level and nature of the patient's activity, and the quality of rapport developed. A depressed patient, for example, may be downcast, with poor eye contact, a furrowed brow, slow motor activity, and poor rapport.

Speech

Recording the **content** of the patient's speech is deferred until the 'Thoughts' section of the MSE. The patient's speech is assessed by considering:

Rate and quantity: Copious speech that is hard to interrupt is 'pressure of speech', which occurs in mania. Slow, sparse, or monotonous speech is described as 'retardation' and may occur in depression or dementia. The combination of slow speech and slow movements is termed 'psychomotor retardation'.

Volume: The patient may speak quietly (depression or paranoia) or loudly (mania or deafness).

Spontaneity: Most people talk spontaneously once they relax, but people with depression, schizophrenia, or anxiety may find it difficult.

Mood

First, assess subjective mood, by asking the patient, 'How are you feeling in your spirits/mood?'

Then, assess objective mood, which includes:

The predominant mood(s) during the examination: e.g. depressed, elated, angry, anxious, or suspicious; alternatively, record that the mood was 'unremarkable'

The variability of the mood(s) during the examination: i.e. whether the patient seems emotionally labile (dementia, mania), emotionally flat (depression), or shows normal situational reactivity

Congruity: does the patient's mood 'fit' with his perceptions and thoughts (congruent mood, normal) or does it clash (incongruity of mood, sometimes seen in schizophrenia)

Thoughts

Information about a person's thoughts is mainly derived from their speech, but may also be derived from writing or drawings, or their behaviour. Thoughts are assessed in two stages: form and content.

Form of thought: This is normal if 'words' and 'sentences' are linked together unremarkably, in the logical way that we usually take for granted. It is abnormal if these links are unusual (such as words or phrases being linked by puns or rhymes, as in the 'flight of ideas' seen in mania) or absent (such as shifts to another, unrelated phrase, which the patient struggles to explain, as in 'loosening of associations', seen in schizophrenia).

Content of thought: The interviewer should ask specifically about (a) depressive thinking including suicidality, (b) obsessions, and (c) delusions.

Depressive thinking: Questions address current helplessness, hopelessness, and guilt. Screen for current suicidal ideation with 'Do you feel as though you would rather not wake up in the morning?' and 'Are you having any thoughts about harming yourself at the moment?' If so, further questions are required, such as 'Have you considered how you might end your life?' and 'Have you got any plans to carry out your ideas?' Asking about suicidal thoughts can be difficult, but is essential.

Obsessions: These are recurrent, intrusive thoughts, images, impulses, or actions that occur despite attempts to suppress them. The interviewer can ask whether the patient is experiencing any thoughts which are repetitive and intrusive, but do not make logical sense. Obsessional phenomena appear to originate from the patient's own mind, rather than from outside his/her head. Obsessional actions such as rechecking are detected by 'Do you have to do any things over and over again?'

Delusions: A delusion is a belief that is firmly held on inadequate grounds, and which is not a conventional belief held by others from a similar cultural background. To a patient, a delusion is identical to any strongly held belief, and it is therefore pointless to ask whether they have any delusions. Rather, delusions become evident on speaking to other people, or by following up elements of the history—once revealed, the patient is asked sympathetically to expand on these beliefs. Fixity of belief must be tested, by tactfully but firmly suggesting an alternative interpretation of the evidence.

Perceptions

Abnormalities of perception include distortions, illusions, and hallucinations.

Distortions

Manic patients may report that perceptions such as colours are more intense during manic phases; and depressed patients may report that the world appears more grey. Changes in hearing sensitivity (hyperacusis/hypoacusis) may be an indication of either physical disorder or psychiatric disorder, such as mood disorder.

Illusions

These occur when the patient misinterprets normal stimuli. When walking alone (and therefore anxious) through a park at night (and therefore sensorily impaired), it is normal to occasionally 'see' something alarming rather than the bush that is actually there.

Hallucinations

A hallucination is a sensory experience perceived in the absence of an external stimulus. Hallucinations are usually auditory or visual in form, although olfactory, gustatory, or somatic hallucinations are sometimes described. Auditory hallucinations usually indicate psychotic illness, whereas visual hallucinations are more common in physical disorders, including dementia, and drug/alcohol intoxication or withdrawal. Ask sensitively about hallucinations by starting with a screening question such as 'Some people experience things that might not actually be there—have you had anything like that?' Then ask whether the patient is experiencing 'voices' from outside their head, or people, objects, sounds, or lights that others cannot see. Are auditory hallucinations second person (voices speaking to you) or third person (voices speaking about you, a first-rank symptom of schizophrenia)? Some people misinterpret their own mind's 'voice' as an auditory hallucination, and so attempt to distinguish whether the perceptions are coming from within ('pseudohallucinations') or from without the patient's head (true hallucinations).

Cognition

If there is any suspicion of cognitive impairment (e.g. patient or corroborant mention poor concentration, poor memory, or a history of head injury or alcohol abuse), or if the patient is over 50 years old, an appropriate cognitive screen should be conducted to assess the following domains: orientation, attention, language, memory ('short-term' and 'long-term'), executive function, praxis, and visuospatial skills. The **Mini-Mental State Examination (MMSE)** is the most widely used screening test of cognitive function. A **clock-drawing test** may also be helpful to detect problems with praxis or executive functioning. Depending on the findings, detailed assessment by a specialist may be required.

Insight

The 'psychiatric' concept of 'insight' is similar to that of concordance. How does the patient explain or understand his difficulties, and how does he view treatments, including self-management? How similar is the patient's understanding to that of those treating him?

How to present the psychological history and examination

The method of presentation will clearly depend upon the setting and the time available. Although a psychiatric assessment may be long and complex, the effective clinician will distil this into something much briefer and more easily comprehensible. A simple approach is to:

1. summarize the **key** points in the history and examination
2. present the preferred diagnosis and differential diagnosis, with a brief justification for each
3. comment on the nature and degree of the main risks

Further Reading

Semple D and Smyth R. 'Psychiatric assessment', in Semple D and Smyth R, eds, *Oxford Handbook of Psychiatry* (3rd edition), 2013. Oxford University Press.

6 Confidentiality

Anna Rathmell

Introduction

There is a strong public perception that healthcare professionals can be trusted to keep medical information confidential. This trust is the key to patients' feeling comfortable with their doctors and being honest about the nature of their medical complaints and is therefore essential for the provision of a good healthcare system. However, this obligation to respect medical confidentiality is not, as is sometimes believed, absolute and there are circumstances where breaching confidentiality may be morally the best course of action and legally required.

Basic concepts

Ethical principles

The importance of medical confidentiality is underpinned primarily by two ethical principles. The first is respect for patient autonomy, or the right of a patient to have control over his own life and in this context to decide who should have access to his personal medical information. The second is a consequentialist idea that there is a duty to bring about the best possible consequences. A great deal of public trust is invested in the medical profession, and breaching medical confidentiality could result in a loss of this trust. Patients who do not trust their doctors may feel less inclined to divulge information about their condition, making it more difficult for them to be treated, the ultimate consequence being a lower standard of health care.

When has confidentiality been breached?

Confidentiality has been breached once a patient has been identified. A patient may be identified either by name or as a result of the nature of the information that has been divulged, for example, if the description of a patient's skin complaint means that he can then be identified by those who see him. If a patient has given valid consent for release of the information, however, this is not considered to be a breach of confidentiality. It is worth mentioning that something as simple as a note above a patient's bed saying 'Diabetic Diet', or a whiteboard displaying the names of patients on a ward could potentially be a breach of confidentiality.

Consent for disclosure of confidential information

In most circumstances, express consent should be obtained from the patient before disclosing his personal medical information (see Chapter 7). There are situations in which consent to sharing information about a patient can be implied. For example, patient information is routinely shared amongst members of a healthcare team without the need for express consent. However, information discussed within the team should be on a need to know basis, and each member of the team has a duty to keep the information confidential outside of this setting.

If an adult patient lacks competence to give consent to release of confidential information, then doctors should act in the patient's 'Best Interests' under the Mental Capacity Act 2005. It would normally be considered to be in a patient's best interests for information about his medical condition to be discussed with carers or close relatives. However, patients who are incompetent have the same legal rights for information about them to be kept confidential, and the same legal protection from unjustified breaches of confidentiality.

Minors over the age of 16 are assumed to be competent to give or refuse consent for disclosure of medical information. Minors below the age of 16 are assumed to be incompetent to give or refuse consent for disclosure of medical information, unless they are assessed as being 'Gillick competent' (See Chapter 7 for further information on Gillick competence). However, in contrast to the situation with competent adults, doctors have a legal obligation to act in the best interests of a competent minor. This means that, if a doctor believes that it is in the competent minor's best interests for confidential information to be shared but the minor refuses consent, then it would generally be considered lawful for the doctor to disclose the information.

Doctors should normally discuss medical information about minors below the age of 16 with their parents. However, if a Gillick competent minor refuses consent for disclosure of information to their parents and it is in the minor's best interests for the parents not to be informed, then information may be withheld from the parents.

Balancing public interests

The law looks mainly at patient confidentiality from the perspective of 'public interests' rather than from the perspective of the individual patient. Article 8 of the Human Rights Act 1998 (HRA) establishes that individuals do have a 'private' right to confidentiality. However this right is not absolute and the public interest in maintaining confidentiality is so strong that, in the context of medical confidentiality, the HRA is of little significance. Therefore, when deciding whether or not a breach in confidentiality is justified, it is necessary to weigh up the public interest in breaching confidentiality versus the public interest in not breaching confidentiality.

The General Medical Council (GMC) offers guidance on when and how a breach of patient confidentiality may be justified. The three main points are as follows:

1. Disclosure of confidential information without consent would normally be justified only in order to prevent risk of death or serious harm to the patient or others. Preventing damage or theft of property would not normally be sufficient reason to breach confidentiality.
2. Disclosure of confidential information should only be made to an appropriate authority.
3. The patient should be informed before disclosure of his confidential information.

While there is a wide range of situations when a doctor must use his own judgement as to whether or not a breach of confidentiality is justified, there are some situations when there is a legal obligation for doctors to breach confidentiality, and some situations when a doctor should not breach confidentiality.

Some situations when doctors are legally obliged to breach confidentiality are as follows:

- notifiable diseases: Public Health (Control of Diseases) Act 1984 (Notifiable Diseases)
- termination of pregnancy: Abortion Act 1967
- births and deaths: Births and Deaths Registration Act 1953
- to the police, on request, name and address (but not clinical details) of someone alleged to be guilty of certain road traffic offences: Road Traffic Act 1988
- certain treatments for infertility: Human Fertilisation and Embryology Act 1990, modified by the Human Fertilisation and Embryology (Disclosure of Information) Act 1992
- suspected terrorist activities: Terrorism Act 2000
- search warrant signed by circuit judge
- under court orders

Disclosure of confidential information in these circumstances should only be made to specific authorities.

Doctors should not normally breach confidentiality in the following circumstances:

- prevention of minor harms to others
- prevention of minor crime (e.g. to property) or to help conviction in the case of minor crimes
- providing information leading to the identity of a patient being treated in a genitourinary clinic for any sexually transmitted disease
- providing reports or fill in forms (e.g. to insurance companies) disclosing confidential information without the patient's consent
- to satisfy someone's curiosity
- 'casual breaches' (e.g. gossip, or carelessly leaving patient notes on the train, etc.)

It would however be unwise for a doctor to lie, for example, to police or insurance companies. Instead, it might be sensible simply to refuse to discuss a patient's confidential medical information.

An important case

W v Egdell **[1990]**

W was a patient detained in a secure hospital as a potential threat to public safety after he killed five people and wounded two others. He was diagnosed with schizophrenia and treated with medication. After ten years in the secure hospital, he applied to a mental health review tribunal to be discharged or transferred to a regional secure unit, with a view to eventually being discharged. W's solicitors instructed a psychiatrist, Egdell, to examine W and write a report which they hoped would support W's application. However, Egdell's report strongly opposed W's discharge or transfer, instead suggesting he have further treatment. When W's solicitors received the report, they withdrew their application. They did not send a copy of the report either to the tribunal or to the hospital caring for W. When Egdell realized this, he contacted the medical director of the hospital and sent a copy of his report to the hospital and to the Secretary of State, who then passed it on to the tribunal.

When W discovered that confidential information about his condition had been disclosed, he made a claim for breach of confidentiality. However, it was held that the public interest in disclosure of the report outweighed the public interest in keeping the findings in Egdell's report confidential. Egdell had relevant information about W's condition which, had he kept it to himself, would have deprived the hospital and the Secretary of State of information which was relevant to public safety.

W v Egdell established four important principles with respect to breaches of confidentiality, which should be considered along with the GMC guidance (see 'Balancing public interests'):

1. There must be a serious risk of danger to the public or an individual to justify disclosure of confidential information.
2. The courts take GMC guidance on confidentiality very seriously.
3. Disclosure should only be to appropriate people with a legitimate interest in the information.
4. Only the minimum amount of information necessary to prevent the risk of danger should be disclosed.

Common issues

The consequences of breaching patient confidentiality

A patient who feels that a doctor has breached confidentiality may pursue his complaint in one or more of the following ways:

- by making a complaint to the doctor himself or, in the case of a trainee doctor, to the doctor's supervising consultant
- by complaining to the doctor's employer, for example, to the hospital in which the doctor works
- by taking his grievance to the GMC; this is a more likely course of action than the patient taking the case to court
- by taking the case to court; note that the courts pay particular attention to the GMC guidance on confidentiality

Casual breaches of confidentiality

Most breaches of confidentiality are accidental or careless, for example, leaving patient notes on a train or being overheard in a lift. These casual breaches of confidentiality are taken extremely seriously by both the courts and the GMC and could well be considered to constitute serious professional misconduct.

Use of patient records

Either disclosure of patient information for audit or research purposes should be anonymized or express consent should be obtained from the patient. When using patients or pictures of patients as case studies in textbooks and clinical papers, express consent should again be sought. Even if the patient cannot be identified, it would be wise to obtain consent wherever possible.

Disclosure after death

Doctors have an obligation to maintain patient confidentiality after a patient has died. However, information may be disclosed in order to assist a coroner with his duties.

Some legal/ethical dilemmas

A 35-year-old patient has been recently diagnosed with epilepsy and regularly suffers from seizures. Although advised that he should inform the DVLA and not continue to drive, it is apparent that he is ignoring that advice, despite the risks to himself and to other road users. What should I do?

Under these circumstances, the GMC advises that every effort should be made to persuade the patient to inform the DVLA and to give up driving voluntarily. If the patient continues to drive, you would be justified in breaching patient confidentiality in the public interest in order to prevent risk of death or serious harm. In this case, you would need to speak in confidence to the medical adviser at the DVLA, disclosing only the minimum amount of patient information necessary. You should also inform the patient of your decision to speak to the DVLA and document your actions in the patient's notes.

A patient has been admitted to A & E with a gunshot wound to the leg. However, he denies being shot and refuses to speak to the police. Should we inform the police and, if so, what information should we give them?

GMC advice states that the police should be informed if anyone arrives at a hospital with a gunshot wound; however, initially, you should not usually identify the patient. Once the patient is well enough to speak to the police, he should be asked whether he is willing to do so. If he refuses to speak to the police and refuses consent to disclosure of confidential information, you may be justified in disclosing information, but only if there are grounds for believing that it would be in the public interest in order to prevent risk of death or serious harm either to the patient or others to do so.

I am a GP and one of my patients, a 40-year-old man, has been recently diagnosed with HIV. Although he claims to be taking his medication, which will reduce the risk of transmission, and says that he is using appropriate contraception, he is refusing to tell his wife that he has HIV. His wife is also one of my patients. Should I inform her?

In cases of this nature, the GMC advises that there are grounds for disclosure of information if there is a serious and identifiable risk to a specific individual who, if not so informed, would be exposed to infection. You should make every effort to persuade your patient either to inform his wife or to consent to you informing her. However, if he still refuses, you may consider it necessary to inform her in order to protect her from a risk of death or serious harm. In this situation, you should advise your patient of your intentions and document this in his medical notes.

Further Reading

General Medical Council guidance on confidentiality: (http://www.gmc-uk.org/guidance/ethical_guidance/confidentiality.asp)

7 Consent

Anna Rathmell

Introduction

In contemporary medicine, the traditional paternalistic model of healthcare has largely been replaced with a model which focuses on patient autonomy and the right of patients to have as much control as possible over decisions relating to their medical care. In English law, this has led to the concept of informed consent and the right of patients to withdraw their consent at any time, even if they have previously given consent or signed a consent form.

Basic concepts

Informed consent

For consent to be valid under English law, three criteria must be met.

- The patient must be **informed**. They should be given general information about the purpose and nature of the procedure, the risks and benefits, and any reasonable alternatives.
- The patient must also be **competent** (have legal **capacity**) to understand the information given to him.
- The consent must be **voluntary**, that is, the patient must not have been coerced.

Consent would normally be express. However, in certain circumstances, it can be implied, for example, when a patient holds out his arm to have blood taken.

Battery and negligence

Legal cases relating to consent for medical procedures normally focus on battery (touching without consent) or, more frequently, negligence.

A doctor can be sued for battery if he has not given the patient information about the specific procedure that he undertakes. For example, if consent has been given for removal of an ovarian cyst, and the doctor performs a hysterectomy, then this could constitute a battery, for which damages would be awarded. The patient would not need to prove that any harm was caused as a result of the battery.

For a doctor to be found liable in negligence, a claimant would need to show that the doctor was in breach of his duty of care. In the context of consent, this would mean showing that the doctor had not provided some relevant information about the procedure. However, in contrast to battery, the claimant would also need to show that harm was caused as a result of the lack of information. In other words, the patient would need to convince the court that had he been properly informed (e.g. of the risk of paralysis following a spinal operation), he would not have consented to the procedure, and so the procedure would not have taken place and no harm would have resulted (in this example, the patient would not have suffered paralysis).

In general, in the context of medical negligence, if a doctor has 'acted in accordance with the practice accepted as proper by a responsible body of medical men skilled in that particular art', he will not be found negligent. This is known as the 'Bolam test'. However, in determining the level of information required for consent to be valid, the courts are increasingly moving away from the Bolam test and are expecting doctors to provide patients with more information, at a level that a 'prudent' patient would require.

Patients who lack capacity, and the Mental Capacity Act 2005

In English law, a person over 16 years of age is assumed to have capacity unless it can be shown to the contrary. Under the Mental Capacity Act (Section 3(1)), a person lacks capacity if he is unable to do at least one of the following:

- **understand** the information relevant to the decision
- **retain** that information
- **use** or **weigh** that information as part of the process of making the decision
- **communicate** his decision (whether by talking, using sign language, or any other means)

Capacity relates to the ability of the patient to make a particular decision, not to the patient as a whole (see '*Re C* [1994]'). Furthermore, a patient does not lack capacity simply because he makes a decision that could be considered by others to be unwise (Mental Capacity Act, Section 1). If a patient is assessed as lacking capacity to make a decision, then, under the Mental Capacity Act, there is a duty to take all practicable steps to enhance his capacity in order to enable him to make that decision.

Under the Mental Capacity Act (Section 9), it is now possible for a person (the 'donor') with capacity to appoint another person (the 'donee') as a **Lasting Power of Attorney (LPA)**. This enables the donee to make decisions for the donor about specified matters of personal welfare, including medical treatment, should the donor lose capacity in the future. Under the Mental Capacity Act, it is also possible for people with capacity to make **Advance Decisions** to refuse treatment at a future point when they may lack capacity (Mental Capacity Act, Sections 24–26). An Advance Decision can also relate to life-sustaining treatment if it is stated to that effect in writing specifying 'even if life is at risk', signed, and witnessed.

Patients who lack capacity and who do not have an LPA or an Advanced Decision should be treated in their 'Best Interests' (Mental Capacity Act, Section 4). The Mental Capacity Act gives guidance as to how a patient's best interests should be assessed, including encouraging the patient's participation in the decision as far as is practicable, considering the patient's past and present wishes, feelings, beliefs, and values, and consulting those with an interest in his welfare. The General Medical Council (GMC) also offers guidance in this area.

Minors (<18 years old)

Minors aged 16 or 17 are presumed to have capacity to consent to treatment unless it can be shown otherwise. If, however, a minor refuses to consent to treatment that a doctor believes is in the patient's best interests, then someone with parental responsibility can consent on his behalf. If no one with parental responsibility is willing to give consent, then the doctor should approach the court for assistance. In an urgent situation where consent is not forthcoming from the minor or from those with parental responsibility, treatment that is immediately necessary to prevent the minor from coming to serious harm should be given without consent. In reality, most doctors would be reluctant to enforce treatment on a competent 16- or 17-year-old unless it were an emergency situation. If a minor aged 16 or 17 lacks capacity, he should be treated in his best interests, preferably with consent from someone with parental responsibility.

Minors under 16 years of age are presumed not to have capacity to consent to medical treatment. However, if the doctor assesses them as being 'Gillick competent' (see '*Gillick v West Norfolk and Wisbech Area Health Authority* [1985]'), then they should be treated as for minors aged 16 or 17. Consent for treatment of minors under 16 years of age who are not Gillick competent should be obtained from someone with parental responsibility (usually the parents). Consent is only required from one person with parental responsibility. Even if one parent refuses to consent to a procedure, it would be lawful to proceed with treatment, provided that consent has been obtained from the other parent and provided that the procedure is in the patient's best interests. If all those with parental responsibility refuse consent, then the doctor has three options:

- It is lawful to not give treatment to a minor, providing that failure to treat is not significantly against the minor's interests, for example, if those with parental responsibility do not want to consent to a vaccination for their child. However, it is worth being aware that should the doctor be subsequently sued for negligence in not treating the minor, it would not be a defence that those with parental responsibility had refused consent.
- If to not give treatment would be significantly against the minor's interests, then the doctor should apply to the court for a 'specific issue order'. This can be obtained within a matter of hours.
- As for minors aged 16 or 17, if treatment is immediately necessary to prevent serious harm to the minor, then this should be administered, even if consent cannot be obtained.

Cases

Re C [1994]

C was a paranoid schizophrenic patient who had developed gangrene in his foot. The consultant recommended that C should have his leg amputated below the knee, as it was considered that his chances of survival without the amputation would only be 15%. C refused the operation, saying that he would rather die with two feet than live with one. The hospital questioned C's capacity to make this decision and so an application for an injunction was made to the court on Cs behalf, preventing the hospital from carrying out the amputation without C's express written consent.

It was held that, although C was a diagnosed schizophrenic, he was able to understand, believe, and use the relevant information in order to come to a decision as to whether or not he wanted to have his leg amputated. In other words, he did have capacity to refuse consent in relation to this matter.

Re C effectively incorporated into English common law the criteria for capacity, which were then amended to form the four legal criteria as specified in the Mental Capacity Act (see 'Patients who lack capacity, and the Mental Capacity Act 2005').

Re C also established that a general reduction in capacity does not necessarily mean that the patient lacks capacity in all areas of his life. Whether a patient lacks capacity relates to the specific decision to be made and not to the patient as a whole.

Gillick v West Norfolk and Wisbech Area Health Authority [1985]

The Department of Health and Social Security had issued a circular to area health authorities containing advice that, under certain circumstances, doctors could give contraception advice and treatment to children under the age of 16 without parental knowledge or consent.

Mrs Gillick sought assurance from her local health authority that her daughters would not be given such advice and treatment before the age of 16. The health authority refused to give such assurance and so Mrs Gillick brought an action against the health authority and the Department of Health and Social Security, arguing that the advice contained in their circular was unlawful.

The case went to the House of Lords where it was decided against Mrs Gillick. Lord Scarman said, 'the parental right to determine whether or not their minor child below the age of 16 will have medical treatment terminates if and when the child achieves a sufficient understanding and intelligence to enable him or her to understand fully what is proposed'.

This case has led to the concept of 'Gillick competence', that is, children under the age of 16 to whom Lord Scarman's judgement applies may give consent to medical treatment. It is unlikely that a child under the age of 12 would be assessed as 'Gillick competent'.

Common issues

Documenting consent

Most hospitals have procedures and guidance in place regarding the taking and documenting of consent. Legally, however, the most important thing is that consent is valid and informed, not whether the patient has signed a consent form or who has obtained consent from the patient. The consent form is useful legally in that it provides evidence that consent has been given. It is also useful as part of an official process to ensure that consent is taken prior to a medical intervention.

The GMC guidance is that responsibility for taking consent can be delegated by the doctor providing the medical treatment to another team member, provided that this team member is suitably trained and qualified and has sufficient knowledge of the proposed investigation or treatment and understands the risks involved. However, overall responsibility for ensuring that consent has been given lies with the doctor undertaking the procedure.

What should the patient be told about risks, benefits, and alternative treatments?

The GMC offers guidance on this. In summary, patients should be given information about common adverse effects and serious adverse effects, even if the likelihood of the serious adverse effect is very small. Even if the patient prefers not to discuss these aspects of their treatment, it would be very unwise to proceed without informing him of the key risks and benefits. If a patient specifically asks for detailed information on risks, benefits, or alternatives, then this information should be given as honestly and fully as possible.

Unexpected findings

If a surgeon makes an unexpected finding during the course of an operation, for example, if, during an appendectomy for which the patient has consented, he discovers an ovarian tumour, he would be unwise to remove the tumour at this stage, even if this would be in the patient's best interests. Although, ethically, removal of the tumour might be the right thing to do, it would only be justified legally if there were good reasons as to why the operation could not be performed at a later stage with the patient's explicit consent. For example, if a delay in the operation would expose the patient to significantly increased risk of death or serious harm. The surgeon could, of course, take the legal risk of removing the tumour on the grounds that he knows the patient well enough to consider legal action very unlikely.

What is the role of the family of an adult (>18 years of age) who lacks capacity?

Unless they have been appointed as an LPA (see 'Patients who lack capacity, and the Mental Capacity Act 2005'), family members have no legal powers to make medical decisions on behalf of an adult who lacks capacity. However, the Mental Capacity Act obliges doctors to act in the best interests of patients who lack capacity. This involves considering patient's previous wishes and values before they lost capacity, and relatives may be in the best position to provide evidence of this. The Mental Capacity Act also specifies consulting a range of people with an interest in the patient's welfare, and this range would most likely include family members.

Some legal/ethical dilemmas

A healthy 3-year-old man has been admitted into A & E with a gunshot wound to the abdomen. His wife says that they are both Jehovah's Witnesses and that her husband has made an Advanced Decision refusing a blood transfusion under any circumstances. Although this Advanced Decision is not in writing, she is quite insistent that both she and her husband would be most distressed at the idea of him receiving blood. The patient has lost a lot of blood and it is now apparent that he will require a blood transfusion immediately in order to save his life. Should we proceed with the transfusion or comply with the patient's and his wife's wishes?

In order for an Advance Decision refusing treatment to be valid and applicable to life-sustaining treatment, it needs to be in writing, stating 'even if life is at risk', signed, and witnessed. This patient has no such written statement and therefore should be treated under the Mental Capacity Act in his best interests. This would involve consultation with the patient's wife, as she will probably have a good insight into the patient's previous wishes and values; however, her opinion does not carry any legal weight. Under these circumstances, since you cannot be sure of the patient's wishes and given the urgent nature of the situation, it would be wise to proceed with the blood transfusion and save the patient's life.

An 84-year-old woman with Alzheimer's disease has been admitted to hospital with suspected pneumonia. She seems unaware of her surroundings and does not recognize her daughter, who has brought her in to hospital. She is very confused and is refusing blood tests and IV antibiotic treatment. Her daughter says that her mother has a fear of needles. It is clear that the patient lacks capacity to consent to this approach to her medical care; however, she is refusing to cooperate. How much force can we impose in order to act in her best interests?

For restraint (use of force or threats) of a patient to be lawful under the Mental Capacity Act (Section 6), the doctor must reasonably believe that restraint is necessary in order to prevent harm to the patient. In addition, the use of restraint must be proportionate to the likelihood and seriousness of that harm. In this situation, where the proposed treatment has been assessed as being in the patient's best interests, it would be necessary to evaluate whether or not the blood tests and IV antibiotics being proposed are necessary to prevent harm to the patient and, if so, to use proportionate restraint to get her to comply.

Further Reading

General Medical Council: *Consent Guidance: Patients and Doctors Making Decisions Together* (http://www.gmc-uk.org/guidance/ethical_guidance/consent_guidance_index.asp)

PART 2

Assessment of symptoms
and presenting problems

8 Palpitation

Patrick Davey

Definition of the symptom

Palpitation is a symptom defined as unpleasant awareness of the heartbeat and is typically described by patients as a disagreeable sensation of pulsation or movement in the chest or adjacent areas. Palpitations can be due to cardiac arrhythmias or a broad range of other disorders. This chapter addresses the differential diagnosis of palpitations as well as the main causes, the specific clues indicating the presence and nature of an arrhythmia, diagnostic tests, therapies available, prognosis, and dealing with uncertainty.

Differential diagnosis

The main causes of palpitations are listed in Box 8.1. Most patients with palpitations are managed in primary care (see Table 8.1).

Context

Palpitations are very common, and probably affect most people at some time during their lives. They comprise 10% of new referrals to cardiology clinics. They can be due either to an appreciation of the normal heartbeat (by far the commonest cause), or an arrhythmia (Box 8.1). When patients present to medical care, and these are very much the minority of those with symptoms, it is usually because they have given rise to concern in the patients' mind that they may have a serious cardiac illness. Clearly, occasionally, this is the case. Much more frequently, either there is no cardiac abnormality at all or there is a low-grade arrhythmia, not associated with any underlying heart disease or impact on outlook. The key to management is to establish the diagnosis rapidly and, usually, reassure the patient. Sometimes psychological support is necessary. Occasionally, though usually more to reassure the patient, it is necessary to undertake some investigation to exclude any underlying heart disease. Very rarely, a dangerous arrhythmia, or serious underlying heart condition comes to light, needing appropriate specialist therapy—this, however, is very much the exception, and certainly not the rule.

Box 8.1 Main causes of palpitations

Cardiac arrhythmias
Supraventricular/ventricular extrasystoles
Supraventricular/ventricular tachycardias
Bradyarrhythmias: severe sinus bradycardia, sinus pauses, second-and third-degree atrioventricular block
Anomalies in the functioning and/or programming of pacemakers and ICDs

Structural heart diseases
Mitral valve prolapse
Severe mitral regurgitation
Severe aortic regurgitation
Congenital heart diseases with significant shunt
Cardiomegaly and/or heart failure of various aetiologies
Hyperthrophic cardiomyopathy
Mechanical prosthetic valves

Psychosomatic disorders
Anxiety, panic attacks
Depression, somatization disorders

Systemic causes
Hyperthyroidism, hypoglycaemia, postmenopausal syndrome, fever, anaemia, pregnancy, hypovolaemia, orthostatic hypotension, postural orthostatic tachycardia syndrome, pheochromocytoma, arteriovenous fistula

Effects of medical and recreational drugs
Sympathicomimetic agents in pump inhalers, vasodilators, anticholinergics, hydralazine
Recent withdrawal of β-blockers
Alcohol, cocaine, heroin, amphetamines, caffeine, nicotine, cannabis, synthetic drugs
Weight reductions drugs

Reproduced with permission from Raviele A, Giada F, Bergfeldt L, et al., Management of patients with palpitations: a position paper from the European Heart Rhythm Association, Europace, volume 13, issue 7, pp.920-34, copyright © 2011 Oxford University Press .

Table 8.1 Common causes of palpitations in primary and secondary care

In primary care	%	In secondary care	%
Non-arrhythmic palpitations • anxiety • hyperventilation syndromes • caffeine excess • thyrotoxicosis • phaeochromocytomas	70%	Ventricular and supraventricular extrasystoles	30%
Ventricular and supraventricular extrasystoles	25%	Non-arrhythmic palpitations	30%
Supraventricular tachycardias	3%	Atrial fibrillation	20%
Other arrhythmias, including atrial fibrillation	2%	Supraventricular tachycardias	10%
		Other arrhythmias, including ventricular tachycardia	10%

Approach to diagnosis

Though the key to the diagnosis is to obtain an ECG during an attack, many clues to the underlying diagnosis can be obtained from the demographics, family history (especially if the patient is young), knowledge of whether there is any underlying heart disease, exact description of the symptoms, and simple tests such as a 12-lead ECG.

Demographics: Young patients, especially if female, are much more likely to have non-arrhythmic symptoms than older male patients are. Patients with known anxiety symptoms are also less likely to have arrhythmic palpitations.

Family history: A family history of palpitations is without any diagnostic value whatsoever, despite the value placed on this by patients. However, a high-level danger alert signal is finding sudden cardiac death in a young first-degree family member—young meaning <40 years for men, <50 years for females—and the younger they are, the more worried one is that there is either a genetic disorder of cardiac ion channels (a channelopathy) or myocardium (e.g. hypertrophic cardiomyopathy).

Heart disease: The presence of heart disease substantially increases the chance that palpitations relate to ventricular tachycardia, a potentially dangerous rhythm disturbance. The more substantial the cardiac illness, the greater the worry—so, mild left ventricular hypertrophy due to hypertension only mildly increases the risk of ventricular tachycardia, whereas substantial left ventricular dysfunction due to a remote myocardial infarction substantially increases the chance of finding ventricular tachycardia. If syncope is present, then there is considerable concern, and aggressive investigations to determine whether intermittent ventricular arrhythmias are present should be undertaken urgently.

Exact nature of the symptoms: Use the symptoms listed in Table 8.2 to determine whether or not you think an arrhythmia is present; then, try and determine which arrhythmia this might be. Unless you have clearly demonstrated what is going on, refrain from being categoric with the patient; tell them what you think the diagnosis is, but do explain that there is some uncertainty.

Red-flag features: These are features which increase the likelihood of a dangerous arrhythmia, and mandate further cardiac assessment. Red flags are: palpitations associated with chest pain, breathlessness or syncope; palpitations provoked by exercise; a family history of cardiomyopathy or sudden death; signs of structural heart disease or heart failure; and an abnormal 12-lead ECG.

Specific clues to the presence of an arrhythmia

There are numerous clues in the history to the diagnosis (Table 8.2).

Specific clues to the nature of the arrhythmia

Extrasystoles (ectopic beats): The patient either feels the beat itself (irregular palpitations, with a normal overall heart rate)—'like the car hiccoughing'—or the beat after the ectopic, which is of increased strength—'the heart misses a beat, then restarts with a thud'.

Supraventricular tachycardia: Supraventricular tachycardia (SVT) is instantaneous-onset, rapid, regular palpitation, of defined but usually brief duration (few minutes), sometime stopped by vagotonic manoeuvres, which the patient has discovered for themselves (e.g. coughing, straining, cold drinks, breath holding). Rarely, post-event polyuria occurs.

Atrial fibrillation: Atrial fibrillation is sudden-onset, fast, irregular palpitation (unlike the irregular palpitations with a normal heart rate of ectopy).

Ventricular tachycardia: Ventricular tachycardia is sudden fast regular palpitation (just like an SVT), but sometimes (not always) accompanied by additional symptoms (dizziness, frank syncope). The real clue is finding a family history of sudden death, an abnormal ECG suggesting a channelopathy, or known cardiac disease.

Key diagnostic tests

The absolute key to diagnosis is to obtain an ECG during an attack—how easy this is depends on the frequency and duration of symptoms (Table 8.3). In addition, all patients should have a 12-lead ECG obtained between attacks, as this can give key clues to the presence of pro-arrhythmic conditions, such as Wolff–Parkinson–White (WPW) syndrome, hereditary long-QT syndrome, Brugada syndrome, or any underlying heart disease. A normal 12-lead ECG between attacks makes a dangerous arrhythmia unlikely.

Other diagnostic tests

These depend on the presumed diagnosis. Most patients should have thyroid function tests, a full blood count, and a biochemical screen performed, to ensure there is no non-cardiac illness

Table 8.2 Clues to the presence of an arrhythmia

	Non-arrhythmic palpitations	Arrhythmic palpitations
Characteristic phrase	Heavy (sometimes slow and regular) thudding	Racing heart rate (sustained arrhythmia); 'fluttering' (ectopics)
Situation	Sometimes when overtly anxious, often not	Not usually related to any stress
Diurnal variation	Rare	Usually none, though ectopic beats more common in the evening/ at night
Onset	Slow—over many minutes	Instantaneous
Offset	Often poorly recalled, otherwise, gradual wearing off	Usually instantaneous, sometimes not recalled
Duration	Often poorly recalled, many hours or all day, sometimes several days	Well defined and remembered, often minutes, though can be seconds, or hours
Heart rate during the attack	Usually normal or near normal	Usually very fast
Associated symptoms during the attack	Often many, though rarely any particular disease-related symptoms complex	Usually none, sometimes breathlessness, angina, very rarely syncope
Associated symptoms after the attack	Often many symptoms remote from an attack—especially tiredness, often rather diffuse, free-floating symptoms	Often no symptoms remote from the attack, rarely symptoms from underlying heart disease
Ability to answer a direct question clearly and in a focused manner	Very poor, often answers a question by expressing a new symptom	Usually very good
Inter-attack ECG	Usually normal	Usually normal, but may show a variety of abnormalities indicating arrhythmia propensity (delta wave, long-QT interval, Brugada syndrome) or underlying cardiac illness (Q waves, etc.)
Physical examination	Normal	Usually normal

Table 8.3 Frequency and duration of symptoms during an arrhythmia

Frequency	Duration	Test
Few minutes	>1 month	Depends on probability of serious arrhythmia; if very low (normal inter-attack ECG, no cardiac disease), consider doing no further investigations; if probability of serious arrhythmia higher, consider either invasive evaluation or an implantable loop recorder
Few minutes	Every fortnight	Cardiac memo (simple ECG machine loaned to the patient for a few weeks)
Few minutes	Every week	7 day ECG recording
Few minutes	Every day	24 hour ECG
>30 minutes	Any frequency	Attend Emergency Dept at any time of day or night for a 12-lead ECG

presenting as palpitations. If the presumed diagnosis is non-cardiac palpitations, a few patients also need urine tests to exclude phaeochromocytoma (catecholamine secreting with paroxysmal secretion: patients usually have intermittent symptoms of palpitations, sweating, or overwhelming anxiety, and many will have lost weight). If there is a possibility of serious heart disease, appropriate tests may include a cardiac ultrasound, exercise stress test, and so on.

If obtaining an ECG at the time of palpitation proves elusive, and a definitive ECG diagnosis is needed, in patients with no red-flag features, a smartphone device (monitor and app) that allows the recording of a single channel ECG can be very helpful. This technology is likely to be increasingly used. In patients with red-flag features (e.g. associated syncope, abnormal resting ECG, left ventricular dysfunction and/or known ischaemic heart disease), then a very small leadless ECG recording device can be implanted subcutaneously in the left chest near the heart. Such devices are typically 1x2x0.5 cm in size, and have battery lives of 2–3 years. They can be remotely interrogated and store all significant brady- or tachy-arrythmias. Implantation of an ECG loop recorder is very rarely indicated in the assessment of palpitation in the absence of red-flag features.

Introduction to therapy

Unless there is a signal that there is a dangerous arrhythmia present, often the best approach is simply to reassure the patient, on the basis of a presumptive diagnosis from the history, that either that their symptoms are likely to be non-arrhythmic, and so benign, or that they probably represent a non-dangerous arrhythmia. Most patients, either without arrhythmias or with brief arrhythmias (e.g. ectopic beats) responds to such reassurance. Patients with a presumptive diagnosis of an SVT should be taught vagotonic manoeuvres. If these approaches are unsuccessful, then beta blockers can often be effective (often given for only a few months). They are both effective for non-arrhythmic palpitations and very good for most arrhythmias and, unless there are any of the usual contraindications, they are very safe.

Prognosis

Unless a dangerous arrhythmia is present, which is most unlikely, the prognosis is for a normal life expectancy. The vast majority of

patients with a normal inter-attack 12-lead ECG fall into this category. However, be aware of the following:

- In those with ventricular extrasystoles, occasionally there is underlying heart disease, which clearly must be detected and treated.
- In those with atrial fibrillation, life may be shortened (by stroke) unless appropriate anticoagulation is given. If you suspect this diagnosis, go to some lengths to prove or disprove this, as it is crucial to give anticoagulation if the benefits outweigh the risks.
- If you suspect a channelopathy, or know there is underlying heart disease, the prognosis may be seriously decreased. These patients need specialist cardiac workup.

How to handle uncertainty in the diagnosis of this symptom

If you cannot prove the diagnosis, that is, obtain an ECG during an attack, then take steps to exclude:

- WPW syndrome with an obvious delta wave
- channelopathies (in practice, done by ensuring that there is no family history of sudden cardiac death in young relatives, and the inter-attack 12-lead ECG is normal)
- underlying heart disease (from the history, physical examination, and echocardiography; most cases have an abnormal inter-attack ECG)
- atrial fibrillation (irregular fast palpitations)

The patients who remain (who comprise the overwhelming majority) are extremely unlikely to have any arrhythmia that affects prognosis and, even without any diagnostic ECG, can usually be managed by reassurance and, if needed, low-dose beta-blocker therapy.

Further Reading

Gale CP and Camm AJ. Assessment of palpitations. *BMJ* 2016; 352: h5649.

Raviele A, Giada F, Bergfeldt L, et al. Management of patients with palpitations: A position paper from the European Heart Rhythm Association. *Europace* 2011; 13: 920–34.

Steinberg JS, Varma N, and Cygankiewicz I. ISHNE-HRS expert consensus statement on ambulatory ECG and external cardiac monitoring/telemetry. *Heart Rhythm* 2017; 14: e55–e96.

9 Acute chest pain

Jonathan Timperley and Sandeep Hothi

Definition of the symptom

Acute chest pain constitutes pain (or any unpleasant sensation) in the chest that has been present for less than 2 weeks, and in many cases for less than a few hours. Patients with acute chest pain usually (but not always) present as an emergency to hospital as they are aware that there may be an immediately life-threatening cause. The main issue with acute chest pain is therefore the differentiation of the serious causes from the benign ones, so that patients with life-threatening illness can be treated early and effectively, and those with benign chest pain can be safely discharged early.

Differential diagnosis in primary care and secondary care

Box 9.1 outlines the differential diagnosis in primary care and secondary care, ordered by probability.

Context

Acute chest pain is a common and typically frightening symptom. The main diagnosis to be considered (although certainly not the only one) is an acute coronary syndrome (ACS), with all its attendant dangers, as opposed to the main diagnosis in chronic chest pain, which is stable angina. These diagnostic differences explain the momentum of the illness and so the speed at which diagnosis and treatment should occur—in chronic chest pain, diagnosis and treatment can occur at a relatively leisurely rate, as complications from stable angina usually occur at a relatively low rates whereas, in acute chest pain, time is of the essence, as many conditions are associated with early death; even if initially it appears that the patient with acute chest pain is well,

---

Box 9.1 Diagnosis in primary care and secondary care, ordered by probability

Common
- non-specific chest pain
- gastro-oesophageal chest pain
- musculoskeletal pain, including chest wall trauma
- acute coronary syndromes
- stable angina:
  - coronary disease +/− anaemia
  - aortic stenosis

Uncommon
- pleurisy, due to:
  - pneumonia
  - pulmonary embolism
  - pneumothorax
  - pericarditis
  - viral pleurisy
- chest manifestations of subdiaphragmatic illness:
  - cholecystitis
  - dyspeptic syndromes

Rare
- aortic syndromes, including aortic dissection
- oesophageal rupture
- viral chest wall infection, herpes zoster and simplex

---

life-threatening complications can occur quickly and indeed often do so. This means that, in acute chest pain, a rapid diagnosis must occur, preferably within minutes and certainly within a few hours. However, the diagnosis may prove elusive and, given that the time window for effective therapy is often small, sometimes, indeed, quite often, empiric therapy must sometimes be given without complete confidence over the diagnosis. Such 'blind' therapy is certainly appropriate in many situations—however, you should always weigh up the risks versus the benefits—for example, it is 2 am, you may believe the likely diagnosis is a pulmonary embolus (PE), and for many patients it is appropriate to give a heparin-type anticoagulant even if the diagnosis is not as yet proven. However, if the patient also has a profound microcytic anaemia, which could be due to chronic gastrointestinal blood loss, heparin may provoke brisk and therefore dangerous gastrointestinal bleeding. What should one do? This is but one example of uncertainty in diagnosis—for the cause of the chest pain as well as comorbidities increase the risk of therapy. Such uncertainty is difficult both for physicians and patients, but nonetheless is the very real-world situation in which we find ourselves. This does mean that if the diagnosis is not clear, the physician must have a strategy that deals effectively with uncertainty. Individual clinicians will develop this for themselves as they become more experienced; often discussing the problem with other clinicians allows one to frame the situation in such a way that the solution becomes obvious. If initial discussions within your unit have not led to a solution, then discuss the problem outside the unit with specialist physicians—in the aforementioned case, titrate the risk of the possible PE (is there evidence of haemodynamic instability such that immediate therapy is needed?) against the risk of gastrointestinal bleeding (and if you don't know what the risk is, ask a senior gastroenterologist).

Approach to diagnosis

The main aim of management is to quickly diagnosis and treat all conditions—both those that are benign (to ensure early and safe discharge), and those that are dangerous and require immediate treatment, sometimes of a very complex nature.

In terms of thinking about the diagnosis, it may be helpful to answer the questions 'What is the most likely diagnosis?', 'How do I diagnose this?', and 'What is the most likely dangerous diagnosis, and how do I exclude this?' If the most likely diagnosis is disproven by investigation, move on to the next most likely diagnosis. The most dangerous diagnosis is often either an ACS or PE; occasionally, such diagnostic doubt exists that both need to be excluded. Aortic syndromes are rare, they often not top of the diagnostic list, and they are easily forgotten, so it is helpful to always ask oneself in patients with undiagnosed pain whether this could be an aortic syndrome. Sometimes the diagnosis cannot be readily made, but one can risk stratify the patient anyway.

In order to develop a model of how we approach diagnosis generally, it is always helpful to remember the words of the great cardiologist JW Hurst on how to make a diagnosis:

Step 1: Obtain the history, perform the physical examination, obtain a resting ECG, and a obtain chest X-ray. These four methods, used properly, will enable us to come to a reasonable conclusion about most patients.
Step 2: The data collected by using the history, physical examination, resting ECG, and chest X-ray must be interrelated so that the whole of the parts give an understanding of the patient's problem that is greater than each of the individual parts considered separately.

Step 3: The data collected by the four methods mentioned in Step 1 should enable the physician to state the diagnosis with certainty or formulate the problem so precisely that it is possible to think clearly about it and develop plans related to it

Step 4: If the diagnosis is not clear, it is then necessary to ask whether the remaining questions should be solved. Will clearer answers really improve the care of the patient?

Step 5: If the answer is no, clearer answers to various questions will not assist in the care of the patient, then doctoring with all its meaning should be implemented. If the answer is yes, clearer answers will assist in the care of the patient, then one must determine if the questions raised are clearly stated. As a rule, the question should be one or more of the following. Is there a structural abnormality? Is cardiac performance or myocardial contractility abnormal? Is there an electrical abnormality? Is myocardial ischaemia present?

Step 6: If further workup can be justified and the questions are clearly stated, it is then possible to choose the technique that is most likely to answer the question. It is not necessary to perform all tests that might answer the question. It is adequate to choose the technique that gives a result with the highest predictive value.

This is as clear an exposition of diagnostic thinking as you will come across—and in this situation, like most others, it tells us that relatively simple data used correctly enable the diagnosis to be made and appropriate therapy instituted—and this is something that should not be forgotten in this age of increasingly sophisticated investigation and treatment.

In terms of Step 1, you need to know what the possible diagnoses are (Box 9.1) and what the key diagnostic clues are (see 'Specific clues to the diagnosis').

If the diagnosis cannot be made immediately, follow Hurst's approach—which single investigation is required to make the most likely diagnosis and exclude the most dangerous diagnosis? For example, you think the diagnosis is benign musculoskeletal chest pain, but the most likely dangerous diagnosis is PE. There is no test for musculoskeletal chest pain—fine; for PE, a D-dimer test with or without CT pulmonary angiography (CTPA) is required.

Sometimes even the best clinicians working within real-world systems cannot make the diagnosis—in this situation, it is helpful to risk stratify the patient (see Table 9.1).

Specific clues to the diagnosis

The history, physical examination (including pulse oximetry), and simple investigations via a chest X-ray and a 12-lead ECG should lead to the correct diagnosis or diagnostic and therapeutic strategy. Establish key points from the demographics and history to determine the initial chance of coronary disease versus other illness, and then consider the specific nature of the pain, along with associated symptoms. In the examination, **in all patients,** look for symptoms and signs of heart failure, PE, aortic dissection, and pulmonary sepsis. Synthesize this data to reach a working diagnosis, then prove it.

ACS

The key to the diagnosis is to ascertain whether historically the pain is myocardial ischaemia; if it is, and it occurs at rest, then the diagnosis is likely to be an ACS; if it lasts longer than 20 minutes, it is likely there is myocardial infarction. How is myocardial ischaemia diagnosed from the history? In some patients this is easy—half of patients with infarction have preceding angina (retrosternal chest pain, not present at rest, provoked by effort, building up and necessitating discontinuation of effort, relieved within 1–2 minutes of rest). These patients now present with pain similar to their effort angina (although more intense and prolonged) but occurring at rest. These patients are easy to diagnose. Another group easy to diagnose are those with previous proven symptomatic coronary disease such as myocardial infarction. Ask if their current pain is similar to their previous pain (this is most helpful when they have had previous proven and unambiguous infarction). Beware, however, that what patients felt may have been proven symptomatic coronary disease may not, in fact, have been this (e.g. a remote diagnosis of angina made by a non-cardiologist without specialist review or supportive data). Accordingly, always ask how the previous diagnosis of angina or infarction was made,

Table 9.1 Short-term risk of death or non-fatal myocardial ischaemia in patients with unstable angina

Feature	High Risk (At least 1 of the following features must be present)	Intermediate Risk (No high-risk feature but must have 1 of the following features)	Low Risk (No high- or intermediate-risk feature but may have any of the following features)
History	Accelerating tempo of ischemic symptoms in preceding 48 hrs	Prior MI, peripheral or cerebrovascular disease, or CABG; prior aspirin use	
Character of pain	Prolonged ongoing (>20 min) rest pain	Prolonged (>20 min) rest angina, now resolved, with moderate or high likelihood of CAD	New-onset CCS Class III or IV angina in the past 2 wk with moderate or high likelihood of CAD
		Rest angina (<20 min or relieved with rest or sublingual NTG)	
Clinical findings	Pulmonary edema, most likely related to ischemia	Age >70 y	
	New or worsening MR murmur		
	S_3 or new/worsening rales		
	Hypotension, bradycardia, tachycardia		
	Age >75 y		
ECG findings	Angina at rest with transient ST-segment changes >0.05 mV	T-wave inversions >0.2 mV	Normal or unchanged ECG during an episode of chest discomfort
	Bundle-branch block, new or presumed new	Pathological Q waves	
	Sustained ventricular tachycardia		
Cardiac markers	Markedly elevated (eg, TnT or TnI >0.1 ng/mL)	Slightly elevated (eg, TnT >0.01 but <0.1 ng/mL)	Normal

Abbreviations: CABG, coronary artery bypass graft surgery; CAD, coronary artery disease; CCS, Canadian Cardiovascular Society; MI, myocardial infarction; MR, mitral regurgitation; NTG, glyceryl trinitrate (nitroglycerin).

Reproduced with permission from Committee Members, Eugene Braunwald et al., ACC/AHA Guidelines for the Management of Patients With Unstable Angina and Non–ST Segment Elevation Myocardial Infarction:Executive Summary and Recommendations: A Report of the American College of Cardiology/American Heart Association Task Force on Practice Guidelines (Committee on the Management of Patients With Unstable Angina), Circulation, Volume 102, Issue 10, Copyright © 2000 Wolters Kluwer Health, Inc. Source: National Heart, Lung, and Blood Institute; National Institutes of Health; U.S. Department of Health and Human Services.

and satisfy yourself that you are comfortable with this diagnosis. You can also use this approach in reverse—if patients have had negative investigations for coronary disease in the past, for example, a normal coronary angiogram, and now present with symptoms identical to those that led to the negative investigations, then it is unlikely that they have myocardial ischaemia.

This approach then leaves a group of patients in whom one cannot early on from the history alone categorically state what the pain is due to. However, there are clues from the history and physical examination (Table 9.2).

Duration of pain: Pain lasting a few seconds is unlikely to be anything serious; conversely, pain lasting many hours **in the setting of a completely normal ECG and normal troponin levels** is also unlikely to be an ACS. Typical angina pain in an ACS lasts a number of minutes, up to 20–30, but rarely longer. In addition, recurrence of pain is usual in an ACS; this means that an isolated episode of pain is unlikely to be an ACS.

Radiation: ACS pain often—but not always—radiates. Radiation of pain to the right arm increases the probability of ACS more than radiation to the left arm although radiation to the right arm is less common than to the left.

Absence of posture dependence, or worsening with respiration: Either absence of posture dependence or worsening with respiration reduces the chance of ACS. Posture dependence (better lying down, worse sitting forwards) may suggest pericarditis, and respiration dependence indicates the pain is pleuritic, for which there is a differential diagnosis (see 'PE').

Associated symptoms: Nausea, sweating, or sense of impending doom—all these increase the chance of infarction.

Physical examination in suspected ACS

The physical exam is rarely productive in ACS, but should always be carried out thoroughly. Look for signs of risk factors such as age, nicotine staining to the hands, lined face indicating smoking status, evidence of hyperlipidaemia (tendon xanthomata especially), high blood pressure, and bruits or lost pulses (feel all pulses, listen over the carotids and femorals), and perform a fundoscopy (for hypertensive and/or diabetic damage) and a urine dipstick test (for glucose and protein). Look for evidence of complications of an ACS—especially heart failure (e.g. jugular venous pressure, peripheral oedema, convincing lung crepitations), and especially a heart operating more stiffly (a third heart sound, probably the most reliable of all signs in ACS, provided the patient is listened to during pain). Look for murmurs, which are occasionally relevant to an ACS (e.g. indicating mitral regurgitation) but are usually more relevant to the overall management (e.g. indicating bystander aortic valve disease in a patient with an ACS).

The key diagnostic test in suspected ACS

The key diagnostic test in suspected ACS (see 'Key diagnostic tests') is an ECG that is initially diagnostically unambiguous (rare) or (more likely) one that changes sequentially in a pattern characteristic of an ACS. The latter characteristic means that ECGs should be repeated frequently. Furthermore, an ECG must always be taken whenever a patient has pain, as some ACSs only show changes, such as transient ST depression (common) or ST elevation (less likely, but indicating a need for immediate angiography), at that time. Ongoing chest pain with a resolutely normal ECG decreases greatly the chance of an ACS (although beware that circumflex territory ischaemia can be electrocardiographically silent—so, if the standard 12-lead ECG is normal, always ask for posterior leads (leads V7, V8, and V9) to be taken). In this situation, consider alternative serious diagnoses such as PE or aortic dissection.

PE

PE is a very common diagnosis. The key to diagnosis is eliciting risk factors from the history, such as recent (within 4–6 weeks) long-distance travel, age, female sex, use of the oral contraceptive pill, immobility, recent surgery, obesity, and cancer (although many patients have none of these factors), and then diagnosing one of the three distinct syndromes with which PE can present:

Table 9.2 Likelihood of myocardial infarction in patients presenting to the Emergency Dept with acute chest pain unrelated to trauma and unexplained by the chest radiograph, based on analysis of data from multiple studies

Finding	Sensitivity (%)	Specificity (%)	Likelihood Ratio* if Finding Is Present	Absent
History				
Male sex	59–72	24–61	1.3	0.7
Age				
<40 years	4	81	**0.2**	—
40-59 years	34	—	NS	—
≥60 years	47–74	54–68	1.5	—
Sharp pain	8–16	59–70	**0.3**	1.3
Pleuritic pain	3–6	74–82	**0.2**	1.2
Positional pain	3–11	75–87	**0.3**	1.1
Relief of pain with glyceryl trinitrate	35–92	12–59	NS	NS
Physical Examination				
Hand gestures				
Levine sign (placing a clenched fist against the sternum)	7	87	NS	NS
Palm sign (placing the extended palm against the sternum)	32	63	NS	NS
Arm sign (gripping the left arm)	18	83	NS	NS
Pointing sign (pointing to a single point on the chest with 1 or 2 fingers)	2	95	NS	NS
Chest wall tenderness	3–15	64–83	**0.3**	1.3
Diaphoretic appearance	28–53	71–94	2.2	0.7
Pallor	70	49	1.4	0.6
Systolic blood pressure <100 mm Hg	6	98	**3.6**	NS
Jugular venous distention	10	96	2.4	NS
Pulmonary crackles	20–38	82–91	2.1	NS
Third heart sound	16	95	**3.2**	NS
Electrocardiogram				
Normal	1–13	48–77	**0.2**	1.5
Nonspecific ST changes	5–8	47–78	**0.2**	1.4
ST elevation	31–56	97–100	**22.3**	0.6
ST depression	20–62	79–96	**3.9**	0.8
T wave inversion	9–39	84–94	2.0	NS

NS, not significant. *For interpretation of Likelihood Ratios (LR), see Chapter 1. LR if finding present = positive LR; LR if finding absent = negative LR.

The findings increasing the probability of myocardial infarction the most are new ST elevation (LR = 22.3) or ST depression (LR = 3.9) on the ECG. The only findings decreasing the probability of myocardial infarction in these studies are pain that is pleuritic (LR = 0.2), positional (LR = 0.3), or sharp (LR = 0.3); a normal electrocardiogram (LR = 0.2); chest wall tenderness (LR = 0.3); and age younger than 40 years (LR = 0.2).

Reprinted from *Evidence-Based Physical Diagnosis*, Third Edition, McGee S, Diagnosing Myocardial Infarction, EBM BOX 47-2, pp. 416-417, Copyright 2012, with permission from Elsevier.

Pleuritic chest pain, laterally (retrosternal pleuritic chest pain is more likely due to pericarditis): Fever and cough increase the chance of pneumonia causing the pleurisy; their absence increases the chance of PE being the cause (or, possibly, viral pleurisy being the diagnosis).

Breathlessness as the dominant feature (with or without pleuritic chest pain): Breathlessness, often with a tachycardia, no wheeze or reduction in peak flow, and a clear chest X-ray, is the hallmark of a PE. Finding hypoxaemia and an increase in the alveolar–arterial gradient further increases the probability of PE. Remember that many patients with underlying diseases making them breathless—such as heart failure or COPD—can have a PE complicating their underlying illness. It is easy, when such patients come in to hospital more breathless, to assume that it is a deterioration in their underlying illness; have a low threshold for ordering PE-directed investigations in these patients, unless there is unambiguous evidence that their breathlessness reflects their underlying illness (e.g. increasing airflow obstruction in COPD—more wheeze and lower peak flow—and radiological left heart failure in chronic heart failure patients).

Haemodynamic collapse: Haemodynamic collapse is usually of sudden onset, with marked breathlessness and, on examination, pallor (from reduced cardiac output), sinus tachycardia (a key finding) or atrial fibrillation, reduced blood pressure, hypoxaemia, raised venous pressure, possibly a right ventricular heave, clear lung fields, and an ECG showing sinus tachycardia (or atrial fibrillation), and some rightward shift in the QRS axis. There is no postural blood pressure drop (no volume loss; part of the differential diagnosis of shock), usually no fever (no sepsis), the lungs are clear, and lying flat is not an issue (no left heart failure, so cardiogenic shock unlikely). Any patient with haemodynamic collapse requires an immediate diagnosis and appropriately directed treatment. If the diagnosis is not immediately obvious, a cardiac ultrasound is likely to help direct therapy (see 'Introduction to therapy'); in PE causing shock, a dilated poorly functioning right heart is found, sometimes with a thrombus still present in the right atrium. The left heart is often small and compressed by the septum, which then is operating as a right ventricular structure.

Aortic dissection

The diagnostic clues are observing risk factors (features of Marfan syndrome or related connective tissue illness; hypertension; age; family history), and pain that is consistent with the diagnosis (retrosternal pain, sometimes tearing, often not, often radiating up to the neck and then into the back). The pain is persistent (i.e. lasts many hours). Examination may be normal (common), only show hypertension, or show complications of dissection, such as tamponade (**the key sign to look for**), aortic regurgitation, or damage from the intimal flap blocking the arterial blood supply to organs—hemiplegia (carotid artery), paraplegia (spinal artery), abdominal pain (mesenteric ischaemia), flank pain (renal ischaemia), or leg pain (femoral ischaemia). A chest X-ray is usually unhelpful (most dissections do not have widened mediastina, and most widened mediastina on chest X-ray are due to other causes, principally obesity), although occasionally diagnostic changes are seen, such as aortic dilatation, or left pleural effusion (suggesting aortic leak into the left pleural space). The ECG is often normal, or shows left ventricular hypertrophy (from long standing hypertension); occasionally a dissection presents as a myocardial infarct (usually inferior, as dissection of the left main stem is usually instantly fatal). The diagnostic test is a CT aortogram with contrast; occasionally, a transthoracic echo is diagnostic in showing the aortic flap, although more usually it 'only' shows pericardial fluid, or nothing. A transoesophageal echo has **no role** outside a cardiothoracic centre in diagnosing acute dissection (it is an invasive procedure that can result in transient hypertension and extension of the dissected aortic flap—**it should only be carried out** in cardiothoracic centres in the anaesthetic room with the surgical team standing by to proceed if positive).

Pneumothorax

The key here is sudden-onset, unilateral, pleuritic chest pain, often with breathlessness. The physical examination is usually unrewarding; in tension pneumothorax hypotension occurs, with tracheal deviation (away from the side with the pneumothorax). The chest X-ray is diagnostic.

Pneumonia

Most patients present with a clear pneumonic syndrome—unwell for a few days, with perhaps a preceding flu-like illness or viral sore throat, fever, cough, malaise, and pleuritic chest pain. By definition, those that end up causing diagnostic doubt in the assessment of chest pain may have atypical features, such as no fever (more likely in the elderly, or immunosuppressed) or no cough (elderly, those on opiates, or with advanced cerebrovascular disease). The clue to the diagnosis in these cases is the chest X-ray, along with blood tests, particularly markers of inflammation.

Oesophageal pain

Oesophageal pain typically occurs in two different manifestations:

Oesophagitis, often in the presence of gastro-oesophageal reflux: Symptoms include a retrosternal burning discomfort that is worse on lying down and is relieved by antacids, including milk; reflux (burning discomfort passing from the epigastrium upwards) may also be present. There are no diagnostic tests, although cardiac investigations obviously are normal. Endoscopy is usually not useful, as oesophagitis can coexist with coronary disease, and so proving the diagnosis by itself does not exclude the more serious diagnosis of an ACS (see 'Musculoskeletal chest pain').

Oesophageal spasm: Oesophageal spasm provokes a pain remarkably similar to myocardial ischaemia (retrosternal tightness, of an unpleasant quality, persistent). The first clue indicating that the pain is due to oesophageal spasm rather than myocardial ischaemia is the demographics being against myocardial ischaemia; the second clue is there being no preceding angina, as there is **never** any preceding angina in the case of oesophageal spasm; the third clue is patients having had recurrent attacks of similar pain always at rest over the years (often with repeated negative cardiac investigations); and the fourth clue is that the ECG and the troponin level remain normal, despite prolonged pain. There can, however, be diagnostic doubt, and in some cases coronary angiography may be indicated to rule out a cardiac cause for symptoms.

Musculoskeletal chest pain

Typically, musculoskeletal chest pain occurs in the setting of unusual or prolonged effort using the arms, or prolonged coughing. However, often there is no preceding unusual effort. Pain is unilateral and often left-sided (as patients worry more about pain in the left chest, and so seek medical help more frequently). It may be sharp ('like a knife') or dull. Typically, it lasts for hours, and is often exacerbated by turning the chest round. There may be point tenderness. All of these features increase the chance of the diagnosis being musculoskeletal pain; however, even if clinically the diagnosis is musculoskeletal pain, coronary-artery-directed tests may be necessary, as occasionally an ACS and musculoskeletal pain coexist (perhaps as patients with an ACS may repetitively rub their chest wall in a fruitless attempt to relieve their cardiac symptoms, thereby provoking a musculoskeletal component to their symptoms).

Chest pain of uncertain aetiology

Chest pain of uncertain aetiology is a not-uncommon diagnosis, where the historical features share some of the features of several different diagnostic groups. In this situation the pragmatic approach is (1) determine the risk of coronary disease from the extant risk factors and (2) if there is a significant risk, risk stratify the patient (see 'Philosophical approach') and then proceed along a pathway to exclude both an ACS and PE (see 'Key diagnostic tests' and 'Other diagnostic tests').

Philosophical approach

As one proceeds along this journey, diagnoses are thrown up, and the key to reaching the correct diagnosis is not just to use the clues from the individual features, but to combine them so that the combination of data is more powerful than any individual factor (Hurst Step 2; see 'Approach to diagnosis'). The key question to ask as you proceed with data gathering is 'Does the new information increase or decrease the chance of my first (and other) diagnoses?'. For example, take a 56-year-old patient with new retrosternal chest pain, being seen in the A & E department, and whose examination shows some chest wall tenderness. Chest pain in A & E has a 30% chance of being an ACS; this chance is increased by age (for most patients the dominant risk factor) and male sex, along with coronary risk factors.

Our patient is younger than most, so the incidence is lower (use the demographics—they are a powerful diagnostic tool). Chest wall tenderness lessens this chance (it is not necessary to know by how much new data adjust, probably, merely the direction of change). Now, factor in a normal presentation ECG, and a normal ECG at 12 hours (further lessening the chance of ACS). The probability that the patient has an ACS is now very small. Although this is a simple example, you should get used to using data in this fashion, and not blindly going to the one positive test (e.g. troponin), believing that it has made the diagnosis for you, as it rarely has!

Table 9.2 shows features of the history that increase or decrease the probability of acute infarction.

Key diagnostic tests

The key to diagnosing the cause of acute chest pain is to use the following simple tests, to understand them, and, where necessary, to repeat them often:

The 12-lead ECG: This is the most important test. This must be done at presentation and then at least four times over a 12-hour period, which is probably the minimum duration for admission for anyone with any realistic chance of having an ACS. There are many features to look for:

ECG changes at presentation: ST elevation of a typical shape (convex upwards) in the distribution of a coronary artery usually indicates ST-elevation myocardial infarction (STEMI) and often trumps other findings; however, bear in mind that not all ST elevation is due to an STEMI (pericarditis, physiological ST elevation, bundle branch block, and Brugada syndrome are all in the differential). ST depression, particularly if marked and not in the lateral leads (where it may indicate left ventricular hypertrophy, digoxin use, or ischaemia) has a high chance of indicating ischaemia. Tachycardia is an important but non-specific finding—always think PE, left ventricular failure, or sepsis (the clinical exam and chest X-ray help distinguish these diagnoses).

Dynamic ECG changes: Dynamic ECG changes are a hallmark of an ACS, and **must** be looked for—all patients should have ECGs at regular intervals (how frequently is unclear; certainly, however, every 4 hours, and whenever pain recurs). The interpretation of fluctuating ECGs over time is not unambiguous, although most will have an ACS. However, be aware that there are many ACSs where dynamic ECG changes do not occur, and bear in mind that not all dynamic ECG changes mean an ACS—for example, a large PE can over a few hours give rise to T-wave inversion anterolaterally, looking remarkably similar to a left anterior descending (LAD) syndrome ECG.

Tachycardia: Tachycardia could indicate left heart failure, pulmonary embolism, sepsis, anxiety, or volume depletion, or just be a non-specific response to pain.

Left ventricular hypertrophy: left ventricular hypertrophy greatly increases the risk of a serious cause underlying the pain, such as coronary disease, aortic syndromes, or aortic valve disease.

Old Q waves: Old Q waves likewise usually indicate established coronary disease, and raise the probability that current symptoms reflect a new coronary event.

Troponin: Troponin is a sensitive marker of cardiac damage or stress. While sequential rises in troponin are the hallmark of an ACS, many patients with severe coronary disease have normal troponins, and many patients with small rises in troponin do not have coronary disease but rather one of the following:
• renal failure, a very common cause of small troponin rises
• a PE, where the extent of troponin rise relates to prognosis
• a cardiac arrhythmia—many patients with atrial fibrillation or a supraventricular tachycardia develop a small rise after prolonged tachycardia
• myocarditis
• stress ('takotsubo') cardiomyopathy

The clues to all these other causes of troponin rise are usually fairly obvious—the one that is most difficult to diagnose can be a PE, and it is worth noting that, if a patient with chest pain and a troponin rise has a coronary angiogram that is normal, this certainly does not mean that they have a healed ruptured coronary plaque; they may have a PE. The moral is, don't stop the diagnostic process at angiography; if the angiogram is normal, often the diagnosis of acute decompensated coronary disease has been disproved and you must restart the diagnostic process with the following:

D-dimer levels: This test can be used to decrease the chance of PE (if the level is normal), but is rarely useful in increasing the chance of PE.

Chest X-ray: A chest X-ray is the key investigation (along with the ECG) in evaluating chest pain. Common abnormalities have already been described in 'PE', 'Aortic dissection', 'Pneumothorax', and 'Pneumonia'. Some key points, however, should be made:
1. If the chest X-ray is normal, consider PE or early pneumonia, in addition to considering the result to be genuinely normal.
2. Do not use the chest X-ray to alter the probability of aortic dissection; many dissections do not have widened mediastina, and virtually all widened mediastina are not due to dissection (obesity is the common explanation).
3. A chest X-ray is useful in diagnosing pneumonia, but a normal chest X-ray does not rule the diagnosis out; it merely decreases the chance of the diagnosis being pneumonia.
4. Always, if possible (using digital technology), compare the current chest X-ray with previous ones.

Nuclear cardiology imaging techniques: In many units, this is the mainstay of diagnosis and risk stratification in chronic stable angina. However, nuclear cardiology has a role in the assessment of acute chest pain:

Standard SPECT MPS: The SPECT (single-photon emission computed tomography) MPS (myocardial perfusion scan) is the standard nuclear scan, done both at rest (which allows remote infarction to be diagnosed) and with stress (from exercise—the preferred method—or by pharmacological methods, using adenosine or its analogues, or dobutamine), which provides quantification for the volume of inducible ischaemia present. The test is done on an expedited basis, within a few days of presentation with acute chest pain. The test is fairly reliable in diagnosing infarction and ischaemia, and provides data on prognosis.

Immediate rest SPECT MPS: In this version of the test, a radioactive isotope is injected during or within 2 hours of chest pain. If the scan is completely normal, by implication no infarction or volume ischaemia is present and the risk of immediate (1–2 weeks) events is low enough to allow hospital discharge. The patient returns for the stress component of the study, which provides data on risk stratification and the need for angiography.

Immediate scanning using infarction-seeking isotopes: This test remains largely investigative.

CTPA: CTPA is a crucial test that is increasingly useful in the assessment of acute chest pain. It should be ordered immediately as soon as PE is suspected, and preferably carried out with a few hours of acute hospital admission. Not only does it establish whether PE is present, but it assesses the quantity of PEs, thereby establishing the risk of haemodynamic collapse and thus determining how aggressive therapy should be (thrombolysis vs heparin alone) and where the patient should be monitored. CTPA also provides data on the presence of pneumonia, concomitant lung disease (e.g. emphysema), aortic disease, and the extent of coronary calcification, a strong predictive factor for coronary disease. Accordingly, even if CTPA excludes PE, it often moves the management forwards.

Coronary angiogram: A coronary angiogram is the key test in ACS, and very useful diagnostically in those in whom non-invasive investigations have failed to firmly establish the diagnosis. Most patients with an ACS have a coronary angiogram, to risk stratify and as a prelude to revascularization (percutaneous or surgical). However, many physicians underestimate its role in diagnosis. If there are significant risk factors for coronary disease, and the pain could be cardiac, and no alternative explanation has emerged, often a coronary angiogram provides a quick and **relatively** safe means of determining whether coronary disease is present. The risks are about 1 in 1000 of a serious adverse complication (heart attack, stroke, death).

Other diagnostic tests

All patients admitted with chest pain should have:

- a full blood count; anaemia can provoke angina, a raised white-cell count may indicate infection (e.g. pneumonia) or PE, and a high platelet count may indicate a haematological process giving rise to an ACS
- a full biochemical profile, to assess renal function, which is always critical in all hospitalized patients, and liver function, which may be abnormal because of complications of cardiac or respiratory illness or because the prime pathology is subdiaphragmatic (e.g. gall bladder disease)
- tests for inflammatory markers, such as C-reactive protein (CRP) and the erythrocyte sedimentation rate
- tests for lipid levels (especially cholesterol) and random glucose

Introduction to therapy

The aim of therapy is to improve prognosis, and relieve symptoms. It is easy to give directed therapy once you know what the diagnosis is, what the exact nature of any comorbidities are, and how they impact therapy, but it can be extremely difficult when the differential diagnosis remains broad and when therapies for some possible diagnoses can easily exacerbate other possible diagnoses (e.g. dual antiplatelet therapy if an ACS is top of the differential but an aortic dissection is Number 2!). How does one approach this?

- First, use the quickest means possible to establish the diagnosis: frame your question (see Hurst's steps in 'Approach to diagnosis'), think of the single test required to establish the diagnosis, and then get this test **immediately** if the condition could be life-threatening. For example, if you think the diagnosis is PE, order CTPA to be done then and there—that is, the afternoon of admission, not routinely, in a few days' time.
- Perform a clinical and investigative screen for comorbidities, especially falls, dementia, COPD, renal failure, and anaemia; establish in your own mind how these impact both diagnosis and therapy.
- If your definitive investigative tool is not available (e.g. out-of-hours CTPA is rarely available, and the same is true for coronary angiography for most chest pain, except STEMI), then use what imaging you have (e.g. out-of-hours cardiac ultrasound often provides useful data on diagnosis and risk both for ACS and PE).
- Do not believe that you MUST give therapy; if you do not know what the diagnosis is, then risk assess the patient **as if** they had an ACS or PE using standard scores (e.g. TIMI for ACS; for PE, the absence of tachycardia, with significant hypoxaemia and ECG changes, indicates lower—although not low—risk). If your risk stratification establishes low risk, and comorbidities substantially raise the risk of empiric therapy, withhold therapy until you can establish the diagnosis.
- Give empiric therapy for your Number 1 diagnosis—if it does not conflict with other possible diagnosis, give full treatment as appropriate. ACS will benefit from dual antiplatelet therapy if there are ECG changes or raised troponin; if neither is present, give mono-antiplatelet therapy (and low-molecular-weight heparin (LMWH) thromboprophylaxis as appropriate). Do not rush in with aspirin/clopidogrel/LMWH in chest pain with a normal ECG and negative troponin, as even if they have an ACS they will not benefit, and the potential to do harm is significant given that the diagnosis may easily not be an ACS (negative early investigations).
- Modify your treatment using common sense; for example, profound dementia and frequent falls implies you should not rush in with aggressive antiplatelet and anticoagulant therapy.
- If you think the diagnosis could be an ACS or PE but anaemia is present, and you cannot get diagnostic imaging (CTPA), then use what information you have and adopt a sensible approach to treatment.

Prognosis

Prognosis in chest pain depends on the diagnosis. Therein lies the problem; if you know the diagnosis, all well and good; risk prediction scores for each illness are available and give you the outcome. However, if you don't know the diagnosis, you have more limited data on prognosis. As most chest pain whose cause is not immediately apparent is either benign or due to an ACS, most strategies in A & E concentrate on excluding an ACS. This is entirely valid, but one must consider the alternative diagnoses, as these strategies are unhelpful in risk stratifying, for example, aortic dissection, pneumonia, or cancer causing rib pain. This emphasizes the need to always think about the diagnosis (e.g. benign chest pain), not the syndrome (e.g. troponin-negative chest pain). Most A & E strategies are designed to identify low-risk patients who can be safely discharged, for outpatient workup if necessary. What strategies are helpful?

- Consider the diagnosis using a standard history/examination/simple investigation approach. Often, this will allow one to be guided away from a chest-pain algorithm.
- All patients with chest pain must have an ECG (done immediately, and then frequently, e.g. at hourly intervals for the first 4–6 hours) and basic blood tests (full blood count, biochemistry, CRP). All patients need chest X-rays. Some patients need D-dimer tests. Do a highly selective troponin at presentation, and one 3 hours later.
- If the diagnosis is not clear after a few hours observation, you will be in a position to risk stratify even if you do not have a diagnosis. If patients are well (no arrhythmias or haemodynamic compromise) and oxygenated normally (no evidence of PE), with all pulses intact, no aortic regurgitation (no evidence of aortic dissection), no evidence of heart failure (from exam and chest X-ray), a normal ECG that remains normal, two negative highly selective troponins, and one negative CRP, then they fall into a low-risk category and they may be discharged with reasonable safety, provided, of course, that you have organized appropriate outpatient follow-up and investigation (this is the responsibility of the A & E clinician).
- Pitfalls in risk stratifying patients with chest pain in A & E include failing to address key factors in the history, failing to notice mild hypoxaemia (PE), failing to recognize that the ECG must be normal or near normal for low risk (fixed ECG abnormalities immediately raise the risk profile, sometimes massively, as in fixed, deep, anterolateral T-wave inversion, which often indicates a high-risk proximal LAD stenosis), failing to look at the chest X-ray (pneumothorax, heart failure)—and, above all, failing to consider a diagnosis of aortic dissection.
- Handling uncertainty in the diagnosis of this symptom is often not easy; however, remember that the greatest risk a patient with a life-threatening condition causing their chest pain faces is being sent home from A & E. Hence, if you have diagnostic doubt about the cause of the chest pain, it is always reasonable to admit the patient for further observation and investigation.

Further Reading

Pollak P and Brady W. Electrocardiographic patterns mimicking ST Segment elevation myocardial infarction. *Cardiol Clin* 2012; 30: 601–15. http://dx.doi.org/10.1016/j.ccl.2012.07.012.

Rybicki FJ, Udelson JE, Peacock WF, et al. Appropriate utilization of cardiovascular imaging in emergency department patients with chest pain: a joint report of the American College of Radiology Appropriateness Criteria Committee and the American College of Cardiology Appropriate Use Criteria Task Force. *J Am Coll Cardiol.* 2016; 67: 853–79.

Vafaie M, Biener M, Mueller M, et al. Analytically false or true positive elevations of high sensitivity cardiac troponin: A systematic approach. *Heart* 2014; 100: 508–14.

10 Chronic chest pain

Jonathan Timperley and Sandeep Hothi

Definition

Chronic chest pain constitutes pain (or discomfort, or indeed any sensation recognized by the patient as being 'not normal') in the chest; the hallmark is that it has been present for a significant time, usually months (to allow differentiation from acute chest pain and acute coronary syndromes (ACSs)). The main question to answer in the management of chronic chest pain is 'Are we dealing with chronic stable angina?'. The aim of having an arbitrary time period in the definition is to try and separate out patients with ACSs (see Chapter 9); this is not always possible in practice and, not infrequently, a diagnosis of an ACS (or other life-threatening condition) is made in those presenting with chronic chest pain—in other words, you need to keep your diagnostic wits about you when approaching chronic chest pain.

Differential diagnosis

Table 10.1 lists the usual causes that are included in the differential diagnosis.

Context

Chronic chest pain is common and may present in primary or secondary care. In both settings, it is important to determine whether chest pains relate to ischaemic heart disease (IHD), another life-threatening cause, or another illness. While IHD is the commonest life-threatening cause, it is not the only life-threatening cause (e.g. chronic pulmonary emboli), so do not restrict your differential diagnosis to the heart alone.

Approach to diagnosis

In thinking of the diagnosis, it is helpful to approach the differential diagnosis systematically:

- First, **think demographically**: 'What are the common causes of chest pain for the age/sex of the patient in front of me?'; in particular, use age and sex to estimate the probability of coronary disease, then adjust the probability by taking into account risk factors for coronary disease. Young females are unlikely to have coronary disease (they have musculoskeletal pains, gastrointestinal pains, breast pains, and, more rarely, pulmonary emboli), whereas older men who smoke and have diabetes are very likely to have coronary disease. Put another way, estimate a preclinical assessment probability of coronary disease (and other causes) using demographics and coronary disease risk factors. Always ask women if they are on the oral contraceptive pill; ask all patients about risk factors for thromboembolic lung disease.
- Second, as for all illness, **use the specific clinical features** to refine your differential diagnosis (see 'Specific clues to the diagnosis'). This is important; elderly patients commonly have coronary disease, but it is not responsible for their symptoms; so with all patients, you must answer the questions 'Do they have coronary disease' and 'If so, is it relevant to the symptoms' (in other words, 'do they have angina?').
- Third, **think anatomically**: 'What are the common causes for chest pain in the anatomical area that my patient experiences symptoms?'; for example, stable angina is usually felt retrosternally (as are many gastrointestinal causes of pain), whereas muscular pain is often felt around the left breast (pain sited here provokes more anxiety in lay patients than right-sided discomfort, and so lasts longer). Back pain radiating anteriorly is often due to

entrapment neuropathy. Ask whether the pain moves around—angina does not move between episodes, whereas musculoskeletal and non-cardiac chest pain does. Pain moving around the chest is described as 'flitting'; angina does not flit, nor does gastrointestinal pain. Most flitting chest pain is benign; rarely, it relates to pleurisy due to autoimmune disease.
- Fourth, **use an investigation (where possible) to confirm the diagnosis** (see 'Key diagnostic tests' and 'Other diagnostic tests') and, where relevant, to exclude the most likely serious diagnosis.
- Finally, **ask for all patients what their risk is of cardiac death**; if coronary disease is present, use standard models (e.g. Duke nomogram; see Chapter 89) to predict death. If you do not think coronary disease is present, ask the following questions:
  - **First**, what is the risk of a cardiac event occurring (using risk prediction charts based on standard risk factors (Table 10.2))?
  - **Second**, in those patients in whom you do not know if coronary disease is present, ask yourself the question 'If coronary disease were to be present, what would the prognosis be?'. This can then really clarify in your mind whether you should order an investigation with risk/cost (e.g. coronary angiography)—for example, if symptoms are infrequent (so there are no symptomatic grounds for intervention), and prognosis, if coronary disease were present, is good, there may be no grounds to undertake coronary angiography, and the patient can be managed medically.

The specific clinical features are ascertained by taking a careful history. The following should be determined:

The character of the pain, including its quality and location/radiation: Angina has a deep-seated quality that, once experienced, is rarely forgotten. If patients have had a previous myocardial infarct, specifically ask if the current symptoms, while differing in severity, have the same quality as the infarct.

The location of the pain: This is helpful, but not as diagnostic as many patients and doctors think. In most cases, angina is felt retrosternally, but this is not true for all cases; in some, angina is felt laterally or, indeed, in the shoulder alone. In most cases, pleurisy is felt laterally, gastrointestinal pain is felt retrosternally, and musculoskeletal pain is felt in the left chest—these are all generalizations and there are many exceptions. Nonetheless, location is a clue as to aetiology although do not use it to the exclusion of other factors.

Time course of symptoms: Inquire about the frequency, severity, and duration of the symptoms (pain lasting seconds is never serious)—first, to determine how intrusive the problem is to the patient and, if so, how important symptom relief is as opposed to diagnosis (clarity in this area is crucial for subsequent management); and, second, to estimate risk—infrequent anginal symptoms often indicate a low risk process, whereas intrusive symptoms are more likely to indicate severe coronary disease, placing the patient at higher risk of infarction and early death. A change in symptoms is also of relevance, as a worsening of chronic angina symptoms (becoming more severe, more frequent, or more easily provoked) often indicates progressive pathology warranting escalation of investigation and management (see Chapter 9).

Provoking and relieving factors: Crucially, one must be quite clear about the relationship with effort, but also ascertain any relation with food or lying flat (suggesting a gastrointestinal pathology), and upper arm movement (suggesting a musculoskeletal problem). It is above all the relationship with effort that allows chest pain to be diagnosed as angina in character, and you must completely understand this in all patients you see with chronic chest pain (see 'Stable angina').

Table 10.1 Differential diagnosis of chronic chest pain

	Condition	Frequency	Specific clinical clues	Diagnostic test	Traps
Cardiac	Chronic stable angina	Very common in specific groups	See text; a syndrome of chest pain provoked by effort and rapidly and totally relieved by rest; if the relationship with exercise is absent, the pain is not chronic stable angina	Confirmation of coronary disease, angiographically or by functional study	Stable angina can be caused by (1) coronary disease, (2) aortic stenosis, (3) pulmonary hypertension, or (4) (rarely) syndrome X (inadequate coronary vasodilator reserve)
	ACS	Common	Similar quality pain to stable angina, occurring at rest	Evidence of myocardial necrosis (enzymes) and coronary angiography	Myocarditis and takotsubo cardiomyopathy may present in a fashion similar to ACS; do not label troponin rises due to renal failure, or tachyarrhythmia (e.g. AVNRT) as an ACS
	Pericarditis	Not rare	Retrosternal pain, worse on inspiration, and on lying	None; typical ECG changes sometimes help	Exclude significant pericardial effusion by cardiac ultrasound; most but not all pericarditis is benign
Respiratory	Pleurisy	Common	Lateral pain, worse with inspiration	None	Always actively diagnose the cause of pleurisy—usually infection—but you must actively exclude pulmonary embolus
	Airways pain	Common	Deep internal discomfort, often associated coughing, worse on effort	Spirometry	Airways discomfort due to COPD may coexist with angina due to coronary disease (smoking causes both)
Gastrointestinal	GORD	Common	Retrosternal burning pain (reflux)	OGD, relief with PPIs	Oesophageal spasm can have symptoms identical to ACS, and this may need to be excluded
	Dyspeptic syndromes	Very common	Epigastric discomfort	Usually relief with PPIs	
	Peptic ulcer disease	Very common	Intrusive epigastric discomfort	OGD, relief with antacids	
	Gallbladder disease	Common	Pains usually occur episodically, felt in the epigastrium (bile duct pain), or right upper quadrant (cholecystitis)	Abdominal ultrasound	Beware: gall bladder stones are very common, and other pathologies may coexist with them
	Chronic pancreatitis	Rare	Severe epigastric pain	CT abdomen	Alcohol excess is very common; such patients often have multiple comorbidities and are at risk of coronary disease
Musculoskeletal pain	Arthritis	Common	Position or movement dependence to pain	No diagnostic test	Often improves with time or NSAIDs
	Non-specific musculoskeletal pain	The most common cause of pain	Many features; most commonly pain moving around chest, of variable duration, sometimes tender	No diagnostic test	May coexist with coronary disease, which usually therefore needs excluding in those at risk
Neurological	Entrapment neuropathy	Common	Back pain radiating anteriorly, lasts for hours at a time, not effort dependent	No diagnostic test; supportive data from finding spinal arthritis	As there is no diagnostic test for this, such patients may also need to have coronary disease ruled out
	Zoster	Rare	Very severe pain, usually only present for a few days	Rash, once it has occurred!	Usually not in the differential diagnosis of chronic chest pain; post-herpetic neuralgia, rarely; the history is diagnostic
Other	Cancer	Rare	Usually severe, localized pain	Imaging and histology	All patients with chest pain MUST have a chest X-ray, mainly to rule out malignancy

Abbreviations: ACS, acute coronary syndrome; AVNRT, atrioventricular nodal re-entrant tachycardia; CT, computed tomography; ECG, electrocardiogram; GORD, gastro-oesophageal reflux disease; NSAIDs, non-steroidal anti-inflammatory drugs; OGD, oesophagogastroduodenoscopy; PPIs, proton-pump inhibitors.

Table 10.2 Clinical pretest probabilities in patients with stable chest pain symptoms

Age	Typical angina		Atypical angina		Non-anginal pain	
	Men	Women	Men	Women	Men	Women
30–39	59†	28†	29†	10*	18†	5*
40–49	69†	37†	38†	14*	25†	8*
50–59	77‡	47†	49†	20†	34†	12*
60–69	84‡	58†	59†	28†	44†	17†
70–79	89§	68‡	69‡	37†	54†	24†
>80	93§	76‡	78‡	47†	65†	32†

Note: Probabilities of obstructive coronary disease shown reflect the estimates for patients aged 35, 45, 55, 65, 75, and 85 years.

* Patients with a pretest probability <15% can be managed without further testing.

† Patients with a pretest probability of 15%–65% could have an exercise ECG, if feasible, as the initial test. However, if local expertise and availability permit a non-invasive imaging-based test for ischaemia, this would be preferable, given the superior diagnostic capabilities of such tests. In young patients, radiation issues should be considered.

‡ Patients with a pretest probability of 66%–85% should have a non-invasive imaging functional test for making a diagnosis of stable coronary artery disease.

§ For patients with a pretest probability >85%, one can assume that stable coronary artery disease is present. They need risk stratification only.

Adapted with permission from Task Force Members, 2013 ESC guidelines on the management of stable coronary artery disease, *European Heart Journal*, Volume 34, Issue 38, Copyright © 2013 Oxford University Press.

Specific clues to the diagnosis

Stable angina

The absolute key to diagnosing chronic stable angina is its relationship to effort (Table 10.3); pains must not be present before effort, must occur reliably on similar levels of effort (earlier if going uphill, when the weather is cold, or after eating), must build up such that continued effort at the same intensity becomes increasingly difficult, and must resolve completely within a minute or so of rest. Pain with these characteristics is termed 'anginal chest pain'. It often means angina due to obstructive coronary disease, but may indicate aortic stenosis, pulmonary hypertension, asthma (a common cause of this symptom), and, very rarely indeed, the very much over-diagnosed syndrome X. Thus, the diagnosis of anginal chest pains is an **interim** diagnosis until the pathological substrate can be determined. In many regards, therefore, it is analogous to **fever**; no one has a final diagnosis of fever. Likewise, no one should have a final diagnosis of angina; rather, the diagnosis should be 'angina due to obstructive coronary disease (or whatever)'. How can you discriminate between the different causes of angina? The following all help: coronary disease risk factors; typicality, or otherwise, of the pain (see Table 10.3, for obstructive coronary disease); physical examination (aortic stenosis, sometimes pulmonary hypertension); and cardiac ultrasound (pulmonary hypertension– aortic stenosis is diagnosed prior to the ultrasound). Chronic chest pain is often classified according to its similarity, or otherwise, to angina, which NICE defines as chest pain which:

- presents as a constricting discomfort in the front of the chest, or in the neck, shoulders, jaw, or arms
- is precipitated by physical exertion
- is relieved by rest or glyceryl trinitrate tablets within about 5 minutes

Table 10.3 Clues to the diagnosis of effort angina using the presence and nature of effort-dependent symptoms

	Present before effort	Leads to effort stopping	Time to resolution following effort
Angina	No	Yes	1–2 minutes
Musculoskeletal chest pain	Often	Sometimes	>20 minutes
Non-cardiac chest pain	Often	No	Substantial, sometimes days

Chest pain exhibiting all three of these features is defined as **typical angina**; chest pain exhibiting two of these features is defined as **atypical angina**; and chest pain exhibiting only one or none of the features is defined as **non-anginal chest pain**.

Unstable angina/acute coronary syndromes

Half of patients with an ACS (see Chapter 90) have preceding-effort angina: they have clear-cut effort-dependent symptoms, now occurring at rest. The diagnosis here is easy. In half, the ACS comes out of the blue; however, in these patients their symptoms, at most, have only been going on for a few weeks—which, by definition, excludes patients with chronic chest pain (where symptoms need to have been present for a few months). Have a high index of suspicion that episodic new chest pain (<2 weeks) in someone at risk of coronary disease could be an ACS—and beware: in these patients, there may be little or no effort dependence to the pain. Age and other coronary risk factors increase the chance that new chest pain is an ACS, whereas multiple previous contacts with physicians and many current symptoms decrease the chance of ACS.

Musculoskeletal pain

Surprisingly, a history of onset clearly related to musculoskeletal injury is rarely present. Upper body movement exacerbates pains, and so may using a particular limb (e.g. the left arm). Pains last a long time, not the minutes that stable angina does, and can last days. The chest wall may be tender to palpation, although this is far from universal. Ninety-nine per cent of musculoskeletal pains are benign and no underlying pathology is found; however, very rarely, musculoskeletal chest pains are due to a cancer eroding a rib or similar structure—the clue here is the localized area of the pain, the unremitting severity of the pain, and systemic features (e.g. malaise and weight loss). A history of previous malignancy is clearly a clue that should not be ignored. One reason for carrying out a full blood count and full biochemical profile in those with chest pain is to look for clues to such systemic illness. As rib metastases are difficult to see on plain chest X-ray, if their presence remains possible despite negative plain film imaging, consider ordering a bone scan.

Neuropathic pain

This is typically a sharp, shooting pain, often with a dermatomal or peripheral nerve distribution. There may be a history of onset after surgery, herpes zoster, and other causes of peripheral neuropathy, such as diabetes mellitus.

Gastrointestinal pains

Gastrointestinal pains may be due to the following:

Peptic ulcer disease: This may cause epigastric pain before eating, or at night (said to occur with duodenal ulcers), or pain related to meals (said to indicate gastric ulcers).

Gastroesophageal reflux disease: This causes a burning sensation which is felt in the retrosternal area or epigastrium, or regurgitation of acid or bile. Oesophageal spasm can be identical to the pain of myocardial ischaemia—a severe retrosternal pain lasting many minutes, and associated with diaphoresis and sometimes fear. The pain is not effort dependent (so the differential is an ACS rather than chronic stable angina). The clue is that, by the time patients present, they have often had many episodes going back years, unlike the case with ACS.

Biliary disease: In this case, symptoms are usually restricted to being subdiaphragmatic; rarely, they may be prominent above the diaphragm.

Respiratory causes of chest pain

Airways disease and pleurisy (infective or thromboembolic in origin) are common causes of abnormal chest sensations. In patients with chest pain due to airways disease, symptoms may be worse on effort ('tightness in the chest'), leading to confusion with angina due to coronary disease—one clue in favour of airways disease is the presence of marked breathlessness (patients usually mention this first rather than the chest tightness), which is rare in angina unless:

- there is severe, multivessel coronary disease—multiple risk factors are usually present, and the standard exercise test is usually very abnormal

- in those with impaired left ventricular function, which can be suspected from the history (previous myocardial infarction) and abnormal resting ECG
- in those with diabetes, in whom, de facto, there is a high pretest probability of coronary disease, indicating a preexisting need for high-level coronary-directed investigations

Other clues are:

Asthma: This is episodic wheeze, with breathlessness. The clue is usually the demographics, together with the prominence of breathlessness as a symptom.

Chronic obstructive pulmonary disease: In the history, the long progressive history of increasingly intrusive breathlessness is a good clue, backed up by the demographics, smoking history, and examination (hyperinflated lungs, poor air entry, wheeze) and confirmed by spirometry.

Non-cardiac chest pain

By this vague term, cardiologists mean 'pain that doesn't come from the heart, and doesn't have specific features allowing a more specific diagnosis' (so it is not musculoskeletal pain, which is diagnosed using the features previously outlined). It is a useful term for medical professionals, although patients find its use challenging. Cardiologists mean by its use 'pain that historically is not anginal (no effort dependence) and for which appropriate coronary (and other cardiac) investigations have been negative'. It means pain that is benign prognostically and does not require cardiac drugs for treatment, or cardiologists for management. Patients with frequent hospital attendances due to non-cardiac chest pain benefit from cognitive behavioural therapy.

Key diagnostic tests

Blood tests

A full blood count, biochemical profile, thyroid function, cholesterol (and HDL/LDL subfraction), glucose, and triglyceride tests are all mandatory.

Resting ECG

In most patients with chronic chest pain, the resting ECG is normal and neither increases nor decreases the post-test probability of IHD. In a very few, there are diagnostic changes—evidence of an old Q-wave infarction, or ST/T-wave changes strongly associated with coronary disease (such as symmetrical pan-anterior T-wave inversion). Minor ECG changes in the elderly are rarely of any diagnostic utility. Occasionally, the ECG raises the possibility of another pathology—gross left ventricular hypertrophy suggests hypertension (usually obvious from the history and examination—and, of course, strongly correlated with the development of coronary disease), aortic stenosis (in this case, the exam is diagnostic), or, if neither are present, hypertrophic cardiomyopathy. A normal resting ECG does not exclude coronary artery disease, and this is the category into which most patients fall.

Chest X-ray

A chest X-ray is mandatory for all presenting with chronic chest pain, although this test rarely helps diagnostically. Usually normal (post-test IHD probability unchanged), it occasionally shows an increase in the size of the cardiac silhouette (in high-BMI individuals, this is not associated with cardiomegaly whereas, in thin patients, a large cardiac silhouette may mean poor ventricular function or a pericardial effusion). Rarely, it shows a neoplasm, often caused by the same risk factors as coronary disease (smoking, age), as the cause of the chest pain.

Exercise ECG

In an exercise ECG, patients are exercised using a standard protocol on a motorized treadmill while an ECG is recorded. The test has varying specificity and sensitivity (see Table 10.3 and Figure 10.1), being least accurate in young women without typical angina, and most accurate in older men with typical angina. While conduction blocks on the ECG, and pacemakers, make the ECG difficult to interpret, the most helpful aspect of the exercise ECG is the accurate documentation of

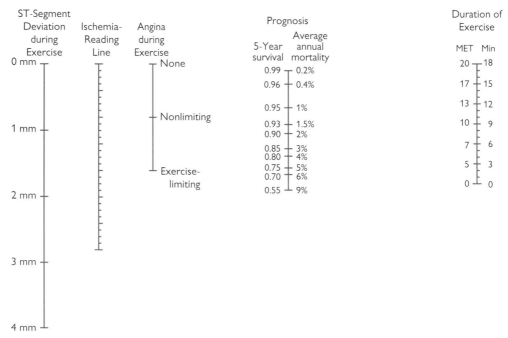

Figure 10.1 Nomogram of the prognostic relations embodied in the treadmill score. Determination of prognosis proceeds in five steps. First, the observed amount of exercise-induced ST-segment deviation (the largest elevation or depression after resting changes have been subtracted) is marked on the line for ST-segment deviation during exercise. Second, the observed degree of angina during exercise is marked on the line for angina. Third, the marks for ST-segment deviation and degree of angina are connected with a straight edge. The point where this line intersects the ischaemia-reading line is noted. Fourth, the total number of minutes of exercise in treadmill testing according to the Bruce protocol (or the equivalent in multiples of resting oxygen consumption (METs) from an alternative protocol) is marked on the exercise-duration line. Fifth, the mark for ischaemia is connected with that for exercise duration. The point at which this line intersects the line for prognosis indicates the 5-year survival rate and average annual mortality for patients.

Reproduced with permission from Mark DB, Shaw L, Harrell FE et al Prognostic value of a treadmill exercise score in outpatients with suspected coronary artery disease. N Eng J Med 1991: 325:849–53.

exercise capacity, a variable strongly associated with prognosis. Thus, even where the ECG is unreliable, useful data can emerge from a well-conducted treadmill test.

Resting echocardiography

A resting echocardiography is rarely helpful by itself in diagnosing the cause of chest pain (very occasionally, it shows regional wall motion abnormalities suggestive of coronary disease), but often is very helpful in determining prognosis in a range of different diagnostic possibilities (the key measure is left ventricular function). Rarely, it shows unsuspected defects (aortic stenosis, hypertrophic cardiomyopathy).

Functional and anatomical imaging

Imaging used to investigate coronary artery disease may be **functional**, in which case it is used to assess possible reductions in myocardial perfusion and function in response to exertion or pharmacologically induced stress. Imaging may also be **anatomical**, in which case it is used to look for radiographic evidence of coronary artery obstruction. The advantage of functional imaging is that it permits detection of physiologically relevant obstructions, in contrast to anatomic imaging (see Chapter 87).

Stress echocardiography

Stress echocardiography uses echocardiography to examine the heart after it has been stressed by a pharmacological agent (usually dobutamine). Abnormal features are stress-induced decreases in wall thickening, regional wall motion hypokinesia/akinesia/dyskinesia, or compensatory hyperkinesis. Obesity and lung disease degrade the quality of the echocardiographic windows and may render the test unusable, though ultrasound contrast agents may cirumvent this. Data shows that stress echocardiography is more accurate than the exercise ECG alone in detecting coronary disease, and about as accurate as myocardial perfusion scintigraphy.

Myocardial perfusion scintigraphy

Myocardial perfusion scintigraphy uses a radioactive tracer (thallium-201 or technetium-99) to determine myocardial perfusion at rest (defects may indicate previous infarction) and during stress (exertional or pharmacological), when inducible defects not present on the rest scan usually indicate myocardial ischaemia. Areas of inducible ischaemia represent areas at risk for future infarction, and their extent correlates to the prognostic benefit and hence need for revascularization. This test offers superior prognostic information, compared to exercise testing, and is also diagnostically useful where resting ECG abnormalities degrade exercise ECG interpretation. Patients with a negative myocardial perfusion scintigraphy result are at low risk for significant coronary artery disease events, although this result does not exclude coronary artery disease being present.

CT calcium scoring

This uses CT scanning to assess the degree of calcification of the coronary arteries (expressed as the Agatston score). A negative test (zero calcium) has a 96%–100% negative predictive value. The more calcium there is, the greater the chance of flow-limiting coronary disease; however, because of this probabilistic relationship, the test cannot positively diagnose coronary disease; it can only estimate the chance of coronary disease, and this is rarely sufficient in clinical practice.

CT coronary angiography

CT coronary angiography, where intravenous contrast is detected by CT imaging, is used to assess the patency of the coronary lumen. It requires a regular heart (so atrial fibrillation is an exclusion) and bradycardia (which is achieved with beta blockers, or ivabradine in patients with reversible airways disease); good luminal images are only obtained in those without extensive coronary calcification (so old age, renal failure, and diabetes are relative exclusions). It is likely to be useful in selected subgroups, although its exact role is still to be determined.

Coronary angiography

Currently, coronary angiography is the gold standard for diagnosing coronary artery disease. The test is invasive (a catheter is passed through the radial or femoral artery to the aortic root) and costly; risk and cost must be balanced against benefit. The risk is about a 1 in 1000 chance of a major adverse complication, including stroke, myocardial infarct, and death (higher in the elderly, diabetics, those with previous stroke, and those with extensive vascular disease). A significant stenosis is ≥70% obstruction of an epicardial coronary artery. All coronary disease carries an adverse prognosis, although in many the risk is surprisingly small and best approached medically. In the few with chronic stable angina with extensive disease (left main disease, disease in all three major epicardial coronary arteries, or disease in the proximal portion of the left anterior descending coronary artery), the prognosis is less good, and improved by early revascularization—for many, the main aim of angiography is to diagnose and treat such severe coronary disease.

Oesophago-endoscopy

Investigations aimed at identifying gastrointestinal causes of chest pain include oesophago-endoscopy. This test enables the direct visualization of inflammation, ulcers, strictures, and both benign and malignant lesions. It also allows tissue sampling for histology. A trial of a proton-pump inhibitor may constitute a diagnostic test for gastro-oesophageal reflux disease (GORD). Ambulatory oesophageal pH monitoring can aid in the diagnosis of GORD. In suspected dyspepsia with no alarm features suggesting malignancy, a positive serology for *Helicobacter pylori* may influence antimicrobial therapy.

Other diagnostic tests

Cardiac magnetic resonance imaging is increasingly used for the assessment of cardiac structure, tissue characterisation, prior infarction, as well as functional assessment during a stress MRI.

Introduction to therapy

Stable angina

Lifestyle advice, such as recommending that the patient attain an ideal weight and engage in high-intensity exercise programmes, together with dietary advice (e.g. consumption of oily fish, low amounts of animal fats, and modest amounts of alcohol) should be provided. Medical therapy is through the use of aspirin (or clopidogrel), lipid-lowering drugs (statins), and angiotensin-converting enzyme (ACE) inhibitors. Symptomatic relief is through the reduction of myocardial oxygen demands via beta blockers, and coronary vasodilatation with nitrates. In three-vessel or left main-stem disease, CABG is the preferred choice for revascularization. Patients with other discrete lesions may be treated with percutaneous coronary intervention if symptoms are refractory on maximum medical therapy.

Musculoskeletal pain

Musculoskeletal pain should be treated with reassurance and very occasionally analgesia.

Gastrointestinal pain

Gastrointestinal pain often responds to proton-pump inhibitors.

Prognosis

Prognosis depends on the diagnosis and extent of the problem. Patients with a negative myocardial perfusion scintigraphy, exercise ECG, stress MRI or stress cardiography result are at a lower risk of future cardiac events than those with a positive result. However, it must be noted that, as with many tests, the sensitivity and specificity of these tests is not 100%, and so an understanding of the probabilistic nature involved in their interpretation is important in determining the relevance of a test result for a particular patient. Where non-invasive investigations are performed but the results are equivocal, formal angiography should be considered to assess for coronary artery disease.

How to handle uncertainty in the diagnosis of this symptom

In this area, more than in most, uncertainly can and does occur, to the frustration of both the patient and clinician. Uncertainty can revolve around diagnosis, response to treatment, and prognosis. For diagnostic uncertainty, depending on the situation, always clarify in your own mind whether you think angina is present on the basis of the history, as this is the key to management. It is entirely permissible to diagnose non-cardiac chest pain, and still undertake coronary-directed tests to clarify cardiac prognosis. However, be clear with patients as to why you are doing tests, particularly if the tests are invasive, as confusion can easily arise and patients may subsequently not understand that, while they have coronary disease and chest pain, the two are not related, something you thought was the case from the outset. Inform patients when you think symptoms are non-cardiac but the investigations to date haven't ruled out severe coronary disease and you need to know more. Be very clear with patients that you believe that, even if you find coronary disease, it does not relate to symptoms. If you find coronary disease, but cannot decide clinically if it is relevant to symptoms, demonstrate myocardial ischaemia (e.g. via myocardial perfusion scintigraphy, fractional flow reserve—see Chapter 87) before proceeding to revascularization. In a very few patients, you may have to undertake revascularization to see if it helps their symptoms; again, be clear with patients that there is a significant possibility that symptoms are non-cardiac **before** revascularization so that, if revascularization fails to improve symptoms, your patients are not surprised. If patients do not respond to treatment, re-evaluate the history so that you are clear as to whether you have been barking up the wrong tree—are you treating angina with proton-pump inhibitors? Are you treating musculoskeletal chest pain with nitrates? The clue to treatment failure is usually in a thorough re-evaluation of the history; occasionally, you may have to introduce empiric therapy as a therapeutic trial, but be clear with patients that this is what you are doing. Cardiac prognosis is usually easy to estimate from the demographics, a knowledge of left ventricular function, and functional (e.g. exercise stress testing (see 'Key diagnostic tests')) or anatomic (e.g. coronary angiography) data. However, you should be very clear with patients that cardiac prognosis is a probabilistic issue, and this is the main difficulty that patients have in understanding outlook—they may have an extraordinary good prognosis, but still die tomorrow, or a terrible prognosis, but live 10 years—you must convey this probabilistic aspect. This comes down to good doctoring.

Further Reading

Chambers JB, Marks EM, and Hunter MS. The head says yes but the heart says no: what is non-cardiac chest pain and how is it managed? *Heart* 2015; 101: 1240–49. doi:10.1136/heartjnl-2014-306277.

Montalescot G, Sechtem U, Achenbach S et al. 2013 ESC guidelines on the management of stable coronary artery disease. *Eur Heart J* 2013; 34: 2949–3003.

National Institute for Health and Care Excellence. *NICE Guideline CG95: Chest Pain of Recent Onset: Assessment and Diagnosis.* 2010. Last updated: November 2016. Available at https://www.nice.org.uk/guidance/cg95 (accessed 8 Jan 2018).

11 Hypotension

Jonathan Timperley and Sandeep Hothi

Definition of symptoms

Hypotension is defined as a systolic arterial blood pressure of less than 90 mm Hg, or a diastolic arterial pressure of less than 60 mm Hg. Hypotension may lead to shock (the hallmark of which is clinical evidence of inadequate blood supply to critical organs), but does not inevitably do so.

Differential diagnosis

The causes of hypotension may be broadly divided by their pathophysiological mechanism and are shown in Table 11.1.

Context

There is substantial inter-individual variability in mean arterial blood pressure and the range of tolerated blood pressures. Thus, while hypotension has multiple possible causes, its effects will depend on the rapidity of onset, the absolute blood pressure, and the difference between the patient's usual blood pressure and its current level. Bearing this in mind, mild hypotension may be observed in the outpatient setting due to drug therapy and not warrant hospital admission. At the other extreme, hypotension may result in organ hypoperfusion and failure, causing critical illness.

Approach to diagnosis

The first issue is to decide whether the person with hypotension is stable and can be investigated and managed slowly, or unstable with signs of organ hypoperfusion ('shock'). For the latter, the diagnostic approach is made simultaneously with management; the priority is to support the circulatory system and affected organs while the diagnosis is established. Diagnostic features are elicited from the history, examination, and investigations, while circulatory and organ support are provided as needed. Assessment typically follows an ABCDE approach, which often identifies life-threatening causes requiring immediate treatment (e.g. tension pneumothorax) and, if not, will usually give strategic direction to further investigation and therapy.

In any acute illness, the presence of hypotension is a poor prognostic sign, and as such, is a feature of many early warning scores. If hypotension induces organ hypoperfusion, then the condition of shock exists. Organ hypoperfusion results in abnormal organ function, as follows:

Cerebral hypoperfusion: anxiety, aggressiveness, altered mental state, altered level of consciousness
Renal hypoperfusion: reduced urine output, acute kidney injury

Cardiac hypoperfusion: may result in myocardial ischaemia if there is preexisting coronary disease
Liver hypoperfusion: ischaemic hepatitis
Skin hypoperfusion: pallor, poor capillary return; sweating is a marker of sympathetic activation and often occurs in hypovolaemic or cardiac causes of shock

As shock can rapidly progress to irreversible organ failure and death, it is critically important to treat immediately according to the most likely cause. Diagnostic testing should be done if this does not delay treatment (e.g. echocardiography, if it can be performed immediately at the bedside) but, if waiting for diagnostic tests will lead to an unacceptably delay (e.g. in situations occurring in the middle of the night), you may have to treat 'blindly' if you feel the patient is deteriorating rapidly and time does not allow your preferred investigation to be performed. This means that treating shock, while distressing for patients, who are critically unwell and may die, and their relatives, can also be very stressful for clinicians, as your level of diagnostic certainty is often much lower than usual, magnifying your anxiety.

Specific clues to the diagnosis

In the stable patient, run through the usual diagnostic possibilities; however, many cases relate to an interaction between age, drugs, and possibly autonomic failure. Elicit whether the hypotension relates to posture, for example, occurs when the patient is standing upright (orthostatic hypotension), or after the patient has been standing still for a prolonged period of time (e.g. neurocardiogenic syncope). Always establish the drug history. Ask about recent weight loss (as this often leads to lowered blood pressure)—and, if present, determine the reason for the weight loss. Determine whether conditions giving rise to autonomic neuropathy are present (e.g. age, diabetes, neurodegenerative conditions).

In the acute setting, the history often provides the best clues as to cause and indicates whether this is likely to be sepsis (fever; pain in appropriate organs; travel history; etc.), hypovolaemia (often obvious blood or excess fluid coming from an orifice), or cardiac (e.g. known cardiac disease, or major risk factors for ischaemic heart disease/pulmonary embolism).

Examination of those in shock

Those in shock have a reflex sinus tachycardia; determine if the heart rate is proportionate to the clinical state, and, if not, consider whether tachy- or bradyarrhythmias are contributing. Sustained ventricular tachycardia is a not uncommon cause of shock; atrial fibrillation rarely causes shock unless the heart rate is very high (>220, as in pre-excited atrial fibrillation in Wolff–Parkinson–White syndrome), or severe left ventricular dysfunction is present. Look for evidence of valvar heart disease in the pulse—slow rising (aortic stenosis) or collapsing (aortic regurgitation). A raised jugular venous pressure may indicate heart failure, but can indicate pericardial tamponade, pulmonary embolism, and, rarely, pneumothorax (although here the signs are dominated by gross respiratory distress). The apex beat, if displaced, gives information about the chronicity of heart failure (it takes time for the heart to enlarge). For those with keen ears, a third or fourth heart sound may be heard in those with left ventricular dysfunction. A pericardial rub is rarely heard in tamponade; bibasal crepitations often indicate heart failure, although they sometimes indicate bronchopneumonia (bronchial breathing is a more reliable guide to lobar pneumonia), reduced air entry (in asthma or COPD), or pulmonary oedema. In severe pulmonary oedema, it may be impossible to hear the heart sounds because of the loud chest sounds. Cardiac

Table 11.1 Causes of hypotension		
Hypovolaemia	**Cardiac pump failure**	**Vasodilatation**
Haemorrhage	Extrinsic (obstruction to inflow/outflow)	Sepsis
Intra-abdominal pooling	Tension pneumothorax	Anaphylaxis
Fluid loss (from kidney, gut, and skin)	Cardiac tamponade	Drug-induced
	Pulmonary embolism	Adrenal insufficiency
	Intrinsic	Autonomic failure
	Ischaemic heart disease	
	Cardiomyopathy	
	Valve disease	
	Arrhythmia	

murmurs may be present and reflect valvar heart disease underlying shock (e.g. critical aortic stenosis, severe mitral regurgitation).

Specific clues to diagnosis

Myocardial ischaemia/infarction

There may be known angina or heart failure. Ischaemic chest pain is often (not always) present (retrosternal heavy chest pain); this must be differentiated from the pain of pleurisy (respiration-dependent breathing, lateralized), which may indicate a pulmonary embolus or pleural involvement in a pneumonic process (do not forget empyema in this situation). Examining those with shock due to ischaemic heart disease often reveals a cool patient with high heart rate, low blood pressure, weak (low volume) pulse, raised jugular venous pressure, quiet heart sounds, and bibasal crackles. The main clue to the diagnosis is provided by the ECG (myocardial ischaemia sufficient to cause shock is almost always manifest as gross ECG changes, although left bundle branch block can, of course, obscure them). Echocardiography, where available, is diagnostic.

Pulmonary embolism

There may be shortness of breath, pleuritic chest pain (may be absent), swollen tender calf, or risk factors for thromboembolism. The chest examination may be normal. The main clue is in the risk factors for venous thromboembolism (cancer, recent surgery, etc.), and the finding of a cool patient with high heart rate, marked tachypnoea, low blood pressure, sometimes a raised jugular venous pressure, hypoxaemia, but otherwise normal cardiorespiratory exam, a clear chest X-ray, and an ECG normal, aside from sinus tachycardia (sometimes atrial fibrillation).

Tension pneumothorax

Look for sudden onset pleuritic chest pain and breathlessness, chest trauma, mechanical ventilation, and deviated trachea, with absent breath sounds on the affected side.

Hypovolaemia

Look for loss of skin turgor, dry mucous membranes, and prolonged capillary refill time with cool peripheries. Postural hypotension (sit the patient forwards in their bed) may be marked. Signs of the underlying cause may be present, as follows:

Ruptured abdominal aortic aneurysm: This is indicated by abdominal tenderness with a pulsatile, central mass and bruising in the flanks. There may be loss of peripheral pulses with aortic dissection

Gastrointestinal bleed: There may be a history of haematemesis, maleana, rectal bleeding, abdominal pain, and use of NSAIDs, steroids, or anticoagulants. Signs of anaemia on physical examination may be present. It is important to perform a rectal examination in suspected **gastrointestinal** bleeds, looking for melaena.

Dehydration: There may be a history of diarrhoea, vomiting, burns, or heat exhaustion. Often, however, the affected patients are elderly, and dehydration has crept up on them; the shock relates to this along with sepsis.

Sepsis

In septic shock, there is hypotension with vasodilation and warm peripheries. If shock is untreated and progresses, the peripheries may become cold as myocardial depression sets in. There may be features of the underlying infection.

Anaphylaxis

Anaphylaxis is characterized by shortness of breath, an urticarial rash, wheezing, and swelling of the tongue and lips. There may have been a clear trigger and a previous history of anaphylaxis and allergy. An allergy alert tag may be present.

Adrenal insufficiency

Adrenal insufficiency presents in a myriad of ways. Symptoms include fatigue, weight loss, nausea, vomiting, and postural hypotension. There may be increased pigmentation of the palmar creases, lips, scars, and mucous membranes. A history of long-term steroid use with sudden cessation may also be suggestive. Addisonian crisis is

severe adrenal insufficiency with profound hypotension or coma. However, no diagnostically useful signs may be present. **This means that, in all cases of undiagnosed shock, it is reasonable to give replacement steroids in case this is the first presentation of undiagnosed adrenal failure.**

Neurological clues

Recent spinal surgery suggests spinal shock. There may be a history of diabetes mellitus (autonomic neuropathy) or Parkinsonian features (multiple system atrophy).

Drug history

A full history of prescribed and non-prescribed medications and drugs must be elicited, along with the actual doses taken.

Key diagnostic tests

ECG

An ECG is a critically useful test in shock. It may indicate:

Arrhythmia: You must always ask yourself whether any arrhythmia is sufficient to cause shock, as arrhythmias can complicate many causes of shock (e.g., atrial fibrillation is common in cardiogenic shock, regardless of the cause, and also in pulmonary embolism). A tachycardia is a common physiological response in most cases of hypotension.

Myocardial ischaemia or infarction: If infarction is the cause, then usually the ST/T changes are gross. If the changes are subtle, you must decide whether myocardial ischaemia is genuinely causative, or a bystander.

Other features may be present with other causes. For instance, if gross left ventricular hypertrophy is present, you should urgently consider whether aortic stenosis is the cause. In pulmonary embolism, there may be evidence of right heart strain (right axis deviation, right bundle branch block, or anterior T-wave inversion), although, more commonly, the ECG only shows sinus tachycardia. With cardiac tamponade there may be low amplitude QRS voltages and sinus tachycardia.

Full blood count

Check for anaemia secondary to bleeding causing hypotension. With acute blood loss, the mean corpuscular volume will remain unchanged, while chronic blood loss causes iron-deficiency anaemia with microcytosis.

Partial thromboplastin time/activated partial thromboplastin time

In hypotension due to bleeding, the coagulation must be checked by using the partial thromboplastin time or the activated partial thromboplastin time test. Where these are abnormal, the fibrinogen level should also be checked.

Urea and electrolytes

Hypotension of any aetiology can cause prerenal failure. Hyponatraemia and hyperkalaemia, in the setting of hypotension, can be suggestive of adrenal insufficiency.

C-reactive protein level and white blood cell count

The C-reactive protein level and white blood cell count is often, but not always, elevated in sepsis. In severe rampant sepsis, these tests may initially be normal, only becoming rather dramatically abnormal hours or indeed days later, way beyond the time they would have been of diagnostic use. The central message is that, if you suspect sepsis, take blood cultures, give broad-spectrum antibiotics immediately, and do not be put off by finding initially normal inflammatory markers.

Chest X-ray

This may show the cause of shock (e.g. pneumothorax), be highly suggestive (the globular heart of pericardial effusion is very characteristic), or may offer pointers, such as findings of cardiac failure (e.g. pulmonary oedema, cardiomegaly, Kerley B lines, upper lobe diversion, or pleural effusions, all of which would strongly suggest that cardiac disease underlies the shock). Hypotension due to chest sepsis may show consolidation and possibly a parapneumonic effusion. The chest radiograph may be normal with pulmonary embolism; very rarely, it reveals a reduction of vascular markings, a wedge-shaped infarction, or a small effusion.

Echocardiogram

This is perhaps the single most useful test in patients with shock of uncertain aetiology—while not always diagnostic, it can substantially increase (left ventricular dysfunction/valvar lesion, pericardial effusion) or lessen the chance of shock being cardiac in origin (vigorous left ventricular function without pericardial fluid greatly lessens the chance of cardiac shock—it does not remove it though; e.g. severe acute mitral regurgitation can present with shock and transthoracic echo appearances which are virtually normal), and it often offers clues to the presence of pulmonary embolus (right ventricular dilatation/dysfunction). It informs about right heart pressures (from inferior vena cava calibre and its change with respiration), which gives information about volume status. Table 11.2 shows typical echocardiographic findings in hypotension of different aetiologies.

Other diagnostic tests

Abdominal ultrasound

An abdominal ultrasound can reveal dilatation and rupture of the abdominal aorta, as well as free fluid in the abdomen. If a ruptured abdominal aortic aneurysm is seriously suspected, or if there is severe abdominal pain without a diagnosis, immediate CT is the investigation of choice, with the emphasis being on immediate.

Troponin T or I

Troponin T or I is elevated with myocardial necrosis (but also in pulmonary embolism, arrhythmias, and renal failure). Only rarely does the immediate troponin provide a categorical diagnosis; often, it provides pointers. However, most patients with shock have rapidly deteriorating renal function and widespread organ hypoperfusion (including of the heart), both of which may give rise to very non-specific, but large rises in troponin. Do not rely on troponin to establish the cause of shock.

D-dimers

D-dimer levels are elevated with thrombus, infection, pregnancy and malignancy; they are also elevated post-operatively and with an inflammatory response. A negative test is reassuring in patients with a low or moderate pretest probability of pulmonary embolism. Again, this test is rarely helpful in shock, as many sick patients, from whatever cause, have large rises in D-dimers. If a pulmonary embolus is seriously suspected, do the most immediately available test, a CT pulmonary angiogram if possible. If the patient is too sick, do a transthoracic cardiac ultrasound instead. Treat until you can establish the diagnosis, with thrombolytics, if necessary.

Adrenocorticotropic hormone stimulation test

Plasma cortisol is measured before and after injection of a synthetic form of adrenocorticotropic hormone to assess for an appropriate release of cortisol by the adrenal glands. This test is of no use in the acute situation. If there is any possibility that hypoadrenalism underlies shock, immediately take a blood sample for cortisol and give intravenous hydrocortisone, continued until either an alternative diagnosis emerges or the patient is stable. Once the patient is stable, usually a few days later, perform a short synacthen test.

Introduction to therapy

There is a difference in the speed of investigation and treatment, depending on the clinical settings (e.g. an elderly patient with postural hypotension and mild symptoms on multiple blood-pressure-lowering agents, vs a patient with post-operative septic shock in secondary care).

In otherwise stable patients in primary care, treatment of the underlying cause is initiated. Thus, in the case of drug-induced hypotension, the offending drug dose may be stopped, reduced in dose, or changed to alternative treatment.

In treating shock, the aim is to maintain adequate tissue perfusion. A rapid assessment of the patient is required with assessment and securing of the airway, assessment of adequacy of breathing, and also of integrity of the circulatory system (the ABC approach; see 'Further Reading'). Oxygen is administered where required. A straight leg raise will help redistribute circulatory volume in hypovolaemia. Intravenous access is obtained and blood taken for analysis and group and save, or crossmatching. Intravenous fluid resuscitation is performed to restore circulatory fluid volume and central venous pressure (unless the patient is in cardiogenic shock). Monitoring should be instituted to include continuous ECG monitoring, urine output, pulse rate, blood pressure, respiratory rate, and pulse oximetry; this usually mandates that a patient, at a minimum, should be on a high-dependency ward, although transfer to an intensive care unit may be necessary. Urine output is a sensitive indicator of cardiac output and will aid management of fluid balance. In some cases, central venous pressure and invasive arterial pressure monitoring are required. The main stay of therapy in most cases of shock, except cardiogenic shock, is fluid replacement. This can be performed with by initially giving a rapid 250–500 ml fluid challenge of colloid or crystalloid fluid. If blood loss is the presumed cause, then blood should be used (the order of preference is crossmatched blood, type-specific blood, O-negative blood). Where there is coagulopathy and haemorrhage, the coagulopathy should be appropriately corrected.

In patients with cardiogenic shock, the heart cannot produce a blood pressure sufficient to maintain adequate tissue perfusion. Usually, there is an increased left atrial pressure and pulmonary oedema. Fluids given here will exacerbate the situation (except for

Table 11.2 Echocardiographic findings in hypotension					
	IVC	**LV size**	**LV contraction**	**RV size**	**RV contraction**
Hypovolaemia	Flat	Small	Increased	Small	Increased
Sepsis	Flat	Normal or large	Normal or reduced	Normal or large	Normal or reduced
LV dysfunction due to ischaemia	Normal or dilated	Large	Reduced regionally or globally	Normal	Normal (unless associated RV infarction)
Acute major pulmonary embolism	Dilated	Normal or small	Normal or increased	Large	Reduced
Cardiac tamponade	Dilated	Normal	Normal or increased	Normal	Diastolic free wall collapse
RV infarction	Dilated	Normal or large if associated LV inferior MI	Normal or reduced if associated inferior MI	Large	Reduced

Abbreviations: IVC, inferior vena cava; LV, left ventricular; MI, myocardial infarction; RV, right ventricular.

Adapted from Chambers and Sprigings. *Acute Medicine: A practical guide to the management of medical emergencies*, 4th edition, Chapter 9, p57, Wiley-Blackwell, Oxford, UK, Copyright © 2007.

those rare patients with predominant right ventricular infarction usually complicating an inferior infarct, as they do benefit from fluids). Instead, immediate treatment is with IV diuretics, opiates (also beneficial for myocardial infarction pain). The use of inotropes is controversial; they may have a place where there is reversible pathology or as a bridge to definitive treatment. There is no evidence that they improve outcome. Mechanical circulatory support (intra-aortic counterpulsation balloon pumping, left ventricular assist devices) has a role in highly selected patients with reversible pathology. In those with acute myocardial infarction, immediate percutaneous coronary intervention has an important role, improving the dreadful outcome, although the prognosis of cardiogenic shock remains poor, despite all therapies. Patients considered to have a reasonable outcome may also require ventilatory support.

In patients with anaphylaxis and hypotension, immediate intramuscular (IM) adrenaline is given, the legs elevated, hydrocortisone IV or IM, and chlorphenamine 10 mg IV or IM. The causal antigen should be removed, where possible, and intravenous fluids given. Nebulized bronchodilators are used if bronchospasm is present. Adrenaline IM can be repeated every 5 minutes, if required. Where the airway is threatened, formal intubation and ventilation may be required with rapid assistance from an anaesthetist and critical care; an ENT surgeon should be present to assist, if required.

In septic shock, a septic screen should be sent (blood, urine, and wound cultures, inflammatory markers, full blood count, and biochemical screen, and usually blood gases, for pH, lactate, and pO_2 and pCO_2 levels), IV resuscitation should be initiated, and broad-spectrum antibiotics should be given promptly. Vasoconstrictor agents (e.g. noradrenaline or adrenaline) should be used when appropriate.

Prognosis

The mortality is variable depending on the cause. Approximate figures of mortality for the major types of shock are 60% in cardiogenic shock, 70% in ruptured aortic aneurysm, 30% in septic shock, and <1% in anaphylaxis. When hypotension is secondary to hypovolaemia, once this is corrected, the mortality is dependent on the underlying cause.

How to handle uncertainty

In the acute setting, the clinical presentation should provide clues to differentiate between cardiogenic shock and other types of shock. Echocardiography is a critically useful investigation, where available, if the diagnosis is unclear, and helps differentiate between acute severe pulmonary embolism, cardiogenic shock, valvular heart disease, and hypovolaemia. In non-cardiogenic shock, initial fluid resuscitation may be performed while the cause is being determined.

Further Reading

Francis GS, Bartos JA, and Adatya S. Inotropes. *J Am Coll Cardiol* 2014; 63: 2069–78.

Lancellotti P, Price S, Edvardsen T, et al. The use of echocardiography in acute cardiovascular care: Recommendations of the European Association of Cardiovascular Imaging and the Acute Cardiovascular Care Association. *Eur Heart J Cardiovasc Imaging*. 2015; 16: 119–46. http://ehjcimaging.oxfordjournals.org/content/ejechocard/16/2/119.full.pdf

Mackenzie DC and Noble VE. Assessing volume status and fluid responsiveness in the emergency department. *Clin Exp Emerg Med* 2014; 1: 67–77. http://dx.doi.org/10.15441/ceem.14.040

Singer M, Deutschman CS, Seymour CW, et al. The Third International Consensus definitions for sepsis and septic shock (Sepsis-3). *JAMA* 2016; 315: 801–10.

Task force of the European Society of Intensive Care Medicine. Consensus on circulatory shock and hemodynamic monitoring. *Intensive Care Med* 2014; 40: 1795–1815. doi: 10.1007/s00134-014-3525-z

12 Acute breathlessness

Jonathan Timperley and Sandeep Hothi

Definition of the symptom

Acute breathlessness or dyspnoea is the new onset of an unpleasant awareness of breathing, at rest or at a level of exercise, which did not previously cause symptoms. It is often associated with other symptoms—including wheeze, cough, chest pain, and palpitation—which, together with the patient's comorbidities, help shape the differential diagnosis.

Differential diagnosis

The differential diagnosis of acute dyspnoea may be organized by system; some common causes are given in Table 12.1.

Context

Acute breathlessness is a frequent reason for presentation to the emergency department, and a common problem complicating the hospital course of inpatients. Decompensated heart failure, exacerbations of asthma or COPD, pneumonia, and pulmonary embolism account for 80% of diagnoses. In older patients, acute breathlessness often results from multiple interrelated pathologies (e.g. pneumonia on a background of COPD, triggering acute atrial fibrillation).

Approach to diagnosis

Acute breathlessness may herald diseases which can lead to death in minutes or hours. It is therefore crucial to assess if the patient is critically ill using simple physiological variables, such as blood pressure, heart rate, respiratory rate, arterial oxygen saturation, and conscious level, as described in detail in Chapter 149. If these observations indicate critical illness, the approach to the diagnosis and management should follow the methods outlined in Chapter 149.

If the patient is not critically ill and there are no immediate threats to life, then a focused history should be taken (see Box 12.1), followed

Table 12.1 Differential diagnosis of acute breathlessness

System	Structures	Examples of disease	Chapter reference
Respiratory	Upper and lower airways, lung parenchyma and pleura	Acute epiglottitis	Chapter 128
		Angioedema	Chapter 299
		Anaphylaxis	Chapter 75
		Asthma	Chapter 133
		Aspiration pneumonitis	Chapter 129
		Chronic obstructive pulmonary disease (COPD) exacerbation	Chapter 134
		Large airway obstruction: foreign body, tumour, blood	Chapter 17
		Pneumonia	Chapter 129
		Non-cardiogenic pulmonary oedema (adult respiratory distress syndrome)	Chapter 139
		Pleural effusion	Chapter 143
		Pneumothorax	Chapter 131
		Vocal cord dysfunction	Chapter 17
Cardiac	Heart and pericardium	Decompensated chronic heart failure	Chapter 92
		Acute heart failure: • acute coronary syndrome with extensive left ventricular ischaemia or infarction • acute severe mitral or aortic regurgitation (e.g. due to infective endocarditis) • acute myocarditis • stress cardiomyopathy	Chapter 91
		Cardiac tamponade	Chapter 107
Pulmonary circulation	Pulmonary arteries and arterioles	Pulmonary embolism (of thrombus, fat, or amniotic fluid)	Chapter 101
Chest wall and diaphragm	Structural and neuromuscular disorders	Diaphragmatic paralysis	Chapter 129
		Flail chest	Chapter 143
		Stroke	Chapter 227
		Guillain–Barré syndrome	Chapter 47
		Myasthenia gravis	Chapter 44
		Myopathies and muscular dystrophies	Chapter 235
		Tetanus	Chapter 307
Blood	Red cell mass	Acute severe blood loss	Chapter 38
Toxic/metabolic		Sepsis	Chapter 309
		Diabetic ketoacidosis	Chapter 184
		Poisoning: salicylate, ethylene glycol, methanol	Chapter 339
		Advanced renal failure	Chapter 162
Other causes		Psychogenic factors	Chapter 241

Box 12.1 Focused history taking in acute breathlessness

- context and time-course of breathlessness
- associated symptoms: wheeze, cough, chest pain, palpitation, orthopnoea (seen in heart failure, diaphragmatic paralysis, ascites, morbid obesity)
- usual effort tolerance and recent change (e.g. distance walked on the flat, number of stairs climbed without stopping, ability to manage activities of daily living unaided; see MRC dyspnoea scale)
- known cardiorespiratory disease
- previous acute exacerbations of chronic obstructive pulmonary disease (COPD) or asthma requiring hospital admission/ non-invasive ventilation/mechanical ventilation
- requirement for home-nebulized bronchodilator and/or long-term oxygen therapy
- previous diagnosis of heart failure, coronary artery disease, myocardial, or valve disease
- risk factors for venous thromboembolism
- other major comorbidities
- current medications
- smoking history
- occupational/environmental exposure to smoke, fumes, toxins/ animals, or birds
- travel history

Table 12.2 The DECAF Score

Variable	Score
Dyspnoea eMRCD 5a eMRCD 5b	 1 2
Eosinopenia (<0.05 × 10⁹/l)	1
Consolidation	1
Acidaemia (pH <7.3)	1
Atrial fibrillation	1
Total DECAF Score	6

Abbreviations: DECAF, dyspnoea, eosinopenia, consolidation, acidaemia, and atrial fibrillation; eMRCD, extended MRC dyspnoea scale.

Note: The extended MRC dyspnoea scale dichotomizes Stage 5 according to whether the patient can wash and dress independently (5a) or not (5b).

Reproduced from *Thorax*, John Steer, John Gibson, Stephen C Bourke, The DECAF score: predicting hospital mortality in exacerbations of chronic obstructive pulmonary disease, volume 67, pp.970-6, copyright © 2012 with permission from BMJ Publishing Group Ltd.

by clinical examination and appropriate investigations. Nonetheless, it may be appropriate to initiate some treatment and investigations simultaneously with the history and examination. High-flow oxygen may be given by mask. Further oxygen therapy should be administered in accordance with British Thoracic Society guidelines. It should be remembered that, although many acutely dyspnoeic patients are hypoxic, hypoxia per se does not correlate with dyspnoea. Patients may remain breathless despite correction of hypoxia. If there is wheeze, or a history of asthma/COPD, peak flow should be measured and compared to the patient's predicted or known normal reading, and a beta-2 agonist given by oxygen-driven nebulizer. If not already done, the patient should be attached to a pulse oximeter to measure

arterial oxygen saturation, ECG and blood pressure monitors, and IV access obtained. Arterial blood gases, pH, and lactate should be measured, and 12-lead ECG and chest radiography performed.

Key diagnostic tests

All patients with acute breathlessness should have a chest radiograph, 12-lead ECG, and measurement of arterial blood gases, including lactate concentration. A full blood count and biochemical profile (including glucose) should be measured. If sepsis is suspected, blood culture should be taken and C-reactive protein or procalcitonin levels measured. Additional culture samples should be taken according to the suspected diagnosis and clinical findings.

The **chest radiograph (CXR)** establishes if the patient has pleural disease (effusion or pneumothorax) or pulmonary parenchymal disease, which may be focal or diffuse. Marked enlargement of the cardiac silhouette may reflect pericardial effusion or advanced valve/myocardial disease. Acute breathlessness with a clear CXR is seen in upper and lower airways disease, pulmonary embolism, sepsis, and metabolic acidosis.

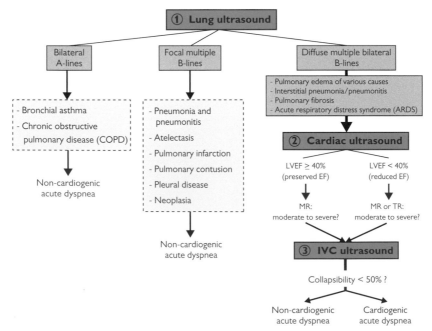

Figure 12.1 Algorithm for the diagnosis of acute dyspnoea based on lung–cardiac–inferior cava-integrated ultrasound; LVEF, left ventricular ejection fraction; MR, mitral regurgitation; TR, tricuspid regurgitation; IVC, inferior vena cava.

Kajimoto K, et al. Rapid evaluation by lung-cardiac-inferior vena cava (LCI) integrated ultrasound for differentiating heart failure from pulmonary disease as the cause of acute dyspnea in the emergency setting. *Cardiovascular Ultrasound* Volume 10, Issue 49 Copyright © Kajimoto et al.; licensee BioMed Central Ltd. 2012.

Table 12.3 DECAF Score and inhospital mortality

DECAF Score	n	Inhospital mortality, %	Sensitivity*	Specificity*	30-day mortality, %
0	201	0.5	1	0	1.5
1	291	2.1	0.99	0.24	3.8
2	226	8.4	0.93	0.59	11.9
3	125	24	0.73	0.84	27.2
4	57	45.6	0.42	0.96	45.6
5	20	70	0.15	0.99	70
6	0	NA	NA	NA	NA

*For inhospital mortality: positive test result = score ≥ corresponding DECAF score; DECAF 0–1 = low risk; 2 = intermediate risk; ≥3 = high risk.

Abbreviations: DECAF, dyspnoea, eosinopenia, consolidation, acidaemia, and atrial fibrillation.

Reproduced from *Thorax*, John Steer, John Gibson, Stephen C Bourke, The DECAF score: predicting hospital mortality in exacerbations of chronic obstructive pulmonary disease, volume 67, pp.970-6, copyright © 2012 with permission from BMJ Publishing Group Ltd.

The **12-lead ECG** may reveal signs of acute myocardial ischaemia or infarction (ST depression or elevation, new left bundle branch block), or evidence of structural heart disease. Sinus tachycardia is the most common ECG abnormality associated with pulmonary embolism; features of right heart strain (right axis deviation, new right bundle branch block, anterior T-wave inversion) may not be present despite major embolism. The ECG may also demonstrate arrhythmia, acute atrial fibrillation being the most commonly encountered.

The **arterial blood gases and pH** establish if the patient has type 1 or type 2 respiratory failure, and also characterize the acid–base status, which carries diagnostic and prognostic information. Please see chapters 135 and 149 for further information on the assessment and management of respiratory failure.

Other diagnostic tests

Ultrasonography of the lungs, heart, and inferior vena cava

Ultrasonography of the lungs, heart, and inferior vena cava can identify pleural and pulmonary parenchymal disease, exclude cardiac tamponade, and provide evidence for or against a diagnosis of heart failure or acute major pulmonary embolism (see Figure 12.1). Pocket-sized ultrasound devices (e.g. Vscan, GE Healthcare) are now available which allow a screening ultrasound examination to be done in a few minutes, as part of the clinical assessment.

Plasma brain natriuretic peptide

Plasma brain natriuretic peptide (BNP) is an important test in the diagnosis of chronic heart failure, but is less helpful in the patient with acute breathlessness. A raised plasma BNP level by itself cannot discriminate between acute, acute-on-chronic, or chronic heart failure, or between left or right ventricular dysfunction. Cor pulmonale and right ventricular dysfunction from acute pulmonary embolism are both causes of a raised BNP, with plasma levels in cor pulmonale typically in the range of 100–500 pg/ml. A patient with chronic heart failure may be acutely breathless because of acute non-cardiac (rather than cardiac) disease. Accepting these limitations, measurement of plasma BNP is a useful

screening test in the patient acute breathlessness, levels <100 and >500 pg/ml having high negative and positive predictive values for heart failure.

Plasma D-dimer

Plasma D-dimer is a degradation product of cross-linked fibrin and gives a measure of endogenous fibrinolysis. A normal level of plasma D-dimer excludes pulmonary embolism in patients in whom the clinical probability is low to moderate. A raised level is seen in a wide range of conditions including sepsis and aortic dissection, and is therefore not diagnostic of venous thromboembolism.

Plasma cardiac troponin I or T levels

Plasma cardiac troponin I or T levels are often measured to exclude acute coronary syndrome as the cause of acute breathlessness. However, troponin release may also occur in pulmonary embolism, myocarditis, stress cardiomyopathy, supraventricular arrhythmias, and sepsis, amongst others conditions, and the plasma troponin level therefore must be interpreted in the light of clinical, ECG, and echocardiographic features.

CT of the chest

CT of the chest will often be diagnostic in acute breathlessness, and has a greater yield than plain radiography. However, the need to lie flat for the scan may not be possible for some patients, and this should be considered when requesting CT, particularly if the same information can be obtained from other modalities performed at the bedside, such as chest ultrasonography or echocardiography.

Further investigation will be guided by the differential diagnosis.

Introduction to therapy

Supportive therapy for the critically ill patient is discussed in Chapter 149. Specific therapy is directed by the working diagnosis.

Prognosis

This depends on the diagnosis, its severity, the patient's comorbidities, and initiation of prompt appropriate therapy. Prognostic scores have

Table 12.4 Prognostic factors for calculating the acute heart failure index

Demographics	Past medical history	Vital signs	Laboratory	ECG	Radiography
Gender	• Coronary artery disease* • Angina • PCI • Diabetes • Lung disease	• Pulse • Systolic blood pressure • Respiratory rate • Temperature	• Blood urea nitrogen • Sodium • Potassium • Creatinine • Glucose • White blood cell count • Arterial pH	• Acute myocardial infarction† • Myocardial ischaemia†	• Pulmonary congestion • Pleural effusion

* As determined by self-report, or if medical records were available, review of the patient's records.

† ECG interpretations were made by the emergency medicine attending physician.

Abbreviations: PCI, percutaneous coronary intervention.

Reproduced from *Emergency Medicine Journal*, James Hsiao, Michelle Motta, Peter Wyer, Validating the acute heart failure index for patients presenting to the emergency department with decompensated heart failure, volume 29, copyright © 2012 with permission from BMJ Publishing Group Ltd.

been developed for an acute exacerbation of COPD (DECAF score; see Tables 12.2 and 12.3), acute heart failure (acute heart failure index; prognostic variables shown in Table 12.4), community-acquired pneumonia (CURB-65 (http://www.mdcalc.com/curb-65-severity-score-community-acquired-pneumonia/)), and pulmonary embolism (Pulmonary Embolism Severity Index (http://www.mdcalc.com/pulmonary-embolism-severity-index-pesi/)).

Further Reading

Francis GS, Felker GM, and Tang WHW. A test in context: Critical evaluation of natriuretic peptide testing in heart failure. *J Am Coll Cardiol* 2016; 67: 330–37.

Lancellotti P, Price S, Edvardsen T, et al. The use of echocardiography in acute cardiovascular care: Recommendations of the European Association of Cardiovascular Imaging and the Acute Cardiovascular Care Association. *Eur Heart J Cardiovasc Imaging* 2015; 16: 119–46.

National Institute for Health and Care Excellence. *Nice Guidelines (CG 187) 2014: Acute Heart Failure: Diagnosing and Managing Acute Heart Failure in Adults.* 2014. Available at https://www.nice.org.uk/guidance/cg187 (accessed 02 March 2017).

13 Chronic breathlessness

David Sprigings, Andrew Jeffrey, Phil Barber, and Nigel Clayton

Definition

The act and sensation of breathing are at the interface between the conscious and the subconscious mind; breathing is an unconscious process, but one which enters consciousness in healthy people in some circumstances, notably during and after exercise. Chronic breathlessness (dyspnoea) can be defined as an unpleasant awareness of breathing at a level of exercise which would not cause symptoms in a healthy person of the same age (or which did not previously cause symptoms), persisting for more than 1 month. It can be graded according to the Medical Research Council dyspnoea scale (Table 13.1). Breathlessness may be accompanied by other symptoms such as chest tightness, cough, or wheeze, which, together with the patient's comorbidities and risk factors for specific diseases, help shape the differential diagnosis.

Differential diagnosis

The differential diagnosis, organized by system, is given in Table 13.2.

Context

Chronic breathlessness is highly prevalent—a survey of people aged 70 and over living at home in a South Wales town found that almost one-third had breathlessness of MRC grades 3–5—and one of the commonest presenting symptoms in primary and secondary care. It usually reflects cardiopulmonary disease, but a broad range of disorders, from anaemia to neuromuscular disease, needs to be considered (Table 13.2). More than one disorder is present in around 20% of patients (e.g. the combination of COPD and heart failure). In addition, obesity and physical deconditioning are often contributory factors, and may be the sole cause of exertional breathlessness. Anxiety states may cause breathlessness and other somatic symptoms, but psychogenic breathlessness is a diagnosis of exclusion and may, of course, coexist with organic disease. Breathlessness is also a major symptom in the terminal phase of many cardiorespiratory diseases.

Approach to diagnosis

Asthma, COPD, heart failure, and interstitial lung disease (ILD) are the final diagnoses in around 80% of patients presenting with chronic breathlessness. One approach is therefore to consider these four diagnoses, together with an additional category of 'Something else', in all patients. Initial probabilities of these disorders, based on age, sex, and risk factor profile, are then adjusted up or down in the light of further information derived from the history and examination, to yield a judgement as to whether each diagnostic category is probable, possible, or unlikely. These assessments are further revised when the results of screening investigations are known. As an example, Table 13.3 summarizes the information relevant to the probabilities of asthma and COPD in a patient with chronic breathlessness associated with wheeze.

Specific clues to the diagnosis

There is considerable overlap between clinical features of the many diseases which can cause chronic breathlessness, and the symptom may reflect the cumulative effect of more than one disease. Consequently, clinical diagnosis should be regarded as provisional, with its aim being to establish a differential diagnosis which can be tested and refined by investigation.

Important clues to the diagnosis are the mode of onset of breathlessness; its duration, pattern, and periodicity; precipitating or aggravating factors; and accompanying symptoms. Breathlessness of psychogenic origin tends to be 'patternless', occurring unpredictably and often at rest. Breathlessness of organic origin is more predictable, and the pattern clinically coherent, often closely and reliably linked to exertion but sometimes variable or episodic, especially in asthma. Orthopnoea (breathlessness in the recumbent position) and nocturnal dyspnoea are characteristic of heart failure (although their absence does not exclude the diagnosis) but are also common in COPD. Orthopnoea is also found in diaphragmatic paralysis, severe ascites, and morbid obesity.

Other relevant aspects of the history in suspected cardiac, respiratory, or neuromuscular disease are covered in detail in Chapters 87, 126, and 220. The psychological status of the patient should also be assessed. This will include asking about significant stressors in the patient's life, and the disability caused by the symptoms. Fear generated by the sensation of breathlessness, and frustration at the associated disability, can significantly worsen symptoms.

The examination findings define the physiological status of the patient and allow diagnostic hypotheses suggested by the history to be tested (Chapter 1). General examination should include an overall impression of the patient's health, assessment of muscle bulk and nutrition, and thyroid status. The presence or absence of conjunctival pallor, cervical lymphadenopathy, finger clubbing, and peripheral oedema are all relevant. Respiratory rate and pattern, arterial oxygen saturation by pulse oximetry, peak flow rate, heart rate and blood pressure, and height and weight (with calculation of body mass index) should be measured.

Features to note in the respiratory examination are the quality of the voice and cough, the tracheal position, and the presence of chest wall abnormalities such as kyphosis, scoliosis, or hyperinflation. Percussion and auscultation may reveal signs of pleural disease, and focal or diffuse crackles and wheezes. Breathlessness due to asthma or COPD typically causes a wheeze audible with the stethoscope but this can be absent even in severe airflow limitation, so that objective measurements (by peak flow rate and spirometry) are essential.

The cardiac examination should include assessment of the jugular venous pressure, palpation of the carotid pulse and precordium, and auscultation of the heart. A raised jugular venous pressure and a displaced apex beat both increase the likelihood of an elevated left ventricular end-diastolic pressure and impaired left ventricular systolic function (positive likelihood ratios 4–8). However, the absence

Table 13.1 Medical Research Council dyspnoea scale	
Grade	**Degree of breathlessness related to activities**
1	Not troubled by breathlessness except on strenuous exercise
2	Short of breath when hurrying or walking up a slight hill
3	Walks slower than contemporaries on level ground because of breathlessness, or has to stop for breath when walking at own pace
4	Stops for breath after walking about 100 m or after a few minutes on level ground
5	Too breathless to leave the house, or breathless when dressing or undressing

Adapted from British Medical Journal, Fletcher CM, Elmes PC, Fairbairn MB et al The significance of respiratory symptoms and the diagnosis of chronic bronchitis in a working population, volume 2, pp. 257-66 copyright © 1959 with permission from BMJ Publishing Group Ltd.

Table 13.2 Differential diagnosis of chronic breathlessness

System	Structures	Examples of disease	Cross reference
Respiratory	Upper and lower airways, lung parenchyma and pleura	Asthma	Chapter 133
		Chronic obstructive pulmonary disease	Chapter 134
		Interstitial lung disease	Chapter 139
Cardiac	Heart and pericardium	Arrhythmias	Chapters 118, 119
		Left ventricular systolic or diastolic dysfunction	Chapter 39
		Valve disease	Chapter 11
		Coronary artery disease	Chapter 90
		Congenital heart disease	Chapter 88
		Constrictive pericarditis	Chapter 108
Pulmonary circulation	Pulmonary arteries and arterioles Pulmonary veins	Pulmonary arterial hypertension	Chapter 100
		Chronic thromboembolic pulmonary hypertension	Chapter 100
		Pulmonary veno-occlusive disease	Chapter 217
Chest wall and diaphragm	Structural and neuromuscular disorders	Kyphoscoliosis	Chapter 149
		Phrenic nerve palsy	Chapter 135
		Myasthenia gravis	Chapter 44
		Myopathies and muscular dystrophies	Chapter 235
Blood	Red cell mass	Anaemia	Chapter 37
Other causes		Thyroid disorders	Chapter 186
		Obesity	Chapter 336
		Physical deconditioning	Chapter 92
		Psychogenic factors	Chapter 241

of these signs and others (e.g. third heart sound, lung crackles) does not significantly reduce the likelihood of heart failure. In summary, abnormal cardiac signs are diagnostically useful if present, but normal cardiac function cannot be inferred from their absence.

Neuromuscular disorders such as myasthenia gravis or myopathies are rare and easily missed causes of chronic breathlessness: they should be considered in the patient with an unexplained restrictive defect.

Key diagnostic tests

Investigation for chronic breathlessness has three stages (Table 13.4). All patients should have Stage 1 or screening tests—chest radiography, electrocardiography, spirometry, and blood tests. When combined with clinical information, the data from these tests should allow the organ system responsible for symptoms to be identified with reasonable accuracy, and provide the basis for an intelligent selection of further tests.

Table 13.3 Features supporting a diagnosis of asthma or COPD in the patient with chronic breathlessness and wheeze

Consider asthma	Consider COPD
Age <40 years	Age >40 years
Smoker or non-smoker	Smoker, with >20 pack-years consumption
Symptoms following exposure to allergens such as grass pollen or animals	Gradual onset of symptoms
Intermittent or seasonal variation in symptoms	Symptoms including cough present on most days
Cough at night or on exercise	Cough worse in morning
Family history of asthma, eczema, hay fever	Industrial exposure to coal/cotton dust
Occupational exposure to dusts, chemicals, or fumes	Pursed lip breathing/prolonged expiration
Variability in serial peak flow measurements >15%	Barrel-shaped chest
FEV$_1$ improves >12% and >200 ml following bronchodilator or steroid therapy	PEF <85% predicted with little variability in serial measurements
	Little or no improvement in FEV$_1$ following bronchodilator or steroid therapy

Stage 1 tests

Chest radiography

The site of pathology is frequently evident on the chest radiograph (CXR), which may reveal structural abnormalities in extra-pulmonary tissues (e.g. deformities of the thoracic cage, rib fractures, diaphragmatic weakness); pleural pathology (pneumothorax, pleural effusion), and gross disease of the pulmonary parenchyma (ILD), consolidation, pulmonary oedema, soft tissue growth).

A CXR is often unhelpful in characterizing airways disease, subtle pathology of the lung parenchyma, and pulmonary vascular disease. Although disease at these sites may be suspected from the clinical assessment, the absence of abnormal findings on the CXR should alert the clinician to consider these diseases more carefully.

Electrocardiography

The ECG defines the cardiac rhythm: tachyarrhythmias (e.g. atrial fibrillation or flutter) and bradyarrhythmias (e.g. sinus bradycardia due to sinus node dysfunction, complete heart block) may be the sole cause of chronic breathlessness or may exacerbate other causes. The ECG also gives indirect information about cardiac structure which shapes the differential diagnosis: relevant abnormalities include pathological Q waves (indicative of previous myocardial infarction), evidence of right ventricular hypertrophy (which may reflect congenital heart disease or pulmonary hypertension) or left ventricular hypertrophy (seen in hypertrophic cardiomyopathy or aortic valve disease), and left bundle branch block (often present in dilated cardiomyopathy). In essence, any ECG arrhythmia or other abnormality warrants transthoracic echocardiography.

Spirometry

Basic spirometry requires the patient to take a maximal breath in, followed by a forced and complete expiration into the spirometer, yielding a volume–time curve. The most common indices recorded are the forced expiratory volume in 1 s (FEV$_1$), the vital capacity (FVC), which is the volume of air exhaled from the point of maximum inspiration, and the ratio of FEV$_1$ to FVC (FEV$_1$/FVC). Psychogenic breathlessness typically produces an effort-limited and variable configuration, while the spirometry of organic disease is usually highly reproducible.

Spirometry allows the categorization of lung disease into obstructive, restrictive, or mixed physiology. Airflow obstruction,

Table 13.4 Investigation in chronic breathlessness		
Stage 1: Screening tests	**Stage 2: Further tests to confirm, refine, or reject possible diagnoses**	**Stage 3: Additional tests which may be needed in individual cases**
Chest radiography	Transthoracic echocardiography	Bronchoscopy
Electrocardiography	High-resolution CT of the chest	Lung biopsy
Spirometry	Pulmonary function testing	Cardiac catheterization
Blood tests	Six-minute walk test with measurement of oxygen saturation	Direct coronary angiography
	Non-invasive tests for coronary artery disease	Transoesophageal echocardiography
		MRI of the heart
		Tests for chronic pulmonary thromboembolism
		Cardiopulmonary exercise testing
		Tests for neuromuscular disease

diagnosed when the FEV_1/FVC ratio falls below the lower limit of normal (Figure 13.1), is due to airway narrowing or obstruction. Common causes of airflow obstruction are COPD, asthma, bronchiectasis, cystic fibrosis, endobronchial tumour, vocal cord dysfunction, and goitre.

Restrictive physiology is characterized by reduced lung volumes. Common causes of restrictive physiology are pulmonary fibrosis, obesity, kyphoscoliosis, neuromuscular disease, and heart failure.

Spirometry typically demonstrates a proportionally reduced FVC and FEV_1, with normal or even increased FEV_1/FVC ratio, indicating reduced lung volume with no airflow obstruction. Most desktop spirometers use a simple algorithm to interpret test data. An FVC below the lower limit of normal will usually be interpreted as restrictive disease (reduced lung volume). In patients with COPD and asthma, a forced expiration is usually accompanied by airway collapse, resulting in a significantly reduced FEV_1 and FVC. The spirometer will

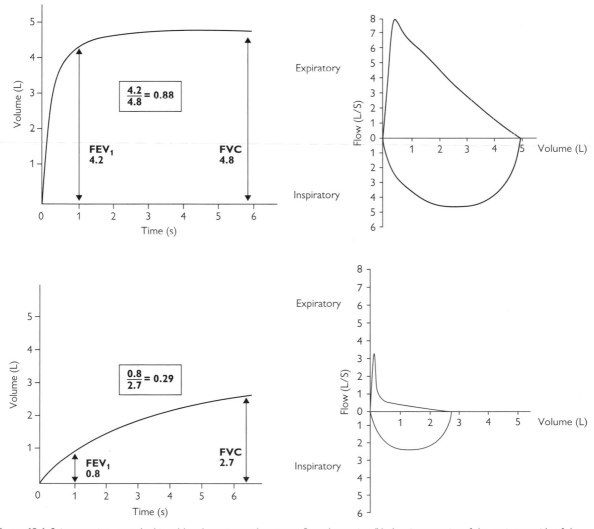

Figure 13.1 Spirograms in a normal subject (a) and a patient with severe airflow obstruction (b), showing scooping of the expiratory side of the flow/volume curve due to airway collapse. It is often stated that airflow obstruction is diagnosed when the FEV_1/FVC ratio falls below 0.7. This is misleading and can lead to over-diagnosis of obstructive physiology in elderly patients, and under-diagnosis in young patients, as the FEV_1/FVC ratio is dependent on age, height, and sex.

often interpret this as mixed disease (small lungs with obstruction) which can be misleading. In COPD, the total lung capacity (TLC) may well be within normal limits, or even increased due to reduced elastic recoil. A measurement of TLC will correctly identify restriction, normal lung volume, or hyperinflation. Where TLC is below the lower limit of normal, then restrictive disease should be considered. Where TLC is above the upper limit of normal, but the FEV_1/FVC ratio is below the lower limit of normal, hyperinflation should be considered. Determination of TLC and other derived lung volumes requires referral to a specialist lung function laboratory.

In diaphragmatic weakness, the restrictive defect is more severe when the patient is supine. With mild diaphragmatic weakness or unilateral paralysis, seated FVC is typically 10%–30% greater than supine FVC; with bilateral diaphragmatic paralysis, it is 30–50% greater.

Blood tests

Given the limitations of clinical assessment of haemoglobin concentration, all patients should have a full blood count done. A biochemical profile should be done to screen for chronic kidney and liver disease, and as a baseline before therapy. If heart failure is possible, plasma brain natriuretic peptide (BNP) (or the equivalent NT-pro-BNP) should be measured. Thyrotoxicosis and hypothyroidism can cause or contribute to chronic breathlessness, and measurement of plasma thyroid stimulating hormone level as a screen for these disorders should be done in patients over 50 or with clinical features of, or risk factors for, these diseases.

Full blood count

Exertional breathlessness is a common symptom of anaemia, although its severity depends on the severity of the anaemia, the time course of its development, and the cardiorespiratory status of the patient. Interpretation of the full blood count is discussed in detail in Chapter 278.

BNP

BNP was so named as it was first isolated from brain tissue. However, the primary source of BNP in plasma is the heart. Ventricular wall stress is the stimulus to synthesis of pre-pro-BNP in cardiomyocytes. After synthesis, the peptide is cleaved first to pro-BNP, then to the biologically active BNP and the inactive amino-terminal fragment, NT-pro-BNP. Measurement of plasma BNP or NT-pro-BNP concentrations substantially improves the accuracy of the diagnosis of chronic heart failure. A plasma BNP level of <100 pg/ml makes heart failure very unlikely (<2%). At levels between 100 and 400 pg/ml, the probability of heart failure is around 75%; judgement as to a diagnosis of heart failure depends on clinical features (e.g. previous myocardial infarction, raised jugular venous pressure, symptoms improved by diuretic). A level of >400 pg/ml gives a probability of heart failure of >95%. Plasma BNP concentration is higher in men than women, increases with age and the degree of chronic kidney disease, and is decreased by obesity.

Further diagnostic tests

Stage 2 tests

Stage 2 tests (Table 13.4) are those typically needed to confirm, refine, or reject possible diagnoses: these include echocardiography, measurement of transfer factor, and high-resolution CT of the chest.

Echocardiography

Transthoracic echocardiography (TTE) provides extensive information about cardiac structure and function and also allows estimation of right atrial and pulmonary artery systolic pressures (Box 13.1). TTE can therefore identify many of the cardiac disorders which may cause chronic breathlessness, and screen for pulmonary hypertension. An important limitation of TTE is that high-quality images cannot be obtained in all patients (e.g. those with body mass index >30, chest wall deformities, or severe COPD). The quality of the images, and the accuracy of their interpretation, also depends on the skill of the operator. A complete study typically takes around 30 minutes to perform. Pocket-sized ultrasound devices (e.g. Vscan, GE Healthcare) are now available which allow a screening echocardiogram to be done in a few minutes, as a component of the physical examination.

Box 13.1 Information derived from transthoracic echocardiography

- presence or absence of congenital abnormalities (e.g. atrial septal defect)
- left ventricular systolic function (global and regional)
- left ventricular diastolic function (inferred from the pattern of mitral inflow, tissue Doppler data, and left atrial size)
- evidence of right ventricular pressure- or volume-overload (indicative of pulmonary hypertension and/or a left-to-right shunt)
- valve function
- estimation of right atrial pressure and pulmonary artery systolic pressure (derived from the size and respiratory change in the inferior vena cava, and the velocity of tricuspid regurgitation)
- pericardial function and the presence of pericardial effusion
- presence and characteristics of pleural effusion

Measurement of transfer factor (diffusing capacity)

When spirometry does not identify the cause of chronic breathlessness, further information may be gained from measuring the transfer factor for carbon monoxide (TLCO). TLCO reflects the function of the alveolar capillary membrane. The patient is required to exhale completely, followed by a maximal inhalation of 0.3% CO, 0.3% CH_4 (or 14% helium), 21% O_2, and balanced N_2. The breath is held for 10 s to allow diffusion of inhaled CO. During exhalation, the expired gas concentration is continuously monitored, and the plateau of expired alveolar gas concentrations measured once dead space has been cleared. Comparing inspired and expired CO and CH_4 concentrations allows the determination of TLCO and effective alveolar volume (V_A). Dividing TLCO by V_A gives the KCO or transfer coefficient. Component parts of the diffusion equation can be used to determine the likely disease process (Table 13.5).

High-resolution CT of the chest

CXR is a useful screen for parenchymal lung disease, but has limited accuracy in the detection and categorization of ILD (false-negative and false-positive rates around 20%). High-resolution CT of the chest (HRCT) has greater accuracy (false-negative and false-positive rates <5%) for ILD, and should be done if the chest radiograph suggests ILD, or if the features on clinical assessment or lung function testing point to ILD, but the CXR is normal (e.g. inspiratory crackles; restrictive physiology on spirometry; normal spirometry but exercise-induced fall in oxygen saturation). Findings on HRCT, when integrated with clinical

---

Table 13.5 Typical disease changes in the transfer factor for carbon monoxide (TLCO) and its components

	TLCO (mmol/min/kPa)	Effective alveolar volume, V_A (l)	Transfer coefficient, kCO (mmol/min kPa⁻¹ l⁻¹)
Emphysema	↓	N or ↓	↓
Lung fibrosis	↓	↓	N or ↓
Anaemia	↓	N	↓
Polycythaemia	↑	N	↑
Vasculitis	↓	N	↓
Mild asthma	↑	N	↑
Extra-pulmonary restriction	↓	↓	↑
Intra-pulmonary haemorrhage	↑	N	↑
Neuromuscular weakness	↓	↓	↑

Data from Hughes JMB. The single breath transfer factor (TL,CO) and the transfer coefficient (KCO): a window onto the pulmonary microcirculation. Clin Physiol & Func Im 2003; 23: 63–71. Pellegrino R, Viegi G, Brusasco V, et al. Interpretative strategies for lung function tests. Eur Respir J 2005; 26: 948–968. Plummer AL. The carbon monoxide diffusing capacity: clinical implications, coding, and documentation. Chest 2008; 134: 663–667.

data, have high diagnostic accuracy as regards the specific cause of ILD, and can guide the type and site for lung biopsy if indicated.

Stage 3 tests

Stage 3 tests are the additional tests which may be needed in individual cases, but would generally not be done before Stage 2 tests. Further discussion of investigation in suspected cardiovascular, respiratory, and neuromuscular disease can be found in Chapters 87, 126, and 220, respectively.

Introduction to therapy

Most patients with chronic breathlessness will have one or more long-term conditions, and need evidence-based management of the underlying cause or causes, ideally delivered by an integrated clinical network that spans primary and secondary care. They are typically vulnerable to acute exacerbations (e.g. from disease flare, super-added infection, arrhythmia, or pulmonary embolism), and should have ready access to specialist care to deal with these. Other elements of management may include immunization against influenza and pneumococcal infection, help with smoking cessation, long-term oxygen therapy, optimization of nutritional state, cardiopulmonary rehabilitation, and psychological support. Opioids can be used to relieve breathlessness of any cause, if the underlying disease cannot be alleviated.

Prognosis

This depends on the specific disease or diseases responsible and their severity and response to treatment. Models to predict prognosis have been constructed for some diseases (e.g. Seattle Heart Failure Model, available online at https://depts.washington.edu/shfm/?width=1093&height=615; the BODE index for COPD, https://www.mdcalc.com/bode-index-copd-survival; and the GAP risk assessment system for idiopathic pulmonary fibrosis https://www.mdcalc.com/gap-index-idiopathic-pulmonary-fibrosis-ipf-mortality).

How to handle uncertainty

If the cause of breathlessness remains unclear, the history should be retaken and the patient re-examined. The CXR and other imaging should be reviewed. Any Stage 2 tests that have not already been done should be requested. Diagnoses that can easily be missed include ILD, atrial septal defect, constrictive pericarditis, pulmonary hypertension, and neuromuscular disorders.

Cardiopulmonary exercise testing (CPET) provides detailed respiratory data in addition to the clinical and cardiovascular data obtained from the standard exercise test. CPET is useful if the cause of chronic breathlessness is still obscure despite Stage 1 and Stage 2 tests, or if multiple possible causes are present and quantification of the contribution of each (including physical deconditioning) is needed.

Further Reading

Guazzi M, Adams V, Conraads V, et al. EACPR/AHA Joint Scientific Statement: Clinical recommendations for cardiopulmonary exercise testing data assessment in specific patient populations. *Eur Heart J* 2012; 33: 2917–27.

Parshall MB, Schwartzstein RM, Adams L, et al. An official American Thoracic Society statement: Update on the mechanisms, assessment, and management of dyspnea. *Am J Respir Crit Care Med* 2012; 185: 435–52.

14 Peripheral oedema

Jonathan Timperley and Sandeep Hothi

Definition of the symptom

Peripheral oedema is a palpable swelling caused by increased interstitial fluid in soft tissues.

Differential diagnosis

Peripheral oedema can be due to local or systemic disease. Fluid distribution between capillaries and the interstitium is governed by Starling forces. The lymphatic system returns excess fluid and protein from the extracellular, interstitial space to the blood stream. Thus, interstitial oedema may arise from factors that increase capillary pressure or permeability, factors that reduce plasma colloid osmotic pressure, factors that impede lymphatic drainage, or a combination of these causes (Table 14.1).

Context

Peripheral oedema may be acute or chronic, and unilateral or bilateral. Mild bilateral ankle oedema may frequently be due to chronic venous disease or benign causes, including gravitational force (e.g. after a long-haul flight); pregnancy; drugs (e.g. dihydropyridines); and obesity. At the other end of the spectrum, peripheral oedema may be due to severe acute or chronic illness.

Approach to diagnosis

Causes needing urgent treatment, such as venous obstruction or thrombosis, organ failure, pre-eclampsia, compartment syndrome, obstruction of the superior vena cava, and necrotizing fasciitis, must be identified. Additionally, a distinction must be made between obesity, lymphoedema, lipoedema, and lipolymphoedema (Table 14.2).

Table 14.1 Causes of peripheral oedema

Cause	Examples
Increased capillary pressure due to renal retention of sodium and water	Primary renal disorders (including nephrotic syndrome)
	Heart failure
	Cirrhosis
	Drug-induced (e.g. NSAIDs, steroids)
	Pregnancy and pre-eclampsia
Increased capillary pressure due to increased venous pressure	Heart failure
	Compression of superior or inferior vena cava, or of iliac veins
	Deep vein thrombosis
	Chronic venous insufficiency
Increased capillary permeability	Allergic reaction
	Infection (e.g. cellulitis)
	Trauma
	Burn
Decreased plasma oncotic pressure	Malabsorption syndrome
	Nephrotic syndrome
	Critical illness
	Liver failure
Impaired lymphatic drainage	Lymph node damage from surgery or radiotherapy
	Lymphatic or lymph node involvement by cancer or infection
	Primary lymphoedema

Lymphoedema may be primary or secondary to a number of causes, including regional lymph node dissection, neoplastic infiltration of lymphatic channels, radiotherapy-induced fibrosis, surgery involving the removal of lymph nodes or channels, and filariasis. Lipoedema is a disorder of adipose tissue with fat distribution that differs from that seen in obesity, and differs from lymphedema in a number of ways. It is usually bilateral, spares the feet, is painful, bruises easily, is orthostatic, and resolves after rest until the late stages.

Specific clues to the diagnosis

Specific clues to the diagnosis are as follows:

- Rapid onset of oedema is seen with venous thrombosis, infection, allergy, and compartment syndrome.
- Pre-eclampsia needs urgent identification and management and is suspected in a pregnant female with proteinuria and hypertension.
- A history of ischaemic heart disease or of liver or renal disease suggests heart, liver, or renal failure, respectively. A history of malignancy or radiotherapy raises the possibility of secondary lymphoedema.
- The drug history may reveal changes in medication (e.g. dihydropyridine antagonists, beta blockers, corticosteroids, oestrogen, progesterone, NSAIDs, glitazones) associated with the onset of oedema.
- The physical examination may also reveal diagnostic clues. On general inspection, there may be features of hypothyroidism (see Chapter 186). An elevated BMI and large neck may exist in sleep apnoea with pulmonary hypertension. The skin has brawny induration in chronic lymphoedema, and haemosiderosis in venous insufficiency.
- Examination of the lower extremities should document the presence or absence of pitting oedema. Both limbs should be compared for any asymmetry, epidermal and dermal changes, ulcers, discoloration, tenderness, cords, and venous prominence. The extent of oedema may be assessed by its height.
- The urine dipstick will show significant proteinuria in nephrotic syndrome, and proteinuria or haematuria in glomerulonephritis.
- Cardiovascular examination may reveal bradycardia, tachycardia, a raised jugular venous pressure, murmurs of valve disease, or third or fourth heart sounds of heart failure. A tender, swollen calf suggests deep vein thrombosis (DVT).
- Pitting oedema occurs with DVT and venous insufficiency. Myxoedema and lymphoedema are non-pitting.
- Respiratory examination may reveal coarse crepitations of underlying lung disease (such as COPD or bronchiectasis) that may result in cor pulmonale. It may also demonstrate fine inspiratory crepitations of either pulmonary fibrosis or pulmonary oedema.
- Abdominal examination may demonstrate ascites, a pelvic mass, a palpable kidney (consider polycystic kidney disease), hepatomegaly, and stigmata of chronic liver disease.

Key diagnostic tests

Where a local cause is suspected (because of unilateral limb swelling or abnormal skin), request a duplex scan and a D-dimer test, to investigate for DVT.

A suspected systemic cause may be detected by the following:

Biochemical profile: urea and electrolytes, a liver function test (LFT), and a thyroid-stimulating hormone test, to assess renal, liver, and thyroid function, respectively; the LFT will provide the serum albumin level

Urinalysis: for detection of proteinuria; if significant proteinuria is present on urinalysis, a 24-hour urinary collection permits

Table 14.2 Differentiating between obesity, lipoedema, lymphoedema, and lipolymphoedema

	Obesity	Lipoedema	Lymphoedema	Lipolymphoedema
Gender	Male or female	Almost always female	Male or female	Almost always female
Time at onset	Childhood onwards	Typically age 10–30 years	Childhood (primary), adult (secondary)	Usually age 30 years onwards
Family history	Common	Common	Only for primary	Occasionally
Effect of dieting	Positive	None	None	None
Effect of elevation	None	Minimal	None	Helpful until fibrosis occurs
Pitting oedema	Absent	Minimal	May stop as fibrosis develops	Usually present to some extent
Easy bruising	No	Yes	No	Yes
Pain	None	In legs	None in early stages	In legs
Area	Generalized	Bilateral legs, sometimes arms	Feet first then legs, often unilateral	Usually bilateral lower limbs, feet eventually affected, Stemmer's sign positive
Positive Stemmer's sign	Absent	Absent	Present	Present

A positive Stemmer's sign is the inability to lift a thickened fold of skin at the base of the second toe or finger.

Adapted from *Advances in Skin & Wound Care*, Fife CE, Maus EA, Carter MJ. Lipedema: a frequently misdiagnosed and misunderstood fatty deposition syndrome, volume 23, pp. 81-92, copyright ©2010 Wolters Kluwer Health, Inc.

quantification of urinary protein loss; measurement of the albumin-to-creatinine ratio will also be important

Albumin-to-creatinine ratio: to quantify the degree of urinary albumin loss

ECG: may suggest cardiovascular disease

Chest X-ray: may demonstrate cardiorespiratory disease

Plasma BNP: will be elevated in heart failure

Echocardiography: to assess for evidence of ventricular dysfunction, tricuspid valve disease, pulmonary hypertension, and pericardial effusion; this will permit diagnosis of heart failure as well as assess for possible causes (e.g. valve disease, regional wall motion abnormalities)

Chest X-ray: to assess for cardiomegaly, malignancy, and coexisting pulmonary oedema

D-dimer test: useful where a DVT is suspected, unless the clinical probability of DVT is high, in which case, definitive imaging should be performed

Other diagnostic tests

Other diagnostic tests include:

Serum lipids: in suspected nephrotic syndrome

Ultrasound: essential in a unilaterally swollen leg in which a DVT is suspected; ultrasound or other imaging of the abdomen is indicated where a pelvic mass is suspected

Computed tomography: this may be used to search for evidence of malignancy, local venous obstruction, and pulmonary disease

Lymphoscintigraphy: where lymphoedema is suspected, this test seeks to identify abnormalities of lymphatic drainage; it involves the administration of radiolabelled large molecules (macromolecules or colloids) into the interstitial space; their movement through lymphatics and lymph nodes is characterized by external gamma cameras

Right heart catheterization: may rarely be required in investigation of suspected pericardial restriction or restrictive cardiomyopathy

Introduction to therapy

Therapy is as follows:

- Venous insufficiency is treated with elevation of the leg and compression stockings. Compression stocks are contraindicated in the presence of arterial insufficiency.

- Lymphoedema is difficult to treat. Options include exercise, elevation, compression, manual lymphatic drainage, and surgery.
- The mainstay of initial treatment for heart failure is diuretic therapy. The underlying cause of heart failure will need directed treatment (e.g. consideration of surgery for valve disease; secondary prevention and possible revascularization in ischaemic heart disease).
- Renal failure will require referral to a nephrologist to treat the specific disorder.
- Liver failure is treated by general and specific principles (see Chapters 209 and 210 on liver disease).
- A DVT is treated with anticoagulation—initially with heparin (usually subcutaneous low molecular weight) and then with warfarin.
- Cellulitis is treated with appropriate antimicrobial therapy.
- Pre-eclampsia requires urgent obstetric involvement to achieve blood pressure control and consideration of early delivery.
- Compartment syndrome requires urgent fasciotomy and debridement.

Prognosis

The prognosis is dependent on the underlying aetiology. An untreated DVT is dangerous due to the risk of pulmonary embolus (PE). Approximately 29%–50% of patients with untreated DVT will develop a PE. The prognosis in heart, liver, and renal failure is generally poor, as described in Chapters 91 and 92, 209 and 210, and 162, respectively.

How to handle uncertainty in the diagnosis of this symptom

Where the aetiology is unclear, it is important to exclude acutely serious conditions (DVT, cellulitis, compartment syndrome, necrotizing fasciitis, pre-eclampsia, acute heart/renal liver failure) in the first instance. Chronic systemic conditions must also be considered.

Further Reading

Kerchner K, Fleischer A, and Yosipovitch G. Lower extremity lymphedema update: Pathophysiology, diagnosis, and treatment guidelines. *J Am Acad Dermatol* 2008; 59: 324–31.

15 Murmur

Jonathan Timperley and Sandeep Hothi

Definition

A murmur is an abnormal sound heard on auscultation of the heart or great vessels due to turbulent blood flow in or near the heart. A bruit is an abnormal sound arising from turbulent flow in a blood vessel.

Aetiology

Murmurs arise from turbulent flow in the heart or great vessels. This may occur because of a structural abnormality of the heart, or increased flow across normal cardiac structures (e.g. innocent flow murmur in pregnancy; the tricuspid flow murmur which may be heard in atrial septal defects with a large left-to-right shunt). Turbulence occurs when laminar blood flow is disrupted. The point at which this occurs is when the velocity exceeds the Reynolds number (Re), predicted by

$$Re = \frac{(\bar{v} \cdot D \cdot \rho)}{\eta},$$

where $\bar{v}$ = mean velocity, ρ = density, D = the diameter of the vessel, and η = viscosity. Thus, high blood velocities and reduced viscosity promote turbulence and hence murmurs.

Murmurs are classified by their timing in relation to the cardiac cycle as systolic, diastolic, or continuous (Box 15.1).

Systolic murmurs are due to:

- obstruction to outflow from the right or left ventricle, at the sub-valvar, valvar, or supravalvar level
- mitral or tricuspid regurgitation
- ventricular septal defect

Diastolic murmurs are due to:

- aortic or pulmonary regurgitation
- abnormal flow across the mitral or tricuspid valves (stenotic valve or increased diastolic flow)

Continuous murmurs, heard in systole and diastole, are due to:

- an abnormal connection between the aorta and the pulmonary artery (e.g. patent ductus arteriosus)
- an abnormal connection between an artery and a vein (e.g. arterio-venous fistula)

Context

Murmurs are a common finding on examination. Murmurs may be organic, functional, or innocent. Organic murmurs are caused by intrinsic cardiac disease. Functional murmurs are due to perturbations which are present in the circulation but which are due to non-cardiac causes. Innocent murmurs can arise from cardiac or non-cardiac sources but are not due to a recognized disease. Systolic murmurs are heard in up to 50% of adults. More than 90% of young adults and around 50% of older adults with a systolic murmur have a structurally normal heart on echocardiography (i.e. an innocent murmur). Diastolic or continuous murmurs always indicate structural disease. The finding of a diastolic murmur, or a new systolic murmur, in an ill patient with fever raises the possibility of infective endocarditis. Anaemia, pregnancy, and thyrotoxicosis may result in a high-output state with a functional (flow) murmur. A pericardial rub can be mistaken for a heart murmur.

Approach to diagnosis

The findings on auscultation need to be placed in relation to the history, other features of the examination, and the ECG. Key examination findings relevant to interpretation of the murmur are:

- pulse rate and rhythm
- arterial blood pressure and pulse pressure
- carotid pulse upstroke and volume
- location and quality of apex beat (note that the apex beat is impalpable in 50% of patients)
- presence of left parasternal lift
- signs of heart failure
- arterial oxygen saturation
- heart sounds
- assessment of JVP
- palpation of liver
- presence of peripheral oedema

The technique of auscultation typically begins with the patient recumbent. The murmur of mitral stenosis is best heard with the patient lying on their left side, using the bell of the stethoscope. Aortic regurgitation is heard best with the patient sitting forwards with their breath held in expiration.

A careful analysis of the characteristics of the murmur aids diagnosis. Key features are:

- timing, in relation to the cardiac cycle (see 'Aetiology')
- intensity, graded from very soft to very loud (e.g. using the Levine grading system, which grades the intensity of murmurs from 1 to 6)
- pitch: high, low, or mixed
- location where the murmur is loudest, and its radiation
- effects of dynamic manoeuvres: various physical manoeuvres can bring about characteristic changes in some murmurs

---

Box 15.1 Timing of murmurs in relation to the cardiac cycle

Systolic murmur

Mid-systolic murmur
- aortic stenosis

Pansystolic murmur
- mitral regurgitation
- tricuspid regurgitation
- ventricular septal defect

Late systolic murmur
- mitral valve prolapse

Diastolic murmur

Early diastolic murmur
- aortic regurgitation
- pulmonary regurgitation

Mid-diastolic murmur
- mitral stenosis
- tricuspid stenosis

Continuous murmur (rare presentation)
- patent ductus arteriosus
- arteriovenous fistula
- venous 'hum'

Murmurs vary with respiration. Murmurs that arise from right-sided lesions increase in intensity with inspiration, while left-sided murmurs are unaltered or decrease in intensity. In expiration, the opposite changes occur. Deep expiration brings the base of the heart closer to the chest wall and makes auscultation of aortic regurgitation and pericardial rubs easier.

The strain phase of a Valsalva manoeuvre reduces the intensity of most murmurs but increases the intensity of murmurs due to hypertrophic cardiomyopathy (HCM). Moving from standing to squatting produces an increase in venous return and increases arterial blood pressure. As a result, most murmurs increase in intensity, except those due to HCM; these reduce in intensity because of increased ventricular size and reduced obstruction to flow. Moving from squatting to standing produces the opposite changes. Handgripping (an isometric exercise) increases systemic vascular resistance and increases the intensity of mitral regurgitation, but reduces the intensity of aortic stenosis because of reduced pressure gradient across the aortic valve. The murmur of HCM becomes softer.

Specific clues to the diagnosis

See Table 15.1 for specific clues to the diagnosis.

Key diagnostic tests

All patients with a murmur should have an ECG. If the murmur has the characteristics of an innocent murmur and the ECG is normal, echocardiography is not mandatory. In all other patients with a murmur, transthoracic echocardiography (TTE) should be performed.

Other diagnostic tests

Other diagnostic tests are as follows:

Transoesophageal echocardiography: This allows better ultrasound imaging where TTE gives inadequate imaging due to limited windows.
Chest X-ray: This may demonstrate cardiomegaly, pulmonary oedema, aortic root dilatation, valvar or valve-related calcification, and prosthetic heart valves.
Blood tests: Where infective endocarditis is suspected, multiple sets of blood cultures should be taken. In addition, a full blood count,

C-reactive protein, ESR and biochemical profile should be checked. BNP will be elevated where a valve lesions results in heart failure. Thyroid function tests should be checked where a high-output flow murmur of thyrotoxicosis is suspected.
Contrast TTE/transesophageal echocardiogram: Echocardiography with contrast permits the assessment of intra-cardiac shunts, including patent foramen ovale or an atrial septal defect.
Cardiac MRI: This permits assessment of cardiac structure, haemodynamics, and function. It permits higher spatial resolution than echocardiography.
Cardiac catheterization: This permits assessment of coronary artery disease in patients being considered for valvular surgery, as well as enabling the measurement of valve gradients and saturation measurements that might identify the site of intra-cardiac shunts.

Introduction to therapy

The management of specific valve and congenital heart lesions is addressed elsewhere. Innocent murmurs need no specific treatment. Mild to moderate valve lesions may be managed by surveillance echocardiography.

In the UK, routine antibiotic prophylaxis for patients with valvular or congenital heart disease is no longer recommended by NICE for dental procedures, or procedures involving the genitourinary, gastrointestinal, or respiratory tracts. They do recommend appropriate antibiotics if a procedure involves a potentially or actually infected gastrointestinal or genitourinary tract.

Prognosis

The prognosis is that of the cause of the murmur. For instance, innocent flow murmurs have a good prognosis, while symptomatic aortic stenosis without intervention has a poor prognosis.

How to handle uncertainty in the diagnosis of this symptom

Transthoracic echocardiography is the key diagnostic test. Occasionally, this can be non-diagnostic, and further information is required. In this case, transoesophageal echocardiography will usually provide the required information.

Table 15.1 Characteristics of different murmurs

Murmur	Cardiac abnormality	Examination findings	Specific clues to the diagnosis
Mid-systolic	*None: innocent murmur*	–	–
Mid-systolic	Aortic stenosis	Narrowly split or reversed S2, harsh mid-systolic murmur, loudest upper right sternal edge radiating to carotids, quiet second heart sound; intensity increased by squatting	Slow rising pulse, slow volume pulse, narrow pulse pressure, left ventricular hypertrophy on 12-lead ECG; exertional chest pain/dyspnoea/syncope
Mid-systolic	Hypertrophic cardiomyopathy with left ventricular outflow tract obstruction	Mid-systolic murmur loudest at apex and left lower sternal edge; intensity decreased by squatting; does not usually radiate to the neck; may be pansystolic murmur at apex (associated mitral regurgitation)	There may be a family history; ECG: left ventricular hypertrophy; septal hypertrophy; ventricular ectopics
Early diastolic	Aortic regurgitation	A2 may be soft; decrescendo, high-pitched early diastolic murmur loudest at left sternal edge; its duration is increased by increasing severity of aortic regurgitation; there may be an Austin–Flint murmur (low-pitched, mid-diastolic, apical murmur); collapsing pulse, wide pulse pressure	–
Mid-diastolic	Mitral stenosis	Mitral facies, signs of pulmonary hypertension with loud P2; loud S1, opening snap, then low-pitched, mid-diastolic murmur, loudest at apex with patient in left lateral position, with presystolic accentuation if in sinus rhythm; murmur intensity increased by exercise	On 12-lead ECG, may have atrial fibrillation, right bundle branch block, right axis deviation
Pansystolic	Mitral regurgitation	Soft or absent S1, pansystolic murmur loudest at the apex, radiating to the axilla; there may be an S3	Hyperdynamic apex, may be displaced with chronic regurgitation
Pansystolic	Tricuspid regurgitation	Pansystolic murmur loudest at lower left sternal edge, increasing with respiration	Giant 'v' wave and rapid 'y' decent in jugular venous pressure, pulsatile liver, peripheral oedema

Further Reading

Nishimura RA, Otto CM, Bonow RO, et al. 2014 AHA/ACC Guideline for the Management of Patients with Valvular Heart Disease: A report of the American College of Cardiology/American Heart Association Task Force on Practice Guidelines. *J Am Coll Cardiol* 2014; 63: e57–e185.

The Joint Task Force on the Management of Valvular Heart Disease of the European Society of Cardiology (ESC) and the European Association for Cardio-Thoracic Surgery (EACTS). Guidelines on the management of valvular heart disease (Version 2012). *Eur Heart J* 2012; 33: 2451–96.

16 Cough

Jacky Smith

Definition of the symptom

A cough is an explosive forced expiratory manoeuvre, usually against a closed glottis and gives rise to a characteristic sound. Acute cough is defined as a cough of less than 3 weeks duration, and chronic cough, of more than 8 weeks duration.

Differential diagnosis

Coughing is a symptom of broad range of upper and lower respiratory tract diseases. Common causes in patients presenting to secondary care with cough as an isolated symptom are shown in Box 16.1.

Context

Acute cough is the commonest presenting symptom in primary care and by far the most frequent cause is viral respiratory tract infection. Most sufferers do not seek medical care; it has been estimated that 50% self-medicate with over-the-counter therapies and only 50% of these consult with their general practitioner, most often because of persistent/severe coughing or concern about a more serious illness.

The prevalence of chronic cough has been estimated as between 11% and 20% of the general population. Women are more frequently affected than men and associations have been reported with smoking, a diagnosis of asthma and symptoms of gastro-oesophageal reflux disease. The main effect of coughing is on quality of life and this is particularly prominent in chronic cough patients who not infrequently develop physical complications such as chest pain, retching and vomiting, hoarseness, incontinence, sleep disturbance, and syncope. In addition psychological distress and social embarrassment are often features.

Approach to diagnosis

Acute cough

The majority of patients presenting to primary care will have an acute cough and the diagnosis is made based upon a symptoms typical of

---

Box 16.1 Common causes of cough seen in secondary care

Acute cough
- acute bronchitis
- pneumonia
- inhaled foreign body

Chronic cough
- cough-variant asthma
- gastro-oesophageal reflux disease
- rhinosinusitis
- eosinophilic bronchitis
- COPD
- bronchial carcinoma
- bronchiectasis
- angiotensin-converting-enzyme inhibitor therapy
- pulmonary tuberculosis
- interstitial lung disease
- heart failure

---

a viral upper respiratory tract infection. Such cases are benign and self-limiting and require no specific investigation or treatment; there is insufficient evidence to suggest that over-the-counter cough medicines are effective. The key is to identify the very small number of individuals in whom acute coughing indicates a serious underlying illness. Further investigation is required if there is a suspicion from the history or examination of an inhaled foreign body or a neoplasm, or if a prominent systemic illness is present. Specific symptoms requiring further investigation are:

- haemoptysis
- fever
- breathlessness
- chest pain
- weight loss

The remainder of this chapter will deal with chronic cough.

Chronic cough

The overall approach to patients should consist of:

1. the diagnosis and treatment of underlying conditions that may explain cough
2. investigations and trials of therapy targeting the known common conditions associated with chronic cough
3. interventions to help control coughing in unexplained or treatment-resistant cough

Several respiratory societies have produced specific detailed algorithms to aid diagnosis and management of chronic cough (see 'Further reading').

Specific clues to the diagnosis

Chronic cough

Specific clues to the diagnosis of chronic cough are as follows:

- Many patients report coughing on minor exposure to environmental irritants and temperature changes and in relation to eating, talking, or laughing; however, there is little evidence to support the notion that these features are suggestive of any particular diagnosis.
- Expectoration of sputum suggests a primary pulmonary pathology.
- Additional symptoms of asthma, gastro-oesophageal reflux, or rhinosinusitis may suggest the diagnosis and should direct trials of therapy.
- Responses to previous therapeutic trials might help narrow possible diagnoses.
- Physical examination may identify signs suggestive of specific conditions associated with chronic cough, such as chronic obstructive lung diseases, bronchiectasis, interstitial lung disease, heart failure, or lung cancer. However, often there are no specific findings.

Key diagnostic tests

Key diagnostic tests are as follows:

Chest radiography: This is mandatory in all patients with chronic cough or with acute cough with atypical symptoms or signs. In respiratory clinics, up to 31% of chest X-rays are abnormal and help establish the diagnosis.
Spirometry: This is mandatory in chronic cough.
Bronchoscopy: This is mandatory in patients with chronic cough where a foreign body or neoplasm is suspected.

If the history/examination and these key diagnostic tests reveal abnormalities that could account for the cough, then these abnormalities should be appropriately investigated to establish a diagnosis, and treatment commenced. Should no abnormality be identified or the cough prove resistant to therapy for the established diagnosis (assuming a response is expected), then subsequent investigations and therapeutic trials should be targeted at the known common causes of chronic cough (see 'Other diagnostic tests').

Other diagnostic tests

The identification of the cause of a chronic cough often hinges on the success of specific therapeutic trials. Diagnostic testing can be useful, but access to some of these specialist tests varies, and approaches should be adapted to local circumstances. The following therapeutic trials/investigations can be helpful in diagnosing and managing chronic cough.

Asthma syndromes

Cough-variant asthma is defined as asthma presenting with an isolated cough; classical symptoms of wheezing and breathlessness are absent.

Investigations

Spirometry may show evidence of airway obstruction reversible with bronchodilators. If spirometry is normal/near normal, then bronchial provocation testing with methacholine or histamine is more useful; a negative test excludes cough-variant asthma but mildly positive tests are common in chronic cough in the absence of other features of asthma.

Induced sputum examination for eosinophilic inflammation contributes to the diagnosis but is rarely available outside of the research setting. If a bronchoscopy is performed, washing of the proximal airways may identify such inflammation. Eosinophilic inflammation in the absence of a positive bronchial provocation test suggests a diagnosis of eosinophilic bronchitis.

Therapeutic trial

Asthma syndromes generally respond well to treatment with corticosteroids, and the cough should resolve following a 2-week course of 30 mg prednisolone. It must be remembered that asthma syndromes are not the only steroid-responsive causes of cough and therefore, if the symptoms return when treatment is converted to inhaled corticosteroids, an alternative diagnosis should be sought.

Gastro-oesophageal reflux disease

Some patients with chronic cough respond well to acid-suppressing therapy; however, it remains unclear how such patients can be prospectively identified.

Investigations

Although reflux disease may be assessed by gastroscopy, 24-hour pH monitoring, and 24-hour pH/impedance monitoring, currently no particular parameter from any of these investigations has been shown to predict a positive response to a particular therapy. Laryngeal appearances to diagnose reflux are also of questionable value in chronic cough.

Therapeutic trial

Proton-pump-inhibitor treatment (the equivalent of 20–40 mg omeprazole twice daily for 8 weeks, before meals) is well tolerated and improves cough in some patients, although randomized controlled trials have been disappointing. The role of more aggressive acid suppression such as the addition of H2 receptor antagonists or the use of prokinetic agents and baclofen is less clear, as is the role of anti-reflux surgery.

Rhinosinusitis

Upper airways diseases are also a common cause of chronic cough. In the past, these were referred to as 'post-nasal drip syndromes', based on the suggestion that secretions dripping into the larynx provoked coughing, but there is little evidence supporting this mechanism.

Investigations

ENT referral/examination and sinus imaging may be useful in patients with prominent upper airway symptoms and where chronic sinus disease is suspected. Examination of the throat may also reveal tonsillar hypertrophy, which can contribute to chronic cough.

Therapeutic trial

Although evidence from randomized controlled trials is lacking, a 1-month trial of topical nasal corticosteroids is recommended in patients where rhinitis is suspected. Antibiotic therapy and decongestants may also be helpful for sinusitis.

In patients in whom targeted investigations and/or therapeutic trials have been unhelpful, the following investigations should be considered:

High-resolution CT of the thorax: This may reveal interstitial lung disease or bronchiectasis not visible on the chest X-ray. Scanning should be performed at the outset, however, if auscultation of the chest suggests such a diagnosis.
Bronchoscopy: This may find rare causes of chronic cough such as tracheomalacia, tracheobronchopathia osteochondroplastica, and endobronchial amyloidosis, which are difficult to diagnose without airway examination.
Sleep studies: Obstructive sleep apnoea (OSA) patients commonly report chronic coughing, and case reports suggest that, in patients presenting with chronic cough and found to have OSA, positive airway pressure therapy might improve coughing.

Introduction to therapy

Generally, therapy for chronic cough should be the appropriate treatment of the underlying cause and may be established as part of the diagnostic process. However, it is increasingly recognized that many patients have either unexplained cough (no identifiable cause) or treatment-resistant cough (no response to therapy for identified potential causes). Unfortunately, effective, well-tolerated antitussive therapies are lacking. Some patients benefit from low-dose amitriptyline (10 mg daily) or low-dose morphine sulfhate (5–10 mg twice daily) but side effects (especially with morphine) are common. Supportive therapies, such as speech and language therapy to teach cough control/suppression, incontinence services, and treatment of anxiety and depression, should also be considered.

Prognosis

Little is known about the prognosis of chronic cough. However, data from one specialist clinic showed that, over a 7-year follow-up, 14% of patients with chronic cough resolved and 40% had a significant improvement.

How to handle uncertainty in the diagnosis of this symptom

Patients with chronic cough can be challenging to manage, especially where no cause or multiple potential causes of cough are identified. These patients benefit from review in a specialist cough clinic.

Further Reading

Smith JA and Woodcock AN. Chronic cough. *N Engl J Med* 2016; 375: 1544–51.

17 Wheeze

Andrew A. Jeffrey

Definition of the symptom

A wheeze is a high-pitched musical sound which reflects airflow obstruction. It may be monophonic or polyphonic, and may be heard during inspiration, expiration, or both phases of respiration. Stridor is the term used to describe wheeze which is louder over the neck than the chest, and may be audible without a stethoscope.

Differential diagnosis

The differential diagnosis of wheeze is given in Table 17.1.

Context

Wheezing is typically associated with breathlessness, and may present as an acute or chronic problem. It is most often due to asthma or chronic obstructive pulmonary disease.

Approach to diagnosis

If wheezing is associated with respiratory distress or other evidence of critical illness, the approach to the diagnosis and management should follow the method outlined in Chapter 126.

In stable patients, a detailed history should be taken, with particular attention to the speed of onset of wheezing, trigger factors, and history of atopy. The clinical features, measurement of peak expiratory flow, and spirometry will usually differentiate between possible diagnoses.

Specific clues to the diagnosis

Asthma

The commonest cause of wheeze is bronchospasm in the context of asthma. The patient, or those around them, may be aware of noisy breathing occurring usually in association with laboured breathing and a sensation of chest tightness or heaviness. In asthma this symptom occurs at rest and in response to specific triggers as well as on exertion. Asthma usually starts in childhood or early adult life, although it can present at any age. The peak expiratory flow rate (PEFR) is significantly reduced when wheeze is present. There is usually a rapid response to short-acting bronchodilator therapy.

Table 17.1 Causes of wheeze by anatomical site of airflow obstruction

Extra-thoracic upper airway (nose, mouth, pharynx, larynx, and upper trachea)	Intra-thoracic upper airway (lower trachea, and bronchi >2 mm in diameter)	Lower airways (bronchi <2 mm in diameter, and bronchioles)
Anaphylaxis	Tracheal disorders	Asthma
Vocal cord disorders	Foreign body aspiration	Chronic obstructive pulmonary disease
Laryngeal disorders	Mucus deposits in large airways	Pulmonary oedema
Tracheal disorders, including extrinsic compression by large goitre	Endobronchial tumours	Bronchiectasis
	Bronchomalacia	Cystic fibrosis

Pulmonary oedema

So-called cardiac asthma results from the narrowing of small airways by mucosal oedema caused by high pulmonary-capillary pressure. This is a relatively uncommon presentation of pulmonary oedema, as other symptoms normally predominate. However, wheeze can occasionally be a dominant feature and hard to differentiate from bronchial asthma. In its character, the wheeze in pulmonary oedema is almost identical to that caused by bronchospasm. As it can occur at rest, particularly in bed at night, the history shares features with asthma as well. The onset of wheeze in an older patient should trigger a search for risk factors, symptoms, and signs of cardiac disease, as well as for asthma. The PEFR can be reduced in pulmonary oedema and so a single low reading is not diagnostic; however, the classical diurnal variation in PEFR is not seen. A raised level of plasma BNP will be found in a patient with wheeze due to cardiogenic pulmonary oedema.

Chronic obstructive pulmonary disease

Wheeze can be found in airflow obstruction, which is usually due to chronic bronchitis. It occurs frequently on exertion or during exacerbations when a degree of bronchospasm is also present due to mucosal oedema. Patients often report frequent 'winter bronchitis'. Onset is later in life and almost invariably in cigarette smokers. No diurnal variation in PEFR occurs.

Vocal cord dysfunction

Vocal cord dysfunction (VCD) is a relatively common problem resulting from an involuntary increase in muscle tone in the laryngeal muscles. In some, this can result in paradoxical narrowing of the laryngeal opening during inspiration, resulting in **inspiratory** wheeze. It occurs relatively commonly in patients with asthma and can be interpreted by the patient as part of the symptoms produced by their asthma, but one that does not respond to bronchodilator therapy and is often not associated with chest tightness. They can present with difficult to control asthma. It is vital in taking the history to establish where in the respiratory cycle (i.e. during inspiration or expiration) that wheezing occurs and to consider VCD in all such patients. Flow-volume loops can sometimes show a characteristic 'flutter' pattern with VCD. Direct observation of the cords during breathing is essential to rule out more sinister laryngeal pathology and can be diagnostic in VCD, but, as the problem varies over time, the diagnosis can be difficult to prove.

Other causes

A simple whistling noise from mucus in airways occurs in the context of a productive cough and usually clears or changes with coughing. Bronchomalacia is a rare disorder in which the cartilage in the major airways softens, resulting in their collapse during expiration (intrathoracic) or inspiration (extra-thoracic). Diagnosis is by bronchoscopy or CT chest with inspiratory and expiratory views

Key diagnostic tests

The key diagnostic tests are:

- measurement of PEFR, before and after inhaled bronchodilator
- spirometry, before and after inhaled bronchodilator (including measurement of the flow-volume loop if extra-thoracic or intra-thoracic upper airway obstruction is suspected)
- chest radiography

Other diagnostic tests

Other diagnostic tests are:

- nasendoscopy/laryngoscopy
- bronchoscopy
- CT of the chest/neck
- provocative tests for asthma

Introduction to therapy

Supportive therapy for the critically ill patient with respiratory failure is discussed in Chapter 135. Specific therapy is directed by the working diagnosis.

Prognosis

The prognosis depends on the cause.

How to handle uncertainty in the diagnosis of this symptom

If the clinical features suggest extra-thoracic upper airway obstruction, refer to an ENT surgeon for consideration of nasendoscopy/laryngoscopy. For suspected intra-thoracic disease, arrange bronchoscopy or a chest CT.

Further Reading

Bohadana A, Izbicki G, and Kraman SS. Fundamentals of lung auscultation. *N Engl J Med* 2014; 370: 744–51.

Boulet L-P and O'Byrne PM. Asthma and exercise-induced bronchoconstriction in athletes. *N Engl J Med* 2015; 372: 641–8.

18 Haemoptysis

Rakesh Panchal

Definition of the symptom

Haemoptysis is the expectoration of blood or blood-stained sputum resulting from haemorrhage into the respiratory tract. Massive haemoptysis (5% of cases) is usually defined as >600 ml in 24 hours.

Differential diagnosis

See Table 18.1 for the differential diagnosis of haemoptysis.

Context

Haemoptysis is a common and non-specific symptom. It can vary from blood-streaked sputum to massive, life-threatening haemorrhage. Haemoptysis may originate from the bronchial arteries (90%), pulmonary arteries (5%), or non-bronchial collaterals. Haemoptysis causing haemodynamic instability and/or respiratory compromise is a medical emergency. Unexplained haemoptysis may herald a serious underlying lung condition and therefore requires a thorough diagnostic workup. The majority of patients can be safely investigated and managed as outpatients. Urgent workup or inpatient management will be determined by the rate and severity of bleeding, and knowledge of either the source of bleeding and/or the underlying condition.

Approach to diagnosis

It is important to distinguish haemoptysis from epistaxis or haematemesis.

A focused history is the key to diagnosis:

Demographics: In patients from the Indian subcontinent or sub-Saharan Africa, a diagnosis of tuberculosis or post-tuberculous bronchiectasis is more likely while, in the West, bronchiectasis or lung cancer is more common.

Smoking: A high-pack-year history of smoking in the context of haemoptysis and other red-flag symptoms such as cough, dyspnoea, chest pain, and weight loss is suggestive of lung cancer.

Volume of haemoptysis: Bronchiectasis and pulmonary haemorrhage typically present with moderate-to-severe bleeding, whereas lung cancer and bronchitis cause mild-to-moderate bleeding.

The clinical examination may be normal, but the following signs may be found:

Nasal signs: Nasal crusting or dried blood may be found in Wegener's granulomatosis (granulomatosis with polyangiitis).

Superior vena cava obstruction: Swelling of the face and neck with fixed elevation of the jugular venous pressure may be found in lung cancer.

Auscultation of the chest: Bronchial breath sounds may be heard in pneumonia or tuberculosis, while coarse crepitations may be heard in bronchiectasis.

Specific clues to the diagnosis

See Table 18.2 for specific clues to the diagnosis.

Key diagnostic tests

Key diagnostic tests are as follows:

Chest radiograph: This is the first investigation of choice, as it may help localize the bleeding site to, for example, a mass lesion, or regions showing consolidation, bronchiectasis, or diffuse interstitial shadowing in vasculitides. In approximately 20%–46% of cases, the chest radiograph will be non-diagnostic.

Blood tests: These should be taken to evaluate haemoglobin, platelet count, and clotting profile (full blood count, international normalized ratio, and activated partial thromboplastin time). If vasculitis or a pulmonary–renal syndrome is suspected, renal and liver function tests as well as antineutrophil cytoplasmic antibodies (ANCAs), autoantibodies, and antiglomerular basement membrane (anti-GBM) antibodies should be requested. All patients should be grouped and saved.

Sputum: In patients at risk for lung cancer, sputum should be sent for cytology; in suspected tuberculosis or pneumonia, it should be sent for Gram stain, stain for acid-fast bacilli, and culture.

CT scan: This is now performed in the majority of unexplained causes of haemoptysis and should be done prior to bronchoscopy, as it directs the bronchoscopist to the likely source of bleeding and therefore increases the potential yield. High-resolution CT should be requested if bronchiectasis is suspected. Contrast-enhanced CT may help in identifying vascular lesions such as arteriovenous malformations. Request for a CT with bronchial artery circulation

Table 18.1 Differential diagnosis of haemoptysis			
Primary care		**Secondary care**	
Infection • bronchitis (25%) • pneumonia (10%) • tuberculosis (8%)	60%–70%	Bronchiectasis	38%
Lung cancer	25%	Mycetoma/aspergilloma	16%
Cardiac haemoptysis	5%	Lung cancer	10%
(pulmonary venous or arterial hypertension; left ventricular failure, mitral stenosis, pulmonary embolism, and, more rarely, congenital heart disease with Eisenmenger syndrome)		Tuberculosis	8%
		Pneumonia	6%
		Pulmonary vasculitis	2%
		Others	8%

Note: Twenty per cent of haemoptyses are **cryptogenic**.

Table 18.2 Specific clues to the diagnosis	
Clues	**Likely diagnosis**
Age	<40 years: bronchiectasis and mitral stenosis >40 years: lung cancer
Fever; rusty-coloured, purulent sputum	Pneumonia, especially *Streptococcal pneumoniae*, or tuberculosis
COPD, cachexia, smoker	Lung cancer
History of lung disease: childhood respiratory illness, tuberculosis, pneumonia, etc.	Bronchiectasis
Major risk factors for venous thromboembolism + haemoptysis	Pulmonary embolism
Fever, weight loss, sinus/nasal symptoms, haematuria, skin rash, eyes, joint, CNS involvement	Vasculitis, e.g. Wegener's granulomatosis (granulomatosis with polyangiitis).

will provide a 'road map' of dilated tortuous bronchial arteries that may be targeted by an interventional radiologist for embolization if a bronchiectatic cavity or aspergilloma is suspected (see 'Other diagnostic tests').

Bronchoscopy: Bronchoscopy, pending CT, is useful as both a diagnostic and therapeutic modality. It enables the anatomical source of the haemoptysis to be directly visualized and allows tissue biopsies or bronchial washes to be taken. From a therapeutic perspective, it allows injection of a bleeding tumour with a vasoconstrictor (e.g. adrenaline) or tamponade via a catheter (e.g. a Fogarty catheter). Many clinicians believe bronchoscopy should be performed in all cases of haemoptysis.

Urinalysis: Microscopic haematuria in the presence of frank haemoptysis should encourage investigations to confirm or refute pulmonary–renal syndrome.

Other diagnostic tests

Subsequent investigations will depend on the presumed underlying diagnosis:

CT pulmonary angiogram: Do this if pulmonary embolism is suspected.

Echocardiography: This will identify moderate/severe pulmonary hypertension or mitral valve disease if suspected as a cause of haemoptysis.

Bronchial artery angiography and embolization (BAE): This technique has both diagnostic and therapeutic benefits. If bleeding is from a bronchial artery, it will identify a mesh of dilated or tortuous vessels surrounding, for example, a bronchiectatic cavity or an aspergilloma. It is best performed during an episode of bleeding in order to maximize the chances of identifying the bleeding source. Abnormal vessel embolization is performed using glue or coils. This technique is only carried out in specialist centres, usually by experienced interventional vascular radiologists, with a success rate in the range of 73%–98%. Complications include transient chest pain which is often ischaemic in origin and, more seriously, a 1% risk of spinal cord ischaemia if the embolized bronchial artery gives rise to the anterior spinal artery.

Pulmonary function tests: In genuine causes of pulmonary haemorrhage, the gas transfer (KCO) will be elevated, reflecting the increased oxygen-carrying capacity of blood present in the alveoli. This may be useful in confirming haemoptysis, provided the other causes of a raised KCO are excluded.

Introduction to therapy

Non-massive haemoptysis is managed conservatively, provided there is no haemodynamic instability or respiratory compromise. The key is to identify and treat the source. If the haemoptysis is persistent or troublesome, then in the absence of severe renal failure an antifibrinolytic such as tranexamic acid may be prescribed either orally (500 mg three times daily, or 15–25 mg/kg two to three times daily) or intravenously (0.5-1.0 g three times daily).

Massive haemoptysis is a medical emergency and must be managed in the same manner as a gastrointestinal (GI) haemorrhage (e.g. variceal bleeding). Resuscitation (intravenous fluids) and airway protection are the first priority. Early anaesthetic input is important, and the patient may need to be admitted to a high-dependency or intensive care unit. If the bleeding source is known, then the patient should be positioned with the bleeding side down to protect and prevent overspill into the unaffected lung. Nebulized adrenaline (5–10 ml of 1:10 000) acts as a vasoconstrictor and may be used under these circumstances. Patients with ongoing massive haemoptysis should be intubated with a large endotracheal tube to allow bronchoscopy and suction. Alternatively, a double-lumen endotracheal tube may be passed to protect the unaffected lung. Early bronchoscopy is advisable as it allows identification of the bleeding source and instillation of topical adrenaline (5–10 ml of 1:10 000) or lavage with iced 0.9% saline to induce vasoconstriction, or tamponade using a balloon catheter. Rigid bronchoscopy is preferable for balloon tamponade but is often done by thoracic surgeons in tertiary centres in the UK. It also allows laser or electrocautery treatment in endoscopically visible tumours.

If haemostasis is achieved, the most effective non-surgical treatment, depending on the likely cause, is BAE (see 'Other diagnostic tests'). However, for select cases (e.g. rebleeding despite BAE; localized bronchiectasis; trauma; hydatid cysts; arteriovenous malformations; thoracic aneurysm and aspergilloma) surgery (e.g. by lobectomy) remains the procedure of choice because it is curative.

Prognosis

In 20%–33% of cases, no source of bleeding is identifiable. This is called **cryptogenic haemoptysis** and has a good prognosis, with resolution of bleeding within 6 months of evaluation. Non-massive haemoptysis has a mortality ranging from 7%–30%. However, in massive haemoptysis the mortality can reach 80% and such an encounter is often a terrifying experience for both clinician and patient alike.

How to handle uncertainty in the diagnosis of this symptom

The majority of cryptogenic haemoptyses can be managed by reassurance; however, it is important to have considered and excluded vasculitides such as Wegener's granulomatosis, microscopic polyangiitis, or Goodpasture's if there is any evidence of systemic disease. Patients may occasionally state that 'blood appeared in my mouth'; if you believe the patient has had a bleed but are unsure if it is haemoptysis, then a thorough history for possible upper respiratory tract (e.g. epistaxis) or upper GI symptoms (dyspepsia, reflux, vomiting, melaena, etc.) should be sought, and referral to either an ENT or a gastroenterologist for possible nasal or upper GI endoscopy should be considered.

Further Reading

Larici AR, Franchi P, and Occhipinti M. Diagnosis and management of hemoptysis. *Diagn Interv Radiol* 2014; 20: 299–309.

Khalil A, Fedida B, Parrot A, et al. Severe hemoptysis: From diagnosis to embolization. *Diagn Interv Imaging* 2015; 96: 775–88.

19 Pleural effusion

Seamus Grundy

Definition of the presentation

A pleural effusion is a collection of fluid within the space between the visceral and parietal pleura. Pleural effusions can be unilateral or bilateral, and differentiation of this can aid with creating a differential diagnosis.

Differential diagnosis

All unilateral pleural effusions require further investigation within a secondary care setting. Bilateral pleural effusions in the setting of known heart failure can be safely treated without further investigations unless the effusions are markedly asymmetric or there are symptoms suggestive of an alternative aetiology.

Context

Pleural effusion is a common clinical problem which can present both to primary and secondary care. In healthy individuals, the pleural space contains approximately 10–15 ml of pleural fluid. Pleural effusions can be caused by many different disease processes. However, the process by which fluid accumulates can be divided into transudative or exudative. Transudative effusions (Table 19.1) occur in the presence of normal pleura and are caused by increased oncotic or hydrostatic pressures. Exudative effusions (Table 19.2) are associated with abnormal pleura and are caused by either increased pleural fluid production due to local inflammation or infiltration or by decreased fluid removal which is caused by obstruction of the lymphatic drainage system.

Patients may be entirely asymptomatic or they may present with breathlessness, particularly if the effusion is large. Other symptoms include a cough and systemic symptoms such as weight loss, anorexia, and fever. Chest pain is suggestive of inflammation/infiltration of the parietal pleura and points towards malignancy or empyema.

It is crucial to illicit the underlying diagnosis rapidly with a minimum of invasive tests in order to allow appropriate management of the causative disease process.

Approach to diagnosis

The initial assessment of a patient with a pleural effusion requires a thorough medical history with particular attention to the following:

Systemic symptoms: High fevers are suggestive of parapneumonic effusion/empyema or tuberculosis. Weight loss/anorexia points towards malignancy or empyema.
Past medical history: In particular, look for previous malignancy or systemic diseases which can be associated with pleural effusion.
Occupational history: Asbestos exposure can cause both malignant mesothelioma and benign asbestos-related pleural effusion. The

Table 19.1 Transudative pleural effusions

- Congestive heart failure
- Cirrhosis
- Nephrotic syndrome
- Peritoneal dialysis
- Hypothyroidism
- Pulmonary embolism (in 10–20% of cases)
- Malignancy (in 5% of cases)

Reproduced with permission from Sprigings D, Chambers JB. *Acute Medicine*, fourth edition, Wiley-Blackwell, Oxford, UK, Copyright © 2008.

Table 19.2 Exudative pleural effusions

- Parapneumonic effusion and empyema
- Malignancy
- Pulmonary embolism
- Congestive heart failure after diuretic therapy
- Mesothelioma
- Tuberculosis
- Rheumatoid arthritis and systemic lupus erythematosus
- Esophageal rupture
- Pancreatitis
- Postcardiotomy syndrome
- Drug-induced
- Chylothorax

Reproduced with permission from Sprigings D, Chambers JB. Acute Medicine, fourth edition, Wiley-Blackwell, Oxford, UK, Copyright © 2008.

temporal relationship with the asbestos exposure is important, with mesothelioma often having a lag time of decades whereas benign asbestos-related effusion normally presents within 10 years of asbestos exposure.

The patient should be examined with close attention being paid to the presence of any palpable lymph nodes, cachexia, and peripheral oedema suggestive of either congestive cardiac failure or a low-protein state. Auscultation of the lungs will reveal diminished breath sounds over the pleural effusion, with stony dullness to percussion.

Specific clues to the diagnosis

Specific clues to the diagnosis are as follows:

Exudate vs transudate: Pleural fluid can be defined as exudative or transudative, according to the concentration of protein and/or lactate dehydrogenase (LDH) within the fluid. Light's criteria have a sensitivity of 97% and a specificity of 80% for diagnosing an exudate (Table 19.3).
Unilateral vs bilateral pleural effusion: A unilateral pleural effusion invariably requires further investigation to determine the underlying pathological process. Bilateral pleural effusions in the presence of a history consistent with left ventricular dysfunction can safely be managed with medical treatments for heart failure without further tests. However, if the effusions are treatment resistant, further investigations should be pursued.
Pleuritic chest pain: The presence of pleuritic chest pain implies involvement of the parietal pleura. This almost invariably suggests that the effusion is exudative in nature and most likely infectious or malignant, although pulmonary embolism with associated lung infarction is an important differential.

Key diagnostic tests

The diagnostic workup of a patient with a pleural effusion should be systematic and based upon clinical judgement and results of initial investigations (see Figure 19.1).

Pleural fluid

In most cases, a sample of pleural fluid should be obtained. This should be analysed for the following:

Biochemistry: Protein and LDH should be measured to define whether the effusion is transudative or exudative. The pH of the fluid should

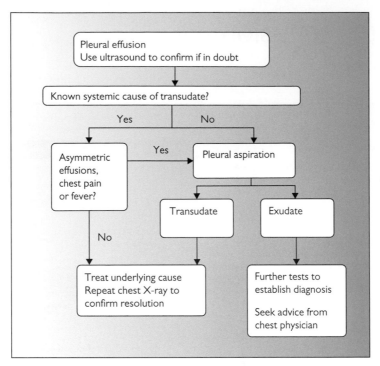

Figure 19.1 Management of pleural effusion.

Reproduced with permission from Sprigings D, Chambers JB. *Acute Medicine*, fourth edition, Wiley-Blackwell, Oxford, UK, Copyright © 2008.

be measured, particularly when pleural infection is suspected. If the pH is <7.2, an intercostal drain should be inserted.

Microbiology: Routine bacterial culture and alcohol/acid fast bacilli should be performed to assess for the presence of bacterial infection or tuberculosis.

Cytology: A sample should be assessed for the presence of malignant cells. A differential cell count can also be helpful. A lymphocyte count >80% is suggestive of tuberculosis. If initial tests are non-diagnostic, a repeat cytology sample can improve the sensitivity for malignant effusions.

See Tables 19.3 and 19.4 for overview of pleural fluid analyses.

Table 19.3 Pleural fluid analysis (1)

Test	Comment
Visual inspection	Blood-stained effusion (pleural fluid hematocrit 1–20% of peripheral hematocrit) is likely to be due to malignancy, pulmonary embolism or trauma
	Purulent fluid signifies empyema
Protein and lactate dehydrogenase (LDH)	These are the only tests needed if the effusion is likely to be a transudate
	Pleural fluid LDH correlates with the degree of pleural inflammation
	Exudative pleural effusions have a protein concentration >30 g/L
	If the pleural fluid protein is around 30g/L, Light's criteria are helpful in distinguishing between a transudate and exudate. An exudate is identified by one or more of the following: • Pleural fluid protein to serum protein ratio >0.5 • Pleural fluid LDH to serum LDH ratio >0.6 • Pleural fluid LDH more than two-thirds the upper limit of normal for serum LDH

Reproduced with permission from Sprigings D, Chambers JB. Acute Medicine, fourth edition, Wiley-Blackwell, Oxford, UK, Copyright © 2008.

Table 19.4 Pleural fluid analysis (2): Additional tests for exudative pleural effusion

Test	Comment
Pleural fluid pH and glucose (check these if a parapneumonic or malignant pleural effusion is suspected. Send sample in heparinized syringe for measurement of pH in blood gas analyzer)	Low pH (<7.3)/low glucose (<3.3 mmol/L) pleural fluid may be seen in: • Complicated parapneumonic effusion and empyema • Malignancy • Rheumatoid or lupus pleuritis • Tuberculosis • Esophageal rupture
Cytology (total and differential cell count; malignant cells)	Neutrophilia (>50% cells) indicate acute pleural disease
	Lymphocytosis is seen in malignancy, tuberculous pleuritis and in pleural effusions after CABG
	The yield of cytology is influenced by the histological type of malignancy: >70% positive in adenocarcinoma, 25–50% in lymphoma, 10% in mesothelioma
Microbiology (Gram stain and culture; markers of tuberculosis (TB))	Send fluid for markers of TB if TB is suspected or there is a pleural fluid lymphocytosis
Other tests depending on the clinical setting (e.g. amylase, triglyceride)	Elevated pleural fluid amylase is seen in acute pancreatitis and esophageal rupture
	Check triglyceride level if chylothorax is suspected (opaque white effusion); chylothorax (triglyceride >1.1 g/L) is due to disruption of the thoracic duct by trauma or lymphoma

CABG, coronary artery bypass graft.

Reproduced with permission from Sprigings D, Chambers JB. Acute Medicine, fourth edition, Wiley-Blackwell, Oxford, UK, Copyright © 2008.

Pleural biopsy

If the initial tests do not provide a firm diagnosis, then a pleural biopsy should be obtained. This can be taken 'blind' with an Abrams needle; under radiological guidance, with a cutting biopsy needle; or at thoracoscopy. The only indication for Abrams biopsy is a suspected tuberculous effusion, as the sensitivity for malignant effusions with a blind biopsy is almost half that with either radiologically guided biopsy or thoracoscopy.

Introduction to therapy

The management strategy for a pleural effusion is aimed at relieving symptoms and treating the underlying pathology. In the case of transudative effusions, effective treatment of the causative process is normally all that is required.

Removal of pleural fluid can be achieved in two ways: therapeutic thoracocentesis or intercostal drain insertion. An intercostal drain should only be inserted once a diagnosis has been achieved, as complete drainage of the pleural space may inhibit the ability to perform thoracoscopy. The only urgent indication for intercostal drain is empyema or parapneumonic effusion with a pleural fluid pH <7.2. If a patient is very breathless, and a diagnosis has not been made, then withdrawal of up to 1 litre of pleural fluid by thoracocentesis will relieve symptoms. The vast majority of pleural procedures should be performed at times when the hospital is well staffed and by experienced practitioners. If an effusion is recurrent or the patient has trapped lung, making effective pleurodesis impossible, a long-term indwelling pleural catheter can be sited. This allows the patient to drain off fluid on a regular basis to relieve symptoms.

Malignant pleural effusions, both mesothelioma and metastatic, require a management strategy aimed at reducing symptoms and optimising quality of life. Pleural fluid can be controlled with pleurodesis via intercostal drain, talc poudrage via thoracoscopy or insertion of in-dwelling pleural catheter. There is currently no clear evidence to define the optimal approach and so patients should be given a choice.

Pleural infection should be treated initially with empirical antibiotics guided by local policy. The bacteriology of pleural infection differs between community acquired and hospital acquired infection. Anaerobes often co-infect the pleural space thus anaerobic antibiotic cover should be continued even if an aerobic bacteria is cultured.

Prognosis

The prognosis of a patient with a pleural effusion is dependent upon the underlying pathology. The life expectancy for patients with malignant pleural effusion or mesothelioma is poor, with a 2-year survival rate of approximately 20%, whereas most patients with a parapneumonic effusion or empyema will make a full recovery with appropriate antibiotics.

Dealing with diagnostic uncertainty

Even if the comprehensive investigation pathway previously described in this chapter is followed, there will always be a small proportion of cases in which a definitive diagnosis cannot be made. It is crucial in cases like these to review thoroughly the case history and revisit any possible symptoms which could suggest malignancy outwith the pleural space. If no underlying pathology is found, a diagnosis of idiopathic pleural effusion is made. Most idiopathic pleural effusions follow a benign course, although some will later turn out to be malignant and so all cases should receive regular follow-up.

A particular challenge can be differentiating the histology of mesothelioma from other tumours such as adenocarcinoma. Often, despite extensive immunohistochemical stains, it is impossible to say with certainty what the primary tumour is. In this situation, a multidisciplinary approach is essential to conclude the final diagnosis and management plan.

Further Reading

Debiane LG and Ost ED. Advances in the management of malignant pleural effusion. *Curr Opin Pulm Med* 2017; 23:317–22.

Light RW. The Light criteria: the beginning and why they are useful 40 years later. *Clin Chest Med* 2013; 34: 21–26. http://dx.doi.org/10.1016/j.ccm.2012.11.006.

Sahn SA. Getting the most from pleural fluid analysis. *Respirology* 2012; 17: 270–7.

CHAPTER 19 **Pleural effusion**

20 Chylothorax

Anjali Crawshaw

Definition of the disease

Chylothorax is an accumulation of lymphatic fluid in the pleural space due to obstruction or injury of the thoracic duct.

Aetiology of the disease

Malignant disease causing obstruction of the thoracic duct accounts for more than 50% of cases; lymphoma is the most common cause. Non-malignant causes are rare. Trauma to the thoracic duct can result from mediastinal surgery, most commonly oesophagectomy. The causes of chylothorax are given in Box 20.1.

Typical symptoms of the disease, and less common symptoms

Dyspnoea and tachypnoea are common, as with pleural effusion of any aetiology. Pleuritic pain and fever are uncommon unless due to underlying disease, as chyle does not irritate the pleural surface.

Demographics of the disease

Chylothorax can occur at any age. There is no gender difference.

Box 20.1 Causes of chylothorax

Congenital
- atresia of the thoracic duct
- pleural thoracic duct fistula

Traumatic
- blunt/penetrating injury
- surgical:
  - oesophagectomy
  - lymph node excision
  - radical neck dissection
  - pneumonectomy
  - aortic repair
  - sympathectomy
- other iatrogenic:
  - subclavian vein catheterization
  - lumbar arteriography

Neoplasms
- lymphoma:
  - non-Hodgkin's
  - Hodgkin's
- benign tumours
- post-radiotherapy

Miscellaneous
- diseases affecting the lymph vessels:
  - sarcoidosis
  - amyloidosis
  - lymphangioleiomyomatosis
- yellow nail syndrome

Natural history and complications of the disease

Malnutrition and immunocompromise (T-cell deficiency) result from the loss of chyle, which is rich in proteins, fats, electrolytes, bicarbonate, fat-soluble vitamins, and lymphocytes.

Approach to diagnosing the disease

Clinical examination and chest radiography should suggest the presence of pleural fluid. A pleural-fluid triglyceride level >110 mg/dl is diagnostic of chylothorax. A low pleural-fluid cholesterol level, the presence of chylomicrons, and a high lymphocyte count support the diagnosis. The appearance of the fluid may be misleading, resulting in under-diagnosis of chylothorax: the classic milky appearance is seen in around 50% of cases.

Other diagnoses that should be considered

Empyema is an important differential requiring early recognition and treatment. The pleural-fluid pH will be low (<7.2). Although the fluid may appear cloudy, when centrifuged, the supernatant is clear.

Pseudochylothorax occurs in more chronic pleural effusion and is characterized by a high cholesterol level (typically >200 mg/dl, although it may exceed 1000 mg/dl). The effusion is usually sterile and requires no treatment unless large enough to cause respiratory compromise. Tuberculous effusions account for more than 50% of pseudochylothorax cases.

Other relevant investigations

A full blood count should be performed, and serum electrolytes and albumin should be monitored. A staging CT should be performed to identify the cause unless the chylothorax is clearly iatrogenic. Lymphangiography may be useful where the site of a persistent leak cannot be determined.

Prognosis

Mortality with conservative management of iatrogenic chylothorax approaches 50%, improving to around 10% with aggressive surgical intervention. Malignant chylothorax has a worse prognosis.

Treatment and its effectiveness

The fluid should be drained and the underlying cause should be treated. Where iatrogenic, the leak should be identified and ligated. Nutritional state should be carefully managed with a low-fat diet with medium-chain fatty acids (absorbed directly into portal circulation), and total parenteral nutrition. Where surgery is not possible or appropriate, pleurodesis is often successful. Somatostatin and octreotide have been used successfully to reduce intestinal chyle production and thereby the chyle losses.

Further Reading

Nair SK, Petko M, and Hayward MP. Aetiology and management of chylothorax in adults. *Eur J Cardiothorac Surg* 2007; 32: 362–9.
Schild HH, Strassburg CP, Welz A, et al. Treatment options in patients with chylothorax. *Dtsch Arztebl Int* 2013; 110: 819–26.

21 Difficulty swallowing

Satish Keshav and Alexandra Kent

Definition of the symptom

Dysphagia is a difficulty in the process of swallowing.

Common causes

Dysphagia is an alarm symptom, and therefore requires referral to secondary care for investigation. There are multiple causes, divided into oesophageal, neurological, surgical, and extrinsic obstruction, as shown in Table 21.1. Investigation and treatment of non-oesophageal causes is not covered in detail in this section.

Context

Swallowing is a complex process involving coordination of many nerves and over 50 pairs of muscles and can be divided into oral, pharyngeal, and oesophageal phases. It is important to ascertain whether patients have a problem initiating the swallow (suggesting a neurological cause) or describe a sensation of 'food sticking' (suggesting oesophageal causes). Dysphagia can lead to weight loss and malnutrition; it also predisposes to aspiration pneumonia. Acute dysphagia has an annual incidence of ~13 per 100 000 population and is usually due to food impaction in obstructing lesions or eosinophilic oesophagitis.

Approach to diagnosis

The cornerstone to diagnosing the cause of dysphagia is a careful medical history. It is important to assess whether dysphagia is intermittent or progressive, and ask for associated symptoms, including heartburn, weight loss, haematemesis, coffee-ground emesis, anaemia, regurgitation of food particles, and respiratory symptoms. Furthermore, it is important to determine the type of food that produces dysphagia (solid vs liquid) and the temporal association to symptoms. For example, motility disorders may produce intermittent symptoms, whereas obstructing lesions (cancer, peptic strictures) will be progressive, involving solids before liquids.

Specific clues to the diagnosis

Specific clues to the diagnosis are as follows:

- Cancers causing obstruction will cause progressive dysphagia, from liquids to solids, with no relief from symptoms. Patients often have associated systemic symptoms including weight loss, anaemia, and chest pain, and risk factors such as smoking.
- Patients with peptic strictures will have an underlying history of gastro-oesophageal reflux.
- Achalasia is a progressive disease often developing over months to years, and may be associated regurgitation or chest pain.
- Motility disorders often have an intermittent history, and associated symptoms including chest pain, heartburn, and regurgitation. There may be symptoms of underlying disease, such as scleroderma, dermatomyositis, Sjögren's syndrome, and so on.
- Pharyngeal pouches are slowly progressive and have associated regurgitation and gurgling.
- Patients with eosinophilic oesophagitis are often younger with a history of atopy.

Key diagnostic tests

Any patient suffering dysphagia requires an upper gastrointestinal (GI) endoscopy, to rule out obstructing lesions. Furthermore, this provides the opportunity to obtain oesophageal biopsies to exclude eosinophilic oesophagitis.

Other diagnostic tests

Patients who are felt to be at risk of complications from endoscopic procedures (comorbidities, such as severe heart or lung disease) should undergo a barium swallow, which will identify mucosal lesions and motility disorders such as achalasia. Oesophageal biopsies taken at the time of endoscopy are fundamental to the diagnosis of eosinophilic oesophagitis. In cases of a normal endoscopy and biopsies, patients should undergo oesophageal manometry to identify a motility disorder.

Patients who have a problem initiating swallowing may have a neurological cause. These patients should undergo CT head, assessment by speech and language therapists (SALT) and video fluoroscopy. Assessment by SALT is important to reduce the risk of aspiration.

Table 21.1 Causes of dysphagia		
		Incidence
Oesophageal	Tumours Oesophagitis Eosinophilic oesophagitis Peptic stricture Diverticulum Rings and webs Motility disorders Scleroderma Functional	Most common causes are peptic stricture and oesophagitis; with increasing age, the incidence of dysmotility increases; dysphagia in juveniles and young adults is more likely to be due to eosinophilic oesophagitis
Extrinsic compression	Aberrant subclavian artery Cervical osteophytes Enlarged aorta Enlarged left atrium Mediastinal mass	Rare
Surgical	Laryngectomy Pharyngectomy Oesophagectomy Head and neck surgery	Rare
Neurological	Stroke or traumatic brain injury Multiple sclerosis Myasthenia gravis Myopathy (dermatomyositis, myotonic dystrophy) Poliomyelitis Cervical brace Cervical spondylosis Motor neuron disease (e.g. amyotrophic lateral sclerosis) Parkinson's disease and other degenerative disorders Cerebral palsy	Increasing with age
Other	Age, ventilator dependency	

Introduction to therapy

Therapy is dictated by the underlying diagnosis:

- Strictures can be treated with endoscopic balloon dilatation, although cancerous strictures have a significantly higher risk of perforation, compared to benign peptic strictures. Patients suffering with oesophageal cancers unsuitable for surgical resection or curative procedures may gain symptomatic relief from placement of an oesophageal stent.
- Oesophagitis and peptic strictures require high-dose therapy with proton-pump inhibitors.
- Achalasia is treated with smooth muscle relaxants, botulinum toxin, balloon dilatation, or surgical myotomy.
- Eosinophilic oesophagitis responds to elimination diets and/or topical steroids in the majority of patients.

Prognosis

Overall prognosis is highly dependent on the underlying diagnosis. However, in most conditions, relief of dysphagia is achievable.

How to handle uncertainty in the diagnosis of this symptom

It is important to take a detailed history, as patients may misinterpret their symptoms, for example, describing 'difficulty in swallowing' when their main symptom is pain on swallowing (odynophagia). Standard tests may yield no clear diagnosis. Dysmotility in the early stages can be subtle, and tests may be negative. However, with time, symptoms may worsen, and subsequent testing may reveal a diagnosis previously not established. Rarely, pseudoachalasia, which is caused by an infiltrating tumour in the gastric cardia, may be misdiagnosed or missed.

Further Reading

Johnston BT. Oesophageal dysphagia: a stepwise approach to diagnosis and management. *Lancet Gastroenterol Hepatol* 2017; 2: 604–09.

22 Haematemesis

Satish Keshav and Alexandra Kent

Definition of the symptom

Haematemesis is the vomiting of fresh or altered blood.

Common causes

Haematemesis is almost exclusively dealt with in the hospital setting, as it is a medical emergency (see Box 22.1). Mallory–Weiss tear, which typically occurs after prolonged vomiting and retching, usually is of small volume, without haemodynamic compromise, and is usually self-limiting, may be recognized as such and not always referred to secondary care. Rare causes of haematemesis are unlikely to be encountered by most general practitioners. No cause for the haematemesis is found in 17% of cases, despite investigation. Endoscopy in the emergency setting can be difficult, and lesions may be missed. The Mallory–Weiss tear may have healed by the time endoscopy is performed, and Dieulafoy lesions may only be transiently visible. Haemoptysis and vomiting of red-stained food can be mistaken for haematemesis, possibly accounting for some cases where a diagnosis is not established.

Context

Upper gastrointestinal haemorrhage (UGIH) has an incidence of 50–150 cases per 100 000 population. Upper gastrointestinal bleeds have a 10% mortality rate, and as such should be treated as a medical emergency. The airway, breathing, and circulation (ABC) should be **immediately** assessed in all patients, as this reflects intravascular volume and the presence of ongoing bleeding. However, the physiological response to blood loss can mask signs and symptoms until >40% of the intravascular volume has been lost. Despite the use of proton-pump inhibitors (PPIs), admission rates for peptic ulcer haemorrhage have increased in older age groups, probably related to increased use of antiplatelet agents and anticoagulants. Further reductions in mortality and morbidity may be prevented by the rising age of the population.

The commonest cause of haematemesis is peptic ulceration, accounting for nearly 50% of cases. Risk factors include the use of NSAIDs, including aspirin; *Helicobacter pylori* infection; smoking; and alcohol use. Ninety per cent of duodenal ulcers, and 70% of gastric ulcers, are associated with *H. pylori*, and eradication is integral to treatment. Excess alcohol consumption has doubled the incidence of variceal bleeding over the past 10 years; this condition carries a high mortality that is related to underlying portal hypertension and liver disease/cirrhosis.

Rapid access to specialist care and emergency endoscopy are desirable, although this standard of care is not yet universally available in the United Kingdom. Integrated management by the acute medical and gastroenterology teams is, however, critically important, whatever the local service structure.

Approach to diagnosis

History and examination will often give clues to the underlying cause of bleeding. If possible, be certain that the blood was vomited rather than coughed up. Was it a large or small volume, and was there evidence of volume depletion, such as feeling faint, weak, sweaty, or unwell? The list of medications can identify precipitants (e.g. aspirin, NSAIDs), medications likely to worsen bleeding (e.g. aspirin, warfarin, clopidogrel), and medications that may mask signs of intravascular depletion (e.g. beta blockers).

Examination should ascertain the level of cardiovascular compromise: level of consciousness, breathing, pulse rate, blood pressure, and postural hypotension. It should also include a rectal examination to check for melaena, the presence of which confirms significant UGIH. Signs of chronic liver disease suggest that variceal bleeding is more likely. This can be torrential and life-threatening and therefore enhanced care is appropriate: for example, early referral to gastroenterology, rapid replacement of blood, attention to comorbidity such as sepsis, and intensive nursing care. Nonetheless, peptic ulceration remains a major cause of haemorrhage even in those with portal hypertension, accounting for 20%–40% of bleeding episodes.

It is important to remember that the circulating haemoglobin level will not fall after haematemesis until the patient has replaced their lost circulating volume with plasma. Therefore, the first test in the emergency setting may be completely or nearly normal. This should not be regarded as reassuring!

Specific clues to the diagnosis

Establishing that haematemesis has occurred may require endoscopy if non-invasive tests are negative. There is no wholly satisfactory alternative to this, although passage of a nasogastric tube, followed by gastric lavage with a few hundred millilitres of saline, may be helpful in some circumstances. A negative lavage may allow the medical team to search more efficiently elsewhere for the cause of hypotension and anaemia, for instance. Endoscopy also allows a diagnosis to be made of the cause of haematemesis. Clues to the underlying diagnosis are shown in Table 22.1. The advantage of rapid or immediate endoscopy is that it also enables therapy to be administered.

Box 22.1 Causes of haematemesis

Common
- duodenal ulcer*
- gastric ulcer
- oesophageal varices*
- Mallory–Weiss tear

Infrequent
- vascular malformations:
  - Dieulafoy lesions
  - gastric antral vascular ectasia (GAVE)
  - angiodysplasia
- upper gastrointestinal cancer oesophagitis*
- gastroduodenal erosions

Rare
- haemobilia
- aortoenteric fistula

* Common with excess alcohol.

Table 22.1 Causes of upper gastrointestinal haemorrhage

Diagnosis	Symptoms, signs, clues
Peptic ulcer disease	Dyspepsia
	Smoking/alcohol/caffeine
	Medications: aspirin, NSAIDs
Varices	Excess alcohol consumption
	Signs of chronic liver disease or portal hypertension
Mallory–Weiss tears	Vomiting prior to haematemesis
Upper gastrointestinal cancers	Weight loss, dysphagia, early satiety, anaemia, older age (>50 years)
Haemobilia	Recent endoscopic retrograde cholangiopancreatography
	Gallstones
Aortoenteric fistula	Aortic aneurysm surgery, signs of endovascular infection

Table 22.2 Rockall score				
Variable	Score			
	0	1	2	3
Age	<60	60–79	>80	
Shock	No shock Systolic BP >100 Pulse <100	Systolic BP >100 Pulse >100	Systolic BP <100	
Comorbidity	None	None	Cardiac failure Ischaemic heart disease Any major comorbidity	Renal failure Liver failure Disseminated malignancy
Diagnosis	Mallory–Weiss tear No lesion and no SRH	All other diagnoses	Malignancy of GI tract	
Major signs of recent haemorrhage	None or dark spot		Blood in upper GI tract Adherent clot Visible or spurting vessel	

Mortality rates (%) as related to initial Rockall score								
Initial risk score	0	1	2	3	4	5	6	7
Mortality	0.2	2.4	5.6	11	24.6	39.6	48.9	50

Key diagnostic tests

Upper GI endoscopy can be used to diagnose the cause of bleeding and provide therapy for ongoing bleeding. The risk of endoscopy must be weighed against the benefit, especially in the elderly and those with underlying cardiorespiratory disease. As a rule, the patient should have adequate fluid resuscitation with a haemoglobin level above 8 g/dl before endoscopy is attempted. Aspiration of gastric contents including blood can cause life-threatening aspiration pneumonia, and therefore the airway must be adequately safeguarded in all patients, and this may necessitate prophylactic endotracheal intubation and ventilation in some cases.

Other diagnostic tests

Visceral angiography and radionuclide scanning rely on rapid bleeding to identify the source. These are an alternative or adjunct to endoscopy, particularly where the endoscopy has not provided a diagnosis. If angiography is performed, it should be performed in a setting that allows therapeutic intervention, such as embolization of a bleeding vessel.

Introduction to therapy

Immediate therapy includes assessing, protecting, and maintaining the airway, breathing, and circulation; fluid resuscitation; and replacement of blood. Postural hypotension may be the first sign of intravascular depletion. Once the patient's condition has been stabilized and their condition assessed, early upper GI endoscopy should be arranged and performed.

Patients thought to have bleeding varices should immediately receive intravenous terlipressin (a somatostatin analogue) prior to endoscopy. If varices are confirmed at endoscopy, terlipressin should be continued for 72 hours (2 mg four times daily).

Thrombocytopenia and coagulopathy should be corrected where necessary: aim to maintain platelets above 40, and administer 10 mg of vitamin K in addition to fresh frozen plasma where necessary. In portal hypertension due to liver disease it can be impossible to maintain normal coagulation status, which should not be pursued at all cost. Give broad-spectrum antibiotics in people with cirrhosis, as non-specific bacteraemia is a recognized risk factor for variceal haemorrhage, possibly by increasing portal venous pressure.

PPIs are an important part of the treatment of non-variceal UGIH. PPIs raise the gastric pH, improving platelet function and coagulation. Patients requiring endoscopic therapy for bleeding ulcers should receive a PPI infusion (80 mg stat, then 8 mg/hour for 72 hours). All patients with peptic ulcers should be tested and treated for *H. pylori*.

Prognosis

The risk of death from UGIH is approximately 10%, and most deaths occur in the elderly with more than one medical condition. This reflects the fact that bleeding is usually self-limiting or can be controlled endoscopically and medically. However, depleted physiological reserves and comorbidity mean that an episode of UGIH can be fatal. These observations have been incorporated into a prognostic score that is general use and which allows some prioritization of the use of endoscopy and other resources (see Table 22.2).

The risk of recurrent peptic ulceration can be obviated by appropriate eradication of helicobacter infection, and by the use of acid suppressants in those on aspirin or NSAIDs. The risk of variceal haemorrhage remains high for as long as the underlying disease, such as liver cirrhosis, remains. Mallory–Weiss tears do not generally recur.

How to handle uncertainty in the diagnosis of this symptom

Haematemesis is potentially life-threatening, and early referral to specialist gastroenterology and endoscopy is advisable. A non-typical history in a patient without evidence of cardiovascular compromise allows time to check for a fall in haemoglobin after a period of a few days—if this does not occur, then significant UGIH is unlikely.

Further Reading

National Institute for Health and Care Excellence. Acute upper gastrointestinal bleeding in over 16s: management. Clinical guideline [CG141]. 2012. Last updated: August 2016. https://www.nice.org.uk/guidance/cg141?unlid=12238505320161021273O.

23 Acute abdominal pain

Satish Keshav and Alexandra Kent

Definition of the symptom

Acute abdominal pain is pain which is below the chest and above the pelvic brim and which has been present for ≤4 weeks. However, typically, patients present within hours of the onset of pain.

Common causes

Acute abdominal pain is a relatively frequent presenting complaint. The diagnosis of irritable bowel syndrome requires that abdominal pain or discomfort be chronic—however, every illness has to start at some point! The differential diagnosis does not differ much in primary and secondary care, although patients in hospital are probably more likely to be prone to iatrogenic illnesses such as pancreatitis, intestinal ischaemia, and *Clostridium difficile*-associated colitis. A list of differential diagnoses is presented in Table 23.1.

Context

Acute abdominal pain can be severe, and prompt patients to seek urgent medical attention. It can also be associated other symptoms that provide clues to diagnosis, such as vomiting, diarrhoea, haematuria, or vaginal discharge. All of these must be taken into account in planning diagnosis and therapy.

Abdominal pain can be separated into three types:

Visceral pain: This originates from the abdominal viscera, which is innervated by autonomic nerves. They respond to distension and contraction. Pain is usually poorly localized, with foregut structures causing upper abdominal pain, midgut structures causing periumbilical pain, and hindgut structures causing lower abdominal pain.

Somatic pain: This corresponds to pain in the parietal peritoneum, which is innervated by somatic nerves. Somatic pain is sharp

Table 23.1 Causes of acute abdominal pain			
		Primary care	**Secondary care**
Common	Gastrointestinal disease	Gastroenteritis and food poisoning	Gastroenteritis and food poisoning
		Dyspepsia/peptic ulcer disease	Dyspepsia/peptic ulcer disease
		Cholelithiasis and cholangitis	Cholelithiasis and cholangitis
		Diverticulitis	Diverticulitis
		Pancreatitis	Pancreatitis
		Mesenteric adenitis (children)	Mesenteric adenitis (children)
		Appendicitis	Appendicitis
		Hepatitis	Hepatitis
	Non-gastroenterological causes	Dysmenorrhoea	Dysmenorrhoea
		Polycystic ovary syndrome	Polycystic ovary syndrome
		Endometriosis	Endometriosis
		Pelvic inflammatory disease	Pelvic inflammatory disease
		Urinary tract infection	Urinary tract infection
		Nephrolithiasis	Nephrolithiasis
Uncommon	Gastrointestinal disease	Intestinal obstruction, e.g. hernia, adhesions	Intestinal obstruction, e.g. hernia, adhesions
		Inflammatory bowel disease	Inflammatory bowel disease
		Peritonitis	Peritonitis
		Mesenteric angina	Mesenteric angina
	Non-gastroenterological causes	Ischaemic heart disease	Ischaemic heart disease
		Basal pneumonia	Basal pneumonia
		Herpes zoster	Herpes zoster
		Abdominal cutaneous nerve entrapment syndrome (ACNES)	Abdominal cutaneous nerve entrapment syndrome (ACNES)
		Abdominal aortic aneurysm	Abdominal aortic aneurysm
		Diabetic or alcoholic keto-acidosis	Diabetic or alcoholic keto-acidosis
Rare	Gastrointestinal disease	Sigmoid or caecal volvulus	Sigmoid or caecal volvulus
		Liver abscess	Liver abscess
		Intra-abdominal abscess	Intra-abdominal abscess
		Ischaemic colitis	Ischaemic colitis
	Non-gastroenterological causes	Ectopic pregnancy	Ectopic pregnancy
		Acute porphyria	Acute porphyria
		Opiate withdrawal	Opiate withdrawal
		Factitious abdominal pain (can be more common in e.g. children)	Factitious abdominal pain (can be more common in e.g. children)

and well localized, and is triggered by irritation, infection, or inflammation.

Referred pain: This is pain perceived in an area (usually a superficial area) which is different from the site of origin. This is thought to be due to the dermatome of the perceived pain arising from the same spinal segment that innervates the underlying abdominal structure.

It can be difficult to differentiate between pain arising from pelvic structures and pain originating from abdominal structures. Therefore, the physician should keep both in mind.

Approach to diagnosis

For information on how to approach the diagnosis, see Figure 23.1 for pain localization.

Specific clues to the diagnosis

A clear history can direct the physician to the underlying cause. Important characteristics include:

Localization and referred location: See Figure 23.1; gallbladder disease is commonly referred to the right shoulder/scapula, whereas splenic or pancreatic pain can be referred to the left shoulder. Pancreatitis, perforated duodenal ulcers, and ruptured aortic aneurysm are classically referred through to the back.

The nature of the pain: Renal and biliary colic are characterized by waves of severe constricting pain, whereas intestinal obstruction usually causes waves of dull pain, and both can be associated with vomiting. Dull colicky pain, which becomes increasingly severe, is common with pancreatitis, mesenteric ischaemia, and strangulated obstructions. Appendicitis characteristically starts with dull, peri-umbilical pain which localizes to the right iliac fossa when the parietal peritoneum is affected. Tearing severe pain is more in keeping with a ruptured aortic aneurysm.

Recurrent pain: Recurrent pain is more common with diverticulitis, gallstones, renal colic, biliary colic, or gynaecological problems, as these are often recurring problems.

Severity: Severe pain is more common with perforation, peritonitis, mesenteric ischaemia, or pancreatitis.

Onset: A sudden onset of pain is more in keeping with a sudden event, including perforated viscus, renal stone, ruptured aneurysm, ruptured ectopic pregnancy, or testicular or ovarian torsion.

Clinical examination will give important clues to the diagnosis, in particular, the severity of the condition. Serious conditions may be associated with tachycardia, hypotension, pallor, and sepsis. The abdominal examination is essential to check for signs of peritonism (tenderness,

guarding, rebound tenderness, rigidity) or obstruction (absent or tinkling bowel sounds, tympanic percussion note, distension).

Key diagnostic tests

Perforation and ruptured aortic aneurysms are rapidly fatal conditions unless treatment is instituted early. Other serious conditions, including obstruction, pancreatitis, and mesenteric ischaemia, also require rapid diagnoses. CT should be performed early and will be effective at diagnosing these and the majority of other abdominal conditions. Discuss whether or not enteral contrast is indicated or feasible. Intravenous contrast is usually administered. CT scanning has reduced the number of diagnostic laparotomies performed for acute abdominal pain.

Abdominal and pelvic ultrasound may be preferable to CT scanning in many cases—for example, for checking for gallstones, and to reduce the radiation dose in young people and potentially pregnant females. However, pregnancy should not preclude CT scanning in urgent or emergency situations.

Other diagnostic tests

Other diagnostic tests include the following:

Abdominal plain X-rays: These are particularly useful for patients with suspected obstruction (dilated bowel and air–fluid levels), perforation (free air seen under the diaphragm), and acute colitis (thickened bowel wall; check for toxic dilatation).

Urinalysis: This should be performed in all women of childbearing age, to exclude pregnancy (ectopic pregnancy). Renal colic normally causes haematuria. Acute porphyria is associated with urinary porphyrins.

Stool cultures: Stool cultures should be sent for bacterial pathogens, amoebiasis, *C. difficile* toxin, and parasites, ova, and cysts.

Blood tests: A greatly raised amylase or lipase level indicates acute pancreatitis, while upper gastrointestinal disease such as peptic ulcer may be associated with a minor elevation. Patients with acute or chronic pancreatitis may also only have modestly elevated pancreatic enzyme levels. A drop in haemoglobin can confirm a haemorrhagic cause of shock (e.g. ruptured aortic aneurysm, bleeding peptic ulcer).

Ultrasound scan: An ultrasound scan is often a more useful investigation for biliary disease, providing more detail about the biliary tree and presence of gallstones.

Endoscopy: This can aid in the diagnosis of dyspepsia and peptic ulcer disease.

Diagnostic laparoscopy: Diagnostic laparoscopy may be necessary where other tests do not provide a firm diagnosis, and where symptoms persist.

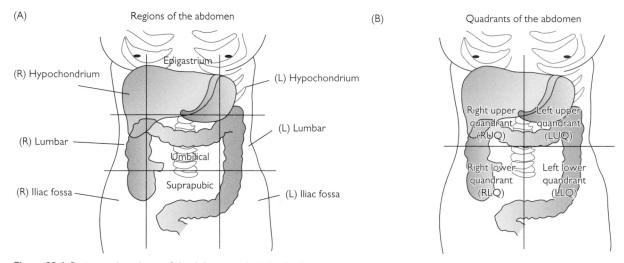

(A) Regions of the abdomen

(R) Hypochondrium — Epigastrium — (L) Hypochondrium

(R) Lumbar — Umbilical — (L) Lumbar

(R) Iliac fossa — Suprapubic — (L) Iliac fossa

(B) Quadrants of the abdomen

Right upper quandrant (RUQ) — Left upper quandrant (LUQ)

Right lower quandrant (RLQ) — Left lower quandrant (LLQ)

Figure 23.1 Regions and quadrants of the abdomen, and pain localization.
Adapted with permission from Mark Harrison, Revision Notes for the FRCEM Primary, Second Edition, Figure A.4.1, Oxford University Press, Oxford, UK, Copyright © 2017.

Introduction to therapy

Patients presenting with severe acute abdominal pain should be kept nil by mouth and treated with intravenous fluids, analgesics (usually opioids), and antibiotics until the diagnosis is clear, or symptoms resolve. The most serious causes of acute abdominal pain (perforation, peritonitis, obstruction, ruptured aortic aneurysm) will require urgent surgical intervention to remove the cause and repair associated damage. However, many other causes also require surgical care (e.g. appendicitis, ectopic pregnancy, torsion, strangulated herniae), and therefore early surgical referral is prudent. Pancreatitis and hepatitis may require intensive supportive care, and treatment, where possible, for the underlying cause. Dyspepsia and peptic ulcer disease respond to antacids and antisecretory therapy.

Prognosis

Most causes of acute abdominal pain resolve, either spontaneously or with appropriate therapy. Patients are often in severe pain, and terrified of a catastrophic outcome. Adequate analgesia and calm, competent, and urgent professional medical attention are critically important.

How to handle uncertainty in the diagnosis of this symptom

Some causes of acute abdominal pain can be catastrophic, and these should be diagnosed rapidly and treated, or excluded by appropriate testing. Other causes are either self-limiting or will reveal themselves as the illness evolves. For example, shingles may be unapparent initially, and then becomes clear when cutaneous vesicles appear in dermatomal pattern. Similarly, acute abdominal pain caused by biliary colic may occur before elevation in liver enzymes, which may be apparent the next day. Consider at all times that the primary pathology may lie outside the abdomen—especially checking for pneumonia and myocardial ischaemia.

Further Reading

Gans SL, Pols MA, Stoker J, and Boermeester MA, On behalf of the expert steering group. Guideline for the diagnostic pathway in patients with acute abdominal pain. *Dig Surg* 2015; 32: 23–31. http://www.karger.com/Article/FullText/371583.

24 Chronic abdominal pain

Satish Keshav and Alexandra Kent

Definition of the symptom

Separating chronic and acute abdominal pain is often difficult, and an arbitrary time limit of 4 weeks is often used. However, many chronic conditions (e.g. chronic pancreatitis) can cause relapsing symptoms, which may be acute during each episode.

Common causes

The common causes of abdominal pain are given in Table 24.1.

Context

The perception of abdominal pain varies between individuals and is influenced by their personality, cultural background, and psychosocial factors. Introspection, awareness of health issues, and stress increase the chance of perceiving abdominal pain as a medical complaint, and the chance of seeking medical attention. Pain receptors in the abdomen respond to chemical and mechanical stimuli. Stretch is the commonest mechanical stimulus to the viscera, although distension, torsion, and contraction are also sensed. Chemical receptors are stimulated by inflammation and infection, and this stimulation leads to the production of various substances, including serotonin, bradykinin, substance P, prostaglandins, and histamine. There are inter-individual differences in pain perception, with some people (e.g. patients with irritable bowel syndrome) being more sensitive to painful stimuli.

Chronic abdominal pain occurs in 9%–15% of all children, and is present on questioning in 75% of adolescents and 50% of adults who are otherwise healthy. It is often a non-specific symptom that alone has a poor sensitivity for organic disease. Usually, it is the associated symptoms, and/or abnormal blood tests, that direct the doctor to a diagnosis.

Table 24.1 Causes of chronic abdominal pain

Common	Gastrointestinal disease	Dyspepsia
		Irritable bowel syndrome
		Cholelithiasis
		Inflammatory bowel disease (stricturing)
	Non-gastroenterological causes	Pelvic (gynaecological) disease, e.g. fibroids, ovarian cysts (common in primary care but rare in secondary care)
Uncommon	Gastrointestinal disease	Chronic pancreatitis
		Diverticular disease
	Non-gastroenterological causes	
Rare	Gastrointestinal disease	Lactose intolerance
		Abdominal migraine
		Eosinophilic gastroenteritis/colitis
		Mesenteric ischaemia
		Abdominal endometriosis
	Non-gastroenterological causes	Familial Mediterranean fever
		Acute intermittent porphyria
		Hereditary angioedema
		Painful rib syndrome

Approach to diagnosis

It is important to differentiate between organic disease (related to pathological abnormalities) and functional disease (no identifiable cause). Pain relieved by defaecation is a classic symptom of irritable bowel syndrome, and certain symptoms make an organic disease more likely: weight loss; fever; dehydration; electrolyte abnormalities; haemodynamic compromise; gastrointestinal blood loss; malnutrition; and anaemia. A change in bowel habit is useful, although a bowel habit varying between constipation and diarrhoea is more suggestive of functional disease. Patient age is influential, with functional disease more common in young adults. Although the most common diagnoses in older patients are benign (diverticular disease, constipation), the fear of cancer influences many presentations and is an important diagnosis to exclude. Differentiating the overall time course is also useful, separating conditions that cause intermittent/relapsing pain from those that cause constant pain. Furthermore, a long history of pain is unlikely to be related to a neoplastic process.

Specific clues to the diagnosis

Specific clues to the diagnosis are the following:

Medications: It is important to take a clear prescription history, as many medications can be associated with abdominal pain, or conditions associated with abdominal pain. For example, opioid-based medications are commonly associated with constipation; NSAIDs and aspirin are associated with peptic ulcer disease; and bisphosphonates are associated with oesophagitis and oesophageal ulceration. Other medications (e.g. metformin) can directly cause abdominal pain.

Alcohol intake: patients with excessive alcohol consumption are at risk of pancreatitis, peptic ulcer disease, and alcoholic hepatitis, all of which can be associated with abdominal pain. Peptic ulcer disease will often have a characteristic story more in keeping with dyspepsia (see 'Dyspepsia'). Chronic pancreatitis is classically associated with a central persistent abdominal pain, worsened by oral intake, and radiating though to the back. Patients with alcoholic hepatitis usually have a more acute history, jaundice, and associated signs of liver dysfunction (raised liver enzymes, thrombocytopaenia, prolonged prothrombin time, etc.).

Site of pain: This can direct the physician to the underlying pathology:
- Right upper quadrant pain can be related to liver, pancreatic, and biliary tract disease.
- Left upper quadrant pain is less common and can be associated with disease of the spleen or colon. Epigastric pain is associated with gastric, pancreatic, or oesophageal disease.
- Right lower quadrant pain can relate to appendiceal, terminal ileal, or colonic disease.
- Left lower quadrant pain is more often associated with diverticular disease or other colonic diseases. Lower abdominal pain can also be caused by pelvic pathology, whereas renal disease usually causes loin pain.

Previous surgery: This can lead to surgical adhesions, placing patients at risk of subacute and acute bowel obstruction.

Background medical history: Patients with risk factors for, or the presence of, vascular disease are at an increased risk of mesenteric ischaemia. It can be associated with pain after eating ('mesenteric angina'), nausea, vomiting, and weight loss. Abdominal migraine more commonly occurs in patients who suffer from classic migraine, although this is not a prerequisite.

Dyspepsia: Pain related to acid is characteristically described as 'burning', usually in the epigastric region and radiating retrosternally. It is often worse when lying or bending over, and can be precipitated by meals, caffeine, or alcohol. Associated symptoms include acid reflux, water brash, nausea, or vomiting.

Inflammatory bowel disease: Inflammatory bowel disease is associated with diarrhoea, blood per rectum, abdominal mass, raised inflammatory markers, and anaemia.

Constipation: Constipation is associated with infrequent defaecation, incomplete evacuation, and hard stools.

Lactose intolerance: Lactose intolerance is associated with bloating and diarrhoea and is precipitated by dairy products.

Giardiasis: Giardiasis is associated with bloating and diarrhoea.

Pelvic disease: Pelvic disease is associated with pelvic pain, dyspareunia, dysmenorrhoea, menorrhagia, and abnormal vaginal bleeding. Pelvic inflammatory diseases can be associated with vaginal discharge and/or fever.

Hereditary angioedema: Hereditary angioedema is associated with intermittent swelling of the face or throat.

Muscular pain: This is pain that is precipitated by exercise and worsened by physical activity, with tender muscles.

Key diagnostic tests

Simple blood tests are a first-line investigation and can rapidly direct the doctor to the diagnosis, and influence further investigations. These should include a full blood count, haematinics (vitamin B_{12}, folate, ferritin/iron studies), urea, creatinine, electrolytes, liver chemistry, inflammatory markers (C-reactive protein/erythrocyte sedimentation rate), thyroid function, amylase, glucose, calcium, and coeliac serology.

Other diagnostic tests

Young people with chronic abdominal pain and a normal initial screen can often be diagnosed as having a functional disorder. This especially applies to patients who meet the Rome III criteria for irritable bowel syndrome. However, patients ≥50 years old almost always require further investigation to exclude a malignant process, since these occur in increasing frequency in these age groups. Associated symptoms will help direct investigations, as they will give clues as to the underlying cause. Additional investigations that should be considered include:

Colonoscopy: This is useful for patients with associated change in bowel habit. It allows direct visualization of the colon to identify abnormal lesions and diverticular disease, and provides the ability to obtain mucosal biopsies.

Gastroscopy: This can be used to visualize the upper gastrointestinal tract, to diagnose oesophageal, gastric, or duodenal inflammation or ulceration. It can also obtain biopsies to diagnose coeliac disease, eosinophilic infiltration, or the presence of *Helicobacter pylori* infection.

Ultrasound scan: This is good for visualizing the biliary tree, and diagnosing gallstones.

CT scan: This will provide clear views of all the intra-abdominal organs and can also be used to diagnose less common conditions, such as surgical adhesions. Often, a pelvic CT will be performed at the same time in order to view the pelvic organs. CT scans can be combined with angiography to visualize the mesenteric circulation and identify arterial narrowing and venous thromboses.

Laparoscopy: This is often reserved for patients with severe pain with signs or symptoms of organic disease. As a diagnostic technique, it is used far more commonly to diagnose gynaecological conditions causing chronic pain. Laparoscopy in abdominal problems is usually reserved for providing treatment, such as laparoscopic cholecystectomy, or laparoscopic fundoplication.

Lactose-hydrogen breath test: A lactose-hydrogen breath test can be performed to diagnose lactose intolerance. It is usually reserved for patients with a clear history of intolerance to dairy products.

Specific conditions: Specific conditions to look for are as follows:

  Acute intermittent porphyria is a rare, autosomal dominant condition characterized by a deficiency of the enzyme porphobilinogen deaminase, which is involved in haem synthesis. A deficiency in haem synthesis results in the metabolite porphobilinogen

accumulating in the cytoplasm. Attacks are characterized by abdominal pain, muscle weakness, neuropathies (motor, sensory, autonomic), headaches, and psychiatric symptoms. Seizures can occur. It is diagnosed by elevated urinary porphobilinogen.

Familial Mediterranean fever is an inherited inflammatory disorder which can present with abdominal attacks of pain. Diagnosis is based on characteristic attacks of pain, and genetic testing is now available.

Hereditary angioedema is an autosomal dominant disorder of C1 inhibitor (C1-INH) deficiency. There are three types, with differing complement levels that can aid diagnosis:

  Type 1: C1-INH low, C2 low, C4 low, C1q normal
  Type 2: C1-INH normal or raised (but dysfunctional), C2 low, C4 low, C1q normal
  Type 3: C1-INH normal, C4 normal

Introduction to therapy

Therapy in patients with chronic abdominal pain is varied, depending on the underlying diagnosis. A large number of patients will be diagnosed with functional pain related to irritable bowel syndrome or functional dyspepsia. Amitriptyline or imipramine is frequently effective for treating pain in the absence of an identified physical cause. In organic disease, treatment aimed at the underlying disease should lead to resolution of abdominal pain. Examples of the effect of therapeutic intervention include proton-pump inhibitors in dyspepsia, steroids in inflammatory bowel disease, and laparoscopic dissection of surgical adhesions. Specific treatment of disease is summarized below:

Diverticular disease: high-fibre diet and/or laxatives to avoid constipation; antibiotics for episodes of acute diverticulitis

Dyspepsia: antisecretory therapy (proton-pump inhibitors, H2 antagonists), dietary adaptations, Nissen's fundoplication

Cholelithiasis: dietary adaptation (avoid fatty food), cholecystectomy

Chronic pancreatitis: analgesics, alcohol abstinence, treatment of exocrine insufficiency with enzyme supplements

Eosinophilic gastroenteritis: corticosteroids, food elimination diet

Mesenteric ischaemia: percutaneous angioplasty, endarterectomy; no effective medical therapy exists

Familial Mediterranean fever: colchicine

acute intermittent porphyria: glucose, analgesics, high-carbohydrate diet, supportive therapy

Hereditary angioedema: supportive therapy during attacks, androgenic agents (danazol, stanozolol), tranexamic acid, C1-INH infusions prior to interventional procedures

Prognosis

Compared to causes of acute abdominal pain, chronic abdominal pain has a lower mortality, but a greater morbidity related to pain, hospital admissions, and time off work. Many conditions are relapsing, associated with severe, and often unpredictable, attacks. Organic diseases, with specific efficacious treatments (gallstones, peptic ulcer disease) have an overall good prognosis, with resolution of pain with appropriate therapy. Functional diseases have the potential to cause far more morbidity, with far less effective treatment, although symptoms are rarely lifelong. It is common for functional symptoms to recur at times of stress and/or concomitant illness.

How to handle uncertainty in the diagnosis of this symptom

The main uncertainty associated with chronic abdominal pain lies in the decision between organic and functional disease. However, pain occurring in isolation is not common, and associated symptoms can aid diagnosis and investigation choice. Generally, a full blood screen and abdominal CT will exclude the majority of conditions. The unusual diagnoses, such as acute intermittent porphyria or familial Mediterranean fever, present with characteristic attacks and are unlikely to be the cause in a patient presenting with abdominal pain alone. If there are no associated symptoms, and blood and imaging tests are normal, then a functional disorder is the most likely diagnosis.

Further Reading

Makharia GK. Understanding and treating abdominal pain and spasms in organic gastrointestinal diseases: Inflammatory bowel disease and biliary diseases. *J Clin Gastroenterol* 2011; 45: S89–S93.

Vermeulen W, De Man JG, Pelckmans PA, and De Winter BY. Neuroanatomy of lower gastrointestinal pain disorders. *World J Gastroenterol* 2014; 20: 1005–20.

25 Dyspepsia

Satish Keshav and Alexandra Kent

Definition of the symptom

Dyspepsia is a term encompassing several symptoms of the upper gastrointestinal (GI) tract), including acid reflux, heartburn, nausea, vomiting, and abdominal pain or discomfort.

Common causes

The majority of patients presenting to their GP with dyspepsia will be suffering with gastro-oesophageal reflux disease (GORD) and will respond to a course of antisecretory therapy (proton-pump inhibitors (PPI) or H2 antagonists). Of those who are referred onto secondary care and then subsequently undergo endoscopy, the cause is GORD (40%), functional or non-ulcer dyspepsia (40%), peptic ulcer disease (13%), or upper GI cancer (3%). Ten per cent of the population will have a hiatus hernia; this is a condition where a defect in the diaphragm allows part of the stomach to move into the chest. It can cause weakness in the lower oesophageal sphincter and be associated with GORD. However, many patients with a hiatus hernia do not suffer with dyspepsia. Functional dyspepsia is a condition characterized by dyspepsia symptoms, with no endoscopic evidence of acid damage, and normal oesophageal pH studies. It is thought to be due to oesophageal hypersensitivity and, as such, is usually poorly responsive to acid-related therapies.

Context

Up to 40% of the population suffer with dyspepsia; 5%–10% will consult their GP, and 1% will undergo endoscopic assessment. Over-the-counter medications cost patients £100 million annually, and prescribed drugs cost the NHS over £463 million annually. There is a steady rise in incidence with increasing age. *Helicobacter pylori* is present in 40% of the UK population, with many individuals acquiring the infection in childhood and remaining asymptomatic. It has been associated with peptic ulcer disease and distal gastric cancer.

Approach to diagnosis

A clear history should be taken, to identify the following alarm symptoms and factors contributing to symptoms:

Alarm symptoms: progressive weight loss, GI bleeding, iron deficiency anaemia, dysphagia, persistent vomiting, or an epigastric mass
Medications: NSAIDs, antiplatelet agents, bisphosphonates, nitrates, calcium channel antagonists, theophyllines, and steroids
Lifestyle: obesity, alcohol, coffee, chocolate, and fatty foods have all been associated with acid reflux
Psychological disorders: patients with functional dyspepsia are more likely to have psychological disorders

Specific clues to the diagnosis

Alarm symptoms have a poor positive predictive value for diagnosing upper GI cancer, but should still instigate an urgent referral. Patients with persistent symptoms despite PPI therapy will usually have functional dyspepsia, although this assumption should not be made in older patients.

Key diagnostic tests

H. pylori tests

H. pylori can be assessed by serology, faecal antigen test, or C-urea breath tests.

Endoscopy

Endoscopy should be reserved for those with alarm symptoms or suspicious radiological investigations. However, patients over 55 years with persistent symptoms, previous gastric ulcer or surgery, a family history of gastric cancer, a continuing need for NSAIDs, or pernicious anaemia should also be referred for endoscopic assessment.

There is no evidence for endoscopic screening for Barrett's oesophagus in patients with dyspepsia, as the absolute risk of adenocarcinoma is less than 1 in 1000. Furthermore, 40% of patients with Barrett's-associated adenocarcinoma are asymptomatic.

Other diagnostic tests

Oesophageal pH studies can identify between patients with pathological acid exposure and those with functional dyspepsia. This investigation involves placement of a pH probe 5 cm above the lower oesophageal sphincter. This can be achieved either by placement of a naso-oesophageal probe or a wireless capsule (less readily available). This procedure is usually reserved for patients with typical symptoms of GORD but who are failing to respond to a trial of PPI; those contemplating anti-reflux surgery; or patients with persistent GORD symptoms after anti-reflux surgery. Multichannel intra-luminal impedance is a newer oesophageal investigation which measures electrical resistance within the oesophagus, and can provide information regarding bolus transport within the oesophagus. When combined with a pH study, it can identify acid and non-acid reflux episodes.

Introduction to therapy

Lifestyle measures, such as weight loss, reduced alcohol intake, and smoking cessation, are integral to treatment. Raising the head of the bed may reduce nocturnal acid reflux. Dyspepsia is invariably a relapsing remitting condition. Medications used for dyspepsia include:

Antacids/alginates: These contain calcium carbonate, aluminium, or magnesium, and work by neutralizing gastric acid and inhibiting the proteolytic enzyme pepsin. They can relieve the symptoms of dyspepsia, although there is no evidence that they can heal peptic ulcers.
PPIs: These block the hydrogen–potassium pump in the gastric lining, and can relieve symptoms and promote ulcer healing.
H2 antagonists: These block the histamine H2 receptors in the gastric mucosa, reducing acid secretion, relieving symptoms, and promoting ulcer healing.
Misoprostol: This is a synthetic prostaglandin analogue, reducing acid secretion and promoting ulcer healing.

Initial treatment for dyspepsia should be test and treat for *H. pylori* and/or empirical PPI treatment for 1 month. PPI can be continued at the lowest dose necessary to control symptoms. Those unresponsive to PPI should be offered H2 antagonists or prokinetic therapy. The only curative treatments are *H. pylori* eradication and anti-reflux surgery. The most common surgical procedure is a Nissen's fundoplication, which is usually performed laparoscopically. However, long-term outcomes from surgically and medically treated patients are not statistically different.

Functional dyspepsia can be harder to treat, and is usually poorly responsive to acid-blocking therapy. Psychological therapies have shown a modest, but short-lived response. Some patients respond to tricyclic antidepressants such as amitriptyline, although there is little evidence to support this treatment strategy.

Prognosis

Persistent acid exposure in the oesophageal can lead to the development of columnar-lined epithelium (Barrett's oesophagus). This is more common in patients with a history of reflux, and is seen in 1.4% of endoscopies. The main concern with Barrett's oesophagus is the association with adenocarcinoma, developing in 1% of patients. Consequently, patients diagnosed with Barrett's oesophagus should undergo endoscopic screening, based upon the degree of dysplasia seen in the columnar cells.

How to handle uncertainty in the diagnosis of this symptom

The vast majority of patients with dyspepsia have benign disease, especially given the low incidence rates of oesophageal and gastric cancer. Despite this, a large number of patients undergo potentially unnecessary upper GI endoscopy due to persistent symptoms. In young patients, it is worthwhile giving a 2-month course of high-dose PPI prior to initiating investigations, as this will significantly increase the healing rate of peptic ulcers.

Further Reading

National Institute for Health and Care Excellence. *NICE Guidelines (CG 184) 2014: Dyspepsia and Gastro-Oesophageal Reflux Disease: Investigation and Management of Dyspepsia*. 2014. Available at https://www.nice.org.uk/Guidance/CG184 (accessed 16 Feb 2017).

26 Abdominal mass

Satish Keshav and Alexandra Kent

Definition of the symptom

Abdominal mass describes a visible or palpable swelling which is located in the abdomen and is abnormal. It may arise from one of the internal organs, such as an enlarged liver or spleen, or from musculoskeletal structures such as a floating rib; alternatively, it may be a hernia containing mesenteric or visceral tissue.

Common causes

Abdominal mass is an uncommon presenting complaint, except where patients notice a hernia. Frequently, the herniation is intermittent or minor, and can be missed on examination. Organomegaly and neoplastic masses can be hard to detect until they are large, and the question of whether or not there really is a mass frequently has to be settled by imaging such as ultrasound or CT scanning. A list of potential diagnoses is shown in Table 26.1.

Context

The significance of an abdominal mass depends to a great extent on the context in which is it is discovered—for example, did the patient notice a swelling and become consumed with a fear of cancer? Reassurance may be all that is required. Is cosmetic appearance critically important? If so, even a benign lesion may need to be assessed for potential correction. Was the discovery incidental? Or might it be related to a pathological process that has led to the examination? For example, in a patient with long-standing fatigue and mildly deranged liver tests, splenomegaly may indicate portal hypertension and cirrhosis, and may prompt a liver biopsy to establish the diagnosis.

Approach to diagnosis

There are several features of a palpable mass that can help develop a differential diagnosis:

- Where is the mass?
- What is the relationship of the mass to surrounding abdominal structures?
- Is the mass tethered to the skin or underlying structures, or is it freely mobile? (A fixed mass suggests a malignant or inflammatory process.)

Table 26.1 Causes of abdominal mass	
Common	Hernia: femoral, inguinal, umbilical, epigastric
	Lipoma
	Faecal loading in constipation
	Pregnancy
	Aneurysmal dilation of the aorta
	Uterine leiomyoma
	Obstructed urinary bladder
Uncommon	Hepatomegaly
	Splenomegaly
	Enlarged kidney: e.g. hydronephrosis, polycystic kidney
	Intra-abdominal lymphoma
	Abscess: diverticular, appendix, hepatic, Crohn's disease
	Pancreatic pseudocyst
	Abdominal and pelvic tumours
Rare	Unusual tumours such as sarcomas
	Exostoses and healed fractures

- What is the consistency (hard, firm, soft)? (A hard liver mass is possibly indicative of cancer; a firm liver mass is possibly indicative of cirrhosis; a soft liver mass is possibly a lipoma.)
- Is the mass tender? (This is typical of inflammation.)
- Is the mass pulsating? Could this be an aneurysm?
- Has the mass developed slowly or quickly? (Tumours will develop more gradually, whereas infection or inflammation can develop quickly.)
- Is the mass present all the time, or is it intermittent? (Hollow organs can fill and empty.)
- Are there associated symptoms such as weight loss, change in bowel habit, jaundice, and so on?

Specific clues to the diagnosis

The site and nature of the abdominal mass can give huge clues as to the underlying cause:

Abdominal aortic aneurysm: a pulsating mass around the umbilicus
Colon cancer: a mass anywhere in the abdomen
Crohn's disease: a tender mass anywhere in the abdomen; associated raised inflammatory markers (C-reactive protein (CRP), erythrocyte sedimentation rate (ESR))
Diverticular abscesses: tender masses, classically located in the left lower quadrant
Gallbladder cancer or cholangiocarcinoma: a moderately tender, irregularly shaped right upper quadrant mass
Gastric cancer: causes a mass in the left upper abdomen in the stomach area (epigastric) if large
Hepatic cancer: hard irregular mass or hepatomegaly in the right upper quadrant
Hepatomegaly: a mass which is located in the right costal margin and epigastric area and moves down on inspiration
Hydronephrosis: a smooth, spongy-feeling ballottable mass in one or both flanks
Ovarian cysts or cancer: cause often smooth masses above the pelvis in the lower abdomen, arising from either side
Pancreatic abscess or pseudocyst: causes irregular masses in the upper abdomen in the epigastric area
Renal cancer: occasionally causes smooth, firm, non-tender, ballottable abdominal masses, in the flanks
Splenomegaly: palpated in the left upper quadrant, with the organ moving down on inspiration
Uterine leiomyoma (fibroids): can cause a round, lumpy mass above the pelvis in the lower abdomen
Urinary retention: a firm, often tender, mass in the suprapubic area; in extreme cases, it can extend as far up to the umbilicus
Volvulus: can cause a mass anywhere in the abdomen

Key diagnostic tests

If the history and examination do not identify the cause unequivocally, then ultrasound scanning and CT scanning are the key tests. Solid tumours may require percutaneous or laparoscopic biopsy.

Other diagnostic tests

Other imaging studies, such as magnetic resonance scanning, can provide valuable information, particularly for hepatobiliary and pancreatic masses. The presence of gastric or colonic masses may necessitate upper endoscopy or colonoscopy, respectively. Similarly, masses in the liver may necessitate endoscopic or laparoscopic investigation of the gastrointestinal and genito-urinary tract to search for a primary source of metastasis or infection. Blood tests may give information about underlying organ function or disease states. For example, a raised white-cell count would be consistent with an abscess, and CRP and the ESR will be raised in infective and inflammatory processes. Tumour markers have poor sensitivity and specificity for diagnosing tumours, although, for instance, a highly elevated CA19-9 antigen or S100 antigen would favour the diagnosis of pancreatic and ovarian tumours, respectively. Carcinoembryonic antigen (CEA), for colo-rectal cancer, and alpha-fetoprotein (AFP), for hepatocellular cancer, are similarly useful to indicate the direction for further investigation.

Introduction to therapy

When organomegaly is due to systemic disease such as infection or tumour, the approach is clearly different to that taken when the mass itself is a problem. Making a clear and definite diagnosis is key to reassuring patients and allowing a reasonable dialogue about the risks and benefits of surgery, for example. The dialogue should include a discussion of the risk of failure from hernia repair, and the relative risk of strangulation and other complications of hernia. For some masses, watchful waiting is the appropriate strategy. This is true, for example, for small aortic aneurysms, lymphadenopathy of uncertain significance, and solid tumours when it is unclear if they are benign or malignant.

Prognosis

Given the long list of differential diagnoses, the majority of patients with an abdominal mass will have a benign cause, and prognosis. Those with underlying neoplasm have a worse prognosis, because palpable neoplastic masses are more likely to be more advanced.

How to handle uncertainty in the diagnosis of this symptom

Thorough investigation of a mass that might signify serious underlying pathology is critical. A reasonable approach when there remains doubt is to identify the most likely diagnoses which merit treatment and which, if untreated, could cause morbidity or mortality. Once these have been systematically explored and excluded, watchful waiting may be offered.

Further Reading

Chen DY and Uzzo RG. Evaluation and management of the renal mass. *Med Clin North Am* 2011; 95: 179–89.
Dufay C, Abdelli A, Le Pennec V, et al. Mesenteric tumors: Diagnosis and treatment. *J Visc Surg* 2012; 149: e239–e251.

27 Constipation

Satish Keshav and Alexandra Kent

Definition of the symptom

Patients and doctors often define constipation differently. The normal frequency of defaecation is once every 3 days to three times per day, and constipation may be defined as abnormally infrequent defaecation. In addition, patients may describe hard stools, the need to strain at stool, a sense of blocked defaecation, the need to digitally or otherwise assist defaecation, or a sense of incomplete evacuation. A change in the normal pattern and frequency for the particular patient is pertinent.

Causes of constipation

There are numerous causes of constipation, and most can be encountered in both primary and secondary care. More abstruse diagnoses are more likely to be made after investigations in secondary care. Potential causes, grouped under headings, are shown in Table 27.1. Patients seen in secondary care will have causes that are similar to those of patients seen in primary care, but are usually referred when they become resistant to routine treatment or there is a need to exclude underlying pathology. Many cases are referred in order to alleviate patients' fears of an underlying cancer.

Table 27.1	Causes of constipation	
Common	Diet related	Low fibre intake
		Low fluid intake
		Low food intake
		Constipation is often due to changes in normal dietary habits
	Drug related	Opioids
		Iron supplements
		Anticholinergics
		Psychotropics
	Constitutive	Slow-transit constipation
		Old age
	Functional	Stress-related (usually transient)
		Irritable bowel syndrome (constipation predominant or mixed)
	Neurological	Parkinson's disease
		Stroke
	Endocrine disease	Hypothyroidism
		Hyperparathyroidism
Uncommon	Primary intestinal disease	Colorectal cancer
		Benign colonic stricture
		Ileus (post-operative, severe illness, electrolyte disturbance)
	Neurological	Spinal cord injury
		Multiple sclerosis
	Electrolyte disturbance	Hypercalcaemia
		Hypokalaemia
		Hypomagnesaemia
Rare	Primary intestinal disease	Volvulus
		Chronic idiopathic pseudo-obstruction (CIPO; Ogilvie's syndrome)
		Pelvic floor dysfunction
		Anorectal obstruction due to rectocele or intussusception

In patients with chronic constipation without an evident cause, irritable bowel syndrome (IBS) is the cause in 59%, pelvic floor dysfunction in 25%, slow transit in 13%, and a combination of pelvic floor dysfunction and slow transit in 3%.

Context

One UK survey found that 8.5% of women defined themselves as being constipated, and 8.2% had constipation meeting the Rome III criteria for IBS (see Chapter 205 for criteria). A larger survey (1892 adults) found that 39% of men and 52% of women reported straining at stool on over a quarter of occasions. Constipation affects twice as many women as men, with a higher prevalence in pregnant women. Prevalence is also greater in the elderly, affecting ~20% in the community.

Approach to diagnosis

A careful history is necessary to check diet, drugs, comorbidity, and symptoms that give clues as to a potential underlying cause for constipation. It is important to assess what each patient considers to be their normal bowel habit, and the effect of any change on their quality of life. Most patients feel that the effectiveness of laxatives declines with time. This is particularly true for stimulant laxatives such as senna.

Specific clues to the diagnosis

Specific clues to the diagnosis are as follows:

Colonic tumour: weight loss, rectal bleeding, tenesmus, iron deficiency anaemia, positive faecal occult blood
Volvulus: acute onset, abdominal pain
IBS: bloating, abdominal cramps, intermittent diarrhoea
Neurological causes: symptoms and signs of underlying disease
Drug-related causes: opiates, anticholinergics, antipsychotics, iron supplements
Hypothyroidism: weight gain, fatigue, cold intolerance, brittle hair, dry skin, myalgia, arthritis
Pelvic floor dysfunction: having undergone vaginal delivery, being multiparous, digital evacuation of stool, difficulty with evacuation

Key diagnostic tests

The key diagnostic test varies depending on the circumstances. Colonic transit studies help to confirm that evacuation is delayed and, in the acute setting, an abdominal X-ray may demonstrate faecal loading of the colon. Examination of the perineum, anus, and rectum to check for local disease, including excessive descent of the perineum associated with pelvic flood dysfunction, is too often omitted. Patients frequently present because they or their medical attendants are concerned about the possibility of colorectal cancer. This can be settled by optical or virtual (CT) colonoscopy. A study in patients undergoing colonoscopy to investigate constipation revealed cancers in 1.4%, and large or advanced adenomatous polyps in 4.3%.

Other diagnostic tests

Other diagnostic tests are:

Screening blood tests: These include thyroid function, biochemical profile, and fasting glucose.
Rectal manometry and special studies to delineate functioning of the pelvic floor: In these tests, a probe is passed into the rectum and

measures the strength of the anal sphincters during various retention and defaecation manoeuvres. A balloon is passed and blown up with increasing volumes of air while the patient's resulting sensations are assessed. This can give information about the rectum's sensitivity during defaecation, and the patient's response.

Introduction to therapy

Apart from the rare circumstance of being able to correct an underlying cause for constipation, therapy is aimed at optimizing diet, reducing factors that cause constipation, and offering laxatives, which are usually highly effective.

Diet may need to be assessed by a qualified dietician to ensure that the optimal amount of fluid and fibre is ingested. Too much insoluble fibre can worsen rather than ameliorate the symptom. Various laxatives are available. Patients often prefer what they see as gentle, natural remedies, such as cracked linseed and syrup of fig, which are good sources of soluble fibre. Osmotic laxatives such as polyethylene glycol and lactulose are highly effective, and do not wane in efficacy over time. Lactulose tends to aggravate bloating and flatulence. Stimulant laxatives such as glycerol suppositories, bisacodyl, and senna are also highly effective in the short term. Stool softeners such as docusate sodium are useful for patients complaining of hard, painful stool. Enemas such as phosphate and mineral oil may be helpful in the acute setting.

Obstructed defaecation due to dysfunction of the pelvic floor may require reconstructive surgery, although biofeedback therapy may also be effective in milder cases. In this therapy, patients are taught to retrain their muscles for defaecation, and trials have shown a response in up to 80% of patients compared to a response to laxatives in 21% of patients.

Prognosis

Constipation due to underlying organic disease often resolves with treatment for the underlying condition. The majority of patients will respond to dietary changes and laxatives. Constipation due to IBS or pelvic floor dysfunction can be more difficult to treat, and patients will often adapt their diet and laxative use to suit themselves. In extreme cases, patients may undergo a subtotal colectomy for relief of symptoms.

How to handle uncertainty in the diagnosis of this symptom

The main uncertainty is approaching a patient with constipation is in deciding how intensively symptoms should be investigated. Often, there is a long history, and investigations provide little that affects management. Fear of cancer is often present, and should be addressed. If the risk is low, for instance, in a young person with near normal and unchanged bowel habits, then appropriate reassurance, rather than inappropriate testing, should be offered. Generally, any person who is over 50 years of age and presenting with a change in bowel habit should undergo investigations to exclude an underlying colorectal cancer.

Further Reading

Bharucha AE, Pemberton JH, and Locke GR 3rd. American Gastroenterological Association technical review on constipation. *Gastroenterology* 2013; 144: 218–38.

28 Acute diarrhoea

Satish Keshav and Alexandra Kent

Definition of the symptom

Acute diarrhoea is the abrupt onset of a change in bowel habit, with the passage of an unusually high volume of stool (greater than the normal of 200 ml per day), and/or increased bowel frequency of bowel opening (greater than the normal of up to three times per day).

The main causes of diarrhoea and infectious diarrhoea

Table 28.1 outlines the main causes of diarrhoea, and Table 28.2 outlines the main causes of infectious diarrhoea. In the UK, acute infectious diarrhoea is most commonly viral in aetiology; *Campylobacter jejuni* is the commonest bacterial pathogen.

Context

Infectious diarrhoea is the commonest cause of acute diarrhoea worldwide, responsible for 3 million deaths per year in children under 5 years in the developing world, mainly due to dehydration. In England, 20% of adults suffer an intestinal infection each year. The majority of infections will cause a benign, self-limiting illness. The overall incidence of infectious diarrhoea appears to be reducing, although under-reporting may bias numbers.

Diarrhoea can be caused by two different mechanisms:

1. impaired fluid, electrolyte, and/or nutrient absorption: this can be due to impaired epithelial transport, impaired water and sodium transport in the colon, incompletely absorbed nutrients (e.g. lactose intolerance), or increased transit time
2. increased intestinal secretion of fluid and nutrients: this is mainly caused by secretory enterotoxins

Often, these two processes coexist.

Approach to diagnosis

The most important factor in diagnosing the cause of diarrhoea is a thorough history, detailing contact history, travel, food/dietary history, medications, recent antibiotics, associated symptoms (fever, vomiting, weight loss), and risk factors, including extremes of age or immunosuppression. Physical examination is often unhelpful is ascertaining a cause, but is important to assess the state of hydration and general well-being.

Table 28.1 Causes of acute diarrhoea

Common	Infectious diarrhoea
	Drug-induced, e.g. laxatives, antacids
	Diverticulitis
	Antibiotic-associated diarrhoea
	Toxigenic *Clostridium difficile* infection
Uncommon	Inflammatory bowel disease
Rare	First presentation of coeliac disease
	Pancreatic insufficiency
	Endocrinopathy, including carcinoid syndrome
	Acute abdomen, e.g. appendicitis, intussusception
	Chemotherapy/radiation-induced enteritis
	Ingestion of toxins, e.g. copper, tin, daffodils, mistletoe

Table 28.2 Causes of infectious diarrhoea

Bacteria	Viruses	Parasites
Diarrhoeagenic *Escherichia coli*	Rotavirus	Protozoans
Campylobacter jejuni	Norovirus (calicivirus)	• *Cryptosporidium parvum*
Vibrio cholerae O1	Adenovirus (Serotype 40/41)	• *Giardia intestinalis*
Vibrio cholerae O139*		• *Microsporidia**
Shigella spp.	Astrovirus	• *Entamoeba histolytica*
Vibrio parahaemolyticus	Cytomegalovirus*	• *Isospora belli**
Bacteroides fragilis		• *Cyclospora cayetanensis*
Campylobacter coli		• *Dientamoeba fragilis*
Campylobacter upsaliensis		• *Blastocystis hominis*
Non-typhoidal *Salmonellae*		Helminths
		• *Strongyloides stercoralis*
Clostridium difficile		• *Angiostrongylus costaricensis*
Yersinia enterocolitica		• *Schistosoma mansoni*
Yersinia pseudotuberculosis		• *Schistosoma japonicum*

* These agents are no longer reported in the Indian subcontinent.

Data from Farthing M, Salam MA, Lindberg G, Dite P, Khalif I, Salazar-Lindo E, et al. Acute diarrhea in adults and children: a global perspective. J Clin Gastroenterol 2013; 47: 12–20.

Specific clues to the diagnosis

Infectious diarrhoea will often be accompanied by systemic symptoms such as fever, nausea, vomiting, and abdominal pain. The following factors can help narrow down the identity of the infectious agent:

Travel: Enterotoxic *Escherichia coli* is the leading cause of traveller's diarrhoea, although *Rotavirus* spp., *Shigella* spp., *Salmonella* spp., and *Campylobacter* spp. are prevalent worldwide and should be considered in any returning traveller. The highest risk area is Africa, followed by Central and South America and Eastern Europe. North America and Europe have had documented major outbreaks of giardiasis and cryptosporidiosis, following contamination of water supplies.

Food contamination: Ingestion of undercooked or contaminated food is a common etiological factor. Contaminated meat often contains *Clostridium perfringens*, *Campylobacter* sp., *Salmonella* sp., or enterohaemorrhagic *E. coli* (EHEC), whereas dairy products are associated with *Campylobacter* and *Salmonella*, and eggs are associated with *Salmonella*. Seafood often contains *Vibrio* spp., astroviruses, or *Plesiomonas shigelloides*.

Animal exposure: Cats and dogs are associated with carriage of *Campylobacter* spp.

Water exposure: Swimming in seawater, freshwater, or swimming pools is also a risk factor for intestinal infection, and *Giardia* spp., *Cryptosporidium* spp., and *Entamoeba* spp. are resistant to water chlorination.

Institutions: Some organisms, including rotaviruses, *Campylobacter* spp., *Shigella* spp., *Giardia* spp., astroviruses, caliciviruses, and *Cryptosporidium* spp., will spread quickly in institutions.

Further factors which can aid diagnosis

Infectious diarrhoea will often present with a very acute onset, compared to inflammatory bowel disease or diverticular disease, which usually have a longer onset of symptoms, and are thus discussed in Chapter 29. Further factors which can aid diagnosis are:

Associated symptoms: Diverticulitis is often accompanied by abdominal pain (which is often left-sided) and fever.
Nutritional depletion: Patients with inflammatory bowel disease may present complaining of acute diarrhoea, but other factors, such as anaemia, weight loss, and hypoalbuminaemia, may indicate a more chronic disease.

Key diagnostic tests

Infection is the commonest cause of acute diarrhoea, and so stool microscopy and culture should be the first-line investigation. Enteroinvasive bacteria will cause leucocytes to be shed into the stool. Different culture mediums are required to isolate bacteria and, subsequently, the microbiologist should be provided with any helpful medical history, such as contact or exposure. A diagnosis of *C. difficile* requires detection of Toxin A via an enzyme-linked immunosorbent assay.

Other diagnostic tests

Rotavirus and adenovirus antigens can be detected by enzyme immunoassay, although the false-negative rate for rotaviruses approaches 50%. The stool anion gap can be calculated in order to differentiate between osmotic and secretory diarrhoea, with levels >100 mOsm/kg being consistent with osmotic diarrhoea. The false-positive rate of stool microscopy and culture means that at least three stool samples should be examined. An abdominal X-ray should be performed in patients who are unwell, to exclude perforation, to assess the extent of colitis, and for toxic dilatation. In patients with persistent symptoms and negative stool examinations, a lower gastrointestinal (GI) endoscopy examination can be performed to obtain mucosal biopsies, although these are more useful when performed in the first 72 hours of infection.

Introduction to therapy

Fluid replacement

Fluid and electrolyte replacement is the cornerstone of therapy. Glucose-based oral rehydration solutions are extremely effective, taking advantage of the active carrier-mediated sodium–glucose co-transport. The ideal solution should have a low osmolarity (210–250 mmol/l) and a sodium content of 50–60 mmol/l. This means that the majority of commercially available drinks are far less suitable as rehydration agents. In more extreme cases, intravenous fluids can be given and will usually reverse any metabolic acidosis associated with the illness.

Antibiotics

The use of antibiotics in GI infections is controversial. In infections that are improving with conservative therapy, antibiotics will often be avoided. Antibiotic therapy should be considered for patients with immunosuppression, malignancy, or cardiac disease; with valvular, vascular, or orthopaedic prostheses; or at the extremes of age. Antibiotics are indicated in shigellosis, *V. cholerae* infections, pseudomembranous enterocolitis, and parasitic infection. However, they should be considered in cases of persistent yersinia infections and early in the course of campylobacter, aeromonas, and plesiomonas infections. Antibiotic therapy, in general, reduces the severity and length of symptoms.

Probiotics

The evidence for the use of probiotics is limited. They have been shown to shorten the length of rotavirus illnesses and bacterial illnesses in children by 1 day.

Antidiarrhoeal therapy

The use of anti-motility agents (usually loperamide) is contentious, associated with fears of increasing the risk of toxic dilatation and increasing the faecal carriage of enteropathogens. Studies have usually used loperamide in combination with antibiotic therapy with some success, and few doctors would be prepared to treated infective diarrhoea with loperamide alone. New antisecretory agents are in development.

Prognosis

The majority of patient will recover from acute diarrhoeal illnesses with no long-term complications. However, it is well recognized that GI infections can precipitate irritable bowel syndrome. *Yersinia enterocolitica* and *C. jejuni* have been associated with Reiter's syndrome, which may present with painful swollen joints. *C. jejuni* infection is the commonest cause of Guillain–Barré syndrome. Haemolytic uraemic syndrome is an important although uncommon complication of shigellosis and EHEC infection.

How to handle uncertainty in the diagnosis of this symptom

Infectious diarrhoea will often have signs or symptoms of underlying infection (fever, leucocytosis, raised inflammatory markers), and a combination of stool samples and mucosal biopsies will often pinpoint a pathogen. In patients with worsening symptoms, empirical antibiotics can be given after liaison with the local microbiologist. However, the majority of patients will improve with conservative therapy.

Further Reading

DuPont HL. Acute infectious diarrhea in immunocompetent adults. *N Engl J Med* 2014; 370: 1532–40.
Leffler DA and Lamont JT. *Clostridium difficile* infection. *N Engl J Med* 2015; 372: 1539–48.

29 Chronic diarrhoea

Satish Keshav and Alexandra Kent

Definition of the symptom

Diarrhoea is defined as the passage of more than three stools per day or a stool weight >400 g/day, and duration ≥4 weeks is regarded as chronic.

Differential diagnosis

The list of possible causes of chronic diarrhoea is long, and likely to be incomplete as many rare conditions may present unusually with diarrhoea as part of the symptom complex (Table 29.1). The key to the diagnostic process is to consider the context in which the presentation occurs, and the most likely causes. Colorectal cancer rarely presents only with diarrhoea, although this is frequently the diagnosis which is most feared and the one which might prompt attendance in primary and secondary care. Most patients will be referred to secondary care for investigations, but their ongoing care will be provided by the GP.

Context

Four to five per cent of the Western population suffers from diarrhoea, with irritable bowel syndrome (IBS) being the commonest cause in 20–40 year-old patients. It is the commonest reason for referral to secondary care gastroenterology clinics. In the absence of

Table 29.1 Causes of chronic diarrhoea	
Common	Irritable bowel syndrome
	Post-infectious irritable bowel syndrome
	Diet related: excessive fruit, non-digestible carbohydrate sweeteners, excessive caffeine intake
	Iatrogenic drug related: e.g. proton-pump inhibitors, metformin, antibiotics
	Coeliac disease
	Microscopic colitis
	Diverticular disease
	Giardiasis
Uncommon	Inflammatory bowel disease
	Lactose intolerance
	Pancreatic insufficiency
	Small bowel bacterial overgrowth
	Chronic infection, e.g. cryptosporidiosis, microsporidiosis, parasitic worm infestation (especially in immunocompromised)
	Autonomic neuropathy (e.g. diabetes mellitus, alcohol, uraemia, amyloid)
	Colonic or ileal resection
	Bile acid malabsorption
	Post-cholecystectomy diarrhoea
	Endocrine disease (e.g. hyperthyroidism, Addison's disease, hypoparathyroidism)
Rare	Factitious diarrhoea and laxative abuse
	Colorectal cancer (rarely presents with diarrhoea)
	Villous adenoma of the colon
	Ischaemic colitis
	Hormone-secreting tumours (e.g. carcinoid, VIPoma, gastrinoma)
	Villous adenoma of the colon
	Factitious diarrhoea and laxative abuse
	Fabry's disease

rectal bleeding, loss of weight, or abnormal blood tests, it is unlikely to be due to a serious illness.

Approach to diagnosis

The patient's age helps in deciding the direction of investigation. Patients who are ≥50 years old should undergo colonic imaging to check for colorectal cancer. Although colorectal cancer is unlikely to present with diarrhoea only, this is an anxiety for patients and referrers and, with the likely introduction of colorectal cancer screening in asymptomatic adults over the age of 50 years, it seems prudent to screen those who have symptoms.

The history will give clues to the likely diagnosis. It is important to compare current symptoms to what the patient considers to be their usual bowel habit. Specific triggers should be sought; commencing new medications, recent surgery, travel, food poisoning or infection, and stress should all be checked. The help of a dietician examining the patient's food diary can be invaluable in identifying excessive or inadequate fibre intake, excessive caffeine, and potential dietary triggers such as lactose or gluten.

Examination should include the perineum, anus, and rectum, checking for evidence of inflammatory bowel disease; constipation and faecal impaction with paradoxical diarrhoea; and corroborative evidence of diarrhoea with excoriation of the perianal skin. Is the patient malnourished or dehydrated? Is there evidence of hyperthyroidism?

Specific clues to the diagnosis

Specific clues to the diagnosis are as follows:

Weight loss/rectal bleeding: These are alarm symptoms irrespective of the patient's age, necessitating urgent investigations due to their association with inflammatory bowel disease and colorectal cancer.
Previous surgery: Bowel resection can lead to diarrhoea due to reduced water absorption (colonic resection), bile salt or fat malabsorption (terminal ileal resection), decreased transit time, or small bowel bacterial overgrowth. Ten per cent of patients develop diarrhoea post cholecystectomy.
Systemic disease: Multiple diseases can be associated with diarrhoea, through various mechanisms. Such diseases include diabetes, thyrotoxicosis, vasculitis, scleroderma, hypoparathyroidism, Addison's disease, and amyloidosis.
Pancreatic disease: Diarrhoea in a patient with a history of excess alcohol consumption or pancreatitis may be due to pancreatic exocrine insufficiency, and resultant fat malabsorption.
Recent travel: Giardiasis is more common following travel to the USA or Eastern Europe, whereas amoebiasis is endemic to western and southern Africa, South Asia, South America, and Mexico.
Family history: There is a strong familial association recognized in colorectal cancer, inflammatory bowel disease, and coeliac disease.
Medication history: Four per cent of cases are drug related, and symptoms may develop some weeks or months after commencing new medications.

Key diagnostic tests

The key test in this diagnosis rests entirely on the context. IBS accounts for the majority of presentations, and it is helpful to be able to make this clinical diagnosis confidently and positively without recourse to excessive testing that can serve to heighten anxiety and reaffirm the patient's suspicion that 'they still can't find what is wrong'. In other contexts, it is critically important to check for inflammatory bowel disease or colorectal cancer, and here either colonic imaging or colonoscopy and biopsy are the key tests. Coeliac disease and thyrotoxicosis frequently present with diarrhoea. In both cases, the key test can be performed on a blood sample, with no need for colonoscopy, although many physicians consider it necessary to confirm the diagnosis of coeliac disease with duodenal biopsy.

Other diagnostic tests

Other diagnostic tests are as follows:

Faecal fat levels: Steatorrhoea can be confirmed from a 3-day stool collection or on spot stool samples, although further tests are required to determine the underlying cause.

Faecal elastase levels: Pancreatic insufficiency can be diagnosed by the finding of reduced faecal elastase levels.

SeHCAT nuclear medicine scan: Bile salt malabsorption can be diagnosed with this test, which checks for reduced retention of an exogenously administered labelled bile acid.

Glucose or lactulose hydrogen breath tests: These test for small bowel bacterial overgrowth.

Gut hormone levels: This test requires a fasting blood sample and tests for levels of gastrin, vasoactive intestinal peptide, pancreatic polypeptide, glucagon, and neurotensin. For accurate gastrin levels, H2 antagonists should be stopped 24 hours prior to the test, and proton-pump inhibitors stopped 6 days prior to the test.

Barium follow-through/MRI small bowel: This can identify small bowel diverticula, entero-enteric fistulae, or terminal ileal disease.

Enteroscopy: This is not often required; it is usually reserved for identifying small bowel lesions seen on radiological examination.

Urinary 5-hydroxyindoleacetic acid: This is raised in patients with carcinoid syndrome.

Lactose hydrogen breath test: This can be used to diagnose lactose intolerance.

Introduction to therapy

Therapy is dictated by the underlying diagnosis, and dealt with in the appropriate section. Symptomatic relief of diarrhoea can be readily achieved using loperamide, diphenoxylate, or codeine phosphate. Codeine is best avoided because of its sedating and potentially addictive properties. Loperamide is well tolerated and can be used in the long term if needed. Table 29.2 gives a summary of treatment strategies for each condition. Advice from a dietician can be extremely helpful for patients requiring dietary modification in IBS, and for those with coeliac disease and therefore needing to follow a strict gluten-free diet.

Prognosis

Organic causes of diarrhoea usually respond to therapy, while IBS can be harder to treat. Patients often learn to cope with their symptoms,

Table 29.2 Treatment of diarrhoeal conditions

Condition	Treatment options
Inflammatory bowel disease	5-ASA, steroids, immunosuppression, anti-TNFα therapy
Coeliac disease	Gluten-free diet
Irritable bowel syndrome	Dietary modification, optimized fibre intake, antidiarrhoeals
Diverticular disease	High fibre diet, colonic resection
Giardia, amoebiasis	Antibiotics
Microscopic colitis	Budesonide, bismuth, 5-ASA
Post-cholecystectomy syndrome	Cholestyramine, loperamide
Bile acid malabsorption	Cholestyramine
Pancreatic insufficiency	Pancreatic enzyme supplements
Bacterial overgrowth	Antibiotics
Vasculitis	Steroids, immunosuppression
Hormone-secreting tumours	Resection, octreotide, chemotherapy

Abbreviations: 5-ASA, 5-aminosalicylic acid; TNFα, tumour necrosis factor alpha.

using loperamide and other antidiarrhoeals to maintain social and professional lives.

How to handle uncertainty in the diagnosis of this symptom

Care should be taken not to over-investigate patients with IBS. However, patients with continuing weight loss, anaemia, or persistently raised inflammatory markers may require intensive investigation, and referral to specialist and tertiary care. Changes from microscopic colitis and inflammatory bowel disease can be patchy, and systemic inflammatory conditions can remit spontaneously temporarily, so that repeated investigation may be necessary when the first tests are normal. In difficult cases, in-hospital assessment of diarrhoea may be necessary to quantify stool volume and to determine if diarrhoea is dependent on oral intake or not. Secretory diarrhoea due to endocrinopathy and secretory tumours of the bowel continues even when the patient does not eat or drink, while diarrhoea due to malabsorption or inflammation tends to be improved when oral intake ceases.

Further Reading

Ford AC, Lacy BE, and Talley NJ. Irritable bowel syndrome. *N Engl J Med* 2017; 376: 2566–78.
Schiller LR. Definitions, pathophysiology, and evaluation of chronic diarrhoea. *Best Pract Res Clin Gastroenterol* 2012; 26: 551–62.

30 Rectal bleeding

Satish Keshav and Alexandra Kent

Definition of the symptom

Rectal bleeding (haematochezia) refers to the passage of bright red blood per rectum.

Differential diagnosis

The differential diagnosis of rectal bleeding, ordered by probability, is shown in Table 30.1.

Context

Rectal bleeding is a common symptom, affecting all age groups, with the highest incidence in the sixth and seventh decades and associated with a higher mortality and morbidity with increasing age. Epidemiological studies have shown rectal bleeding to occur in nearly 1% of hospital admissions. Bleeding stops spontaneously in 80% of cases, although rebleeding occurs in 25%. The majority of patients will present to their general practitioner and will be referred to colorectal or gastroenterology outpatient clinics. Massive lower gastrointestinal (GI) bleeding is a medical emergency.

Approach to diagnosis

The initial approach to patient care should be assessment of their haemodynamic stability, including vital signs. The most important diagnosis to be excluded is colorectal cancer, especially in older (>50 years) patients. Associated GI symptoms may narrow the differential diagnosis (weight loss, abdominal pain), although many causes of bleeding may be otherwise asymptomatic (angiodysplasia, polyps). A concise history and examination should significantly narrow the differential diagnosis.

Specific clues to the diagnosis

Clues to the diagnosis of rectal bleeding are given in Table 30.2.

Key diagnostic tests

Endoscopic evaluation by flexible sigmoidoscopy or colonoscopy is the key test and allows biopsies to be taken from abnormal lesions. Bleeding lesions can be treated endoscopically by sclerotherapy or cauterization; in these instances, biopsies are usually deferred until active bleeding has settled. Brisk lower GI bleeding usually precludes effective endoscopy and treatment, and CT scanning with or without angiography may be necessary in the acute situation. In elderly patients in whom rectal bleeding is not causing haemodynamic

Table 30.2 Clues to the diagnosis of rectal bleeding

Diagnosis	Comorbidities and background	Symptoms and signs
Diverticular disease	Diverticulitis	Left iliac fossa pain, constipation
Inflammatory bowel disease	Family history	Diarrhoea, abdominal pain, fatigue, weight loss, extra-intestinal manifestations
Neoplasia	Family history, smoker	Weight loss, constipation, change in bowel habit
Arteriovenous malformations/ angiodysplasia	Aortic stenosis	Asymptomatic
Ischaemic colitis	Ischaemic heart disease, peripheral vascular disease, diabetes, hypertension, hyperlipidaemia	Severe abdominal pain, bloody diarrhoea
Radiation proctitis	Previous pelvic radiotherapy	–
Solitary rectal ulcer		Constipation, straining, mucus per rectum
Haemorrhoids	Constipation	Pruritus ani, mucus, palpable lump
Anal fissure	Constipation	Pain on defaecation
Fistula-in-ano	Previous anorectal abscess, inflammatory bowel disease	Visible fistula, perianal discharge, pain, swelling
Upper gastrointestinal bleed	Recent NSAID/aspirin use, excess alcohol	Haematemesis, dyspepsia

compromise, a CT scan may be preferable, to identify possible causes (e.g. diverticular disease) or exclude serious pathologies (e.g. malignancy).

Other diagnostic tests

Brisk bleeding may obscure endoscopic views. Diagnostic tests can usually be deferred until bleeding has settled and patients have received pre-endoscopic bowel purgatives. In cases where bleeding is torrential with associated haemodynamic compromise, mesenteric angiography may identify the bleeding site, and allow embolization of the responsible vessel.

Each patient should be assessed individually; many patients presenting with lower GI bleeding are elderly and/or frail, and endoscopy may be difficult. In such cases, radiological imaging (abdominal CT, barium enema) may exclude diagnoses such as neoplasia or diverticular disease, with more invasive tests avoided unless bleeding persists.

Introduction to therapy

The stability of the patient and rate of bleeding dictate the initial approach to patient care, with restoration of intravascular volume

Table 30.1 Causes of rectal bleeding

Common	Infrequent	Rare
Haemorrhoids (affects 4% of the population)	Inflammatory bowel disease Fistula-in-ano	Radiation proctitis Ischaemic colitis
Anal fissure	Arteriovenous malformations/ angiodysplasia	Solitary rectal ulcer
Divericular disease		
Neoplasia (distal colorectal cancer, polyps)	Massive upper gastrointestinal bleed	

Note: In ~10% of cases, the cause of bleeding is not found.

being the most important objective. Patients require surgery more often when bleeding is due to a lower GI source than when it is due to an upper GI source, and patients requiring ≥4 units of blood in the first 24 hours have a 50% chance of requiring surgery.

Specific therapeutic options are as follows:

Haemorrhoids: stool softeners, high-fibre diet, band ligation, local injection

Solitary rectal ulcer: endoscopic treatment of active bleeding ulcer using endoscopic adrenaline injection or cauterization

Diverticular disease: The majority of cases will stop bleeding spontaneously; some centres advocate endoscopic adrenaline injection, although endoscopic therapy does incur a higher risk of colonic perforation. Persistent bleeding usually leads to surgical resection.

Arteriovenous malformation: usually endoscopically cauterized using argon plasma coagulation

Radiation proctitis: Bleeding points can be treated endoscopically using argon plasma coagulation. Other rectal therapies, including steroids, 5-aminosalicylic acid (5-ASA), or sucralfate, are less effective.

Inflammatory bowel disease and colorectal cancer: see Chapters 203 and 204, respectively.

Prognosis

Rectal bleeding is a common symptom and as such has a poor positive predictive value for diagnoses such as colorectal cancer. The majority of patients will have a benign diagnosis.

How to handle uncertainty in the diagnosis of this symptom

Since rectal bleeding is associated with colorectal cancer, all patients age ≥50 years, or <50 years and without an obvious cause for bleeding, should have a test to exclude colon cancer. In patients with normal investigations and stable haemoglobin, rectal bleeding is usually due to local anorectal causes, which may not require further treatment.

Further Reading

Gralnek IM, Neeman Z, and Strate LL. Acute lower gastrointestinal bleeding. *N Engl J Med* 2017; 376: 1054–63.

Jacobs D. Hemorrhoids. *N Engl J Med* 2014; 371: 944–951.

31 Jaundice

Satish Keshav and Alexandra Kent

Definition of the symptom

Jaundice, also known as icterus, is the yellowish discolouration seen in skin, mucous membranes, and sclerae when the plasma bilirubin concentration is >40 μmol/l.

Differential diagnosis

The differential diagnosis of jaundice, ordered by probability, is shown in Table 31.1.

Context

As erythrocytes are destroyed, haemoglobin is broken down, releasing haem, which is further broken down to produce bilirubin. This bilirubin, referred to as 'free', 'indirect', or 'unconjugated', binds to albumin and is transported to the liver, where it is conjugated with glucuronic acid and becomes water soluble. It is then excreted in the bile into the small intestine. In the colon, it is metabolized by bacteria to urobilinogen and then stercobilinogen, and is subsequently oxidized to stercobilin. Stercobilin gives stool its brown colour. A small amount of urobilinogen is absorbed from the intestine and excreted in the urine, giving urine its yellow colour. Eighty per cent of bilirubin comes from haemoglobin, and the remainder comes from breakdown of other iron-containing proteins, such as myoglobin and cytochromes.

Jaundice may arise from increased production of bilirubin, for instance, in haemolysis; from reduced conjugation of bilirubin in the liver, as in Gilbert's syndrome; or from reduced excretion of bilirubin via bile, as in intra-hepatic cholestasis. Jaundice also occurs when the flow of bile is obstructed, for instance, by gallstones. In these cases, hepatic function might not be impaired profoundly, although, again, the disease process causing biliary obstruction, such as malignancy, may be advanced by the time jaundice is apparent.

Approach to diagnosis

The initial approach is to determine if the jaundice is pre-hepatic, intra-hepatic, or post-hepatic.

Pre-hepatic jaundice

Causes of pre-hepatic jaundice include conditions such as sickle cell anaemia, spherocytosis, glucose-6-phosphate dehydrogenase deficiency, and haemolytic uraemic syndrome, which associated with an increased rate of haemolysis and thus lead to an increased production of unconjugated bilirubin. Serum bilirubin will be unconjugated and, since unconjugated bilirubin is not water soluble, there will be no bilirubin in the urine.

Hepatic jaundice

Conditions leading to a reduction in the capacity of the liver to metabolize and excrete bilirubin cause hepatic jaundice. All causes of acute hepatitis can cause hepatic jaundice in which bilirubin is usually conjugated. Inherited conditions that affect bilirubin metabolism include Gilbert's syndrome, and Types I and II Crigler–Najjar syndrome, in which reduced levels, or a total lack, of glucuronosyltransferase causes unconjugated hyperbilirubinaemia, and Dubin–Johnson and Rotor syndromes, which are caused by defective bilirubin excretion, with conjugated hyperbilirubinaemia.

Post-hepatic jaundice

Post-hepatic jaundice is also known as obstructive jaundice, as it is caused by a blockage within the biliary system, resulting in failure of biliary drainage. The blockage prevents bile from being excreted into the gastrointestinal tract, and the stool subsequently becomes pale. Urine darkens due to the excess bilirubin being excreted into the urine. Causes of post-hepatic jaundice include gallstones, pancreatic tumours, pancreatic cysts, cholangiocarcinomas, and, in neonates, biliary atresia.

Hepatic impairment

It is important to determine the extent of hepatic impairment associated with jaundice by measuring serum transaminases, prothrombin time, and albumin, and by checking clinically for evidence of hepatic dysfunction. This can vary from virtually none, for example, in Gilbert's syndrome or massive haemolysis, to fulminant liver failure in other instances. Management is very much guided by the degree by the degree of hepatic impairment.

Specific clues to the diagnosis

As described in 'Context', changes in urine and stool colour can be used to predict whether hyperbilirubinaemia is pre- or post-conjugation: unconjugated bilirubin is not water soluble and therefore the bilirubin will pass into the GI tract, and the urine will not change colour; in contrast, conjugated bilirubin is water soluble, and the excess bilirubin passes into the urine as it cannot drain out of the liver, so stool becomes paler, and urine darker. The following factors also give clues as to the underlying diagnosis:

Pain: Impacted gallstones causing biliary obstruction will be associated with biliary colic and classically right upper quadrant abdominal pain.

Alcohol intake: This suggests liver injury and raises the possibility of more chronic liver damage and cirrhosis.

Weight loss: Pancreatic tumours classically present as painless obstructive jaundice, and may well have associated symptoms such as weight loss and cachexia.

Viral symptoms: The viral illnesses which most commonly cause acute jaundice are hepatitis A and infectious mononucleosis (glandular fever). Hepatitis A often presents with fever, fatigue, diarrhoea, anorexia, nausea, and abdominal pain. Glandular fever presents with fatigue, sore throat, fever, arthralgia, and lymphadenopathy. Many other viruses can cause jaundice, including the hepatitis B virus, the hepatitis E virus, cytomegalovirus, and so on.

Medications: The commonest causes of drug-induced hepatitis are co-amoxiclav, flucloxacillin, chlorpromazine, and drugs used for antituberculosis therapy. Any recent changes to medications should be noted, as liver derangement is a common side effect.

Table 31.1 Causes of jaundice

Common	Infrequent	Rare
Gilbert's syndrome	Hepatic metastases from cancer	Inherited disorders of bilirubin metabolism
Drug-induced jaundice		
Viral hepatitis	Pancreatic cancer	
Alcoholic hepatitis/alcoholic liver disease	Haemolysis	Cholangiocarcinoma
		Pancreatic cysts/ pseudocysts
Cirrhosis of the liver		
Cholelithiasis		

Key diagnostic tests

With respect to liver chemistry, classically, the alkaline phosphatase and gamma-glutamyl transferase levels are elevated in post-hepatic (obstructive) causes of jaundice, whereas the transaminases are elevated in hepatic causes. Acute cholelithiasis and cholangitis can, however, be associated with markedly raised transaminases.

The most important test is to perform is an ultrasound scan of the biliary tract, to determine if there is biliary obstruction. Ultrasonography can diagnose biliary obstruction, gallstones, pancreatic masses, biliary tree dilatation, and liver echogenicity.

Prothrombin time and albumin concentration provide a measure of hepatic synthetic function, which is particularly important in acute jaundice where there is concern about liver failure.

Other diagnostic tests

The following blood tests may give further information regarding the cause of jaundice:

Unconjugated and conjugated bilirubin: This test can ascertain whether the rise in bilirubin occurs before or after conjugation in the liver.

Tests for haemolysis: Haemolysis can be confirmed from a blood film, a reticulocyte count, haptoglobin levels, the lactate dehydrogenase test, and/or the Coombs test.

Viral serology: Hepatitis A IgM is positive in acute hepatitis A (IgG is not diagnostic). Infectious mononucleosis is diagnosed by the presence of Epstein–Barr virus IgM, or the heterophile antibody test (the monospot test). Infectious mononucleosis may also be associated with thrombocytopaenia, raised transaminases, and a raised erythrocyte sedimentation rate.

If an ultrasound is inconclusive, magnetic resonance cholangio-pancreatography (MRCP) can provide clear views of the biliary tree, and is safer than endoscopic retrograde cholangiopancreatography (ERCP). However, ERCP may be required to allow removal of obstructing stones, or relief of a stricture by stenting, and to aid diagnosis by obtaining biopsies or biliary brushings.

Introduction to therapy

Treatment of jaundice is dependent on the underlying cause. ERCP involves passing an endoscope into the duodenum and intubating the sphincter of Oddi; the test is used to identify the site and cause of obstruction, and potentially to relieve it by removal, stenting, and, or sphincterotomy. Treatment of pancreatic cancer and cholangiocarcinoma will be decided by a multidisciplinary team, including oncologists and gastroenterologists.

Non-obstructive jaundice requires treatment aimed at the underlying disease. Viral illnesses are usually self-limiting. Treatment of drug-induced jaundice depends on the causative medication. The majority of drug-induced jaundice require removal of the offending agent and close monitoring for signs of liver failure. Alcoholic liver disease and alcoholic hepatitis require supportive treatment with laxatives, nutrition, and an investigation into underlying precipitant of decompensation (e.g. toxins, infection, constipation, GI bleed).

Prognosis

The prognosis is as follows:

- The overall prognosis of a patient with jaundice depends on the underlying disease process.
- Patients with obstructive jaundice from gallstones usually respond well to ERCP treatment, with further episodes being prevented by a cholecystectomy.
- The presence of ascending cholangitis worsens the prognosis, but the early institution of antibiotics can resolve sepsis.
- The elderly, and patients with cardiovascular disease, always have a poorer prognosis from cases of obstructive jaundice.
- Pancreatic and cholangiocarcinoma have an overall poor prognosis.
- Viral causes of jaundice usually recover with conservative treatment.
- Drug-induced jaundice, if caught late, can be fatal due to the associated liver failure.

How to handle uncertainty in the diagnosis of this symptom

The most important diagnosis to exclude is obstructive jaundice, as patients can rapidly deteriorate due to associated ascending cholangitis. In the setting of fever and obstructive jaundice, it is safer to advocate early antibiotics if ascending cholangitis is a possible diagnosis. A combination of blood tests and radiological investigations usually provides a clear diagnosis, and the commonest cause in patients with no additional symptoms or signs is Gilbert's syndrome.

Further Reading

Addley J and Mitchell RM. Advances in the investigation of obstructive jaundice. *Curr Gastroenterol Rep* 2012; 14: 511–19.

Kathpalia P and Ahn J. Assessment of jaundice in the hospitalized patient. *Clin Liver Dis* 2015; 19: 155–70.

32 Ascites

Ehoud Shmueli

Definition of the symptom

Ascites is the accumulation of fluid within the peritoneal cavity.

Differential diagnosis

The differential diagnosis of a swollen abdomen includes obesity, large bowel obstruction, and huge liver, ovarian, or mesenteric cysts. Differentiation from ascites is by physical examination and imaging. Most patients with ascites usually have a known diagnosis of cirrhosis, malignancy, or heart failure.

Context

For patients newly presenting with ascites, the diagnostic problem is usually to differentiate between cirrhosis and malignancy. For patients with established liver disease, ascites represents a deterioration of their liver function, the development of a hepatocellular carcinoma, or another complication. Worsening of preexisting ascites may be due to spontaneous bacterial peritonitis. In malignancy, ascites denotes the development of peritoneal deposits or massive liver metastases.

Approach to diagnosis

The diagnosis may be obvious from the context, but can be confirmed with imaging and a diagnostic paracentesis. The serum–ascites albumin gradient (SAAG; [ascitic fluid albumin] − [serum albumin]) reflects portal pressure, and is the key diagnostic test. A SAAG >11 g/l indicates portal hypertension, and therefore probably cirrhosis. A SAAG <11 g/l excludes portal hypertension, and therefore the ascites is not caused by cirrhosis. The SAAG can be determined almost immediately and will guide further investigation.

The causes of ascites according to the SAAG

The causes of ascites are shown in Tables 32.1 and 32.2.

Key diagnostic tests

Diagnostic paracentesis

In obvious ascites, this should not wait for the ultrasound scan. Severe thrombocytopenia and impaired clotting are only relative contraindications. Bleeding is a rare complication of paracentesis. Patients with an international normalized ratio greater than 2.0 can receive fresh frozen plasma prior to the procedure, although it is not clear that this is absolutely necessary. Patients with a platelet count lower than $20 \times 10^3/\mu l$ should receive an infusion of platelets before the procedure.

Ascitic fluid should routinely be analysed as shown in Tables 32.3, 32.4, and 32.5.

Imaging

Abdominal ultrasound is usually the first imaging to confirm the diagnosis, image the liver, and determine patency of the portal vein. CT scanning of chest–abdomen–pelvis should follow a finding of a low SAAG.

Laparoscopy

If, in a low-SAAG ascites, CT scanning and cytology fail to provide a diagnosis, a diagnostic laparoscopy will be the next step. Typical findings are tuberculous or malignant peritoneal deposits.

Table 32.1 High serum–ascites albumin gradient (11 g/l or greater, denoting portal hypertension)

Cause	Comment
Cirrhosis (about 80% of patients)	Stigmata of chronic liver disease
	Clear yellow fluid
	Albumin concentration usually <10 g/l
	Protein concentration is <25 g/l
Alcoholic hepatitis	Recent alcohol intake of 10 units or more per day
	Jaundice
	Hepatomegaly—often tender
	Moderately raised alanine aminotransferase
	Neutrophilia
Spontaneous bacterial peritonitis	Should be considered in any patient with advanced cirrhosis who deteriorates from any cause
	The fluid may or may not look cloudy
	The neutrophil count in ascitic fluid is >250/ mm³
	The protein concentration is <10 g/l
Budd–Chiari syndrome	Acute liver failure and ascites in the context of myeloproliferative disease, hypercoagulable states, or hepatocellular carcinoma
	Diagnosis is by imaging
Portal vein thrombosis	Can complicate cirrhosis
	In the absence of liver disease, consider pancreatic pathology, myeloproliferative disorders, hypercoagulable states, and abdominal sepsis or surgery
Cardiac failure	Including severe tricuspid regurgitation, and constrictive peritonitis
	Total ascites protein concentration is usually >25 g/l, which helps differentiate it from cirrhosis
Massive liver metastases	Usually obvious on abdominal ultrasound

Other diagnostic tests

Tests for levels of CA19-9, carcinoembryonic antigen, and alpha-fetoprotein may be useful if the primary malignancy is not obvious. A CA-125 test should not be requested, as it is always high in ascites, regardless of the cause. In high-SAAG ascites, serology for the hepatitis B and C viruses, an autoantibody screen, and iron studies should be requested.

Introduction to therapy

Ascites with portal hypertension

Patients with alcoholic cirrhosis are often also fond of salt. They can improve dramatically with abstention from alcohol, and with salt restriction. The latter involves three instructions to patients:

avoid adding salt in cooking or before eating

avoid obviously salty foods, such as crisps, salted nuts, and some cheeses

avoid or take care with pre-prepared or 'fast foods'

Failure to comply with salt restriction is a frequent cause of 'diuretic failure'

Most patients require diuretic therapy starting with 100 mg spironolactone and 40 mg furosemide per day. The doses can be

Table 32.2 Low serum–ascites albumin gradient (<11 g/l denoting normal portal pressure)

Cause	Comment
Peritoneal deposits	From ovary, breast, colon, lung, pancreas, or liver, and occasionally mesothelioma
	CT may be normal
	Overall cytology is positive in 50%–100%, but usually negative in mesothelioma
	The neutrophil count in ascitic fluid may be >250/ mm³, but there is a predominance of lymphocytes in the total white-cell count
	Spontaneous bacterial peritonitis is rare in malignant ascites, but secondary bacterial peritonitis from perforation should be considered in the context of fever and pain
Peritoneal tuberculosis	Abdominal pain and ascites developing over several months
	About one-third of patients may have signs of old TB on a chest X-ray
	The majority of patients have an ascitic white-cell count of 150–4000 mm³, with a lymphocytic predominance
	Diagnosis usually requires laparoscopy and biopsy of the white peritoneal deposits
Nephrotic syndrome	Peripheral oedema usually dominates the picture
	Proteinuria greater than 3.0–3.5 g in 24 hours, or spot urine protein:creatinine ratio of >300–350 mg/mmol
Pancreatitis	Protein concentration is usually >30 g/l, and there is a high amylase concentration often >1000 IU/l
Meigs syndrome	Benign solid ovarian tumour associated with ascites and pleural effusion that disappear after tumour removal
Chylous ascites	Disruption of the lymphatic system
	Ascitic triglycerides should be >2.26 mmol/l, or twice serum levels

titrated upwards to a maximum of 400 mg spironolactone and 160 mg furosemide per day. Amiloride 10–40 mg can be substituted for spironolactone if gynaecomastia is a problem but it is less effective.

There is no limit to the daily weight loss of patients who have significant oedema. Once the oedema has resolved, 0.5 kg is probably a reasonable daily maximum.

NSAIDs, beta blockers, angiotensin-converting-enzyme inhibitors, and angiotensin receptor II blockers can all impair the effectiveness of diuretic treatment in ascites by reducing renal perfusion and function. Hyponatraemia (<120 mmol/l), a rising creatinine, or encephalopathy are indications for stopping diuretic therapy and using large-volume paracentesis.

At large volume, paracentesis human albumin solution (HAS) is usually infused to prevent hypovolaemia, although the necessity for this remains controversial. Approximately 8 g of albumin are infused per litre of ascites drained (100 ml of 20% HAS contains 20 g of albumin).

Transjugular intra-hepatic portosystemic shunt (TIPS) is used to decompress the portal circulation in patients who require frequent large-volume paracentesis. Hepatic encephalopathy, portal vein

Table 32.3 Appearance

Clear or straw-coloured	Uncomplicated ascites; deeply jaundiced patients will have a darker coloured ascites
Cloudy	Infection
Milky	Chylous ascites
Bloody	Traumatic tap causes a heterogeneously bloody specimen
	Malignancy causes a homogenously bloody specimen

Table 32.4 Biochemistry

SAAG*	SAAG reflects portal pressure
	>11 g/l = portal hypertension
	<11 g/l = no portal hypertension
Protein	<10 g/l is a risk for spontaneous bacterial peritonitis
	>10 g/l with more than 250/mm³ neutrophils should prompt suspicion of bowel perforation
	>25 g/l and an SAAG of >11 g/l suggests heart failure
Glucose (not required routinely)	A low glucose occurs with malignancy
	An undetectable glucose may occur with bowel perforation
Ascitic fluid:serum LDH ratio (not required routinely)	<0.4 in uncomplicated cirrhotic ascites
	Approaches 1.0 in spontaneous bacterial peritonitis
	May be greater than 1.0 in perforation or malignancy
Amylase (not required routinely)	High, often >1000 IU/ml in pancreatic ascites

Abbreviations: SAAG, serum–ascites albumin gradient; LDH, lactate dehydrogenase.
*SAAG = [ascitic fluid albumin] − [serum albumin].

thrombosis, and heart failure are contraindications to TIPS. Hepatic encephalopathy occurs in up to 30% of patients who receive a TIPS; hence, it is used mostly as a last resort and usually in younger patients with less severe liver dysfunction and who are thus less likely to become encephalopathic.

Ascites from peritoneal carcinomatosis

This is treated with repeated large-volume paracentesis. Unlike the case for patients with ascites due to portal hypertension, in patients with peritoneal carcinomatosis, large volumes of fluid can be removed without fear of haemodynamic problems, and HAS infusion is not required. Diuretics do not work unless there is also portal hypertension from hepatic metastases.

Prognosis

This depends on the cause but, in general, malignancy-associated ascites carries a prognosis of 1–4 months. Patients who develop ascites as a complication of cirrhosis have a 50% 2-year mortality. However, patients with alcoholic cirrhosis who stop drinking can do surprisingly well.

How to handle uncertainty in the diagnosis

The diagnosis of newly presenting ascites is often unclear. The stigmata of liver disease can be subtle, an alcoholic history may be hidden, malignancy may not be apparent on CT, and the admitting

Table 32.5 Microbiology and pathology

Cell count	>500 WBCs or >250 neutrophils/mm³ suggests infection.
	A predominance of lymphocytes suggests TB or malignancy
Gram stain	Rarely positive
Culture (not required routinely)	A repeat sample of 20 ml ascitic fluid in blood culture bottles (10 ml/bottle) before antibiotics are stated gives the best chance of obtaining a culture
Cytology (not required routinely)	If malignancy is suspected, send 50 ml

Abbreviations: WBC, white blood cell.

clinician may have forgotten to request an ascitic albumin concentration. A high Ca-125 can lead clinicians in the wrong direction. The SAAG is the key test. A high-SAAG ascites will usually indicate cirrhosis. A low-SAAG ascites most commonly indicates a malignancy.

About 5% of patients may have a combination of causes for the ascites, such as cirrhosis plus malignancy or tuberculosis, and it is important to be open to that possibility.

Further Reading

Pericleous M, Sarnowski A, Moore A, Fijten R, and Zaman M. The clinical management of abdominal ascites, spontaneous bacterial peritonitis and hepatorenal syndrome: a review of current guidelines and recommendations. *Eur J Gastroenterol Hepatol* 2016; 28: e10–18.

33   Chylous ascites

Ehoud Shmueli

Definition of the symptom

Chylous ascites is ascites that has a cloudy or milky appearance due to a high level of triglycerides (>2.26 mmol/l).

The causes of chylous ascites

The causes of chylous ascites are given in Table 33.1.

Table 33.1 The causes of chylous ascites

Cause	Comment
Cirrhosis	Due to rupture of serosal lymphatics spontaneously or due to hepatocellular carcinoma; SAAG > 11 mg/l
Neoplastic: lymphoma, and any malignancy disrupting the lymphatics	The diagnosis may be obvious from the history; SAAG < 11 mg/l
Complex surgery or trauma: involving the retroperitoneum, e.g. abdominal aortic aneurism repair or retroperitoneal node dissection	Lymphatic disruption during surgery or following trauma causes chylous ascites in the first post-operative week; chylous ascites occurring weeks/months after surgery is due to adhesions or other extrinsic lymphatic compression
Congenital: yellow nail syndrome; primary lymphatic hypoplasia, or hyperplasia; intestinal lymphangiectasia	The most common cause in children
Infection: Tuberculosis, filariasis	The most common cause in developing countries
Inflammatory causes: Radiotherapy, pancreatitis, retroperitoneal fibrosis	Causing fibrosis of the lymphatics
Right heart failure, constrictive pericarditis	Impaired drainage of lymph; SAAG > 11 mg/l
Nephrotic syndrome	Unknown pathogenesis
HIV associated	Kaposi's sarcoma, mycobacterium avium intracellulare

Abbreviations: SAAG, serum–ascites albumin gradient.

Context

Chylous ascites is very rare and is due to disruption of the lymphatic system. The cause may be clear from the history; in developed countries, the differential rests between cirrhosis and malignancy, especially lymphoma. In developing countries, tuberculosis or filariasis is more likely.

Key diagnostic tests

Check triglycerides (should be >2.26 mmol/l, or twice serum levels) and exclude infection. Lymphocytes should predominate; neutrophils indicate infection. Request culture, cytology, and albumin concentration. The serum–ascites albumin gradient (SAAG) is calculated as follows: SAAG = [ascitic fluid albumin] − [serum albumin]. A SAAG >11 g/l indicates portal hypertension. A SAAG <11 g/l indicates that there is no portal hypertension. Low-SAAG chylous ascites should be investigated by CT scanning for tumour and, if necessary, laparoscopy for tumour, tubercle deposits, or lymphatic leaks. Lymphangiography and lymphoscintigraphy can detect abnormal retroperitoneal nodes, leakage from dilated lymphatics, fistulization, and patency of the thoracic duct.

Treatment

Treatment is directed to the cause. Cirrhosis is treated in the usual way. In malignancy, repeated large-volume paracentesis may be necessary. A high-protein low-fat diet with orlistat (a lipase inhibitor) reduces chyle flow by restricting long-chain triglyceride availability to the intestinal lymph ducts. If malnourished, add medium-chain triglycerides that are absorbed and transported directly to the liver via the portal vein, avoiding the lymphatics. Avoid medium-chain triglycerides in severe cirrhosis, as they precipitate hepatic encephalopathy. Somatostatin or analogues with a low-fat diet or total parenteral nutrition close lymphatic leaks following surgery and relieve symptoms in malignancy.

Further Reading

Feldman M, Friedman LS, and Brandt LJ. *Sleisenger and Fordtran's Gastrointestinal and Liver Disease* (10th edition), 2015. Elsevier Saunders.

34 Swelling in the neck

John Newell-Price, Alia Munir, and Miguel Debono

Definition of the symptom

Swelling in the neck is defined as the presence of a swelling in or around the neck; this swelling can involve any structure with in this anatomical region. A number of conditions may present with a swelling or lump in the neck. A detailed history and examination, defining the site of the swelling is paramount in reaching a diagnosis.

The differential diagnosis

Table 34.1 and Box 34.1 outline the differential diagnosis, ordered by probability.

Context

The commonest cause of neck swelling is enlarged lymph nodes secondary to infection, of which non-specific infection is most common (followed by infectious mononucleosis, TB, syphilis, toxoplasmosis, and cat scratch fever). But the second most common cause is secondary metastatic deposits, then lymphoproliferative diseases, and sarcoid. Even when only one lymph node is palpable, the adjacent nodes are invariably diseased.

Approach to diagnosis

History

To determine **generalized** aetiology, ask about malaise, weight loss, fever, rigours, infectious disease, and travel history to indicate an infective cause.

To determine **local** causes, ask about pain in the mouth, sore throats, ulcers, nasal discharge, blockage of the airway, problems swallowing, changes in voice, difficulty breathing, and skin lesions.

In non-specific **inflammatory lymphadenopathy**, recurrent bouts of tonsillitis are common. The majority of patients are young; age <10 years, pyrexia, anorexia, and a painful lump are common. Typically, lymph nodes may be tender and hot, and firm but not fixed.

With **tuberculous lymphadenitis and abscess**, upper cervical lymph nodes are commonly affected. Children, young adults, the elderly, immigrants, and those who are immunosuppressed are commonly affected. A neck lump appears with or without pain; if abscess formation occurs, the lump may become painful. It may discharge. There may be signs of TB in the lungs, other lymph nodes, and urinary tract. Typically, nodes are not hot and may be firm and matted together. An abscess may feel fluctuant. Consider associated HIV infection.

Box 34.1 Midline neck swellings

Common
- thyroid swellings
- thyroglossal cyst

Uncommon
- lymph nodes
- sublingual dermoid cyst
- plunging ranula
- pharyngeal pouch
- subhyoid bursa
- carcinoma of the larynx/trachea/oesophagus

Carcinomatous lymphadenopathy is seen most often in patients over the age of 50 (the exception being papillary carcinoma of the thyroid, which occurs in younger adults). Upper deep cervical nodes drain lesions above the hyoid bone. Middle and lower deep cervical lymph nodes drain the thyroid and larynx, and supraclavicular lymphadenopathy indicates thoracic or abdominal disease. Lymph nodes may be non-tender and hard, and may be fixed.

Lymphoma presents with a painless lump or lumps, with systemic symptoms, typically, malaise, weight loss, pallor, itching, and periodic fevers (Pel–Ebstein). There may also be bone pain. Typically, lymph nodes are described as rubbery.

If **thyroid goitre** is suspected, take a history to determine thyroid status, ask about a change in appearance, intolerance to hot or cold temperatures, tremor, palpitations, change in appetite or bowel habit, dyspnoea, chest pain, irritability, and, in females, a change in the menstrual cycle. Also ask about any eye symptoms, in particular, staring or protruding eyes and difficulty closing eyelids (exophthalmos), and double vision (ophthalmoplegia). Swelling of the conjunctive (chemosis) may be present, as may pain secondary to corneal ulceration. An enlarged thyroid in Graves' disease is typically diffusely enlarged and moves on swallowing.

Other, rarer, neck masses include carotid body tumours, cystic hygromas, pharyngeal pouch, sternomastoid tumour, and cervical rib.

Examination

The neck is divided into the anterior triangle (bounded by the anterior border of the sternocleidomastoid, the lower edge of the jaw, and the midline) and the posterior triangle (bounded by the posterior border of the sternocleidomastoid, the anterior edge of trapezius, and the clavicle). The differential diagnoses for swellings in these regions are listed in Table 34.1.

Specific clues to the diagnosis

Specific clues to the diagnosis are:

- history and age of the patient
- 75% of lateral neck masses in patients aged >40 are caused by malignant tumours
- in the absence of overt signs of infection, a lateral neck mass is metastatic squamous cell carcinoma or lymphoma until proven otherwise

Table 34.1 Lateral neck swellings

	Anterior triangle	Posterior triangle
Lymph nodes	Lymph nodes Cold abscess	Lymph nodes Cold abscess
Salivary glands	Submandibular swelling Parotid swelling	
Cystic structure	Branchial cyst	Cystic hygroma
Vascular structures	Carotid body tumour Carotid body aneurysm	Subclavian artery aneurysm
Other	Sternomastoid tumour	Tumour of clavicle

Key diagnostic tests

Depending on clinical suspicion, the key diagnostic tests are:

- full blood count
- urea and electrolytes
- liver function tests
- bone chemistry
- thyroid function tests
- inflammatory markers
- Ziehl–Neelsen stain (also known as the acid-fast stain)
- TB PCR
- HIV test
- fine-needle aspiration, with or without neck ultrasound; in experienced hands, this technique is accurate, inexpensive, and can be performed in the clinic for histological diagnosis

Other diagnostic tests

Other diagnostic tests are:

- chest X-ray
- CT neck; thorax and abdomen, if indicated

Introduction to therapy

Therapy will depend on the underlying diagnosis. Liaison with other specialists may be recommended as follows:

Tuberculosis: Refer to infectious disease team to start a 6-month course of chemotherapy and offer HIV test.
Malignancy: Tissue diagnosis will be required, as will liaison with surgeons and oncologists for consideration of surgery, chemotherapy, and radiotherapy.
Lymphoma: Refer to medical oncologists/haematologists for consideration of chemotherapy.
Thyroid disease: Refer to endocrinologists for management of hyper- or hypothyroidism. Thyroid malignancies require thyroidectomy and referral to oncology for joint management. Radioiodine therapy may be required. Chronic suppression of TSH is standard practice.

Prognosis

The prognosis will depend upon the underlying diagnosis:

Tuberculosis: Tuberculosis, if untreated, kills two-thirds of affected people; however, with treatment, the mortality rate is <5%.
Head and neck cancer: Early head and neck cancers have high cure rates; however, 50% present with advanced disease, and probability of cure is inversely proportional to the size of the tumour and to the extent of regional node involvement.
Lymphoma: Indolent non-Hodgkin's lymphoma has a good prognosis, with a median survival of 10 years; however, if it is advanced, it is not curable. High-grade lymphomas are more aggressive but more chemo-responsive, with a median survival of 2 years. Overall cure rates for Hodgkin's lymphoma are around 75%–80%. For young people at an early stage of the disease, cure rates approach 100%.
Thyroid malignancy: Thyroid conditions are mostly benign. Of the thyroid malignancies, papillary thyroid carcinoma and follicular thyroid carcinoma carry a 97% cure rate; medullary thyroid carcinoma is usually more aggressive and has a worse prognosis but is rarer; anaplastic thyroid carcinoma is aggressive, and the prognosis is poor, with a mean survival of 6 months from diagnosis.

How to handle uncertainty in the diagnosis of this symptom

Retake the history and re-examine the patient. Arrange an ultrasound or a CT if these have not already been done. Refer to an ENT surgeon.

Further Reading

Perros P, Colley S, Boelaert K, et al. Guidelines for the management of thyroid cancer: Third edition. *Clin Endocrinol* 2014; 81(Suppl 1): 1–122.
Rosenberg TL, Brown JJ, and Jefferson GD. Evaluating the adult patient with a neck mass. *Med Clin North Am* 2010; 94: 1017–29.

CHAPTER 34 **Swelling in the neck**

35 Splenomegaly and other disorders of the spleen

Chris Bunch

The spleen

The spleen is a predominantly lymphoid organ, normally about the size of a clenched fist (11 cm in length; 150–200 g) located beneath the diaphragm in the left upper abdomen. It has a dual role as a filter for the circulation, and a primary lymphoid organ in its own right. About three-quarters of its volume is a matrix of capillaries and sinuses (the red pulp), through which blood is able to percolate slowly and come into contact with fixed macrophages, which are able to remove senescent or damaged red cells, or other particulate matter such as bacteria. An important function is maintenance of red-cell integrity: the spleen is able to remove red-cell inclusions or damaged portions of membrane. The slow circulation through the spleen leads to a 'pooling' effect, with up to one-third of circulating platelets and 5% of red cells present in the spleen at any one time. The degree of pooling increases with splenomegaly.

The lymphoid tissue is organized into scattered follicles (the white pulp), which have a particularly important role in initiating primary humoral immune responses and antibody (IgM) synthesis.

In the fetus, both the liver and the spleen are major sites of haemopoiesis, but this reduces rapidly and the bone marrow becomes predominant after birth. However, in certain infiltrative bone marrow disorders, such as myelofibrosis, chronic myeloid leukaemia, and polycythaemia vera, extramedullary haemopoiesis can return to these organs.

Splenomegaly

The spleen commonly enlarges when either its filtration function is increased—as in haemolysis—or it is stimulated by infection or inflammation. It may also be involved in myeloproliferative and lymphoproliferative neoplasias. Common causes are listed in Box 35.1.

Hypersplenism

Increased splenic pooling and phagocytic activity may accompany any cause of splenomegaly, leading to a variable degree of anaemia, thrombocytopenia, or neutropenia out of proportion to any expected from the underlying cause of splenomegaly. Splenectomy may be of benefit if symptoms of the cytopenias are a problem.

The combination of splenomegaly, neutropenia, and long-standing seropositive rheumatoid arthritis is known as **Felty's syndrome**. Patients are particularly prone to infection because of the neutropenia.

Splenectomy

The spleen is probably most often removed surgically because of trauma, but may be removed electively in a number of haematological conditions (Box 35.2). Awareness of the risks of overwhelming pneumococcal sepsis (see 'Overwhelming post-splenectomy infection') has led to a more cautious approach to splenectomy in most situations.

Hyposplenism

Loss of splenic function due to its removal, congenital absence, damage from conditions such as sickle cell disease, or atrophy in coeliac disease (Box 35.3) produces characteristic changes in the blood, reflecting mainly the loss of the spleen's function in maintaining red-cell integrity. The red cells show Howell–Jolly bodies, acanthocytes,

---

Box 35.1 Causes of splenomegaly

Infections, esp.:
- chronic bacterial infections
- glandular fever
- rubella
- brucellosis
- subacute bacterial endocarditis
- malaria
- kala azar

Inflammatory disorders
- rheumatoid arthritis
- systemic lupus erythematosus
- sarcoidosis

Malignancy
- lymphomas
- leukaemias
- myeloproliferative disorders, e.g. polycythaemia vera, chronic granulocytic leukaemia
- **not** carcinomas, as a rule

Increased 'work' (phagocytic activity)
- haemolytic anaemias

Congestion
- portal hypertension

Storage disorders
- Gaucher's disease

---

and target cells; there may also be a mild monocytosis, lymphocytosis, and thrombocytosis.

There are no entirely reliable tests for diagnosing or excluding functional hyposplenism. Most but not all patients will have the aforementioned blood film changes; in addition, phase contrast microscopy of red cells may reveal pits in the membrane which would normally lead to removal of the cell by a functional spleen. Cross-sectional or ultrasound imaging will usually reveal absence of the spleen or a significant reduction in its size.

Overwhelming post-splenectomy infection

Overwhelming post-splenectomy infection (OPSI), that is, overwhelming sepsis with pneumococci (or, less commonly, haemophilus or meningococci) is a rare but devastating late complication of splenectomy, and also occurs in those who have lost splenic function for other reasons, such as sickle cell disease. This risk is low

---

Box 35.2 Common indications for splenectomy

- trauma
- hereditary spherocytosis
- chronic idiopathic thrombocytopenia
- hypersplenism
- for diagnosis of splenomegaly, when cause cannot otherwise be determined

---

Box 35.3 Causes of functional hyposplenism

- splenectomy
- splenic irradiation
- therapeutic splenic embolization
- coeliac disease
- sickle cell disorders
- chronic graft-vs-host disease

(less than 1%), but is considerably higher in children, reflecting perhaps relatively immature immunity. It may be lower in those who have had splenectomy for trauma, although such patients are not normally followed up as assiduously. There is some evidence that the traumatized spleen may seed sufficient splenic tissue into the abdominal cavity for some splenic function to be retained.

In its early stages, post-splenectomy infection is indistinguishable from any other febrile illness of acute onset, but its subsequent course may fulminate within 24–48 hours, so early recognition is essential. For this reason, various approaches to prophylaxis have been recommended:

Immunization: All individuals with absent or dysfunctional spleens should be fully immunised according to the national schedule (see below). Immunization should preferably be undertaken before splenectomy, as the spleen may be important for a satisfactory response, but if this is not possible it should still be offered after the operation

Prophylactic antibiotics: Adults (>16) at high risk of pneumococcal infection should be prescribed life-long prophylactic antibacterials. High-risk patients include the following:

- greater than 50 years of age;
- history of previous invasive pneumococcal disease;
- * splenectomy for underlying haematological malignancy, particularly in the context of ongoing immunosuppression.

Penicillin is usually recommended (250 mg, once or twice daily) but erythromycin is a satisfactory alternative.

Life-long antimicrobial prophylaxis for all hyposplenic patients is no longer recommended.

Contingent antibiotics: All hyposplenic patients not on prophylaxis should have a ready supply of antibiotic (amoxicillin or erythromycin) to take at the very first sign of any febrile illness. Most such situations will not be serious, but it is not worth taking the risk of waiting to see. This approach requires close co-operation of the general practitioner in maintaining a fresh supply of antibiotics.

Patient education is important, and patients should be encouraged to wear an alert bracelet or carry a card with relevant details (see Further Reading). It is important also that they understand the need for prompt treatment of any febrile illness.

Other infections in hyposplenic patients

Patients with functional hyposplensim are also at increased risk of infection from tick-borne organisms (e.g. babesiosis, Lyme disease), rickettsial diseases and malaria. Appropriate advice should be given to those contemplating travel to endemic areas for such conditions.

Further Reading

Public Health England. Immunisation of individuals with underlying medical conditions 2013. Last updated 29 September 2016 — see all updates. Available at: https://www.gov.uk/government/uploads/system/uploads/attachment_data/file/566853/Green_Book_Chapter7.pdf

Public Health England. Splenectomy: leaflet and card 2015. Available at: https://www.gov.uk/government/publications/splenectomy-leaflet-and-card

Rubin LG and Schaffner W. Care of the asplenic patient. *N Engl J Med* 2014; 371: 349–56.

36 Lymphadenopathy

Chris Bunch

Lymph nodes

Lymph nodes are small, bean-shaped structures generally a few milli-metres in size, distributed widely throughout the body and assuming a major role in the immune system. There are several hundred lymph nodes, networked by lymphatic channels and the blood stream and organized into anatomical groups, for example, cervical, subman-dibular, hilar, mediastinal, axillary, para-aortic, inguinal, and so on. They are composed principally of lymphocytes and macrophages.

Lymph draining from the tissues percolates through lymph nodes, coming into contact with lymphocytes and macrophages, which will respond to the presence of foreign antigen by proliferation and pro-duction of antibody and sensitized cells.

Lymphadenopathy

Peripheral lymph nodes are not normally palpable except in thin individuals. Enlargement of lymph nodes is called lymphadenopa-thy, important causes of which are shown in Box 36.1. It is impor-tant to distinguish between reactive lymphadenopathy, which is usually an appropriate response to infection or inflammation, and malignant or neoplastic lymphadenopathy. This is often possible on clinical grounds, but biopsy may be required if lymphadenopathy is persistent or progressive over several weeks and is not associated with other evidence of infection. Surgical excision biopsy gives the most reliable information, and histological examination can be sup-plemented by immunological or molecular analysis as required. Fine-needle-aspiration cytology is simpler and more rapid, but does not yet have the accuracy of surgical biopsy.

Clinical assessment of lymphadenopathy should include full examination of all superficial lymph node groups: cervical (anterior and posterior), occipital, submandibular, supraclavicular, axillary, epitrochlear, inguinal, and femoral. Note should be taken of their size, texture (soft, hard), mobility, and attachment as well as the number of enlarged glands in each group. Abnormally large iliac or abdominal nodes may also be palpable in thin individuals.

Radiologically, lymphadenopathy is best assessed by CT scanning. PET scanning can indicate metabolic activity in enlarged lymph nodes and can be helpful in monitoring effects of treatment in malignant lymph nodes.

Box 36.1 Causes of lymphadenopathy

Inflammatory

Suppurating
- pyogenic infection

Non-suppurating
- infection
- rheumatoid arthritis
- systemic lupus erythematosus
- dermatopathic (draining skin affected by e.g. psoriasis or eczema)

Granulomatous
- tuberculosis
- histoplasmosis
- toxoplasmosis
- sarcoidosis
- syphilis

Malignant
- secondary carcinoma, melanoma, or sarcoma
- lymphoma
- leukaemia

Congenital
- lymphangiomas
- cystic hygroma

Further Reading

Alitalo K. The lymphatic vasculature in disease. *Nat Med* 2011; 17: 1371–80.

Eisenmenger LB and Wiggins RH III. Imaging of head and neck lymph nodes. *Radiol Clin N Am* 2015; 53: 115–32.

37 Anaemia

Chris Bunch

Definition

Anaemia denotes a reduction in the circulating haemoglobin (Hb) level or red-cell count below that which is normal for the individual's age and sex.

There are, however, wide individual and population differences in the levels of Hb and the red-cell count, so absolute criteria for diagnosing anaemia are difficult to define. A more functional definition is a state in which the circulating red-cell mass is insufficient to meet the oxygen requirements of the tissues, although this is also subject to wide variation, and is influenced by other factors such as the presence of cardiovascular or lung disease.

Anaemia may be graded as severe (less than 60 g/L), moderate (60–90 g/L), or mild (between 90 g/L and the lower limit of normal).

Context

Anaemia is common and may be a primary problem or a feature of a wide variety of other conditions (Box 37.1). Its presence in these should be unsurprising, and further investigation is only warranted if there are unusual features or it does not improve with treatment of the underlying condition.

Box 37.1 Principal causes of anaemia (with examples)

Primary anaemia
- blood loss
- deficiency anaemias:
  - iron deficiency
  - B_{12} deficiency
  - folate deficiency
- defective haemoglobin production:
  - thalassaemias
  - lead poisoning
- haemolytic anaemia, congenital:
  - haemoglobinopathies (haemoglobin S, haemoglobin C)
  - red-cell enzyme defects (glucose-6-phosphate dehydrogenase, pyruvate kinase)
  - red-cell membrane defects (spherocytosis, elliptocytosis)
- haemolytic anaemia, acquired:
  - autoimmune haemolytic anaemia
  - paroxysmal nocturnal haemoglobinuria
  - poisoning

Secondary anaemia
- anaemia of chronic disease:
  - infection
  - inflammatory disorders
  - malignancy
- marrow failure:
  - leukaemia
  - myelodysplasia
  - myeloproliferative disorders
- renal failure
- liver disease
- endocrine disorders:
  - hypothyroidism
  - hyperthyroidism
  - adrenal insufficiency

In primary care, a general practitioner can expect to encounter one new case of anaemia every month; most of these will be mild or moderate anaemias due to blood loss/iron deficiency, or the anaemia of chronic disease.

Approach to the diagnosis

Anaemia is neither a symptom nor a disease. The function of Hb is to transport oxygen to the tissues. Actual tissue oxygen delivery is also influenced by several other factors, for example, blood flow (itself influenced by cardiac output and vascular resistance) and the oxygen affinity of Hb, which can be varied adaptively to a significant degree.

The clinical consequences of anaemia are thus variable and depend upon the degree to which the body has compensated for a falling Hb level: it may be entirely asymptomatic or may cause varying degrees of tiredness and fatigue. Moderate-to-severe anaemia is likely to exacerbate symptoms and signs of any coexisting cardiac or respiratory disease, such as angina, dyspnoea, and heart failure.

There are no specific clinical signs of anaemia: some pallor of the mucous membranes is usual in moderate-to-severe anaemia. Jaundice accompanies significant haemolysis (with haemoglobinuria, if haemolysis is intravascular) and a 'lemon-yellow' tinge is characteristic of megaloblastic anaemias. Glossitis and cracking of the corners of the mouth (angular cheilosis) may occur in deficiency anaemias, and nail changes (koilonychia) are characteristic of severe iron deficiency.

Anaemia is usually classified in terms of the average red-cell size (mean corpuscular volume (MCV)) as **normocytic** (MCV 80–100 fl), **microcytic** (MCV less than 80 fl), or **macrocytic** (MCV greater than 100 fl).

Microcytic anaemias

Small red cells indicate inadequate haemoglobinization of the red cell, and are the hallmark of iron-deficient erythropoiesis and the thalassaemias. Lesser degrees of microcytosis are also seen in the anaemia of chronic disease (infections, inflammation, malignancy), and sideroblastic anaemias.

Macrocytic anaemias

Minor degrees of macrocytosis are common in alcohol excess and pregnancy, and are usually of no consequence unless associated with anaemia, when causes include liver disease, haemolytic anaemia (reflecting a high proportion of reticulocytes, which are larger than normal red cells), hypothyroidism, myeloma, and myelodysplasia. Significant macrocytosis (MCV > 110 fl) is characteristic of megaloblastic erythropoiesis (B_{12} or folate deficiency). An MCV greater than 120 fl is usually an artefact due to red-cell clumping in vitro, which can occur in autoimmune haemolytic anaemias.

Normocytic anaemias

As the MCV is an average of the red-cell size distribution, there is considerable overlap between micro- and macrocytic anaemias, and anaemias with a normal MCV. Causes include blood loss, renal failure, anaemia of chronic disease, haemolytic anaemia, bone marrow failure, myelodysplasia, and haematological malignancies.

Specific clues to the diagnosis

A full blood count will be a routine investigation in a wide range of clinical situations, and will reveal anaemia if it is present. In individuals with unexplained tiredness, fatigue, or pallor, the result will often be reassuring.

Key diagnostic tests

The key diagnostic test for anaemia is the full blood count (see Chapter 278), and the important parameters are the Hb level, red-cell count, and MCV. Other red-cell parameters—packed cell volume, or haematocrit; mean cell Hb levels, and mean cell Hb concentration—are calculated from these but are of relatively little use clinically.

The reference range for Hb varies slightly between laboratories but, for adults in developed countries, Hb levels between 120 and 160 g/L would generally be considered normal in females, and between 140 and 180 g/L for males. The difference in Hb levels between adult males and females reflects higher levels of androgens (which stimulate erythropoiesis) in males.

Other diagnostic tests

Specific tests for specific anaemias are described in the relevant chapters.

Introduction to therapy

The principles of treatment in anaemia are to correct any deficiencies if present, treat any underlying conditions, and, as a last resort, to consider red-cell transfusion, but only if the anaemia is moderate or severe, symptomatic, and unlikely to respond to the first two approaches. In selected situations, for example, renal disease and cancer, administration of recombinant erythropoietin may be useful.

Prognosis

The prognosis in anaemia is dependent on the cause and the prognosis of any underlying condition. Simple deficiency anaemias are usually easily corrected. On the other hand, congenital anaemias such as sickle cell disease and thalassaemias are essentially incurable, and homozygous forms are life shortening. More details are available in the relevant chapters.

How to handle uncertainty in the diagnosis of anaemia

The diagnosis of anaemia is based on the Hb concentration, which is normally accurate and reproducible. However, there are situations where this may give an inaccurate or misleading picture. In addition, the Hb concentration may vary in an individual by as much as 10 g/L from day to day.

Blood for the full blood count should be taken with care: prolonged tourniquet pressure may give rise to slight haemoconcentration and an artefactual rise in the Hb level, while taking blood from an arm that also has a running intravenous infusion in place commonly leads to haemodilution and an abnormally low Hb level. Samples may deteriorate if delayed in transit to the laboratory.

The clinical context is important: for example, Hb levels are commonly slightly reduced in the elderly for no easily discernible reason. It is unwise to label such patients as anaemic on the basis of a single Hb estimation.

Further Reading

DeLoughery TG. Microcytic anemia. *New Engl J Med* 2014; 371: 1324–31.

Gangat N and Wolanskyj AP. Anemia of chronic disease. *Semin Hematol* 2013; 50: 232–8.

Lopez A, Cacoub P, Macdougall IC, and Peyrin-Biroulet L. Iron-deficiency anaemia. *Lancet* 2016; 387: 907–16.

CHAPTER 37 **Anaemia**

38 Bruising and bleeding

Nicola Curry and Raza Alikhan

Definition of the symptom

The amount of blood that leaks from a blood vessel into the subcutaneous tissue will determine the size and description of a lesion. Minute amounts of blood producing pin-point red lesions <2 mm in size are described as petechiae, larger lesions (2 mm–1 cm) are purpura, and bruises (ecchymoses) tend to be >1 cm.

Differential diagnosis in primary care and secondary care

Box 38.1 gives examples of the causes of bruising and bleeding that are likely to present in primary and secondary care, as well as causes relating specifically to neonates and children.

Context

Bruising is extremely common and a normal response to injury. Perception of what is a normal level of bruising is subjective and it can be difficult to differentiate a patient with 'normal' bruising from a patient who has bruising due to a mild bleeding disorder.

However, spontaneous bruising or bruises that seem incongruent to the degree of injury experienced must be taken seriously. Therefore, it is important that you assess your patient globally before providing reassurance that their symptoms are not worrying.

Approach to the diagnosis, and specific clues to the diagnosis

It can be helpful to categorize patients with bruising/bleeding into two clinical groups: those who have no other symptoms, in whom the cause is likely to be either a normal response to injury, or an isolated platelet disorder or clotting factor deficiency; and those who have additional symptoms, in whom haematological disease (e.g. thrombocytopenia due to bone marrow infiltration) or systemic disease (e.g. connective tissue disorder) is more likely.

The history is the most important part of the assessment of a patient who presents with bruising or bleeding. The main considerations to make are:

- the accompanying symptoms
- the timescale of the symptoms
- the site of bruising or bleeding
- the severity of the problem

Accompanying symptoms

Try to get a feel for whether the patient has an isolated bleeding problem, or whether their symptoms are a manifestation of a wider problem. Ask about accompanying fatigue (anaemia), increased infection (leucopenia), lymphadenopathy, joint pains, and so on. Be guided by the history.

Timescale of the symptoms

It is important to determine whether the problem has been a lifelong one or whether it started recently, to differentiate between inherited or acquired disease. If the history suggests an inherited disease, ask whether there is a family history of bleeding. Inherited bleeding disorders can be X-linked (haemophilia), autosomal dominant (some forms of von Willebrand's disease), or autosomal recessive (some factor deficiencies

---

Box 38.1 Causes of bruising and bleeding likely to present in primary and secondary care, and causes relating specifically to neonates and children

Primary care

- 'easy bruising'
  - no underlying diagnosis
  - elderly
  - steroid therapy
- drugs
  - antiplatelet agents
  - anticoagulants
- systemic disease
  - liver disease, including alcoholic liver disease
  - uraemia
  - thyroid disease
  - Cushing's disease
  - autoimmune disease
- thrombocytopenia
  - in particular, immune thrombocytopenia purpura
- von Willebrand's disease
- haemophilia A
- haemophilia B

Secondary care

- drugs
  - antiplatelet agents
  - anticoagulants
  - heparin
- systemic disease
  - liver disease
  - uraemia
- sepsis/disseminated intravascular coagulopathy
- thrombocytopenia
  - platelet destruction
    - immune thrombocytopenia purpura
    - disseminated intravascular coagulopathy
    - thrombotic thrombocytopenia purpura
    - haemolytic uraemic syndrome
  - reduced production of platelets
    - marrow failure
    - marrow infiltration
- von Willebrand's disease
- haemophilia A
- haemophilia B
- vasculitis
- collagen disorders

Causes relating specifically to neonates and children

Neonates

- sepsis/disseminated intravascular coagulopathy
- congenital infection (TORCH):
  - toxoplasmosis
  - other (syphilis)
  - rubella
  - cytomegalovirus
  - herpes simplex virus
- vitamin K deficiency
- immune thrombocytopenia purpura

Box 38.1 (Continued)
- neonatal alloimmune thrombocytopenia
- haemophilia

Childhood
- immune thrombocytopenia purpura
- leukaemia
- inherited bleeding disorders
- non-accidental injury

and various platelet diseases). It may therefore, in some circumstances, be important to ask whether the patient's parents are related other than by marriage. If the problem started recently, ask whether the symptoms relate temporally to any new medications, or new activities.

Site of bruising or bleeding

Epistaxis

Bleeding from the nose is one of the most common symptoms of platelet disorders and von Willebrand's disease. It is also a common symptom of hereditary haemorrhagic telangiectasia. However, a large number of the population also suffer from nosebleeds. If the bleeding is confined to a single nostril, it is more likely due to a localized abnormality rather than a coagulopathy. Epistaxis during childhood is also common and tends to disappear after puberty. The need to seek medical advice, nasal packing, cautery, or transfusions must be sought from the history.

Gums

Spontaneous bleeding from the gums is another common symptom of a platelet disorder or von Willebrand's disease. Bleeding from the gums after tooth brushing may be normal or abnormal, depending on the presence or absence of gingival disease and the type of toothbrush employed.

Skin

Is the bleeding response excessive or in keeping with the degree of trauma to the skin? Spontaneous bruising is likely to be pathological. It is sometimes difficult to elicit a history of trauma from a patient; therefore, the location of a bruise can help in deciding if bruising is traumatic. In general, bruises following trauma arise at bony surfaces and on the arms and legs. Bruising arising on the back or trunk are likely to be spontaneous or due to minimal trauma.

Tooth extraction

This is often the first and only significant haemostatic challenge a person faces. The need for packing, suturing, or transfusions may be significant and indicate the presence of an underlying bleeding disorder.

Haematemesis

It is important to look for an anatomical cause. Defects in haemostasis may arise in patients with liver disease or oesophageal varices, or who are on aspirin.

Haemoptysis

As with haematemesis, it is important to look for an anatomical cause.

Menorrhagia

Menorrhagia is defined as the loss of more than 80 ml of blood per cycle. It is often difficult to assess the severity of blood loss from the history or by the number of sanitary towels used. Pictorial menstrual charts have been found to be useful in quantifying blood loss. If no gynaecological cause is present, it is important to look for platelet disorders and, specifically, von Willebrand's disease.

Pregnancy

It is important to take a detailed history of bleeding both during pregnancy and in the post-partum period. The need for transfusions,

dilatation and curettage, iron therapy, and/or hysterectomy needs to be documented.

Haemarthroses

Spontaneous joint bleeds are a feature of haemophilia (see Chapter 284).

Umbilical stump bleeding

Delayed bleeding from the umbilical stump is a feature suggestive of Factor XIII deficiency, but may also occur in haemophilia.

Severity of the problem

As a general rule, the more severe the symptom, the more severe is the bleeding disorder. The following points suggest further investigation is required:

- recurrent bleeding (i.e. more than three times at one site of the body)
- more than two sites of the body affected at one time
- unusual bleeding following a routine operation/childbirth, particularly if a blood transfusion is required
- iron deficiency anaemia secondary to blood loss
- bleeding lasting more than 30 minutes and requiring intervention (such as nasal packing)

Key diagnostic tests

The following tests should be performed as a screen for patients with increased bruising and bleeding symptoms:

- full blood count and film
- coagulation profile (prothrombin time, activated partial thromboplastin time, fibrinogen)

Any abnormality that arises in these tests can then guide you to your next investigation.

If the history suggests a systemic cause for the bleeding, consider checking:

- urea and electrolytes
- liver function tests
- thyroid function tests
- an autoantibody screen

Other diagnostic tests

If you have a patient with a suspected bleeding disorder, it is often best to refer them to a haematologist. The specialized testing is often only available in haemophilia centres (see Chapter 273). These tests include:

- coagulation factor assays (Factor VIII, Factor IX, and Factor XI)
- von Willebrand's disease screen (FVIII:C, vWF:Ag, vWF:RiCof)
- platelet analysis:
  - platelet aggregometry and nucleotide testing
  - electron microscopy
  - flow cytometry
- DNA analysis

Introduction to therapy

Treatment for patients with symptoms of bruising will depend on the underlying diagnosis. Many patients will require simple reassurance that their bruising is not clinically concerning and that no active intervention is required.

For those patients that are bruising because of a systemic disorder, symptoms can be ameliorated by treating the underlying disease.

When drugs such as aspirin or warfarin are the cause of the symptoms, the risks and benefits of continuing or stopping the drug must be weighed up.

Whatever the cause of the bleeding, simple instructions can be given to reduce risks of further bleeding:

- avoidance of intramuscular injections
- avoidance of antiplatelet/anti-inflammatory/anticoagulant drugs, if possible
- avoidance of contact sports in severe bleeding disorders
- informing any physician/dentist, prior to an invasive procedure, of the bleeding history and, if possible, seeking advice from a haematologist

Patients with inherited bleeding disorders, and those with significant acquired bleeding disorders, should be treated by a haemophilia centre so that, at times of significant haemostatic challenge (such as childbirth or surgery), they are managed appropriately and safely.

Prognosis

It is impossible to provide specifics regarding prognosis, as this will entirely depend on the underlying cause of the bleeding and the severity of the disease.

How to handle uncertainty in the diagnosis of this symptom

Bruising is a very difficult symptom to diagnose with accuracy. Therefore, uncertainty is common.

The simple rule to follow is, don't ignore bruising/bleeding if:

- a patient has systemic symptoms
- it is spontaneous or recurrent
- it has required active intervention to halt it
- it has led to the need for iron replacement or blood transfusion

These types of symptoms require urgent attention. Less convincing evidence of disease can be investigated at a more leisurely pace and, indeed, underlying pathology may not be found.

Further Reading

British Society for Haematology: Haemostasis and Thrombosis Guidelines. Available at: http://www.b-s-h.org.uk/guidelines/?category=Haemostasis+and+Thrombosis&p=1&search=#guideline-filters__select__status.

Rydz N and James PD. Why is my patient bleeding or bruising? *Hematol Oncol Clin North Am* 2012; 26: 321–44.

World Federation of Hemophilia: *About Bleeding Disorders* (http://www.wfh.org/en/page.aspx?pid=1282)

39 Transient loss of consciousness

Jonathan Timperley and Sandeep Hothi

Definition of the symptom

Transient loss of consciousness (TLoC) is characterized by a rapid, transient, and complete loss of consciousness of short duration with spontaneous, complete recovery. Syncope is a specific type of TLoC caused by transient, global, cerebral hypoperfusion.

Differential diagnosis

TLoC may be traumatic or non-traumatic. Causes of non-traumatic TLoC include syncope, epilepsy, psychogenic causes, and other, rarer causes. Causes of syncope are shown in Box 39.1.

Context

TLoC is common and affects up to half the population at some point in their lives. It accounts for approximately 3% of A & E attendances and 1% hospital admissions; with etiologies ranging from benign conditions and clinical courses on the one hand, and up to 33% mortality on the other when there is underlying cardiac structural disease. The incidence of TLoC rises with age, particularly beyond the age of 70 years. The diagnostic process can be difficult, investigations can be costly, and even potentially serious conditions may be difficult to diagnose early.

Approach to diagnosis

The first aim is to confirm a diagnosis of TLoC (see 'Definition of the symptom'), and then to determine if there are features predictive

---

Box 39.1 Causes of syncope

Reflex (neurally mediated)
- vasovagal
  - emotional stress
  - orthostatic
- situational
  - micturition
  - coughing, sneezing
  - post-exercise
- carotid sinus hypersensitivity

Orthostatic hypotension
- drug induced
- hypovolaemia
- primary autonomic failure
- secondary autonomic failure

Cardiovascular
- arrhythmia
  - bradyarrhythmias (sinus node dysfunction; atrioventricular block)
  - supraventricular and ventricular tachyarrhythmias
- structural heart disease
  - stenotic valve disease
  - cardiomyopathies
- acute major pulmonary embolism
- severe pulmonary hypertension

Data from Task Force for the Diagnosis and Management of Syncope of the European Society of Cardiology (ESC), volume 30, p. 2631, Copyright © 2009 *Eur Heart Journal*

Box 39.2 History taking after syncope

Questions regarding circumstances prior to the attack:
- position (supine, sitting, or standing)
- activity (rest, change in posture, during or after exercise, during or immediately after urination, defaecation, cough, or swallowing)
- predisposing factors (e.g. crowded, warm, prolonged standing, postprandial) and precipitating factors (fear, pain, neck movements)

Questions about the onset of the attack:
- nausea, vomiting, abdominal discomfort, feeling cold, sweating, aura, neck or shoulder pain, blurred vision, dizziness
- palpitations

Questions about the attack (eyewitness):
- way of falling, skin colour, duration of loss of consciousness, breathing pattern, movements, duration of movements, onset of movements in relation to fall, tongue biting

Questions about the end of the attack:
- nausea, sweating, feeling cold, confusion, muscle aches, skin colour, injury, chest pain, palpitations, urinary or faecal incontinence

Questions about the background:
- family history of sudden death, cardiomyopathy, or fainting
- previous cardiac disease
- neurological history
- metabolic disorders
- medication and other drugs, including alcohol
- if recurrent syncope, information about recurrences including time from first event and frequency of events

Data from Task Force for the Diagnosis and Management of Syncope of the European Society of Cardiology (ESC), volume 30, p. 2631, Copyright © 2009 *Eur Heart Journal*

---

of a high risk of cardiovascular events or death. The presence of the following features makes syncope highly likely: complete loss of consciousness; rapid loss of consciousness; spontaneous and full recovery; and loss of postural tone. If any of these features are absent, a non-syncopal cause of TLoC should be considered.

The account of a witness, if available, is of importance. This, together with the patient's account, will be required to build a description of events from before the episode through to the recovery. Thus, the features in the Box 39.2 should be elicited.

Specific clues to the diagnosis

History

The duration of TLoC due to syncope is typically in the region of 20 seconds, and rarely up to a few minutes. A previous history of episodes of TLoC and their descriptions may help confirm the diagnosis as well as establishing the frequency and impact upon the patient's life.

Myoclonic jerks can occur after the onset of syncope, but only last for seconds; in contrast, during epilepsy, they occur simultaneously with the onset of loss of consciousness and usually last minutes.

Neurally mediated syncope is suggested by the absence of cardiac disease; multiple episodes; and onset after prolonged standing or after exertion, head rotation, or specific situational triggers.

Orthostatic hypotension is suggested by TLoC after standing; the recent start of drugs causing hypotension; TLoC in hot, crowded places; autonomic neuropathy; Parkinson's disease; and TLoC associated with standing after the cessation of exercise. Cardiac syncope is suggested by structural cardiac disease, exertional symptoms, palpitations, or an abnormal ECG.

Features suggesting epilepsy include prodrome, tongue biting, unilateral head rotation during the event, prolonged jerking of the limbs, and postictal confusion. Tongue biting (especially of the lateral tongue) is very rare in syncope. Its presence strongly suggests the diagnosis of epilepsy.

The previous medical history may reveal conditions predisposing to TLoC, such as known heart disease, Parkinson's disease, and epilepsy. The drug history may identify a cause, for instance, antihypertensives, diuretics, antiarrthymic drugs, QT-prolonging drugs, or alcohol. The family history may reveal a familial predisposition to a specific cause for TLoC, such as inherited cardiac or neurological diseases. A family history of sudden death or syncope is therefore important, whether the diagnosis is certain or not.

Physical examination

Measurement of vital signs may identify abnormalities of heart rate and/or blood pressure. A postural blood pressure should be checked: a decrease in systolic pressure of 20 mm Hg or more, or 10 mm Hg diastolic, within 3 minutes of standing, is significant and represents orthostatic hypotension.

Cardiovascular examination may reveal an irregular pulse, a diminished pulse volume in severe aortic stenosis, a bradycardia, or a tachycardia. On auscultation there may be a mid-systolic murmur with aortic stenosis or hypertrophic cardiomyopathy; there may be a malar flush and diastolic murmur with mitral stenosis.

Neurological examination should, by definition, demonstrate no permanent de novo neurological abnormalities causing TLoC. There may, however, be neurological deficits secondary to neurological injury sustained during injury caused by the loss of consciousness. There may also be features of Parkinson's disease or autonomic neuropathy and its causes (multiple system atrophy, diabetes mellitus, Lewy body dementia, amyloidosis, renal failure, spinal cord lesions).

Key diagnostic tests

Key diagnostic tests are:

ECG: conduction abnormalities, ventricular pre-excitation, ventricular or atrial arrhythmias, long or short QT intervals, ST- or T-wave changes, pathological Q waves, Brugada syndrome

Blood tests: full blood count, to exclude anaemia, and blood glucose, to exclude hypoglycaemia

Other diagnostic tests

Other diagnostic tests are:

TSH level: Where tachyarrhythmias or bradyarrhythmias are identified, the TSH level should be checked to exclude hyperthyroidism and hypothyroidism (bradycardia).

Urea and electrolytes: These must also be checked; hypokalaemia is associated with tachyarrhythmias and acquired long-QT syndrome; hyperkalaemia may also cause ventricular arrhythmias.

Echocardiography: This test may reveal aortic or mitral stenosis, aortic dissection, or left ventricular systolic dysfunction.

Carotid sinus massage: Carotid sinus massage (CSM) is performed by applying pressure to the carotid sinus (the point of bifurcation of the common carotid artery) while recording the heart rate and blood pressure to identify symptomatic bradycardia or hypotension. Carotid sinus hypersensitivity (CSH) is diagnosed when CSM causes a pause of 3 or more seconds or a reduction in systolic blood pressure of 50 mm Hg or more. This must be performed with resuscitation facilities to hand in case of asystole. CSH in the presence of a history of syncope is highly suggestive of carotid

sinus hypersensitivity as the cause of TLoC. Complications include a small risk of stroke. CSM should be avoided in patients with a history of TIA, recent stroke (3 months), or carotid bruits.

ECG monitoring: Cardiac monitoring (in hospital) is appropriate in patients considered high risk for cardiac arrhythmia as the cause of TLoC in the immediate phase after presentation. Other forms of monitoring include Holter monitoring (up to 48 hours recording), external event recorder (applied by the patient when palpitations occur), or implantable event recorder (over 3 years monitoring). The selection of these forms of monitoring is based on the frequency of episodes of TLoC.

Short Synacthen test: This test is done when adrenal insufficiency is suspected to cause orthostatic hypotension.

Orthostatic challenging: A change in posture from supine to upright results in venous pooling and reduced venous return. In the normal situation, compensatory mechanisms act to minimize consequent hypotension and syncope. Abnormalities may be cardioinhibitory response (reflex bradycardia), vasodepressor response (reflex hypotension), or both, in such patients. Two forms of test exist to identify significant hypotension and syncope caused by a change in posture. The first involves a change from supine to standing, where the blood pressure is measured in the supine position and then on standing (commonly known as postural blood pressure, described in 'Physical examination'. The second method is known as tilt-table testing. In this test, the patient has blood pressure and heart rate monitoring while being put into a head-up tilt, to assess for neurally mediated syncope. It is thus useful in assessing for neutrally mediated orthostatic hypotension. False positives may be seen in other forms of neurally mediated syncope as well as sinus node dysfunction.

EEG: This is useful in suspected epilepsy rather than as a test for the investigation of syncope.

CT head: This is performed to exclude injury secondary to TLoC when there is suspected head injury, and to exclude structural brain abnormality where a new diagnosis of epilepsy is considered.

CT pulmonary angiogram: This is done where pulmonary embolism is suspected.

Transoesophageal echocardiography/CT/MR aorta: These are done to exclude aortic dissection.

Exercise testing: This is done to assess syncope during or post exertion.

Cardiac catheterization: This is done to exclude myocardial ischaemia or ischaemia-induced arrhythmias.

Introduction to therapy

Patients must be advised not to drive while awaiting specialist review; the relevant driving guidelines must be consulted. Depending on the patient's occupation, modification of working patterns may be needed, such as working at height or operating machinery. Lifestyle advice should be given, including avoidance of triggers, and modification of behaviours that might be dangerous.

Neurally mediated syncope and orthostatic hypotension

In terms of lifestyle advice, education and reassurance should be given that the condition is quite benign. Advice of the identification and avoidance of triggers is also important. Cessation of exacerbating factors, such as specific drugs, should be advised. Education in recognizing prodromal symptoms will enable the patient to perform manoeuvres to prevent progression to TLoC (e.g. physical counterpulsation manoeuvres that cause a rise in blood pressure). Tilt training may reduce TLoC caused by reflex orthostatic hypotension. An adequate intravascular volume should be aimed for by sufficient fluid intake (2–3 l/day) and ~10 g salt per day, in the absence of hypertension.

Compression stockings can help reduce gravitational venous pooling. Physical counterpressure may be useful if patients have prodromal symptoms that can be used as warnings. Midodrine (an alpha agonist) may be of help in chronic autonomic failure, and the mineralocorticoid fludrocortisone may also be helpful. Especially if the patient is unable to adequately increase their fluid and salt intake. In severe cases of TLoC due to reflex syncope with a cardioinhibitory response revealed on tilt testing, permanent pacing may be indicated.

Carotid sinus syndrome

In carotid sinus syndrome, when TLoC is caused by a predominant cardioinhibitory response, permanent cardiac pacing is the treatment of choice.

Cardiac arrhythmia

Permanent pacing is indicated in sinus node dysfunction causing bradycardia as well as atrioventricular block with symptoms. Syncope caused by atrioventricular reentrant tachycardia, atrioventricular nodal reentrant tachycardia, or atrial flutter is ideally treated by ablation. Antiarrhythmic therapy is used while awaiting ablation or following failed ablation.

For ventricular tachycardia (VT) or ventricular fibrillation (VF), any proarrhythmic drugs must be stopped. An implantable cardioverter defibrillator (ICD) is indicated in VT with a reduced ejection fraction, or VT/VF without reversible causes. Ablation may be considered in a structurally normal heart. Revascularization should be considered in ischaemic arrhythmias.

Structural heart disease

Where TLoC is secondary to underlying structural heart disease, treatment is aimed at the specific abnormality as well as an aim to reduce the risk of future events. Treatment thus varies but includes, for instance, surgery for severe aortic stenosis, revascularization, and secondary prevention for myocardial ischaemia and anticoagulation for pulmonary embolism. An ICD may be indicated where the risk for arrhythmia remains high despite optimum management (see 'Further reading').

Epilepsy

Treatment should be directed by an expert and includes antiepileptic drugs and driving advice.

Prognosis

Situational and vasovagal syncope usually follow a benign course. The EGSYS 2 (Guidelines in Syncope 2) study demonstrated that, in patients presenting to the emergency department with TLoC, a higher mortality was observed in those with an abnormal ECG and/or heart disease, seen in 82% of those who died.

In general, features suggestive of a serious condition need rapid assessment, include an abnormal ECG, signs of heart failure, exertional TLoC, cardiac murmur, family history of sudden cardiac death or cardiac disease, and unexplained or new breathlessness.

How to handle uncertainty in the diagnosis of this symptom

Where the diagnosis remains unclear despite appropriate investigations, psychogenic pseudosyncope and psychogenic non-epileptic seizures should be considered. These are particularly likely if TLoC events are variable in their nature, prolonged, or accompanied by other unexplained physical features. In addition, an implantable loop recorder will determine if a cardiac arrhythmia is the underlying causes in cases of recurrent, unexplained TLoC.

Further Reading

National Institute for Health and Clinical Excellence: *Transient Loss of Consciousness ('Blackouts') Over 16s. Clinical Guideline CG109* https://www.nice.org.uk/guidance/cg109)

Shen W-K, Sheldon RS, Benditt DG, et al. 2017 ACC/AHA/HRS guideline for the evaluation and management of patients with syncope: a report of the American College of Cardiology/American Heart Association Task Force on Clinical Practice Guidelines and the Heart Rhythm Society. *J Am Coll Cardiol* 2017; 70: e39–110.

Wieling W, Thijs RD, van Dijk N, et al. Symptoms and signs of syncope: A review of the link between physiology and clinical clues. *Brain* 2009; 132: 2630–42.

40 Coma

David Sprigings

Definition

Coma is a pathological state of unconsciousness from which a patient cannot be roused to wakefulness by stimuli. The comatose patient has closed eyes and no speech, and lacks both wakefulness and awareness, the two clinical dimensions of consciousness. The level of consciousness can be graded using the Glasgow Coma Scale (GCS), based on eye-opening, verbal, and motor responses to stimuli (Table 40.1). Coma is defined as a score of 8 or below on the GCS.

Differential diagnosis

Coma reflects dysfunction of the brainstem reticular system and its thalamic projections (the neuronal basis of wakefulness), or diffuse injury of both cerebral hemispheres. A unilateral lesion of a cerebral hemisphere (e.g. haemorrhagic stroke) will not cause coma unless there is secondary compression of the contralateral hemisphere or brainstem. Coma may be due to systemic or primary intracranial disease. Often both mechanisms and both etiologies are involved (e.g. alcohol intoxication complicated by head injury; opioid poisoning complicated by respiratory arrest with resultant hypoxic-ischaemic brain injury). Excluding head trauma, the commonest causes of coma are poisoning, stroke, and metabolic disorders. Box 40.1 summarizes the causes of coma (defined in this study as a GCS score of 10 or below for >30 minutes) in a series of 938 medical patients presenting to two urban emergency departments in Sweden; the data are probably representative of the case in the UK as well. Over half the cases of poisoning involved alcohol, either alone or in combination with sedative drugs. Poisoning was the cause of coma in 80% of patients under 40, but only 11% of those over 60.

Context

Over 70 causes of coma are recognized, ranging from the common disorders in Box 40.1 to rarities such as cerebral fat embolism following long-bone fracture or hyperammonaemic coma complicating ornithine transcarbamylase deficiency (an X-linked urea cycle disorder). However, the age of the patient, the comorbidities present, the setting in which coma occurs, and the examination findings generally limit the differential diagnosis to a handful

Box 40.1 Causes of non-traumatic coma seen in an emergency department

- poisoning (38%)
- focal neurological lesion (24%)
- metabolic or diffuse cerebral disturbance (21%)
- seizures or postictal state (12%)
- psychogenic (1%)
- cause not defined (4%)

Adapted by permission from BMJ Publishing Group Limited. Forsberg S, et al. Coma and impaired consciousness in the emergency room: characteristics of poisoning versus other causes, *Emerg Med Journal*, volume 26, pp.100-2, copyright © 2009.

of diseases. The common causes of coma by context are given in Table 40.2.

Approach to diagnosis

Coma is a medical emergency, because a comatose patient is at high risk of permanent brain injury or death, caused either by the

Table 40.1 Grading of level of consciousness using the Glasgow Coma Scale*

Points	Eye opening (E)	Best verbal response (V)	Best motor response (M)
6	–	–	Obeys commands
5	–	Orientated	Localizes pain
4	Spontaneous	Confused	Withdraws to pain
3	To speech	Words	Flexes to pain
2	To pressure	Sounds	Extends to pain
1	None	None	None

* The score is expressed both as its components (e.g. E2, V1, M4) and sum (e.g. Glasgow Coma Scale (GCS) 7). By definition, a patient in coma will have a score of E < 3, V < 3, and M < 5. In a patient with an endotracheal tube in place, preventing assessment of verbal response, the modifier 'T' is attached to the score (e.g. E2, M4; GCS 6T). The accuracy and reliability of the measurement of the GCS score are influenced by technique and experience.

Adapted from Teasdale G, Maas A, Lecky F, et al. The Glasgow Coma Scale at 40 years: Standing the test of time *Lancet Neurol* 2014; 13: 844–54, with permission from Elsevier.

Table 40.2 Causes of coma by context

Patient group	Causes to consider*
Emergency department patient under 40	Poisoning with alcohol and/or other psychoactive substances
	Postictal state
	Hypoglycaemia
	Traumatic brain injury
	Carbon monoxide poisoning
Emergency department patient over 40	Stroke
	Subdural haematoma
	Hypoxic-ischaemic brain injury following cardiac arrest
	Postictal state
	Hypoglycaemia
	Respiratory failure
	Traumatic brain injury
	Poisoning with alcohol and/or other psychoactive substances
	Carbon monoxide poisoning
Medical inpatient	Respiratory failure
	Stroke
	Subdural haematoma (e.g. following fall in hospital)
	Liver failure
	Septic encephalopathy
Surgical inpatient	Respiratory failure
	Opioid intoxication
	Septic encephalopathy
Patient with cancer	Raised intracranial pressure due to brain or meningeal metastases
	Opioid intoxication
	Hypercalcaemia
	Hyponatraemia

*This is not an exhaustive list, but highlights those causes which are commonly seen in the given context.

underlying disorder or the secondary effects of coma. Stabilization of the airway, breathing, and circulation, and exclusion of hypoglycaemia, are the first priorities before diagnosis is explored further. In coma, the reflexes which protect the airway (pharyngeal (gag) and tracheal (cough) reflex, mediated via cranial nerves IX and X) are impaired or lost, and endotracheal intubation to protect the airway should be discussed with an anaesthetist. It is particularly important that the patient's airway is protected during neuroimaging, when supine positioning of the patient and relative isolation during scanning increase the risk of airway compromise. Blood glucose should be checked by stick test at the bedside, and hypoglycaemia corrected. Seizures should be treated. If Wernicke's encephalopathy is suspected (e.g. coma with eye signs in the setting of chronic alcohol abuse and malnutrition, recurrent vomiting or after gastrointestinal surgery), give thiamine intravenously (before the administration of glucose). When opioid poisoning or the use of benzodiazepine in hospital (e.g. for procedural sedation) is suspected as the cause of coma, the appropriate antidote (naloxone/flumazenil) should be given.

Having dealt with these priorities, the cause of coma must be determined, as the quicker this is treated, the better is the outcome. Clinical assessment together with neuroimaging will usually identify the likely cause or causes. As a general rule, the absence of meningeal signs or focal neurological abnormalities indicates a systemic cause of coma (usually toxic or metabolic). However, some intracranial diseases (e.g. hypoxic-ischaemic brain injury, bilateral subdural haematomas) may not give rise to meningeal or focal signs. Conversely, focal signs do not necessarily indicate a primary intracranial cause of coma: they may be the consequence of secondary pathology (e.g. cerebral herniation with brainstem compression complicating cerebral oedema due to fulminant hepatic failure), may reflect previous unrelated disease (e.g. stroke) or may be seen in certain metabolic disorders (e.g. hyperglycaemic or hyperammonaemic states).

The history

The history is the richest source of information relevant to the diagnosis and needs to be gathered from all available sources, including ambulance personnel, family and friends, GP and hospital records, and the patient's belongings. The patient's age and comorbidities, and the setting and time course of loss of consciousness provide the most important clues. Current medications, history of previous or recent alcohol/substance abuse, and travel history (to determine whether infectious diseases acquired abroad (e.g. malaria) should be included in the differential diagnosis) must be established. Additional questions may of course be relevant in particular circumstances.

The examination

The examination of the comatose patient has general and neurological aspects. Findings on neurological examination contribute to diagnosing the mechanism and cause of coma, determine immediate management, and serve as a reference point against which neurological progress can be measured.

The general examination

The general examination begins with assessment of airway, breathing, and circulation, and measurement of body temperature. Severe hypertension suggests raised intracranial pressure (or, rarely, hypertensive encephalopathy) as the cause of coma. A rapid comprehensive examination should then be done, including checking for signs of head injury (e.g. scalp laceration or bruising; bleeding from an external auditory meatus or from the nose) and possible complications of coma (e.g. pressure injury of skin or muscle; corneal abrasions; inhalation pneumonia). If there are signs of head injury, additional cervical spine injury should be suspected until proven otherwise: the neck must be immobilized in a collar and X-rayed before testing for neck stiffness and the oculocephalic response.

The neurological examination

The neurological examination should include documentation of the level of consciousness using the GCS, examination of the eyes and fundi, testing for neck stiffness, and examination of the limbs.

Examination of the eyes

The position of the eyes; the size and symmetry of the pupils; the response of the pupils to bright light; the corneal reflex; and the oculocephalic response should be observed (Table 40.3).

The fundi

The fundi should be examined for spontaneous venous pulsation (which, if present, excludes raised intracranial pressure), papilloedema, and retinal haemorrhages. Subhyaloid and vitreous haemorrhage may be seen in aneurysmal subarachnoid haemorrhage.

Testing for neck stiffness

Neck stiffness is an important sign of meningeal irritation, and may be seen in bacterial meningitis, meningoencephalitis, subarachnoid haemorrhage, cerebral or cerebellar haemorrhage with extension into the subarachnoid space, and cerebral malaria. In any of these conditions, neck stiffness may be lost with increasing depth of coma.

The limbs

Limb tone, response to painful stimuli, tendon reflexes, and plantar responses should be examined. Consistent asymmetry between right- and left-sided findings usually indicates a structural cause for coma, although symmetrical findings do not exclude this. Limb tone is generally normal or reduced in toxic/metabolic coma (an exception is neuroleptic malignant syndrome, which is characterized by bilateral limb rigidity). An extensor plantar response usually indicates a structural lesion in the motor pathway (cerebral cortex, subcortex, brainstem, or spinal cord). However, bilateral extensor plantar responses

Table 40.3 Diagnostic significance of eye signs in the comatose patients

Sign	Significance
Conjugate deviation of the eyes	Seen with cerebral hemisphere lesions (eyes and head deviated away from the hemiplegic side) and pontine lesions (towards the hemiplegic side); also a feature of focal epilepsy
Dysconjugate deviation of the eyes	Indicates brainstem dysfunction (either primary brainstem lesion or secondary compression) or III/VI nerve lesion
Roving eye movements	Seen in toxic/metabolic coma (may be absent in deep coma); indicate an intact brainstem
Pupillary size and response to light	Small unreactive pupils are seen in opioid poisoning and pontine lesions, and fixed mid-point pupils in midbrain lesions; fixed dilated pupils are seen with central herniation and severe hypoxic-ischaemic brain injury; asymmetric pupillary size and response to light indicate brainstem dysfunction or III nerve lesion (compression of III nerve by uncal herniation results in ptosis, pupillary dilatation, reduction, and eventual loss of light reflex and deviation of the eye laterally and downwards)
Corneal reflex	A normal response bilaterally (eyelid closure and upward deviation of the eyes) indicates normal function of the midbrain and pons; the corneal reflex may be lost in deep coma due to a toxic/metabolic cause; loss of the corneal reflex is associated with loss of the cough reflex
Response to rotation of the head	Normal reflex eye movements (both eyes rotate counter to movement of the head) indicate normal brainstem function; abnormal eye movements may be seen in brainstem lesions and Wernicke's encephalopathy

may be seen transiently after tonic–clonic seizures. Hemiplegia with a contralateral III palsy may be seen with a unilateral cerebral hemisphere mass lesion complicated by uncal herniation and brainstem compression.

Other signs

Other signs are as follows:

- Multifocal myoclonus (brief, random, asynchronous jerks in limb, trunk, or facial muscles) suggests a toxic/metabolic cause.
- Myoclonic twitches of facial muscles and fingers may be seen in non-convulsive status epilepticus.
- Focal or general seizures may complicate many systemic and primary intracranial diseases causing coma.

Specific clues to the diagnosis

The cause of coma may be obvious (e.g. documented ingestion of alcohol and psychoactive medication in a young patient; coma following prolonged cardiorespiratory arrest). However, in many cases, the cause or causes of coma are less clear. The neurological signs allow patients to be placed in one of three subsets (Box 40.2) which constrain the differential diagnosis and establish priorities in management and therapy (e.g. urgency of neuroimaging; need for empirical antimicrobial therapy).

Key diagnostic tests

Key diagnostic tests are:

Blood glucose: This should be checked immediately at the bedside, and confirmed by laboratory testing.

CT: This should be done urgently in all patients, unless there is a clear toxic cause of coma in a younger patient, with no features pointing

---

Box 40.2 Clues to the diagnosis of coma from the neurological findings (less common or rare causes are placed in parentheses)

No meningeal or focal signs
- toxic/metabolic disorders
- hypoxic-ischaemic brain injury
- postictal state
- septic encephalopathy
- (cerebral venous sinus thrombosis)
- (bilateral subdural haematomas)
- (cerebral vasculitis)
- (cerebral fat embolism)

Meningeal but no focal signs
- subarachnoid haemorrhage
- bacterial meningitis
- meningoencephalitis
- (cerebral malaria)

Focal signs
Cerebral hemisphere signs
- trauma
- cerebral infarction
- mass lesion (haematoma, neoplasm, abscess)
- (cerebral venous sinus thrombosis)
- (acute demyelinating encephalomyelitis)

Brainstem signs
- trauma
- brainstem infarction or haemorrhage
- cerebellar infarction or haemorrhage
- posterior fossa mass lesion causing hydrocephalus
- Wernicke's encephalopathy
- (brainstem encephalitis)
- (central pontine myelinolysis)
- (basilar artery thrombosis)

---

to additional disease. CT is very sensitive for intracranial haemorrhage (sensitivity for subarachnoid haemorrhage, 95%; for other intracranial haemorrhage, >95%) and will identify mass lesions, hydrocephalus, marked cerebral oedema, and large cerebral hemisphere ischaemic strokes. Non-contrast CT may be normal in patients with meningitis or meningoencephalitis; early ischaemic stroke, especially of the brainstem or cerebellum; diffuse axonal injury from trauma; hypoxic-ischaemic brain injury; and white matter disorders (e.g. central pontine myelinolysis).

Examination of the cerebrospinal fluid: This test (assuming no contraindication to lumbar puncture) should be done in patients with a normal CT scan and in whom coma remains unexplained, to rule out intracranial infection.

Other key tests: Other key tests are measurement of arterial blood gases and pH; full blood count; a coagulation screen; and a biochemical profile. A toxicology screen and measurement of plasma paracetamol and salicylate levels should be done if poisoning is possible.

Other diagnostic tests

Other diagnostic tests are:

MRI: This should be done if CT and other tests do not establish the cause of coma, or a cause to which CT is insensitive is suspected.

EEG: This is indicated if the clinical findings suggest non-convulsive status epilepticus or if the cause of coma remains unclear after neuroimaging and other tests.

Other tests: Other tests such as blood culture, measurement of adrenal and thyroid function, measurement of plasma osmolality (raised in poisoning with ethanol, ethylene glycol, isopropyl alcohol, or methanol), measurement of plasma ammonia (raised in hepatic encephalopathy, valproate poisoning, and ornithine transcarboxylase deficiency), and measurement of red-cell transketolase level (reduced in Wernicke's encephalopathy due to thiamine deficiency) may be helpful in specific circumstances.

Introduction to therapy

Patients with coma should be nursed in a high-dependency or intensive care unit. As well as specific treatment directed at the underlying cause, supportive care of the comatose patient, including stabilization of the airway, breathing, and circulation, correction of hypoglycaemia or hyperglycaemia, treatment of seizures if present, correction of fever or hypothermia, and anticipation and prevention of the complications of coma (e.g. use of pressure mattress and positioning/turning to prevent pressure injury of skin and muscle) should be performed. Induced hypothermia can improve the neurological prognosis for coma after cardiac arrest. Thiamine and other B vitamins should be given intravenously (before the administration of glucose) if Wernicke's encephalopathy is possible (e.g. in the setting of chronic alcohol abuse, hyperemesis, or refeeding syndrome). If bacterial meningitis or viral meningoencephalitis is possible (because of fever and meningism), empirical antimicrobial therapy (with cefotaxime (plus ampicillin in patients over 55 or at increased risk of *Listeria* infection) and aciclovir) should be started immediately, after taking blood for culture. An urgent neurosurgical opinion should be sought if CT shows a structural cause for coma.

Prognosis

Patients in coma may make a complete recovery (e.g. after poisoning with psychoactive drugs), survive with varying degrees of brain injury (including the vegetative state), or die from brain death or systemic disease. The prognosis largely depends on the cause of coma, and is poor when due to major structural brain disease. For a given cause, the depth of coma and the status of brainstem reflexes influence prognosis (better with normal brainstem function).

In patients with coma after cardiac arrest, the neurological findings in the first 24 hours do not allow a firm prognosis to be made. However, if pupillary or corneal reflexes are absent at 24 hours, or motor responses are absent at 72 hours, the prognosis is very poor.

How to handle uncertainty in the diagnosis

Coma versus psychogenic unresponsiveness

Psychogenic unresponsiveness should be considered if there is a resistance to passive eye opening, the avoidance of stimuli, a response to stimuli discordant with the assessed level of consciousness, and a history of non-epileptic seizures or other functional disorders. The diagnosis should not be made simply because the existing investigations are normal. Appropriate consideration should always be given to the possibility of additional organic pathology, which should be assessed and investigated according to the principles discussed in this chapter.

Coma versus brain death

Brain death may follow coma because of the primary and secondary effects of the underlying disease or diseases. In brain death, brainstem reflexes and respiratory function (response to arterial carbon dioxide level >8.0 kPa) are absent. There are no motor reflexes. In the UK, brainstem death can be confirmed on the basis of clinical examination by two experienced doctors. When performed, EEG shows electrocerebral silence, and evoked potentials are absent. A PET scan or a functional MRI shows absent cortical metabolism.

Further Reading

Edlow JA, Rabinstein A, Traub SJ, et al. Diagnosis of reversible causes of coma. *Lancet* 2014; 384: 2064–76.

Teasdale G, Maas A, Lecky F, et al. The Glasgow Coma Scale at 40 years: Standing the test of time *Lancet Neurol* 2014; 13: 844–54.

41 Delirium (acute confusional state)

David Sprigings

Definition

Delirium (from the Latin *delirare*, to deviate from the furrow when ploughing, and hence to be crazy or rave) is a functional brain disorder characterized by disturbances of consciousness, attention, and cognition which develop over a period of hours to days, and often fluctuate during the day. Delirium can reflect a primary neurological disorder, substance intoxication or withdrawal, an adverse effect of drugs (especially those with an anticholinergic effect), or a systemic disorder such as sepsis. The term 'acute confusional state' is often used synonymously with delirium, although delirium is preferred (as confusion is not specific to delirium, and its definition is imprecise). Delirium may be associated with a range of associated clinical features including increased or decreased psychomotor activity (hyperactive and hypoactive variants), hallucinations and delusions, and efferent sympathetic hyperactivity. Delirium with pronounced psychomotor and sympathetic hyperactivity is more often seen in younger patients with alcohol or substance intoxication/withdrawal (delirium tremens), but no cause is specific to a clinical subtype.

Delirium is distinguished from dementia (with which it may coexist, as dementia is a major risk factor for delirium) by its speed of onset (over hours or days), and its reversibility with correction of the underlying cause. In some patients, however, delirium may be followed by long-term cognitive impairment, suggesting that the pathophysiology of delirium overlaps with that of dementia.

Differential diagnosis

Several neuropsychiatric disorders may give rise to abnormal consciousness, language, memory, or behaviour, and thus enter the differential diagnosis of delirium (Table 41.1).

Context

Delirium is present on hospital admission in around 15% of older patients (age over 65), and develops after admission in a further 20%, making it the commonest complication of hospitalization in this age group. In patients of all ages, delirium may reflect a primary neurological disorder, or substance intoxication/withdrawal. In older patients, it can be caused by a wide range of systemic disorders (most commonly infection) or medications, especially those with an anticholinergic effect. Delirium predisposes to injury, falls, dehydration, malnutrition, incontinence, and pressure ulceration, and thus

> **Box 41.1 Major risk factors and precipitants of delirium**
>
> *Major risk factors*
> - dementia
> - age over 65
> - current hip fracture
> - severe illness
>
> *Common precipitants*
> - infection
> - medications, especially with those with an anticholinergic or psychoactive effect
> - electrolyte disorders
> - alcohol intoxication or withdrawal
> - major surgery
> - urinary retention or faecal impaction
> - sleep deprivation
>
> Data from NICE, Delirium: prevention, diagnosis and management, 2010 nice.org.uk/guidance/cg103

significantly increases morbidity and mortality. Given these adverse consequences, prevention of delirium is of high importance; studies suggest that 30%–40% of cases are preventable, and multicomponent intervention (see 'Introduction to therapy') has been shown to reduce the incidence in vulnerable patients.

Delirium can be conceived as the interaction between risk factors which predispose to delirium (brain vulnerability), and precipitants which trigger it. Common risk factors and precipitants are shown in Box 41.1; the interval between onset of precipitant and delirium is typically >24 hours. A postulated model of the neuronal pathophysiology underlying delirium is illustrated in Figure 41.1. In highly vulnerable patients, such as those with dementia, a relatively minor precipitant such as a urinary tract infection may cause delirium. Often, several precipitants act in concert. Causes of delirium to consider in particular patient groups are summarized in Table 41.2.

Major surgery is a common precipitant of delirium in older patients, with rates of up to 50% after cardiac surgery and surgery for hip fracture. Delirium typically appears 2–7 days post-operatively, when plasma levels of inflammatory and catabolic mediators reach their peak, consistent with these having a causal role.

Table 41.1 Differential diagnosis of delirium	
Diagnosis	**Comment**
Dementia	Delirium and dementia often coexist, as dementia is a major risk factor for delirium; dementia is characterized by the gradual onset of impairment of memory, impairment of the execution of activities of daily living, and impairment of social behaviour; there is no clouding of consciousness
Acute functional psychosis (manic or schizophrenic)	In acute functional psychosis, hallucinations, if present, are typically auditory, whereas in delirium they are typically visual or tactile; assume a diagnosis of delirium rather than acute functional psychosis if the patient is older than 40 with no previous psychiatric history, there is a history of alcohol or substance abuse, there are major medical comorbidities, there is disorientation, clouding of consciousness, or decreased alertness, or if physiological observations are abnormal
Non-convulsive status epilepticus	In non-convulsive status epilepticus, there are often mild clonic movements of the eyelids, face, or hands, or simple automatisms; the EEG is abnormal
Transient global amnesia	In transient global amnesia, there is an abrupt onset of antegrade amnesia without clouding of consciousness or loss of personal identity; cognitive impairment is limited to amnesia, and there are no focal neurological or epileptic signs; symptoms resolve within 24 hours
Fluent (receptive) dysphasia	Speech is fluent but with meaningless words, unnecessary phrases, and nonsensical grammar; there is no clouding of consciousness

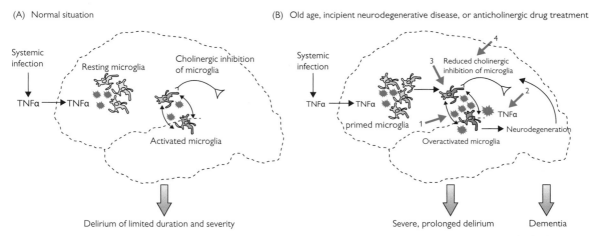

(A) Normal situation

(B) Old age, incipient neurodegenerative disease, or anticholinergic drug treatment

Delirium of limited duration and severity

Severe, prolonged delirium   Dementia

Figure 41.1 Neuronal pathophysiology underlying delirium: A postulated model based on clinical and research observations. (A) In the normal situation, peripherally produced pro-inflammatory cytokines, such as tumour necrosis factor alpha (TNFα) can enter the brain and activate microglia that produce inflammatory mediators affecting neuronal functioning, thus causing delirium. However, cholinergic inhibition controls microglial activation and thereby limits the severity and duration of delirium. (B) In old age, incipient neurodegenerative disease, or anticholinergic drug treatment, microglia might already be primed, which leads to overactivation on new stimuli. If cholinergic inhibition also fails, because of either preexisting neurodegeneration or use of drugs with anticholinergic effects, neuroinflammation could spin out of control, leading to severe prolonged delirium that can become associated with dementia. The green arrows indicate four ways in which control could be re-established over activated microglia: (1) direct inhibition of microglial activation by anti-inflammatory treatment (e.g. minocycline); (2) inhibition of the effects of cytokines (e.g. anti-TNFα); and augmentation of inhibitory cholinergic control by (3) nicotine-receptor ligands (e.g. anabasine) or (4) other cholinomimetic drugs (e.g. cholinesterase inhibitors).

Reprinted from *The Lancet*, Volume 375, Gool WA, van de Beek D, Eikelenboom P. , Systemic infection and delirium: when cytokines and acetylcholine collide, pp.73-75, Copyright 2010, with permission from Elsevier.

Approach to diagnosis

There are two aspects to the diagnosis of delirium: recognition of the syndrome, and identification of its cause or causes. Any patient with an abnormal mental state may have a disease which is an immediate threat to life (e.g. respiratory failure), and therefore exploration of the diagnosis should be preceded by a rapid assessment of the patient to ensure that the airway, breathing, and circulation are not compromised. Blood glucose should be measured and hypoglycaemia excluded.

Recognition of delirium requires examination of the mental state and establishing the antecedent history by talking to family members, carers, or hospital staff. Mental state examination should include tests of attention, orientation, and memory and can be done in a few minutes with the 10-item abbreviated mental status examination, or equivalent (Box 41.2). The Confusion Assessment Method (CAM) instrument is an alternative and simpler method of confirming a diagnosis of delirium, with a sensitivity and specificity of >90% when compared to a diagnosis based on the criteria of the *Diagnostic and Statistical Manual of Mental Disorders, 4th Edition, Text Revision* (a recognized standard) (see Inouye et al., 1990). Using CAM, the diagnosis of delirium requires an acute onset and fluctuating course, with evidence of reduced attention together with disordered thinking or an altered level of consciousness.

Given the broad range of disorders which may underlie delirium, identification of the cause requires a comprehensive assessment of the patient. Of particular importance in the history are the presence

Table 41.2 Causes of delirium by context

Patient group	Causes to consider*
Older patient in the emergency department	Acute infection
	Adverse effect of medication
	Electrolyte disorder
	Stroke
	Subdural haematoma
Younger patient in the emergency department	Alcohol intoxication
	Poisoning with cocaine, amphetamine, or other psychoactive drugs
	Primary neurological disorder (e.g. encephalitis)
Older patient with delirium after surgery	Acute infection
	Adverse effect of medication
	Urinary retention
	Faecal impaction
Patient from psychiatric hospital	Neuroleptic malignant syndrome
	Primary neurological disorder (e.g. encephalitis)
Patient with alcohol dependence	Alcohol intoxication or withdrawal
	Wernicke's encephalopathy
	Liver failure
	Acute infection (e.g. pneumonia, spontaneous bacterial peritonitis)
Patient with cancer	Adverse effect of medication (e.g. opioid toxicity)
	Brain or meningeal metastases
	Electrolyte disorder (e.g. hyponatraemia, hypercalcaemia)
	Paraneoplastic effect

* This is not an exhaustive list, but highlights those causes which are commonly seen in the given context.

> **Box 41.2 Examination of the mental state in suspected delirium (abbreviated mental status examination)**
>
> - Age
> - Time (to nearest hour)
> - Address for recall at end of test—this should be repeated by the patient to ensure it has been heard correctly: 42 West Street.
> - Year
> - Name of hospital
> - Recognition of 2 people (e.g. doctor, nurse)
> - Date of birth (day and month sufficient)
> - Year of 2nd World War
> - Name of present monarch
> - Count backwards 20–1
>
> Each correct answer scores one mark. The healthy elderly score 8–10.
>
> Reproduced with permission from Qureshi KN, Hodkinson HM., Evaluation of a ten-question mental test in the institutionalized elderly, *Age and Ageing*, volume 3. pp.152-7, copyright © 1974 Oxford University Press

of other systemic or neuropsychiatric symptoms; comorbidities which may be systemic (e.g. chronic obstructive pulmonary disease, diabetes, chronic liver disease), neurological (e.g. dementia, parkinsonism), or psychiatric; a complete list of current and recent medications; and enquiry about alcohol or substance abuse. In addition to assessment of the mental state and conscious level, the examination should include assessment of the airway, breathing, and circulation; measurement of body temperature; abdominal findings; and testing for neck stiffness, lateralized weakness, tendon reflexes, and plantar responses. Blood glucose should be checked at the bedside by stick test.

Specific clues to the diagnosis

Delirium is under-diagnosed in hospital, particularly in patients with the hypoactive variant. Patients with major risk factors for delirium (Table 41.2) should be screened on admission by mental state examination. Delirium should also be suspected in patients with:

- abnormal cognitive function (confusion, impaired concentration, slow responses to questions—the patient described as a 'poor historian')
- abnormal mood ('depression' developing in hospital)
- abnormal perception (visual or auditory hallucinations)
- abnormal behaviour (hyperactivity or hypoactivity (restlessness, agitation, or reluctance to mobilize); unwillingness to eat or drink; abnormal sleep–wake cycle)
- abnormal social behaviour (withdrawal from social contact; unwillingness to cooperate with care—the patient described as 'uncooperative' or 'difficult')

Key diagnostic tests

Delirium is a diagnosis based on clinical findings. There is no laboratory test for delirium, although investigation is usually needed to establish the cause or exclude other diagnoses (Table 41.1). As a general rule, all patients with delirium should have a full blood count, a biochemical profile, a C-reactive protein test, and urinalysis.

Other diagnostic tests

Other diagnostic tests are:

Neuroimaging (by CT or MRI): This is indicated if delirium followed a fall or head injury; if there are new focal neurological signs; if there is papilloedema or other evidence of raised intracranial pressure; if the patient has cancer or HIV–AIDS; if the patient's behaviour prevents adequate neurological examination; or if no systemic cause for the delirium is apparent.

Examination of the cerebrospinal fluid: This should be done (assuming no contraindication to lumbar puncture) if meningitis or encephalitis is suspected; if the patient is febrile and no systemic focus of infection is found; or if the cause of delirium remains unclear.

Electroencephalography: This is indicated if non-convulsive status epilepticus or encephalitis is suspected, or no cause for delirium is apparent. It may be useful in distinguishing delirium from psychosis.

Introduction to therapy

The major elements in the therapy of delirium are:

- identification and treatment of the underlying cause
- comprehensive supportive care (summarized in Table 41.3), with avoidance of physical restraint, and anticipation and prevention of complications of delirium
- avoidance of unnecessary medications, especially those with anticholinergic effect

Short-term (1 week or less) therapy with haloperidol (in a dose of <3 mg daily) or olanzapine (the latter is contraindicated in patients with dementia) can be used if patients are distressed or are likely to injure themselves or others.

Table 41.3 Interventions to prevent delirium	
Clinical factor	**Preventive intervention**
Cognitive impairment or disorientation	• Provide appropriate lighting and clear signage. A clock (consider providing a 24-hour clock in critical care) and a calendar should also be easily visible to the person at risk. • Reorientate the person by explaining where they are, who they are, and what your role is. • Introduce cognitively stimulating activities (for example, reminiscence). • Facilitate regular visits from family and friends.
Dehydration or constipation	• Encourage the person to drink. Consider offering subcutaneous or intravenous fluids if necessary. • Seek advice if necessary when managing fluid balance in people with comorbidities (for example, heart failure or chronic kidney disease).
Hypoxia	• Assess for hypoxia and optimise oxygen saturation if necessary.

Immobility or limited mobility	• Encourage the person to:
	  – mobilise soon after surgery
	  – walk (provide walking aids if needed – these should be accessible at all times).
	• Encourage all people, including those unable to walk, to carry out active range-of-motion exercises.

Infection	• Look for and treat infection. • Avoid unnecessary catheterisation. • Implement infection control procedures in line with 'Infection control' (NICE clinical guideline 2).
Multiple medications	• Carry out a medication review for people taking multiple drugs, taking into account both the type and number of medications.
Pain	• Assess for pain. Look for non-verbal signs of pain, particularly in people with communication difficulties. • Start and review appropriate pain management in any person in whom pain is identified or suspected.
Poor nutrition	• Follow the advice given on nutrition in 'Nutrition support in adults' (NICE clinical guideline 32). • If the person has dentures, ensure they fit properly.
Sensory impairment	• Resolve any reversible cause of the impairment (such as impacted ear wax). • Ensure working hearing and visual aids are available to and used by people who need them.
Sleep disturbance	• Avoid nursing or medical procedures during sleeping hours, if possible. • Schedule medication rounds to avoid disturbing sleep. • Reduce noise to a minimum during sleep periods[4].

[4] See 'Parkinson's disease' (NICE clinical guideline 35) for information about sleep hygiene.

From National Institute for Health and Clinical Excellence (2010) CG 103 Delirium: diagnosis, prevention and management. London: NICE. Available from http://guidance.nice.org.uk/CG103 Reproduced with permission.

Prognosis

As compared to matched controls, patients with delirium have increased hospital morbidity and mortality rates, longer lengths of stay, higher readmission rates, and poorer cognitive and functional status during the year after hospital admission.

How to handle uncertainty in the diagnosis

The differential diagnosis of delirium is given in Table 41.1, where those clinical features discriminating delirium from other neuropsychiatric disorders are highlighted. Bear in mind that delirium can complicate any of these disorders (e.g. a patient treated for an acute functional psychosis may develop delirium due to neuroleptic malignant syndrome). If in doubt, assume a diagnosis of delirium, and look for an underlying acute illness, pending a detailed collateral history from family members, carers, or hospital staff.

Further Reading

Inouye SK, van Dyck CH, Alessi CA, et al. Clarifying confusion: The confusion assessment method: A new method for detection of delirium. *Ann Intern Med* 1990; 113: 941–8.

Marcantonio ER. Delirium in hospitalized older adults. *N Engl J Med* 2017; 377:1456–66.

42 Seizures

Dirk Bäumer

Definition

Seizures are transient neurological events caused by abnormal excessive or synchronous neuronal activity in the brain. This can arise from a localized brain region, causing focal seizures, or simultaneously from both hemispheres, leading to generalized seizures. Epilepsy is the tendency to develop recurrent seizures and is usually diagnosed after two or more unprovoked seizures.

Clinical types of primary generalized seizures include tonic–clonic convulsions, absence seizures (manifesting as a brief impairment of consciousness with no or minimal motor manifestations), and myoclonic jerks. The onset of primary generalized epilepsies occurs in childhood, adolescence, or young adulthood, and may be associated with photosensitivity.

Focal (or partial) seizures present with paroxysmal motor, sensory, autonomic, or psychic manifestations, corresponding to the following sites of origin:

Motor cortex: contralateral clonic or tonic movements, commonly of hand or face due to large area of representation; sometimes spread of seizure activity (Jacksonian march)
Sensory cortex: tingling or numbness, again commonly affecting hand or face
Visual cortex: flashing lights, geometrical figures
Temporal lobes: rising epigastric sensation, fear, depersonalization, smell, strange feeling in the head

If full awareness is maintained, the seizures are simple partial seizures. Complex partial seizures are focal seizures with impairment of consciousness. They often start as a simple partial seizure (which is then called an aura) before awareness becomes impaired, and manifest as motor arrest or motionless staring, followed by automatisms such as lip smacking, chewing or hand movements, or more complex behaviour. Complex partial seizures frequently arise from the temporal lobes, but can arise from other parts of the brain. Simple and complex partial seizures can secondarily generalize into tonic–clonic seizures. Status epilepticus is defined as seizures of any type lasting for >30 minutes or recurring repeatedly without recovery of consciousness.

Differential diagnosis

Paroxysmal neurological symptoms occur in a large number of conditions, and the differential diagnosis depends on the type of presentation (see Table 42.1).

Context

Seizures will affect between 5% and 10% of the population at some time in their life. This can be in the form of isolated or acute symptomatic seizures during an acute medical or neurological illness, or as part of an epilepsy syndrome. Epilepsy has a point prevalence of 5–10/1000 persons. Some people with epilepsy also have non-epileptic, psychologically mediated attacks (dissociative seizures), although most people with non-epileptic attacks do not have epilepsy.

Common presentations in the acute medical take include:

- seizures or other paroxysmal events in a patient with known epilepsy
- first seizure
- seizure in the context of an acute medical or neurological illness

Table 42.1 Differential diagnosis of seizures and other paroxysmal events

Loss of consciousness	Syncope • reflex • orthostatic hypotension • cardiac arrhythmia • obstruction to the circulation Metabolic disturbance (e.g. hypoglycaemia) Intoxication Daytime sleep attacks Non-epileptic/psychogenic
Paroxysmal motor disorder	TIA • basal ganglia ischaemia • shaking TIAs Movement disorders • tics • myoclonus • chorea • tremor Tonic spasms (e.g. in MS) Sleep disorders • hypnagogic jerks • periodic limb movements • REM parasomnia
Paroxysmal sensory disorder	TIA Migraine with aura
Paroxysmal behaviour disturbance	Psychiatric disease • panic attacks • hysterical fugue • episodic dyscontrol • acute psychotic episode Acute encephalopathy (metabolic/toxic) Transient global amnesia Basilar migraine Sleep disorders
Drop attacks without loss of consciousness	Spinal cord disease Cataplexy Third ventricular colloid cyst Idiopathic drop attacks

Approach to diagnosis

Step 1: Establish whether or not the paroxysmal event was a seizure. For past events, this distinction lies solely in the history taken from the patient and, whenever possible, from an eyewitness. If no witness is with the patient, a telephone call to a person who saw what happened is more useful than any diagnostic test.
Step 2: Further define the type of seizure by analysis of the seizure semiology and use of the EEG (see 'Key diagnostic tests'). Is there more than one seizure type? Aim to define a syndrome.
Step 3: Establish the underlying aetiology. Demographic features can point to a likely cause, but investigations are needed to establish the cause of seizures (see 'Key diagnostic tests').

Specific clues to the presence of seizures

Ask the patient and witnesses what happened before, during, and after the event, bearing in mind that no single feature in the history is completely specific for the presence of a seizure. A common difficulty is to distinguish between epileptic seizures, syncope (loss of consciousness due to a global reduction in cerebral blood flow), and non-epileptic events (Table 42.2).

Table 42.2 Differential diagnosis of seizures, syncope, and non-epileptic attacks

Timing	Feature	Seizure	Syncope	Non-epileptic attack
Before	Precipitating factors	Uncommon Sleep deprivation, alcohol Specific trigger in reflex epilepsies (rare)	Pain, emotion, standing, Valsalva Exercise or none (cardiac)	Stressful circumstance
	Prodrome	Non-specific warning in some Aura (part of seizure)	Tiredness, sweating, nausea, visual disturbance (brief hallucinations and tunnel vision), muffled hearing	None or symptoms of anxiety
During	Onset	Sudden	Often gradual	Gradual
	Duration	1–3 minutes	1–30 seconds	Minutes to hours
	Facial appearance	Blue/cyanosed Frothing at mouth	Pale	Normal
	Eyes	Open, or clonic eyelid movements	Open, turned up	Closed, resists eye opening
	Movement	Synchronous rhythmic limb movements	None, can have brief convulsion (less than 15 seconds), myoclonus, and tonic flexion or extension	Asynchronous, waxing and waning, pelvic thrusts
	Tongue biting	Common, lateral tongue biting	Rare	Occasionally, tip of tongue
	Incontinence	Common	Uncommon	Uncommon
After	Recovery	Slow Headache, myalgia, fatigue	Rapid	Variable
	Injury	Common	Uncommon	Uncommon
	Confusion	Prolonged	Brief	None (maybe emotional)

Specific clues to the nature of seizures

Specific clues to the nature of seizures are as follows:

- Is this an acute symptomatic seizure? Ask about preceding febrile illness and look for meningism and rash (meningitis, encephalitis?), trauma (head injury), and signs of alcohol or substance intoxication or withdrawal.
- If patients present with generalized tonic–clonic seizures, search for additional seizure types suggestive of a generalized epilepsy syndrome. For example, a young adult with absences and myoclonus in addition to generalized tonic–clonic seizures might have juvenile myoclonic epilepsy. There might be a family history.
- Are seizures preceded by other symptoms (motor, sensory, autonomic, psychic) that could represent focal seizures? For example, a rising sensation from abdomen to chest before a convulsion would indicate medial temporal lobe focal seizures.
- Does the physical examination show features of a syndrome known to be associated with epilepsy, for example, a neurocutaneous syndrome, or focal signs such as weakness or reflex asymmetry, which point towards an underlying structural lesion?
- The age of onset will narrow the differential diagnosis (Table 42.3).

Table 42.3 Differential diagnosis of seizures according to age

Age	Aetiology
Neonates and infants	Birth injury/hypoxia Metabolic disorder Infantile spasms
Childhood	Febrile convulsions Metabolic disorder Developmental disorder Primary generalized epilepsy
Adolescence and early adulthood	Primary generalized epilepsy Trauma Drugs/alcohol Neoplasm
Middle age	Trauma Neoplasm Metabolic disorders (renal/liver failure, electrolyte abnormalities)
Late life	Stroke Degenerative disease Neoplasm

Key diagnostic tests

Key diagnostic tests are as follows:

Blood tests: In the acute setting, rule out hypoglycaemia, electrolyte abnormalities (Na^+, Ca^{2+}, Mg^{2+}), and infection (full blood count, C-reactive protein). Check renal and liver function to look for precipitant factors and guide therapy. The creatine kinase is often raised. Perform a toxicology screen.

ECG: Rhythm disturbance can mimic seizures. In particular, look at the PR interval (heart block) and QTc time.

Neuroimaging: MRI of the brain is the imaging modality of choice to detect epileptogenic lesions and should be performed in any patient with suspected epilepsy unless contraindicated. A CT brain is not sufficiently sensitive, but can be helpful in emergency presentations to rule out gross underlying pathology.

EEG: An EEG may be helpful to make an accurate diagnosis of the epilepsy type and to distinguish between focal and generalized epilepsies. Epileptiform discharges (sharp waves, spikes, spike-and-wave forms, polyspikes) are present in ~55% of interictal EEGs in patients with epilepsy, so a negative EEG does not rule out epilepsy. The sensitivity is higher in the sleep EEG. Normal people may have non-specific abnormalities (10%) and rarely epileptiform changes (<1%).

Other diagnostic tests

Other diagnostic tests are as follows:

Serum prolactin levels: Serum prolactin levels rise after generalized tonic–clonic and complex partial seizures of non-frontal origin and can be helpful if obtained within 20 minutes, but are not of sufficient sensitivity or specificity to be generally recommended

EEG video telemetry: The prolonged, simultaneous recording of EEG and video is useful when there is diagnostic uncertainty about the nature of paroxysmal attacks, and in the workup for epilepsy surgery, to unequivocally establish the site of onset in focal epilepsies.

Introduction to therapy

Therapy is as follows:

Emergency treatment: Convulsions not subsiding after 5–10 minutes should be treated as potential status epilepticus, using locally agreed guidelines.

General advice: Give general advice about avoiding potentially danger- ous situations such as swimming or bathing, lifestyle measures such as avoiding triggers like sleep deprivation and excessive alcohol intake, and the need to cease driving.

Antiepileptic treatment: Generally, antiepileptic treatment is deferred after the first seizure, unless imaging and/or EEG show features suggest a high risk of recurrence. Antiepileptic drugs are chosen according to seizure and epilepsy type as well as comorbidities:

- Sodium valproate is a reasonable first choice for primary general- ized epilepsies, and carbamazepine for focal seizures, but treat- ment needs to be tailored to the patient.
- All anticonvulsant drugs increase the risk of fetal anomalies. Sodium valproate in particular increases the risk of neural tube defects. Therefore, it is not recommended as first-line treatment in women of childbearing age (consider lamotrigine or levetiracetam).
- All women on anticonvulsant drugs and contemplating preg- nancy should also be prescribed high-dose folic acid 5 mg daily for several months before conception. Some agents interfere with the oral contraceptive pill (in particular, enzyme inducers such as carbamazepine) and, in women of childbearing age, this may influence the choice of either the contraception method or the anticonvulsant drug.

Prognosis

The risk of recurrence after a single seizure is about 50%, and about 70% after a second one. It is higher when congenital or acquired brain abnormalities are present, and lower when the seizure had an acute precipitant. Approximately 70% of epilepsy patients become seizure-free with medication. Epilepsy is associated with excess mortality, related to the underlying cause, to the seizures them- selves (causing accidents or leading to status epilepticus), and to suicide. Sudden unexpected death in epilepsy (SUDEP) is rare but important.

How to handle uncertainty in the diagnosis of seizures

This is common after one isolated event, and it is better to leave the diagnosis open than to attach a diagnostic label. If paroxysmal events recur and uncertainty remains, revisit the history, try to get an eyewitness and ask for a (mobile-phone) video recording of the event. A repeat sleep EEG can be helpful. In some cases, uncertainty about the diagnosis remains even after prolonged ambulatory and video telemetry monitoring.

Further Reading

Glauser T, Shinnar S, Gloss D, et al. Evidence-Based Guideline: Treatment of Convulsive Status Epilepticus in Children and Adults: Report of the Guideline Committee of the American Epilepsy Society. *Epilepsy Curr* 2016; 16: 48–61.

National Institute for Health and Clinical Excellence. *NICE Guidelines (CG137): Epilepsies: Diagnosis and Management.* 2012. Available at http://www.nice.org.uk/guidance/cg137?unlid=191027622016 12141566 (accessed 22 Feb 2017).

43 Difficulty speaking (including dysphasia and dysarthria)

Dirk Bäumer and Melanie Lord

Definitions

Difficulty speaking can arise from a problem with speech content, or the production of speech due to defective articulation or alteration of the voice (see Box 43.1)

Differential diagnosis

Differential diagnosis of dysphasia syndromes

Subdividing dysphasias may help in neuroanatomical diagnosis. Language is a function of the left hemisphere in the majority of people (even when they are left-handed). The main language areas border the Sylvian fissure: a receptive area is located in the inferior parietal and posterior superior temporal lobe and includes Wernicke's area. Lesions here cause problems in understanding written and spoken language, but also faulty (paraphasic) but fluent language output. An expressive region subserving motor aspects of speech is located in the posterior inferior frontal lobe (Broca's area) and adjacent insula. Lesions here cause non-fluent, agrammatic speech with relatively intact comprehension. These two main regions (receptive and expressive) are linked via the arcuate fasciculus. Several distinct aphasia syndromes are recognized with damage to either core language centre or their connections, but rarely occur in the pure form (Table 43.1). In addition, because neuronal networks underlying language have interconnected and overlapping functions, there is often incomplete correlation of symptoms with lesion site.

Lesions in the periphery of the peri-Sylvian area can cause dysphasia syndromes with markedly intact repetition that otherwise look like Broca's or Wernicke's dysphasia. These are called transcortical motor and transcortical sensory aphasias.

Differential diagnosis of dysarthria

In analogy to limb weakness, dysarthria can result from pathology of the muscle, neuromuscular junction, lower motor neuron, and upper motor neuron, as well as the extrapyramidal and cerebellar control of articulation. Mixed pathology, for example, of the lower and upper motor neurons or of the upper motor neuron and cerebellum, is common.

Context

Dysphasia commonly occurs in anterior circulation stroke. Occlusion of the superior branch of the middle cerebral artery causes Broca's aphasia; occlusion of the inferior branch is likely to cause aphasia of the Wernicke type. Posterior circulation stroke can occasionally cause dysphasia by involvement of the dominant posterior thalamus (mixed transcortical aphasia).

Intra-cerebral haemorrhage, primary or metastatic tumours, brain abscess, or encephalitis can equally cause dysphasia. depending on their localization. Anomic aphasia in particular can be an early sign of Alzheimer's disease and is the main feature of the language-variant forms of frontotemporal dementia.

Dysarthria also occurs in cerebrovascular disease. Because the bulbar muscles on each side are innervated by both motor cortices, unilateral stroke of the cerebral hemispheres usually causes only mild or transient dysarthria. Bilateral involvement of the corticobulbar tract as in widespread cerebrovascular disease or multiple sclerosis causes spastic ('pseudobulbar') dysarthria.

The dysarthria of amyotrophic lateral sclerosis (motor neuron disease) can be spastic or a combination of upper and lower motor neuron bulbar dysfunction. Lower motor neuron and neuromuscular dysarthria (flaccid or 'bulbar' dysarthria) commonly occur in motor neuron disease (progressive bulbar palsy) and myasthenia gravis. Other causes include primary muscle disease (oculopharyngeal muscular dystrophy, myotonic dystrophy, inclusion body myositis, polymyositis) and spinobulbar muscular atrophy (Kennedy syndrome). Guillain–Barré syndrome and botulism are causes of acute bulbar weakness. Diphtheria and bulbar poliomyositis are now rare.

Multiple lower cranial nerve palsies can give rise to dysarthria and dysphonia. They can result from infectious or malignant meningitis, compression by tumours (including nasopharyngeal carcinoma, neurofibromas, meningiomas, and lymphomas), structural abnormalities of the craniocervical junction such as platybasia or the Chiari malformation, or inflammatory conditions such as vasculitis or sarcoidosis.

Ataxic dysarthria occurs in multiple sclerosis, stroke, after anoxic encephalopathy, and in a large number of degenerative disorders affecting the cerebellum. Hypokinetic dysarthria occurs in Parkinson's disease, whereas hyperkinetic dysarthria is common in dystonia and Huntington's disease. Stuttering is usually a developmental problem giving rise to spasms in the articulatory muscles, but can occasionally occur in patients recovering from aphasic disorders, or as an early sign of left-hemisphere lesions such as gliomas.

Box 43.1 Definitions

Dysphasia is impairment of production and/or comprehension of spoken or written language.

Dyslexia is difficulty reading.

Dysgraphia means difficulty writing.

Dysarthria is defective articulation with otherwise normal language function.

Dysphonia is an alteration of the voice due to a laryngeal problem.

The prefix 'a-' (as in 'aphasia') means complete loss of the respective function but, in practice, is often used interchangeably with 'dys-'.

Paraphasia relates to the use of malformed or inappropriate words which can be **semantic** (using the wrong word, e.g. 'fork' for 'spoon') or **phonemic** (using a wrong sound within a word, e.g. 'shoon' for 'spoon').

Neologisms are non-existent word forms. Together with paraphasias, they are characteristic of jargon **aphasia**.

Mutism is the complete failure of speech output, caused by a severe language disorder, anarthria, or psychiatric disturbance.

Dysphagia means difficulty swallowing, which often accompanies dysarthria and dysphonia.

Stuttering and **stammering** are used synonymously to characterize dysfluent speech with sound repetitions (e.g. 'b-b-b-book'), blocks, and prolongations, the latter being mainly of initial sounds.

Table 43.1 Main types of dysphasia

Type of dysphasia	Speech	Comprehension	Naming	Repetition	Lesion
Broca	Non-fluent Laboured Phonemic paraphasia	Relatively intact Problems at sentence level	Poor	Impaired	Anterior to Sylvian fissure
Wernicke	Fluent Devoid of meaning Jargon Neologisms, semantic paraphasias	Very impaired	Poor	Impaired	Posterior to Sylvian fissure
Global	Non-fluent, mute	Very impaired	Poor	Impaired	Extensive peri-Sylvian
Conduction	Fluent	Relatively intact	Poor	Severely impaired	Broca–Wernicke connections
Anomic	Fluent Word-finding difficulties	Relatively intact	Poor	Spared	Left hemisphere, non-localizing

Approach to diagnosis

The first step in assessing the patient with difficulty speaking is to decide whether the problem is one of articulation or of speech content. Systematically assess spontaneous speech, comprehension, naming, and repetition using the following steps; at this stage, try to decide if a major aphasia or dysarthria type is present (Tables 43.1 and 43. 2):

Step 1: Major communication difficulties with altered speech content will become apparent quickly while taking the history and engaging the patient in conversation. Assess spontaneous speech for alterations of articulation (is it slurred or indistinct?) and decide whether it is fluent or non-fluent. Does the patient use long phrases (with, say, more than five words)? Are there paraphasic errors or neologisms? Consider whether there is evidence of more widespread cognitive alteration indicating a delirium (with altered awareness, distractibility, fluctuating attention, and disorientation) or dementia.

Step 2: Test comprehension: start with single words ('point to the bed, the chair, the window'), then sentences of increasing complexity ('touch the watch with your finger', 'take this paper, fold it in half, then put it on the floor').

Step 3: Ask the patient to name objects. Are there phonemic or semantic paraphasias? Is the right answer given when presented with a choice (in Broca's, not in Wernicke's).

Step 4: Test repetition. Tongue twisters such as 'British constitution' can accentuate dysarthria. Repetition of lingual, labial, and velar consonants ('la-la-la', 'me-me-me', 'k-k-k') can then point to the major articulation problem. Repetition of meaningless phrases such as 'no ifs, ands, or buts' is impaired in most dysphasia syndromes, but preserved in transcortical aphasia and anomic aphasia.

Step 5: A comprehensive assessment includes assessing reading and writing. These are usually disrupted in parallel with spoken language, but there are rare situations when a dissociative deficit occurs. For example, a patient with pure word mutism cannot speak, but is able to write. Problems with reading or writing unrelated to core language function can occur in disorders of visual perception and praxis.

Next, look for associated signs to reach a neuroanatomical diagnosis:

Step 6: In patients with dysphasia, look for an associated hemiparesis, hemisensory loss, or visual field defect. Test other dominant hemisphere functions: calculation (read numbers, arithmetic operations) and praxis ('blow out a candle', 'salute', 'use a toothbrush', copy of meaningless hand gestures).

Step 7: In dysarthric patients, examine the cranial nerves, with particular attention to eye movements and ptosis; observe symmetrical palatal elevation; look at the tongue in the floor of the mouth to see fasciculations; observe tongue movements; and test the jaw jerk. Ask the patient to cough. Look for proximal weakness (neck flexion) and upper or lower motor neuron signs, as well as cerebellar signs in the limbs.

Step 8: Look for clues to the aetiology: examine the cardiovascular system for causes of stroke (hypertension, atrial fibrillation, endocarditis, etc.). Look for signs of systemic illness (weight loss, rash, lymphadenopathy).

Consider the time course of symptoms, and the context of the history, to narrow down the possible pathological differential diagnosis. Sudden onset dysphasia is probably due to stroke, whereas an insidious history might indicate malignant disease or neurodegeneration. Further investigations are often needed (see 'Other diagnostic tests'). Finally, look for complications, such as aspiration

Table 43.2 Main types of dysarthria

Dysarthria	Speech	Other findings	Lesion
Flaccid (neuromuscular, 'bulbar')	Breathy, nasal, indistinct consonants	Nasal escape Flaccid/fasciculating tongue Lax lips Drooling May have associated dysphagia and dysphonia	Muscle or neuromuscular junction Lower motor neuron (lower brainstem nuclei or cranial nerves)
Spastic (Upper motor neuron, 'pseudobulbar')	Slow, stiff, harsh voice, monotonous, 'plum in mouth'	Stiff, slow tongue Brisk jaw and facial jerks Impaired emotional control (pseudobulbar affect)	Corticobulbar connections, usually bilaterally
Extrapyramidal: hypokinetic	Soft, monotonous, slow or rapid and cluttered, festinant	Low volume (hypophonia) Hypomimia	Basal ganglia Parkinson's disease
Extrapyramidal: hyperkinetic	Variable rate and loudness, distorted vowels, sudden stoppages of speech	Dystonia Chorea	Basal ganglia
Ataxic	Irregular, explosive, staccato, unnatural separation of syllables Excess and equal stress (scanning if combined with spasticity)	Poor coordination of speech and respiration	Cerebellum

pneumonia, and associated respiratory compromise needing rapid intervention.

Specific clues to the nature of dysphasia

In the acute setting, dysphasia syndromes often do not easily fit into the categories shown in Table 43.1 and instead present a mixed type. Associated findings might point to the site of the lesion:

- A (right-sided) brachiofacial hemiparesis is often associated with anterior lesions (Broca), as is a degree of orofacial dyspraxia and mild dysarthria, because cortical areas in control of the bulbar musculature may be involved. There may be ipsilateral (left) arm dyspraxia.
- A homonymous hemi- or quadrantanopia can accompany posterior lesions (Wernicke).
- Hemiparesis, hemisensory loss, and hemianopia accompany global aphasias.

When dysphasia is progressive, with few other signs, consider a dementia, if there is no lesion on the scan.

Specific clues to the nature of dysarthria

Specific clues to the nature of dysarthria are as follows:

- In neuromuscular/bulbar dysarthria, look for symptoms and signs of myasthenia gravis: is there diurnal variation in symptoms? Double vision? Droopy eye lids? Look for fatigable ptosis, ophthalmoplegia, jaw weakness, deterioration of speech over time, neck weakness, and fatigable proximal limb weakness.
- In an acute syndrome with facial weakness, particularly bilaterally, look for absent deep tendon reflexes and sensory features—could this be part of Guillain–Barré syndrome?
- If there are multiple cranial nerve palsies, think about malignant infiltration/meningitis or inflammatory conditions.
- Is the tongue wasted and fasciculating? Look for other signs of motor neuron disease—weakness and wasting in the limbs, with normal or brisk reflexes.
- In upper motor neuron/spastic dysarthria, look for evidence of stepwise progression and history of strokes—is this cerebrovascular disease?
- Optic atrophy, internuclear ophthalmoplegia, cerebellar signs, and signs suggestive of spinal cord disease (e.g. para- or tetraparesis, sensory level) point towards multiple sclerosis.
- Frequent falls, symmetrical rigidity, and impaired vertical eye movements occur in progressive supranuclear palsy.
- A patient who is completely mute might have a severe global aphasia, be anarthric, have a frontal lobe syndrome with akinetic mutism, a severe extrapyramidal syndrome, or a psychogenic problem (e.g. catatonia).

Key diagnostic tests

Brain imaging is needed to clarify the nature of lesions in dysphasia. It is also helpful in dysarthria to reveal widespread vascular disease, demyelination, cerebellar atrophy, or lesions of the brainstem or skull base.

Other diagnostic tests

Other diagnostic tests are as follows:

- Neurophysiology with nerve conduction studies and EMG can help to show a neuropathy, or signs of denervation, as in motor neuron disease.
- CSF examination is indicated in suspected Guillain–Barré syndrome or malignant meningitis.

- Acetylcholine receptor antibodies are assayed in suspected myasthenia gravis.

Introduction to therapy

A number of different specific therapies may be needed, depending on the underlying cause (e.g. thrombolysis for acute ischaemic stroke). Speech and language therapy can often help with symptomatic management of dysphasia and dysarthria.

Therapy for dysphasia

A cognitive neuropsychological language processing model can be useful to assess areas of language comprehension and expression which are relatively impaired and intact and analyse individual patterns at single word/sentence level. Impairment-based therapy aiming to improve underlying language processing may be effective, including after the spontaneous recovery period. If central semantics (i.e. the store of word meanings) is significantly impaired, this is likely to be an effective area to target, as it impacts on comprehension and expression. This may be achieved, for example, by repeated spoken/written word to picture matching. It is important to select and work on a core vocabulary of greatest relevance to the patient. Depending on prognosis, therapy is likely to focus to a greater or lesser extent on using supportive communication techniques (e.g. the use of gesture, drawing, phonological/graphemic cueing to assist with word-finding difficulties). Using computer therapy and working with a patient's family can increase the frequency of therapy activities and improve outcome.

Therapy for dysarthria

There is some evidence that intensive oromotor and articulation exercises can help increase range and rate of movement of muscles to improve the intelligibility and quality of speech. This is most useful in non-progressive conditions (e.g. after stroke or traumatic brain injury).

Therapy particularly for progressive dysarthrias (e.g. in motor neuron disease) focuses on compensatory strategies to maximize intelligibility (e.g. using a slow speech rate, segmenting multisyllabic words, taking frequent breaths, managing fatigue). As the condition progresses, communication aids are usually introduced to supplement speech or as the main form of communication (e.g. an alphabet board; voice output communication aids, such as the Lightwriter™; or software packages on laptops or phones which can be accessed via a keyboard, switch, or eye gaze).

Prognosis

This depends on the nature of the underlying pathology. After stroke, most spontaneous recovery from dysphasia usually occurs within the first three months. Initial severity of the dysphasia is the single best predictor of outcome. Severe dysphasias might evolve into other dysphasia types; for example, a patient with severe global aphasia at the onset might develop Broca's with time. Overall, left-handedness is a positive prognostic marker.

How to handle uncertainty in the diagnosis

It is often difficult to put a dysphasia or dysarthria into a neat diagnostic category, and mixed types occur. In this case, focus on symptoms and signs in addition to the speech difficulty to reach a diagnosis.

Further Reading

Hillis AE. Aphasia: Progress in the last quarter of a century. *Neurology* 2007; 69: 200–13.

44 Weakness

Cris S. Constantinescu and Su-Yin Lim

Definition of the symptom

Motor weakness is a decrease in muscle strength leading to an inability of a muscle or group of muscles to perform its usual function.

Differential diagnosis

The differential diagnosis of motor weakness ordered by probability is detailed in Box 44.1.

Various causes of motor weakness (Box 44.1) may be encountered in the primary and secondary care setting. Acute onset weakness is more frequently encountered in secondary care, whereas weakness of an insidious onset can present to both primary and secondary care.

CNS lesions may be caused by vascular disorders (haematoma, ischaemia), tumours, cysts, infections, cavitation/syrinx (spinal cord and brainstem), inflammation, or demyelination. Lesions in the brainstem are often vascular, inflammatory/demyelinating, or malignant in origin.

The list of conditions causing weakness associated with a generalized polyneuropathy is extensive and includes Guillain–Barré Syndrome (GBS), neuropathies associated with the vasculitides and connective tissue disorders, multifocal motor neuropathy, nutritional deficiencies (B_{12}, thiamine), drug or toxin-induced weakness (vinca alkaloids, isoniazid, heavy metals), malignancy (infiltrative and paraneoplastic), renal failure, endocrine disorders (hypothyroid or hyperthyroid), sarcoidosis, diabetes, paraprotein-related weakness, and amyloidosis. The most common hereditary neuropathy is Charcot–Marie–Tooth disease (CMT, or hereditary motor and sensory neuropathy).

Conditions that can affect the peripheral nerves in an asymmetrical pattern giving rise to a multiple mononeuropathy include vasculitides, connective tissue diseases, diabetes, sarcoidosis, Lyme disease, malignant infiltrative disease, HIV, and hepatitis C infection. Disorders of the cervical, brachial, or lumbosacral plexus can be caused by trauma, malignant infiltrative disease, vasculitis, infections (e.g. Lyme disease,

HIV) or may be idiopathic (e.g. neuralgic amyotrophy, known as brachial neuritis or Parsonage–Turner syndrome when it involves the brachial plexus).

Diseases of the muscles may be primary (muscular dystrophies) or secondary (thyroid myopathy, drug-induced myopathy) in origin, be associated with metabolic disorders (e.g. glycogen storage diseases) or mitochondrial disorders (Kearns–Sayre syndrome, chronic progressive external ophthalmoplegia, MELAS syndrome), or be part of a systemic inflammatory disorder (polymyositis, dermatomyositis). Disorders of the neuromuscular junction may be antibody mediated (myasthenia gravis, Lambert–Eaton myasthenia syndrome (LEMS)) or toxin induced (botulism). The main anterior horn cell disorders are motor neuron disease (MND), poliomyelitis, and spinal muscular atrophy.

Context

The origin of weakness may be localized to upper motor neurons, lower motor neurons (including nerve roots, nerve plexuses, and peripheral nerves), anterior horn cells, neuromuscular junctions, or muscles. The upper motor neurons responsible for voluntary movement consists of the neurons located in the motor cortex and corticospinal (or pyramidal) tracts and their various connecting interneurons. The lower motor neurons originate in the anterior horn of the spinal cord. On leaving the spinal cord, the lower motor neurons become organized into plexuses (cervical, brachial, and lumbosacral), subsequently forming peripheral nerves which synapse with the muscle cell membrane at the neuromuscular junction. In the brainstem, the lower motor neurons in the cranial nerve motor nuclei innervate the muscles responsible for eye movements, speech, and swallowing.

Approach to diagnosis

Clinical history

The patient's description of weakness must first be clarified and differentiated from malaise, lassitude, or fatigue, although fatigue itself is frequently present in neuromuscular diseases. A thorough history should include details of the onset and time course (acute, subacute, or chronic), pattern (e.g. generalized, hemiparetic, paraparetic, or monomelic; distal or proximal; symmetrical or asymmetrical; focal or multifocal), progression or worsening of symptoms, associated symptoms, past medical history, family history, drug history, travel history, and social history. Patients may volunteer examples of functional impairment pointing towards a pattern of weakness; for example, difficulty rising from a chair or from squatting may indicate proximal muscle weakness, whereas difficulty opening jars or tripping may indicate distal weakness in the upper limbs.

A general medical evaluation should be done, with particular attention paid to respiratory and cardiovascular function, skin changes, thyroid function, skeletal deformities, and the presence of lymphadenopathy, fever, or weight loss.

Examination

Examination of the motor system should include an assessment of muscle bulk, tone, strength, reflexes, and gait. Other associated neurological features such as cranial nerve dysfunction, visual field detects, speech abnormalities, ataxia, sensory disturbance, and musculoskeletal deformities should be sought.

Muscle bulk

Atrophy with fasciculations may appear within a few weeks of onset of weakness caused by a polyneuropathy. Fasciculations may

---

Box 44.1 Causes of motor weakness and main differential diagnoses

Cause of motor weakness
- central nervous system disorders
- peripheral nerve disorders
- neuromuscular junction disorders
- muscle disorders
- anterior horn cell disorders

Main differential diagnoses
- acute stroke or TIA
- brain tumour (primary or metastatic)
- demyelination (e.g. multiple sclerosis)
- generalized polyneuropathy (various causes)
- multiple mononeuropathy (various causes)
- plexopathy (various causes)
- myasthenia gravis
- botulism
- Lambert–Easton myasthenic syndrome
- muscular dystrophies
- other myopathies (various causes)
- motor neuron disease; amyotrophic lateral sclerosis
- poliomyelitis

be localized in a radiculopathy. Muscle hypertrophy may be seen in some muscular dystrophies (e.g. pseudohypertrophy of the calf muscles, a classical finding).

Tone

Flaccid weakness point to a lower motor neuron disorder. However, acute upper motor neuron disorders can present with a flaccid weakness at onset. Hypertonia in upper motor neuron disorders appear days or weeks later, typically resulting in a 'clasp-knife' rigidity. Ankle clonus may be elicited in upper motor neuron disorders.

Strength

Muscle strength may be assessed manually by muscle resistance testing or by functional testing. Strength is usually graded using the 6-point BMRC (British Medical Research Council) scale (Table 44.1). Functional testing such as tiptoe and heel walking can be used to evaluate distal lower limb power, whereas the patient's ability to stand from sitting unaided reflects proximal muscle power. Grip strength can be quantitatively assessed using a dynamometer.

Typically but not always, pyramidal weakness of the upper limbs has a predilection for extensors over the flexor muscles, whereas in the lower limbs the flexors are weaker than the extensors. Testing for a pronator drift is useful for eliciting a mild pyramidal weakness.

Pattern and distribution of weakness

Table 44.2 summarizes the most common patterns of weakness which help localize the site of the lesion.

Reflexes

Tendon reflexes are diminished or absent in lower motor neuron disorders and exaggerated in upper motor neuron disorders. In lower motor neuron disorders, the distribution of the diminished reflexes can help to localize the lesion. For instance, a diminished/absent ankle jerk could indicate a lesion of the S1 nerve root or the sciatic nerve on the same side.

A spinal cord lesion may cause tendon reflexes to be diminished at the level of the lesion, but exaggerated below it. The plantar response is typically extensor in upper motor neuron disorders.

Tendon reflexes are preserved in myasthenia gravis (MG) and botulism but are reduced or absent in LEMS. In LEMS, facilitation of reflexes (appearance after repeated muscle contraction) is characteristic.

Tendon reflexes may be preserved or reduced in myopathies.

Gait

A waddling gait is typical of proximal muscle weakness. A high-stepping gait is seen in ankle dorsiflexion weakness (foot drop). A scissoring gait, caused by a tendency to adduct both hips, occurs in a spastic paraparesis.

Specific clues to the diagnosis

Symptom onset and time course

Sudden onset of weakness without warning is suggestive of a vascular cause such as an ischaemic or haemorrhagic stroke.

Table 44.1 Strength grading using the 6-point BMRC (British Medical Research Council) scale

BMRC scale	Evaluation
0	No movement observed
1	Flicker or trace of movement observed
2	Active movement with gravity eliminated
3	Active movement against gravity
4	Active movement against resistance
5	Normal strength

Adapted from Medical Research Council Aids to the examination of the peripheral nervous system, Memorandum no. 45, Her Majesty's Stationery Office, London, 1981. Used with the permission of the Medical Research Council.

Subacute onset over days is typical of GBS, vasculitic neuropathy, polymyositis, and acute CNS demyelination (e.g. multiple sclerosis, inflammatory myelitis).

A more insidious onset with progressive symptoms over weeks to months is seen in space-occupying lesions such as tumours and vascular malformations, neurodegenerative conditions such as MND, neurosarcoidosis, and many peripheral nerve diseases. Progression over years can be seen in certain muscular dystrophies.

Fluctuating weakness is characteristic of MG and mitochondrial and metabolic muscle disorders, where it is precipitated by activity.

Weakness caused by vasculitis, chronic inflammatory demyelinating radiculoneuropathy (CIDP), multiple sclerosis (MS), or porphyria may demonstrate a relapsing pattern.

A childhood history of poor motor skills or slow development point towards a hereditary or genetic cause of weakness, such as hereditary spastic paraparesis, muscular dystrophy, and various forms of CMT.

Involvement of the motor system only

Sensory signs are absent in myopathies, neuromuscular junction disorders, pure motor neuropathies, and anterior horn cell disease (e.g. MND), although some patients may complain of mild sensory symptoms. A pure motor neuropathy should be differentiated from MND. Variants of GBS, lead toxicity, and a subtype of CMT may present with a pure motor neuropathy.

Involvement of the sensory system

In upper motor neurons, sensory signs may be seen in cerebral, brainstem, and spinal cord lesions. In lower motor neurons, sensory signs are present in peripheral nerve disorders, including radiculopathies, plexopathies, mononeuropathies, and the various causes of polyneuropathies.

Involvement of the autonomic nervous system

Autonomic disturbance (e.g. orthostatic hypotension, cardiac arrhythmias, pupillary dysfunction, urinary retention) is often present in some polyneuropathies (e.g. in GBS, amyloidosis, and diabetes), LEMs, and botulism.

Involvement of the cranial muscles

An upper motor neuron pattern of facial weakness (forehead sparing) is seen in brainstem lesions of various causes. A lower motor neuron pattern of facial weakness is seen in vasculitis, neurosarcoidosis, Lyme disease, GBS, MG, botulism, HIV infection, myotonic dystrophy, mitochondrial myopathies, the fascioscapulohumeral and oculopharyngeal forms of muscular dystrophy, and idiopathic Bell's palsy.

Bulbar weakness causing dysarthria and dysphagia occurs in brainstem lesions, MND, GBS, MG, botulism, myotonic dystrophy, muscular dystrophy (oculopharyngeal form), thyroid myopathy, and inflammatory myopathies. Wasting and fasciculations of the tongue raises a strong suspicion of MND.

Weakness of the extraocular muscles giving rise to an ophthalmoplegia may be present in brainstem disorders, variants of GBS (e.g. Miller Fisher syndrome), MG, botulism, mitochondrial myopathies, and the oculopharyngeal form of muscular dystrophy.

Involvement of the sphincter muscles

Sphincteric disturbance (urinary retention and loss of anal tone) with a sensory level is highly suggestive of a spinal cord lesion.

Sphincteric disturbance with 'saddle' anaesthesia and lower limb weakness is suggestive of a lesion of the conus medullaris or cauda equina. Conus medullaris lesions tend to present with bilateral mixed upper motor neuron and lower motor neuron signs (brisk knee jerks and absent ankle jerks, occasionally with fasciculations) whereas cauda equina lesions present with lower motor neuron signs which are often unilateral or bilateral and asymmetrical.

Involvement of the respiratory system

Neuromuscular disorders may present with respiratory dysfunction due to diaphragmatic and respiratory muscle weakness.

Table 44.2 Weakness patterns that help localize the site of the lesion

UMN or LMN signs	Distribution of weakness	Likely location of lesion
UMN	Hemiparesis	Contralateral cerebral hemisphere
	Hemiparesis with cranial nerve deficits	Brainstem
	Tetraparesis	Spinal cord (cervical)
	Tetraparesis with cranial nerve deficits	Brainstem
	Paraparesis of the lower limbs	Spinal cord (thoracic)
LMN	All four limbs, facial, ocular, and bulbar weakness	Neuromuscular junction
	All four limbs, predominantly proximal weakness	Muscle (myopathy, dystrophy)
	All four limbs, predominantly distal weakness	Peripheral nerves (peripheral neuropathy)
	Facial, ocular, and bulbar	Cranial nerves (cranial neuropathy)
	Focal, asymmetric (single limb)	Nerve root (radiculopathy), plexus (plexopathy), or peripheral nerve (mononeuropathy)
	Multifocal, asymmetric (more than one limb)	Peripheral nerves (multiple mononeuropathy)
Mixed UMN and LMN	All four limbs with bulbar and facial weakness but no ocular involvement	Anterior horn cell
	Paraparesis of the lower limbs	Conus medullaris

Abbreviations: LMN, lower motor neuron; UMN, upper motor neuron.

Symptoms include dyspnoea, orthopnoea, and morning headaches and, if severe, may result in respiratory arrest. Acute onset of respiratory failure is seen in GBS, MG, and botulism, whereas a gradual, progressive worsening is seen in MND and the muscular dystrophies (Duchenne, myotonic dystrophy, and limb-girdle forms).

Damage to the spinal cord may result in diaphragmatic weakness (C3–C5) and intercostal muscle weakness (T1–T11).

Respiratory muscle function may be assessed at the bedside by asking the patient to cough or sniff (diaphragmatic function), observing for paradoxical abdominal movements on inspiration, and measuring their forced vital capacity (FVC). Elective intubation should be considered if FVC falls below 15 ml/kg.

Lesions of the brainstem can adversely affect respiratory function through depression of the respiratory drive.

Other signs and symptoms

Muscle pain or myalgia can occur in an inflammatory myopathy and myotonic dystrophy. Neuropathic pain often occurs with a vasculitic neuropathy, radiculopathy, and compressive neuropathy. Shoulder pain is usually present in brachial neuritis. Back pain is a typical feature of cord compression but may also appear in GBS.

Myotonia is the slow relaxation of skeletal muscle after contraction (e.g. with handgrip), typically seen in myotonic dystrophy. Other features characteristic of this condition include frontal balding and temporalis wasting (myotonic facies), cataracts, cardiac arrhythmias, and cardiomyopathy

Muscle cramps and exercise intolerance may indicate a metabolic myopathy, mitochondrial myopathy, or a myotonic dystrophy.

Trophic changes may be present in peripheral nerve disorders. A skin rash is often a hallmark of a vasculitic process or may be associated with a connective tissue disorder.

Drug and social history

Chronic alcoholism and malabsorption syndromes predispose to subacute combined degeneration of the spinal cord (vitamin B_{12} deficiency) and a thiamine deficiency-related sensory–motor neuropathy. Injecting drugs users are at risk of botulism and embolic strokes. Patients on statins or steroids can rarely suffer from a drug-induced myopathy. Certain cytotoxic chemotherapy drugs (e.g. vinca alkaloids) can be associated with a sensory–motor peripheral neuropathy.

Key diagnostic tests

Medical imaging

CT is useful in the emergency setting, such as when an intra-cerebral bleed, ischaemic stroke, solid tumour, or acute cord compression is suspected to be the cause of weakness. Magnetic resonance imaging, however, is preferable over CT as a diagnostic aid due to the superior image resolution and sensitivity to soft tissue pathology. The finding of weakness with a possible upper motor neuron origin or weakness affecting the cranial muscles should prompt an MRI of the relevant segment of the neuroaxis. MRI is also useful in demonstrating nerve root impingement in radiculopathies, inflammation, or compression in plexopathies and to identify subclinical changes or the pattern of affected muscles in myopathies.

CSF analysis

Barring contraindications to lumbar puncture, CSF analysis may be undertaken to aid the diagnosis of an inflammatory, infective, or malignant cause of weakness affecting the central nervous system or spinal roots. In the context of weakness, raised CSF protein is seen in infections, intra-cerebral haemorrhage, malignant infiltration, and inflammatory disorders such as GBS, CIDP, and MS. Oligoclonal bands have a relatively high specificity for MS, although they may also be present in vasculitis of the CNS, neurosarcoidosis, Lyme disease, and viral infections.

Neurophysiological studies

Electromyography (EMG) may aid in the differentiation between weakness of a neuropathic cause or a myopathic origin and can assist in localizing the lesion in a plexopathies, radiculopathies, or mononeuropathies. Findings in MND characteristically reflect denervation (fibrillation potentials, giant motor unit potentials, and positive sharp waves) and reinnervation changes (increased jitter). Myopathies typically demonstrate spontaneous activity with fibrillations, positive sharp waves, and low-amplitude polyphasic action potentials of a short duration.

Nerve conduction studies can differentiate axonal from demyelinating peripheral neuropathies. In demyelination, distal motor latency is prolonged and motor conduction velocity is slowed. In axonal neuropathies, the compound muscle action potential is reduced but the distal motor latency and conduction velocity can be preserved. In nerve entrapment, there is slowing of nerve conduction at the site of compression.

Repetitive nerve stimulation is performed in suspected myasthenic syndromes, showing characteristic decrement in the compound muscle action potential in MG and an increment in LEMS.

Somatosensory, visual, and brainstem auditory evoked potentials are useful in the assessment of CNS conduction, particularly in cases of suspected MS.

Nerve and muscle biopsy

Peripheral nerve biopsy (usually sural or radial nerve) is indicated where a vasculitic or neoplastic cause of a peripheral neuropathy is suspected. Muscle biopsy (usually quadriceps) is performed in cases of suspected myositis, muscular dystrophy, and mitochondrial and metabolic myopathies, aided by immunostaining and electron microscopy.

CHAPTER 44 **Weakness**

Other diagnostic tests

In generalized polyneuropathies, tests that need to be considered include antiganglioside antibodies (in suspected GBS), thyroid function, fasting blood glucose, vitamins A, E, and B_{12}, erythrocyte sedimentation rate, antinuclear antibodies (ANA), antineutrophil cytoplasmic antibody (ANCA), serum electrophoresis, and serum angiotensin-converting enzyme (ACE).

Creatine kinase (CK) is released by muscles during breakdown. CK levels are raised in inflammatory and immune myopathies, Duchenne dystrophy, and Becker dystrophy. However, CK may also be increased in Afro-Caribbeans in the absence of pathology. Trauma, sepsis, or exercise can also increase CK levels.

Tests for metabolic and mitochondrial myopathies include serum and CSF lactate, urinary organic acids, and serum and urine carnitine levels.

In MG, anti-acetylcholine antibodies and/or muscle-specific kinase (MuSK) antibodies may be present. To aid in the diagnosis further, an edrophonium test can be performed, consisting of an intravenous bolus injection of edrophonium, a short-acting acetyl-cholinesterase inhibitor, which causes a brief but marked improvement of symptoms in patients with the condition.

Paraneoplastic causes of weakness are very rare and can take the form of a myelitis, motor neuropathy, myopathy, or a neuromuscular junction disorder. The underlying pathogenesis is believed to be autoimmune. However, in most cases, an antibody is not identified. Voltage-gated calcium channel antibodies are associated with LEMS, a neuromuscular junction disorder which may present as a paraneoplastic syndrome. A skeletal survey, chest and abdominal CT, or whole-body PET may help localize a malignancy in a suspected paraneoplastic syndrome.

Genetic tests are conducted in suspected hereditary neuropathies and myopathies, usually guided by the history, examination, and clinical findings. Techniques include cytogenetics, DNA mutation tests, and microarrays.

Introduction to therapy

Therapy is tailored to treating the underlying cause of weakness and symptoms that arise from it. Neurosurgical intervention may be sought for compressive or space-occupying lesions of the brain and spinal cord. Therapy for ischaemic stroke comprises of antiplatelet therapy, anticoagulation therapy, thrombolytic therapy (where indicated), secondary prevention, and neurorehabilitation. Disease activity in inflammatory and immune-mediated conditions may be controlled by steroids and/or immunosuppressants. Malignant tumours may be treated with surgical debulking, radiotherapy, and/or chemotherapy, depending on tumour type and location.

Supportive therapy in the form of mechanical ventilation may be required for patients with respiratory muscle weakness. Enteral feeding via a gastrostomy or jejunostomy should be considered in those with bulbar weakness who are at risk of aspiration. Skeletal muscle relaxants (such as baclofen and tizanidine) are used to treat spasticity and recurrent muscle spasms. Regular Botox injections can help relieve spasticity and dystonias. Further supportive care is provided by physiotherapists and occupational therapists.

Specific treatments

GBS is treated with intravenous immunoglobulin (IVIg) typically at a dose of 0.4 g/kg day^{-1} for 5 days, or plasma exchange. Therapy is generally indicated if the patient is no longer able to walk. IVIg is preferred over plasma exchange, as it is much easier to administer. Patients require regular monitoring of their respiratory function (FVC) and cardiovascular function (cardiac rhythm and blood pressure).

CIDP can be treated with long-term corticosteroids, intravenous immunoglobulins, or plasma exchange. In patients who cannot have the aforementioned therapy or fail to respond adequately to them, immunosuppressive therapy (such as azathioprine and mycophenolate mofetil) may be considered.

Treatment for MND is largely supportive and consists of physiotherapy, occupational therapy, nutritional support, respiratory support, and social support. Riluzole 50 mg orally twice a day may extend survival modestly, although it has not been shown to improve strength or quality of life.

Treatment strategies for MG depend on the severity of symptoms, the age of the patient, the presence of a thymoma, and other related comorbidities. Patients with mild symptoms may require only symptomatic therapy with an anticholinesterase drug (i.e. pyridostigmine). For those who remain symptomatic on anticholinesterases or have more generalized weakness, treatment with corticosteroids is usually initiated along with bone and gastric protection. Immunosuppressive therapy (e.g. azathioprine) is often used as a steroid-sparing agent and for those who do not adequately respond to pyridostigmine and steroids. Thymectomy may be considered in seropositive patients under 60 years of age, and in all patients with thymoma. In a myasthenic crisis, plasma exchange or IVIg is used as acute therapy.

Treatment for MS is predominantly with immunomodulatory drugs such as glatiramer acetate, interferon beta, and natalizumab, which aim to reduce relapse rates. High-dose corticosteroids are used in the management of acute relapses to aid in the recovery rate.

No specific therapy is available for the majority of the hereditary and metabolic neuromuscular disorders. Treatment is supportive.

Prognosis

Prognosis largely depends on the cause of the motor weakness, treatment, and the presence/absence of complicating factors. In many causes of neuromuscular weakness, prognosis is poorer in patients who have cardiorespiratory involvement and in those who acquire the disease at an older age. Nonetheless, the prognosis for many such disorders has vastly improved with the use of ventilatory support, cardiac intervention, antibiotics, and immunosuppressive and immune-modulatory treatments. Prognostic factors for specific conditions are discussed as follows.

Poorer prognosis in GBS is associated with older age, ventilator dependency, campylobacter infection, and axonal neuropathy. Mortality is as high as 8%. One-third of patients have significant residual disability despite treatment.

The vast majority of CIDP patients (90%) respond well to therapy. However, at least 50% relapse within 4 years, and less than a third achieve remission off treatment.

The prognosis of MND remains very poor. Mean survival time from diagnosis is 2 years in the classical form. Prognosis is worse in patients who are older and those with a rapid decline following initial diagnosis.

Poor prognostic factors in MS include older age of onset, male sex, progressive course at onset, early residual disability, short inter-relapse interval, and high early relapse rates. The majority of patients with relapsing–remitting MS eventually demonstrate secondary progression.

How to handle uncertainty in the diagnosis of this symptom

Not infrequently, investigative test results do not correlate with the clinical examination findings of weakness. The approach to this issue is to retake the clinical history and carefully re-examine the patient, either noting any inconsistencies or confirming one's earlier findings. Neurological signs and symptoms have a tendency to evolve over a period of time, often becoming clearer or more distinct as the illness progresses.

Tests results including imaging findings should be re-evaluated in the correct context. Diagnostic tests performed too early or in mild disease states may yield normal results. Examples include the frequent finding of a normal CT scan in an acute stroke, and normal cerebrospinal fluid markers with normal electrophysiological readings in early GBS.

Alternative diagnoses are often worth considering. Migraines and epilepsy can present with episodes of brief motor dysfunction which can mimic TIAs or strokes. In the elderly, fractures and joint dislocation may present with painless loss of limb function.

Non-neurological or non-organic muscle weakness is commonly encountered in the clinical setting. This could be considered if inconsistencies are demonstrated in the history, and examination findings with the clear presence of strong indicators of a somatization disorder in the patient's past medical history (which is usually notable for abnormal illness behaviour), their social history (substance abuse and self-harm are often evident,) and their mental state (frequently coexisting depression, anxiety, or a personality disorder).

Further Reading

Kress JP and Hall JB. ICU-acquired weakness and recovery from critical illness. *N Engl J Med* 2014; 370: 1626–35.

Pfeffer G, Povitz M, Gibson GJ, et al. Diagnosis of muscle diseases presenting with early respiratory failure. *J Neurol* 2015; 262: 1101–14.

Wiles CM. Pyramidal weakness. *Pract Neurol* 2017; 17: 241–42. doi:10.1136/practneurol-2016-001584

45 Tremor and other abnormal movements

Susanne Schneider, Alexander Schmidt, Kailash P. Bhatia, and Peter G. Bain

Definition of the symptom

Tremor is a rhythmic involuntary oscillatory movement of a body part most commonly affecting the hands and arms but other body parts can also be affected including the legs, head, jaw, chin, palate, voice, and trunk.

Differential diagnosis

The broad differential diagnosis in primary and secondary care is shown in Table 45.1, ordered in decreasing probability.

Context

Tremor is the most common movement disorder. Estimates of the prevalence of tremor vary widely and range up to about 20% of the general population. It is more common in the elderly. For the most common type of tremor, essential tremor (ET), an annual incidence has been reported to be 23.7 per 100 000; and a prevalence of 0.4 to 6% has been reported for those over 40 years, and of 12% for those over 70 years.

There are multiple ways to classify tremor, for example, by clinical features, by tremor frequency, by aetiology, and so on. The International Movement Disorders Society classifies tremor according to the behavioural state in which it occurs, namely, at rest or on action, as this can give a clue towards the aetiology. The most common cause of rest tremor is idiopathic Parkinson's disease (PD). Action tremor comprises postural tremor (when the arms are outstretched) and kinetic tremor (during movement; this includes intention tremor which occurs during a goal-directed movement like the finger–nose test). The most common causes of action tremor are ET and cerebellar dysfunction resulting from different causes. Task-specific tremors are brought on by or are most prominent during a specific task, for example, hand tremor during writing or when playing a particular musical instrument.

Approach to diagnosis

The key to the diagnosis of different forms of tremor is the clinical examination of patients. As a first step, patients should be examined at rest for tremor of arms, legs, and the head. The arms should be relaxed and fully supported on chair rests to observe for rest tremor.

Next, the patients are instructed to hold their arms outstretched in front of them, which will bring out the postural component of tremor—sometimes after a pause (as in PD). Dystonic posturing may be present in the hands, arms, shoulder, or neck and indicates a dystonic tremor syndrome. The finger–nose test will disclose intention tremor, as in cerebellar disease. Further useful tests include writing, which brings on primary task-specific writing tremor, or drawing a spiral, which documents the tremor. Holding a cup or pouring water from one glass into another demonstrates the functional impact of arm tremor. If slowness or fatiguing of movements on repetitive finger and foot tapping is present, a parkinsonian disorder should be considered. A broad-based gait in addition to intention tremor can hint towards a cerebellar disorder.

Specific clues to the diagnosis

There are several specific clues from the medical history and clinical examination to the underlying diagnosis of different tremor types.

In primary care, common causes of tremor include:

- drugs (e.g. dopamine-blocking agents, antidepressants, lithium, sympathomimetic agents, antiasthmatics, sodium valproate, and other antiepileptics)
- toxins (e.g. amphetamines, caffeine, nicotine, alcohol)
- medical and metabolic conditions (e.g. hyperthyroidism); the presence of associated symptoms like diarrhoea, weight loss, or palpitations can help to confirm the diagnosis

A physiological form of tremor is seen in all healthy people during muscle activation and is a fine postural tremor with frequencies ranging from <6 Hz (in children) to 13 Hz (in adults). Normally, it does not interfere with daily activities but it can become aggravated in stressful situations, for example, from the anxiety before a public performance (enhanced physiological tremor), and in chronic anxiety states. In addition, many drugs and conditions will aggravate a preexisting physiological tremor. It is treated by reassurance, avoidance of the triggering factors, and treatment of any underlying anxiety disorder.

In secondary care, causes of tremor include (ordered in decreasing probability):

- ET
- PD
- atypical parkinsonism

Table 45.1 Differential diagnosis of tremor			
Patient seen in primary care	**Probability**	**Patient seen in secondary care**	**Probability**
Drug-induced tremor (e.g. via dopamine-blocking agents, antidepressants, lithium, sympathomimetic agents, antiasthmatics (beta agonists), sodium valproate, or other anticonvulsants)	Common	Essential tremor	Common
		Parkinson's disease	
		Dystonic tremor	
Toxin-induced tremor (e.g. via caffeine, nicotine, alcohol)		Cerebellar tremor	
Tremor due to medical conditions (e.g. hyperthyroidism)		Atypical parkinsonism	
Enhanced physiological tremor			
Essential tremor	Less common	Psychogenic tremor	Less common
Parkinson's disease		Orthostatic tremor	
Cerebellar tremor		Peripheral neuropathies	
Atypical parkinsonism		Holmes tremor	
Holmes tremor		Wilson's disease	
Other (see less common causes of secondary care)		Palatal tremor	
		Chin tremor	
		Other (see common causes of primary care)	

- cerebellar tremor
- dystonic tremor
- Holmes tremor
- fragile X syndrome / FXTAS (Fragile X associated tremor ataxia syndrome)
- peripheral neuropathy
- Wilson's disease
- orthostatic tremor
- palatal tremor
- tremor of the chin and the lower jaw
- psychogenic tremor

ET

ET comes into consideration in patients of all ages, many with a positive family history of tremor. It is characterized by a symmetrical 4–12 Hz postural and kinetic tremor of the arms. In severe cases, the head and the voice may be also affected. Age of onset peaks in the second and sixth decades. Exclusion criteria are the presence of other neurological signs or a history of recent neurological trauma, a sudden onset, an isolated position- or task-specific tremor, and an isolated tremor of the voice, chin, tongue, or legs. Many patients (40%–75%) note improvement after alcohol intake but rebound worsening hours later is typical. A positive family history is common (50%–70%) and genetic linkage has revealed three regions of interest (2p22–25, 3q13, and 6p23) but no specific gene mutation has yet been reported. The location of the oscillator of ET also remains unknown but dysfunction of the cerebellum, the thalamus, and brainstem regions including the inferior olive, the nucleus coeruleus, and the red nucleus is suggested.

PD

PD should be considered in elderly patients where the tremor is present at rest. Although PD is a relatively common disorder, it is rare in community general practice, with a prevalence of about 100 to 150 cases per 100 000. The tremor typically presents as an asymmetric rest tremor, with a pill-rolling motion between the thumb and the index finger at rest at a frequency of 4–6 Hz being characteristic. An additional postural tremor at the same frequency or slightly faster is seen in over 50% of patients. Other features, including hypomimia, slowness and fatiguing of repetitive finger movements, small handwriting, slow gait, postural instability, and rigidity, support the diagnosis but may be subtle in the tremor-dominant variant of PD.

Atypical parkinsonism

Other parkinsonian disorders apart from PD, so-called atypical parkinsonism, may also present with tremor, but are rare. Although rest tremor is present in 30%–40% of patients with multisystem atrophy, a typical pill-rolling rest tremor (as in PD) is seen in only 8% of cases. In other atypical parkinsonian conditions like corticobasal degeneration and progressive supranuclear palsy, resting tremor is seen in approximately 20% of cases but again typical rest tremor (of PD) is not seen.

Cerebellar tremor

Cerebellar tremor, typically seen in multiple sclerosis, manifests as a low-frequency, coarse, terminal tremor during a goal-directed movement. Additional postural tremor may be present. Rest tremor is usually absent. Other signs of cerebellar disease may be present including ataxic gait, nystagmus, dysarthria with slurred or saccadic speech, hypometria, and dysdiadochokinesis. Causative lesions on imaging may be found within the cerebellum, particularly in the superior cerebellar peduncle and the dentate nucleus, as well as the afferent and efferent tracts but a clear correlation between location of the lesion and tremor features may not be ascertained. Other causes of cerebellar tremor include cerebellar infarction, spinocerebellar degeneration, and Friedreich's ataxia.

Dystonic tremor

Dystonic tremor is often present in patients with different types of dystonia. For example, patients with spasmodic torticollis often have tremor in addition causing a head shake. Sometimes tremor may even be more prominent than the dystonia, resulting in possible confusion with the diagnosis of ET. Tremor can be present in the part that is also affected with dystonia (dystonic tremor) or in

a part of the body that is separate from that affected by dystonia (dystonia-associated tremor). Head tremor in association with cervical dystonia is the most common presentation but the arms are also often involved, typically by a postural tremor that worsens during the performance of fine tasks. Patients often describe a sensory trick to improve their dystonia or dystonic tremor, for example, touching themselves lightly in the face or the neck (geste antagoniste) to control cervical dystonia. A broad range of tremor frequencies has been found (mainly less than 7 Hz).

Dystonic tremor may also have a resting component and may then be confused with PD tremor (discussed in the recent literature under the eponym SWEDDs (subjects without evidence of dopaminergic deficits)). It is thus important to carefully assess patients with a resting tremor for true bradykinesia and subtle signs of dystonia.

Holmes tremor

Holmes tremor is usually a unilateral or an asymmetrical tremor caused by lesions in the midbrain or thalamus. It typically consists of a combination of resting tremor, postural tremor, and severe intention tremor. Common causes include vascular lesions (e.g. Benedikt's syndrome), and toxoplasmosis in HIV-positive patients.

Fragile X syndrome

Fragile X syndrome is a trinucleotide-repeat disorder and the most common cause of inherited mental retardation. Recently, the permutation expansion (55–200 CGG repeats) has been related to the 'fragile X-associated tremor/ataxia syndrome' (FXTAS). The main clinical features are intention tremor and cerebellar ataxia, affecting men over 50 years. It may therefore be confused with multiple system atrophy in the elderly. Cognitive decline, parkinsonism, peripheral neuropathy, and autonomic dysfunction may be seen in FXTAS and these may be clinical clues towards this diagnosis. MRI brain scans show a characteristic appearance, with an increased T2 signal in the middle cerebellar peduncles and around the dentate nuclei.

Peripheral neuropathy

Peripheral neuropathies, particularly chronic inflammatory demyelinating neuropathies (especially during relapses), immunoglobulin M chronic paraproteinaemic demyelinating neuropathy, and the hereditary motor and sensory neuropathy type 1, are differential diagnoses of upper limb action tremor (postural and kinetic). Tremor can occur in the absence of sensory loss. Frequency is between 3 and 6 Hz in hand muscles.

Wilson's disease

Wilson's disease should be excluded in any patient with tremor under 50 years old. Other features that suggest this condition are dysarthria, dystonia, and parkinsonism. Serum caeruloplasmin is low in these patients (<20 mg per decilitre) and a Kayser–Fleischer ring of the cornea is visible in 99.3% of patients on slit lamp examination.

Orthostatic tremor

Orthostatic tremor is a distinct disorder defined by a high frequency (13–18 Hz) tremor of the leg muscles (quadriceps and gastrocnemius) when standing and is sometimes not visible but palpable only. Patients may report subjective unsteadiness during stance which is absent when walking.

Palatal tremor

Palatal tremor is defined by rhythmic contractions of the levator or tensor veli palatini muscle (1.5–3 Hz). Synchronous ear clicks accompany the movements in some patients.

Tremor of the chin and lower jaw

Tremor of the chin and the lower jaw (hereditary geniospasm) is a rare condition with autosomal dominant inheritance and early onset.

Psychogenic tremor

Psychogenic tremor is a positive diagnosis. Suggestive features include sudden onset, static course, spontaneous remission, clinical inconsistencies with distractibility of tremor frequency, lack of responsiveness to treatment, somatizations, presence of psychiatric disease, and secondary gain.

Key diagnostic tests

Key diagnostic tests for the underlying diagnosis of different tremor types are routine blood tests, which should include those for thyroid function, liver function, and kidney function, as well as electrolyte status and protein electrophoresis. Serum caeruloplasmin and copper assays should be performed in all patients under 50 who present with tremor, to exclude Wilson's disease.

Other diagnostic tests

Other investigations used mainly in secondary care include electrophysiological investigations, particularly electromyography and accelerometry studies, which can help to evaluate tremor characteristics like frequency, amplitude, and coherence. Differentiation of ET and dystonic tremor from tremor due to PD or Parkinson-plus syndromes is facilitated by new imaging techniques (like dopamine transporter (DaT) SPECT or fluorodopa PET) used to visualize presynaptic dopaminergic neuron integrity, which is reduced in PD but normal in ET and dystonic tremor. Cerebral imaging methods (CT and MRI) and lumbar puncture can also help to identify tremor-causing diseases.

Introduction to therapy

Mild tremor does usually not require treatment. However, as severe tremor has an impact on the quality of life and daily activities, different drugs have been investigated for their efficacy to improve tremor. Overall, symptomatic drug treatment is unsatisfactory, as exemplified by the long list of drugs mentioned in the literature to improve tremor. In ET, a non-selective beta blocker, particularly propranolol or primidone (or a combination of them), are recommended as first-line treatments, with a Class A level of evidence. Other beta blockers may also reduce tremor but are usually less effective than propranolol. There is no difference between the long-acting and the normal formulation of propranolol. It is advisable to titrate propranolol or primidone carefully upwards to minimize side effects when these drugs are utilized. Second-line anti-ET drugs include benzodiazepines, topiramate, and gabapentin (Class B and C evidence). In PD, levodopa and dopamine agonists (like pramipexole or ropinirole) are first-line treatments for tremor, bradykinesia, and rigidity. Anticholinergics and beta blockers may also be considered, especially in tremor-dominant PD. Treatment of cerebellar tremor is more difficult. Clonazepam or beta blockers may be helpful. Botulinum toxin injections are helpful in dystonic tremor and may improve tremor of head, jaw, chin, palate, and voice when oral drugs are ineffective.

Surgical intervention may be considered in patients with disabling drug-resistant tremors. The thalamus, which is involved in tremorgenesis of various tremor types, is the traditional target (particularly the ventral intermediate nucleus). However, the zona incerta is now considered the most effective target for suppressing most tremors. Historically, thalamotomy played a role but has now largely been replaced by deep brain stimulation (DBS) because of fewer adverse effects and greater functional benefits following DBS. Suppression of tremor by DBS ranged from 68% to 89% in patients with ET and from 71% to 94% in patients with PD. In multiple sclerosis, DBS tends to be less successful and is associated with a greater risk of adverse events. Most recently, noninvasive magnetic resonance-guided focused ultrasound has also been proposed for treatment of disabling tremor.

Prognosis

The prognosis of tremor depends on the underlying disease. In most tremor types, the life expectancy is normal. However, depending on tremor severity, it can be very disabling and socially embarrassing. The uncontrollable shakiness of the hands forces 15%–25% of patients with ET to retire prematurely, 60% of patients choose not to apply for a job or a promotion, and up to 55% of patients do not go shopping alone because of the tremor. If other neurological signs are present on clinical examination (e.g. slowness or fatiguing of movements, a broad-based gait) and parkinsonian or cerebellar disorders are suspected, the prognosis may be significantly impaired. Consequently, these patients need specialist neurologic workup.

How to handle uncertainty in the diagnosis of this symptom

Uncertainty in the diagnosis of tremor is rare, as this symptom is easy to recognize. However, establishing the correct aetiology of a particular tremor type may be very difficult, even for movement disorder specialists. If a detailed medical history and clinical examination of patients in combination with routine blood tests does not lead to a diagnosis, a specialist neurologic workup is needed.

Further Reading

Donaldson I, Marsden CD, Schneider SA, et al. *Marsden's Book of Movement Disorders*, 2012. Oxford University Press.
Schneider SA, Deuschl G. Medical and surgical treatment of tremors. *Neurol Clin*. 2015 Feb;33(1):57–75

46 Gait disorders

Richard Abbott

Introduction

Gait problems can arise from a number of different causes ranging from primary neurological to locomotor conditions. Prevalence increases with age, and causation is often multifactorial. Falls are a frequent consequence.

Definition of gait disorder

A gait disorder is an abnormality in the manner of walking; it results from a loss of smoothness, symmetry, or synchrony of movement patterns.

Patterns of gait disorder

Neurological and non-neurological patterns of gait disorder are given in Box 46.1.

Context

Difficulty with walking is a relatively common clinical problem, and the causation is often self-evident. Leg deformity resulting from previous trauma, and hemiparesis caused by a recent stroke, are examples. In a less simple scenario, pattern recognition may allow spot diagnosis by the experienced clinician. However, a full history and examination will usually be required to back up initial observation, and the presence of additional neurological signs, for example, nystagmus in the patient with a wide-based gait, will corroborate suspicions of cerebellar disease.

The clinical impressions may need to be followed by further investigations but the direction taken will be guided by the initial clinical assessment. More complex gait analysis techniques are rarely required for diagnosis but can be used as an aid to treatment and prognosis.

Approach to diagnosis

A detailed history is essential but, even prior to taking this, the opportunity will arise to watch the patient on entering the room. Observe whether they are accompanied and whether they require a walking aid. Do not assume that a patient in a wheelchair cannot walk, as there may be some other reason for the wheelchair, such as reduced exercise tolerance or painful feet! In the ambulant patient, watch progress closely; observe the general demeanour, stance, and posture, look for asymmetry of limb movement, and assess whether balance appears to be an issue. Listening closely may also herald the high step and flop of a dropped foot or the dragging of a spastic leg.

While the history is being taken, the opportunity will arise to assess behaviour, personality, and mood, to observe the presence of involuntary movements, and to assess the speech. The presence of dysarthria, dysphonia, or dysphasia will hint strongly at the presence of a neurological disorder and also be a pointer to the neurological system involved.

Neurological examination will follow and it is often convenient to examine gait at the outset before the patient is disrobed and asked to climb onto the examining couch. A suggested approach to routine gait examination is to ask the patient to proceed as in Box 46.2.

Extrapyramidal problem

Observe rising from a low chair, an activity which may prove difficult. Problems in initiating gait, as well as slow movements, flexed posture, and reduced arm swing are seen with parkinsonism. Festination, a tendency to topple forwards when walking, may occur.

Observe walking through a doorway, an activity which may induce freezing. Perform the 'pull test' to look for postural instability, which is demonstrated by the patient taking a step backwards when a gentle pull is exerted (retropulsion).

Labyrinthine imbalance

The Unterberger stepping test is a variant of Romberg's test which can be performed in patients with vertigo and who are suspected of having vestibular pathology. The patient is asked to walk on the spot with eyes closed and arms outstretched for 30 seconds. Rotation to either the right or the left by more than 40 degrees is abnormal and indicates underaction of the ipsilateral labyrinth.

Proximal muscle weakness (myopathy)

A 'waddling'-type gait is typically caused by pelvic instability. The patient will have difficulty rising from a low chair. Ask him to stand from a sitting position with his arms folded. This will prevent him from pushing himself up using his arms, an accessory movement used to overcome the lower limb weakness. In more severe cases,

---

Box 46.1 Neurological and non-neurological patterns of gait disorder

Neurological
- peripheral (motor)
- peripheral (sensory)
- hemiplegic
- spastic
- extrapyramidal
- cerebellar
- frontal
- myopathic

Non-neurological
- locomotor (antalgic)
- non-organic
- cautious gait

Box 46.2 Routine gait examination

1. Have the patient stand on a narrow base, with his feet together, his arms at his side, and eyes open; can he stand unsupported?
2. Have the patient close his eyes (Romberg test); loss of balance indicates a deficit of proprioception.
3. Have the patient stand on each leg in turn with eyes open; the unsteadiness may be lateralized.
4. Have the patient walk briskly the length of the room and observe the nature of his gait. Look for the presence of a wide-based gait. If the patient is mildly ataxic, have him walk in a circle, to exaggerate any deficit.
5. Have the patient walk as if on a tightrope (tandem gait, or heel–toe walking); even mild ataxia inhibits this manoeuvre.

Depending upon the findings or suspected site of the pathology, the examination can be extended accordingly.

ask the patient to rise from the supine position. He will need to pull himself up using a support or, alternatively, exhibit the Gower manoeuvre whereby he pulls himself up from the floor by 'walking up' his own body.

Specific clues to diagnosis

Peripheral motor weakness

Essentially, the gait difficulty will arise due to flaccid foot drop leading to a 'high step and flop' gait. Weakness of the dorsiflexors combined with reduced muscle tone necessitates a higher step in order to provide clearance of the toes from the ground when stepping. As the foot returns to the floor, it will slap down in a poorly controlled manor. The patient will tend to stub the toes when walking and finds difficulty with clearance when climbing stairs. Examination of the limb may reveal typical lower motor neuron signs, such as muscle wasting and areflexia. Long-standing pathology, such as, for example, hereditary motor and sensory neuropathy (Charcot–Marie–Tooth) may be associated with profound distal wasting and pes cavus.

Peripheral sensory loss

Loss of touch sensation in the feet will impair the ability to feel the ground when walking and the patient may say it is like walking on air or rubber. The patient will walk in a hesitant manor and balance may be affected. If, in addition, as is frequently the case, proprioception is lost, then sensory ataxia will result. Gait may be high stepping, as the patient is unaware of the exact position of the floor, and may stamp down as the foot reaches the floor. The gait is wide-based and significantly worse in the dark, when visual clues are no longer available. A positive Romberg test will differentiate from other causes of ataxia, and formal testing of proprioception will reveal impairment. As the pathology lies in the posterior spinal columns, vibration sense in the feet will also be impaired.

Hemiplegic gait

Due to the imbalance in muscle tone, the flexors are stronger in the affected arm while the extensors are stronger in the leg. The leg will tend to adduct at the hip, and the foot tends to plantar flex and invert. Knee flexion is weak. To overcome a tendency to catch the foot when walking, the limb circumducts at the hip as the leg moves forwards.

Spastic gait

The legs are stiff and inflexible and the feet will appear to be dragged along. The gait is slow and there is poor clearance of the foot from the ground. Foot drop may occur due to greater weakness of the dorsiflexors than the plantar flexors, but flopping is not seen because of the increase in motor tone. In severe cases of diplegia, such as may occur with cerebral palsy or hereditary spastic paraplegia, 'scissoring' may occur due to the exaggerated tone in the hip adductors. Milder forms of spasticity may only manifest after the patient has been walking for some distance. Examination typically reveals increased tone, hyperreflexia, and extensor plantars. Clonus may be evident.

Extrapyramidal

Idiopathic Parkinson's disease (IPD) is asymmetric at outset, and motor features commonly commence in the upper limb. Gait becomes affected when the ipsilateral leg is involved. The gait then appears almost hemiplegic, but the reduced arm swing and tremor are characteristic. The increase in tone has the typical cogwheeling feature, and pyramidal signs are absent. Instability, gait initiation problems, falls, et cetera, are features seen later as the disease progresses.

Gait and balance problems occurring early in the course of an extrapyramidal disease should arouse suspicions of an alternative diagnosis to IPD. Backward falls, for instance, occur early in the course of progressive supranuclear palsy and should trigger a close examination of the eye movements looking for upward gaze palsy. Likewise, early development of autonomic features such as impotence or postural hypotension may point to a diagnosis of multisystem atrophy. Vascular pseudoparkinsonism often affects gait, but facial expression and upper limb function may be normal—so-called lower-body parkinsonism.

Cerebellar disease

Charcot's triad of cerebellar disease is nystagmus, dysarthria, and intention tremor. Ataxia should, of course, be added to this. Gait is typically wide-based and, if the cerebellar lesion is lateralized, staggering will occur towards the ipsilateral side. Midline or chronic pathology may not be lateralized, but gait and speech involvement (scanning speech) are usually prominent.

Frontal pathology

Chronic bilateral frontal lobe pathology can lead to profound gait difficulty which can be mistaken for parkinsonism. Gait initiation failure, shuffling, and disequilibrium may be seen, but other typical extrapyramidal features, such as reduced arm swing, cogwheel rigidity, and tremor, are lacking. Unlike in Parkinson's disease (PD), the gait is wide-based. Small vessel vascular disease and normal pressure hydrocephalus are good examples.

Myopathic gait

A myopathic gait is typically waddling, with a swaying, wide-based characteristic and often with pronounced lumbar lordosis. The presence of myopathic facies, nasal speech, and proximal upper limb weakness may accompany the typical history of difficulty getting out of the bath or turning over in bed. A family history is important.

Non-neurological gait disorders

Locomotor disorders

These are common, particularly in the elderly, where degenerative joint disease is a frequent comorbidity with neurological disease. This can lead to confusion. As a generalization, pain is unlikely to exist with a pure neurological problem. For example, a patient with PD may state that his leg feels 'stiff'. Is he referring to increased tone due to his PD or does he mean pain and joint stiffness due, for instance, to osteoarthritis of his knee?

Low-back pathology is also a common explanation for gait difficulty. This can, not infrequently, have a non-organic basis.

Non-organic (functional) gait disorders

Non-organic gait disorders are not uncommon in neurological clinics and should be suspected when the gait pattern does not fit with an expected pattern, and 'hard' neurological signs are lacking. Often, the patient arrives in a wheelchair. When asked to stand, the patient may be reluctant but on, rising, may appear to dramatically lose balance only to stagger against a supporting object, never actually toppling to the ground. Another common presentation is the dragging leg, whereby the patient will move forwards apparently pulling the involved leg behind him with the limb externally rotated. Again formal examination fails to reveal convincing neurological signs such as wasting or reflex abnormalities. Give-way weakness may be apparent.

Cautious gait

Cautious gait is seen in patients with a previous history of falls. There may be an underlying neurological condition, such as gait apraxia, but many patients are merely afraid that they will fall again, and have lost their confidence. They will rise fearfully from a chair and show extreme reluctance to standing without gripping disproportionately strongly on the arm of a chair or the supporting carer. Gait initiation appears difficult and, when steps are finally taken, the gait is broad-based, the patient constantly expressing the desire to grab onto a support. Physiotherapy is often dramatically helpful in restoring confidence and full recovery.

Diagnostic tests

The pattern of clinical presentation should be a clear guide as to how investigation should proceed. By using the descriptions of gait pattern already described, it should be possible in most cases to decide in which neurological system the pathology lies. Thus, neurological imaging with MRI can target the brain in patients with clear-cut upper motor neuron signs, cerebellar disease, or features of gait apraxia. Spinal MRI will be appropriate in patients who exhibit spasticity without features suggestive of cerebral involvement.

More complex imaging tools are sometimes used. An example would be a form of SPECT scanning (123-I-FP-CIT DaT), which is a form of functional imaging used to study patients with suspected extrapyramidal disease and who exhibit a deficiency of dopamine neurotransmission.

Electromyography will be normal in CNS disease but is the investigation of choice for peripheral nerve disorders. It will distinguish axonal from demyelinating peripheral neuropathy, and neuropathic from myopathic pathology. Evoked potential studies are used when central conduction pathways are to be evaluated.

A useful tool in the neurological armamentarium is lumbar puncture, which is used selectively when pressure measurement or CSF analysis is likely to be diagnostically helpful. Examples would be CSF protein elevation in demyelinating neuropathy, or the presence of oligoclonal IgG in multiple sclerosis.

Blood tests may reveal a suspected diagnosis such as, for example, vitamin B_{12} deficiency or thyroid disorder; measurement of creatine phosphokinase may point to muscle disease. Alternatively, DNA analysis may define the genetic basis of the condition.

Therapy

The availability of treatment will depend upon the underlying cause of the gait problem. Many neurological conditions are not amenable to intervention, but an accurate diagnosis will aid ongoing management and prognosis.

Drug treatment may be symptomatic rather than curative, the use of antispasticity drugs being a good example. Other drug treatments, such as levodopa for PD, are both symptomatically and diagnostically beneficial. Vitamin B_{12} treatment for subacute combined degeneration of the spinal cord, on the other hand, will significantly improve the condition and prevent recurrence.

Timely neurosurgical intervention in the appropriate case can have dramatic benefit upon gait and balance. Examples of where this might apply are posterior fossa tumours, normal pressure hydrocephalus, and cervical myelopathy.

Many conditions which impair gait are not amenable to curative intervention and are progressive in nature. Patients can be helped by acquiring an accurate diagnosis and a management plan, assisted by appropriate supportive therapies.

How to handle uncertainty in diagnosis

Gait disorders follow characteristic patterns as described. Experience and increasing familiarity with modes of presentation will make diagnosis easier. Atypical or variability of function should raise the suspicions of a non-organic disorder. Full neurological examination will normally display appropriate physical signs which corroborate the initial clinical impression.

Subsequent investigations should be targeted at confirming the diagnosis suspected following detailed clinical examination. A blunderbuss approach using tests uncritically may uncover the answer by chance, but is expensive and usually inconvenient and uncomfortable for the patient.

Further Reading

Jankovic J. Gait disorders. *Neurol Clin* 2015; 33: 249–68.

Pirker W and Katzenschlager R. Gait disorders in adults and the elderly: A clinical guide. *Wien Klin Wochenschr* 2017; 129: 81–95. Open access, available at doi: 10.1007/s00508-016-1096-4.

47 Sensory loss

Sarah Stoneley and Simon Rinald

Definition of sensory loss

Sensory loss relates to any alteration in perception of external stimuli such as pain, temperature, touch, or perception

Context

The presentation of sensory loss can be extremely varied and is frequently accompanied by motor dysfunction. To effectively assess and diagnose sensory disorders, an understanding of the relevant functional anatomy is required.

Neuroanatomy basics

To experience sensation, our body requires a stimulus to be detected. The sensory information is relayed via peripheral nerves, plexus, roots, and dorsal horns into the spinal cord and transmitted in either the dorsal columns or spinothalamic tracts to the brain. Sensory loss can be caused by pathology anywhere along this pathway. The sensory innervation of the skin is depicted in Figure 47.1.

The detection of cutaneous sensation begins with free nerve endings or end organs in the skin. Sensory information is divided into touch, proprioception, vibration, temperature, and pain, and

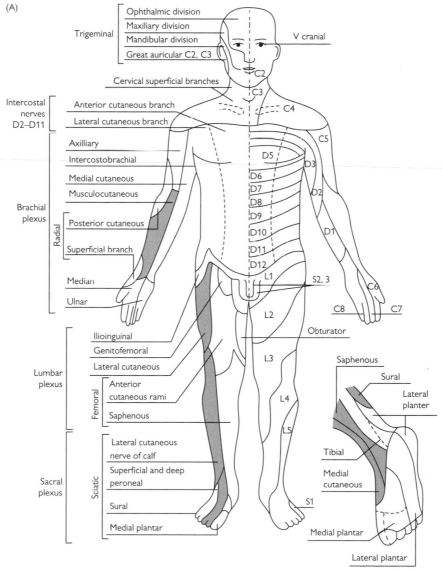

Figure 47.1 Sensory innervation of the skin. Cutaneous areas of distribution of spinal segments and sensory fibres of the peripheral nerves: (a) anterior and (b) posterior views.

Reproduced with permission from Walton J, Brain's Diseases of the Nervous System, Tenth Edition, Oxford.

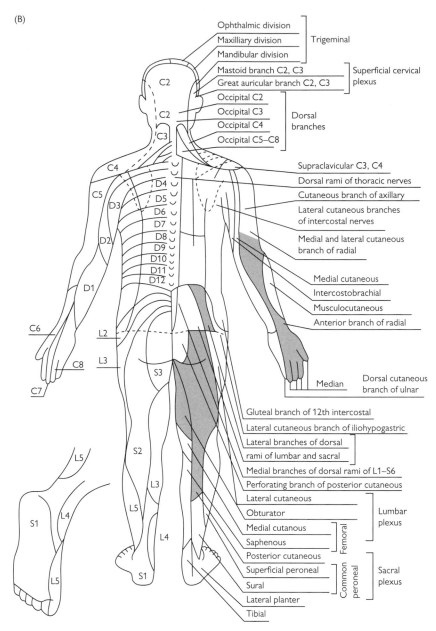

(B)

Ophthalmic division
Maxilliary division — Trigeminal
Mandibular division
Mastoid branch C2, C3 — Superficial cervical plexus
Great auricular branch C2, C3
Occipital C2
Occipital C3
Occipital C4 — Dorsal branches
Occipital C5–C8
Supraclavicular C3, C4
Dorsal rami of thoracic nerves
Cutaneous branch of axillary
Lateral cutaneous branches of intercostal nerves
Medial and lateral cutaneous branch of radial
Medial cutaneous
Intercostobrachial
Musculocutaneous
Anterior branch of radial
Median — Dorsal cutaneous branch of ulnar
Gluteal branch of 12th intercostal
Lateral cutaneous branch of iliohypogastric
Lateral branches of dorsal rami of lumbar and sacral
Medial branches of dorsal rami of L1–S6
Perforating branch of posterior cutaneous
Lateral cutaneous
Obturator — Lumbar plexus
Medial cutanous
Saphenous — Femoral
Posterior cutaneous
Superficial peroneal — Common peroneal — Sacral plexus
Sural
Lateral planter
Tibial

Figure 47.1 (Continued)

each is transmitted to the brain differently. The first difference occurs at the level of the sensory nerve fibres. Large, extensively myelinated fibres (A-α and A-β) covey touch and pressure. Small, sparsely myelinated (A-δ) and unmyelinated (C) fibres covey temperature and different qualities of pain sensation.

In the spinal cord, the dorsal or posterior columns relay touch/pressure, proprioception (joint position sense), and vibration sense. These fibres synapse in the nuclei cuneate and gracile of the medulla, then cross, and ascend to the contralateral thalamus and sensory cortex via the medial lemnisci of the brainstem. The spinothalamic tracts convey pain and temperature to the contralateral sensory cortex. In contrast to the fibres in the dorsal columns, these fibres decussate to the contralateral spinothalamic tract typically within one to three levels of their entry into the cord, via the ventral white commissure. The ultrastructural organization of the spinal tracts is also important with respect to sensory dysfunction. At increasingly higher levels, crossing spinothalamic fibres are added to the medial aspect of the ascending tract, such that sacral fibres lie lateral to cervical fibres. The opposite situation exists in the dorsal columns.

In the thalamus, and particularly in the 'sensory homunculus' of the postcentral gyrus of the parietal lobe, representations of the face and hand are juxtaposed and subserved by disporportionally large areas of brain.

Approach to the diagnosis

The initial aim is to localize the lesion within the nervous system. Both the nature of the sensory symptoms and the parts of the body involved are important in this respect. A differential diagnosis can then be compiled which directs appropriate investigations.

Sensory disturbance can either be a complete loss (anaesthesia) or a reduction (hypoaesthesia) in the ability to perceive the sensory input. Dysaesthesia is an abnormal increase in the perception of normal sensory stimuli. Hyperalgesia is an increased sensitivity to normally painful stimuli, and allodynia is the perception of usually innocuous stimuli as painful.

A complete loss of sensation is likely to be due to a CNS problem, while a tingling/paraesthesia (large fibre) or burning/temperature (small fibre) sensation is likely due to an acquired peripheral nervous system problem. Shooting, electric-shock-like pains suggest radicular pathology, a tight-band spinal cord dysfunction. Positive sensory *symptoms* are usually absent in inherited neuropathies, even in the context of significant deficits on examination. It is also clear that patients often have great difficulty in satisfactorily describing abnormal sensory sensations when they are present

The history also gives the first pointer to the distribution of the sensory syndrome: which limb(s) is it in, which side is it on, whether it is proximal or distal, symmetrical or asymmetrical. A report of a 'numb' or 'dead' limb may reflect weakness and should not be taken at face value. Ask specifically about any motor, bladder, bowel, and autonomic dysfunction. The tempo of onset and duration of symptoms may be indicative of the nature of the pathology. A near instantaneous development of maximal deficit suggests a vascular cause; progression over seconds implies epilepsy; over minutes, migraine; over days, multiple sclerosis; over weeks, neoplasia. Other parts of the history—such as additional generalized seizures, headaches, prior optic neuritis, weight loss—can back up this initial impression.

An appropriate neurological examination is important. Even with apparently purely sensory problems, however, it is almost always best to leave the sensory examination to last. For example, the reflex pattern may be more useful in 'localizing the lesion' than the sensory examination itself. Ideally, an hypothesis for the potential expected sensory abnormalities will have already been established on the basis of history and other aspects of the examination. Sensory examination is difficult and subjective, and can be tiring and confusing for both you and the patient. Approaching it blindly, without any thought to the possible differential diagnosis, is more likely to confuse than clarify the situation. Be wary of attaching great significance to unexpected minor qualitative differences, especially in pinprick. The most useful and reliable information is usually obtained by working from an area of abnormality to normality—having first demonstrated to the patient what 'normal' is.

Specific clues to the diagnosis

Having established an hypothesis, the expected abnormality can now be specifically sought. Common patterns of sensory loss and their causes are as follows.

Glove and stocking loss

Glove and stocking sensory loss is primarily a result of peripheral polyneuropathy.

Length-dependant axonal neuropathy

Length-dependant axonal neuropathy, sometimes called 'dying back' polyneuropathy, is the most common pathology. There is symmetrical damage to the axons of peripheral nerves, and the furthest extremities of the longest peripheral nerves are affected first (i.e. those in the feet). As the symptoms reach mid-calf, symptoms begin in the fingers, giving the glove and stocking distribution. Vibration is affected first and reflexes (especially at the ankles) are diminished as these are dependent on the largest fibres, which are usually primarily and predominantly affected. There are several causes, including diabetes, alcohol, vitamin B_{12} deficiency, drugs, syphilis, HIV, uraemia, chemotherapy, and connective tissue diseases. Despite extensive investigations, a large majority of these cases remain idiopathic.

Demyelinating neuropathies

Demyelinating neuropathies are suggested clinically by globally depressed reflexes and weakness out of proportion to wasting. Although the sensory loss is often length dependent, weakness is usually more pronounced proximally.

Guillain–Barré syndrome

Guillain–Barré syndrome is an acute, inflammatory, demyelinating polyradiculoneuropathy. It often begins with back pain and paraesthesia of the hands and feet, although hard sensory *signs* are much less frequently found. The symmetrical weakness ascends from the legs to the arms, and often then to the cranial nerves and respiratory muscles. Most commonly, the limb weakness affects proximal more

than distal muscles. Areflexia is characteristic. There may also be autonomic dysfunction. There is a history of a recent infection, particularly a diarrhoeal or respiratory illness, in around 70% of cases. It is fatal in 3%–10% cases, and one-third of cases require admission to the ITU with respiratory failure. Treatment is with immunomodulatory therapy such as plasmapheresis or intravenous immunoglobulin (IVIg), which can shorten the duration of the disease.

Chronic inflammatory demyelinating polyradiculoneuropathy

Chronic inflammatory demyelinating polyradiculoneuropathy (CIDP) progresses over more than 8 weeks, or has a relapsing and remitting course. Typical features are those of a demyelinating neuropathy. Positive sensory symptoms and preferential loss of vibration and proprioceptive sensation are also common. Nerve conduction studies are mandatory for diagnosis. Steroids and IVIg are the mainstays of treatment.

Paraproteinaemic neuropathies

Paraproteinaemic neuropathies can be clinically indistinguishable from CIDP. Other cases have a **distal acquired demyelinating symmetrical (DADS)** phenotype—with slowly progressive, distal, and symmetric sensory loss, sensory ataxia, tremor, and little if any weakness—particularly in the presence of an IgM paraprotein and anti-MAG antibodies. Sometimes length-dependent axonal polyneuropathies are associated with a paraprotein. Whether this is pathologically relevant or simply an occasional coincidental finding remains uncertain.

POEMS syndrome

POEMS syndrome (polyneuropathy, organomegaly, endocrinopathy, monoclonal gammopathy, skin changes) is a fortunately rare, haematologically benign, but neurologically and systemically malignant disorder. The neuropathy is of a mixed demyelinating and axonal type, affects motor and sensory nerves, and spreads aggressively from distal to proximal regions, sparing autonomic function and the cranial nerves. In addition to the core features noted in the acronym, other elements such as ascites, pulmonary oedema, thrombosis, and renal failure may be seen. It is associated with elevated levels of certain cytokines, most notably vascular endothelial growth factor (VEGF). Potent immunomodulatory therapy with cytotoxic agents, or even bone marrow transplant, is required to halt progression.

Inherited neuropathies

Inherited neuropathies can be either axonal or demyelinating, and present at an earlier age with foot deformities and motor loss. Patients frequently have few if any positive sensory symptoms.

Small fibre neuropathies

Small fibre neuropathies are characterized by predominant pain and other positive sensory symptoms such as paraesthesia and allodynia. Deficits in pain and temperature sensation can be seen but, as large fibres are not involved, vibration, proprioception, and the deep tendon reflexes are spared, and nerve conduction studies are normal. Thermal threshold testing and skin biopsy (assessing intra-epithelial nerve fibre density) are used for diagnosis.

Sensory level

Sensory loss below a certain dermatomal level implies spinal cord pathology. Such pathology usually additionally affects motor function and causes abnormalities of tone and of the deep tendon reflexes (see Chapter 233). Anterior compression or anterior spinal artery infarction predominantly affects pain and temperature conveyed by the spinothalamic tracts. In such cases, sacral and dorsal column involvement is associated with pathology affecting a larger cross-sectional area of the cord, and hence a poorer prognosis. Hemisection of the cord (Brown–Séquard syndrome), is where the ipsilateral side of the body has vibration, weakness, and reduced proprioception, and the contralateral side has reduced pinprick and temperature— reflecting the differing anatomical pathways of the corticospinal tract and dorsal columns.

Suspended sensory level

Symmetrical sensory loss involving several contiguous dermatomes, with normal sensation above and below, is also caused by spinal cord pathology. In this case, the lesion lies in the central cord, taking out the decussating fibres of the spinothalamic tracts as they cross via the ventral white commissure (ventral to the central canal). This gives an isolated loss of pain and temperature sensation, typically beginning 1–2 dermatomes below the affected cord level. There may be additional weakness and/or reflex changes if the anterior horn cells or other tracts are involved. The classical situation is a cape-distribution deficit caused by a syrinx affecting cervical levels, but central cord syndromes related to multiple sclerosis are more common. Rarely, suspended sensory loss can be caused by ependymoma or central glioma.

Hemisensory disturbance

Hemisensory loss suggests contralateral disease in the brainstem, thalamus, or cerebral cortex. If the affected side of the face is opposite to the affected side of the body, the lesion is the brainstem (Wallenberg/lateral medullary syndrome). Thalamic infarcts give a contralateral sensory deficit. If the sensory cortex is affected, there is usually a small part of the body affected; there may be aphasia, neglect, or cortical sensory loss. Multiple sclerosis, stroke, and space-occupying lesions are important causes. Migraine and functional disorders can also present with hemisensory loss. With many of these pathologies, more patchy, discrete deficits involving parts of a limb, the face, or the trunk can also be seen.

Discrete abnormalities in a single limb

Mononeuropathies

Mononeuropathies result in symptoms and signs confined to a single nerve distribution. These are often caused by local compression. Common upper limb examples are median nerve (carpal tunnel), ulnar nerve (entrapment at the elbow), and radial nerve ('Saturday night palsy' causing wrist drop). Lower extremity examples are peroneal, femoral, and lateral cutaneous nerve of the thigh. There may only be small areas of paraesthesia due to the overlap of dermatomes. Multiple nerves are affected by **mononeuritis multiplex**, further described in 'Multifocal deficits' and most strongly associated with the vasculitides.

Plexopathies

Plexopathies affect the brachial or lumbosacral plexus. They often begin with excruciating pain felt over the plexus, followed by the development of sensory loss and weakness not confined to a single peripheral nerve or nerve root territory. Often these are dissociated—weakness in one or more myotomes with sensory loss in other dermatomes can be a clue. There is an association with diabetes, but many cases are idiopathic. Most are monophasic and steroids may help recovery. Bilateral plexus involvement is not uncommon. Infiltration from lymphoma or breast cancer, and radiation damage, are more serious and progressive causes.

Radiculopathies

Radiculopathies are lesions affecting the nerve root and are usually caused by either intervertebral disc herniation or narrowing of the foramina due to spondylosis, carcinomatosis, or focal extramedullary tumours. Neuropathic pain radiating along a limb is suggestive. Infection (varicella, Lyme disease, CMV) and particularly autoimmune/inflammatory causes (CIDP) often affect multiple levels. Usually, dermatomes and myotomes are involved.

Multifocal deficits

Other pathologies can initially have more patchy sensory involvement, sometimes developing an apparent length-dependent appearance as they progress.

Mononeuritis multiplex

Mononeuritis multiplex is characterized by painful asymmetrical motor and sensory loss involving damage to at least two separate peripheral nerves. Most often, the common peroneal or tibial nerves are affected first. As the condition progresses, it becomes less multifocal and more symmetrical, when it can begin to mimic a length-dependent process. In over half of all cases, mononeuritis multiplex

is caused by a systemic vasculitic process which incorporates the vasa nervorum. Diabetes, rheumatoid arthritis, atherosclerotic disease, HIV, and sarcoidosis are other notable causes.

Hereditary neuropathy with liability to pressure palsies

Hereditary neuropathy with liability to pressure palsies (HNPP) can produce a similar clinical picture to mononeuritis multiplex. Critically, however, the peripheral nerve dysfunction in HNPP is caused by compression and improves spontaneously thereafter, unlike vasculitic mononeuritis multiplex, which when untreated is relentlessly progressive.

Sensory ganglionopathies

Sensory ganglionopathies are rare. They are caused by the degeneration of the dorsal root ganglia. They present with sensory ataxia, absent reflexes, and sensory loss. Proximal and distal regions are affected, often asymmetrically. The trunk, face, and perineum may be involved. Crucially, given the site of the pathology, there is no weakness. They are associated with Sjögren's syndrome and paraneoplastic causes such as small cell lung cancer with anti-Hu antibodies.

Key diagnostic tests

It is important to take blood and check the full blood count, routine biochemistry, B_{12} and folate, glucose, thyroid function, cholesterol, and inflammatory markers. Protein electrophoresis, ideally with immunofixation, and a chest X-ray complete a reasonable battery of first-line screening tests for length-dependent, axonal, polyneuropathies. The yield of further tests in this situation is low. Nerve conduction studies may be useful for single nerve lesions, multiple mononeuropathies plexopathies, and radiculopathies. If CNS problems are suspected, then an MRI is usually indicated. Further tests may be required, depending on the diagnosis suspected (e.g. paraneoplastic antibodies for suspected paraneoplastic neuropathy, CSF protein measurement in CIDP/Guillain–Barré syndrome).

Therapy

Therapy depends on the cause of the problem and ranges from supportive for some conditions to aggressive treatment such as neurosurgery and immunosuppression for others. Physiotherapy will play a big role in all diagnoses where there is accompanying motor loss. Foot care is important, particularly in the context of diabetic peripheral neuropathy. If there is an underlying cause, this should be identified and treated. Some mononeuropathies, radiculopathies, and spinal cord and brain lesions may be amenable to surgery but, otherwise, treatment is supportive. Often, the neuropathic pain experienced will need addressing with agents such as tricyclics or gabapentinoids.

Prognosis

Prognosis depends on the individual cause. Peripheral neuropathies are usually slowly progressive, while some radiculopathies and mononeuropathies may improve with conservative management alone. Sensory ganglionopathies may herald an untreatable and rapidly progressive small cell lung tumour. Neurosurgical decompression for radiculopathies and myelopathy is performed to prevent further deterioration and/or improve pain, although sometimes improvement can be seen. Damage to the brain by stroke may improve with physiotherapy and rehabilitation.

How to handle uncertainty

Most uncertainty can be eliminated by following the basic neuroanatomical principles detailed in this chapter. Once the distribution and nature of the sensory disturbance has been delineated, the site of pathology should be apparent. Reference to a dermatome chart can help, particularly for discrete abnormalities which may be caused by damage to a single nerve or root.

Difficulties tend to arise when the sensory exam does not 'make sense'. There is sometimes a temptation to immediately equate this to a functional disorder. This may be the reason, but there are traps for the unwary. As ever, a functional diagnosis is best supported by clear positive signs. Characteristically, functional sensory loss has very sharply demarcated boundaries. Individual complete sensory loss affecting the whole circumference of a single limb—typically, an arm below the shoulder or a leg below the groin—is an anatomical impossibility. Hemisensory disturbance with a sharp demarcation between normal and abnormal falling absolutely in the midline is again suggestive. Dermatomes overlap in the midline; thus, in organic pathology, a transition to normal sensation begins before the midline is reached. A sensory level on the trunk should be higher posteriorly than anteriorly. Vibration sensation splitting the shin or skull is not reliable.

Labelling a symptom functional simply because the examination findings appear inconsistent or do not absolutely fit a textbook description risks misdiagnosis, however. Anatomical variation, difficulty in performing the examination, and the over-reporting of minor, insignificant differences by the well-meaning patient can all confound the situation.

In the extreme example, a clear neurological diagnosis has already been established following history and completion of the motor examination, which then appears to be contradicted by subsequent sensory findings. It is worth pausing to give thought to the possibility of a second pathology, but experience suggests excluding the discrepant sensory findings from the diagnostic formulation is sometimes the correct approach.

Further Reading

Callaghan BC, Cheng HT, Stables CL, et al. Diabetic neuropathy: Clinical manifestations and current treatments. *Lancet Neurol* 2012; 11: 521–34.

Donaghy M. 'The clinical approach', in Donaghy M, ed., *Brain's Diseases of the Nervous System* (12th edition), 2009. Oxford University Press.

Gwathmey KG, Burns TM, Collins MP, et al. Vasculitic neuropathies. *Lancet Neurol* 2014; 13: 67–82.

Yuki N and Hartung H-P. Guillain–Barré syndrome. *N Engl J Med* 2012; 366: 2294–304.

48 Headache

Paul Davies

Definition of headache/head pain

Headache is a pain in the head, with the pain being above the eyes or the ears, behind the head (occipital), or in the back of the upper neck. It may be secondary to numerous disorders such as meningitis (secondary headaches) or be a disorder in and of itself, such as migraine and cluster headache (primary headaches). Primary headaches are benign, diagnosed entirely on the history, and form the major morbidity in the problem of headache. They often exist in episodic and chronic forms. Secondary headaches may be acute or chronic, and benign or serious. Only some require investigation for their diagnosis.

In chronic headache management, it can be helpful to remember the International Association for the Study of Pain's definition of chronic pain: 'an unpleasant sensory and emotional experience associated with actual or potential tissue damage, or described in terms of such damage' (see http://www.iasp-pain.org/Taxonomy). Patients' ideas and emotions (e.g. a fear of more serious disease, or frustration and anger from a failure to adequately understand or treat their pain) are often important components in the clinical problem.

Context

Headache is one of the most common of all complaints and affects most people at some stage during their lives. Much is self-diagnosed and managed adequately, if not optimally. Migraine is the most common severe form of primary headache; it affects about 6 million people in the UK in the age range 16–65 years, and costs the UK almost £2 billion a year in direct and indirect costs. Over 100 000 people are absent from work or school every working day because of migraine. Tension-type headache, although less severe than migraine, is more prevalent and results in as great a societal burden, causing as many days lost from work as migraine does.

Healthcare professionals often find the diagnosis of headache difficult, and often patients worry about serious but rare causes of headache, such as brain tumour. Often, it is difficult to explain benign headache, and patients with chronic benign headache may journey through opticians and eye, ENT, or neurology clinics, searching, in vain, for the cause or cure.

Migraine is under-diagnosed and under-treated. Sadly, much headache can be a result of inappropriate medical treatment (e.g. frequent opiate treatment of migraine, leading to medication overuse headache). Advances in headache treatment now mean most sufferers can be helped.

Approach to the diagnosis

Diagnosis of the headache syndrome is the first step in managing the patient, and recognizing serious causes of headache is paramount. Patients may present with acute, subacute, or chronic headache and, with there being over 200 medical causes of headache, making the correct diagnosis of headache can be challenging. Taking a good history is the key to the diagnosis of all headaches, and the only tool the clinician has for the diagnosis of most of them. Perhaps no other symptom in medicine is so heavily dependent on an accurate and detailed history for headache diagnosis and patient management. Some patients recognize more than one headache type, and a separate history should be taken for each. A comprehensive history may not be obtained at the first consultation. Questioning may vary depending on the clinical situation but serious causes of headache, although rare, even in a casualty setting, must not be missed.

Since a benign headache syndrome is the most likely diagnosis, a good awareness of these conditions, particularly the most common,

Table 48.1 Common headache types and their estimated lifetime prevalence

Headache type	Estimated lifetime prevalence (%)
Primary headache	
Tension-type headache	72
Episodic	69
Chronic	3
Migraine without aura	9
Migraine with aura	6
Cluster headache	0.3
Primary stabbing headache	1
Secondary headache	
Substances (not alcohol) or their withdrawal	3
Hangover headache	72
Non-cephalic infection	63
Metabolic disorder	22
Disorders of the sinuses	15
Head trauma	4
Disorders of the cranium/neck/eyes	3
Vascular disorders	1
Non-vascular cranial disorders	0.5

is essential (see 'Common diagnoses', but detail is beyond the scope of this chapter). For most patients, further investigations are redundant but many are investigated nonetheless.

Common diagnoses

Some common headache types, looking particularly at primary and secondary care, are shown in Tables 48.1 and 48.2.

Is there a serious cause for headache?

In general, if headache is the only symptom and it has been going on for more than 3 months in a well patient with no neurological abnormalities, then it is very unlikely there will be a serious cause. A short headache history, without the stereotypical pattern of primary

Table 48.2 Diagnosis of headache types in primary and secondary care

Diagnosis in primary care	Diagnosis in secondary care
Primary headache syndromes	
24% of total headache presentations: • migraine: 73% • tension-type headache: 23% • cluster headache: 4%	General neurology clinics: GPs refer 3% of headache patients Emergency room: About 1% of all referrals are for headache; majority of cases are migraine
Secondary headache syndromes	
6% of total headache presentations: • 'sinus' headache: 83%	General neurology clinics: Most cases are benign Emergency room: As in general neurology clinics but more haemorrhage and meningitis

Note: Most patients presenting to primary care with headache (4.4% of *total* consultations) are not diagnosed. Headache accounts for about 30% of new patient general neurology referrals.

Box 48.1 Causes of a 'thunderclap' headache

- subarachnoid haemorrhage
- cough headache (may or may not be benign)
- orgasm headache (should be investigated for possible intracranial haemorrhage unless it has occurred three or more times in that situation and no other)
- reversible cerebral vasoconstriction syndrome
- cerebral venous sinus thrombosis (although the onset is usually more chronic, causing headache and papilloedema)

headache disorders and with the pain being the only or major feature may not give much to go on. It is the features of that pain that help diagnosis. Red flags are now a key part of headache management guidelines; the key red flags are:

- sudden onset, severe headache ('thunderclap')
- persistent morning headache with nausea
- new onset headache in the elderly person
- headache only with actions which alter CSF pressure
- steadily worsening headache
- posturally related headache
- headache with immunosuppression/cancer

Sudden onset, severe headache ('thunderclap'): Intracranial bleeding?

The term 'thunderclap' is used to describe headache that is severe at onset and perhaps worsens a little over the next few seconds or so. Subarachnoid haemorrhage is the archetypical example but there are several other causes (see Box 48.1).

Persistent morning headache with nausea: Raised intracranial pressure?

Many migraine sufferers wake up with migraine headache and associated nausea but attacks last no more than 3 days (by definition). Persistent morning headache, especially with nausea, can be due to raised intracranial pressure but there may be other causes (see Box 48.2).

New onset headache in the elderly person: Consider temporal arteritis

Temporal arteritis must not be overlooked but benign headaches in the elderly are very common. About 5% of migraine presents over the age of 50 years. Temporal arteritis is extraordinarily rare below the age of 50 years.

Headache only with actions which alter CSF pressure: Posterior fossa disorder?

A number of headaches may relate, in essence, to carrying out a Valsalva manoeuvre. Some can be due to structural abnormalities such as a Chiari malformation, where the cerebellar tonsils lie low and extend into the foramen magnum, thereby acting as a 'plug' when intracranial pressure increases. Some have no detectable underlying cause. Investigation with MRI (not CT, as this does not show the foramen magnum very well) should be considered in all cases. Cough headache is headache occurring not only with coughing but perhaps with sneezing or bending over (as in tying your shoe laces). Benign forms of headache may respond to propranolol or indometacin.

Box 48.2 Some causes of morning headaches

- migraine
- medication overuse headache
- hangover headache
- sleep apnoea
- carbon monoxide poisoning
- nocturnal seizures

Steadily worsening headache: Could it be due to some form of growth, such as skull metastases?

Chronic headache which has gone on for more than 3 months, with no other symptoms, in a well person, and where the clinical examination is normal is unlikely to have any serious cause. However, worsening headache could, rarely, be due to skull bone metastases, and so worsening headache may need investigation.

Posturally related headache: Consider low intracranial pressure or a colloid cyst of the third ventricle (rare)

Headaches following a lumbar puncture are well known and characteristically are improved quite quickly by lying down and worsened by getting upright. Such headaches can occur spontaneously from a tear of the dura (usually cervical) due to arthritis. These headaches often have characteristic MRI appearances which greatly aid their diagnosis. They may settle spontaneously; otherwise, a lumbar blood patch (even if it is a cervical leak!) can be very effective treatment.

Headache with immunosuppression/cancer

Immunosuppression from HIV, monoclonal antibody treatments, or the use of steroids may modify the presentation of intracranial pathology. The threshold for investigation should be lowered in patients with such types of immunosuppression.

If a serious cause for headache has been considered and ruled out, then what is the diagnosis?

Is it a primary or secondary headache?

All primary headaches and most secondary headaches are diagnosed on the history. Primary headaches are usually stereotyped and are considered to come in episodic and chronic forms (e.g. episodic tension-type headache and chronic tension-type headache). Some people recognize combined headaches such as migraine and tension-type headache. Perhaps a total of six diagnoses account for the vast majority of benign headaches (primary headaches: tension-type headache, migraine, and cluster headache; secondary headaches: medication overuse headache and (although controversial) cervicogenic headache). Determining headache periodicity (e.g. cluster headache), duration (e.g. 4–72 hours in migraine; see Box 48.3), and frequency, as well as the laterality of pain (see Table 48.3), are often key to forming the diagnosis.

Migraine pain generally builds up slowly over 30 minutes or more and, at its peak severity, patients like to keep still; in contrast, in cluster headache, the pain comes on rapidly and patients are restless. In chronic tension-type headache, the pain is dull and often 'band-like' and responds poorly to analgesics. Premonitory symptoms (previously called prodromal symptoms) only occur in migraine and may be overlooked unless specifically sought, as they are often rather vague symptoms such as tiredness with frequent yawning. Migraine aura comes in many forms but is usually visual and stereotyped and lasts 20–30 minutes before the headache starts (migraine with aura, previously termed classical migraine). Most migraine is without aura (previously termed common migraine). Careful enquiry about analgesic consumption will minimize the risk of overlooking medication overuse headache.

Box 48.3 Some causes of chronic daily headache (lasting ≥4 hours/day)

Primary headaches
- chronic migraine
- chronic tension-type headache
- new daily persistent headache
- hemicrania continua

Secondary headaches
- medication overuse headache
- post-traumatic headache
- cervical spine disorders

Table 48.3 Illustration of some key pain factors (duration, attack frequency, and lateralization) in headache diagnosis; internationally accepted diagnostic criteria exist for each headache condition (see http://www.ihs-headache.org/)

Pain duration	Attack frequency	Lateralized?	Diagnosis
Constant or near-constant	No attacks	Not usually	Chronic daily headache (headache on most days for at least 3 months for which no underlying cause has been found). See Box 48.3 for causes.
4–72 hours	Up to 3/week	Often	Migraine
15–180 minutes	Up to 8/day	Always	Cluster headache
<1 sec	Up to 100s/day	Usually	Idiopathic stabbing headache
Rare diagnoses			
Continuous	No attacks	Always	Hemicrania continua
2–45 minutes	1–40	Yes	Chronic paroxysmal hemicrania
1–30 minutes	1–30	Yes	Episodic paroxysmal hemicrania
15–30 minutes	1–3/night	Sometimes	Hypnic headache
5–250 seconds	Up to 30/hr	Yes	SUNCT (Short-lasting neuralgiform headache with conjunctival injection and tearing)

Reproduced with permission from Headache Classification Committee of the International Headache Society, The International Classification of Headache Disorders, 3rd edition (beta version), *Cephalalgia*, volume 33, pp.629-808 Copyright © SAGE.

Key diagnostic tests

Where there are red flag features, further investigation (usually CT in the A & E setting, MRI otherwise) is required, although significant pathology may not be found. Where there are no red flag features, if a specific diagnosis is not made, then the question of whether to do a brain scan may arise. Reports from headache clinics show that extremely few serious causes of headache found on scanning were unsuspected. Certainly, there is no place for routine scanning. Where asymptomatic groups of patients have had routine MRI head scans, significant pathology can be found in about 1%. Explaining to a patient that their arachnoid cyst is not the cause of their headache can be problematic.

Other diagnostic tests

The erythrocyte sedimentation rate is very helpful in suspected temporal arteritis, and the temporal artery biopsy can be diagnostic. Following normal imaging and, in particular, having ruled out venous sinus thrombosis, a lumbar puncture showing a raised opening pressure (>30 cm of water, if the patient is obese) but with normal constituents may confirm a diagnosis of idiopathic intracranial hypertension. CT scanning or plain X-rays of the sinuses may show sinus inflammation but this may not necessarily be the cause of headache. At least normal results exclude sinusitis, which is vastly over-diagnosed. MRI head scanning shows characteristic changes in low CSF pressure headache and has facilitated the diagnosis of spontaneous intracranial hypotension.

An introduction to therapy

Where recognizable pathology is found, the diagnosis and treatment options are usually clear. When no recognizable disease process is found, the situation can be more difficult but diagnosis should follow accepted diagnostic criteria, and treatment be evidence based. We know that as doctors we are more ready than patients to treat headache and we do not explain enough. Part of the problem is that we have terms, such as chronic tension-type headache, which we ourselves don't understand, even though we can recognize and manage the conditions associated with these terms. In approaching therapy, we need to know what the patient wants, be it just reassurance, explanation, treatment, or a brain scan. Furthermore, we must consider whether their goals are realistic.

Therapy of the different headache syndromes is beyond the scope of this chapter. Migraine (as it is the most common) and cluster headache (as it is the most painful primary headache syndrome) therapy will be outlined. Headache treatment can often be considered along the lines of:

- trigger identification and avoidance
- optimal acute attack treatment
- prophylaxis

Trigger identification and avoidance

Migraine may have many triggers. Common ones include relaxation after mental (or sometimes physical stress); menstrual or hormonal triggers (in women); problems with sleep (lack or excessive); environmental factors (e.g. bright light, strong smells); and dietary factors (e.g. missing meals; eating chocolate, cheese, or citric products; drinking alcohol). Carbon monoxide poisoning as a cause of intermittent headache must not be overlooked. Posture or repetitive movement may be important in cervicogenic headache. Alcohol triggers headache in about 50% of cluster sufferers (but only during the bout).

Optimal acute attack treatment

Migraine

Most people obtain adequate migraine relief from over-the-counter medications. Those who don't could be prescribed analgesic/anti-inflammatory agents with or without an anti-emetic. Soluble preparations work best. Suppository formulations should be considered in those who have a lot of nausea and vomiting (although some patients have diarrhoea). Ideally, any medication should be trialled three times before concluding on efficacy. Triptans have revolutionized the treatment of migraine. There are seven now available in the UK. Sumatriptan remains the market leader and is now available over the counter. There are two nasal sprays and one injection kit. Not everyone responds to triptans, and some only respond to the sumatriptan injection.

Cluster headache

The most effective therapies for cluster headaches are sumatriptan by injection, and high-flow oxygen. Sometimes sumatriptan or zolmitriptan nasal sprays can be effective but, in general, oral triptans are too slow in onset to be helpful. There is no place for analgesics such as opiates in the treatment of cluster headache.

Prophylaxis

Migraine

When trigger factors have been addressed and acute therapy optimized, prophylactic treatment should be considered if more treatment is required or if heavy reliance on acute therapy could lead to medication overuse headache.

The first-line agents for prophylaxis include:

Beta blockers: Propranolol is used the most. Evidence indicates that efficacy starts at 80 mg/day but it is sometimes initiated at lower doses. Efficacy may take several weeks to establish and a slow upward titration in dosage should be considered if there is a lack of response. Atenolol and metoprolol are also commonly used.

Sodium valproate: This is firmly established as a prophylactic agent. Generally, the starting dose is 300 mg twice daily, with a view to 600 mg twice daily later if the lower dose is ineffective.

Topiramate: This is a more recent addition to the prophylactic agent repertoire. It must be introduced slowly (25 mg every 2 weeks), with a target dose of 50 mg twice daily.

Other agents: A number of other agents, such as pizotifen, calcium blockers (e.g. verapamil), and flunarazine may be used.

Cluster headache

First-line treatment for episodic cluster headache includes verapamil, steroids, and lithium. For chronic cluster headache, verapamil and lithium are commonly used.

Alternative treatments

Many patients look at alternative medicine, perhaps due to a lack of support or efficacy from conventional medicine. Often, the evidence base for alternative treatments is poor. Treatments that are recently introduced include botulinum toxin injections for chronic migraine with or without medication overuse, and occipital nerve stimulation.

Prognosis

Prognosis is determined by the diagnosis. Primary headache syndromes are not curable. Treatment is aimed at symptom control. Migraine, in general, improves with age but in women may start at the menopause or worsen at this time. Migraine usually disappears during pregnancy (especially during the last two trimesters) but may soon return post delivery. In many sufferers, episodic migraine can move into a chronic form. Factors driving this transformation are now beginning to be understood.

Cluster headache, like migraine, can be a lifelong condition but tends to improve with age. In women, the effect of pregnancy on cluster headache has not been well studied.

How to handle uncertainty in the diagnosis of this symptom

Uncertainty in diagnosis is usually due to an uncertain headache history. Specifically asking about red flag features in this situation is a priority. A thorough examination may then be all you can do at that consultation. If there are no red flags, then it may be best to give the patient a dedicated headache diary to complete, and then arrange a timely review. Merely asking the patient to record their own symptoms is unlikely to be too revealing.

The question of scanning commonly arises. The worried patient and the uncertain doctor can be enlightened by an MRI head scan but asymptomatic pathology may be seen in about 1% or more of scans and create additional problems. In general, relevant pathology revealed on brain imaging is seldom unsuspected.

Further Reading

Charles A. Migraine. *N Engl J Med* 2017; 377: 553–561.

Headache Classification Committee of the International Headache Society. The International Classification of Headache Disorders, 3rd edition. *Cephalalgia* 2013; 33: 629–808.

Steiner TJ, MacGregor A, and Davies PTG. *Guidelines for All Healthcare Professionals in the Diagnosis and Management of Migraine, Tension-Type Headache, Cluster Headache and Medication-Overuse Headache* (3rd edition) (1st revision), 2010. British Association for the Study of Headache (http://www.bash.org.uk/wp-content/uploads/2012/07/10102-BASH-Guidelines-update-2_v5-1-indd.pdf)

49 Loss of vision

Susan Mollan and Alastair Denniston

Definition of the symptom

Loss of vision describes reduction in vision that cannot be corrected by glasses or contact lenses. Patients who complain of changes in their vision may have loss of visual acuity, distorted vision, or visual field loss.

The World Health Organization (WHO) classifies visual impairment as blindness or low vision. Blindness is defined as visual acuity of less than 3/60 in the better eye (ICD-10:54 visual impairment categories 3, 4, and 5). Low vision is present when the visual acuity is less than 6/18 but equal to or better than 3/60, in the better eye (ICD-10 categories 1 and 2).

Differential diagnosis

The aetiology of permanent visual loss is diverse and depends on the region studied. No large studies have documented referral practices within primary and secondary care. In the UK, visual impairment registration data shows the leading causes to be 'degeneration of the macula and posterior pole' (including age-related macular degeneration (AMD)), glaucoma, diabetic retinopathy, optic atrophy, and cataract.

Context

In the UK, 2.5% of the population have some degree of visual impairment which is not correctable by glasses. Worldwide, cataract is the leading cause of poor vision (48%), followed by glaucoma (12%), and AMD (9%). In developed countries, AMD is the commonest cause, followed by diabetes-related eye diseases.

Any degree of visual loss can be a great concern. Patients with sudden changes in vision tend to present acutely, whereas gradual loss may not be noticed, particularly when it is unilateral.

Approach to diagnosis

Visual loss may indicate serious systemic pathology that requires timely medical intervention. A structured history will help narrow the differential diagnosis.

Is it transient or persistent?

Transient loss of vision is generally due to a temporary or subcritical vascular event, and is often a sign of impending systemic vascular pathology (Table 49.1). Persistent loss of vision suggests a more permanent insult (Table 49.2).

Was it sudden or gradual?

Sudden loss of vision is usually vascular in origin, caused by either an occlusion or a haemorrhage (Table 49.2). Gradual loss of vision is usually due to degenerations or depositions (Table 49.3).

Does it affect one or both eyes?

Unilateral events indicate a local cause, whereas bilateral involvement may suggest a systemic process (e.g. giant cell arteritis (GCA) or migraine).

Central or peripheral visual field loss?

Central blurring suggests macular pathology. Unilateral peripheral loss may arise from a vascular retinal event (e.g. branch retinal vein occlusion (BRVO) or branch retinal artery occlusion (BRAO)), optic nerve pathology (e.g. glaucoma, non-arteritic anterior ischaemic optic neuropathy (AION)), or other retinal disease (e.g. retinal detachment). Bilateral peripheral loss can result from retinal or optic nerve disease, and any lesion involving the optic tracts to the visual cortex.

Any pain?

Ocular pain usually indicates disease at the front of the eye (e.g. anterior uveitis, keratitis, primary angle closure glaucoma). Painless loss of vision is typically due to disease of the posterior part of the eye (e.g. cataract; macular and other retinal problems; optic nerve disease). Note that optic neuritis and GCA can present with or without pain.

Associated timing?

Cortical ('spoke-like') cataracts can cause glare from headlights at night or in bright sunlight. Episodes of eye pain with 'haloes' occurring in dim light conditions may suggest angle closure glaucoma.

Previous eye surgery or disease

Common post-operative problems include thickening of the posterior capsule after cataract surgery ('posterior capsule opacification').

Drug history

Drugs which can cause reversible or permanent visual changes include chlorpromazine, clofazimine, corticosteroids, ethambutol, hydroxychloroquine/chloroquine, isotretinoin, sildenafil, tamoxifen, thioridazine, topiramate, and vigabatrin.

Table 49.1 Differential diagnosis of transient visual loss					
Diagnosis	**Eye**	**Duration**	**Vision**	**Other features**	**Ocular examination**
Headaches with visual aura (migraine)	Bilateral; any age	Minutes up to less than 1 hour	Resolves completely with or without headache	Zigzags, flashing, or scintillating scotoma	Normal
Amaurosis fugax	Unilateral; age >50 years	Seconds to minutes	Resolves completely	Atrial fibrillation, carotid bruit, or heart murmur	Likely normal; refractile emboli may be seen in vasculature
Transient visual obscurations	Bilateral or unilateral; any age	Minutes	Resolves completely	Raised intracranial pressure symptoms	Papilloedema; enlargement of physiological blind spot

Table 49.2 Differential diagnosis of sudden persistent visual loss

Diagnosis	Typical presentation	Visual loss	Other features	Fundal examination
Vascular				
'Wet' age-related macular degeneration	Unilateral; age >55 years; female > male	Variable (mild to HM)	Distorted vision; distorted Amsler grid	Large central macula changes with or without haemorrhage
Branch retinal vein occlusion	Unilateral; age >65 years (15% <45 years)	Normal or mild reduction	Horizontal visual field defect	Flame-shaped haemorrhages and CWS in one quadrant
Central retinal vein occlusion	Unilateral; age >65 years (15% <45 years)	Moderate (6/36–HM)	RAPD +	360° flame-shaped haemorrhages and CWS
Central retinal artery occlusion	Unilateral; age >50 years	Severe (CF-PL)	RAPD +	Normal optic disc; retina is pale with 'cherry red spot' of the macula
Branch retinal artery occlusion	Unilateral; age >50 years	Normal or mild reduction	Horizontal visual field defect	Refractile emboli may be seen in arterioles
Giant cell arteritis (Arteritic AION)	Unilateral; can progress rapidly to bilateral involvement; age >55 years	Severe (amaurosis fugax precedes visual loss in 25%)	RAPD +; tender temporal arteries; new onset headache, malaise, weight loss, and jaw claudication	Swollen optic nerve and CWS
Non-arteritic AION	Unilateral; age >50 years	Variable (normal to severe (NPL))	RAPD +/−; 'altitudinal' visual field defect	Segmental or diffusely swollen optic disc
Vitreous haemorrhage	Unilateral; any age	Variable	History of diabetes	Hazy fundal view
Structural				
Angle closure glaucoma	Unilateral; any age	Moderate to severe	Pain ++; nausea and vomiting	Red eye; cloudy cornea; poorly reactive pupils
Retinal detachment	Unilateral; any age	Variable	Flashing lights, floaters, and shadow	Retina bowing forwards
Inflammatory				
Anterior uveitis	Unilateral; any age	Variable	Red, painful, photosensitive eye	Red eye
Posterior uveitis	Unilateral or bilateral; any age	Moderate to severe	Floaters	Hazy view with haemorrhages and retinal changes
Central serous retinopathy	Unilateral; age: 20–50 years	Moderate	Red desaturation; distortion or scotoma on Amsler grid	Disturbance at macula
Demyelinating				
Optic neuritis	Unilateral; age: 15–45 years	Severe (HM to PL)	Discomfort on eye movement; RAPD +; red desaturation	Optic nerve may or may not be swollen
Degenerative				
Macular dystrophies	Bilateral; variable age groups	Variable	Positive family history	Alteration of macula architecture

Abbreviations: AION, anterior ischaemic optic neuropathy; CF, counting fingers; CWS, cotton-wool spot; HM, hand movements; NPL, no perception of light; PL, perception of light; RAPD, relative afferent pupillary defect.

Specific clues to the diagnosis

Both transient and permanent sudden visual loss can indicate significant pathology (Tables 49.1 and 49.2). There should be a high index of suspicion for GCA as it can present with an arteritic AION, amaurosis fugax, a vascular occlusion (arterial or venous), or double vision. An important distinction is whether the visual loss was sudden or gradual. Sudden loss tends to indicate a more serious event (Table 49.2) than a gradual reduction does (Table 49.3). An exception is diabetic maculopathy, where macular oedema may cause gradual loss but requires urgent treatment.

Functional visual loss is a diagnosis of exclusion and requires careful ophthalmic assessment, as it can coexist with genuine pathology.

Key diagnostic tests

Visual acuity

When testing for visual acuity, use the patient's distance correction (glasses or contact lenses). Here, a pinhole test is invaluable: punch a 1 mm hole in a card and then hold the card in front of the patient's eye while other eye is occluded, and recheck vision. If the vision improves, it is likely that there is a refractive error or a non-urgent condition present (Table 49.3).

'Swinging flashlight' test

A swinging flashlight can be used to detect a relative afferent pupillary defect (RAPD). The normal response when a bright light is shone into one eye is for both pupils to constrict symmetrically. Swing the torch to the other eye, and the pupils will remain the same, or constrict minimally. An RAPD is present if the pupil dilates to a larger size. Both pupils will then constrict when the light is shone back in the unaffected eye. This test is only positive when there is severe retinal and optic nerve injury (Table 49.2) in one eye.

Confrontational visual fields

Some patients report unilateral loss of vision even though both eyes are affected. This is common in homonymous hemianopia, where patients may only notice the loss in the eye where the temporal field is affected. Defects respecting the horizontal midline (i.e. superior or inferior defects) represent a hemispheric vascular event (e.g. BRVO, AION) or glaucoma. Defects respecting the vertical midline represent a neurological lesion such as a stroke or compressive lesions. Central defects are caused primarily by AMD. In any macular disease, patients get a positive scotoma (i.e. a 'spot' in the vision is seen and reported). Conversely, in optic nerve disease, a negative scotoma is present, but not reported (i.e. the defect is not 'seen' by the patient, but can be detected on examination).

Table 49.3 Differential diagnosis of gradual visual loss

Diagnosis	Typical presentation	Vision	Other features	Ocular examination
Degenerative				
Cataract	Bilateral; age >50 years	Pinhole improvement	Glare reported	Red reflex is dulled centrally or dark opacities seen
Dry or atrophic age-related macular degeneration	Bilateral; age >50 years	Reduction with pinhole; affected by ambient lighting	Distorted vision; distorted Amsler grid	Yellow drusen deposits or pigmentary changes at macula
Macular hole	Unilateral (20% bilateral involvement); age >50 years	Reduction with pinhole	Distortion or central scotoma on Amsler grid	Macula disturbance may be seen
Corneal disease	Bilateral; any age	Pinhole improvement; may vary through day	Can present with pain	Corneal opacity may be seen
Hereditary retinal disease (e.g. retinitis pigmentosa)	Bilateral; any age	Variable	Positive family history	Abnormal retinal appearance (e.g. pigmentation)
Vascular				
Diabetic maculopathy	Unilateral or bilateral; any age	Mild-to-moderate loss	Distortion noticed on Amsler grid	Exudates and microaneurysms at macula
Inflammatory				
Intermediate uveitis	Bilateral (often asymmetric)	Variable	Increasing floaters	Hazy fundal view and macula changes
Other				
Compressive lesions of the optic pathways	Unilateral or bilateral; any age	Variable; reduced colour vision	Visual field defects	Normal or pale optic nerves
Refractive errors	Bilateral; any age	Pinhole improvement	None	Normal

Other diagnostic tests

Colour vision test

A colour vision test checks optic nerve function. If no formal tests (e.g. Ishihara pseudo-isochromatic plates) are available, ask the patient to assess the colour quality of a bright red object (e.g. the top of a red pen or bottle). A relative difference between the eyes indicates pathology affecting the optic nerve (e.g. optic neuritis).

Amsler grid

The Amsler grid test checks macular function. The chart is a 10 cm grid, split into 0.25 mm^2 squares, with a central dot for the patient to fixate on. Distortion will be reported if macular pathology exists (AMD or macular oedema). A central scotoma may be detected in optic nerve disease.

Blood tests

In suspected GCA, the erythrocyte sedimentation rate (ESR) and C-reactive protein level (CRP) will be raised and, in the majority of GCA cases, a thrombocytosis will be present. However, some cases of temporal artery biopsy-proven GCA have normal inflammatory markers. Conversely, there are many other causes of a raised ESR and CRP (e.g. infection, malignancy, and other types of vasculitis).

Introduction to therapy

The aetiology of visual loss is diverse, and the majority of cases will need primary care input to manage the systemic risk factors, and timely input from specialist ophthalmic services. Routine referrals can be made for cataracts and posterior capsular opacification when the visual loss interferes with the patient's quality of life. The management of loss of vision is shown in Table 49.4.

Prognosis

Prognosis depends on the working diagnosis. WHO estimates that up to 75% of all visual impairment is preventable or treatable.

Table 49.4 Management of loss of vision

Diagnosis	Management
Amaurosis fugax	Exclude GCA; perform complete cardiovascular and neurological examinations; direct referral to transient ischaemic attack clinic for carotid imaging; perform modifications of risk factors and consider antiplatelet therapy, if it is not contraindicated
Arterial occlusion (CRAO and BRAO)	Discuss with local eye services urgently, as occasionally treatment within 24 hours can dislodge the emboli; exclude GCA; complete a cardiovascular examination
GCA	Immediate high-dose intravenous corticosteroid therapy to prevent loss of sight in other eye; often managed jointly by ophthalmology and rheumatology
Optic neuritis	The majority of patients resolve spontaneously, with recovery starting within 10 days; corticosteroids do not alter the long-term visual prognosis, but may hasten recovery
Retinal detachment	Urgent ophthalmic assessment for treatment
Vein occlusions (CRVO and BRVO)	Perform a complete cardiovascular examination; uncontrolled diabetes mellitus, hypertension, GCA, and hyperviscosity syndromes must be identified and managed; consider antiplatelet therapy if it is not contraindicated; refer to ophthalmic outpatient department
Vitreous haemorrhage	Urgent ophthalmic assessment (e.g. to exclude retinal detachment)
'Wet' AMD	Urgent referral to local rapid-access AMD clinic

Abbreviations: AMD, age-related macular degeneration; BRAO, branch retinal artery occlusion; BRVO, branch retinal vein occlusion; CRAO, central retinal artery occlusion; CRVO, central retinal vein occlusion; GCA, giant cell arteritis.

How to handle uncertainty in the diagnosis of this symptom

As loss of vision can be a sign of serious pathology, discuss your full history and examination findings with a local ophthalmologist or emergency eye department.

Further Reading

Biousse V and Newman NJ. Ischemic optic neuropathies. *N Engl J Med* 2015; 372: 2428–36.

Denniston AKO and Murray PI. Oxford Handbook Of Ophthalmology (3rd edition), 2014. Oxford University Press.

50 The red eye

Susan Mollan and Alastair Denniston

Definition of the symptom

'Red eye' is a term used to describe the colour of the conjunctiva when there is either dilation of the blood vessels (hyperaemia) or a ruptured blood vessel (subconjunctival haemorrhage). It can be characterized by its distribution:

- diffuse (generalized hyperaemia, which can be superficial or deep)
- focal (hyperaemia only in one sector)
- circumcorneal (hyperaemia at the junction of the cornea and conjunctiva)

Differential diagnosis

There is a multitude of different etiologies that present with 'red eye'. It is seen and managed in all healthcare settings, including optometry services. Table 50.1 presents conditions that can usually be successfully managed in the primary care environment, and others that need immediate or elective management in more specialized services.

Context

Red eye is one of the commonest ophthalmic complaints. Although the majority of causes are self-limiting and treated in the primary care setting, some cases require early and urgent assessment by the ophthalmologist. Even in the absence of specialist equipment, a careful history and general examination will crystallize a diagnosis and identify those conditions that are potentially sight threatening.

Approach to diagnosis

A structured history and examination will differentiate between benign and sight-threatening pathology. The following information is particularly useful:

- onset
- any subjective change in vision, and whether it clears on blinking
- any known precipitations (such as contact lens wear; infectious contacts; hay fever; chemical injury; history of trauma, DIY, grinding, or drilling)

- associated features (such as pain, discharge, and photophobia (see Table 50.2))
- previous eye surgery or disease

The key to diagnosis is to determine whether there is any effect on the vision, as any significant reduction of vision suggests serious pathology (see 'Key diagnostic tests'). Many healthcare professionals feel uncomfortable examining the eye; however, even a simple external examination can provide diagnostic clues, such as preauricular lymphadenopathy (associated with viral conjunctivitis), periocular eczema (associated with atopic conjunctivitis), or acne rosacea (commonly associated with blepharitis and marginal keratitis).

A bright torch can be used to assess the clarity of the cornea and highlight if a white spot (infiltrate or abscess) is present. It can also assess pupil reactions (brisk or sluggish). Gently pull down the lower lid to look at the distribution of hyperaemia and assess the mucus or discharge collecting on the inside of the lower lid and in the fornix. On the inside of the lower lid is the palpebral conjunctiva, and it is here that papilla or follicles can be seen (swollen and irregular). In the primary care setting, a direct ophthalmoscope can give a useful magnified view (dial in the +10 dioptre lens). Instil fluorescein drops and use a blue light or blue filter on the direct ophthalmoscope to highlight any stains caused by corneal epithelial defects (seen in abrasions and ulcers).

Specific clues to the diagnosis

Most bilateral red eye is due to ocular surface disease, which generally causes mild foreign body discomfort and transient blurring of vision that clears on blinking. A unilateral painful red eye with reduced vision is an indicator of more serious pathology (Table 50.2).

Key diagnostic tests

The key to diagnosis is to determine whether there is any effect on the vision. If a vision chart is available, test the vision with the patient's normal distance glasses or contact lenses, each eye separately.

If no chart is available, consider using any text that is available (such as a book (tests near visual acuity levels N6–N8) or newspaper (tests N6)). Test each eye in turn. Remember, patients who normally wear reading spectacles should use these for the test.

Table 50.1 Causes of red eye

	Primary care	Secondary care
Eyelids	Blepharitis (chronic inflammation of the eyelids) Floppy eyelid syndrome	Molluscum contagiosum
Conjunctiva	Subconjunctival haemorrhage Allergic conjunctivitis Bacterial conjunctivitis Viral conjunctivitis Chemical injury Inflamed pterygium or pingueculum	Atopic conjunctivitis Vernal conjunctivitis Chlamydial conjunctivitis Neonatal conjunctivitis (ophthalmia neonatorum) Inflammatory conjunctivitis (ocular mucous membrane pemphigoid; graft-vs-host disease) Neoplastic conjunctivitis (squamous cell carcinoma) Chemical injury
Cornea	Foreign body Abrasion Dry eye syndrome	Microbial/bacterial keratitis Marginal keratitis Viral keratitis
Sclera	Episcleritis	Scleritis
Anterior segment		Uveitis Angle closure glaucoma

Table 50.2 Clues to the diagnosis of red eye

Diagnosis	Visual acuity	Location	Redness	Pain/discomfort	Type of discharge	Other features
Blepharitis	Normal	Bilateral	Mild/diffuse	Mild	–	Crusty lids
Dry eye syndrome	Normal	Bilateral	Mild/diffuse	Mild	Watery +/–	Foreign body sensation
Bacterial conjunctivitis	Normal	Bilateral	Diffuse	Mild	Purulent discharge	Foreign body sensation
Viral conjunctivitis	Normal	Bilateral	Diffuse	Mild	Watery ++	Preauricular lymph nodes
Allergic conjunctivitis	Normal	Bilateral	Diffuse	Mild	Watery +/stringy mucus	Itch
Subconjunctival haemorrhage	Normal	Unilateral	Confluent area of haemorrhage	None to mild	None	–
Inflamed pterygium or pingueculum	Normal	Unilateral (sectoral)	Focal	None to mild	None	Other eye has fibrovascular tissue in same distribution
Episcleritis	Normal	Unilateral (sectoral)	Focal or diffuse (superficial)	None to mild	None	–
Corneal abrasion or foreign body	Normal or reduced	Unilateral	Focal or diffuse	Mild to moderate	Watery	History of trauma (e.g. from DIY/grinding)
Marginal keratitis (sterile ulcer)	Normal	Unilateral	Focal	Moderate	Watery +/–	Associated with blepharitis and acne rosacea
Bacterial keratitis (corneal ulcer)	Reduced	Unilateral	Diffuse	Moderate to severe	Watery +/– or purulent	Photophobia; history of contact lens wear or trauma
Viral keratitis/dendritic ulcer	Reduced	Unilateral	Diffuse	Moderate	Watery	Photophobia; dendritic ulcer
Chemical injury	Reduced	Unilateral or bilateral	Diffuse	Severe	Watery	History of contact with chemicals
Uveitis	Reduced	Unilateral	Diffuse or circumcorneal	Moderate to severe	Watery	Photophobia; irregular pupil
Scleritis	Normal or reduced	Unilateral	Diffuse and deep	Severe	None	Associated systemic diseases
Acute angle closure glaucoma	Reduced	Unilateral	Diffuse or circumcorneal	Severe	Watery	Photophobia; hazy cornea; poorly reactive pupil

Other diagnostic tests

Routine laboratory tests are generally not necessary; however, other diagnostic tests include:

- cultures, which must be taken in all neonates and immunocompromised patients
- conjunctival scrapings for Giemsa stain and or direct chlamydial immunofluorescence for chlamydial conjunctivitis
- samples taken from corneal ulcers by the attending ophthalmologist, for microbiology (as appropriate)

Scleritis requires a full evaluation for associated systemic disease.

Introduction to therapy

The following points regarding therapy should be noted:

- redness itself should not be treated without a specific diagnosis
- any patient with red eye should not wear contact lenses
- non-ophthalmologists should refrain from prescribing topical steroids without prior consultation: topical steroids can induce corneal melts, glaucoma, and cataracts
- treatment of the common causes of red eye is outlined in Tables 50.3 and 50.4

Immediate ophthalmic input is required in certain conditions to prevent loss of sight:

- any chemical burn should have copious irrigation with normal saline before direct referral to accident and emergency or eye department
- conjunctivitis in children under 1 month old (ophthalmia neonatorum) is a notifiable disease and needs immediate referral to the local eye department for culture and management
- contact-lens-related keratitis or a severe mucopurulent bacterial conjunctivitis is a potentially sight-threatening condition and should be referred promptly

Table 50.3 Treatment of common causes of red eye

	Condition	Treatment
Eyelids	Blepharitis	Lid hygiene, warm compress, and lubrication is the main advice given; however, there is insufficient evidence for recommendation of any one regimen
Conjunctiva	Subconjunctival haemorrhage	Reassurance; the red eye will resolve within 2 weeks; lubrication
	Allergic conjunctivitis	Avoidance of the allergen; systemic antihistamines and topical antihistamines or a mast cell stabilizer
	Bacterial conjunctivitis	Usually self-limiting; however, use of topical antibiotic is associated with a quicker clinical and microbiological resolution; as it is contagious, advise hygiene measures
	Viral conjunctivitis	Usually self-limiting; lubrication; as it is contagious, advise hygiene measures
	Chemical injury	Immediate normal saline irrigation until pH normalizes; then, emergency referral
	Inflamed pterygium or pingueculum	Lubrication
Cornea	Foreign body	Removal of foreign body; antibiotic ointment
	Abrasion	Antibiotic ointment; patching has not been proven to be of benefit
	Dry eye syndrome	Lubrication
Sclera	Episcleritis	Lubrication

Table 50.4 Advice for the patient on lubrication and antibiotic therapy

Treatment	Advice
Lubrication	Use topical artificial tear supplements frequently throughout the day, and an ointment at night can be prescribed to relieve mild-to-moderate discomfort
Topical antibiotic	Should be administered at least every 2 hours, then at a reduced frequency as the infection is controlled; continue 48 hours after healing
Ointment antibiotic	Should be used at night (when using drops during the day) or 3–4 times/day if used alone

Prognosis

Prognosis depends on the presumed diagnosis. Conditions where the vision is not affected are mostly self-limiting, and the prognosis is good. In conditions where vision is affected, prompt referral may well help limit the potential visual damage.

How to handle uncertainty in the diagnosis of this symptom

The patient should be referred for slit lamp examination if there is any of the following:

- loss of vision
- moderate-to-severe pain
- severe purulent discharge
- any corneal involvement
- history of previous herpetic eye disease
- lack of response to treatment

Further Reading

Sundaram V, Barsam A, Barker L, et al. *Training in Ophthalmology*. 2016. Oxford University Press.

51 Hearing loss

James Ramsden

Definition of the symptom

Poor hearing is defined by the patient but affects the ability to hear sounds and discriminate speech. This usually presents with reduced clarity ('why are they all mumbling'), absent sounds ('I can't hear the birds') or communication difficulties ('Granny is going deaf'). In children, this can often present as behaviour difficulties at school or home, without complaints from the child. As a rule of thumb, 20 dB HL (decibels Hearing Level) is taken as the lower limit of normal hearing.

Differential diagnosis

A side-by-side comparison outlining the differential diagnosis in primary care and secondary care, ordered by probability, is shown in Table 51.1.

Context

Hearing loss is a common complaint in primary care. It causes communication difficulties and substantially reduces quality of life. While most causes of hearing loss can be managed in primary care without specialized investigation, the clinician should be aware of rare, but serious, causes, which would need investigation. Furthermore, the correction of hearing loss is usually straightforward and rewarding.

Approach to diagnosis

Simple in-office tests can establish the likely cause of hearing loss, and direct further management. Few patients require sophisticated investigation.

Several particularly important points should be appreciated to guide diagnosis and treatment:

- Unilateral hearing loss suggests pathology, and a cause should be sought.
- Hearing loss must be divided into conductive hearing loss (CHL) and sensorineural hearing loss (SNHL). CHL is caused by sound not reaching the cochlear (abnormality of the ear canal, tympanic membrane, middle ear, or ossicles), whereas SNHL is a condition affecting the cochlear or auditory (eighth cranial) nerve. This division is most easily achieved in the office by use of a 512 Hz tuning fork (see 'Specific clues to the diagnosis') and confirmed with a pure tone audiogram (PTA).
- Hearing loss may be accompanied by other cardinal signs of ear disease, such as otalgia (pain), discharge from the ear, vertigo, facial nerve palsy, and tinnitus, which guide the diagnosis.

Other factors which determine the differential diagnosis include:

Age: In young children, middle ear effusion related to immature Eustachian tube function is the most common cause of hearing loss.

More than 60% of children will have a period of reduced hearing related to middle ear effusions following an upper respiratory tract infection at some point during childhood, although less than 5% fail to resolve spontaneously within 3 months. In the elderly, presbycusis is the most common cause of hearing loss, with a progressive high-frequency SNHL.

Previous ear surgery: A previous history of ear surgery may suggest a conductive-middle-ear cause for the hearing loss.

Medical history: Some conditions predispose to hearing loss. These include Wegener's granulomatosis (middle ear involvement), vasculitis (cochlear artery involvement), syphilis (dizziness and hearing loss), meningitis, and many neurological conditions.

Noise-induced hearing loss: Even many years later, noise-induced hearing loss (NIHL) due to industrial or military noise exposure can cause subsequent hearing loss, with a characteristic loss greatest at 4 kHz, although it will often progress to affect other frequencies.

Medication history: Some medications are ototoxic. These include aminoglycosides such as gentamicin/streptomycin, which can cause irreversible vestibular and cochlear toxicity, especially if renal excretion is impaired or loop diuretics are co-administered. An X-linked mitochondrial genetic susceptibility to aminoglycosides can lead to cochlea injury after a single dose. Other common potentially ototoxic medications include cisplatin, carboplatin, vancomycin, macrolides, loop diuretics, aspirin, and quinine.

Family history: The presence of other members of the family with deafness at ages <50 suggests a genetic cause, of which the most common would be otosclerosis.

Specific clues to the diagnosis

The most important diagnostic step is to establish whether the hearing loss is SNHL or CHL. This can be tested with a tuning fork. In the Rinne test, the degrees of air conduction (AC) and bone conduction (BC) are determined by placing a 512 Hz tuning fork beside the ear, and on the mastoid bone behind the ear, respectively. It is important to firmly press the tuning fork onto the mastoid bone to ensure good BC. Normally, AC > BC. If AC < BC, then there is a CHL on that side. This should be confirmed by placing the tuning fork on the vertex (Weber's test). If there is CHL, then the sound should localize to the affected ear. Other clues to the diagnosis of SNHL and CHL are given in Tables 51.2 and 51.3.

The other important diagnostic step is to examine the external canal and tympanic membrane. If there is wax occluding the view, it should be removed by syringing or microscope-assisted clearance. No assessment is complete until the pars tensa and pars flaccida of the tympanic membrane has been visualized.

Key diagnostic tests

The tuning fork tests just described will guide the clinician. Other important tests include:

PTA: This should be conducted by an experienced audiologist and will give air-conduction and/or bone-conduction thresholds. Masking allows the testing of each ear independently.

Tympanometry: This allows the compliance of the tympanic membrane to be assessed, as well as, indirectly, determine middle ear pressure. It can confirm the diagnosis of middle ear effusion, perforated tympanic membrane, or reduced middle ear pressure.

Speech audiogram: Speech perception is the most important function of hearing, and tests of speech discrimination can aid diagnosis.

Table 51.1 Causes of hearing loss	
Primary care	**Secondary care**
Wax	Presbycusis
Presbycusis	Noise-induced hearing loss
Otitis externa	Middle ear effusion
Acute otitis media	Otosclerosis
Perforated tympanic membrane	Cholesteatoma/chronic otitis media
Noise-induced hearing loss	Congenital
Otosclerosis	Vestibular schwannoma
Cholesteatoma/chronic otitis media	Ototoxicity
Congenital	Meniere's disease

Table 51.2 Clues to the diagnosis of sensorineural hearing loss

Sensorineural hearing loss	Diagnosis	Other features
Gradual onset, patient over 60, bilateral symmetrical SNHL	Presbycusis	Sloping hearing loss with high-frequency loss, normal canal, and normal tympanic membrane; consider NIHL if occupational/military exposure to >85 dB without ear defenders
Sudden SNHL, usually unilateral	Idiopathic SNHL; better outcome with course of steroids; normal TM	Needs MRI to exclude vestibular schwannoma (rare, but can present with sudden SNHL)
SNHL from birth, may be uni- or bilateral	Congenital SNHL	If severe and bilateral, may require cochlear implantation
Unilateral SNHL with vertigo	Meniere's disease (>1 attack) Labyrinthitis Vestibular schwannoma	MRI to exclude vestibular schwannoma
Bilateral rapidly progressive SNHL	Autoimmune inner ear disease Ototoxicity	May respond to steroids; check recent medication very carefully
SNHL after trauma	Cochlea injury; usually associated with severe vertigo	Much more likely if facial nerve also injured

Abbreviations: MRI, magnetic resonance imaging; NIHL, noise-induced hearing loss; SNHL, sensorineural hearing loss; TM, tympanic membrane.

Other diagnostic tests

It is unusual to require further tests. If there is asymmetrical SNHL, then MRI of the vestibular–cochlear nerve is required to exclude a vestibular schwannoma, although only ~1% of patients prove to have a vestibular schwannoma.

Table 51.3 Clues to the diagnosis of conductive hearing loss

Conductive hearing loss (CHL)	Diagnosis	Other features
CHL with itching in ear, pain, swollen canal, scanty discharge	Otitis externa	Often starts following water exposure to ears
CHL with severe pain, profuse mucoid discharge, pyrexia	Acute otitis media	Duration <2 weeks
CHL with profuse discharge, smell, granulations, or perforated tympanic membrane	Chronic otitis media with or without cholesteatoma Tumour of ear canal (rare)	Duration >3 months
CHL with effusion, usually painless	Otitis media with effusion, commonest in children	If fails to spontaneously resolve, may require treatment
CHL with wax	May be all of above or just simple wax	Wax alone does not cause more than a mild hearing loss
CHL with recent trauma	Haemotympanum CSF leak, if skull fracture Ossicular disruption	Haemotympanum is the commonest and should resolve over a few weeks
CHL with no abnormality seen, especially if family history	Otosclerosis	Usually asymmetrical; commonest cause of adult CHL with normal tympanic membrane

If there is chronic discharge and suspected chronic otitis media with or without cholesteatoma, or an unexplained CHL, then CT of the temporal bone may be indicated, although interpretation of the findings requires specialist skills and a synthesis of clinical and radiological findings.

Specialist tests such as stapedial reflexes or vestibular tests are rarely helpful.

Introduction to therapy

The treatment depends on the diagnosis.

Wax may be safely treated by irrigation, although it is important to be gentle to avoid trauma to the tympanic membrane and to use body temperature water to avoid a caloric effect causing vertigo. It is important to avoid irrigation if there is a history of previous perforated ear drum or a single hearing ear.

If the hearing loss is caused by infection and discharge, then topical treatment (e.g. with ciprofloxacin ear drops) combined with dry mopping is much more effective than systemic antibiotic treatment.

Many ototopical ear drops, except quinolone drops such as ciprofloxacin, are potentially ototoxic if they enter the middle ear. Evidence suggests that there is little risk from a short course of drops in an inflamed middle ear, as the thickened middle ear mucosa does not permit the entry of chemicals to the inner ear. Extreme caution should be used with long courses (>5 days) of potentially ototoxic drops in ears with perforated tympanic membranes if there is no obvious discharge.

SNHL is best treated with a digital hearing aid, of which there are various types specific to different losses. Severe/profound bilateral SNHL not benefiting from hearing aids may require cochlear implantation.

CHL treatment depends on the cause. Common options include digital hearing aid. If it is not possible to fit an aid because of chronic discharge or abnormalities of the ear canal, then a bone-conduction hearing aid (or a bone-anchored hearing aid, which is osseointegrated) may be appropriate. Middle ear effusions may be treated with grommet insertion. Otosclerosis can be corrected by stapedotomy, and ossicular abnormalities by ossicular chain reconstruction.

With all hearing loss, however, the most important ear is the better hearing ear, as hearing disability is largely determined by the air-conduction threshold of the best ear.

Prognosis

The prognosis depends upon the pathology.

How to handle uncertainty in the diagnosis of this symptom

Important points to remember when assessing an ear are as follows:

- Sudden SNHL should be promptly assessed and treated in an ENT department (same day).
- Unilateral symptoms require a search for pathology, and this may require specialist input.
- Unilateral SNHL needs to have a vestibular schwannoma excluded.
- If a patient has only one hearing ear, then be very careful.
- If the parents think a child is deaf, or the child is not speaking words by the age of 18 months, then the child needs paediatric audiological assessment.
- If there is hearing loss with other symptoms such as facial nerve palsy, fever, vertigo, or altered behaviour, then look for other conditions, including complications of middle ear infections. Otogenic infection is still the most common cause of temporal lobe brain abscesses, which can be surprisingly silent clinically.

Further Reading

Sajjadi H and Paparella MM. Meniere's disease. *Lancet* 2008; 372: 406–14.
Schreiber BE, Agrup C, Haskard DO, et al. Sudden sensorineural hearing loss. *Lancet* 2010; 375: 1203–11.

52 Facial pain

Paul Davies

Definition of facial pain

Facial pain occupies the area below the orbitomeatal line, above the neck and anterior to the pinnae. It comes in many forms and may or may not be accompanied by other symptoms. It may be acute, subacute, or chronic, arise from local pathology (e.g. dentition, parotid gland, sinus), be referred from other structures (e.g. pain behind the eye may be due to cervical spondylosis or sphenoidal sinusitis) or be part of a neurological syndrome such as trigeminal neuralgia or persistent idiopathic facial pain (previously termed atypical facial pain).

Differential diagnosis

There is a wide differential diagnosis (Box 52.1). As with headache, serious causes are rare. Some benign conditions are particularly painful (trigeminal neuralgia, cluster headache) but have effective treatment. Most facial pain is dealt with in primary care.

Context

Facial pain is common in primary and secondary care. The site of the pain and its associated features makes the diagnosis obvious in many cases. In secondary care patients with facial pain are commonly seen by ophthalmologists, maxillofacial surgeons, ENT surgeons, and neurologists.

Sometimes localizing the causative pathology is difficult. Facial pain is transmitted via the trigeminal nerve. The central pain pathway then descends to the upper cervical spinal cord to connect with cervical afferents. This trigeminocervical complex then passes rostrally to higher pain centres. It is this complex anatomy which explains referred pain. However, pain remains ipsilateral to its cause. Pain just above the eye, without other diagnostic features, might imply frontal sinusistis but amongst other causes a cervical origin is possible. The physical signs may be diagnostic, for example, orbital pulsation and bruit, as in carotico-cavernous fistula. Often, investigations are essential to confirm a diagnosis or exclude alternatives

Box 52.1 Causes of facial pain

Local pathology
- dental pathology
- sinus (e.g. sinusitis, trauma, carcinoma)
- nose (e.g. nasal injury, upper respiratory tract infection)
- ear (e.g. otitis externa and media)
- mastoiditis
- parotid gland (e.g. parotitis, calculi, obstruction, tumour)
- eye (e.g. glaucoma)
- temporomandibular joint
- temporal arteritis

Neurological causes
- trigeminal neuralgia
- persistent idiopathic facial pain
- cluster headache
- migraine
- tension-type headache (can occur as a facial pain)
- post-herpetic neuralgia
- neck-related (cervicogenic) pain

Approach to the diagnosis

Taking a good history is the start to every diagnosis and may be the only information available for the diagnosis of many. The history for a diagnosis of trigeminal neuralgia or cluster headache is unique, and there are no abnormal findings on examination or investigation. On the other hand, persistent idiopathic facial pain does not have a unique history and so a focused examination and, if necessary, investigations (both of which should be normal) are needed for the diagnosis. Sometimes the physical signs may be diagnostic, for example, bilateral parotid swelling in mumps, or the typical rash of herpes zoster. Investigations can be helpful in excluding diagnoses; for example, clear sinuses on X-ray or CT examination exclude sinusitis as a cause of pain. but may be misleading (e.g. a CT scan showing marked sinus disease does not necessarily explain the cause of pain).

Deciding whether the pain is due to focal pathology is essential and dictates the referral pathway.

Demographics

Dental problems may occur at any age. Persistent idiopathic facial pain is a condition of middle-aged women. Cluster headache is predominantly a condition of males, with peak age of onset in the 20s and 30s. Trigeminal neuralgia is typically a condition of the elderly and, if it occurs in young people, consider an underlying cause (e.g. demyelination at the trigeminal nerve root entry zone). Teeth grinding as a cause of jaw pain is more common in anxious people. Shingles and post-herpetic neuralgia are more common in the elderly. Sometimes it relates to immunosuppression. A history of Paget's disease or myeloma may make you consider bone pathology as a cause of pain. Mumps may occur for the first time in adults. Sarcoidosis is associated with parotid disease. Polymyalgia rheumatica overlaps with temporal arteritis. Systemic conditions may be relevant to the diagnosis of the facial pain.

Specific clues to the diagnosis

Specific clues to the diagnosis are nearly always in the history:

Severity: Severity of pain can be difficult to judge but trigeminal neuralgia, cluster headache, and dental abscess pain is severe. The first two conditions, very treatable if not curable, do not respond to analgesics. Persistent idiopathic facial pain and tension-type headache (which may be behind the eyes or across the nose rather than more typically a headache) are mild but persistent pains and do not respond well to over-the-counter analgesics.

Duration: The duration of the pain is often the key to the diagnosis. Trigeminal neuralgia is a brief shooting but repetitive pain, with each paroxysm lasting 1–4 seconds. Short-lasting neuralgiform headache with conjunctival injection and tearing (SUNCT) paroxysms are 5–250 seconds long. Cluster headache is 15–180 minutes long. Sometimes, particularly when trigeminal neuralgia is very active, a constant similarly localized facial pain may also occur due to a trigeminal nerve 'wind-up' phenomenon. This can also occur in very active cluster headache. Facial migraine is not common, considering how common migraine is in the population; the pain is, by diagnostic criteria, 4–72 hours in duration. Idiopathic facial pain is constant or near-constant.

Pain frequency: Trigeminal neuralgia may relapse and remit with varying frequency. During cluster headache bouts, pain attacks can occur up to eight times a day (often at night).

Triggering: Triggering (e.g. touching the face/talking, in trigeminal neuralgia; chewing, as in temporomandibular joint dysfunction; or jaw pain on chewing (claudication) in temporal arteritis) may be a characteristic feature. In cluster headache, alcohol may be a trigger, in up to 50% of sufferers, but only during the cluster bout. Pain onset is generally abrupt. In facial migraine, some link to stress or hormonal factors may be seen and, typically, migraine pain builds up slowly to peak severity in 30–60 minutes.

Periodicity of the pain: Trigeminal neuralgia may remit and relapse, whereas episodic cluster headache has typical periodicity (e.g. pain recurs frequently often at night over several weeks or months then remits for a year or so). It may be seasonally linked. Morning jaw pain may be from teeth grinding at night and be relieved by a tooth guard.

Unilaterality of the pain: Some conditions are strictly unilateral; for example, bilateral trigeminal neuralgia is very rare and suggests serious intracranial disease; cluster headache is always unilateral, although it may change sides between attacks. Some conditions are often unilateral but not uncommonly may be bilateral (e.g. idiopathic facial pain). Cervicogenic headache is a term used to describe pain which is felt on the head or face but which is due to pathology in the (usually upper) cervical spine. Its existence is not disputed but its frequency, characteristics, and treatment remain controversial—at least amongst neurologists. It is often a unilateral persistent pain.

Site of pain: The site of pain is important. Trigeminal neuralgia is nearly always in Divisions 2 or 3 of the trigeminal nerve. If a pain with similar characteristics is around the eye, and associated with marked tearing, consider SUNCT. Cluster headache is usually centred around one eye but may occur in the jaw (so-called lower-half headache) and it may spread even to the neck and shoulder. Pain over the nose, particularly if worsened by wearing glasses, is often tension-type headache.

Associated features: Associated features—depression in idiopathic facial pain; redness; watering/running of the ipsilateral eye and/ or nostril during a cluster headache attack— can be revealing. However, they may potentially mislead (e.g. nasal discharge ipsilateral to cluster headache versus sinus disease).

Key diagnostic tests

Tests are done to try and confirm or rule out a diagnosis of structural disease as a cause of pain. Some are not completely accurate and may have to be repeated; for example, early in temporal arteritis, the erythrocyte sedimentation rate may be normal. Many conditions have no diagnostic tests (e.g. trigeminal neuralgia, cluster headache, migraine). MRI is usually the imaging modality of choice but bone is not well seen on MRI. For suspected sinusitis, sinus X-ray or CT scanning can help. Dental X-rays may be important.

Introduction to therapy

The diagnosis leads to prognosis and treatment. Ideally, the cause of the problem should be treated (e.g. use steroids for temporal arteritis, and antibiotics for a dental abscess). Sometimes the cause is never found or the diagnosis rests largely on tests having excluded a cause (e.g. idiopathic facial pain). Sometimes there is a cause, for example, an aberrant artery causing trigeminal neuralgia, but it may not be best to start off by treating it. If there is no specific therapy, then symptomatic therapy, doing nothing, or learning to cope with the condition are the only alternatives.

Prognosis

The prognosis depends on the diagnosis. Even if there is no cure for the problem, telling patients what they have got and giving them a good understanding of the condition is key to successful management. Cure may not be a realistic goal for neurological causes of facial pain such as cluster headache and trigeminal neuralgia but there are many treatment options, and such patients should be managed by specialists in that area.

How to handle uncertainty in the diagnosis

As with headache management, ruling out serious pathology (and convincing the patient that it has been done) is the first step. Uncertainty at this stage should lead to investigation or referral onwards. A good knowledge of the benign conditions (the majority of causes of facial pain) and a clear history from the patient is needed for a certain diagnosis (e.g. trigeminal neuralgia and cluster headache). Sometimes poor historians need to be instructed on keeping a diary of symptoms, and then a timely review may reveal the diagnosis. Sometimes asking patients to read up about the suspected diagnosis can be helpful (e.g. a suspected cluster headache sufferer may read accounts of that condition on the cluster headache UK charity website (http://ouchuk.org/home). Basing a diagnosis on a trial of treatment is potentially misleading and can be dangerous. A good response to steroids can occur in temporal arteritis as well as facial pain due to cervical spondylosis. However, a lack of response to subcutaneous sumatriptan should lead to a reappraisal of the diagnosis of cluster headache.

Sometimes it is the patient who is uncertain of the diagnosis. Problems with management arise particularly when patients are not convinced of the benign nature of their condition and when 'the cause' has not been demonstrated to their satisfaction. This can be particularly true for patients with idiopathic facial pain.

Persistent idiopathic facial pain (atypical facial pain) is associated with psychiatric morbidity. As with trigeminal neuralgia-like symptoms, it can be associated with previous dental procedures. Sometimes it is hard to know which came first.

Further Reading

Siccoli MM, Bassetti CL, and Sándor PS. Facial pain: Clinical differential diagnosis *Lancet Neurol* 2006; 3: 257–67.
Zakrzewska JM and Linskey ME. Trigeminal neuralgia. *BMJ* 2014; 348: g474.

53 Dizziness

Linda Luxon and Louisa Murdin

Definition of the symptom

'Dizziness' as defined by the Barany Society refers to a sensation of disturbed or impaired spatial orientation without a false or distorted sense of motion. It is distinguished from vertigo, which is the sensation of self-motion when no self-motion is occurring or the sensation of distorted self-motion during an otherwise normal head movement. However, patients using this term may be referring to many different sensations. Its inherent subjectivity can make it hard for sufferers to describe their experience and for clinicians to translate the history into a differential diagnosis. A systematic approach is therefore required, and patients complaining of dizziness should be strongly encouraged to describe the sensation further.

Table 53.1 shows the causes of dizziness encountered in secondary care, although the ranking will vary according to the age of the patient.

Context

Dizziness is one of the commonest presenting symptoms in primary care; 5 in 1000 per year visit their GP for symptoms classified as 'vertigo', and 10 in 1000 per year visit their GP for dizziness or giddiness, according to statistics from The Royal College of General Practitioners/Office for National Statistics. It is a major cause of chronic ill health, with an associated reduction in quality of life. There are major economic and social implications associated with dizziness, since it is a frequent cause of inability to work and attendant social benefits claims.

Approach to diagnosis

The most valuable part of the assessment is the history. First, the symptom itself needs clarification: is the patient describing vertigo, light-headedness, disorientation, or something else? Vertigo is suggestive of an audiovestibular disorder, whereas a cardiac cause of dizziness is more likely to be experienced as light-headedness. Patients may experience many types of dizziness, and each should be characterized. It is crucial to clarify the time course of the symptom. Is this a single acute presentation, a recurrent episodic disorder, a continuous symptom, or some combination of these? The onset of the disorder, associated symptoms, and triggering/relieving factors should also be recorded.

Physical examination should begin with a careful assessment of blood pressure, especially in the elderly, in whom postural hypotension, often secondary to antihypertensive drugs, is a common cause

of dizziness. To maximize sensitivity, patients should lie down for at least 10 minutes before the first reading is made. Blood pressure should then be recorded immediately on standing and then again after 3 minutes of standing. Neuro-otological examination comprises examination of the external ear and otoscopy; eye movement examination assessing horizontal and vertical gaze, smooth pursuit, saccades, and characterization of nystagmus; a head-thrust test (see 'Specific clues to the diagnosis'); a Romberg test; gait assessment; and positional testing. One commonly used positional test is the Dix–Hallpike manoeuvre. In this test, the patient starts in a sitting position with legs extended along the couch. The head is turned 45° towards the side to be tested. The patient is then moved quickly to a supine position, and any resulting nystagmus is observed. The patient is then restored to a sitting position, with any further nystagmus noted. This manoeuvre is used to diagnose benign paroxysmal positional vertigo (BPPV). The nystagmus of the commonest type of BPPV (canalolithiasis of the posterior canal) is torsional and geotropic (upper pole of the eye beating towards the ground) with a latency of a few seconds. It fatigues (lessens in intensity with repeated manoeuvres) and can reverse on assumption of the seated posture. Other types of positional nystagmus are less common, and are seen in BPPV of the horizontal or anterior canals, vestibular migraine, and central vestibular disorders.

Specific clues to the diagnosis

Associated symptoms are frequently useful in pinpointing the diagnosis, and should be specifically sought. Hearing loss, tinnitus, and aural fullness are all suggestive of an otological disorder. Migrainous headache, phono- and photophobia, motion sickness, childhood episodes of dizziness/vomiting, and a family history may point towards vestibular migraine, one of the commonest causes of recurrent episodic vertigo. Cerebellar signs and symptoms such as intention tremor, dysarthria, past-pointing, saccadic hypermetria, broken smooth pursuit, and central-type nystagmus (e.g. bidirectional or vertical nystagmus) are helpful in localizing the problem to the CNS and will require further investigation.

The head-thrust test is a particularly useful test, both in the acute care and outpatient settings. This test involves asking the patient to fixate on a target, such as the bridge of the examiner's nose, while a passive high-velocity rotation of the head is made in the horizontal plane. If the vestibulo-ocular reflex is intact, the patient will be able to maintain visual fixation during these movements. If the vestibulo-ocular reflex is disrupted, as by a peripheral vestibular lesion, then the patient will be unable to maintain fixation. The examiner will then see

Table 53.1 Causes of dizziness encountered in secondary care		
Common	**Uncommon**	**Rare**
Vestibular neuritis/labyrinthitis	Ménière's disease	Tumour
Drugs	Bilateral vestibular failure	Foramen magnum compression (e.g. Arnold–Chiari malformation)
Psychological disorder (e.g. panic disorder)	Post-traumatic vertigo	Neurovascular compression
Cardiac arrhythmia/valvular disease/outflow obstruction/carotid sinus disease	Multiple sclerosis	Autoimmune inner ear disease (systemic or localized)
Postural hypotension	Posterior circulation vascular disease	Superior semicircular canal dehiscence
Benign paroxysmal positional vertigo	Haematological: anaemia, hyperviscosity	Genetic disorders (e.g. episodic ataxias)
Vestibular migraine	Metabolic: hypoglycaemia	Vestibular paroxysmia

a 'catch-up' saccade in the contralateral direction when the head is rotated towards the lesion.

One rare but distinctive presentation is that of dizziness triggered by loud sounds or increases in intracranial pressure, the so-called Tullio phenomenon, which can be caused by superior semicircular canal dehiscence.

Key diagnostic tests

The correct diagnostic test will depend on the information provided by the history and examination. Blood tests can diagnose anaemia, hypoglycaemia, and inflammatory or autoimmune disorders. If a cardiac cause is suspected, then ambulatory ECG recording and echocardiography may be required. For neurological disorders, imaging is usually required, and frequently MRI scanning. Magnetic resonance angiography can also be helpful in cases where vascular disease is suspected.

In suspected vestibular disorders, caloric testing is the cornerstone of diagnosis. Water is irrigated sequentially into each external ear canal at 30°C and 44°C, and the vestibular response (duration or maximum slow phase velocity of the induced nystagmus) is recorded. The information obtained can be used to identify and lateralize a peripheral vestibular disorder. Pure tone audiometry can also be used to characterize a hearing loss such as the low-frequency hearing loss of Ménière's disease and identify more subtle subclinical deficits.

Other diagnostic tests

Specialist neuro-otological centres can further characterize vestibular disorders with techniques such as eye movement recordings, video head impulse testing, rotating chairs, vestibular evoked myogenic potentials, and platform posturography. Tilt-table and other autonomic function testing can be helpful where autonomic neuropathies are suspected.

Introduction to therapy

Therapy will be guided by an appropriate diagnosis.

In **acute peripheral vestibular pathology** (e.g. vestibular neuritis/labyrinthitis), the experience of severe dizziness *per se* can be extremely frightening and distressing for patients. In many cases, patients who can be reassured that there is no sinister pathology will experience a reduction in symptom intensity. Vestibular suppressant drugs (e.g. cinnarizine, cyclizine) and anti-emetics (e.g. prochlorperazine) are frequently used in the acute phases of an illness to alleviate symptoms. However, studies on animals have suggested that prolonged use of these medications can slow down recovery that occurs through cerebral compensation for a peripheral deficit. Most experts would therefore recommend that use of these medications is strictly limited to management of acute symptoms only, aiming for a maximum period of use of 1 week.

For **BPPV**, particle-repositioning manoeuvres are an extremely satisfying (for both patient and clinician) and effective treatment. Such patients should **not** be treated with medication. The Epley and modified Semont manoeuvres are both in common use in clinical practice for the treatment of posterior canal disease.

For **vestibular migraine**, acute and prophylactic medications can be used, and principles are similar to those used in other kinds of migraine. Careful consideration needs to be given to the timing of vestibular rehabilitation therapy in patients with migraine since frequent headaches can interfere with recovery and with adherence to exercise programmes.

For **Ménière's disease**, treatment in the acute phase comprises vestibular suppressants and anti-emetics, frequently by absorption through the buccal membrane. Betahistine is sometimes used, but convincing evidence either for or against its efficacy is lacking. Many experts recommend a low-salt diet and/or diuretics such as bendroflumethazide, but, again, the evidence base is currently weak. Trials of intra-tympanic medications such as gentamicin or dexamethasone are underway. Preliminary results suggest some benefit, but with an attendant risk of adverse effects such as infection, perforation of the tympanic membrane, and hearing loss.

It is also known that, for peripheral vestibular disorders, physical activity is important in recovery, and patients should be encouraged to mobilize as soon as is practical. Customized vestibular rehabilitation programmes supervised by an appropriately trained therapist have been shown to be beneficial, with maximum benefit sustained when the programme is begun early.

Patients with chronic dizziness can frequently develop secondary psychological symptoms and disorders, especially related to anxiety, panic, agoraphobia, and depression. For successful recovery from a vestibular disorder, it is essential that such disorders are acknowledged and addressed appropriately, either through medication or through psychotherapy such as cognitive behavioural therapy.

Prognosis

The prognosis depends greatly on the underlying cause, ranging from the self-limiting or eminently treatable (e.g. BPPV) to conditions which can cause progressive problems over many years (e.g. Ménière's) to the acute and life-threatening (cerebellar haemorrhage). For vestibular disorders, prognosis in general is better when conditions are identified and treated early, before the development of maladaptive physical or psychological responses.

How to handle uncertainty in the diagnosis of this symptom

One of the principle aims of assessment is to identify the minority of patients presenting with dizziness or vertigo, who have a potentially serious or life-threatening condition such as cerebellar haemorrhage or posterior fossa tumour. Careful examination for cardiac abnormalities, central neurological signs, and, where appropriate, imaging can render such conditions highly unlikely. Once such conditions have been excluded, patients may be treated expectantly, with regular reviews, to identify new diagnostic features which may become apparent during the natural history of the disorder, such as the hearing loss of Ménière's disease or the headache of migraine. Patients with chronic subjective dizziness, and no physical disorder identified after appropriate assessment, can be managed with a combination of physical and psychological therapy to address activity levels and maladaptive behaviours. Selective serotonin reuptake inhibitors appear to be helpful in some cases.

Further Reading

Bronstein, A. (ed.). *The Oxford Textbook of Vertigo and Imbalance*, 2013. Oxford University Press.

Luxon LM. 'Vertigo and imbalance', in Donaghy M, ed., *Brain's Diseases of the Nervous System* (12th edition), 2010. Oxford University Press.

54 Disorders of sleep

Sophie West

Definition of the symptom

Typically, disorders of sleep cause disturbance either to the sufferer or to their bed partner. If total sleep time is reduced, this may lead to problems with excessive daytime sleepiness, which can affect work, driving, concentration, and relationships. 'Sleepiness' implies an intrusive desire to fall asleep, caused by some form of sleep deprivation or sedative drugs; this is different from 'tiredness', which implies general fatigue, lethargy, and exhaustion and which is caused by a range of conditions, including depression, chronic disease, or a busy lifestyle.

Adults sleep on average for 8 hours per night. Normal sleep consists of periods of deep or slow-wave sleep, interspersed with shorter periods of dreaming or rapid-eye-movement (REM) sleep. Periods of REM sleep lengthen towards the morning and hence some people remember their dreams on waking. Different disorders of sleep can affect any of these sleep stages.

Differential diagnosis

Snoring is very common and many people seek help from primary care. It is important to determine if there is any suspicion of obstructive sleep apnoea (OSA). So called simple snorers are those with intrusive snoring, but no suggestion of OSA. Much less commonly, narcolepsy or parasomnias (sleep disorders associated with abnormal behaviours, such as sleep walking) occur. Conditions in which the day–night cycle is disturbed include phase shift disorder, shift work disorder, and circadian rhythm disorder.

Context

Sleep disorders are common but in most people are transient (e.g. sleep disorders related to jet lag, shift work, or stress). Attention to good sleep patterns (or 'sleep hygiene') minimizes sleep problems for most people. Good sleep hygiene includes a regular bedtime; regular wake time; minimal caffeine, nicotine, and alcohol consumption, particularly in the evening; a bedtime wind-down routine; avoidance of stimulatory 'blue-light' activities at bedtime, such as use of the television, computer, or mobile telephone; and avoidance of daytime naps in order to promote sleep at bedtime.

Approach to diagnosis

A careful sleep history, including details of snoring, witnessed apnoeas, sleep patterns, restless legs, night-time behaviour, and a quantification of daytime sleepiness will usually give clear pointers to the diagnosis. It is not uncommon for people who are seen in specialist sleep clinics for suspicion of a sleep disorder to have fundamental sleep hygiene issues causing their problems. Dealing effectively with these can be invaluable.

Daytime sleepiness can subjectively be given a value using a tool such as the Epworth sleepiness score, an 8-point questionnaire referring to a person's current way of life, in which they ascribe a score to how likely they are to doze off in certain situations.

Specific clues to the diagnosis

OSA: The patient complains of unrefreshing sleep, daytime sleepiness, and possibly a sensation of choking at night. The bed partner complains of loud snoring, witnessed apnoeas, and restless sleep. There is a strong association with obesity, and a collar size of greater than 17 inches. Symptoms worsen with weight gain. Sleep studies show repeated episodes of apnoea, and oxygen desaturation, terminated by an arousal or awakening, occurring possibly hundreds of times a night.

Central sleep apnoea: This is also known as Cheyne–Stokes respiration, or periodic breathing. There is reduced ventilation during sleep, without evidence of upper airway obstruction, as well as absence of respiratory effort, and apnoeas. It is much less common than OSA. The bed partner may complain of witnessed apnoeas.

Restless legs syndrome: This encompasses a range of sensory symptoms affecting the legs (or, less commonly, the arms) and which are characteristically uncomfortable, creating an overwhelming urge to move the limbs. Movement relieves the sensation, as long as the movement continues. Symptoms are worse at rest and in the evening and night. Can occur at any age; symptoms are mild at first but progress with age. Restless legs may be primary (either idiopathic or familial (with positive family history in 60%–90%)) or secondary (occurring during pregnancy; due to iron-deficiency anaemia, end-stage renal disease, or peripheral neuropathy). The pathophysiology is not completely understood; it is predominantly a CNS disorder, with dopaminergic dysfunction in subcortical systems. Patients have a reduced concentration of ferritin and increased transferrin in their CNS, despite normal serum ferritin levels. Diagnosis is clinical. Neurological examination and neurophysiological tests are normal (including EMG and nerve conduction studies); these are not usually required for diagnosis.

Periodic leg movements during sleep: Periodic leg movements during sleep (PLMS) occur in 80%–90% of restless leg sufferers. Polysomnography using anterior tibial electrodes demonstrates involuntary repetitive movements—stereotypical flexor withdrawal reflex movements of the limbs, lasting up to 5 seconds and occurring every 5–90 seconds. Approximately one-third of these movements are associated with a cortical arousal, and thus interrupted sleep and daytime sleepiness can occur. The partner's sleep is often affected by the recurrent limb movements.

Narcolepsy: This is severe irresistible daytime sleepiness and cataplexy, a sudden loss of muscle tone triggered by strong emotions such as laughter or anger. It typically affects face muscles, head control, and knees. Sleep paralysis, hypnagogic and hypnopompic hallucinations, vivid dream recall, and difficulty differentiating dreams from reality may also occur. Short naps are refreshing. It typically presents in adolescence or early adulthood with excessive daytime sleepiness. It may not be recognized or diagnosed for years. It is caused by deficient hypocretin (or orexin) secretion from the hypothalamus. The DQB1 0602 allele predisposes towards narcolepsy and is identified in 85%–90% of narcolepsy patients. Diagnosis is with polysomnography, primarily to exclude other sleep disorders, and multiple sleep latency testing, which typically shows sleep-onset REM within 15 minutes. Low hypocretin levels are found in the CSF, although lumbar puncture not usually necessary in patients with clear history of cataplexy.

Idiopathic hypersomnia: This is persistent daytime sleepiness despite adequate sleep. Affected individuals sleep for longer than 11–12 hours on 24-hour sleep monitoring. They also take long naps of 1–2 hours, which are typically unrefreshing. The cause of idiopathic hypersomnia is unclear. Polysomnography is normal.

REM behaviour disorder: This is one of the parasomnias. Loss of normal muscle atonia during REM sleep leads to dream-enacting behaviours, which are often violent, with shouting, or the bed partner being hit. Typically occurs in over-50s, but can occur after treatments with tricyclic antidepressants, fluoxetine, or monoamine oxidase inhibitors, and after alcohol withdrawal. Polysomnography is not essential to make the diagnosis, but loss of muscle atonia during REM is noted. This disorder maybe a precursor to Parkinson's disease. Treatment is with clonazepam at bedtime. Tolerance can develop, and intermittent drug holidays are advised.

Sleepwalking: This is common in young children, and occurs in 3%–4% adults. It is a so-called arousal disorder, with incomplete waking. It occurs during slow-wave sleep. There is limited emotional or autonomic activation, but motor activity, which ranges from sitting in bed fiddling with covers to walking downstairs and opening the front door, is observed. Treat with good sleep routines, safety measures (door lock, stair gate, etc.), and nocturnal sedation, if required.

Circadian rhythm sleep disorders: These include jet lag, shift work sleep disorder, and delayed sleep phase syndrome.

Key diagnostic tests

It may be appropriate to perform an overnight sleep study to clarify events. A variety of studies can be performed, such as polysomnography, with full sleep staging via EEG; limited sleep study, predominantly looking at respiratory and cardiovascular signals; actigraphic monitoring, using small devices to determine periods of activity and rest, showing circadian rhythms, and screen for restless legs. Sleep diaries can be helpful to determine the exact day/night pattern a patient has and how much sleep they are getting. Usually, referral to a physician with an interest in sleep disorders (usually in respiratory medicine or neurology) is appropriate to arrange diagnostic tests.

Other diagnostic tests

These depend on the likely sleep disorder. It is important to exclude hypothyroidism in those patients suspected of having OSA or daytime sleepiness. As there is a strong correlation of OSA with obesity and type 2 diabetes, it is sensible to check blood glucose also. In restless legs, check ferritin levels.

Introduction to therapy

For symptomatic OSA, continuous positive airway pressure is the mainstay of treatment. The positive pressure applied acts as a 'splint' to the upper airway, preventing upper airway obstruction, apnoeas, and hence awakenings. Sleep is improved and daytime sleepiness is resolved. Patients should inform the DVLA of the diagnosis. A mandibular advancement device may be appropriate for those with mild OSA or simple snorers.

In restless legs and PLMS, patients should strive for good sleep hygiene and avoid aggravating factors such as sleep deprivation and standing or sitting for prolonged periods. Diuretics, antidepressants (especially tricyclics), calcium channel antagonists, phenytoin, and anti-emetics can aggravate symptoms. Iron replacement should occur if levels are low or low normal. Drug treatment may be required if simple measures have not helped and/or sleep is being disturbed. The dopamine agonists pramipexole, ropinirole, and transdermal rotigotine are used first line. Second-line treatments include levodopa, gabapentin, carbamazepine (particularly if pain is a feature), clonazepam, and opiates.

In narcolepsy, the first-line treatment is modafinil, a long-acting wake-promoting drug. Second-line drugs include methylphenidate and amphetamines. Specific treatment for cataplexy may be required if this is particularly problematic, usually with non-sedating antidepressants. Regular sleep–wake cycles are encouraged, with attention to standard sleep hygiene issues. Patients should inform the DVLA of the diagnosis.

Prognosis

Sleep disorders are not usually life limiting, but predominantly cause morbidity due to daytime sleepiness. Appropriate treatment can resolve this, but accurate and correct diagnosis is essential. Treatment which does not resolve symptoms should prompt further investigation, as two sleep disorders with different etiologies, such as narcolepsy and OSA, can often coexist.

How to handle uncertainty in the diagnosis of this symptom

If the diagnosis is not clear, involving a sleep specialist can be helpful. While a person has daytime sleepiness, either due to an uncertain diagnosis or prior to effective treatment, they should not drive, to protect both themselves and other road users. Driving is permitted when satisfactory control of symptoms is achieved.

Further Reading

American Academy of Sleep Medicine. *International Classification of Sleep Disorders* (3rd edition), 2014. American Academy of Sleep Medicine.

Greenstone M and Hack M. Obstructive sleep apnoea. *BMJ* 2014; 348: g3745.

Scammell TE. Narcolepsy. *N Engl J Med* 2015; 373: 2654–62.

55 Haematuria

Aron Chakera, William G. Herrington, and Christopher A. O'Callaghan

Definition of the symptom

Haematuria is the presence of blood in the urine. Haematuria may be either macroscopic (frank or visible haematuria) or detectable only on urine dipstick (microscopic or non-visible haematuria).

Differential diagnosis

See Table 55.1 for the differential diagnosis of haematuria in primary and secondary care.

Context

Frank haematuria can appear quite dramatic and usually leads patients in the community to seek medical attention. The high incidence of urinary tract infections as an underlying cause means that patients often have associated dysuria and frequency. Significant haematuria can lead to clot formation in the urinary tract and obstruction. The resulting symptoms are equivalent to those from obstruction due to stones (see Chapter 166). Microscopic haematuria is usually noted as an incidental finding.

Approach to diagnosis

Frank haematuria always requires further investigation usually necessitating fast-track referral to the urology department to exclude underlying malignant disease (unless a secondary cause is obvious). Usual initial investigations include a CT urogram and flexible cystoscopy.

Patients with microscopic haematuria should be questioned to determine whether it is a new finding (e.g. the persistent benign haematuria of thin basement membrane disease), and whether there is a family history of haematuria. A full urological and gynaecological history should be taken and any recent renal trauma noted. Examination should include inspection for evidence of bleeding elsewhere, (which may be consistent with over-anticoagulation or other bleeding diathesis), and palpation for renal masses or an enlarged prostate. Patients

older than 40 are usually referred to the urology service in most centres to exclude malignancy (as for macroscopic haematuria).

A dipstick should always be performed with both micro- and macroscopic haematuria. Haematuria with positive leukocytes and nitrites is consistent with a urinary tract infection. Urine microscopy may reveal dysmorphic red blood cells with glomerular bleeding. The presence of coexisting proteinuria occurs with glomerulonephritis. In acute cases, red blood cell casts may be present (see Chapter 157, Figure 157.1(b)). Serial urine collections for cytology should be performed where there is a high index of suspicion of urothelial malignancy.

Blood tests to document renal function and clotting parameters should be done routinely and, if bleeding is heavy, blood should be grouped and saved.

Specific clues to the diagnosis

Long-standing microscopic haematuria, associated with raised serum IgA levels and episodes of frank haematuria with upper respiratory tract infections, is characteristic of IgA nephropathy (see Chapter 159). Thin basement membrane disease is often familial, and is associated with persistent (usually microscopic) haematuria, and normal renal function. A family history of deafness and progressive renal impairment suggests Alport's syndrome. The presence of loin pain or a renal angle mass should raise the suspicion of renal cell cancer. Metastatic disease primarily occurs in the liver and lungs, and can lead to shortness of breath or jaundice.

Severe colicky loin pain radiating towards the groin is a feature of ureteric obstruction, which may be related to stone disease (see Chapter 166), or a clot obstructing the ureter. Infections invariably result in irritative symptoms with frequency and urgency.

Key diagnostic tests

A urine dipstick is essential to confirm the presence of blood in the urine and whether there is any protein, or evidence of infection.

A coagulation profile should be requested if a bleeding diathesis is suspected and the renal function should normally be determined.

Investigations for urinary tract malignancy include a CT urogram and cystoscopy.

Immunological tests are indicated if a glomerulonephritis seems likely, and a renal biopsy may be performed in these cases.

Conditions mistaken for haematuria/other causes of dark urine include:

- myoglobinuria
- porphyria
- medications that discolour urine (e.g. rifampicin)
- heavy beetroot consumption (discolours urine)

Other diagnostic tests

Urine microscopy may help determine the source of bleeding (dysmorphic red cells from the glomerulus). Urine cytology can be performed if urothelial malignancy is suspected.

Introduction to therapy

The management of haematuria is entirely dependent on cause. Malignant diseases of the renal tract are usually treated with surgery and/or chemotherapy, depending on the stage and the patient's functional status. Benign causes of haematuria (e.g. thin basement membrane disease) require reassurance only. However, as most patients

Table 55.1 A side-by-side comparison outlining the differential diagnosis in primary care and secondary care, ordered by probability

Primary care	Secondary care
Macroscopic	Macroscopic
Infection	Post-instrumentation, e.g. catheterization
Stone	Post-biopsy
Anticoagulation	Anticoagulation
Cysts	Post-surgery
Tumours	
Microscopic	Microscopic
IgA nephropathy	Glomerulonephritis
Thin basement membrane disease or Alport's syndrome	(Exclude myoglobinuria)
Infection	
Benign prostatic hypertrophy	
Glomerulonephritis	
Stone	
Tumour	
(Exclude menstrual bleeding)	

receive a clinical diagnosis without proceeding to renal biopsy (as the risks of biopsy are thought to outweigh the benefits of a definitive diagnosis), it is prudent to monitor renal function over time. Renal tract infections or stones should be treated as discussed in Chapters 158 and 166, respectively.

Prognosis

Uncomplicated stones or infections generally have a good prognosis, although patients may suffer from repeated attacks. Renal cell cancers confined to the kidney and completely excised also carry a good prognosis. Microscopic haematuria in association with thin basement membrane disease is a benign condition. However, IgA nephropathy, the major differential diagnosis for thin basement membrane disease, causes progression to end-stage renal disease in up to 40% of patients.

How to handle uncertainty in the diagnosis of this symptom

The major area of uncertainty is the need for urological investigation in younger patients presenting with microscopic haematuria.

In this group, the risk of underlying malignancy is low and the tests are invasive (cystoscopy) and require exposure to ionizing radiation. Decisions should be made on an individual basis.

Further Reading

Margulis V and Sagalowsky AI. Assessment of hematuria. *Med Clin N Am* 2011; 95: 153–9.

National Institute for Health and Care Excellence (NICE). Suspected cancer: recognition and referral. NICE guideline [NG12]. 2015. Last updated: July 2017. https://www.nice.org.uk/guidance/NG12/chapter/1-Recommendations-organised-by-site-of-cancer#urological-cancers.

Wyatt RJ and Julian BA. IgA nephropathy. *N Engl J Med* 2013; 368: 2402–14.

56 Oliguria and anuria

Aron Chakera, William G. Herrington, and Christopher A. O'Callaghan

Definition of the symptom

Oliguria is defined as a urine output of less than 400 ml in 24 hours, and is a marker of kidney injury (see KDIGO classification of acute kidney injury in adults in Chapter 162, Table 162.1). Anuria is the complete absence of urine production. Some sources consider a serum creatinine that increases by 100 µmol/l day^{-1} to represent an 'anuric rate of rise', a rise consistent with the absence of any meaningful renal function. Normal urine production is approximately 0.5 ml/kg h^{-1}.

Differential diagnosis in primary care and secondary care

Oliguria can be caused by any factor that affects renal function, or the free passage of urine down the urinary tract. Complete anuria most commonly occurs in men as a consequence of bladder outlet obstruction from an enlarged prostate. It can also arise in patients who have a single functioning kidney which then becomes obstructed or loses its vascular supply. Other causes of complete anuria to be considered are:

- anti-glomerular basement membrane (GBM) disease (Goodpasture's)
- bilateral renal vascular occlusion/aortic occlusion
- massive rhabdomyolysis

See Table 56.1 for a side-by-side comparison outlining the differential diagnosis in primary care and secondary care, ordered by probability.

Context

Oliguria occurs commonly in hospitalized patients, is usually secondary to impaired renal perfusion, and is often predictable. The elderly and more unwell patients, for example, those in critical care settings, are most at risk. The presence of oliguria tends to reflect the severity of the underlying disease processes. The commonest cause of complete anuria is bladder outflow obstruction from an enlarged prostate. This may be precipitated by prostatitis or constipation in a

patient with benign prostatic hypertrophy. In catheterized patients, a blocked catheter must be excluded.

Approach to diagnosis

The causes of oliguria can be considered anatomically, and divided into prerenal, renal (intrinsic), or post-renal etiologies. Obstructive causes should be excluded early, and the history should focus on symptoms suggesting prostatic disease or bladder or bowel dysfunction. In women, a gynaecological history should be taken. A detailed list of all current medications should be sought, including over the counter preparations, asking specifically about NSAIDs. In hospitalized patients, fluid balance, operative notes, and anaesthetic notes should be reviewed, blood pressure recordings checked for episodes of hypotension, and current medications documented. Examination should include an accurate assessment of intravascular fluid balance, focusing on capillary refill, pulse, blood pressure (both supine and standing, if possible), jugular venous pressure, and any evidence of pulmonary oedema. The presence of peripheral oedema does not correlate well with intravascular fluid status. The abdomen should be palpated to exclude an enlarged bladder, and the kidneys balloted. Enlarged kidneys, for example, secondary to hydronephrosis, will sometimes be palpable. If there is a urinary catheter in situ, it should be flushed if there is any concern that it may be blocked. Investigations will be guided by the results of the history and examination, but will usually include a renal tract ultrasound, to exclude significant hydronephrosis or obstruction. For thin individuals, experienced ultrasonographers or radiologists can usually assess renal perfusion and flow characteristics within the renal artery and vein.

Specific clues to the diagnosis

A palpable bladder or distended bladder on ultrasound suggests an obstructive aetiology. The presence of a rash, neuropathy, or joint involvement, particularly if associated with active urinary sediment (e.g. blood and protein) or constitutional symptoms, may suggest an underlying immune aetiology. Documented hypotension, administration of IV contrast or treatment with NSAIDs, angiotensin-converting-enzyme inhibitors, or angiotensin II receptor blockers should raise suspicion of ischaemic renal injury. The passage of cola-coloured urine (associated with red-cell casts on microscopy), may indicated a rapidly progressive glomerulonephritis. There may be concurrent haemoptysis from pulmonary haemorrhage. Dipstick evidence of haematuria without the presence of red blood cells on microscopy may represent myoglobinuria; the serum creatinine kinase should be checked.

Key diagnostic tests

Key diagnostic tests include serial measures of renal function (urea and creatinine), including urgent assessment of potassium if acute renal failure is suspected. A dipstick urinalysis should always be performed, and the urine should be examined by microscopy and, if appropriate, sent for culture. A renal tract ultrasound will help exclude post-renal causes and can often provide information on renal perfusion.

Other diagnostic tests

If intrinsic renal disease is suspected, immunological tests should be requested (see Chapter 159) and a renal biopsy may be indicated. Complete anuria in the absence of post-renal obstruction requires

Table 56.1 A side-by-side comparison outlining the differential diagnosis in primary care and secondary care, ordered by probability

Primary care	Secondary care
Benign prostatic hypertrophy obstruction	Acute tubular necrosis
Drugs • NSAIDs • ACE-I/ARB	Hypotension (renal hypoperfusion) • Post-operative • Haemorrhage • Cardiac diseases • Sepsis
Dehydration • Gastroenteritis	Drugs • NSAIDs • ACE-I/ARB • Aminoglycosides • Chemotherapy agents • Contrast
Autoimmune diseases	Emboli

Abbreviations: ACE-I, angiotensin-converting-enzyme inhibitor; ARB, angiotensin II receptor blocker; NSAIDs, non-steroidal anti-inflammatory drugs.

urgent renal vascular imaging, a serum creatinine kinase test, and assessment for anti-GBM antibodies.

Introduction to therapy

As the presence of oliguria or anuria is a marker for significant renal disease, initial therapy should be directed at identifying and treating any life threats. Major problems include pulmonary oedema, hyperkalaemia, and metabolic acidosis. These should be treated as discussed in Chapters 139, 173, and 178, respectively.

Where patients are stable, close observation is indicated, with regular review of fluid balance, urine output, and renal function. Any potentially nephrotoxic medication should be stopped and the doses of other medications adjusted for the degree of renal impairment. The rate of change of renal function with time should be noted, and evidence of ongoing decline or of worsening clinical state should prompt referral to specialist renal services (or intensive care) for consideration of renal replacement therapy if indicated.

Prognosis

The development of oliguria or anuria is associated with increased morbidity and mortality. The vast majority of cases in hospital are secondary to inadequate renal perfusion, leading to acute tubular necrosis. If treated early, the prognosis in these cases may be good, but tends to depend on the severity of the underlying condition(s) leading to renal impairment. Oliguria secondary to obstruction recovers rapidly if the onset was acute. Chronic obstruction can result in permanent renal impairment. Details of outcomes from particular syndromes can be found in Part 6.

How to handle uncertainty in the diagnosis of this symptom

In many cases, the cause of oliguria is multifactorial. As post-renal causes can usually be readily excluded following examination and an ultrasound if needed, where diagnostic uncertainty persists, management should focus on optimizing renal perfusion and function. This includes avoiding nephrotoxins, preventing obstruction, and supporting renal perfusion, while seeking an underlying cause(s). Where investigations have been inconclusive, a renal biopsy may help establish a diagnosis.

Further Reading

Kidney Disease: Improving Global Outcomes (KDIGO) Acute Kidney Injury Work Group. KDIGO clinical practice guideline for acute kidney injury. *Kidney Inter Suppl* 2012; 2: 1–138.
National Institute for Health and Care Excellence. Acute kidney injury: prevention, detection and management. Clinical guideline [CG169]. 2013. https://www.nice.org.uk/guidance/cg169?unlid=429931086201692925215.

57 Polyuria

Aron Chakera, William G. Herrington, and Christopher A. O'Callaghan

Definition of the symptom

Polyuria describes the passage of more than 3 l of urine a day. This is an arbitrary definition, and the term is commonly applied to patients who are complaining of passing larger than normal volumes of urine. As water excretion is tightly regulated by the body to maintain normal osmolality, water excretion varies greatly depending on intake. Polyuria may be physiological or pathological.

Major causes of polyuria

The causes of polyuria can be divided into:

- excessive fluid intake (e.g. polydipsia)
- exposure to diuretic compounds (e.g. furosemide, hyperglycaemia, hypercalcaemia)
- failure of renal tubular water reabsorption (diabetes insipidus, chronic kidney disease, or recovering acute tubular necrosis)

Table 57.1 outlines the differential diagnosis of polyuria in primary and secondary care, ordered by probability.

Diabetes insipidus is a rare but important cause of polyuria as it is may be readily treatable. It results from a failure of vasopressin, also known as antidiuretic hormone (ADH), to regulate collecting duct water reabsorption. It can be caused by damage to the hypothalamus or pituitary gland (central diabetes insipidus) or resistance to its action (nephrogenic diabetes insipidus) (see Table 57.2.)

Context

A patient with polyuria often presents with nocturia, urination overnight that disturbs sleep. It is usually accompanied by polydipsia (to maintain normal fluid balance). In hospital the commonest causes of polyuria are diuretic therapy and recovery from an acute kidney injury (e.g. acute tubular necrosis or obstruction). This polyuric phase can result in an impressive diuresis (8–10 l/day) before tubular cells recover their ability to concentrate urine. During this period, patients are vulnerable to dehydration and may require intravenous fluid replacement. Following pituitary surgery, the urine output should be closely monitored for evidence of new diabetes insipidus.

Approach to diagnosis

Polyuria can be confirmed by collecting urine for 24 hours. In catheterized patients, a urine output that is persistently above 125 ml/h suggests polyuria.

Table 57.1 Major causes of polyuria

Primary care	Secondary care
Diuretic medications	Recovery from acute tubular necrosis
Compounds with diuretic effects, e.g. alcohol, tea, and coffee	Recovery from obstructive renal failure
Diabetes mellitus	Central diabetes insipidus, e.g. post neurosurgery or trauma
Chronic kidney disease	
Diabetes insipidus	Rare endocrine causes, e.g. Addison's disease
Psychogenic polydipsia	

Table 57.2 Causes of diabetes insipidus

Central diabetes insipidus	Nephrogenic diabetes insipidus
Pituitary surgery/trauma	Lithium
Pituitary infiltration (tumour/sarcoid)	Hypercalcaemia
	Hypokalaemia
Post-meningitis/encephalitis	Tubulointerstitial diseases
	Congenital

Specific clues to the diagnosis

The onset and severity of the polyuria may provide important clues to the diagnosis. Intermittent polyuria suggests an exogenous cause, and a careful drug and dietary history may uncover the causative agent. Transient polyuria also occurs with supraventricular tachyarrhythmias, and any history of palpitations should be noted. Diabetes mellitus should be considered in patients with a history of progressive polyuria with a prodrome of weight loss or recurrent infections (e.g. candidiasis or urinary tract infections).

Diabetes insipidus most commonly occurs following neurosurgical procedures involving or near to the pituitary gland. Central diabetes insipidus is usually characterized by a sudden onset.

Key diagnostic tests

If diabetes insipidus is suspected, blood and urinary osmolality are requested. Urine osmolality will be inappropriately dilute (<250 mOsm/l) despite a high blood osmolality. A water deprivation test will help differentiate diabetes insipidus from psychogenic polydipsia and central and nephrogenic diabetes insipidus (see Chapter 175). In psychogenic polydipsia, urine will become concentrated during water deprivation, whereas it will not with diabetes insipidus. Central diabetes insipidus responds to the administration of synthetic vasopressin (desmopressin), whereas nephrogenic diabetes insipidus does not.

Urinary frequency can be an indicator of polyuria. However, bladder irritation is a more common cause of urinary frequency and results in the passage of regular small volumes of urine that do not amount to 3 l a day. The commonest cause is a urinary tract infection (see Chapter 158).

Other diagnostic tests

Diabetes mellitus is confirmed by a random blood sugar above 11.1 mmol/l or a fasting plasma glucose above 7.0 mmol/l. Serum creatinine, electrolytes, and calcium measurement may be useful. Diabetes insipidus can cause hypernatraemia.

Addison's disease causes hyponatraemia and hyperkalaemia and, if suspected, early morning cortisol and short tetracosactide tests should be performed.

Introduction to therapy

Treatment of the underlying cause of polyuria may resolve the problem. Normoglycaemia will halt the diuresis in diabetes mellitus. Cranial diabetes insipidus may be effectively treated with intranasal synthetic vasopressin (desmopressin). Careful dosing is required to avoid overcorrection. Nephrogenic diabetes insipidus is more difficult to treat.

Prognosis

Polyuria does not carry a poor prognosis in itself. Most of the causes are treatable. In the case where treatment is limited, compensatory polydipsia can maintain normal fluid balance.

How to handle uncertainty in the diagnosis of this symptom

The diagnosis is usually straightforward. Diagnostic uncertainty may arise in patients with psychogenic polydipsia as it can mimic diabetes insipidus. The water deprivation test is helpful under these circumstances.

Further Reading

Jakes AD and Bhandari S. Investigating polyuria. *BMJ* 2013; 348: 34–9.
Robertson GL. Diabetes insipidus: Differential diagnosis and management. *Best Pract Res Clin Endocrinol Metab* 2016; 30: 205–18.

58 Dysuria

Jackie Sherrard and Graz Luzzi

Definition of the symptom

The term dysuria denotes painful urination, or disturbance of urination.

Differential diagnosis

In adults, the differential diagnosis differs to some extent between males and females, age of the patient and sexual behaviour (Table 58.1).

Context

Dysuria is most often caused by inflammation of the urethra. In males, the main differential diagnosis is between urinary tract infection (UTI) and sexually acquired urethritis.

Although UTI may be diagnosed in all age groups, the likelihood of UTI as the cause of dysuria increases with age and in sexually inactive men. Urethritis rarely causes urinary frequency, and so this associated symptom suggests UTI as the cause of dysuria. Dysuria associated with urethritis is often mild and may take the form of irritation or itching during urination; the exception is dysuria associated with herpes simplex virus (HSV) which may be very painful and can provoke urinary retention.

In females, dysuria is most commonly associated with UTI and much less commonly with sexually acquired urethritis. For anatomical reasons, vulvitis may be associated with dysuria because of involvement of the urethra in the inflammatory process.

Approach to diagnosis

Adult males

A thorough history should be taken, to include:

- duration and abruptness of onset (severe dysuria with abrupt onset is more suggestive of UTI than urethritis)
- associated symptoms, which are helpful in distinguishing between UTI and urethritis; associated frequency and haematuria are suggestive of UTI; associated urethral discharge is very suggestive of urethritis, although purulent urethral discharge is described in UTI caused by *E. coli*
- a full sexual history, covering at least the previous 3 months, including type of sexual intercourse (vaginal, oral, rectal) and use of condoms

A careful physical examination should be conducted, focusing on the genital area, lower abdomen, and inguinal regions.

- Urethritis is suggested by urethral meatal reddening (inflammation) and/or urethral discharge (gonorrhoeal urethritis is typically purulent; the discharge from urethritis caused by chlamydia or *Mycoplasma genitalium* is typically clear or turbid). UTI may be associated with bladder (suprapubic) or renal (loin) tenderness.
- Acute epididymitis typically causes unilateral, painful, tender swelling of the epididymis or testicle.
- Acute prostatitis typically presents with symptoms of UTI, pain of prostatic origin (penile tip and perineum), a swollen, tender prostate on rectal examination, and systemic symptoms (fever, malaise, sometimes rigors).

Adult females

A thorough history should be obtained, to include:

- duration and severity of symptoms (severe dysuria suggests UTI or genital herpes)
- associated symptoms, including frequency, vulval itching or pain, and vaginal discharge
- a full sexual history, covering at least the last 3 months, including type of sexual intercourse (vaginal, oral, rectal) and use of condoms

A careful physical examination should be conducted, focusing on the vulva, vagina, pelvis, and inguinal areas.

- Vulvitis is characterized by diffuse reddening of the vulval skin, which may be swollen and fissured in severe cases. Candidal vulvovaginitis, *Trichomonas vaginalis* infection, and vulval eczema can all cause this appearance.
- Primary vulval HSV infection causes a severe vulvitis with multiple, very tender, shallow ulcers around the introitus, and inguinal lymphadenopathy.
- Other skin conditions (which may present with characteristic appearances) can involve the vulva, including lichen sclerosus, lichen planus, lichen simplex chronicus, and vulval intra-epithelial neoplasia.

Specific clues from immediate investigations

See Table 58.2 for specific clues from immediate investigations, including key diagnostic tests.

Specific clues to other diagnoses

Males

Urethral stricture or bladder outlet obstruction

Clues indicating urethral stricture or bladder outlet obstruction include difficulty initiating urination (hesitancy), poor urine flow, and need to strain. Urethral stricture is now a rare complication of urethritis; bladder outlet obstruction is most commonly caused by benign prostatic hyperplasia.

Table 58.1 Causes of dysuria in males versus females	
Males	**Females**
Urinary tract infection	Urinary tract infection
Urethritis • chlamydia • gonorrhoea • *Mycoplasma genitalium* • genital herpes	Urethritis • chlamydia • gonorrhoea • genital herpes
Urethritis associated with • epididymitis • prostatitis	Urethral syndrome
Urethral obstruction • urethral stricture • meatal skin conditions (e.g. lichen sclerosus) • urethral carcinoma or other malignancy (extremely rare)	Interstitial cystitis
Other causes of urethral irritation/ inflammation • soaps, e.g. shower gel, spermicide	Vulvitis • *Candida* • eczema and other inflammatory skin conditions

Table 58.2 Investigatory clues as to the different diagnoses of dysuria

Diagnosis	Urine dipstick	Gram-stained urethral smear	Urine culture	Other diagnostic tests
Urinary tract infection	Leucocytes+ Nitrite+ Blood+/−	+/− for leucocytes	+	
Urethritis • gonorrhoea • chlamydia • *Mycoplasma genitalium*	Leucocytes +/− Nitrite − Blood −	+ for leucocytes (Gram-negative diplococci in gonorrhoea)	−	Chlamydia NAAT; *Neisseria gonorrhoeae* culture or NAAT; NAAT for *Mycoplasma genitalium*
Genital herpes	Leucocytes +/− Nitrite − Blood −	+/− for leucocytes	−	HSV detection by PCR
Vulvitis	Leucocytes +/− Nitrite − Blood +/−	Not indicated	−	Candida culture (vaginal swab)

Abbreviations: HSV, herpes simplex virus; NAAT, nucleic acid amplification test; PCR, polymerase chain reaction.

Meatal stenosis

A clue indicating meatal stenosis is reduced meatal size (it may be pinhole size); meatal stenosis may be idiopathic or related to a penile skin disorder, especially lichen sclerosus. Typical appearance includes pallor, scarring, telangiectasia, and areas of erythema.

Epididymitis

Epididymitis is usually acute onset, with painful swollen epididymis; it may involve the whole testicle (reactive hydrocele) and is rarely bilateral. It may be associated with urethritis or dysuria. In men aged <35 years, it is usually sexually acquired (chlamydia is the commonest cause). In older age groups, it is usually a complication of UTI (positive urine culture).

Prostatitis

For clues indicating acute prostatitis, see 'Approach to diagnosis'. Chronic bacterial prostatitis typically causes recurrent UTI caused by the same organism (clue: same antibiotic sensitivities). Chronic pelvic pain syndrome (commonly called prostatitis) is a non-infective cause of penile and perineal pain in men and may be associated with mild urinary disturbances including dysuria and variable or reduced urine flow.

Other diagnostic tests

For uncomplicated presentations of urethritis and UTI, additional diagnostic tests are not generally indicated, although recurrent UTI may require further investigation of the urinary tract by imaging. If there are associated symptoms suggestive of lower urinary tract obstruction, these should be investigated further by uroflowmetry and urinary tract ultrasound (for residual bladder volume). These would most often be undertaken after referral to a urologist.

Presentations of lower urinary tract malignancy that may cause disturbance of urinary flow, including bladder carcinoma in situ (with prostatic invasion), prostate cancer, and urethral cancer are mostly diagnosed by urologists and present very rarely to genitourinary medicine or sexual health departments.

Introduction to therapy

In general, treatment is indicated for a presumptive diagnosis of UTI or urethritis (presumed chlamydial) based on the history and results of the urine dipstick test, until the results of the chlamydia nucleic acid amplification (NAAT) test and urine culture are known.

In males, treat presumptive UTI with a minimum of 7 days of a suitable antibiotic such as trimethoprim or amoxicillin (depending on local policy, which is based on prevailing antibiotic resistance patterns) while awaiting the results of urine culture and sensitivities; non-specific urethritis (presumed chlamydial until NAAT result is known) should be treated with 1 doxycycline 100mg twice daily for 7 days. Advise avoidance of sexual intercourse for at least 1 week, until the results are known and until after the sexual partner has also been treated.

Purulent urethritis (presumed gonorrhoea until proved otherwise) should be referred to a specialist service such as a genitourinary medicine or sexual health clinic, for microscopy of a urethral smear and culture or NAAT test. There is well-documented resistance to all available treatments for gonorrhoea, so follow-up is essential. If treated presumptively, intramuscular ceftriaxone 500 µg in 1% lignocaine together with azithromycin 1 g orally as a single dose should be used. If these are unavailable, ciprofloxacin 500 mg single dose can be given but this is associated with a significant risk of treatment failure.

In females, presumptive UTI should be treated with 3 days of a suitable antibiotic such as trimethoprim or amoxycillin (depending on the local policy) while awaiting the results of urine culture and sensitivities. Dysuria presumed secondary to vaginitis should be treated empirically with anticandidal therapy while waiting for results (e.g. with 150 mg fluconazole oral single dose or clotrimazole 500 mg vaginal pessary single dose).

Complicated infections (acute epididymitis, acute prostatitis, suspected chronic bacterial prostatitis) require specific investigation and longer courses of antibiotic treatment, appropriate to the condition involved. Suspected urethral stricture or other cause for outflow obstruction, unexplained persistent urethral symptoms following treatment, or suspected interstitial cystitis should be referred to urology.

Prognosis

Prompt treatment of UTI and urethritis usually leads to rapid resolution of symptoms within a few days (usually 1–3 days). Failure to treat the sexual partner of patients with sexually acquired urethritis is associated with a risk of reinfection and recurrence of symptoms.

Delayed treatment of UTI may lead to complications, including acute epididymitis, acute prostatitis, and septicaemia. Delayed treatment of chlamydial urethritis may lead to complications including chlamydial epididymitis and urethral stricture (rare). Delayed treatment of urethral gonorrhoea may lead to complications, including abscess formation in the accessory glands of the genital tract, gonococcal epididymitis or prostatitis, and disseminated gonococcal infection.

How to handle uncertainty in the diagnosis of this symptom

Not infrequently, the cause of dysuria remains uncertain when the results of tests are available (when urethral smear, urine culture, and tests for chlamydia and gonorrhoea are all negative). In the absence of associated features, the prognosis is generally good, and these patients should be reassured.

Persistent dysuria with associated features (unexplained microscopic haematuria, urethral bleeding, bladder symptoms) should always be followed up with further investigations, especially in older age groups. Appropriate, timely referral to urology may be indicated for consideration of urethrocystoscopy and investigations to exclude benign prostatic hyperplasia, prostate carcinoma, and interstitial cystitis.

Further Reading

Hooton TM. Uncomplicated urinary tract infection. *New Eng J Med* 2012; 366: 1028–37.

Horner P, Blee K, O'Mahony C, et al. *2015 BASHH UK National Guideline on the management of non-gonococcal urethritis.* British Association for Sexual Health and HIV. Available at https://www.bashhguidelines.org/media/1146/ngu-update-05_2017-final.pdf (accessed 7 March 2017).

59 Urinary incontinence

Simon Jackson and Natalia Price

Definition of the symptom

Urinary incontinence is the complaint of any involuntary leakage of urine. It can be classified as:

Stress urinary incontinence: This is involuntary leakage of urine on effort, exertion, sneezing, or coughing.

Urge urinary incontinence: This is involuntary leakage of urine accompanied by, or immediately preceded by, a strong desire to pass urine (void). Urgency with or without urge urinary incontinence and usually with frequency and nocturia is also defined as overactive bladder syndrome (OAB).

Mixed urinary incontinence: The involuntary leakage of urine associated with both urgency and exertion, effort, sneezing, or coughing. Usually, one of these is predominant; that is, either the symptoms of urge incontinence, or those of stress incontinence, are most bothersome.

Overflow incontinence: This occurs when the bladder becomes large and flaccid and has little or no detrusor tone or function. It is usually due to injury or insult, occurring post surgery or post-partum. The bladder simply leaks when it becomes full.

Incontinence due to a fistula: This is incontinence resulting from a vesicovaginal, ureterovaginal, or urethrovaginal fistula.

Congenital incontinence: This is incontinence due to congenital causes (e.g. ectopic ureter).

Differential diagnosis/secondary causes

The following causes of urinary incontinence should always be considered:

- urinary tract infection
- bladder outflow obstruction; uncommon in women unless there is past pelvic or incontinence surgery, but common in men, due to prostatic enlargement; severe constipation can also cause bladder outflow obstruction
- psychological and metabolic causes of polydipsia and polyuria, such as diabetes mellitus, diabetes insipidus, or excessive fluid consumption
- neurological abnormalities (spinal cord injuries, spina bifida, multiple sclerosis, and other causes of upper motor neuron disorders)
- drugs (e.g. loop diuretics)

Context

Urinary incontinence is a common problem throughout the world. In the UK, there are more than 3.5 million sufferers. Patients are categorized according to their symptoms into stress, mixed, or urge urinary incontinence. Overall, half of all incontinent women complain of pure stress incontinence and 30%–40% have mixed symptoms of stress and urge incontinence. Women with mixed urinary incontinence, who have an involuntary leakage associated with urgency and also with exertion, are treated according to the most troublesome symptom. Initial treatment should commence on this basis.

Approach to diagnosis

History

History taking in urinary incontinence guides the investigation and management, by evaluating symptoms, their progression, and their impact on lifestyle, including how daily life and social, personal, and sexual relationships are affected.

The onset of urinary symptoms and their duration and severity should be recorded. The predominant bother symptom (e.g. urgency, urge incontinence, or stress incontinence) should be identified. As different underlying conditions cause similar urinary symptoms, history alone is a poor predictor of pathophysiology.

Colorectal symptoms and genitourinary prolapse should be asked about. Accompanying symptoms that may indicate a more serious diagnosis and which require referral, such as haematuria, persisting bladder or urethral pain, or recurrent urinary tract infection (UTI), should also be identified from the history.

Clinical examination

Clinical examination should include an abdominal examination to exclude abdominal mass or palpable bladder, a bimanual examination to exclude pelvic mass, and a vaginal examination. Neurological assessment of the lower limbs and perineum is required if a neurological cause is suspected.

Vaginal examination should include an assessment of urethral and bladder neck descent on straining, anterior vaginal wall mobility, and concurrent uterovaginal prolapse. An assessment of pelvic floor strength should be made in women with urinary stress incontinence. Vaginal examination is performed to palpate the levator ani muscles. Pelvic floor strength is graded 0 to 5 on a modified Oxford scale, and endurance (i.e. length of time of maximum contraction) and number of repeated contractions are also recorded.

Specific clues to the diagnosis

Specific clues to the diagnosis are as follows:

- From the history, explore possible etiological factors and ask about neurological disease, past obstetric trauma, and previous gynaecological and urological surgery.
- If polyuria is present, exclude secondary causes (e.g. diabetes mellitus, diabetes insipidus, or hypercalcaemia). However, most patients will have primary polydipsia, and simple advice regarding fluid restriction is sufficient to resolve urinary frequency.
- The predominant symptom (e.g. urgency, urge incontinence, or stress incontinence) should be identified.

Key diagnostic tests

Key diagnostic tests are as follows:

Urinalysis: Reagent strip testing of urine for leukocyte esterase, nitrates, protein, blood, and glucose is a sensitive and cheap screening test.

Urine culture: Perform urine microscopy and culture for those with a positive screening test result. Exclusion of infection is mandatory, as symptoms of detrusor overactivity overlap with those of UTI.

Residual check: A post-void residual check should be carried out (either ultrasound scan or catheterization) if there are symptoms suggestive of incomplete bladder emptying.

Urinary diary: Diagnosis is assisted with the use of a frequency/volume chart (urinary diary). This is a simple and practical method of obtaining objective quantification of fluid intake, functional bladder capacity, and voiding behaviour. Frequency and times of voiding, voided volumes, and leakage episodes (day and night) are all recorded for at least 24 hours and typically 3 days.

Urodynamic investigations: These include uroflowmetry, post-void residual measurement, and cystometry. It is important that any clinician referring a patient for such tests has an understanding of what the tests entail and the indications for it. Clinical indications for urodynamic assessment are:

- complex mixed urinary symptoms (urge incontinence and stress incontinence)
- symptoms suggestive of detrusor overactivity unresponsive to pharmacotherapy
- voiding dysfunction with incomplete bladder emptying
- neuropathic bladder disorder (videourodynamics preferred)

Other diagnostic tests

Imaging of the urinary tract

Imaging of the lower urinary tract is not routinely justified in all women presenting with urinary symptoms, but should be targeted at specific indications. The available diagnostic procedures include:

Ultrasonography: This is used to (1) exclude incomplete bladder emptying; (2) check for congenital abnormalities, calculi, and tumours; and (3) detect cortical scarring of the kidneys.

X-ray: Plain abdominal X-ray film is useful for screening for foreign bodies and calculi.

Intravenous urography: This is indicated in women with neuropathic bladder or suspected congenital or acquired abnormalities (e.g. uterovaginal fistulae).

Micturating cystourethrography: This is useful to demonstrate bladder and urethral fistulae, vesicoureteric reflux, and anatomical abnormalities of the lower urinary tract, such as urethral diverticula.

CT: This can detect and characterize solid renal masses as well as renal tract calculi, renal and perirenal infections, and associated complications.

MRI: This remains a research technique for incontinence and prolapse, due to cost and availability. It is mainly used for characterization of renal or pelvic masses, and tumour staging.

Introduction to therapy

Urge urinary incontinence

Start with the simplest of conservative therapies and progress through to treatments that are more radical, if necessary. Reducing fluid intake, if the urinary diary suggests this is excessive, and cutting caffeine out of the diet often has a dramatic effect. This simple advice may be all that is required to cure frequency and urgency. Drugs (e.g. diuretics and antipsychotics) altering bladder function should be reviewed.

Bladder training should be offered as first-line treatment to patients with OAB, often in combination with anticholinergic therapy. The three main components of bladder training are patient education, timed voiding with systematic delay in voiding, and positive reinforcement. The patients should be asked to resist the sensation of urgency and void according to a timetable. A self-completed urinary diary should be used to monitor the times of voids. Continence rates of up to 90% have been reported but the cure rates could be considerably lower than this.

Pharmacological suppression of detrusor overactivity with anticholinergics (antimuscarinics) is the most widely used treatment. Anticholinergic drugs block the muscarinic receptors that mediate detrusor smooth-muscle contraction and have a direct, relaxing effect on the detrusor muscle. There are a number of drug treatments available, which differ in their selectivity for various muscarinic receptors; some drugs have additional actions, such as direct smooth-muscle effects. In postmenopausal women with vaginal atrophy, intravaginal oestrogens can be tried for OAB symptoms.

Surgery is recommended for intractable detrusor overactivity only when medical and behavioural therapy has failed. Procedures such as bladder distension, detrusor myomectomy, and augmentation cystoplasty have limited efficacy and high rates of complication. Permanent urinary diversion is occasionally indicated in women with intractable incontinence.

Some new treatments, such as intra-vesical botulinum toxin injections, neuromodulation, and sacral nerve stimulation are showing considerable promise. Botulinum toxin A may revolutionize OAB

management. It blocks neuromuscular transmission, causing the affected muscle to become weak. The toxin is injected cystoscopically under local or general anaesthesia into the detrusor muscle in 10–30 different locations, sparing the trigonum. Cure, or improvement rates of 60%–93%, has been reported at initial follow-up. The duration of response to a single dose is on average 9 months (range 3–12 months). The most common complication is voiding dysfunction and urinary retention (5%–20%), resolving as the effect of the treatment wears off. This treatment shows promise as a therapy for overactive bladder symptoms, but little controlled-trial data exist on benefits and safety.

Neuromodulation and sacral nerve stimulation provide continuous stimulation of the third sacral spinal nerve root via an implanted electrical pulse generator and improves the ability to suppress detrusor contractions. It is being used increasingly in the treatment of refractory detrusor overactivity. Overall, neuromodulation has a 30%–50% clinical success rate. It is a very expensive treatment, as the implant alone costs approximately £10 000. Insertion of the implant is an invasive procedure, and lifelong follow-up is required.

Stress urinary incontinence

Conservative treatment is usually initiated in primary care. This involves treating the symptoms of stress incontinence, for example, through adjustment of lifestyle (weight reduction if BMI > 30; smoking cessation; treatment of chronic cough and constipation), pelvic floor exercises, and pharmacotherapy.

Pelvic floor exercise is an appropriate first-line treatment for most women. The aim of pelvic floor exercise is to promote the woman's awareness of her pelvic floor muscles and to improve their contractility and coordination. Wherever possible, an appropriately trained physiotherapist should make an assessment of the pelvic floor musculature.

Surgery for stress urinary incontinence is considered when conservative measures have failed and the woman's quality of life is compromised. It is important to be clear about the underlying cause of the incontinence, as the effects of surgery are largely irreversible. The options depend on the woman's fitness for anaesthesia and whether there is any coexisting prolapse. Burch colposuspension used to be a 'gold-standard' procedure for many years, with a success rate of 85%–90%. The retropubic space is entered through a small suprapubic incision, and two or three permanent sutures are placed on either side of the bladder neck to the corresponding ileopectineal ligament. This procedure can also be performed laparoscopically. There are also a variety of 'sling' procedures that can be performed abdominally or vaginally, with rectus sheath, fascia lata, or synthetic materials. The commonest of these is the tension-free vaginal tape procedure, which has a success rate of between 80% and 90%.

Injectables or bulking agents are appropriate, if previous surgery has failed or in very elderly patients. Various compounds, including collagen, have been used, with success rates of around 50%.

Complications for all these procedures include post-operative voiding difficulty, bleeding, infection, de novo detrusor overactivity, and suture or mesh erosion (in 'sling' procedures).

Prognosis

Incontinence can be cured or significantly improved in most women, providing they are appropriately investigated and treated. However, for a small number of women, a cure may be impossible. For this group, containment with pads, devices, or even catheters may be the most appropriate therapy. Bladder catheterization (using an intermittent or indwelling urethral or suprapubic catheter) should be considered for patients in whom persistent urinary retention is causing incontinence, symptomatic infection, or renal dysfunction, and in whom this cannot otherwise be corrected. Clean intermittent self-catheterization is a technique that can be taught to patients or carers (e.g. by a continence nurse) to facilitate bladder emptying in case of urinary retention with large residuals. This may relieve overflow incontinence.

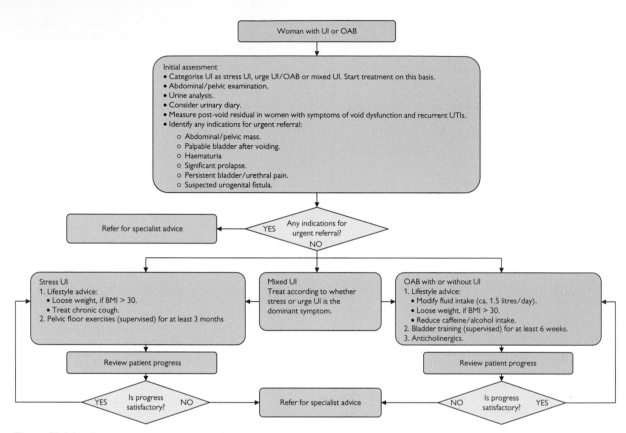

Figure 59.1 Initial assessment and management of women with urinary incontinence.

Data from Urinary incontinence in women: management, NICE clincial guideline cg717, 2013 nice.org.uk/guidance/cg171.

How to handle uncertainty in the diagnosis of this symptom

Figure 59.1 illustrates the initial steps in diagnosis and assessment of women with urinary incontinence, and shows the conservative management steps to be undertaken before referring for specialist advice on surgical management.

Further Reading

Abrams P, Cardozo L, Khoury S, et al. Incontinence. International Consultation on Urological Diseases, 4th International Consultation on Incontinence, Paris July 5–8, 2008. Available at http://www.icud.info/PDFs/Incontinence.pdf (accessed 8 March 2017).

National Institute for Health and Care Excellence (NICE). Urinary incontinence in women: management. Clinical guideline [CG171] 2013. Last updated: November 2015. https://www.nice.org.uk/guidance/cg171.

60 Faecal incontinence

Udi Shmueli

Definition of the symptom

Faecal incontinence (FI) is the recurrent uncontrolled passage of faecal material.

It is important to subdivide it into passive leakage, when the patient is unaware of stool loss, and urge incontinence, when there is insufficient time to reach the toilet. The inadvertent escape of flatus and partial soiling of undergarments with liquid stool is graded as minor incontinence, and the involuntary excretion of solid faeces as major incontinence.

Context

Estimates of the prevalence of FI vary widely in studies, depending on the definition used and the population studied, but about 2% of adults are incontinent of faeces about once a week. The problem increases with age to affect up to a third of residential and nursing home patients. It is a highly embarrassing problem that patients try to hide, and avoid talking about to their spouse or their doctor. The presenting complaint may be diarrhoea, a change in bowel habit, or with the symptoms of irritable bowel syndrome and it may take direct questioning to elucidate the problem.

Approach to diagnosis

A careful history is the key to diagnosis. Establish if there is passive leakage, when the patient is unaware of stool loss until the underpants are actually soiled, or urge incontinence, when the patient is aware of the need to defecate but has insufficient time to reach the toilet. Determine the frequency and severity of the FI and if there has been a change in bowel habit, which would require further investigation. Move on to a general history, including any obstetric and surgical history, and concentrate on the presence or absence of neurological or spinal disorders, diabetes, cognitive impairment, behavioural abnormalities, or physical impairment that might impair access to the toilet. Apply your finding to Table 60.1 to obtain a differential diagnosis.

Physical examination of the abdomen perianal area and rectum is essential, looking for rectal or anal tumours, inflammatory change, faecal impaction, fistulae, or rectal prolapse. Assess anal sensation, resting tone, and squeeze pressure. Gaping of the anus when the buttocks are parted or the inability to contract the anus on command suggests significant sphincter damage or neurological problems. Be aware, however, that, unless there is a gross abnormality, digital examination is a poor determinant of sphincter integrity and function.

Specific clues to the diagnosis

With urge incontinence, it is essential to establish if the patient has had a change in bowel habit to looser stools, as this would require further investigation. Diarrhoea that responds to small doses of loperamide is likely to be functional, but may still need to be investigated. Be aware that a patient with urge incontinence may actually be constipated, even if complaining of frequent defaecation. In a constipated patient, physical activity or a gastrocolic reflex after eating may bring on an urgent call to stool, with incontinence in those unable to reach a toilet in time. Sometimes the only clue to constipation is a history of unsatisfying defaecation with small hard stools or mucous. An abdominal X-ray is occasionally necessary to demonstrate a colon loaded with stool.

Table 60.1 Common causes of faecal incontinence

Causes	Mechanisms
With mainly urge incontinence	

External anal sphincter dysfunction
  Vaginal delivery
  Surgery for fistulae
  Haemorrhoidectomy
  Other trauma
	Direct trauma to the anal sphincters; damage to the pudendal nerve by stretching of the pelvic floor during pregnancy

Inflammatory conditions
  Ulcerative colitis
  Crohn's disease
  Radiation proctitis
	Inflammation of the rectal mucosa causes a much more urgent call to stool; chronic inflammation and fibrosis can reduce rectal compliance; diarrhoea, which may be of large volume

Functional faecal incontinence	As part of an irritable bowel syndrome, often with a prominent gastrocolic reflex; defined as faecal incontinence with abnormal functioning of normally innervated and structurally intact muscles
Other physical or behavioural problems	The patient may be unable or unwilling to reach the toilet in time
With mainly passive incontinence	
Constipation Common in the elderly, institutionalized and inactive people, or those taking strong analgesics	Passive leakage due to inhibition of the internal sphincter; they may also complain of diarrhoea (due to overflow) and deny any possibility that they are constipated; constipation may also be associated with a prominent gastrocolic reflex, which in the poorly mobile may lead to urge incontinence

Neuropathy and spinal injury
  Multiple sclerosis
  Diabetes
  Spinal trauma
  Pregnancy causes partial denervation of the pelvic muscles and anal sphincter by stretching and compressing the pelvic floor
	Diminished sensation and diminished or absent external sphincter activity to oppose bowel contraction; exacerbated in multiple sclerosis by constipation with overflow; exacerbated in diabetes by diarrhoea due to autonomic neuropathy, metformin, or small bowel bacterial overgrowth

Internal anal sphincter dysfunction	Degeneration of unknown cause; radiotherapy (e.g. for prostate or cervix); systemic sclerosis

With passive incontinence, it is vital to look for faecal impaction by rectal examination, even if there are factors in the history such as radiotherapy that may explain the problem.

Key diagnostic tests

Endoscopic assessment of the rectosigmoid mucosa is recommended in most patients. Diarrhoea must be appropriately investigated. Endoscopy may not be necessary in constipation unless there are alarm symptoms such as bleeding, weight loss, or a family history of bowel cancer.

Other diagnostic tests

These are used in patients with suspected sphincter damage who do not respond to simple treatment.

The internal and external anal sphincters can be imaged by endo-anal ultrasound and MRI. Small defects are common and may not be related to symptoms. Large sphincter defects may be amenable to surgical repair, but patients with additional neurological damage do less well with surgery. Dynamic MRI can also demonstrate pelvic floor motion.

Anorectal manometry is performed with a catheter assembly that includes a balloon positioned in the rectum and pressure transducers in the anal canal. A low resting anal pressure suggests dysfunction of the internal anal sphincter. A reduced squeeze pressure is associated with external anal sphincter dysfunction. Impaired sensation means that techniques such as biofeedback are unlikely to be successful.

The pudendal nerve is tested by stimulation with a glove-mounted electrode while the anal sphincter EMG response is measured. A prolonged conduction time indicates pudendal nerve damage. EMG recordings of the anal sphincter detect proximal neurogenic or myopathic lesions.

Introduction to therapy

Treatment will depend on the underlying cause and the severity of the symptoms. Most patients will be improved by medical therapy aimed at restoring normal bowel habits. Constipated patients should have aggressive therapy with laxatives, and usually enemas or suppositories.

Loperamide is used in patients with loose stools and occasionally in patients with normal stools and FI, as hard stools are easier to retain. Loperamide will slightly increase internal sphincter tone in addition to reducing bowel frequency, but the dose of loperamide has to be carefully titrated in order to avoid constipation. Loperamide can be taken before bed for people with night-time or early morning problems, before physical activity, or before meals for those with a prominent gastrocolic reflex. Patients with a prominent gastrocolic reflex may also benefit from hyoscine or mebeverine.

Another approach is for the patient to use rectal suppositories or a self-administered micro enema to clear out the rectum in the morning, or before going out. This may prevent significant incontinence and enhance confidence.

A toilet access 'Just Can't Wait' card and a 'RADAR' key to allow access to 'disabled' toilets in the National Key Scheme can be obtained from the Bladder & Bowel Community, who also provide patient information including information on continence products.

Perianal hygiene is vital. The anus should be cleaned with water whenever possible and dried by gentle dabbing. Barrier creams such as zinc oxide or calamine can help prevent skin damage. Irritation may be due to a fungal infection or dermatitis and should be treated with appropriate creams.

Patients should be encouraged to strengthen the anal sphincters with pelvic floor exercises, such as repeatedly tightening and relaxing the anus.

Patients who fail to improve with medical therapy should be referred to specialist centres, where a range of investigation and treatment techniques are available. These include biofeedback therapy, sacral nerve stimulation, and surgery.

Surgical intervention is occasionally necessary but caries the risk of worsening the incontinence. The best results are with a relatively simple overlapping repair to a single defect in the external anal sphincter, or an abdominal rectopexy to repair a rectal prolapse, as this may restore internal sphincter function. However, patients with internal sphincter defects, pudendal nerve neuropathy, multiple defects, or external sphincter atrophy are unlikely to benefit from surgery. A colostomy is used in severe FI when other treatments have failed.

Prognosis

If the underlying problem is functional incontinence, constipation, inflammatory bowel disease, or other resolvable bowel disturbance problems, then most patients will be helped by medical therapy. Patients with sphincter disruption or neurological problems and severe FI are less likely to improve sufficiently with simple measures and will benefit from an early referral to a specialist centre.

How to handle uncertainty with this symptom

Patients are afraid to socialize or leave the house for fear of embarrassing incontinence. They are reticent to talk about their problem even to their partner. They lose self-confidence and self-esteem. They need and welcome the opportunity to discuss their problem with a sensitive healthcare professional, if only to 'fine-tune' their coping strategies.

Further Reading

Bladder & Bowel Community (https://www.bladderandbowel.org/)

Bharucha AE, Dunivan G, Good PS. et al. Epidemiology, pathophysiology, and classification of fecal incontinence: State of the Science Summary for the National Institute of Diabetes and Digestive and Kidney Diseases (NIDDK) Workshop. *Am J Gastroenterol* 2015; 110: 127–36.

National Institute for Health and Care Excellence. *Faecal Incontinence: The Management of Faecal Incontinence in Adults*. 2007. Available at http://www.nice.org.uk/Guidance/CG49 (accessed 8 March 2017).

61 Vaginal discharge

Jackie Sherrard and Graz Luzzi

Definition of the symptom

Vaginal discharge may be a normal feature (physiological discharge). However, as a symptom, the term is used to denote vaginal discharge which is excessive in quantity or abnormal in appearance, consistency, or odour. Causes of vaginal discharge are given in Table 61.1.

Context

Vaginal discharge is the result of secretions produced from glands in the vaginal and the cervical mucosae. It is a common presenting symptom and may be caused by a range of physiological and pathological conditions. All women have physiological discharge starting a year or two before puberty and ending after the menopause. During the menstrual cycle, concentrations of oestrogen and progesterone vary, leading to alterations in the quantity and type of cervical mucus. Prior to ovulation, oestrogen concentration increases, altering cervical mucus from non-fertile to fertile (clearer, wetter, stretchy, and slippery). After ovulation, oestrogen concentration decreases and progesterone concentration increases; cervical mucus becomes thick and sticky and hostile to sperm. The amount of discharge varies from woman to woman, as do perceptions of what is normal. However, there are also a number of conditions, both infective and non-infective, that may give rise to pathological vaginal discharge. Many of the

symptoms and signs are non-specific, and a number of women may have other conditions such as vulvar dermatoses or allergic reactions as a cause of their symptoms.

A normal physiological discharge is a white or clear, non-offensive discharge that varies with the menstrual cycle. Sexual arousal, pregnancy, and using the oral contraceptive pill are typically associated with an increase in 'normal' vaginal discharge.

Three common infections are associated with vaginal discharge—bacterial vaginosis, candidiasis, and trichomoniasis. Infections with other organisms such as *Chlamydia trachomatis* and *Neisseria gonorrhoeae* may cause vaginal discharge due to cervicitis.

Approach to diagnosis

A full sexual history (to assess STI risk) and clinical history should be sought, with a particular note of the nature of the discharge (what has changed, odour, onset, duration, colour, consistency) and associated symptoms (may include itch, superficial dyspareunia, or dysuria), or symptoms suggestive of upper reproductive tract infection (e.g. abdominal pain, deep dyspareunia, abnormal bleeding, dysuria, pyrexia). Also consider concurrent medications (e.g. recently starting, changing, or stopping hormonal contraceptives, antibiotics, corticosteroids), and medical conditions (e.g. diabetes, immunocompromised state).

Specific clues to the diagnosis

Symptoms suggesting that discharge is abnormal include:

- a discharge that is heavier or thicker than usual
- greyish, greenish, yellowish, or blood-tinged discharge
- offensive smelling discharge

Vaginal infections are suggested by a discharge accompanied by vulval or vaginal itching, burning, rash, or soreness, the presence of genital sores or ulcers, abdominal pain or pain on intercourse, and a recent change in sexual partner, a new partner, or concurrent symptoms in a sexual partner.

Infective, non-sexually transmitted causes of vaginal discharge

There are two infective, non-sexually transmitted causes of vaginal discharge:

Bacterial vaginosis: Bacterial vaginosis is due an overgrowth of anaerobic bacteria and occurs and remits spontaneously. It typically presents as a thin, profuse, and fishy-smelling discharge without itch or soreness, and may cause dyspareunia.

Candidiasis: Candidiasis is more common in pregnant women and those with diabetes mellitus, recent antibiotic treatment, or immunosuppression. The characteristic symptoms are thick, white, non-offensive discharge associated with vulval itch and soreness. It may cause mild dyspareunia and external dysuria, and on examination there may be vulval and/or vaginal erythema, oedema, and fissuring.

Infective, sexually transmitted causes of vaginal discharge

Chlamydia trachomatis, Neisseria gonorrhoeae, and *Trichomonas vaginalis* can all present with vaginal discharge:

Chlamydia trachomatis: This is asymptomatic in 80% of women but may cause a copious purulent vaginal discharge due to cervicitis. The woman may complain of post-coital and/or intermenstrual

Table 61.1 Causes of vaginal discharge, listed according to age and pregnancy status	
Prepubertal	Physiological
	Allergic dermatitis
	Vulval dermatitis
Reproductive age	Non-sexually transmitted infection: • bacterial vaginosis • *Candida* infections
	Sexually transmitted infection: • *Chlamydia trachomatis* • *Neisseria gonorrhoeae* • *Trichomonas vaginalis*
	Cervical polyps and ectopy
	Vulval dermatitis
	Physiological
	Foreign bodies, e.g. retained tampon
	Erosive lichen planus
	Genital tract malignancy (cancer of cervix, cancer of uterus, ovarian cancer)
	Fistulae
Pregnancy	Physiological
	Non-sexually transmitted infection: • *Candida* infections common in pregnancy (30%–40%) • bacterial vaginosis
	Sexually transmitted infection: • *Chlamydia trachomatis* • *Neisseria gonorrhoeae* • *Trichomonas vaginalis*
Postmenopausal	Atrophic vaginitis
	Cervical polyps and ectopy
	Desquamative inflammatory vaginitis
	Vulval dermatitis
	Genital tract malignancy (cancer of cervix, cancer of uterus, ovarian cancer)
	Fistulae

bleeding. Chlamydia infection may be complicated by pelvic inflammatory disease.

Neisseria gonorrhoeae: This is asymptomatic in up to 50% of women but may present with a purulent vaginal discharge due to cervicitis. Other symptoms include dysuria and intermenstrual bleeding. Gonorrhoea may be complicated by pelvic inflammatory disease.

Trichomonas vaginalis: This may cause an offensive yellow vaginal discharge, which is often profuse and frothy, and may be associated with vulval itch and soreness, dysuria, abdominal pain, and superficial dyspareunia.

Non-infective causes of vaginal discharge

The following are non-infective causes of vaginal discharge:

Allergic reactions: Diagnosis is suspected on taking the history (e.g. use of irritant chemicals in douching, contact with latex and semen).

Retained foreign bodies: These are usually tampons or condoms and result in a foul-smelling serosanguinous discharge. The diagnosis is confirmed on examination.

Cervical polyps and ectopy: These tend to be asymptomatic but there may be increased discharge and intermenstrual bleeding. The diagnosis is made on speculum examination.

Genital tract malignancy: The presentation varies and, in some cases, a persistent vaginal discharge not responding to conventional treatment may be the first clue. The diagnosis is made on examination and biopsy.

Fistulae: A history of trauma or surgery is suggestive. There may be a foul or feculent discharge in association with recurrent urinary tract infections.

Key diagnostic tests

Exclusion of infective and other causes can help confirm that a vaginal discharge is physiological. Patients complaining of discharge should have an examination of the external genitalia for evidence of vulvitis or ulcers, and a speculum examination to allow inspection of the vagina and cervix and to undertake appropriate investigations.

A woman presenting with symptoms suggestive of bacterial vaginosis or vulvovaginal candidiasis can be treated without taking swabs at first presentation, if she is at low risk for STIs and without symptoms indicative of upper reproductive tract infection. However, a woman complaining of vaginal discharge should be investigated if she requests investigation; is deemed to be at increased risk of STIs; has symptoms indicative of upper genital tract infection; is postnatal, post-miscarriage, post-abortion, or within 3 weeks of intrauterine contraceptive device insertion; or if previous treatment has failed.

Initial investigations outside a GUM clinic include:

- a high vaginal swab to identify bacterial vaginosis, candida infections, and *Trichomonas vaginalis*
- endocervical or vulvovaginal swab for DNA amplification test to diagnose gonorrhoea
- endocervical or vulvovaginal swab for a chlamydial DNA amplification test to diagnose *Chlamydia trachomatis*
- vaginal pH testing (using narrow range pH paper) is a quick, cheap, and simple test that can help discriminate between bacterial vaginosis (pH 4.5 or above) and vulvovaginal candidiasis (pH <4.5)

Other diagnostic tests

In a woman at risk of STIs, it is prudent to offer a full screen, including testing for blood borne viruses and syphilis serology. Further tests will depend upon the findings on examination, and may include patch testing for allergies, or biopsy of suspicious lesions.

Introduction to therapy

General principles include good basic personal hygiene (cleanliness without the use of douches and perfumed chemical agents), with avoidance of tight synthetic clothing. Where it is decided that the discharge is physiological, the woman may need careful explanation of this, and reassurance regarding the absence of pathology.

Infective, non-sexually transmitted vaginal discharge

The following are therapies for infective, non-sexually transmitted causes of vaginal discharge:

Bacterial vaginosis: The recommended treatment is oral metronidazole (400–500 mg twice daily for 5–7 days).

Candidiasis: Vaginal imidazole preparations (e.g. clotrimazole, econazole, miconazole) or fluconazole 150 mg orally are equally effective in the treatment of vulvovaginal candidiasis. Avoid oral azole regimens in pregnancy, due to potential teratogenicity. Vulval antifungals (in addition to oral or vaginal regimens) can be used if women have vulval symptoms. Latex condoms, cervical caps, and diaphragms may be damaged by azole-containing local preparations.

Infective, sexually transmitted vaginal discharge

Patients with infective, sexually transmitted vaginal discharge should be referred to the GUM clinic (unless your practice has the appropriate expertise and access to local treatment protocols and partner notification). Patients need to be fully screened for concurrent STIs and treated as is appropriate, and partners will need to be identified, screened, and treated too:

Chlamydia trachomatis: First-line therapy includes doxycycline 100 mg twice daily for 7 days (contraindicated in pregnancy) and azithromycin 1 g orally in a single dose.

Gonorrhoea: Therapy includes ceftriaxone intra-muscularly as a single dose.

Trichomonas vaginalis: Metronidazole 2 g orally in a single dose or metronidazole 400–500 mg twice daily for 5–7 days.

Non-infective causes of vaginal discharge

The following are therapies for non-infective causes of vaginal discharge:

Allergic reactions: Treatment includes identifying and removing the cause.

Retained foreign bodies: These can usually be removed with a sponge forceps or similar instrument. A short course of antibiotics may be needed if the object was there long enough to cause secondary infection.

Cervical polyps and ectopy: In this case, excision of larger symptomatic or suspicious looking polyps may be necessary.

Prognosis

The prognosis is as follows:

- Bacterial vaginosis has a 70%–80% cure rate after one course of treatment (but commonly recurs).
- Candida has a cure rate of 80%–95%.
- Trichomoniasis has a 95% cure rate.
- The finding of an STI should prompt patient education, screening for other infections, and sexual contact tracing for testing and appropriate management to prevent reinfection.

How to handle uncertainty in the diagnosis of this symptom

In women who experience intermittent symptoms, it may be necessary to see them acutely when they are symptomatic to establish the diagnosis. Where no cause is found for discharge, and examination is normal, a woman often needs careful explanation of the nature of physiological discharge and reassurance regarding the absence of pathology.

Some women suffer with recurrent discharge and, in general, the advice is the same as for the initial presentation, although it is prudent to go through the symptoms, signs, and examination process rigorously to ensure coexistent pathology hasn't been missed (e.g. an STI in the case of a patient being treated for bacterial vaginosis) and explore personal hygiene habits that may contribute to the disruption of normal vaginal flora (such as douches). Finally, be alert to possible underlying associated problems such as diabetes, immunosuppression, or concurrent antibiotic administration and for psychosexual problems and depression that can be associated with recurrent episodes of vaginal discharge.

Further Reading

BASHH. *Management of Vaginal Discharge in Non-Genitourinary Medicine Settings*, 2012. Joint British Association for Sexual Health & HIV and Faculty for sexual and reproductive health guideline (http://www.bashh.org/guidelines).

Sherrard J, White D, and Donders G. European (IUSTI/WHO) guideline on the management of vaginal discharge. *Intl J STD AIDS* 2011; 22: 421–9.

62 Joint pain

Pippa Watson

Definition of the symptom

When a patient complains of pain confined to a joint or joints, they are said to have **arthralgia.** If, in addition, there is swelling of the joint, tenderness of the joint line to palpation, and limitation of movement, the patient is said to have an **arthritis.** It is important to establish if an arthritis is **inflammatory** or **non-inflammatory**, as this affects the differential diagnosis. Soft tissue swelling of the joint, the presence of a joint effusion, increased temperature of the joint, erythema of overlying skin, and early morning stiffness of at least 30 minutes duration are signs of an inflammatory arthritis.

Differential diagnosis

Joint pain (arthralgia) may reflect trauma, degenerative and inflammatory arthritis, inflammation of extra-articular tissues, systemic infection, or an allergic reaction to medication. The causes of acute arthralgia in primary and secondary care are shown in Table 62.1

Context

A history of trauma should prompt consideration of diagnoses such as fracture or ligament damage. Other conditions which can mimic monoarthritis include bursitis or tendonitis. It is always vital to consider the diagnosis of septic arthritis because of the serious consequence of late or missed diagnosis. Systemic upset, fever, severe pain, and grossly restricted range of movement of the joint raise the possibility of this diagnosis, and should trigger urgent referral to a specialist.

It is useful to make the distinction between septic arthritis, where there is infection in a joint, and reactive arthritis, where a joint becomes inflamed in response to infection elsewhere. Septic arthritis is usually the result of haematogenous spread, but may result from adjacent osteomyelitis. Reactive arthritis can occur in response to sexually transmitted infections, when it may result in the classical triad of arthritis, conjunctivitis, and non-specific urethritis. It may also be triggered by a range of viral or bacterial infections.

Approach to diagnosis

Pattern recognition is important in determining the cause of a hot joint. A thorough history and examination will often provide the necessary information to make a diagnosis.

Table 62.1 Causes of acute arthralgia in primary and secondary care

	Primary care (% of cases)	Secondary care (% of cases)
Gout/pseudogout	77	66
Monoarticular presentation of inflammatory arthritis	15	20
Reactive arthritis	5	10
Haemarthrosis	2	3
Septic arthritis	1	1
Monoarticular presentation of connective tissue disease or vasculitis	<1	1

Key factors in the history

Key factors in the history are as follows:

Demographics: Premenopausal women are extremely unlikely to suffer from gout, while conditions such as pseudogout and septic arthritis are more common in the elderly.

The time course of symptom onset: Symptom onset may be acute, chronic, relapsing, flitting, migrating, or additive. Attacks of gout typically develop over a matter of hours. The onset of septic arthritis is usually fairly rapid but can have a more insidious onset in elderly or immunosuppressed patients.

The number of joints involved and the pattern of involvement: Determining the number of joints involved (monoarticular, oligoarticular, polyarticular, spinal involvement) and the pattern of involvement (symmetrical vs non-symmetrical; small joints, large joints, or mixed; upper limb vs lower limb predominant) is important because, although the knee is frequently affected by all conditions, some conditions have a predilection for certain joints (e.g. gout and the first metatarsophalangeal joint). Screen for involvement of other joints, past or present. Patients with gout or pseudogout will often have a previous history of similar attacks. Morning stiffness lasting for longer than an hour is a classical feature of inflammatory arthritis. Patients with rheumatoid arthritis will often have pain involving the hands. Those with ankylosing spondylitis may report lower back or buttock pain (suggestive of sacroiliitis). It is, however, important to remember that crystal arthritis and infection can occur as a secondary problem in preexisting inflammatory and degenerative arthritis.

The presence of systemic upset: Fever and malaise makes the diagnosis of septic arthritis more likely. Other risk factors for infection should also be screened for, notably, diabetes, immunodeficiency/immunosuppression, previous joint replacement, and underlying inflammatory arthritis.

A history of current or recent infection: This is important, as it may indicate a septic or reactive arthritis. Care must be taken to screen for common infections (urinary, respiratory tract), and particularly sexually transmitted diseases, which are frequently associated with reactive arthritis. This should include asking about recent unprotected sexual intercourse and vaginal or urethral discharge. Age should not be a discriminating factor for taking a sexual history.

Systemic enquiry: It is always worth performing a screen for involvement of other systems: skin, cardiovascular, respiratory, gastrointestinal, and neurological. Connective tissue disorders and vasculitis may present with a hot joint.

Past medical history: Psoriasis or inflammatory bowel disease can be pointers towards seronegative inflammatory arthritis. A history of haemophilia, von Willebrand's disease, or anticoagulation raises the possibility of haemarthrosis. Although relatively rare, a past history of TB should prompt consideration of this as a cause of septic arthritis.

Key features on examination

Key features on examination are as follows:

Fever: Fever is usually present in septic arthritis.
Severely restricted movement of a joint: This indicates serious pathology, and should prompt urgent referral to a rheumatologist.
Involvement of other joints: Conditions such as pseudogout invariably develop on a background of osteoarthritis.
Involvement of other systems: A careful examination may pick up further clues as to the likely diagnosis. Expose the patient fully and look for psoriatic plaques, tophi, and rheumatoid nodules or pustules (gonococcus).

Specific clues to the diagnosis

Table 62.2 outlines specific clues which can aid diagnosis.

Key diagnostic tests

Further investigation is not always indicated. For example, a patient with previous gout who develops acute pain and swelling of his ankle and is systemically well could sensibly be treated with a course of NSAIDs, and advice to rest the affected joint.

Joint aspiration and synovial fluid analysis are extremely useful, and comprise the key investigation when the problem is a single hot joint. Joint aspiration is mandatory if septic arthritis is suspected, and is desirable in cases of suspected gout, pseudogout, or haemarthrosis. As well as being a key diagnostic test, aspiration often provides symptomatic benefit. Wherever possible, drain the joint to dryness, as this will reduce pain and improve function.

Large joint aspiration, especially of the knee, is relatively safe. However, when undertaking joint aspiration, it is important to first consider a couple of factors. Look carefully for the presence of cellulitis, or psoriasis, which may affect the skin overlying a joint. It is never desirable to enter a joint through abnormal skin and, whenever possible, an alternate route should be taken. Similarly, if a patient is taking an oral anticoagulant, or is suspected of having coagulopathy, check a clotting screen before proceeding. If in doubt, seek advice from a specialist. Fluid should be aspirated and sent to microbiology for an urgent Gram stain, microscopy, and sensitivity. Fluid should also be sent to cytology for polarized light microscopy, looking for crystals of gout or pseudogout.

In cases in which further investigation is felt to be necessary, blood tests provide a useful adjunct to synovial fluid analysis. Consider performing the tests outlined in Table 62.3.

A plain radiograph must always be performed if there is a history of trauma, and may also yield diagnostic clues to the presence of other conditions (see Table 62.4).

Other diagnostic tests

Further investigations will be guided by the history and examination, and likely diagnosis (see Chapter 264). Other tests which may be helpful include X-rays of the hands and feet if involvement of these joints is revealed by the history or examination. A full sexually

Table 62.2 Specific clues to the diagnosis of acute joint pain			
Condition	**Common sites**	**Features in history**	**Features on examination**
Osteoarthritis	Weight-bearing joints; hips, knees; first CMC/MTP joints and DIP joints in hands; neck/lumbar spine	Insidious onset; lack of morning stiffness; pain worse after activity; previous trauma; weight gain	May be bony swelling, e.g. Bouchard's or Heberden's nodes; pain and crepitus on movement of a joint
Rheumatoid arthritis	Hands; involvement tends to be symmetrical; MCP joints, PIP joints, and wrists	Morning stiffness >1 hour; joint pain and swelling	May be rheumatoid nodules, typically at elbows/pressure points; 'boggy swelling'; joint effusions
Seronegative inflammatory arthritis: • psoriatic • enteropathic • reactive • ankylosing spondylitis	Hands (including DIP joints) and large joints; spine and sacroiliac joints may be affected	Recent infection; psoriasis; inflammatory bowel disease; alternating buttock pain; morning stiffness >1 hour	Asymmetrical arthritis; psoriatic plaques/nail changes; limited spinal movement; sacroiliitis; dactylitis; enthesitis; conjunctivitis/uveitis
Polyarticular/chronic tophaceous gout	Hands, large joints, first MTP joint	Family history; high alcohol/protein intake; diuretic use	Gouty tophi, particularly on ears, elbows, hands, or feet
Connective tissue diseases: • SLE • scleroderma	Hands, arthralgia more common than arthritis, may be tenosynovitis	Female gender; Raynaud's disease; skin rash; skin thickening; difficulty swallowing	Malar or photosensitive rash; sclerodactyly; correctable ulnar deviation (Jaccoud's arthropathy)
Vasculitis: • Henoch–Schonlein purpura • Wegener's granulomatosis • Churg–Strauss syndrome	Any	Systemic features, e.g. fever, malaise, weight loss	Rash; lung/abdominal/renal/neurological signs; blood/protein on urine dipstick
Septic arthritis	Any, most commonly knee or hip	Fever and systemic upset; marked pain and inability to move the affected joint	High temperature; haemodynamic compromise; single hot and swollen joint with grossly restricted movement
Gout	First MTP joint, knee, ankle, wrist, elbow	Previous attacks; family history; high alcohol intake or high purine diet; diuretic use; typically sudden onset (hours)	Joint typically erythematous and exquisitely tender; gouty tophi on affected joint, ears, elbows, or hands (in chronic gout)
Pseudogout	Knee, ankle, wrist, shoulder	Osteoarthritis; previous attacks; associated infective trigger, e.g. urinary infection or dehydration	Nodal osteoarthritis; nodal osteoarthritis; crepitus on joint examination
Monoarticular presentation of generalized arthritis (e.g. rheumatoid or psoriatic arthritis)	Any; frequently knee or hip	History of inflammatory arthritis; involvement of other joints; morning stiffness	Synovitis of other joints; rheumatoid nodules; psoriatic plaques or nail changes; dactylitis
Reactive arthritis	Any; frequently knee or hip	History of recent infection; vaginal/urethral discharge or diarrhoea; eye involvement	Conjunctivitis/uveitis; fever; vaginal/urethral discharge; sacroiliitis
Haemarthrosis	Any	Haemophilia/von Willebrand's disease or anticoagulant use; history of bleeding after minor procedures, e.g. tooth extraction	Bruising around the affected joint

Abbreviations: CMC, carpometacarpal; DIP, distal interphalangeal; MCP, metacarpophalangeal; MTP, metatarsophalangeal; PIP, proximal interphalangeal; SLE, systemic lupus erythematosus.

Table 62.3 Investigations ordered for the diagnosis of acute joint pain, with their justifications

Blood test	Reason for performing test
Blood cultures	Diagnosis of bacteraemia in suspected septic or reactive arthritis
FBC	Raised WCC in infection; reduced Hb in chronic disease, e.g. rheumatoid arthritis
Clotting screen; PT/APTT	May be prolonged in patients on warfarin or with bleeding disorders
ESR and CRP	Raised in systemic inflammation
Plasma urate	Raised in cases of gout (although caution required, as it may not be elevated during acute attack)
Plasma creatinine	Screen for renal involvement in systemic disease; also important to consider renal function before prescribing NSAIDs
Liver function tests	Screen for hepatic involvement
Rheumatoid factor/ anti-CCP antibody	May be positive in patients with rheumatoid arthritis
ANA, ANCA	Only indicated if features in the history/ examination suggest the possibility of underlying connective tissue disease or vasculitis

Abbreviations: ANA, antinuclear antibody; ANCA, antineutrophil cytoplasmic antibody; APTT, activated partial thromboplastin time; CCP, cyclic citrullinated peptide; CRP, C-reactive protein; ESR, erythrocyte sedimentation rate; FBC, full blood count; Hb, haemoglobin; NSAIDs, non-steroidal anti-inflammatory drugs; PT, partial thromboplastin time; WCC, white-cell count.

transmitted disease screen, including throat and genital swabs, is essential where reactive arthritis is suspected or there is a history of high-risk behaviour. If there are features to suggest the presence of connective tissue disease or vasculitis, a chest radiograph and urinalysis/urine microscopy must also be performed. More detailed imaging of a particular joint using CT or MRI may be useful if there is uncertainty about the diagnosis. CT scans are particularly good for looking at bone, while MRI is the modality of choice for soft tissue.

Introduction to therapy

Septic arthritis

Patients with septic arthritis should be referred to the on-call orthopaedic team for urgent review and admission. Management usually involves urgent washout of the affected joint and prolonged treatment with IV and subsequently oral antibiotics.

Idiopathic peripheral inflammatory arthritis (seropositive or seronegative rheumatoid arthritis)

Once a diagnosis of inflammatory arthritis has been given, disease-modifying anti-rheumatic drugs (DMARDs) should be started with minimal delay. These include methotrexate, sulfasalazine, leflunomide, hydroxychloroquine, and azathioprine. Many authorities now advocate early aggressive combination therapy with monitoring for

Table 62.4 Radiographic features of diseases leading to acute joint pain

Condition	Features on radiographs
Septic arthritis	Likely to be normal on presentation or may show osteopenia in surrounding bone; late changes include rapid joint destruction
Gout	Soft tissue swelling and juxta-articular erosions (areas of punched-out bone)
Pseudogout	Features of underlying osteoarthritis (joint space narrowing, osteophytes, subchondral cysts, and sclerosis); chondrocalcinosis
Rheumatoid arthritis	Erosions (areas of punched-out bone)

potential side effects such as bone marrow suppression and drug-induced hepatitis. In the appropriate clinical setting, the treatment can be stepped up to include the use of biological agents such as anti-tumour necrosis factor (anti-TNF) therapy (etanercept, adalimumab, infliximab, certolizumab, golimumab), B-cell depletion therapy (rituximab), and IL-6 blockade (tocilizumab).

Connective tissue disorders and vasculitis

There are a variety of connective tissue disorders and vasculitic syndromes, each of which require a tailored approach to treatment, depending on organ involvement. Careful and frequent follow-up allows the clinician to react appropriately to any changes in disease expression. These diseases require early specialist input to direct management. Aggressive immunosuppression may be required, as well as a range of supportive measures in the event of threat to vital organs.

Crystal arthropathies

Treatment of crystal arthropathies can be divided into two sections: the acute flare and chronic prophylaxis. The acute flare is conventionally treated with NSAIDs, colchicine, or steroids. The exact choice depends on patient-related factors such as renal function, cardiovascular disease, gastrointestinal disease, and diabetes. Chronic prophylaxis is only available to treat gout. Uric-acid-lowering therapy with allopurinol (or febuxostat, if the patient is allergic to allopurinol), a xanthine oxidase inhibitor, is the treatment of choice. It is necessary to titrate the dose of allopurinol to achieve a serum uric acid level in the lower half of the normal range. Uricosuric drugs such as sulfinpyrazone and probenecid drugs, which increase renal uric acid excretion, are generally less safe and less effective and therefore used less often. Other forms of crystal arthritis are managed by symptom control of recurrent acute flares.

Spondyloarthropathies

In the presence of purely axial disease, NSAIDs and physiotherapy have been found to be of marked benefit. DMARDs only have an impact if there is accompanying peripheral joint involvement. Where there is inadequate response to full conservative drug and non-drug measures, it is possible to escalate treatment to use anti-TNF therapy.

Prognosis

Outcomes are very variable, depending on the cause of the inflammation. Most cases will settle after a period of time with appropriate treatment. Even cases of septic arthritis can, if managed well, have good outcomes, with return to normal function. Once movement returns to an affected joint, if there has been a prolonged period of reduced activity, patients often benefit from a course of physiotherapy to help build up affected muscles.

How to handle uncertainty in the diagnosis of this symptom

Proper assessment of a patient with a hot joint requires a good history and examination. The key is not to miss a septic arthritis. Any patient suspected of having this condition must be referred urgently for further evaluation in hospital.

Removal of synovial fluid is extremely useful and should be undertaken whenever possible as it is useful therapeutically, and diagnostically.

Make sure that the patient is aware of the likely diagnosis and the anticipated duration of symptoms, and encourage them to seek further review if things don't settle as expected.

Further Reading

Russell AS and Ferrari R. 'Clinical presentation and diagnosis of rheumatic disease' in *Oxford Textbook of Medicine*, (5th edition), 2011. Oxford University Press.

Singh JA, Saag KG, Bridges SL Jr, et al. 2015 American College of Rheumatology Guideline for the treatment of rheumatoid arthritis. *Arthritis Rheumatol* 2016; 68: 1–26.

63 Muscle pain

Parthajit Das and Rachel Jeffery

Definition of the symptom

Muscle diseases constitute a large group of hereditary and acquired disorders, collectively referred to as **myopathy**. Symptoms of myopathy are muscle pain, muscle cramps or spasms, stiff or rigid muscles, and muscle weakness.

Muscle pain, or **myalgia**, is by far the most common presentation. Although most myalgia will be benign and self-limiting, it can be a reflection of underlying serious illnesses which may lead to significant morbidity. It is important to differentiate myalgia from **myopathy** (muscle disease) and **myositis** (inflammatory myopathy).

A muscle is said to be in **spasm** when it contracts involuntarily. When the spasm is forceful and sustained, it becomes a **cramp**. Muscle cramps commonly occur with dehydration, with electrolyte abnormalities (hypokalaemia, hypocalcaemia, or hypomagnesaemia) and in neurological conditions such as Parkinson's disease, motor neuron disease, radiculopathies, and polyneuropathies. They are not usually associated with primary muscle diseases.

A successful clinical approach to a patient with a muscle pain is based on a thorough medical history and clinical examination to establish the pattern and nature of the muscle symptoms.

Approach to diagnosis

What is the time course of symptoms?

The time course of the onset of myalgia can be indicative:

Acute-onset myalgia: With prominent constitutional symptoms, acute-onset myalgia suggests viral or bacterial infections or inflammatory disease, (inflammatory arthritis, connective tissue disease, vasculitis). In the older patient (>50 years), myalgia involving the neck, shoulders, and upper arms (+/− buttocks, hips, thighs) raises the possibility of polymyalgia rheumatica.
Subacute onset myalgia: This is usually seen in drug-induced myalgia (e.g. from statins) and can occur weeks to months after initiating therapy.
Chronic-onset myalgia: This is seen in endocrine myopathies, nutritional deficiency (vitamin deficiency), and chronic widespread musculoskeletal pain syndrome (fibromyalgia).

What is the distribution of muscle pain?

The distribution of muscle pain can be indicative:

Localized myalgia: Common causes are strenuous exercise or overuse. Other causes include soft tissue disease (local trauma, tendonitis, bursitis), compartment syndrome, and complex regional pain syndrome.
Generalized myalgia: This is most commonly seen in viral illnesses. When prolonged, it may suggest metabolic myopathy, inflammatory myopathy, nutritional deficiency related muscle disease (e.g. vitamin D deficiency), other autoimmune rheumatic diseases (SLE, systemic sclerosis) or chronic pain syndrome (fibromyalgia).
Referred pain: Pain can be referred to the upper limb from the neck and shoulder joint, and to the lower limb and thigh from the spine and hip joints.
Proximal muscle pain: This is a feature of inflammatory muscle disease (especially dermatomyositis), endocrine myopathy, and vitamin D deficiency.

Is there associated muscle weakness?

Associated muscle weakness can be indicative of a number of conditions:

- Muscle weakness can occur with chronic disuse, neurological disorder, and muscle disease and it can be difficult to distinguish between these on examination alone.

- Neuropathies, inflammatory myopathies, toxic myopathies, and endocrine myopathies may present with pain and weakness.
- Patients with 'true' muscle weakness will struggle to perform specific tasks such as rising from sitting without support, raising their head off the pillow, walking upstairs, lifting their arm above the shoulder, combing their hair, or holding a glass of water.
- Muscle wasting can occur with muscle weakness (an exception is Duchenne muscular dystrophy with calf hypertrophy), disuse, and lower motor neuron lesions.
- Involvement of pharyngeal, thoracic, diaphragmatic, or sphincteric muscles indicates systemic disease and can be life-threatening.

Is there associated muscle stiffness?

Associated muscle stiffness can be indicative of a number of conditions:

- Muscle pain along with stiffness is usually associated with inflammatory muscle disease.
- There is muscle stiffness with weakness in myositis (as seen in polymyositis and dermatomyositis).
- There is muscle stiffness without weakness in polymyalgia rheumatica and fibromyalgia (non-inflammatory chronic pain syndrome).
- Parkinson's disease can also present with muscle pain and stiffness.

Does the clinical picture suggest an inflammatory or non-inflammatory myopathy?

Features suggestive of inflammatory muscle disease are:

- symmetrical proximal muscle weakness
- stiffness

Features suggestive of non-inflammatory muscle disease are:

- a family history of myopathy (storage diseases, genetic myopathies and neuropathies)
- muscle weakness/cramps worsened by exercise or dietary change, for example, fasting or excess carbohydrate intake (metabolic myopathies)
- drug history (statins, zidovudine, alcohol, steroid, vincristine, colchicines, etc.)
- muscle atrophy, hypertrophy, or myotonia (e.g. Duchenne and Becker's muscular dystrophy, myotonic dystrophy)
- fasciculation and other neurological signs

Are there clinical signs pointing to a specific aetiology of myopathy?

A thorough examination may reveal important clues as to the aetiology of myopathy, such as:

- cushingoid habitus, steroid purpura (exogenous steroids or Cushing's disease)
- myxoedema changes (thyroid disease); hyperpigmentation (Addison's disease)
- malar rash (SLE); sclerodactyly, digital infarcts, telangiectasia, (systemic sclerosis); heliotrope rash, Gottron's papules, mechanic's hands, calcinosis (dermatomyositis); livedo reticularis, purpura, digital infarcts (vasculitis)
- joint involvement (degenerative or inflammatory joint disease)
- absent peripheral pulses (peripheral vascular disease, arteritis, compartment syndrome)

Box 63.1 Causes of a raised creatine kinase level

Traumatic causes
- trauma
- crush injury
- electrical injury

Non-traumatic causes

Infection
- bacterial pyomyositis
- systemic bacterial infection
- viral infection
- falciparum malaria

Electrolyte abnormalities
- hypokalaemia
- hypophosphataemia

Immune mediated
- dermatomyositis
- polymyositis

Drugs/toxins (common causes)
- statins
- colchicine
- alcohol
- cocaine
- amphetamine

Metabolic disorders
- myophosphorylase deficiency
- phosphofructokinase deficiency
- carnitine palmitoyltransferase deficiency

Others
- status epilepticus
- coma of any cause with muscle compression
- compartment syndrome
- acute myocardial infarction
- hypothermia
- diabetic ketoacidosis and hyperosmolar non-ketotic
- hyperglycaemia
- hypothyroidism
- neuroleptic malignant syndrome
- malignant hyperthermia
- drowning
- prolonged strenuous exercise

- lymphadenopathy/hepatosplenomegaly (infectious disease: EBV, HIV; autoimmune rheumatic disease: SLE, sarcoidosis)
- evidence of malignancy (which can be associated with inflammatory muscle disease)

Key diagnostic tests

All patients with muscle pain should have the following tests:

- full blood count, which may show the anaemia of chronic inflammatory disease, leucopenia (SLE, HIV), or thrombocytopenia (SLE)
- erythrocyte sedimentation rate and C-reactive protein
- biochemical profile
- plasma creatine kinase level (see Box 63.1)
- thyroid function tests
- urinalysis and urine microscopy (to screen for myoglobinuria and evidence of vasculitis)
- chest radiography (consolidation, malignancy, interstitial lung disease, pleural or pericardial effusions, hilar lymphadenopathy, pseudofractures)

Further investigation

Further investigation will be directed by the clinical features and findings on key diagnostic tests:

- spirometry, if there is systemic involvement or respiratory symptoms (reduced forced vital capacity with diaphragmatic weakness; requires close monitoring and ventilatory support if compromise results)
- infection screen (blood cultures, HIV, hepatitis serology, borrelia)
- cortisol level, dexamethasone suppression test (Cushing's disease), tetracosactide test (Addison's), parathyroid hormone level
- autoantibodies (antinuclear antibody (ANA), extractable nuclear antigen antibody (ENA), anti-double-stranded DNA antibody (dsDNA), rheumatoid factor, anti-citrullinated protein antibody (anti-CCP); antineutrophil cytoplasmic antibody (ANCA), if vasculitis suspected)
- echocardiography (assess myocardial function re possible cardiac involvement, ischaemic, cardiomyopathy, pericardial effusion, valvular abnormality)
- MRI scan brain and/or spine (exclude central neurological cause)
- electromyography and nerve conduction studies (helpful to distinguish primary muscle disease, neuropathy, or inflammatory myopathy)
- MRI muscles, T2-weighted/fat-suppressed STIR sequence (can show muscle inflammation, atrophy, or fat infiltration and guide best site for muscle biopsy)
- muscle biopsy; open sample is best (for diagnosis of primary muscle disease and inflammatory myositis)

See Parts 10 and 12 for disease-specific information.

Further Reading

Kyriakides T, Angelini C, Schaefer J, et al. EFNS review on the role of muscle biopsy in the investigation of myalgia. *Eur J Neurol* 2013; 20: 997–1005.
Manji H, Connolly S, Kitchen N, et al. *Oxford Handbook of Neurology* (2nd edition), 2014. Oxford University Press.

64 Low back pain

Elaine Buchanan and Chris Lavy

Definition of the symptom

Low back pain (LBP) is pain arising from the structures of the lumbar spine, including joints, discs, connective tissue, and nerves. Symptoms include pain and muscle tightness or stiffness, with or without referral of pain to the legs.

Differential diagnosis

Most (95%) of LBP is managed in primary care; the rest is managed in secondary care (see Table 64.1).

Context

LBP affects nearly everyone at some point in their life and has an annual prevalence of around 40%. It is less common in children but from age 16 onwards the point prevalence for all age groups is around 25%. Many experience milder persisting symptoms interspersed with exacerbations, and 7% of adults have persisting LBP, which restricts function. With an aging and less fit population, this situation is unlikely to improve.

LBP is one of the most prevalent musculoskeletal conditions presenting to healthcare. It accounts for 4% of all GP consultations and 5% of all NHS specialist referrals. The main reasons for seeking healthcare are to gain an understanding of the problem, to obtain a prognosis, and for symptom relief.

LBP is the leading cause of occupational disability and missed workdays. Although not more prevalent, it is most bothersome in the working age population and accounts for 13.5% of UK incapacity benefit.

Degenerative changes of lumbar spinal structures are commonly found in both asymptomatic and symptomatic populations. The relationship between radiological findings and specific diagnoses is weak.

The key to management is to identify and refer onwards the minority with serious and surgical presentations and to reassure, advise to remain active, and provide symptomatic relief for the others.

Approach to diagnosis

The approach to diagnosis includes the following:

- history, and examination of back, neurology in legs, and abdomen
- exclude non-spinal causes of back pain (e.g. disease of the kidneys or abdominal aorta, gynaecological disease)
- categorize spinal back pain into:
  - serious spinal pathology (e.g. fracture, neoplasm, inflammatory disease, cauda equina syndrome, infection)
  - non-specific LBP (NSLBP)
  - radicular pain
  - neurogenic claudication

The information needed to categorize patients is mainly found in the subjective history.

Serious spinal pathology

It is important to first identify or rule out the possibility of serious spinal pathology. Delayed or misdiagnosis has a major impact on patient survival, quality of life, and clinical outcome and may result in medical negligence litigation. Red flags (Box 64.1) are recommended internationally as a system for screening for serious spinal pathology. It is important to remember that the presence of one red flag is common but the incidence of serious spinal pathologies is rare. Independently, some red flags are more predictive than others and should always result in further investigation. The predictive utility of other red flags is individually low but significantly increases when used in combination.

Inflammatory back pain

Inflammatory back pain is worse after prolonged rest and relieved by exercise. It is therefore worse in the morning and is associated with prolonged morning stiffness of the back of greater than 30 minutes (often several hours). Occasionally, there is an associated peripheral inflammatory arthritis, which helps to clarify the underlying inflammatory pathophysiology. Inflammatory arthritis of the spine is referred to as spondyloarthritis or spondylitis. The commonest cause of spondyloarthritis is ankylosing spondylitis—a condition typically causing chronic inflammation of both sacroiliac joints (sacroiliitis) and associated with progressive calcification of the spinal ligaments, resulting in

---

Table 64.1 Low back pain diagnosis in primary and secondary care, in order of frequency

Diagnosis in primary care	Frequency (%)	Diagnosis in secondary care	Frequency (%)
Non-specific low back pain	80	Neurogenic claudication	35
Radicular pain	10	Radicular pain	30
Neurogenic claudication	7	Non-specific low back pain	25
Serious spine pathology	3	Serious spine pathology	10

Box 64.1 Red flags in screening for serious spinal pathology

Strong red flags (always investigate)
- past history of cancer
- unexplained weight loss >10% of body weight
- widespread neurology
- known osteoporosis
- erythrocyte sedimentation rate >50, packed cell volume <30
- under age 16
- recent significant trauma
- penetrating wound near spine
- recent bacterial infection

Weak red flags (but which in combination raise suspicion)
- age 16–20
- age >50
- non-mechanical pain
- thoracic pain
- local pain or tenderness
- past history of steroids
- past history of substance abuse
- immunosupression
- clinician judgment
- >1/12 duration, no response to treatment

Cauda equina syndrome (emergency referral)
A combination of:
- saddle anaesthesia
- recent onset of bladder dysfunction
- recent onset of faecal disturbance
- reduced anal tone

Note: MRI is the investigation of choice.

Box 64.2 Yellow, blue, and black flags for identifying people at increased risk of non-specific low back pain

Yellow flags (personal risk factors)

Thoughts
- negative thinking
- dysfunctional belief about pain, prognosis and cure
- health anxiety

Feelings
- emotional distress (anxiety, depression)
- fear of movement or damage

Behaviours
- passive coping strategies
- healthcare shopping without effect

Blue flags (occupational risk factors)

Employee
- high physical job demands
- low expectation of return to work
- low job satisfaction
- belief that work is harmful

Workplace
- lack of employer support
- lack of work modification

Black flags (social risk factors)
- financial and compensation issues
- interpretation of media reports
- reaction of friends and family
- social dysfunction
- national/workplace policies

progressive spinal fusion. Inflammatory spinal pain should be referred for evaluation by a specialist multidisciplinary rheumatology team. Several other diseases associated with HLA-B27 can also present with spinal or sacroiliac inflammation:

- psoriatic arthritis (spondylitis type)
- reactive arthritis
- arthritis related to inflammatory bowel disease (associated with Crohn's disease and ulcerative colitis)
- undifferentiated spondyloarthritis (may have several features of the conditions in this list)

In addition to articular symptoms, these patients often have enthesitis at multiple sites (e.g. Achilles tendon insertion, plantar fascia).

NSLBP

The largest diagnostic group is NSLBP, where it is back pain that dominates. Symptoms may or may not be referred to the leg, but are not associated with any neurological abnormality. Currently there is no reliable system for subclassification of NSLBP. Psychosocial factors are more predictive of long-term LBP related disability than biomedical factors. The use of yellow, blue, and black flags to classify factors (Box 64.2) is an internationally recognized method of identifying people at increased risk. The most effective psychosocial screening employs a battery of questionnaires (self-reported disability, health beliefs, and emotional distress) used in combination with a thorough consultation. Early identification of those at risk, at 6–8 weeks from onset, is fundamental, to prevent disability becoming established. Spinal imaging may exclude other pathology but does not influence the diagnosis, management, or outcome in NSLBP.

Radicular pain

Leg-dominant pain referring in a dermatomal distribution is categorized as radicular pain and there may also be neurological deficits of sensation, power, or reflexes, correlating with the symptomatic dermatome. It is important to look for signs of cauda equina syndrome, saddle anaesthesia, bladder/bowel disturbance, and anal tone. A positive straight leg raise is suggestive of disc protrusion but low specificity limits its usefulness. Early spinal imaging (around 6 weeks) is helpful in patients who wish to proceed to invasive management. The commonest cause of radicular pain is disc herniation.

Neurogenic claudication

Neurogenic claudication secondary to spinal stenosis results in leg-dominant symptoms which severely restrict walking but are eased by sitting. The leg symptoms are commonly non-dermatomal and described as cramp, heaviness, or generalized lower-limb weakness. Many patients have a good range of spinal flexion, normal straight leg raise, and intact neurology. Spinal imaging is clinically helpful in patients with concerning neurological deficits and in those having had symptoms for greater than 6 months and who wish to consider invasive management.

Specific clues to the diagnosis

See Table 64.2 for specific clues to the diagnosis.

Table 64.2 Specific clues to the diagnosis of non-specific low back pain, radicular pain, neurogenic claudication, and serious pathologies

	Non-specific low back pain	Radicular pain	Neurogenic claudication	Serious pathology
Age	>16 years	>18 years	Developmental stenosis at >30 years; acquired stenosis at >50 years	Any age, but especially at <16 and >55 years
Onset	Variable	Variable	Gradual	Variable
Back pain	Yes	Leg pain dominates	Leg pain dominates	Yes
Leg pain	Back pain dominates	Unilateral, dermatomal; most commonly L5 or S1	Foramenal stenosis: unilateral and dermatomal; canal stenosis: bilateral and non-dermatomal	Dependant on location of pathology
Activity	Mechanical pattern	Mechanical pattern	Worse with walking and standing; eases with sitting	Variable
Lumbar range of movement	Global restriction	Restricted forward flexion	Restricted extension	Variable
Neurological deficit	No	Correlating with the affected nerve root	Neurological signs at or below the stenotic level	Dependant on location of pathology
Straight leg raise	Normal	Reduced	Normal	Variable
Saddle anaesthesia	Nil	Possible in cauda equina syndrome	Rare	Dependant on location of pathology
Bladder/bowel dysfunction	Nil	Possible in cauda equina syndrome	20% report bladder dysfunction	Dependant on location of pathology

Table 64.3 Imaging of choice compared with diagnostic categories duration of pain

Diagnostic category	Duration	Imaging of choice
Past history of cancer	Any	Limited MRI whole spine
Leg-dominant pain (moderate or severe)	>6 weeks	Full MRI lumbar spine
Under age 16	Any	Limited MRI thoracolumbar spine
Acute deformity in older people	Any	Limited MRI thoracolumbar spine
Neurogenic claudication (moderate or severe)	>6 months	Full MRI lumbar spine
Inflammatory spinal disease	Any	Limited MRI; thoracolumbar and sacrum
Non-specific low back pain	Only after optimal conservative management	Limited MRI lumbar spine
Infection	Any	Limited MRI thoracolumbar
Painful osteoporotic collapse	Any	Limited MRI thoracolumbar with axial views through level of collapse

Key diagnostic tests

Diagnostic tests are only useful if they change the diagnosis, management, or outcome of LBP (Table 64.3). It is the correlation between symptoms, clinical findings, and diagnostic tests that is important. This is especially relevant because of the prevalence of abnormal imaging findings in the asymptomatic population.

When diagnostic tests are clinically indicated, MRI is the gold standard for investigating most pathologies. It is superior at demonstrating soft tissue, more sensitive at differentiating between neoplastic disease, infection, and osteoporotic spinal pathologies, and images more planes, compared to other radiology tests. CT is the best for investigation of bony pathologies and in patients where MRI is contraindicated.

Limited MRI (sagittal T1 and STIR images) is a highly sensitive and cost-effective investigation for suspected serious spinal pathologies and potential surgical candidates with back dominant pain. Full MRI (sagittal and axial T1 and T2 images) is indicated for patients with clinical signs of cauda equina or radicular involvement, who are potential candidates for surgery or therapeutic spinal injection.

A warning: in patients with lower limb weakness, with a past history of cancer or upper motor neuron lesions, it is important to scan the whole spine. We have seen too many patients with paraplegia who have only had lumbar spine imaging.

In contrast, the clinical value of diagnostic tests for NSLBP is limited by the high prevalence of spinal degenerative radiological findings in asymptomatic individuals. Imaging does not change the diagnosis, management, or outcome for patients with NSLBP but is associated with higher healthcare costs. There is a morbidity associated with the communication of radiological findings, which may result in increased anxiety or delay return to normal activities. Surgical rates have been shown to be higher when imaging rates are higher, but no better clinical outcomes are achieved.

Other diagnostic tests

In a small number of patients, diagnostic tests, in addition to imaging, help with differential diagnosis. Nerve conduction studies are useful where a neurological weakness is found on examination, but not explained by spinal imaging. Nerve root blocks are informative for surgical planning where potentially significant nerve root pathology exists at more than one level on MRI. Although occasionally used, the popularity of discography has reduced because of low specificity and because it may hasten disc degeneration.

In addition to imaging, laboratory tests can be useful where cancer, infection, or inflammatory disease is suspected.

Introduction to treatment

UK, European, and American guidelines clearly outline evidence-based management of acute and chronic non-specific LBP with or without radicular pain or neurogenic claudication.

The only surgical emergencies are cauda equina syndrome and pathologies resulting in cord compression.

In the absence of concerning red flags, acute LBP with or without leg pain is usually self-limiting. Early management includes reassurance and medication. Return to normal activities is actively encouraged. Patient information, such as *The Back Book*, should reinforce self management.

Persisting non-specific LBP is a condition we can treat but not cure. Modern management emphasizes self-care. Evidence-based patient information and pain relief are key. For those who continue to seek healthcare, exercise and manual therapy, are recommended. These interventions have evidence of small-to-moderate benefit. In patients with persisting disability and/or distress, who have not responded to the initial core therapies, referral to an intensive combined physical and psychological programme (CPPP) is recommended. CPPP optimizes quality of life and the potential to return to some form of meaningful work. A small number of those who have severe pain post CPPP may be considered for spinal fusion. Fusion offers small-to-moderate benefit in some patients who have not been helped by CPPP, but the complication rate is high (16%). NICE NG59 recommend that fusion should only be offered as part of a randomised controlled trial.

In radicular pain due to disc herniation and persisting beyond 6 weeks, surgery offers quick relief of leg pain and return to function. Early surgery is also recommended for those with progressive neurological deficit. Therapeutic injections, including nerve root blocks and epidurals, are useful in patients with severe leg pain but who are not suitable for surgery. The success rate of injection is only around 50%. Decisions regarding invasive treatment should take account both the fact that benefits may be relatively short term and the tendency for patients to improve either with or without intervention.

Although evidence is limited, conservative treatment for neurogenic claudication have been shown to be beneficial. When severe symptoms persist beyond 6 months, surgical decompression can be helpful in improving quality of life. The benefits of surgery however tend to tail off after 2 years.

Prognosis

In general, the clinical course of acute NSLBP and radicular pain is favourable: 80% of patients who present for healthcare during an acute attack improve sufficiently to return to normal activities within the first 6 weeks, and stop consulting healthcare within 3 months. Further improvement beyond 6 weeks is slower, and 62% continue to have symptoms at 1 year. Back pain symptoms commonly fluctuate over time, and recurrences of variable severity are common.

Around 7% of those with NSLBP are at risk of long-term pain-related disability. Without CPPP, people who have established LBP-related disability have a very bleak long-term prognosis.

Neurogenic claudication has an unfortunate long-term prognosis in that 70% will have persisting symptoms of a similar severity, 15% will improve, and 15% will worsen over time.

How to handle uncertainty in the diagnosis of this symptom

The only certainty with back pain is that most of us will get it. First, it is essential to minimize risk by identifying the small number with serious pathology, through:

- use of red flags to raise diagnostic suspicion of serious spinal pathology
- early referral or investigation of those concerning red flags
- remembering that most of those with red flags will not have serious spinal pathology
- keeping diagnosis under review for those who continue to seek healthcare

Thereafter, we can be confident that the risk of overlooking serious spinal pathology is highly unlikely. For the remainder, diagnostic uncertainty is the norm; thus, symptom-based classifications are used. It is the symptomology that drives management decisions. It is good management that optimizes outcome. Note that:

- conservative management is appropriate for most LBP
- the presence of leg-dominant pain with or without neurological deficits will more likely be suitable for an invasive procedure
- in leg-dominant pain, a strong correlation between the clinical presentation and diagnostic imaging improves diagnostic certainty
- non-specific LBP is a diagnosis by exclusion; despite extensive research, correlations between diagnostic imaging and symptomology remain weak and, while diagnostic theories have been proposed, no gold-standard test exists

Further Reading

Chou R, Qaseem A, Snow V, et al. Diagnosis and treatment of low back pain: A joint clinical practice guideline from the American College of Physicians and the American Pain Society. *Annals of Int Med* 2007; 147: 478–91.

Maher C, Underwood M, and Buchbinder R. Non-specific low back pain. *Lancet* 2017; 389: 736–47.

National Institute for Health and Care Excellence. *Low Back Pain and Sciatica*. 2016. Available at https://www.nice.org.uk/guidance/ng59/evidence/full-guideline-assessment-and-noninvasive-treatments-pdf-2726158003.

Qaseem A, Wilt TJ, McClean RM, and Forciea MA. Noninvasive treatments for acute, subacute, and chronic low back pain: A clinical practice guideline from the American College of Physicians. *Ann Intern Med* 2017; 166: 514–30.

65 Painful leg

Benjamin Bloch and David Sprigings

Definition of the symptom

The leg (more accurately called the lower limb) extends from the gluteal region to the foot. Pain in the leg may reflect disease of its constituent bones, joints, soft tissues, or neurovascular supply, or be referred from diseases of the spine.

Differential diagnosis

The differential diagnosis of leg pain is given in Table 65.1.

Table 65.1 Differential diagnosis of leg pain

Tissue/ structure	Acute leg pain	Chronic leg pain
Skin and subcutaneous tissues	Erysipelas Cellulitis Necrotizing fasciitis Hypersensitivity reaction to insect sting or bite Contact dermatitis	Ulceration (venous, arterial, or mixed aetiology) Post-phlebitic syndrome
Arteries	Acute ischaemia	Chronic ischaemia Popliteal artery entrapment syndrome
Veins	Superficial thrombophlebitis Deep vein thrombosis Phlegmasia cerulea dolens	Post-phlebitic syndrome
Nerves	Acute neuropathies, including Guillain-Barre syndrome Acute radiculopathies Herpes zoster	Chronic neuropathies Peroneal nerve entrapment Neurospinous claudication
Muscles	Localized • strain injury (partial tear) • contusion injury (direct impact) • intramuscular haematoma • intramuscular abscess • tendon rupture • compartment syndrome Generalized • systemic infection • acute myositis • acute vasculitis	Localized • chronic exertional compartment syndrome Generalized • metabolic, inflammatory, or nutritional-deficiency myopathies • autoimmune rheumatic diseases (e.g. SLE) • polymyalgia rheumatica • fibromyalgia
Joints	Fracture Meniscal or ligamentous injury Acute arthritis Acute bursitis Ruptured Baker (popliteal) cyst (may complicate rheumatoid arthritis or osteoarthritis of the knee)	Osteoarthritis Chronic inflammatory arthritis
Bones	Subperiosteal haematoma Fracture Osteomyelitis	Primary or metastatic cancer Infection Stress fracture Medial tibial stress syndrome Loosened hip or knee replacement Osteomyelitis

Context

Acute leg pain (symptoms present for <2 weeks) is a medical emergency, as it may signify disease (e.g. acute ischaemia, necrotizing fasciitis, deep vein thrombosis) which is a threat to life or the viability of the limb.

Approach to diagnosis

Diagnosis begins with determining whether pain is felt in one leg or both, its principal site and radiation, and the time course of symptoms. Establish if there has been preceding trauma or fall and if the patient is known to have arterial disease, diabetes, or other systemic disease. Are there risk factors for venous thrombosis (see Chapter 101)? Has the patient had previous surgery to the leg? Is there associated weakness, sensory impairment, back pain, or sphincter disturbance?

General examination should include standard physiological observations. Is the patient febrile? Is there evidence of haemodynamic instability (which may reflect sepsis or pulmonary embolism)? Does the patient look well, acutely ill, or chronically unwell? The legs should be examined systematically (Table 65.2), front and back, comparing one side with the other.

Specific clues to diagnosis

Skin and subcutaneous tissues

Cellulitis

Cellulitis is an acute, spreading, bacterial infection of the dermis and subcutaneous tissue, usually complicating a wound, ulcer, or primary skin disorder. Other predisposing factors include previous episodes of cellulitis, lymphoedema, and vein harvest for coronary artery bypass grafting. Involved skin is erythematous, tender, warm, and swollen, without sharp demarcation from surrounding areas.

Erysipelas

Erysipelas is a more superficial infection of the dermis and epidermis. It is clinically distinguished from cellulitis by a more clearly demarcated border.

Table 65.2 Examination of the leg

Tissue/ structure	Diagnostic features
Skin and subcutaneous tissues	Swelling; oedema; discolouration; rash; blister, ulcer or abscess formation; tenderness; induration; crepitus; temperature difference; lymphangitis
Arteries	Arterial pulses normal, reduced, or absent; femoral bruit; prolonged capillary refill; ischaemic lesions of the feet
Veins	Superficial thrombophlebitis; localized tenderness over the deep veins
Nerves	Muscle power; tendon reflexes; light touch and pinprick sensation
Muscles	Localized or diffuse swelling or tenderness
Joints	Swelling around the joint; presence of effusion; increased temperature of the joint; reduced range of movement; instability; tenderness
Bones	Alignment (normal, angled, or rotated); localized swelling; localized tenderness

Necrotizing fasciitis

Necrotizing fasciitis, a rapidly progressive infection of the deep fascia and muscle, is rare but should be suspected in an ill patient with severe leg pain disproportionate to the physical signs. The skin may be very tender, with blue-black discolouration and blistering.

Arteries

Acute ischaemia

Acute ischaemia is recognized by leg pain and paraesthesiae, with absent arterial pulses. The skin distal to the occlusion is cool and may be pale or mottled. Causes of acute limb ischemia include acute thrombosis of a limb artery or bypass graft; embolism from the heart or a proximal arterial aneurysm; aortic dissection with involvement of the limb artery; and trauma (e.g. arterial puncture or cannulation). Findings on neurological examination (sensory loss/muscle weakness) and Doppler assessment of arterial and venous flow stratify the degree of ischaemia and guide further management. If acute limb ischaemia is suspected, give heparin 5000 units intravenously over 5 minutes, followed by an IV infusion, and seek urgent advice from a vascular surgeon.

Chronic ischaemia

Chronic ischaemia may be asymptomatic or may present with intermittent claudication: pain, aching, muscle stiffness, or fatigue of the affected areas on exercise and relieved by a few minutes' rest. In aortoiliac disease, symptoms typically occur in the buttocks, thighs, and calves. In superficial femoral artery disease, the calves only are affected. Features distinguishing intermittent claudication from other causes of chronic leg pain associated with exercise are shown in Table 65.3.

Veins

Deep vein thrombosis

Deep vein thrombosis (DVT) should be considered in every patient with leg pain, and may complicate other disorders such as cellulitis.

Table 65.3 Differential diagnosis of intermittent claudication

Condition	Location	Prevalence	Characteristic	Effect of exercise	Effect of rest	Effect of position	Other characteristic
Calf IC	Calf muscles	3% of adult population	Cramping, aching discomfort	Reproducible onset	Quickly relieved	None	May have atypical limb symptoms on exercise
Thigh and buttock IC	Buttocks, hip, thigh	Rare	Cramping, aching, discomfort	Reproducible onset	Quickly relieved	None	Impotence. May have normal pedal pulses with isolated iliac artery disease
Foot IC	Foot arch	Rare	Severe pain on exercise	Reproducible onset	Quickly relieved	None	Also may present as numbness
Chronic compartment syndrome	Calf muscles	Rare	Right, bursting pain	After much exercise (jogging)	Subsides very slowly	Relief with elevation	Typically heavy muscled athletes
Venous claudication	Entire leg, worse in calf	Rare	Tight, bursting pain	After walking	Subsides slowly	Relief speeded by elevation	History of iliofemoral deep vein thrombosis, signs of venous congestion, edema
Nerve root compression	Radiates down leg	Common Sharp lancinating pain	Induced by sitting, standing, or walking	Often present at rest	Improved b change in position	History of back problems. Worse with sitting. Relief when supine or sitting. Not intermittent	
Symptomatic Baker cyst	Behind knee, down calf	Rare	Swelling, tenderness	With exercise	Present at rest	None	Not intermittent
Hip arthritis	Lateral hip, thigh	Common	Aching discomfort	After variable degree of exercise	Not quickly relieved	Improved when not weight bearing	Symptoms variable. History of degenerative arthritis
Spinal stenosis	Often bilateral buttocks, posterior leg	Common	Pain and weakness	May mimic IC	Variable relief but can take a long time to recover	Relief by lumbar spine flexion	Worse with standing and extending spine
Foot/ankle arthritis	Ankle, foot, arch	Common	Aching pain	After variable degree of exercise	Not quickly relieved	May be relieved by not bearing weight	Variable, may relate to activity level and present at rest

Abbreviations: IC, intermittent claudication.

Reprinted from *Journal of Vascular Surgery*, Volume 61, issue 3, Society for Vascular Surgery practice guidelines for atherosclerotic occlusive disease of the lower extremities: Management of asymptomatic disease and claudication , Michael S. Conte et al., pp. 2S-41S.e1, Copyright 2015 with permission from Elsevier.

2) *Adapted from Journal of Vascular Surgery*, Volume 45, issue 1, InterSociety Consensus for the Management of Peripheral Arterial Disease (TASC II), L. Norgren, W.R. Hiatt, J.A. Dormandy, M.R. Nehler, K.A. Harris, F.G.R. Fowkes, pp. S5-67 Copyright 2007, with permission from Elsevier.

Table 65.4 Wells score to determine the clinical probability of deep vein thrombosis

Variable	Points
History	
Active cancer (treatment on-going, or within previous 6 months, or palliative)	1
Paralysis, paresis or recent plaster immobilization of the legs	1
Recently bed-ridden for more than 3 days, or major surgery within 4 weeks	1
Examination	
Entire leg swollen	1
Calf swelling by >3 cm when compared with asymptomatic leg (measured 10 cm below tibial tuberosity)	1
Pitting edema (greater in the symptomatic leg)	1
Localized tenderness along the distribution of the deep venous system	1
Collateral superficial veins (non-varicose)	1
Alternative diagnosis	
Alternative diagnosis as likely or more likely than DVT?	−2
Clinical probability (prevalence of DVT)	Score
Low (<5%)	0 or less
Intermediate	1–2
High (>60%)	>3

Abbreviations: DVT, deep-vein thrombosis.

Reprinted from The Lancet, Volume 350, issue 9094, Philip S Wells,David R Anderson,Janis Bormanis,Fred Guy,Michael Mitchell,Lisa Gray,Cathy Clement,K Sue Robinson,Bernard Lewandowski, Value of assessment of pretest probability of deep-vein thrombosis in clinical management, pp. 1795-1798, Copyright (1997), with permission from Elsevier.

The Wells score (Table 65.4), based on specific features in the clinical assessment, is a validated method of determining the probability of DVT. This guides investigation (see Chapter 101).

Phlegmasia cerulea dolens

Phlegmasia cerulea dolens is a syndrome due to extensive iliofemoral DVT with occlusion of collateral veins. This results in a marked increase in capillary pressure in the leg, with resultant fluid extravasation. The leg is painful, grossly swollen, and cyanotic. Venous gangrene may develop.

Nerves

Peripheral neuropathy

Pain may be a feature of many peripheral neuropathies (see Chapter 234), notably those due to diabetes and alcohol.

Spinal disorders with referred pain

Spinal disorders with referred pain should be considered if no pathology is evident in the leg: these include isolated nerve root compression with radiculopathy, and spinal stenosis with neurospinous claudication (see Chapter 233).

Muscles

The assessment of muscle pain is discussed in Chapter 63.

Acute generalized muscle pain

Acute generalized muscle pain with prominent constitutional symptoms is most commonly due to systemic infection.

Chronic generalized muscle pain

Chronic generalized muscle pain is seen in metabolic, inflammatory, and nutritional-deficiency myopathies, autoimmune rheumatic diseases (e.g. systemic lupus erythematosus), and patients with chronic pain syndromes such as fibromyalgia.

Polymyalgia rheumatica

Polymyalgia rheumatica typically presents in a person aged over 50 (peak incidence between 70 and 80) with bilateral aching and morning stiffness in the neck, shoulders, upper arms, hips, and thighs. The pain is exacerbated by activity, and is often associated with systemic features including fever, malaise, and weight loss. The erythrocyte sedimentation rate is typically at least 40 mm per hour.

Compartment syndrome

Compartment syndrome is defined as increased pressure within a myofascial space (most often tibial), compromising the circulation and function of tissues within that space. It typically follows trauma, particularly fractures, crush injuries, and burns, but can also follow IV drug administration or arterial puncture. Unrelieved, it causes acute ischaemia and thus threatens the viability of the limb. In a patient at risk, if there is pain which is worse on stretching the muscles within the affected compartment, there should be a high clinical suspicion of compartment syndrome and immediate orthopaedic review should be sought. The diagnosis can be confirmed with compartment pressure monitoring, and the treatment is emergent decompression of the affected compartment by fasciotomy.

Bones and joints

The assessment of acute joint pain is discussed in Chapter 62.

Septic arthritis

Septic arthritis is usually the result of haematogenous spread, but may result from adjacent osteomyelitis. Systemic upset, fever, severe pain, and grossly restricted range of movement of the joint raise the possibility of this diagnosis, and should trigger urgent referral to an orthopaedic surgeon. Diagnosis should be made by prompt aspiration of the joint (before antibiotic treatment is commenced).

Reactive arthritis

Reactive arthritis may be triggered by a range of viral or bacterial infections, and can occur in response to sexually transmitted infection, giving the triad of arthritis, conjunctivitis, and non-specific urethritis.

Hip pain

Pain arising from the hip joint typically gives rise to groin pain, which can radiate to the knee, but may be felt only around the knee. Hip pain is usually due to osteo- or inflammatory arthritis, but can result from bony metastases or stress fractures in athletes. The hip is a deep joint and is difficult to palpate. The greater trochanter is felt laterally, and tenderness here may indicate trochanteric bursitis. Movement should be assessed in flexion, extension, abduction, adduction, and internal and external rotation. If there is a significant effusion, such as in septic arthritis, then the hip is held flexed, abducted, and externally rotated, as this position maximizes capsular volume, and any movement is extremely painful. In fractured neck of femur, the typical presentation is with a shortened, externally rotated leg, but this is not always seen.

Knee pain

Pain arising from the knee joint generally localizes to the joint lines around the knee, or more anteriorly in patellofemoral problems. It may be associated with an effusion. Knee pain in younger patients is usually due to injury to the menisci and ligaments, but may also result from patella dislocation, osteochondral fracture, or avulsion fracture. In older patients (>50 years), arthritis is the major cause of knee pain. Look for the presence of an effusion or for a boggy swelling of the pre- or infrapatellar areas; the latter may be consistent with a bursitis. Feel for warmth compared with the other side. Tenderness may be felt over the joint lines. Move the knee and compare it with the other side, particularly with respect to extension; when the unaffected knee can hyperextend but the affected knee does not, this represents a loss of extension. There may be audible or palpable crepitus on movement.

Ankle pain

Pain arising from the ankle joint is generally felt as a band over the anterior surface of the ankle. The ankle has stabilizing ligamentous structures—the medial deltoid ligament and the lateral ligament complex. Both of these may be damaged as a result of trauma and can give rise to pain in the chronic situation.

Foot pain

The foot is a complex structure consisting of the hindfoot (calcaneus and talus), midfoot (tarsal bones), and forefoot (metatarsals and phalanges). In cases of foot pain, careful clinical examination should give you clues as to where the pain is arising, with maximal tenderness over the affected area. Morton's neuroma may be associated with a 'Mulder's click' sign on compression of the metatarsal heads.

Long bone pain

Pain arising from the long bones—the femur and tibia—is uncommon, and may be caused by primary or metastatic tumours, infection, stress fractures, and loosened hip or knee replacements.

Key diagnostic tests

Diagnostic tests are determined by the likely pathology (Table 65.5). Additional tests needed for management may include measurement of a full blood count, C-reactive protein, erythrocyte sedimentation rate, biochemical profile, creatine kinase, and blood glucose. Blood culture should be done if systemic sepsis is suspected.

Introduction to therapy

Therapy is determined by the working diagnosis.

Prognosis

The prognosis for viability of the leg and survival depend on the causative disease, the speed with which the diagnosis is made, and the response to treatment. Many causes of acute leg pain need multidisciplinary management to achieve a good outcome, and the appropriate surgical opinion should be promptly sought.

How to handle uncertainty

Uncertainty most commonly arises from leg pain without characteristic clinical features. In patients with no abnormal signs evident, consider DVT, small-fibre neuropathies, bone disease, and referred pain from the spine.

Table 65.5 Diagnostic tests in leg pain	
Suspected site of disease	**Key diagnostic tests**
Skin and subcutaneous tissues	Microscopy and culture of samples from areas of ulceration
	Plain radiography if suspected gas in tissue or underlying fracture, osteomyelitis or foreign body
	Ultrasonography, CT, or MRI if suspected necrotizing fasciitis
Arteries	Duplex scan
	Angiography (CT or direct)
Veins	Duplex scan
	Measurement of plasma D-dimer (to rule out low-probability deep vein thrombosis)
Nerves	Nerve conduction studies
	MRI of lumbosacral spine
Muscles	Ultrasonography
	MRI
	Measurement of plasma creatine kinase
Joints	Plain radiography (in anteroposterior and lateral views)
	Joint aspiration if effusion present
	CT or MRI if suspected fracture not revealed by plain radiographs
Bones	Plain radiography (in anteroposterior and lateral views)
	CT or MRI if suspected pathology not revealed by plain radiographs

Further Reading

Creager MA, Kaufman JA, and Conte MS. Acute limb ischemia. *N Engl J Med* 2012; 366: 2198–206.
Von Keudell AG, Weaver MJ, Appleton PT, et al. Diagnosis and treatment of acute extremity compartment syndrome. *Lancet* 2015; 386: 1299–310.

66 Leg ulcers

Emily Davies and Susan Cooper

Definition of the symptom

Leg ulcers are defined as open wounds, usually below the knee, persisting for more than 6 weeks.

Differential diagnosis

Over 80% of leg ulcers are managed in primary care, and the majority of these are due to venous disease. The causes are outlined in Table 66.1.

Context

Leg ulcers are a common and costly problem. Treatment of leg ulcers places a significant financial burden on healthcare providers and uses a substantial amount of medical resources. Estimated costs to the NHS are £300–600 million per annum. Studies have found that venous ulcers affect 2% of the population in Western countries. The prevalence of leg ulcers is increasing as the population ages, with an estimated 3.6% of the population over the age of 65 affected.

Approach to diagnosis

The key to making an accurate diagnosis is taking a detailed medical history, examination of the ulcer and surrounding skin, and measurement of the ankle–brachial pressure index (ABPI). It is also important to remember that many ulcers are of mixed origin.

History

The incidence of venous ulcers increases with age. Patients with arterial ulcers are often men over the age of 40 with a sedentary lifestyle. It is important to enquire about previous deep-vein thrombosis, varicose veins, knee or hip surgery, trauma, smoking history, diabetes mellitus, hypertension, and hyperlipidaemia. The clinician should ask about symptoms of intermittent claudication or rest pain.

Site of the ulcer

The site of the ulcer can be a pointer towards venous, arterial, or neuropathic disease. Venous ulcers are typically on the medial gaiter region of the lower leg. Arterial ulcers are typically seen on the toes, foot, and ankle. Neuropathic ulcers classically present at pressure sites. Other key features of the different types of ulcer are outlined in 'Specific clues to the diagnosis'.

Surrounding skin

There are numerous signs in the surrounding skin which can provide useful clues towards the different types of ulcers, including haemosiderin pigmentation, varicose eczema, atrophie blanche, venous flare, lipodermatosclerosis, calluses, shiny atrophic skin and loss of hair. The temperature of the skin should be noted.

ABPI

Measurement of the ABPI is useful to assess for arterial disease. An index >0.8 is considered normal, but one <0.8 would imply a degree of arterial disease. Results should be interpreted in conjunction with the examination findings, as falsely high readings may be obtained if the arteries are calcified.

Specific clues to the diagnosis

As outlined in 'Approach to diagnosis', there are many clues in the history and examination to help with the diagnosis; these are outlined in Table 66.2. Pain is not usually a helpful diagnostic indicator, as both arterial and venous ulcers can be extremely painful.

Key diagnostic tests

Arterial and venous duplex ultrasound is the preferred method of investigation for assessing vascular structure and function. This will highlight any abnormalities of the vascular anatomy and blood flow which might be amenable to surgical intervention.

Other diagnostic tests

Other diagnostic tests are as follows:

Skin biopsy: This should be a deep incisional biopsy to include both the ulcer margin and the bed; it should be taken if the ulcer is not healing, is in an atypical site, or has any suspicious features of neoplasia (e.g. rolled edge, overgranulation). It should be sent for histological evaluation and also for fungal and mycobacterial culture if the ulcer has not started to heal after 3 months of treatment.

Swabs for bacterial microscopy and culture: These should be taken if infection is suspected. All open wounds will be colonized, so it is important only to treat if there are clinical (increased temperature, pain, fever) and/or laboratory (raised white-cell count and C-reactive protein) signs of infection.

Full blood count: A full blood count should be taken to investigate for factors that might be contributing to the ulceration, such as anaemia, polycythaemia, and infection (elevated white-cell count).

Urine dipstick: This should be taken to screen for diabetes mellitus.

Coagulopathy screen: This should be done particularly in young patients and should include Protein C, Protein S, Factor V Leiden, Antithrombin III, and lupus anticoagulant.

Additional laboratory tests: Additional laboratory tests that might be considered would include serum albumin, ferritin, erythrocyte sedimentation rate, antinuclear antibodies, rheumatoid factor, hepatitis B and C, cryoglobulins, and cryofibrinogen.

Patch testing: Patients with chronic leg ulcers often develop an allergic contact dermatitis, commonly to an antibacterial agent, preservative, or rubber chemicals. Patients in whom a contact allergy is suspected should be referred for patch testing.

Table 66.1 The causes of leg ulcers

Causes of leg ulcers	%
Venous disease	70
Mixed venous/arterial disease	12.5
Arterial disease	7.5
Diabetic/neuropathic	5
Vasculitis	5
Neoplasms	<1
Haematological disorders	<1
Infections	<1
Others including: • pyoderma gangrenosum • rheumatoid arthritis • scleroderma • necrobiosis lipoidica • Martorell's ulcer (hypertensive ulcer)	<1

Table 66.2 The clinical features of venous, arterial, and neuropathic ulcers

	Venous	Arterial	Neuropathic
History	DVT Phlebitis Varicose veins Previous leg injury Knee/hip/major abdominal surgery	Smoking Diabetes mellitus Hypertension Hyperlipidaemia Hyperhomocystinaemia Intermittent claudication Rest pain	Diabetes mellitus Other rarer causes include drugs, alcohol, spinal cord lesions, hereditary sensory and motor neuropathy, and leprosy
Site	Medial gaiter region of the lower leg	Toes, foot, and ankle	Pressure sites
Ulcer	Irregular borders Sloping edge Slough in wound bed	'Punched out' Necrotic base Deep, pale base	'Punched out'
Exudate	Often high volume	Often low volume	Usually low volume
Surrounding skin	Haemosiderin pigmentation Varicose eczema Atrophie blanche Venous flare Lipodermatosclerosis	Shiny Atrophic Loss of hair Cool	Calluses
Other findings	Leg oedema often present Varicose veins Obesity Lymphoedema in long-standing cases	Weak/absent peripheral pulses Prolonged capillary refill time (>3–4 seconds)	Peripheral neuropathy with decreased sensation

Introduction to therapy

Treatment depends on the underlying cause of the ulcer as well as some common principles, such as treating any infection, controlling pain, and correcting factors such as anaemia, which may contribute to poor wound healing. It is also important that any problems in the surrounding skin are treated. For example, varicose eczema should be treated with emollients and topical steroid.

The choice of dressing depends on the nature of the wound; the degree of exudate; odour; and ulceration. The ideal dressing should provide a moist wound environment to accelerate healing and there are many alternatives with different properties available. Sterile maggots are sometimes used to debride slough and necrotic tissue from wounds.

The management strategy for venous ulceration is elevation, exercise, and graduated sustained compression (usually aim for 30–40 mm Hg at the ankle).**Weight loss is important in overweight patients.** Pentoxifylline is sometimes used to accelerate healing. Sclerotherapy is a useful non-surgical procedure. Vascular surgery (to superficial veins and perforators) and skin grafts are also suitable treatments for some patients. A sympathectomy is occasionally used for intractable arterial ulcers, especially those due to small vessel disease.

Patients with arterial leg ulcers should be assessed by a vascular surgeon, as the main aim of treatment is to re-establish an adequate arterial supply. Risk factors such as smoking, weight loss, control of hypertension, and reducing cholesterol should be addressed.

The management of diabetic neuropathic ulcers involves optimizing diabetic control, treating associated arterial disease, aggressive debridement, off-loading pressure with a non-weight bearing regime, and prompt treatment of any infections.

Other, rarer causes of leg ulcers have specific treatments, such as topical and systemic steroids or ciclosporin for pyoderma gangrenosum.

Prognosis

The recurrence rate for venous ulceration can be greater than 70%. There is a higher recurrence rate in patients with ulcers for more than 1 year. A large wound area, ABPI < 0.8, and history of venous ligation or stripping are also associated with a poorer prognosis.

Wearing support stockings by day, keeping active, and elevation of the legs are all important strategies to reduce the risk of recurrence. It is also important to keep the skin well hydrated with emollients to help maintain good barrier function.

Between 16% and 37% of patients with arterial ulcers require an amputation. The higher rate reflects those who did not undergo revascularization. The risk of amputation is also higher in patients with diabetes and a larger ulcer size; 14%–24% of patients with diabetic neuropathic ulcers will require amputation. Poor glycaemic control, diabetes for more than 10 years, male gender, and associated cardiovascular, renal, or retinal complications are all risk factors. Addressing these risk factors and taking great care to avoid injury (e.g. use of good-fitting shoes) will help reduce the need for amputation.

How to handle uncertainty in the diagnosis of this symptom

If a leg ulcer is not responding to usual treatments, is in an unusual site, or has atypical features, always consider other causes such as neoplasia, vasculitis, pyoderma gangrenosum, infection, and hypercoagulable states. A skin biopsy for histology and culture and more focused blood tests may help with diagnosis.

Further Reading

Healthcare Improvement Scotland. *Management of Chronic Venous Leg Ulcers: A National Clinical Guideline*. Available at http://www.sign.ac.uk/pdf/sign120.pdf (accessed 12 Mar 2017).

Singer AJ, Tassiopoulos A, and Kirsner RA. Evaluation and management of lower-extremity ulcers. *N Engl J Med* 2017; 377: 1559–567.

67 Limb ischaemia

David Ratliff

Definition

Acute limb ischaemia is defined as a decrease in the arterial blood flow, over a period of minutes to days, which threatens the viability of the limb. Presentation is within 2 weeks of the onset of symptoms. **Chronic limb ischaemia** (presentation >2 weeks after the onset of symptoms) can be divided into **critical ischaemia**—a potential threat to limb viability, with ischaemic rest pain, ischaemic ulcers, or gangrene—and **non-critical ischaemia**, which may be symptomatic (typically with claudication) or asymptomatic.

Differential diagnosis

See Box 67.1 for a list of the different causes of limb ischaemia.

Context

Acute limb ischaemia

Acute limb ischaemia is usually caused by embolic occlusion or in situ thrombosis of a native vessel or arterial bypass graft. The leg is affected in >80% cases. Over the past 20 years, embolic occlusion has become rarer, owing to the increased use of anticoagulation for thromboprophylaxis in atrial fibrillation, while in situ thrombosis is now more common, as the prevalence of peripheral arterial disease has increased. In contrast, acute arm ischaemia is usually due to embolism from the heart. Cardiac sources of embolism include left atrial thrombus as a consequence of atrial fibrillation, left ventricular mural thrombus following myocardial infarction or in dilated cardiomyopathy, valve vegetations due to infective endocarditis, and left atrial myxoma.

Chronic limb ischaemia

Chronic limb ischaemia is most commonly due to atherosclerotic arterial disease. Segmental lesions causing stenosis or occlusion are usually localized in the large and medium-sized vessels. The leg is much more often affected than the arm.

Approach to diagnosis

History

Sudden onset of severe pain in the leg or arm, with evidence of impaired circulation, is typical of acute ischaemia. The insidious progression of intermittent claudication of the buttocks, thighs, or calves over several months or years indicates chronic lower limb ischaemia. The symptoms of limb ischaemia in a heavy smoker (typically male) under 40 years of age raise the possibility of Buerger's disease, thromboangiitis obliterans. Other causes to consider are given in Box 67.1.

Examination

Assess the limb for reduced sensation and movement, the cardinal features of acute ischaemia. An acutely painful cold limb with reduced or absent sensation is due to acute ischaemia until proven otherwise. Assess the limb muscles for tenderness or rigidity.

Inspect the lower legs and feet. Marked pallor, hair loss in the pretibial area, tissue loss, ulceration, or gangrene occurs in chronic lower limb ischaemia. Critical lower limb ischaemia is indicated by a positive Buerger's sign (elevation pallor with venous guttering, followed by dependency rubor).

Assess the capillary refill time (return of capillary circulation after blanching produced by pressure). This is a useful assessment of the peripheral circulation and is normally <4 seconds.

Assess the skin temperature with the dorsum of the hand. A clearly marked change of temperature may reveal the site of arterial occlusion.

Box 67.1 Causes of limb ischaemia

Acute ischaemia
- embolic occlusion
- thrombosis of a diseased artery or arterial bypass graft
- trauma (including arterial cannulation)
- aortic or arterial dissection

Chronic ischaemia
- atherosclerotic arterial disease
- Buerger's disease (thromboangiitis obliterans), and other types of arterial disease (e.g. polyarteritis nodosa, Takayasu's arteritis)
- popliteal artery aneurysm with secondary thromboembolism
- popliteal artery entrapment
- arterial thoracic outlet syndrome
- embolic occlusion
- congenital or acquired coarctation of the aorta

Assess the pulses in the limbs, grading them as normal, reduced, or absent. In the arm, palpate the subclavian, axillary, brachial, radial, and ulnar pulses and, in the leg, the femoral, popliteal, posterior tibial, and dorsalis pedis pulses. A reduced or absent pulse indicates severe stenosis or occlusion of the proximal artery.

Listen for a bruit over the subclavian artery in the supraclavicular fossa, over the iliac artery in the iliac fossa, over the femoral artery in the groin, and over the superficial femoral artery in the thigh.

Measure the blood pressure in both arms, and examine the heart.

Specific clues to the diagnosis

The symptoms of acute limb ischaemia are pain and paraesthesiae, followed rapidly by reduced sensation and movement and subsequent muscle swelling and rigidity. Tissue necrosis typically occurs after 6 to 12 hours of acute ischaemia, although this is influenced by the location of the occlusion and the degree of collateral circulation.

Patients with chronic lower limb ischaemia usually have long-standing symptoms and will describe intermittent claudication (from the Latin *claudicare*, to limp or be lame), the equivalent of angina of the leg. Patients complain of pain, aching, muscle stiffness, or fatigue of the affected areas during exercise but which is relieved quickly by rest. In aortoiliac disease, symptoms typically occur in the buttocks, thighs, and calves. In superficial femoral artery disease, the calves only are affected. The differential diagnosis of intermittent claudication is given in Chapter 104.

In critical lower limb ischaemia, rest pain occurs. It usually involves the toes or foot in a stocking distribution and is relieved by dependency of the limb (hanging the foot out of bed at night), which increases perfusion pressure.

Key diagnostic tests

Non-invasive tests

Non-invasive tests provide an accurate vascular assessment and objective evidence of the severity of the disease, and are the initial investigations of first choice:

- ankle–brachial pressure index at rest and after exercise (walk test on a treadmill) (Figure 67.1).
- arterial duplex scan (ultrasonography with colour-flow imaging)

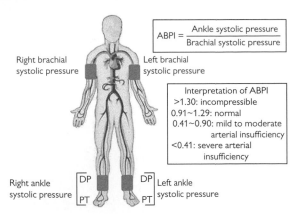

ABPI = Ankle systolic pressure / Brachial systolic pressure

Right brachial systolic pressure

Left brachial systolic pressure

Interpretation of ABPI
>1.30: incompressible
0.91~1.29: normal
0.41~0.90: mild to moderate arterial insufficiency
<0.41: severe arterial insufficiency

Right ankle systolic pressure

DP

PT

DP

PT

Left ankle systolic pressure

Figure 67.1 Measurement of ankle–brachial pressure indices; ABPI, ankle–brachial pressure index; DP, dorsalis pedis artery; PT, posterior tibial artery.

Xiaoyun Li, Ling Wang, Chi Zhang, et al., "Why Is ABI Effective in Detecting Vascular Stenosis? Investigation Based on Multibranch Hemodynamic Model," The Scientific World Journal, vol. 2013, Article ID 185691, 10 pages, 2013. doi:10.1155/2013/185691.

Angiography

The following angiographic techniques show the site and extent of the arterial disease, and provide a road map for treatment:

- CT angiogram
- MR angiogram
- catheter-based angiogram (potentially therapeutic as well as diagnostic)

Other diagnostic tests

Other diagnostic tests are:

Electrocardiography: This defines the cardiac rhythm and is a screen for structural heart disease.

Echocardiography: This should be done if embolic occlusion is suspected from the history or if abnormalities are found on cardiac examination or electrocardiography.

Introduction to therapy

Acute limb ischaemia

As soon as the diagnosis of acute ischaemia is made, the patient should be given 5000 IU heparin intravenously (to prevent propagation of thrombus) and referred for a vascular specialist opinion as an emergency. Balloon embolectomy under local anaesthesia is the standard treatment for emboli. Patients with preexisting vascular disease will often require emergency angiography and treatment by percutaneous thrombolysis, angioplasty, or reconstructive surgery.

Chronic limb ischaemia

Patients with atherosclerotic peripheral arterial disease should be treated with aspirin 75 mg daily and a statin, even if their cholesterol level is within the normal range. Vascular risk factors should be managed, with advice on smoking cessation and optimal control of hypertension and diabetes. Regular foot care is very important for patients with diabetes; such patients should be referred promptly for treatment in a multidisciplinary diabetic foot clinic should any problem develop.

A graduated exercise programme is the initial treatment for mild to moderate leg claudication. Angioplasty is offered to patients with disabling symptoms. It is carried out under local anaesthesia and is effective, with a low risk of serious complications (1%–2%). Lower limb reconstructive vascular surgery is indicated for patients with severe restrictive claudication or critical ischaemia not suitable for treatment by angioplasty.

Prognosis

In acute limb ischaemia, limb loss and mortality are high. Acute arm ischaemia carries less risk to life and limb than acute leg ischaemia. Prompt recognition and treatment of the cause is the key to reducing mortality.

Claudication is a relatively benign symptom and carries a very low rate of limb loss in patients with good control of vascular risk factors, but a high mortality from cardiovascular disease.

How to handle uncertainty in the diagnosis of this symptom

Most patients can be diagnosed by careful history taking and clinical examination, and there is no substitute for this. Non-invasive tests are valuable adjuncts to the clinical assessment.

Further Reading

Creager MA, Kaufman JA, and Conte MS. Acute limb ischemia. *N Engl J Med* 2012; 366: 2198–206.

National Institute for Health and Care Excellence. *Peripheral Arterial Disease: Diagnosis and Management.* 2012. Available at https://www.nice.org.uk/guidance/cg147?unlid=10358203332017218368 (accessed 13 Mar 2017).

68 Rashes

Christine Soon

Definition of the symptom

Rash is a term used to describe the appearance of discolouration of areas of the skin. It can be due to any factor and can be different colours. It is a generic term and by itself does not confer any true meaning without further elaboration.

Differential diagnosis

There are numerous causes for rashes to appear. A useful way to think about rashes is to start with the description. Common terms used to describe rashes are:

Macule: a flat area of discolouration of the skin; ≤5 mm wide
Papule: a raised area of discolouration of the skin; a palpable, raised lump ≤5 mm wide
Patch: a flat area of skin, >5 mm in diameter
Plaque: a raised area of skin, ≥5 mm in diameter
Purpura: discolouration due to extravasation of red blood cells; found in the skin or mucous membranes, 2 mm–1 cm in diameter
Petechia: a small purpuric lesion <2 mm in diameter
Ecchymosis: a large area of extravasation of blood, >1 cm in diameter; more commonly called a bruise
Nodule: a lump >5 mm in diameter
Vesicle: a fluid-filled lesion which can come out in crops (e.g. in chicken pox); generally, 1–3 mm in diameter
Bulla: a large, fluid-filled lesion

Context

Rashes are very common and most people will have had a few episodes of rashes in their life. It is one of the most common presentations to a GP practice. The key to correctly diagnosing and identifying a rash lies in the ability to describe it correctly and recognizing the context in which it occurs.

Most rashes are transient and will clear on their own accord. Many are linked with concurrent viral or bacterial infections. The most common rashes seen, especially in childhood, include chicken pox, impetigo, hand, foot and mouth, glandular fever, and viral exanthem.

More persistent and troublesome rashes include eczema and psoriasis; they are common, and their severity ranges from mild to serious.

Drug eruptions, for example, rashes occurring as a result of exposure to certain medications (e.g. from an allergy to penicillin), are also very commonly seen.

Approach to diagnosis

Description, distribution, and duration of the eruption are key to the diagnosis of rashes. Family history medication history, concurrent illnesses, and past medical history are also very relevant.

Demographics

Children are very prone to viral infections and atopic eczema. Older patients are more likely to have a drug-related rash.

Family history

Often patients with eczema or psoriasis have a family history of similar conditions. A history of atopy such as asthma or hay fever is also very relevant in eczema.

Concurrent illnesses

The presence of a concurrent illness, such as an upper respiratory tract infection, can be very helpful in the diagnosis of a rash. Guttate psoriasis can be triggered by a concurrent upper respiratory tract infection. Hay fever and asthma indicate an atopic tendency. Individuals with atopic tendencies are more likely to have eczema. Headaches, photophobia, and meningeal stiffness in association with a rash could mean meningitis.

Past medical history

Patients may have previously experienced a similar rash, which has recurred; for example, psoriasis tends to recur with intercurrent periods of stress, whether physical or mental. Past history of a drug allergy is very important.

Drug history

The drug history is a crucial part of the diagnosis of a rash. Many rashes are linked with medications. Angiotensin-converting-enzyme (ACE) inhibitors are known causes of angioedema, and NSAIDs can cause urticaria. Minocycline and amiodarone can cause grey pigmentation of the skin. Calcium channel antagonists can cause a photosensitive rash.

Social history

The patient's occupation and hobbies can give very important clues towards their diagnosis. A rash that gets better when the patient is off work or on holiday may be linked to the individual's occupation. Hobbies may lead to exposure to allergens, which could trigger a contact dermatitis response. Social contacts maybe relevant, especially in infectious conditions, such as a chicken pox outbreak in a playgroup.

Having taken a careful, thorough history, it is time to examine the patient. Ask the patient to remove clothing and check the distribution of the rash. The next step is to try to describe the rash and try to see if it fits a pattern. The mucous membrane should not be forgotten.

Specific clues to the diagnosis

Symptoms (e.g. the rash being pruritic, painful, asymptomatic) are crucial to the diagnosis of the rash. Signs such as dryness, scaliness, or flakiness are also important, as is the exact distribution of the rash (see Table 68.1).

Key diagnostic tests

Usually, no diagnostic test is necessary to diagnose a rash. However, a skin biopsy can be helpful when the diagnosis is uncertain. Depending on the differential diagnosis, a bacterial or viral swab of the skin, skin scraping, hair plucking, or nail clipping may be carried out.

Introduction to therapy

Therapy is as follows:

- For short-term, transient rashes (e.g. secondary to viral infections), no treatment is usually necessary other than treatment for the underlying infection.
- Moisturizers are the mainstay of treatment for eczema and most dry skin conditions; topical steroid therapy is helpful for

Table 68.1 Common diagnoses and their distribution

Common diagnoses	Distribution	Description
Atopic eczema	Flexures of the limbs	Dry, red, itchy patches
Psoriasis	Extensors of the limbs, scalp, umbilicus, behind ears, nails, genital areas	Scaly, red plaques, often very thick, nail pitting, onycholysis
Lichen planus	Extensor surfaces of wrists, mucous membranes, nails, trunk	Violaceous papules with whitish streaks called Wickham's striae
Chicken pox	Trunk and limbs, mucous membranes	Erythematous patches with vesicles; intensely itchy; crusts at later stages
Urticaria	All over body	Very itchy; each individual lesion tends to come and go over 24 hours; can be associated with angioedema
Meningococcal septicaemia	Anywhere over body; usually starts with lower limbs	Purpura and petechiae, spreads rapidly
Mycosis fungoides	Trunk	Scaly, atrophic patches
Vasculitis	Usually lower legs first	Purpura and petechiae
Drug eruption	Several different presentations; a common presentation to hospital is widespread on trunk and limbs	Can be maculopapular, urticaria, lichen planus-like, vasculitic
Erythema multiforme	Palms, soles, trunk; mucous membranes may be involved	Target lesions, patches, and plaques
Bullous pemphigoid	Trunk and limbs	Bullae and erythematous patches

inflammatory dermatoses such as eczema and lichen planus; vitamin D$_3$ analogues, coal-tar-based treatments, and topical steroid therapies are all helpful in psoriasis.

- Conditions such as severe bullous pemphigoid may require systemic immunosuppressants such as prednisolone at the initial stages and then azathioprine; tetracycline antibiotics and nicotinamide have also been shown to be helpful.
- In vasculitis, treatment would depend on the type and underlying cause.
- Phototherapy can be helpful for widespread psoriasis, eczema, and mycosis fungoides.
- Biologics are used for severe psoriasis not responsive to disease-modifying antirheumatic drugs (DMARDs).

Prognosis

The prognosis for most rashes is very good. The majority of rashes will clear within a few weeks. Chronic skin conditions such as eczema and psoriasis tend to persist, although their severity tends to vary and some patients do have clear periods. Atopic eczema often clears in childhood but may recur under the correct conditions. Although rare, serious rashes such as toxic epidermal necrolysis and meningococcal septicaemia are associated with fatality.

How to handle uncertainty in the diagnosis of this symptom

Uncertainty in the diagnosis of this symptom can be handled as follows:

- Retake the history and ensure that a comprehensive history has been obtained: for example, a patient with multiple, itchy, red ring-shaped patches could have tinea; does the patient have a pet or had other contact with animals?
- Look for other hidden signs; check nails, scalp, behind the ears, and other often-overlooked areas.
- Ask about recent travel and contacts.
- A sexual history might be helpful.
- A systemic examination may be crucial in giving further clues.
- A skin biopsy can be sent, not just for histology but also for immunofluorescence if immunobullous conditions such as bullous pemphigoid or pemphigus are suspected.

Further Reading

Morris-Jones R. *ABC of Dermatology* (6th edition), 2014. Wiley-Blackwell.
Venning V. 'Clinical approach to the diagnosis of skin disease' in Warrell DA, Cox TM, and Firth JD, eds, *Oxford Textbook of Clinical Medicine* (5th edition). Oxford University Press.

69 Blistering rashes

Emily Davies

Definition of the symptom

A blister is a fluid-filled, circumscribed elevation of the skin. By convention, blisters are divided by size; blisters less than 0.5 cm wide are called vesicles, and those greater than 0.5 cm wide are called bullae. A blistering rash is used to describe any skin condition which morphologically consists of vesicles or bullae. Vesicles more than 48 hours old may evolve into pustules (pus-filled lesions). Pustular eruptions have not been included in this chapter.

Secondary lesions include erosions (partial loss of epidermis), which may occur when a superficial blister ruptures or is scratched, and ulcers (loss of epidermis and superficial papillary dermis), which may occur either as part of the blistering process or secondary to infection.

Differential diagnosis

Eczema, infections, and oedema are the commonest causes of blistering seen in primary care (see Table 69.1).

Context

Blisters can be caused by a number of different mechanisms: it can be due to friction, skin fragility, or oedema; it can be secondary to infectious agents or drugs; it can be toxin mediated; or it can occur via autoimmune attack. Bullous pemphigoid is the commonest immunobullous disease in Western Europe and will be covered in detail in Chapter 252.

Approach to diagnosis

A detailed medical history is important. Preceding symptoms such as itch (sometimes can precede blistering by several months in bullous pemphigoid), systemic upset (fever, malaise), atopic history, and allergies should be recorded. A detailed drug history should be taken and other factors such as recent sunburn, injuries (portal of entry for cellulitis), or insect bites should be noted.

All of the skin should be examined, including the hair, nails, and mucous membranes. It should be noted if the blistering is localized or generalized, and the size of the blisters. The presence of pustules, erosions, ulcers, and any evidence of infection (crusting, weeping, increased heat) should be documented.

The skin should be palpated for tenderness, and Nikolsky's sign checked (positive when gentle rubbing of the skin at the edge of a blister results in extension of the blister). This is almost always positive in toxic epidermal necrolysis and pemphigus and is used to distinguish pemphigus vulgaris from bullous pemphigoid. Any changes in the surrounding skin such as oedema or eczema should also be looked for. In addition, baseline observations, that is, temperature, pulse, and blood pressure, should be assessed. Investigations can then be targeted, depending on these initial findings.

Table 69.1 The differential diagnosis of blistering rashes in primary and secondary care

Diagnosis in primary care	%	Diagnosis in secondary care	%
Acute eczema: • irritant/allergic contact dermatitis • pompholyx	40	Acute eczema: • irritant/allergic contact dermatitis • pompholyx	40
Bacterial infections: • impetigo • staphylococcal scalded skin syndrome • cellulitis	20	Bacterial infections: • impetigo • staphylococcal scalded skin syndrome • cellulitis	30
Viral infections: • herpes zoster • herpes simplex • varicella • hand, foot, and mouth	10	Viral infections: • herpes zoster • herpes simplex • varicella • hand, foot, and mouth Fungal infections: • tinea pedis	10
Secondary to oedema	10	Secondary to oedema	15
Insect bite reactions	5	Immunobullous disorders such as bullous pemphigoid and pemphigus	10
Cold/thermal injury (e.g. sunburn)	5	Erythema multiforme Stevens–Johnson syndrome Toxic epidermal necrolysis	5
Fungal infections: • tinea pedis	5	Insect bite reactions Cold/thermal injury (e.g. sunburn)	
Erythema multiforme Stevens–Johnson syndrome Toxic epidermal necrolysis Immunobullous disorders such as bullous pemphigoid and pemphigus Others: • lichen planus • psoriasis • vasculitis • lupus erythematosus • drug reactions • porphyria cutanea tarda	5	Others: • lichen planus • psoriasis • vasculitis • lupus erythematosus • drug reactions • porphyria cutanea tarda	

Specific clues to the diagnosis

Table 69.2 outlines diagnostic features which may help to differentiate the different conditions.

It is important to remember that any blistering disorder can be complicated by secondary bacterial infection, which may confuse the clinical picture.

Key diagnostic tests

These will depend on the differential diagnosis formed after initial history and examination, but the following would be recommended on most patients:

- skin biopsy for histology (fresh blister)
- skin swabs for bacterial and viral microscopy and culture

- full blood count
- C-reactive protein

The key to diagnosing immunobullous disorders such as Bullous pemphigoid and pemphigus is direct and indirect immunofluorescence. Direct immunofluorescence is performed on a sample of perilesional skin and demonstrates deposition of immunoglobulins and complement. Indirect immunofluorescence is performed on serum and detects circulating immunoglobulins.

Other diagnostic tests

Other tests may be warranted, depending on the provisional diagnosis, such as patch testing if an allergic contact dermatitis is suspected. Fungal microscopy and culture should be carried out in cases

Table 69.2 Diagnostic features which may help to differentiate the different conditions

Diagnosis	Age	Site	Examination findings	Symptoms	Other information
Acute eczema	Any	Any	Acutely inflamed skin with vesicles	Itch /pain	Background of eczema; often recurrent; there may be a history of contact with an irritant or allergen; often there is secondary staphylococcus infection
Impetigo	Children	Frequently face	Large bullae, become cloudy and then rupture to form honeycrusts; healing from the centre gives rise to circinate lesions	None	Contagious; only some impetigo is bullous; often localized
Staphylococcal scalded skin syndrome	Children	Widespread	Skin tenderness, fever and widespread superficial blistering erythema which evolves into large painful areas where the superficial epidermis has stripped off	Pain	Toxin mediated; mucous membranes not affected
Cellulitis	Adults	Any, but often leg (usually unilateral)	Hot, red, and tender	Pain	Portal of entry
Varicella (chicken pox)	Any age, usually children	Widespread	Malaise and upper respiratory tract symptoms followed by a widespread papulovesicular eruption	Itch	Scalp involvement characteristic
Herpes zoster	Older adults	Dermatomal	Erythema and grouped vesicles (may be haemorrhagic)	Preceding burning pain	
Herpes simplex	Any	Face, lips, and genitals	Occurs in roughly the same place each time	Preceding tingling or burning pain	Recurrent
Hand, foot, and mouth	Children	Hands, feet, and mouth	Small grey vesicles, with a halo of erythema on the hands and feet with small erosions of the buccal mucosa	Oral lesions may be painful	
Oedema	Older adults	Legs bilateral	Pitting oedema with blisters and weeping	Discomfort	Often associated with congestive cardiac failure, low albumin, or other medical causes
Tinea pedis	Adults	Feet, often unilateral	Scale, erythema, and a vesiculopustular eruption	Itch	Nails may be affected
Insect bite reaction	Any	Usually lower legs	Bullae on an erythematous base; often linear configuration	Itch	Inflammatory papules may also be present
Erythema multiforme	Any	Usually acral; may be mucous membrane involvement	Erythematous macules/plaques with a central bulla and marginal ring of vesicles	None	Recurrent attacks are often secondary to herpes simplex
Stevens–Johnson syndrome/ toxic epidermal necrolysis	Any	Widespread	Tender, erythematous skin which develops widespread erosions	Pain	Marked mucous membrane involvement Spectrum of severity Usually due to a drug
Porphyria cutanea tarda	Older adults	Sun-exposed sites—dorsa of hands	Presents with skin fragility, blisters, and milia	Pain	Often associated with high alcohol intake in men or oestrogen-containing tablets in women
Bullous pemphigoid	Elderly	Usually widespread	Tense bullae and sometimes urticated plaques	Itch/pain	Often prodrome of pruritus for several months before the onset of blisters
Cold/heat injury	Any	Any	Acute erythema and blisters	Pain	Usually clear history, e.g. sunburn

of possible tinea pedis. Patients with possible porphyria cutanea tarda should have blood and urine porphyrins measured.

Introduction to therapy

Treatment depends on the underlying cause of the blistering, as well as some common principles, such as treating any secondary infection and controlling any pain or pruritus with appropriate analgesia and sedating antihistamines (at night) if required:

- Acute eczemas should be treated by removing any possible allergen or irritant and then topical therapy with emollients, soap substitutes, and an appropriate strength topical steroid.
- Bacterial infections, including toxin-mediated staphylococcal scalded skin syndrome (SSSS), require appropriate antibacterial treatment, topically, orally, or intravenously, depending on the extent of involvement and any systemic upset; it is important that family members do not share towels with the patient, as SSSS is highly contagious.
- Varicella, in most immunocompetent individuals, does not require active treatment, but soothing emollients can help with the itch. Herpes zoster and simplex may be treated with oral or intravenous acyclovir.
- The offending drug should be removed in all cases of drug reactions, although it may take several weeks or even months for the rash to resolve.
- Treatment for oedema blisters needs to be targeted at managing the cause of the oedema.
- Clinicians should be alert for signs of secondary bacterial infection in all blistering rashes; patients should be advised to keep their nails short to limit damage from scratching the skin.

Prognosis

Once treated, most causes of blisters, such as acute vesicular eczemas and infections, usually resolve over a couple of weeks. More persistent causes of blistering are the immunobullous disorders, which have a remitting and relapsing course.

How to handle uncertainty in the diagnosis of this symptom

If a blistering eruption is not responding to an initial treatment (e.g. antibiotics for suspected bullous impetigo), always consider a biopsy through an intact blister, for histology, and of perilesional skin, for direct immunofluorescence, in case the patient has an immunobullous disorder. In addition, always retake a drug history, including over-the-counter and herbal remedies, as well as medications which are just taken occasionally, in case a drug reaction is the cause.

Most blistering reactions, although dramatic in appearance, are localized and short-lived. It is important not to miss the rarer, more persistent blistering conditions which need specific targeted treatment.

Further Reading

Creamer D, Walsh S, Dziewulski P et al. UK guidelines for the management of Stevens–Johnson syndrome/toxic epidermal necrolysis in adults. *Br J Dermatol* 2016; 174: 1194–227.

70 Photosensitive rashes

Jane McGregor

Definition of the symptom

Clinical photosensitivity is an abnormal reaction of the skin to sun exposure. This can present in many ways, including sunburn, urticaria, itching, pain, and the development of skin rashes as diverse as skin necrosis and eczema.

Differential diagnosis

The majority of the common reactions to sun exposure, including sunburn, polymorphic light eruption, and solar urticaria are managed in general practice (Table 70.1). The rare photodermatoses require specialist investigation and are usually managed in the specialist centres.

Context

Sunburn is the commonest form of photosensitivity. When this is seen in the context of overexposure, then symptomatic relief with emollients and hydration, sometimes with oral or topical steroids, is all that is required. When the degree of sunburn seems disproportionate to the exposure, then drug phototoxicity should be considered (many drugs are potentially phototoxic). Easy sunburn in children should raise the possibility of the very rare condition known as xeroderma pigmentosum (a DNA-repair-deficient condition which results in premature development of skin cancer and early death). This is not an easy diagnosis to make and children with suspected sunburn after minimal exposure should be referred to a specialist.

Polymorphic light eruption (PLE) is the second most common form of photosensitivity. It affects about 10% of the population, predominantly women. The history is usually clear, namely, the patient develops an itchy papular eruption a few hours after sun exposure, and only on sun-exposed sites. It can occur in the context of systemic lupus erythematosus, and this should be considered and investigated.

Other forms of photosensitivity are very rare, but any patient presenting with pain (erythropoetic protoporphyria), itching (polymorphic light eruption, urticaria, chronic actinic dermatitis), or a skin rash of any other type following sun exposure should be referred to a specialist for investigation.

Approach to diagnosis

The key to making a diagnosis of photosensitivity is to take a very careful history. This should include any seasonal variation in the symptoms, the time after exposure that the reaction occurs (minutes, hours, days), the nature of the reaction (pain, itching, rash), and the duration of symptoms (minutes, hours, weeks or months). Since many forms of photosensitivity are acute and transient, there may be no rash to examine at the time of the consultation.

If a skin rash is present, then either the consultation has occurred soon after the episode of photosensitivity, or the eruption is chronic. Careful observation should include details of cut-off, that is, sparing of non-exposed sites, and the nature of the rash (urticaria, papules, nodules, excoriation, blistering, skin thickening, eczema, etc.).

Specific clues to the diagnosis

Specific clues to the diagnosis are shown in Table 70.2.

Key diagnostic tests

The diagnosis is a clinical one in many cases, so the history and clinical examination are paramount. First, there should be an accurate assessment of photosensitivity, and then there are tests (see 'Other diagnostic tests') which can be used to confirm a diagnosis in some specific cases.

Other diagnostic tests

Photosensitivity can be objectively demonstrated in selected cases by using a monochromator light testing procedure—this is time consuming, expensive, and only available in specialist centres. It is useful in confirming a diagnosis of chronic actinic dermatitis and in defining the causal wavelengths in solar urticaria.

Patch testing is required in patients with chronic actinic dermatitis, as concomitant contact allergies are common.

Lupus serology (antinuclear antibody (ANA), anti-double-stranded DNA (ds DNA), and extractable nuclear antigen antibody tests) is mandatory in patients suspected of having photosensitivity associated with both cutaneous and systemic lupus erythematosus. It should also be undertaken in any patient presenting with classical features of polymorphic light eruption, before undertaking phototherapy.

Porphyrin analysis (blood, urine, faeces) is required to confirm a diagnosis of the cutaneous porphyrias, including in erythropoetic protoporphyria.

Human leukocyte antigen (HLA) testing can be helpful in supporting a diagnosis of the rare condition known as actinic prurigo. HLA DRB1 is present in 90% of patients (compared with 30% of the general population), and 60% of these will have the rare HLA BRB1 0407 haplotype.

DNA repair can be estimated in ex vivo fibroblasts (requires a skin biopsy)—a defect confirms a diagnosis of the very rare xeroderma pigmentosum—but this requires a specialist opinion first.

Introduction to therapy

Therapy depends on the diagnosis (see Table 70.3).

Prognosis

Prognosis depends on diagnosis (see Table 70.4).

Table 70.1 The causes of photosensitive rashes in primary and secondary care

Diagnosis in primary care	%	Diagnosis in secondary care	%
Sunburn • overexposure • drug phototoxicity	 75% 25%	Sunburn • overexposure • drug phototoxicity • xeroderma pigmentosum	 10% 80% 10%
Polymorphic light eruption	70%	Polymorphic light eruption	30%
Solar urticaria	80%	Solar urticaria	20%
Other photodermatoses (rare) Managed in the specialist centres			

Table 70.2 Clues to the diagnosis of photosensitive dermatoses

Symptoms	Investigation	Diagnosis	Recommendations
Itching and whealing	Routine bloods (usually normal); porphyrin analysis (EPP can present with urticaria); history and examination	Wheals indicate solar urticaria	If sun avoidance and antihistamines are insufficient, will require referral to specialist
Itching and papules	Lupus serology to exclude lupus	Polymorphic light eruption	If sun avoidance and antihistamines are insufficient, will require referral to specialist
Itching, papules, nodules, and excoriations	HLA testing	Actinic prurigo (rare)	Refer to specialist
Pain and/or scarring	Exclude porphyria	Hydroa vacciniforme	Refer to specialist
Eczema at sun exposed sites	Patch test to exclude airborne or other contact allergies	Chronic actinic dermatitis	Refer to specialist
Sunburn	Consider drug phototoxicity; consider XP in child	–	Withdraw drug and review; refer to specialist for opinion and further investigation
Blistering and skin fragility	Porphyrin analysis, liver function tests, ferritin and alpha feto protein	Cutaneous porphyria (porphyria cutanea tarda or variegate porphyria)	Refer to specialist
Erythema (redness) or scaling, annular eruption	Lupus serology: ANA, anti-dsDNA, ENA	Cutaneous lupus or photosensitivity in systemic lupus erythematosus	Refer to specialist

Abbreviations: ANA, antinuclear antibody; anti-dsDNA, anti-double-stranded DNA antibody; ENA, extractable nuclear antigen antibody; EPP, erythropoietic protoporphyria; HLA, human leukocyte antigen; XP, xeroderma pigmentosum.

Table 70.3 Therapy in the different diseases causing photosensitive dermatoses

Diagnosis	Investigations	Therapy	Other recommendations
Sunburn	Consider drug phototxicity (withdraw drug if relevant); consider XP in child with easy sunburn (rare)	Emollients, topical or oral steroids for a few days, hydration	Advise on sun protection; refer to specialist
Polymorphic light eruption	Lupus serology to exclude lupus as a cause	Sunblock and sun avoidance measures; phototherapy (desensitization programme)	Refer to specialist if simple measures are insufficient
Actinic prurigo	HLA testing	Sun block and sun avoidance; phototherapy desensitization; thalidomide	Refer to specialist
Hydroa vacciniforme	Clinical diagnosis of exclusion	Sunblock and sun avoidance; phototherapy desensitization; immunosuppression	Refer to specialist
Solar urticaria	Clinical diagnosis may be supported (if necessary) by phototesting in specialist centres to define precipitating wavelengths	Antihistamines and sun avoidance; phototherapy desensitization; photophoresis; immunosuppression	Refer to specialist if simple measures are insufficient
Chronic actinic dermatitis	Clinical diagnosis supported by monochromator phototesting	Sun avoidance; topical steroids; oral immunosuppression	Refer to specialist
Cutaneous porphyrias	Clinical diagnosis supported by porphyrin analysis; look for haemochromatosis (in PCT)	Sun avoidance; avoidance of precipitating factors (e.g. alcohol, oestrogens, etc.); venesection (if ferritin raised); low-dose hydroxychloroquine	Refer to specialist

Abbreviations: HLA, human leukocyte antigen; PCT, porphyria cutanea tarda; XP, xeroderma pigmentosum.

Table 70.4 Prognosis of different photosensitive dermatoses

Diagnosis	Prognosis
Sunburn	Good outlook if infrequent; long-term consequences include increased risk of melanoma and non-melanoma skin cancer
Drug phototoxicity (sunburn)	Good outcome if drug identified and withdrawn; usually no further sequelae
Xeroderma pigmentosum	Patients at 1000x risk for melanoma and non-melanoma skin cancer; some xeroderma pigmentosum complements develop neurological complications; patients need specialist care and continued, lifelong vigilance; death from metastatic skin cancer common
Polymorphic light eruption	Usually self-limiting; patients may remit after several years but some are photosensitive for life; with desensitization, they can live a reasonable life outside during summer
Solar urticaria	Often self-limiting; can be very disabling if symptoms not adequately controlled
Actinic prurigo	Usually well controlled with therapy; most children grow out of this condition but it occasionally persists into adulthood
Hydroa vacciniforme	May self-limit; some cases persist into adulthood; lifelong scarring
Chronic actinic dermatitis	Can be very disabling, and severity may limit exposure outside, even with therapy; rarely remits
Porphyrias	Depends on type; risk of liver damage and hepatoma

How to handle uncertainty in the diagnosis

Photosensitivity can be a surprisingly difficult symptom to elicit, especially in the chronically photosensitive patient who may not be aware of the relationship with sun exposure. If in doubt, even if you have elicited a good history for photosensitivity, refer to a specialist—making a specific diagnosis and subsequent management can be challenging.

Further Reading

European Dermatology Forum: Guidelines on the photoderma-toses. http://www.euroderm.org/edf/index.php/edf-guidelines/category/3-guidelines-on-photodermatoses

Gruber-Wackernagel A, Byrne SN, and Wolf P. Polymorphous light eruption: clinic aspects and pathogenesis. *Dermatol Clin* 2014; 32: 315–34.

71 Itching

Christine Soon

Definition of the symptom

Itching, also known as pruritus, is an unpleasant sensation on the skin that leads to an urge to scratch the skin in order to obtain some relief from the symptom.

Differential diagnosis in primary care and secondary care

There are many causes of itching. More common ones are listed in Table 71.1.

Context

Itching is a very common symptom and nearly everyone will have experienced it in his or her lifetime. Most itching is temporary and resolves quickly. It can be a response to a physical stimulus, such as an insect bite. However, chronic itching can be debilitating and it is often helpful to find the cause and treat it accordingly. Most patients with eczema will have experienced itching that requires treatment of their condition. It is the most common symptom of an inflammatory skin condition.

Approach to diagnosis

An accurate and detailed history is crucial to diagnose the cause. History should include age of onset, duration of symptom, distribution of symptom, family history, drug history, contact history, any associated systemic symptoms, and social history.

Examination is crucial, and care must be taken to document any rash on the skin and its distribution. Areas that may give clues to the diagnosis include the scalp, genital areas, mucosal surfaces, and nails.

Specific clues to the diagnosis

Babies, toddlers, and young children are more likely to have seborrhoeic dermatitis and atopic eczema. A detailed family history of

Table 71.1 Common causes of itching

Directly related to skin	Systemic causes of itching
Dry skin	Chronic renal failure
Eczema, including atopic eczema, seborrhoeic dermatitis, pompholyx, contact dermatitis, asteatotic eczema, gravitational eczema, irritant eczema	Biliary obstruction
	Haematological malignancies such as lymphomas and leukaemias
Psoriasis	Iron deficiency anaemia
Urticaria	Polycythaemia
Lichen planus	Thyroid dysfunction
Lichen simplex	Medications
Tinea	
Scabies	
Varicella	
Bullous pemphigoid	
Pityriasis rosea	
Folliculitis	
Lichen sclerosus	
Dermatitis herpetiformis	
Fleas	
Lice	
Insects such as mosquitoes	

atopy should be sought. History of age of onset of symptom and any accompanying rash is important. The distribution of the rash is also important. Seborrhoeic dermatitis commonly occurs on the scalp, in the skin folds, and in the nappy area. It may be accompanied by crusting on the scalp.

Atopic dermatitis tends to occur on flexor surfaces of the limbs. There may be a history of sleep disturbance caused by the itching. Widespread eczema occurring at weaning age may indicate intolerance to certain foods. In adults who present with eczema, but without a previous history of atopic eczema, a careful contact history should be sought to elicit any possible underlying allergen; for example, a cashier presenting with hand eczema may have an allergy to nickel present in coins. It is also common to see irritant eczema secondary to occupational causes such as frequent handwashing in medical and nursing staff, use of harsh detergents in pot washers and hairdressers, and constant wet work in bar staff. Asteatotic eczema tends to present in older individuals, especially on the lower limbs. This is associated with very dry skin leading to a crackled egg appearance.

Psoriasis tends to have two peak ages of presentation: in the late teens and in the 50s. Patients often have a family history, and typical erythematous scaly well-demarcated plaques distributed on the extensor aspects of the limbs, lower back, scalp, behind the ears, and umbilicus. Nails and genital areas can also be involved. Nails may be brittle and demonstrate onycholysis, pitting, thickening, and discolouration. There may be associated arthropathy.

There are many causes of urticaria. Acute urticaria can be caused by a reaction to medications, foods, and plants, and viral, bacterial, and helminth infections. There may also be associated angioedema. Urticaria is often intensely itchy. Dermographism may be present. Each urticated lesion resembles an erythematous raised papule or plaque, which typically lasts for less than 24 hours. Physical stimuli such as heat, cold, water, pressure, sun, and exercise can also be implicated. It is often hard to find a cause for chronic urticaria. Occasionally, a systemic cause such as thyroid disease may be implicated.

Lichen planus tends to present as violaceous, flat-topped polygonal papules. White streaks, known as Wickham's striae, may be seen on the papules and on the oral mucosa. There may be nail pitting.

In infestations, such as with scabies, lice, fleas, or bedbugs, the culprit may be detectable with the naked eye. Scabies is intensely itchy and tends to occur in outbreaks in institutions such as residential and nursing homes for the elderly, and hospitals. Patients may have a widespread rash with lots of excoriations. Burrows may be seen.

Lice and their eggs may be seen in hair-bearing areas. Fleas may also be present in the patient's pets. In infestations, there may be other close contacts who are affected.

Varicella, also known as chickenpox, can cause intense itching in the acute phase. A history of contact with affected people or of outbreaks in the school or nursery will help to point towards the diagnosis. In UK, varicella is a common childhood illness. It is self-limiting. It typically occurs centripetally before spreading to the limbs. Lesions ranging from vesicles, papules, and pustules may be seen. Mucosal surfaces are often affected. The lesions then crust over.

Folliculitis appears as inflamed hair follicles often with pustules. Infection, occlusion, irritation, and certain drugs can cause it. It is common and can be seen often in women who shave their legs, and in beard areas of men.

Dermatitis herpetiformis presents as intensely itchy vesicles and papules on the limbs and the buttocks. It is associated with coeliac disease. It is important to take a gastrointestinal history if this diagnosis is suspected.

Bullous pemphigoid presents as blisters in older patients. There is often underlying erythema and itching.

Lichen sclerosus commonly affects the genital areas and presents as a white, crinkled patches. It can be intensely itchy. Ecchymoses may be present. In about 10% of cases, extra-genital areas may be affected, although these do not appear to be as itchy.

Lichen simplex is used to describe an area of lichenified skin caused by repeated rubbing or scratching. It is often seen on the nape of the neck, the upper shoulders, lateral aspect lower limbs, and wrists. It can be linked with stress.

If the patient's skin appears normal with no obvious signs of dryness or inflammation, a pruritus screen should be conducted to look for underlying causes. A systemic examination including checking for hepatosplenomegaly, and lymphadenopathy should be performed. A careful drug history should also be taken. Pregnancy and postmenopause are times associated with a higher incidence of itching in women.

Key diagnostic tests

In inflammatory skin conditions, a skin biopsy will usually confirm the diagnosis. However, this is often unnecessary as the diagnosis may be obvious from the clinical appearance. If allergic contact dermatitis is suspected, patch tests should be carried out.

In pruritus of unknown cause, blood tests, including full blood count, urea and electrolytes, liver function tests, immunoglobulins, iron levels, thyroid function tests, lactate dehydrogenase, and serum electrophoresis, should be carried out.

Other diagnostic tests

Depending on the findings of the pruritus screen, a chest X-ray, renal ultrasound, hepatic ultrasound, gastroscopy, colonoscopy, bone marrow biopsy, and CT of the chest, abdomen, and pelvis may be necessary. A blood film may be useful. Prick tests may be carried out to confirm the suspected trigger of acute urticaria.

Introduction to therapy

Treatment of itching will depend on the underlying cause. In conditions associated with dry skin, such as eczema and psoriasis, emollients are the mainstay of treatment. These need to be applied regularly and frequently. It is useful to stop soap and replace it with an emollient bath oil or shower cream. Avoidance of placing irritants such as lamb's wool next to the skin of affected individuals can be very helpful. In allergic contact dermatitis, patch tests should be carried out and the relevant allergens avoided. Education and counselling will be very important here.

Topical steroids of varying strengths are usually used in inflammatory skin conditions. Coal-tar-based treatments and vitamin D analogues can be helpful in psoriasis. Occlusion can be helpful for lichen simplex. Immunomodulators such as tacrolimus and pimecrolimus are often used in place of topical steroids, especially on the face.

Sedating antihistamines are often used in individuals whose itching wakes them from sleep. Care should be taken to ensure that they do not interact with other medications the patient may already be on.

Non-sedating antihistamines such as fexofenadine are useful in the treatment of urticaria. In acute urticaria and angioedema with a known trigger, avoidance of the trigger is recommended. If systemic symptoms such as wheeze and hypotension are present, nebulizers, systemic steroids, and even adrenaline may have to be administered.

Phototherapy can be useful in intractable itchy conditions associated with renal failure. It is also often used for itching linked with other causes. It is an established treatment for eczema and psoriasis.

Systemic medications such as oral prednisolone are used in severe cases of skin inflammation. Immnosuppressants such as methotrexate and ciclosporin are also used.

In psoriasis, biologics such as anti-tumour necrosis factor inhibitors are increasingly used.

Infestations can be treated with insecticides. Often, close contacts of the affected individual will need to be treated as well. In cases of bedbugs, the premises may also need to be treated. Pets may also need to be treated if they have fleas. Education about infestations is important to prevent recurrence. Head lice and scabies can spread particularly easily if close contacts are not treated.

Varicella can be treated with aciclovir, which can be helpful if given within 24 hours of the rash appearing.

Treatment of the underlying condition is important in systemic illnesses. It can, however, be very difficult as the underlying condition may be very hard to treat. This is the case in chronic renal failure.

Prognosis

Itching associated with infestations is relatively easy to cure. The aim would be to eradicate the responsible organism and ensure adequate measures are taken to prevent recurrence. Patients should be warned that they might itch for a few weeks even after successful eradication, especially post scabies.

Itching associated with viral infections such as varicella tends to resolve once the acute infection is over. There is now a vaccine for varicella.

Most urticarias tend to resolve within 6 weeks. Chronic urticaria, however, may take months or years to resolve. If there is a known trigger, avoiding it will generally treat the condition.

There is no cure for eczema or psoriasis. Treatment is aimed at controlling the disease and reducing the symptoms. However, in allergic contact dermatitis, avoidance of the allergen may cure the condition. Although patch tests are exceedingly helpful, allergens are not always easy to identify.

The prognosis for itching associated with systemic illnesses is harder to predict. Treating the underlying cause will hopefully help with the itching, but this is not always possible and, occasionally, itching persists despite treatment of the cause.

How to handle uncertainty in the diagnosis of this symptom

Diagnosing an itch is usually very straightforward, as patients will generally give a very good description of this symptom. Excoriations and scratch marks may be seen on physical examination.

Diagnosing the cause of the itch can be very challenging, especially if there is no obvious skin inflammation. It is crucial to take a detailed history. It is very easy to miss important clues such as medication started around the first onset of the itch. A systemic examination may be helpful, and blood tests to rule out common causes should be performed. If there is an associated rash, a skin biopsy could be carried out. In some cases, no cause can be found.

Although psychogenic itching should only be diagnosed after other causes have been ruled out, it can occasionally be very obvious from the history. In delusions of parasitosis, sufferers complain of parasites infesting their skin. They may present with numerous excoriations and may bring along samples of crusts, scabs, and hair, which they have removed from their skin. The skin may be dry from overuse of antiseptics and other cleaning agents that have been applied in attempts to eradicate the parasites. There may be a history of psychiatric illness. Treatment is not easy, and antipsychotics are often necessary.

Itching can be more common during pregnancy and menopause. It is also more common in the elderly, as dry skin is more common in this age group. It is, however, important to bear in mind other causes and to take steps to rule them out, if appropriate. AIDS and anorexia nervosa are also linked with itching.

In a patient with widespread intractable itching for which no cause can be found, it may be prudent to continue follow-up, as itching has been reported to precede haematological malignancies by a number of years.

Further Reading

Berger TG, Shive M, and Harper M. Pruritus in the older patient: A clinical review. *JAMA* 2013; 310: 2443–50.

Yosipovitch G and Bernhard J. Chronic pruritus. *N Engl J Med* 2013; 368: 1625–34.

72 Lumps and bumps

Rubeta Matin, Jane McGregor, and Catherine Harwood

Definition of the symptom

A skin 'lump or bump' is taken here to refer to a lesion on the skin that an individual recognizes as something new or unusual. It comprises a heterogeneous group and presents in many guises, usually to primary care. Common causes of 'lumps and bumps' include warts, moles, skin tags, dermatofibromas, lipomas, epidermoid cysts, and, of course, melanoma and non-melanoma skin cancers. Distinguishing malignant from non-malignant is not always straightforward. Maintaining a low threshold for referral into secondary care is wise, especially for pigmented lesions, but also for those lesions where there is no obvious diagnosis. Occasionally, a lump in the skin may have arisen from an internal source, such as a metastasis or lymph node. In this section, we describe only primary cutaneous lesions and classify them according to their origin.

Differential diagnosis

The differential diagnosis in primary care and secondary care, ordered by probability, is outlined in Table 72.1.

Context

Approximately 25% of all consultations in primary care are skin related, and a significant proportion of these are 'lumps and bumps'.

Table 72.1 Two tables, side by side, outlining the differential diagnosis in primary care and secondary care, ordered by probability

	Diagnosis in primary care	Diagnosis in secondary care
Infective (most common)	Viral wart Molluscum contagiosum Skin abscess (bacterial)	Skin abscess (bacterial, deep fungal, mycobacterial)
Benign (common)	Fibroepithelial polyps (skin tag) Seborrhoeic keratosis (basal cell papilloma) Dermatofibroma Epidermoid ('sebaceous') or acne cyst Lipoma Melanocytic naevus Pyogenic granuloma Haemangioma (e.g. Campbell de Morgan spot) Sebaceous gland hyperplasia Keloid/hypertrophic scar	Fibroepithelial polyps (skin tag) Seborrhoeic keratosis (basal cell papilloma) Dermatofibroma Epidermoid ('sebaceous') or acne cyst Lipoma Melanocytic naevus Pyogenic granuloma Haemangioma (e.g. Campbell de Morgan spot) Sebaceous gland hyperplasia Keloid/hypertrophic scar
Malignant (less frequent)	Precancerous lesion (e.g. actinic keratosis, Bowen's disease) Non-melanoma skin cancer (e.g. basal cell carcinoma, squamous cell carcinoma) Melanoma Cutaneous metastasis	Non-melanoma skin cancer (e.g. complex or facial basal cell carcinoma, squamous cell carcinoma, keratoacanthoma, Kaposi's sarcoma, appendageal tumours, sarcomas (e.g. dermatofibrosarcoma protuberans), Merkel cell carcinoma, cutaneous lymphoma) Melanoma

The majority of these will be benign, but skin cancer is common and should always be considered in the differential of any new or changing lump, particularly in an adult and presenting on sun-exposed skin. Melanoma in particular is an aggressive skin cancer but, in its early stages, when it is curable, the signs indicating malignancy, such as irregular outline, irregular pigmentation, or growth, can be subtle. It is important to take a careful history and not to dismiss concerns about changing moles, as early detection is essential to improved survival outcomes.

Occasionally, patients are troubled by the cosmetic appearance of a lump, or by itching or bleeding from trauma, and may request removal of the lesion.

Approach to diagnosis

History

A detailed history of the lesion should be taken, including:

- when the lesion was first noticed, how long it has been there, and whether or not it is changing with time
- the site of the lesion—whether it is on sun-exposed or non-exposed sites, and whether it is single or multiple (multiple lesions are less likely to be malignant)
- the nature of the lesion if it is changing (e.g. changing in colour, contour, or elevation)
- any associated symptoms, such as itch or ulceration; be wary of patients attributing skin lesions to an injury which is slow to heal—this is a cardinal sign of skin malignancy
- previous treatment, if any
- risk factors (e.g. previous history of precancerous or cancerous lesions; see Chapter 259, Table 259.2)
- recreational or occupational exposure to UV
- family history of skin cancer
- immunosuppression

Examination

Inspection

The following features should be assessed and documented:

- site (where on the body—sun exposed or non-exposed skin—and where in the skin—e.g. is it epidermal, dermal, subcutaneous, or vascular?)
- size (a visual estimate)
- border (regular, irregular)
- colour (pigmented or non-pigmented; erythematous; flesh-coloured)

Palpation

Assess for:

- tenderness
- consistency (e.g. is it soft, firm, hard, translucent, pulsatile, or compressible?)
- relationship to other structures (e.g. origin and attachment)

Examination of other sites

Examine other sites as necessary. Examine regional lymph nodes, if skin cancer is suspected. In addition, examine the rest of the body for similar lesions.

Specific clues to the diagnosis

See Box 72.1 for specific clues to the diagnosis of lumps and bumps.

Box 72.1 Specific clues to the diagnosis of lumps and bumps

Non-pigmented lesions

Cyst (e.g. epidermoid, pilar, and acne type)
- well-circumscribed, deep nodule within dermis on trunk/scalp
- fluctuant, mobile, cystic lesion
- central punctum may be visible (epidermoid cysts)
- similar cysts may occur in individuals with acne after damage to hair follicles

Actinic keratosis
- scaly, red lesion on chronically sun-exposed sites (e.g. face, hands)
- often multiple

Non-melanoma skin cancer
1. Basal cell carcinoma
   - slowly growing erythematous patch (superficial subtype), papule, or nodule (nodular or morphoeic subtypes) on sun-exposed areas
   - can ulcerate
   - may also be pigmented (see 'Pigmented lesions')
2. Squamous cell cancer
   - hyperkeratotic and/or ulcerated lesion on chronically exposed skin
   - often tender and with relatively rapid growth

Lipoma
- soft, mobile, subcutaneous nodule
- usually long-standing and asymptomatic

Dermatofibroma
- firm, hard papule situated in the dermis
- 'like a button'
- commonly on legs
- usually history of insect bite/minor trauma
- may also be pigmented (see 'Pigmented lesions')

Neurofibroma
- skin-coloured, pink, or red papule or nodule appearing anywhere on the skin after puberty
- if multiple, check for clinical signs of neurofibromatosis (e.g. axillary freckling; see Chapter 224)

Infective lesions
1. Viral wart
   - human papillomavirus infection of the epidermis
   - a small, papilliferous nodule, often multiple, on fingers or toes
   - a filiform lesion has finger-like projections and is commonly seen on the face
   - a plane wart is flat-topped and may koebnerize
   - may also be pigmented (see 'Pigmented lesions')
2. Molluscum contagiosum
   - pox virus infection of the skin
   - usually affects children
   - small, 1–5 mm white or pink umbilicated papule
   - may koebnerize
   - in adults, suggestive of immunosuppression

Pigmented lesions

Seborrhoeic keratosis
- warty-looking lesion with 'stuck-on' appearance
- may have grey/yellow, greasy appearance which may be mistaken for pigment
- solitary or multiple, on face and trunk
- common in late adulthood

Dermatosis papulosa nigra
- found in Asian/black skin
- histologically identical to a seborrhoeic wart
- may present on cheeks
- inherited as an autosomal dominant trait

Melanocytic naevus and atypical naevus
- a mole can be pigmented or skin-coloured
- a mole with variable colour/abnormal features is atypical
- multiple atypical naevi comprise a risk factor for melanoma

Basal cell carcinoma (nodular subtype)
- occasionally, a basal cell carcinoma is heavily pigmented and can be confused with a melanoma
- a typical rolled edge should suggest the diagnosis

Kaposi's sarcoma
- small, red-brown/purple macule or papule which grows to form nodules and plaques
- mainly observed in patients with HIV/AIDS and iatrogenically immunosuppressed individuals (see Chapter 296)

Melanoma
- a changing or new mole with irregular contours or pigment*
- may occur at any site
- a low index for referral should be maintained

Dermatofibroma
- pink-brown nodule, often with darker circumference
- can be mistaken for compound naevus but firmer on palpation, and squeezing lesion from the side results in puckering of the surface
- may also be unpigmented (see 'Non-pigmented lesions')

Vascular lesion
1. Pyogenic granuloma
   - rapidly growing
   - often at site of injury, particularly digits, lips
   - bleeds profusely if traumatized
2. Campbell de Morgan spots (cherry angiomas)
   - multiple small bright red/purple papules on trunk and proximal limbs in >35-year-olds

Viral wart
- common warts are firm, rough, skin-coloured, or brown papules with black pinpoint dots on the surface
- plane warts may often be pigmented
- may also be unpigmented (see 'Non-pigmented lesions')

*ABCDE criteria (**A**symmetry, **B**order irregularity, **C**olour variation, **D**iameter > 6 mm, **E**levation) are used to identify early melanomas.

Key diagnostic tests

For the majority of common skin lumps and bumps, a diagnosis can be made after a careful history and examination, and no further investigations are required. Where malignancy is suspected, or the diagnosis is not certain, then referral to a dermatologist in secondary care is recommended. Dermoscopy (epiluminescence microscopy) is used as an adjunct by trained specialists, especially when assessing pigmented lesions.

In cases of diagnostic uncertainty or suspected skin malignancy, histological examination is mandatory. Sometimes a diagnostic biopsy is indicated, with a view to obtaining histological diagnosis before making definitive management decisions. In other cases, such as small tumours or suspected melanoma, a primary excision is recommended, with narrow excision margins taken in the first instance. Shave biopsies should be avoided in these circumstances, as it may not be possible to assess excision margins or stage the lesion. In addition, an incorrect diagnosis can occur due to sampling error. Incisional or punch biopsy (a core of skin tissue up to 6 mm in diameter) is occasionally acceptable, for example, in the differential diagnosis of lentigo maligna of the face, of acral melanoma, or of a very large tumour where primary excision and closure would not be possible. Table 72.2 details the different biopsy techniques and their applications.

Other diagnostic tests

Clinical photography of individual lesions can be helpful for monitoring lesions where there is uncertainty regarding change. Total body mole mapping is used for individuals with a large number of moles, as they may have an increased risk of malignant change. The images created can then be used as part of an individual's skin cancer surveillance programme. As the incidence of melanoma is increasing

Table 72.2 Different biopsy techniques and their applications

Biopsy technique	Use
Incisional biopsy (small part of lesion removed)	To establish a diagnosis before definitive treatment is instigated
Punch biopsy (up to 6 mm core diameter of skin lesion is removed)	To remove very small lesions
Curettage	To removing superficial (epidermal) lesions such as seborrhoeic keratoses, viral warts, and actinic keratoses
Excision	To remove a lesion in its entirety (usually a malignancy); allows the pathologist to examine the periphery and adequacy of removal

and individuals are becoming more aware of the need to detect skin cancer early, mole mapping is an expanding field. Mole mapping can be undertaken using conventional photographic mapping or digital dermoscopic imaging. In the former, a series of standardized photographic images (taken by qualified medical photographers) of body regions are taken to generate a complete map of the skin. Images are printed on photographic paper, or stored on a computer/CD-ROM. Dermoscopic images allow recording of a more detailed image of the mole. Digital devices standardize images for magnification and illumination and can accurately record moles. Most digital dermoscopic systems have integrated computer software which can provide a risk analysis of how suspicious a mole is. Independent published research has repeatedly shown limitations in the diagnostic ability of these systems, and the interpretation of any changes seen is best performed by a trained specialist.

For infective lesions, swabs can be taken to identify any causative bacteria by Gram stain and culture. Viruses can be identified by electron microscopy, culture, or PCR. Occasionally, blood testing is indicated; for example, multiple infected boils may raise the possibility of diabetes, whereas resistant viral warts/mollusca in adults may alert the clinician to immunosuppression. Radiological imaging (e.g. ultrasound scans) may be used to assist the diagnosis of subcutaneous lumps, especially if diagnostic fine-needle aspiration is planned. CT and MRI may be used in selected cases to delineate structures prior to surgery.

Introduction to therapy

Treatment of lumps and bumps depends on their cause. In many cases, skin lesions are benign or self-limiting (e.g. molluscum), and no treatment is required. Request for removal by the patient may be made because of the cosmetic appearance (intradermal naevi, skin tags, Campbell de Morgan spots, seborrhoeic warts, etc.). Histological examination of any lesion removed is mandatory.

Benign lesions

Seborrhoeic keratoses

Seborrhoeic keratoses do not require any treatment. If they are repeatedly traumatized, treatment options include cryotherapy, curettage and cautery, and excision.

Epidermoid cysts

Epidermoid cysts, which are well-defined, keratin-containing cysts, are subject to recurrent infection and can rupture, resulting in subsequent fibrosis and scarring. Cysts may be surgically excised in their entirety, with the sac lining intact to prevent future recurrence. Active infection should be treated prior to surgical intervention.

Actinic keratoses

Spontaneous regression is reported in 15%–25% of cases of actinic keratosis over a 1-year period. Common treatment modalities for individual lesions include cryotherapy, curettage, and cautery. Surgical intervention includes excision or shave excision/curettage.

It has the benefit of providing histological diagnosis and is useful in the management of larger, tender indurated lesions when distinction from a non-melanoma skin cancer is required. For multiple lesions, fluorouracil cream, 5% imiquimod cream and ingenol mebutate are useful, but result in transient inflammation. Diclofenac 3% gel (Solaraze®) is also useful in milder cases or when fluorouracil/imiquimod is not tolerated. When there are multiple actinic keratoses or they are confluent at sites of poor healing or exhibit poor response to standard therapies, photodynamic therapy (combination of dedicated light source and photosensitizing cream with active agent 5-aminolaevulinic acid) may be helpful.

Infective lesions

Viral warts

Treatment of warts depends on the age of the patient and the number of lesions present. In young children, the best treatment is conservative management, as lesions generally resolve spontaneously. In older children and adults, topical keratolytics, 5% imiquimod cream, cryotherapy, and curettage and cautery are some of the treatment options available.

Molluscum contagiosum

Trauma to individual lesions can result in resolution. In children these eventually resolve spontaneously over 6–24 months.

Vascular lesions

Pyogenic granuloma

These vascular lesions grow very rapidly and can arise at the site of trauma. Distinction from amelanotic melanoma is important and therefore, where possible, surgical excision is the best management. Other options include deep shave excision with cautery to the base.

Suspected skin cancers

For skin cancers, the treatment of choice is usually surgical, so that excision margins can be assessed and documented. In the majority of cases, this procedure will be curative. In the UK, basal cell carcinomas with low-risk features (depending on anatomical site, size, and histological subtype) can be excised in primary care by trained surgeons who are members of the local skin cancer multidisciplinary team (LSMDT). Basal cell carcinomas with high-risk features should be referred into secondary care for further management, usually surgery. In selected cases, radiotherapy may be used, either as primary or adjunct therapy. All suspected squamous cell carcinomas should be referred into secondary care for surgery.

All suspected melanomas should be referred into secondary care (LSMDT) for further management. After primary excision, a further wide local excision is undertaken which reduces the risk of local recurrence, although it does not alter eventual outcome. Management of skin cancers is detailed further in Chapter 259.

Prognosis

Benign lesions

Most benign skin lesions cause no health hazard but may cause significant morbidity in terms of anxiety or cosmesis. Diagnosis of some skin lesions can alert the clinician to systemic or inherited disease (e.g. boils and diabetes; multiple epidermoid cysts before puberty, and polyposis coli (Gardner's syndrome) or Gorlin syndrome; adult mollusca/viral warts, and immunosuppression/HIV infection; adenoma sebaceous and tuberous sclerosis; and neurofibromas and neurofibromatosis).

Malignant and premalignant lesions

Actinic keratoses

Actinic keratoses are low-risk lesions, 25% of which will remit spontaneously without treatment. They have potential to progress to squamous cell cancers (estimated risk <1% per annum, latent period 10 years). Actinic keratoses are a biological marker of UV damage and, in the UK, an estimated 25% of Caucasians over 65 years old will develop at least one actinic keratosis. The presence of multiple actinic keratoses is a risk factor for both non-melanoma and melanoma skin cancer (Madan et al., 2010).

Skin cancers

The prognosis of skin cancers is discussed in Chapter 259.

How to handle uncertainty in the diagnosis of this symptom

When there is diagnostic uncertainty, referral to a specialist dermatologist, trained in the diagnosis and management of skin lesions, is recommended. Lesions suspected to be squamous cell carcinoma or melanoma should be referred urgently and, in the UK, this is governed by the 2-week wait rule for assessment by local screening services, which are usually run by dermatologists.

Further Reading

Madan V, Lear JT, and Szeimies RM. Non-melanoma skin cancer. *Lancet* 2010; 375: 673–85.
Marsden JR, Newton-Bishop JA, Burrows L, et al. Revised U.K. guidelines for the management of cutaneous melanoma 2010. *Br J Dermatol* 2010; 163: 238–56.

73 Falls

Adam Darowski

Definition of the symptom

A fall is an involuntary event that results in coming to rest at a lower level. Most falls occur while standing or walking. Some people fall off a chair or out of bed, particularly in hospitals and care homes, when transferring is a time of particular risk.

A side-by-side comparison outlining the differential diagnosis in primary care and secondary care, ordered by probability, is given in Table 73.1.

Context

Adults fall at a rate of about 35% each year. This rate increases in later life, so that about 50% of people aged 80 years fall each year. It is not just the number of falls that changes with increasing age, but the unexpected circumstances in which they occur and their more severe consequences. With ageing, the body become more frail, fragile, osteoporotic, and weaker. The damage may be physical, but also psychological, with fear of falling (and family anxiety) limiting activities and causing increased dependency.

Fall-related injuries (particularly head injuries and hip fractures) consume a large fraction of the health budget. They are more common, and result in more occupied hospital bed days than do any of stroke, heart disease, or cancer. They are the most common cause of moving into a care home: 25% of all social care in the UK is due to the consequences of hip fracture. The 58 244 hip fractures that occurred in England in 2005–6 would have cost £1.4 billion pounds in health and social care in their first year, and resulted in about 17 000 deaths. The cost of fall-related injuries in the US in 2000 was estimated to be $19 billion.

Falls can be classified into four main groups:

- accidents—slips and trips—as occur at any age; if such accidents recur, an underlying cause should be sought
- illness: falling can be the presentation of almost any illness in the elderly; commonly, infections present with falls
- an intrinsic tendency to fall because of impairments of gait, balance, or vision; this may be because of neurological or musculo-skeletal degeneration, or due to disability caused by illness (most commonly stroke, Parkinson's disease) or the effects of medicines or alcohol
- paroxysmal events:
  - syncope and presyncope
  - seizures
  - vascular events (stroke, myocardial infarction, pulmonary embolus)
  - vertigo
  - rarities (e.g. cataplexy)

In general, falls are multifactorial. Most falls are simple accidents, as occur throughout life. When falls occur in people who are physically sprightly, an accident or some paroxysmal event is the probable cause.

Most recurrent falls occur in people with some degree of impaired balance, poor gait, and poor vision. It is thought probable that an age-related degeneration of proprioceptive function is the main cause of the unsteadiness seen in later life. This combines with muscular weakness due to lack of exercise, to the muscle loss of ageing, and to weight loss from any cause. In addition, pathological changes in the white matter in the brain cause disruption of cerebral pathways, slowing reaction times. The patient may have other neurological diseases—stroke and Parkinson's disease are common causes of falling, together with a wide variety of other neurological problems. Movements are made around joints that may be arthritic and painful, which may give way; prosthetic joints do not provide proprioceptive inputs to the brain. The whole system becomes deprived of adequate sensory input, weaker, slower, and less accurate. What might have been a stumble or a moment of imbalance becomes a fall.

One reason that falls are important is that they lead to fractures. Patients who fall require an osteoporosis assessment.

The nonsense term 'mechanical fall' provides closure through pseudodiagnosis and should be avoided.

Approach to diagnosis

The diagnosis is usually with a thorough history and a practised ear. A falls history can be very time consuming, and may involve extensive detective work to establish all the facts. The history is in three parts: the narrative, direct questioning, and corroboration.

The narrative

The narrative is the patient's account, elicited by an open question: what happened to you? It is likely to give you the patient's interpretation of events, and should not be the end of your enquiries.

Direct questioning

Direct questioning aims to establish several things:

- The scale of the problem: how long have unexpected falls being happening, and how many falls have here been? Are falls becoming more frequent? Has something happened to provoke them (new medication, illness, injury)?
- Is the story that of syncope, which is common, or of presyncope, which is extremely common? People seen to be unconscious deny it in about 30% of cases, so the history cannot always exclude syncope reliably. Was syncope followed by a secondary seizure?

Table 73.1 A side-by-side comparison outlining the differential diagnosis in primary care and secondary care, ordered by probability

Falls occurring in the community	Falls in hospital or care homes
Most falls have multiple causes, with an event occurring in a susceptible individual.	
Accidents	Illness
Poor gait and balance: • sedative or hypotensive medications • neurological disability • weight loss and weakness	Syncope and presyncope
Syncope and presyncope: • hypotension and orthostatic hypotension, carotid sinus hypersensitivity, vasovagal syndrome, medication effects • bradycardias or tachycardias	Impaired balance
Seizures	
Other paroxysmal events	
Illness	Accidents
	About 40% are confused due to delirium or dementia
	About 40% occur trying to get to the toilet

- Are the falls stereotyped? What did the patient experience? Were there any symptoms beforehand or afterwards? Does the patient experience postural giddiness or vertigo?
- What was the patient doing just before the fall and at the time of the fall? Where were they? Were they sitting or standing? If standing, had they just stood up? Had they just got out of bed? Were they turning at the time? Was it unequivocally an accident?
- What were the consequences of the fall? Was there a fracture, head injury, or soft tissue damage? Has this resulted in loss of confidence in walking?
- A drug history and the indications for all the drugs: anything that acts on the CNS roughly doubles the chances of a fall. Any drug that affects the pulse or blood pressure may cause syncope or presyncope. Many people are taking antidepressants, antianginals, and antihypertensives that they no longer need, or in doses that are too big.

Corroboration

Corroboration from a witness to a fall, from a family member, or from GP or hospital records usually shows that the problem of falling is of longer duration and more frequent than the patient has volunteered. A witness may be able to confirm whether the patient lost consciousness, and for how long. Unconsciousness in syncope is brief—less than a minute—unless it is followed by a secondary seizure, which is common. More prolonged unconsciousness (as distinct from amnesia), or coming round confused or disorientated are suggestive of a seizure. Commonly, the patient remembers coming round in the ambulance or in hospital, but witnesses describe only a short period of unconsciousness.

Falls in hospital

Falls in hospitals are commonly due to delirium and agitation. They occur most frequently in the setting of someone trying to find a toilet in an unfamiliar environment, weakened by an illness. The use of hypotensive and sedating medications contributes to the falls risk. Orthostatic hypotension is common in patients who are dehydrated on multiple medications. Patients in hospital need an appropriate walking aid and proper footwear as soon as they are admitted and can try to walk. They need their glasses and hearing aids. They may need bed rails to keep them safe when unsupervised. Some falls risk has to be accepted during the process of rehabilitation.

Specific clues to the diagnosis

Specific clues to the diagnosis are as follows:

- In patients who are sprightly, the chances of syncope are greater. In frailer patients who have an obvious gait and balance problem, it cannot be assumed to be the cause of their fall, and syncope and presyncope need to be considered.
- Syncope in the elderly is most commonly due to a drop in blood pressure. The resting blood pressure may be low but, more commonly, the patient will have one of three syndromes of paroxysmal hypotension: orthostatic hypotension, vasovagal syndrome, or vasodepressor carotid sinus hypersensitivity. These are all very common. These conditions are usually due to the side effects of drugs, to autonomic dysfunction, or to both.
- Syncope may also be due to a rhythm disorder, such as heart block, cardioinhibitory carotid sinus hypersensitivity, fast atrial fibrillation, or any other bradycardia or tachycardia.
- Presyncope is caused by a brief reduction in cerebral blood flow and is due to the same causes that can cause a feeling of faintness or weakness, and loss of postural tone without loss of consciousness.
- Confusion on coming round or prolonged unconsciousness suggests a seizure.
- Any illness in an older person can cause falls. Most commonly, this is an infection.
- A history of neurological disease, and examination findings to confirm it, commonly reveal Parkinson's disease, a stroke that has gone undiagnosed, or a peripheral neuropathy. A large number of other neurological conditions present as falls.

- Any disease causing slow weight loss will result in falls due to muscular weakness. The first presentation of malignancy is commonly with falls.

Postural giddiness is a difficult symptom to interpret. Standing up causes a sudden reduction in sensory inputs to the brain—with proprioceptive input only from the feet telling the patient where the ground is, as well as sudden changes in visual fixation, and momentary changes in vestibular function. These combine to produce giddiness. Orthostatic hypotension also causes giddiness, but more commonly is asymptomatic. Less than half of postural giddiness is due to orthostatic hypotension.

Almost everyone who has giddiness will have it on standing. The key question with giddiness is whether it occurs when the patient is lying down (benign positional vertigo, cerebral white matter disease) or sitting (rhythm disturbance, vestibular disease).

Key diagnostic tests

Key diagnostic tests are as follows:

- Cardiovascular, musculoskeletal, and neurological examinations should be performed. Is the patient in sinus rhythm? Always check the lying and standing blood pressure, looking for a systolic drop of >20 mm Hg from lying to standing, using a manual sphygmomanometer. Are there signs of aortic stenosis?
- An assessment of mobility should be performed. This can be done on several levels of complexity.
- Most simply, an assessment of gait should be performed, looking at step length and regularity, and whether the patient looks stable. Perform a Romberg's test, with the patient having both feet together and then one foot in front of the other (tandem standing).
- Someone who can stand on their tip toes with their arms extended and their eyes closed for 5 seconds is unlikely to have any significant neurological abnormality causing falls.
- Tests should be done to look for infection (white-cell count, C-reactive protein, urine stick testing, chest X-ray), even if infection is not clinically apparent.

Other diagnostic tests

Patients with syncope should have an ECG, and Holter monitoring for at least a week. An echocardiogram is necessary if there are murmurs, to exclude aortic stenosis. Tilt-table testing adds less than might be expected (many false positives; elderly patients with syncope have multiple abnormalities on tilt testing of uncertain relevance). A good history often does away with the need for tilt testing.

A low level of vitamin B_{12} (<250 ng/l) is an important, curable cause of orthostatic hypotension.

Further balance assessments include:

- timed get up and go: in this assessment, the patient gets up from a chair, walks 3 m, turns around, and then goes to sit down again; a normal time for this is less than 12 seconds
- the Berg balance score: this is a validated balance score (no gait component), with marks out of 56; it correlates well with risk of future falls

All patients who fall need an osteoporosis assessment. Use the FRAX score, a WHO-validated tool for the assessment of the risk of fracture over the next 10 years (http://www.shef.ac.uk/FRAX/tool.jsp).

Introduction to therapy

Treatment is aimed at the underlying cause:

- If syncope is the underlying cause, therapy may consist of a pacemaker, antiarrhythmic treatments, or may be withdrawal or dose reduction of culprit medication.
- Impaired gait and balance is treated with rehabilitation involving exercises that challenge balance and which need to continue for 6 months. The patient should be referred to the local falls service. Fear of falling is treated with group therapies through a day hospital.

- The provision of appropriate walking aids and exhortation to use them greatly improves safety, particularly in the hospital setting, where lack of such an aid is a major cause of falls.
- Drug hygiene involves an examination of all medication acting on the nervous and cardiovascular systems, and checking their indication and dosage. Commonly, patients are prescribed tablets they no longer need.
- Patients need an occupational therapy assessment, including a review of their home and their care arrangements.

Prognosis

When syncope is due to a rhythm disorder, it can usually be treated successfully. When it is due to hypotension, it may be possible to reduce the drug burden. Orthostatic hypotension responds poorly to treatment, but some patients improve with fluid expansion using fludrocortisone or slow sodium. A low B_{12} level needs to be treated.

Falls due to balance disorders can be reduced in frequency by exercise programmes. Education aimed at heightening awareness of falls and improving safety improves confidence and function.

Falls assessments can reduce the number of falls by about a third and, in some patients, prevent them altogether.

How to handle uncertainty in the diagnosis of this symptom

Falls have multiple causes. It is rarely clear which of the many factors is the most important one in a given patient. What is treatable should be treated, and the patient should be referred on for further assessment by a falls service. It has to be accepted that a patient's life cannot always be made completely safe. The patient commonly has her own perception of her falls risk, and may not always agree to an assessment, let alone intervention.

Further Reading

National Institute for Health and Care Excellence. *Falls in Older People: Assessing Risk and Prevention*. 2013. Available at http://www.nice.org.uk/guidance/CG161 (accessed 29 Mar 2017).

Pirker W and Katzenschlager R. Gait disorders in adults and the elderly: A clinical guide. *Wien Klin Wochenschr* 2017; 129: 81–95. Open access, available at doi 10.1007/s00508-016-1096-4.

74 Immobility ('Off legs')

Adam Darowski

Definition of the symptom

Immobility is a progressive or a sudden deterioration in the ability to walk. Table 74.1 gives a side-by-side comparison of the differential diagnoses in primary care and secondary care, ordered by probability.

Context

Immobility is one of the 'geriatric giants', and can be the presentation of any illness. Poor mobility during hospital stay is a marker of poor outcomes. Patients with poor mobility when in hospital have a much higher mortality and a prolonged length of stay, tend to have a decline in their functional status, and are more likely to require discharge to a care home. About 16% of people aged over 70 years in a medical take are immobile, with another 32% having impaired mobility. They require prompt treatment of their underlying medical conditions and help getting back on their feet as soon as possible to prevent the consequences of immobility.

Table 74.1 A side-by-side comparison of the differential diagnoses in primary care and secondary care, ordered by probability

Immobility presenting to hospital	Immobile at home
Immobility can be the presenting feature of virtually any illness in an elderly patient.	
Important to exclude diagnoses requiring urgent treatment:	
Cord compression: urgent MRI if there is any doubt	
Fracture: hip and pelvic fractures can be missed easily	
Acute polyneuropathy (Guillain–Barré syndrome)	
Stroke requiring thrombolysis	
Intracranial haemorrhage	
Usually not a single cause: predisposing factors with an intercurrent illness	Rapid onset: fall related injury, infection, vascular event
Infection is the proximate cause in >50% Usually chest, urine, gut, or skin, but occult infection common (biliary, cardiac, brain, diverticular)	Slow deterioration; multiple factors Chronic disability due to old injury or illness Arthritis: osteoarthritis, most commonly of the hip and knee Rheumatoid disease, gout, other arthritides
Recent fall with or without bony injury	Muscular weakness: • disuse atrophy • weight loss • 'sarcopaenia of ageing' • neuropathy, root lesions
Intracerebral lesion: • subdural haematoma, stroke • primary or secondary cerebral tumours	Obesity
Joint pain: • exclude septic arthritis, gout, pseudogout by joint aspiration • trauma, flare up of osteoarthritis, other joint disease	Dementia, depression, anxiety, fear of falling
Metabolic: • commonly dehydration, renal failure, diabetes, hyponatraemia • rarely hypercalcaemia, Addison's	Chronic neurological disease: • previous stroke • parkinsonism • neuropathies • cervical myelopathy

Immobility presenting to hospital	Immobile at home
Sedating medications: • tricyclic antidepressants • antipsychotics • benzodiazepines Drugs affecting circulation, causing bradycardia, hypotension, or orthostatic hypotension: • antihypertensives • antianginals • tricyclics • serotonin-norepinephrine reuptake inhibitors • phenothiazines	Infections: • difficult to diagnose in the patient's home
Disability from neurological disease: • previous stroke • parkinsonism • any other (multiple sclerosis, motor neuron disease, cervical myelopathy, neuropathies) Gait apraxia, painful neuropathy	
Lack of mental ability/will to walk • dementia, delirium • depression, personality disorder, conversion disorder	
Back pain: • degenerative disc disease • osteoporotic collapse • malignancy: secondaries usually from breast, bronchus, prostate, kidney, gut, thyroid	
Cardiovascular disease: • severe orthostatic hypotension • profound bradycardia or hypotension	
Obesity, deconditioning, muscular weakness	

Approach to diagnosis

Ensure this is not a disorder of consciousness (delirium, postictal, or drugged). Are they ill? Are they hypothermic? Are they hypoglycaemic, severely hyponatraemic, or uraemic? Is this the consequence of trauma? Can they understand instructions?

Do they have a cardiovascular problem—reasonably well while lying down, but unsteady on getting up? This is an uncommon cause for immobility (and the diagnosis is usually obvious) except for people who have such severe orthostatic hypotension that they cannot stand (or sometimes even sit) without severe symptoms.

The patient is usually old, frail, deaf, dysphasic, dysarthric, and often delirious or demented. It may not be possible to obtain a history from the patient. Such people are known to others; contact family, GP, district nurse, carers, and neighbours to get an assessment of the patient's normal function and recent history. A good history of how the patient came to be immobile and of the patient's usual level of function provides the framework for everything else in this case.

Satisfy yourself that the patient does not have cord compression (leg weakness, sensory loss, bowel, bladder, reflexes, sensory level—MRI spine), intracranial haemorrhage (are they hypertensive, do they take aspirin or warfarin, was there a head injury) or a fracture of the hip or pelvis (history may not be available; X-rays may be normal initially; they may need MRI). These conditions are uncommon causes of immobility, but may require urgent treatment.

Infection is the most probable diagnosis, and no test excludes it. Fever (often missed—sublingual and tympanic measurements are insensitive tests for fever, measured using inadequate instruments—ignore a 'normal' temperature), raised white blood cell count (normal in 50% of febrile older people) and a raised C-reactive protein (not specific for infection; raised with any inflammation or tissue damage) are all markers of underlying infection. Ensure the urine has been tested, examine the chest, and obtain a chest X-ray. Remove any bandages on the legs to check for cellulitis.

Is the history of a sudden deterioration (consider stroke), or chronic? What is the normal level of function (Does the patient do their own shopping? Do they walk out of the house? Are they housebound? Do they use the stairs? Are they mostly chairfast? Do they use a walking stick or a walking frame?) to assess how great is the change. What support do they have at home?

Are there symptoms of other diseases (cough, sputum, dysuria, frequency, chest pains, dyspnoea, diarrhoea)? Is there a history of neurological disease, or could this be a first presentation (Parkinson's, stroke, neuropathy, any other)?

Assess hydration status. If in doubt, consider supplementary IV fluids, if safe to do so.

Specific clues to the diagnosis

Do not expect there to be a single unifying diagnosis. There will be predisposing factors and possibly a proximate cause.

If the patient can cooperate, can they move their legs freely? If practical, try to get the patient to stand. This will exclude many musculoskeletal and neurological diagnoses, or make them more obvious.

Check for metabolic and cardiovascular causes, and for markers of infection. In an older person, pneumonia sufficient to cause immobility may produce no respiratory symptoms or signs (consolidation may not be visible behind the heart on a chest X-ray).

If leg movement is impaired, then a full neurological examination followed by appropriate imaging is required. Stroke is usually associated with neurological signs, but may present as immobility without obvious signs. Subdural haematoma commonly presents without any neurological signs. Have a low threshold for requesting a CT of the brain. Look for signs of Parkinson's disease.

Key diagnostic tests

Key diagnostic tests are as follows:

- pelvic X-rays and spinal MRI, if indicated, to exclude surgical causes
- CT of the brain, to look for intracranial lesions
- chest X-ray, to look for chest infection (and other pathologies)
- urea, electrolytes, glucose, and calcium; dehydration may be a cause of immobility or a consequence of poor access to fluids while immobile; if the patient is dehydrated, are renally excreted drugs (atenolol, angiotensin-converting enzyme (ACE) inhibitors) making things worse?
- stick testing of urine (if normal does not exclude infection), midstream specimen of urine, blood cultures
- blood count and C-reactive protein may point to an inflammatory cause; however, normal results do not exclude infection, and raised ones do not confirm it

- liver function tests; a raised bilirubin and alkaline phosphatase point to biliary disease
- prostate specific antigen in men, to exclude a significant prostatic carcinoma (weight loss, spinal metastases)

Other diagnostic tests

The use of other diagnostic tests is determined by the clinical findings and the results of initial tests. Other diagnostic tests are:

- X-rays of injured or painful areas, lateral of spine if vertebral collapse is suspected
- nerve conduction studies for neuropathies
- urine and plasma osmolality; urinary sodium; Synacthen test for hyponatraemia
- tests for weight loss: gastroscopy, CT colon

Introduction to therapy

Therapy is aimed at the underlying diagnoses, and at the immobility. Immobile patients require assessments by physiotherapists and occupational therapists as soon as possible. They will probably require additional support at home on discharge, which takes time to arrange and requires forward planning to prevent delays in hospital. Many patients wish to go home, but domiciliary rehabilitation, while desirable, is not readily available, and even then is rarely of adequate intensity.

Prognosis

The outcome depends upon the underlying diagnosis and the previous functional level. Where immobility is due to an infection (that has been treated successfully), walking improves over a week or two. Patients with fall-related trauma require several weeks to regain whatever function will recover.

For every day the patient is left immobile, they will require several days to recover their lost function. Vigorous rehabilitation prevents them becoming weaker, shortens length of hospital stay, and increases their chances of getting back to their own home.

How to handle uncertainty in the diagnosis of this symptom

It is important to establish there is no condition requiring urgent treatment. What is left is a mixture of metabolic, infective, neurological, musculoskeletal, and chronic diseases, and drug-side effects. Always bear in mind occult infection, and have a low threshold for giving antibiotics on empirical grounds. It is very easy to miss a significant infection in an older person.

Stop as many tablets as you can safely, and reconsider their need.

Further Reading

British Geriatrics Society. *Fit for Frailty: Consensus Best Practice Guidance for the Care of Older People Living with Frailty in Community and Outpatient Settings*. 2014. http://www.bgs.org.uk/campaigns/fff/fff_full.pdf (accessed 14 Mar 2017).

Marcantonio ER. Delirium in hospitalized older adults. *N Engl J Med* 2017; 377:1456–466.

75 Suspected anaphylaxis

Siraj Misbah

Definition of the symptom

A type I IgE-mediated systemic allergic reaction is characterized by a constellation of symptoms which are due to widespread histamine release and which comprise acute-onset urticaria, angioedema, bronchospasm, and hypotension. While a mild reaction may be limited to localized urticaria and or angioedema, a full-blown allergic reaction associated with systemic features is best described as anaphylaxis. The term 'anaphylactoid', previously used to denote non-IgE-mediated systemic allergic reactions, is no longer recommended for use.

Differential diagnosis

Other disorders which share some of the clinical features of anaphylaxis may occasionally cause diagnostic confusion. In most cases, a good history will help distinguish anaphylaxis from syncope, disorders associated with flushing (carcinoid), disorders associated with excessive endogenous histamine release (systemic mastocytosis), panic attacks, and angioedema due to C1-inhibitor deficiency or drug allergy.

Although no precise figures are available, the majority of allergic reactions are managed in primary care.

The differential diagnosis in primary and secondary care is given in Table 75.1.

Context

There has been a dramatic increase in the overall burden of allergic disease, including anaphylaxis, over the past two decades. The underlying explanation for this phenomenon, as enunciated in the hygiene hypothesis, has been attributed to the skewing of immune responses to the Th2 group of 'allergy-prone' lymphocytes due to poor infection-driven priming of Th1 lymphocytes. Although the hygiene hypothesis is unlikely to be the sole explanation for the upsurge in allergic disease, epidemiological trends over the past several decades clearly document an inverse relationship between the incidence of infectious diseases and the incidence of Th2-driven autoimmune disease.

The increasing incidence of anaphylaxis has prompted the introduction of evidence-based management guidelines by the UK Resuscitation Council and the Royal College of Physicians.

Approach to diagnosis

Anaphylaxis is a clinical diagnosis based primarily on the history and the recognition that one or more of the clinical features mentioned in 'Definition of the symptom' has developed acutely (evolving over minutes to a few hours) following exposure to a potential triggering agent.

Specific clues to the diagnosis

Although there are no symptoms or signs that are specific for anaphylaxis, the occurrence of acute-onset bronchospasm and/or hypotension accompanied by cutaneous signs of histamine release in the form of angioedema and urticaria is highly suggestive of a systemic allergic reaction. Many patients who have experienced anaphylaxis describe a sense of impending doom as part of the clinical picture.

A clearly identifiable trigger (foods, drugs, insect venom stings) preceding the reaction by minutes provides a strong pointer to the diagnosis but this would not be apparent in the case of idiopathic anaphylaxis. The diagnosis of idiopathic anaphylaxis should only be made after careful consideration of known causes of anaphylaxis.

Key diagnostic tests

Mast cell activation and degranulation is a key event responsible for the clinical features of anaphylaxis. Of the many biomarkers of mast cell and basophil activation, the demonstration of elevated plasma or serum tryptase levels up to 3–4 hours after the event constitutes strong supportive evidence of anaphylaxis. Elevated tryptase levels are particularly associated with anaphylaxis associated with drugs or injection of insect venom. It is uncommon to find elevated tryptase levels in the case of food-induced anaphylaxis or in the absence of hypotension. Consequently, a normal tryptase level does not exclude a diagnosis of anaphylaxis.

Tryptase can also be measured in post-mortem blood samples and, if significantly elevated, points to anaphylaxis as being a possible cause of sudden, unexplained death. Although large amounts of histamine are also released during anaphylaxis, its short half-life of 10–15 minutes makes plasma histamine assays impractical in a routine laboratory. While elevated tryptase and histamine levels are strong clues suggestive of anaphylaxis, they are unable to pinpoint the cause of the reaction.

Other diagnostic tests

Based on the clues elicited in the history, potential triggers (drugs, foods, insect venom) should be selected for measurement of allergen-specific IgE and the performance of skin tests. The optimal time for performance of these tests is approximately 3–4 weeks after the episode, to avoid the possibility of false-negative results.

Introduction to therapy

The immediate injection of adrenaline (0.5 ml of a 1:1000 solution) is the single most important intervention in the treatment of anaphylaxis. In the vast majority of cases, the intramuscular route of administration should be used. Because of the risk of potentially lethal arrhythmias, intravenous adrenaline is reserved for the treatment of intractable anaphylaxis in an intensive-care setting. Attention to the airway, and the use of oxygen, fluid replacement, parenteral antihistamines, steroids, and bronchodilators are important additional measures that may be required in individual patients.

Lack of efficacy of adrenaline is usually due to either a delay in injection or use of suboptimal doses on a milligram per kilogram basis. Anaphylaxis in patients on long-term beta-blocker therapy may prove to be refractory to adrenaline due to its inability to interact with the

Table 75.1 Differential diagnosis		
Triggers	**Approximate percentage of diagnoses in primary care (%)**	**Approximate percentage of diagnoses in secondary care (%)**
Idiopathic	30	30
Food (e.g. nuts, eggs, milk, shellfish)	20	20
Insect venom (e.g. bee, wasp)	20	10
Drug (e.g. beta-lactam antibiotics)	20	30
Latex	10	10

Table 75.2 Anaphylactic shock

Clinical features	**History** (1) Premonitory aura—apprehension, light-headedness, dizziness, tingling or itching of skin (2) Facial, tongue or throat swelling (3) Stridor or wheeze (4) Syncope or collapse (5) Exposure to precipitant—foodstuffs (e.g. peanuts), hymenopteran stings, drugs (e.g. parenteral penicillins)
	Examination (1) Cyanosis (2) Hypotension (3) Facial, tongue, or throat swelling (4) Stridor or wheeze (5) Urticaria, angio-oedema, skin erythema, or extreme pallor
Immediate management	(1) Stop any potential causative agent immediately (2) Oxygen—high flow, with reservoir bag if needed, to achieve Pao_2 >92% (3) Adrenaline (epinephrine) Give 0.3–0.5 ml of 1:1000 adrenaline (0.3–0.5 mg) intramuscularly into lateral thigh, repeated every 5–10 min as needed If this is ineffective, or if the patient is about to die: Give 5 mg adrenaline (5 ml of undiluted 1:1000 adrenaline) nebulized with oxygen, and Make up 1:100 000 preparation of adrenaline by diluting 0.5 mg adrenaline (0.5 ml of 1:1000 adrenaline) to total of 50 ml with 0.9% saline and give at 0.5–1.5 ml/min, titrated according to clinical response (4) Fluid—give balanced salt solution or 0.9% saline, 10–20 ml/kg, as rapid IV infusion if patient is hypotensive Second line therapy—can be considered after cardiorespiratory stability has been achieved (but no strong evidence that they are required): (5) H_1-blocker, eg. chlorphenamine 10–20 mg IV, repeated up to 40 mg in 24 h (change to oral when patient tolerates) (6) H_2-blocker, e.g. ranitidine 50 mg IV three times daily (change to oral when patient tolerates) (7) Steroid, e.g. hydrocortisone 1.5–3 mg/kg IV, then repeated four times daily (change to oral prednisolone 40 mg daily when patient tolerates) (8) β_2-Agonist, e.g. salbutamol 5 mg (repeated as necessary) via oxygen-driven nebulizer if bronchospasm is a persistent problem
Key investigations	**To establish the diagnosis:** (1) Anaphylaxis is a clinical diagnosis (2) Mast cell tryptase—immediately after resuscitation, after 1–2 h, and after 24 h (or convalescent)
	Other important tests: ECG, chest radiograph, electrolytes, renal function, arterial blood gases (depending on context)
Further management	(1) Patients must be observed for 4–6 h after full recovery before discharge from immediate medical care (2) Determination of allergen (if any)—refer to allergy services; advice regarding avoidance; MedicAlert bracelet (3) Instruction regarding self-injection of adrenaline and supply of appropriate medication

Reproduced with permission from Warrell et al. *Oxford Textbook of Medicine*, fifth edition, Oxford University Press, Oxford, UK, Copyright © 2010.

beta 1 and beta 2 adrenergic agonist receptors, which mediate (along with alpha 1 adrenergic vasoconstrictor effects) the beneficial effects of adrenaline. In such cases, glucagon should be considered in view of its cardiac inotropic effects.

Once patients are successfully rescued from anaphylaxis, it is essential that all patients undergo careful assessment by an allergist or immunologist to determine the trigger by testing for allergen-specific IgE antibodies and/or skin testing. Where a clear trigger is identified, long-term risk reduction is based on avoidance of the trigger.

For insect-venom-induced anaphylaxis, long-lasting protection can be achieved by desensitization immunotherapy, which involves the sub-cutaneous injection of the relevant purified venom over a period of 3–5 years. In cases where the trigger is unknown or where its avoidance is difficult, such as in severe nut allergy, patients should be provided with self-injectable adrenaline and trained in its use.

The recognition and management of anaphylaxis is summarized in Table 75.2

Prognosis

Where the trigger for anaphylaxis has been conclusively identified and appropriate avoidance measures instituted, recurrence of ana-phylaxis is unusual. For patients with insect-venom allergy, desensiti-zation offers a success rate of approximately 90% in reducing the risk of anaphylaxis with future stings. In contrast, the long-term progno-sis for patients with idiopathic anaphylaxis is uncertain because the underlying trigger(s) are unknown and, consequently, it is difficult to devise avoidance measures. In such patients, the possibility of under-lying mastocytosis must be considered and investigated appropri-ately, using serum tryptase and bone marrow biopsy.

How to handle uncertainty in the diagnosis of anaphylaxis

Uncertainty in the diagnosis of anaphylaxis may occur in the absence of a clear history or where a patient has anaphylaxis-like symptoms due to another disorder (see Table 75.1). If a rise in serum tryptase has been documented, this would provide useful supportive evidence of mast cell degranulation suggestive of anaphylaxis.

Where uncertainty does exist, it is important to acknowledge it and undertake a thorough review of the history.

Further Reading

Jones SM and Burks AW. Food allergy. *N Engl J Med* 2017; 377: 1168–176.

Lieberman PL. Recognition and first-line treatment of anaphylaxis. *Am J Medicine* 2014; 127: S6–S11.

Simons FER, Ebisawa M, Sanchez-Borges M, et al. 2015 update of the evidence base: World Allergy Organization anaphylaxis guidelines. World Allergy Organization Journal 2015; 8:32. (Open access) DOI 10.1186/s40413-015-0080-1.

76 Fever

Emma Wall and Graham Cooke

Definition of the symptom

Fever is a rise in core body temperature, which is measured at the tympanic membrane, of greater than 37.8°C and which is one standard deviation beyond the upper limit of the normal range.

Common causes of fever

Common causes of fever are shown in Table 76.1.

Context

Febrile illness comprises approximately 1%–2% of Emergency Department presentations to UK hospitals. Fever has many causes, of which bacterial and viral infections are the most common (Table 76.1). Rare but important causes of fever include systemic fungal infections, tuberculosis, malaria, HIV (both seroconversion and chronic infection), autoimmune diseases (such as SLE and temporal arteritis), malignancies (such as lymphoma), parasitic infestations, and reactions to drug therapy or allergens.

Fever may be experienced for weeks to months without an identifiable cause. In one definition, fever of unknown origin (FUO), or pyrexia of unknown origin (PUO), is a recorded fever of greater than 38.0°C–38.5°C that has been present for more than 3 weeks or is still present after more than 1 week of investigation. Where a cause is identified, infection accounts for approximately one-third of causes of PUO, with another third being due to collagen vascular diseases (commonly temporal arteritis), and the last third to malignancies (commonly lymphoma). A significant number of patients with PUO have no identifying diagnosis, but this group has an overall good prognosis.

Approach to diagnosis

The most important aspect of the approach to a patient with fever is to take a full and detailed history. This should include all current and preceding symptoms, but also a detailed travel, occupational, and sexual history, contacts with any known infection or febrile symptoms in close contacts, any illicit or non-prescribed drug use, and unusual localizing symptoms. The importance of this cannot be overstressed, particularly for diseases associated with a specific risk factor. For example, the majority of deaths from malaria in the UK are due to delay or failure to suspect the diagnosis, which requires an adequate travel history and high index of suspicion.

A thorough and systematic physical examination of all the major organ systems is also essential; for example, subtle rashes, insect bites, masses, murmurs, respiratory crackles, and other physical signs may not have been noticed by the patient, and will lead towards a diagnosis in the majority of cases.

Specific clues to the diagnosis

Most clues towards the diagnosis of fever are obtained from the history. The following are particular diagnostic clues:

Travel: An enormous spectrum of diseases causing fever can be acquired through travel; the most important to recognize promptly is malaria. When necessary, advice from a tropical specialist should always be sought when investigating a febrile returning traveller.

Drug use: The use of all illicit drugs is associated with risks specific to the substance of abuse. Intravenous drug users particularly are at risk of deep-tissue, blood-borne infections which commonly present as a febrile illness.

Pattern of fever: Degree of fever can be divided into high grade (measured core body temperature >38.5°C) and low grade (measured core body temperature 37.6°C–38.5°C). Fever can also present as a relapsing or periodic symptom. Traditionally, there has been great emphasis on patterns of fever; however, while fever patterns can be helpful in suggesting a diagnosis, high-quality evidence in support of their use in diagnosis is lacking. Table 76.2 gives classical examples of diseases that have an associated fever pattern. However, this table is not comprehensive, and no pattern is sensitive or specific.

Weight loss: This is a particularly sinister symptom to accompany a complaint of fever. Malignancies, HIV infection, and tuberculosis are common in this scenario, along with amoebic liver abscesses and endocarditis, amongst others.

Key diagnostic tests

Where the source of fever is clinically apparent (e.g. pneumonia), then tests may be limited to screen for causes of that infection. FUO/PUO should only be used as a working diagnosis once initial common causes have been ruled out, and basic investigations as

Table 76.1 Common causes of fever in primary and secondary care

Primary care	Patients admitted to hospital	Hospital inpatients
Upper and lower respiratory tract infection, including otitis media and sinusitis	Lower respiratory tract infection including exacerbation of chronic obstructive pulmonary disease (COPD) and pneumonia	Hospital-acquired pneumonia Ventilator-associated pneumonia
Urinary tract infection	Urinary tract infection, including pyelonephritis	Catheter-associated urinary tract infection
Gastrointestinal infection	Severe gastrointestinal infection	Norovirus infection *Clostridium difficile* diarrhoea
Skin and soft tissue infection	Severe skin and soft tissue infection	Surgical-site infection
	Non-infectious causes of fever (e.g. inflammatory and neoplastic diseases)	Central-line-associated bloodstream infection Prosthetic-device-associated infection

Table 76.2 Classical patterns of fever and associated aetiology

Fever pattern	Associated aetiology
High grade	Bacterial sepsis, typhoid fever, *Plasmodium falciparum* malaria, systemic viral infections e.g. influenza, lymphoma
Low grade	Infective endocarditis, tuberculosis, bacterial abscesses/collections, malignancies other than lymphoma, HIV infection and associated opportunistic infections, collagen vascular diseases
Relapsing (every 1–3 days)	*Plasmodium vivax* malaria, rickettsial infections, autoimmune diseases, parasitic infections
Periodic	Inherited febrile tendencies (e.g. familial Mediterranean fever), juvenile rheumatoid arthritis, adult-onset Still's disease, Crohn's disease, and Behçet's syndrome

Box 76.1 Initial investigation of a patient with unexplained fever

- blood cultures:
  - two sets of 10 ml each where possible (three, if bacterial endocarditis is suspected)
- microbiological assessment of any body tissues where the source of the fever is suspected:
  - Gram and auramine staining
  - bacterial, tuberculosis, and fungal culture
  - 16S/18S ribosomal PCR
  - appropriate antibody screening, depending on the patient's history
- septic screen, for tissue culture and sensitivity:
  - throat swab
  - urine dip and culture
  - stool microscopy and culture
  - high vaginal swab
  - lumbar puncture
- a blood film examined for malarial parasites in any febrile patient with a history of travel to a relevant area, however brief or distant to the presenting complaint
- HIV serology plus p24 antigen testing
- basic imaging:
  - chest radiography
  - abdominal and pelvic ultrasonography
  - echocardiography
- inflammatory markers:
  - C-reactive protein
  - erythrocyte sedimentation rate
  - these tests are highly sensitive for the presence of inflammation, but have poor specificity
- autoimmune screen:
  - rheumatoid factor
  - antinuclear antibody
  - antineutrophil cytoplasmic antibody
  - complement
  - anti-streptolysin O test
  - lactate dehydrogenase
  - immunoglobulins
- serology following relevant exposure
  - e.g. *Borrelia burgdorferi* following a tick bite
  - consult with a specialist

detailed in Box 76.1 completed as deemed necessary by the thoughtful clinician. Fever in an immune-suppressed patient is a specialist area, and expert advice should be sought.

Other diagnostic tests

The tests outlined in 'Key diagnostic tests', when performed appropriately, will yield a diagnosis in the majority of patients. The following further investigations into the cause of a fever may be performed when indicated clinically or diagnostic uncertainty persists:

- contrast-enhanced CT or MRI scan of a relevant area (commonly brain/spinal cord/bone/joints/chest/abdomen/pelvis)
- bone-marrow aspirate and trephine
- liver biopsy
- lymph-node biopsy
- transoesophageal echocardiography
- radiolabelled white-cell scan
- radioisotope bone scan
- whole-body FDG-PET scan

Introduction to therapy

Empirical broad-spectrum antibiotic therapy should always be started when a patient presents with fever and signs of sepsis (see Chapter 152) or other serious infection, such as meningitis, where delay in initiating therapy may be harmful to the patient. The choice of drug should be made according to local guidelines or following advice from a medical microbiologist. When a source is found, this must be controlled with appropriate antibiotics or other treatment, such as surgical intervention, when necessary.

In a situation when the patient is not seriously unwell, and a clear, treatable cause is not immediately apparent, then empirical antibiotic therapy may be withheld pending the results of appropriate cultures, serology, or other tests, following close discussion with either a clinical infection specialist or a medical microbiologist. This is to allow time for a thoughtful diagnostic approach and directed therapy based on culture results.

Symptomatic fever may be relieved, if causing distress to the patient, with antipyretics during the diagnostic period, although there is no clear evidence to demonstrate noxious effects of fever per se, or of the clinical benefit of relieving symptoms on illness duration. Paracetamol may be used safely to reduce fever in most cases without significantly altering the inflammatory response, and may be superior to aspirin in endotoxaemia. However, equivalent effects have been seen in upper respiratory infections. In severe sepsis, there is some data to suggest that aggressive therapeutic management of the febrile response with paracetamol may be harmful, and alternative measures may be required to cool the patient. Ibuprofen is potentially more potent than paracetamol in reducing symptomatic fever in children and in adults with malaria, but data in other causes of fever is lacking. Ibuprofen is used in children, in whom the risk of Reye's syndrome outweighs any potential benefit of antipyretic treatment with aspirin.

Prognosis

The prognosis from most infectious causes of fever in the immunocompetent is excellent, with the exception of septicaemia associated with the systemic inflammatory response syndrome (see Chapter 152). It is otherwise impossible to give a prognosis for the entire range of the causes of fever, and much depends on the medical comorbidities of the individual patient. Conditions such as diabetes, chronic kidney disease, malignancies, and connective tissue diseases are associated with significantly higher risk of infection and a worse prognosis.

How to handle uncertainty in the diagnosis of this symptom

When the cause of fever is not immediately apparent, there are clear pathways for investigation, as previously outlined. The importance of regularly revisiting the history with the patient and relatives, and repeated detailed clinical examination, must be emphasized. Details from any previous medical notes and laboratory tests must be obtained, as these often contain highly relevant information. Consultation with an infection specialist may provide guidance and suggest alternative important investigations and management.

Further Reading

Horowitz HW. Fever of unknown origin or fever of too many origins? *N Engl J Med* 2013; 368: 197–9.

77 Hyperthermia

Matt Wise and Paul Frost

Definition of the symptom

As homeotherms, humans maintain their core temperature between 36°C–38°C, and this occurs despite variation in metabolic activity and environmental temperature. Elevation of core body temperature due to an increase in the thermoregulatory set point, but with intact thermoregulatory mechanisms, is called fever (see Chapter 76). By contrast, an elevation in core body temperature due to thermoregulatory failure with a normal thermoregulatory set point is called hyperthermia.

Differential diagnosis

Hyperthermia is a defining feature of a number of potentially life-threatening conditions (heat illnesses; Box 77.1).

Context

Hyperthermia occurs when heat production exceeds heat loss. Heat is primarily produced as a result of metabolic activity and this can be dramatically increased during exertion. Additionally, when ambient temperatures exceed 39°C, heat can be transferred from the environment. Thermoregulation is controlled by the preoptic nucleus in the anterior hypothalamus, principally by regulation of cutaneous blood flow and sweat production. Consequentially heat loss occurs mainly through the skin as a result of radiation, evaporation, conduction, and convection. Behavioural adaptation to heat, for example, removing clothing or seeking shade from the sun, is also very important. If these thermoregulatory mechanisms fail then hyperthermia ensues.

Although there is wide variation in individual tolerance to hyperthermia, in general, a core body temperature above 42°C for >8 hours is life-threatening, while death is virtually inevitable at temperatures above 45°C. Death occurs as a result of multiple organ failure due to the direct effects of the thermal injury and a massive inflammatory response to the heat stress. Therefore, hyperthermia should be viewed as a medical emergency requiring immediate intervention.

Globally, the most common heat illnesses are heat exhaustion and heat stroke, and these are major causes of morbidity and mortality. These illnesses represent a continuum of disease ranging from mild (heat exhaustion) to total (heat stroke) failure of thermoregulation. Heat exhaustion is characterized by sweating, muscle cramps, fatigue, vomiting, headaches, dizziness, and fainting. These symptoms may also occur in heat stroke but, in addition, neurological signs such as confusion, seizures, and coma predominate. Not surprisingly, the incidence of these illnesses increases in regions with a high ambient temperature. While the diagnosis of these conditions may be straightforward, hyperthermia may complicate a variety of rarer illnesses (Box 77.1). Knowledge of these is essential, as successful management of hyperthermia is dependent on identification and treatment of the underlying cause.

Approach to diagnosis

Temperature, either taken orally or, more commonly, at the tympanic membrane, is one of the first measurements carried out on newly admitted patients. Therefore, patients with pyrexia are usually identified quite rapidly.

Clearly, definitive management of pyrexia requires identification of the underlying cause, but it is important to remember that patients with hyperpyrexia (>41.5°C) need immediate treatment, regardless of the aetiology.

As a general rule, hyperpyrexia is usually associated with a heat illness rather than a condition causing fever. Occasionally, the pattern of temperature elevation, for example, the intermittent fever seen in malaria, or the remittent fever observed in infectious endocarditis, will suggest an infectious aetiology. However, this is rare and, most often, there are no pathognomonic features (duration, extent, or pattern) of an elevated temperature per se that will reliably identify the underlying disease or distinguish hyperthermia from fever. As such, a meticulous history is required to differentiate the many causes of fever (infection, cancers, immunological causes, drugs, tissue infarction, pulmonary thromboembolism, etc.; see Chapter 76) from a heat illness.

Particular attention should be paid to the general circumstances around the admission, as this can frequently lead to the diagnosis; for example, the case of an athlete who collapses during an endurance event on a hot day, or of a witnessed overdose with the 'recreational' drug MDMA (3,4-methylenedioxy-N-methamphetamine).

Specific enquiry should be made about conditions known to cause heat illnesses, for example, endocrine or neuropsychiatric disease; culprit drugs such as neuroleptic agents or dopamine antagonists; a family history of malignant hyperthermia, or risk factors for heat exhaustion such as immobility, decreased fluid intake, or poor housing (lack of air-conditioning or ventilation).

Eliciting symptoms of 'heat illnesses' is frequently diagnostically unrewarding, as they are typically non-specific, often resembling those due to viral illness, such as, for example, myalgia, fatigue, nausea, vomiting, and irritability. However, CNS symptoms such as hallucinations, odd behaviour, delirium, or confusion are important because, in the context of recent heat exposure, the combination of CNS symptoms and hyperthermia is strongly suggestive of heat stroke. CNS examination is crucial, as a plethora of signs, including seizures, reduced level of consciousness, opisthotonus, pupillary abnormalities, and cerebellar dysfunction, can occur in heat stroke. Moreover, extrapyramidal effects, (choreiform movements, cogwheel rigidity, oculogyric crisis, dyskinesia, and festinating gait) are characteristic of neuroleptic malignant syndrome (NMS).

Signs of automonic dysfunction (tachycardia, tachypnoea, diaphoresis, incontinence, and hypertension) may also be seen in NMS, and these should also be sought.

Specific clues to the diagnosis

In all cases, the core temperature is typically, but not invariably, elevated to 38°C–42°C.

Heat exhaustion/heat stroke

Specific clues to heat exhaustion/heat stroke are:

- high ambient temperature (heat wave)
- reduced ability for behavioural adaptation to heat (extremes of age, mental incapacity, physical immobility)

Box 77.1 Causes of hyperthermia

- heat exhaustion
- heat stroke
- malignant hyperthermia
- neuroleptic malignant syndrome
- drug-induced hyperthermia
- hormonal hyperthermia
- hypothalamic dysfunction
- neuropsychiatric hyperthermia

- limited acclimatization (tourist)
- recent vigorous exercise (athletes, military training)

Malignant hyperthermia

Specific clues to malignant hyperthermia are:

- anaesthesia with known trigger drugs (depolarizing muscle relaxants and inhalational agents)
- the following events occurring during the first 30 minutes of anaesthesia:
  - inexplicable increase in heart rate
  - inexplicable hypertension
  - inexplicable increase in end-tidal CO_2
  - inexplicable increase in oxygen consumption
  - generalized muscular rigidity

Neuroleptic malignant syndrome

Specific clues to neuroleptic malignant syndrome are:

- use of neuroleptic drugs (phenothiazines, butyrophenones, and thioxanthines)
- muscular rigidity
- autonomic instability
- altered mental status

Drug-induced hyperthermia

Specific clues to drug-induced hyperthermia are:

- history of overdose of salicylates
- history of drug abuse with:
  - cocaine
  - MDMA
  - amphetamines

Hormonal hyperthermia

Specific clues to hormonal hyperthermia are clinical and laboratory features of:

- thyrotoxicosis (thyroid storm)
- phaeochromocytoma
- Addison's disease
- hypoglycaemia
- hyperparathyroidism

Hypothalamic dysfunction

Central (hypothalamic) thermoregulatory failure is rare. However, after exclusion of other causes of hyperthermia, hypothalamic dysfunction (via infection, cerebrovascular accident, tumour, granulomatous disease) should be considered.

Neuropsychiatric hyperthermia

Specific clues to neuropsychiatric hyperthermia are:

- clinical features suggestive of status epilepticus (known epilepsy, witnessed seizures, or post-ictal state)
- delirium tremens (history of drug or alcohol withdrawal)
- lethal catatonia (mutism, psychotic excitement, echolalia, muscular rigidity)

Key diagnostic tests

Key diagnostic tests are:

- core body temperature (tympanic, rectal, or oesophageal)
- tests providing evidence of organ damage and shock (which can occur in all heat illnesses):
  - creatine kinase (if elevated, suggests rhabdomyolysis)
  - liver enzymes (if elevated, suggests liver damage)
  - full blood count (will show haemoconcentration secondary to dehydration)
  - clotting screen (to exclude disseminated intravascular coagulopathy)
  - urea and electrolytes (to exclude acute kidney injury)
  - blood glucose (to exclude hypoglycaemia as a feature of acute liver failure)
  - arterial blood gas (to exclude type A lactic acidosis)
  - urinalysis (to exclude haematuria and myoglobinuria)
- halothane caffeine contracture test (to exclude malignant hyperthermia)
- capnography (elevated end-tidal CO_2 indicates malignant hyperthermia)
- drug toxicity screen (to exclude hyperthermia secondary to overdose or drug abuse)
- thyroid function tests; plasma and urinary catecholamines and metanephrines; cortisol; calcium; and parathyroid hormone (to exclude endocrinopathy associated with hyperthermia)
- MRI and CT of the brain (to exclude CNS disease causing hypothalamic dysfunction)
- lumbar puncture (to exclude CNS disease causing hypothalamic dysfunction)
- electroencephalography (to detect subclinical seizures)

Other diagnostic tests

Blood cultures and other microbiological samples should be taken as indicated by clinical history and examination (infection is an important differential diagnosis of heat illness).

Introduction to therapy

The following points should be noted:

- Heat illnesses can be life-threatening and, in all but the most minor cases of heat exhaustion, senior assistance should be sought.
- An airway, breathing, and circulation (ABC) approach should be taken so as to rapidly establish a safe airway, ensure adequate ventilation, and restore circulating blood volume
- Multi-organ failure is likely, so the patient should be managed in an intensive care unit or high-dependency ward.
- In cases of hyperpyrexia (>41.5°C), immediate cooling is required; a variety of methods are available (although all of these methods are successful, the patented devices seem to be the most efficient):
  - evaporative cooling; this relies on spraying the body with tepid (15°C) water while cooling with air flow from large fans; this technique has been successfully deployed on victims of heat stroke at the annual Hajj (Muslim pilgrimage to Mecca)
  - iced water immersion
  - rapid intravenous administration of cold (4°C) Hartmann's solution (30 ml/kg of ideal body weight), followed by surface cooling using ice or cold packs
  - patented devices (water-circulating external cooling devices, air-circulating external cooling devices, and intravascular cooling systems)
  - cardiopulmonary bypass
- Dantrolene is a muscle relaxant that works by blocking the release of calcium from the sarcoplasmic reticulum, thus reducing the amount of heat produced by the muscles. This drug is recommended as a specific therapy for malignant hyperthermia and NMS.
- Dopamine agonists (to treat hyperthermia) and benzodiazepines (to treat muscular rigidity) have been used for NMS.
- Definitive treatment requires identification and management of the underlying cause but, in cases of hyperpyrexia, ascertaining the diagnosis should not delay cooling.

Prognosis

The mortality rate for heat stroke has been reported to range from 10% to 70%. While some of this is attributable to comorbidity and increasing age, higher death rates were reported in those patients when treatment was delayed for more than 2 hours. In the 1960s, the mortality rate for malignant hyperthermia was 80%. Today, with earlier recognition and the use of dantrolene, the mortality rate is around 10%. The key message is that heat illnesses are all potentially lethal and that prognosis can be improved by early recognition and instigation of timely and effective treatment.

How to handle uncertainty in the diagnosis of this symptom

Provided the core temperature has been measured accurately, there is little uncertainty in the diagnosis of hyperthermia. Uncertainty resides in diagnosing the underlying cause. This requires a meticulous history and examination as well as appropriate investigations. However, this process should not delay treatment of life-threatening hyperpyrexia.

Further Reading

Atha WF. Heat-related illness. *Emerg Med Clin N Am* 2013; 31: 1097–108.

Perry PJ and Wilborn CA. Serotonin syndrome vs neuroleptic malignant syndrome: A contrast of causes, diagnoses, and management. *Ann Clin Psychiatry* 2012; 24: 155–62.

Rosenberg H, Pollock N, Schiemann A, Bulger T, Stowell K. Malignant hyperthermia: a review. *Orphanet J Rare Dis* 2015; 10: 93. doi:10.1186/s13023-015-0310-1

Definition

Hypothermia is defined by a core body temperature of <35.0°C, and may be further characterised as mild (32.0°C–34.9°C), moderate (28.0°C–31.9°C), or severe (<28.0°C). Primary hypothermia is the result of environmental exposure, while in secondary hypothermia there is an underlying medical condition which perturbs thermoregulation.

Differential diagnosis

The number of cases of hypothermia and the aetiology of the underlying cause are greatly influenced by the local environment. Common characteristics of people with hypothermia are given in Box 78.1. Many individuals die of hypothermia without coming into contact with healthcare professionals.

Mild hypothermia (32.0°C–36.0°C) has used as a therapeutic modality in intensive care for traumatic brain injury, to lower intracranial pressure, although a recent, large, multicentre trial suggested that its use may actually increase mortality. It has also been used following out-of-hospital cardiac arrest, to improve neurological outcomes. However, recently, a large, international, multicentre trial found that 36.0°C was equally as effective as 33.0°C in relation to death and poor neurological outcome. International guidelines, therefore, recommend maintaining a constant temperature between 32.0°C–36.0°C in unconscious survivors of out-of-hospital cardiac arrest. Hypothermia and even hypothermic circulatory arrest are also used during cardiac surgery and aortic root replacement surgery.

Box 78.1 Common characteristics of people with hypothermia

Found outside

Urban
- young male
- alcohol use
- drug intoxication
- deliberate self-harm
- mental illness
- homelessness
- assault

Extra-urban
- young male
- water pursuits
- water immersion
- outdoor pursuits
- primary exposure
- trauma (falls)

Found inside
- elderly
- stroke
- endocrine disorders:
  - diabetes (common)
  - hypothyroidism
  - hypopituitarism
  - adrenal insufficiency
- infection
- self-neglect
- fall or immobility

Context

It is difficult to know exactly how many individuals are affected by hypothermia because the number of estimated cases greatly exceeds officially recorded numbers. Many individuals succumb to hypothermia without ever coming to the attention of healthcare workers until after death. The prevalence varies enormously, depending on environmental and economic circumstances. It is commoner in cold or rapidly changing climates, or in areas where there is a focus on pursuits such as mountaineering, fell-walking, or outdoor water sports. Alcohol, drugs, and mental illness are important etiological factors in patients found hypothermic in urban areas and reflect local socio-economic demographics.

The diagnosis is obvious when a patient is discovered cold after being lost on a mountain or pulled from prolonged immersion in water. Individuals, particularly when found inside, pose more of a diagnostic challenge when suffering from mild hypothermia as they may be confused, dysarthric, ataxic, or dizzy. These findings may raise the possibility the patient is suffering from a stroke, diabetic complication, or infection. However, the patient's clinical findings may be the result of primary hypothermia or secondary hypothermia related to sepsis, hypoglycaemia, or stroke.

Clinical findings in hypothermia

Mild hypothermia

The clinical findings for mild hypothermia are:

- shivering
- hypertension
- tachycardia
- tachypnoea
- confusion (e.g. paradoxical undressing)
- dysarthria
- ataxia
- apathy
- diuresis

Moderate hypothermia

The clinical findings for moderate hypothermia are:

- the patient is not shivering (at this stage, the shivering stops)
- hypotension
- bradycardia
- hypoventilation
- stupor
- hyporeflexia
- dilated pupils
- sluggish pupillary reflexes

Severe hypothermia

The clinical findings for severe hypothermia are:

- coma
- apnoea
- absent reflexes, including pupillary reflexes
- muscle rigidity mimicking rigor mortis
- ventricular fibrillation (VF) or asystole may occur spontaneously

Approach to diagnosing hypothermia

All patients admitted to hospital have a temperature recorded, so a diagnosis of hypothermia may be quickly established. Oral temperature is not an accurate representation of core temperature.

A low-reading thermometer should be used to accurately record core temperature. Core temperature can be recorded with a tympanic, rectal, or oesophageal thermometer. Oesophageal temperature most accurately reflects core temperature during rewarming. Recording core temperature is extremely important in the prehospital setting to prevent an additional decrease (after-drop) of core temperature, which can occur following rescue and is often the cause of post-rescue collapse.

Specific clues to diagnosis

Patients with hypothermia will not complain that they are cold and may be confused or comatose. Nevertheless, temperature is measured on all hospital admissions and so the diagnosis should not be overlooked. If the temperature is recorded as <35.0°C, a low-reading thermometer must be used.

Key diagnostic tests

The majority of investigations in hypothermic patients are focused on causes of secondary hypothermia:

- CT head, to exclude:
  - intracerebral, subdural, or extradural haemorrhage
  - traumatic brain injury
  - haemorrhagic or ischaemic stroke
  - empty sella syndrome
  - pituitary tumour
- blood glucose, to exclude:
  - hypoglycaemia
  - diabetic ketoacidosis (acute hypothermia can elevate plasma glucose)
- toxicology plasma or urine (to exclude accidental or intentional self-harm), to exclude the presence of:
  - alcohol
  - benzodiazepines
  - opiates
  - gamma-hydroxybutryric acid
  - barbiturates
  - carbon monoxide
  - paracetamol
  - salicylate
  - tricyclic antidepressants
  - phenothiazines
  - ethylene glycol
- blood, urine, sputum, ascites, or CSF culture, in suspected sepsis
- imaging:
  - radiographs or CT in suspected trauma
  - a chest radiograph, to look for aspiration pneumonia, community-acquired pneumonia, or fractured ribs
- endocrine tests:
  - thyroid function
  - Synacthen test
- ECG, which will show features such as:
  - J waves
  - bradycardia
  - conduction delays
  - atrial or ventricular arrhythmias

Introduction to therapy

Prehospital care

The principle aims of treatment in prehospital care are to:

- prevent heat loss
- rewarm the core temperature
- avoid precipitating VF

In mild hypothermia, wet clothing should be removed and replaced with dry clothing; the patient should be made to exercise, to keep warm; and the peripheral limbs should be massaged. Giving alcohol to the patient may drop the core temperature further and should be avoided.

Moderate-to-severe hypothermia requires core rewarming, which may be achieved with humidified, warmed (42.0°C) oxygen in the prehospital environment. VF can occur spontaneously below 30.0°C, so the patient should be kept in the horizontal position. Unnecessary movement or intervention should be avoided, as this may precipitate VF, which is resistant to drugs and defibrillation unless the core temperature is raised to above 30.0°C. Core temperature, vital signs, and ECG readings should be monitored.

Hospital care

Patients who are comatose should be intubated and mechanically ventilated with warmed, humidified oxygen. Central access must be established, as peripheral cannulation is difficult, and flow to the central circulation is variable. Wet clothing should be removed, if not done previously, and an ECG monitor attached. Core temperature must be monitored. Manipulation of the patient should be kept to a minimum if a cardiac rhythm is present, as needless intervention or movement of the patient can precipitate VF. If the patient has no palpable pulse for >45 seconds, CPR should be initiated. Defibrillation, vasoactive drugs, including adrenaline and atropine, and cardiac pacing are largely ineffective unless the core temperature exceeds 30.0°C. Thus, if initial defibrillation for VF is unsuccessful, further defibrillation and drugs should be withheld until the core temperature exceeds 30.0°C. Importantly, repeated administration of drugs at temperatures below 30.0°C leads to accumulation and toxicity. Life-threatening trauma should be excluded either as the cause or a complication of the patient's hypothermia and should be treated accordingly. An inspection should be made for frostbite.

Mild hypothermia has a good prognosis in the absence of an underlying medical condition, and treatment is aimed at reducing further heat loss. Patients can be left to passively rewarm in mild hypothermia by moving to a warm, dry environment and being allowed to shiver. Rewarming is slow by this method and relies on normal endocrine function and adequate energy stores. Active external rewarming with forced air warming blankets has been used in such cases, but caution should be exercised, as this technique can reduce core temperature further. It is preferable to use warmed, humidified oxygen or warmed fluids at 40.0°C–42.0°C.

It is uncertain how quickly the patient should be rewarmed in moderate-to-severe hypothermia. Only techniques aimed at increasing core temperature should be used. An oesophageal temperature probe most closely correlates with cardiac temperature during rewarming and should be monitored in preference to rectal or tympanic temperature, when available.

Increasing the core temperature

The following may be used to increase the core temperature:

- humidified, warmed oxygen
- warmed intravenous fluid (Hartmann's solution may increase already elevated lactate levels, as liver metabolism of lactate is impaired in hypothermia)
- gastric, peritoneal, thoracic, or bladder lavage with warm fluids
- haemofiltration or haemodialysis
- intravascular cooling devices developed for therapeutic hypothermia in the intensive care unit, as these also can be used to rewarm hypothermic patients
- cardiopulmonary bypass may be required for core rewarming in severe cases

Complications following return to normal temperature

The following complications may occur after the core temperature has returned to normal:

- arrhythmia
- pulmonary oedema
- hypotension
- infections, including pneumonia
- pancreatitis
- rhabdomyolysis
- severe electrolyte disturbance

Prognosis

Prognosis depends principally on the severity of hypothermia and the presence of any underlying medical condition. In previously fit individuals with no trauma, prognosis is excellent, providing after-drop is avoided and the patient does not sustain VF. Mortality is extremely high in severely hypothermic patients with trauma or an underlying medical condition such as sepsis or stroke. In one study of patients admitted to urban hospitals in the west of Scotland over a winter period, one-half had an underlying medical condition, and mortality was 31%.

How to handle uncertainty in the diagnosis of hypothermia

There should be little diagnostic uncertainty of hypothermia in a hospital setting because all patients have their temperatures recorded. If a temperature <35.0°C is measured, a low-reading thermometer should be used to accurately record a low core temperature. However, a number of diagnostic uncertainties surround hypothermia. The following points should be noted:

- If there is no response to rewarming, suspect sepsis or an endocrine disorder.
- Be sure to exclude an underlying medical condition, such as diabetes, stroke, sepsis, trauma, and intoxication with drugs or alcohol.
- As coagulation tests and blood gases are performed at 37.0°C, patients may show clinical evidence of bleeding but have normal laboratory coagulation results, because enzymes are temperature dependent. Coagulopathy resolves with correction of core temperature. Uncorrected blood gas analysis is recommended.
- Severe hypothermia mimics death and it can be difficult to know when to stop resuscitation. Patients have survived with intact neurological function when core temperatures as low as <15.0°C have been documented. If the chest is frozen or there is an injury incompatible with survival, resuscitation should not be attempted. Resuscitation may be abandoned when the core temperature exceeds 32.0°C and there is no response to advanced cardiac life support.

Further Reading

Bernhardt V and Babb T. Exertional dyspnoea in obesity *Eur Respir Rev* 2016; 25: 487–95

Paal P, Gordon L, Strapazzone G, et al. Accidental hypothermia—an update. *Scand J Trauma Resusc Emerg Med* 2016; 24: 111. doi:10.1186/s13049-016-0303-7.

Truhlář A, Deakin CD, Soar J, et al. Cardiac arrest in special circumstances. *Resuscitation* 2015; 95: 148–201.

79 Fatigue

Trudie Chalder and Matteo Cella

Definition of the symptom

Fatigue is a term used to describe difficultly in sustaining physical or mental effort. It should be distinguished from weakness, which is an inability to generate normal muscular strength. Fatigue is a natural signal to reduce or stop physical activity, but also a common subjective experience which may escalate to a significant health complaint as either a primary or a secondary (or supporting) symptom to an existing condition.

Differential diagnosis

Fatigue is the one of the commonest symptoms experienced by the general population. Approximately 25% of patients attending their general practitioner complain of fatigue. However, only 10%–15% of these patients will receive a diagnosis of a physical illness (see Tables 79.1 and 79.2).

Context

Fatigue is a common and natural experience in everyday life; nonetheless, it is a somehow vague and imprecise concept, difficult to measure, and with a broad range of possible etiologies. Patients generally describe fatigue with terms such as tiredness, exhaustion, or weariness. Fatigue may be associated with pain, aches, anxiety, low mood, irritability, and frustration. Moderate fatigue can occur as a result of stressful situations or illness, and in these settings is usually transient. Extreme and persistent levels of fatigue are associated with high levels of disability, limitations in mental, physical, and social functioning, and considerable social and economic impact because of increased consumption of healthcare and absenteeism from work. Prevalence studies find 25%–30% of patients in general practice complaining about fatigue, while as many as 30%–50% reported symptoms of fatigue in the general population at large.

A severe, incapacitating, chronic fatigue that is not caused by an underlying medical condition can be diagnosed as chronic fatigue syndrome (CFS). CFS has been reported with a prevalence of 0.1%–2.6% in the community and in primary-care-based studies, depending on the criteria used. Women are at higher risk of developing CFS than men are. Although many patients report a viral infection prior to the onset of chronic fatigue, no physiological link has been established which could be solely responsible for the onset of the illness. To date, CFS is conceptualized mainly as a disorder with a mixed

Table 79.1 Differential diagnosis of fatigue in primary and secondary care

Diagnosis in primary care	%	Diagnosis in secondary care	%
Physical illnesses: • anaemia • emphysema • asthma • arthritis • cancer • diabetes • viral infection • multiple sclerosis	10	Chronic fatigue syndrome	50
Sleep problems	5	Physical illnesses (after appropriate tests)	10
Depression, anxiety, and stress	20	Depression or anxiety	25
Chronic fatigue syndrome	10	Sleep problems	5
Other psychological causes	10	Other psychiatric illnesses	5
Other secondary fatigue	45	Other secondary fatigue	5

Table 79.2 Abnormal blood results in people presenting with fatigue

Test	%
Haemoglobin	5
White blood cell count	4
Erythrocyte sedimentation rate/plasma viscosity	8
Urea	9
Electrolytes	2
Glucose (serum or urine)	2
Thyroid-stimulating hormone/thyroxine	4
Monospot	10

aetiology in which psychological and physical factors are thought to work together to predispose an individual to develop chronic fatigue, and to precipitate and perpetuate the illness.

Approach to diagnosis

One of the key aspects in assessing fatigue is to ascertain whether the fatigue is a manifestation of an underlying medical condition. When fatigue is a symptom within the context of a medical condition, it is likely that, by treating the main illness, the fatigue severity will recede. This type of fatigue is sometimes referred to as secondary fatigue, as it is not the patient's primary complaint and it is the product of a clear, medical condition. Multiple sclerosis, cancer, and a number of endocrine, inflammatory, and immune disorders are known to cause secondary fatigue.

When fatigue is medically unexplainable, a diagnosis of CFS can be considered. CFS can be diagnosed in individuals who report signs of persistent and debilitating fatigue for at least 6 months. In addition to this criterion, routine laboratory tests (e.g. full blood count, erythrocyte sedimentation rate, renal, liver, and thyroid function, and urinary protein and glucose) and a physical and mental state examination need to be performed in order to rule out any other possible explanation for the fatigue. In 1994, the Centers for Disease Control (CDC) operationalized the criteria for the diagnosis of CFS. According to these criteria, a diagnosis of CFS can be made when patient presents with persistent or relapsing fatigue which starts with a definite onset, remains unexplained after clinical evaluation, produces a marked decline in the patient's previous level of occupational and social activities, and lasts for at least 6 months. In addition, patients should present with at least four of the following eight possible subjective complaints: muscle pain, joint pain, headaches, sore throat, tender lymph nodes, unrefreshing sleep, post-exertional malaise, and impaired short-term memory and concentration. According to the CDC criteria, conditions such as morbid obesity, drug or alcohol abuse, and psychiatric disorders such as psychosis, dementia, and eating disorders would invalidate the diagnosis of CFS, whereas conditions such as non-psychotic depression, anxiety disorder, and somatoform disorder would be consistent with a CFS diagnosis.

Although CFS is the most frequently used diagnostic label to identify a pathology of unexplained and debilitating fatigue, this condition is sometimes referred to by alternative terms, including myalgic encephalomyelitis, chronic fatigue and immune dysfunction syndrome, or post-viral fatigue syndrome.

Specific clues to the diagnosis of chronic fatigue

There is currently no diagnostic test or pattern of tests that can assist the diagnosis of CFS. Specialists generally carry out investigations for

Table 79.3 Aspects that should be taken into consideration for a diagnosis of chronic fatigue syndrome

	Secondary fatigue	Primary fatigue or chronic fatigue
Viral infection	Acute or remission phase	Fully remitted
Situation	May be linked to treatment due to side effects of drugs	May be linked to levels of activity and/or stress
Weekly variation	Often improvement	Stable
Onset	With medical condition	Sometimes with viral infections but not necessarily
Duration	Variable	More than 6 months
Cognitive symptoms	Sometimes	Often
Associated symptoms	Variable	Pain, sleep problems, concentration and memory problems
Comorbid diagnosis	Unspecific	Depression, IBS, anxiety, fibromyalgia, pain
Physical examination	Could be positive to a medical illness	Normal
Laboratory tests	Could be positive to a medical illness	Negative to medical conditions
Beliefs	Sometimes catastrophic	Fear of engaging in activity Focus on symptoms Somatic illness attributions Catastrophizing Perfectionism

unusual patterns in the patient's history (e.g. pronounced weight loss, foreign travel), look for any abnormality in symptom presentation (e.g. no cognitive symptoms), and carry out a physical examination and basic laboratory tests to screen for other possible explanations for fatigue. Nevertheless, acute and debilitating fatigue is also present in a number of conditions as a secondary symptom. Table 79.3 attempts to summarize some of the aspects that should be taken into consideration for a diagnosis of CFS and may be helpful in distinguishing fatigue as a primary complaint from secondary fatigue.

Key diagnostic tests

As the diagnosis of chronic fatigue is achieved by 'exclusion' of other possible explanations of fatigue, all the investigations to be conducted are aimed at confirming the absence of a condition that could account for the abnormal levels of fatigue. The first step for the diagnosis of CFS is a comprehensive clinical investigation comprising a detailed history and physical examination. Further, a number of laboratory investigations are recommended in order to exclude underlying medical conditions. Recommended laboratory investigations are full blood count, erythrocyte sedimentation rate or C-reactive protein, urea and electrolytes, thyroid function tests, and urine for protein and sugar. It may be also helpful to consider the following: rheumatoid factor, Epstein–Barr serology, antinuclear factor, and serological tests for cytomegalovirus, Q fever, toxoplasmosis, and HIV.

In addition to the physical examination, a psychiatric screening needs to be conducted to exclude the presence of a major psychiatric condition. Fatigue is a common complaint in mental disorders and, where it can be fully explained by a specific psychiatric disease, a diagnosis of CFS should not be made. However, a number of psychiatric conditions, particularly depression, anxiety, and somatoform disorder, commonly occur as comorbid features of CFS.

Introduction to therapy

To date, evidence suggests that behavioural interventions are the most effective treatment strategies for fatigue symptoms. In particular two approaches, cognitive behavioural therapy (CBT) and graded exercise therapy (GET), have been shown to be effective in reducing fatigue symptoms, disability, and fatigue-associated complaints. CBT involves the use of specific techniques to alter and modify thoughts and actions that maintain and exacerbate fatigue-related behaviour. These strategies involve planned activity and rest, sleep management, activity monitoring, cognitive restructuring for unhelpful beliefs, and challenging of unhelpful assumptions.

GET involves an individually tailored, structured exercise programme aimed at gradually increasing the level of aerobic activity. The suggested exercise is usually walking, and patients are advised not to exceed the prescribed exercise duration or intensity.

Pharmacological intervention specifically targeting fatigue-related symptoms is per se unwarranted by research evidence. Medication acting against viral persistence or targeting immune function does not show a sizable reduction in fatigue levels in CFS patients. Similarly, treating chronic fatigue with antidepressants does not produce marked improvement on fatigue, but such treatment is often justified and helpful in treating frequently associated mood disorders.

There is insufficient evidence to recommend dietary supplementation, interferon, evening primrose oil, or intramuscular magnesium as a treatment for CFS. Prolonged rest cannot be recommended as a treatment of chronic fatigue, as this strategy may in fact perpetuate or increase fatigue in people recovering from viral infection.

In the case of secondary fatigue (e.g. related to cancer or multiple sclerosis), both CBT and GET can help alleviate the symptoms and associated disability.

Prognosis

The prognosis of fatigue is variable and depends largely on the condition responsible for the fatigue exacerbation. If an organic condition can be ascertained and fatigue is a clear by-product of such a condition, recovery from the condition will most likely result in an improvement of fatigue symptoms, although not always.

Prognosis of CFS shows considerable variability, but it is never associated per se with an increased risk of mortality.

In the case of untreated CFS, full recovery is rare and only a small proportion of individuals report improvement in symptoms. CBT and GET improve fatigue and disability in about 50%, and two studies showed that about 25% make a full recovery at 2 and 5 years after a course of CBT. Poor prognostic outcomes are associated with psychiatric comorbidity, while good prognostic outcomes are associated with low severity of fatigue symptoms, illness attribution style which is not physical, and a sense of control over symptoms. CFS is associated with significant disability and dysfunction both at home and at work, with rates of CFS-related unemployment as high as 37%. For CFS patients seen in primary care, symptom improvement is more commonly reported than full recovery.

How to handle uncertainty in the diagnosis of this symptom

Fatigue is a common symptom shared by many disorders. It is therefore important to initially assess the aetiology of the symptoms; in particular, clarify if the fatigue is the result of a medical condition or is medically unexplained. Laboratory tests, medical examination, and specialists' opinions may be helpful in the first instance to establish the cause of fatigue. If criteria for the diagnosis of CFS can be satisfied, the patient should be introduced to fatigue management strategies and referred to specialist clinics.

Further Reading

Clark, LV, Pesola, F, Thomas, JM, Vergara-Williamson, M, Beynon, M, and White, PD. Guided graded exercise self-help plus specialist medical care versus specialist medical care alone for chronic fatigue syndrome (GETSET): a pragmatic randomised controlled trial. *Lancet* 2017; 390: 363–73.

80 Unintentional weight loss

Satish Keshav and Alexandra Kent

Definition of the symptom

Unintentional weight loss refers to weight loss that is not voluntary, and can reflect serious underlying pathology. It can be caused by inadequate nutritional intake, increased metabolism, malabsorption, or a combination of these factors. Weight loss of 5% of body weight over 6–12 months should be investigated. Cachexia is a complex syndrome in which loss of body mass (fat and protein) cannot be reversed nutritionally, that is, is due to underlying disease processes inducing catabolism, rather than to inadequate nutritional intake.

The differential diagnosis in primary care and secondary care

Box 80.1 outlines the differential diagnosis in primary care and secondary care, ordered by probability.

Context

Body weight is determined by the combination of metabolic rate, calorie intake, and activity levels. Clinically relevant weight loss is considered to be ≥5% of body weight over 6–12 months; ≥10% weight loss can lead to physiological impairment (e.g. impaired immune system, increased infections), and ≥20% leads to organ dysfunction. Men reach their maximum weight in the fifth decade, and women in their sixth. Beyond this, natural weight loss is usually due to declining muscle mass, with the redistribution of muscle mass in the extremities, leading to greater truncal fat stores.

Approach to diagnosis

Patients will often have had their weight documented at previous, possibly unrelated, outpatient clinics, or the GP may have previous weights

---

Box 80.1 Differential diagnosis in primary care and secondary care, ordered by probability

Common
- coeliac disease
- systemic disease causing wasting and disordered metabolism (e.g. diabetes mellitus, thyrotoxicosis, tuberculosis, lymphoma, HIV, emphysema, heart failure)
- medications that suppress appetite or cause nausea and food aversion (e.g. opiates, amphetamines, antibiotics, chemotherapeutics)
- poor dentition and oral ulceration
- social isolation and poverty
- disseminated malignancy (e.g. from breast, lung, prostate)

Uncommon
- chronic pancreatitis and pancreatic insufficiency
- Crohn's disease and ulcerative colitis (less frequently)
- oesophageal dysmotility (especially in the elderly)
- mucocutaneous candidiasis
- psychiatric disease, including depression and anorexia nervosa (begging the question of intentionality)

Rare
- Upper gastrointestinal malignancy (especially oesophageal and gastric cancer)

---

documented in their records. It is important to attempt to quantify and confirm weight loss as it is often very subjective. Furthermore, the initial consultation should identify the most likely physiological cause of weight loss: malabsorption, increased metabolism, catabolism, and so on. It is important to ask the patient the following questions:

- How much weight have you lost?
- When did the weight loss begin?
- Over what period of time has the weight loss occurred?
- Are you eating less?
- How is your appetite?
- Have you changed your diet?
- Are you on any new medications?
- Are you doing more exercise?
- Have you been unwell recently?
- Do you have any underlying medical problems?
- Have you been feeling more stress or anxiety than usual?
- Have you had constipation or diarrhoea?
- Are there any additional symptoms?

Twenty-five per cent of patients with cancer suffer from anorexia, and up to 60% have cachexia. Weight loss is common in patients with lung and gastrointestinal cancers, especially of the oesophagus, stomach, and pancreas. Conversely, weight loss is rare in breast or prostate cancer, unless there is disseminated disease.

Specific clues to the diagnosis

True weight loss is often apparent, with the patient's clothes hanging loosely, although this may not be obvious in patients who originally had a high BMI. Specific questions which can aid diagnosis include:

- Do you have any dental problems or mouth sores?
- Do you have occasional uncontrollable hunger with palpitations, tremor, and sweating? (This suggests hyperthyroidism.)
- Do you have increased sensitivity to cold or heat? (This suggests thyroid dysfunction.)
- Do you have increased thirst or are you drinking more? (This suggests diabetes mellitus.)
- Are you urinating more than usual? (This suggests diabetes mellitus.)
- What medications/drugs are you taking? (The use of diuretics, laxatives, alcohol, and illicit drugs can lead to weight loss.)
- Do you feel low? Do you suffer with poor sleep? (This suggests depression.)
- Are you pleased or concerned with the weight loss? (This question may help differentiate between pathological and psychological weight loss.)

Age will immediately influence the differential diagnosis, with cancers being more common in patients over 50 years. Younger patients are more likely to suffer from malabsorption. Patients with weight loss related to chronic disease will invariably be aware of the chronic disease diagnosis, although it is often important to ensure weight loss is not related to a coincidental pathology. With elderly patients, assess how they obtain their food, especially in those with ill health or reduced mobility. Shopping and preparing meals may be problematic, and poor dentition or ill-fitting dentures may make chewing difficult. Social support, such as 'Meals on Wheels', may be a simple measure that will prevent further weight loss.

Key diagnostic tests

Key diagnostic tests are as follows:

Full blood count: Normocytic anaemia may occur with chronic disease, and renal failure. Malabsorption can result in microcytic or macrocytic disease, depending on the underlying cause, and the nutritional deficiency. A full blood count should be accompanied by haematinics to identify the cause of anaemia. Combined iron and folate deficiency is usually due to untreated coeliac disease. Iron deficiency anaemia should be considered a sign of gastrointestinal disease unless there is a clear alternative diagnosis.

Erythrocyte sedimentation rate (ESR) and/or C-reactive protein (CRP): These inflammatory markers, when raised, are non-specific indicators of disease, malignancy, infection, or connective tissue disorder.

Urea, creatinine, and electrolytes: These tests are used to exclude renal failure and Addison's disease.

Fasting blood glucose: This is used to exclude diabetes mellitus.

Albumin: Albumin levels can reflect nutritional intake, although they can also be reduced in chronic disease.

Liver function tests, clotting screen: These are used to exclude liver failure.

Thyroid function tests: These are used to exclude hyperthyroidism.

Chest X-ray: This is used to exclude malignancy and tuberculosis.

Coeliac serology: This is used to exclude coeliac disease.

CT scan: Patients (especially those >50 years) with weight loss of unknown cause and with no specific clues to the diagnosis, will invariably undergo a CT scan of the chest, abdomen, and pelvis, to exclude underlying malignancy.

Other diagnostic tests

Further investigations depend on the associated symptoms, which direct you to the body system likely to be responsible for the weight loss. For example, weight loss and microcytic anaemia suggest a gastrointestinal cause, and would be investigated by a gastroscopy and colonoscopy (either endoscopically or radiologically). Patients with non-specific abdominal or pelvic pain may be referred for an abdominal and pelvic CT scan. Bone pain would initiate X-rays and/or a bone scan. Patients with progressive weight loss and for whom you are suspicious of an unidentified underlying malignancy may benefit from a PET scan.

Overall, potential further investigations include:

- HIV serology
- an autoimmune disease screen
- screening for tumour markers (these are not sensitive for detecting cancer, but may help direct investigations)
- endoscopic examination
- ultrasound scan
- CT scan
- MRI
- PET scan

Introduction to therapy

Clear documentation of the patient's weight is necessary, to set a benchmark for future reviews. Inpatients can be weighed once or twice a week, in order to provide the overall trend, and outpatients should have a weight documented every time they attend the hospital clinic. Food diaries are useful resources, helping the doctor or dietician assess the average oral intake and dietary balance of nutrients. Food diaries can also be used to correlate food intake with symptoms; this is a useful process in patients with gastrointestinal symptoms.

The mainstay of management for weight loss is directed at treating the underlying cause and providing nutritional support. Improving a patient's general health will improve their appetite. Specific electrolyte and nutritional supplements (e.g. potassium, folate, vitamin B_{12}) can be replaced. Patients who are severely malnourished may

---

> **Box 80.2 Refeeding syndrome**
>
> This condition usually occurs after 3–4 days feeding in a malnourished patient. The underlying cause is the shift from fat to carbohydrate metabolism, which leads to increased insulin release and the resultant cellular uptake of phosphate. Patients characteristically develop hypophosphataemia, although many electrolyte disturbances can occur. This, in turn, can lead to neurological, cardiological, muscular, and haematological disturbances. Patients should be closely monitored as nutrition is reinstituted, and phosphate replacement should be given as required.

benefit from intravenous therapy, with vitamin and/or iron infusions. Any patient who recommences feeding after a period of poor intake should be monitored for refeeding syndrome (see Box 80.2).

Consideration should be given to the patient's environment, and their ability to obtain and prepare food. If they lack interest in food and have an inability to eat, weight loss is almost inevitable. Approaching these problems often requires a multidisciplinary team, with community support and social services. Finally, patients may benefit from enteral supplementation via a nasogastric tube or percutaneous gastrostomy. This is necessary in patients with neuromuscular problems that cause dysphagia, and may be a temporary measure in patients with nutritional deficiencies, to allow continuous feeding through the night. Placement of these feeding tubes does not prevent normal eating and drinking.

Prognosis

It is well recognized that underweight patients have a greater incidence of complications and higher mortality. Although prognosis is hugely related to the underlying diagnosis, overall recovery will be reduced in an undernourished patient. Specific complications associated with abnormally low weight include infection, depression, poor wound healing, oedema, muscle wasting, fatigue, weakness, and subsequent immobility.

How to handle uncertainty in the diagnosis of this symptom

Weight loss is a subjective symptom, but is considered to be an 'alarm sign', due to the association with malignancy and overall poor health. Therefore, it is not a symptom to be ignored. If no cause is found after initial investigations, radiological imaging should be performed in order to exclude underlying malignancy. Many patients are unable to quantify their weight loss, and clearly documenting weight is extremely important for confirming the patient's complaint. Associated symptoms will help direct the need for investigations and the most appropriate ones. Although monitoring weight will confirm the diagnosis, it is inappropriate to delay investigations

Further Reading

Bosch X, Monclús E, Escoda O, et al. Unintentional weight loss: Clinical characteristics and outcomes in a prospective cohort of 2677 patients. *PLoS ONE* 2017; 12: e0175125. https://doi.org/10.1371/journal.pone.0175125

Palesty JA and Dudrick SJ. Cachexia, malnutrition, the refeeding syndrome, and lessons from Goldilocks. *Surg Clin North Am* 2011; 91: 653–73.

81 Obesity: differential diagnosis

John Newell-Price, Alia Munir, and Miguel Debono

Definition of the symptom

Obesity is defined as a body mass index (BMI; calculated as the weight in kilograms divided by the square of the height in metres) of 30 or above (Table 81.1). While BMI is the most commonly used measure of obesity, the waist to height ratio correlates better with visceral obesity.

The differential diagnosis of obesity in primary care and secondary care

Box 81.1 shows the differential diagnosis of obesity in primary care and secondary care, ordered by probability.

Context

The International Obesity Task Force has recently estimated that at least 1.1 billion adults are overweight worldwide. It is only in less than 1 out of every 100 cases that a medical cause for obesity is found. Usually, a patient becomes obese in the setting of recent lifestyle changes, such as eating more calories than is necessary or increasing the amount of alcohol intake or the use of drugs of abuse. Reducing the total amount of physical activity and leading a sedentary lifestyle are other important and frequent causes for this problem. If the amount of calories provided by the daily food intake is more than the calories one burns off, the body will store the energy as fat, resulting in obesity. In a smaller number of cases, a medical cause may be responsible. Obesity-related syndromes like Laurence–Moon–Biedl syndrome may be inherited, while a number of endocrine disorders, like Cushing's syndrome or hypothyroidism, or disorders affecting the hypothalamus may also cause obesity. The diagnosis of obesity may be easily made in clinic by measuring BMI or waist circumference. The consequences of obesity are serious. Approximately 50% of all hypertension is secondary to obesity, and the heart may also be harmed by obesity-induced chronic volume overload and ischaemic heart disease. Insulin-related changes are the most damaging. Obesity contributes strongly to the pathophysiology of type II diabetes and its consequences. Furthermore, obese patients have higher rates of stroke, osteoarthritis, obstructive sleep apnoea, gastro-oesophageal

reflux, chronic liver disease, and infertility. Obesity increases the incidence of some cancers (e.g. breast, prostate, and colorectal). The psychological and social effects of obesity are also important, and include higher rates of depression and anxiety, and reduced employment.

Approach to diagnosis

On becoming obese, one gradually develops mild symptoms which become more severe on worsening of the obesity. Initially, patients may complain of breathlessness, increased sweating, difficulties coping with sudden physical activity, and increasing lethargy, especially at the end of the day. Some patients complain of back pain and joint pains. Eating behaviour and physical activity should be assessed.

Complications of obesity should be identified by history, examination, and investigations. Psychosocial distress and lifestyle, environmental, social, and family factors—including a family history of overweight and obesity—and comorbidities should be covered.

Specific points in the history and on examination for medical causes of obesity should be identified (e.g. family history of autoimmune disorders or hereditary syndromes, signs of endocrine disorders), and a drug history should be taken.

Healthcare professionals should use their clinical judgement to decide when to measure a person's height and weight.

Box 81.1 Differential diagnosis of obesity in primary and secondary care (ordered by probability)

Primary care
- exogenous obesity
  - lifestyle related
- constitutional obesity
  - family history
  - polygenic
  - 20%–40% of all obesity cases
- drug induced
  - glucocorticoids
  - phenothiazines
  - combined oral contraceptive

Secondary care
- endocrine-related causes
  - <1% of all obesity cases
  - hypogonadism
  - polycystic ovary syndrome
  - hypothyroidism
  - Cushing syndrome
- hypothalamic-related causes
  - <1% of all obesity cases
  - trauma (base of skull injury)
  - midbrain tumours affecting hypothalamus
  - inflammation (meningitis, encephalitis)
- rare genetic disorders
  - <1% of all obesity cases
  - Laurence–Moon–Biedl syndrome
  - Prader–Willi syndrome

Table 81.1 The World Health Organization international classification of body weight, according to body mass index

Classification	BMI(kg/m²)
Underweight	**<18.50**
Severe thinness	<16.00
Moderate thinness	16.00–16.99
Mild thinness	17.00–18.49
Normal range	**18.50–24.99**
Overweight	**≥25.00**
Pre-obese	25.00–29.99
Obese	**≥30.00**
Obese class I	30.00–34.99
Obese class II	35.00–39.99
Obese class III	≥40.00

Reprinted from BMI classification, World Health Organization http://apps.who.int/bmi/index.jsp?introPage=intro_3.html.

Specific clues to the diagnosis

The following medical causes need to be excluded:

- hypothyroidism (indicated by increasing lethargy, constipation, cold intolerance, menorrhagia, hoarseness)
- hypogonadism (indicated by small testes, decreased body and facial hair, a high-pitched voice, gynaecomastia, muscle weakness)
- polycystic ovary syndrome (PCOS; indicated by hirsutism, acne, oligomenorrhoea)
- Cushing's syndrome (indicated by myopathy, easy bruising, thin skin, purple striae, hypertension)
- hypothalamic disorders (indicated by visual field defects, signs of multiple pituitary hormone deficiencies, a history of trauma or meningitis, insomnia, disorders of thirst, appetite, temperature regulation)

Key diagnostic tests

Tests should exclude causes and complications. All patients who are obese should have the following tests:

- fasting glucose test
- oral glucose tolerance test
- lipid profile
- blood pressure test

One should consider taking the following tests only when there is a high clinical index of suspicion:

- thyroid function tests (for hypothyroidism)
- luteinizing hormone, follicle-stimulating hormone (in women); 9 am testosterone (in men); sex hormone binding globulin, free androgen index (for hypogonadism, PCOS)
- overnight dexamethasone suppression test; to be used only if there is a high clinical index of suspicion (for Cushing's syndrome; see 'Specific clues to the diagnosis').

Other diagnostic tests

If clinically indicated, the following tests may also be performed:

- MRI pituitary/hypothalamus
- pituitary function tests
- ECG, echocardiogram, elective stress test; consider these tests if the patient complains of cardiac type-chest pain or shortness of breath
- sleep study; consider this test if the patient shows symptoms suggestive of obstructive sleep apnoea
- joint X-rays (osteoarthritis)

Introduction to therapy

More than half the adult population is obese or overweight, and a large proportion will need help with weight management. The aim of treatment is to lose weight, with the aim of improving physical health and ameliorating psychological well-being and quality of life. Losing weight is a long-term commitment which may be hard, and one should be encouraged to try and maintain excellent calorie control. Managers and health professionals should ensure that preventing and managing obesity is a priority. The NICE guidelines for obesity in 2006 suggested the following lines of management for these patients:

- lifestyle change
- dietary control
- exercise
- weight loss groups
- drugs
- surgery

Lifestyle change

Lifestyle management should be implemented as follows:

- Assess the patient's readiness to make lifestyle changes.
- Explore barriers to lifestyle changes.
- Tailor lifestyle advice according to the patient's social background.
- Encourage the patient's workplace/school to provide opportunities to eat a healthy diet and be physically active.
- Advise the patient to check weight periodically.

Dietary control

One should aim to lose 0.5–1.0 kg (1–2 lb) of weight per week, which usually means eating 500 to 1000 calories less than before. The ideal approach is to reduce intake of saturated fat and refined carbohydrates. Fruit, vegetables, fibre-rich foods, and unrefined carbohydrates should make up the bulk of the diet. A food diary to record the food one eats is recommended. Portion size should be controlled, and breakfast is recommended.

Exercise

To prevent obesity, most people should be advised to do 45–60 minutes of moderate-intensity activity per day, particularly if they do not reduce their energy intake. Types of activities recommended are ones that can be incorporated into everyday life, such as walking, gardening, or supervised walking programmes. One should also reduce the total time of inactivity.

Weight loss groups

Weight loss groups are recommended if they are based on achieving a balanced healthy diet, encourage regular physical activity, and expect people to lose no more than 0.5–1 kg (1–2 lb) a week.

People with certain medical conditions should check with their GP or hospital specialist before starting a weight-loss or exercise programme.

Drugs

Orlistat should be prescribed only as part of an overall plan for managing obesity in adults in patients with a BMI of 28.0 kg/m² or more and with associated risk factors, or a BMI of 30.0 kg/m² or more. Therapy should be continued beyond 3 months only if the person has lost at least 5% of their initial body weight since starting drug treatment.

Surgery

Bariatric surgery is recommended as a treatment option for adults with obesity if all of the following criteria are fulfilled:

- they have a BMI of 40 kg/m² or more, or a BMI between 35 kg/m² and 40 kg/m² and other significant disease (for example, type 2 diabetes or high blood pressure) that could be improved if they lost weight
- all appropriate non-surgical measures have been tried but have failed to achieve or maintain adequate, clinically beneficial weight loss for at least 6 months
- the person has been receiving or will receive intensive management in a specialist obesity service
- the person is generally fit for anaesthesia and surgery
- the person commits to the need for long-term follow-up

Bariatric surgery is also recommended as a first-line option (instead of lifestyle interventions or drug treatment) for adults with a BMI of more than 50 kg/m² and in whom surgical intervention is considered appropriate.

Prognosis

In England, over 9000 deaths per year are caused by obesity alone. Being obese can take up to 9 years off one's life span. Obesity increases one's risk of developing a number of complications. Mortality rates for men and women at least 50% above average weight are increased approximately twofold and, if diabetes is present, may increase fivefold in males and eightfold in females. Patients with a BMI >29 kg/m² have a quadrupled risk of developing ischaemic heart disease. Weight loss reduces risk of developing diabetes and improves diabetes control; in addition, every 1 kg of weight loss leads to a fall in blood pressure of 1–2 mm Hg.

How to handle uncertainty in the diagnosis of this symptom

Diagnosis of obesity is straightforward and should not cause any uncertainty. However, management of obesity is not easy and requires a combined multidisciplinary effort from healthcare authorities, carers, family members, and the patients themselves.

Further Reading

Heymsfield SB and Wadden TA. Mechanisms, pathophysiology, and management of obesity. *N Engl J Med* 2017; 376: 254–66.

National Institute for Health and Care Excellence. *Obesity: Identification, Assessment and Management*. 2014. Available at https://www.nice.org.uk/guidance/cg189 (accessed 15 Mar 2017)

82 Self-harm

Roger Smyth

Definition of the symptom

Self-harm refers to self-poisoning or self-injury, regardless of the apparent purpose of the act. The term self-harm is preferred to the older terms **parasuicide/attempted suicide** (which suggests an intent to die which might not have been present) and **deliberate self-harm** (because self-harm may also occur without deliberate intent in dissociative states). Self-harm includes a wide range of behaviours, including poisoning with drugs, poisoning with toxic chemicals, cutting, mutilation, jumping from heights, jumping in front of moving vehicles, and attempted drowning, shooting, asphyxiation, and hanging.

Conventionally excluded from definitions of self-harm are (1) habitual behaviours where the harm is incidental to the primary purpose of the act (e.g. tobacco smoking, recreational drug use), (2) behaviour where the aim is adornment and where there is at least subcultural acceptance (e.g. tattooing, piercing, decorative scarring) and, (3) where the individual lacks capacity to understand the behaviour (e.g. self-injurious behaviour in patients with a learning disability).

Self-harm is a behaviour with a wide range of possible motivations, including a genuine wish to die with fortuitous survival, an attempt to escape an intolerable situation or emotional state, the relief of symptoms, the communication of distress, the relief of tension or anxiety, or an attempt to manipulate others. Self-harm can become a habitual behaviour in some individuals in response to ongoing psychological or social stressors.

The prevalence of self-harm, and the relative frequency of the method chosen, vary between counties and between population subgroups. The relative frequencies of the method chosen will also vary between those who do and those who do not seek hospital treatment.

Within the UK, among self-harm patients presenting to hospitals, roughly 75%–90% of cases will involve self-poisoning (the vast majority of these by prescribed or over-the-counter medication), approximately 10% will involve self-injury by laceration to limbs or torso, and less than 5% will involve more violent methods of self-injury. Conversely, in patients who do not seek hospital treatment following self-harm, self-laceration is the most common method.

Methods of self-harm also show considerable variation by age, gender, and country of origin, although, consistently, cutting and violent methods are found to be commoner in males than in females. In self-poisoning, the particular medication or combination of medications taken varies by country and within countries over time, as prescribing patterns and fashions change. Currently in the UK, overdose of paracetamol accounts for more than half of the cases of self-harm with medication.

Context

Self-harm is a behaviour which can lead to medical presentation, rather than a symptom in itself. The importance of self-harm is its association with later completed suicide and with the presence of mental disorder. There is also an association with psychosocial stresses of all kinds.

The period after a self-harm episode offers an opportunity for positive intervention to reduce suicide risk, diagnose and manage mental disorder, or to direct the patient to appropriate sources of practical or psychological help. Following immediate medical or surgical management of the self-poisoning or self-injury, a psychosocial assessment should be carried out.

While a minority of cases of self-harm are individuals with a clear intent to die, the majority reflect other motivations or combination of motivations. These may be unclear and mixed and change with time, depending on when the assessment takes place. Key themes are often communication with others (e.g. of distress), escape from intolerable symptoms or an intolerable situation, attempts to influence the behaviour of others, and relief of tension or anxiety.

Approach to diagnosis

Usually the fact that poisoning or injury is self-inflicted is obvious and will readily be admitted by the patient. There may occasionally be diagnostic confusion with accidental self-harm (e.g. in children or confused elderly) or with accidental overdoses of drugs taken for therapeutic effect. Careful and empathic history taking can clarify the situation here; be alert to the risk of a patient who has a clear intent to die and is concealing his or her intent to try again.

Provisions for the assessment of patients following self-harm vary, with some centres providing on-site specialist mental health nurses or psychiatric liaison services. All clinicians should, however, be competent in carrying out basic risk assessment and assessment of mental state sufficient to allow initial management and appropriate onward referrals.

The diagnostic issues in the self-harm patient group are (1) distinguishing between those patients with previous or ongoing suicidal intent, and those without; (2) determining the presence or absence of mental disorder and, if present, its diagnosis; and (3) assessing currently active psychological or social stressors for which intervention could usefully be carried out.

The key method used in establishing the underling meaning of the act is an empathic and thorough clinical interview. This should cover the nature and purpose of the act itself, review any symptoms of mental disorder, and establish the psychosocial context in which the act took place.

Specific clues to the diagnosis

When considering whether there is or was suicidal intent, the patient's account of their actions and the intent behind them is paramount. The examiner should explore the nature of the act, the patient's beliefs about the probable outcome, the amount of pre-planning, the presence of final acts (e.g. setting one's affairs in order, leaving a suicide note), and the route by which the patient has now come to medical attention. Intent to die is associated with violent methods, methods of high lethality, final acts, and precautions to avoid detection.

A majority of patients with self-harm will merit a diagnosis of mental disorder; the diagnosis rate will depend on the diagnostic method used. Common mental disorders seen in those with self-harm are depressive illnesses, personality disorders, drug and alcohol problems, and anxiety disorders. Functional psychoses such as schizophrenia are rarer but may be associated with bizarre self-harm related to delusions. Mental disorder is diagnosed clinically by examination of the current mental state and exploration of the patient's history (see 'Definition of the symptom').

Key diagnostic tests

Diagnostic tests appropriate to the method of self-harm should be carried out. Many units will also routinely screen for paracetamol and salicylate levels in those with self-poisoning. In psychiatric assessment following self-harm, the single most important diagnostic instrument is the clinical interview, which will include assessment of suicide risk, inquiry about symptoms of mental disorder, and a full psychosocial assessment.

Other diagnostic tests

A variety of assessment instruments are available, usually developed in research populations, which can aid clinicians in assessing patients after self-harm. They are generally self-report or clinician-rated structured clinical interviews producing a score validated against at-risk populations. Examples include the Beck Suicide Intent Scale, the Beck Hopelessness Scale, the Reasons for Living Inventory, and the Suicide Assessment Checklist (see Table 82.1). No currently available assessment instrument replaces clinical assessment, but such instruments may be helpful as screening tools, research tools, and for use in service audit.

A problem with the use of this type of instrument in the self-harm population is that, although the future risk of completed suicide is significantly raised compared with the general population, the absolute risk remains low. Currently validated rating scales are therefore poor at predicting future completed suicide. They generally have more success in identifying the group at risk of repeat self-harm.

Introduction to therapy

The first priority in management is the medical or surgical care of the patient, appropriate to their condition. Consultation with psychiatric services may occur early to clarify the situation regarding use of the Mental Health Act, and questions of capacity to refuse treatment.

The subsequent management will vary depending on the type of self-harm and the suicidal intent, and presence or otherwise of mental disorder. For patients with clear ongoing suicidal intent or severe mental disorder, transfer to inpatient psychiatric care (under the Mental Health Act, if necessary) is often required. For patients with mental disorder, there will be discussion with the mental health services about appropriate review and follow-up. Patients without mental disorder or ongoing suicidal intent but with ongoing psychosocial stressors can often be usefully referred on to appropriate services (e.g. social services, relationship counselling, bereavement counselling, citizens advice, women's aid, domestic abuse services, or drug treatment services).

Prognosis

The rates for completed suicide in the period following self-harm are 0.5–2.0% in the first year. Between 10% and 20% of cases of self-harm will repeat in the subsequent year. The prognosis relates strongly to the type of mental disorder.

How to handle uncertainty in the diagnosis of this symptom

These patients will inevitably arouse anxiety in the treating team, not so much because of diagnostic uncertainties or difficulty in physical management but because of the risk of completed suicide and the possible presence of mental disorder. This may give rise to doubt about individual competence to manage these cases and uncertainty about how to proceed. This anxiety is best assuaged by a carefully taken and empathic history, documentation of decisions made, and discussion of selected cases with specialist services.

In a minority of cases, considerable additional anxieties are caused when the patient refuses treatment or absconds after initial assessment. Here, the anxiety arises because of uncertainty as to whether to accept the patient's desire not to be treated (and the risk of negative outcomes as a result), or proceed with treatment (with attendant worries about the legal basis for, and legal risks of, such actions).

For patients who refuse treatment, the issue is that of capacity to refuse treatment and whether there is evidence of a mental disorder impairing judgement. Lack of capacity to refuse medical treatment cannot be assumed on the basis of any previous diagnosis of mental disorder but should be assessed on a case-by-case basis. In brief, to have the capacity for medical treatment decisions, the patient must be able to understand and retain memory of the proposed treatment, believe and understand the information regarding the risks of having the treatment and those of not having the treatment, and be able to weigh up the information in order to arrive at a decision. Mental disorder, intoxication, acute distress, and the physical consequences of self-harm can all negatively affect capacity.

The law and the correct use of different aspects of the law is unclear in this area. Many clinicians would view it as reasonable to treat an incapable patient in an emergency setting under common law, while later considering the use of the Mental Health Act (to detain the patient in hospital and legally prevent them from leaving)

Table 82.1 The Beck Suicide Intent Scale, the Beck Hopelessness Scale, the Reasons for Living Inventory, and the Suicide Assessment Checklist

Name	Source	Structure	Content
Beck Hopelessness Scale	Beck et al. 1974a	20 items, self-report	Inventory covering three aspects of hopelessness: thoughts about the future, motivation, and expectations
Beck Suicide Intent Scale	Beck et al. 1974b	20 items, clinician rated	Assessment of current suicidal intent via examination of objective circumstances of most recent episode, and self-report of the patient's beliefs regarding risk
Suicide Assessment Checklist	Rogers et al. 1990	21 items, clinician rated	Contains items covering patient social and demographic features and psychological and psychosocial status
Reasons For Living Inventory	Linehan et al. 1983	48 items, self-report	Assessment of patient's reasons for wanting to live, in a series of subcategories of beliefs, responsibilities, fears, and moral objections

Beck, A., Weissman, A., Lester, D., et al. (1974a) The measurement of pessimism: the hopelessness scale. Journal of Counselling and Clinical Psychology, 42(6), 861–865.

Beck, A.T., Schuyler, D. & Herman, J. (1974b) Development of suicidal intent scales. In The Prediction of Suicide (eds A.T. Beck, H.C. Resnick & D. Lettieri), pp. 45–56. Bowie, MD: Charles Press.

Linehan, M.m. & Goodstein, J.L. (1983) Reasons for staying alive when you are thinking of killing yourself: the reasons for living inventory. Journal of Counselling and Clinical Psychology, 51, 276–286.

Rogers, J.R., Alexander, R.A. & Subich, L.M. (1994) Development and psychometric analysis of the Suicide Assessment Checklist. Journal of Mental Health Counselling, 16, 352–368.

Beck, A., Weissman, A., Lester, D., et al. (1974a) The measurement of pessimism: the hopelessness scale. Journal of Counselling and Clinical Psychology, 42(6), 861–865.

Beck, A.T., Schuyler, D. & Herman, J. (1974b) Development of suicidal intent scales. In The Prediction of Suicide (eds A.T. Beck, H.C. Resnick & D. Lettieri), pp. 45–56. Bowie, MD: Charles Press.

Linehan, M.M. & Goodstein, J.L. (1983) Reasons for staying alive when you are thinking of killing yourself: the reasons for living inventory. Journal of Counselling and Clinical Psychology, 51, 276–286.

Rogers, J.R., Alexander, R.A. & Subich, L.M. (1994) Development and psychometric analysis of the Suicide Assessment Checklist. Journal of Mental Health Counselling, 16, 352–368.

and incapacity law (to authorize medical treatment in an incapable patient). The extent to which detention under the Mental Health Act can authorize purely physical treatment is debatable.

Further Reading

Hawton K and Van Heeringen K. (2009). Suicide. *Lancet* 2009; 373: 1372–81.

Hawton K and Witt KG (2009). Taylor Salisbury TL, et al. Psychosocial interventions following self-harm in adults: A systematic review and meta-analysis. *Lancet Psychiatry* 2016; 3: 740–50.

National Institute for Health and Care Excellence. *Self-Harm in Over 8s: Long-Term Management.* 2011. Available at http://www.nice.org.uk/guidance/cg133 (accessed 15 Mar 2017).

National Institute for Health and Care Excellence. *Self-Harm in Over 8s: Short-Term Management and Prevention of Recurrence.* 2004. Available at http://www.nice.org.uk/guidance/cg16 (accessed 15 Mar 2017).

83 Alcohol intoxication

Satish Keshav and Palak Trivedi

Definitions

Alcohol intoxication occurs when the quantity of alcohol (ethanol) consumed exceeds one's tolerance for the substance, with consequent impairment of the individual's mental and physical functional status. **Alcohol abuse** is a broad term for general ill health (mental, social, and/or physical) resulting from the repetitive, compulsive, and uncontrolled consumption of alcoholic beverages. Manifestations of alcohol abuse include a failure to fulfil one's responsibilities, resulting in loss of employment, personal relationships, or finances. **Alcohol dependence** is a condition which arises as a result of alcohol abuse and occurs when an individual continually uses alcohol, despite significant areas of dysfunction, with evidence of physical dependence.

Alcohol withdrawal syndrome is the set of symptoms and physical signs observed when an individual reduces or abruptly stops alcohol consumption after prolonged periods of excessive intake; it is largely due to the development of a 'hyperexcitable' central nervous system. **Delirium tremens** (also known as 'DTs') is the most severe form of alcohol withdrawal; it manifests as altered mental status, hallucinations, and sympathetic overdrive, which may progress to cardiovascular collapse if left untreated.

Etiopathogenesis of alcohol abuse

Contributors to alcohol abuse are complex and are likely a combination of psychosocial factors, societal and economic factors, and genetic and biological factors.

Psychosocial factors

Psychosocial factors include risk-taking, expectancies, sensitivity, tolerance, personality and psychiatric comorbidity, a family history of alcoholism, childhood neglect, and physical or sexual abuse.

Societal and economic factors

Peer-pressure influences and inaccurate perceptions of the risks of alcohol abuse represent some of the commonest reasons for alcohol abuse amongst younger individuals. Moreover, the relatively cheap price of alcoholic beverages (e.g. in the UK the current price of grocery store cider is cheaper than that of bottled water) and easy availability further contributes to the development of pathological drinking behaviour.

Genetic and biological factors

Genetic and biological factors can influence alcohol absorption and metabolism, alcohol intoxication, alcohol withdrawal, and delirium tremens.

Alcohol absorption and metabolism

Twenty per cent of ethanol is absorbed into the bloodstream directly from the stomach, and 80% from the small intestine. The longer the alcohol remains in the stomach, the more slowly it will be absorbed. This explains the sobering effect of food, which slows the process of emptying the stomach contents and hence the absorption of alcohol. When alcohol is taken with food, absorption is generally complete in 1–3 hours, with blood alcohol concentration reaching a peak 20–60 minutes after ingestion. Once alcohol is absorbed, it is converted to acetaldehyde. The liver metabolizes about 90% of consumed alcohol, and the lungs excrete about 5% during exhalation. Another 5% is excreted into the urine. Alcohol metabolism involves three discrete enzymes: the microsomal cytochrome P450 isoenzyme CYP2E1, the cytosol-based enzyme alcohol dehydrogenase, and the peroxisome catalase system. Acetaldehyde is then converted to acetate. Genetic polymorphisms coding for alcohol dehydrogenase, as well as the frequency at which ethanol is consumed and absorbed, also affect the speed of metabolism of alcohol.

Alcohol intoxication

Chronic ethanol exposure has been found to alter the phosphorylation of intra-cerebral GABA receptors, which consequently alters receptor function. Alcohol also inhibits the glutamate pathway, and long-term ingestion results in increased receptor turnover and synthesis. Several other neurotransmitter systems in the brain, including opiates, serotonin, and dopamine are also affected; increased opiate levels help explain the euphoric effect of alcohol ('alcohol reward effect'), while its effects on GABA receptors mediate the anxiolytic and sedative effects. Alcohol also enhances the function of components of several other neurotransmitter systems, including glycine, serotonin, and nicotinic acetylcholine receptors.

Alcohol withdrawal and delirium tremens

When ethanol is withdrawn, a functional decrease in the inhibitory neurotransmitter GABA is seen. Ethanol also acts as an NMDA receptor antagonist, causing the loss of inhibitory control of excitatory neurotransmitters such as norepinephrine, glutamate, and dopamine, as well as adrenergic hypersensitivity of the limbic system and brainstem. This results in the clinical manifestations of ethanol withdrawal. Past episodes of withdrawal lead to increased frequency and severity of future episodes, and persons who abuse alcohol over the long term are more prone to alcohol withdrawal syndrome than persons who have been drinking for only short periods of time. Opiate receptors are increased in the brains of recently abstinent alcoholic patients, and the number of receptors correlates with cravings for alcohol.

Symptoms of alcohol intoxication, alcohol dependence, and alcohol withdrawal

Symptoms of alcohol intoxication

The signs and symptoms of alcohol intoxication include confusion, aggression, and seizures (the latter more common with withdrawal). Cardiovascular effects include tachycardia and dysrhythmias, peripheral vasodilatation, and volume depletion. Respiratory effects such as reduced airway sensitivity to foreign material and reduced ciliary clearance may also be seen, and reduced respiratory rate may be noted in cases of severe alcohol poisoning. Acute alcohol intoxication can cause upper gastrointestinal symptoms such as nausea and vomiting, and a dysfunction of oesophageal, gastric, and duodenal motility is also commonly recognized. An increase in duodenal propulsive waves toward the ileum results in increased transit of intestinal contents, contributing to the diarrhoea seen in alcoholics.

The effects of alcohol vary widely from person to person. The following factors may account for differences in how alcohol affects one person more than another:

Habituation: Prior experiences with alcohol in long-time, heavy drinkers may result in blood alcohol concentration levels that would normally be fatal for the casual drinker. Conversely, a novice drinker may have severe symptoms with the ingestion of a moderate amount of alcohol. As a person's drinking habit increases, the liver will increase its capacity to metabolize alcohol, and the brain becomes used to frequent, even constant, high blood alcohol concentrations.

Concomitant medication/drug ingestion: The effects of alcohol are enhanced if a person is taking sedatives, and are altered by other medications which affect the metabolism of alcohol (e.g. metronidazole, nitrofurantoin, isoniazid, nitrates).

Blood alcohol concentration is commonly expressed in percentages or milligrams per decilitre, whereby 0.1% is equal to 100 mg/dl. Although there is a tremendous variation from person to person, and not all people exhibit all the effects, the following scale serves as a guide to blood alcohol concentration and its effects on a typical social drinker:

- Serum levels <25 mg/dl are associated with a sense of warmth and well-being.
- Levels between 25 and 50 mg/dl give rise to euphoria and decreased judgement.
- Levels of 50–100 mg/dl can lead to incoordination and decreased reaction time and reflexes. Ataxia may be noticeable.
- Cerebellar dysfunction (i.e. ataxia, slurred speech, nystagmus) is seen with 100–250 mg/dl.
- Coma can occur at levels >250 mg/dl, and respiratory depression, loss of protective reflexes, and death can occur with levels >400 mg/dl.

Symptoms of alcohol dependence

Alcohol dependence is recognized via the following criteria, which were incorporated into the fourth edition of *Diagnostic and Statistical Manual of Mental Disorders* (DSM-IV):

- tolerance
- withdrawal symptoms when attempts at abstinence are made
- the consumption of larger amounts of alcohol over time, or for longer periods than intended; in addition, larger quantities of alcohol being needed to achieve the subjective desired effect
- persistent desire or unsuccessful efforts to cut down on alcohol use
- the majority of the individual's time being spent on obtaining alcohol or recovering from its effects
- social, occupational, and recreational pursuits being given up or reduced because of alcohol use, or revolving around activities central to alcohol
- continued use of alcohol, despite knowledge of alcohol-related harm (physical or psychological)

Symptoms of alcohol withdrawal

Alcohol withdrawal can be classified based on the following symptoms and signs, which develop in a temporal manner:

Minor: These usually occur after a short interval (6–24 hours) following the last drink. Symptoms include tremor, anxiety, nausea, vomiting, and insomnia.

Major: These occur 10–72 hours after last drink and can manifest as hallucinations (usually visual but can be auditory), hypertension, diaphoresis, and global tremulousness.

Seizures: These are generalized motor seizures which tend to occur within the first 6–48 hours after withdrawal. They usually occur only once or twice and generally resolve spontaneously

Delirium tremens: This is the most severe form of alcohol withdrawal and can occur 3–10 days following the last drink, with a peak incidence around Day 5. Symptoms are characteristically worse at night and include agitation, global confusion, disorientation, hallucinations, altered perception and visual illusions, formication, paranoia, autonomic hyperactivity (hypertension, diaphoresis, and tachycardia), and fever. Delirium tremens should be distinguished from alcoholic hallucinosis, the latter occurring in approximately one-fifth of hospitalized alcoholics but without a risk of significant mortality. In contrast, delirium tremens carries up to 15% mortality with treatment, and 35% mortality without treatment.

Demographics of the disease

Alcohol abuse

Alcohol represents the oldest and most diffuse substance of abuse. The full economic cost of alcohol abuse in European countries is estimated to be 2%–5% of gross national product. Alcohol intoxication is becoming increasingly recognized in the teenage population, both in Europe and the United States. A large group of patients may present with ethanol intoxication as their sole problem but many others have it as part of a larger picture. The morbidity is often from co-ingested substances or coexisting injuries and illnesses. Alcohol intoxication is common in modern society, and some studies suggest more than half of all trauma patients are intoxicated with ethanol at the time of arrival to the emergency department. Alcohol is also commonly taken as part of suicide attempts. Europe has the highest levels of alcohol consumption and alcohol-related harm in the world, with a total economic cost of around €125 billion per year. Alcohol use alone causes is responsible for 10% of total disability-adjusted life years lost, and the harm to self and others inflicted by alcohol exceeds that caused by cocaine and heroin. Alcohol consumption is markedly skewed, and determining the exact percentage of the UK population with alcohol-related disorders is difficult. Studies suggest that alcohol abuse is most prevalent between the ages of 15 and 24, and epidemiological data from the United States estimate that 12% of the North American population are affected with alcoholism. Approximately three-quarters of such patients never receive medical treatment.

Alcohol withdrawal and delirium tremens

Approximately 50% of alcohol-dependent persons develop significant withdrawal symptoms necessitating pharmacological intervention upon cessation of alcohol intake. Fewer than 5% of patients with ethanol withdrawal progress to DTs. The influence of gender in the rates of development of severe alcohol withdrawal is not clear. Currently recognized risk factors for alcohol withdrawal include:

- prior ethanol withdrawal seizures ('kindling')
- race; black patients have a lower risk of developing withdrawal than white patients do
- previous history of delirium tremens
- concurrent illness
- daily heavy and prolonged ethanol consumption
- greater number of days since last drink
- severe withdrawal symptoms at presentation
- prior attempts at detoxification
- intense craving for alcohol

Natural history and complications of the disease

People who have been drinking heavily for several days or weeks may have withdrawal symptoms after the acute intoxication has subsided. Excessive consumption of large amounts of alcohol persistently can lead to the development of memory loss, blackouts, and pathological drunkenness symptoms. Alcoholism is significantly associated with suicide and violence, with rates approaching 80% and 60%, respectively, as a result of alcohol abuse. Long-term persistent consumption also leads to several deleterious biological health effects; these include traumatic injury, ketosis, hypoglycaemia, hypertriglyceridaemia, hyperuricaemia, insulin resistance, and the following types of end-organ damage:

- alcoholic liver disease (fatty liver, acute alcoholic hepatitis, or chronic liver disease; 10% of alcoholics develop cirrhosis over 10 years)
- cardiomyopathy
- acute and/or chronic pancreatitis
- dementia
- cerebellar degeneration

Chronic alcoholism may also lead to malnutrition and hypovitaminosis. A commonly recognized complication is that of thiamine deficiency, which, if left untreated, can lead to the development of Wernicke's encephalopathy. This is characterized clinically by the presence of:

- disordered ocular motility, including nystagmus (commonest abnormality), bilateral lateral rectus palsies, disorders of conjugate gaze, and, less frequently, pupillary abnormalities, ptosis, scotomata, and anisocoria
- truncal and gait ataxia, often as a presenting symptom; this is a combination of vestibular paresis (most often in the acute state), polyneuropathy, and cerebellar damage
- encephalopathy characterized by a global confused state, disinterest, inattention, and agitation; stupor and coma are uncommon

When persistent deficits are present, patients with Wernicke's encephalopathy may progress and develop Wernicke–Korsakoff syndrome. Academically, this represents two distinct syndromes, with potentially reversible features as part of Wernicke's encephalopathy, and persistent and irreversible findings of dementia constituting Korsakoff's syndrome. Moreover, individuals with Wernicke–Korsakoff syndrome may have additional abnormalities detectable on clinical assessment, including painless vision loss, diplopia, a wide-based, short-stepped gait, inability to walk or stand without assistance, apathy and indifference, paucity of speech, hallucinations, agitation, anterograde and retrograde amnesia (incomplete), and confabulation.

Approach to diagnosis

Although not a substitute for careful history taking, a range of validated questionnaires can be used to screen for alcohol misuse behaviour and alcohol dependence. These include the Alcohol Use Disorders Identification Test (AUDIT), a 10-item screening tool developed by the World Health Organization (https://www.drugabuse.gov/sites/default/files/files/AUDIT. pdf), the Fast Alcohol Screening Test (http://www.effectivepi. co.uk/files/FAST%20&%20other%20AUDIT%20questions_EPI%20 version%20Mar%2009.pdf), and the T-ACE Screening Tool (http:// www.mirecc.va.gov/visn22/T-ACE_alcohol_screen.pdf). A commonly used method for assessing (and treating) patients with suspected alcohol withdrawal is the Clinical Institute of Withdrawal Assessment for alcohol (CIWA-Ar) scale (http://umem.org/files/ uploads/1104212257_CIWA-Ar.pdf). While valuable as a clinical tool, the 67-point scoring system may not be practical to use on a day-to-day basis. A more concise model is the Glasgow Modified Alcohol Withdrawal Score (http://qjmed.oxfordjournals.org/ content/qjmed/105/7/649.full.pdf). Although easier to use, this model requires the patient to have been abstinent for a minimum of 8 hours before administering treatment.

Other diagnoses that should be considered

A detailed alcohol history is of paramount importance in the assessment of any individual presenting with altered mental status. However, alcohol intoxication predisposes patients to other causes of altered consciousness such as head trauma, and one must also be vigilant to consider other substance abuse which, when ingested may cause a similar presentation. Diagnostic overshadowing is common in alcohol-intoxicated patients, who require a thorough workup to exclude other pathophysiological processes (see Box 83.1).

The differential diagnosis of delirium tremens includes Wernicke–Korsakoff syndrome, and thiamine replacement therapy should be instituted in all patients suspected of alcoholism (see 'Treatment and its effectiveness'). Additional differentials of Wernicke–Korsakoff syndrome may include:

- temporal lobe epilepsy
- transient global amnesia
- concussive head injury
- Lewy-body dementia
- third ventricle ('ball–valve') tumour
- meningoencephalitis

Box 83.1 Differential diagnosis of alcohol intoxication

Metabolic causes
- hypoglycaemia
- diabetic ketoacidosis
- alcohol ketoacidosis
- hyperosmolar non-ketotic coma
- Wernicke–Korsakoff syndrome
- hypothermia

Systems failure
- acute liver failure
- acute renal failure

Stroke
- stroke
- subdural haematoma
- subarachnoid haemorrhage

Sepsis
- meningitis
- encephalitis

Other substance misuse
Use of:
- barbiturates
- benzodiazepines
- ethylene glycol and methanol
- other sedative–hypnotics
- heroin or other opioids
- cocaine

Miscellaneous
- hypoxia
- dehydration

'Gold-standard' diagnostic tests

Gold-standard diagnostic tests are as follows:

For alcohol intoxication: In alcohol intoxication, the blood alcohol level is grossly elevated. Alternatives such as field-sobriety tests ('breathalysers') are less accurate.

For alcohol dependence: Alcohol dependence is diagnosed based on three out of seven of the DSM-IV criteria (see 'Symptoms of alcohol dependence').

For alcohol withdrawal and delirium tremens: Although a single diagnostic test for alcohol withdrawal does not exist, a history of pathological drinking behaviour prior to hospital admission is suggestive of the diagnosis when combined with the classical clinical features of alcohol withdrawal.

Other relevant investigations

The extent of the diagnostic workup depends partly on the history as well as the clinical presentation. Although it is often difficult, the quantity of alcohol and the type of beverage consumed, the time course of symptoms, circumstances, and eventual injuries are important to ascertain. Physical examination must include an analysis of vital signs as well as nutritional status, hydration, and alcoholism-related signs, as well as features of alcohol-induced end-organ damage such as chronic liver disease. Physical assessment must be repeated frequently, often in order to follow up acute alcohol intoxication-related alterations. Evaluation for traumatic head injury is vital, and exclusion of an acute subdural haemorrhage with CT scanning may be necessary for the newly diagnosed alcoholic patient with altered mental status. The following additional investigations centre on assessing evidence of alcohol-induced end-organ damage as well as ruling out other serious metabolic or infectious etiologies which may be masked by the alcohol history:

Serum glucose: Hypoglycaemia is not uncommon, particularly in younger patients with alcohol intoxication.

Electrolytes, renal, liver function, and coagulation studies: These are used to look for signs of dehydration and end-organ damage.

Serum salicylate and paracetamol (acetaminophen) levels: In intentional suicidal ingestions, the presence of other toxic substances must be determined.

Blood gas analysis: A determination of the pH is important when polysubstance ingestion or ketoacidosis is suspected. The pCO_2 is useful in assessing respiratory depression; pH also can help exclude co-ingestion of methanol and ethylene glycol.

Serum osmolality: The osmolar gap can provide information about the ethanol concentration in the blood as well as give clues when suspecting the ingestion of other alcohols.

Full septic screen: CSF analysis may also be necessary if cause of altered mental state remains unclear.

Serum thiamine levels: These have been used in case reports to confirm Wernicke–Korsakoff syndrome. However, studies have not directly examined the correlation between a critical serum thiamine level and the development of the disease; thus, this test is seldom performed.

Prognosis

Only a quarter of patients with alcohol dependence receive medical treatment, yet after one year more than 50% of patients are still dependent or continue to experience symptoms related to chronic alcoholism. Continued consumption of alcoholic beverages, even in small quantities, increases the chances of relapse in an individual with previous alcohol dependence. According to the World Health Organization, morbidity attributable to alcohol in countries with an established market economy is 10.3% of disability-adjusted life years, second only to that of tobacco (11.7%). Although cardiovascular disease is one of the commonest causes of death relating to alcohol, 10% of all alcoholics develop cirrhosis over 10 years, with liver disease being responsible for 70% of the 'directly attributed' mortality from alcohol. Conversely, alcohol causes around 80% of deaths from liver disease, and trends in liver mortality reflect trends in overall alcohol-related harm. Another common cause of death in alcoholics is suicide (18% of alcoholics), the risk of which increases the longer a person drinks. This is likely a combination of alcohol causing physiological distortion of brain chemistry, as well as social isolation. In fact, over 25% of suicides in adolescents are related to alcohol abuse.

Treatment and its effectiveness

The management of a patient with acute alcohol intoxication is dependent upon the patient's current mental status and consciousness level, and whether there is an extensive background history of chronic alcohol dependence. Initial treatment should include medically stabilizing the patient by assessing respiratory, circulatory, and neurological systems. A patient intoxicated to the point of psychosis is considered a medical emergency because of the risk of unconsciousness, withdrawal seizures, and delirium tremens.

Patients with alcohol dependence require a multifaceted approach assessing biological and psychosocial factors, both those predisposing to the patient's current status of ill health as well as those likely to contribute to perpetuating the cycle of continued alcohol consumption and its associated consequences. In the acute setting, management focuses on stabilizing the patient, excluding other serious differential diagnoses, identifying and treating alcohol-induced end-organ damage (e.g. acute alcoholic hepatitis, alcoholic pancreatitis), the prevention and treatment of withdrawal symptoms, and preventing the development of Wernicke–Korsakoff syndrome.

Prophylactic thiamine replacement can be offered orally or parenterally to heavy or harmful drinkers. The latter is the preferred option in those patients attending the emergency department.

Those at high risk of withdrawal seizures, vulnerable patients, and adolescents/children under the age of 16 should be offered admission to hospital.

In states of established alcohol withdrawal, benzodiazepines should be offered. Practice varies from institution to institution but the ultimate aims are to follow a 'symptom-triggered' regimen; using the minimum dosage required to abolish withdrawal symptoms while simultaneously recognizing features of breakthrough. A common starting regimen is chlordiazepoxide 40 mg four times daily, tapering down to 5 mg four times daily gradually over a period of 5 days (e.g. 40 mg four times daily on Day 1, 30 mg four times daily on Day 2, etc.). Diazepam is also used as an alternative in some centres.

Patients presenting with established features of delirium tremens may warrant parenteral therapy. Lorazepam and haloperidol are currently used in UK clinical practice, although neither has UK marketing authorization for this indication.

The key to reducing the long-term burden of alcohol-related diseases is prevention and early identification of pathological drinking behaviours. A person-centred approach is advocated, taking into account an individual's needs, preferences, and capabilities. Abstinence is the goal of all preventative measures. Many people, in particular those with severe problems and complex comorbidities, do not appear to benefit from treatment and/or frequently lose contact with healthcare services. One common approach is to offer intensive residential rehabilitation. However, the evidence on the effectiveness of residential rehabilitation is uncertain, as many of the more severely ill alcoholics are not entered into clinical studies. As a result, clinical opinion is divided on the benefits of residential rehabilitation, with some authorities suggesting that those who benefit are a 'motivated and selected group' who may do just as well with intensive community treatment, but this too is currently limited in availability.

Harmful drinkers with mild alcohol dependence should be offered psychological support with cognitive behavioural therapy or social-network therapy. Younger patients also benefit from multicomponent programmes (multidimensional family therapy, brief strategic family therapy, functional family therapy, or multisystemic therapy). The latter approach is also advocated for those with significant comorbidities and/or limited social support. Following successful withdrawal in individuals with moderate-to-severe alcohol dependence, the National Institute of Clinical Excellence recommends that pharmacological therapy be prescribed in combination with psychological approaches. The following agents are generally only effective when used in combination with psychological therapies:

Acamprosate: As chronic alcohol consumption inhibits NMDA and consequently leads to the overproduction of NMDA receptors, sudden abstinence will cause the excessive numbers of NMDA receptors to be more active. This leads to the symptoms of delirium tremens, and excitotoxic neuronal cell death. Alcohol withdrawal also induces a surge in release of excitatory neurotransmitters like glutamate, which in turn activates NMDA receptors. The exact mechanism of action of acamprosate is unknown but it is believed to possess 'dual function properties' which block glutamatergic NMDA receptors while activating GABA receptors. By reducing the excessive NMDA activity which occurs at the onset of alcohol withdrawal, acamprosate can also reduce or prevent withdrawal-related neurotoxicity. Compared with placebo, acamprosate reduces drinking frequency and effectively increases abstinence in patients with alcoholism.

Naltrexone: This drug functions as an opioid antagonist, thus preventing the 'euphoric' effects which follow alcohol consumption. It is effective in reducing cravings for alcohol, and a number of studies have demonstrated its efficacy in reducing the frequency and severity of relapse to drinking. Patients must be abstinent for 5–7 days before naltrexone can be administered.

Disulfiram: This drug blocks aldehyde dehydrogenase in the liver and thus inhibits the metabolism of acetaldehyde. Continued alcohol consumption leads to increased concentrations of acetaldehyde, resulting in an unpleasant reaction characterized by flushing, nausea, hypotension, and palpitations. In addition, disulfiram prevents the conversion of intracerebral dopamine to noradrenaline. Studies have shown that oral disulfiram was not significantly different from placebo in preventing relapse to alcohol consumption nor was the rate of discontinuation different between the two groups. However, in comparison with acamprosate and naltrexone, disulfiram is more likely to increase the time until participants first drink alcohol again, and is effective in reducing rates of heavy drinking, the amount of alcohol consumed, and the number of drinking days.

Other pharmacological agents: Other pharmacological agents which have been trialled in alcohol dependence include SSRIs, baclofen, and the anticonvulsants topiramate and gabapentin. These agents have less evidence supporting their use in preventing relapse to drinking, and are not currently licensed in the UK.

Further Reading

Connor P, Haber PS, and Hall WD. Alcohol use disorders. *Lancet* 2016; 387: 988–98.

Friedmann PD. Alcohol use in adults. *N Engl J Med* 2013; 368: 365–73.

McPherson A, Benson G, and Forrest EH. Appraisal of the Glasgow assessment and management of alcohol guideline: A comprehensive alcohol management protocol for use in general hospitals. *Q J Med* 2012; 105: 649–56.

National Institute for Health and Care Excellence. *Alcohol-Use Disorders: Diagnosis, Assessment and Management of Harmful Drinking and Alcohol Dependence.* Available at https://www.nice.org.uk/guidance/CG115 (accessed 15 Mar 2017).

Vonghia L and Leggio L. Acute alcohol intoxication. *Eur J Int Med* 2008; 19: 561–7.

84 Intravenous drug use

Bryan Timmins

Definition of the symptom

Intravenous drug use (IVDU) is the unlawful self-administration of a psychopharmacologically active substance by the intravenous route. Opioids such as heroin (diamorphine), buprenorphine (especially in France), and morphine (usually medicinal morphine sulfate ground into powder and suspended in partial solution) are the drugs most commonly taken intravenously. Amfetamine sulfate, cocaine, and increasingly crack cocaine (especially in Latin America) and short-acting benzodiazepines such as temazepam and lorazepam are also frequently injected. Single drug use is rare and many users will experiment with different compounds and may have comorbid alcohol abuse or dependency and major psychiatric disorders such as depression and schizophrenia or schizoaffective disorder.

Context

Home Office data identify 0.5 million intravenous drug users (IDUs) in the UK, with 2001 prevalence data ranging from 1.2%–2%. The global estimate is 11.6 million, with 1.1 million in Western Europe and 1.6 million in North America alone. The number of IDUs has been increasing for 30 years, although smoking of heroin and snorting or smoking of cocaine and its derivative crack cocaine are more prevalent and often act as a gateway to intravenous use. The increase in the intravenous use of opioids in particular is believed to be due to law enforcement driving up prices and reducing the potency of drugs reaching the street dealers. Abusers are then tempted into getting the best effect they can by injecting rather than smoking heroin. In addition, the increased availability of clean needles and syringes via exchange services may have encouraged higher numbers of users to experiment with intravenous and subcutaneous drug use.

Approach to diagnosis

An open-minded and non-judgemental approach will encourage honest disclosure of drug type and amounts and frequency of use. You must emphasize your impartiality and, unless otherwise required by law, the confidentiality of any admission of drug use.

The patient needs to trust the clinician and to feel respected even if his or her lifestyle is obviously harmful. Most regular drug users will know that they are risking their health, and an approach based upon motivational interviewing techniques will facilitate accurate diagnosis and treatment.

Specific clues to the diagnosis

If confronted with an unusual group of signs or symptoms, especially in a younger person, allow yourself to consider the possibility and then ask tactfully about alcohol and drug habits. Clinicians faced with unexplained medical complications may not recognize the patient as a current or former drug user and may feel uncomfortable asking about illegal activities for fear of angering the patient. A negative drug screen should not be taken as evidence that a patient is not actively using drugs, and not all IDUs are regular users or even drug dependent.

A history of IVDU can usually be obtained from the patient or reliable collateral sources. These include previous A & E records, family, friends, community mental health and drug treatment teams, general practice records of care, police national computer records, and police intelligence reports.

Physical examination will usually reveal stigmata of repeated venepuncture in readily accessible sites such as the antecubital fossae.

Bruising from extravasation thrombophlebitis and venous ulceration are less common with older experienced drug abusers, especially where needle exchange services operate (only approximately 25% have access to exchange services). Many regular users will have thrombosed easily accessible sites and moved onto injecting saphenous, femoral, cervical, and even genital veins.

IDUs experience suppressed appetite, malnutrition, and self-neglect. Personal care may be poor, minor cuts and abrasions may be untreated, and clothing may be dirty and contain items used in the preparation of injections (e.g. citric acid powder and syringes, needles, and burned spoons). Staff should take care with any blood-contaminated items found. The patient may also hide drugs in body cavities and, depending on the type of drug, the amount of it, and the security of its wrapping, these drugs may affect the clinical state at the time of assessment or later during the care pathway. Be particularly alert to collapsed patients received from airports, as they may have ingested large quantities of drugs. Patients under arrest who suddenly collapse may also have swallowed excessive amounts to avoid conviction for supplying drugs. Such patients, fearful of criminal consequences, may conceal their use from the clinical team. The author encountered one case where nursing colleagues discovered that heroin, which had been wrapped in cling film, was hidden beneath the foreskin of a prisoner who had been admitted to the ITU for ventilatory arrest believed due to asthma. Removal of the drug was followed by prompt recovery.

Unexplained bizarre behaviour or significant neuropsychiatric manifestations may be caused by drug intoxication or withdrawal reactions and by related problems such as epileptic seizure, traumatic brain injuries, encephalopathies, and sepsis. A large proportion of IDUs have hepatitis C (70%), compared to the background population prevalence of 0.7%, and many female addicts are also involved in prostitution. Of the known HIV cases outside sub-Saharan Africa, 30% are due to IDUs. The health impact of hepatitis C and sexually transmissible diseases such as syphilis is considerable and may be delayed by decades. Patients may by then have moved out of drug abuse and be reluctant to acknowledge their previous habits. Early genotypes of hepatitis C were circulating amongst prison populations of addicts from the mid-1970s. The author has diagnosed several patients who presented up to 30 years after IVDU with chronic fatigue states and slight but persistently raised alanine aminotransferases.

Key diagnostic tests

Key diagnostic tests are as follows:

- a mental state examination, including a structured cognitive assessment (e.g. a Mini–Mental State Examination (MMSE))
- urine, saliva, and serum drug testing (see Table 84.1): NB: a positive result does not imply drug dependency

Other investigations

Other investigations include:

- urea and electrolytes
- liver functions tests
- a viral hepatitis screen
- C-reactive protein
- full blood count
- blood cultures
- plain chest X-ray for pulmonary fibrosis due to talc granulomatosis, then possibly CT scan for pulmonary fibrosis
- 12-lead ECG (methadone causes QTc prolongation), and echocardiography if infective endocarditis suspected

Table 84.1 Drug testing in urine samples

Drug or its metabolite(s)	Duration of detectability in urine samples
Amphetamines, including methylamphetamine and MDMA detectable	up to 2 days
Benzodiazepines: • Ultra-short-acting (half-life 2h) (e.g. midazolam) • Short-acting (half-life 2–6h) (e.g. triazolam) • Intermediate-acting (half-life 6–24h) (e.g. temazepam, chlordiazepoxide) • Long-acting (half-life 24h) (e.g. diazepam, nitrazepam)	@ 12hrs @ 24hrs @ 2–5 days @ 7 days
Buprenorphine and metabolites	@ 8 days
Cocaine metabolites	@ 2–3 days
Methadone (maintenance dosing)	7–9 days (approximate)
Codeine, dihydrocodeine, morphine, propoxyphene heroin is detected in urine as the metabolite morphine)	Up to 48 hours

Reproduced from Department of Health (England) and the devolved administrations (2007). Drug Misuse and Dependence: UK Guidelines on Clinical Management. London: Department of Health (England), the Scottish Government, Welsh Assembly Government and Northern Ireland Executive.

• baseline EEG, if seizure suspected
• CT scan brain if the Glasgow Coma Scale is reduced or cerebral abscess suspected

Other diagnostic tests

Other diagnostic tests include counselling, and HIV/other STD testing. Hair samples are now routinely used as forensic evidence in the courts to reveal past use of drugs and can identify type and duration of use; however, they are insensitive to recent use.

Introduction to therapy

Therapy begins with developing the patient's trust in the clinical team and is maintained by honesty and open collaboration, even if the patient's initial response is not positive. Many patients vacillate about the need to stop or change their ingrained habits and can be greatly influenced to do so by trained counsellors employing motivational interviewing techniques. Most healthcare systems have access to dedicated drug treatment services, and patients are able to get general healthcare advice, support for drug cessation or substitution (e.g. methadone and buprenorphine), and follow-up monitoring, as well as a host of psychosocial and welfare advocacy. There are specific agencies working with vulnerable groups such as prostitutes, those with dual-diagnosis mental disorders, and young offenders, often with the compulsion of court orders and probation services. Referral to specialist services (usually within the local mental health network) as per the National Institute for Health and Care Excellence (2007a, b) guidelines on drug misuse is strongly encouraged.

The management of acute and secondary complications such as sepsis, hepatitis, and HIV are beyond the scope of this chapter, and the reader is directed to the relevant sections of this book. There is no evidence that active IVDU reduces the efficacy of antiviral treatments, and nearly all attempts to treat IDUs yield benefits in hard outcomes such as mortality.

Subtle yet significant long-term benefits can be achieved, particularly if lifestyles and risk taking can be shaped by contact with services. Those who stay in touch with treatment agencies, even if still using, have a much greater chance of eventually giving up their habit. Services have generally more impact if they are adaptable enough to seek out and engage addicts without being restricted to conventional outpatient settings. Visiting needle exchange points and offering health checks and general advice about common complications such as leg ulcers can result in simple effective improvements, such as the use of NSAIDs and paracetamol instead of opiates for ulcer pain.

The management of acute withdrawal reactions depends on the type and strength of drug a patient has been using. Street drugs are often diluted and mixed with inert fillers, such as starch, cellulose, and talc, by drug suppliers who usually have no experience or knowledge of the basic chemistry of the drug or possible harm caused to the users by their choice of filler. Embolic events can easily arise when drugs not intended for intravenous use are injected in suspension. Pulmonary fibrosis due to talc-induced granulomas can develop insidiously and become massive, with associated pulmonary hypertension and right-sided cardiac failure. This can be further complicated by infective endocarditis.

The difficulty in calculating equivalent pharmaceutical doses based on users' accounts of their habit is due largely to the varying purity of street drugs, especially heroin. Patients often report amounts based on cost alone (e.g. the popular £10 bag). Unintentional overdoses with resulting respiratory depression are often encountered by IV heroin users when either their own tolerance has been reduced by enforced abstinence, perhaps following a period in prison or hospital, or if the supplier sells a stronger batch of the drug.

In acute clinical settings, the decision to start a substitution regime or manage a withdrawal reaction should not be made without a multidisciplinary review. The safest approach is to add nothing other than supportive measures such as fluids and vitamins, especially thiamine, and to treat specific complications as they arise. Heroin and amphetamine withdrawal are unpleasant but not life-threatening. Poorly calculated substitution attempts, especially with methadone, can kill. All staff should be aware that drug abuse may occur on the wards, and patients who are expecting withdrawal symptoms may have brought drugs in or have them delivered during their admission.

Benzodiazepine abusers are at risk of extreme agitated withdrawal reactions similar to delirium tremens and may develop epileptic seizures. A safe approach is to substitute with oral diazepam at a sufficient dose to suppress agitation and autonomic arousal. The dose can then be reduced by one-eighth every two weeks.

Occasionally, a functional psychotic disorder such as schizophrenia will be encountered, although many patients experience brief polymorphic psychotic symptoms such as transient hallucinations, paranoid feelings, and short-lived delusions. Some may react dangerously, attempting to flee tormenting images or being commanded by voices to jump through windows. Careful nursing in well-lit settings, with reassurance and judicious use of diazepam or antipsychotic drugs such as olanzapine, which is available in both oral and intramuscular forms, or risperidone, under guidance from liaison psychiatrists or following hospital rapid tranquilization policies, can help avoid unnecessary distress and risk of injury.

Prognosis

The outcome for IV drug abusers as a group is poor, with up to 50% dying prematurely from a range of physical conditions. The annual mortality is estimated at 2.2%. The UK has one of the worst records for IDU deaths in Europe: 1500 died in England alone in 2005. In one study, 22.3% of deaths were due to overdose, 14% were due to chronic liver disease, and 10.2% were due to accidents. The population also suffers from a very high rate of mental disorder and suicide. The criminal association of drug use brings many into conflict with their families, leading to rejection, social isolation, and, particularly for women, sexual exploitation and child neglect. Surveys identify up to 78% of street prostitutes have used heroin, with 63% claiming their drug use as the reason for prostitution.

There is a general decline in prevalence of IVDU with age, and an associated reduction in mortality in each age group. The highest risk group remains the young, inexperienced IV abusers below the age of 25, as these are 11.5 times more likely to die prematurely. The estimated third who leave drug use permanently remain at higher risk of late complications such as cirrhosis and mental illness, particularly depressive disorders and alcohol abuse.

How to handle uncertainty in the diagnosis of this symptom

The main issue with diagnosing IV drug abuse is to consider the diagnosis. Once considered, there is less likely to be uncertainty about confirming IV drug misuse. The patient usually knows what they have used and for how long and probably what risks they have been exposed to. Whether they will admit this to a clinician or even to themselves depends upon many factors outside the clinician's control. Any legal proceedings, especially if this involves family courts and child access, can result in denial, as can the shame of making an admission in front of families or friends. Patients who are receiving methadone may be at risk of having their script withheld if they are found to have used heroin and may conceal use for this reason.

Doubt about the cause of psychotic episodes often results in delaying the formal diagnosis of mental illnesses such as schizophrenia and can lead to long periods of inadequate treatment for this disorder in particular. The diagnosis may be delayed for months or years before positive drug testing or an admission or disclosure of use by a collateral source occurs.

Further Reading

Aldridge RW, Story A, Hwang SW, et al. Morbidity and mortality in homeless individuals, prisoners, sex workers, and individuals with substance use disorders in high-income countries: A systematic review and meta-analysis. *Lancet* 2018; 391: 241–50.

Degenhardt L and Hall W. Extent of illicit drug use and dependence, and their contribution to the global burden of disease. *Lancet* 2012; 379: 55–70.

National Institute for Health and Care Excellence. *Drug Misuse in Over 16s: Opioid Detoxification*. 2007a. Available at http://www.nice.org.uk/Guidance/CG52 (accessed 16 Mar 2017).

National Institute for Health and Care Excellence. *Drug Misuse in Over 16s: Psychosocial Interventions*. 2007b. Available at https://www.nice.org.uk/guidance/cg51 (accessed 16 Mar 2017).

Wurcel AG, Merchant EA, Clark RP, and Stone DR. Emerging and underrecognized complications of illicit drug use. *Clin. Infect. Dis.* 2015; 61; 1840–9.

PART 3

Cardiovascular disorders

85 Normal function of the cardiovascular system

Manish Kalla and Neil Herring

Cardiac physiology

The cardiac cycle: The ECG, blood flow, and heart sounds

The cardiac cycle represents the electromechanical events that take place from one heartbeat to the next. This is divided into two phases: relaxation of the ventricle, or diastole, which allows the heart to fill with blood, and contraction of the ventricle, or systole. Knowledge of this cycle is essential for understanding the cardiovascular examination at the bedside.

Electrical impulses generated by spontaneous depolarization of the sinoatrial node in the high right atrium initiate a cycle. This is followed by atrial depolarization, generating a P wave on the ECG. The P wave is followed by small rise in atrial pressure and, as there are no valves between the right atrium, the superior vena cava, and the jugular vein, this causes the A wave of the jugular venous pulse (JVP). There is a delay of 0.12–0.2 seconds until ventricular depolarization, largely due to slow atrioventricular (AV) node conduction, allowing more time for the ventricles to fill.

Ventricular depolarization is responsible for the QRS segment of the ECG, and occurs briefly before the rise in ventricular pressure caused by contraction. Pressure rises rapidly, leading to closure of the AV valves and thus generating the first heart sound. A further increase in pressure occurs over 0.02–0.03 seconds to generate enough force to open the aortic and pulmonary valves. This phase is known as isovolumetric contraction, as there is an increase in tension with no change in ventricular volume. Ejection of blood occurs once the ventricular pressure exceeds the aortic (80 mm Hg) or the pulmonary artery pressure (8 mm Hg) for the left and right ventricles, respectively.

Ventricular repolarization or relaxation in preparation for the next contraction is represented by the T wave on the ECG. This corresponds with relaxation and a rapid fall in pressure. The higher pressure in the aorta and the pulmonary artery then closes the aortic and pulmonary valves, generating the second heart sound. A brief period of relaxation then occurs without change in ventricular dimension; this is known as isovolumetric relaxation.

During ventricular systole, continuous venous return fills the atria, leading to an increase in atrial pressure (the V wave of the JVP). Once atrial pressure is higher than the ventricular pressure at the start of diastole, the AV valves open, leading to ventricular filling. Eighty per cent of ventricular filling occurs rapidly by passive flow, and is sometimes associated with a quiet, third heart sound, with a final 20% generated by atrial contraction in the healthy adult. Atrial contraction is sometimes associated with a quiet, fourth heart sound, especially during exercise, when the diastole shortens and ventricular filling by atrial contraction becomes more important. This sequence repeats with each heartbeat and is summarized in Figure 85.1.

Control of cardiac output

Cardiac output is the volume of blood ejected into the aorta by the left ventricle each minute, while venous return is the volume of blood returning to the right atrium each minute. These volumes must be balanced to avoid congestion of blood. Cardiac output at rest is approximately 5.6 l/min for males, and 4.9 l/min for females, but is influenced by basal metabolic rate, age, and body size. In clinical practice, cardiac output is often defined in terms of cardiac index to adjust for the influence of body surface area (3 l/min m⁻² for a 70 kg

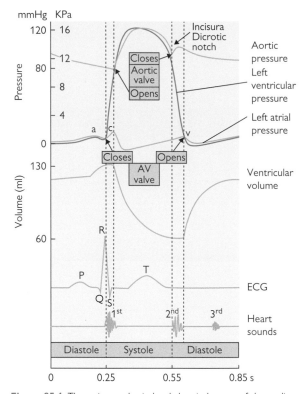

Figure 85.1 The major mechanical and electrical events of the cardiac cycle; AV, atrioventricular.

Reproduced with permission from Gillian Pocock and Christopher D Richards, *Human Physiology*, Third Edition, Oxford University Press, Oxford, UK, Copyright © 2006.

adult). Cardiac index increases rapidly in childhood (4 l/min m⁻²), and then declines with increasing age (2.4 l/min m⁻²).

The contractile properties of any muscle are also dependent upon the degree of tension applied prior to contraction, and the resistance against which the contraction takes place. For the heart, the former is the preload, which is dependent on venous filling pressure, and the latter is the afterload, which is the pressure in the aorta. Significant disruption to both these parameters occurs in disease states, leading to changes in cardiac output and function.

Venous return and control of cardiac output: The Frank Starling law, and Bainbridge effects

Cardiac output is controlled locally by changes in venous return, which in turn affects stroke volume (volume ejected per contraction) and heart rate. The Frank Starling law describes how stroke volume adapts to changes in venous return. An increase in venous return causes increased left ventricular (LV) end diastolic volume. The resulting ventricular dilatation causes an increase in force generation, thereby emptying the increased return (see Figures 85.2 and 85.3). Right atrial stretch caused by volume loading results in increases in heart rate driven by the sinoatrial node. This is the Bainbridge effect. However, if the heart is excessively stretched, heart valves leak and

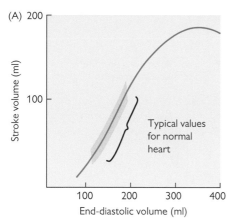

Figure 85.2 The relationship between end-diastole volume and stroke volume, determined using an isolated heart–lung preparation.

Reproduced with permission from Gillian Pocock and Christopher D Richards, *Human Physiology*, Third Edition, Oxford University Press, Oxford, UK, Copyright © 2006.

contractile performance is impeded, as it becomes less efficient at converting circumferential tension into radial pressure (the law of Laplace).

The role of the autonomic nervous system

Cardiac output is also controlled by the autonomic nervous system to maintain blood pressure in response to short-term haemodynamic disturbance via the baroreflex, or increase cardiac output during exercise (see Figure 85.4). Sympathetic stimulation increases inotropic (force of contraction) and chronotropic (heart rate) performance. Stroke volume can double and heart rate can increase up to 200 beats/min (depending on age), with up to a six- to sevenfold increase in cardiac output in elite athletes. A reduction in sympathetic stimulation has the converse effect. Parasympathetic stimulation via the vagus nerve can cause a strong slowing of heart rate, and even transient standstill, with a subsequent slow escape rhythm during ongoing stimulation. Contractile function can also be reduced up to 30%. The greater chronotropic effect is explained by the greater parasympathetic innervation of atrial tissue, as compared to the ventricles.

Vascular physiology

The circulatory system's function is to provide blood flow to body tissues and remove waste products. The rate at which blood is

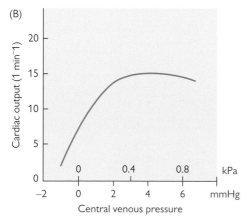

Figure 85.3 The relationship between cardiac output and central venous pressure in the intact heart.

Reproduced with permission from Gillian Pocock and Christopher D Richards, *Human Physiology*, Third Edition, Oxford University Press, Oxford, UK, Copyright © 2006.

delivered is closely regulated to maintain optimum conditions for cellular and organ function. Each vascular structure in the circulation fulfils a specific role for which it is adapted. Arteries transport blood under high pressure to tissues and divide into terminal branches called arterioles, which control the flow of blood into capillaries. Capillaries allow exchange of blood constituents across their membranes and the interstitial fluid. Capillary outflow enters venules, which coalesce to form veins. Veins transport blood back to the heart and also act as major capacitance or storage vessels in the circulation. Blood pressure also changes with transition between each of these circulatory vessels (see Figure 85.5).

Control of local blood flow

For a given perfusion pressure (arterial–venous pressure), individual organ beds can regulate their own blood flow, depending on metabolic need, by modulating the local resistance to blood flow. A constant flow is needed to maintain capillary pressure, which ensures adequate solute transport without causing oedema. This autoregulation process is mediated by changes in arteriolar radius. Resistance to flow is inversely proportional to the radius raised to the fourth power; therefore, halving the radius of the vessel can compensate for a 16-fold increase in perfusion pressure. This allows vascular beds to maintain capillary flow between perfusion pressures ranging from 50–150 mm Hg.

The cellular mechanisms that underlie this process include:

Metabolic vasodilatation: Hypoxia, acidosis, and metabolites caused by low perfusion lead to vasodilatation in arteriolar smooth muscle cells.

Myogenic vasoconstriction: In regions of high perfusion pressure (e.g. the feet), capillary pressure nears venule rather than arteriolar levels. Increased vascular tone is mediated by wash out of vasodilatory metabolites, and stretch-dependent Ca^{2+} entry into arteriole smooth muscle.

The vascular endothelium also contributes to local regulation of blood flow. These mechanisms are crucial for maintaining adequate blood flow in the event of vessel vasodilatation in an organ bed. This could potentially 'steal' blood from other beds supplied by the same feeding artery. A change in shear stress in the affected and feeder vessels result in an endothelial-dependent vasodilatation throughout the vascular tree. This process is mediated by changes in endothelial-derived relaxation (for example via nitric oxide) and hyperpolarization, as well as endothelial-derived vasoconstriction (for example via endothelin).

Capillary transfer

Capillaries constitute the microcirculation and are responsible for nutrient transport and removal of waste products. This purpose is reflected by capillary wall structure, which is constructed of a single-cell layer of highly permeable endothelial cells. Capillary inflow is controlled by arteriolar tone and local factors (as previously described), thereby allowing each tissue to control flow in relation to need.

Particles continually diffuse between the plasma and the interstitial fluid, with overall filtration determined by the differences in the hydrostatic pressure and the osmotic pressure exerted by proteins (colloid or oncotic pressures) on each side of the capillary barrier, as well as the filtration coefficient (a property of the barrier itself). This relationship between these 'Starling forces' is shown in Figure 85.6.

If the sum of these forces is positive, fluid filtration across the capillary wall will occur; if it is negative, absorption will take place. Capillary hydrostatic pressure can be elevated due to raised venous pressure in congestive heart failure, or secondary to a deep vein thrombosis, leading to tissue swelling and oedema. Conversely, tissue swelling can also occur if capillary colloid pressure is reduced, as occurs in nephrotic syndrome or liver failure. The filtration coefficient can be increased due to the release of local inflammatory mediators, which increase capillary permeability.

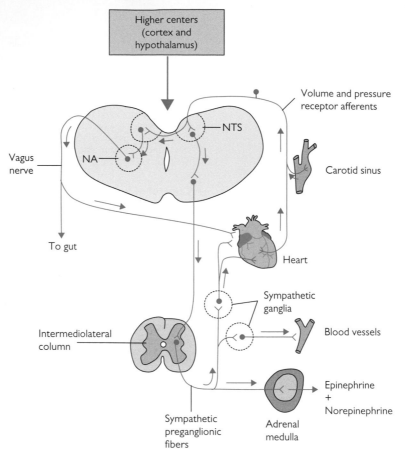

Figure 85.4 A highly simplified schematic diagram to show the sympathetic and parasympathetic innervation of the cardiovascular system.
Reproduced with permission from Gillian Pocock and Christopher D Richards, *Human Physiology*, Third Edition, Oxford University Press, Oxford, UK, Copyright © 2006.

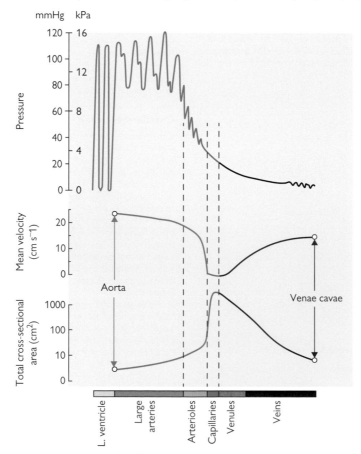

Figure 85.5 The changes in blood pressure and the velocity of blood flow in the various parts of systemic circulation.
Reproduced with permission from Gillian Pocock and Christopher D Richards, *Human Physiology*, Third Edition, Oxford University Press, Oxford, UK, Copyright © 2006.

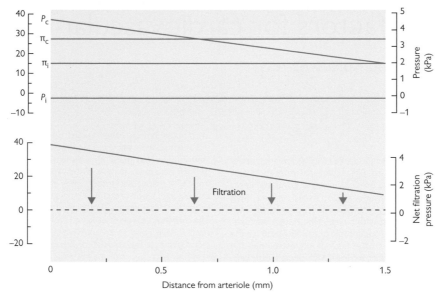

Figure 85.6 The factors that determine the direction of fluid movement across the wall of a capillary in the skin of the hand. P_c capillary hydrostatic pressure, P_i interstitial hydrostatic pressure, π_c capillary oncotic pressure, π_i interstitial oncotic pressure.

Reproduced with permission from Gillian Pocock and Christopher D Richards, *Human Physiology*, Third Edition, Oxford University Press, Oxford, UK, Copyright © 2006.

Integrated cardiovascular control

Arterial blood pressure (ABP) is described in terms of systolic (SBP) and diastolic (DBP) blood pressure. These values differ from LV systolic pressure due to the elastic properties of arteries. In the young adult, blood pressure is typically in the region of 120/80 mm Hg (SBP/DBP). ABP varies beat to beat, has diurnal variation, and responds acutely to stress and exercise. ABP can be defined as the product of cardiac output and total peripheral resistance (TPR), and the control of cardiac output has previously been discussed. Autoregulatory processes in each organ system underpin the local control of TPR, while overall control of cardiac output, TPR, and ABP encompasses short-term baroreflex-dependent mechanisms, and long-term mechanisms linked to renal perfusion and regulation of fluid volume and osmolarity.

Short-term or beat-to-beat changes in ABP are monitored by arterial baroreceptors in the aortic arch and carotid sinus, which influence cardiovascular autonomic control. These mechanisms do not set ABP but control fluctuations by adjusting cardiac output and TPR, while resetting of its operating pressure allows an increase in ABP and heart rate during exercise. The baroreceptors respond to the rate of change of transmural pressure during systole. A drop in ABP results in reduced stretch, which results in reduced afferent traffic via the ninth and tenth cranial nerves to the central cardiac and vasomotor centres. The efferent response increases sympathetic activity and decreases vagal tone, leading to positive chronotropy and inotropy, and increased sympathetic activity leads to vasoconstriction of resistance arterioles. The increase in cardiac output and TPR thereby restores ABP to its original level. An increase in ABP is adjusted by the converse effect.

Long-term regulation of ABP is coupled to renal perfusion, blood volume, and osmolarity. These mechanisms are important during cardiovascular shock and salt-sensitive hypertension. An increase in central blood volume is sensed by cardiopulmonary baroreceptors that mediate a reflex vasodilatation and release of atrial natriuretic peptide to cause natriuresis. Conversely, the juxtaglomerular apparatus in the kidney releases rennin in response to reduced arteriolar perfusion pressure, a reduced sodium load in the distal convoluted tubule, and sympathetic nerve stimulation. Renin catalyses the first step in the production of angiotensin II, which acts as a potent vasoconstrictor, potentiates norepinephrine release from sympathetic nerve terminals, and promotes aldosterone release from the adrenal cortex. Aldosterone acts upon the distal convoluted tubule and collecting ducts of the nephron to promote sodium and water reabsorption. Central hypothalamic osmoreceptors can also alter blood volume by detecting and responding to a 2%–3% change in blood osmolarity. They strongly influence the release of antidiuretic hormone, which promotes reabsorption of water at the collecting ducts of the kidney, and promote the perception of thirst to encourage fluid intake.

Further Reading

Herring N and Wilkins R. *Basic Science for Core Medical Training*, 2015. Oxford University Press.

Herring N and Paterson DJ. *Levick's Introduction to Cardiovascular Physiology* (6th edition), 2018. CRC Press.

Amitava Banerjee and Kaleab Asrress

Introduction

The most prevalent cardiovascular diseases (CVDs) are atherosclerotic, affecting all arterial territories. Figure 86.1 illustrates the major contributors to CVD, showing the predominance of coronary artery disease (CAD) and cerebrovascular disease (stroke and transient ischaemic attack). Globally, every year 7.3 million people die from CAD, and 6.2 million from stroke, with far-reaching associated costs.

Over 50 years of large-scale epidemiologic studies such as the Framingham and INTERHEART studies have firmly established the commonest or 'traditional' risk factors for CVD; namely, smoking, hypertension, diabetes mellitus, hypercholesterolaemia, and a family history of CVD. The 'risk-factors approach' to CVD looks at these factors, individually and in combination, in the causation of disease (Figure 86.2). The complex causation pathways involve interplay of individual factors, whether genetic or environmental. More recently, there has been increasing interest in 'epigenetics' or the way in which the environment interacts with genes in the process underlying CVD.

Traditional risk factors

Blood pressure

Much of our current understanding about the role of blood pressure in CVD can be attributed to decades of high-quality research from the Framingham study. This was established in 1949 with the aim of securing epidemiological data on atherosclerotic and hypertensive CVD. Their first major report, after 14 years of follow-up of a cohort of 5127 subjects, showed that elevated blood pressure was a major risk factor for CAD, as well as for all forms of stroke. This link has

been made in many other studies; however, the lower limit of where this risk becomes apparent was more difficult to establish. A major contribution was made by Lewington and colleagues (2002), who performed a meta-analysis of individual data for over 1 million adults from 61 prospective studies. They showed that, throughout middle and old age, blood pressure is strongly and directly related to stroke, ischaemic heart disease, and overall mortality, without any evidence of a threshold, down to at least 115/75 mm Hg. Many interventional studies have gone on to shown that treatments aimed at reducing blood pressure are associated with improved outcomes.

Age

The risk of coronary heart disease (CHD) increases markedly with age. Some of this can be explained by a worsening in risk factor profile with increasing age. For example, in most populations, serum total cholesterol increases as age increases. In men, this increase usually levels off around the age of 45–50 years, whereas, in women, the increase continues sharply until the age of 60–65 years. Blood pressure also tends to increase with age. The increases in blood pressure are explained in part by increasing BMI and obesity. These observations provide an example of the importance of interaction between risk factors in determining overall cardiovascular risk. When all major risk factors are accounted for, however, increasing age remains an independent predictor of adverse cardiovascular outcomes.

Gender

There is a marked difference in CHD, with all major epidemiological studies showing higher risk in men. Among middle-aged people, the incidence of CAD is approximately two times more common in men

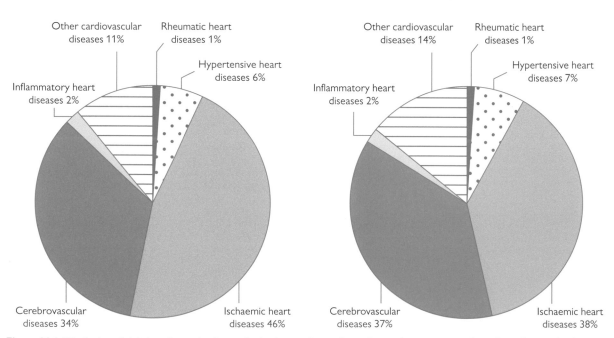

Figure 86.1 Distribution of global cardiovascular disease deaths due to ischaemic heart diseases (coronary artery disease), cerebrovascular diseases, and other types of cardiovascular diseases in males (left panel) and females (right panel).

Reproduced, with the permission of the publisher, from Mendis, S., Puska, P. & Norrving, B. (Eds) *Global Atlas on Cardiovascular Disease Prevention and Control*. Geneva, World Health Organization, 2011 (Figures 4 & 5, Page 4 http://whqlibdoc.who.int/publications/2011/9789241564373_eng.pdf?ua=1).

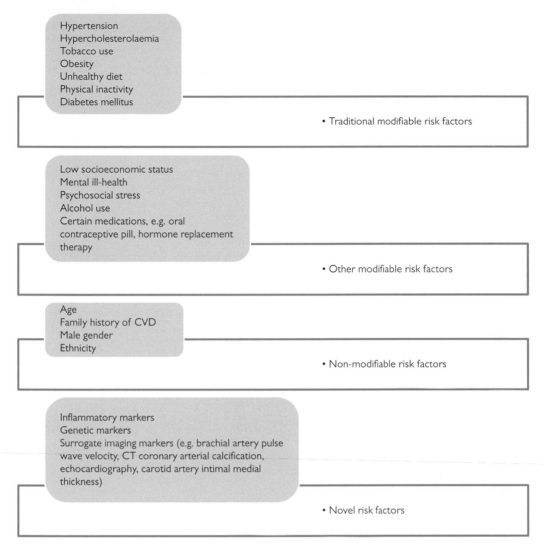

Figure 86.2 Risk factors for coronary artery disease and other cardiovascular disease (CVD).

- Traditional modifiable risk factors

Hypertension
Hypercholesterolaemia
Tobacco use
Obesity
Unhealthy diet
Physical inactivity
Diabetes mellitus

- Other modifiable risk factors

Low socioeconomic status
Mental ill-health
Psychosocial stress
Alcohol use
Certain medications, e.g. oral
contraceptive pill, hormone replacement
therapy

- Non-modifiable risk factors

Age
Family history of CVD
Male gender
Ethnicity

- Novel risk factors

Inflammatory markers
Genetic markers
Surrogate imaging markers (e.g. brachial artery pulse
wave velocity, CT coronary arterial calcification,
echocardiography, carotid artery intimal medial
thickness)

than in women, with mortality being five times greater, with this sex ratio varying between populations. In a large prospective Finnish study of 14,786 subjects, equating to 156,095 person-years of follow-up, it was found that the sex differences in measured cardiovascular risk factors explained nearly half of the observed sex difference in CHD incidence and mortality, with the difference in the HDL/total cholesterol ratio being the major determinant of the difference in risk.

Lipids

Once again, the Framingham study led the way in establishing the importance of lipid abnormalities in increasing CVD. They showed that serum cholesterol and lipoprotein levels were powerfully related to the subsequent rate of CHD. Most of the risk can be attributed to elevated LDL, with HDL being protective. Data on the link with stroke were more difficult to establish. This was primarily due to the fact that many of the early trials did not distinguish between haemorrhagic and thromboembolic stroke, as well as the difficulty in establishing the diagnosis by imaging in very large studies, some of which predated routine use of CT scanning in stroke patients. The Multiple Risk Factor Intervention Trial of 350,977 subjects showed that there is an inverse relation between serum cholesterol level and the risk of death from haemorrhagic stroke, but its public health impact is overwhelmed by the positive association of higher serum cholesterol levels with death from non-haemorrhagic stroke and total CVD. Several interventional trials have consistently shown that treatment with

statins, resulting in lower LDL, results in reduced cardiovascular risk. In subsequent years, interest focused on the importance of the lipid-transporting apolipoproteins. ApoB transports all potentially atherogenic very low-density lipoprotein, intermediate-density lipoprotein, and LDL particles, and ApoA-I transports and acts as the major anti-atherogenic protein in the HDL particles. The INTERHEART study showed that a raised ApoB:ApoA-I ratio was the strongest risk factor for predicting adverse cardiovascular risk. Contemporary guidelines on lipid management remain predominantly targeted at reducing LDL.

Diabetes mellitus

There is overwhelming evidence of the link between all forms of diabetes mellitus (DM) and cardiovascular risk, and DM is an independent risk factor for several forms of CVD. Furthermore, diabetics suffering with CVD have a worse prognosis than non-diabetics. Cardiovascular sequelae of DM include CHD, stroke, peripheral arterial disease, nephropathy, retinopathy, neuropathy, and cardiomyopathy. Type 2 DM is the most prevalent form, arising from a combination of insulin resistance and the defective secretion of insulin by pancreatic beta cells. Due to the aging population, increasing prevalence of obesity, and sedentary lifestyle, which all predispose to type 2 DM, the global burden of diabetes mellitus is increasing at an alarming rate. The metabolic syndrome encompasses a cluster of metabolic risk factors associated with increased risk for type 2 DM and

CVD. Insulin resistance, in the absence of overt DM, is increasingly recognised as an independent risk factor for CVD, as well as playing an important role in the pathophysiology of the metabolic syndrome.

Smoking

The association between smoking and CVD was first established in large epidemiological studies, including the Framingham study and the British Doctors Study. It can result in a sevenfold increase in the risk of peripheral arterial disease, and at least a twofold increase in risk of CAD. It has a greater impact on acute, typically thrombotic, events than on atherogenesis; this effect is most marked in young and middle-aged adults, in whom smoking is responsible for approximately 50% of premature acute myocardial infarctions. Numerous studies have demonstrated a substantial decrease in CHD mortality associated with smoking cessation, as compared to that associated with continuing smokers, with this diminution in risk occurring relatively soon after cessation of smoking. Similar rapid decreases in risk with smoking cessation are also seen for ischemic stroke.

Family history

A positive family history has long been associated with increased risk of CVD. However, when individual risk factors are accounted for, the impact becomes significant less. For example, in the INTERHEART study, when adjustments are made for the nine risk factors (smoking, raised ApoB/ApoA-I ratio, history of hypertension, abdominal obesity, psychosocial factors, daily consumption of fruits and vegetables, regular alcohol consumption, and regular physical activity), the attributable risks to the populations studied only rose from 90.4% to only 91.4%, indicating that, although family history is an independent risk factor for myocardial infarction, most of the associated risk burden can be accounted for through the other risk factors studied.

Ethnicity

Cardiovascular risk varies by ethnic group. Relative to white subjects, Afro-Caribbeans and people of African descent have high incidence of stroke and end-stage renal failure, whereas CHD is less common. On the other hand, South Asians (from the Indian subcontinent) have a higher incidence of CHD. Although a different genetic make-up might, in part, explain such differences, environmental and modifiable factors relating to diet and lifestyle play an important role. What remains clear is that, on a population survey, hypertension and diabetes were raised two- to threefold in South Asians, Caribbeans, and West Africans in Britain; with obesity being above national targets in all ethnic groups. These have to be borne in mind when developing public health policies.

Alcohol

Moderate alcohol consumption is believed to be protective against CHD, with a J-shaped relationship; the lowest risk is seen among light-to-moderate drinkers, and higher rates are seen among abstainers and heavy drinkers. This is complicated by the observation that this relationship is significantly affected by ethnicity, gender, type of alcoholic beverage, and pattern of alcohol intake. In a prospective study in African Americans, no J-shaped curve was found; instead, there was no beneficial effect, and mortality increased with increasing average consumption of more than one drink a day. Similar patterns were seen in a study of Indian men. In the INTERHEART study, alcohol use was protective against myocardial infarction in the entire study population (recruited from 52 countries around the globe), although it was harmful amongst Indians. The protective effect of alcohol is strongest in studies conducted in Mediterranean countries, where drinking habits are typically characterized by the use of daily constant amounts of alcohol mainly in the form of wine, while in Northern Europe and in the United States, alcohol is commonly consumed during the weekend in the form of beer and spirits. Data on whether this observation is due to the form of alcohol consumed or pattern of consumption remain unclear.

Diet

There is extensive evidence about the role of nutrition in CVD, through a direct influence on atherogenesis or effects on other risk factors such as lipid levels, blood pressure, and glucose metabolism. As an example, Table 86.1 summarizes the impact

Table 86.1 Impact of specific dietary and lifestyle changes on favourable lipid profile

Lifestyle intervention to improve lipid profile[1]	Magnitude of effect[2]	Level of evidence[3]
Reduce dietary saturated fat	+++	A
Increase dietary fibre	++	A
Reduce dietary cholesterol	++	B
Utilize functional foods enriched with phytosterols	+++	A
Reduce excessive body weight	+++	A
Utilize soy protein products	+	B
Increase habitual physical activity	+	A
Utilize red yeast rice supplements	+	B
Reduce alcohol intake	+++	A
Use alcohol with moderation	++	B
Reduce total amount of dietary carbohydrate	++	A
Utilize supplements of n-3 polyunsaturated fat	++	A
Quit smoking	+	B

Adapted from 2011 ESC guidelines on the management of dyslipidemias.
[1] Reduce total cholesterol or LDL, reduce triglycerides, or increase HDL levels.
[2] Standard deviation of daytime systolic blood pressure; +++ = general agreement on the effects on lipid level; ++ = less pronounced effects on lipid levels, although the weight of evidence/opinion is in favour of efficacy; + = conflicting evidence, where the efficacy is less well established by evidence/opinion.
[3] Level of evidence A = derived from multiple randomized clinical trials or meta-analyses; B = data derived from a single randomized clinical trial or large non-randomized studies.

of dietary intake and specific lifestyle on lipid levels. When the global patterns of dietary intake are studied, an unhealthy diet, assessed by a simple dietary risk score, increases the risk of acute myocardial infarction and accounts for approximately 30% of the population-attributable risk.

Body weight

Body weight is closely related to several traditional cardiovascular risk factors, including hypertension, age, insulin resistance, social factors, and lipid profile. When these are taken into account, obesity, particularly abdominal obesity, remains an independent risk factor for CVD. The attributable risk is much higher in high- and middle-income countries, where the risk can be greater than that associated with smoking. Weight reduction and physical exercise programmes have been shown to result in improvement in risk both in primary and secondary prevention of CVD.

Psychosocial factors

There is a large body of evidence showing that psychosocial factors increase cardiovascular risk. As well as interacting negatively with many traditional risk factors, they also increase risk independently. These include low socio-economic status, education, deprivation, lack of social support, social isolation, stress, and depression. In addition to increasing the risk of a first event, these factors also worsen prognosis, as well as acting as a barrier to treatment compliance and efforts to improved lifestyle. There is also evidence of the beneficial effects of psychosocial interventions for patients with CVD.

Table 86.2 provides a summary of the major determinants of cardiovascular risk.

Table 86.2 A summary of the major determinants of cardiovascular risk

Hypertension	Family history
Age	Ethnicity
Gender	Alcohol intake
Lipid profile	Diet
Smoking	Waist circumference
Diabetes mellitus	Psychosocial factors

Non-traditional risk factors

The risk factors just summarized can account for the vast majority of the attributable risk to CVD. The majority of primary and secondary prevention measures are aimed at addressing these. There are, however, a whole host of other recognized or emerging markers of increased cardiovascular risk. As many of these are much newer, our understanding of their mechanisms for increasing risk, whether they are casual or an effect of another process, remains up for debate. A summary of these factors is presented in this section.

It has long been recognized that **systemic inflammation** increases the risk of CVD. These observations were first made in sufferers of inflammatory disorders such as rheumatoid arthritis and SLE. Certain traditional risk factors such as hypertension and overt DM are more common in autoimmune inflammatory disorders, although this does not account for all of the excess risk. There has been intensive work assessing global biomarkers of inflammation in CVD. Several have been shown to predict increased cardiovascular risk, including **C-reactive protein**, **fibrinogen**, **D-dimers**, and **homocysteine** levels. These may serve alongside traditional risk factors to identify individuals at increased risk of cardiovascular events, as well as being potential targets for intervention.

JUPITER, a large randomized trial, has shown the benefit of using statin therapy in apparently healthy individuals with elevated high-sensitivity C-reactive protein levels, resulting in a significant reduction in major cardiovascular events. This shows the importance of continuing to look above and beyond traditional risk factors to identify patients at increased cardiovascular risk, with the aim of identifying proportions of the population that may benefit from risk factor modification. A variety of additional markers that reflect various elements of the complex systems governing inflammation, including pro- and anti-inflammatory cytokines, mediators of cellular adhesion, and matrix degradation enzymes, continue to be studied and may offer mechanistic insight as well as therapeutic potential.

Other biomarkers associated with increased cardiovascular risk include high haemoglobin levels, tissue plasminogen activator, and serum amyloid A; angiotensin-converting enzyme polymorphism; elevated von Willebrand factor levels; elevated gamma-glutamyltransferase levels; and overexpression of receptor activator of nuclear factor-kappa B ligand.

Genetic factors

CVD risk, including all the risk factors described so far, is ultimately determined by genetic factors, environmental factors, and the interaction between the two. Large-scale genome-wide association studies have identified several gene loci underlying susceptibility to CAD, and similar strategies are being employed in ischaemic stroke. This information has been used to develop genetic risk scores to identify individuals at increased risk, although the clinical utility and cost effectiveness of such scores are currently debated. What is clear is that there is limited association between these identified gene polymorphisms and traditional risk factors, suggesting that they act through previously unidentified pathways and thus providing new avenues for research into prevention and treatment strategies. Similarly, the epigenetics governing the interaction of genes with environmental factors in determining gene expression is increasingly recognized as important in contributing to cardiovascular risk, offering potential for earlier prevention and novel therapeutic options.

Further Reading

Hippisley-Cox J, Coupland C, and Brindle P. Development and validation of QRISK3 risk prediction algorithms to estimate future risk of cardiovascular disease: prospective cohort study. *BMJ* 2017; 357: j2099. (The QRISK®3-2017 risk calculator is available online at https://qrisk.org/three)

Khera AV, Emdin CA, Drake I, et al. Genetic risk, adherence to a healthy lifestyle, and coronary disease. *N Engl J Med* 2016; 375: 2349–58.

Lewington S, Clarke R, Qizilbash N, et al. Age-specific relevance of usual blood pressure to vascular mortality: A meta-analysis of individual data for one million adults in 61 prospective studies. *Lancet* 2002; 360: 1903–13.

National Institute for Health and Care Excellence. *NICE Guideline CG181: Cardiovascular disease: risk assessment and reduction, including lipid modification. 2014 Last updated: September 2016.* Available at https://www.nice.org.uk/guidance/cg181.

Yusuf S, Rangarajan S, Teo K, et al. Cardiovascular risk and events in 17 low-, middle-, and high-income countries. *N Engl J Med* 2014; 371: 818–27.

87 Diagnosis and investigation in suspected heart disease

Colin Forfar

Introduction

The past 20 years have seen significant changes in both the demographics and natural history of many cardiovascular diseases. Important reductions in case-fatality rates (such as in acute coronary syndromes) have resulted from improved diagnostics and treatment options and better understanding of natural history. For others (such as infective endocarditis), improvements have been limited and disappointing. While advances in therapy and the scientific evidence underpinning treatments have been crucial, the importance of accurate diagnosis has remained a key element for progress.

Many of the principles needed for diagnosis are constant: the pre-eminence of a focused accurate history, complete physical examination, and timely and relevant investigation endures. It is essential to have a secure knowledge of the strengths and limitations of interpretation of a frequently bewildering array of tests. Progress in this field has been rapid; advances in ultrasound, scintigraphy, and cardiac magnetic resonance stand out at the interface between structure and function central to good patient care.

History taking

Chest pain

There are few areas in acute medicine where accurate and informed history taking has such dominance in clinical assessment. Despite chest pain being one of the commonest reasons for hospital referral and emergency admission, the importance of a comprehensive history is frequently overlooked. **Myocardial ischaemia** presents in both stable and acute forms, the latter acute coronary syndromes comprising unstable angina, ST-elevation myocardial infarction, and non-ST-segment elevation myocardial infarction. Ischaemic chest pain is likely to be associated with an enzyme rise if lasting more than 15 minutes and if associated with autonomic upset, including nausea/vomiting, sweating, and collapse. Stable angina has predictable triggers (effort, emotion), relief within minutes of rest, and exacerbation by effort performed postprandially, uphill, or in cold windy conditions. Discomfort or pain may be central within the anterior chest but variations and radiation to back arms and neck/jaw are common. The history must be placed in context with careful review of cardiovascular risk factors (Table 87.1). These explain at least 90% of acute coronary events.

The pain of **acute pericarditis** has a sharper quality, with positional variation usually worst on lying and on inspiration. An intercurrent viral prodrome is common, and fever and a friction rub may aid diagnosis. Although **acute aortic dissection** is a much less common diagnosis, its pain is often of instant onset, is very severe, and may progress from the anterior chest to the back as the dissection spreads. Awareness of this diagnosis should prompt immediate investigation and emergency treatment. Aortic dissections are usually spontaneous; risk factors include hypertension, Marfan syndrome, and other hereditary and congenital aortopathies. **Musculoskeletal chest pain** may be a diagnosis of exclusion but is preferred as a positive diagnosis. It is localized, positional, and variable in intensity and onset, may have point tenderness, and is rarely associated with systemic upset. Reassurance, patient explanation, simple analgesia, and avoidance of unnecessary investigation all facilitate effective management. **Pleuritic pain** usually has a clear inspiratory trigger and associated lung symptoms, while **oesophageal pain** causes burning central discomfort associated with food and acid reflux.

Table 87.1 Independent risk factors for cardiovascular disease

		Hazard ratio
Modifiable	Smoking	2.9
	Hyperlipidaemia (ApoB; Apo-I)	3.3
	Hypertension	1.9
Potentially modifiable	Diabetes	2.4
	Psychosocial factors	2.7
	Obesity	1.6
Protective	Alcohol	0.9
	Regular exercise	0.9
	Diet (fruit and vegetables)	0.7

Adapted from *The Lancet*, Volume 364, issue 9438, Yusuf S, Hawken S, Ounpuu S, on behalf of the INTERHEART Study Investigators, Effect of potentially modifiable risk factors associated with myocardial infarction in 52 countries (the INTERHEART study): case-control study, pp. 937-52, Copyright (2004), with permission from Elsevier.

Non-cardiac chest pain should be an uncommon conclusion on history, as this diagnosis limits focused investigation and often encourages inappropriate tests.

Breathlessness

Precise history taking allows the separation of cardiogenic from non-cardiogenic causes in most cases. Restriction of exercise capacity should be carefully documented in both a time-defined and a patient-specific context; orthopnoea, paroxysmal nocturnal dyspnoea, and symptoms of congestion provide strong clues to a cardiogenic cause; fatigue may be prominent. **Heart failure** is no more than a symptom complex and demands a cause, whether that cause is systolic or diastolic pump dysfunction or is secondary to valvular or extracardiac causes (Box 87.1). The history will identify the dominance of left or right heart symptoms, whether they are congestive and associated with fluid retention or the result of impaired forward flow. It is important to remember that physical limitation may result from transient as well as persistent ventricular dysfunction, as seen, for example, in exertional breathlessness as an angina equivalent in a patient with multivessel coronary artery disease.

Symptoms of fluid retention, whether pulmonary or peripheral, follow activation of the renin–angiotensin–aldosterone cascade and a renal response, as well as arterial vasoconstriction. Understanding of the complex mechanisms involved has promoted many therapeutic advances in medical treatment.

Palpitations

Awareness of one's heart beating is common, and most causes are benign, reflecting **ectopic heart beats** or **situational tachycardia** with, for example stress, exercise, caffeine, or alcohol. Each can usually be identified by a careful history and asking the patient to describe or tap out their sense of the rhythm change. It is rarely necessary and frequently inappropriate to investigate such individuals beyond history examination and ECG. Over-investigation can promote somatization.

Paroxysmal arrhythmias, including **regular supraventricular tachycardia**, are often of sudden onset and may be associated with sweating, chest tightness, and altered consciousness. Duration,

Box 87.1 Principle causes of the syndrome of cardiac failure

Ventricular dysfunction (systolic dominates)
- ischaemic heart disease
- hypertensive heart disease
- dilated or hypertrophic cardiomyopathy
- restrictive cardiomyopathy

Valvular disease
- aortic stenosis and/or regurgitation
- mitral stenosis and/or regurgitation
- rarely, pulmonary or tricuspid disease

Congenital heart disease
- left-to-right shunt lesions (ventricular septal defect, atrial septal defect, persistent ductus, truncus arteriosus)
- obstructive lesions (aortic stenosis, coarctation, pulmonary stenosis)
- complex (cyanotic) disease (tetralogy of Fallot, Eisenmenger reaction, pulmonary and tricuspid atresia, palliated syndromes)

Extra-cardiac disorders
- endocrine (hyper- and hypothyroidism, phaeochromocytoma, acromegaly, hypercalcaemia)
- constrictive pericarditis
- severe anaemia, high-output states

Combination
- renal failure
- COPD
- pulmonary hypertension

Box 87.2 Common causes of syncope

Cardiovascular
- bradycardia (sinus pause, atrioventricular block)
- tachycardia (ventricular or supraventricular)
- structural (fixed: aortic stenosis; dynamic: hypertrophic cardiomyopathy, right ventricular outflow tract obstruction (RVOTO), myxoma)
- channelopathy (e.g. long-QT syndrome, Brugada syndrome)

Neurally mediated
- vasovagal syncope
- carotid sinus hypersensitivity
- reflex (cough, micturition)
- autonomic (central: multisystem atrophy, parkinsonism; peripheral: diabetic)

Neurological
- cerebrovascular disease
- migraine
- neuropsychiatric

block or sinus arrest, will result in syncope. Both ventricular and supraventricular tachyarrhythmias may also cause loss of consciousness. Cardiovascular adaptive mechanisms after arrhythmia onset determine whether consciousness is lost. Ventricular tachycardia causing loss of consciousness is a potentially life-threatening event, and urgent investigation to determine the cause and the possible presence of structural cardiac disease is essential. Substrates include various structural cardiac diseases, both genetic and acquired, as well as less common channelopathies.

Examination

The periphery, pulse, and blood pressure

Careful general examination will always pay dividends. **Cyanosis** (whether central or peripheral) reflects arterial desaturation in the relevant arterial bed and may be secondary to alveolar dysfunction, right-to-left shunting at the cardiac or pulmonary level, or localized hypoperfusion. **Tachypnoea** and **orthopnoea** may suggest interstitial lung oedema of cardiac origin. **Peripheral vasoconstriction** and delayed capillary filling may reflect a low cardiac output. Examination of the hands may reveal **pallor** (anaemia), **finger clubbing** (hypoxaemia), or **splinter haemorrhages** (vasculitis or embolism). **Skin rashes** or **conjunctival haemorrhage** may also reflect vasculitis or embolism. Peripheral pulse examination assesses **rate, rhythm, pulse volume** (normal, increased or decreased), and **character** (slow, normal, or rapid upstroke), as well as **presence and synchronicity** in upper and lower limbs. An abrupt drop in cardiac output and blood pressure with inspiration (so-called pulsus paradoxus) may indicate cardiac tamponade from a pericardial effusion compressing the right heart and impeding diastolic filling of the left ventricle. **Hepatosplenomegaly, ascites, peripheral oedema, or vascular bruits** may point to a number of primary cardiac diagnoses. General systematic medical examination is rarely a wasted endeavour. For example, a patient with chest pain may have evidence of hypercholesterolaemia (arcus lipidus, skin xanthelasma, or tendon xanthoma), peripheral vascular disease, or evidence of chronic tobacco use.

Blood pressure is recorded after a short rest period, at the brachial artery, using a sphygmomanometer and suitably sized cuff, and while the patient is sitting or semi-recumbent. The standard for diastolic measurement is disappearance of heart sounds (so-called Korotkoff V), unless there is more than 10 mm Hg difference between this and sound muffling (Korotkoff IV) when both are recorded. Three readings over at least 15 minutes or at intervals provide a better reflection of overall pressure and prognosis and should form the minimum to describe a diagnosis of hypertension or guide the need for changes in antihypertensive therapy. Ambulatory home or automated 24-hour blood pressure monitoring is widely used to further define average levels and thresholds for treatment.

frequency, triggers, and associations (e.g. polyuria) give clues to diagnosis. Loss of consciousness is an important association that should always be investigated. **Atrial fibrillation** may be of sudden onset and variable rate and duration and may occur with or without established cardiovascular disease. The irregularity may be prominent or not apparent but investigation is required to establish cause and the need for rhythm-stabilizing or antithrombotic therapies.

Ventricular tachycardia is associated with structural heart disease in most cases and requires full investigation and treatment determined by appropriate risk stratification. Antiarrhythmic therapy must be safe, targeted, and effective. For those at high risk, device therapy allowing both anti-tachycardia pacing and defibrillation therapy has been a substantial step forwards.

Syncope

Transient loss of consciousness may reflect cardiovascular, neurological, or neurally mediated mechanisms (Box 87.2). A prodrome of sweating, light-headedness, yawning, and altered hearing or vision is typical in simple **vasovagal syncope**. Trigger factors (pain, distress, unpleasant images) may be present. Injury and incontinence are unusual. The history provides the greatest clue to diagnosis and guides simple management advice: most importantly, for the patient to lie flat (if needed, with legs in the air) and perform isometric exercises to block the stimulation of vagal efferents from ventricular mechanoreceptors responding to adrenergic stimulation and emptying of the ventricles. **Carotid baroreceptor hypersensitivity** reflects abnormal activation of the reflex involved in blood pressure control through afferent, central, or efferent pathways and may be elicited by stimulation of the baroreceptor pathway via carotid artery massage; profound bradycardia or a period of asystole may follow. **Central autonomic dysfunction**, seen in long-standing diabetes and certain neurodegenerative conditions, can cause postural syncope and presyncope resulting from orthostatic hypotension. Antihypertensive drugs can be associated with postural hypotension.

Cardiac syncope may follow paroxysmal bradycardia or tachycardia sufficient to cause abrupt loss of cardiac output. The classical Stokes–Adams attack requires rapid but transient loss of consciousness and posture with early recovery and no ictal features. Ventricular standstill for 7 seconds or longer, from complete atrioventricular

The jugular venous pulse

Despite ready evaluation at the bedside and considerable information content, the **jugular venous pulse (JVP)** is frequently inadequately or incorrectly assessed. Given the absence of valves in the jugular veins and superior vena cava, and the normal variation in right atrial pressure with respiration, assessment of venous pressure should be described qualitatively but accurately rather than quantitatively and inaccurately.

The most useful element is **whether the JVP is elevated and abnormal**. To determine this, the patient should be relaxed, semi-recumbent at 45°, and with the head supported. At this angle, neck venous pulsation should not be visible above the clavicle. If it is, then a suitable description will reflect its height against relevant landmarks and patient position: appropriate descriptors might say, for example, 'venous pressure visible at base of neck at 45°' or 'venous pressure halfway up the neck at 45°' or 'venous pressure beyond the angle of the jaw sitting upright', reflecting mild, moderate, or severe elevation, respectively. If the neck venous pulsation is not easily visible at 45°, the patient should be repositioned to be either flatter or more upright, depending on suspicions. While the presence of hepatojugular reflux can be helpful in defining a low-normal level, it is not a substitute for careful observation of the neck with suitable angled lighting to facilitate visualization of pulsation. Venous pulsation is rarely palpable unless very high and is usually obliterated by light pressure.

Waveform can be most useful diagnostically. The internal jugular vein is more reliable for this purpose, although the external vein has utility provided it is not obstructed. **Presystolic pulsation** (timed from the carotid pulsation on the opposite side) reflects the atrial contraction waveform (a wave). It may point to elevated right heart pressures from left ventricular disease, pulmonary hypertension, or pulmonary valve stenosis. It is, of course, absent in atrial fibrillation. **Systolic pulsation** occurs with ventricular contraction (v wave) and reflects tricuspid valve regurgitation. External restriction to ventricular filling such as occurs in constrictive pericarditis results in rapid but truncated ventricular filling in the presence of elevated filling pressure and a rapid so-called x and y descent after the a and v waves, respectively. Inspiration causes a paradoxical increase in venous pressure, whereas it usually falls. Intermittent surges in JVP **(cannon waves)** reflect atrial contraction against a closed tricuspid valve from ectopy, usually ventricular or AV dissociation, such as complete heart block.

The precordium

The position of the **apex beat** reflects the most inferior and lateral impulse of the heart against the chest wall and defines clinical cardiomegaly, provided there is no chest deformity and the mediastinum is central. The normally positioned apex beat is within the midclavicular line and the fifth intercostal space. The impulse may be **tapping** (reflecting a palpable first heart sound seen in rheumatic mitral stenosis), **diffuse** (reflecting underlying ventricular dysfunction), **heaving** (reflecting pressure loading from hypertension or aortic stenosis), **thrusting** (reflecting volume loading such as mitral or aortic regurgitation), or **rocking/dyskinetic** (usually reflecting previous myocardial infarction). It may also be impalpable. A **parasternal lift** suggests right ventricular loading. The presence of any thrills (palpable murmurs) should be recorded, whether apical or basal, and whether systolic or, occasionally, diastolic. The latter is unusual and often associated with a shortened diastole; it is easily mistaken without careful timing of the cardiac cycle.

Heart sounds should be recorded for number, type, and timing within the cardiac cycle. The **first** and **second** sounds reflect closure of AV valves (mitral and tricuspid) and outlet valves (aortic and pulmonary), respectively. The second heart sound commonly splits with inspiration, as the right ventricular systole prolongs with increased venous return, and closure of the pulmonary valve is delayed. Paradoxical splitting of the second sound (split in expiration and single in inspiration) occurs when left ventricular activation is delayed (as seen in left bundle branch block (LBBB) or severe left ventricular systolic dysfunction). The **third** and **fourth** sounds are low-pitched, best heard with the bell, and occur in mid- and late diastole, respectively. Both are ventricular filling sounds. The third sound

usually signifies ventricular dysfunction, although it is physiologically in the young. The fourth sound is presystolic and often reflects a relatively stiff heart, such as that seen in hypertension. **Valve clicks** may be systolic or diastolic, reflecting opening of diseased mitral (diastolic and apical), aortic (systolic and basal), or pulmonary (systolic and less audible) valves from acquired (rheumatic mitral) or congenital (aortic or pulmonary) disease.

Heart murmurs should be documented as to timing within the cardiac cycle (systole and diastole are easily separated by palpation of the carotid pulse), site, radiation, duration, quality, and intensity. They reflect the turbulence of blood passing through the heart as a result of stenosed or regurgitant valves or outflow chambers, or as a result of abnormal connections between different chambers. The intensity of a murmur reflects a complex interplay between pressure gradient and blood flow, and does not necessarily reflect the functional significance of the lesion. For example, a small ventricular septal defect may generate a loud, harsh, but localized systolic murmur close to the left sternal border as a result of a high pressure gradient between the ventricles throughout systole but with low blood flow, whereas severe aortic stenosis with impaired left ventricular contraction (a life-threatening situation) may result in a rather quiet ejection murmur at the base and neck. A large atrial septal defect may create a substantial shunt from the left to the right atrium but this does not per se cause a murmur, as the pressure gradient is very small. High flow results from the compliance of the right-sided chambers. In this condition, turbulence and a systolic murmur are caused by increased flow across the right ventricular outflow tract; occasionally, a mid-diastolic murmur is caused by enhanced flow across the tricuspid valve.

Mitral regurgitation causes a pansystolic or mid–late systolic murmur located at the apex and radiating towards the axilla. Severity correlates to an extent with murmur intensity unless there is major structural disruption of the valve, such as that seen after myocardial infarction. There are many causes of mitral regurgitation (Box 87.3) but mitral valve prolapse and calcific degeneration of the mitral valve apparatus are most prevalent in the Western world. Clinical cardiomegaly and a thrusting apex beat reflect the severity of valve regurgitation. Intervention (repair or replacement) is based primarily on symptoms or evidence of progressive left ventricular enlargement. **Mitral stenosis** is usually of rheumatic origin. The first heart sound may be loud as a result of abrupt closure of thickened but still mobile leaflets. Left ventricular filling causes a rumbling, low-pitched, apical mid-diastolic murmur after valve opening (opening snap), with presystolic accentuation if sinus rhythm (and hence atrial contraction) persists.

Aortic stenosis causes an ejection systolic murmur which is located at the base and commonly radiates to the neck and apex. In an adult with acquired calcific disease, findings of clinical left ventricular hypertrophy, a narrowed pulse pressure, a slow-rising carotid pulse, and a soft or absent closing sound are all clues to severity of obstruction, and their presence mandates further investigation. **Aortic regurgitation** causes a high-pitched decrescendo murmur usually best heard upright in held expiration, at the lower left sternal edge. Again, severity does not necessarily relate to the intensity or duration of the murmur. With severe aortic regurgitation, high left ventricular filling pressure (which can approach aortic diastolic pressure) may soften the murmur in late diastole. Peripheral evidence of chronic aortic regurgitation, such as a collapsing pulse, nail-bed pulsation, and several other eponymous signs all reflect a chronically enhanced left ventricular stroke volume and reduced diastolic pressure. A pulse may be described as bisferious (or double impulse) in the presence of both stenosis and regurgitation.

Hypertrophic obstructive cardiomyopathy typically produces an ejection systolic murmur increasing in intensity in late systole as the severity of left ventricular outflow tract obstruction increases. The pulse may have a jerky character. Associated mitral regurgitation is common. Murmurs originating from the right side of the heart are less common. **Tricuspid regurgitation** is best diagnosed from assessment of the JVP but results in a soft systolic murmur at the base. **Pulmonary stenosis** produces an ejection systolic murmur at the base, more to the upper left sternal edge but often radiating to the back. An opening systolic click is common. **Pulmonary**

Box 87.3 Causes of mitral regurgitation

Mitral leaflet prolapse (chordal rupture)
- congenital/genetic
- Marfan syndrome
- Ehlers–Danlos syndrome
- osteogenesis imperfecta

Papillary muscle dysfunction secondary to ischemic heart disease (IHD)
- myocardial infarction with partial or complete rupture
- myocardial infarction or IHD with chronic with papillary muscle stunning or hypocontraction

Functional secondary to mitral annulus dilatation
- IHD
- dilated cardiomyopathy

Rheumatic heart disease

Vasculitis/inflammatory
- SLE
- polyarteritis nodosa
- other arteritides

Infective
- bacterial endocarditis

Other
- degenerative (calcific)
- atrial myxoma
- hypertrophic cardiomyopathy
- endocardial tumours (rare)

regurgitation is more common than is clinically apparent, although it is rarely of clinical significance. However, it may be a dominant issue in some forms of treated congenital heart disease, such as after repair of the tetralogy of Fallot or of right ventricular outflow tract obstruction.

The chest

In the appropriate clinical setting, basal crackles (crepitations) with tachypnoea suggest interstitial pulmonary oedema. Wheeze is, of course, most commonly secondary to obstructive airways disease but occasionally reflects bronchospasm from left heart failure. Evidence of chronic pulmonary disease is helpful to place cardiac disease in context.

General

A focused general examination of a patient with suspected cardiovascular disease is always rewarding. Many genetic diseases with important cardiovascular involvement may be recognized at the bedside (Table 87.2). Despite the considerable utility of both simple and sophisticated investigations in suspected cardiovascular

Table 87.2 Systemic genetic diseases with important cardiovascular involvement

Condition	Cardiovascular manifestations
Marfan syndrome	Aortic root dilatation/dissection; aortic and mitral regurgitation
Myotonic dystrophy	Atrial (ventricular) arrhythmias; heart block/conduction disease
Duchenne dystrophy	Cardiomyopathy; ECG changes
Becker dystrophy	Cardiomyopathy; ECG changes
Familial hypercholesterolaemia	Ischaemic heart disease
Osteogenesis Imperfecta	Aortic and mitral regurgitation
Haemochromatosis	Congestive cardiomyopathy
Down's syndrome	Atrioventricular septal defects; pulmonary hypertension: tetralogy of Fallot
DiGeorge syndrome	Tetralogy of Fallot; ventricular septal defect; aortic arch anomalies
Fabry's disease	Cardiomyopathy; hypertension

disease, as discussed in 'Investigation of cardiovascular disease', it is both poor quality and wasteful medical practice to rely on tests without careful consideration of all relevant clinical signs. Accurate interpretation of these signs not only points to the correct diagnosis but allows focused and valuable investigation and earlier and more effective treatment for the individual. The art of medicine must never be subordinate to overzealous application of its science.

Investigation of cardiovascular disease

ECG

With surface traces of human heart activation in use for over a century, the **standard 12-lead ECG** (Figure 87.1) retains great utility, with virtues of availability, ease, and speed of recording and standardization.

The electrical signature created from bipolar (limb leads I, II, and III), complex bipolar (limb leads aVr, aVl, and aVf) and 'unipolar' (chest or V leads) recordings are primarily of value in the detection of **rhythm disturbances, activation changes, hypertrophy**, and **ischaemia/infarction**. However, they may also provide clues to several genetic cardiac abnormalities, such as **long-QT syndrome** or **Brugada syndrome**, and inherited muscle diseases—either cardiospecific ones, such as **hypertrophic cardiomyopathy**, or ones that are primarily skeletal but with cardiac involvement, such as **myotonic dystrophy** or the **dystrophinopathies**.

The basic PQRST waveform reflects atrial activation from the sinus node (P wave), conduction across the atrium and delay through the AV junction (PR interval), ventricular activation (QRS), and repolarization (ST segment and T wave).

Rhythm disturbances

Ectopic activity may be of atrial, junctional, or ventricular origin and is rarely of clinical significance. Frequent atrial ectopic activity may be associated with both paroxysmal **atrial tachycardia** and **atrial fibrillation.** In the latter, atrial activation becomes chaotic, and mechanical function of the atrium is largely lost (Figure 87.2).

Atrial flutter usually persists and follows a re-entrant pathway, commonly within the right atrium. The typical flutter waves have a cycle length of 200 milliseconds, giving a rate of 300 bpm. The ventricular rate is dependent on refractoriness of the AV junction, which may conduct at 3:1, 2:1, or even 1:1, giving ventricular rates of 100, 150, and 300 bpm, respectively. **Regular supraventricular tachycardia** results from either an abnormal AV junction with zones of slow conduction **(atrioventricular nodal re-entrant tachycardia)** or the presence of an abnormal pathway separate from the junction **(atrioventricular re-entrant tachycardia)**, which may or may not be discerned on the surface ECG, depending on its site and antegrade conduction properties (Figure 87.3).

Ventricular tachycardia may be paroxysmal or sustained. The threat depends on the speed and duration of the arrhythmia, the extent of associated structural cardiac disease, and the clinical syndrome. Syncope or presyncope is always significant. Most ventricular tachycardia of left ventricular origin occurs as a result of a zone of slowed or blocked conduction from scar tissue, for example, after myocardial infarction (Figure 87.4). Ventricular tachycardia originating from the right ventricle may reflect scarring or infiltration of the body or outflow tract, as seen, for example, in arrhythmogenic right ventricular cardiomyopathy.

Activation changes

Conduction delay may occur at atrial, junctional, or ventricular levels and is classified according to type and resulting rhythm. Impulse delay from the sinus node or into the atrium (sinoatrial disease) results in pauses in atrial activity. The presence of an accessory pathway separate from the AV node and inserting into ventricular muscle may produce a short PR interval and slurred upstroke to the QRS deflection **(Wolf–Parkinson–White syndrome)**. **Heart block** may be first degree, where the PR interval is above 200 milliseconds; second degree, where AV conduction intermittently fails with incremental **(Wenckebach)** or fixed **(Möbitz)** AV delay on conducted beats; or complete, resulting in an escape ventricular rhythm of narrow or

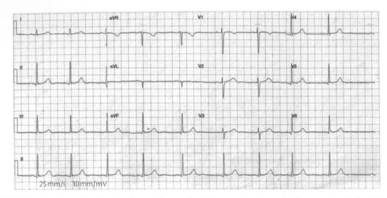

Figure 87.1 The normal ECG. The leads are displayed in four columns. In addition, a rhythm strip (conventionally lead II) runs along the bottom of the ECG. The ECG is usually recorded at a paper speed of 25 mm/s, and at a sensitivity of 10 mm/mV, but these settings can be adjusted on most ECG machines, if required.

Reproduced with permission from Houghton and Gray, Electrocardiography in *Oxford Textbook of Medicine*, Oxford University Press, Oxford UK.

broad (Figure 87.5) configuration. Conduction abnormalities below the AV junction result in **right bundle branch block (RBBB)** or **LBBB**, with characteristic ECG signatures. In RBBB, delayed activation of the right side results in QRS delay at or beyond 120 milliseconds, and delayed activation of the right side. With LBBB, the usual left-to-right septal depolarization is lost, and left-sided activation is delayed. ST depression and T-wave inversion reflect abnormal repolarization when depolarization is abnormal, and have little diagnostic value. Pathological Q waves in the presence of LBBB, however, do reflect myocardial infarction.

Hypertrophy

The standard criterion for electrocardiographic evidence of **left ventricular hypertrophy** is the presence of an R wave >11 mm in height in aV1 (90% specificity), or the sum of the heights of the S wave in V1 or V2 and the R wave in V5 or V6 being greater than 35 mm (75% specificity). However, both criteria lack sensitivity. The presence of repolarization changes (asymmetrical ST depression and T-wave inversion; the so-called strain pattern) enhances both the sensitivity and the specificity of the voltage criteria. Nonetheless, caution is needed in interpretation, especially in the young or those with a narrow chest.

Right ventricular hypertrophy shifts the frontal axis to the right and increases right ventricular activation, giving an increase in the R wave in right-sided leads, and a prominent S wave on the left.

Ischaemia/infarction

The hallmark for acute myocardial infarction is ST-segment elevation of 1 mm or more in two contiguous standard leads, or 2 mm

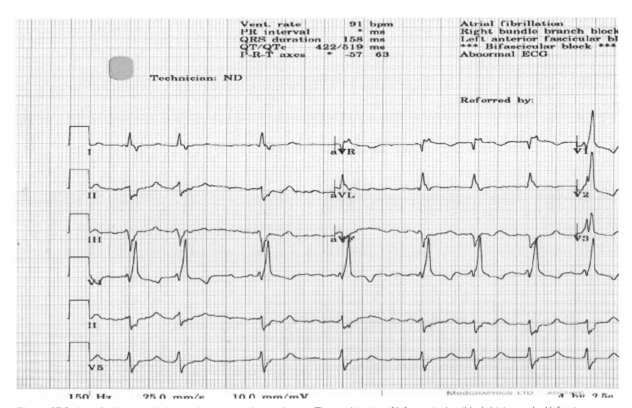

Figure 87.2 Atrial fibrillation with abnormal intraventricular conduction. The combination of left anterior hemiblock (giving marked left axis deviation) and complete right bundle branch block (delayed activation of the right ventricle resulting in an rsR' pattern in V1 and broad S wave in leads I and V6) is one form of bifascicular block.

Reproduced with permission from Ali Khavandi *Essential Revision Notes for Cardiology KBA*, Oxford University Press, Oxford, UK, Copyright © 2014.

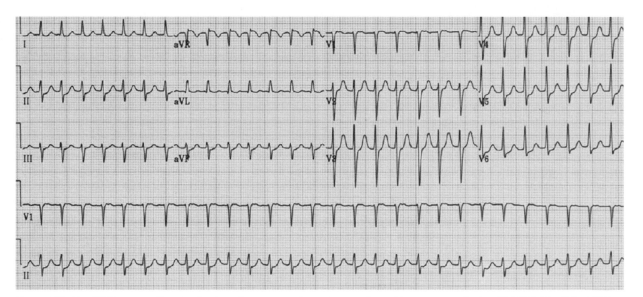

Figure 87.3 Usual ECG pattern of junctional tachycardia suggestive of an atrioventricular nodal re-entrant mechanism (AVNRT). The 12-lead ECG shows a regular narrow complex tachycardia (sweep speed 25 mm/s). Note the pseudo r′ in V1, and the accentuated S waves in II, III, aVF, which are suggestive of AVNRT.

Reproduced with permission from Ali Khavandi *Essential Revision Notes for Cardiology KBA*, Oxford University Press, Oxford, UK, Copyright © 2014.

or more in the chest leads. The cornerstone of immediate diagnosis of this emergency is provided by the history and the 12-lead ECG (Figure 87.6). Emergency coronary reperfusion, preferably by coronary angioplasty, thrombus extraction, and stenting, has become the gold standard for care and should be delivered as quickly as possible at an appropriate heart attack centre. Most but not all ST-elevation myocardial infarction ECG patterns evolve over hours to days into pathological Q waves and T-wave inversion, but overlap with non-ST-elevation infarction is considerable.

Myocardial ischaemia usually changes the repolarization signature in the ECG, causing ST-segment depression and variable T-wave changes. ST elevation is less common. Exercise ECG (see 'Additional

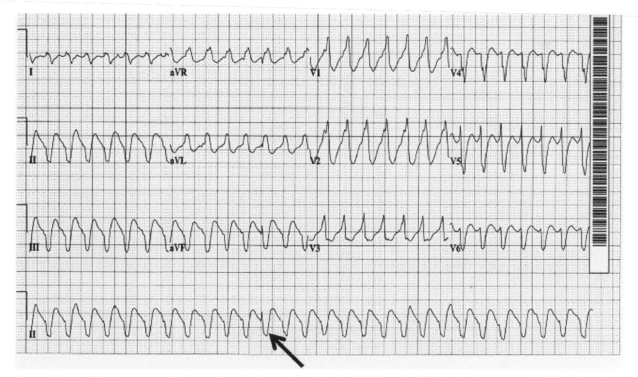

Figure 87.4 An ECG showing several diagnostic features of ventricular tachycardia (VT). First, the QRS duration is approximately 200 ms. Second, there is a fusion beat (indicated by the arrow), which demonstrates independent P wave activity. Third, the morphology of the ECG is 'RBBB-like' (i.e. similar to that seen in right bundle branch block: positive in V1, negative in V6) but the appearance is highly atypical, with a deep S wave in V6, suggesting that the left ventricle is the origin of the VT. Fourth, the inferior leads are negative, further localizing the origin of the VT to the inferior portion of the left ventricle. Fifth, the aVR is positive, and the frontal ECG axis is 210°.

Reproduced with permission from Ali Khavandi *Essential Revision Notes for Cardiology KBA*, Oxford University Press, Oxford, UK, Copyright © 2014.

CHAPTER 87 **Diagnosis and investigation in suspected heart disease**

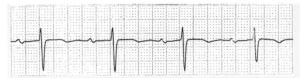

Rhythm strip 1—first degree heart block.

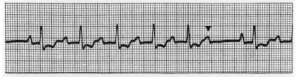

Rhythm strip 2—second degree heart block Möbitz type I.

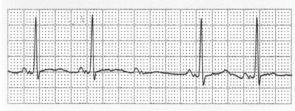

Rhythm strip 3—second degree heart block Möbitz type II.

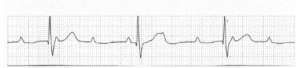

Rhythm strip 4—third degree (complete) heart block.

Figure 87.5 Rhythm strips showing atrioventricular conduction abnormalities.

Reproduced with permission from David A. Warrell, Timothy M. Cox, and John D. Firth, *Oxford Textbook of Medicine*, Latest update: May 2017, Figures 16.4.7, 16.4.7.8, 16.4.7.9, and 16.4.7.10, Oxford University Press, Oxford, UK, Copyright © 2017.

applications of ECG') is particularly useful, as changes are temporary and reflect the imbalance between supply and demand as the latter is increased through increases in heart rate and blood pressure.

Additional applications of ECG

Symptom-limited **treadmill or bicycle exercise testing** has considerable utility in the evaluation of patients with suspected symptomatic angina and in evaluating the prognosis in patients with established ischaemic heart disease. Parameters of value include symptoms, exercise capacity, systolic blood pressure, and ECG changes. Importantly, treadmill exercise ECG has limited, if any, utility in the evaluation of non-cardiac chest pain and should not be used as a 'rule out' where there is genuine diagnostic uncertainty after careful history and examination. In patients with suspected angina, the development of 1 mm horizontal or downsloping ST depression in two or more leads has 75% specificity and sensitivity for myocardial ischaemia; using ≥2 mm of ST depression as the criterion for diagnosis increases specificity but reduces sensitivity. Patients who are unable to exercise to within 90% of their predicted heart rate maximum for whatever reason should either undergo alternative testing for suspected ischemic heart disease or be regarded as being at high risk. Careful clinical supervision throughout the test and in recovery is essential, with interval assessment of systolic blood pressure. The diagnostic value of the ECG is often greatest in early recovery.

Ambulatory 24- or 48-hour ECG recording utilizes a solid-state or analogue recording device, typically with three chest leads, and is valuable for suspected tachy- or bradyarrhythmias, especially those that are transient or associated with altered consciousness. Ventricular tachycardia, atrial fibrillation, and various conduction blocks may be demonstrated and direct treatment. This analysis is, however, relatively labour- intensive and should not be used when the history strongly suggests simple ectopy and examination, and the ECG is normal.

Several **ECG event recording** devices are available and can be helpful for evaluating less frequent events suggestive of an arrhythmia. They do, however, require patient activation, and recording quality may be a limitation. For rare but potentially serious rhythm disturbances, an **implantable loop recorder** may be considered. These devices are relatively expensive, and their battery life is limited to several months, but they can be activated after a clinical event (e.g. on recovery from loss of consciousness) or programmed to record suspected tachy- or bradyarrhythmias (Figure 87.7).

Echocardiography

Few technologies in medicine have advanced as dramatically as **transthoracic echocardiography (TTE)** and **transoesophageal (TOE) echocardiography.** Both use high-frequency sound to penetrate tissues and reflect sound according to acoustic impedance.

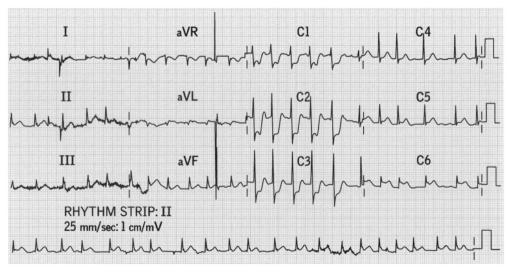

Figure 87.6 Acute posterolateral ST-segment elevation myocardial infarction.

Reproduced with permission from Longmore, Wilkinson, Baldwin and Wallin, Oxford *Handbook of Clinical Medicine*, ninth edition, Oxford University Press, Oxford, UK, Copyright © 2014.

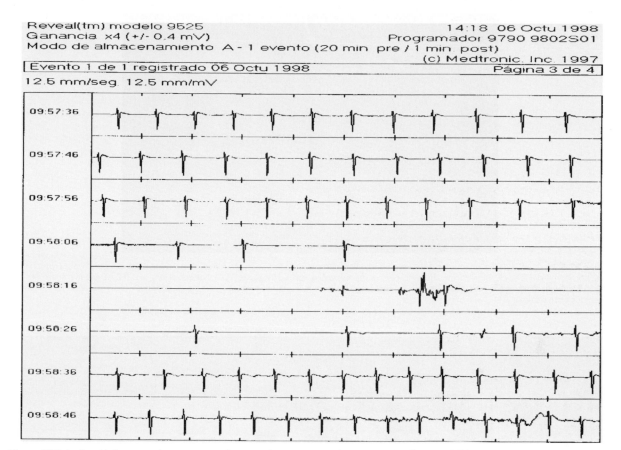

Reveal(tm) modelo 9525
Ganancia x4 (+/- 0.4 mV)
Modo de almacenamiento A - 1 evento (20 min pre / 1 min post)

14:18 06 Octu 1998
Programador 9790 9802S01
(c) Medtronic, Inc. 1997

Evento 1 de 1 registrado 06 Octu 1998
Página 3 de 4
12.5 mm/seg. 12.5 mm/mV

Figure 87.7 Implantable loop recorder registration of syncope due to paroxysmal sinus arrest. An 80-second ECG registration taken by an implantable loop recorder during an episode of syncope. A gradual slowing of sinus rhythm is followed by an asystole of about 15 seconds before an escape rhythm starts.

Reproduced with permission from Lucas Boersma et al., Value of the implantable loop recorder for the management of patients with unexplained syncope, *Europace*, Volume 6, Issue 1, Copyright © 2004 Oxford University Press.

Bone or air-filled structures such as the lung reflect sound and prevent penetration to deeper structures—hence the importance of a suitable acoustic window for good quality images. The Doppler shift principle allows quantification of blood or tissue velocity as a result of frequency shift of reflected sound moving towards or away from the receiving transducer. TOE utilizes the proximity of the oesophagus and stomach to the heart to eliminate acoustic interference. Three-dimensional reconstruction may provide added detail of valve structure and function.

Standard TTE allows long-axis, short-axis, apical, subxiphoid, and, if needed, suprasternal images of the heart. The technique is safe, simple, reproducible, and inexpensive, although it requires technical skill for image generation and interpretation. Atrial and ventricular dimensions at end-systole and diastole, myocardial thickness, systolic and diastolic function, valve function, and proximal great vessel structure can all be reliably determined in most patients. TTE should be a routine investigation in suspected valvular, myocardial, or congenital heart disease. A comprehensive TTE evaluation will take 20 minutes, and central physician-accessible image recording is becoming routine. However, there remains a place for limited study where only specific questions need to be answered, such as, for example, the presence of left ventricular hypertrophy in a hypertensive, or follow-up of known valvular heart disease.

TOE is usually performed with throat anaesthesia and under light sedation as needed. It has advantages of avoiding limited transthoracic windows and having close proximity to the heart and great vessels. Specific adult applications include detailed valve function, for example, accurate assessment of site and extent of anterior and posterior mitral valve regurgitation; valve detail, such as identification of vegetations in suspected endocarditis; and perioperative use for monitoring ventricular and valve performance during and after cardiac surgery. Appropriate training and expertise is essential to maximize the information content of the investigation, particularly with the routine use of multiplane imaging. However, the procedure is invasive to a degree and should not be regarded as a substitute for careful clinical evaluation and TTE.

Stress echocardiography utilizes the changes in myocardial contraction as a result of induced ischaemia to identify the extent and severity of myocardial perfusion abnormality. Epicardial coronary anatomy is not defined but the functional significance of disease, important for prognosis, is indicated through observation of initially increased (without ischaemia) then hypocontractile (ischaemic) regional wall motion as myocardial oxygen demand is increased by intravenous inotrope infusion (commonly dobutamine). Infarcted areas remain thinned and akinetic or dyskinetic. Good TTE windows are essential for accurate diagnosis. Changes in global ventricular function can also be determined.

Nuclear scintigraphy

Intravenous injection of a radiolabelled chemical allows analysis of myocardial perfusion and/or myocardial function via a gamma camera, either by single-photon emission CT (SPECT; using thallium-201) or multiple-gated acquisition (using technetium-99m). SPECT imaging with sestamibi or tetrofosmin is useful in defining the extent and territory of coronary perfusion abnormality (Figure 87.8), guiding both prognosis and intervention threshold in patients with single or multivessel coronary artery disease, as well as identifying those in the low-risk group for which intervention on prognostic grounds would not be justified. The radiolabels used have a short physical and biological half-life. Several stress protocols are used, including treadmill or bicycle

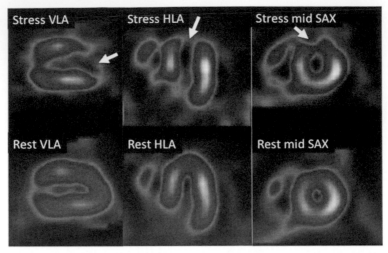

Figure 87.8 Myocardial perfusion imaging with single-photon emission computed tomography (SPECT): An example of inducible hypoperfusion in the anterior wall and apex. Panels, from left to right, show representative vertical long-axis (VLA), horizontal long-axis (HLA), and mid short-axis (SAX) slices, with stress above rest. The white arrows show a perfusion defect which is present on the stress slices but which resolves at rest. Please see colour plate section.

Reproduced with permission from Warrell, Cox and Firth, *Oxford Textbook of Medicine*, fifth edition, Oxford University Press, Oxford, UK, Copyright © 2010.

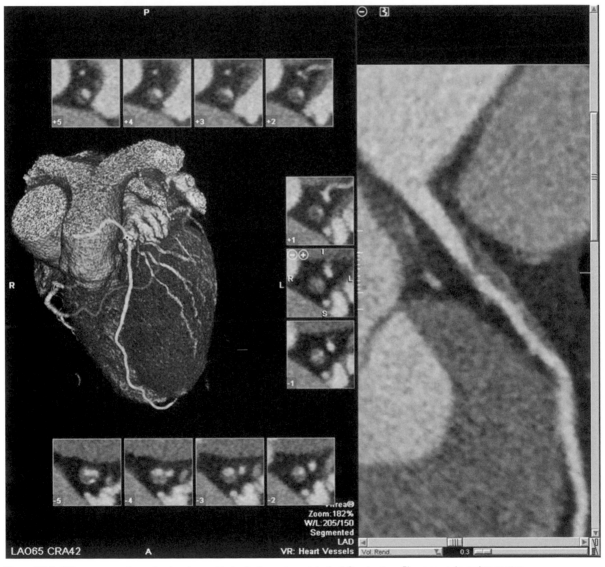

Figure 87.9 CT coronary angiography showing a critical soft plaque stenosis in the left main stem. Please see colour plate section.

Reproduced with permission from Warrell, Cox and Firth, *Oxford Textbook of Medicine*, fifth edition, Oxford University Press, Oxford, UK, Copyright © 2010.

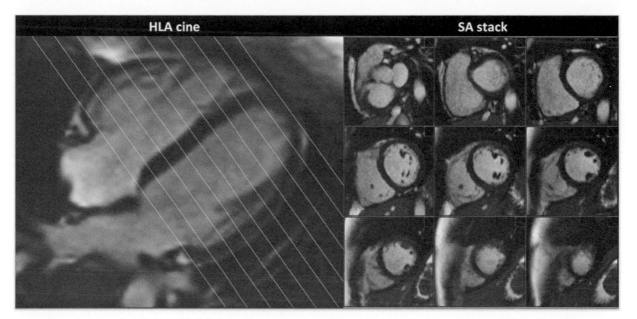

Figure 87.10 End-diastolic still images from multiple contiguous short-axis steady-state free precession (SSFP) cines which encompass the left ventricle, from base to apex. Note the position of the short-axis (SA) slices marked on the still frames of the end-diastolic horizontal long-axis (HLA) cine image, and the excellent delineation of the myocardium from the blood and the surrounding tissue.

Reproduced with permission from Warrell, Cox and Firth, *Oxford Textbook of Medicine*, fifth edition, Oxford University Press, Oxford, UK, Copyright © 2010.

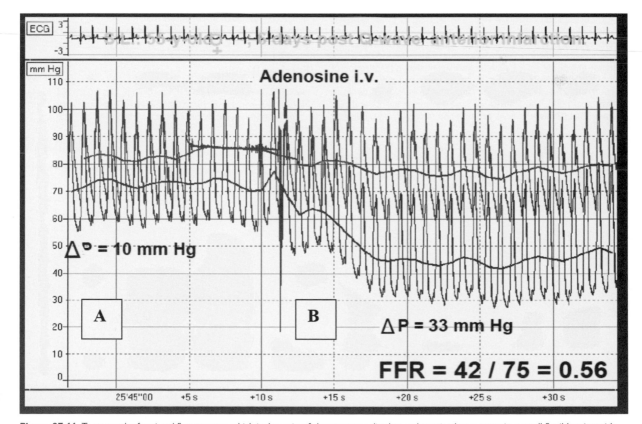

Figure 87.11 To assess the fractional flow reserve, which is the ratio of the pressures distal to and proximal to a stenosis, a small flexible wire with two separate pressure sensors is placed across a candidate coronary artery stenosis. Under resting conditions (A), there is only a 10 mm Hg gradient (ΔP) across the lesion but, under maximal hyperaemia ('adenosine i.v.'; B), the gradient increases markedly to 33 mm Hg, with a mean distal-to-proximal pressure ratio of 0.56. Thus, in this case, the fractional flow reserve indicates the presence of a functionally significant stenosis, and coronary angioplasty is indicated; FFR, fractional flow reserve; i.v., intravenous. Please see colour plate section.

exercise, as well as pharmacological 'stress' with either inotropic agents, such as dobutamine, or vasodilators, such as dipyridamole or adenosine. The latter two agents highlight relative perfusion defects in ischemic myocardium through the enhancement of perfusion in non-ischaemic areas. Injection of the radiochemical is typically undertaken at peak stress, with images acquired shortly thereafter compared to those acquired after a period of rest and re-equilibration.

The most valuable use of myocardial perfusion imaging is in assessing risk in patients with established ischemic heart disease and recurrent chest pain, and in determining risk in patients with intermediate probability of symptomatic coronary heart disease.

CT scanning

Contrast-enhanced CT has offered detailed images of cardiac structure and anatomical relationships for several decades. Well-established applications include evaluation of the great vessels, such as, for example, for identifying suspected aortic dissection or a major pulmonary embolism, or evaluating an aortic aneurysm or coarctation, but recent advances in signal processing and improvements in resolution have made coronary angiography a reality. Reasonable anatomical detail of proximal and mid-sized epicardial coronary vessels can be obtained with modest radiation exposure and avoidance of further investigation in suitably selected patients (Figure 87.9).

Cardiac magnetic resonance

Few technologies in medicine have advanced as rapidly as the application of cardiac magnetic resonance imaging (CMRI) to aid understanding of both structure and function of the human heart. By using a pulsed radiofrequency wave in the presence of a strong magnetic field, it is possible to create high-quality images in any plane, from the signal generated from the hydrogen nuclei in water and fat molecules. Spectroscopy adds the ability to obtain additional signals from phosphorus and other nuclei, thus affording insights into the metabolic state of cardiac tissue.

Although capital costs are high, and acquisition times relatively long, the technology allows detailed assessment of molecular structure, anatomical relationships, and myocardial perfusion without the use of ionizing radiation. Signal-processing techniques and the use of contrast-enhancing agents such as gadolinium allow identification of myocardial scar, tissue oedema, and assessment of valve regurgitant fraction and stenosis severity. Advanced techniques, such as 'four-dimensional flow', and the use of hyperpolarizing agents and high magnetic field strengths hold promise for future understanding of disease pathogenesis. In the space of a few years, CMRI has become an invaluable and increasingly available tool for cardiologists, and an essential element for managing ischaemic, congenital, and valvular heart disease. Indeed, while it lacks the availability and relative simplicity of ultrasound, it has better signal-to-noise characteristics and will undoubtedly develop considerably in the coming years. An example of an image obtained via a current CMRI technique, steady-state free precession imaging, is shown in Figure 87.10.

Invasive assessments

Recognition that injection of iodinated contrast into cardiac structures, including the coronary arteries, can be safely performed now enjoys a 50-year history and remains a centrepiece of cardiovascular investigation and therapy. The modern cardiac laboratory should offer both diagnostic and treatment facilities, preferably 24/7, with a skilled team available to assess haemodynamics, anatomy, structure, and function, as well as offer planned and emergency reperfusion therapy for acute ST-elevation and non-ST elevation myocardial infarction and chronic stable angina. The rapid expansion of 'minimally invasive' procedures for the treatment of both congenital and acquired valvular disease, as well as expansion of interventional electrophysiology procedures, has meant that the 'cathlab' has become the home of diverse subspeciality interests in cardiology, and the hub of a cardiac centre. The role of invasive diagnostics will continue to decline as non-invasive technologies develop further, limited to an extent by more sophisticated applications such as coronary lesion-specific functional assessments (e.g. pressure-wire fractional flow reserve (see Figure 87.11) and new techniques for assessing coronary microcirculation, such as flow reserve and microvascular resistance. However, there remains a place for invasive haemodynamic assessment for the diagnosis of several cardiac conditions, including valve diseases, such as mitral stenosis, and constrictive and restrictive cardiomyopathy, and for diagnostic coronary angiography in dilated cardiomyopathy and left ventricular dysfunction, when an ischemic aetiology is suspected. Consequently, it is premature to write the obituary of the skilled cathlab diagnostic cardiologist.

Further Reading

Hurst JW. *The Canterbury Tales* and cardiology. *Circulation* 1982; 65: 4–6.
Murphy JG and Lloyd MA (eds). *Mayo Clinic Cardiology: Concise Textbook* (4th edition), 2012. Mayo Clinic Scientific Press.

88 Congenital heart disease in adults

Liz Orchard

Introduction

Congenital heart disease is the most common congenital abnormality, affecting 0.8% of births. There have been major advances in both the surgical and interventional treatment of congenital heart disease, with about 85% of patients surviving into adulthood. It is estimated that there are about 250 000 adults with congenital heart disease in the UK, and the number of adults with congenital heart disease now exceeds the number of children. As these patients live longer, the likelihood of them developing problems in later life increases. Despite this, there are fewer adult congenital cardiologists than paediatric cardiologists in the UK, and thus it is increasingly likely that general cardiologists and physicians will manage these patients either acutely or in outpatients. Cardiologists need to have an understanding of the complex physiology of these patients, in case they develop complications which require immediate treatment, such as heart failure, arrhythmias, thrombosis, or endocarditis.

Congenital heart disease can be divided into simple and complex lesions. Simple lesions include atrial septal defect (ASD), ventricular septal defect (VSD), patent ductus arteriosus (PDA), coarctation of the aorta, and left ventricular outflow tract lesions. More complex lesions include transposition of the great arteries (TGA), tetralogy of Fallot, single ventricle/Fontan physiology, pulmonary atresia/VSD or pulmonary atresia/intact septum, and Ebstein's anomaly of the tricuspid valve.

Simple congenital heart disease

Ventricular Septal Defect (VSD)

A VSD is a direct communication between the right and left ventricles, and is the commonest form of congenital heart disease, accounting for about 20% of all lesions (see Figures 88.1 and 88.2). The size of the VSD and the degree of pulmonary vascular resistance determine the degree and direction of the right to left shunt.

VSDs can be described by position: muscular VSD (completely enclosed by muscle; 10%–15% of VSDs), perimembranous VSD (partly enclosed by the fibrous continuity between aortic and tricuspid valves; 80% of VSDs), or doubly committed VSD (partly enclosed by the fibrous continuity between aortic and pulmonary valves; 5% of VSDs). VSDs are also described according to size: it is 'restrictive' or 'small' when the defect limits the amount of blood flow between the left and right ventricles and therefore does not produce left ventricle dilatation, and is 'non-restrictive' when the defect is moderate or large (pulmonary flow:systemic flow > 1.5:1), leading to markedly increased pulmonary flow, initially with left ventricle dilatation, and failure to thrive and, if untreated, to the development of pulmonary hypertension.

Restrictive defects are not normally operated on unless the patient has suffered from infective endocarditis or has developed aortic regurgitation from prolapse of a leaflet. Non-restrictive VSDs are normally operated on in childhood to prevent the development of Eisenmenger syndrome (irreversible pulmonary hypertension due to a large systemic-to-pulmonary artery shunt).

Clinical findings for VSD

Patients with VSD have a holosystolic murmur—the smaller the defect, the louder the murmur. The apex is displaced if there is a significant shunt. P2 is loud if there is pulmonary hypertension.

Atrial Septal Defect (ASD)

An ASD is a communication between the right and the left atrium, and can be a secundum ASD (within the oval fossa; 75% of ASDs); a primum ASD, or partial atrioventricular septal defect (AVSD;

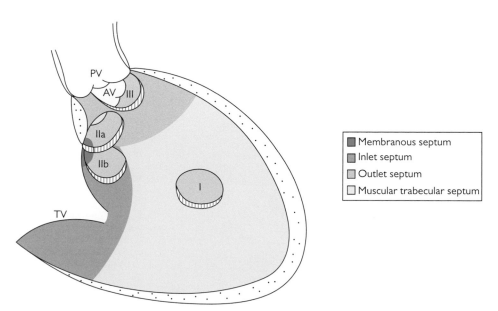

Figure 88.1 Schematic representation showing the sites of different types of ventricular septal defects (VSDs). The heart is in cross-section, viewed from the right ventricular aspect. I, muscular VSD; IIa, perimembranous outlet VSD; IIb, perimembranous inlet VSD; III, doubly committed subarterial VSD; AV, aortic valve, seen through VSD; PV, pulmonary valve; TV, tricuspid valve.

Reproduced with permission from Warell, Cox & Firth, *Oxford Textbook of Medicine*, Fifth Edition Oxford University Press, Oxford, UK, Copyright © 2012.

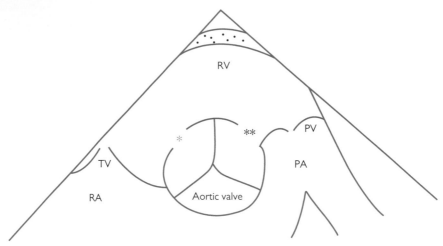

Figure 88.2 Schematic representation of the transthoracic echocardiographic parasternal short-axis view, to demonstrate sites of ventricular septal defects (VSDs); ** indicates the site of doubly committed subarterial VSD—the aortic and pulmonary valves are in continuity and form the roof of the VSD; * indicates the site of subaortic perimembranous VSD; PA, pulmonary artery; PV, pulmonary valve; RA, right atrium; RV, right ventricle; TV, tricuspid valve.

Reproduced with permission from Warell, Cox & Firth, *Oxford Textbook of Medicine*, Fifth Edition Oxford University Press, Oxford, UK, Copyright © 2012.

common atrioventricular junction with a cleft in the left atrioventricular valve; 10%–15% of ASDs); a sinus venosus ASD (communication between the superior or the inferior vena cava and the left atrium); or a coronary sinus ASD, where there is a connection between the left atrium and coronary sinus (see Figure 88.3).

Clinical presentation of ASD

Symptoms of an ASD include dyspnoea, palpitations, or a stroke due to a paradoxical embolism. If ASD is left untreated, excessive pulmonary blood flow leads to right heart dilatation. Signs of ASD include a pulmonary-flow murmur, a fixed, split, second heart sound, and cyanosis if there is a right to left shunt.

Complications of ASD

Complications of ASD include arrhythmia, which can present even after surgery; right heart failure; and paradoxical emboli. If ASDs are diagnosed in childhood, and the shunt is >2:1, they are generally repaired before school age. If they are repaired when the patient is <25 years old, then the patients should have normal long-term survival.

Atrioventricular Septal Defect (AVSD)

An AVSD is a communication at the junction of the atria and ventricles (see Figure 88.4). It can be classified as follows:

Complete: primum ASD and non-restrictive VSD, with a five-leaflet atrioventricular valve; >75% of patients with complete AVSD have trisomy 21
Intermediate: primum ASD and restrictive VSD, with abnormal but separate atrioventricular valves
Partial: ostium primum ASD, with a cleft in the mitral valve

Clinical findings for AVSD

As with other left-to-right shunts at the atrial or ventricular level, complete AVSDs are normally repaired in early infancy to prevent the development of Eisenmenger syndrome. Partial AVSDs are normally repaired in early childhood. Repaired AVSDs can still develop problems with mitral or tricuspid regurgitation or stenosis, subaortic stenosis, atrial arrhythmias, or complete atrioventricular block

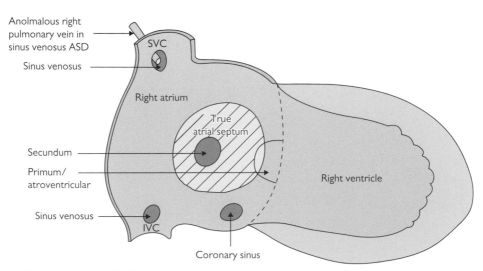

Figure 88.3 Sites of atrial septal defects. The shaded area delineates the true atrial septum. Sinus venosus and coronary sinus defects are therefore not strictly atrial septal defects, although they permit shunting at atrial level; ASD, atrial septal defects; IVC, inferior vena cava; SVC, superior vena cava.

Reproduced with permission from Warell, Cox & Firth, *Oxford Textbook of Medicine*, Fifth Edition Oxford University Press, Oxford, UK, Copyright © 2012.

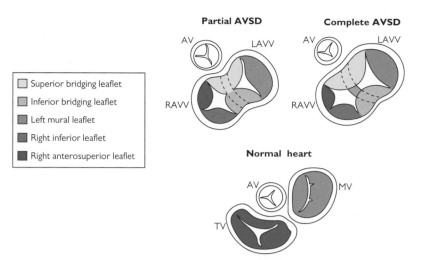

Partial AVSD

AV LAVV

RAVV

Complete AVSD

AV LAVV

RAVV

- ☐ Superior bridging leaflet
- ☐ Inferior bridging leaflet
- ☐ Left mural leaflet
- ☐ Right inferior leaflet
- ☐ Right anterosuperior leaflet

Normal heart

AV MV

TV

Figure 88.4 Schematic representation of the atrioventricular junction in atrioventricular septal defect (AVSD). Short-axis view, seen from the atrial aspect. In both forms of AVSD, there is a common atrioventricular valve ring guarded by five valve leaflets. In the partial defect, the superior and inferior bridging leaflets fuse to create two separate valve orifices. This fusion does not occur in complete AVSD, so there is a common valve orifice; AV, aortic valve; LAVV, left atrioventricular valve; MV, mitral valve; RAVV, right atrioventricular valve; TV, tricuspid valve.

Reproduced with permission from Warell, Cox & Firth, *Oxford Textbook of Medicine*, Fifth Edition Oxford University Press, Oxford, UK, Copyright © 2012.

PDA

PDA is a remnant of the fetal circulation, connecting the proximal left pulmonary artery to the descending aorta distal to the left subclavian artery. Its significance depends on the size of the duct, with large ducts leading to increased pulmonary blood flow and left atrial and ventricular dilatation, with the long-term development of pulmonary vascular disease and Eisenmenger syndrome.

Clinical findings for PDA

Patients with a PDA have a continuous murmur which is holosystolic, and diastolic loudest at the left upper sternal edge. If Eisenmenger syndrome develops, there is a differential cyanosis between upper and lower limbs. PDA can present with an acute endarteritis and should be closed if there is endarteritis or left ventricle volume overload; it can be closed percutaneously with a device.

Coarctation of the aorta

Coarctation of the aorta is a narrowing of the aorta, normally at the isthmus (site of the ductus arteriosis). In neonates/infants, it can present as an emergency when closure of the duct leads to underperfusion of the lower half of the body, and prostaglandins are required in order to maintain perfusion prior to operative correction. In adults it can present as an uncommon cause for hypertension which is resistant to treatment (see Figure 88.5). Coarctation can be associated with hypoplastic aortic arch, anomalies of head and neck vessels, intra-cerebral berry aneurysms, and a bicuspid aortic valve (50% of patients).

Investigations for coarctation of the aorta

Investigations for coarctation of the aorta include an ECG for left ventricular hypertrophy, an echo which will demonstrate a narrowed descending aorta with increased velocity, and a chest X-ray; in the latter, look for rib notching due to the erosion of the inferior edge of the ribs by dilated intercostal arteries. CT and MRI will give detailed information of the coarctation site.

Repair of coarctation

Coarctation is normally repaired in childhood by subclavian flap repair or end-to-end anastomosis. Patients who have undergone these procedures can develop aneurysms at the site of repair; these require intervention to prevent rupture. Patients with primary coarctation presenting in adulthood can be treated by direct stenting, due to the surgical risk of repair, from long-standing collateral vessels. Post repair these patients often remain hypertensive, despite adequate luminal patency, and there is little data on best medical therapy for hypertension.

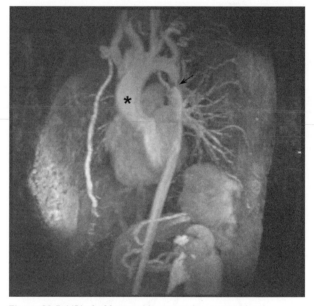

Figure 88.5 MRI of a 20-year-old woman who presented with hypertension. There is a severe discrete coarctation (indicated by the arrow), multiple tortuous collaterals, and a dilated ascending aorta (indicated by the asterisk) associated with a bicuspid aortic valve.

Reproduced with permission from Warell, Cox & Firth, *Oxford Textbook of Medicine*, Fifth Edition Oxford University Press, Oxford, UK, Copyright © 2012.

Left ventricular outflow tract lesions

Left ventricular outflow tract lesions can be:

- subvalvar, if there is discrete fibrous membrane or a tunnel below the valve
- valvar, if there is a bicuspid aortic valve (this affects 2% of the population and is associated with an abnormality of aortic root tissue)
- supravalvar, if there is aortic narrowing at the sinotubular junction (this is associated with Williams syndrome)

Clinical findings for left ventricular outflow tract lesions

Symptoms of left ventricular outflow tract lesions include dyspnoea on exertion, angina, and syncope if there is severe obstruction.

Clinically, patients may have a slow rising pulse, low pulse pressure, and ejection click if the valve is pliable, with an ejection systolic murmur. Treatment of subvalvar or supravalvar obstruction is with surgical resection.

Valvar stenosis can be treated with either surgical valvotomy or resection, or balloon dilatation, and depends on the age of the patient at presentation, and the pliability of the valve (pliable valves can be balloon dilated and this is the preferred treatment in childhood). Treatment is warranted for:

- relief of symptoms
- severe aortic stenosis (peak gradient of 80 mm Hg, or valve area <0.5 cm²/m² on echocardiography)
- catheter peak gradient of 60 mm Hg
- an abnormal ECG response to exercise

In adults, aortic valve replacement is considered the best treatment.

Complex congenital heart disease

Transposition of the Great Arteries (TGA)

In TGA, the aorta arises from the right ventricle, and the pulmonary artery from the left ventricle; this condition can be simple or complex (i.e. associated with other lesions such as VSD; see Figure 88.6). Simple transposition is not compatible with life, due to the circulation being in parallel, unless mixing of the circulation occurs (e.g. via an ASD).

Two types of operation are undertaken for TGA:

Atrial switch: In this procedure, the Senning or Mustard procedure (see Figure 88.7; also see 'Surgical procedures'), the atrial blood is redirected so that the right ventricle receives pulmonary venous blood, making it the systemic ventricle; the left ventricle receives systemic venous blood. Most adults who have undergone repair for TGA have had this operation. However it has now been replaced by the arterial switch.

Arterial switch: In this procedure, the aorta and the pulmonary artery are 'switched' to the correct position, and the coronary arteries are reimplanted (see 'Surgical procedures').

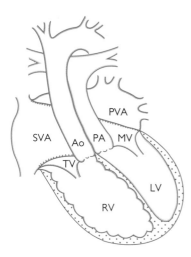

Figure 88.7 Repair of complete transposition of the great arteries, via atrial switch (using the Senning procedure or the Mustard procedure); Ao, aorta; LV, left ventricle; MV, mitral valve; PA, pulmonary artery; PVA, pulmonary venous atrium; RV, right ventricle; SVA, systemic venous atrium; TV, tricuspid valve.

Reproduced with permission from Warell, Cox & Firth, *Oxford Textbook of Medicine*, Fifth Edition Oxford University Press, Oxford, UK, Copyright © 2012.

Complications post atrial switch

Most complications occur post atrial switch and include:

- atrial tachyarrhythmia (atrial re-entrant tachycardia) and bradyarrhythmia (sinus node dysfunction) secondary to extensive atrial surgery
- right ventricle dysfunction, and failure of the systemic right ventricle
- tricuspid regurgitation
- risk of sudden death
- obstruction of systemic or pulmonary venous pathways ('baffle obstruction')

Post-atrial switch patients are complex to manage; their arrhythmias often require ablation, and they need a thorough assessment of right ventricle dysfunction and the severity of tricuspid regurgitation, and this can be difficult to obtain. However, the final pathway for a failing systemic right ventricle is transplantation.

Complications post arterial switch

There is 88% 15-year survival post arterial switch; however, complications include:

- pulmonary stenosis
- dilatation of the neo-aortic root, with aortic regurgitation
- coronary ostia stenosis due to reimplantation

Congenitally corrected TGA

In congenitally corrected TGA (ccTGA), the ventricles are inverted, the systemic venous return reaches the pulmonary artery via the left ventricle, and the pulmonary venous return enters the right ventricle and is pumped to the aorta; therefore, the circulation is 'physiologically' corrected (see Figure 88.8). It is a rare condition: ccTGA cases constitute <1% of all cases of congenital heart disease. In addition, 95% of ccTGA cases are associated with other lesions (e.g. VSD, pulmonary stenosis, aortic stenosis, AVSD, Ebstein's anomaly of the tricuspid valve).

Complications of ccTGA

If ccTGA is not associated with other abnormalities, it can present late in life. However, complications include development of heart block, systemic ventricular failure, and tricuspid regurgitation.

Management of ccTGA

Management of ccTGA includes pacing and the use of angiotensin-converting enzyme (ACE) inhibitors and diuretics for right ventricular dysfunction. Tricuspid valve replacement is

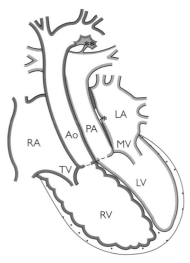

Figure 88.6 Schematic representation of complete transposition of the great arteries (discordant ventriculo-arterial connections). The pulmonary and systemic circulations are completely separate once the arterial duct and foramen ovale close. Without intervention, the condition is not compatible with life; Ao, aorta; LA, left atrium; LV, left ventricle; MV, mitral valve; PA, pulmonary artery; RA, right atrium; RV, right ventricle; TV, tricuspid valve; * patent arterial duct; ** patent foramen ovale.

Reproduced with permission from Warell, Cox & Firth, *Oxford Textbook of Medicine*, Fifth Edition Oxford University Press, Oxford, UK, Copyright © 2012.

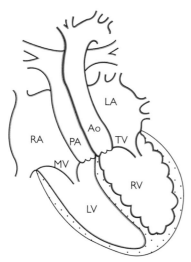

Figure 88.8 Schematic representation of congenitally corrected transposition of the great arteries (discordant atrioventricular and ventriculo-arterial connections). The circulation is congenitally physiologically 'corrected' in that systemic venous blood reaches the pulmonary artery (via the left ventricle) and pulmonary venous blood reaches the aorta (via the right ventricle); Ao, aorta; LA, left atrium; LV, left ventricle; MV, mitral valve; PA, pulmonary artery; RA, right atrium; RV, right ventricle; TV, tricuspid valve.

Reproduced with permission from Warell, Cox & Firth, *Oxford Textbook of Medicine*, Fifth Edition Oxford University Press, Oxford, UK, Copyright © 2012.

undertaken for severe tricuspid regurgitation, and transplantation is performed for end-stage right ventricle dysfunction. Children presenting with tricuspid regurgitation can be considered for an anatomical repair via either a double switch (atrial and arterial switch) or a combined Senning–Rastelli operation (see 'Surgical procedures').

Tetralogy of Fallot

In tetralogy of Fallot, anterocephalad deviation of the outlet septum leads to hypertrophy of septoparietal trabeculations, and right ventricular outflow tract obstruction (RVOTO)/pulmonary artery obstruction (see Figure 88.9).

This produces:

- VSD
- right ventricle hypertrophy
- aortic override

The timing and presentation of patients in infancy depends on the severity of the RVOTO, as a significant obstruction leads to early cyanosis. Tetralogy of Fallot is associated with 22q deletion in 15% of patients, with the presence of a right aortic arch in 25% of patients, and with coronary artery abnormalities in 10% of patients. Patients are offered primary repair before 18 months of age (VSD closure, relief of RVOTO—sometimes with patch enlargement of pulmonary valve annulus), but neonates who are symptomatic with cyanosis are palliated with a Blalock–Taussig (subclavian-to-pulmonary artery) shunt (see 'Surgical procedures').

Complications of tetralogy of Fallot

The following complications are seen with tetralogy of Fallot:

- pulmonary regurgitation with right ventricle enlargement and dysfunction
- RVOTO—at the infundibular, pulmonary valve, or branch pulmonary level
- aneurysmal dilatation of the right ventricular outflow tract (predisposes to ventricular tachycardia)
- residual VSD
- aortic regurgitation +/− aortic root dilatation
- arrhythmia:
  - atrial: scar-related intra-atrial re-entrant tachycardia
  - ventricular: associated with right ventricle dilatation; a QRS duration >180 milliseconds is a marker for sustained ventricular tachycardia

Management of tetralogy of Fallot

Pulmonary valve replacement is recommended for patients with severe pulmonary regurgitation; the replacement can be either surgical or percutaneous.

The development of arrhythmia requires a thorough haemodynamic and electrophysiological assessment.

Single ventricle circulation

The term 'single ventricle circulation' encompasses many complex congenital abnormalities; however, in all of them, the pulmonary and the systemic venous returns drain into a functional single ventricle that then pumps to both the pulmonary artery and the aorta (see Figure 88.10).

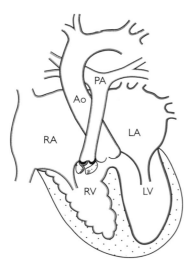

Figure 88.9 Schematic representation of tetralogy of Fallot. Anterocephalad deviation (indicated by the asterisk) of the outlet septum creates a ventricular septal defect, subpulmonary stenosis, aortic overriding of the crest of interventricular septum, and secondary right ventricular hypertrophy; Ao, aorta, LA, left atrium, LV, left ventricle, PA, pulmonary artery, RA, right atrium, RV, right ventricle.

Reproduced with permission from Warell, Cox & Firth, *Oxford Textbook of Medicine*, Fifth Edition Oxford University Press, Oxford, UK, Copyright © 2012.

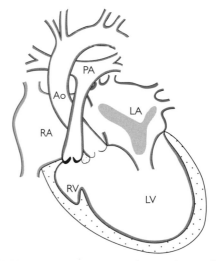

Figure 88.10 Schematic representation of tricuspid atresia. Systemic venous blood leaves the right atrium via an atrial septal defect and mixes with pulmonary venous blood in the left atrium. The left ventricle thus supports both the systemic and pulmonary circulations, and the patient is cyanosed. The rudimentary right ventricle does not play a functional role; Ao, aorta; LA, left atrium; LV, left ventricle; PA, pulmonary artery; RA, right atrium; RV, right ventricle.

Reproduced with permission from Warell, Cox & Firth, *Oxford Textbook of Medicine*, Fifth Edition Oxford University Press, Oxford, UK, Copyright © 2012.

There is also a more rudimentary ventricle, with the functional ventricle being either of left or right morphology. However, due to the complexity of the anatomy, a biventricular repair is not surgically possible.

The anatomical configurations of a single ventricle defect include:

- tricuspid atresia (rudimentary right ventricle)
- unbalanced AVSD
- a double-inlet left ventricle, often with transposition and pulmonary stenosis
- pulmonary atresia with a hypoplastic right vesicle

The Fontan procedure, used to repair single ventricle circulation, was originally a direct right atrium to pulmonary artery anastomosis; however, due to complications, patients now undergo a total cavopulmonary connection. This procedure combines a Glenn anastomosis (superior vena cava to the pulmonary artery connection), which is performed before the patient is 1 year of age, and a connection from the inferior vena cava to the pulmonary artery, which is created either via a lateral tunnel (using the atrial wall) or through an extra-cardiac conduit and is made when the patient is around 5 years old (see Figure 88.11; also see 'Surgical procedures').

Complications of single ventricle circulation

Complications associated with single ventricle circulation are:

- arrhythmias:
  - atrial re-entrant tachycardia (commonly)
  - sinus node dysfunction
- thromboembolic events

- right atrial dilatation, and hepatic dysfunction due to high hepatic venous pressure
- protein-losing enteropathy (intestinal protein loss leading to low serum protein, peripheral oedema, and ascites)
- ventricular dysfunction
- obstruction/leak of Fontan pathway
- systemic venous collateralization
- failing Fontan

Survival at 15- to 20-years after the Fontan procedure ranges from 60 to 85%, and is influenced by the underlying cardiac diagnosis. Further interventions (e.g. Fontan revision, pacemaker implantation) are commonly needed.

Eisenmenger syndrome

Eisenmenger syndrome arises due to excess pulmonary blood flow from a left to right shunt leading to the development of irreversible pulmonary vascular disease. The shunt can occur at atrial, ventricular or arterial level, and with the development of pulmonary hypertension, the shunt reverses to right to left and cyanosis occurs. Patients with Down's syndrome are at increased risk of developing Eisenmenger physiology. The over-all incidence is reducing, due to early diagnosis of congenital heart disease and consequently earlier surgery, with better outcomes.

Complications of Eisenmenger syndrome

The complications associated with Eisenmenger syndrome are:

- the development of iron deficiency

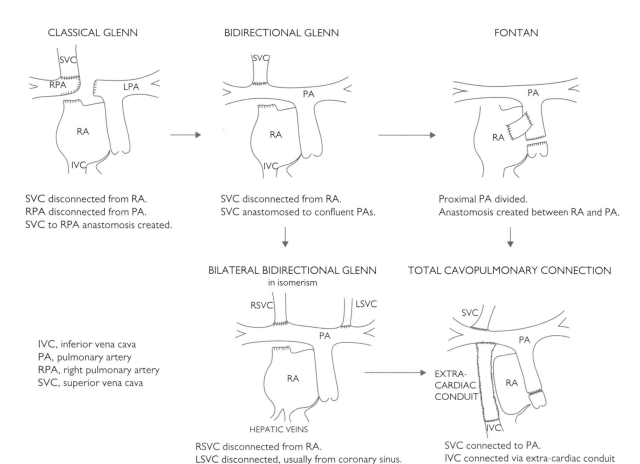

Figure 88.11 Evolution of the Fontan and total cavopulmonary connection operations; IVC, inferior vena cava; PA, pulmonary artery; RPA, right pulmonary artery; LSVC, left superior vena cava; RSVC, right superior vena cava; SVC, superior vena cava.

Reproduced with permission from Warell, Cox & Firth, *Oxford Textbook of Medicine*, Fifth Edition Oxford University Press, Oxford, UK, Copyright © 2012.

- thromboembolism (pulmonary/cerebral emboli), despite an increased bleeding risk
- hyperviscosity due to secondary erythrocytosis
- arrhythmias (supraventricular or ventricular)
- sudden cardiac death
- bacterial and viral infections (endocarditis, cerebral abscess, and pneumonia)
- gallstones and cholecystitis
- gout
- acne

Treatment includes avoiding dehydration, hypovolaemia, and nephrotoxic drugs. Avoid general anaesthesia and non-cardiac surgery, if possible, and any general anaesthesia should be performed by a cardiac anaesthetist. Consider pulmonary vasodilator therapy (e.g. non-selective endothelin receptor antagonists), once the patient has been referred to a pulmonary hypertension centre.

Ebstein's anomaly of the tricuspid valve

In Ebstein's anomaly, the tricuspid valve has an abnormal structure and position, with apical displacement of the valve. This leads to atrialization of the right ventricle, with a dilated right atrium, and a valve that may become severely regurgitant. Most cases are associated with an ASD or patent foramen ovale, which may result in some cyanosis; 25% of patients have associated Wolff–Parkinson–White syndrome.

Presentation of Ebstein's is variable, depending on the degree of leaflet displacement and the amount of right ventricle dysfunction and tricuspid regurgitation. Management should include closure of the atrial shunt, and tricuspid valve surgery, if very regurgitant, before the right ventricle starts to fail; but this operation is complex and requires specialist surgical input.

Cyanosis

Cyanosis occurs when there is a right to left shunt or decreased pulmonary blood flow and is clinically detectable when saturations drop below 85%. Cyanosis can be associated with low, normal, or high pulmonary vascular resistance.

Complications of cyanosis

The complications associated with cyanosis are:

- the development of secondary erythrocytosis, which is a physiological adaptation to hypoxia in order to increase oxygen-carrying capacity; it may cause hyperviscosity symptoms but is not associated with an increased risk of cerebrovascular accident; previously, venesection was recommended for therapy but now it is known that it causes iron deficiency and so is not beneficial
- thrombocytopenia
- coagulopathy (haemorrhage or thrombosis); often very difficult to manage
- renal impairment (due to glomerular proteinuria); can lead to iatrogenic renal decompensation if the patient is dehydrated or given nephrotoxic agents
- cerebrovascular accidents due to paradoxical emboli, and cerebral abscess
- acne
- gout
- pigment gallstones

Emergencies in adult congenital heart disease patients

Adult congenital heart disease patients are at risk from specific emergencies, including:

- haemoptysis:
  - This is a major cause of death, especially if pulmonary hypertension is present.
  - The patient will need resuscitation.
  - Lower the blood pressure, as pulmonary artery pressure is equivalent to systemic blood pressure—use beta blockade.
  - Intubate if the bleeding is uncontrolled.

- An urgent CT chest is needed to determine the source of the bleeding; causes can be in situ pulmonary artery thrombosis, bleeding from pulmonary arteriovenous malformations, or collaterals and infection.
  - Management issues to consider include IV access with an air filter, due to risk of paradoxical embolism in cyanotic patients.
- tachyarrhythmias:
  - These can be either atrial or ventricular.
  - These are poorly tolerated and require cardioversion.
  - DC cardioversion is often safer than drug treatment.
- cerebral abscess

In addition, it is important to:

- avoid vasodilators, as these may increase cyanosis
- avoid iatrogenic renal dysfunction
- maintain haemoglobin post-operatively, to maintain adequate oxygen carrying capacity

Surgical procedures

Arterial switch

Arterial switch is an operation used to repair TGA, in which the great arteries are 'switched' (see 'TGA'). It involves moving the coronary arteries from the aortic root to the neo-aorta.

Blalock–Taussig shunt

In a classical Blalock–Taussig shunt, there is a direct end-to-side anastomosis of the subclavian artery to the pulmonary artery. In a modified Blalock–Taussig shunt, there is a graft from the subclavian artery to the pulmonary artery.

Glenn shunt

In a Glenn shunt, an anastomosis of the superior vena cava to the pulmonary artery is created.

Fontan procedure

This is a palliative operation for patients with single ventricle physiology, where blood from the systemic veins return to the lungs without passing through the subpulmonary ventricle (see 'Single ventricle circulation'). There are three versions of this operation:

Classic Fontan: in this version, a direct connection is made between the right atrium and the pulmonary artery

Björk modification: in this version, a valved conduit is made between the right atrium and the right ventricle

Total cavopulmonary connection: in this version, a connection is made from the inferior vena cava to the pulmonary artery via either a lateral tunnel or an extra cardiac conduit, with anastomosis of the superior vena cava to the pulmonary artery (Glenn shunt)

Mustard/Senning operation

The Mustard/Senning operation is an atrial switch, used to repair TGA (see 'TGA'). Venous blood is 'baffled' across to the contralateral ventricle by using synthetic material (Mustard) or fashioning an atrial wall (Senning).

Norwood operation

Divided into stages, the Norwood operation is used to repair a hypoplastic left heart and the associated hypoplastic aortic root and ascending aorta. Stage I, which is performed in neonates, involves the reconstruction of the aorta by using the pulmonary valve and trunk to create a neo-aorta, with the pulmonary blood supply being from a modified Blalock–Taussig shunt. In Stage II, which is performed in patients <1 year old, the Blalock–Taussig shunt is taken down and a bidirectional Glenn operation is performed. In Stage III, which is performed when the patient is <5 years old, the Fontan circulation is completed.

Rastelli operation

The Rastelli operation is used to repair TGA, VSD, and pulmonary stenosis (see 'TGA' and 'VSD'). The VSD is closed by a patch connecting the left ventricle to the aorta, with a conduit from the right ventricle to the pulmonary artery.

Further Reading

Baumgartner H, Bonhoeffer P, De Groot NM, et al. European Society of Cardiology guidelines for the management of grown-up congenital heart disease (new version 2010). *Eur Heart J* 2010; 31: 2915–57.

Bhatt AB, Foster E, Kuehl K, et al. Congenital heart disease in the older adult: A scientific statement from the American Heart Association. *Circulation* 2015; 131: 1884–931.

89 Chronic stable angina

Cheerag Shirodaria and Sam Dawkins

Definition of the disease

Chronic stable angina is a condition where patients experience symptoms of chest pain of a particular character (e.g. angina pectoris; see 'Typical symptoms and less common symptoms') on effort only, due to atherosclerotic coronary artery disease. The hallmarks of stable angina are as follows:

- There must be stable atherosclerotic coronary artery disease (but see 'Other diagnoses that should be considered'), resulting in luminal narrowing(s) in one or more of the major epicardial coronary arteries. Such atheroma can be detected using appropriate technology (see '"Gold-standard" diagnostic test' and 'Acceptable alternatives to the gold standard'). Not all angina chest discomfort is due to atherosclerotic coronary disease—some is due to aortic stenosis, and some to hypertrophic cardiomyopathy; rarely, pulmonary hypertension is the cause.
- Symptoms must have been present for some time, say, arbitrarily, 2–3 months, as opposed to the case for angina of acute coronary syndromes, where symptoms have been present only for a few weeks at most—see Chapter 90. This time limit is important, as it allows the differentiation of symptoms from coronary obstruction due to coronary atheroma (generally a stable pathology, with a lower risk of infarction) from symptoms of coronary obstruction due to atheroma with superadded thrombus, which can be quite unstable and lead suddenly to total coronary obstruction with all its attendant risks.
- Symptoms must be stable, that is to say, from day to day, roughly similar levels of effort must be required for provocation. The pathological translation of this is that the degree of coronary obstruction is stable, as opposed to the rapidly changing coronary obstruction found in acute coronary syndromes.

Typical symptoms and less common symptoms

The hallmarks of angina are (1) its relationship with exercise, (2) the nature of the pain, and (3) its duration. All must be present for diagnosis; if they are not, atypical angina or non-cardiac chest pain is diagnosed, symptoms which have a lower chance of being due to obstructive coronary disease (see Chapter 10).

The relationship of the pain with exercise

Reliable provocation of symptoms by exercise and rapid relief by rest is the hallmark of angina. Symptoms are **never** present before exercise, build up during exercise, and are **fully relieved** by 2 minutes' rest. Angina pectoris occurs when myocardial oxygen demand exceeds supply; atherosclerotic coronary obstruction, unless very severe, has no impact on resting coronary blood flow, but reduces the increase in coronary blood flow during exercise, explaining the effort dependence of symptoms. If oxygen demand exceeds supply, ischaemic metabolites build up, are sensed, and produce the feeling of angina. Angina can occur without exercise in situations with tachycardia, as tachycardia (1) increases myocardial oxygen demand and (2) reduces myocardial blood flow, as coronary blood flow occurs during diastole, and an increased heart rate reduces the proportion of time spent in diastole. Tachycardia due to an arrhythmia (e.g. atrial fibrillation, supraventricular tachycardia) is sufficiently profound to cause angina in those with less severe coronary disease. However, although the tachycardia associated with emotional stress can provoke angina, as the tachycardia and changes in myocardial oxygen demand and supply are relatively mild, patients need to have severe coronary disease for emotional stress to provoke angina. Put another way, those with angina during emotional stress often have angina on fairly minimal effort, and one should have a low threshold for angiography in such patients.

The nature of the pain

Angina is often described as discomfort, pressure, or tightness in the chest, rather than as pain. It can radiate to the jaw, either arm, and less commonly to the back. Patients cannot usually localize the pain precisely and may diffusely rub their hand over the anterior chest wall, indicating the general area of discomfort; if they place a finger precisely at the site of pain, ischaemia is unlikely to be the cause. Two **atypical symptoms** may occur in some: (1) breathlessness, rather than angina (this is common in the elderly, and diabetics, and is termed 'angina equivalent'; the clues to angina are the effort dependence of symptoms, the rapid relief by rest, and the presence of coronary disease risk factors); and (2) effort intolerance without specific features (usually this is due to age, physical deconditioning, arthritis, or other factors; however, rarely, it relates to coronary disease—the clue is that the alternative diagnoses have usually reduced exercise capacity over years, whereas coronary disease can reduce exercise capacity over just a few months).

Some patients interpret the pain as being gastrointestinal in origin, and use phrases such as 'burning'; alternatively, they interpret it as being arthritis, particularly if symptoms are felt around the shoulder; as always, the clue to the real diagnosis is the effort dependence of symptoms, and relief with rest.

The duration of the pain

In chronic stable angina, pain does not last more than a few minutes. If it occurs during exercise, patients rest, or take glyceryl trinitrate, thus rapidly relieving symptoms. Pain that lasts longer is either due to an acute coronary syndrome (the clue is that the prolonged pain is similar in quality to previous angina, although longer lasting and may be more severe) or, conversely, not due to a coronary problem at all (random episodes of prolonged pain going back many months lasting ≥20–30 minutes and never related to exercise). Far and away, the commonest cause of prolonged chest pain is non-cardiac pain.

Classification of angina severity

Angina severity is classified using a scale devised by the Canadian Cardiovascular Society (see Table 89.1).

Demographics and etiology of the disease

Stable angina in nearly all cases relates to atherosclerotic coronary artery disease, which in turn relates to the various risk factors for atheroma, including age (the most important factor), diabetes, obesity (especially centripetal), smoking, hypertension, poor genes (sometimes seen as an adverse family history of documented coronary disease in first-degree relatives ≤65 years old (coronary death or coronary revascularization only), male gender, psychosocial stress, and dyslipidaemia. A diet high in fruits and vegetables, moderate alcohol intake, and exercise are protective, and relevant on a population basis. The biology of atheroma is complex; in essence, cholesterol enters the vessel wall (this is a normal physiological process), is trapped (perhaps as it has been altered by smoke products), and excites an inflammatory response, resulting in the formation of scar tissue and the atheromatous plaque. This can build up by extension of this process, or by incorporation of super-added thrombus, so narrowing the lumen.

Table 89.1 Angina severity scale	
Grade	**Definition**
I	Ordinary physical activity, such as walking or climbing stairs, does not cause angina. Angina occurs with strenuous, rapid, or prolonged exertion at work or recreation.
II	Slight limitation of ordinary activity. Angina occurs on walking or climbing stairs rapidly, walking uphill, walking or climbing stairs after meals, or in cold, in wind, or under emotional stress, or only during the few hours after awakening. Angina occurs on walking more than 2 blocks on the level and climbing more than 1 flight of ordinary stairs at a normal pace and in normal condition.
III	Marked limitations of ordinary physical activity. Angina occurs on walking 1 to 2 blocks on the level and climbing 1 flight of stairs in normal conditions and at a normal pace.
IV	Inability to perform any physical activity without discomfort—anginal symptoms may be present at rest.

Reproduced with permission from L Campeau, Letter: Grading of angina pectoris, *Circulation*, Volume 54, Issue 3, p522, Copyright © 1976 Wolters Kluwer Health, Inc.

Complications

The major complications in chronic stable angina are myocardial infarction and/or sudden death. On average, the annual incidence is 1% but prognosis varies widely. Factors associated with an adverse prognosis are (1) multiple risk factors for coronary disease, especially if they cannot be controlled (e.g. smoking; diabetes is strongly associated with a worse outcome); (2) symptoms on low levels of effort; (3) impaired left ventricular function, especially if the ejection fraction is <40%; (4) extensive coronary disease involving all three major coronary arteries; (5) proximal coronary disease affecting the left main stem or proximal left anterior descending coronary artery; and (6) increasing age.

A few patients develop the following complications:

Arrhythmias: The commonest is atrial fibrillation, which is serious due to its thromboembolic risk. Most patients presenting with atrial fibrillation in middle age and beyond need to have coronary disease excluded.

Heart failure: This is not rare in chronic coronary disease and has a number of different etiologies and treatments:

- Chronic coronary disease increases the fibrous content of the heart, making it stiffer and leading to diastolic heart failure—the clue is good left ventricular systolic function, absence of critical coronary disease, and a raised biomarker for heart failure, such as BNP.
- Chronic coronary disease, if severe, can lead to a reduction in resting coronary blood flow—often this results in myocardial infarction but, in a few, the reduction in blood flow can be compensated for by cells shutting down energy expensive functions, such as contractile functions; that is, the heart can hibernate. The heart then enlarges and systolic performance falls away. Patients usually present with a history of progressive breathlessness over several months; the clue is that, on echocardiography, left ventricular wall thickness remains good, the ECG does not show Q waves, and angiography shows critical coronary disease. It can be difficult, however, to fully determine whether the myocardium is hibernating or dead—cardiac magnetic resonance (lack of scar tissue) and a myocardial perfusion scan (tracer uptake) may distinguish between these two possibilities. Revascularization improves hibernating myocardium, but not a scarred heart.
- Critical proximal multivessel coronary disease can result in heart failure—such patients often present with life-threatening pulmonary oedema. When the acute episode has been treated, good left ventricular function is found echocardiographically and troponin levels are only minimally elevated, but angiography shows either left main or severe three-vessel coronary artery disease.
- There may be isolated disease affecting a papillary muscle; the commonest is disease in the circumflex coronary leading to ischaemia or infarction, papillary muscle dysfunction, and severe mitral regurgitation, presenting as pulmonary oedema. Outside the episode, there may be very little mitral regurgitation, and normal left ventricular function. Angiography usually shows disease limited to the circumflex coronary artery.

Approach to diagnosing the disease

The principle is one valid for most diseases: reach a diagnosis from the history, exclude other possible causes of angina from the physical examination (particularly aortic stenosis and other causes of left ventricular outflow tract obstruction, and also, where possible, pulmonary hypertension), and confirm the diagnosis using an appropriate test (see '"Gold-standard" diagnostic test'). Always in your own mind decide whether the patient is experiencing angina before you order tests—if you do not do so, you will not know what to do with the results! Once you have diagnosed chronic stable angina, assess left ventricular function (usually done echocardiographically), then make an assessment of the severity of the coronary disease—there are many ways to do this, and part of the skill of the clinician is to decide which test is appropriate for which patient. Once you know the diagnosis, how intrusive symptoms are, left ventricular function, and coronary extent, you can plan the best management, be it medical alone or revascularization also.

Other diagnoses that should be considered

The other causes of anginal chest pain include aortic stenosis, pulmonary hypertension, and cardiomyopathy with left ventricular outflow tract obstruction. Asthma and COPD can give rise to similar symptoms. Other causes of chronic chest pain include musculoskeletal pain, various gastrointestinal pains (including gastroesophageal reflux disease, oesophagitis, peptic ulcer disease, and dyspeptic syndromes; very rarely, biliary pain is felt predominantly in the chest), non-cardiac chest pain, and pain referred from the back, due to either degenerative back disease or entrapment neuropathy. Pain from metastatic deposits is a very rare cause of pain, occasionally seen.

'Gold-standard' diagnostic test

The gold standard for assessing coronary arteries is coronary angiography but this test is far from perfect. It is an anatomical test, assessing coronary artery luminal diameter in the resting artery, rather than a functional test measuring ischaemia. This is an important difference, as the anatomical appearances of the severity of the luminal narrowing only have a modest relationship with the impairment in coronary artery function. Most narrowings that are ≥90% of the luminal diameter impair coronary blood flow, whereas most that are ≤50% do not. However, in between, it is difficult to predict whether the arterial narrowing impedes blood flow or not. In other words, while as a generalization the more severe the narrow in an artery appears angiographically, the more likely it is to reduce peak blood flow, there are many exceptions—angiographically minor narrowings can have very major functional impacts and, perhaps surprisingly, angiographically severe narrowings can have very modest impacts on function. It is the degree of functional impairment that relates to symptoms and to prognosis—it is the functionally most damaged arteries that are most likely to have plaque rupture and so provoke a myocardial infarct. This means that, in chronic stable angina, it is more difficult to decide whether to undertake revascularization based on the angiogram than it is in an acute coronary syndrome, where the main aim of percutaneous coronary intervention is to stabilize an unstable segment of artery with plaque rupture and superadded thrombus—and usually the trouble with the artery has been diagnosed by the finding of an elevated troponin and ECG changes, allowing localization of the affected artery. In chronic stable angina, it is important to demonstrate ischaemia prior to revascularization, and this can be done by a variety of investigations.

Acceptable alternatives to the gold standard

For many patients, a non-invasive diagnostic strategy is appropriate. Those with a high pretest probability of coronary artery disease should undergo angiography as the first-line investigation, as should some with equivocal or conflicting results from non-invasive testing. A low threshold for angiography is appropriate in those with known coronary disease, previous acute coronary syndrome, or revascularization.

Exercise tolerance testing is a useful inexpensive means to assess suspected coronary disease. A treadmill or a bicycle is used for incremental exercise. Exclusions to exercise tolerance testing include the physical incapacity to exercise, left bundle branch block, and pre-excitation (e.g. Wolff–Parkinson–White syndrome). Ideally, the test should be carried out while the patient is off anti-anginal medication.

There are several endpoints: the patient reaching ≥85% maximum heart rate (where, for men, the maximum heart rate is 220 − age and, for women, the maximum heart rate is 210 − age) without symptoms (a negative test); limiting chest pain or diagnostic ECG changes (ST depression >2 mm, ST elevation >1 mm); or a sustained fall in systolic blood pressure (>10 mm Hg). The duration of exercise, development of chest pain, and extent of ECG changes are used to risk stratify patients, for example, by using the Duke treadmill score.

Exercise testing is inaccurate in low risk or asymptomatic individuals, as false positives outweigh genuine positives, rendering the test poorly specific; in addition, false negatives are also common in this group, rendering the test poorly sensitive. Patients at high risk of having coronary artery disease (from the history and risk factors) should be referred for angiography, as exercise tolerance testing will not provide any further information.

Coronary CT angiography (CTA) is a non-invasive test currently undergoing rapid development and evaluation. High-resolution, three-dimensional pictures of the heart and great vessels are produced during coronary CTA, allowing demonstration of luminal architecture, and so the presence of coronary artery disease. It is particularly useful in evaluating the patency of coronary bypass grafts. In order to obtain optimal image quality, the subject's heart rate should be <60 bpm, which is achieved by using either beta blockers or ivabradine.

Investigations useful for the demonstration of myocardial ischaemia

Dobutamine stress echocardiography (DSE) or a **myocardial perfusion scan (MPS)** is used if the exercise test is not possible or is inaccurate (resting ECG changes, left bundle branch block). They are also of particular use in asymptomatic patients with diabetes. The choice between these modalities generally depends on staff and equipment availability; their accuracy is comparable.

In DSE, baseline transthoracic echocardiography is carried out prior to starting a dobutamine infusion (which increases heart rate and contractility), and then echocardiography is repeated as the heart rate increases and during recovery. Myocardial contractility is impaired where there is coronary ischaemia (regional wall motion abnormality). Regional wall motion abnormalities at rest are likely to be due to infarcted muscle, which will not benefit from revascularization.

In an MPS, exercise or a coronary vasodilator (adenosine or dipyridamole) is used to increase myocardial blood flow; then, a radioactive isotope (technetium or thallium) is injected, which is taken up by the myocardium in proportion to myocardial blood flow. The heart is then imaged using a CT gamma camera, allowing reconstruction of a three-dimensional image of the heart. It is then possible to determine if there are differences in uptake between different areas of the heart, in other words, if areas of the heart are supplied by stenosed arteries. The scans are undertaken at rest (allowing diagnosis of previous myocardial infarction), and following stress, to determine areas of ischaemia

A fractional flow reserve (FFR) technique, using pressure wires and adenosine vasodilatation, can also be used (see Chapter 97).

Other relevant investigations

A resting ECG should be performed in patients presenting with chronic chest pain; this is to provide evidence of previous infarction, or left ventricular hypertrophy (associated with hypertension and coronary disease). Occasionally—though rarely—there is evidence of an acute coronary syndrome. The resting ECG is usually normal in chronic stable angina.

Resting transthoracic echocardiography is appropriate in chronic chest pain to exclude valve disease or cardiomyopathy, and to examine left ventricular function in breathless patients. Patients with ECG abnormalities such as left bundle branch block or ECG evidence of a previous myocardial infarction should also undergo echocardiography.

A chest X-ray should be undertaken in patients with angina, mainly to exclude other smoking- and age-related diseases that may impact on angina treatment, and, ; occasionally, suspected valve disease, heart failure, or suspected pulmonary disease.

Prognosis and how to estimate it

Prognosis in chronic stable angina is variable but overall annual mortality is 1%, as is risk of non-fatal myocardial infarction. Patients at higher risk are those with multiple cardiovascular risk factors, multi-vessel disease, proximal stenosis, severe angina, or reduced left ventricular function.

Treatment and its effectiveness

The aims for treating angina are to treat symptoms and improve prognosis. Beta blockers are the first-line treatment, and further agents should be added if anginal symptoms persist.

Drugs to improve symptoms

Drugs used to improve symptoms are:

- short-acting nitrates:
  - These relieve angina.
  - Glyceryl trinitrate spray and sublingual tablets have rapid onset (1–4 minutes) and last for 15–30 minutes.
  - They cause vascular smooth muscle relaxation, systemic vasodilatation (reducing afterload and cardiovascular work), and coronary vasodilatation (improving myocardial oxygen delivery) and reduce preload through venodilatation.
  - Side effects include flushing, headache, dizziness, and hypotension.
  - Nitrates taken prior to planned exertion can increase exercise capacity.
  - Patients should seek medical advice should angina not improve 5 minutes after one glyceryl trinitrate spray.
- longer-acting nitrates:
  - These can be used for patients with frequent symptoms.
  - Isosorbide dinitrate acts for 4–8 hours, and isosorbide mononitrate for 6–12 hours.
  - Nitrate tolerance develops quickly, and having a nitrate-free period each day prevents this.
- calcium channel blockers:
  - The longer-acting dihydropyridines (e.g. amlodipine) cause coronary and systemic vasodilatation through vascular smooth muscle relaxation.
  - These drugs, and more so the short-acting dihydropyridine nifedipine, cause a reflex tachycardia and so are often used in conjunction with beta blockers.
  - The non-selective calcium channel blockers (verapamil and diltiazem) also cause vascular smooth muscle relaxation and additionally have a negative effect on heart rate and myocardial contractility, which reduces myocardial oxygen demand still further.

Approaches used to improve the prognosis

Approaches used to improve the prognosis are:

- the use of aspirin
- aggressive risk factor modification:
  - Reduce blood pressure to ≤130/80 mm Hg.
  - Use statins to achieve a target LDL cholesterol level of ≤2.6 mmol/l.
  - Offer patients assistance with smoking cessation and dietary advice.

- the use of angiotensin-converting enzyme (ACE) inhibitors (or angiotensin receptor blockers)
  - These should be considered in patients with a history of myocardial infarction, chronic kidney disease, diabetes, or heart failure.

Drugs that have an effect on both symptoms and prognosis

Drugs that have an effect on both symptoms and prognosis are:

Beta blockers: These reduce myocardial oxygen demand by reducing contractility, heart rate, and blood pressure; they also improve oxygen supply through a reduction in heart rate, thus lengthening diastole and therefore the time for myocardial perfusion. Regular use results in reduced frequency of anginal attacks and increased exercise tolerance. In patients who have had a previous myocardial infarction, or in systolic heart failure, beta blockers have prognostic benefit.

Nicorandil: This is a potassium-channel activator that causes venous and arterial vasodilatation. It also has a modest effect on prognosis.

Exercise

The importance of regular exercise in patients with chronic stable angina should not be underestimated. A regular exercise programme improves exercise tolerance and aids weight loss. In lower-risk patients, a programme of regular exercise can be as effective as revascularization, both in terms of exercise capacity and event-free survival, at considerably lower cost.

Revascularization

Diagnostic angiography with a view to revascularization (percutaneous coronary intervention or coronary artery bypass grafting) should be considered in patients with severe angina which is significantly affecting quality of life despite medical therapy, or in those with high-risk markers.

Prevention

See Chapter 343.

Further Reading

Montalescot G, Sechtem U, Achenbach S, et al. 2013. ESC guidelines on the management of stable coronary artery disease. *Eur Heart J* 2013; 34: 2949–3003.

National Institute for Health and Care Excellence. *Stable Angina: Management.* 2011. Last updated: August 2016. Available at https://www.nice.org.uk/guidance/cg126?unlid=110029818201733224941 (accessed 20 Mar 2017).

90 Acute coronary syndromes

Cheerag Shirodaria and Sam Dawkins

Definition of the disease

The term 'acute coronary syndrome' (ACS) includes unstable angina, ST-elevation myocardial infarction (STEMI), and non-ST-elevation myocardial infarction (NSTEMI). The difference between these three syndromes is as follows:

- In STEMI and NSTEMI, there is evidence of myocardial necrosis, as evidenced by raised cardiac enzymes, specifically, the very sensitive cardiac biomarker troponin. STEMI is diagnosed when the ECG shows persisting ST elevation in an appropriate territory consistent with STEMI, whereas, in NSTEMI, there can be any or no ECG changes, or very transient self-limiting ST elevation.
- In unstable angina, there is no myocardial necrosis, and troponins are normal. The ECG is as for NSTEMI and often shows no change, ST depression, or T-wave inversion.

The prognoses in STEMI and NSTEMI are identical; unstable angina has a better prognosis than either STEMI or NSTEMI.

Typical symptoms and less common symptoms

A patient with an acute coronary syndrome usually presents with ischaemic chest pain. A careful history should establish the nature of pain. Ischaemic chest pain usually comes on over minutes, rather than second or hours, and is often described not as a pain but rather a pressure or tight band around the chest. The pain is usually poorly localized, and patients are unable to put a finger on the precise location. If there is radiation, it is classically to the throat and the left arm, although pain radiating to the right or both arms is more strongly predictive of myocardial ischaemia. Symptoms associated with the pain can be variable. Nausea, indigestion, and an unpleasant taste in the mouth are associated with gastro-oesophageal reflux but these can also be features of myocardial infarction. Equally, an improvement in the pain with glyceryl trinitrate spray does not necessarily indicate cardiac disease. Sweating is more strongly predictive of cardiac disease and is generally not associated with gastro-oesophageal disease.

Certain patients are more likely to have atypical symptoms. Those with diabetes mellitus tend to have less severe pain and may present with the complications of silent myocardial infarction (including heart failure or confusion). Female patients are more likely to use words such as 'sharp' or 'burning' to characterize their pain.

Demographics and etiology of the disease

Coronary artery disease remains the largest cause of mortality and morbidity in industrialized countries. Increasing age, positive family history, male gender, and smoking all increase the risk of atherosclerosis. Other risk factors include diabetes mellitus, dyslipidaemia, hypertension, lack of exercise, and obesity (especially centripetal 'abdominal' obesity), and psychosocial stress.

Natural history

The pathological process that leads to acute coronary syndrome begins with atherosclerosis, which is a disease of the vessel intima, due to cholesterol and lipid deposition and the infiltration of inflammatory cells. This leads, in mature lesions, to a lipid-rich core enclosed by a fibrous cap within the vessel intima. Plaques may occlude the vessel lumen, or may become 'unstable', when increased inflammatory activity causes weakening of the fibrous cap. Plaque rupture may lead to mural thrombosis and acute vessel occlusion, or downstream showering of emboli to occlude the microvessels. These pathological events result in a continuous spectrum of clinical syndromes, from stable angina, to unstable angina, to myocardial infarction.

Complications of ACS

Complications associated with ACS are as follows:

Arrhythmias: Arrhythmias are common in ACS:
- Atrial fibrillation commonly complicates ACS, and is associated with more severe coronary disease.
- Ventricular tachycardia can complicate ACS, in which case it is often associated with remote myocardial infarction (producing an 'arrhythmogenic' scar) with new myocardial ischaemia—and it is the two together that are necessary for such ventricular arrhythmias.
- Ventricular fibrillation complicates ACS and, indeed, the commonest cause of sudden cardiac death is ventricular fibrillation related to myocardial ischaemia. It occurs in up to 30% of ACS, although, as this occurs usually very early on, it is now not common in patients once they reach hospital and receive modern therapy.
- Heart block can complicate myocardial ischaemia, especially when the right coronary artery is involved.

Myocardial rupture: Myocardial rupture was previously a relatively common cause of death in ACS. Traditional teaching was that this occurred 2–7 days post myocardial infarction, and could be either of the free wall, resulting in cardiac tamponade and immediate death, or internal, resulting in a ventricular septal defect; the low pressure in the right ventricle would result in blood shunting from the left ventricle into the right ventricle, so diminishing systemic cardiac output and resulting in prominent right heart failure. The clues to the development of a ventricular septal defect are a patient becoming less well, though happy to lie flat; peripheral oedema; and a loud pansystolic murmur along the left sternal edge. Cardiac ultrasound is diagnostic; angiography confirms the diagnosis and diagnoses the extent of coronary disease. Surgical repair can be life-saving. Mortality is high.

Heart failure: Heart failure can be due to several mechanisms:
- the death of contractile tissue, related to the size of the myocardial infarction
- hibernation of contractile tissue (see Chapter 92)
- papillary muscle dysfunction, usually due to circumflex territory ischaemia—this can result in torrential mitral regurgitation; severe pulmonary oedema, so that the patient automatically sits bolt upright; and profound hypoxaemia; the murmur of mitral regurgitation is usually absent or very quiet; cardiac ultrasound is usually diagnostic; treatment is immediate intubation, angiography, and surgery; even in the best units, mortality is high

Pericarditis: Pericarditis usually only complicates a full-thickness ('Q-wave') myocardial infarct rather than other forms of ACS.

Dressler's syndrome: Dressler's syndrome (see Chapter 109) is rare, and usually only with larger infarcts (full-thickness Q wave).

Some 30% of patients die during a myocardial infarct—of these deaths, some 70%–80% occur in the first few hours, usually before patients reach hospital. Put another way, patients who reach hospital are immediately in a better prognostic group, as they have survived this early death rate. Treatments (see 'Treatment and its effectiveness') to improve the prognosis of those reaching hospital are vital, but perhaps overall of less importance than encouraging patients with possible ACS to come to hospital early.

Approach to diagnosing the disease

The general approach is to diagnose an ACS from the history, use the examination to exclude complications or other important possible diagnoses, and confirm the diagnosis with the ECG and biomarkers. See also Chapters 9 and 10.

History

About half of patients with an ACS have previous stable angina now complicated by an ACS. Diagnosis here is easy; they have had effort-related ischaemic chest pain, usually only on good levels of exercise, then often a period of symptoms on increasingly mild effort, culminating in rest pain, usually lasting >20 minutes and not responding to glyceryl trinitrate. Likewise, some patients have had a previous **proven** ACS; they present with symptoms similar to those for the last ACS. The diagnosis here is also easy. The difficulty arises when patients present 'out of the blue', and the diagnosis here can be difficult, as the pain may be atypical, or confused with gastrointestinal (or other) causes of pain, or masked by other symptoms (breathlessness, malaise, confusion, 'off legs') that have a very broad differential diagnosis. As an ACS is so common, it not infrequently presents in an atypical fashion or in the elderly, in whom dementia may render the history unreliable. It is important, therefore, to have a high index of suspicion in any adult presenting to hospital with appropriate risk factors and symptoms that are not immediately diagnosed as something else, and which just might represent an ACS. In these patients, undertake standard tests to exclude an ACS (sequential ECGs, biomarkers), always bearing in mind that the interpretation of these tests will require a much broader differential than in those presenting with typical symptoms.

Investigations

ECG

The ECG is the crucial investigation in suspected ACS. It should be carried out at presentation, every 2–3 hours, and whenever there is chest pain.

If the ECG remains resolutely normal despite prolonged rest pain, the chances of an ACS are significantly reduced—one diagnosis to beware of is circumflex coronary artery disease, which can present with an ACS with a normal ECG, as this part of the heart can be electrically quiet. However, many high-risk ACSs are excluded if the troponin remains negative despite repeated measurements. Put another way, most circumflex territory ACSs, despite possibly having normal or near normal ECGs, have abnormal troponins.

If the ECG shows fixed abnormalities (but see 'Other diagnoses that should be considered in possible ACS') that do not change, then the chance of an ACS is probably neither increased nor decreased. If the ECG shows signs classically associated with a high-grade coronary stenosis, such as pan-anterior (or inferior), **deep** T-wave inversion, the chances of an ACS have increased very substantially—however, even pan-anterior T-wave inversion (an ECG so highly correlated with a high-grade stenosis in the proximal portion of the left anterior descending (LAD) coronary artery that it has been termed a 'LAD-syndrome ECG') is not universally due to high-grade coronary disease, and similar ECGs can be seen with pulmonary emboli (quite commonly), takotsubo cardiomyopathy (much more common than once realized—see 'Other diagnoses that should be considered in possible ACS') and hypertrophic cardiomyopathy (a much less likely diagnosis). The basic principle, as in virtually all investigations, remains that one should use the investigation to increase or decrease the probability of the disease in question, and not absolutely rely on any one test to diagnose the illness, unless you know that test to be completely reliable.

If the ECG shows 'dynamic' ST changes (i.e. the ST segments go down—or up—over time), it is likely that there is an ACS and, in particular, a high-risk ACS (although there are many exceptions—and, in particular, beware that hyperventilation can result in ST-segment shift).

Troponin (or other biomarkers)

Biochemical markers are both used in the diagnosis of myocardial infarction and also have prognostic value once the diagnosis has been made (from the degree of the elevation). Troponin is a regulatory enzyme that is found almost exclusively in cardiac muscle; there are two subtypes, T and I. Serum troponin rises with myocardial damage, and the extent of elevation correlates with the size of infarction. Troponin levels start to rise 3–4 hours post myocardial infarction, reach a peak over the next 12 hours, and return to undetectable levels after around 10 days. For this reason, a single negative troponin results does not exclude myocardial infarction and it is important to make sure a further sample is taken 6–12 hours after admission and after any subsequent episodes of chest pain.

There are many causes of a troponin rise, other than an ACS. Correlation with the clinical condition of the patient, in addition to serial troponin measurements and measurement of renal function, helps to correctly diagnose myocardial infarction as the cause of a troponin rise (see Table 90.1). As is true of most tests, minor deviations from normal are common and result in the most diagnostic doubt. You should be most aware that **small rises in troponin do not make the diagnosis of an ACS**. You must use all the clinical clues to determine whether patients with small increases in troponin have an ACS or some other condition. It is only when the troponin is very elevated that you can be reasonably sure the test is diagnostic of ACS.

If the ECG remains normal, troponin is not elevated, and symptoms settle, then patients fall into a low-risk category, even if they have unstable angina. Most such patients can be safely discharged and undergo expedited outpatient evaluation.

Other diagnoses that should be considered in possible ACS

Chest pain with positive troponin

See Table 90.1. Exclude **renal failure** as a cause of elevated troponin, in which case the differential is that of chest pain with negative troponin. The commonest alternative of chest pain with raised troponin is a **pulmonary embolus**, which remains in the differential even when the troponin is negative.

Stress (takotsubo) cardiomyopathy is an increasingly recognized cause of chest pain and raised troponin in women. The typical case involves a middle-aged woman who has had an emotional event (an argument, bad news, etc.). Ischaemic-sounding chest pain develops and patients present rapidly to hospital (perhaps as the vast majority of those affected are women—men with chest pain present late to hospital). The ECG sequentially develops changes that look like those for a proximal LAD lesion, that is to say, pan-anterior T-wave inversion, and the troponin is mildly raised. At angiography (which must happen as the differential diagnosis is an acute coronary event), the coronary arteries are shown to be smooth and unobstructed. However, a left ventriculogram demonstrates the classic abnormality of this condition, which is akinesis of the anteroapical and distal inferior wall of the left ventricle, a contractile abnormality beyond the distribution of a single coronary artery. The contractile abnormality can be profound, with overall left ventricular function sometimes being severely impaired (although contraction in the unaffected segments is normal or even hyperdynamic). Treatment is with angiotensin-converting enzyme (ACE) inhibitors, and beta blockers, to improve left ventricular function. Prognosis is generally good; even in the absence of treatment, left ventricular function returns to normal within a few months. Complications are rare, but the occasional patient does die during the acute episode, usually of arrhythmias. The exact pathophysiological mechanism remains obscure.

Chest pain with negative troponin

One cause of chest pain with negative troponin is unstable angina, the clues to which are in the history, and often from an abnormal

Table 90.1 Non-coronary conditions with troponin elevations

	Frequency as a cause of troponin elevation	Notes
Renal failure (either acute or chronic)	Universal	The commonest cause of mild–moderate troponin elevations in acute medical admissions (commoner than ACS); very few have an ACS—the clue to an ACS is a changing troponin despite stable (albeit abnormal) renal function; if the renal function is changing, it is difficult to diagnose ACS from changing troponin—rely more on the history and ECG
Tachyarrhythmia	Common	Sustained (20–30 mins) of tachyarrhythmia very commonly results in elevated troponin in the absence of an ACS; this is very common with SVT (where heart rates are in 160–190 bpm), and not rare with AF; arrhythmias should be >140 bpm to result in raised troponin
Pulmonary embolus	Common	Troponin rises with a pulmonary embolus are very common; the extent of rise correlates to the severity of right ventricular strain, and so to the size of the pulmonary embolus, and the outcome
Acute left ventricular failure	Common	Any cause of acute left ventricular failure will give moderate elevations in troponin even when no ACS is present—diagnose an ACS here on the basis of the history (ischaemic chest pain), ECG changes, and if troponin rises are substantial
Inflammatory disease (e.g. myocarditis or myocardial extension of endocarditis/pericarditis)	Common	Very frequent in myocarditis—clues are tachycardia and heart failure; common in pericarditis, where it indicates some myocarditis (and has implications for recommending exercise restriction until the patient is better)
Acute neurological disease (e.g. stroke, subarachnoid haemorrhage)	Not rare	Like major ECG changes (e.g. pan-anterior T-wave inversion), troponin elevations are not rare in subarachnoid haemorrhage; their extent correlates with the severity of the neurological insult
Cardiac contusion (e.g. from deceleration injury (RTC), ablation, insertion of a new pacing lead, cardioversion, or endomyocardial biopsy)	Common	Usually easily diagnosed from the history
Critically ill patients (especially those with respiratory failure or with sepsis)	Common	Troponin rises (just like ECG changes) are common in critical illness, and it can be difficult to determine whether this reflects the illness, or a complicating ACS—if doubt exists and diagnosis alters treatment, coronary angiography may be necessary
Drug toxicity (e.g. Adriamycin, 5-fluorouracil, Herceptin)	Not common	Probably common in those suffering cardiac toxicity from these drugs, but rare in those not suffering cardiac toxicity
Aortic dissection	Rare	These do occur, although usually the etiology is fairly clear
Aortic valve disease		
Hypertrophic cardiomyopathy		
Infiltrative diseases (e.g. amyloidosis, haemochromatosis, sarcoidosis, scleroderma)		
Hypertensive crisis		
Hypothyroidism	Rare	Occurs, but very rarely seen in acute admissions

Abbreviations: ACS, acute coronary syndrome; AF, atrial fibrillation; bpm, beats per minute; ECG, electrocardiography; RTC, road traffic collision; SVT, supraventricular tachycardia.

ECG, either at presentation or over the next few hours. If patients are troponin negative, have **persistently** normal ECGs, their pain settles, and there is no other obvious alternative diagnosis, they fall into a very good prognostic group, even if they have unstable angina. However, many patients presenting with prolonged chest pain, normal ECGs, and negative troponin do not have any cardiac illness.

Aortic dissection, oesophageal rupture, and other causes

Additional diagnoses that should be considered include:

- aortic dissection; this rare, but still seen several times a year in most units (see Chapter 103)
- oesophageal rupture; this is usually obvious from a history of vomiting followed by severe chest pain
- causes that lead to raised troponin levels but do not relate to the heart (see Table 90.1)

'Gold-standard' diagnostic test

The diagnosis will often be settled by coronary angiography. The advantage of this technique is that it can be diagnostic and lead to the therapeutic procedure of percutaneous coronary intervention (PCI).

Acceptable diagnostic alternatives to the gold standard

In reality, coronary angiography is usually not required to make the diagnosis, as this can be made on the basis of clinical symptoms, ECG, and troponin:

STEMI: In STEMI, the history and ECG are sufficient to make the diagnosis. Coronary angiography is helpful, as it is the essential prelude to PCI, a procedure associated with marginally improved survival compared to thrombolysis.

The rest of the acute coronary syndrome spectrum: For the rest of the acute coronary syndrome spectrum, a combination of history, examination, ECG, and cardiac biomarkers can be used to make the diagnosis. If, despite this, the diagnosis remains in doubt, it can be clarified by using invasive or non-invasive tests. Not infrequently, however, patients have major comorbidities, and introducing empirical therapy is appropriate—an approach should always be guided by an experienced cardiologist, preferably an interventional cardiologist. Put another way, it is important that interventional cardiologists see all patients with possible ACS, regardless of the patient's age or comorbidity, to ensure that the largest number of patients benefit from appropriate medical therapy and, where relevant, targeted interventional therapy.

Imaging

It is also possible to diagnose an ACS using nuclear cardiology techniques—radioactive technetium is injected (at ≤2 hours of chest pain) and then the heart is imaged with a CT gamma-radiation-detecting camera. If the scans are normal, myocardial perfusion is normal and this excludes most high-risk ACS cases—provided ECGs and biomarkers remain negative, these patients can be safely discharged to return the following day for the stress component to evaluate any ischaemic burden. In other words, a normal post-chest-pain scan does not exclude coronary disease; it does, however, risk stratify the patient and exclude most immediately life-threatening forms of coronary disease.

Occasionally, cardiac magnetic resonance is used to diagnose infarction (by finding scar tissue in the distribution of a coronary artery) in situations where differentiation from myocarditis is important and cannot be made using traditional techniques. Likewise, cardiac ultrasound is used to look for evidence of regional wall motion abnormalities indicating coronary artery disease.

Other relevant investigations

The aim of additional investigation is to determine:

- the size of the myocardial infarct (troponin, and cardiac ultrasound)
- the presence of other illness impacting on cardiac management; renal function is important, as are general blood tests to exclude anaemia and determine if there is any ill health (diagnosed from low albumin), cancer (raised inflammatory markers/abnormal liver/bone function tests), or infection
- glucose and cholesterol

Prognosis and how to estimate it

The prognosis in ACS is determined by many factors, including age, renal function, comorbidity, extent of coronary disease, vessel affected by the acute lesion (left main and proximal left anterior descending artery lesions have higher risk), left ventricular function, presence of heart failure, and extent of biomarker release. These factors are combined in a number of widely available scoring systems, including TIMI (http://www.mdcalc.com/timi-risk-score-ua-nstemi/) and GRACE (http://www.outcomes-umassmed.org/grace/acs_risk/acs_risk_content.html).

Treatment and its effectiveness

The aims of treatment in ACS are to relieve symptoms and improve prognosis—however, the issue is complicated, as it is not always apparent who has an ACS, so the diagnostic process sometimes needs to run in parallel with the therapeutic process. Furthermore, angiography is not appropriate for all, most often on account of comorbidity, when the prognostic element may be removed from the equation. There also can be controversies about the best approach to revascularization in NSTEMI and unstable angina and, in particular, which patients should have PCI and which should have a coronary artery bypass graft (CABG).

Treatment for STEMI

All patients should receive immediate pain relief (morphine), aspirin (in the ambulance), and clopidogrel (or similar). Oxygen is commonly given. The occluded artery needs to be opened immediately. Thrombolysis with intravenous thombolytics is effective but primary (i.e. first-line treatment, ≤30 minutes of presentation) PCI is slightly more so and thus is now the standard treatment. Following the opening of the occluded artery, any bystander disease may be treated by PCI or CABG, depending on the exact anatomy and patient preference. Bystander revascularization usually takes place after recovery from the initial infarct, although there is increasing evidence that this should be done as early as possible.

Treatment for NSTEMI

Provide pain relief, dual antiplatelet agents (see 'Drugs'; aspirin and clopidogrel), heparin (or similar), and beta blockers (or similar).

Angiography is used to risk stratify high-risk NSTEMI to determine which artery has an acute lesion, and the extent of the coronary disease. PCI to acute thrombotic lesions has been shown to reduce reinfarction and death rates (discussed in Chapter 97).

Drugs with an important role in ACS

Drugs with an important role in ACS include:

Aspirin: Aspirin causes the irreversible inhibition of the COX-1 enzyme, which inhibits production of thromboxane A2, a powerful platelet aggregator released by activated platelets and leading to platelet activation. Aspirin in ACS reduces the risk of infarction and death. The first dose should be chewed or given in dispersible form to ensure a rapid onset of action. Unless contraindicated, aspirin should be continued for the rest of the patient's life.

Clopidogrel: Clopidogrel (a thienopyridine) prevents platelet aggregation via inhibition of an ADP receptor ($P2Y_{12}$), and has an additive effect in combination with aspirin. It reduces the risk of death, further myocardial infarction, and urgent revascularization, but with an increased bleeding risk. Prognostic benefit is restricted to high-risk patients. Clopidogrel should be given for 1 year following an ACS. Newer thienopyridines such as prasugrel can also be used with particular benefit in patients undergoing primary PCI, due to its quick onset of action. However, prasugrel must be used with caution in patients over 65 or under 60 kg, due to an increased risk of bleeding.

Ticagrelor: Ticagrelor is more effective than clopidogrel and is increasingly used, especially in diabetic patients.

Anticoagulation drugs: Anticoagulation with low-molecular-weight heparin reduces the death rate and further myocardial infarction. Direct thrombin inhibitors and fondaparinux, a selective inhibitor of factor Xa, have similar actions. The low-molecular-weight heparins (e.g. enoxaparin, dalteparin) are the most commonly used anticoagulants in ACS. They reduce the risk of angina, myocardial infarction, and death. They do not require anticoagulant monitoring and have less risk of heparin-induced thrombocytopenia, compared with unfractionated heparin. There is no benefit to prolonged heparin treatment.

Beta blockers: Beta blockers are important in ACS, acting through several mechanisms. They are negatively chronotropic (so reducing myocardial oxygen demand) and prolong diastole, improving coronary artery perfusion. They reduce ventricular tachyarrhythmias and sudden death. In the long term, beta blockers have a role in ventricular remodelling and thus their use can lead to an improvement in ventricular function. In patients with COPD, beta blockers are often withheld because of a perceived risk of bronchospasm. The benefits of beta blockers outweigh this risk in the majority of COPD patients, as most have largely fixed airways obstruction; cardioselective beta blockers should be given in patients with mild-to-moderate airways disease.

Glycoprotein IIb/IIIa inhibitors: Glycoprotein IIb/IIIa inhibitors such as abciximab and tirofiban block the final common pathway of platelet activation by binding to fibrinogen and, under high shear conditions, to von Willebrand factor, thus inhibiting the bridging between activated platelets. In patients at intermediate to high risk, particularly patients with elevated troponins, ST depression, or diabetes, either eptifibatide or tirofiban for initial early treatment can be used in addition to oral antiplatelet agents. In high-risk patients not pretreated with glycoprotein IIb/IIIa inhibitors and proceeding to PCI, abciximab has been shown to reduce the combination of death and myocardial infarction or need for urgent revascularization at 30 days.

Angiotensin-converting enzyme (ACE) inhibitors: ACE inhibitors reduce the incidence of further myocardial infarction and sudden death post myocardial infarction. They also improve ventricular remodelling if ventricular function is impaired. They should be used in STEMI patients. In NSTEMI, an ACE inhibitor should be started in those with diabetes, chronic kidney disease, hypertension, or a left ventricular ejection fraction of ≤40%; it is not unreasonable to consider starting an ACE inhibitor in patients outside these groups. The drug should be started prior to hospital discharge. An angiotensin II receptor blocker should be started in patients who cannot tolerate an ACE inhibitor (usually due to cough).

Statins: Statins should be started in high dose in ACS (e.g. atorvastatin 80 mg every day) and continued for 1–2 years, after which time conventional-dose statins are used.

Hypoglycaemic drugs: patients with hyperglycaemia on admission have a worse outcome, whether they are known to have diabetes mellitus or not. Indeed, much type II diabetes mellitus is diagnosed during an admission for ACS. There is debate on how to manage hyperglycaemia here. Intensive glucose control, while controlling hyperglycaemia, may put the patient at risk of hypoglycaemia, which has a negative impact on outcome. The pragmatic approach is to institute insulin therapy in diabetic patients with an elevated blood glucose on admission, but to use oral agents in those patients with moderately raised blood glucose.

Further Reading

Ibanez B, James S, Agewall S, et al. 2017 ESC Guidelines for the management of acute myocardial infarction in patients presenting with ST-segment elevation. Eur Heart J 2018; 39: 119–77.

Reed GW, Rossi JE, Cannon CP. Acute myocardial infarction. *Lancet* 2017; 389: 197–210.

Roffi M, Patrono C, Collet J-P, et al. 2015 ESC Guidelines for the management of acute coronary syndromes in patients presenting without persistent ST-segment elevation. *Eur Heart J* 2016; 37: 267–315.

91 Acute heart failure

Kazem Rahimi

Definition of the disease

Heart failure is a clinical syndrome characterized by an inadequate cardiac output for the needs of the body in the absence of low filling pressures, and reflects abnormal cardiac structure or function. Although various definitions for acute heart failure (AHF) exist, here AHF is defined as new-onset heart failure or an acute exacerbation of chronic heart failure, requiring urgent therapy. Patients with AHF typically have clinical features of organ hypoperfusion, with or without pulmonary and peripheral oedema.

Aetiology of the disease

It is best to think of AHF in a two-stage manner: first, there is a cardiac substrate; second, there may be a cardiac or non-cardiac event provoking acute deterioration. Identifying and treating all underlying and contributory causes is central to the management of AHF.

Underlying cardiac causes

Underlying cardiac causes include:

- acute coronary syndromes
- hypertensive heart disease
- valvular disease (especially if acute, such as acute valvar regurgitation due to endocarditis)
- cardiomyopathies
- myocarditis
- pericardial diseases

Provoking causes

Provoking causes include:

- cardiac causes such as atrial fibrillation (which requires an underlying cardiac substrate to lead to heart failure, i.e. atrial fibrillation by itself does not cause heart failure)
- volume overload (e.g. from a rapid blood transfusion or excess intravenous fluid)
- severe anaemia, especially if acute (e.g. from a gastrointestinal bleed)
- hypoxia (e.g. caused by acute exacerbation of COPD)
- infection, especially if a sepsis syndrome is present (septicaemia)
- thyrotoxicosis
- medications (e.g. NSAIDs, glitazones)
- intoxications (e.g. from heroin, barbiturates, etc.)
- nutritional (thiamine deficiency)
- lack of adherence to chronic treatment (this is particularly common)

Typical symptoms of the disease and less common symptoms

Dyspnoea is the most common presenting symptom. Typically, this has been present on effort for some time, and now occurs at rest. However, in a minority of cases, AHF reflects the sudden deterioration of cardiac function (e.g. due to a myocardial infarct, or acute myocarditis). Such patients clearly may be completely well until an hour or two before their acute presentation with respiratory distress. A postural dependence to breathlessness (orthopnoea) is common. A small minority of patients present with symptoms from hypotension or frank shock. With acute coronary syndrome being a major cause for AHF, chest pain is commonly found at presentation. Other common symptoms and findings include cough, haemoptysis, agitation and, in severe cases, drowsiness (due to hypoxia, hypercapnia), and multi-organ failure. Symptoms often resemble those of acute respiratory disorders due to pneumonia and asthma, especially if there is underlying chronic lung disease, and this clearly can pose a diagnostic challenge to clinicians.

Demographics of the disease

Accurate estimates of the prevalence of AHF are not available, partly because of reporting of the underlying causes of this syndrome. European data suggests that AHF accounts for at least 5% of all hospital admissions and complicates the admission of a much larger patient population. With the wide spectrum of the underlying causes, patient demographics are highly heterogeneous, but patients are usually elderly with considerable cardiovascular and non-cardiovascular comorbidities. In one European registry, the mean age of patients admitted to hospital for heart failure was 70 years, and half were women. The majority of people admitted to hospitals with AHF are known to have chronic heart failure and only 15%–20% are incident presentations of heart failure. About 25% of patients are hypertensive at presentation (systolic blood pressure >160 mm Hg) and <10% are hypotensive. Half of AHF patients have a relatively preserved left ventricular systolic function. These patients tend to be older, are more likely to be women, and are more likely to present with severe hypertension and atrial arrhythmias.

Natural history and complications of the disease

The clinical course of AHF is highly variable. On average, people improve rapidly and can be discharged after a short hospital stay (median hospital duration in the US registries is about 5 days). The average hospital mortality rate ranges from a low of 4% (with large regional variations) to up to 20% in the small subgroup of AHF patients who present with hypotension and renal failure (<5% of the AHF population). Those who are discharged from hospital are at substantial risk of readmission and death. Readmission rate is about 30% at 60 to 90 days after discharge, and mortality ranges from 5% to 15%. Post-discharge outcomes seem to be similar for those with preserved and reduced systolic function; however, the epidemiology of the former group is less well described.

Approach to diagnosing the disease

Diagnosis is based on the amalgamation of the presenting symptoms, the physical examination, and simple clinical findings, especially the chest X-ray, and BNP. In essence, to diagnose AHF, the combination of acute breathlessness (or equivalent) with the physical findings of left heart failure (pulmonary oedema), an abnormal ECG, a raised biomarker, and abnormal cardiac substrate is required. Accordingly, a number of investigations can help confirm the diagnosis and identify the underlying cause or precipitant.

Physical findings include the following:

General: General findings are obvious breathlessness with tachypnoea, cyanosis, pallor, sweating, and cold skin (due to sympathetic nervous system activation).

Cardiovascular: Cardiovascular findings are raised jugular venous pressure, tachycardia, gallop rhythm due to a third heard sound, murmurs (functional mitral regurgitation is very common; alternatively, the murmur of any underlying valvar lesion), hepatomegaly, peripheral oedema, and hyper- or hypotension.

Respiratory: Respiratory findings include wheeze, crackles, and pleural effusion.

Chest X-ray: Chest X-ray findings include dilated and prominent upper lobe vessels, alveolar oedema ('bat's wings'), interstitial oedema (Kerley B lines), and pleural effusion with or without cardiomegaly. Isolated right pleural effusion can be due to heart failure, whereas isolated left pleural effusion is not.

ECG: An ECG may show acute ischaemic changes, left ventricular hypertrophy, bradycardia or tachycardia, atrial fibrillation/flutter, ventricular arrhythmias, broad QRS complexes, or signs of pericardial tamponade. A normal ECG makes the diagnosis of heart failure, especially with systolic dysfunction, very unlikely.

Laboratory tests: Patients with AHF should have a full blood count, serum electrolytes, creatinine, glucose, liver function tests, and urine analysis. In people with untreated mild-to-moderate heart failure, marked abnormalities of the blood count or electrolytes are uncommon. However, mild hyponatraemia, hyperkalaemia, and abnormal renal function are commonly encountered. Natriuretic peptides (BNP/NT-pro-BNP) are raised as a biochemical correlate for increased myocardial wall stress and left ventricular filling pressures. Evidence for their use in the acute setting is less established, but average values are usually much higher than in patients with chronic heart failure. Despite their high negative predictive value, they may not be raised in AHF at the time of admission if blood samples are taken immediately after symptom onset (in particular during flash pulmonary oedema or acute mitral regurgitation). Mild elevations of cardiac troponin are common, even in the absence of coronary events or myocarditis. While raised troponin levels are almost always a marker of myocardial tissue damage, they may be difficult to interpret in the context of chronic renal impairment, where mild chronic elevations of troponin levels are common. Here, serial measurements might be useful.

Echocardiography: Echocardiography plays a central role in making the diagnosis. Lack of any evidence for structural or functional heart disease on cardiac ultrasound makes the diagnosis of heart failure extremely unlikely. It allows assessment of heart chamber sizes, left ventricular ejection fraction (LVEF) and regional wall motion abnormalities, diastolic function, myocardial thickness, pericardial effusion, valvular function, and pulmonary arterial pressure. Approximately 50% of AHF patients have a relatively preserved systolic function (LVEF > 45%–50%); there are a number of acronyms for this condition, a common one being heart failure with preserved ejection fraction.

Cardiac MRI may be an alternative to echocardiography in those with poor echocardiographic windows or when characterization of the tissue is particularly important, such as in suspected myocarditis or an infiltrative myocardial disease.

Arterial blood gas analysis: The usual finding is of hypoxaemia with hypocapnia due to hyperventilation; pCO_2 levels may be normal or elevated due to exhaustion (or in less severe cases). Metabolic alkalosis is often a sign of diuretic toxicity.

Other diagnoses that should be considered

AHF is a syndrome, and investigations should include tests for underlying causes. The differential diagnosis includes pulmonary infection, chronic obstructive pulmonary disease or asthma, chest sepsis, pulmonary infiltrative processes, and, very occasionally, fluid overload duet to renal dysfunction. In people presenting with hypotension, alternative causes of shock should be considered (pulmonary emboli being a leading cause). Since multimorbidity is the rule rather than the exception in those with heart failure, the presence of alternative diagnoses usually does not definitely rule out heart failure, and sometimes assessment of response to empiric therapy might be useful.

'Gold-standard' diagnostic test

There is no single gold-standard diagnostic test. However, for a secure diagnosis, appropriate symptoms, a chest X-ray clearly showing pulmonary oedema, raised biomarkers, and a very abnormal cardiac ultrasound secure the diagnosis. The fewer of these features that are present, the less secure is the diagnosis.

Acceptable diagnostic alternatives to the gold standard

Appropriate symptoms responding rapidly to diuretics is sometimes regarded as diagnostic.

Other relevant investigations

Diagnostic investigations include BNP, cardiac ultrasound, and coronary angiography, if proximal/multivessel coronary artery disease is not unlikely; with ST-segment elevation myocardial infarction, angiography should be done immediately; for non-ST-segment elevation myocardial infarction, it should be done once the patient is stabilized. C-reactive protein is valuable in most patients as a pointer to underlying infection.

Investigations to assess the response to therapy, and the 'sickness' of the patient, include ECG monitoring, pulse oximeter measurements, urinary catheterization, arterial line, and central venous line. Daily assessment of patient weight is the most effective method for documenting effective diuresis. Insertion of a pulmonary artery catheter is unnecessary for the diagnosis and management of AHF and can be lethal. Tissue Doppler echocardiography offers an alternative non-invasive means of estimating the pulmonary capillary pressures and left ventricular filling pressures.

Prognosis and how to estimate it

Many scoring systems for the evaluation of the prognosis of patients admitted with AHF exist. The selection of the method will depend on the availability of data for risk estimation and the type of outcome to be predicted. In a US-based study, the strongest independent predictors of inhospital death were higher age, lower systolic blood pressure, and higher blood urea nitrogen levels. Other factors with some predictive value were a higher heart rate, lower blood sodium levels, presence of chronic obstructive pulmonary disease, and non-black race. Interestingly, the predictive value of the model was independent of the left ventricular systolic function. However, the model was based on total mortality, with no information on cause-specific mortality or long-term post discharge outcomes.

Treatment and its effectiveness

Treatment can be divided into three stages: the early stage, the intermediate stage, and the final stage.

Early stage

In the early stage, immediately after presentation, the goal is to achieve haemodynamic stability, relieve symptoms, and restore organ perfusion.

Intermediate stage

The intermediate stage is about identifying the underlying cause of heart failure with targeted intervention. In general, evidence for the immediate management of AHF is mostly empiric, with many recent trials showing disappointing results. Patient should undergo immediate airway and fluid status assessment, and intravenous access should be secured. Fluid removal with loop diuretics, and preload and afterload reduction with vasodilators, are the mainstay of therapy. The intensity and combination of vasodilator and diuretics depends on the patient's haemodynamic status (i.e. blood pressure and degree of fluid overload). In patients with new-onset AHF, an initial dose of furosemide is 40 mg IV, or bumetanide 1 mg IV may suffice. However, patients with chronic oral diuretic dose should be given double or at least equivalent dose to their usual therapy as an IV injection, and those with renal failure or large volume overload are also likely to need higher doses or a continuous infusion. The total dose of furosemide should, however, if possible, remain <120 mg in the first 6 hours, with monitoring of the urinary output. In non-responders, a combination of a loop diuretic with thiazide diuretics (e.g. metolazone 2.5 mg) is preferable to higher doses of loop diuretics alone (to increase response rate and to avoid toxicity). Intravenous glyceryl trinitrate is the most widely used vasodilator. It should be avoided in AHF patients with a systolic blood pressure of <90 mm Hg.

Patients with hypotension and signs of organ hypoperfusion (reduced urinary output, liver dysfunction, somnolence, lactic acidosis) or those with congestion, despite vasodilators and diuretics, may need inotropes. Their use should be kept as brief as possible because of the potential risk of myocardial injury, despite acute improvement in the haemodynamic status. Vasodilating inotropes such as dobutamine, milrinone, and levosimendan are commonly used. Inotropes with a more prominent vasoconstricting effect are less commonly used. Current guidelines give preference to dopamine over alternative vasopressors (noradrenaline and adrenaline), with the recommendation that such agents should be reserved for special circumstances (sepsis and cardiac resuscitation). However, these recommendations have been challenged by recent trial evidence showing no significant difference between dopamine and noradrenaline.

Hypoxic patients should be given oxygen to maintain arterial oxygen saturation >95% (>90% in COPD patients). However, routine use of oxygen in people with normal oxygen saturations should be avoided because of the potential risk of aggravating ischaemia.

Non-invasive ventilation (NIV) may be required for people with respiratory failure (persistent respiratory distress or respiratory acidosis with or without hypoxia). Usual settings are a positive end expiratory pressure of 5–7.5 cm H_2O, with an FiO_2 of ≥40%. However, evidence for the efficacy of NIV is limited. Patients presenting in cardiogenic shock or severe pulmonary oedema may require intubation and mechanical ventilation. Indication for mechanical ventilation (usually more than one factor required) includes:

- exhaustion
- hypoxaemia (oxygen partial pressure <8 kPa, or arterial saturation <93%)
- hypercapnia (oxygen partial pressure >8 kPa)
- acidosis (pH <7.2)
- failure to respond to NIV

A number of new and old pharmacological treatments for AHF exist, with little evidence for their safety and efficacy. Notably, digoxin may have a role for the management of people with AHF and reduced systolic function, even in the absence of atrial fibrillation. In some patients, analgesia and sedation may be required. Intravenous morphine in boluses of 2.5–5.0 mg is usually administrated to patients with severe AHF who present with restlessness, anxiety, or chest pain. Morphine should be combined with antiemetics (e.g. metoclopramide 5–10 mg).

Treatment in the intermediate stage includes treatments for the underlying cause of heart failure, such as antihypertensive medication, rate control, coronary intervention, valve operation, and so on. Ultrafiltration may be used for those with excessive fluid overload and renal impairment. Intra-aortic balloon pump and left ventricular assist devices may be used in more severe cases as bridging or for a short period of time until recovery, although the evidence for their effectiveness is limited.

Final stage

The final pre-discharge stage aims to initiate long-term chronic therapy prior to discharge. The principle underlying chronic heart failure drug therapy is neuroendocrine blockade; in the early days of heart failure treatment, therapy was directed towards increasing the inotropic state of the heart, that is, its contractility. All these drugs (with the exception of digoxin) led to an increase in mortality when used chronically (i.e. they are harmful). Later work clarified that the neuroendocrine activation seen in chronic heart failure (i.e. increases in epinephrine, norepinephrine, and other vasoconstrictors, including endothelin, etc.) was deleterious, and neuroendocrine blockade with angiotensin-converting enzyme (ACE) inhibitors (or angiotensin-receptor blockers), beta blockers, or mineralocorticoid antagonists (spironolactone, eplerenone) improves outcome, especially if these agents are used in combination. Generally, it is recommended that patients with AHF who are already on medication for chronic heart failure should continue with these during the acute admission whenever possible and, if needed, at a reduced dose. Prior to discharge, the patient should have made a successful transition from intravenous to oral medication, with arrangements for early follow-up after discharge. Many patients will have a significant improvement of their symptoms, but acute treatment usually will not completely abolish symptoms. Plans should be in place for long-term intervention with complex pacing devices, such as an implantable cardioverter defibrillator or a cardiac resynchronization therapy device, if appropriate, and for longer-term lifestyle interventions, including exercise.

Further Reading

National Institute for Health and Care Excellence. *Acute Heart Failure: Diagnosis and Management*. Available at https://www.nice.org.uk/guidance/cg187/resources/acute-heart-failure-diagnosis-and-management-35109817738693 (accessed 23 Mar 2017).

The Task Force for the diagnosis and treatment of acute and chronic heart failure of the European Society of Cardiology (ESC). 2016 ESC Guidelines for the diagnosis and treatment of acute and chronic heart failure. *Eur Heart J* 2016; 37: 2129–200.

92 Chronic heart failure

Kazem Rahimi

Definition of the disease

The European Society of Cardiology defines heart failure as a clinical syndrome in which patients have all of the following features (see Table 92.1):

- symptoms typical of heart failure, such as:
  - breathlessness
  - fatigue
  - ankle swelling
- signs typical of heart failure, such as:
  - tachycardia
  - tachypnoea
  - pulmonary crackles
  - pleural effusion
  - raised jugular venous pressure
  - peripheral oedema
  - hepatomegaly
- objective evidence of a structural or functional abnormality of the heart at rest, such as:
  - cardiomegaly
  - third heat sound
  - cardiac murmurs
  - abnormality on the echocardiogram
  - raised natriuretic peptide concentration

Heart failure results in activation of the sympathetic nervous system and the renin–aldosterone–angiotensin system, and release of a number of hormones, such as natriuretic peptides and cytokines, including tumour necrosis factor amongst others. While neurohormone activation is initially compensatory and helps in the short term to maintain circulatory needs, ultimately, it has detrimental effects on the myocardium and compromises its function further. These mechanisms are, therefore, therapeutic targets to improve symptoms and lessen the risk of death.

Aetiology of the disease

Chronic heart failure is a clinical syndrome that is caused by a cardiac pathology, but may be acutely precipitated by a number of cardiac and/or non-cardiac conditions. For specific causes, see Chapter 91, 'Aetiology of the disease'. The major differences between acute and chronic heart failure are in:

Timing: Chronic heart failure is often present for months, whereas acute heart failure progresses rapidly over minutes to hours.

Severity: Acute heart failure causes symptoms at rest, whereas chronic heart failure usually does not.

Manifestation: Acute heart failure largely manifests as left heart failure (pulmonary oedema), whereas chronic heart failure generally manifests as peripheral oedema (right heart failure).

Typical symptoms of the disease, and less common symptoms

Breathlessness, tiredness, and fatigue are characteristic symptoms, but assessment of these, in particular in the elderly, requires skills and experience. Since many patients with chronic heart failure can present with rapidly worsening symptoms, many of the symptoms described in Chapter 91 also apply to chronic heart failure. However, a key difference is that the chronicity of long-standing heart failure leads to the other major complications that of cardiac cachexia, a complex syndrome driven by several pathophysiological mechanisms including cytokine activation (tumour necrosis factor, interleukins, etc.), which leads to muscle loss and, in turn, underlying fatigue and many other symptoms. Visible cachexia is a grim prognostic sign.

Demographics of the disease

Aging populations and the improved survival rates from acute cardiovascular events continue to contribute to a growing prevalence of heart failure in most high-income countries (data from low- and middle-income countries are very limited). In the UK, about 1% of the population suffers from chronic heart failure, but the prevalence increases rapidly with age, affecting about 7% of the population aged 75 years or more. Patient demographics are highly heterogeneous, but patients tend to be elderly with considerable cardiovascular and non-cardiovascular comorbidities, such as coronary artery disease, diabetes, renal dysfunction, depression, cognitive impairment, and respiratory diseases. In one community-based cohort study, the average age of people with heart failure was about 75 years, with similar distributions for men and women. However, women, the elderly, and those with hypertension or diabetes are more likely to have preserved systolic function (ejection fraction > 45%–50%).

Natural history and complications of the disease

Advances in diagnosis and management of heart failure have led to a steady decline in morbidity and mortality during recent years.

Table 92.1 Definition of heart failure with preserved (HFpEF), mid-range (HFmrEF), and reduced ejection fraction (HFrEF)

Type of HF		HFrEF	HFmrEF	HFpEF
CRITERIA	1	Symptoms ± Signs[a]	Symptoms t Signs[a]	Symptoms ± Signs[a]
	2	LVEF <40%	LVEF 40%–49%	LVEF ≥50%

	3	–	1. Elevated levels of nauiuretic peptides[b];
			 2. At least one additional criterion:
			   a. relevant structural heart disease (LVH and/or LAE),
			   b. diastolic dysfunction (for details see Section 4.3.2).
				1. Elevated levels of natriuretic peptides[b];
				 2. At least one additional criterion:
				   a. relevant structural heart disease (LVH and/or LAE),
				   b. diastolic dysfunction (for details see Section 4.3.2).

Abbreviations: BNP, brain natriuretic peptide; HF, heart failure; HFmrEF, heart failure with mid-range ejection fraction; HFpEF, heart failure with preserved ejection fraction; HFrEF, heart failure with reduced ejection fraction; LAE, left atrial enlargement; LVEF, left ventricular ejection fraction; LVH, left ventricular hypertrophy; NT-pro-BNP, N-terminal brain natriuretic peptide.
[a]Signs may not be present in the early stages of HF (especially in HFpEF) and in patients treated with diuretics.
[b]BNP >35 pg/ml and/or NT-pro-BNP >125 pg/ml.

Reproduced with permission from Piotr Ponikowski et al., 2016 ESC Guidelines for the diagnosis and treatment of acute and chronic heart failure, *European Heart Journal*, May 2015, ehw128; DOI: 10.1093/eurheartj/ehw128 Copyright © 2015 Oxford University Press.

However, patients with heart failure remain at substantial risk of adverse outcomes; these include:

Death: Overall, 50% of patients are dead at 4 years, which makes heart failure much worse than many other serious illnesses, such as breast or colon cancer. Death may occur from progressive heart failure, arrhythmias, or complications of the underlying illness (e.g. further myocardial infarction).

Recurrent hospitalization: This can be from exacerbations of heart failure, arrhythmias, or the more general health impacts. Heart failure is a debilitating condition that has profound implications for the individuals who are affected by it, in terms of life expectancy and quality of life. In addition, heart failure is associated with a substantially increased risk of recurrent admissions to hospitals, putting a heavy burden on health services.

Poor quality of life: This is partly from the heart failure itself, which leads to disabling breathlessness, fatigue, and loss of muscle; but it is also the result of how heart failure interacts with the other diseases which are often associated with it, such as COPD; immobility (and so breathlessness, from physical deconditioning)

from severe arthritis; obesity; and cerebrovascular disease, particularly dementia.

Approach to diagnosing the disease

The approach to diagnosis of chronic heart failure involves a two-stage process. The goal of the first stage is to confirm or refute heart failure. Once diagnosis has been established, further investigations are required to elicit the underlying cause of the heart failure.

The European Society of Cardiology proposes an algorithm for the diagnosis of chronic heart failure, acknowledging that most of its recommendations are based on expert opinion (Figure 92.1). Components of the algorithm are clinical examination, ECG, chest X-ray, echocardiography, and measurement of blood levels of natriuretic peptides (e.g. BNP or NT-pro-BNP). The order or combination of tests depends on local accessibility and costs.

Echocardiography is usually the most useful method for evaluating systolic and diastolic dysfunction. It also can identify or narrow possible underlying cause of chronic heart failure. A completely normal

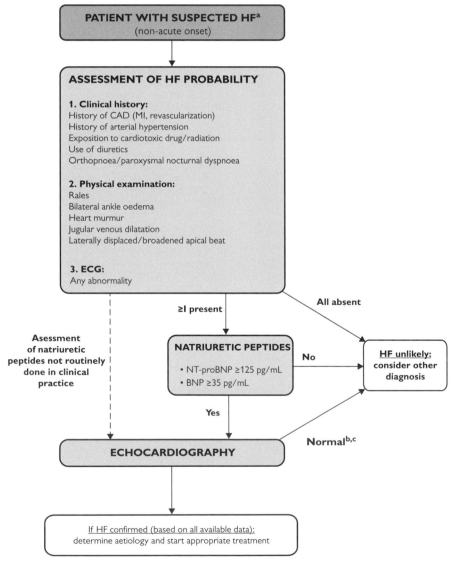

Figure 92.1 Diagnostic algorithm for a diagnosis of heart failure of non-acute onset; BNP, B-type natriuretic peptide; CAD, coronary artery disease; HF, heart failure; MI, myocardial infarction; NT-proBNP, N-terminal pro-B type natriuretic peptide; [a]patient reporting symptoms typical of HF; [b]normal ventricular and atrial volumes and function; [c]consider other causes of elevated natriuretic peptides.

Reproduced with permission from Piotr Ponikowski et al., 2016 ESC Guidelines for the diagnosis and treatment of acute and chronic heart failure, *European Heart Journal*, May 2015, ehw128; DOI: 10.1093/eurheartj/ehw128 Copyright © 2015 Oxford University Press.

ECG makes chronic heart failure, in particular with systolic dysfunction, very unlikely (<10%). Chest X-ray allows assessment of pulmonary congestion and may demonstrate important pulmonary or thoracic causes of dyspnoea. Plasma concentrations of natriuretic peptides can help in establishing the diagnosis and may provide additional useful information for staging and guiding further management.

Other diagnoses that should be considered

The differential diagnosis includes pulmonary infection, COPD, or asthma and restrictive lung disease (e.g. caused by obesity); renal dysfunction and other causes of oedematous states such as chronic venous thromboembolism; and liver cirrhosis. Immobility and obesity by themselves can lead to profound peripheral oedema. Calcium channel blockers likewise underlie some oedematous states. Often, however, many of these other diseases/conditions coexist, and it can be difficult to determine how many of the symptoms are from heart failure and how many from the comorbidities, including depression and physical deconditioning, which themselves are therapeutic targets

'Gold-standard' diagnostic test

The confirmation of the diagnosis of chronic heart failure requires both clinical and objective evidence. While no gold standard exists, the triad of appropriate symptoms plus a raised biomarker (e.g. BNP) and a sufficiently abnormal echocardiography is commonly considered to meet diagnostic criteria.

Acceptable diagnostic alternatives to the gold standard

A suggestive clinical situation, with raised biomarkers but relatively normal cardiac ultrasound, may be acceptable (e.g. in the case of heart failure with preserved ejection fraction). For screening in primary care, the tactic is to exclude heart failure, by ECG and BNP; heart failure is very unlikely here and so echocardiography is not justified, unless either or both of these tests are abnormal, in which case echocardiography with or without specialist evaluation is appropriate.

Other relevant investigations

Other relevant investigations include:

Tests to investigate for myocardial ischaemia: All patients require ischaemia risk evaluation (this is done using the pretest probability; see Chapter 89). Given the typical demographics of heart failure, most patients require tests evaluating ischaemia (e.g. nuclear myocardial perfusion scans and/or coronary angiography. If severe, proximal, multivessel coronary disease is found, then tests for hibernating myocardium (viable heart muscle whose function improves after revascularization) are indicated; there are no perfect tests for hibernation, but nuclear isotope scanning (SPECT) using either technetium-99m or thallium, or, better still, 18F-labelled glucose analogues, imaged using PET, may be helpful. Cardiac MRI also has a role.

Tests to evaluate arrhythmia risk and presence: Arrhythmia risk is evaluated mainly by estimation of ejection fraction, and arrhythmia presence from symptoms, office ECGs, and 24-hour ECGs. Occasionally, implantable reveal devices are used.

Right heart catheterization: This is not uncommonly used, mainly to investigate the degree and site of pulmonary hypertension, but also to diagnose pericardial constriction and intracardiac shunts.

Cardiac MRI: This is used, independently of its role in evaluating hibernation, mainly to very accurately assess ventricular function (especially when there are poor echocardiographic windows), to diagnose subtle changes (e.g. right ventricular cardiomyopathy), to understand the pattern and mechanism of left ventricular hypertrophy further, and to distinguish cardiomyopathy from infarction.

Transoesophageal echocardiography: This may have some incremental value over transthoracic echocardiography (e.g. in people with inadequate transthoracic echocardiographic windows) and allows a more accurate assessment of valve dysfunction and morphology.

Exercise testing: Exercise testing, with or without measurement of gas exchange, is very useful in documenting exercise capacity and physical fitness, as some patients complain bitterly of symptoms which objective testing fails to confirm. It is also useful in evaluating whether exercise-induced arrhythmias, particularly ventricular arrhythmias, are present.

Pulmonary function tests: These are indicated to exclude lung disease and follow up patients on amiodarone.

Holter ECG: This is indicated as part of an arrhythmia workup, especially in hypertrophic cardiomyopathy.

Myocardial biopsy: This is usually only used when amyloid heart disease is under consideration.

Genetic testing: This may also be useful to gain further insight into causes of heart failure and to better plan further management.

Prognosis and how to estimate it

As a chronic condition, heart failure affects patients' quality of life and reduces their life expectancy. Several statistical tools for prediction of risk of death and readmissions have been reported. Most prognostic scores are based on readily available data such as age, severity of symptoms, ejection fraction, heart rate, blood pressure, BNP levels, and renal function. On average, patients are at high risk of death and hospitalization soon after the initial diagnosis, and about 50% of patients will die within four years of the initial diagnosis.

Treatment and its effectiveness

The goals of treatment are symptom relief, avoidance of hospitalization, and the prevention of premature death. Treatment of acute heart failure is described in Chapter 91. Pharmacological treatment is the cornerstone of heart failure in patients with left ventricular systolic function (evidence for effective therapy in patients with preserved systolic function is limited). Pharmacological treatment should be complemented by other measures, including lifestyle changes concentrating on physical fitness and ideal weight. In selected patients, device therapy and surgery have a role.

Therapy for systolic dysfunction

Therapy for patients with systolic dysfunction (left ventricular ejection fraction < 40%) includes the following:

Angiotensin-converting-enzyme (ACE) inhibitors: Use of ACE inhibitors is the first-line therapy in people with systolic heart failure. ACE inhibitors have been shown to be highly effective in reducing mortality (up to 40% relative risk reduction), have modest positive effects on quality of life, and reduce hospital admission due to worsening heart failure. Potential adverse effects include cough, worsening renal function, hyperkalaemia, and symptomatic hypotension. A certain rise in blood creatinine levels (up of 50% from baseline or about 250 μmol/l) is expected after the initiation of ACE-inhibitor use and is not an indication for treatment withdrawal.

Angiotensin-receptor blockers (ARBs): The efficacy of ARBs is similar to that of ACE inhibitors; however, because of higher costs, the use of ARBs is usually limited to patients intolerant of ACE inhibitors because of cough. ARBs can be used concomitantly with ACE inhibitors in patients who remain symptomatic despite optimal therapy with ACE inhibitors and beta blockers and who are unable to tolerate aldosterone antagonists.

Beta blockers: Beta blockers are also first-line therapy, together with ACE inhibitors, in patients with systolic dysfunction, regardless of the underlying cause. Treatment with beta blockers reduces mortality by about a third, improves symptoms, and prevents hospitalization. Beta blockers may need to be withdrawn in people presenting with severe systemic hypoperfusion, but many people admitted to hospital with heart failure can continue with a smaller dose of their usual beta-blocker therapy and it should be initiated in cautiously in people with no beta-blocker therapy at the time of admission to hospital. Unlike asthma, COPD is not a contraindication to beta-blocker use. The use of beta blockers should be avoided in people with high-degree heart block in the absence of a permanent pacemaker. Many patients with systolic heart failure have chronic asymptomatic hypotension; beta blockers should not be withheld in these patients.

Aldosterone antagonists: Aldosterone antagonists are recommended in all patients who have severe systolic heart failure (ejection fraction ≤ 30%) but remain symptomatic (New York Heart Association (NYHA) Class II or IV) despite treatment with a diuretic, an ACE inhibitor (or ARB), and a beta blocker. However, triple therapy consisting of an ACE inhibitor, an ARB, and an aldosterone antagonist should be avoided because of the risk of renal dysfunction and hyperkalaemia. Breast tenderness and/or enlargement can occur with spironolactone treatment. In such cases, spironolactone should be replaced by eplerenone.

Hydralazine and isosorbide dinitrate (H-ISDN): In symptomatic patients, H-ISDN may be used as an alternative to ACE inhibitors or ARBs (e.g. because of intolerance), or in addition to them, if patients remain symptomatic despite treatment with an ACE inhibitor, a beta blocker, and an ARB or an aldosterone antagonist. The most common side effects of H-ISDN are headache, dizziness, and nausea. Arthralgia is less common (about 10%).

Sacubitril-valsartan: The combination of an angiotensin-receptor blocker and neprilysin inhibitor (ARNI), sacubitril-valsartan, can be used in place of an ACE-inhibitor or ARB in patients with heart failure due to LV systolic dysfunction (ejection fraction 35% or less) who remain symptomatic (in NYHA classes II-IV) despite a stable dose of one or other of these therapies. Adverse effects of sacubitril-valsartan include hypotension, hyperkalaemia, and renal failure.

Diuretics: Diuretics can provide rapid relief of dyspnoea and fluid retention. The lowest dose needed to achieve the dry weight is used. In severe cases of fluid retention, a loop diuretic may need to be combined with other classes of diuretics under close monitoring of blood electrolytes. Diuretics should be reduced in dose and, if possible, withdrawn in people without evidence of fluid retention, to avoid renal dysfunction and dehydration.

Other medications: Digoxin is usually recommended in patients with symptomatic heart failure or in those with fast atrial fibrillation. Digoxin has been shown to improve symptoms and to reduce hospital admission for worsening heart failure, but there is no evidence to suggest that digoxin has an impact on survival. It can be prescribed in addition to a beta blocker. Unlike studies in the general population, there is no evidence that antiplatelet agents and statins reduce cardiovascular events in people with heart failure.

Implantable cardioverter defibrillators (ICDs): ICDs are recommended for patients who survive an unprovoked episode of ventricular fibrillation or sustained ventricular arrhythmia, and for primary prevention in people who have been identified as NYHA Class II or III, have an ejection fraction that is persistently 35% or less despite optimal medical therapy, and who are expected to survive for at least 1 year with a reasonable quality of life.

Cardiac resynchronization therapy (CRT): CRT can improve quality of life and reduce admissions to hospital by achieving a more synchronous contraction of the left ventricle. Current European Society of Cardiology guidelines recommend CRT (Class I indication) for symptomatic patients with heart failure in sinus rhythm with a QRS duration >130 ms, and LBBB morphology, and a LVEF <35% despite optimum medical therapy; CRT should be considered (Class IIa) for those with QRS duration >150 ms and non- LBBB morphology. Patients in permanent atrial fibrillation can also benefit from CRT, but in this group, it may be necessary to ablate the AV node to ensure biventricular pacing occurs most of the time. Most patients for whom CRT is indicated also qualify for an ICD. An ICD component can be added to CRT by using a right ventricular ICD lead and a CRT defibrillator generator (CRT-D) instead of a standard CRT pacemaker (CRT-P). However, the additional benefit of CRT- D over CRT- P is uncertain, and the best choice of device for the individual patient is the subject of current research. Cardiac device therapy is discussed in chapter 121.

Other interventions: The role of other interventions, such as coronary revascularization, cardiac transplantation, and left ventricular assist devices, is less straightforward and often requires a case-by-case decision. Lifestyle modifications, such as restriction of sodium intake, are often recommended, but with little evidence for their effectiveness. Aerobic physical activity, however, can improve functional capacity and quality of life, based on limited trial evidence.

Disease management strategies: Disease management strategies, such as patient education and nurse-led monitoring, can be effective, but the optimal content of such programmes is uncertain and is likely to depend on the availability of resources at the local level. Palliative care for patients with refractory symptoms despite optimal medical therapy is recommended.

Therapy for preserved left ventricular ejection fraction

No specific treatment has been shown equivocally to reduce morbidity and mortality in patients with preserved left ventricular ejection fraction (left ventricular ejection fraction ≥ 40%). Diuretics are commonly used for symptom control. There is some evidence to suggest that verapamil and nebivolol may have beneficial effects in this patient population. In clinical practice, treatment is commonly targeted at the underlying causes of heart failure, such as hypertension or atrial fibrillation.

Further Reading

Metra M and Teerlink JR. Heart failure. *Lancet* 2017; 390: 1981–95.

The Task Force for the diagnosis and treatment of acute and chronic heart failure of the European Society of Cardiology (ESC). 2016 ESC Guidelines for the diagnosis and treatment of acute and chronic heart failure. *Eur Heart J* 2016; 37: 2129–200.

Yancy CW, Jessup M, Bozkurt B, et al. ACC/AHA/HFSA focused update of the 2013 ACCF/AHA guideline for the management of heart failure: a report of the American College of Cardiology/American Heart Association Task Force on Clinical Practice Guidelines and the Heart Failure Society of America. *Circulation* 2017; 136: e137–e161.

93 Aortic stenosis

Patrick Davey and Jim Newton

Definition of the disease

Aortic stenosis is characterized by thickening and reduced mobility of the aortic valve leaflets and results in restriction to the blood flow from the left ventricle to the aorta, and secondary left ventricular hypertrophy (Figure 93.1).

Symptoms

A normal trileaflet aortic valve opens to an orifice area of 3 cm². Symptoms do not usually develop until the valve area is <1.0 cm², although they may occur earlier in the presence of common comorbidities, such as coronary artery disease (found in 25%–50% of patients with moderate or severe aortic stenosis). Stenotic valves with an orifice area <1 cm² allow sufficient cardiac output at rest, but do not allow normal arterial perfusion during exercise.

Exertional breathlessness is typically the first symptom, followed by effort angina. Syncope on exertion is an ominous symptom. Sudden death is a rare presentation of asymptomatic aortic stenosis, but becomes more prevalent as symptoms occur and the left ventricle fails.

The valve area and symptoms in aortic stenosis are given in Table 93.1.

Demographics and aetiology of aortic stenosis

The commonest cause of aortic stenosis is calcific degeneration of a structurally normal trileaflet valve. This is a disease process similar to atherosclerosis and is associated with hyperlipidaemia, diabetes, renal failure, and increasing age. Early inflammation due to endothelial damage leads to lipid deposition, which promotes fibrosis and calcification. Patients usually present around the seventh decade of life

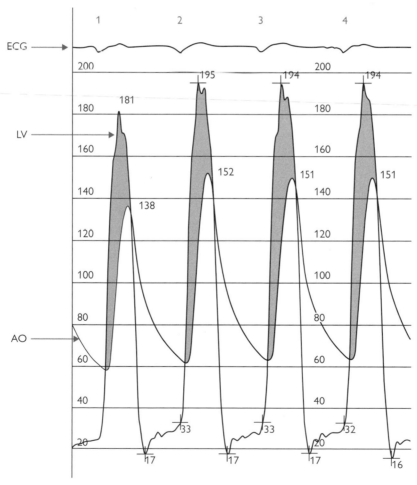

Figure 93.1 Simultaneous measurement of the pressure in the left ventricle (LV) and that in the aortic root (AO), with the classic finding of aortic stenosis shown as the difference in pressure between the two in systole (normal individuals should have no pressure drop between the left ventricle and the aortic root in systole).

Table 93.1 Valve area and symptoms in aortic stenosis

Classification	Symptoms	Valve area	Peak pressure drop (mm Hg)
Normal	–	>3.0 cm²	0–10
Mild aortic stenosis	–	1.5–2.0 cm²	10–40
Moderate aortic stenosis	– (+ if comorbidities)	1.0–1.5 cm²	40–60
Severe aortic stenosis	++	<1.0 cm²	>60
Critical aortic stenosis	+++	<0.8 cm²	> 80

Note: The insidious onset of symptoms can be difficult to elicit in the elderly, as they reduce their daily activities to compensate; formal assessment of their exercise capacity may prove very useful.

and, overall, it is the most common form of valvular heart disease in the Western world.

Up to 2% of the population are born with a bicuspid aortic valve. Although not stenotic at birth, altered flow dynamics and shear stress promote premature leaflet degeneration, and patients present with stenosis around the fifth decade of life. Important associations include Turner's syndrome, aortic coarctation, and aortic root dilation. The latter is due to both altered post-stenosis flow and abnormal collagen with the aortic media; 10% of cases are genetic and related to NOTCH1 gene mutations.

Rheumatic fever can affect the aortic valve as well as the mitral valve, with a similar process involving leaflet thickening and commissural fusion, and subsequently significant stenosis, usually when the patient is in the third to fifth decades of life.

Natural history of the disease

Aortic stenosis is a slowly progressive disease with a long asymptomatic phase, as cardiac output is maintained by secondary left ventricular hypertrophy. The valve orifice area reduces by a mean of 0.12 cm²/year, and the pressure drop across the stenotic valve increases by 4–6 mm Hg per year—therefore it takes around 10 years to progress from mild to severe stenosis. Symptoms usually develop insidiously, although some patients present in established heart failure or with sudden syncope.

Complications of aortic stenosis

The principle complication of aortic stenosis is left ventricular failure occurring when the ventricle can no longer overcome the afterload, leading to myocyte apoptosis and fibrosis.

Patients with aortic stenosis are also at risk of:

- atrial fibrillation (can prompt sudden deterioration)
- atrioventricular conduction disease (due to calcific infiltration)
- infective endocarditis
- myocardial infarction (even with normal coronary arteries)
- sudden death (higher risk if symptoms or left ventricle dysfunction)
- Heyde's syndrome (colonic angiodsyplasia and coagulation factor destruction)

Approach to diagnosing the disease (including diagnostic pitfalls)

The diagnosis should be suspected in patients with either typical symptoms or murmur, or both. The physical examination is usually diagnostic, and the most common signs are:

- a loud ejection systolic murmur heard at the base of the heart and radiating to the aortic area and carotids; the loudness of the murmur correlates with severity if left ventricular function is normal
- decreased intensity of the second heart sound (aortic valve closure) due to reduced valve compliance
- a slow-rising arterial pulse (may also be found in elderly patients with stiff vasculature)

The left ventricle hypertrophies in response to stenosis and usually leads to typical ECG changes with increased voltages and lateral T-wave inversion. These changes may regress as the ventricle develops fibrosis and fails later in the disease. However a normal ECG is unusual in severe aortic stenosis.

Clinical examination is accurate in the majority of patients, but can be unreliable in patients with poor ventricular function and insufficient forward flow to generate an obvious murmur.

Other diagnoses that should be considered

The symptoms of effort dyspnoea, angina, or syncope have a broad differential diagnosis (see Table 93.2).

The murmur of aortic stenosis can be confused with other murmurs, usually those arising from the left ventricular outflow tract:

Innocent flow murmur: This is usually less intense and with a normal second heart sound and pulse character.
Hypertrophic obstructive cardiomyopathy: In this case, the murmur arises from the anterior mitral valve leaflet encroaching on the left ventricular outflow tract during systole. The murmur is more prominent in late systole, and the second heart sound is usually normal. An additional clue is that, during squatting, there is a reduction in the murmur, which increases immediately afterwards. Additional mitral regurgitation due to mitral valve distortion is common.
Subvalvar stenosis: This is due to a congenital membrane located below the aortic valve and which obstructs left ventricular outflow; it is rare and typically presents in childhood.
Eccentric mitral regurgitation: Eccentric mitral regurgitation can be directed onto the underside of the aortic root and mimic the radiation of aortic stenosis. However, the murmur is pansystolic, the quality of the carotid pulse is normal, and the second heart sound is preserved.

'Gold-standard' diagnostic test

The gold-standard test for aortic stenosis is invasive confirmation of a pressure difference between the left ventricle and the aortic root. This is achieved by passing a catheter retrogradely across the aortic valve into the left ventricle; the catheter is then withdrawn while recording pressure. The aortic valve area can be derived from the pressure drop across the valve. This test is rarely performed, as echocardiography is usually sufficient, and crossing a stenotic aortic valve carries a risk of provoking systemic emboli and stroke. The measurement of aortic root pressure is influenced by blood pressure and can underestimate the true pressure drop. It is now only used when the cardiac ultrasound is non-diagnostic, or has produced discordant data.

Acceptable diagnostic alternatives to the gold standard

Standard transthoracic echocardiography is diagnostic in the majority of cases. The structure of the aortic valve, the degree of calcification, and the degree of valve thickening are assessed with 2D imaging. Doppler echocardiography allows measurement of the velocity of blood in the left ventricular outflow tract and across the stenosis; from this measurement, the valve orifice area can be derived. In addition, the degree of adaptive left ventricular hypertrophy can be quantified, as can both systolic and diastolic function. Additional valve disease, such as mitral regurgitation, can be identified or excluded.

Table 93.2 Symptoms of effort dyspnoea, angina, or syncope

	Effort breathlessness	Effort angina	Effort syncope
In the young	Asthma	Syndrome X	Vasomotor (usually post-effort)
		Pulmonary hypertension	Pulmonary hypertension
In the middle-aged or elderly	COPD	Coronary disease	Arrhythmias; usually ventricular tachycardia, or supraventricular tachycardia + poor left ventricular function
	Heart failure from any other cause		
	Anaemia		
	Physical deconditioning		

The velocity of blood flow across the stenotic orifice is related not only to the degree of stenosis but also to the stroke volume and the force of ventricular contraction. In patients with a low stroke volume—due either to small body size, or poor ventricular function—the pressure drop measured by echocardiography may not be in the severe category even if severe aortic stenosis is present. This can be overcome by increasing the stroke volume by peripheral infusion of dobutamine and reassessing the Doppler data as stroke volume is normalized. An alternative scenario is when the valve appears to open poorly and severe stenosis is suspected but, when the stroke volume is improved, the increased force of flow opens the valve and non-severe aortic stenosis is confirmed—so-called pseudo-severe stenosis, where poor left ventricular function is the main issue.

Other relevant investigations

The similarity of the pathophysiology of aortic stenosis to that of atherosclerosis warrants an assessment of atherosclerosis risk factors in all patients, although interventions with statins and antihypertensives have not yet been shown to influence disease progression.

Many patients will claim to be asymptomatic, but in reality have reduced their physical activity in response to early symptoms. In such patients, exercise treadmill testing can be used to quantify effort capacity, heart rate, and blood pressure response to exertion and symptoms. Such testing is safe in severe aortic stenosis, if there are no unstable symptoms or heart failure.

In patients proceeding to surgical aortic valve replacement, coronary angiography is performed in almost all cases, to exclude significant coronary disease warranting concomitant coronary artery bypass grafting.

Plasma brain natriuretic peptide (BNP) can be measured in patients where symptoms are of uncertain aetiology, such as in patients with multiple comorbidities. A normal BNP should prompt screening for an alternative cause of dyspnoea.

If transthoracic imaging is insufficient, then the following alternative imaging investigations may be performed:

Transoesophageal echocardiography: This provides improved visualization of valve anatomy and disease but limited accuracy of Doppler assessment.
Computed tomography: This can identify valve anatomy and degree of calcification but cannot measure flow or easily assess left ventricular function.
Cardiac MRI: This can assess valve anatomy but not calcification, and is accurate for flow assessment and quantification of ventricular function.

Prognosis and how to estimate it

The prognosis is related to symptoms. Asymptomatic patients have a good prognosis with a low risk of sudden death or major complications. Patients with effort dyspnoea survive on average for 5 years without intervention; those with angina, only 3 years. Heart failure is an ominous symptom, with death by 12 months without definitive intervention. Prognosis after successful intervention is primarily related to the patient's age and additional comorbidities.

Treatment and its effectiveness

Patients who are genuinely asymptomatic and have normal left ventricular function can be reviewed intermittently after education on general cardiac health, the need to promptly report symptoms, and advice on reducing the risk of endocarditis. No medical therapy has yet been shown to influence disease progression.

Patients with symptoms and severe aortic stenosis must be referred for surgical aortic valve replacement, if this can be performed at acceptable risk. Even patients in their eighties can safely undergo aortic valve replacement if there are minimal comorbidities and good left ventricular function, although the recovery time will be prolonged. The overall operative death risk is 2%–4%, and patients afterwards return to a normal, age-matched life expectancy.

Patients with symptomatic, severe aortic stenosis and who are at high risk for surgical aortic valve replacement should be considered for transcatheter aortic valve implantation. The minimally invasive nature of the procedure promotes more rapid recovery, as formal sternotomy is avoided, although the procedural risks are similar to those for surgical valve replacement. Outcomes are excellent in selected patients with appropriate anatomy, compared to those for medical therapy or high-risk surgical valve replacement.

Balloon valvuloplasty can be performed as rescue therapy in patients with severe aortic stenosis, poor left ventricular function, and heart failure, if definitive intervention is likely to be feasible if cardiac function recovers.

Further Reading

Nishimura RA, Otto CM, Bonow RO, et al. 2017 AHA/ACC focused update of the 2014 AHA/ACC guideline for the management of patients with valvular heart disease: a report of the American College of Cardiology/American Heart Association Task Force on Clinical Practice Guidelines. *Circulation* 2017. doi:10.1161/CIR.0000000000000503.

Otto CM and Prendergast B. Aortic-valve stenosis: From patients at risk to severe valve obstruction. *N Engl J Med* 2014; 371: 744–56.

CHAPTER 93 **Aortic stenosis**

94 Aortic regurgitation

Kazem Rahimi

Definition of the disease

Aortic regurgitation is the diastolic reflux of blood from the aorta into the left ventricle, across the aortic valve.

Aetiology of the disease

Aortic regurgitation can be caused by either damage to or dysfunction of the aortic valve leaflets or as a consequence of distortion or dilatation of the aortic root.

Disorders of the aortic valve leaflets

The following are disorders of the aortic valve leaflets:

- rheumatic heart disease
- infective endocarditis
- degenerative valve disease
- traumatic or iatrogenic leaflet rupture or paravalvular damage
- congenital abnormalities (e.g. bicuspid aortic valve, subarterial ventricular septal defect, subaortic stenosis)
- rheumatoid arthritis
- SLE (Libman–Sacks endocarditis)

Disorders of the aortic root

The following are disorders of the aortic root:

- aortic root dilatation (e.g. from Marfan syndrome, osteogenesis imperfecta, syphilis, ankylosing spondylitis, Reiter's syndrome)
- proximal aortic dissection
- systemic hypertension

Primary disorders of the aortic valve leaflets are falling in incidence. In developed countries, aortic regurgitation due to root pathology now accounts for >50% of cases in those undergoing surgery. Acute aortic regurgitation is usually caused by infective endocarditis or aortic dissection.

Typical symptoms of the disease, and less common symptoms

Chronic aortic regurgitation may remain asymptomatic for decades, owing to compensatory enlargement of the left ventricle. During this phase, patients may only report awareness of a pounding heart as a result of the increased left ventricular stoke volume. Failure of the heart's compensatory mechanisms over time leads to the development of dyspnoea and fatigue. Patients may also report palpitations (due to sinus tachycardia or extrasystoles) and non-specific chest discomfort. Typical angina is rare and is likely to reflect concomitant coronary artery disease.

Acute aortic regurgitation usually presents with acute severe dyspnoea due to pulmonary oedema.

Demographics of the disease

The prevalence of aortic regurgitation depends on age and the severity of the condition. Aortic regurgitation of any degree (even trace aortic regurgitation) is uncommon before age 50. In a population-based cohort of the Framingham Heart Study, the prevalence of moderate-to-severe aortic regurgitation was 0.5%, 0.6%, and 2.2% in men at ages 50–59, 60–69, and 70–83, respectively. The corresponding rates in women were 0.2%, 0.8%, and 2.3%.

Natural history, and complications of the disease

The prognosis of chronic aortic regurgitation is highly dependent on the presence of symptoms. The average annual rate of onset of symptoms is <6% in chronic asymptomatic patients. This may be somewhat higher in those with aortic root dilatation or bicuspid aortic valve. Without valve replacement, symptomatic patients are at substantial risk of death.

Approach to diagnosing the disease

The physical examination of patients with chronic severe aortic regurgitation is usually abnormal and establishes the diagnosis. The increased stroke volume results in abrupt distension of the peripheral arteries and an elevation in systolic blood pressure. Reflux of blood into the left ventricle then leads to a rapid fall in pressure, with quick collapse of the arteries and a low diastolic blood pressure, which may approach zero in severe disease. The net effect is a wide pulse pressure, which is manifested on examination as a 'water hammer' or Corrigan pulse. A number of eponymous signs related to the wide pulse pressure have been described.

The apex beat in chronic aortic regurgitation is laterally displaced and hyperdynamic. A high-pitched decrescendo diastolic murmur is usually present but can easily be missed unless the patient is examined sitting forward with breath held in end-expiration. In very severe regurgitation with ventricular decompensation, the murmur may become soft or even absent. While the intensity of the murmur does not correlate well with the severity of aortic regurgitation, its timing and duration may be useful for grading the severity. An early onset of the murmur with extension through most of the diastole suggests severe aortic regurgitation.

While the ECG and chest radiograph are usually abnormal in patients with severe aortic regurgitation, definitive diagnosis is achieved with echocardiography. Echocardiography allows assessment of aortic valve leaflet and aortic root structure, severity of aortic regurgitation, left ventricular size and function, and the presence of any other cardiac abnormalities. Serial measurements can be useful for evaluation of changes that may occur over time. The severity of aortic regurgitation is classified according to a combination of echocardiographic measures (see Table 94.1).

Transoesophageal echocardiography (TOE) affords better views of the valve and, in particular, of the aortic root. Real-time 3D TOE or cardiac MRI can be of further assistance in difficult cases. Cardiac catheterization is rarely required, although coronary angiography is usually performed in patients being considered for surgical treatment.

Since onset and progression of symptoms is usually gradual, patients may be sedentary and feel relatively asymptomatic. In such cases, exercise testing may be useful to assess effort tolerance.

Other diagnoses that should be considered

The bounding pulse and wide pulse pressure (without a diastolic murmur) may accompany other conditions, such as thyrotoxicosis, fever, anaemia, pregnancy, patent ductus arteriosus, liver cirrhosis, Paget's disease of the bone, multiple arteriovenous fistulae, and, in elderly patients, systolic hypertension due to increased stiffness of the aorta and major arteries.

Table 94.1 Echocardiographic measures used to classify the severity of aortic regurgitation

| | Severity | | |
	Mild	Moderate	Severe
Vena contracta*	<0.3 cm	0.3–0.6 cm	>0.6 cm
Jet width in LVOT	<25% LVOT	25–65% LVOT	>65% LVOT
Descending aorta flow	Brief early diastolic flow	–	Holosystolic flow reversal
Pressure half time^	>500 ms	500–200 ms	<200 ms
Regurgitant volume	<30 ml	30–60 ml	>60 ml
Left ventricle size#	Normal		Moderate or severe dilatation with no other cause

*May be unreliable if jet is not circular.

^ In chronic aortic regurgitation, equalization of pressure across the valve may lead to underestimation of aortic regurgitation severity.

#In acute aortic regurgitation, ventricle size is usually normal.

Note that the more abnormal the valve morphology, the broader the regurgitant jet on colour flow, and the louder the regurgitant Doppler signal, the more severe the regurgitation.

Abbreviations: LVOT, left ventricular outflow tract.

Reproduced with permission from Patrizio Lancellotti et al., European Association of Echocardiography recommendations for the assessment of valvular regurgitation. Part 1: aortic and pulmonary regurgitation (native valve disease), *European Heart Journal*, Volume 11, pp.223-244, Copyright © 2010 Oxford University Press.

Table 94.2 The prognosis of patients with aortic regurgitation

	Prognosis (% per year)
Asymptomatic	
Preserved LV systolic function, LVESD <40 mm	0*
Preserved LV systolic function, LVESD 40–50 mm	6*
Preserved LV systolic function, LVESD >50 mm	19*
Impaired LV systolic function	>25†
Symptomatic	
NYHA Class II	6‡
NYHA Class III/IV	>25‡

* Progression to symptoms, LV dysfunction, or death.

† Progression to symptoms.

‡ Mortality.

Abbreviations: LV, left ventricular; LVESD, left ventricular end-systolic diameter; NYHA, New York Heart Association.

Data from The Joint Task Force on the Management of Valvular Heart Disease of the European Society of Cardiology (ESC) and the European Association for Cardio-Thoracic Surgery (EACTS), Guidelines on the management of valvular heart disease (version 2012), *European Heart Journal*, volume 33, pp.2451-2496 Copyright © 2012 Oxford University Press.

'Gold-standard' diagnostic test

Echocardiography confirms the diagnosis.

Acceptable diagnostic alternatives to the gold standard

Cardiac MRI and invasive aortography may be useful in quantifying the degree of aortic regurgitation when clinical and echocardiographic findings are discordant.

Other relevant investigations

Blood BNP and NT-pro-BNP levels show some correlation with severity of aortic regurgitation and presence of symptoms, and they may play a role for the assessment of progression of the disease.

Prognosis and how to estimate it

The prognosis of patients with aortic regurgitation is determined largely by symptom status and by left ventricular size and function (see Table 94.2).

More recent data suggest that quantification of aortic regurgitation fraction measured by cardiac MRI may be better at discrimination of clinical deterioration. Patients with a regurgitant fraction of >33% are highly likely to progress to surgery within <3 years.

Treatment and its effectiveness

Asymptomatic patients with mild or moderate chronic aortic regurgitation do not require treatment unless there is coexistent systemic hypertension. Asymptomatic patients with severe aortic regurgitation or progressive ventricular enlargement may benefit from vasodilator therapy (angiotensin-converting enzyme (ACE) inhibitors, hydralazine, or nifedipine), although supportive evidence is limited.

Diuretics may palliate symptoms, but should not be used to defer the need for valve surgery. Beta blockers are relatively contraindicated on theoretical grounds because their prolongation of diastole leads to an increased regurgitant volume. Asymptomatic patients require frequent clinical review to assess for symptoms, progression of aortic regurgitation, and left ventricular size and function. The frequency of follow-up depends on the cause of aortic regurgitation and its severity, and varies from every 3–5 years for mild aortic regurgitation, to every 3–6 months for asymptomatic severe aortic regurgitation.

Waiting for the patient to develop exercise intolerance or dyspnoea may result in some degree of irreversible left ventricular dysfunction, with an increased perioperative risk. Therefore, surgery is recommended, even in subgroups of asymptomatic patients presenting with (moderate or) severe aortic regurgitation. Indications for surgery in asymptomatic patients include:

- left ventricle ejection fraction < 50%, or left ventricular end-systolic diameter > 50 mm, or left ventricular end diastolic diameter > 70 mm
- aortic root dilatation > 55 mm (> 50 mm if bicuspid valve or Marfan syndrome; lower thresholds are recommended in those with Marfan and additional risk factors, such as strong family history of dissection, rapid increase in size, planned pregnancy)
- in those undergoing coronary artery bypass graft, aortic regurgitation is at least moderate, and progression is likely

Symptomatic patients should undergo surgery to repair or replace the aortic valve for both symptomatic and prognostic indication. Valve-sparing aortic root surgery is increasingly used in expert centres. This technique may be particularly suitable for younger patients with less valve calcification and no retraction of the cusps.

Further Reading

Baumgartner H, Falk V, Bax JJ, et al. 2017 ESC/EACTS Guidelines for the management of valvular heart disease. *Eur Heart J* 2017; 38: 2739–91

Nishimura RA, Otto CM, Bonow RO, et al. 2014 AHA/ACC Guideline for the management of patients with valvular heart disease: A report of the American College of Cardiology/American Heart Association Task Force on Practice Guidelines. *J Am Coll Cardiol* 2014; 63: e57–e185.

95 Mitral regurgitation

Kazem Rahimi

Definition of the disease

Mitral regurgitation (MR) is the reflux of blood from the left ventricle into the left atrium as a result of dysfunction of the mitral valve. MR can result from abnormalities of any part of the mitral valve apparatus (valve leaflets, annulus, chordae tendineae, and papillary muscles), or dilatation/disease of the left ventricle

Aetiology of the disease

In the developed world, rheumatic heart disease is now uncommon, and the major causes of MR are degenerative mitral valve disease and ischaemic heart disease. Mitral annular calcification is a common finding in the elderly. It is often associated with mild to moderate MR but is unlikely to cause severe MR.

Disorders of the mitral valve apparatus

Disorders of the mitral valve apparatus include:

- degenerative mitral valve disease (also called myxomatous mitral valve disease or mitral prolapse, defined as movement by one or both mitral leaflets of at least 2 mm beyond the long-axis annular plane); degenerative disease can lead to leaflet redundancy, thickening, or thinning, and to lengthening or rupture of the chordae
- rheumatic heart disease
- infective endocarditis
- papillary muscle rupture complicating acute myocardial infarction
- disorders caused by traumatic damage to the chordae or leaflets (e.g. via balloon valvotomy)
- congenital disorders (e.g. mitral valve cleft)
- drug-induced disorders (e.g. via ergotamine, cabergoline)
- disorders due to connective tissue disorders (e.g. Marfan syndrome, Ehlers–Danlos syndrome, osteogenesis imperfecta, pseudoxanthoma elasticum, psoriatic arthritis, SLE)

Diseases of the left ventricular myocardium

The following are the diseases of the left ventricular myocardium:

- dilatation of the left ventricle, due to ischaemic heart disease with previous myocardial infarction or dilated cardiomyopathy
- hypertrophic cardiomyopathy

Typical symptoms of the disease and less common symptoms

The development of symptoms in MR depends on a number of factors:

- severity of MR
- rate of progression
- degree of pulmonary hypertension
- heart rate and rhythm
- additional valve or ventricular disease

In isolated mild-to-moderate MR, forward cardiac output remains normal. Hence, patients are often asymptomatic. Even with chronic, severe MR, most patients remain asymptomatic until there is left ventricular failure, pulmonary hypertension, or atrial fibrillation. The most common symptoms are exertional dyspnoea and fatigue, due to the combination of an inadequate cardiac output, and pulmonary hypertension. Another common clinical presentation is intermittent or persistent atrial fibrillation.

Acute MR typically presents with acute severe dyspnoea due to pulmonary oedema.

Demographics of the disease

MR is the most common valve lesion, accounting for one-third of all cases of valve disease. Estimates of the prevalence of MR depend on the method of assessment. The widespread use of colour Doppler echocardiography, a sensitive technique for detecting valvular regurgitation, has increased the recognition of this lesion: trivial (physiological) MR is detectable in up to 70% of healthy adults. MR of greater than mild severity on colour Doppler echocardiography affects about 19% of men and women, while moderate or severe MR has been reported in 1.9% and 0.2% of the population, respectively. However, the prevalence increases with age, with moderate or severe MR being present in about 6% of people aged 75 years or more.

Natural history and complications of the disease

The principal complication of MR is left ventricular failure as a consequence of increased workload and cardiac dilatation. Pulmonary hypertension and right-sided heart failure in advanced stages is also common. This evolution generally occurs over many years, even decades, depending upon the severity of the regurgitant lesion and the cardiovascular response to the regurgitant volume. Other complications include atrial and ventricular ectopy, atrial fibrillation (about 5% per year), systemic embolism due to left atrial thrombus, infective endocarditis (<1% over 5 years), and sudden cardiac death (rare).

The heterogeneity of the underlying causes of MR makes the assessment of its natural history challenging. Most robust data are based on cohorts of patients with mitral valve prolapse, but they may be applicable to some other MR groups. Based on these data, the mortality risk increases with systolic dysfunction (ejection fraction < 50%), left atrial enlargement (>40 mm), atrial fibrillation, pulmonary hypertension, and age.

Approach to diagnosing the disease

MR is usually suspected from the clinical signs and confirmed by echocardiography. However, additional information may be helpful in the identification of complications and assessment of the risk.

Clinical signs

The following are clinical signs of MR:

Arterial pulse: It may be reduced in volume, but is usually brisk in upstroke, reflecting the decreased left ventricular ejection time. It may give the impression of a bounding pulse, similar to that seen with aortic regurgitation, but the pulse pressure is normal with MR.
Palpation: The apex beat may be laterally displaced due to cardiac enlargement. In severe MR, a thrill might be palpable.
Auscultation: The first heart sound is diminished (failure of the mitral leaflets to close properly), and the second heart sound is split (decrease in left ventricular ejection time leading to an early A2, and pulmonary artery hypertension leading to an increased and delayed P2). A third heart sound may be audible in severe MR. The characteristics of the systolic murmur of MR are variable and depend on the aetiology, severity, and direction of the

regurgitant jet. The classical murmur is a high-pitched, pansystolic murmur which is loudest at the apex and radiates to the axilla and back.

ECG

ECG may show signs of left atrial enlargement (broad P wave in Lead II, biphasic in V1), left ventricular hypertrophy, or right ventricular hypertrophy in the presence of pulmonary hypertension. Atrial fibrillation is common in chronic severe MR.

Chest X-ray

The commonest finding in chronic severe MR is enlargement of the cardiac silhouette due to left ventricular dilatation. Other abnormalities, such as mitral annular calcification, displaced left main bronchus, pulmonary arterial enlargement, or pulmonary oedema, may be present.

Echocardiography

Echocardiography is essential for identifying the aetiology of MR and grading its severity. Other important echocardiographic features are left atrial size, left ventricle size and systolic function, and pulmonary artery pressures. Left atrial size is usually increased. Left ventricular size and systolic function are normal early in the disease course, but progressive ventricular dilation and a decline in ejection fraction occur with chronic severe MR. Serial studies permit measurement of changes in ventricular dimensions or left ventricular ejection fraction. Standard transthoracic imaging is usually diagnostic, but 3D echocardiography or transoesophageal imaging may offer additional insight when information from transthoracic imaging is limited. The severity of MR is classified according to a combination of echocardiographic measures (many of which have their potential pitfalls mandating a combined assessment; see Table 95.1).

Other diagnoses that should be considered

Differential diagnosis includes other causes of heart failure. The following additional causes of pansystolic murmur should be considered:

Table 95.1 Echocardiographic measures

	Severity		
	Mild	Moderate	Severe
Vena contracta*	<0.3 cm	0.3– 0.6 cm	>0.6 cm
Jet area (Nyquist 50–60 cm/s)#	<4 cm² or <20% left atrium	Variable	>10cm² or >40% left atrium
PISA radius (Nyquist 40 cm·s)*	<0.4 cm	0.4–1 cm	>1 cm
Pulmonary vein flow~	Systolic dominant	Systolic blunting	Systolic flow reversal
Mitral inflow§	A wave dominant	Variable	E wave dominant and >1.2 m/s
Continuous wave Doppler#	Soft, mild density, parabolic	Variable	Dense and triangular shape
Regurgitant fraction^	<30%	30%–50%	>50%
EROA (via PISA)^	0–20 mm²	20–40 mm²	>40 mm²

* May be unreliable if jet is not circular or patient in atrial fibrillation.
# Multiple or eccentric jets and enlarged atrium may lead to underestimation of severity.
^ Severity may be underestimated in eccentric jets.
~ Severity may be overestimated if jet directed towards pulmonary vein.
§ Depends on preload and can be affected by other factors, such as mitral stenosis. They can all vary with the volume status, heart rate, and blood pressure. Note that the more abnormal the valve morphology, the broader the regurgitant jet on colour flow, and the louder the regurgitant Doppler signal, the more severe the regurgitation.
Abbreviations: EROA, effective regurgitant orifice area; PISA, proximal isovelocity surface area.

Reproduced with permission from Patrizio Lancellotti et al., European Association of Echocardiography recommendations for the assessment of valvular regurgitation. Part 2: mitral and tricuspid regurgitation (native valve disease), *European Heart Journal*, Volume 11, pp.307-332, Copyright © 2010 Oxford University Press.

- tricuspid regurgitation: murmur increases on inspiration, abnormal jugular venous pressure
- ventricular septum defect: murmur radiated to the right sternal edge

'Gold-standard' diagnostic test

Echocardiography confirms the diagnosis.

Acceptable diagnostic alternatives to the gold standard

Cardiac MRI and cardiac catheterization may have some value in some cases, for example, when the clinical and echocardiographic features are discordant.

Other relevant investigations

The complex relationship between the valve leaflets, annulus, papillary muscle system, and ventricular wall mean that the regurgitant volume can vary significantly with heart rate, loading conditions, and ischaemia. Consequently, the true extent of mitral regurgitation is difficult to assess and quantify during a resting study. Exercise echocardiography may allow assessment of MR and pulmonary artery pressure during stress.

Prognosis and how to estimate it

The prognosis of patients with MR depends on severity of the lesion, the presence or absence of systems, underlying aetiology, and degree of left ventricular dysfunction. The prognosis of patients with chronic severe MR can be estimated by the left ventricular size. When the end-diastolic dimension is less than 60 mm, and the end-systolic dimension is less than 40 mm (as measured by echocardiography), patients have a benign prognosis. Patients with a left ventricular end-diastolic dimension greater than 70 mm, end-systolic dimension greater than 45–47 mm, or a left ventricular ejection fraction less than 50%–55% are commonly classified as decompensated, and have a poor long-term prognosis, even with surgical treatment. Measurement of regurgitant fraction by cardiac MRI may provide another useful risk marker. People who are in the transitional status from compensated to decompensated have a good outcome with surgical treatment.

Treatment and its effectiveness

Medical management

Surgery is the mainstay of management of severe MR associated with symptoms and/or left ventricular impairment, and should be considered in all patients. Medical therapy should not be used to defer the need for surgery, but may be applicable for temporary symptomatic relief or palliation in those unsuitable for intervention. Diuretics are commonly used to reduce fluid overload. Angiotensin-converting enzyme (ACE) inhibitors, beta blockers, and aldosterone antagonists are indicated in those with left ventricular systolic dysfunction. Other antihypertensives may be required in those with a high blood pressure. Oral anticoagulation may be indicated if patient is in atrial fibrillation.

Surgical management

Evidence for the best timing of the surgery is limited to observational studies. Based on these studies, it is generally believed that corrective surgery (valve repair or replacement) should be performed in people with chronic MR before reaching the decompensated status stage where the myocardium is unlikely to recover and the operative risk is substantial.

In asymptomatic severe MR, therefore, surgery should be considered if there is:

- evidence of left ventricular dysfunction (ejection fraction < 60% and/or end-systolic volume > 45 mm)
- normal left ventricular systolic function with pulmonary hypertension (systolic pulmonary artery pressure greater than 50 mm Hg)

- normal left ventricular systolic function and new-onset atrial fibrillation.

Surgery is also indicated in chronic severe MR if symptomatic and if the ejection fraction > 30% and the end-systolic diameter < 55 mm. In people with severe left ventricular dysfunction and/or a dilated left ventricle, however, surgery should be considered if symptoms are refractory to medical therapy and the likelihood of valve repair is high.

People with acute symptomatic severe MR should undergo immediate surgical intervention.

Weighing the benefits or early surgery (before the development of left ventricular dysfunction) against the small operative risks in individual patients is often difficult. In the absence of robust evidence, approaches commonly depend on local expertise and the likelihood of valve repair.

Whenever possible, valve repair techniques such as annuloplasty, resection of prolapsing segments, or the use of adjunctive artificial chord replacement, are preferred to traditional valve replacement. Valve repair preserves all of the functional components of the native valve and avoids the use of a prosthetic heart valve with its attendant complications. In certain groups of patients, such as those with severe calcification or degeneration of the mitral valve or those with widespread prolapse of both leaflets, mitral valve repair is not an option. In such cases, valve replacement with preservation of the subvalvular apparatus is usually performed. Emerging technologies such as percutaneous valve implantation or clipping may offer an alternative to those at high risk of surgery in the future.

Valve surgery may be accompanied by other surgical procedures, such as ablation therapy for atrial fibrillation or removal of the left atrial appendage to remove a potential source of embolism. Cardiac resynchronization therapy may be beneficial to patients with severe functional MR.

Further Reading

Baumgartner H, Falk V, Bax JJ, et al. 2017 ESC/EACTS Guidelines for the management of valvular heart disease. *Eur Heart J* 2017; 38: 2739–91

Nishimura RA, Otto CM, Bonow RO, et al. 2014 AHA/ACC Guideline for the management of patients with valvular heart disease: A report of the American College of Cardiology/American Heart Association Task Force on Practice Guidelines. *J Am Coll Cardiol* 2014; 63: e57–e185.

96 Miscellaneous valvar pathology: Mitral stenosis, pulmonary stenosis, and tricuspid regurgitation

Kazem Rahimi

Mitral stenosis

Definition of mitral stenosis

Mitral stenosis is obstruction to inflow of blood from left atrium to left ventricle at the level of the mitral valve. Non-valvar causes of left ventricular inflow obstruction include left atrial tumours and cor triatriatum.

Aetiology of mitral stenosis

Mitral stenosisis usually due to rheumatic disease, although a positive history cannot be elicited in over 40% of such patients. Other systemic inflammatory conditions (e.g. SLE and endomyocardial fibrosis) can lead to mitral stenosis. Congenital mitral stenosis is rare.

Typical symptoms of mitral stenosis, and less common symptoms

The symptoms are primarily related to the severity of the valvular stenosis. The normal mitral valve orifice has a cross-sectional area of about 5.0 cm². Mitral valve area has to fall by around a half before the onset of symptoms. However, many patients with severe mitral stenosis (valve area < 1 cm²) deny symptoms because they adapt and reduce their level of activity as the stenosis slowly progresses. Typical symptoms are (exertional) dyspnoea and fatigue. If right heart failure ensues, it may be accompanied by oedema and ascites. In many patients, pregnancy, emotional stress, tachycardia, or infection may trigger the initial symptoms and lead to pulmonary oedema. Patients may also present with other symptoms, such as haemoptysis (rupture of anastomosis between pulmonary and systemic veins), dysphagia, thromboembolism, or hoarseness (due to atrial enlargement).

Demographics of mitral stenosis

Mitral stenosis is now rare in Western societies due to the declining incidence of rheumatic fever. Worldwide, it remains an important cause of cardiovascular morbidity and mortality due to the higher prevalence of rheumatic fever in developing countries. The incidence and prevalence of mitral stenosis is therefore geographically highly variable, with the prevalence ranging from 100 cases per 100 000 population in India to 1 case per 1 000 000 in the US. Women are 2–3 times more likely to present with mitral stenosis (despite similar rates of rheumatic fever among men and women).

Natural history and complications of mitral stenosis

The natural history of mitral stenosis is largely based on cohorts of patients with rheumatic heart disease. Rheumatic mitral stenosis has an asymptomatic latent period of 16 –40 years from the initial episode of rheumatic fever to the onset of symptoms. The mean age of presentation is between 40 and 50 years. A long asymptomatic period is associated with good prognosis. Prognosis deteriorates dramatically once symptoms develop:

- New York Heart Association (NYHA) Class I–II: 10-year survival > 80%
- NYHA Class III: 10-year survival = 40%
- NYHA Class IV: 5-year survival < 20%

Serial assessment in such patients suggests a gradual narrowing of the valve area of 0.1–0.3 cm²/year. Left untreated, severe mitral stenosis typically leads to death from pulmonary hypertension and heart failure (65%), systemic embolism (20%), pulmonary embolism (10%), or infection and endocarditis.

Approach to diagnosing mitral stenosis

Physical examination gives clues to the diagnosis, which is then usually confirmed with echocardiography. However, additional investigations may be helpful in the identification of complications and assessment of the risk.

Clinical signs of mitral stenosis

The clinical signs of mitral stenosis are as follows:

General findings: General findings may include malar flush (mitral facies), small volume pulse, atrial fibrillation, V wave in jugular venous pressure, tapping apex beat, palpable first heart sound, apical diastolic thrill, and left parasternal heave (indicating right ventricular hypertrophy).

Auscultation: There is a loud S1 (if in sinus rhythm), accentuated P2, opening snap (maximal in expiration at the apex and only if leaflets still mobile and not heavily calcified), low-pitched rumbling mid-diastolic murmur, and early diastolic murmur of pulmonary regurgitation. Signs of coexistent other valvular diseases are likely to be present.

ECG in mitral stenosis

ECG may show bifid P waves (left atrial enlargement), tall, peaked P waves (pulmonary hypertension), or atrial fibrillation. Right axis deviation and right bundle branch block indicative of right ventricular enlargement may also be present.

Chest X-ray in mitral stenosis

The most likely abnormalities on a chest X-ray are left atrial enlargement (double silhouette along the right heart border and horizontal left bronchus) and pulmonary congestion.

Echocardiography in mitral stenosis

Transthoracic echocardiography is diagnostic. Classical findings in mitral stenosis are restricted opening of the mitral valve leaflets, with the doming of the anterior leaflet leading to a typical 'hockey stick' configuration in the parasternal long-axis view. The severity of mitral stenosis is assessed by measurement of valve area, either directly or indirectly using Doppler flow measurements (see Table 96.1).

Other diagnoses that should be considered aside from mitral stenosis

The differential diagnosis for the symptoms is broad, and includes many forms of heart and lung disease. For the signs, the murmur of left ventricular inflow obstruction can also be caused by an atrial myoxoma, a left atrial thrombus causing ball-valve obstruction, or a tumour. These are all rare.

Table 96.1 Doppler flow measurements

	Severity		
	Mild	Moderate	Severe
Mean pressure gradient*	<5 mm Hg	5–10 mm Hg	>10 mm Hg
Systolic pulmonary artery pressure	<30 mm Hg	30–50 mm Hg	>50 mm Hg
Valve area†	1.5–2.5 cm²	1.1–1.5 cm²	<1.0 cm²

* Useful in patients in sinus rhythm and a heart rate of 60–80 bpm.
† Valve area is usually overestimated if calculated with the pressure half-time (PHT) equation. A PHT >220 should be interpreted as severe mitral stenosis, irrespective of the calculated valve area. Severe tricuspid regurgitation leads to underestimation of severity, and severe mitral regurgitation to its overestimation. In atrial fibrillation, an average of 2–3 cycles should be used.

European Journal of Echocardiography (2009) 10, 1–25 doi:10.1093/ejechocard/jen303 EAE/ASE RECOMMENDATIONS Echocardiographic assessment of valve stenosis: EAE/ASE recommendations for clinical practice.

'Gold-standard' diagnostic test for mitral stenosis

Echocardiography is the main diagnostic test to diagnose and assess the severity of mitral stenosis.

Acceptable diagnostic alternatives to the gold standard test for mitral stenosis

Transoesophageal echocardiography is often performed for the assessment of the suitability of the valve for balloon valvuloplasty (Wilkins score) and to rule out intracardiac thrombus. Cardiac catheterization allows accurate assessment of the haemodynamics and is often used when echocardiographic findings are inconclusive, or prior to balloon valvuloplasty.

Other relevant investigations for mitral stenosis

Cardiac MRI may have some merit in cases of diagnostic uncertainty.

Prognosis for mitral stenosis, and how to estimate it

Prognosis is associated with the severity of disease and presence of symptoms (see 'Natural history and complications of the disease'). There are no validated prognostic tools for discrimination of future risk.

Treatment of mitral stenosis, and its effectiveness

Medical management of mitral stenosis

Patients who are asymptomatic with respect to sinus rhythm and normal pulmonary artery pressures require no specific treatment. In those patients with mild symptoms, diuretics can lower left arterial pressure and relieve pulmonary congestion. Control of heart rate with beta blockers, calcium channel blockers, or digoxin, particularly in those who develop atrial fibrillation, is crucial. Electrical cardioversion may also be useful to restore sinus rhythm. Afterload reduction with angiotensin-converting enzyme (ACE) inhibitors is relatively contraindicated. Patients with atrial fibrillation, pulmonary hypertension, or a history of an embolic event require anticoagulation with warfarin. The risk of stroke approaches 10% per year. Thus, anticoagulation to an international normalized ratio of 2.5–3.5 is mandatory unless a major contraindication exists.

Interventional or surgical management of mitral stenosis

If symptoms cannot be controlled easily medically or if asymptomatic pulmonary hypertension develops, mechanical relief of the stenosis should be considered. Typical indications include:

• symptomatic patients with moderate or severe mitral stenosis (<1.5 cm²)
• asymptomatic patients with moderate or severe mitral stenosis (<1.5 cm²), and pulmonary hypertension (>50 mm Hg at rest or >60 mm Hg during exercise)

Indications may be expanded to other groups, such as those with previous thromboembolism, paroxysmal atrial fibrillation, need

for non-cardiac surgery, and early or intended pregnancy. The preferred option is percutaneous balloon valvuloplasty (commissurotomy). The suitability for balloon valvuloplasty depends on (i) valve mobility, (ii) subvalvular thickening, (iii) leaflet thickening, and (iv) degree of valvular calcification; the values for these are combined to give a single score (Wilkins score) for evaluation. In addition to a favourable anatomy, absence of severe mitral regurgitation and absence of thrombus in the left atrium are prerequisites for balloon valvuloplasty. Patients with an unfavourable anatomy or the presence of a thrombus or severe mitral regurgitation should undergo surgical valve repair or replacement.

Tricuspid regurgitation

Definition of tricuspid regurgitation

Tricuspid regurgitation is the reflux of blood from the right ventricle into the right atrium as a result of dysfunction of the tricuspid valve. It can arise from abnormalities of any part of the tricuspid valve apparatus, or dilatation/disease of the right ventricle.

Aetiology of tricuspid regurgitation

Tricuspid regurgitation is commonly functional, that is, it is secondary to non-valvular pathologies leading to dilatation of the right ventricle and annular ring (90%). A primary valve pathology is less common (10%).

Secondary or functional tricuspid regurgitation is usually due to pulmonary hypertension (e.g. caused by mitral valve disease or pulmonary embolism) or right ventricular dilatation and diastolic hypertension with malcoaptation of the tricuspid valve (e.g. atrial septal defect).

Primary tricuspid regurgitation is caused by infective endocarditis, Ebstein's anomaly, carcinoid syndrome, trauma, rheumatic heart disease, ischaemic heart disease with papillary muscle dysfunction, or connective tissue disorders (e.g. Marfan syndrome).

Typical symptoms of tricuspid regurgitation, and less common symptoms

There are no specific symptoms with tricuspid regurgitation alone and usually the symptoms of the underlying cause dominate. Many patients with isolated severe tricuspid regurgitation remain asymptomatic for many years. If symptoms develop, they are usually related to the raised atrial and venous pressures manifesting as pulsation in the neck, and right-sided heart failure with abdominal distension, jaundice, and peripheral oedema.

Demographics of tricuspid regurgitation

A small degree of (physiological) tricuspid regurgitation is present in approximately 70% of normal adults. Physiological tricuspid regurgitation is short in duration and often does not extend throughout systole. Moderate-to-severe tricuspid regurgitation was reported in 15% of adults undergoing echocardiography.

Natural history and complications of tricuspid regurgitation

Information on the natural history of tricuspid regurgitation is limited because of the heterogeneity of its underlying causes which usually dominate the long-term outcome. Severe tricuspid regurgitation can lead to cachexia, cyanosis, jaundice, ascites, and peripheral oedema.

Approach to diagnosing tricuspid regurgitation

Typical clinical findings include signs of right-sided heart failure (raised jugular venous pressure, hepatosplenomegaly, ascites, peripheral oedema) and a characteristic murmur (pansystolic murmur best heard at the right or left midsternal border or at the subxiphoid area, with accentuation during inspiration). The jugular veins may show a distinct 'c–v wave' due to systolic regurgitation into the right atrium. The venous pressure is usually pulsatile and may be confused with the carotid arterial pulse. A murmur may be absent in severe tricuspid regurgitation.

ECG and chest X-ray may give clues to the underlying causes of tricuspid regurgitation (e.g. pulmonary hypertension).

Echocardiography confirms diagnosis and identifies possible aetiology. The right ventricle is usually dilated as is the valve annulus. Doppler colour flow shows the regurgitant jet. A vena contracta width >0.7 cm and systolic flow reversal in the hepatic veins suggest severe tricuspid regurgitation. Other criteria are a dilated inferior vena cava with severely reduced respiratory variation; a dense, triangular-shaped Doppler signal with an early peak; and dilated right heart chambers.

Invasive evaluation via cardiac catheterization may be performed to determine pulmonary vascular resistance or to investigate causes of functional tricuspid regurgitation.

Other diagnoses that should be considered aside from tricuspid regurgitation

Other diagnoses that should be considered in this case are mitral regurgitation and ventricular septal defect.

'Gold-standard' diagnostic test for tricuspid regurgitation

Echocardiography is the 'gold-standard' diagnostic test for tricuspid regurgitation.

Acceptable diagnostic alternatives to the gold-standard test for tricuspid regurgitation

Cardiac MRI is an acceptable diagnostic alternative to echocardiography when diagnosing tricuspid regurgitation.

Other relevant investigations for tricuspid regurgitation

Another relevant investigation for tricuspid regurgitation is right heart catheterization.

Prognosis for tricuspid regurgitation, and how to estimate it

Prognosis depends on the underlying cause of tricuspid regurgitation and its severity. In one study, the survival rates at 1 year for patients with no, mild, moderate, or severe tricuspid regurgitation were 92%, 90%, 79%, and 64%, respectively. Among the subsets of patients without pulmonary hypertension and without left ventricular dysfunction, the association of tricuspid regurgitation with decreased survival was still significant.

Treatment for tricuspid regurgitation, and its effectiveness

There is no established medical therapy for primary tricuspid regurgitation. Diuretics may improve symptoms by reducing the right ventricular volume overload and hepatic congestion. Treatment of pulmonary hypertension (e.g. balloon valvuloplasty for mitral stenosis; pulmonary thromboembolectomy; or the use of vasodilators such as sildenafil or bosentan) can be useful. The value of valve repair (mainly annuloplasty for functional tricuspid regurgitation) is controversial. Generally, in people who have severe tricuspid regurgitation and undergo surgery of left-sided heart disease, annuloplasty is recommended. In mild-to-moderate tricuspid regurgitation, such procedures have not been shown to be beneficial unless there is mitral valve prolapse as, in such patients, myxomatous changes of the tricuspid valve are common and may progress over time.

Pulmonary stenosis

Definition of pulmonary stenosis

Pulmonary stenosis is the thickening and immobility of the pulmonary valve leaflets and leads to the obstruction of blood flow from the right ventricle to the lungs. As a result, there is an increase in pressure within the right heart.

Aetiology of pulmonary stenosis

Pulmonary stenosis is almost always congenital in nature. Associations with sub- or supravalvular stenosis should be considered, and more complex congenital lesions such as Fallot's tetralogy may be present.

Typical symptoms of pulmonary stenosis, and less common symptoms

Pulmonary stenosis may remain asymptomatic over many years as the right ventricle hypertrophies in response to the increased pressure. Once compensatory mechanisms fail, symptoms of dyspnoea, fatigue, and exertional syncope may develop.

Demographics of pulmonary stenosis

Up to 10% of children will have pulmonary stenosis, with a slightly higher rate in females.

Natural history, and complications of pulmonary stenosis

Most patients present in childhood. Isolated pulmonary stenosis has a benign prognosis, for which the survival rate is not significantly different from that of the general population.

Approach to diagnosing pulmonary stenosis

An ejection systolic murmur in the pulmonary area, together with a split-second heart sound and a quiet P2, is usually present. Patients may have a parasternal heave due to right ventricular hypertrophy. In more advances stages, signs of right-sided heart failure (elevated venous pressure, jaundice, peripheral oedema) may be present.

ECG may reveal signs of right-heart enlargement (P pulmonale, right-axis deviation, right ventricular hypertrophy). A chest X-ray may demonstrate dilated pulmonary arteries due to poststenotic dilatation.

Echocardiography confirms the diagnosis and can identify associated abnormalities. Cardiac MRI may provide a more accurate assessment of the valve and its severity, together with right ventricular volume and function. A right-heart catheter is rarely required for making the diagnosis unless intervention is planned or complex heart disease is present.

Other diagnoses that should be considered aside from pulmonary stenosis

It is more common to miss pulmonary stenosis than to mistake it for an alternative diagnosis. However, the murmur may be misinterpreted as indicating aortic stenosis or a ventricular septal defect.

'Gold-standard' diagnostic test for pulmonary stenosis

The 'gold-standard' diagnostic test for pulmonary stenosis is right-heart catheterization.

Acceptable diagnostic alternatives to the gold-standard test for pulmonary stenosis

Echocardiography is an acceptable diagnostic alternative to right-heart catheterization when diagnosing pulmonary stenosis.

Other relevant investigations for pulmonary stenosis.

Another relevant investigation for pulmonary stenosis is cardiac MRI.

Prognosis for pulmonary stenosis, and how to estimate it

Patients with mild pulmonary stenosis have a benign disease that rarely progresses. Overall, patients' long-term outcome is unlikely to be affected by an isolated pulmonary stenosis.

**Treatment for pulmonary stenosis,
and its effectiveness**

There is no established medical therapy for pulmonary stenosis. Balloon valvuloplasty is commonly performed to relieve symptoms and to prevent right heart failure. Alternatively, surgical valvotomy, valve repair, or valve replacement is performed in more complex cases. Balloon valvuloplasty is recommended in symptomatic patients with a peak systolic gradient >30 mm Hg and in asymptomatic patients with peak systolic gradient >40 mm Hg (moderate-to-severe disease). Although the evidence is less well established, because of the excellent outcome of balloon valvuloplasty, this procedure may also be considered in asymptomatic patients with a peak systolic gradient of 30–39 mm Hg.

Further Reading

Baumgartner H, Falk V, Bax JJ, et al. 2017 ESC/EACTS Guidelines for the management of valvular heart disease. *Eur Heart J* 2017; 38: 2739–91

Nishimura RA, Otto CM, Bonrow RO, et al. 2017 AHA/ACC Focused Update of the 2014 AHA/ACC Guideline for the Management of Patients With Valvular Heart Disease: A Report of the American College of Cardiology/American Heart Association Task Force on Clinical Practice Guidelines. *Circulation* 2017; 135: e1159–e1195.

Rodés-Cabau J, Taramasso M and O'Gara PT. Diagnosis and treatment of tricuspid valve disease: current and future perspectives. *Lancet* 2016; 388: 2431–42

97 Percutaneous coronary intervention

Cheerag Shirodaria and Sam Dawkins

Cardiac catheterization

Cardiac catheterization is a procedure by which **information** is obtained from the heart by passing fine plastic tubes (occasionally other instruments) either near to or within the heart, to introduce contrast to cardiac structures to understand their anatomy and function better, to measure pressures, and/or to measure oxygen saturations in different cardiac chambers. It is an extraordinarily useful **diagnostic** procedure. Percutaneous coronary intervention (PCI) is the modern term for an **intervention** on a coronary artery that relieves narrowing. It includes balloon angioplasty and stent insertion. It is a **therapeutic** procedure.

Cardiac catheterization comprises a number of different procedures:

- **coronary angiography**, where dye is injected into coronary arteries, allowing an understanding of their lumen to be made, and the diagnosis of the severity and extent of coronary narrowings
- **left ventricular cine-angiography**, where dye is injected directly into the left ventricle; used to measure left ventricular systolic function and the severity of mitral regurgitation
- **aortography**, where dye is injected into the aortic root, allowing determination of the aortic root size, the severity of aortic regurgitation, and the presence or absence of aortic dissection (this role is now largely superseded by CT aortography)
- **right-heart saturation measurements**, used to determine intra-cardiac shunt location and magnitude
- **pressure measurements of the cardiac chambers**, which give information about left ventricular performance, pulmonary artery pressure, and pulmonary vascular resistance; **simultaneous right- and left-heart pressure measurements** can be used to diagnose pericardial constriction

Cardiac catheterization is an extraordinarily useful technique; however, it is now largely used for coronary angiography in patients with chest pain and who are suspected of having severe coronary disease. The technique allows the operator to visualize the coronary arteries and identify any narrowings (stenosis). If stenoses are identified, a therapeutic intervention, such as balloon angioplasty or deployment of a coronary artery stent (collectively known as PCI), can be carried out.

The procedure is minimally invasive; access is gained to the arterial system via the femoral artery (one-third of procedures), the radial artery (two-thirds of procedures), or brachial arteries (arterial cutdown; rare these days). A fine catheter is passed to the ostium of the left and then the right coronary artery. Once the catheter is in the ostium, an iodine-based contrast agent is injected and X-rays are taken; as X-ray radiation can pass through thoracic structures but not through the contrast agent in the coronary arteries, a negative image of the coronary lumen is obtained. X-rays are taken in multiple projections to delineate the entire length of the coronary arteries.

Interpretation of coronary angiogram

A knowledge of how to interpret the data obtained from coronary angiography is important. The aim of angiography is to delineate anatomy so as to guide treatment, and in particular, to determine how many coronary stenosis are present and their severity.

Coronary lesion severity

Previously, in chronic stable angina, coronary disease severity was classified by the reduction in transluminal diameter caused by atheroma seen angiographically, although debate arose as to whether a ≥50% or a ≥70% reduction was significant. This debate has been settled by invasive studies of coronary function obtained using the fractional flow reserve technique (see 'Other invasive techniques to evaluate coronary arteries'). Not surprisingly, it turns out that achieving symptomatic relief from coronary intervention depends on whether the coronary obstruction interferes with coronary artery function; perhaps more surprisingly, it turns out that functional impairment of coronary flow does not relate precisely to anatomic appearance. One-third of narrowings of 50%–70% severity interfere with function, and two-thirds of narrowings of 70%–90% severity interfere with function. About 96% of stenoses ≥ 90% interfere with function. Put another way, in some patients, surprisingly mild narrowings can interfere with function and, conversely in others, surprisingly severe narrowings may not. If functionally unimportant narrowings are treated by PCI or coronary artery bypass graft (CABG), then patients are exposed to risk and not benefit. Unless the narrowing is severe, information beyond that obtained from angiography is needed to plan optimal treatment in chronic stable angina. Such functional data on the extent of ischaemia can be obtained non-invasively prior to angiography (via nuclear, MRI, or stress echocardiography studies) or by fractional flow reserve at angiography. In acute coronary syndrome (ACS), the severity of the stenosis in the artery with the ruptured plaque is important, as the natural history of tighter narrowings is worse; however, as relatively mild untreated narrowings can still lead to abrupt vessel closure, most operators also treat by PCI angiographic lesions **at the site of the ruptured plaque** of 50%–70%. Increasing evidence suggests that 'bystander' disease (i.e. anatomically significant lesions found at the time of angiography undertaken for an ACS, but themselves not directly responsible for the ACS) should also be treated in ACS patients.

Coronary disease location and extent

Different patterns of coronary disease are seen; these are traditionally classified by the number of major epicardial vessels involved and their location, particularly, whether the left main coronary artery or the proximal portion of the left anterior descending (LAD) artery is involved. Major epicardial vessel involvement is regarded as narrowings within the main epicardial arteries but not in their side branches. Patients may therefore have single-, two-, or three-vessel coronary disease, with or without left main or proximal LAD involvement. The extent of prognostic benefit from CABG relates to the severity of the coronary disease, and patients with left main disease, or proximal LAD or three-vessel coronary disease benefit prognostically from early CABG, a benefit magnified in those with diabetes or impaired left ventricular function. Coronary disease can be classified from the perspective of PCI lesion complexity by using **the Syntax Score** (http://www.syntaxscore.com) derived from a major trial. This takes data from the lesion distribution and outputs a number, with a high score indicating technical complexity for PCI (and thus favouring CABG), and a low score indicating technical ease during PCI (so favouring PCI).

Other invasive techniques used to evaluate coronary arteries

While coronary angiography is by far the most common means of invasively assessing coronary artery disease, there are other complementary techniques available:

Fractional flow reserve: This is used to determine whether narrowings within coronary arteries impede coronary blood flow. In it, a small pressure probe built into a coronary guide wire is passed into a coronary artery, allowing pressure to be measured simultaneously both within the coronary artery beyond the possible narrowing and, using the standard catheter pressure measurement, at the ostium of the coronary artery. The pressure fall over the narrowing is obtained with the artery in its resting state. The artery is then dilated using the coronary vasodilator adenosine, so increasing blood flow. If the lesion is flow limiting, the increase in coronary flow results in an increased pressure drop over the coronary segment being interrogated. A ratio of ≤0.75 in the ratio of proximal to distal pressure indicates a flow limiting lesion; a ratio of ≥0.80 indicates no flow limitation; and a ratio of 0.75–0.80 indicates possible flow limitation.

Intravascular ultrasound (IVUS): In IVUS, a small ultrasound probe is inserted into the coronary artery over a standard guide wire. Ultrasound emissions (20–40 MHz) are made at 90° to the wire to obtain a two-dimensional, cross-sectional image of the artery. The IVUS probe is then withdrawn with a motorized device at the speed of 0.5 mm/s, so imaging a length of coronary artery. IVUS is extremely good at looking at vessel and luminal diameter (to determine how large a stent is needed), plaque burden (to determine whether intervention is needed), and, perhaps its most important use, how well deployed a stent is. The use of IVUS is sometimes limited by vessel calcification.

Optical coherence tomography (OCT): OCT is an emerging technology that uses light rather than ultrasound to image coronary arteries, obtaining a very high resolution; indeed, so much so that it has been called 'virtual histology'. It has yet to find a clinical role, but its scientific role is fast developing.

Percutaneous coronary intervention (PCI)

Early in its development, PCI consisted of percutaneous transluminal coronary angioplasty (PTCA), a procedure in which a balloon was passed over a thin wire ('a guide wire') to the stenosis and inflated to squeeze the material comprising the blockage to the side of the artery, thereby removing luminal obstruction. There were two limitations to this technique:

• high rates of coronary dissection, resulting in acute vessel closure, myocardial infarction, and the need for emergency CABG
• high rates of restenosis following the procedure (up to 25%–40%); the PTCA balloon injures the vessel wall and, as in all tissues injured, scar tissue (neo-intimal proliferation) results. In the case of the coronary artery, such scar tissue results in luminal obstruction, recurrent symptoms, and, in a few cases, myocardial infarction

These issues have largely been dealt with by using **coronary stents**; these are alloy steel slotted metal tubes, deployed within a coronary artery. They seal dissections and substantially reduce the risk of restenosis. Stents used in PCI can either be **bare metal or drug eluting**, in which case the stent is coated with a drug that reduces neointimal proliferation. Stents are thrombogenic and require moderately intense antiplatelet therapy until they are endothelialized (4 weeks for bare-metal stents, 1 year for drug-eluting stents).

Drug-eluting stents are associated with a small increase in the risk of in-stent thrombosis; the risk can be minimized by giving the patient a second antiplatelet agent (e.g. clopidogrel) with aspirin for the first year post-PCI. The coatings most widely used for drug-eluting stents are paclitaxel (an anti-mitotic agent used in cancer chemotherapy) and sirolimus/everolimus (used for immunosuppression in transplant patients). Drug-eluting stents are of greatest benefit in long (>15 mm), narrow (<3 mm), or proximal lesions (left main, proximal LAD), especially in diabetics. They are also commonly used in high-risk PCI. They should only be used in patients who are able to comply with antiplatelet therapy and should be avoided if the patient may undergo major surgery within the year, as post-surgical bleeding is considerably higher in those taking dual antiplatelet agents.

Types of PCI

Primary PCI is now used as a slightly better alternative to thrombolysis and refers to PCI that is carried out as an emergency (<1 hour from hospital presentation) for patients with ST-elevation myocardial infarction (STEMI). **Rescue (salvage) PCI** is PCI carried out in patients who have had thrombolysis but in whom there is clinical evidence of continuing occlusion, such as ongoing pain, or failure of ECG resolution. **Facilitated PCI** is primary PCI carried out soon after thrombolysis, and is most often used when a patient cannot undergo primary PCI within the target time (usually because the patient presents to a hospital that does not offer primary PCI) and so receives thrombolytic therapy first, either in the referring hospital or, increasingly, in the ambulance, and then undergoes primary PCI on arrival at the primary PCI centre.

Drugs used in PCI

All patients undergoing PCI should be on aspirin (or another antiplatelet agent) for life. The use of a thienopyridine agent, such as clopidogrel, greatly reduces the risk of stent thrombosis and is used for most PCI. Ideally, clopidogrel starts ≥5 days before PCI; if PCI is carried out the same day, a large (600 mg) loading dose is used. Clopidogrel is given for 1 month for bare-metal stents, and for 1 year for drug-eluting stents. There are several new inhibitors of platelet aggregation available, such as prasugrel and ticagrelor, and their use will become more commonplace. Prasugrel acts more quickly and inhibits platelet function more reliably than clopidogrel, and is therefore widely used in primary PCI, where quick, reliable antiplatelet therapy is vital. Ticagrelor is superior to clopidogrel in risk reduction following ACS and may become standard therapy whether or not PCI is used.

Glycoprotein IIb/IIIa antagonists, such as abciximab, tirofiban, or eptifibatide, block the final common pathway of platelet aggregation. They are used in high-risk PCI, such as primary PCI for STEMI, or PCI in non-STEMI with a major troponin rise indicating a large thrombin-rich clot within the coronary artery, as the clot may generate a substantial additional thrombus and acute vessel closure when squeezed with a balloon. It is also used if a PCI procedure has not gone well and arterial occlusion due to thrombus formation has occurred.

Anticoagulation is used in PCI. Unfractionated heparin is the standard; the degree of anticoagulation is monitored from serial activated clotting time (ACT) measurements. The target ACT is 250–350 seconds, and 200–250 seconds if a glycoprotein IIb/IIIa antagonist is used. In patients on low-molecular-weight heparin (LMWH), the amount of unfractionated heparin used depends on the time since the last dose of LMWH and procedure complexity. Post-procedure heparin confers no advantage. Bivalirudin is a direct thrombin inhibitor (in part derived from hirudin, a chemical found in the medicinal leech *Hirudo medicinalis*) which gives predictable, although short-acting, anticoagulation and, in primary PCI, improves outcome, compared to heparin.

Indications for PCI

Stable coronary disease

PCI is a useful adjunct to medical therapy in stable angina. Its main use is symptom relief, not prognostic improvement. Patients have different views on the degree of angina that is tolerable; for many, angina on strenuous exertion may be acceptable, but others prefer to be symptom-free. Comorbidity is another consideration prior to PCI. In the few patients where a large area of ischaemic myocardium is identified by non-invasive testing (e.g. myocardial perfusion scanning), PCI is associated with a prognostic benefit. The amount of myocardium that needs to be ischaemic to yield prognostic benefit from PCI depends on the technique measuring ischaemia—for myocardial perfusion scanning, it is ≥10% of the myocardium.

CABG improves prognosis, compared to PCI, in patients with severe coronary disease (e.g. left main stem disease, triple-vessel disease, proximal LAD disease). However, recent advances in stent technology and better angiographic risk stratification (e.g. Syntax score) according to disease pattern have identified patients in whom outcomes with PCI are equivalent to those with CABG. There are institutional issues about selecting the best means of revascularization for an individual patient, with cardiologists being biased towards PCI, and surgeons to CABG. To ensure that patients receive the best evidence-driven treatment, all revascularization decisions (unless obvious) should be made by a multidisciplinary team including a cardiologist and surgeons. Whether revascularization is being considered or not, risk factor modification should be aggressively pursued in all, with the implementation of lifestyle changes (those concerning exercise, weight, smoking, and alcohol being the most important), and the use of statins, an angiotensin-converting enzyme (ACE) inhibitor, and, for many, a beta blocker.

STEMI

Primary PCI is superior to thrombolysis in reducing mortality, stroke, and non-fatal reinfarction in STEMI. It requires significant infrastructure both inhospital (24-hour access to a fully staffed catheterization laboratory) and prehospital (ambulance crews trained to interpret ECGs and/or transmit them to the hospital). The role of PCI in patients with STEMI depends on the local availability of facilities: if primary PCI cannot be delivered within ≤2 hours of first contact (usually for geographical reasons) then thrombolysis, alone or as a bridge to facilitated PCI, is the preferred option. Most ambulance services now record an ECG on initial assessment, and, if an STEMI is identified, transfer the patient directly to the nearest primary PCI centre, reducing the time from first medical contact to coronary reperfusion. In the UK, primary PCI is offered to almost all patients with STEMI.

ACS

Most patients with ACS require angiography and PCI if a suitable target lesion is identified. Determining the urgency (and necessity) of PCI depends on risk, and risk-scoring systems such as GRACE and TIMI (both available as web-based calculators) can aid decision-making. There is evidence to suggest that higher-risk patients benefit from invasive management instead of a conservative strategy; this benefit is greatest in the elderly, so these patients particularly should be considered for early referral for PCI. Patients with haemodynamic instability, severe left ventricular dysfunction, angina despite medical therapy (such as morphine and vasodilators), or sustained ventricular arrhythmias should be referred for immediate angiography and treated with the same urgency as those referred for primary PCI. Patients fulfilling the following criteria should be referred for **early** (≤72 hours) angiography ± PCI: raised troponin, dynamic ST- or T-wave changes, impaired left ventricular function, diabetes mellitus, ongoing angina, previous myocardial infarction or CABG, or PCI within the last 6 months. Patients with no further chest pain, no clinical features of heart failure, no new ECG changes, and no troponin rise are low risk and may be suitable for elective rather than urgent PCI and, in some cases, PCI may not be necessary.

Post-procedure management of PCI

PCI can be carried out as a day-case procedure in patients with stable angina, but must be carried out as an inpatient stay for those with ACS. Post-PCI care is generally straightforward, with most patients requiring observation only. Secondary prevention should always be addressed (or readdressed) during an admission for PCI, and this is a good opportunity to check fasting glucose and lipids, and optimize medication.

Complications of PCI

The mortality rate in all PCI is less than 1%; this risk is considerably lower in elective PCI in patients with stable disease (around 0.1%) and higher in primary PCI (4%). Mortality increases with age. The rate of emergency surgery is 0.07%, and that of stroke is 0.08%, for all PCI.

As patients who receive PCI have undergone an arterial puncture while taking high-dose antiplatelet agents and will usually also be anticoagulated, bleeding is the most common initial complication post-PCI. This can occur at the puncture site, demonstrated by an enlarging haematoma or continued bleeding. This can be treated by applying manual pressure to the site or by using one of the various mechanical devices available for this purpose. In patients who have undergone PCI using femoral access, retroperitoneal haematoma is a possibility and should be considered in patients who are haemodynamically compromised or have a falling haemoglobin post-PCI. This is usually managed conservatively with blood transfusion and reversal of anticoagulation, if appropriate. If a large haematoma forms in continuity with the arterial puncture site, a pseudoaneurysm can form. This is usually detected as a swelling at the puncture site, and diagnosis is confirmed using ultrasound. They can be managed by using ultrasound-guided injection of thrombin. Ensuring an adequate period of manual compression post-procedure can reduce the risk of pseudoaneurysm formation. A haematoma adjacent to arterial and venous puncture sites can lead to arteriovenous fistula formation and can be detected clinically by the presence of a bruit. It is diagnosed using ultrasound and usually requires surgical management.

The contrast agent used in angiography and PCI causes a small rise in the serum creatinine in most patients, and a period of hypotension in the acutely unwell patient can accentuate this rise. In some patients, this can be significant and, in <1%, overt renal failure can be precipitated. Patients at risk of contrast nephropathy are those with preexisting renal disease and diabetes. For this reason, in these patients, the contrast dose should be minimized and the patients should be adequately hydrated before and after the procedure to minimize the risk. If the procedure is not urgent, N-acetylcysteine can be administered in the 48 hours before the procedure to reduce the risk further.

Stent complications

There are two major complications seen with intracoronary stents: thrombosis and restenosis. Broadly speaking, stent thrombosis occurs early (<1 month post-procedure) and restenosis later (>6 months).

The highest incidence of stent thrombosis is in the first 30 days post procedure, usually during the first 48 hours. For this reason, a patient with chest pain in the month following PCI should be evaluated very carefully. Taking clopidogrel dramatically reduces thrombosis risk, and the patient should be carefully counselled on the importance of taking clopidogrel regularly and for the prescribed duration. The current guidance is for patients with bare metal stents to take clopidogrel for 1 month, and those with drug-eluting stents should take it for 1 year. The reason for this difference is that the coating on drug-eluting stents impairs the process of endothelialization of the stent struts and thus increases thrombosis risk. There is an increased risk of very late stent thrombosis (>9 months post-procedure) with drug-eluting stents but this risk is small (<1%). Other factors that increase the risk of stent thrombosis include the use of long stents; stenting a narrow lesion; the presence of bifurcations; and patients having ACS (rather than stable angina).

The other major complication, stent restenosis, is highest with balloon angioplasty. The use of bare metal stents reduces this risk, and the use of drug-eluting stents reduces it further still. Risk factors for stent restenosis are similar to those for thrombosis, and also include preexisting chronic kidney disease and diabetes mellitus.

Further Reading

Byrne RA, Stone GW, Ormiston J, and Kastrati A. Coronary balloon angioplasty, stents, and scaffolds. *Lancet* 2017; 390: 781–92.

Cuisset T, Verheught FWA, and Mauri L. Update on antithrombotic therapy after percutaneous coronary revascularisation. *Lancet* 2017; 390: 810–20.

98 Heart surgery

David Taggart and Yasir Abu-Omar

History

Cardiac surgery is still a relatively young specialty, having developed only in the latter half of the twentieth century with the introduction of extracorporeal circulation or 'cardiopulmonary bypass' (CPB). This initiated the era of open heart surgery, initially allowing the repair of congenital heart defects, then valve replacements, coronary artery bypass grafting (CABG), and, finally, heart transplantation. Over the last two decades, improvements in medical, anaesthetic, and surgical management of patients, allied to refinements in extracorporeal perfusion technology, have resulted in a decreasing mortality and morbidity from heart surgery despite the advanced age and significant comorbidity of many patients. Today, heart surgery continues to improve the prognosis and quality of lives of patients around the world. Surgical techniques and technologies continue to evolve and recent years have witnessed the emergence of, amongst others, the use of long-lasting conduits for CABG procedures, beating-heart ('off-pump') surgery, the use of minimally invasive and robotic techniques, and long-term mechanical circulatory support.

CPB

Although perfusion technology has evolved, the principles of CPB have remained consistent since the earliest clinical application by Gibbon in 1953. By diverting blood from the right atrium to the ascending aorta via a perfusion machine where blood is oxygenated and, if required, cooled, CPB supports the systemic circulation while bypassing the heart and lungs. The heart can then be temporarily paralysed, using biochemical solutions containing a high concentration of potassium, allowing surgery on a still, bloodless operating field. Numerous technological advances have resulted in highly sophisticated perfusion machines and biocompatible circuits, but systemic anticoagulation is still mandatory to prevent blood coagulation on exposure to the extracorporeal circuit. Use of CPB, however, has some drawbacks. Contact of blood with the extracorporeal circuit results in activation of a systemic inflammatory response syndrome which, although usually subclinical, can (rarely) result in end-organ dysfunction or failure. Other limitations include systemic hypoperfusion and microembolization, which may further contribute to end-organ injury.

Surgery for ischaemic heart disease

Despite significant advances in its treatment over the last two decades, including ever-improving medical therapy and interventions where appropriate, coronary artery disease (CAD) remains a major health burden in the developed world. Annually, it accounts for around 95 000 deaths in the UK, making it the most common cause of death (20% of men and 14% of women still die as a consequence of CAD).

CABG is the most common surgical procedure performed on the heart, with over half a million operations carried out worldwide every year. It is the most extensively studied surgical procedure ever undertaken with follow-up data extending to over four decades.

For the last three decades, CABG has remained the 'gold-standard' treatment for patients with multivessel and left main CAD. Despite advances in percutaneous coronary intervention (PCI) with drug-eluting stents, CABG still remains the best therapy in terms of prognosis and relief of symptoms in patients with more extensive CAD. CABG is highly effective in relieving the symptoms of CAD and improving life expectancy in certain anatomic patterns of disease;

these benefits are magnified in diabetic patients as well as those with the most severe disease, demonstrable ischaemia, and especially in the presence of impaired left ventricular function. Furthermore, CABG is a remarkably safe therapy. Improvements in medical, anaesthetic, and surgical management have ensured that its mortality has remained static (below 2% overall and 1% for elective patients) over the last decade, despite being applied in an ever-increasing, ageing, and sicker patient population.

The principle of CABG is to bypass diseased segments of the coronary arteries by using arterial and venous conduits. The most frequently used conduits are the left internal mammary artery (LIMA) and the long saphenous vein. The main drawback of CABG over the long term is vein graft failure, occurring in up to 50% of vein grafts at 10 years, and 75% at 15 years, leading to recurrent angina, myocardial infarction, and death. Whether the widespread use of antiplatelet agents and statins may improve graft longevity and subsequent outcome is unknown.

While the mammary artery is the conduit of first choice, several other conduits have been used with varying results. Performance of conduits is judged on the basis of patency, which ultimately affects clinical outcome. Patient factors, including coronary anatomy, also play an important part in the decision-making process. Figure 98.1 shows some of the graft configurations that may be used in CABG.

Conduits used in CABG

LIMA

The LIMA became the established graft of first choice when its superiority to saphenous vein grafts, with respect to patency rates and improved patient survival, was reported in 1986. The patency rate of the LIMA to the left anterior descending coronary artery, functionally the largest and most important coronary artery, is in excess of 90% at 10 years, in comparison to 50% for vein grafts. This improves survival by around 10% at 10 years, as well as reducing the incidence of recurrent angina, myocardial infarction, and the need for repeat intervention.

Bilateral internal mammary artery

Intuitively, the superior patency rate of the LIMA suggests that use of bilateral internal mammary artery (BIMA) would lead to even greater clinical benefits. To date, the most powerful evidence supporting this comes from a systematic review of observational studies by Taggart and colleagues of over 15 000 patients (Wijns et al., 2010). However, the use of BIMA should be weighed against its potential drawbacks, which include devascularization of the sternum (and hence an increased risk of wound complications, especially in obese diabetic patients), the increased operation time, and the technical challenges associated with its use. A randomized trial involving over 3000 patients (the Arterial Revascularisation Trial) on the use of BIMA versus single internal mammary artery has been completed and is due to be reported in the near future.

Long saphenous vein

The long saphenous vein was first used as a conduit for CABG in the 1960s and, to date, remains the most commonly used conduit. It is usually harvested using an open technique, but minimally invasive approaches are being increasingly utilized with the aim of reducing leg wound morbidity. Its main limitation is a continuing attrition due to the development of atherosclerosis leading to poorer patency rates over the longer term (only 50% at 10 years, and 25% at 15 years) but this may improve with increased use of secondary preventative measures such as antiplatelets and statins.

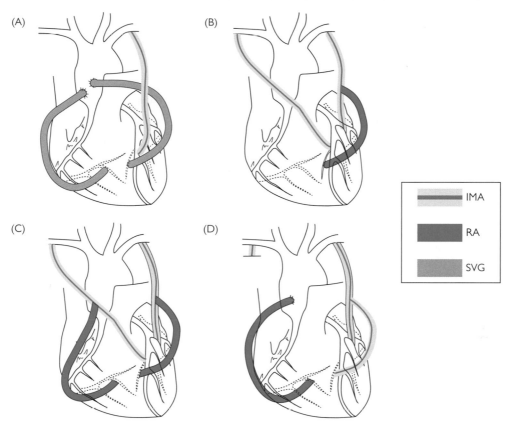

	IMA
	RA
	SVG

Figure 98.1 (A–D) Various graft configurations that can be used in coronary artery bypass surgery; IMA, internal mammary artery; RA, radial artery; SVG, saphenous vein graft.

Reprinted from *Medicine*, Volume 42, edition 9, Yasir Abu-Omar,David P. Taggart, Coronary artery bypass surgery, pp. 527-531, Copyright © 2014), with permission from Elsevier.

Radial artery

This conduit was first used in the 1970s but soon abandoned due to an observed increased risk of morbidity as a consequence of arterial spasm. Improved harvesting techniques, the use of antispasmodics to prevent vasospasm, and the demonstration of the radial artery's superior patency rate, as compared to those for vein grafts, has led to a resurgence of interest in its use as a conduit. Advantages include the low morbidity associated with radial artery harvesting, and avoidance of the need for leg incisions, thus encouraging early post-operative mobilization.

Other conduits

Other conduits, such as the short saphenous and cephalic veins or the inferior epigastric and gastroepiploic arteries, are only rarely used, when other conduits are not available, because of inferior patency rates.

Off-pump coronary artery bypass (beating-heart surgery)

CABG using CPB remains the gold-standard treatment for CAD. Over the past decade, techniques of revascularization on the beating heart without the use of CPB ('off-pump' surgery) have evolved, with an attempt to reduce the potential deleterious effects of extracorporeal circulation.

Around 20% of CABG procedures are currently performed off pump in the Western world but a far higher proportion is performed in the Far East. There is conflicting evidence about the efficacy of off-pump CABG in reducing mortality and/or morbidity, in comparison to that of conventional CABG with CPB. Several but not all trials have reported a significant reduction in morbidity following off-pump surgery in lower-risk patients, while large observational studies in higher risk patients have also reported a reduction in mortality. Furthermore, off-pump surgery potentially allows complete

avoidance of aortic manipulation, especially in patients with severe aortic atherosclerosis, thus reducing the incidence of stroke.

Off-pump surgery is technically more challenging than conventional CABG, and concerns have been expressed about inferior-quality anastomoses leading to reduced graft patency. Off-pump surgery, however, remains a safe and efficacious alternative to conventional CABG in experienced hands and may have the additional advantage of reducing mortality, morbidity, and, particularly, the risk of stroke in older, sicker patients

Surgery for valvular heart disease

Surgery remains the treatment of choice for symptomatic patients with valvular heart disease and results in significant improvements in prognosis and quality of life. The majority of valve lesions are diagnosed using echocardiography to precisely define the valvular lesion (stenosis, regurgitation, or mixed) and identify associated abnormalities (e.g. left ventricular impairment). Indications for surgery in the management of valve disease are discussed elsewhere. In general terms, valve surgery is recommended for all symptomatic patients with severe valve lesions, provided the risk of surgery (as assessed by scoring systems such as EuroSCORE) is not prohibitive. In asymptomatic patients with severe valve lesions, surgery may be advised in specific circumstances (e.g. when valve disease has resulted in left ventricular systolic dysfunction or severe pulmonary hypertension).

Surgical techniques used for valvular heart disease

Techniques to treat aortic valve disease

The mainstay treatment of aortic valve disease is valve replacement using a prosthetic valve. This is a frequently performed procedure with a low mortality (around 2%) and morbidity, and results in a remarkable improvement in prognosis and quality of life. Recent developments include the use of percutaneous aortic valve implantation techniques, but developments are ongoing. Open surgical valve replacement remains the gold standard for many patients. However, Transcatheter Aortic Valve Implantation (TAVI) is a rapidly evolving field, and increasing numbers of patients are undergoing this procedure. Current UK criteria are extremes of age, or co-morbidity rendering the risks of cardiac surgery prohibitively high. However, as technology improves, these criteria are being progressively relaxed, and some patients at lower risk for conventional surgery now undergo TAVI. All patients for aortic valve surgery should be reviewed by a multidisciplinary team prior to intervention to ensure that they receive the best procedure for them.

Techniques to treat mitral valve disease

In mitral valve disease, valve repair rather than replacement is the first-line treatment, particularly in patients with mitral regurgitation. Around 90% of regurgitant valves can be repaired with low mortality (around 1%) and morbidity, and excellent clinical outcome. The technique of repair depends on the underlying pathology and may involve surgery on the leaflets, chordae, or mitral valve annulus. Use of minimally invasive techniques in mitral valve surgery is rapidly gaining in popularity and reduces morbidity by reducing surgical trauma and hospital stay while hastening patient recovery.

Choice of valve prosthesis

When valve replacement is necessary, several prostheses are available, broadly divided into mechanical and biological valves. Choice is dictated by several factors that include patient age and preference and longevity of the valve substitute. Mechanical valves are virtually indestructible and are reserved for the younger age group, but their main disadvantage is the need for lifelong anticoagulation (with around a 1% annual risk of serious bleeding). In contrast, biological valves have a limited lifespan, compared to mechanical valves, but do not necessarily require anticoagulation unless indicated by patient factors, such as the presence of atrial fibrillation. Biological valves are therefore usually reserved for patients over 65–70 years of age and especially because structural deterioration is much faster in these patients than in younger patients. In patients over the age of 70 years, the life expectancy of current biological valves would be expected to be in excess of 90% at 10 years. Infrequent but major complications following valve replacement include haemorrhage (secondary to anticoagulation), thromboembolism, and infection.

Surgery of the thoracic aorta

Surgery of the thoracic aorta has evolved over the last three decades, with improved preoperative assessment, surgical techniques, and perioperative management. It does, however, remain particularly challenging, with a higher risk of mortality and major morbidity particularly affecting the CNS.

Surgery for aortic dissection

Aortic dissection is the commonest thoracic aortic emergency and arises when a tear in the intima allows blood to be directed from the aortic lumen into the media, resulting in the formation of true and false lumens. The dissection may extend distally and compromise perfusion of the aortic side branches, resulting in end-organ ischaemia. It may also extend proximally and result in coronary ischaemia by compromising coronary blood flow. If the false lumen penetrates the adventitia of the aortic wall, it usually results in rupture and immediate death.

Patients present with acute onset chest or back pain, and there may be additional signs of end-organ ischaemia (e.g. stoke, renal failure, bowel infarction, leg ischaemia). Risk factors for aortic dissection include long-standing hypertension, atherosclerosis, connective tissue disorders (e.g. Marfan syndrome), trauma, and iatrogenic factors.

The most commonly used classification of aortic dissection is the following, called the Stanford system:

- Type A: dissection involving the ascending aorta
- Type B: dissection sparing the ascending aorta

The classification of an aortic dissection has very important implications for its treatment. An acute Type A aortic dissection is a surgical emergency with a mortality of up to 90% in the first 48 hours

(many of the patients die before reaching hospital). Prompt resuscitation and blood pressure control is followed by immediate surgical repair, which involves replacement of the ascending aorta with a prosthetic graft to prevent progression and rupture. This procedure may require systemic cooling (usually to 18°C –20°C) and circulatory arrest to construct the distal anastomosis to the arch of the aorta. Type A dissection carries an immediate mortality of around 20% and a high risk of cerebral injury.

Type B aortic dissection is usually managed medically with rigorous blood pressure control and regular follow-up. Intervention is indicated in the presence of life-threatening complications such as imminent rupture or malperfusion. The conventional approach is with surgery, but this is associated with a high risk of mortality and paraplegia secondary to spinal cord ischaemia. There is an increasing trend towards minimally invasive approaches using endovascular grafts which significantly reduce the immediate operative risk and major complications, but with a less durable outcome over the longer term.

Some patients present with chronic dissection of the aorta. Surgery is only indicated in these cases in the presence of persistent symptoms, malperfusion, or aneurysm formation.

Surgery for thoracic aortic aneurysm

Aneurysms of the thoracic aorta have a significant male preponderance and are classed as follows according to the part of the aorta involved:

- ascending
- arch
- descending thoracic
- thoracoabdominal

The aetiology of aortic aneurysms may be degenerative (atherosclerosis), congenital (associated with bicuspid aortic valve disease), due to connective tissue disorders (Marfan and Ehlers–Danlos syndromes), associated with aortic dissection, infective (mycotic), inflammatory (aortitis), or traumatic.

Surgery is indicated for:

- dissection
- rupture
- associated aortic valve disease
- large aneurysms:
  - >5.5 cm for the ascending aorta
  - >6.5 cm for the descending aorta
  - >4.5 cm in patients undergoing concomitant surgery
- aneurysms with a rate of growth of >1 cm/year

Imaging (using contrast CT) is essential in the preoperative evaluation and in planning the operative strategy. The surgical technique depends on the part of the aorta affected and involves replacing the aneurysmal segment of the aorta with a prosthetic graft.

Surgery for heart failure

End-stage heart failure is increasingly prevalent in the Western world, and ischaemic heart disease is the primary cause, affecting over half of all cases. Despite improvement in medical therapy for heart failure, prognosis remains very poor, with a mortality of 30% at 1 year. Surgical techniques continue to evolve in the management of heart failure and include revascularization; mitral valve surgery; mechanical circulatory support and the total artificial heart; and heart transplantation.

Revascularization

Coronary revascularization is a high-risk procedure in this group of patients and is indicated only in those with evidence of significant ischaemia and myocardial viability.

Mitral valve surgery

Left ventricular dilatation may result in significant mitral regurgitation, which is associated with a significant reduction in survival. Mitral valve surgery in selected patient groups has been shown to improve long-term outcome.

Mechanical circulatory support and the total artificial heart

Mechanical support may provide assistance to the failing heart by supporting the left and/or the right ventricles. It is increasingly used in view of limited donor organ availability for heart transplantation. These devices may be used to provide temporary support of the myocardium in acute myocarditis until recovery occurs (bridge to recovery), or until transplantation can be performed (bridge to transplant). Alternatively, these devices may be used for permanent support of patients with end-stage heart failure who are not candidates for transplantation (destination therapy). The technology associated with these devices continues to evolve rapidly, and in the future they will become viable alternatives to heart transplantation.

Heart transplantation

This is the best treatment for suitable patients with end-stage heart failure. Survival following successful transplantation is over 50% at 10 years. It is however limited by donor-organ shortage in an era with increased demand for transplantation.

Summary

Heart surgery offers highly cost-effective symptomatic and prognostic benefits to a broad range of patients with cardiovascular disease. Advances in technology, and scrutiny of results, have allowed for the evolution of cardiac surgical techniques which have translated into direct clinical benefits. Most adult cardiac surgical practice currently centres on the treatment of ischaemic heart disease and valvular disease, but in the future is likely to increasingly focus on mechanical support in patients with heart failure.

Further Reading

Alexander JH and Smith PK. Coronary-artery bypass grafting. *N Engl J Med* 2016; 374: 1954–64.

Nishimura RA, Otto CM, Bonow RO, et al. 2017 AHA/ACC focused update of the 2014 AHA/ACC guideline for the management of patients with valvular heart disease: a report of the American College of Cardiology/American Heart Association Task Force on Clinical Practice Guidelines. *Circulation* 2017. doi: 10.1161/CIR.0000000000000503.

99 Circulatory support therapy

Kazem Rahimi

Introduction

A broad range of acute and chronic conditions reaching from hypovolaemic shock to ventricular tachycardia can present with circulatory failure. Hence, the approach for management of circulatory failure can vary considerably. This chapter focuses on circulatory failure due to pump failure of the heart and builds on general treatment strategies discussed in Chapters 91 and 92. Three major circulatory support therapies are discussed further: pharmacological therapy, balloon pumping, and surgically inserted devices. Treatment of circulatory failure unrelated to pump failure, and general measures such as fluid resuscitation, are beyond the scope of this chapter.

Pharmacological therapy

Pharmacological therapy aims to support myocardial function by increasing myocardial contractility. Currently, three major classes of inotropic agents are described:

- beta agonists: dobutamine, dopamine, adrenaline, noradrenaline
- phosphodiesterase inhibitors (increase contractility by increasing intracellular calcium concentration): amrinone, milrinone, vesnarinone, enoximone
- calcium sensitizers (increase the sensitivity of calcium receptors without increasing the intracellular calcium concentration): levosimendan, pimobendan

These agents differ in many pharmacological respects, both within and among classes. Beta agonists are the oldest and most widely used, albeit least well-studied, inotropic agents. On the basis of some distinctive pharmacological properties, many experts have traditionally given preference to the combination of dobutamine and dopamine over other beta agonists for treatment of systolic heart failure. However, there is little evidence to support such a choice. In fact, in the SOFA-II trial, which compared dopamine with noradrenaline for the treatment of shock (including cardiogenic shock), the use of dopamine was associated with a higher rate of arrhythmic complications, compared to noradrenaline. Similarly, many other promising pharmacological properties of inotropes have failed to translate into measurable clinical benefits. Current recommendations are, therefore, largely based on expert opinion and can be summarized as follows:

- The use of inotropes should be restricted to patients with persistent hypotension (systolic blood pressure <80–90 mm Hg) despite adequate fluid resuscitation and who have evidence of organ dysfunction (somnolence, oliguria, lactic acidosis, worsening renal or liver function) due to systolic heart failure.
- Patients with persistent fluid overload despite intensive diuretic therapy may also benefit from inotropic therapy.
- The use of inotropes should be limited to a minimum to avoid some of their common risks, such as arrhythmia.
- Treatment with inotropes can be used as a bridge to more definitive therapy, such as insertion of assist devices, or heart transplantation, or until circulatory recovery.
- Dobutamine (2–20 µg/kg min⁻¹) is the first choice in low-output states, often in combination with dopamine (1–10 µg /kg min⁻¹).
- The phosphodiesterase inhibitors milrinone and enoximone may have an advantage over beta agonists in patients in whom beta blocker use is maintained. However, they can worsen hypotension due to their significant vasodilating effect, and trial evidence (e.g. from OPTIME-CHF, PROMISE) for many phosphodiesterase inhibitors has been disappointing.

- Calcium sensitizers are considered experimental in the US. Levosimendan has not been shown to be superior to dobutamine in terms of reduction in risk of mortality (SURVIVE trial). The European Society of Cardiology recommends its use as an alternative to other inotropes, in particular if patients are already on a beta-blocker therapy.
- The vasoconstricting beta agonist noradrenaline is usually used in cardiogenic shock (in combination with dobutamine). Adrenaline's use is restricted to cardiac arrest.

The disappointing findings from many trials testing the efficacy and safety of inotropes, despite promising haemodynamic improvement, have challenged the whole concept of improved contractility without modification of energy metabolism, and have led to the hypothesis that the mismatch between energy consumption and energy production may be responsible for the harms caused by these agents. Emerging therapies such as ranolazine or perhexiline improve cardiac performance by modifying substrate utilization from free fatty acids to more efficient fuels like glucose and lactate, and thus provide energy to a myocardium that has run out of fuel. Whether such improvements in the utilization of myocardial energy can translate into clinical benefits is subject to a number of ongoing and planned trials.

Balloon pumping

The intra-aortic balloon pump (IABP), or balloon pumping, is a percutaneously inserted balloon in the descending aorta distal to the left subclavian artery; it inflates in the early diastole (filled with helium gas and triggered by ECG) and deflates in the late systole. IABP is currently the most widely used circulatory assist device. The counterpulsation of the balloon in the diastole has two main desired effects:

- It leads to augmentation of blood pressure during early diastole and hence improved coronary perfusion.
- The rapid deflating of the balloon in late diastole leads to reduced afterload through a vacuum effect and increases myocardial contractility at a lower myocardial energy consumption level.

Measurable haemodynamic effects in the individual patient are highly variable and depend on the exact timing of the balloon inflation and deflation, the volume of the balloon, its position in the aorta, heart rate, rhythm, the compliance of the aorta, and systemic resistance. On average, patients with cardiogenic shock may be expected to show the following haemodynamic changes:

- a decrease in systolic pressure by 20%
- an increase in diastolic pressure by 30%
- a reduction of the heart rate by less than 20%
- a decrease in the mean pulmonary capillary wedge pressure by 20%
- an elevation in the cardiac output by 20%

The evidence for the balance of efficacy and safety of IABP is tenuous. Randomized clinical trials for many of the currently recommended and widely used indications are lacking. Indeed, a meta-analysis of all trials that compared IABP with no IABP showed no difference in 30-day mortality but an increased 6% and 2% risk of bleeding and stroke, respectively, in the 500 patients in the IABP group as compared to the 500 patients in the control group (Sjauw et al., 2009). Planned trials may shed some light on the clinical value of IABP. Guidelines predating this meta-analysis acknowledge the gap in evidence but make recommendations for IABP use for the following indications:

- persistent hypotension (<90 mm Hg) unresponsive to other measures and with signs of end-organ dysfunction

- cardiogenic shock
- pre- and post-complex percutaneous coronary intervention/coronary artery bypass graft in haemodynamically unstable patients or patients with intractable angina
- acute mitral regurgitation or ventricular septal defect, as a bridge to more definitive therapy

IABP should not be used in patients with:

- significant aortic regurgitation
- aortic dissection
- severe peripheral arterial disease
- a high risk of bleeding

As many as 7% of patients experience complications related to IABP, of which a third can be considered as major. Complications include:

- stroke
- limb ischaemia
- perforation of the femoro-iliac arteries
- aortic dissection
- cholesterol emboli (e.g. leading to renal failure)

The use of IABP requires anticoagulation, usually with unfractionated heparin. IABP use should be kept to a minimum. Stepwise weaning, with reduction of the assisted counterpulsations from 1:1 to 1:3 every 3–4 hours, is recommended. After haemodynamic stability for about 4 hours without support (usually after initiation of vasodilators and/or beta blockers), the use of IABP can be withdrawn.

Surgically inserted devices

Surgical devices for mechanical cardiac support are commonly called ventricular assist devices (VADs). They are based on the principle of a parallel 'artificial heart' which bypasses the blood flow away from the ventricle(s) with the use of an extracardiac mechanical pump and improves forward circulatory output and cardiac filling pressures. On the basis of the ventricle(s) being supported, three types of VADs can be differentiated:

- left ventricular assist device (LVAD): this channels blood from the left ventricle or left atrium to the pump and then from the pump to the ascending aorta
- right ventricular assist device (RVAD): this channels blood from the right ventricle or right atrium to the pump and then from the pump to the pulmonary artery
- biventricular assist device: this is a combination of an LVAD and an RVAD

The newer, third-generation VADs (e.g. Heart Ware HVAD, Duraheart, Levacor) are becoming increasing smaller in size and have continuous-flow centrifugal pumps that are magnetically or hydrodynamically levitated with minimal risk of bearing failure, which was seen with older-generation VADs. The net beneficial effect of these rapidly developing devices, however, has not yet been shown in randomized trials, and current recommendations are largely based on expert opinion. VADs are most commonly used as a bridge to transplantation in people with severe heart failure despite optimal medical therapy, or as bridge to recovery in people with severe myocarditis (although the ability to wean off VADs is usually poor). The increased longevity of the devices, reduced post-operative morbidity, and the greater likelihood of patient acceptance have led to some enthusiasm for the use of VADs as destination devices in people with severe left ventricular dysfunction and severe symptomatic heart failure but who are not candidates for transplantation. However, supporting evidence for such an expansion in indication is currently awaited.

Contraindications for VAD support usually include high surgical risk for device implantation, recent or evolving stroke, conditions impairing the ability to manage the device, a coexistent terminal condition, an abdominal aortic aneurysm >5 cm, active systemic infection, fixed pulmonary or portal hypertension, severe pulmonary dysfunction, multisystem failure, inability to tolerate anticoagulation, bleeding disorder, and pregnancy.

Common adverse events include surgical mortality, bleeding, right ventricular failure, infections, thrombosis, device malfunction, and neurological events.

Further Reading

Francis GS, Bartos JA, and Adatya S. Inotropes. *J Am Coll Cardiol* 2014; 63: 2069–78.

Harjola V-P, Mebazaa A, Celutkiene J. Contemporary management of acute right ventricular failure: a statement from the Heart Failure Association and the Working Group on pulmonary circulation and right ventricular function of the European Society of Cardiology. *Eur J Heart Fail* 2016; 18: 226–41.

Levy B, Bastien O, and Bendjelid K. Experts' recommendations for the management of adult patients with cardiogenic shock. *Ann Intensive Care* 2015: 5: 17.

Van Herck JL, Claeys MJ, De Paep R, Van Herck PL, Vrints CJ, and Jorens PG. Management of cardiogenic shock complicating acute myocardial infarction. *Eur Heart J: Acute Cardiovasc Care* 2015; 4: 278–97.

Robert MacKenzie-Ross, Karen K. K. Sheares, and Joanna Pepke-Zaba

Definition of the disease

Pulmonary hypertension (PH) is a haemodynamic and pathophysiological condition defined as mean pulmonary artery pressure ≥25 mm Hg at rest, assessed by right-heart catheterization (8–20 mm Hg is considered normal). A pulmonary capillary wedge pressure measurement of >15 mm Hg indicates a significant pulmonary venous component.

PH is associated with a variety of causes. The current PH classification is helpful in understanding the different etiological, pathological, and treatment approaches (see Box 100.1).

Box 100.1 Updated clinical classification of pulmonary hypertension (Nice, 2013)

1. Pulmonary arterial hypertension
   - idiopathic
   - heritable
     - BMPR2
     - ALK-1, ENG, SMAD9, CAV1, KCNK3
   - drug and toxin induced
   - associated with:
     - connective tissue diseases
     - HIV infection
     - portal hypertension
     - congenital heart diseases
     - schistosomiasis
   - persistent pulmonary hypertension of the newborn
   - pulmonary veno-occlusive disease and/or pulmonary capillary haemangiomatosis
2. Pulmonary hypertension owing to left heart disease
   - Left ventricular systolic dysfunction
   - Left ventricular diastolic dysfunction
   - Valvular disease
   - Congenital/acquired left heart inflow/outflow tract obstruction and congenital cardiomyopathies
3. Pulmonary hypertension owing to lung diseases and/or hypoxaemia
   - COPD
   - interstitial lung disease
   - other pulmonary diseases with mixed restrictive and obstructive pattern
   - sleep-disordered breathing
   - alveolar hypoventilation disorders
   - chronic exposure to high altitude
   - developmental abnormalities
4. Chronic thromboembolic pulmonary hypertension
5. Pulmonary hypertension with unclear multifactorial mechanisms
   - haematologic disorders:
     - splenectomy
     - chronic haemolytic anaemia, myeloproliferative disorders
   - systemic disorders:
     - sarcoidosis
     - pulmonary histiocytosis
     - lymphangioleiomatosis
   - metabolic disorders:
     - thyroid disorders
     - glycogen storage disease
     - Gaucher's disease

   - others:
     - tumoural obstruction
     - chronic renal failure on dialysis
     - fibrosing mediastinitis

http://dx.doi.org/10.1016/j.jacc.2013.10.029

Aetiology of the disease

Different pathological features characterize the diverse clinical PH groups.

Group 1 (pulmonary arterial hypertension (PAH)) displays characteristic changes in the pulmonary artery, including medial hypertrophy, intimal proliferation, adventitial thickening, and plexiform and thrombotic lesions. This reduces the vessel calibre, changing its compliance and diffusion properties.

Group 2 (pulmonary hypertension owing to left heart disease) pathological changes are characterized by enlarged pulmonary veins, pulmonary capillary dilatation, and interstitial oedema.

Group 3 (pulmonary hypertension owing to lung diseases and/or hypoxia) pathological changes predominantly involve medial hypertrophy and intimal obstructive proliferation of the distal pulmonary arteries.

Group 4 (chronic thromboembolic pulmonary hypertension (CTEPH)) is characterized by organized thrombi attached to the pulmonary arterial medial layer, replacing the normal intima. These may completely occlude the lumen or form different grades of stenosis, webs, and bands. In the non-occluded areas, a pulmonary arteriopathy, indistinguishable from changes seen in Group 1 (including plexiform lesions), develops.

Group 5 (pulmonary hypertension with unclear multifactorial mechanisms) includes heterogeneous conditions with different pathological pictures.

In all cases, there is increased pulmonary artery pressure and increased pulmonary vascular resistance affecting the right ventricular workload.

Typical symptoms of the disease, and less common symptoms

Symptoms are nonspecific and often attributed to another cause, leading to late diagnosis. Symptoms start with breathlessness on exertion, progressing to breathlessness on minimal exertion, and ultimately at rest. Other symptoms include fatigue, weakness, angina, presyncope, abdominal distension, and, in advanced cases, peripheral oedema, syncope, arrhythmias, chest pain, and ascites.

If PH is associated with another disease, there will also be symptoms related to this condition.

Demographics of the disease

The aetiology of the PH will determine the demographics. The most frequent causes of PH are common medical diseases (e.g. left heart disease, COPD).

Group 1

The demographics of Group 1 PH are as follows:

Idiopathic PAH: incidence 1 to 3.3 cases per million per year; female predominance

PAH associated with connective tissue disease: predominantly seen with scleroderma (8%–22% prevalence in this group)
PAH associated with HIV: ~0.5% prevalence in the HIV population
Portopulmonary hypertension: prevalence 1%–6% in patients with portal hypertension

Group 2

The prevalence of PH associated with left heart dysfunction is up to 70% in patients with isolated left ventricular diastolic dysfunction, and up to 60% in patients with severe left ventricular systolic dysfunction.

Group 3

The demographics of Group 3 PH are as follows:

PH in patients with COPD: in patients screened for lung volume reduction surgery/lung transplantation (mean FEV_1 24% of predicted), the prevalence is estimated at 40%
PH associated with interstitial lung disease: prevalence is estimated at between 8% and 34%

Group 4

Between 1% and 5% of patients with acute pulmonary embolism progress to CTEPH. However, 25% of patients with CTEPH do not give a history of acute pulmonary embolism.

Natural history, and complications of the disease

Hypoxic vasoconstriction and remodelling of the arterial or venous components of pulmonary circulations will initially increase pulmonary artery pressure and pulmonary vascular resistance. As the disease progresses, cardiac output will fall, leading to right-heart failure, which is the cause of the death in the majority of cases.

Increased right atrial pressure can re-open a foramen ovale, thereby helping to offload the right-heart chambers.

For PH associated with other conditions, the symptoms will intertwine with any symptoms related to the underlying disease process.

Approach to diagnosing the disease

Medical history

The main symptom is progressive exertional breathlessness. Ask about other symptoms (see 'Typical symptoms of the disease, and less common symptoms'). A diagnosis of idiopathic PAH should only be made after excluding other conditions which could contribute to PH.

Important risk factors are:

- use of dieting drugs (aminorex, fenfluramine, dexfenfluramine, benfluorex) .
- history of DVT or pulmonary embolism
- history of splenectomy
- childhood murmurs
- Raynaud's phenomenon, or skin changes

Examination

Depending on the severity, there may be clinical signs of right-heart failure: raised jugular venous pressure (JVP), loud second heart sound, systolic murmur of tricuspid regurgitation, right ventricular heave, peripheral oedema, enlarged pulsatile liver, and/or ascites. The rest of the examination is directed towards the search for underlying causes.

Diagnostic tests

ECG

ECG will be normal in the early disease stage or will show a right ventricular strain pattern: right-axis deviation, a dominant R wave in V1, T-wave inversion in the anterior chest leads, right bundle branch block, or an enlarged P wave in Lead II (P pulmonale).

Chest X-ray

The chest X-ray may be normal, but often shows enlarged central pulmonary vessels, attenuation of the peripheral vessels, and a prominent right-heart border (right atrial enlargement). Look for causes of PH (e.g. lung parenchymal diseases, pulmonary infarcts).

Blood tests

The following blood tests may be used:

- full blood count: this is often normal; polycythaemia suggests congenital heart disease or hypoxic lung disease
- urea and electrolytes, and liver function test: these are often normal; the liver function test could be abnormal from liver cirrhosis or hepatic congestion from right heart failure
- thyroid function testing, hepatitis serology, and HIV testing: these can identify conditions associated with PH
- autoantibody testing: antinuclear antibodies for connective tissue disease (anticentromere for limited scleroderma); up to 40% of patients with idiopathic PAH have elevated antinuclear antibodies
- antiphospholipid antibody testing: this is performed if there is a history of DVT or pulmonary embolism

Arterial blood gases

Arterial blood gases can give an indication of hypoventilation or hypoxia from associated lung diseases.

Other tests

Other useful tests in approaching the diagnosis are lung function testing, echocardiography, ventilation/perfusion scanning, pulmonary angiography, CT, and cardiac MRI (see 'Other relevant investigations').

Other diagnoses that should be considered

Pulmonary valve stenosis and tricuspid valve abnormalities could mimic PH (symptoms of right-heart failure in the absence of pulmonary vasculopathy). A restrictive cardio myopathy or pericardial effusion can cause breathlessness with a raised JVP.

'Gold-standard' diagnostic test

Right-heart catheterization is mandatory for establishing the diagnosis. This test measures the pressure in the pulmonary artery and right heart chambers; cardiac output; and blood oxygen saturations. Blood oxygen saturations can identify left-to-right intra-cardiac shunts.

A vasoreactive challenge (using inhaled nitric oxide, or IV epoprostenol) during right-heart catheterization in patients with idiopathic PAH, heritable PAH, or PAH associated with anorexigen use will identify patients who may benefit from treatment with calcium channel blockers. A positive response is defined by a decrease in the mean pulmonary artery pressure of ≥10 mm Hg, reaching a mean pulmonary artery pressure of ≤40 mm Hg, and having an unchanged/increased cardiac output.

The data from right-heart catheterization gives information required to assess prognosis and to establish a management plan.

Acceptable diagnostic alternatives to the gold standard

Transthoracic echocardiography provides several variables which correlate with right-heart haemodynamics, including pulmonary artery systolic pressure, and should always be performed if PH is suspected. Echocardiographic estimation of pulmonary artery pressure from the tricuspid regurgitant jet is well correlated with right-heart catheterization measurements, but also does give false positive and negative results. The echocardiogram can evaluate the presence of congenital, valvular, or other cardiac conditions.

Other relevant investigations

Blood testing

BNP and N-terminal pro-BNP are useful blood markers of right-heart distension, giving prognostic information. Poor renal function will cause erroneously high results.

Serum uric acid is a marker of impaired oxidative metabolism of ischaemic peripheral tissue. High levels can be a marker of poor survival.

Lung function testing

Full lung function testing in PAH might be within normal range. In advanced cases, it can show a reduced gas transfer with otherwise normal lung volumes. Other lung function changes will suggest other causes for PH (e.g. an obstructive pattern in COPD or an increased transfer factor in left-to-right congenital heart shunts).

V/Q scanning

Normal perfusion in ventilation/perfusion scintigraphy, (V/Q scan), will rule out chronic thromboembolic disease.

CT scanning

High-resolution CT imaging of the thorax can screen for lung parenchymal causes of PH (e.g. fibrosis or emphysema). Interlobular septal thickening is characteristic of left-heart failure, pulmonary veno-occlusive disease. Mosaic perfusion of CTEPH. Contrast CT pulmonary angiography can distinguish pulmonary emboli and cardiac septal defects. CTEPH changes can present as filling defects, webs, bands, and vessel amputation or pruning.

MRI

Cardiac MRI is useful in assessing cardiac function and detecting congenital defects. Magnetic resonance pulmonary angiography can be used as a means of imaging the pulmonary arteries in the evaluation of CTEPH.

Conventional pulmonary angiography

Conventional pulmonary angiography remains the gold standard in imaging the pulmonary circulation in chronic thromboembolic disease.

Exercise testing

The 6-minute walk test is an objective assessment of exercise capacity. This is a submaximal cardiopulmonary exercise test used to monitor exercise capacity and disease progression. Cardiopulmonary exercise testing assessment of peak VO2 and VE/VCO2 has some correlation with pulmonary pressures.

Prognosis and how to estimate it

Historical series give a median survival of 2.8 years for untreated idiopathic PAH. Disease-modifying therapies for PAH have improved survival. Prior to disease-specific therapies, 1-year survival was 68% and 5-year survival was 34%, for patients with idiopathic PAH. With targeted therapies, these rates have improved to 87% at 1 year and to 47%–55% at 5 years, depending on the published series. Scleroderma-associated PAH has a worse prognosis, even with treatment: 3-year survival estimates are 47% without pulmonary fibrosis, and 28% with pulmonary fibrosis. PH in conjunction with COPD is associated with an increased mortality, compared to COPD alone. Survival in PH associated with Eisenmenger syndrome is considerably better.

The following factors are associated with a poor patient prognosis at first presentation:

- PH classified as WHO Functional Class III or IV
- poor performance on a 6-minute walk test (distance <380 m)
- raised BNP or N-terminal pro-BNP level
- enlarged right atrium or a pericardial effusion on echocardiography
- right-heart catheterization showing a reduced cardiac index or low mixed venous oxygen saturations

Medical intervention aims to improve these parameters, with an optimal condition being the PH is classified as WHO Functional Class I or II, and the patient can walk >500 m and has normal BNP/N-terminal pro-BNP levels and echocardiography parameters.

Treatment and its effectiveness

Standard supportive treatments

Supportive treatment is with diuretics, to control oedema from right-heart failure, and oxygen, to correct hypoxia. Anticoagulation has some evidence to support its use, in idiopathic and heritable PAH. Anticoagulation is vitally important in CTEPH.

Calcium-channel blockers (CCBs) have some benefit in patients with idiopathic PAH who have a positive vasoreactive response (<10%; hence, CCBs should not be used except by specialist PH centres). There is no good evidence to support the use of CCBs in other forms of PH.

Specific Group 1 (PAH) drug therapy

Three main drug classes are currently used for specific Group 1 drug therapy: prostanoids (epoprostenol, iloprost, treprostinil sodium), prostenoid receptor agonists (selexipag) endothelin receptor antagonists (bosentan, ambrisentan, macitentan), phosphodiesterase-5 inhibitors (sildenafil, tadalafil), and guanylate cyclase stimulators (riociguat). They have been subject to randomized controlled trials (predominantly in idiopathic PAH, and PAH associated with connective tissue disease), and generally demonstrate improvement in exercise capacity and pulmonary haemodynamics. These study results have been extrapolated to all patients with PAH. These drug therapies have vasoremodelling properties, giving symptomatic improvement, delay disease progression, and improve survival.

It is recommended that these drugs are only prescribed and managed by PH specialist centres. Some combinations of drug therapies have been shown to be beneficial. At present, available therapies are not curative, and new therapeutic targets are actively researched.

Common side effects from these drugs are flushing, headaches, gastrointestinal disturbance, and hypotension. Endothelin-receptor antagonists require monthly liver function monitoring because of liver toxicity. Prostanoids can be delivered by intravenous, nebulized, or subcutaneous routes.

Specific PAH therapies are not recommended for patients in Groups 2, 3, and 5. The current best treatment for these groups is considered optimal treatment of their associated left heart or lung condition.

In Group 4, when possible pulmonary endarterectomy surgery is the treatment of choice. For patients unsuitable for pulmonary endarterectomy surgery (due to surgical inaccessibility or due to significant comorbidities) and patients who still have residual PH following pulmonary endarterectomy surgery riociguat is the only licensed therapy. There is increasing evidence for the role of balloon pulmonary angioplasty playing a role in treatment of CTEPH.

Invasive and surgical treatments

Balloon atrial septostomy

Balloon atrial septostomy is a palliative treatment, performed to offload a failing right ventricle and improve symptoms at the expense of decreased systemic arterial oxygen saturations.

Pulmonary endarterectomy

Pulmonary endarterectomy surgery is considered the treatment of choice for CTEPH. All patients must be carefully screened for surgical suitability. Success is dependent on the extent and location of the organized thrombus and pulmonary haemodynamic severity. After an effective intervention, a dramatic drop in the pulmonary vascular resistance can be expected with a near normalization of pulmonary haemodynamics. The result is improved exercise capacity, pulmonary haemodynamics, and survival.

Lung transplantation

If medical therapy has failed to halt symptom progression, bilateral lung/heart–lung transplantation should be considered. Transplantation offers a potential 'cure' for many forms of PH. The

5-year survival after lung transplantation for PH is similar to survival for all indications for lung transplant.

Further Reading

Galie N, Humbert M, Vachiery JL, et al. 2015 ESC/ERS Guidelines on the diagnosis and treatment of pulmonary hypertension. *Eur Heart J.* 2016: 37: 67–119.

Lau EMT, Giannoulatou E, Celermajer DS, et al. Epidemiology and treatment of pulmonary arterial hypertension. *Nat Rev Cardiol* 2017; 14: 603–14.

Simonneau G, Gatzoulis M, Adatia I, et al. Updated clinical classification of pulmonary hypertension. *JACC* 2013: 62 suppl: D34–41.

Taichman DB, Ornelas J, Chung L, et al. Pharmacologic therapy for pulmonary arterial hypertension in adults: CHEST guideline and expert panel report. *Chest* 2014; 146: 449–75.

101 Venous thrombosis and pulmonary embolism

Karen Sheares and Joanna Pepke-Zaba

Definition of the disease

Venous thromboembolism (VTE) is a condition in which a thrombus forms in a vein, commonly in the deep veins of the leg, causing deep vein thrombosis (DVT). The thrombus may dislodge from the site of origin and be carried into the pulmonary vasculature, causing pulmonary embolism (PE). DVT and PE share similar predisposing factors; however, mortality is greater in those who present with PE than in those who present with DVT. Thrombi may form in other parts of the vasculature; this is covered in Chapter 285.

Aetiology of the disease

The three primary risk factors for development of venous thrombosis are venous stasis, vascular damage, and hypercoagulability (these factors are also known as Virchow's triad). Predisposing factors may be temporary or permanent and include reduced mobility (e.g. neurological disability, hospitalization, or institutional care), medical comorbidity (e.g. chronic cardiac or respiratory failure), surgery (particularly orthopaedic surgery), active cancer or cancer treatment, previous VTE, use of hormone replacement therapy or oestrogen–containing contraception, pregnancy, the presence of indwelling central venous lines, thrombophilias (see Chapter 285), obesity, and varicose veins. In approximately 20%, idiopathic or unprovoked PE may occur.

Typical symptoms of the disease, and less common symptoms

The symptoms of DVT include unilateral leg swelling, calf pain, redness, and warmth. The symptoms in PE are not specific and include dyspnoea, pleuritic chest pain (caused by pleural irritation in pulmonary infarction), retrosternal chest pain (due to right ventricular ischaemia), cough, and haemoptysis. The classic triad of dyspnoea, pleuritic chest pain, and haemoptysis is only seen in a minority.

Patients with PE may be tachypnoeic, tachycardic, and hypoxic, with an elevated jugular venous pressure, a gallop rhythm, a widely split second heart sound due to delayed right ventricular ejection, a tricuspid regurgitation murmur, and possible flow murmurs around the embolic obstructions. With pulmonary infarction, there may be a pleural rub and pyrexia. In severe cases, the right ventricle is unable to match the increase in afterload and so fails, leading to systemic hypotension and shock.

Demographics of the disease

Community studies have reported an annual incidence rate for VTE of 1.4–1.8 per 1000, with that for DVT approximately 1 per 1000, and that for PE about 0.5 per 1000. The incidence of venous thromboembolism rises markedly with increasing age for both sexes; over the age of 75, the annual incidence reached 1 per 100 population. VTE is uncommon in the paediatric population.

Natural history, and complications of the disease

Untreated VTE carries significant morbidity and mortality. In 2005, it was estimated that 25 000 people in the UK die of preventable, hospital-acquired VTE every year.

Proximal DVTs resolve slowly during treatment with anticoagulation, and thrombi remain detectable in 50% after a year, particularly in those with a large initial thrombus or cancer. About 10%–20% of patients with symptomatic DVTs develop severe post-thrombotic syndrome characterized by chronic pain, swelling, and skin ulceration. An estimated 40%–50% of patients with symptomatic proximal DVT develop PE which may be asymptomatic.

About 10% of PEs are rapidly fatal (most clinically unrecognized), and an additional 5% cause death later, despite diagnosis and treatment. There is approximately 50% resolution of PE after 1 month of treatment, and perfusion eventually returns to normal in two-thirds of patients. Between 0.5% and 5.0% of treated patients with PE develop chronic thromboembolic pulmonary hypertension due to poor resolution and/or the development of a distal pulmonary arteriopathy. Untreated patients with chronic thromboembolic pulmonary hypertension have a poor prognosis, with a 3-year survival as low as 10% in patients with a mean pulmonary artery pressure of greater than 30 mm Hg. This is covered in further detail in Chapter 100.

In both DVT and PE, there is a 6%–15% chance of recurrence after a course of anticoagulation. The risk of recurrent thrombosis is higher (i.e. approximately 10% per patient-year) in patients with permanent risk factors, active cancer, and acquired or hereditary thrombophilia.

Approach to diagnosing the disease

The symptoms and signs in acute VTE are not sensitive or specific, and therefore cannot be used to rule in or rule out DVT or PE. However, a key step in all diagnostic algorithms is an assessment of the clinical probability of these disorders.

Several clinical prediction models incorporating predisposing factors, symptoms, and clinical signs have been developed. The Wells prediction models for suspected DVT (see Table 101.1) and PE

Table 101.1 Wells clinical prediction model for DVT	
Clinical Characteristic	**Score**
Active cancer (patient receiving treatment for cancer within the previous 6 mo or currently receiving palliative treatment)	1
Paralysis, paresis, or recent plaster immobilization of the lower extremities	1
Recently bedridden for 3 days or more, or major surgery within the previous 12 wk requiring general or regional anesthesia	1
Localized tenderness along the distribution of the deep venous system	1
Entire leg swollen	1
Calf swelling at least 3 cm larger than that on the asymptomatic side (measured 10 cm below tibial tuberosity)	1
Pitting edema confined to the symptomatic leg	1
Collateral superficial veins (nonvaricose)	1
Previously documented deep-vein thrombosis	1
Alternative diagnosis at least as likely as deep-vein thrombosis	−2

* A score of 2 or higher indicates that the probability of deep-vein thrombosis is likely; a score of less than 2 indicates that the probability of deep-vein thrombosis is unlikely. In patients with symptoms in both legs, the more symptomatic leg is used.

Reprinted from *The Lancet*, Volume 350, issue 9094, Philip S Wells et al., Value of assessment of pretest probability of deep-vein thrombosis in clinical management, pp. 1795–1798, Copyright 199, with permission from Elsevier.

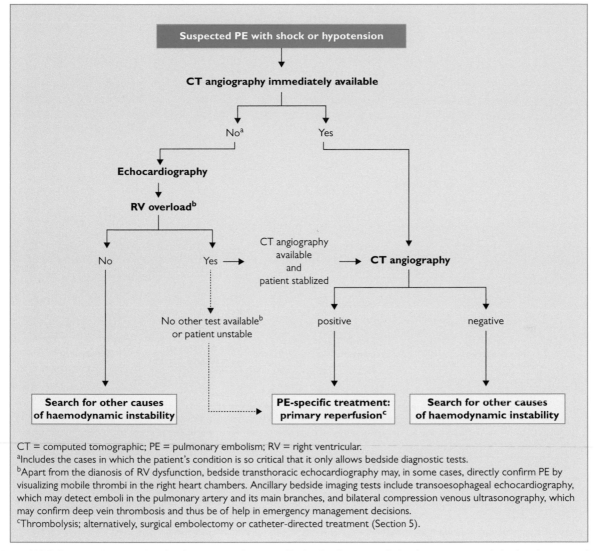

Suspected PE with shock or hypotension

↓

CT angiography immediately available

No[a] — Yes

Echocardiography

↓

RV overload[b]

No — Yes → CT angiography available and patient stablized → **CT angiography**

No other test available[b] or patient unstable

positive — negative

| Search for other causes of haemodynamic instability | PE-specific treatment: primary reperfusion[c] | Search for other causes of haemodynamic instability |

CT = computed tomographic; PE = pulmonary embolism; RV = right ventricular.
[a]Includes the cases in which the patient's condition is so critical that it only allows bedside diagnostic tests.
[b]Apart from the dianosis of RV dysfunction, bedside transthoracic echocardiography may, in some cases, directly confirm PE by visualizing mobile thrombi in the right heart chambers. Ancillary bedside imaging tests include transoesophageal echocardiography, which may detect emboli in the pulmonary artery and its main branches, and bilateral compression venous ultrasonography, which may confirm deep vein thrombosis and thus be of help in emergency management decisions.
[c]Thrombolysis; alternatively, surgical embolectomy or catheter-directed treatment (Section 5).

Figure 101.1 Proposed diagnostic algorithm for patients with suspected high-risk pulmonary embolism (i.e. presenting with shock or hypotension).
Reproduced with permission from Authors/Task Force Members,Stavros Konstantinides et al., 2014 ESC Guidelines on the diagnosis and management of acute pulmonary embolism, *European Heart Journal*, Aug 2014, DOI: 10.1093/eurheartj/ehu283

(see Figures 101.1 and 101.2) have been validated extensively and are the most frequently used.

Each hospital should have a diagnostic algorithm for the investigation of patients with suspected DVT and/or PE; this algorithm will depend on local resources, expertise, and patient population. The National Institute for Health and Care Excellence has proposed algorithms as shown in Figures 101.3 and 101.4. VTE can be safely excluded in patients who have a low pretest clinical probability of VTE and a negative D-dimer, without further diagnostic imaging.

Other diagnoses that should be considered

In the case of a swollen painful leg, cellulitis, myositis, ruptured Baker's cyst, or haematoma may be alternative diagnoses. The differential diagnosis in suspected PE may be wide, including pneumonia; exacerbation of asthma or COPD; acute coronary syndrome; aortic dissection; lung cancer; pneumothorax; fractured ribs; costochondritis, or musculoskeletal pain.

'Gold-standard' diagnostic test

The gold-standard diagnostic test for DVT of the leg is contrast venography. Venography can detect both distal thrombi (in the calf

veins) and proximal thrombi (in the popliteal, femoral, and iliac veins). Venography is invasive, requiring pedal vein cannulation, which may be difficult with swollen legs, and the use of intravenous contrast.

Selective pulmonary angiography is the gold-standard test for PE, showing direct evidence of a thrombus either as a filling defect or as amputation of a pulmonary arterial branch. However, this invasive test has been increasingly replaced by CT pulmonary angiography (CTPA).

Acceptable diagnostic alternatives to the gold standard

The inability to compress the vein lumen during compression venous ultrasonography of the lower limb is diagnostic of DVT and an alternative to venography. DVT usually starts in the calf, and distal emboli that do not extend into proximal veins rarely lead to clinically significant emboli. This has guided the rationale for using serial ultrasonography and it is considered safe to withhold anticoagulation treatment from patients with clinically suspected DVT but who have normal results on compression ultrasonography at the time of presentation and at 1 week later.

CT venography has been used to diagnose DVT in patients with suspected PE, as it can be combined with chest CT angiography. However, it increases the overall detection rate only marginally in patients with suspected PE and adds a significant amount of radiation.

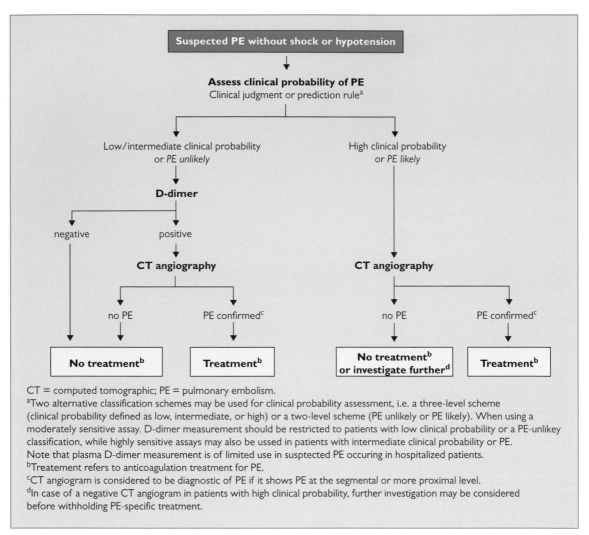

Figure 101.2 Proposed diagnostic algorithm for patients with suspected not high-risk pulmonary embolism.

Reproduced with permission from Authors/Task Force Members,Stavros Konstantinides et al., 2014 ESC Guidelines on the diagnosis and management of acute pulmonary embolism, *European Heart Journal*, Aug 2014, DOI: 10.1093/eurheartj/ehu283

Planar ventilation–perfusion scintigraphy is a well-tolerated and established diagnostic test for suspected PE in patients with normal chest X-rays. It allows identification of hypoperfused segments with normal ventilation, so-called mismatched defects, in PE. A normal test reliably excludes a PE; however, patients with indeterminate results require further investigation. Ventilation–perfusion single-photon emission CT offers three-dimensional views with potentially improved sensitivity and lower non-diagnostic rates.

Multidetector-row CTPA, with its high spatial and temporal resolution and quality of arterial opacification, has improved the sensitivity and specificity of CT in the diagnosis of PE. It allows adequate visualization of the pulmonary arteries up to at least the segmental level and allows assessment of the secondary effects, for example, dilatation of the right-heart chambers, dilatation of the main pulmonary artery, and tricuspid regurgitation. It has become the main thoracic imaging test for investigating suspected PE and also allows the identification of alternative diagnoses. The disadvantages are that the intravenous contrast is nephrotoxic and best avoided in renal failure; some patients are allergic to the contrast; and the radiation burden is approximately 2–6 mSv, compared to 1.1 mSv for perfusion scintigraphy.

Other relevant investigations

Plasma D-dimer is a degradation product of cross-linked fibrin and gives a measure of endogenous fibrinolysis. It has a good negative predictive value and is useful in excluding DVT or PE. Unfortunately, it has a low specificity and is elevated in a wide range of conditions, for example, infection, inflammation, trauma, surgery, and pregnancy. Hence, an elevated D-dimer is not diagnostic of DVT or PE. It should not be measured in patients with a high clinical pretest probability, as it has a low negative predictive value in this population. A variety of different assays are available, each with different sensitivities, specificities, and predictive values. Generally, enzyme-linked immunosorbent assays (ELISA) are more sensitive than latex-agglutination techniques.

The chest X-ray may be normal or show atelectasis, pleural effusion, hypovascularity (Westermark's sign), or wedge-shaped peripheral infarct (Hampton's hump). It is also useful in excluding other causes of dyspnoea and chest pain.

ECG may show signs of right-ventricular strain, such as inversion of T waves in Leads V1–V4, a QR pattern in Lead V1, an S1Q3T3 pattern, and incomplete or complete right bundle branch block. This is useful, but of limited sensitivity. The ECG will exclude myocardial infarction or pericarditis.

Echocardiography may show signs of right-ventricular overload or dysfunction in at least 25% of patients with PE and may be helpful in excluding other diagnoses such as cardiac tamponade, acute valvular dysfunction, and acute myocardial infarction. It rarely enables direct visualization of PE but may reveal thrombus in the right atrium or right ventricle. It has an important role in prognostic stratification.

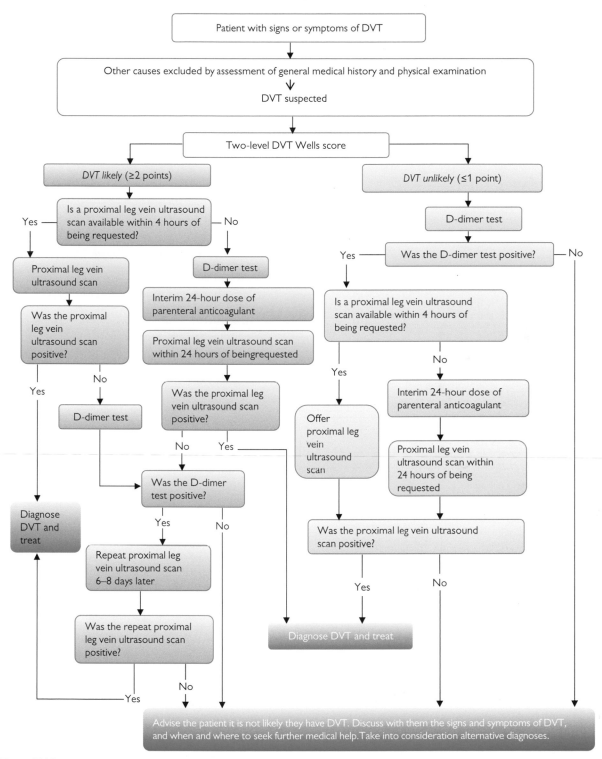

Figure 101.3 Diagnosis of deep vein thrombosis (DVT).

Reproduced with permission from National Institute for Health and Clinical Excellence (2012) Venous thromboembolic diseases: the management of venous thromboembolic diseases and the role of thrombophilia testing. London: NICE. Available from http://guidance.nice.org.uk/CG144. This information was accurate at time of publication, for update information please visit www.nice.org.uk

PE may be associated with hypoxaemia due to ventilation–perfusion mismatch, shunting through areas of collapse and infarction and/or through a patent foramen ovale, and low mixed venous oxygen saturation due to the reduced cardiac output. Up to 20% of patients with PE may have a normal arterial oxygen pressure and a normal alveolar–arterial oxygen gradient.

Routine full blood count and biochemistry might be normal. If pulmonary infarction has occurred, there may be polymorphonuclear leucocytosis, an elevated level of C-reactive protein, and an elevated erythrocyte sedimentation rate.

BNP and its precursor, NT-pro-BNP, are released during myocardial stretch and are markers of ventricular dysfunction.

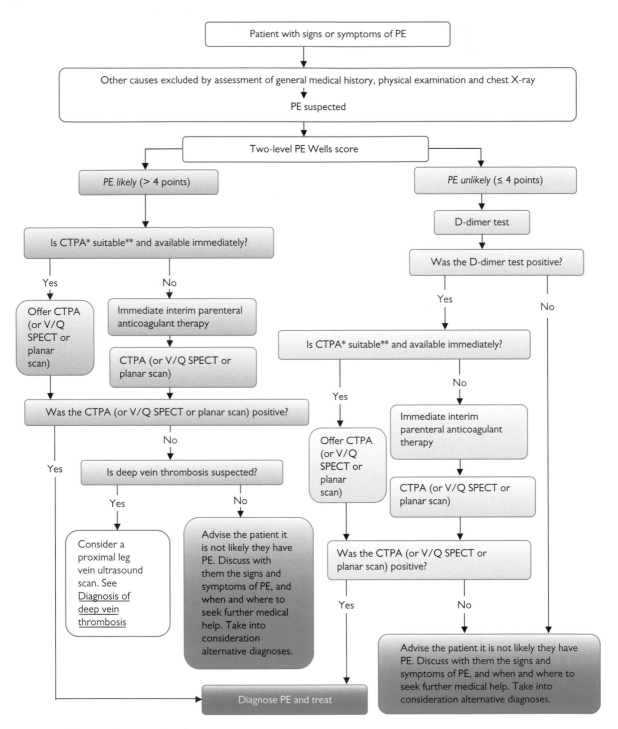

*Computed tomography pulmonary angiogram

**For patients who have an allergy to contrast media, or who have renal impairment, or whose risk from irradiation is high, assess the suitability of V/Q SPECT† or, if not available, V/Q planar scan, as an alternative to CTPA.

†Ventilation/perfusion single photon emission computed tomography

Figure 101.4 Diagnosis of pulmonary embolism (PE).

Reproduced with permission from National Institute for Health and Clinical Excellence (2012) Venous thromboembolic diseases: the management of venous thromboembolic diseases and the role of thrombophilia testing. London: NICE. Available from http://guidance.nice.org.uk/CG144. This information was accurate at time of publication, for update information please visit www.nice.org.uk

Cardiac troponins may be elevated during right ventricular infarction and are associated with increased mortality, even in the subgroup of haemodynamically stable patients with PE.

There is an association between cancer and VTE. Careful history and examination may highlight patients who require further investigations for occult cancer.

Prognosis and how to estimate it

The European Society of Cardiology has suggested that patients with PE can be stratified into three levels of risk of early death, as measured by inhospital or 30-day mortality. This classification system also helps in management. High-risk PE, previously known as massive PE, is characterized by cardiogenic shock or systemic hypotension (systolic blood pressure less than 90 mm Hg or a fall in systolic blood pressure by 40 mm Hg or more, for at least 15 minutes and which is not due to a new-onset arrhythmia, hypovolaemia, or sepsis. This life-threatening situation carries an early mortality of more than 15%. If a patient with suspected high-risk PE is too unstable or CTPA is not immediately available, echocardiography will show indirect signs of acute pulmonary hypertension and right ventricular overload; otherwise, an alternative diagnosis must be sought.

Intermediate-risk (submassive) PE is diagnosed in normotensive patients by evidence of right ventricular dysfunction and /or myocardial injury. Right ventricular dysfunction may be seen on echocardiography, CTPA, ECG, or by an elevation of BNP or NT-proBNP. Myocardial injury can be detected by elevated cardiac troponin levels.

Low-risk (non-massive) PE is diagnosed in haemodynamically stable patients with no evidence of right ventricular dysfunction or myocardial injury, and the risk of early mortality is less than 1%. This has important implications, as these patients may be considered for early discharge if they do not have additional comorbidities.

Treatment and its effectiveness

The aim of anticoagulation in VTE is to prevent death and VTE recurrences while minimizing the risk of bleeding. Patients with DVT or PE are treated with a rapidly acting anticoagulant (unfractionated heparin, low-molecular-weight heparin (LMWH), or fondaparinux) followed by oral vitamin K antagonists (commonly, warfarin). Parental anticoagulants should be stopped when the international normalized ratio is 2.0 or above for at least 24 hours. For patients at a high risk of bleeding and those with severe renal impairment, intravenous unfractionated heparin should be considered for initial treatment. Direct inhibitors of factor Xa or direct thrombin inhibitors are increasingly being used for treatment of VTE.

The duration of anticoagulation is dependent on whether the VTE event was provoked, the presence of temporary or permanent risk factors, previous history of VTE, and bleeding risks. A table giving the possible duration of anticoagulation is shown in Chapter 285. The use of elastic compression stockings reduces the incidence of post-thrombotic leg syndrome.

Patients with high-risk life-threatening PE should be treated with intravenous unfractionated heparin and be considered for early thrombolysis. This has been shown to improve survival, but there is a risk of major bleeding. High-risk patients with PE who have failed thrombolysis or in whom thrombolysis is contraindicated may be considered for surgical embolectomy or percutaneous catheter embolectomy.

Studies with inferior vena cava (IVC) filters have not shown short-term or long- term survival benefits, and there are late complications, in particular, recurrent DVT and the post-thrombotic syndrome. Currently, temporary IVC filters may be used when there are absolute contraindications to anticoagulation and a high risk of VTE recurrence. The IVC filter should be removed as soon as the patient becomes eligible for anticoagulation treatment.

VTE prophylaxis is crucial in reducing the morbidity and mortality of VTE. All medical and surgical patients should be assessed for the risks for VTE and bleeding. Patients should be encouraged to mobilize as soon as possible, avoid dehydration unless clinically indicated, and be considered for mechanical (for example anti-embolism stockings, foot impulse or intermittent pneumatic compression devices) and/or pharmacological prophylaxis (such as LMWH, fondaparinux, or unfractionated heparin).

Pregnancy

PE is a leading cause of maternal death in the UK. Although the relative risk of VTE in pregnancy is elevated four- to sixfold, and this is increased further postpartum, the absolute risk is low, with an overall incidence of VTE in pregnancy and the puerperium of 1–2 in 1000. The clinical features of VTE are similar to those in the non-pregnant state and it is essential to confirm the diagnosis while minimizing radiation exposure to the mother and fetus.

Compression duplex ultrasonography should be undertaken where there is clinical suspicion of DVT. A positive result warrants anticoagulation and makes thoracic imaging unnecessary. If an acute PE is suspected and ultrasonography is negative, CTPA or perfusion scintigraphy may be considered, depending on local availability and discussion with the obstetrician, radiologist and patient. The radiation dose delivered to the fetus during a CTPA is lower than that of perfusion scintigraphy in the first or second trimester, but a CTPA carries a higher radiation dose to maternal breast tissue.

The treatment of VTE in pregnancy is with LMWH or unfractionated heparin, as these do not cross the placenta or are found in breast milk. Warfarin crosses the placenta and is teratogenic.

Further Reading

Di Nisio M, van Es N, and Buller HR. Deep vein thrombosis and pulmonary embolism. *Lancet* 2016; 388: 3060–73.

Konstantinides SV, Torbicki A, Agnelli G, et al. 2014 ESC guidelines on the diagnosis and management of acute pulmonary embolism. *Eur Heart J* 2014; 35: 3033–69.

National Institute for Health Care Excellence. *Venous Thromboembolic Diseases: Diagnosis, Management and Thrombophilia Testing.* 2012. Available at http://www.nice.org.uk/Guidance/cg144 (accessed 28 Mar 2017).

National Institute for Health and Clinical Excellence. *Venous Thromboembolism: Reducing the Risk for Patients in Hospital.* Available at https://www.nice.org.uk/guidance/cg92 (accessed 28 Mar 2017).

Royal College of Obstetricians and Gynaecologists. Thromboembolic disease in pregnancy and the puerperium: Acute management. Green-top Guideline no 37b April 2015.

102 Aortic aneurysm

John Chambers

Definition of the disease

The epidemiology and natural history of thoracic aortic aneurysm (TAA) and abdominal aortic aneurysm (AAA) are different:

- The thoracic aortic diameter is dependent on age and body habitus as well as the level at which it is measured. Average diameters are 2.1 cm/m² for the ascending thoracic aorta, and 1.6 cm/m² for the descending thoracic aorta, giving approximate thresholds for the diagnosis of a TAA of 40 mm and 35 mm, respectively.
- AAAs are defined by a diameter >30 mm and are mainly infrarenal, with only 2%–5% in a suprarenal position.

Aetiology of the disease

Generic risk factors for all aortic disease are age, weakness of the aortic wall, and the arteriosclerotic risk factors: hypertension, dyslipidaemia, smoking, and diabetes. However, for AAA, the main risk factors are age >65, male gender, smoking (>100 cigarettes in a lifetime), and family history, with the other arteriosclerotic factors being less important.

Weakness of the aortic wall as a result of medial necrosis occurs in Marfan syndrome, Ehlers–Danlos syndrome type IV, and Loeys–Dietz syndrome. A bicuspid aortic valve should be regarded as a general thoracic aortopathy and is associated with coarctation, but also dilatation of the ascending aorta as a result of medial necrosis. Pregnancy also causes or exacerbates medial weakness. Vasculitides, especially giant cell arteritis and Takayasu's arteritis, trauma, cocaine, and amphetamines can also weaken the arterial wall. In contradistinction to the usual symmetrical 'fusiform' dilatation of a segment of aorta, a less common 'saccular' aneurysm consisting of an outpouching of the aorta can result from inflammation as a result of syphilis.

Typical symptoms of the disease, and less common symptoms

An aortic aneurysm is usually asymptomatic and an incidental finding on ultrasound scanning or chest X-ray. An enlarging aneurysm causes symptoms depending on its site. A TAA can cause hoarseness from stretching of the recurrent laryngeal nerve, occasionally tracheal or bronchial compression or phrenic nerve paresis leading to breathlessness or cough, or oesophageal compression causing dysphagia. Superior vena cava compression may also occur. Breathlessness and heart failure may also result from aortic regurgitation as a result of aortic root dilatation. An enlarging AAA can cause abdominal, groin, or back pain. Rupture or bleeding of an AAA causes the triad of acute back or abdominal pain (72%), hypotension (45%), and a pulsatile abdominal mass (83%).

Demographics of the disease

TAA is uncommon, with an incidence of six new aneurysms per 100 000 person-years, with median age 65 in men, and 77 in women. Of all degenerative aneurysms, about 5% are TAA, and most of the rest are AAA. The prevalence of AAA in the general population aged 65–79 is 5%–10%. AAA is rare in women or non-smokers, while TAA occurs approximately equally in both sexes, with median age 65 for men, and 77 for women. About 25% with TAA also have infrarenal AAA, while, of those presenting with AAA, only 3.5%–12.0% have TAA.

Natural history, and complications of the disease

TAA can be complicated by rupture or dissection. The mean rate of growth is 1 mm/year and is higher for the descending aorta than for the ascending aorta. The risk of rupture rises rapidly above a threshold of 60 mm for the ascending aorta, and 70 mm for the descending thoracic aorta (Elefteriades, 2002). The total risk of rupture or dissection above these thresholds is 30% for the ascending thoracic aorta, and 40% for the descending thoracic aorta. The risk is 7% per annum when the diameter of the ascending aorta exceeds 60 mm. Other complications of TAA involving the root are aortic regurgitation, and sinus of valsalva rupture. TAA involving the ascending or descending aorta can be complicated by perforation causing mediastinal haematoma.

The mean rate of growth for AAA is 2–5 mm/year, which is faster than for TAA. The annual risk of rupture for AAA is 9% for a diameter of 55–59 mm, 10% for a diameter of 60–69 mm, and 33% for a diameter ≥70 mm. Complications are dissection within the wall of the aneurysm, or rupture, causing retroperitoneal or free peritoneal blood. Intraluminal thrombus formation with distal embolization may cause cold and painful toes, livedo reticularis, and renal failure. Less commonly, embolization of the muscular branches of the lower extremities can cause intermittent claudication. Rare complications are bleeding as a result of erosion into the gastrointestinal tract, and renal dysfunction as a result of ureteric compression.

Approach to diagnosing the disease

TAA is usually detected incidentally on echocardiography, often as a result of investigating aortic regurgitation. It may also be detected on a routine chest X-ray. It must be sought by annual echocardiography in patients with collagen abnormalities (e.g. Marfan syndrome). Similarly, AAA is usually found by screening, which is recommended for AAA in men aged 65–75 who have smoked (US Preventative Services Task Force, 2014). Serial scans are not usually recommended if the aorta is normal, since the risk of a new aneurysm developing by 10 years is low. However, serial studies are recommended, either annually for an aneurysm 30–40 mm in diameter, or 6-monthly for an aneurysm 40–45 mm in diameter.

Other diagnoses that should be considered

TAA may be difficult to differentiate from a mediastinal mass on chest X-ray. The differential diagnosis of a pulsatile abdominal mass on examination includes a tortuous aorta, transmitted pulsation from an abdominal mass, and horseshoe kidney. The differential is easily resolved on imaging. Ruptured AAA must be part of the differential diagnosis of acute abdominal pain or shock; the differential diagnosis also includes pancreatitis and intestinal perforation.

'Gold-standard' diagnostic test

Screening for aortic aneurysm is with echocardiography for TAA, and abdominal ultrasound for AAA. Definitive imaging either to check dimensions or, more usually, as a prelude to intervention should be performed with CT or MRI.

Acceptable diagnostic alternatives to the gold standard

There are no acceptable diagnostic alternatives to the gold standard.

Other relevant investigations

The full range of tests for cardiovascular risk factors should be performed, particularly cholesterol and renal function. Syphilis serology, where relevant, should also be performed. Prior to any surgical intervention, it is usual to assess left ventricular function, and perform some form of non-invasive test to determine the presence and extent of coronary artery disease.

Prognosis and how to estimate it

See 'Natural history, and complications of the disease' for prognosis and how to estimate it.

Treatment and its effectiveness

Small asymptomatic aneurysms are managed medically with routine surveillance. Smoking cessation is essential. Beta blockers lower wall stress as well as absolute blood pressure and reduce the risk of rupture and the rate of dilatation (Judge and Dietz, 2005). There is also preliminary evidence that angiotensin-receptor blockers reduce the rate of progression of aortic dilatation in Marfan syndrome. Statins may reduce the risk of aortic rupture or dissection, particularly in descending thoracic and thoracoabdominal aneurysms (Stein et al., 2013).

Surgery should be considered at a diameter below the threshold beyond which the risk of events climbs. This is 55 mm for the ascending aorta if the aetiology is arteriosclerosis or low-risk bicuspid valve disease, and 50 mm for low risk Marfan syndrome. High-risk features are family history of aortic dissection, aortic diameter increase >3 mm in a year, systemic hypertension, and, for bicuspid valves, the presence of aortic coarctation (Erbel et al., 2014). If high-risk features are present, the threshold for surgery should be lower: 50 mm with a bicuspid aortic valve, or 45 mm for Marfan syndrome (Vahanian et al., 2012). The threshold will also be lower if there is severe aortic regurgitation or if the patient is planning pregnancy. Conversely, higher thresholds may be accepted in patients with significant comorbidity.

For aneurysms of the descending thoracic aorta, including those involving the abdominal aorta (thoracoabdominal aneurysms), the threshold for surgery depends on the aetiology of the aneurysm and whether endovascular stenting is feasible. A diameter of 60 mm is the standard cut-point for surgery (Ziganshin and Elefteriades, 2014) if endovascular stenting is not feasible, and surgical risk is high, for example, because of comorbidities. However, the threshold is 55 mm if there is a collagen abnormality, the aetiology is chronic dissection, or if endovascular stenting is feasible (Hiratzka et al., 2010). The mortality for surgery of TAA is 3%–15%, depending on the case mix, the risk of paraplegia or paraparesis is 3%–10%, and the risk of renal failure is 2%–20% (Ziganshin and Elefteriades 2014). Results are improving with better methods of spinal cord and renal protection, including left heart bypass, CSF drainage, hypothermia, and neuromonitoring.

For AAA, surgery can be considered if the diameter is >55 mm or has increased by >5 mm in a year. Conventional surgery consists of replacement of the diseased aorta with a fabric graft. The mortality is 5% if elective, 25% if symptomatic, and 50% if rupture has occurred.

Endovascular repair using a stent is possible for aneurysms of the descending thoracic aorta and AAA, with a mortality of only 5% in elective cases, an incidence of paraplegia of 2%–3%, and an incidence of renal failure of 1% (Ziganshin and Elefteriades, 2014). However, complications may occur, including endoleaks at either anastomosis; stent migration; perforation of the aorta; or aneurysmal rupture (Ellozy et al., 2003). A repeat procedure is needed in 6%–7% cases, including conversion to open repair in about 1%–2%. The long-term durability of endovascular stents is not known.

Further Reading

Elefteriades JA. Natural history of thoracic aortic aneurysms: Indications for surgery, and surgical versus nonsurgical risks. *Ann Thorac Surg* 2002; 74: S1877–S1880.

Ellozy SH, Carroccio A, Minor M, et al. Challenges of endovascular tube graft repair of thoracic aortic aneurysm: midterm follow-up and lessons learned. *J Vasc Surg* 2003; 38: 676–83.

Erbel R, Aboyans V, Boileau C, et al. 2014 ESC guidelines on the diagnosis and treatment of aortic diseases. *Eur Heart J* 2014; 35: 2873–926.

Hiratzka LF, Bakris GL, Beckman JA, et al. 2010 ACCF/AHA/AATS/ACR/ASA/SCA/SCAI/SIR/STS/SVM guidelines for the diagnosis and management of patients with thoracic aorta disease. *J Am Coll Cardiol* 2010; 55: e27–e129.

Judge DP and Dietz HC. Marfan syndrome. *Lancet* 2005; 366: 1965–76.

Stein LH, Berger J, Tranquilli M, et al. Effect of statin drugs on thoracic aortic aneurysms. *Am J Cardiol* 2013; 112: 1240–5.

US Preventive Services Task Force. *Final Recommendation Statement: Abdominal Aortic Aneurysm: Screening*. June 2014. Available at http://www.uspreventiveservicestaskforce.org/Page/Document/RecommendationStatementFinal/abdominal-aortic-aneurysm-screening (accessed 28 Mar 2017).

Vahanian A, Alfieri O, Andreotti F, et al. 2012. Guidelines on the management of valvular heart disease (version 2012). *Eur Heart J* 2012; 33: 2451–96.

Ziganshin BA and Elefteriades JA. Surgical management of thoracoabdominal aneurysms. *Heart* 2014; 100: 1577–82.

103 Aortic dissection

John Chambers

Definition of the disease

Aortic dissection is the separation of an endothelial flap from the underlying media. The natural history and management depend on the classification of dissection as either Type A, which involves the ascending thoracic aorta, or Type B, which involves only the descending thoracic aorta.

Aetiology of the disease

Risk factors for dissection are age, hypertension, and medial necrosis of the aortic wall. Medial necrosis is a feature of Marfan syndrome and Ehlers–Danlos syndrome type IV, but also occurs with a bicuspid aortic valve and with pregnancy.

Aortic dissection is usually preceded by aortic dilatation leading to an increase in transmural sheer stresses, but the aorta may be minimally dilated in pregnancy or in Marfan syndrome. Dissection occurs as a result of either endothelial damage or rupture of the vasa vasorum, causing an intramural haematoma. Both these events lead to the separation of an endothelial flap from the underlying vessel wall. Approximately 15% of clinically diagnosed acute dissections are caused by intramural haematoma. Dissection can also complicate aortic surgery or instrumentation. Aortic transaction is a separate entity associated with trauma—most commonly, deceleration injuries. Approximately 85% of transactions occur just distal to the origin of the descending thoracic aorta.

Typical symptoms of the disease, and less common symptoms

Dissection is characterized by pain which (a) is instantaneous in onset, (b) tracks along the line of the dissection, and (c) is associated with neurological symptoms. It may also present with unexplained syncope (15%) because of a small acute pericardial bleed. A larger bleed leads to acute tamponade and death.

Demographics of the disease

Dissection is rare and occurs in between 30 and 50 per million population per year, with a peak in the age range 50–65.

Natural history, and complications of the disease

The immediate mortality after acute type A dissection is 40% and, thereafter, the untreated mortality is about 1% each hour for the first 24 hours. Death occurs because of dissection into the pleural cavity or the pericardial space to cause acute tamponade. Early complications are aortic regurgitation and the results of involvement of branch arteries: of the cerebral vessels to cause stroke; of the right coronary artery to cause inferior myocardial infarction; of the iliac vessels to cause lower limb ischaemia; or of the mesenteric or renal arteries. For the few survivors, late complications are aneurysmal dilatation and redissection and heart failure as a result of severe aortic regurgitation. Early complications of type B dissection are rupture and organ or limb ischaemia. Late complications are aneurysmal dilatation leading to rupture.

Approach to diagnosing the disease

Acute dissection is strongly suggested by the symptoms in the presence of either a high-risk predisposing condition (e.g. Marfan syndrome) or high-risk features on the examination (asymmetry of pulses or blood pressure, the immediate diastolic murmur of aortic regurgitation). The chest X-ray may be helpful showing widening of the mediastinum, a double aortic shadow, or left-sided pleural fluid. However, the posteroanterior and lateral films are normal in 50% cases, and the definitive diagnosis is with imaging (see '"Gold-standard" diagnostic test').

Other diagnoses that should be considered

Acute myocardial infarction can be differentiated from dissection because the pain rises to a peak within a minute or so, rather than instantaneously. In infarction there are associated evolutionary changes on the ECG, although, rarely, involvement of acute dissection with the right coronary artery can cause an inferior infarction. This can be suspected by the clinical presentation and widening of the mediastinum on the chest X-ray. Pulmonary embolism is initially differentiated by the clinical setting, hypoxia, and evidence of acute pulmonary hypertension and right ventricular strain on the echocardiogram. Oesophageal rupture also causes severe chest pain, but usually after instrumentation or prolonged vomiting. Other causes of an acute aortic syndrome are intramural haematoma, penetrating ulcer, pseudoaneurysm, and contained or free aortic rupture (usually after trauma).

'Gold-standard' diagnostic test

In suspected acute dissection with a characteristic history, it is possible to make the diagnosis in the emergency room using transthoracic echocardiography in 80% of cases of type A dissection, and 50%–70% of cases of type B dissection. This allows the patient to be referred immediately to a cardiothoracic centre. In cases that are clinically uncertain or where the transthoracic echocardiogram is non-diagnostic, the next step is either transoesophageal echocardiography or CT scanning. A transoesophageal study can be performed in the high-dependency unit or even in the operating theatre.

Acceptable diagnostic alternatives to the gold standard

MRI produces excellent three-dimensional reconstruction of the aorta in chronic disease, and is therefore an alternative to CT scanning, but is rarely suitable for patients presenting acutely.

Other relevant investigations

In patients with acute chest pain, a 12-lead ECG excludes an acute ST-segment elevation, although, in about 2% of all type A dissections, there is involvement of the right coronary artery. ST-segment depression and electrical evidence of left ventricular hypertrophy are commonly seen. Fibrinogen degradation products (FDP) are elevated in dissection as a result of sequestration of blood in the aortic wall. Although it is possible that very high levels (>1600 mg/ml) favour dissection above other causes of chest pain and raised FDP, notably pulmonary embolism, this is not used clinically as a 'rule-in' test. However, a normal FDP concentration is a clinically useful rule-out test, with a negative predictive value of 95% when the clinical likelihood is low (it may occasionally be normal in high-risk patients with intramural haematoma or localized dissections). Coronary angiography not usually necessary and should be avoided because of the risk of damage to the aorta.

Prognosis and how to estimate it

See 'Natural history, and complications of the disease' for prognosis and how to estimate it.

Treatment and its effectiveness

Dissection is treated initially with pain relief and blood pressure lowering, usually with labetalol. Patients should be transferred to a cardiothoracic centre unless surgery is contraindicated by comorbidity. Type A dissections require immediate surgery which carries a risk of about 20% and gives a 3-year survival of 70%. Uncomplicated type B dissections are treated medically since conventional surgical treatment carries an approximately 30% mortality and 20% risk of spinal cord damage. Complicated dissections are treated by endovascular stenting since the results (30-day mortality, 8%; stroke, 8%; and spinal cord ischaemia, 2%) are better than for conventional surgery. Complications include:

- severe pain that continues or recurs
- signs of rupture (large pleural effusion, increasing para-aortic or mediastinal haematoma)
- a fall in urine output; if not due to excessive hypotensive therapy or hypovolaemia, this suggests involvement of the renal arteries and is an ominous sign
- evidence of other branch artery involvement (e.g. abdominal pain with bloody diarrhoea due to ischaemic colitis)

- refractory hypertension
- early aortic expansion

Endovascular stenting is also used in the subacute (2–6 weeks) and chronic (>6 week) phases, indicated by aortic dilatation (diameter ≥ 55 mm, an increase by ≥10 mm acutely, or an annual increase ≥5 mm), refractory hypertension, recurrent symptoms, or failure of the false lumen to thrombose. Stenting is also beginning to be used in patients with acute type B dissections, although this in not established practice. There has been preliminary use of stenting for acute type A dissections in patients who are at unacceptably high risk for conventional surgery (Senay et al., 2007).

Further Reading

Auer J, Berent R, and Eber B. Aortic dissection: Incidence, natural history and impact of surgery. *J Clin Basic Cardiol* 2000; 3: 151–4.

Erbel R, Aboyans V, Boileau C, et al. 2014 ESC guidelines on the diagnosis and treatment of aortic diseases. *Eur Heart J* 2014; 35: 2873–926.

Senay S, Alhan C, Toraman F, et al. Endovascular stent-graft treatment of type A dissection: Case report and review of literature. *Eur J Vasc Endovasc Surg* 2007; 34: 457–60.

Tsai TT, Nienaber CA, and Eagle KA. Acute aortic syndromes. *Circulation* 2005; 112: 3802–13.

104 Peripheral arterial disease

Jeremy Perkins

Definition

Peripheral arterial disease is defined as an alteration to the blood supply to a limb, caused by an occlusion or stenosis in the arteries supplying that limb. The acuteness of the arterial compromise, and its severity and extent, will determine the symptoms experienced by the patient.

Aneurysmal disease is defined as a localized dilatation of an artery and is most commonly seen in the infrarenal abdominal aorta. An infrarenal abdominal aorta is defined as being aneurysmal if its maximum anteroposterior diameter is 3 cm or greater.

Aetiology

The majority of chronic peripheral arterial disease is caused by atherosclerosis. Atherosclerotic plaques cause luminal narrowing of the artery, which becomes progressively narrower with time, and the narrowing may progress to occlusion. Plaque rupture and ulceration in atherosclerotic stenoses of the extra-cranial internal carotid arteries results in embolization to the cerebral circulation, and stroke.

Risk factors for atherosclerosis include age, race, hyperlipidaemia, smoking, hypertension, and diabetes. Rarely, previous radiotherapy, popliteal entrapment, vasculitis, or elevated levels of homocysteine may be implicated.

Acute peripheral arterial disease may be caused by acute or chronic thrombosis, where there are preexisting atherosclerotic stenoses in the arteries, or when embolization from a proximal source causes acute occlusion of the normal arterial supply to a limb. In patients with atrial dysrhythmias, such as atrial fibrillation, the most likely source of embolization is the heart. Trauma—blunt, penetrating, or iatrogenic—for example, transaction of the popliteal artery in knee dislocation caused by a road traffic accident—can cause acute limb ischaemia.

Aneurysm formation is an unspecified disorder of connective tissue.

Symptoms

Limb symptoms are commonest in the lower limb (symptoms occur in the arm in only one out of five cases). The symptoms of acute limb ischaemia are the six P's: pain, pallor, pulseless, paraesthesia, paralysis, and perishing coldness. These may vary, but the greater the degree of paralysis and sensory loss, the more severe the degree of ischaemia. The leg may be deathly white, but is often rather more mottled. Acute on chronic limb ischaemia is often characterized by less severe symptoms, with more minor sensory loss, some pain and coldness with preserved motor function (patients are able to move their foot/toes), but very limited mobility.

Chronic limb ischaemia produces two different sets of symptoms, depending on severity:

Intermittent claudication: Cramping pain is felt in the limb, predominantly the calf, on walking. It occurs after walking a reproducible distance and eases after stopping walking. There is no pain at rest or at night.

Critical limb ischaemia: Rest pain and night pain occur. This pain is felt in the toes and forefoot and not in the calf. It is often relieved by dependency. Tissue loss (ulceration or gangrene) may be present as well.

Carotid artery disease produces symptoms of stroke, transient ischaemic attack (TIA), or amaurosis fugax (transient loss of vision).

These neurological symptoms are focal, allowing localization to one cerebral hemisphere and carotid circulation.

Abdominal aortic aneurysms are usually asymptomatic, and frequently detected as an incidental finding in patients being scanned for other conditions. The major risk is of aneurysm rupture. This may be a cause of sudden death, or present with back, loin, groin, or suprapubic pain, and collapse with the associated signs of hypovolaemic shock. Rarely, aortic aneurysms may embolize, either with a solid embolus causing acute limb ischaemia, or with a shower of fine cholesterol emboli, resulting in fine punctuate areas of tissue loss on the feet or purpuric areas on the legs/feet.

Demographics

Peripheral arterial disease is a common problem. Twenty per cent of people aged 65 or over have some evidence of peripheral arterial disease on clinical examination, and 5% will have symptomatic intermittent claudication. Acute limb ischaemia affects approximately 14/100 000 population per year.

Abdominal aortic aneurysm (AAA) occurs predominantly in men aged 60–65 years. The prevalence of AAA in men aged 56 or over is ~5%, with around 2.5%–3.0% having an aneurysm of 4 cm or larger. Rupture of an AAA accounts for 1%–2% of all deaths for men aged 60 or over in the UK. The National Screening Committee has recommended a national screening programme in England and Wales to be rolled out over the next 3–4 years. This will comprise a single ultrasound scan, offered to all men when they are 65 years old. Patients with aneurysms in the 3.0–5.5 cm range will be entered into a surveillance programme with interval scans, depending on AAA size at initial detection. Patients with an AAA of 5.5 cm or greater will be offered treatment.

Natural history and complications

Acute limb ischaemia carries a high rate of death and limb loss: 25%–40% of patients will die in hospital after an episode of acute limb ischaemia, and amputation rates run as high as 50%. Late presentation (over 24 hours) or delay in treatment beyond 12 hours leads to a poor outcome.

Intermittent claudication is a benign condition that rarely progresses to limb loss. The risk of amputation for a claudicant is ~1% per year. The risk of cardiovascular death is 3–4 times higher than for an age- and sex-matched non-claudicant population. Risk factor management—stopping smoking; control of blood pressure and hypercholesterolaemia; diagnosis and control of diabetes; antiplatelet agents and statin—is important to reduce this excess mortality. In terms of walking performance, one-third of claudicants will remain stable, one-third will improve spontaneously, especially if encouraged to exercise, and one-third will deteriorate so that ~20% will come to some form of intervention.

Critical limb ischaemia is a limb-threatening condition and requires intervention to prevent limb loss. Mortality rates within 1 year of the onset of critical limb ischaemia may approach 30%–50%.

Carotid artery disease may be symptomatic or asymptomatic. Symptomatic carotid artery disease (TIA, amaurosis fugax, or completed stroke) carries a high risk of recurrent events. Patients with a severe symptomatic internal carotid artery stenosis (>60%) have a 20%–30% risk of a further stroke over the subsequent 2–3 years. If the stenosis is asymptomatic, then the risk of stroke is much less, being around 11%–12% over 5 years.

AAAs grow slowly in size, with growth rates related to size. AAAs between 4.0 and 5.5 cm grow ~0.3 cm per year. As the aneurysm increases in size, the growth rate increases also. Treatment is considered when the aneurysm diameter reaches or exceeds 5.5 cm. The

Table 104.1 Risk of rupture of an abdominal aortic aneurysm, according to aneurysm diameter

Size (cm)	Annual rupture risk (%)
<4.0	<0.5
4.0–4.9	0.5–1.0
5.0–5.9	1.0–5.0
6.0–6.9	5.0–15.0
7.0–7.9	15.0–30.0
>8.0	30.0–50.0

major complication of AAA is rupture. The risk of rupture is also size related. The rupture rates are at best a guesstimate, but typically quoted values are shown in Table 104.1.

Overall mortality for ruptured AAA is 80%–90%.

Approach to diagnosing the disease

Diagnosis of acute and chronic limb ischaemia is made on clinical grounds. Acute limb ischaemia is characterized by the absence of pulses, and a varying degree of sensory and motor impairment. The leg may be pale or mottled. The other limb should be examined for comparison. The presence of normal pulses on the other limb suggests embolization as the cause. Absent pulses (including femorals) on both legs, combined with loss of power bilaterally and mottling to the waist, indicate a saddle embolus or acute aortic occlusion.

Areas of fixed mottling distally, extensive skin blistering, and swelling of the foot with muscle rigidity raise doubts about the viability of the limb.

Intervention for acute limb ischaemia should not be delayed for angiography or other investigations, especially where there is significant motor or sensory loss, or calf muscle tenderness.

The diagnosis of intermittent claudication can be made largely on history alone. It is most frequently unilateral and characterized by cramping, gripping pain in the posterior calf or, less commonly, the thigh or buttock. The pain comes on after walking a set distance, which is less when walking uphill or carrying a load. There may be some variability in walking performance, but generally the distance the patient can walk is the same from day to day. It eases rapidly when the patient stops walking, and does not occur at rest or at night. Examination of pulses will confirm the presence of peripheral arterial disease.

Where patients have significant proximal disease, such as a chronic distal aortic occlusion or bilateral iliac occlusion, the leg symptoms may be more general and patients complain of a heaviness or tiredness in the whole leg that prevents them walking.

The presence of pedal pulses excludes the diagnosis of peripheral arterial disease, and the loss of one pedal pulse is not sufficient to cause claudication or critical limb ischaemia.

Handheld Doppler machines can be used as adjunct to clinical diagnosis in peripheral arterial disease to assess arterial signals from pedal arteries and to measure the ankle–brachial pressure index (ABPI). An ABPI >0.8 is normal, values for claudicants typically range from 0.5 to 0.8, and critical ischaemia is commonly associated with an ABPI <0.5. These cut-offs are not absolute and are taken in conjunction with clinical findings.

The neurological symptoms and signs of TIA, stroke, or amaurosis fugax are self-evident. Carotid endarterectomy is considered for patients with severe internal carotid artery stenoses of 60% or greater.

Abdominal aortic aneurysms are mostly asymptomatic and are diagnosed frequently on abdominal ultrasound or CT scans to investigate other pathology. Routine abdominal examination may reveal an enlarged aorta, although sizing of an AAA on clinical examination is unreliable and should be confirmed by additional investigation.

Other diagnoses that should be considered

Nerve trauma, spinal disease, and cerebrovascular accident can all simulate acute limb ischaemia, but the finding of absent pulses is the absolute criterion for acute ischaemia.

Leg pain on walking, the characteristic of intermittent claudication, may occur with other pathology. The major differential diagnosis comes from musculoskeletal disorder. Spinal claudication (from spinal stenosis) produces a more variable restriction on walking, often with back pain and associated numbness or parasthesia distally. Hip and knee osteoarthritis and peripheral neuropathies can cause pain on exercise.

Tissue loss in the toes may result from embolization rather than true critical ischaemia. Severe cardiac disease can cause toe discolouration and ulceration from simple 'pump failure', even with normal arteries in the leg.

'Gold-standard' diagnostic tests and acceptable alternatives

Angiography is infrequently used for diagnostic purposes, and is used when treatment (angioplasty and/or stenting) is required.

Duplex ultrasound scanning is the initial investigation of choice for peripheral arterial disease. Duplex ultrasound may be non-diagnostic in obese patients when looking at the aorta and iliac arteries, or where arteries are very calcified. Magnetic resonance angiography or CT angiography are useful alternatives in this scenario. These are all non-invasive diagnostic methods. Intra-arterial angiography may be necessary to investigate disease in the crural (below knee) arteries.

Carotid artery stenosis is diagnosed using duplex ultrasound or magnetic resonance angiography.

Abdominal aortic aneurysms are diagnosed using ultrasound or CT. CT is the investigation of choice to demonstrate the relationship to the renal arteries and aneurysm morphology if treatment with an endovascular stent graft is being considered.

Other relevant investigations

Patients with carotid artery disease presenting with TIA or stroke require structural brain imaging with CT or MRI to exclude any space-occupying lesion as the cause of their symptoms.

Patients being considered for aortic aneurysm surgery require cardiac investigation, depending on local protocols. Stress investigation with dobutamine stress echocardiography, exercise multigated acquisition scan, exercise myocardial perfusion scanning, or cardiopulmonary exercise testing is often used.

Prognosis and how to estimate it

Acute limb ischaemia carries a high rate of limb loss and mortality. Any delay in presentation and treatment, and the presence of significant comorbidities, will significantly increase limb loss and mortality.

Claudication carries a very low rate of limb loss, but a high mortality from cardiovascular disease (50% at 10 years).

Patients with critical limb ischaemia are a heterogeneous group, usually with significant comorbidities. Mortality approaches 30% at 1 year, and the rate of limb loss without intervention is high. Limb salvage is preferable to amputation where feasible.

The prognosis for AAA is related to rupture risk (see 'Natural history and complications').

Treatment and its effectiveness

Acute limb ischaemia due to arterial embolization requires urgent surgical embolectomy when there is significant motor and sensory loss. Acute on chronic ischaemia, when thrombosis occurs on pre-existing atheromatous disease, may present less severely and allow time for treatment with intrarterial thrombolysis. In all cases of acute ischaemia, mortality is high. Revascularization later than 8–12 hours carries a high rate of limb loss.

Intermittent claudication can be safely managed conservatively where impairment of walking performance is mild to moderate. Pharmacological treatment is generally ineffective. Minimally invasive intervention with angioplasty and/or stenting is the preferred treatment, with results being more durable in the iliac arteries than in the femoral or poplitela arteries. Femoropopliteal bypass grafting may be considered.

Critical limb ischaemia requires revascularization for limb salvage either by percutaneous angioplasty/stenting or by bypass grafting. Bypass grafts are more long lasting and effective the more proximal the recipient artery (i.e. above-knee popliteal versus posterior tibial at the ankle).

Carotid endarterectomy is the treatment of choice for symptomatic carotid artery stenosis with an absolute risk reduction at 2 years of 17% for ipsilateral ischaemic stroke. Carotid stenting has shown worse results, but remains under trial.

AAAs can be repaired by open surgery or endovascular stent grafting. Perioperative mortality and morbidity are reduced from 5% to 2% with endovascular stent grafting, but patients require continuing surveillance to detect potential stent migration or failure.

Further Reading

Creager MA, Kaufman JA, and Conte MS. Acute limb ischemia. *N Engl J Med* 2012; 366: 2198–206.

Gerhard-Herman MD, Gornik HL, Barrett C, et al. 2016 AHA/ACC Guideline on the management of patients with lower extremity peripheral artery disease: a report of the American College of Cardiology/American Heart Association Task Force on Clinical Practice Guidelines. *Circulation* 2017; 135: e726–e779.

Kent CK. Abdominal aortic aneurysms. *N Engl J Med* 2014; 371: 2101–8.

Teraa M, Conte MS, Moll FL, and Verhaar MC. Critical limb ischemia: current trends and future directions. *JAMA* 2016; 5: e002938

105 Raynaud's phenomenon

Kenny Sunmboye and Rachel Jeffery

Definition

Raynaud's phenomenon is characterized by episodic digital ischaemia due to vasospasm causing closure of the small arteries and arterioles of the distal extremities, in response to cold exposure or emotional stimuli. This is manifested clinically by the sequential development of intense pallor of the fingers or toes, cyanosis, and rubor, following cold exposure and subsequent rewarming. These colour changes may be accompanied by paraesthesiae and other sensations, but pain is not usually a prominent feature.

Raynaud's phenomenon is separated into two categories:

- primary (idiopathic): Raynaud's disease
- secondary Raynaud's phenomenon, which may be due to underlying disease or environmental associations (Box 105.1)

Diagnosis

A history of cold, painful hands since childhood or adolescence, especially in females, is suggestive of Raynaud's phenomenon. There

---

Box 105.1 Causes of secondary Raynaud's phenomenon

- rheumatic diseases:
  - systemic sclerosis (occurs in 90% of patients)
  - mixed connective tissue disease (85%)
  - SLE (40%)
  - dermatomyositis or polymyositis (25%)
  - rheumatoid arthritis (10%)
  - Sjögren's syndrome
  - vasculitis
- haematologic diseases:
  - polycythaemia rubra vera
  - leukaemia
  - thrombocytosis
  - cold agglutinin disease (mycoplasma infections)
  - paraproteinaemias
  - protein C deficiency, protein S deficiency, antithrombin III deficiency
  - presence of the factor V Leiden mutation
  - hepatitis B and C (associated with cryoglobulinaemia)
- occlusive arterial diseases:
  - external neurovascular compression, carpal tunnel syndrome, and thoracic outlet syndrome
  - thrombosis
  - thromboangiitis obliterans
  - embolization
  - arteriosclerosis
  - Buerger's disease
- environmental associations:
  - vibration injury
  - vinyl chloride exposure
  - lead exposure
  - organic solvent exposure (e.g. xylene, toluene, acetone, chlorinated solvents)
- neoplastic disease

Box 105.2 Clinical features pointing to secondary Raynaud's phenomenon

- males presenting at any age
- females presenting at age >40
- swollen fingers
- vasculitic changes, ulcers, or loss of finger pulp
- presence of dilated capillaries in the finger nail bed and fold (use of an ophthalmoscope set at +20 and with aqueous clear gel for contact can often pick these up without need for capillaroscopy)
- presence of antinuclear antibodies in titres >1:160, particularly if an anticentrometer pattern is present on immunofluorescence

---

is often a family history. Patients with Raynaud's disease may have hands and feet that are of normal appearance in a warm atmosphere. Hypersensitivity to cold is common. A typical attack may be precipitated by immersion of the hands in cold water, when the digits will first go white, then blue, and finally a dusky red.

There is no specific objective test for Raynaud's phenomenon, but secondary causes need to be excluded. Raynaud's phenomenon that begins in childhood, during the teen years, or in the patient's 20s, is most likely to be primary Raynaud's phenomenon in the absence of overt connective tissue disease symptomatology. Leading clinical features of secondary Raynaud's phenomenon are given in Box 105.2.

Investigations

Investigations of the patient with Raynaud's phenomenon are given in Table 105.1.

Table 105.1 Investigations of the patient with Raynaud's phenomenon

Investigation	Comment
Full blood count	To check for polycythaemia rubra vera, leukaemia, or thrombocytosis
Blood film	To check for leukaemia
Thrombophilia screen (including antiphospholipid screen)	To check for antiphospholipid syndrome, protein C and S deficiency, and factor V Leiden mutation
Hepatitis screen	To rule out hepatitis B and C
Cryoglobulins	To check for cryoglobulinaemia
Serum and urine electrophoresis	To evaluate for paraproteinaemias
ANA and extra-nuclear antibodies	ANA titres >1:160 should raise suspicion, and ENAs may contain connective tissue disease-related antibodies
Rheumatoid factor	May be positive in rheumatoid arthritis or cryoglobulinaemia
Creatinine kinase	To check for poly- and dermatomyositis
Nail fold capillaroscopy	Abnormal in secondary causes of Raynaud's phenomenon related to connective tissue disease

Abbreviations: ANA, antinuclear antibody; ENA, extractable nuclear antigen antibody.

Treatment

The treatment for primary Raynaud's phenomenon (Raynaud's disease) is as follows:

- reassurance, and advice to dress warmly and avoid cold exposure
- ancillary aids: hand and feet warmers, heated gloves and garments
- avoidance of tobacco and aggravating medications such as nonselective beta blockers
- calcium-channel antagonists (nifedipine, diltiazem) may be tried, but can cause more side effects (ankle oedema, facial flushing, headache) than clinical benefit

The treatment for secondary Raynaud's phenomenon is as follows:

- general treatments as listed for primary Raynaud's phenomenon
- treatment of the underlying disorder
- drug treatments tailored to the severity of Raynaud's phenomenon, including calcium-channel blockers, losartan, fluoxetine, prostacyclin analogues, administered intravenously in severe cases with critical digital ischaemia, and newer oral agents such as bosentan and sildenafil for severe Raynaud's phenomenon associated with recurrent digital ulceration

Further Reading

Denton CP and Khanna D. Systemic sclerosis. *Lancet* 2017; 390: 1685–99.

Wigley FM and Flavahan NA. Raynaud's phenomenon. *N Engl J Med* 2016; 375: 556–65.

106 Heart muscle disease (cardiomyopathy)

Kazem Rahimi

Introduction

Cardiomyopathy is defined as disease of heart muscle, and typically refers to diseases of ventricular myocardium. A consensus statement of the European Society of Cardiology (ESC) working group on myocardial and pericardial diseases, first published online in 2007, abandoned the inconsistent and rather arbitrary classification into primary and secondary causes and based its classification on ventricular morphology and function only (Elliot et al., 2008). This classification distinguishes five types of cardiomyopathy: dilated cardiomyopathy, hypertrophic cardiomyopathy, restrictive cardiomyopathy, arrhythmogenic right ventricular cardiomyopathy, and unclassified cardiomyopathies (such as takotsubo cardiomyopathy and left ventricular non-compaction). Each category is further subdivided into familial and non-familial causes.

In a departure from the 1995 WHO classification (Richardson et al., 1996), the ESC consensus statement excludes myocardial dysfunction caused by coronary artery disease, hypertension, valvular disease, and congenital heart disease from the definition of cardiomyopathy. The rationale for this was to highlight the differences in diagnostic and therapeutic approaches of these common diseases, and to make the new classification system more acceptable for the routine clinical use. In addition, in contrast to the American Heart Association scientific statement (Maron et al., 2006), the ESC definition does not consider channelopathies as cardiomyopathies. The sections on cardiomyopathy in this chapter are based on the ESC definition, with a brief reference to channelopathies.

Dilated cardiomyopathy

Definition of dilated cardiomyopathy

Dilated cardiomyopathy (DCM) is defined by left ventricular dilatation and left ventricular systolic dysfunction in the absence of abnormal loading conditions (hypertension, valve disease) or coronary artery disease sufficient to cause global systolic impairment. Right ventricular dilation and dysfunction may be present but are not necessary for the diagnosis. DCM does not require severe left ventricular dilation. Mild dilatation is sufficient to confirm diagnosis if systolic function is severely impaired.

Aetiology of DCM

The list of causes of DCM is extensive, with about 20%–48% of all cases being familial.

Familial causes include:

- genetic mutation (sarcolemma–sarcomere genes)
- mitochondrial dysfunction
- metabolic with storage disturbance
- unknown hereditary causes

Non-familial causes include:

- viral myocarditis (e.g. parvovirus B19) and viral persistence
- non-viral myocarditis (e.g. Chagas disease)
- toxicity (alcohol; drugs such as adriamycin)
- antibodies and autoimmune disease
- non-hereditary infiltrative diseases (e.g. haemochromatosis)
- peripartum
- endocrine causes (e.g. thyrotoxicosis)

- nutritional and electrolyte disturbances: thiamine, carnitine, selenium, hypophosphataemia, hypocalcaemia
- chronic incessant tachycardia (e.g. persistent atrial fibrillation with a rapid ventricular response)

Typical symptoms of DCM, and less common symptoms

Patients with DCM may be asymptomatic. Some may present with features of heart failure, such as exertional dyspnoea, orthopnoea, reduced exercise tolerance, and peripheral oedema. DCM may also manifest with palpitations due to conduction disorders and arrhythmia, thromboembolic complications, or sudden cardiac death.

Demographics of DCM

DCM is the most common cardiomyopathy worldwide. It develops at any age, but is more common in adults. In children, the yearly incidence is 0.57 cases per 100 000 per year overall, but is higher in boys than in girls, in black people than in white people, and in babies younger than 1 year than in children. In adults, DCM is more common in men than in women. The prevalence is estimated at 1 in 2500 individuals, with an incidence of 7 per 100 000 per year. However, these may be an underestimate of true figures, due to underdiagnosis of a disease which can remain asymptomatic.

Natural history, and complications of DCM

The clinical course is largely unpredictable in the individual patient and may depend on the underlying cause. In the absence of more reliable evidence, information gained from studies in the general systolic heart failure population is often extrapolated to the DCM population to predict outcome. Thus, factors such as degree of systolic function and presence of symptoms are thought to correlate with patient's risk of future adverse events. Long-term complications include pump failure, sudden death, arrhythmic events, and systemic embolism.

Approach to diagnosing DCM

The approach to the diagnosis of DCM depends on patient history, and clinical, echocardiographic, or cardiac MRI features of DCM or heart failure, or both. The diagnostic strategy is usually the same as for chronic heart failure (see Chapter 92). In addition, some specific diagnostic tests may be required to elicit the underlying cause of DCM and to tailor treatment accordingly.

Endomyocardial biopsy is recommended to further define the cause of the disease in those presenting with acute or fulminant heart failure of unknown aetiology and who deteriorate rapidly with ventricular arrhythmia and/or heart block, or in patients who are unresponsive to conventional heart failure therapy. In such cases, the histology of heart muscle can be clinically useful to distinguish between disease processes that need alternative treatment strategies, such as storage diseases, malignancies, sarcoidosis, and haemochromatosis. Confirmation of viral myocarditis is sometimes possible with endomyocardial biopsy (but not routinely recommended), as is the identification of virus-negative, immune-mediated myocarditis, which could result in additional treatment such as immunomodulation or immunosuppression therapies. The role of cardiac MRI as a non-invasive technique for the diagnosis of the cause of DCM is evolving rapidly. In particular, a midwall pattern of late gadolinium enhancement suggests DCM.

If the cause of DCM is not apparent, the following studies may be warranted, depending on the potential findings identified in the history and physical examination:

- thyroid function tests, particularly in patients over the age of 65 or in patients with atrial fibrillation
- uron studies (ferritin and total iron-binding capacity) to screen for hereditary haemochromatosis (the absence of other characteristic findings of haemochromatosis does not preclude the diagnosis)
- antinuclear antibody and other serologic tests for lupus
- viral serologies and antimyosin antibody if myocarditis is suspected
- evaluation for phaeochromocytoma
- thiamine, carnitine, and selenium levels

In confirmed familial DCM, screening of first-degree relatives should be considered (yield depending on the cause less than 60%).

Other diagnoses that should be considered in addition to DCM

Diagnosis of DCM requires exclusion of coronary artery disease, hypertension, valvular disease, and congenital heart diseases which are sufficient to explain the degree of left ventricular dilatation and systolic dysfunction. This is, however, often clinically challenging because of the high prevalence of such conditions in the general population.

'Gold-standard' diagnostic test for DCM

Diagnosis requires imaging (e.g. echocardiography, cardiac MRI) to show a dilated left ventricle with or without impaired systolic function.

Acceptable diagnostic alternatives to the gold-standard test for DCM

Any imaging modality that allows assessment of the size of the heart and its function can be considered as an alternative to the 'gold standard'.

Other relevant investigations for DCM

Diagnosis of DCM requires exclusion of other causes of heart failure, such as coronary artery disease, hypertension, valve disease, and congenital heart disease. Exclusion of coronary artery disease in particular may require a coronary angiography.

Prognosis for DCM, and how to estimate it

DCM is a heterogeneous condition, and the prognosis of those affected largely depends on the underlying cause of DCM. Prognostic tools developed for patients with acute or chronic heart failure may be useful in people with DCM.

Treatment of DCM, and its effectiveness

Since DCM accounts for only 10% of all heart failure population, patients with DCM have been naturally underrepresented in many heart failure trials. Current guidelines for treatment of people with systolic heart failure assume that evidence gained form trials conducted in the general heart failure population is similarly applicable to those with DCM. Based on current guidelines, treatment of symptomatic patients should follow the recommendations for patients presenting with acute or chronic heart failure. In brief, diuretics and vasodilators should be used to relieve symptoms in the acute phase. Inotropes and haemodynamic support with medical devices may be necessary in more severe cases presenting with severe hypotension and signs of organ hypoperfusion.

Medical therapy is the mainstay for the long-term therapy of DCM. Angiotensin-converting enzyme (ACE) inhibitors and beta blockers are routinely initiated and complemented with other drugs such as aldosterone antagonists, aldosterone-receptor antagonists, and digoxin. Medical devices, such as cardioverter defibrillators, and cardiac resynchronization therapy are recommended in subgroups of people with systolic heart failure. In people with the most severe symptomatic heart failure despite optimal medical and device therapy, cardiac transplantation (with or without bridging with ventricular assist devices) should be considered. In addition to these general heart failure therapies, treatment of the underlying causes of non-familial DCM can have some disease-modifying effect for certain conditions.

Hypertrophic cardiomyopathy

Definition of hypertrophic cardiomyopathy

Hypertrophic cardiomyopathy (HCM) is defined by increased ventricular wall thickness or mass in the absence of loading conditions (hypertension, valve disease) sufficient to cause the observed abnormality. This definition contrasts with previous definitions which required the absence of intramyocardial storage material as the cause of myocardial hypertrophy, and has the advantage of avoiding the conundrum of not being able to reliably exclude storage disorders in many patients, even with endomyocardial biopsy.

The distribution and severity of left ventricular hypertrophy can vary greatly. The major patterns include:

- asymmetrical septal hypertrophy (80%), with or without left ventricular outflow obstruction
- concentric hypertrophy, with maximal thickening at the level of papillary muscles (8%)
- apical hypertrophy

Aetiology of HCM

Many individuals have familial disease with an autosomal dominant pattern of inheritance (with incomplete penetrance) caused by mutations in genes that encode different proteins serving contractile, structural, and regulatory functions in the cardiac sarcomere. More than 400 mutations in 11 genes have been identified that are associated with HCM. The most common mutations are in the genes that encode beta-myosin heavy chain and cardiac myosin-binding protein C.

Typical symptoms of HCM, and less common symptoms

Most patients have no or only minor symptoms and are often diagnosed during family screening. Common symptoms include palpitations, dyspnoea, angina, and syncope or presyncope.

Demographics of HCM

Left ventricular hypertrophy in the absence of hypertension and valve disease occurs in approximately 1 in 500 in the general population. It affects men and women equally and occurs in many races and countries.

Natural history, and complications of HCM

The clinical course of HCM is variable. It can manifest clinically at any age, with many asymptomatic or mildly symptomatic patients having a normal life expectancy. Others develop progressive symptoms of heart failure despite medical therapy. The degree of hypertrophy can increase in adolescents and young adults but remains usually stable in older adults. Atrial fibrillation occurs in 10%–15% of patients. A small proportion of patients can develop left ventricular dilatation with reduced systolic function. The annual mortality rate is about 1% in adults, and 2% in children.

Approach to diagnosing HCM

Diagnosis is based on family history, physical examination, ECG, and echocardiography. Cardiac MRI is becoming a valuable tool to complement echocardiography. Alternative causes of left ventricular hypertrophy need be excluded. Genetic testing can be useful for confirming the diagnosis and guiding family screening.

Physical examination may be normal. The classic murmur of obstructive HCM is a harsh systolic murmur that increases in intensity with physical or pharmacologic manoeuvers that reduce afterload or preload, or increase ventricular contractility (e.g. the Valsalva manoeuver, or nitrate application).

ECG shows voltage criteria for left ventricular hypertrophy; prominent Q waves in inferior or precordial leads; left axis deviation; and left atrial enlargement. In apical HCM, deep T-wave inversions in precordial leads are often present.

Echocardiography shows left ventricular hypertrophy with a diastolic wall thickness of 15 mm or greater. Other findings include a septal-to-posterior wall ratio of 1.3 or more; a small left ventricular cavity; reduced septal motion and thickening; normal or increased motion of the posterior wall; systolic anterior motion of the mitral leaflets; mitral regurgitation; and partial midsystolic closure of the aortic valve, with coarse fluttering of the leaflets in late systole. In the setting of obstructive HCM, a resting gradient of more than 30 mm Hg and a provocable gradient of more than 50 mm Hg are present, with a late-peaking (dagger-shaped) Doppler signal. Tissue Doppler imaging can detect reduced early diastolic (E′) and systolic (S′) velocities of the myocardium.

Cardiac MRI allows a more accurate assessment of myocardial mass, regional hypertrophy, or wall motion abnormalities. Late gadolinium enhancement may be seen in a patchy intramyocardial distribution or, typically, at the junctions of the interventricular septum and right ventricular free wall.

Cardiac catheterization is usually reserved for assessment of coronary artery disease and assessment prior to surgical or interventional procedures. In the setting of obstructive HCM, there is typically a subaortic outflow gradient on catheter pullback, spike-and-dome pattern of aortic pressure tracing, elevated left atrial and left ventricular end-diastolic pressures and elevated pulmonary capillary wedge pressure. A post-extrasystolic pulse pressure typically increases as a result of increased dynamic obstruction (Brockenbrough sign).

Other diagnoses that should be considered in addition to HCM

Main alternative causes of left ventricular hypertrophy that need to be considered are hypertension, aortic stenosis, athlete's heart, and Fabry's disease.

Athlete's heart is a benign physiological condition caused by long-term athletic training. In athlete's heart, the hypertrophy is usually symmetric and rarely greater than 16 mm. In HCM the left ventricular end-diastolic dimension is usually less than 45 mm and shows signs of impaired relaxation and an enlarged left atrium. In addition, left ventricular hypertrophy does not regress with deconditioning.

Fabry's disease is a rare, multisystem, X-linked recessive glycolipid storage disease. Echocardiography and cardiac MRI can be used to differentiate between Fabry's and HCM, even without any other systemic involvement of the storage disease.

'Gold-standard' diagnostic test for HCM

The gold-standard diagnostic test for HCM is echocardiography.

Acceptable diagnostic alternatives to the gold-standard test for HCM

Cardiac MRI is often used to confirm diagnosis and rule out other causes.

Other relevant investigations for HCM

Screening of first-degree relatives of patients with HCM should be performed. This should include history, physical examination, ECG, and echocardiography. Genetic testing may also be useful in those from families with a known genetic mutation.

Prognosis for HCM, and how to estimate it

The prognosis of the majority of HCM patients is good. The major concern with the disease is sudden cardiac death. Risk factors for sudden cardiac death include:

- prior cardiac arrest or sustained ventricular tachycardia
- family history of sudden cardiac death
- unexplained syncope
- hypotensive blood pressure response to exercise
- nonsustatained ventricular tachycardia on ambulatory monitoring
- identification of a high-risk mutant gene
- massive hypertrophy, with a wall thickness of 30 mm or greater

Outflow tract obstruction per se is not a strong predictor of sudden cardiac death.

Treatment of HCM, and its effectiveness

Asymptomatic patients usually do not require pharmacological therapy. Beta blockers, verapamil, and disopyramide are used to reduce left ventricular contractility, relieve outflow tract obstruction, and improve symptoms. Patients with refractory symptoms due to left ventricular outflow obstruction should be considered for septal myectomy (Morrow procedure) or alcohol septal ablation. An implantable cardioverter defibrillator (ICD) is recommended for survivors of cardiac arrest or sustained ventricular tachycardia and for high-risk patients, who are defined as having two or more of the major risk factors for sudden cardiac death. Dual-chamber pacing has not been shown to be effective in improving symptoms.

Restrictive cardiomyopathy

Definition of restrictive cardiomyopathy

Restrictive cardiomyopathy (RCM) is defined as non-dilated ventricles (one or both) showing a restrictive physiology, that is, a pattern of ventricular filling in which increased stiffness of the myocardium causes ventricular pressure to rise precipitously with only small increases in volume. Hypertrophy is typically absent, although infiltrative and storage diseases such as amyloidosis may cause an increase in left ventricular wall thickness. Systolic function was historically defined as being normal, but many patients have some degree of systolic dysfunction.

Aetiology of RCM

Approximately half of RCM cases are idiopathic without specific histological findings. Identifiable causes are usually due to systemic disorders, but familial causes have been described. Most common causes include:

- amyloidosis
- sarcoidosis
- endomyocardial fibrosis without eosinophilia
- radiation
- chemotherapy such as anthracycline

    Less common causes include:

- haemochromatosis
- Fabry's disease
- carcinoid
- scleromderma
- pseudoxanthoma elasticum
- endomyocardial fibrosis with eosinophilia (Löffler's syndrome)
- metastatic cancer
- advanced stages of HCM, DCM
- familial, mostly autosomal dominant (e.g. mutations in the troponin I gene)

    By definition, restrictive pathologies caused by ischaemic heart disease, valvular disease, or hypertension do not classify as RCM.

Typical symptoms of RCM, and less common symptoms

Most patients present with signs of heart failure (e.g. dyspnoea, peripheral oedema, palpitations, fatigue, weakness, reduced exercise tolerance, hepatosplenomegaly, and ascites). Syncope or presyncope due to orthostatic hypotension or bradycardic events due to conduction disorders are less common. Thromboembolic complications may be the initial presentation.

Demographics of RCM

The exact prevalence of RCM is unknown, but it is probably the least common type of cardiomyopathy in Europe and North America. RCM due to endomyocardial fibrosis, however, is a common cause of heart failure and death in tropical regions, including parts of Africa, Central and South America, India, and other parts of Asia. Idiopathic

RCM is commonly diagnosed in elderly adults and is more common in older women than men.

Natural history, and complications of RCM

The natural history of the RCM is variable and depends on the underlying cause. Most types of RCM are associated with chronic heart failure symptoms and thromboembolic events which determine patient's prognosis.

Approach to diagnosing RCM

Diagnosis is based on clinical findings of heart failure, with supporting evidence from ECG and chest X-ray. Echocardiography is crucial to identify the restrictive physiology. Cardiac catheterization, cardiac MRI, and endomyocardial biopsy can help in confirming the diagnosis and identifying the underlying cause.

ECG

An ECG will show large P waves indicating biatrial enlargement, with unspecific STsegment and T-wave abnormalities. Atrial fibrillation is common. Even in the presence of myocardial thickening (e.g. in amyloidosis), QRS voltage is normal or even low. Infiltration of the conductive system may lead to a prolonged PR interval (or high-degree heart blocks).

Chest X-ray

A chest X-ray usually shows a normal-sized heart with enlarged atria and variable degrees of pulmonary congestion.

Echocardiography

On echocardiography, there is typically biatrial enlargement, with normal-sized ventricles and normal or slightly impaired systolic function. Thickening of the myocardium and valves may be present. The myocardium may show a 'granular' appearance. The endocardium may be involved, showing extensive thrombi in the ventricular apices (common in endomyocardial fibrosis without eosinophilia). Mild pericardial effusion may be present (e.g. in amyloidosis).

Restrictive physiology is assessed by mitral inflow Doppler velocities, tissue Doppler, and speckle tracking. Severe diastolic dysfunction is suggested by a high early diastolic left ventricular filling wave (E wave) with a short deceleration time, and a low late-diastolic filling wave (A wave, if the patient is in sinus rhythm), and decreased isovolumic

relaxation time. Tissue Doppler velocities of the mitral annulus (E′ wave) are reduced (in both systole and diastole), resulting in a high E/E′ ratio. Speckle tracking is less prone to errors and allows a more reliable assessment of filling pattern.

Cardiac catheterization

Cardiac catherization will show a square-root (or dip-plateau) sign, which is characterized by an early diastolic dip quickly followed by a plateau. Usually, the diastolic pressure of both ventricles is elevated, with the highest plateau being in the left ventricle.

Patients may show a spectrum of ventricular filling abnormalities, from a more advanced typical restrictive pattern to a milder form of abnormal relaxation with long isovolumic relaxation time. Measurement of restriction during catheterization and Doppler measures will vary according to the volume status, heart rate, and rhythm.

Other diagnoses that should be considered in addition to RCM

The main differential diagnosis of RCM is constrictive pericarditis (see Table 106.1).

Endomyocardial biopsy or response to pericardiectomy may reveal the definite pathology in some patients.

'Gold-standard' diagnostic test for RCM

Endomyocardial biopsy may show distinctive features of the underlying condition. However, this is often not necessary and can only be considered complementary once restrictive physiology is confirmed.

Acceptable diagnostic alternatives to the gold-standard test for RCM

Acceptable diagnostic alternatives to the gold-standard test for RCM are echocardiography and MRI.

Other relevant investigations for RCM

ECG, cardiac catheterization, CT, and blood investigations (e.g. BNP) can contribute to the diagnostic strategy.

Prognosis for RCM, and how to estimate it

The epidemiology of RCM, as it is a heterogeneous condition, is not well described. In idiopathic RCM, mortality without cardiac

Table 106.1 Features differentiating restrictive cardiomyopathy from constrictive pericarditis

Feature	Favours restrictive cardiomyopathy	Favours constrictive pericarditis
History	Amylodiosis Sarcoidosis	Previous pericarditis Cardiac surgery Uraemia TB Malignancy
Clinical examination	Kussmaul's sign and pulsus pardoxus absent	Kussmaul's sign and pulsus pardoxus present
ECG	Normal or low voltage Conduction abnormalities Pathological Q-waves	Low voltage
Echocardiography	Granular appearance of the myocardium Normal or low normal systolic function No significant respiratory variation of the mitral Doppler velocities Reduced tissue Doppler of mitral annulus (E′ velocity <8 cm/s).	Pericardial thickening (>5 mm) Normal or supranormal systolic function Increased myocardial contractility on tissue Doppler (E′ velocity >12 cm/s) and speckle tracking Paradoxical septal movement, with a D-shaped left ventricle during inspiration
CT	Normal pericardium Ventricular thrombus	Pericardial thickening (>5 mm) or calcification
MRI	Normal pericardium Ventricular thrombus Myocardial tissue characterization consistent with underlying disease (e.g. late gadolinium enhancement)	Pericardial thickening Paradoxical septal movement, with a D-shaped left ventricle during inspiration
Cardiac catheterization	Left ventricular filling pressures are >5–7 mm Hg higher than right ventricular ones, with no significant respiratory variation	Equilibration of filling pressures (mainly during inspiration)
Plasma BNP level	Significantly elevated	Usually normal

transplantation is >50% after manifestation of symptoms. Embolic stroke is a common complication as a consequence of large atria and atrial fibrillation.

Treatment of RCM, and its effectiveness

There is no established treatment for RCM. Treatment of the underlying causes is described elsewhere. Symptomatic treatment is achieved with careful dosing of diuretics to avoid hypovolaemia, and rate control with beta blockers, calcium-channel antagonists, or digoxin. Prophylactic anticoagulant therapy is recommended in RCM patients with enlarged atria even before supraventricular tachycardia has developed. Cardiac transplantation in children with idiopathic RCM should be considered.

Arrhythmogenic right ventricular cardiomyopathy

Arrhythmogenic right ventricular cardiomyopathy, also called arrhythmogenic right ventricular dysplasia, is characterized by a scarred appearance with fibrous or fibrofatty replacement of the right ventricular myocardium and which can also involve the left ventricle. It should be considered in patients who present with ventricular tachycardia with a left branch bundle block configuration in the absence of apparent heart disease. However, ECG can be normal in early years of manifestation. Detailed diagnostic criteria based on ECG, echocardiography, cardiac MRI, family history, and endomyocardial biopsy have been proposed (Marcus et al., 2010) and should be used for diagnosis.

Unclassified cardiomyopathies

Takotsubo cardiomyopathy

Takotsubo, or stress-induced, cardiomyopathy is an increasingly reported diagnosis which is characterized by transient, regional, left ventricular dysfunction in the absence of significant coronary artery disease. It presents usually with an acute coronary syndrome. Pheochromocytoma and myocarditis need to be ruled out. In addition, the absence of left ventricular function recovery after 4 weeks makes the diagnosis unlikely.

Left ventricular non-compaction

Left ventricular non-compaction (LVNC) is a rare type of cardiomyopathy which manifests with heart failure, atrial and ventricular arrhythmias, and thromboembolic events. It is usually characterized by an altered myocardial wall with prominent trabeculae and deep intertrabecular recesses, resulting in thickened myocardium with two layers consisting of compacted and noncompacted myocardium, respectively. The diagnosis of LVNC is usually established by echocardiography. Cardiac MRI, CT, and left ventriculography are other imaging modalities that may be diagnostic or raise the initial clinical suspicion. The differential diagnosis of LVNC includes dilated cardiomyopathy, hypertensive heart disease, apical hypertrophic cardiomyopathy, infiltrative cardiomyopathy, and eosinophilic endomyocardial disease.

Channelopathies

Channelopathies are a group of genetic disorders that are caused by defects in the movement of ions (e.g. sodium, potassium, and calcium) across the cardiac cell membrane. The main types of channelopathies are long-QT syndrome (ECG: prolonged QT interval, and T-wave abnormalities), Brugada syndrome (ECG: ST-segment elevation in Leads V1–V3, and a right bundle branch block pattern in the right precordial leads), and catecholaminergic polymorphic ventricular tachycardia (ECG: premature ventricular contractions, and non-sustained polymorphic VT). Channelopathies usually present with syncope, arrhythmia, and sudden death.

Further Reading

Bozkurt B, Colvin M, Cook J, et al. Current diagnostic and treatment strategies for specific dilated cardiomyopathies. A Scientific Statement From the American Heart Association. *Circulation* 2016; 134: e1–e68.

Corrado D, Wichter T, Link MS, et al. Treatment of arrhythmogenic right ventricular cardiomyopathy/dysplasia: An International Task Force Consensus Statement. *Circulation* 2015; 132: 441–53.

Garcia M. Constrictive pericarditis versus restrictive cardiomyopathy? *J Am Coll Cardiol* 2016; 67: 2061–76.

Gati S, Rajani R, Carr-White GS, and Chambers JB. Adult left ventricular noncompaction: Reappraisal of current diagnostic imaging modalities. *JACC Cardiovasc Imaging* 2014; 7: 1266–75.

Lyon AR, Bossone E, Schneider B, et al. Current state of knowledge on Takotsubo syndrome: A Position Statement from the Taskforce on Takotsubo Syndrome of the Heart Failure Association of the European Society of Cardiology. *Eur J Heart Fail* 2016; 18: 8–27.

Priori SG, Wilde AA, Horie M, et al. HRS/EHRA/APHRS Expert Consensus Statement on the diagnosis and management of patients with inherited primary arrhythmia syndromes. *Heart Rhythm* 2013; 10: 1932–63.

The Task Force for the Diagnosis and Management of Hypertrophic Cardiomyopathy of the European Society of Cardiology (ESC). 2014 ESC Guidelines on diagnosis and management of hypertrophic cardiomyopathy. *Eur Heart J* 2014; 35: 2733–79.

Myxoma

Definition of myxoma

Myxoma is the most common primary tumour of the heart in adults and constitutes about 40% of all cardiac tumours. About 75% –85% of myxomas occur in the left atrium, with another 15% –20% being located in the right atrium. Less than 10% arise in the left ventricle and right ventricle together. Myxomas are usually pedunculated and typically arise from the interatrial septum (and often in the fossa ovalis) via a stalk. Tumours vary widely in size, ranging from 1 to 15 cm in diameter.

Aetiology of myxoma

Myxoma is a tumour of primitive connective tissue, with a gelatinous consistency on histopathological examination. Most cases are sporadic, but about 10% are familial, with autosomal dominant inheritance. Although they are typically benign, local recurrence due to inadequate resection or malignant transformation has been reported.

Typical symptoms of myxoma, and less common symptoms

Symptoms depend on tumour location and are related to intermittent mechanical obstruction of the mitral (or tricuspid) valve, systemic emboli, or paraneoplastic effects. Hence, symptoms can include paroxysmal shortness of breath, cough, haemoptysis, fatigue, and stroke. About a third of patients report fever and weight loss.

Demographics of myxoma

Actual incidence is unknown, but in one study surgical incidence was 1 in 500 000 population per year. Myxomas usually occur between the third and sixth decades of life and are more common in women.

Natural history, and complications of myxoma

The natural history of the disease is not well understood, as most patients undergo surgical removal of the tumour after the initial diagnosis. Complications include stroke, sudden cardiac death, valvular complications, and infection.

Death is typically caused by coronary or systemic embolization, or by obstruction of blood flow at the mitral or tricuspid valve.

Approach to diagnosing myxoma

The approach to diagnosing myxoma includes the following investigations:

History: A positive family history may be present.
Physical examination: A characteristic diastolic 'tumour plop' may be audible.
Chest X-ray: This may reveal atrial calcification.
ECG: This will show left (or right) atrial enlargement.
Echocardiography: This will show a solitary, mostly atrial, tumour, which commonly has an irregular contour. Often a stalk is visible, arising from the interatrial septum.
MRI: Tissue characterization can help to differentiate myxomas from thrombus and lipomas.

Other diagnoses that should be considered aside from myxoma

Other diagnoses that should be considered aside from myxoma are other cardiac tumours, and thrombus. Associated valvular damage needs to be ruled out.

'Gold-standard' diagnostic test for myxoma

The gold-standard diagnostic test for myxoma is histopathology.

Acceptable diagnostic alternatives to the gold-standard test for myxoma

Acceptable diagnostic alternatives to the gold-standard test for myxoma are imaging with echocardiography, and tissue characterization with MRI.

Other relevant investigations for myxoma

Another relevant investigation for myxoma is the erythrocyte sedimentation rate, which may be elevated.

Prognosis of myxoma, and how to estimate it

Tools for the prediction of the risk of complications for myxoma are currently not available, but risk is likely to be related to tumour location, size, and shape. The major risks of left-sided myxomas are stroke and embolic events. Embolism occurs in about 30%–40% of patients, but this may be more common in polypoid than in round tumours (58% vs 0%).

Treatment of myxoma, and its effectiveness

Myxomas are usually removed surgically along with at least 5 mm of surrounding atrial septum. The septum is then repaired, using material from the pericardium. Conduction disorders and atrial arrhythmias may occur after the operation. Recurrences rate is about 5%, but can be about 30% in familial cases. Recurrence after 4 years is uncommon.

Pericardial malignancy

Definition of pericardial malignancy

Pericardial malignancy is defined as malignant involvement of the pericardium, as a primary tumour (less common) or as a secondary tumour which has spread from either a nearby or a distant focus of malignancy.

Aetiology of pericardial malignancy

Secondary tumours

Secondary tumours can involve the pericardium by contiguous extension from a mediastinal mass, nodular tumour deposits from haematogenous or lymphatic spread, or diffuse pericardial thickening from tumour infiltration (with or without effusion). Common causes include lung, breast, or oesophageal cancer, lymphoma, leukaemia, and Kaposi sarcoma. Melanomas have a very high propensity of metastasis to the myocardium (up to 65%).

Primary tumours (extremely rare)

In pericardial malignancy, the primary tumours, which are extremely rare, are mesotheliomas, teratomas, and paragangliomas.

Typical symptoms of pericardial malignancy, and less common symptoms

Pericardial malignancy may be asymptomatic and incidentally diagnosed, or present with shortness of breath, chest pain, reduced exercise tolerance, and/or oedema as the manifestation of pericarditis; pericardial effusion; cardiac tamponade; and/or pericardial constriction.

Demographics of pericardial malignancy

Malignant involvement of the pericardium is detected in 1%–20% of cases in autopsy studies, with similar rates in men and women. It can occur at any age.

Natural history, and complications of pericardial malignancy

The natural history of pericardial malignancy is usually determined by the underlying malignancy, but people with pericardial involvement have a more extensive disease and, hence, a worse prognosis, compared to those without pericardial involvement. Pericardial tamponade may add to the mortality unless promptly detected and appropriately treated.

Approach to diagnosing pericardial malignancy

The diagnostic approach for pericardial malignancy is the same as for the diagnosis of pericardial diseases and includes ECG, echocardiography and other imaging studies, and diagnostic pericardiocentesis with cytology testing. In addition, pericardial biopsy may be necessary. Pericardial effusion as the initial presenting sign of a previously undiagnosed cancer is uncommon. Screening for occult malignancy is recommended for patients who have persistent pericarditis that is unresponsive to anti-inflammatory therapy, and those who present with a new large pericardial effusion or cardiac tamponade.

Other diagnoses that should be considered aside from pericardial malignancy

In addition to pericardial malignancy, alternative causes of pericardial disease should be considered.

'Gold-standard' diagnostic test for pericardial malignancy

The gold-standard diagnostic tests for pericardial malignancy are cytology and histology.

Acceptable diagnostic alternatives to the gold-standard test for pericardial malignancy

For pericardial malignancy, an acceptable diagnostic alternative to cytology and histology is non-invasive imaging, which may guide diagnostic strategy.

Other relevant investigations for pericardial malignancy

Other relevant investigations for pericardial malignancy include CT thorax and PET scan.

Prognosis of pericardial malignancy, and how to estimate it

The life expectancy of patients with symptomatic malignant pericardial effusion is, on average, only 2–4 months. However, the prognosis may be better in certain subsets of patients, such as those with an absence of malignant cells in the pericardium, those with haematologic rather than solid tumours, and those whose primary malignancy is otherwise well controlled.

Treatment of pericardial malignancy, and its effectiveness

In pericardial malignancy, individualized treatment, requiring a detailed consideration of patient's condition and the prognosis of the underlying malignancy, is mandatory. Components of management may include:

- pericardiocentesis, for symptom relief
- prevention of effusion reaccumulation, via pericardial ballooning, pericardial sclerosis, or surgical window pericardiectomy
- pericardiectomy, for management of pericardial constriction
- treatment of the underlying malignancy

Myocardial malignancy

Definition of myocardial malignancy

Myocardial malignancy is defined as the malignant involvement of the myocardium as the result of a primary cardiac tumour (less common) or secondary to spread from a nearby or distant focus of malignancy. Secondary malignancies are not discussed further here (see 'Pericardial malignancy').

Aetiology of myocardial malignancy

Primary malignancies in myocardial malignancy (very rare) are mainly caused by sarcomas (angiosarcoma, rhabdomyosarcoma, leiomyosarcoma, and fibrosarcoma).

Typical symptoms of myocardial malignancy, and less common symptoms

In addition to pericardial involvement (see 'Pericardial malignancy'), the symptoms of myocardial malignancy are related to local obstruction, embolic complications, and rhythm abnormalities. About 75% of primary myocardial tumours have already metastasized at the time of initial diagnosis. Hence, symptoms related to distal metastases may lead to the initial diagnosis.

Demographics of myocardial malignancy

Cardiac sarcomas are extremely rare and, for most types, only isolated case reports have been described.

Natural history, and complications of myocardial malignancy

Sarcomas proliferate rapidly, and cause death through widespread infiltration of the myocardium, obstruction of blood flow through the heart, and/or distant metastases.

Approach to diagnosing myocardial malignancy

The diagnostic approach is based on echocardiography, MRI, and CT, with or without biopsy.

Other diagnoses that should be considered aside from myocardial malignancy

Other diagnoses that should be considered aside from myocardial malignancy are benign tumours, and thrombus

'Gold-standard' diagnostic test for myocardial malignancy

The gold-standard diagnostic test for myocardial malignancy is histopathology.

Acceptable diagnostic alternatives to the gold-standard test for myocardial malignancy

Non-invasive imaging tests are acceptable diagnostic alternatives to histopathology for diagnosing myocardial malignancy.

Other relevant investigations for myocardial malignancy

Other relevant investigations for myocardial malignancy are CT and PET scan.

Prognosis of myocardial malignancy, and how to estimate it

The prognosis of sarcomas is very poor and is not much affected by currently available treatment.

Treatment of myocardial malignancy, and its effectiveness

In the treatment of myocardial malignancy, surgery with or without chemotherapy is often attempted, but the mean survival of treated patients only ranges from 6 to 12 months. Cardiac transplantation and autotransplantation (transplantation after tumour resection ex vivo and reconstruction of the heart) are alternative measures with little evidence for their efficacy.

Cancer treatment and the heart

Radiation therapy is a vital component of modern cancer management. During the course of their treatment, approximately two-thirds of cancer patients receive radiotherapy with either curative or palliative intent. However, radiotherapy may be associated with some unintended harms to the cardiovascular system. This section focuses on cardiac complications of radiotherapy. The effect of chemotherapy on the heart is discussed in Chapter 122.

A few decades ago, the cardiovascular system was considered to be relatively resistant to radiation-induced injury, and little consideration was given to avoidance of the heart during thoracic radiotherapy. During the 1960s, the first reports of patients treated with radiotherapy for Hodgkin's lymphoma, including doses of >30 Gy to the heart, established radiation-induced cardiovascular disease as a distinct entity. However, it was still thought that cardiovascular disease was not induced by cardiac radiation doses of <30 Gy. Over the last 10 years, new evidence from several independent sources has revealed that cardiovascular risks are also increased by much lower doses of radiation. Although modern radiotherapy techniques undoubtedly deliver lower doses to normal tissues, such as the heart, than in previous decades, some degree of cardiovascular radiation exposure remains inevitable.

The pathology of radiation-induced injury to the human cardiovascular system is non-specific to radiation. Irradiation of a substantial volume of the heart to a sufficiently high dose can damage virtually any component of the heart, including the pericardium, myocardium, heart valves, coronary arteries, capillaries, and conducting system. Therefore, radiotherapy can increase the risk of a variety of heart conditions, such as coronary artery disease, pericarditis, restrictive or dilative cardiomyopathy, valvular conditions, and conduction disorders. In modern practice, the majority of these diseases are rarely seen in the first few years following exposure, and usually occur after a latency of many years. Subclinical effects may be detected earlier, but the proportion of cases which progress to clinical disease, and the rate of disease progression, are largely unknown. The incidence that may occur in the future as a result of modern radiation therapy is therefore difficult to predict, particularly as the doses and techniques of radiotherapy have altered substantially over the last half century, and due to a lack of validated dose-response relationships on which to base such predictions. Reduction of cardiac doses of radiotherapy to a minimum is therefore recommended by many experts. Whether treatment with established therapies such as blood pressure lowering or LDL lowering can reduce the risk of radiation-induced heart disease is unknown.

Further Reading

Jain S, Maleszewski JJ, Stephenson CR, et al. Current diagnosis and management of cardiac myxomas. *Expert Rev Cardiovasc Ther* 2015; 13: 369–75.

Maleszewski JJ, Anavekar NS, Moynihan TJ, et al. Pathology, imaging, and treatment of cardiac tumours. *Nat Rev Cardiol* 2017; 14: 536–49.

Mankad R and Herrmann J. Cardiac tumors: echo assessment. *Echo Res Pract* 2016; 3: R65–R77.

The Task Force for the diagnosis and management of pericardial diseases of the European Society of Cardiology (ESC). 2015 ESC Guidelines for the diagnosis and management of pericardial diseases. *Eur Heart J* 2015; 36: 2921–64.

Zamorano JL, Lancellotti P, Muñoz DR et al. 2016 ESC Position Paper on cancer treatments and cardiovascular toxicity developed under the auspices of the ESC Committee for Practice Guidelines: The Task Force for cancer treatments and cardiovascular toxicity of the European Society of Cardiology (ESC). *Eur Heart J* 2016; 37: 2768–801.

108 Cardiac infection

Cheerag Shirodaria and Jim Newton

Endocarditis

Definition of the disease

Endocarditis is inflammation of the endocardium, and is typically infection of valve tissue, most commonly the aortic or mitral valves. Infective endocarditis (IE) is caused by bacterial infection but there are other rare varieties such as fungal and non-IE (in connective tissue disease and malignancy).

Typical symptoms of endocarditis, and less common symptoms

A classical patient with endocarditis will present with chronic fever, malaise, anorexia, and symptoms of heart failure due to progressive valve destruction and regurgitation, often with chronic vasculitic phenomena due to peripheral emboli and immune activation. Alternatively, patients can present with a very brief history of fever and rapid onset of fulminant heart failure due to acute aortic or mitral regurgitation, usually due to staphylococcal infection.

While fever is almost universal in endocarditis, the associated symptoms are varied, and patients can present in numerous ways to a wide range of specialities, such as:

- Neurology (for stroke due to embolic infarction, or intracranial haemorrhage)
- Orthopaedics (for back pain due to discitis)
- Haematology (for chronic anaemia, splenomegaly, lymphadenopathy)
- Nephrology (for renal dysfunction, glomerulonephritis)
- Rheumatology (for vasculitis, arthropathy)
- Elderly care (for confusion, weight loss)
- Ophthalmology (for visual field loss, retinitis, ophthalmitis)

Demographics and aetiology of endocarditis

IE is more common in men, and over half of all cases occur in patients over the age of 60. Most patients who develop IE have underlying acquired or congenital structural heart disease, although endocarditis can occur in completely normal hearts. Risk factors for IE include prosthetic valves, prior endocarditis, renal failure, intravenous catheter, or drug use.

In any patient with a prosthetic heart valve, there is an annual 1% risk of developing endocarditis, the risk being higher in the first year post surgery. High-risk congenital lesions include ventricular septal defects and aortic stenosis, with pulmonary stenosis being at low risk. Rheumatic heart disease has largely been eradicated from the developed world, but should always be considered, particularly in patients from areas where the disease remains endemic. Tricuspid or pulmonary valve endocarditis is usually related to intravenous drug use or the presence of a permanent pacemaker. Patients with chronic renal disease have an increased risk for developing endocarditis due to a higher incidence of calcific valvular heart disease, long-term venous access catheters and, in the case of transplant recipients, long-term immunosuppression.

In the developed world, staphylococcal endocarditis is more common than streptococcal disease, particularly in patients undergoing haemodialysis or with long-term venous catheters. Table 108.1 outlines the microbiological diagnosis of endocarditis.

Cases of endocarditis should be described according to the underlying aetiology, culture results, and treatment status:

- native valve or prosthetic valve
- left-sided or right-sided valve involvement
- device-related infection (e.g. pacemaker)
- community acquired or nosocomial
- active or treated
- relapse or reinfection
- culture positive or negative

Describing a case as 'culture-negative prosthetic aortic valve endocarditis' conveys important information and assists in multidisciplinary management.

Natural history of endocarditis

IE is often described as a subacute illness with a chronic presentation due to streptococcal infection; often, an acute presentation in an elderly patient with staphylococcal infection of a prosthetic valve or degenerative valve lesion is more common.

Presentation is vague with fever and weight loss, and endocarditis is often initially misdiagnosed as a viral illness. With a careful history and clinical examination, paying particular attention to the cardiovascular examination and the ECG, the diagnosis can be made earlier.

Complications of endocarditis

Three-quarters of patients with endocarditis will develop at least one complication during the course of the disease. The most common are heart failure, embolism, infection, renal complications, and iatrogenic complications.

Heart failure

One-third of patients develop heart failure, usually due to leaflet destruction and perforation leading to severe regurgitation. Rarely, physical obstruction of the valve orifice by a large vegetation can occur. Left ventricular damage following coronary obstruction by a large vegetation or a more diffuse septic myocarditis can further contribute to haemodynamic decline.

Embolism

Emboli are common and can be widespread, leading to a wide variety of clinical syndromes, including stroke, myocardial infarction, abscess formation, spinal cord involvement, and solid organ infarction. Right-sided endocarditis is associated with pulmonary embolism and, rarely, with systemic embolism in the presence of a right–left communication (e.g. patent foramen ovale).

Infection

Fever usually settles within a week of starting antibiotics. Persisting fever may suggest a resistant organism or an uncontrolled local infection (e.g. abscess formation), or may be a side effect of the antibiotics themselves. A thorough search for other sources of infection (e.g. infected venous catheters) should be carried out, and further blood cultures obtained. Uncontrolled local infection is most common with aortic valve involvement, and in prosthetic valve endocarditis (>50%). Rarely, mycotic aneurysms may form within the vascular tree and should be suspected in patients with any focal neurological deficit.

Renal complications

Acute renal failure is common and may be caused by acute glomerulonephritis due to immune complex deposition, renal infarction secondary to septic emboli, or the nephrotoxic effect of antibiotics such as aminoglycosides or high-dose penicillin.

Iatrogenic complications

The duration of antimicrobial therapy puts the patient at risk of a number of complications: antibiotic toxicity (e.g. ototoxicity with

Table 108.1 Microbiological diagnosis of endocarditis

Organism	Estimated incidence	Relevant clinical history	Blood cultures	Serology
Staphylococcus aureus	30% of community community-acquired 46% of hospital-acquired	IVDU/IV access devices	Usually positive	Under development (lipid S)
Coagulase-negative staphylococci	5% of native valve endocarditis	Vasectomy/angiography/haemodialysis IVDU	Usually positive	In progress
Viridans streptococci	Up to 58%	Dental abscess/poor oral hygiene	Positive, if no previous antibiotics	In progress
Streptococcus bovis	Up to 12%	Gastrointestinal malignancy/presumed normal heart valves/older patient population	Positive, if no previous antibiotics	None
HACEK	3%	Dental treatment/URTI/IVDU	Most positive in 6 days with high CO_2 concentrations	None
Fungal	Up to 10%	Prosthetic valves/IVDU/immunosuppression/long-term IV lines. Should be performed if multiple risk factors for fungal endocarditis	Filamentous fungi rarely positive, candida commonly positive	Fungal serology not validated for endocarditis
Enterococcus spp.	Up to 10%	Urinary catheter insertion/gastrointestinal malignancy	Positive, if no previous antibiotics	In progress
Brucella spp.	1–4%	Endemic area/contaminated milk consumption	Positive in 80%. May need prolonged incubation	Reference assay = tube agglutination

Coxiella burnetii (Q fever)	3–5%	Farming background/exposure to domestic ruminants/raw milk consumption/previous valvulopathy/endemic area	Rarely positive. Tissue cell culture reported as optimal method	• Major criteria for modified Duke criteria:
				  • Anti-phase 1 IgG >800 and IgA antibody >100 is highly sensitive
				  • Reference assay = microimmunofluorescence

Bartonella	Up to 3%	Homelessness/alcoholism/exposure to cats	Rarely positive	Reference assay = microimmunofluorescence
Legionella	<1%	• Usually an outbreak/institution • Role unclear for prosthetic valves/pneumonia	• Rarely positive IE. Urinary antigen. • Bronchial washings/sputum	• High antibody levels • Reference assay = microimmunofluorescence
Chlamydia	Unknown due to cross-reactivity with bartonella	• Pneumonia • Significance is controversial	Rarely positive. Needs tissue cell culture.	Cross-reaction with *Bartonella* spp. Reference assay = microimmunofluorescence

Abbreviations: IV, intravenous; IVDU, intravenous drug use; URTI, upper respiratory tract infection.

Reprinted from *Journal of Infection*, Volume 47, issue 1, R.W. Watkin, S. Lang, P.A. Lambert, W.A. Littler, T.S.J. Elliott, The microbial diagnosis of infective endocarditis, pp. 1-11, Copyright 2003, with permission from Elsevier.

gentamicin), infection of central venous catheters, and interactions with any oral anticoagulant drug therapy.

Approach to diagnosing endocarditis

Endocarditis is challenging to diagnose and easy to miss. It should be considered in any patient with a fever and no other obvious cause, and blood cultures (taken carefully to avoid contamination) are absolutely key to achieving a diagnosis. Even in acutely ill patients with sepsis and haemodynamic upset, it should be possible to take at least one peripheral blood culture before antibiotic therapy is administered.

One practical strategy is to define the likelihood of endocarditis by utilizing the Duke criteria. IE is probable if there are two major criteria present, or one major plus three minor criteria, or five minor criteria.

The major criteria are:

• positive blood culture with an organism typical for endocarditis
• echocardiographic abnormalities consistent with endocarditis

The minor criteria are:

• predisposing heart condition, or intravenous drug use
• temperature >38.0°C (100.4°F)
• vasculitic injury, such as arterial emboli, mycotic aneurysms
• conjunctival haemorrhage
• atypical positive blood cultures or positive antigens to organisms causing endocarditis
• abnormal echocardiographic findings but no definite endocardial involvement

Other diagnoses that should be considered aside from endocarditis

The list of potential differential diagnoses is large and, given the common finding of a murmur in elderly patients, many patients present with murmur and fever but do not have IE. It is important, however, to always consider the possibility and ensure blood cultures are taken. If fever persists despite antibiotic treatment, consider other sources of infection, either as an alternative diagnosis, or reflecting malignant spread from a cardiac lesion.

'Gold-standard' diagnostic test for endocarditis

The gold-standard diagnostic test for endocarditis is demonstration of vegetations or microorganisms histologically, but this is only practical if the patient is undergoing surgery.

Acceptable diagnostic alternatives to the gold-standard test for endocarditis

In clinical practice, the gold standard is a combination of positive blood cultures and echocardiographic evidence of vegetations. Transoesophageal echocardiography (TOE) is the preferred investigation, as it will identify vegetations in the majority of positive cases, or evidence of valve involvement. Given the invasive nature of TOE, transthoracic echocardiography (TTE) is usually performed first. TTE has reasonable sensitivity for IE, but it can underestimate the size of vegetations, or miss small vegetations (<3 mm). A normal TTE with no vegetations or valve regurgitation makes endocarditis unlikely, but frequently a TOE is required to fully exclude the diagnosis if there is high clinical suspicion.

Echocardiographic abnormalities typical for endocarditis include:

- vegetations: an oscillating intra-cardiac mass on valvular apparatus, in the path of regurgitant jets, or on implanted material in the absence of an alternative anatomic explanation
- abscess cavity or fistula formation
- new partial dehiscence of prosthetic valve
- new valvular regurgitation

All patients with suspected prosthetic valve endocarditis should undergo TOE examination, as the sensitivity of TTE is poor. A negative TOE is reassuring (sensitivity >90%) but a low threshold should be applied to rescanning if the clinical situation changes. For right-sided endocarditis (e.g. pacemaker, intravenous drug use), TTE and TOE are of comparable sensitivity and sensitivity. but both may be required for a full assessment.

Routine serial echocardiography is not recommended but, if there is treatment failure or there are new clinical findings, then repeat imaging is warranted. An increase in vegetation size, or development of an abscess, suggests failure of antimicrobial therapy and warrants consideration of surgical intervention.

Other relevant investigations for endocarditis

Three blood cultures from different sites should be taken, ideally 30 minutes apart, with further samples on subsequent days until a microbe is identified. Draw at least 5 ml for each blood culture bottle with a scrupulous sterile technique as this increases the likelihood of identifying a pathological microbe. Blood cultures can be taken at any time; taking them during a fever does not increase their sensitivity, as the bacteraemia in IE is continuous. Seek assistance from the local microbiologist for further advice on other specialist tests that may be appropriate.

Routine haematology and biochemistry may reveal elevated inflammatory markers (C-reactive protein, erythrocyte sedimentation rate, or white-cell count) and a normocytic anaemia. Baseline assessment of renal and liver function should be performed, to screen for complications of IE and for monitoring during antibiotic therapy.

Patients should have regular ECGs to monitor rhythm and any evidence of atrioventricular block (especially in aortic valve endocarditis), as this may indicate abscess formation and should prompt repeat echocardiography.

Prognosis of endocarditis, and how to estimate it

Estimating the prognosis of endocarditis is difficult, as patients with endocarditis make up a heterogeneous group and often have other comorbidities. Broadly speaking, inhospital mortality with IE is around 15%–20%, with 1-year mortality approaching 40%.

Predictors of higher mortality include increasing age, staphylococcal infection, prosthetic valve endocarditis, and the presence of heart failure. Staphylococcal and fungal infections are also associated with an increased embolic risk. Early surgical intervention is associated with lower mortality.

Treatment of endocarditis, and its effectiveness

Multidisciplinary management, with a team including a cardiologist, a cardiac surgeon, and a microbiologist, is the key to effective management of endocarditis (see Box 108.1).

Antibiotic therapy in endocarditis

Empirical antibiotic therapy (see Table 108.2) should be started early, after blood cultures have been taken. The choice of antibiotic depends on local policy, recent antibiotic exposure, and whether it is native endocarditis or prosthetic valve endocarditis. Once a microbe has been identified, narrow-spectrum antibiotics can be selected and these should continue for at least 6 weeks in prosthetic valve endocarditis, and for between 2 and 6 weeks in native valve endocarditis. Outpatient (or home) antibiotic therapy can be considered in stable patients after the first 2 weeks, if local facilities exist.

Box 108.1 Characteristics of the 'Endocarditis Team'

When to refer a patient with IE to an 'Endocarditis Team' in a reference centre

1. Patients with complicated IE (i.e. endocarditis with HF, abscess, or embolic or neurological complication or CHD), should be referred early and managed in a reference centre with immediate surgical facilities.
2. Patients with non-complicated IE can be initially managed in a non-reference centre, but with regular communication with the reference centre, consultations with the multidisciplinary 'Endocarditis Team', and, when needed, with external visit to the reference centre.

Characteristics of the reference centre

1. Immediate access to diagnostic procedures should be possible, including TTE, TOE, multislice CT, MRI, and nuclear imaging.
2. Immediate access to cardiac surgery should be possible during the early stage of the disease, particularly in case of complicated IE (HF, abscess, large vegetation, neurological, and embolic complications).
3. Several specialists should be present on site (the 'Endocarditis Team'), including at least cardiac surgeons, cardiologists, anaesthesiologists, ID specialists, microbiologists and, when available, specialists in valve diseases, CHD, pacemaker extraction, echocardiography and other cardiac imaging techniques, neurologists, and facilities for neurosurgery and interventional neuroradiology.

Role of the 'Endocarditis Team'

1. The 'Endocarditis Team' should have meetings on a regular basis in order to discuss cases, take surgical decisions, and define the type of follow-up.
2. The 'Endocarditis Team' chooses the type, duration, and mode of follow up of antibiotic therapy, according to a standardized protocol, following the current guidelines.
3. The 'Endocarditis Team' should participate in national or international registries, publicly report the mortality and morbidity of their centre, and be involved in a quality improvement programme, as well as in a patient education programme.
4. The follow-up should be organized on an outpatient visit basis at a frequency depending on the patient's clinical status (ideally at 1, 3, 6, and 12 months after hospital discharge, since the majority of events occur during this period).

Abbreviations: CHD, coronary heart disease; CT, computed tomography; HF, heart failure; ID, infectious disease; IE, infective endocarditis; MRI, magnetic resonance imaging; TOE, transoesophageal echocardiography; TTE, transthoracic echocardiography.

Reproduced with permission from Gilbert Habib, Patrizio Lancellotti, Manuel J. Antunes. Et al., 2015 ESC Guidelines for the management of infective endocarditis, *European Heart Journal*, Volume 36, Issue 44, pp.3075-3123, Copyright © 2015 Oxford University Press

Surgery in endocarditis

The timing of surgery in endocarditis can be difficult; the patients who are the most unwell, and are therefore at highest risk for surgery, may be the most likely to benefit. There are three principal indications for surgery in IE: heart failure, uncontrolled infection, and prevention of embolism.

Heart failure

Heart failure is the most common reason for surgical intervention in IE, whether it is due to acute valve incompetence, fistulae, or valve obstruction by vegetation. Intractable pulmonary oedema or cardiogenic shock is an indication for emergency surgery. If heart failure is less severe, a period of stabilization and intravenous antibiotics prior to surgery may be possible.

Uncontrolled infection

The indications for surgery in endocarditis with uncontrolled infection are as follows:

Ongoing systemic sepsis: If fever persists for more than 7 days despite appropriate antibiotic therapy, urgent surgery is indicated once

Table 108.2 Proposed antibiotic regimens for initial empirical treatment of infective endocarditis in acute severely ill patients (before pathogen identification)[a]

Antibiotic	Dosage and route	Class[b]	Level[c]	Comments
Community-acquired native valves or late prosthetic valves (≥12 months post surgery) endocarditis				
Ampicillin with	12 g/day IV in 4–6 doses			Patients with BCNIE should be treated in consultation with an ID specialist.
(Flu)cloxacillin or oxacillin with	12 g/day IV in 4–6 doses	IIa	C	
Gentamicin	3 mg/kg/day IV or IM in 1 dose			
Vancomycin with	30–60 mg/kg/day IV in 2–3 doses	IIb	C	For penicillin-allergic patients
Gentamicin	3 mg/kg/day IV or IM in 1 dose			
Early PVE (<12 months post surgery) or nosocomial and non-nosocomial healthcare associated endocarditis				
Vancomycin with	30 mg/kg/day IV in 2 doses			Rifampicin is only recommended for PVE and it should be started 3–5 days later than vancomycin and gentamicin has been suggested by some experts. In healthcare associated native valve endocarditis, some experts recommend in settings with a prevalence of MRSA infections >5% the combination of cloxacillin plus vancomycin until they have the final *S. aureus* identification
Gentamicin with	3 mg/kg/day IV or IM in 1 dose	IIb	C	
Rifampicin	900–1200 mg IV or orally in 2 or 3 divided doses			

Abbreviations: BCNIE, blood culture-negative infective endocarditis; ID, infectious disease; IM, intramuscular; IV, intravenous; PVE, prosthetic valve endocarditis.

[a]If initial blood cultures are negative and there is no clinical response, consider BCNIE aetiology and maybe surgery for molecular diagnosis and treatment, and extension of the antibiotic spectrum to blood culture-negative pathogens (doxycycline, quinolones) must be considered.

[b]Class of recommendation.

[c]Level of evidence.

Reproduced with permission from Gilbert Habib, Patrizio Lancellotti, Manuel J. Antunes. Et al., 2015 ESC Guidelines for the management of infective endocarditis, *European Heart Journal*, Volume 36, Issue 44, pp.3075-3123, Copyright © 2015 Oxford University Press

other potential sources of infection have been excluded (e.g. cerebral/renal/spinal abscess).

Uncontrolled local infection: An increase in the size of vegetations, or local abscess/fistula formation, is an indication for urgent surgery.

Resistant organisms: If the infection is likely to be difficult to treat (e.g. a fungal infection; infection from MRSA or Gram-negative organisms), early surgical intervention should be considered.

Prevention of embolism

The risk of embolism during endocarditis is highest earlier in the disease and during the first two weeks of antibiotic therapy. Large vegetations (>10 mm) are associated with a higher risk of embolism and early surgery may be appropriate.

Prevention of endocarditis

Antibiotic prophylaxis for patients at risk of IE, such as those with structural heart disease or prosthetic valves or grafts, has been a controversial area over the last few years. European and North American guidelines broadly agree that high-risk patients (e.g. patients with prosthetic heart valves or previous endocarditis) should have antibiotic prophylaxis for invasive respiratory, gastrointestinal, dental, and genitourinary procedures. However, current UK NICE guidelines do not recommend antibiotic prophylaxis at all, except in gastrointestinal or genitourinary procedures where there is suspected infection. An increasing number of patients with endocarditis have no previous cardiac disease, so identifying those at risk, and targeting antibiotic prophylaxis, can be very challenging. Emphasis on meticulous oral hygiene and regular dental review is important to reduce the incidence of endocarditis.

Acute rheumatic fever

Definition of acute rheumatic fever

Acute rheumatic fever is a disease that follows Group A streptococcal infection (usually presenting as pharyngitis) and develops into a syndrome affecting the joints, heart, skin, and brain.

Aetiology of acute rheumatic fever

The clinical manifestations of acute rheumatic fever are thought to be due to a phenomenon known as molecular mimicry. Following a streptococcal infection, antibodies generated against Group

A streptococcus cross-react with the myosin and membrane proteins in cardiac tissue, causing inflammation which can lead to pancarditis. A similar process is seen in joints, skin, and the brain.

Typical symptoms of acute rheumatic fever, and less common symptoms

For lists of the typical and the less common symptoms of acute rheumatic fever, see 'Approach to diagnosing rheumatic fever'.

Demographics of acute rheumatic fever

Although Group A streptococcal infection is common, acute rheumatic fever is rare in the developed world, partly due to improved living conditions and partly to the routine treatment of pharyngitis with antibiotics. Infection with Group A streptococcus remains a considerable problem in the developing world, resulting in half a million deaths from the infection itself and its sequelae (rheumatic heart disease, glomerulonephritis).

Natural history, and complications of acute rheumatic fever

Acute rheumatic fever presents with fever, myalgia, and arthralgia, which is usually preceded by streptococcal pharyngitis occurring approximately 2 weeks before any other symptoms.

Most patients will develop a carditis, which is often subclinical. Carditis is inflammation affecting all layers of the heart; the most common findings are pericarditis (causing chest pain and a pericardial rub), systolic dysfunction (caused by myocarditis), and mitral or aortic regurgitation. A large-joint polyarthritis is another common finding. Other, rare, findings are subcutaneous nodules (firm, painless nodules, <2 cm in diameter, found over tendons), and erythema marginatum.

Sydenham's chorea is a late manifestation which is seen in around a third of cases. It occurs around 3 months after initial infection, and is a movement disorder characterized by rapid, jerking movements of the limbs and face, associated with emotional instability.

A third of patients will develop chronic rheumatic heart disease. The mitral valve is most commonly affected; initial inflammation becomes a fibrotic process, resulting in the gradual fusion of the mitral valve commissures and shortening of the chordae tendineae. This leads to mitral stenosis.

CHAPTER 108 **Cardiac infection**

Approach to diagnosing acute rheumatic fever

Rheumatic fever is defined by the Jones criteria: a diagnosis is made when a patient has evidence of preceding Group A streptococcal infection, as well as two major, or one major and two minor, criteria:

The major criteria are:

- carditis
- migratory polyarthritis
- subcutaneous nodules
- erythema marginatum
- Sydenham's chorea

The minor criteria are:

- fever
- arthralgia
- elevated inflammatory markers (e.g. erythrocyte sedimentation rate (ESR), or C-reactive protein (CRP))
- leucocytosis
- evidence of heart block on ECG
- evidence of streptococcal infection (e.g. a positive anti-streptolysin O test)
- previous episode of rheumatic fever

Other diagnoses that should be considered aside from acute rheumatic fever

A post-streptococcal reactive arthritis (Reiter's syndrome) is the other main differential diagnosis for acute rheumatic fever, the main difference between the two diagnoses being that the former does not result in a carditis.

'Gold-standard' diagnostic test for acute rheumatic fever

There is no single diagnostic test for acute rheumatic fever, but evidence of Group A streptococcal infection can help to secure a diagnosis. Throat-swab culture may identify the pathogen but, as patients with acute rheumatic fever may present weeks after any pharyngitis has resolved, the culture may be negative. A test for antibodies to Group A streptococcus (e.g. anti-streptolysin O) is more reliable.

Acceptable diagnostic alternatives to the gold-standard test for acute rheumatic fever

Not all patients with acute rheumatic fever will demonstrate an elevated anti-streptolysin O level and, in patients where the clinical suspicion of acute rheumatic fever is high, testing for other streptococcal antibodies (such as anti-DNAse B) should be performed.

Other relevant investigations for acute rheumatic fever

Initial blood tests will demonstrate a leucocytosis with elevated CRP and ESR. The chest X-ray may be normal but, in fulminant disease, it may show cardiomegaly and evidence of pulmonary oedema. ECG may demonstrate A–V block or features consistent with pericarditis. Echocardiography will show evidence of systolic dysfunction and/or valve abnormalities (regurgitation in the acute phase, stenosis, or regurgitation chronically).

Treatment for acute rheumatic fever, and its effectiveness

The risk of developing acute rheumatic fever can be reduced by the prompt antibiotic treatment of Group A streptococcal pharyngitis. The treatment of acute rheumatic fever includes antibiotic therapy to eliminate Group A streptococcal carriage, high-dose aspirin for symptomatic management of arthritis, and, if heart failure is present, conventional medical heart failure therapy.

Patients who develop chronic rheumatic heart disease affecting the mitral valve are at high risk of developing atrial fibrillation and subsequent systemic thromboembolism and should therefore be followed up regularly.

Further Reading

The Task Force for the Management of Infective Endocarditis of the European Society of Cardiology (ESC). 2015 ESC Guidelines for the management of infective endocarditis. *Eur Heart J* 2015; 36, 3075–123 doi:10.1093/eurheartj/ehv319.

Watkins DA, Johnson CO, Colquhoun SM, et al. Global, regional, and national burden of rheumatic heart disease, 1990–2015. *N Engl J Med* 2017; 377: 713–22. doi: 10.1056/NEJMoa1603693

109 Pericardial disease

David Adlam

Definition of the disease

The pericardium forms a continuous sac around the heart, analogous to the pleura surrounding the lungs, and the peritoneum surrounding the abdominal viscera. Between the parietal and visceral layers of the serous pericardium is the pericardial space, which normally contains a small volume of pericardial fluid.

The clinical spectrum of pericardial diseases can be divided into:

- pericarditis, caused by acute inflammation
- pericardial effusion, or fluid accumulation in the pericardial space, which may lead to cardiac tamponade
- constrictive pericarditis, caused by chronic infiltration or inflammation leading to pericardial constriction

Aetiology of the disease

Pericardial inflammation has multiple causes. It can be caused by:

- infection (viral, bacterial, mycobacterial, or, rarely, fungal)
- inflammatory disease (connective tissue disorders, vasculitis)
- metabolic causes (uraemia, hypothyroidism)
- neoplasia (usually infiltrative)
- injury (due to trauma, cardiomyotomy, myocardial infarction, or acute dissection)
- other causes, including unknown causes (in the case of idiopathic pericardial inflammation), rare genetic syndromes, and, more commonly, drugs such as minocycline, which have side effects which can lead to serositis

An autoimmune process may be central to the pathophysiology of 'idiopathic' and, indeed, several other types of pericarditis (including post cardiomyotomy pericarditis, rheumatic pericarditis, and Dressler's syndrome). The nature of the ensuing clinical presentation depends on the cause and duration of the inflammatory process.

Typical symptoms of the disease, and less common symptoms

Symptoms of acute pericarditis

Acute pericarditis is common, accounting for 5%–10% of emergency admissions with chest pain syndromes. The predominant aetiology is viral or idiopathic. Presentation varies, but classically the pain is worse on inspiration and lying flat and is eased by sitting forwards. There may be associated coryzal symptoms and myalgia.

Symptoms of pericardial effusion

Pericardial effusions are often asymptomatic until the rate of fluid accumulation in the pericardial space exceeds the rate at which the pericardium can dilate and remodel. When this occurs, the pressure in the pericardial space rises. When pericardial pressure exceeds that within the cardiac chambers in diastole, cardiac chambers collapse, atrial and ventricular filling are impaired, and pericardial tamponade ensues. Presentation acutely is usually with dyspnoea and/or haemodynamic collapse. When fluid accumulates more gradually, a less acute presentation may occur with worsening effort dyspnoea and signs of right-sided heart failure.

Symptoms of constrictive pericarditis

Chronic constrictive pericarditis often presents insidiously with dyspnoea, oedema, abdominal distension, and ascites, or, rarely, a protein-losing enteropathy.

Natural history, and complications of the disease

Natural history, and complications, of acute pericarditis

Acute pericarditis is usually self-limiting. Reported recurrence rates depend on the population studied and disease definition. In the COPE study (Imazio et al., 2005), reported recurrence of symptoms was 22.5%. Serious sequelae such as multiple severe clinical relapses, pericardial tamponade, or constrictive pericarditis are rare.

Natural history, and complications, of pericardial effusion

Pericardial effusions causing tamponade are a medical emergency, requiring immediate drainage. Those not causing tamponade require careful serial imaging to exclude progression and risk of tamponade.

Natural history, and complications, of constrictive pericarditis

Constrictive pericarditis is progressive if untreated. Pericardectomy is the definitive treatment and, if successful, is associated with good long-term survival.

Approach to diagnosing the disease

Approach to diagnosing acute pericarditis

Acute pericarditis is a clinical diagnosis. Typical symptoms may be accompanied by fever, tachycardia, and, occasionally, a pericardial friction rub.

Approach to diagnosing pericardial effusion

Pericardial effusions causing tamponade may be suspected from the clinical findings. These are classically hypotension, a raised jugular venous pressure (JVP), and quiet heart sounds. The most sensitive reported clinical signs are raised JVP (76%), pulsus paradoxus (82%), tachycardia (77%), and tachypnoea (80%). Pulsus paradoxus, a condition in which the systolic blood pressure falls more than 10 mm Hg during inspiration, is reportedly the most specific clinical sign (80%).

Approach to diagnosing constrictive pericarditis

Constrictive pericarditis causes clinical findings of right-sided heart failure. There is a high venous pressure with rapid x and y descent (Kussmaul's sign of a rise in venous pressure with inspiration may be present), relative hypotension, pleural effusions, peripheral oedema, hepatic congestion, and even ascites. A pericardial knock in early diastole, reflecting abrupt cessation of ventricular filling, is a characteristic but rare finding.

Other diagnoses that should be considered

Other diagnoses that should be considered aside from acute pericarditis

Acute pericarditis has a broad differential diagnosis covering the causes of acute chest pain syndromes. Most importantly, acute coronary syndromes and acute pulmonary embolus must be excluded.

Other diagnoses that should be considered aside from pericardial effusion

Pericardial effusion should be considered in all new presentations of symptoms and signs of right-sided heart failure, especially where there is a history of malignancy. Echocardiographic diagnosis is usually straightforward, once the investigation has been requested.

Other diagnoses that should be considered aside from constrictive pericarditis

Constrictive pericarditis is usually a gradual process and frequently presents insidiously. The diagnosis should particularly be considered in patients presenting with features of right-sided heart failure or ascites, especially where there is a past history of cardiac surgery, tuberculosis, or pericardial effusion requiring drainage.

'Gold-standard' diagnostic test

'Gold-standard' diagnostic test for acute pericarditis

Acute pericarditis is a clinical diagnosis usually made via a combination of typical symptoms, ECG findings, and the exclusion of alternative differential diagnoses.

'Gold-standard' diagnostic test for pericardial effusion

Pericardial effusion and tamponade are usually diagnosed echocardiographically. Pericardial fluid is demonstrated as an echolucent pool (although an acute haemopericardium may be less lucent) surrounding the heart and must be carefully distinguished from a pleural effusion. The principle echocardiographic features of tamponade are chamber collapse (because of their differential diastolic pressures, in a global effusion, the right atrium and then the right ventricle collapse first, with the left ventricle most rarely affected).

'Gold-standard' diagnostic test for constrictive pericarditis

Constrictive pericarditis requires careful echocardiographic assessment, and often cardiac catheterization is needed for definitive diagnosis. Echocardiographic features are of biatrial dilation with normal systolic function. There may be a paradoxical septal movement or a wobble, and the inferior vena cava is dilated without dynamic change in dimensions with respiration. Doppler velocities across the mitral or the tricuspid valve show increased respiratory variation (>25%) with rapid deceleration of the E wave and an absent A wave. At cardiac catheterization, elevation and equalization of chamber end-diastolic pressures are seen, with typical 'dip-and-plateau' patterns.

Other relevant investigations

Other relevant investigations for acute pericarditis

Acute pericarditis is classically associated with ECG findings of widespread scalloped ST-segment elevation with PR depression, although less typical ST and T wave changes may occur. Inflammatory markers and the white-cell count are often elevated. A small increase in troponin is common, with larger elevations occurring when the inflammatory process extends into the myocardium (myopericarditis). There are currently no published data on the relative sensitivity and specificity of particular clinical or laboratory findings.

Other relevant investigations for pericardial effusion

Pericardial effusions may show small complexes on the ECG or rarely electrical alternans where QRS voltage varies on a beat-to-beat basis, although neither finding has sufficient sensitivity and specificity to aid diagnosis. A globular appearance of the heart on chest X-ray carries a reported 89% sensitivity. Assessment of a fluid sample may provide useful diagnostic material to identify the cause of the effusion (for example in malignancy or tuberculous effusions).

Other relevant investigations for pericardial effusion

Constrictive pericarditis may have abnormal chest X-ray and CT imaging, with thickening and/or calcification of the pericardium.

Treatment and its effectiveness

Specific treatments of pericardial inflammation and its sequelae depend on the underlying cause.

Treatment of acute pericarditis

Acute pericarditis can usually be safely treated in an outpatient setting, providing there is no significant pericardial effusion at presentation. Treatment is with NSAIDs such as ibuprofen (300–800 mg, 6–8 hourly) or aspirin (600–650mg, 6 hourly). There are no randomized data demonstrating either the effect or the optimal duration of therapy with NSAIDs. Treatment is usually continued until resolution of symptoms and markers of inflammation. The COPE study (Imazio et al., 2005) demonstrated that the addition of colchicines to NSAIDs leads to more rapid symptom resolution and reduced symptom recurrence. COPE also showed increased recurrence in patients treated with steroids, although this was from a secondary multivariate analysis. Steroids are therefore usually reserved for patients with autoimmune or connective tissue disorders and pericarditis. The data on steroids in tuberculous pericarditis have not demonstrated clear benefit.

Treatment of pericardial effusion

Pericardial effusions causing tamponade require immediate drainage. This is usually performed percutaneously via an apical or subcostal route. Complications are rare (4.7% in a large series), but recurrence is common (up to 27% reported), so follow-up with serial echocardiography is recommended. Outcome relates to the underlying condition, with malignant effusions having a universally poor survival (reported median, 134 days). Recurrent effusions may require a surgical pericardial window or balloon fenestration.

Treatment of constrictive pericarditis

Constrictive pericarditis requires operative pericardectomy. Operative mortality is reported at 6%–12% but, if successful, a good long-term outcome can be expected.

Further Reading

Imazio M, Gaita F, and LeWinter M. Evaluation and treatment of pericarditis: A systematic review *JAMA* 2015; 314: 1498–506.

Ristić AD, Imazio M, Adler Y, et al. Triage strategy for urgent management of cardiac tamponade: a position statement of the European Society of Cardiology Working Group on Myocardial and Pericardial Diseases. *Eur Heart J* 2014; 35: 2279–84. doi:10.1093/eurheartj/ehu217

The Task Force for the diagnosis and management of pericardial diseases of the European Society of Cardiology (ESC). 2015 ESC Guidelines for the diagnosis and management of pericardial diseases. http://www.escardio.org/static_file/Escardio/Guidelines/Publications/PERICA/2015%20Percardial%20Web%20Addenda-ehv318.pdf.

CHAPTER 109 **Pericardial disease**

110 Extrasystoles

Moutaz El-Kadri and George Hart

Definition

An extrasystole is a cardiac electrical impulse (often premature) that is not part of the normal heart rhythm. Extrasystoles most frequently arise from the ventricles and are then called ventricular extrasystoles, or premature ventricular complexes. Less often they originate from the atria, the atrioventricular junction, or rarely from the sinus node—these are termed supraventricular extrasystoles. The term 'bigeminy' refers to an extrasystole every second beat, and 'trigeminy', every third beat. Two successive extrasystoles are called a 'couplet'; three are called a 'triplet'. Extrasystoles with varying morphology are described as 'polymorphic' or 'multifocal', whereas those maintaining the same morphology are termed 'unifocal'.

Aetiology and demographics

Extrasystoles are common in all age groups, including in people with normal hearts, but may also be a marker of cardiac disease. The quoted prevalence of extrasystoles varies greatly, being sometimes as high as 80%, depending on study design. In general, the frequency of ectopy increases with age and is commoner in males. Many factors can provoke extrasystoles, such as:

- cardiovascular factors:
  - acute ischaemia
  - heart failure
  - hypertension (particularly with left ventricular hypertrophy)
  - cardiomyopathies (dilated, hypertrophic, or arrhythmogenic right ventricular)
  - myocarditis
  - cardiac contusion
  - congenital heart disease
  - cardiac channelopathies
  - mitral valve prolapse
- respiratory factors:
  - hypoxia
  - hypercapnoea
  - COPD (mainly supraventricular extrasystoles)
- drugs:
  - digoxin
  - aminophylline
  - β-2 agonists
  - alcohol
  - caffeine
  - tobacco
  - cocaine
- biochemical factors:
  - hypokalaemia
  - hypomagnesaemia
  - hypercalcaemia
- other factors:
  - anxiety
  - exhaustion
  - sleep deprivation

Three mechanisms underlie extrasystoles. Re-entry is responsible for ectopy in many patients with structural heart disease, such as post-infarction scarring; enhanced automaticity is probably the underlying mechanism in acute ischaemia and electrolyte imbalance; and triggered activity is prominent in drug toxicity (digitalis), ischaemia (reperfusion arrhythmias), and right ventricular outflow tract (RVOT) ectopy.

Typical symptoms of the disease

Most extrasystoles are asymptomatic, and are found incidentally during ECG monitoring. When symptomatic, they typically produce palpitations, often characterized as extra or skipped beats (due to the compensatory pause which occurs after an ectopic beat). Less commonly, patients can experience light-headedness, presyncope, and chest or neck discomfort. When associated with severe left ventricular dysfunction or profound sinus bradycardia, frequent extrasystoles can give rise to symptoms of fatigue or hypotension.

Natural history of the disease

Extrasystoles generally become more prevalent with advancing age. In most cases, they produce few or no symptoms and, in these settings, reassurance is probably the best treatment. There is no evidence that suppressing ectopic beats can reduce the risk of more serious arrhythmias or improve overall prognosis, even in patients with heart disease. The Cardiac Arrhythmia Suppression Trial showed that treatment with Class Ic antiarrhythmic agents to suppress ventricular extrasystoles in patients who had sustained myocardial infarction actually increased overall mortality (Echt et al., 1991).

Symptoms may develop if extrasystoles become frequent, sometimes due to provoking factors such as stress, drugs, or electrolyte imbalance. In these circumstances, treatment of the offending cause may be all that is needed to achieve a substantial improvement in symptoms.

Complications

Sustained ventricular arrhythmias such as ventricular tachycardia or ventricular fibrillation can sometimes be triggered by ventricular extrasystoles. This is more likely to occur in the presence of underlying heart disease (e.g. acute myocardial infarction), particularly if ventricular extrasystoles are frequent (e.g. >10/hour) or complex (e.g. polymorphic). Similarly, supraventricular extrasystoles can sometimes precipitate supraventricular (e.g. atrial fibrillation) and, rarely, ventricular tachyarrhythmias.

Patients with ventricular extrasystoles may have an increased risk of sudden cardiac death (SCD), depending on the nature and severity of their intrinsic heart disease.

There is evidence to suggest that reversible left ventricular dysfunction may develop in patients with very frequent ventricular extrasystoles (e.g. >10 000 per 24 hours). The mechanism is not fully understood, but may be due to dyssynchronous contraction of the ventricles. Left ventricular function may be improved in such cases by pharmacological suppression or catheter ablation.

Frequent extrasystoles can sometimes provoke considerable anxiety.

Approach to diagnosing the disease

Diagnosis is normally based on history, examination, and ECG. The history should document the description of the palpitations (frequency, timing, and any triggering factors such as exercise), the presence of syncope or presyncope, coexisting heart disease, and a family history of SCD.

Physical signs are subtle and rarely helpful. Cannon a waves may occasionally be noted in the jugular venous pulse. Peripheral pulse palpation may demonstrate the premature beat (often as a weaker beat) or the compensatory pause (followed by an augmented beat). Extrasystoles are often associated with a reduction in the intensity of the heart sounds and coexisting cardiac murmurs due to reduction in diastolic filling times and volumes.

An ECG recording is usually required to confirm the presence of extrasystoles and to establish their origin. It is important not to attribute palpitations to extrasystoles unless there is a clear correlation between symptoms and extrasystoles on ECG. This may require prolonged periods of monitoring, as well as a detailed symptom diary.

Other diagnoses that should be considered

Frequent extrasystoles may be confused with atrial fibrillation on palpation of peripheral pulses. Furthermore, pulse rate may appear slow during sustained episodes of bigeminy, suggesting a bradyarrhythmia. An ECG should easily establish the correct diagnosis.

'Gold-standard' diagnostic test

An ECG recording demonstrates the presence of extrasystoles. A 12-lead ECG will identify their potential origin and possible underlying cause (e.g. Q waves or long QT). Ambulatory ECG monitoring devices are useful, and a Holter monitor can be used if symptoms occur daily. Patient-activated loop recorders can provide monitoring periods of up to 2 weeks. Implantable loop recorders may also be used (battery life ~2 years).

Typically, ventricular extrasystoles have wide QRS complexes (>120 ms), large T waves in the opposite direction to the QRS complex, and a full compensatory pause. Supraventricular extrasystoles have normal QRS complexes (unless conducted aberrantly), and less than a full compensatory pause. They may completely fail to conduct if the ventricles are still in the refractory period. Atrial extrasystoles are usually associated with abnormally shaped P waves (the PR interval may vary, but is rarely <120 ms). Junctional extrasystoles may have a very short PR interval (<90 ms), no P wave (hidden within the QRS), or a P wave within the ST segment.

Acceptable diagnostic alternatives to the gold standard

Extrasystoles are often seen during electrophysiological studies, during which their exact nature may be identified. However, such an invasive test is rarely warranted to establish the diagnosis.

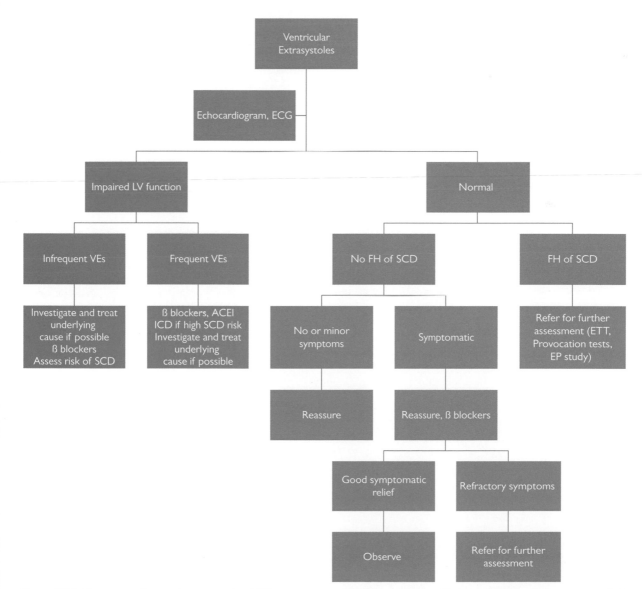

Figure 110.1 Management of ventricular extrasystoles; ACEI, angiotensin-converting enzyme inhibitor; EP, electrophysiology; ETT, exercise treadmill testing; FH, family history; ICD, implantable cardioverter defibrillator; LV, left ventricular; RF, radiofrequency; VEs, ventricular extrasystoles.

Other relevant investigations

Other relevant investigations include:

- 12-lead ECG
- biochemistry: electrolytes (K^+, Mg^{2+}), thyroid function tests, drug levels
- echocardiogram: to assess for structural heart disease and left ventricular function
- exercise stress test: useful in the assessment of complex ectopy and exercise-induced palpitations (catecholamine mediated), and to screen for coronary artery disease If coronary disease is considered to be anything other than low probability, CT coronary angiography or a functional test such as dobutamine stress echocardiography, or myocardial perfusion imaging should be undertaken.

Prognosis

Supraventricular extrasystoles are generally benign and have an excellent prognosis. Similarly, in subjects with no structural heart disease, ventricular extrasystoles appear to carry no adverse prognostic implications. In contrast, ventricular extrasystoles predict an increased risk of mortality in the presence of structural heart disease. The risk of SCD appears to be directly related to the extent of structural damage, although ventricular extrasystoles may simply be just a marker of the severity of the underlying disease rather than an independent risk factor for SCD (since pharmacological suppression of premature ventricular contractions does not improve overall survival). Ventricular extrasystoles elicited during exercise testing, even in apparently normal subjects, appear to imply increased risk over time. RVOT ectopy generally has a good prognosis, whereas right ventricular ectopy in the presence of structural abnormality (such as arrhythmogenic right ventricular cardiomyopathy) has a more sinister prognosis.

Treatment and its effectiveness

No therapy is required for asymptomatic patients. When present, symptoms may be alleviated by reassurance, and treating precipitating causes. If these measures fail, then β blockers may be effective in suppressing extrasystoles, and should normally be first choice (particularly post myocardial infarction or in heart failure). Alternatives include calcium-channel blockers, amiodarone, sotalol, and flecainide (the latter should be avoided post myocardial infarction). Radiofrequency ablation may be considered in refractory cases with symptomatic, frequent, monomorphic ventricular extrasystoles (especially if causing left ventricular impairment), and in cases where ventricular tachycardia is consistently provoked by ventricular extrasystoles of a similar morphology. Patients at high risk of SCD should be considered for implantation of an implantable cardioverter defibrillator (Figure 110.1).

Further Reading

Echt DS, Liebson PR, Mitchell LB, et al. Mortality and morbidity in patients receiving encainide, flecainide, or placebo. *New Engl J Med* 1991; 324: 781–8.

Lee V, Hemingway H, Harb R, Crake T, and Lambiase P. The prognostic significance of premature ventricular complexes in adults without clinically apparent heart disease: A meta-analysis and systematic review. *Heart* 2012; 98: 1290–98.

Lin CY, Chang SL, Lin YJ, et al. An observational study on the effect of premature ventricular complex burden on long-term outcome. *Medicine* (Baltimore). 2017; 96: e5476.

111 Sinus tachycardia

Michael Jones, Norman Qureshi, and Kim Rajappan

Definition of the disease

Sinus tachycardia is a condition of multiple different potential etiologies, characterized by an elevated rate of automaticity of the sinoatrial node, such that the heart rate is elevated. The exact point at which sinus tachycardia meets sinus rhythm is debatable; however, by convention, an upper rate of 100 min^{-1} is accepted for sinus rhythm; >100 min^{-1} denotes sinus tachycardia.

Aetiology of the disease

The commonest cause of sinus tachycardia is enhanced sympathetic drive (catecholamine mediated), which has the secondary effect of increasing the frequency of the automaticity of the sinoatrial node, thus increasing the atrial and ventricular rates. Possible causes include the following:

- fever/septicaemia
- anaemia
- hypovolemia
- hyperthyroidism
- hypotension
- catecholamine overproduction (phaeochromocytoma)
- heart failure
- anxiety states
- pulmonary embolus
- myocardial ischaemia/infarction
- hypoxia/chronic pulmonary disease
- stimulant-drug use (caffeine, nicotine, cocaine, etc.)
- beta-agonist drug use (isoprenaline, salbutamol, etc.)
- anticholinergic drug poisoning (atropine, tricyclic antidepressants, antihistamines, etc.)
- acute beta-blocker withdrawal (rebound sinus tachycardia)

There are two other categories of sinus tachycardia: one comprises inappropriate sinus tachycardia (IST; also termed 'chronic non-paroxysmal sinus tachycardia') and postural tachycardia syndrome (POTS); the other comprises sinus node re-entrant tachycardia (SNRT).

Typical symptoms of the disease and less common symptoms

Sinus tachycardia may be associated with symptoms of palpitations and an elevated heart rate, but it can also be completely asymptomatic. The underlying disease leading to the sinus tachycardia may also cause symptoms in its own right (e.g. acute myocardial infarction, pulmonary embolus, thyrotoxicosis); in addition, sinus tachycardia may worsen the symptoms of underlying conditions (such as heart failure, angina, etc.) through its elevation of the heart rate.

Demographics of sinus tachycardia

Sinus tachycardia is usually present in infants (normal physiology), where the heart rate is between 110 and 150 min^{-1}. The sinus rate then falls progressively with advancing age to the normal range for an adult (<100 min^{-1}).

Natural history, and complications

Generally, correction of the underlying physiological basis of the sinus tachycardia results in a lowering of the sinus rate to 'normal' levels (i.e. correction of hypovolaemia, treatment of sepsis, etc.). In the case of acute beta-blocker withdrawal (the so-called 'rebound' sinus tachycardia), normalization of the sinus rate may take days to weeks, and significant symptoms may require a more gradual down-titration of the beta-blocker dose. In the long term, untreated persistent sinus tachycardia may lead to a tachycardia-related cardiomyopathy, like the other persistent supraventricular tachycardias. This cardiomyopathy is generally reversible with correction of the tachycardia, in the absence of another cause for cardiomyopathy.

Approach to diagnosing the arrhythmia, including clinical clues, through concentrating on the ECG diagnosis

Sinus tachycardia is diagnosed from the 12-lead ECG, and requires that the P-wave morphology match the baseline sinus-rhythm P-wave morphology exactly (see Figure 111.1). This may be difficult to discern if there is no premorbid ECG; nevertheless, a P wave that demonstrates a positive morphology in the inferior limb leads (II, III, and aVF), a negative (or positive) morphology in aVR, and a positive morphology across the precordial leads (V1–V6) is likely to have its origin in the vicinity of the sinus node.

Sinus tachycardia may slow in response to enhanced vagal tone (carotid sinus massage (CSM)), but this is less likely to occur in SNRT than in the other forms of sinus tachycardia. Occasionally, slowing of the sinus rate may be necessary to clearly see the P waves and exclude atrial flutter or atrial tachycardia, when alternate P waves may be superimposed (hidden) in the QRS complexes.

The effect of IV adenosine administration may be to (1) increase AV nodal block and so result in 2:1 or other degrees of AV conduction block, (2) slow the sinus rate slightly, or (3) terminate the tachycardia. As with carotid massage, adenosine administration may assist in identifying any intervening P waves which had been hidden (superimposed) in QRS complexes.

The QRS morphology is usually the same as that seen during sinus rhythm, although aberrant conduction may occur with higher ventricular rates.

Other diagnoses that should be considered

Atrial flutter with 2:1 atrioventricular (AV) conduction may be mistaken for sinus tachycardia, especially if the P waves are hidden (superimposed) inside the QRS complexes. The diagnosis can be clarified by increasing AV nodal blockade (via CSM and/or IV adenosine administration) so that the P wave morphology and atrial rate can be clearly seen. The importance of differentiating sinus tachycardia from atrial flutter lies in the fact that, like multifocal atrial tachycardia, sinus tachycardia is not an indication for consideration of anticoagulation per se, whereas atrial flutter may be, depending on the patient's intrinsic risk (as determined by e.g. the CHADS-Vasc score).

'Gold-standard' diagnostic test

The diagnosis of sinus tachycardia should be able to be made from the surface 12-lead ECG. Very rarely, an invasive electrophysiology (EP) study may be helpful in differentiating sinus tachycardia from other forms of supraventricular tachycardia, where the 12-lead ECG is insufficient to make the diagnosis. At an invasive EP study, the site of origin of the tachycardia can be mapped to the sinus node region, and subsequent radial atrial activation can be demonstrated by activation mapping techniques.

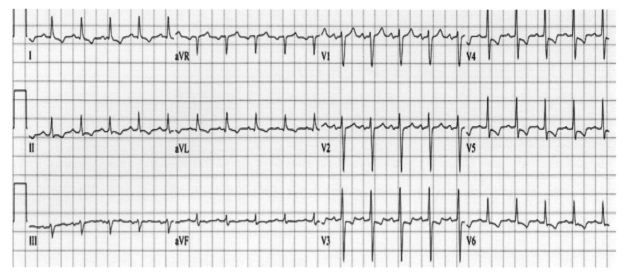

Figure 111.1 Sinus tachycardia ECG; note that the P waves are positive in the inferior and precordial leads and aVL, and negative in aVR. Also, the QRS is normal in width.

Acceptable diagnostic alternatives to the gold standard

Aside from the 12-lead ECG, or invasive EP study, there are currently no other diagnostic tests that can definitively diagnose sinus tachycardia.

Other relevant investigations

As there are a large number of potential etiologies for sinus tachycardia, there are a number of investigations that might need to be considered, in selected cases:

- full blood count, renal function, inflammatory markers (if anaemia, sepsis, hypovolaemia, or electrolyte disturbance is suspected)
- arterial blood gas analysis, D-dimer levels, and possibly lung perfusion scanning (if pulmonary embolus is suspected)
- chest X-ray (if infective or obstructive airways disease, pleural effusion/empyema, or heart failure is suspected)
- thyroid-stimulating hormone level (if hyperthyroidism is suspected)
- cardiac troponin assay (if acute coronary ischaemia is suspected)
- serum toxicology screen (if drug abuse is suspected)
- 24-hour urinary excretion of catecholamines (if phaeochromocytoma is suspected)

Echocardiography should be performed in all cases where sinus tachycardia cannot be readily explained by an obvious underlying pathology, and in cases where structural heart disease or heart failure is suspected.

Other investigations may subsequently be indicated, depending on the results of the initial testing—for example, myocardial perfusion studies or coronary angiography in cases where underlying coronary ischaemia is suspected.

Prognosis

The prognosis of sinus tachycardia is dependent upon the underlying pathology that is present, rather than the tachycardia itself. The exception to this is the possibility of developing a rate-related cardiomyopathy, if the tachycardia goes unnoticed and uncontrolled for a prolonged period of time.

Treatment and its effectiveness

The treatment of sinus tachycardia is essentially the treatment of the underlying condition predisposing to the tachycardia. The tachycardia should rarely ever require treatment per se in the case of an appropriate (reactive or physiological) sinus tachycardia. The syndromes of IST/POTS and SNRT are the exceptions to this rule, and are discussed separately in the following paragraphs.

Treatment of IST and POTS

The uncommon condition IST remains poorly defined, but essentially consists of elevated sinus rates with no apparent cause or physiologic explanation, in the context of normal cardiac structure and function. The mechanism of IST is still debated, but may be a primary 'dysautonomia' (excess sympathetic tone—depressed vagal efferent activity and/or enhanced beta-adrenoceptor sensitivity) that leads to the chronically elevated sinus rates. Alternatively, the sinus node itself may be abnormally sensitive to circulating catecholamines. The diagnosis is one of exclusion, when the potential causes for sinus tachycardia have been excluded, and cardiac structure and function have been assessed and shown to be normal. The prognosis is generally benign, although the symptoms can be very intrusive.

Treatment of IST is difficult and often unsuccessful in alleviating symptoms entirely. Beta blockers and non-dihydropyridine calcium-channel blockers (diltiazem, verapamil) may help in some cases, but both classes of drugs can result in side effects that are more troublesome than the tachycardia. Ivabradine is a newer agent that acts directly upon the sinus node itself (selectively inhibits the I_f current in a dose-dependent manner, which reduces cardiac pacemaker activity, slowing the sinus rate), and has been shown to be beneficial in some cases. Occasionally, catheter ablation (modification) of the sinus node is helpful if other treatments have been unsuccessful or poorly tolerated, but results are mixed, and chronotropic incompetence of the sinus node is a possible complication of this procedure (potentially requiring the implantation of a cardiac pacemaker). Catheter ablation should therefore be considered only as a last option for the management of IST.

POTS is a condition characterized by orthostatic intolerance symptoms, with a rapid increase in heart rate of ≥30 bpm, usually up to ≥120 bpm, but without orthostatic hypotension. Symptoms can be classic orthostatic in nature (light-headedness, dizziness, presyncope, palpitations) and non-orthostatic (bloating, nausea, vomiting, abdominal pain, constipation, diarrhoea, fatigue, migraine, sleep disturbance). Symptoms may be exacerbated by heat and exercise, are worse postprandially, and can intensify during the menstrual period. Females are predominantly affected (female to male ratio, 4:1), between 15 and 50 years of age. The prevalence of POTS is unknown, and the pathophysiology remains unclear, with some studies suggesting the presence of dysautonomia, a hyperadrenergic state, hypovolaemia, and an abnormal rennin–aldosterone response to hypovolaemia in POTS patients. There is considerable overlap between POTS, IST, vasovagal syncope, and chronic fatigue syndrome.

The diagnosis of POTS is made on the basis of a sustained rise in the heart rate of ≥30 bpm, or to ≥ 120 bpm with orthostatic stress (upright tilting), and this is conventionally performed on an automated tilt table.

The evidence base for treating POTS is poor, but treatments that may be of benefit include salt and water supplementation, lower-limb resistance training exercises, and the use of pressure stockings (non-pharmacological approach). Pharmacological therapies which may improve symptoms include fludrocortisone, midodrine, beta blockers, clonidine, pyridostigmine, ivabradine, octreotide, and possibly desmopressin. Decisions regarding therapy are best referred to a specialist service with experience in the management of dysautonomia, as the response to treatments is variable and requires tailoring to each individual patient.

Generally, the long-term prognosis of POTS is benign, with the majority of patients being able to return to normal activities after assessment, and treatment has been instituted.

Treatment of SNRT

SNRT is an uncommon arrhythmia, and is rarely symptomatic. The sinus rate is generally between 100 and 150, with P waves that are identical to normal P waves during sinus rhythm. The QRS is similarly unchanged compared to sinus rhythm, save that rate-related aberrancy may occur at faster sinus rates. The mechanism is thought to be a re-entrant circuit involving the sinus node, and possibly the perinodal tissues. The arrhythmia may be paroxysmal (brief and infrequent or frequent and sustained), or even incessant—in which case, it can be associated with a tachycardia-mediated cardiomyopathy, which is generally reversible with elimination of the tachycardia. The diagnosis can be difficult to make, but essentially relies upon the demonstration of spontaneous paroxysms of rapid sinus rates (which differentiates this condition from other atrial tachyarrhythmias). At electrophysiological studies, SNRT can be induced by programmed atrial extra-stimuli, and terminated in similar fashion; the atrial activation sequence will be shown to be similar to that seen during normal sinus rhythm.

Given the high degree of autonomic innervation of the sinoatrial node, CSM will generally terminate an episode of SNRT, whereas it will result in a gradual slowing and then acceleration of sinus tachycardia (on cessation of the CSM); AV nodal conduction block may also be seen during CSM. This manoeuver can be helpful in differentiating the two conditions. Adenosine, similarly, will usually terminate an episode of SNRT.

Therapy is rarely required for SNRT, but beta blockers, non-dihydropyridine calcium-channel blockers (diltiazem, verapamil), and digoxin may be beneficial. In refractory cases, catheter ablation of the re-entrant circuit may be an appropriate treatment.

Key points

- Sinus tachycardia is an atrial tachyarrhythmia of multiple potential etiologies, characterized by an elevation in the rate of automaticity of the sinus node.

- The P-wave morphology is identical to that of normal sinus rhythm, and QRS complexes are generally identical to those associated with sinus rhythm; however, rate-related aberrancy may occur.
- AV conduction during sinus tachycardia may be 1:1; alternatively, Wenckebach or higher degrees of AV conduction block may be seen. This depends on the intrinsic AV nodal conduction of the patient, and the concomitant use of AV nodal blocking drugs.
- There are three broad categories of sinus tachycardia: (1) sinus tachycardia due to enhanced sympathetic tone (hyper-adrenergic state), (2) IST/POTS, and (3) sinus node re-entrant tachycardia.
- Careful assessment of sinus tachycardia is essential, and a thorough search for an aetiology is required in all cases, so that secondary sinus tachycardia can be differentiated from the other causes of sinus tachycardia (namely IST, POTS, and SNRT); there must also be consideration of potential predisposing conditions.
- The effects of **adenosine** and **CSM or other vagal manoeuvres** are as follows: (1) in secondary sinus tachycardia, IST, or POTS, a transient slowing of the ventricular rate is likely to be seen (the mechanism is increased AV nodal conduction block), but termination of the arrhythmia is unlikely; (2) in SNRT, termination of the tachycardia is more likely.
- The differential diagnosis includes ectopic atrial tachycardia and atypical AV nodal re-entrant tachycardia; however, the P-wave morphology on the 12-lead ECG changes in these latter arrhythmias, thus clearly differentiating the conditions.
- The management of secondary sinus tachycardia is focused on treatment of the underlying cause of the elevated sinus rate.
- The management of IST is more difficult and challenging than that of secondary sinus tachycardia but, in the first instance, non-dihydropyridine calcium-channel blockers or beta blockers are helpful in some cases. Ivabradine is a newer agent that also can control symptoms in many cases.
- The management of POTS is complex, but the initial approach involves salt and fluid repletion, leg exercises, the use of pressure stockings, and fludrocortisone. Midodrine may also be helpful. Referral to a specialist clinic is recommended.
- SNRT rarely produces symptoms and so rarely requires treatment, but non-dihydropyridine calcium-channel blockers, beta blockers, and digoxin are reasonable first choices. Catheter ablation may be appropriate in selected cases.

Further Reading

Femenia, F, Baranchuk A , and Morillo, C. Inappropriate sinus tachycardia: Current therapeutic options. *Cardiol Rev* 2012; 20: 8–14.
Jones PK, Shaw BH, and Raj SR. Clinical challenges in the diagnosis and management of postural tachycardia syndrome. *Pract Neurol* 2016; 16: 431–38.

112 Focal (ectopic) atrial tachycardia

Michael Jones, Norman Qureshi, and Kim Rajappan

Definition of the disease

Focal atrial tachycardia is an atrial arrhythmia arising in either the left or the right atrium, usually faster than 100 min⁻¹ and regular, with a P-wave morphology that is different from the normal P-wave morphology associated with sinus rhythm—the difference in morphology being more pronounced the further away the focus lies from the sinus node.

The ventricular rate is generally fast also, dependent on the nature of the atrioventricular (AV) conduction; 1:1 conduction may be seen, especially in younger patients or patients with accessory pathways capable of very rapid antegrade conduction; alternatively, 2:1, Wenckebach-type, or higher-grade AV block may be seen.

Aetiology of the disease

Focal atrial tachycardia may be the result of three different atrial mechanisms: (1) enhanced automaticity, (2) triggered activity (early after-depolarizations, occurring during the plateau phase of the action potential, or delayed after-depolarizations, occurring during the fourth phase of the action potential), or (3) micro-re-entry (via small, protected area of tissue with conduction slowed to such an extent that tissue recovery occurs in sufficient time for the same wavefront, on re-encountering that tissue, to re-depolarize the tissue repeatedly).

Focal atrial tachycardia may occur in normal hearts, or may be associated with conditions leading to atrial stretch, elevated atrial pressure, inflammation, and fibrosis (scarring), such as chronic hypertension (systemic or pulmonary), cardiomyopathy, ischaemia, infection, and alcohol ingestion. Metabolic conditions such as hypokalaemia and hypoxia may predispose to atrial tachycardia. Stimulant drug abuse (cocaine, amphetamine), and the medications theophylline and digoxin can predispose to focal atrial tachycardia, especially at supratherapeutic levels.

Focal atrial tachycardias arise in specific locations in the atria, due to the particular tissue characteristics of those locations (alterations in myocyte orientation, and the presence of tissue with automaticity properties): in the right atrium (75%), commonest locations include the tricuspid valve annulus, the crista terminalis, the coronary sinus ostium, tissue directly adjacent to the sinoatrial and the atrioventricular nodes, and the right atrial appendage; in the left atrium (25%), the commonest sites of origin include the pulmonary vein antra, the mitral valve annulus, the coronary sinus body, septum, and the left atrial appendage.

Typical symptoms of the disease, and less common symptoms

Most patients experience paroxysmal palpitations as the cardinal symptom of focal atrial tachycardia. Attacks can last for seconds or up to as long as hours. Other patients may present with a cardiomyopathy from incessant atrial tachycardia (i.e. atrial tachycardia present for 90% or more of the time) rather than with palpitations. This cardiomyopathy is often reversible, with successful elimination of the tachycardia. Other symptoms of cardiac disease may manifest more prominently during episodes of atrial tachycardia, including angina and heart failure, owing to the rapid ventricular rates during the atrial tachycardia.

Demographics of focal atrial tachycardia

The overall prevalence of atrial tachycardia is low, and accounts for only 10% of the arrhythmias in patients undergoing electrophysiology studies for supraventricular tachycardias. Men and women are equally affected.

Natural history, and complications

Focal atrial tachycardia usually carries a benign prognosis, and may spontaneously remit over time. The exception to this is incessant atrial tachycardia, which can result in a tachycardia-mediated cardiomyopathy.

Approach to diagnosing the arrhythmia, including clinical clues, through concentrating on the ECG diagnosis

Focal atrial tachycardia is essentially an ECG diagnosis. The arrhythmia is generally of abrupt onset and offset, with an atrial rate of between 100 and 300 min⁻¹, and a P-wave morphology that is unlike that of sinus rhythm. This last point may be difficult to appreciate if the focus of the tachycardia is located adjacent to the SA node (e.g. high cristal atrial tachycardia, which may be indistinguishable from sinus tachycardia on P-wave morphology alone). The episodes may be brief (seconds) or prolonged (days), and changes to the atrial rate tend to be sudden, rather than gradual (as is the case for sinus rhythm). The PR relationship may give clues to the diagnosis of atrial tachycardia, as there is generally a long and variable RP interval during tachycardia, and AV dissociation may be seen. This last point helps differentiate atrial tachycardia from AV nodal re-entrant tachycardia and AV re-entrant tachycardia, where AV dissociation is not seen.

Performance of carotid sinus massage will typically increase AV nodal block (and so reduce ventricular rate), and reveal the P waves more clearly. IV adenosine may have the same effect, but it may also terminate the atrial tachycardia.

The QRS morphology is usually the same as that seen during sinus rhythm, although aberrant conduction may occur with higher ventricular rates. Autonomic tone and the use of concomitant AV nodal blocking medications will determine the ventricular response rate to the atrial tachycardia, which itself generally remains constant during an episode of tachycardia.

On preliminary inspection, the ECG shown in Figure 112.1 might be mistaken for sinus tachycardia, but the morphology and vector of the P waves (indicated by arrows) differ significantly from those of normal sinus P waves. The deeply negative P waves in Leads II, III, and aVF suggest that atrial electrical activation is proceeding caudocranially rather than craniocaudally, and the positive P waves in aVL and aVR suggest a more atrial-septal than free-wall location of the focal atrial tachycardia. This tachycardia may be located in the interatrial septum, coronary sinus os, or the right inferior pulmonary vein antrum. The exact location can be mapped during an electrophysiology study, and the focus ablated.

Other diagnoses that should be considered

Other causes of narrow complex tachycardia should be considered, such as atrial flutter, AV nodal re-entrant tachycardia, and AV re-entrant tachycardia. Sometimes, administration of carotid sinus massage, IV adenosine, or invasive electrophysiology studies are required to make the diagnosis.

'Gold-standard' diagnostic test

While the 12-lead ECG may make and confirm the diagnosis of focal atrial tachycardia, the gold-standard investigation is the electrophysiology study. Pacing manoeuvers that demonstrate VA dissociation,

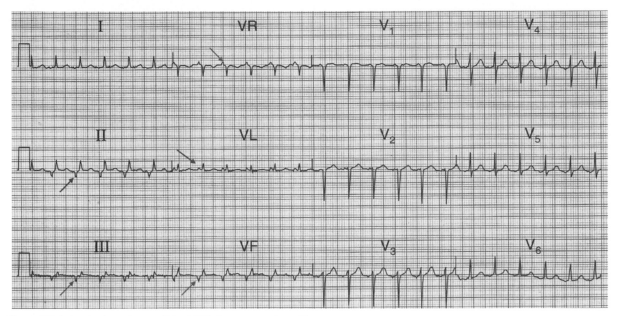

Figure 112.1 Atrial tachycardia on a 12-lead ECG; P waves are indicated by arrows.

and that demonstrate the tachycardia is driven by atrial activity, confirm the diagnosis. Catheter mapping techniques can demonstrate a radial atrial activation pattern from the atrial focus of the tachycardia.

Acceptable diagnostic alternatives to the gold standard

Aside from the 12-lead ECG or invasive electrophysiology study, there are currently no other diagnostic tests that can definitively diagnose atrial tachycardia.

Other relevant investigations

Echocardiography should be performed in all cases, to exclude the presence of structural heart disease (cardiomyopathy, significant valvular lesions, intra-cardiac shunts (an agitated saline study may be required if clinical suspicion of a shunt is high)) and to assess left ventricular size and function, left atrial dimension, pulmonary pressures, right-heart function, and pericardial appearance.

Full blood count and renal function testing may be relevant in certain cases where a predisposing cause is suspected, percutaneous catheter intervention is planned, or antiarrhythmic drug therapy is being considered.

Other investigations may be indicated, depending on the clinical setting. A suspicion of coronary disease or the desire to use Class 1 antiarrhythmic drugs might prompt an exercise treadmill test, a myocardial perfusion scan, or a coronary angiogram. Ambulatory heart rate monitoring (Holter monitoring) may be useful in assessing heart rate variability over a 24-hour period, to help differentiate atrial tachycardia from sinus tachycardia in cases where the P-wave morphology is very similar to sinus rhythm.

Prognosis

The prognosis is generally benign, apart from cases of incessant tachycardia, where a tachycardia-mediated cardiomyopathy may ensue.

Treatment and its effectiveness

Acute treatment

Any underlying or predisposing factors for focal atrial tachycardia should be identified and corrected—for example, hypokalaemia;

hypoxia; or theophylline or digoxin toxicity (anti-digitalis antibodies may be considered). And, as is the case with other tachyarrhythmias, assessment of the patient's haemodynamic state is the first consideration. In cases where haemodynamic compromise is present, acute cardioversion should be attempted—focal atrial tachycardia may respond less well to electrical cardioversion than the other tachyarrhythmias, or may reinitiate soon after cardioversion. In such a situation, chemical cardioversion with a Class III (amiodarone) or Class I (flecainide) antiarrhythmic drug should be considered. If the haemodynamic state is not compromised, vagal manoeuvers or IV adenosine may be administered; these can terminate the tachycardia or, alternatively, slow the ventricular response rate (via increased AV nodal block). Additionally, beta blockers or non-dihydropyridine calcium-channel blockers can be administered, with similar effects of slowing the ventricular response, and occasionally terminating the arrhythmia.

Chronic treatment

The aim of chronic therapy of focal atrial tachycardia is to prevent recurrence of atrial tachycardias and to control the ventricular response rate during atrial tachycardia if it should recur. Generally, beta blockers or non-dihydropyridine calcium-channel blockers are prescribed first, as these are the safest agents available which have reasonable efficacy.

If these agents fail, then consideration of an interventional approach to the management should be given. In an electrophysiology study, focal atrial tachycardias can be mapped to their site of origin in the atria, and ablated successfully and curatively in the majority of cases. The added advantage of this interventional approach is the fact that ongoing suppressive pharmacotherapy is generally not required after the ablation.

If ablation is unsuccessful, or if a particular patient is not a suitable candidate or refuses intervention, then Class III (amiodarone, sotalol) or Class I (flecainide) antiarrhythmic drugs can be tried, but the long-term side effects of these agents (especially their proarrhythmia tendencies) need to be considered in such cases.

Finally, if none of these approaches provide relief from atrial tachycardia, an AV nodal ablation together with the implantation of a permanent pacemaker is a reasonable option. This strategy necessarily renders a patient dependent on their pacemaker; moreover, it dictates repeated (7–10 yearly) pacemaker generator replacements (due to battery depletion) for the life of the patient. Hence, this is a less attractive strategy for younger patients, who would be faced with a future of repeated surgical procedures.

Key points

- Focal atrial tachycardia is a regular atrial arrhythmia, with atrial rates of between 100 and 300 min^{-1}, usually paroxysmal but occasionally incessant in nature, with QRS complexes generally identical to sinus rhythm, but with a different P-wave morphology to sinus rhythm.
- The prognosis of focal atrial tachycardia is generally benign, save when the tachycardia is incessant, and a tachycardia-mediated cardiomyopathy results—this is generally reversible with successful treatment of the tachycardia.
- Ventricular activation during atrial tachycardia may be 1:1; alternatively, Wenckebach or higher degrees of AV conduction block may be seen. This depends on the intrinsic AV nodal conduction of the patient, and the concomitant use of AV nodal blocking drugs
- Atrial rates fluctuate less than sinus rhythm rates, and generally change in sudden steps, rather than gradually as seen with sinus rhythm.
- The effect of **adenosine** and **carotid sinus massage or other vagal manoeuver** is transient slowing of ventricular rate (the mechanism is increased AV nodal conduction block) or, occasionally, slowing and termination of the atrial tachycardia itself.

- Differentials in the diagnosis include sinus tachycardia, atrial flutter, AV nodal re-entrant tachycardia, and AV re-entry tachycardia.
- ECG clues to the diagnosis of focal atrial tachycardia are (1) variable RP interval, (2) AV dissociation/evidence of AV nodal block, and (3) P-wave morphology different from that of sinus rhythm (it may be difficult to ascertain if the focal atrial tachycardia is arising in the high crista terminalis, close to the sinus node itself).
- Focal atrial tachycardia may arise in normal hearts, in patients with atriopathy or in patients with certain metabolic conditions; in addition, certain drug toxicities predispose to focal atrial tachycardia.
- Acutely, the intention of management is to terminate focal atrial tachycardia or control ventricular rate, with consideration of haemodynamic compromise being paramount.
- In the chronic setting, medical therapy or catheter ablation is appropriate, the decision being made on an individual patient basis.
- If all else fails, an AV nodal ablation and implantation of a permanent pacemaker is a reasonable option for treatment, but renders the patient pacemaker dependent for life.

Further Reading

Rosso R and Kistler P. Focal atrial tachycardia. *Heart* 2010; 96: 181–5.

113 Multifocal atrial tachycardia

Michael Jones, Norman Qureshi, and Kim Rajappan

Definition of the disease

Multifocal atrial tachycardia (MAT) is an atrial arrhythmia arising in the left or right atrium, or both, with multiple different P wave morphologies (at least three), with an atrial rate usually faster than 100 min^{-1}. The atrial rhythm may be irregular; however, the defining difference between MAT and atrial fibrillation is the presence of a P wave prior to each QRS complex in MAT (but the absence of P waves in atrial fibrillation). MAT may be compared to sinus rhythm with very frequent polymorphic atrial ectopic beats, and in fact similar pathophysiologic mechanisms underlie both conditions; thus, differentiating one from the other may be difficult—the principle difference is the lack of a single dominant sinus pacemaker in MAT.

Aetiology of the disease

MAT most probably arises as a consequence of abnormal automaticity, or triggered activity, rather than re-entry, given that, during electrophysiology study, programmed electrical stimulation is generally unable to induce or interrupt the arrhythmia.

MAT is associated with significant lung disease in over half of the cases, and is frequently seen on the ECGs of patients admitted with respiratory failure. COPD is the most commonly associated pulmonary condition, most probably through the mechanism of pulmonary hypertension causing right atrial pressure elevation and stretch. Other pulmonary conditions associated with MAT include pneumonia, pulmonary arterial embolus, hypoxia, hypercapnoea, acidosis, autonomic imbalance, and right atrial enlargement. Cardiac disease is also associated with developing MAT, especially conditions leading to elevation of right and left atrial pressures—valvular disease, hypertension, left ventricular systolic dysfunction, and ischemia.

Certain drugs are associated with MAT, including aminophylline, theophylline, and isoprenaline, and other conditions that may predispose to MAT include impaired glucose tolerance, hypokalaemia, hypomagnesaemia, and chronic renal failure.

Typical symptoms of the disease, and less common symptoms

Patients with MAT may experience palpitations; however, they are more likely to be symptomatic of significant pulmonary or cardiac comorbidity, as previously explained. As with focal atrial tachycardia, if MAT is incessant or very frequently present, it may be associated with a tachycardia-mediated cardiomyopathy.

Demographics of MAT

MAT is an uncommon arrhythmia, and is seen on roughly 15 out of 10 000 ECGs performed in hospital patients. Patients are generally elderly, with an average age of approximately 75 years. Respiratory disease is present in 50%–80% of patients with MAT (mainly COPD). MAT is less often seen in the younger age groups but, when it does occur, it is generally associated with a benign prognosis.

Natural history, and complications

Studies have demonstrated that MAT is associated with an inhospital mortality rate of 45%, which is probably attributable more to the severe underlying respiratory and cardiac comorbidities than to the MAT itself. MAT is often preceded by, or progresses to, atrial fibrillation or another atrial tachycardia. MAT occurs far less often than atrial fibrillation.

Occasionally, patients present with a heart rate less than 100 min^{-1} but otherwise fulfil all of the criteria for MAT. This condition should be termed slow MAT or multifocal atrial rhythm. It is not the same rhythm as wandering atrial pacemaker (WAP), as the latter is usually a benign rhythm of stable, healthy patients. Clinical criteria alone thus differentiate slow MAT from WAP: MAT and slow MAT occur almost exclusively in the setting of serious coexisting cardiopulmonary disease, while WAP occurs in healthy individuals.

Approach to diagnosing the arrhythmia, including clinical clues, through concentrating on the ECG diagnosis

MAT is diagnosed on the 12-lead ECG (Figure 113.1), based upon the presence of (1) at least three different P-wave morphologies, (2) evidence of an isoelectric segment between the P waves, and (3) an atrial rate of greater than 100 min^{-1}. The ECG may demonstrate changes consistent with significant pulmonary disease (pulmonary hypertension) in addition to the tachycardia. Performance of carotid sinus massage (should it be considered necessary) may increase atrioventricular (AV) nodal block (and so reduce ventricular rate), and reveal the P waves more clearly. Intravenous adenosine may have the same effect.

The QRS morphology is usually the same as that seen during sinus rhythm, although aberrant conduction may occur with higher ventricular rates. Autonomic tone and the use of concomitant AV nodal blocking medications will determine the ventricular response rate to the atrial tachycardia. Various degrees of AV nodal block are usually observed, given that these patients usually have significant cardiac comorbidity.

This ECG may be initially mistaken as showing atrial fibrillation; however, on close inspection, a definite P wave can be observed before each QRS complex. There are at least three different morphologies of P wave, each with subtly different PR intervals. This is most apparent on Lead V1 in this case. On this 12-lead ECG, AV conduction appears to be 1:1.

Other diagnoses that should be considered

Atrial fibrillation and atrial flutter are the two arrhythmias that should be considered in the differential diagnosis, but the presence of different P waves of different morphologies with isoelectric segments in-between should exclude these two diagnoses in the majority of cases. The importance of differentiating MAT from atrial fibrillation lies in the implications for thromboembolism and stroke risk—MAT is not considered an indication for anticoagulation per se, whereas atrial fibrillation and flutter may be, depending on the patient's intrinsic risk (as determined by the CHADS-Vasc score).

'Gold-standard' diagnostic test

The 'gold-standard' diagnostic test is the electrophysiology study, which may be required in a minority of cases to make the diagnosis. The placement of cardiac catheters inside the atria may demonstrate the multifocal nature of this arrhythmia and, moreover, pacing manoeuvers will enable other mechanisms for supraventricular tachycardia to be excluded.

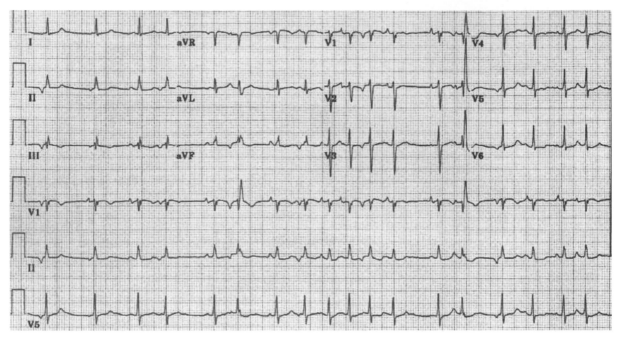

Figure 113.1 Multifocal atrial tachycardia 12-lead ECG.

Acceptable diagnostic alternatives to the gold standard

An acceptable diagnostic alternative to the gold standard is interpretation of the 12-lead ECG in the clinical context.

Other relevant investigations

Given that MAT occurs so frequently in the setting of severe cardiopulmonary disease, investigation and management should focus on coexistent pulmonary and cardiac disease.

Echocardiography should be performed in all cases, to exclude the presence of structural heart disease (cardiomyopathy, significant valvular lesions, intra-cardiac shunts (an agitated saline study may be required if clinical suspicion of a shunt is high), left ventricular size and function, left atrial dimension, pulmonary pressures, right-heart function, and pericardial appearance).

Myocardial perfusion studies or coronary angiography may be indicated in cases where underlying coronary ischaemia is suspected.

Full blood count and renal function should be assessed, in all cases, once again on the basis of the likely underlying cardiopulmonary disease.

Prognosis

MAT is often benign in infants and children, but the prognosis is poor in adults; inhospital mortality from underlying disease (generally respiratory) is between 40% and 60% and, in most cases, advanced age is compounded by severe cardiopulmonary comorbidity.

Treatment and its effectiveness

The main focus of treatment in patients with MAT is of the underlying disease; with improvement in pulmonary or respiratory status, MAT also improves.

Magnesium administration may be an effective treatment, with one study demonstrating a slowing of the heart rate and restoration of sinus rhythm in patients treated with magnesium. Potassium supplementation may have a similar effect.

Verapamil is effective in reducing the degree of atrial ectopy in MAT, and may restore sinus rhythm. Caution has to be exercised in its use, given the potential for hypotension (negative inotropy and

peripheral vasodilatation). Beta blockers (metoprolol) also suppress the atrial ectopy, and reduce AV nodal conduction, thus decreasing the ventricular rate by both mechanisms; however, bronchospasm and decompensated systolic function can complicate the use of beta blockers in these patients.

The limited studies of antiarrhythmic drugs in this condition have failed to demonstrate efficacy, and digoxin does not have a role in the management of MAT. Electrical cardioversion similarly has no role in the treatment of MAT.

In cases of refractory MAT with sustained elevated ventricular rates, in spite of optimal management of underlying cardiopulmonary disease, AV nodal ablation and permanent pacemaker implantation may be appropriate. Given the multifocal nature of MAT, this condition is not considered amenable to catheter ablation of the multiple foci per se, unlike focal atrial tachycardia, where a single atrial focal origin of the tachycardia may be found and successfully ablated.

Key points

The key points concerning MAT are as follows:

- MAT is an atrial arrhythmia, characterized by at least three different P wave morphologies with an isoelectric intervening segment, atrial rates greater than 100 min^{-1}, and QRS complexes generally identical to sinus rhythm.
- MAT generally arises in patients with significant underlying pulmonary or cardiac pathology, the commonest being COPD.
- MAT occurs either as a consequence of enhanced automaticity or triggered atrial activity; it is unlikely to be a re-entrant arrhythmia, given the inability of pacing manoeuvers to induce or terminate MAT.
- Ventricular activation during MAT may be 1:1 or, alternatively, Wenckebach or higher degrees of AV conduction block may be seen. This depends on the intrinsic AV nodal conduction of the patient, and the concomitant use of AV nodal blocking drugs
- The effect of **adenosine**, **carotid sinus massage**, or **other vagal manoeuvre** is transient slowing of the ventricular rate (via increased AV nodal conduction block); termination of the arrhythmia is unlikely.
- Differentials in the diagnosis include sinus rhythm with frequent multifocal atrial extrasystoles, and 'coarse' atrial fibrillation.
- ECG clues to the diagnosis of MAT are (1) irregular atrial rate, (2) P waves of at least three different morphologies, with no single

dominant sinus pacemaker apparent, and (3) a clear isoelectric segment between P waves.

- The management of MAT is essentially the management of the underlying significant respiratory or cardiac disease.
- Non-dihydropyridine calcium channel blockade (e.g. verapamil) and cardioselective beta blockade (e.g. metoprolol) both have efficacy in suppressing the atrial ectopy, and beta blockade reduces AV nodal transmission.
- Magnesium and potassium repletion therapy may be beneficial in suppressing MAT.
- Antiarrhythmic drugs and electrical cardioversion have not been shown to have efficacy in the treatment of MAT

- If heart rates remain elevated and symptoms uncontrolled despite adequate management of the underlying cardiopulmonary disease, AV nodal ablation and permanent pacing may be the appropriate treatment.

Further Reading

McCord J and Rorzak S. Multifocal atrial tachycardia. *Chest* 1998; 113: 203–9.

Schwartz M, Rodman D, and Lowenstein SR. Recognition and treatment of multifocal atrial tachycardia: A critical review. *J Emerg Med* 1994; 12: 353–60.

114 Atrioventricular nodal re-entrant tachycardia

Michael Jones, Norman Qureshi, and Kim Rajappan

Definition of the disease

Atrioventricular nodal re-entrant tachycardia (AVNRT; also known as atrioventricular junction reciprocating tachycardia) is one of the five subtypes of supraventricular tachycardia (SVT), manifesting most commonly as a regular, narrow QRS complex tachycardia, rate 150–250 min⁻¹ (usually 160–180 min⁻¹), occurring paroxysmally, with P waves either not apparent, or seen to follow the QRS complexes.

Aetiology of the disease

AVNRT arises in structurally normal hearts, or in the presence of heart disease. The requirement for AVNRT is the presence of two functionally discrete electrical pathways (Limb A and Limb B in Figure 114.1(A)) within or adjacent to the atrioventricular (AV) node in the low septal right atrium. These pathways are not macroscopically or microscopically visible in tissue section; rather, they comprise tracts of electrically conductive cells that display certain distinct electrophysiological properties. Limb A demonstrates rapid conduction velocity but a slow recovery time, whereas limb B conducts slowly, but recovers more quickly. In the normal situation, impulses travel down both A and B, but as A is faster, this is the route by which activation occurs (His–Purkinje activation, in this case). The impulse does enter the other limb (Limb B), at both ends, and collision occurs (impulse extinguishes in Limb B), owing to the slower conduction velocity in Limb B. Figure 114.1(B) shows what happens when a critically timed premature impulse encounters these pathways—Limb A has not yet recovered, but Limb B has done, so the impulse travels down B to the His–Purkinje system, but it travels slowly, as B can only conduct impulses slowly. The result is prolonged AV conduction (i.e. a long PR interval for that beat). The impulse can then enter Limb A at its distal end, and conduct backwards up Limb A to the atrium, as Limb A has by now recovered from the previous beat. The atrium is thus activated retrogradely via Limb A, and the impulse then re-enters B antegradely, and thus AVNRT is initiated (Figure 114.1(C)).

The exact anatomical location of these pathways is not clear, but they are believed to lie in the region of the inferior inter-atrial septum, adjacent to the tricuspid valve and the coronary sinus os. This region is termed the 'triangle of Koch'; the compact AV node and the fast pathway fibres lie at the apex of this triangle, and the slow pathway fibres run along the right side of the triangle, adjacent to the coronary sinus os. These pathways meet distally in the distal compact AV node, just proximal to the His bundle, and their proximal ends are joined most probably by perinodal atrial tissue.

The association between dual AV nodal pathways and clinical AVNRT is not perfect; the presence of two AV nodal pathways does not necessarily imply AVNRT will occur, and neither can dual AV nodal pathways be demonstrated in all cases of AVNRT.

Typical symptoms of the disease, and less common symptoms

The most common symptom is palpitations, affecting nearly all patients. Other symptoms include dizziness, dyspnoea, chest pain, fatigue, and syncope. The type and severity of symptoms depends in part on the rate of the tachycardia, and the presence of any associated heart disease. AVNRT involves near-simultaneous mechanical activation of the atria and the ventricles and, as a consequence, the contraction of the right ventricle against an open tricuspid valve may result in a pounding sensation in the neck in many patients.

Demographics of the disease

AVNRT represents 50%–60% of SVT cases. It is more common in women (2:1). AVNRT is more likely to occur in younger patients, but can present at any age. The mean age of symptom onset is the third decade.

Natural history, and complications of the disease

Although the natural history of AVNRT is quite variable, the electrophysiological properties of the AV node change over time and, generally speaking, symptoms decrease with advancing age. Given that SVT due to AVNRT is rarely ever incessant but, rather, is paroxysmal in nature, it is not associated with a tachycardia-mediated

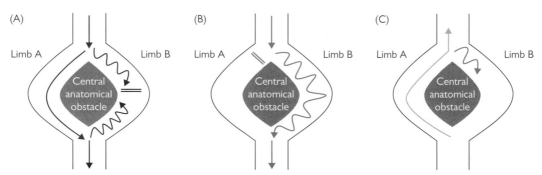

Figure 114.1 (A) Fast and slow pathways, conducting both antero- and retrogradely. In this diagram, the electrical impulse passes quickly down the fast pathway, and back up the slow pathway, meeting the much slower anterograde impulse, so blocking ongoing conduction in the slow pathway. (B) The longer refractory period of the fast pathway means that when a supraventricular extrasystole arrives early, the fast pathway is blocked, as shown here, and the impulse passes down the slow pathway, which has a shorter refractory period. (C) A ventricular extrasystole passes up the fast pathway, but not up the slow pathway, which has depolarized more recently and so is still refractory. This allows the impulse to re-enter the slow pathway from above, triggering a re-entrant arrhythmia.

Reproduced with permission from Yaver Bashir, Timothy R. Betts, and Kim Rajappan, *Cardiac Electrophysiology and Catheter Ablation*, Oxford University Press, Oxford, UK, Copyright © 2010

cardiomyopathy. And, unlike atrial flutter and fibrillation, there is no need for anticoagulation associated with AVNRT, in the absence of another indication for anticoagulation.

Approach to diagnosing the disease (including diagnostic pitfalls)

The ECG during AVNRT demonstrates a regular tachycardia, usually with narrow QRS complexes (which implies that ventricular activation is occurring only over the normal His–Purkinje cardiac conduction system). P waves may not be visible (i.e. completely buried inside the QRS), may be seen in the ST segment, or, less commonly, may be seen after the T wave, usually with a negative vector in the inferior ECG leads. The finding of an 'RsR' pattern in Lead V1 during tachycardia is highly specific for AVNRT (see Figure 114.2). Comparing the tachycardia 12-lead ECG to the sinus rhythm ECG is the easiest way to identify if P waves are visible.

Clues to differentiating AVNRT from the other types of SVT are found in the mode of initiation of the tachycardia—often, AVNRT is seen to initiate after a premature P wave conducts to the ventricles via the slow AV nodal pathway, as the fast AV nodal pathway (the usual route for A–V conduction) has not yet recovered sufficiently from the previous beat to conduct an impulse. The result is a longer PR interval, followed by retrograde atrial activation via the fast AV nodal pathway (which has now recovered), and ongoing AVNRT. The QRS is usually narrow, but may be wide if rate-related left or right bundle branch aberration occurs or, alternatively (and more rarely), in the presence of a bystander accessory A–V connection (bundle of Kent) capable of A–V conduction during AVNRT (termed 'pre-excited AVNRT').

Roughly 10% of patients demonstrate 2:1 A:V block during AVNRT, and only a very small minority show 2:1 V:A (retrograde) block—but, as the P waves are often not apparent, this is usually not seen on the ECG. There can be variation in cycle length (tachycardia rate) during an episode of AVNRT, and this is generally due to variation in the antegrade AV nodal conduction time (slow pathway conduction). QRS alternans can also be seen during AVNRT, again, due to antegrade AV nodal conduction variability.

Another 12-lead ECG clue to diagnosing AVNRT is the finding of alternating long and short PR intervals on a sinus rhythm ECG. Some patients can demonstrate ongoing antegrade conduction down both fast and slow AV nodal pathways, resulting in two QRS complexes for each P wave. This 'two-for-one' phenomenon is rarely seen, and is essentially a non-re-entrant form of AV nodal tachycardia.

Another form of AVNRT, atypical AVNRT, occurs less frequently than the typical AVNRT just described. In atypical AVNRT, antegrade conduction is via a fast or 'intermediate' pathway, and retrograde conduction via the slow pathway (i.e. the same circuit, in reverse). The result is an SVT with a long RP interval (owing to the slow pathway conducting retrogradely in this case). A 'slow–slow' form of AVNRT also exists, but this is rare.

Often, an invasive electrophysiology study is required to make the diagnosis of AVNRT when the ECG diagnosis is not clear.

'Gold-standard' diagnostic test

The gold-standard diagnostic test is the invasive electrophysiology study.

Acceptable diagnostic alternatives to the gold standard

There are currently no other diagnostic tests that can definitively diagnose AVNRT, other than an invasive electrophysiological investigation.

Other relevant investigations

No other specific investigations are routinely indicated; however, some patients may warrant investigation for coronary ischaemia (if chest pain and ischaemic ECG changes are noted during episodes of AVNRT), and echocardiography to exclude structural heart disease (if hypotension, shock, and syncope are prominent features).

Prognosis and how to estimate it

As previously mentioned, the symptom burden tends to decrease with advancing age and, as this is almost never a persistent arrhythmia but rather a paroxysmal SVT, it is not associated with tachycardia-mediated cardiomyopathy. In the absence of heart disease, the prognosis is usually good.

Treatment and its effectiveness

Acute management

Acute management focuses on acutely changing the conduction properties of the slow or fast pathways, to rendering them less favourable to ongoing re-entry. Carotid sinus massage, Valsalva, or other 'vagal' manoeuvers can terminate an episode of AVNRT, by slowing antegrade slow-pathway conduction. They are more successful if performed early after tachycardia onset. The tachycardia may only slow briefly, rather than terminating with these manoeuvers.

If these fail to terminate tachycardia, adenosine is the next and best treatment. It is given by rapid intravenous push (12 mg and then, if necessary, 18 and 24 mg, preferably via a proximal vein), although the drug will still be effective if given at a larger dose (18–24 mg) peripherally. Vagal manoeuvers should be reattempted after adenosine administration, if the drug has been unsuccessful. As with vagal manoeuvers, the effect of adenosine may be to merely slow the tachycardia briefly (reflecting slowing of conduction velocity in the slow AV nodal pathway) rather than terminating it.

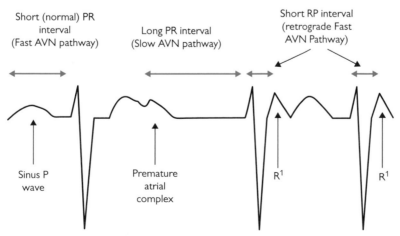

Short (normal) PR interval (Fast AVN pathway)

Long PR interval (Slow AVN pathway)

Short RP interval (retrograde Fast AVN Pathway)

Sinus P wave

Premature atrial complex

R^1

R^1

Figure 114.2 The PR interval duration will depend on whether a fast or slow pathway is used for conduction; AVN, atrioventricular nodal.

Reproduced with permission from Yaver Bashir, Timothy R. Betts, and Kim Rajappan, *Cardiac Electrophysiology and Catheter Ablation*, Oxford University Press, Oxford, UK, Copyright © 2010

CHAPTER 114 **Atrioventricular nodal re-entrant tachycardia**

Alternatives to adenosine for acute termination of AVNRT include intravenous calcium-channel blockers (diltiazem, verapamil) or beta blockers (metoprolol, atenolol, esmolol), but these agents can cause significant negative inotropic side effects and, in the case of beta blockers, can precipitate acute bronchospasm in patients with reactive airways disease.

As is the case for all tachycardias in the setting of haemodynamic compromise, electrical cardioversion (synchronized) is the first treatment of choice.

Class IA, IC, and III antiarrhythmic drugs are rarely ever used for the acute termination of AVNRT, but are effective in slowing retrograde fast-pathway conduction, and thus terminating the tachycardia.

Prevention of recurrences

Digoxin, beta blockade, and calcium-channel blockade are all effective in prevention of recurrent episodes of AVNRT, but these agents need to be taken every day in order to be effective, and so the frequency of episodes would need to justify this approach. Also, the use of these agents is frequently complicated by side effects (fatigue, dizziness, effort intolerance, depression). Similarly, Class IA (procainamide, disopyramide, quinidine), IC (flecainide, propafenone), and III (sotalol, amiodarone) drugs are effective in preventing recurrent episodes of AVNRT, but the side effects of these agents, in particular their tendency to QT-interval prolongation and sudden death, make them less attractive options for the long-term management of AVNRT.

Percutaneous catheter ablation of the slow AV nodal pathway is now an established treatment for recurrent symptomatic AVNRT, and should be offered early in the natural history of the condition. Acute procedural success rates and long-term success rates are around 95%, with no requirement for ongoing medical prophylaxis against further episodes in those successfully treated. The procedure is minimally invasive, and performed by the transvenous route (usually femoral vein) and, as such, can be complicated by vascular injury and perforation, but this is uncommon (~0.5%). The other significant complication of slow pathway ablation for AVNRT treatment is inadvertent compact AV nodal ablation, resulting in complete heart block and the need for emergent permanent pacing. This also is a rare occurrence (~0.5%), but may be a significant consideration, especially in very young patients, for whom a permanent pacemaker would involve numerous device and lead revisions over the ensuing years.

Key points

The key points concerning AVNRT are as follows:

- AVNRT is one of the four types of SVT, the others being atrioventricular re-entrant tachycardia, focal (ectopic) atrial tachycardia, and atrial flutter.

- Symptoms include palpitations, dyspnoea, chest pain, dizziness, and syncope.
- AVNRT results from a re-entrant circuit which is normally made up of two AV nodal pathways with differing conduction and recovery properties and termed the slow and the fast AV nodal pathways.
- Typical AVNRT is an SVT with a short RP interval; retrograde atrial activation is via the faster of the two pathways, and hence P waves are either very closely related to the QRS complexes, or are buried within them (not seen).
- Atypical AVNRT is rare, and is an SVT with a long RP interval; P waves are seen after the QRS complexes. Retrograde atrial activation is via the slow pathway in this case, and antegrade activation of the His bundle is via the fast pathway.
- The QRS will be wide if there is preexisting bundle branch block (apparent on ECGs performed during sinus rhythm), or can be wide if rate-related bundle branch block is encountered during tachycardia, or in the presence of an accessory AV connection. But, generally, the QRS is narrow.
- Clues to the diagnosis of AVNRT involve the suggestion of dual AV nodal pathways at the start of the tachycardia, or on sinus rhythm ECGs. The RSR' pattern in V1 during tachycardia is very specific for typical AVNRT
- Carotid sinus massage, other vagal manoeuvers, and IV adenosine may acutely terminate AVNRT, or may briefly slow the rate only.
- AV nodal blocking drugs are useful for prophylaxis, but side effects often limit the clinical utility of such drugs.
- Percutaneous transvenous catheter ablation of the slow AV nodal pathway is the treatment of choice for most patients with recurrent symptomatic AVNRT, and provides a long-term cure in over 95%. This technique is associated with a ~0.5% risk of adverse outcomes, including the need for a permanent pacemaker, and this needs to be fully discussed with the patient prior to considering this approach.

Further Reading

Page RL, Joglar JA, Caldwell MA, et al. 2015 ACC/AHA/HRS guideline for the management of adult patients with supraventricular tachycardia: a report of the American College of Cardiology/American Heart Association Task Force on Clinical Practice Guidelines and the Heart Rhythm Society. *J Am Coll Cardiol* 2016; 67: e27–115.

115 Atrioventricular re-entrant tachycardia

Michael Jones, Norman Qureshi, and Kim Rajappan

Definition of the disease

Atrioventricular (AV) re-entrant tachycardia (AVRT) is a type of supraventricular tachycardia (SVT), manifesting most commonly as a regular, narrow-QRS-complex tachycardia. It is usually a paroxysmal tachycardia, and is dependent upon the presence of an accessory electrical connection located between the atria and the ventricles (distinct and separate from the AV node–His–Purkinje system) and which is capable of atrioventricular (antegrade) or ventriculoatrial (retrograde) electrical conduction (or both). This pathway, together with the AV node–His–Purkinje system and the atrial and ventricular myocardia, forms a macro-re-entrant circuit that enables AVRT to occur.

AVRT can be **orthodromic (oAVRT; 95% of cases)**, in which case antegrade conduction occurs via the AV node–His–Purkinje system, and retrograde conduction via the accessory pathway; or **antidromic (aAVRT)**, in which case antegrade conduction occurs via the accessory pathway, and retrograde conduction via the AV node–His–Purkinje system. The latter type has a wide QRS complex during tachycardia, as the ventricles are exclusively activated by the accessory pathway and, as such, aAVRT can be mistaken for ventricular tachycardia. A third type of AVRT, termed 'pathway-to-pathway' AV nodal re-entrant tachycardia (AVNRT), is infrequently seen; two accessory pathways form the limbs of the re-entrant circuit, the QRS is fully pre-excited (just as with aAVRT), and the AV node–His–Purkinje system is a bystander (not involved in the tachycardia circuit).

Aetiology of the disease

As previously mentioned, AVRT arises as a consequence of an accessory electrical connection located between the atria and the ventricles and which is capable of electrical conduction in one or both directions. The majority of antegradely conducting (or '**manifest**') accessory pathways can also conduct retrogradely; only 5% of patients have pathways that only conduct antegradely.

A pathway only capable of retrograde conduction is termed '**concealed**', as it cannot be observed (does not manifest itself) on a routine sinus rhythm ECG (no delta wave). Up to 50% of accessory pathways that participate in AVRT can only conduct retrogradely.

The accessory connection can often be seen both macro- and microscopically as a band of myocardial fibres that traverse the annulus fibrosis; the only electrical structure that should normally traverse the annulus is the His bundle. Accessory pathways are believed to be congenital, representing incomplete separation of the atrial and the ventricular myocardia by the developing annulus fibrosis; however, there is also some evidence to suggest that an accessory connection can be acquired later in life.

In patients with AVRT, one or occasionally two or more accessory pathways are present, connecting the atria and the ventricles electrically. The most common location is the posterolateral mitral valve annulus, but other areas include the posteroseptal and anteroseptal spaces, and the tricuspid valve annulus.

During normal sinus rhythm, antegradely conducting accessory pathways may conduct the atrial impulse to the ventricle, where they insert. As this leads to premature activation of that part of the basal left or right ventricle, earlier than it would have been activated via the normal AV node, the 12-lead ECG is altered, with a widening of the QRS; this widening reflects the early basal ventricular activation (termed 'pre-excitation') **which occurs at the same time (i.e. fuses with) activation of the rest of the ventricles by** the **AV node–His–Purkinje system**. This feature is called a **delta wave** and represents a slurring, and usually a shortening, of the PR interval. The extent to which this occurs, or the degree of pre-excitation (i.e. the amount of QRS widening/magnitude of the delta wave), depends on the location of the accessory pathway, the sinus rate, and the electrical conduction properties (velocity) of the atria and the AV node; for example, a left lateral accessory pathway may only encounter an atrial depolarization when the impulse has already conducted through the AV node and depolarized a large volume of the ventricles; thus, the contribution of pre-excitation to the ECG is relatively small in this case. The opposite is true of pathways located close to the sinus node and AV node. It is quite common to see variable degrees of pre-excitation on serial ECGs, given that the relative contribution of the AV node (largely determined by autonomic tone, which is variable) to ventricular activation will vary continuously over time. A distant (i.e. left free wall) accessory pathway that can conduct antegradely but does not manifest any delta waves on the ECG is termed a '**latent**' pathway. Most accessory pathways conduct very rapidly, and recover very rapidly, unlike AV nodal tissue.

During sinus rhythm, concealed accessory pathways (retrogradely conducting-only accessory pathways) do not alter the QRS width, but if premature ventricular complexes (VPCs) occur, retrograde P waves (atrial echo beats) can occasionally be seen following the VPC (as a consequence of retrograde conduction from the ventricle back up the pathway to the atria). These 'atrial echoes' can also be seen occasionally following a normally conducted QRS, and they manifest as a perturbation of the normal ST segment or T wave.

During normal sinus rhythm in a patient with a left-sided accessory pathway capable of bidirectional conduction, the sinus beat activate the ventricles by both the AV node and the accessory pathway, resulting in a fusion of ventricular activation and a delta wave on the surface 12-lead ECG. In the setting of a VPC, atrial activation may occur retrogradely via the accessory pathway, resulting in an atrial echo beat with an unusual P wave appearance, noted as a deflection in the terminal QRS/ST complex.

AVRT arises when an impulse (generally a premature atrial or ventricular depolarization) blocks (fails to conduct through) either the AV node or the accessory pathway, but still manages to conduct via the **other** pathway, often with a slower conduction speed than normal, thus permitting the other pathway (that had initially been unable to conduct the premature impulse) **to recover sufficiently to reconduct the impulse in reverse direction and so initiate tachycardia**.

Most commonly, this situation arises when a premature atrial beat blocks antegradely, completely, in the accessory pathway, manifesting as sudden and complete loss of the pre-excited appearance of the QRS for that beat (i.e. the QRS narrows to normal). The impulse conducts through the AV node, but with delay (a longer PR interval). This electrical delay in the AV node allows the accessory pathway to recover excitability completely, and so it conducts the ventricular depolarization back to that part of the atrium where the accessory pathway inserts. It can then re-enter the AV node antegradely, thus initiating oAVRT.

In oAVRT, a premature left atrial depolarization does not conduct down the accessory pathway (as the pathway is still refractory from the preceding sinus beat) but instead conducts down the AV node–His–Purkinje system, albeit more slowly (i.e. with a longer PR interval). Conduction then spreads through the ventricular myocardium, eventually reaching the basal left ventricle and the location of the accessory pathway. Given that the pathway has, by this time, recovered from its refractoriness, it conducts the impulse backwards to the left atrium, thus initiating oAVRT.

Tachycardia initiation can also occur from the ventricle; a PVC blocks in the His–Purkinje system but conducts backwards up the accessory pathway and activates the atrium, thence eventually activating the AV node, His bundle, and ventricles and consequently initiating oAVRT.

In oAVRT, conduction to the ventricles (the antegrade limb) occurs via the normal AV node–His–Purkinje system, and retrograde conduction to the atria is via the accessory pathway. The reverse situation also arises, although it is less common; this is termed aAVRT. In aAVRT, ventricular activation occurs entirely over the accessory pathway, and the 12-lead ECG is fully pre-excited. The initiation of aAVRT generally results from a premature atrial beat which blocks in the AV node but conducts to the ventricles via the accessory pathway, giving rise to a fully pre-excited 12-lead ECG appearance (the ventricles are entirely activated by the accessory pathway, with no contribution from the AV node). The His–Purkinje system, AV node, and, finally, the atria are then activated retrogradely, thus resulting in aAVRT.

Typical symptoms of the disease, and less common symptoms

The most common symptoms of AVRT are palpitations, dizziness, dyspnoea, chest pain, fatigue, and syncope. As with AVNRT, the type and severity of symptoms depends in part on the rate of the tachycardia, and the presence of any associated heart disease. AVRT tends to be faster than AVNRT, but a great deal of overlap exists. In the case of persistent junctional reciprocating tachycardia (PJRT), owing to the slow conduction properties of the accessory pathway, incessant tachycardia is often present and, if the tachycardia is not diagnosed early, patients may present later in life with symptoms of heart failure from having developed a tachycardia-mediated cardiomyopathy.

Demographics of the disease

AVRT accounts for roughly 35% of all cases of SVT, and is therefore the second most common form of narrow-complex SVT, after AVNRT, which represents 50%–60% of SVT cases. The overall incidence of antegradely conducting accessory pathways detected on ECGs is between 0.01% and 0.31%; however, this does not necessarily correlate with symptomatic tachycardia predisposition. AVRT affects all ages, but the incidence decreases with age, with a mean age of symptom onset in the thirties. The incidence of accessory pathways in first-degree relatives of patients with pre-excitation is 3.4%, significantly higher than in the general population. Although pre-excitation appears to be lost in nearly one-quarter of cases over time, the relationship of this observation to symptom frequency is unclear.

Natural history, and complications of the disease

Of patients with A–V bypass tracts, between 40% and 80% will manifest tachycardias at some stage, with the tachycardia most commonly being oAVRT. aAVRT is much less common and, interestingly, atrial fibrillation or flutter may be the initial arrhythmia noted in 5%–10% of these patients, rather than AVRT.

Up to 50% of patients with AVRT will experience atrial fibrillation at some stage; the reasons for this are not clear. Overt pre-excitation (antegradely conducting accessory pathways) is associated with atrial fibrillation five times more than concealed pathways of a similar location are.

Antegradely conducting accessory pathways are often capable of very rapid and frequent conduction of atrial arrhythmias to the ventricles. This is an important consideration in assessing the potential for the accessory pathway to induce ventricular fibrillation in the setting of atrial fibrillation. Similarly, in the setting of atrial flutter, 1:1 atrioventricular conduction can occur, resulting in ventricular rates of 300 min^{-1}. Ventricular fibrillation and sudden death can occur in a small percentage of these patients. The incidence of sudden death (SCD) in patients with antegrade pre-excitation is quite low, ranging from 0%

to 0.39% annually. Most patients with an accessory pathway and who have survived an aborted episode of SCD have a history of AVRT or atrial fibrillation. The main predictors of risk include the refractory period of the pathway (i.e. how quickly the pathway can recover from one depolarization and conduct another), and the shortest R to R interval seen during atrial fibrillation; an effective refractory period of <250 ms, measured at an electrophysiology study, and a minimum R to R interval less than 250 ms during an episode of atrial fibrillation are considered to be markers of increased risk. Conversely, a pathway that demonstrates intermittent pre-excitation is not likely to be dangerous, as the refractory period and minimum R-to-R intervals are unlikely to be <250 ms if studied at an electrophysiology study. As such, patients of this latter type rarely require an invasive study for the purpose of risk stratification.

Concealed bypass tracts (retrogradely conducting only) can be fast-conducting or (much less commonly) slowly conducting. The former gives rise to paroxysmal SVT with a long RP (and therefore short PR) interval, and the latter can result in constant re-entrant tachycardia and a tachycardia-mediated cardiomyopathy (PJRT is one such type, often seen in children or adolescents).

Accessory pathways can be associated with other congenital cardiac disease, most notably Ebstein's anomaly (which is associated in 10% of cases with pre-excitation). Right-sided accessory connections seem to be much more commonly associated with congenital heart disease than left-sided ones are (45% compared to 5%).

Approach to diagnosing the disease (including diagnostic pitfalls)

AVRT, like AVNRT, manifests most commonly as a regular, narrow-QRS-complex tachycardia on the ECG, with or without apparent P waves. Differentiating AVRT from other types of SVT can be difficult, but there are some additional clues that can suggest AVRT as the diagnosis; for example, the presence of delta waves on the baseline 12-lead ECG favours AVRT, as does a long RP interval. Also, if any periods of AV block are seen (i.e. two or three P waves per QRS complex), this effectively excludes AVRT from the diagnosis, given that AVRT requires the atrium and the ventricle as integral parts of the tachycardia circuit. Atrial tachycardia and flutter, on the other hand, do not require the ventricular myocardium to sustain the arrhythmia (which is confined to the atria); therefore, periods of AV block can be seen during ongoing tachycardia. Often, the only way to firmly establish AVRT as the diagnosis is to perform an invasive electrophysiology study.

Occasionally, antegradely conducting accessory pathways are present in patients who experience other tachycardias, and this can give rise to other forms of 'pre-excited' tachycardia that can make diagnosis challenging. For example, a patient with atrial flutter, atrial tachycardia, or AVNRT may have an antegradely conducting accessory pathway (either manifest or latent during sinus rhythm) which causes a degree of QRS widening during tachycardia, but which is not itself a part of the tachycardia mechanism. Pre-excited atrial fibrillation is another example of a bystander accessory pathway which carries with it certain specific risks needing to be considered, as previously described.

'Gold-standard' diagnostic test

The gold-standard diagnostic test for pre-excitation on the ECG and AVRT is the invasive electrophysiology study.

Acceptable diagnostic alternatives to the gold standard

There are currently no other diagnostic tests that can definitively diagnose AVRT, other than an invasive electrophysiological investigation.

Other relevant investigations

Given the association between accessory pathways and congenital cardiac abnormalities, especially Ebstein's anomaly, echocardiographic investigation should be considered in all patients with accessory pathways, especially right-sided pathways, as the association is stronger here. No other specific investigations are routinely indicated; however, some patients may warrant investigation for coronary ischaemia (if chest pain and ischaemic ECG changes are noted during episodes of AVRT).

Prognosis, and how to estimate it

Over time, some patients lose the pre-excited appearance to their ECG. The likelihood of experiencing symptomatic arrhythmia relates to the age at diagnosis, with older patients less likely to experience AVRT than patients diagnosed with pre-excitation at an early age. The risk of SCD in the setting of atrial fibrillation and an antegradely conducting accessory pathway is discussed in 'Natural history, and complications of the disease'.

Treatment and its effectiveness

Acute management

The immediate treatment for an episode of AVRT should focus on termination. In the first instance, so-called vagal manoeuvers can be tried; for example, the Valsalva manoeuver and carotid sinus massage are often effective in terminating an episode, especially if they are attempted early. Failing these, acute pharmacotherapy can be administered, with the same intention of acutely terminating the arrhythmia. Adenosine is probably the best initial choice of drug, and needs to be administered as a rapid IV bolus via a proximal vein, given the very short plasma half-life of this drug. Adenosine can induce premature atrial extrasystoles, and can reinduce AVRT. Other choices of agent include verapamil, and then flecainide. In the setting of hypotension or haemodynamic instability, DC cardioversion is appropriate, if the other measures have failed or are inappropriate.

In the setting of a wide-QRS tachycardia in a patient suspected of having an accessory pathway, it is important to determine whether or not atrial fibrillation is in fact the underlying arrhythmia—for the reason that any drug which is administered in this situation and which has AV nodal blocking properties (i.e. beta blockers, centrally acting calcium-channel blockers, digoxin, adenosine) will cause AV nodal block, thus preferentially causing ventricular activation to occur exclusively via the accessory pathway (without actually terminating the underlying atrial fibrillation). The effect of this can be the induction of ventricular fibrillation, and SCD. In the situation of an irregular, rapid, wide-complex tachycardia, IV flecainide is the drug of choice, after which DC cardioversion should be chosen as the best management.

Prevention of recurrences

The decision regarding when to institute prophylactic treatment against recurrent SVT episodes is difficult, and essentially depends on the degree to which the symptoms are interfering with a particular patient's life and work. For example, some patients are easily able to terminate episodes rapidly with a vagal manoeuver, without the need for medications or presentations to the emergency room. These patients do not need to take regular prophylaxis against further episodes. On the other hand, if episodes are frequent and intrusive, or cannot be terminated with vagal manoeuvers, beta blockers and non-dihydropyridine calcium-channel blockers are frequently prescribed, given their (relatively) superior safety and side-effect profile when compared to Class I and III antiarrhythmic agents. The benefits of these drugs, on the other hand, may be limited, as they do not affect accessory pathway function directly—rather, they slow AV nodal transit and might possibly (in the case of beta blockers) reduce the catecholamine-mediated premature atrial complexes that can induce episodes of AVRT.

If these agents are ineffective, then Class Ic antiarrhythmic agents (flecainide, propafenone) are the next treatment of choice, but the pro-arrhythmic potential of these drugs (especially in patients with structural or ischaemic heart disease) limits their use. Amiodarone and sotalol are also effective in the long-term prophylaxis of episodes of AVRT, but long-term toxicity, in the case of amiodarone, and pro-arrhythmia, in the case of sotalol (QT prolongation and torsades-de-points risk) make these drugs less attractive for long-term management.

Electrophysiology studies and percutaneous catheter ablation of the accessory pathway is now an established treatment for recurrent symptomatic AVRT, and should be considered early in the natural history of the condition. Acute procedural success rates and long-term success rates are around 95%, with no requirement for ongoing medical prophylaxis against further episodes in those successfully treated. Additionally, the performing of an electrophysiology study enables risk stratification of the pathway. The procedure is minimally invasive, and is performed by the transvenous route (usually via the femoral vein); as such, it can be complicated by vascular injury and perforation, but this is uncommon (~0.5%). The other significant complication of SVT ablation in general terms is inadvertent compact AV nodal ablation, resulting in complete heart block and the need for permanent pacing. This also is a rare occurrence (~0.5%), but may be a significant consideration, especially in very young patients, for whom a permanent pacemaker would involve numerous device and lead revisions over the ensuing years.

Key points

The key points to note about AVRT are as follows:

- AVRT is one type of SVT, the others being AVNRT, focal (ectopic) atrial tachycardia, and atrial flutter.
- Symptoms include palpitations, dyspnoea, chest pain, dizziness, and syncope
- AVRT results from a re-entrant circuit, made up of the AV node and an accessory pathway between the atria and ventricles. The pathway, AV node, and ventricular and atrial myocardia are all integral parts of the re-entry circuit—as such, AVRT can only ever be seen with a 1:1 atrioventricular relationship—**any periods when the A:V or V:A ratio is 2:1 or more excludes AVRT as the diagnosis**.
- The accessory connection can be **manifest** (delta waves on the sinus rhythm ECG), **latent** (no delta waves seem but pathway is still capable of antegrade conduction), or **concealed** (the pathway can only conduct backwards and so is not apparent on sinus-rhythm 12-lead ECG).
- The delta wave represents a **fusion** of ventricular activation events during sinus rhythm, with some taking place via the AV node, and some taking place via the accessory pathway.
- **oAVRT** utilizes the AV node antegradely, and the accessory pathway conducts retrogradely; **aAVRT** does the reverse (antegrade conduction is via the pathway, and retrograde is via the AV node).
- oAVRT is usually a narrow-QRS-complex SVT (unless bundle branch block has occurred), with P waves seen to follow the QRS complexes in a 1:1 relationship. The RP interval is variable, but is usually longer than that seen in AVNRT.
- aAVRT has a wide and fully pre-excited QRS morphology, as all the ventricular activation is taking place via the accessory pathway.
- Certain patients with antegrade-conducting accessory pathways are at a slightly elevated risk of SCD, as a consequence of very rapid conduction of atrial arrhythmias (generally coincidental atrial fibrillation) to the ventricles, thus inducing ventricular fibrillation. The risk marker for this possibility is a minimum R to R interval during atrial fibrillation of <250 ms, and (at electrophysiology study) an accessory pathway refractory period of <250 ms.
- AVRT in the absence of atrial fibrillation or flutter is not considered an indication for anticoagulation per se.
- Carotid sinus massage, other vagal manoeuvers, and IV adenosine may acutely terminate AVRT. Many patients are successfully managed in the long term with self-administered vagal manoeuvers, which terminate episodes of AVRT but do not reduce the frequency of recurrent episodes.
- AV nodal blocking drugs are frequently used for prophylaxis, but efficacy is often low. Class I and III antiarrhythmic agents are effective, but pro-arrhythmic side effects and long-term toxicities make these less attractive long-term management options.

- Percutaneous transvenous catheter ablation of the accessory pathway is the treatment of choice for many patients with recurrent symptomatic AVRT, provides a long-term cure in over 95%, and, at the very least, can risk stratify the accessory pathway. This technique is associated with a ~0.5% risk of adverse outcomes, including the need for a permanent pacemaker. As such, the pros and cons of an invasive approach need to be fully discussed with the patient prior to considering this approach.

Further Reading

Page RL, Joglar JA, Caldwell MA, et al. 2015 ACC/AHA/HRS guideline for the management of adult patients with supraventricular tachycardia: a report of the American College of Cardiology/American Heart Association Task Force on Clinical Practice Guidelines and the Heart Rhythm Society. *J Am Coll Cardiol* 2016; 67; e27–115.

116 Atrial fibrillation

Michael Jones, Norman Qureshi, and Kim Rajappan

Definition of the disease

Atrial fibrillation is a tachycardia arising in the atria, with atrial electrical activity occurring chaotically and continuously, without any effective atrial contraction occurring. The effects of this are an irregular ventricular rate, loss of the atrial contribution to ventricular filling, and the pooling of blood in the atria, thus increasing the risk of thrombus formation. The ventricular rate may be fast, slow, or of normal speed, depending on the state of the patient's atrioventricular conduction.

Atrial fibrillation is classified as paroxysmal (self-terminating within 7 days), persistent (lasting longer than 1 week, or requiring cardioversion to terminate), long-standing (continuous, lasting for ≥1 year when it is decided to adopt a rhythm control strategy), or permanent (cardioversion unable to terminate durably to sinus rhythm).

Aetiology of the disease

Atrial fibrillation can arise in structurally normal hearts ('lone' atrial fibrillation) but, more commonly, it occurs in the setting of structural heart disease, namely, as an atrial myopathic process which can be found at microscopic level, even in lone atrial fibrillation patients. This atriopathy is associated with progressive and diffuse changes in electrical conduction velocity and tissue refractoriness (time to recovery of excitability), which results in non-uniform anisotropic conduction of electrical impulses. Or, to put it another way, the atrial tissue progressively develops diffusely and non-uniformly distributed slowing in electrical conduction velocity, but tissue recovery becomes markedly quicker. The complex, multilayered anatomy of the atrial muscular wall itself increases the electrophysiological significance of this anisotropy. In addition to these factors, there exists a diffusely distributed relative imbalance in cholinergic and sympathetic innervation of the atria. These three factors are currently believed to provide the cellular basis for sustained fibrillatory atrial electrical conduction.

The triggering event for episodes of atrial fibrillation has been shown to be high frequency bursts of electrical activity that arise in the very proximal parts of the pulmonary veins, near to where they enter the left atrium. These electrical discharges conduct out from the pulmonary veins into the left atrium, and initiate an episode of atrial fibrillation. The result is disorganized and constantly changing atrial activation patterns, at 'rates' of between 200 and 500 min⁻¹. The AV node normally conducts sinus rhythm with a 1:1 atrial systole:ventricular systole ratio; during atrial fibrillation, the intrinsic physiology of the AV node protects against 1:1 conduction of the fibrillation waves to the ventricles (which would result in ventricular fibrillation and death if it did occur); nevertheless, the ventricular rates are generally elevated in atrial fibrillation, compared to normal sinus rhythm. During an episode of atrial fibrillation, the sinus node is essentially overdrive-suppressed by the fibrillation (i.e. it is constantly penetrated and reset by the fibrillation waves, and does not discharge).

Medical conditions that predispose to developing atrial fibrillation include chronic hypertension/hypertensive heart disease, ischaemic heart disease, heart failure/dilated cardiomyopathy, rheumatic/valvular heart disease, hypertrophic cardiomyopathy, congenital heart disease, pulmonary embolism, myocarditis, pericarditis, obstructive sleep apnoea, obesity, hyperthyroidism, alcoholism, and a family history of atrial fibrillation (genetic factors).

Typical symptoms of the disease, and less common symptoms

Atrial fibrillation may be (a) completely asymptomatic, (b) symptomatic secondary to predisposing medical conditions (e.g. hyperthyroidism), (c) symptomatic secondary to the sequelae of atrial fibrillation (e.g. left ventricular failure, thromboembolism), or (d) symptomatic directly as a consequence of the atrial fibrillation itself. The latter type can include all of the following symptoms: palpitations, dyspnoea, fatigue, effort intolerance, chest pain, presyncope, syncope, and weakness.

While some paroxysms of atrial fibrillation may be associated with some or all of these symptoms, others are completely asymptomatic, even in the same patient. An important consideration is syncope, which can indicate any of the following: a significant pause after termination of a paroxysm of atrial fibrillation (slow recovery of the sinus node, especially in the elderly); very slow atrioventricular conduction of atrial fibrillation (e.g. in response to excessive AV nodal blocking medication); very rapid atrioventricular conduction in patients with diastolic heart dysfunction, outflow tract obstruction, or rapidly conducting accessory AV connections; or the presence of another arrhythmia, such as ventricular tachycardia, in the setting of left ventricular systolic dysfunction.

Demographics of atrial fibrillation

The overall prevalence of atrial fibrillation is currently around 1%. Atrial fibrillation is more common in men, in all age groups, and the incidence and prevalence increase with age; in those aged over 80, the prevalence is 9%. The overall prevalence appears to be increasing over time.

Natural history, and complications

The natural history of atrial fibrillation is quite variable, and depends to a significant degree on the correction of any predisposing medical conditions (i.e. control of hypertension and hyperthyroidism, correction of valvular heart lesions). Nevertheless, atrial fibrillation tends to progress over time from infrequent to more frequent paroxysms, to persistent episodes requiring cardioversion, and eventually to permanent atrial fibrillation. The expression, 'atrial fibrillation begets atrial fibrillation', refers to the progressive atriopathy and left atrial dilatation that accompany increasing atrial fibrillation burden, such that the electrophysiological abnormalities in atrial myocytes progressively worsen with higher atrial fibrillation burden, and thus predispose to ever more atrial fibrillation. To an extent, the reverse is also true (sinus rhythm begets sinus rhythm, with improvement in the cellular electrophysiological abnormalities).

Untreated, atrial fibrillation may result in (a) no complications (truly silent atrial fibrillation); (b) thromboembolic complications, such as stroke or peripheral arterial or coronary arterial embolization; (c) left ventricular dilatation, impaired systolic contractility, functional mitral incompetence, and heart failure symptoms, especially if ventricular rates have been generally fast (>100 min⁻¹); and (d) progressive slowing of ventricular rates with advancing age (due to degenerative fibrosis of the AV node), resulting in increasing effort intolerance, fatigue, and, eventually, syncope.

Approach to diagnosing the arrhythmia, including clinical clues, through concentrating on the ECG diagnosis

Atrial fibrillation is a clinical diagnosis in the first instance, based upon the examination finding of an irregularly irregular pulse and usually associated with variation in the intensity of the heart sounds and in the intensity (to palpation) of the carotid and radial pulses. Blood pressure is also variable, beat to beat.

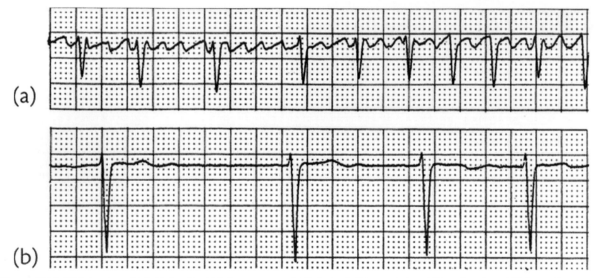

Figure 116.1 ECG showing atrial fibrillation. Panel (a) shows coarse atrial fibrillation (which can mimic atrial flutter), and panel (b) fine atrial fibrillation.

Reproduced with permission from David A. Warrell, Timothy M. Cox, and John D. Firth, *Oxford Textbook of Medicine*, Latest update: May 2017, Figure 16.4.24, Oxford University Press, Oxford, UK, Copyright © 2017.

The diagnosis of atrial fibrillation requires confirmation by ECG in all cases (Figure 116.1); the absence of organized atrial activity (no uniform P waves, although the atrial activation can often appear quite coarse and of high amplitude, especially in Lead V1) is diagnostic. The ventricular response is usually irregular, but may not always be (i.e. in the setting of ventricular pacing in a patient with underlying atrial fibrillation).

Atrial fibrillation should be suspected in patients describing palpitations, dyspnoea, or effort intolerance and who have risk factors for atrial fibrillation, as described in 'Aetiology of the disease'. Patients may not be in atrial fibrillation at the time of clinic review; therefore, ambulatory monitoring should be performed to attempt making the diagnosis. This can take the form of a 24-hour Holter monitor, a ≥2-week external event recorder, or an implantable subcutaneous loop monitor—the choice depending on the frequency of symptoms, and the difficulty and significance of making the diagnosis in each case (i.e. it might not be justified in some patients to proceed to invasive monitoring procedures).

Other arrhythmias may appear irregularly irregular on clinical examination, namely, atrial flutter and atrial tachycardia with variable AV nodal conduction. Prolonged examination should reveal periods of regularity, at different rates; in these cases, however, only the ECG provides a definitive diagnosis.

Other diagnoses that should be considered

Atrial flutter frequently coexists with atrial fibrillation in the same patient, and can produce symptoms which are similar to those of atrial fibrillation. Most other clinical arrhythmias can also produce symptoms similar to those of atrial fibrillation, including supraventricular tachycardia (ectopic atrial tachycardia, multifocal atria tachycardia, AV nodal re-entrant tachycardia, and AV re-entrant tachycardia), and ventricular tachycardia. The ECG provides the definitive diagnosis of atrial fibrillation and distinguishes it from the other tachyarrhythmias.

'Gold-standard' diagnostic test

The gold-standard diagnostic test for atrial fibrillation remains the ECG; the finding of no definite P waves and, frequently, an irregular ventricular rhythm, is diagnostic.

Acceptable diagnostic alternatives to the gold standard

There are currently no other diagnostic tests that can definitively diagnose atrial fibrillation, other than electrocardiographic or invasive electrophysiological investigation.

Other relevant investigations

Echocardiography should be performed in all cases, to investigate for valvular heart disease, hypertensive heart disease, intra-cardiac shunts (an agitated saline study may be required if clinical suspicion of a shunt is high), left ventricular size and function, left atrial dimension, pulmonary pressures, right-heart function, and pericardial appearance. Full blood examination and clotting studies are mandatory, to exclude anaemia and define baseline coagulatory function (important if anticoagulation or antiplatelet therapy is being considered). Renal function and electrolyte testing are essential, as a prelude to the safe use of many relevant medications (angiotensin-converting enzyme (ACE) inhibitors, angiotensin II receptor antagonists, calcium-channel and beta blockers, digoxin, direct rennin inhibitors, diuretics, etc.). Baseline liver function is mandatory also, prior to the institution of vitamin K analogue therapy, or amiodarone/dronedarone therapy.

Other investigations may be indicated, depending on the clinical setting; a suspicion of coronary disease or the desire to use Class I antiarrhythmic drugs might mandate an exercise treadmill test, a myocardial perfusion scan, or a coronary angiogram; the need to assess heart-rate control in long-term rate-controlled atrial fibrillation might require a 24-hour, ambulatory Holter monitor and an exercise treadmill test; alternatively, an invasive electrophysiology study may be required, if pre-excitation is suspected, or if distal conduction system disease is suspected in the context of unexplained syncope. Finally, transoesophageal echocardiography may be indicated in the setting of elective cardioversion, if anticoagulation has been subtherapeutic, to exclude the presence of left atrial appendage thrombus.

Prognosis

The data from the Framingham and other epidemiological studies have suggested a slight reduction in life expectancy in sufferers of atrial fibrillation, but whether this is largely due to the comorbid conditions that predispose to atrial fibrillation is unclear.

If the atrial fibrillation is left untreated, there is an increased risk of thromboembolic events in paroxysmal, persistent, and permanent atrial fibrillation patients, and this risk increases with age, gender, and comorbid conditions. The CHA_2DS_2-VASC scoring algorithm is currently the most widely accepted means of determining the long-term anticoagulation requirements of any individual patient. Treatment with antiplatelet or anticoagulant therapy has a definite and favourable impact on the risk of thromboembolism, but at the cost of a higher risk of bleeding. This bleeding risk profile is slightly improved with newer direct-acting oral anticoagulants (DOAC) anticoagulants (DOAC), such as dabigatran, a direct thrombin inhibitor, or rivaroxaban, apixaban and edoxaban which target Factor Xa directly. Before prescribing long-term anticoagulation, consideration of the bleeding risk and potential for falls must be made. In the case of falls risk and bleeding, recent data suggest that a very high burden of falls is needed before the risks of anticoagulation outweigh the benefits in patients at high risk of stroke.

There are as yet no conclusive data that reverting atrial fibrillation to sinus rhythm and attempting to maintain sinus rhythm in the long term is associated with any improvement in morbidity or mortality in the majority of patients. Trials of drug therapy to maintain sinus rhythm have not demonstrated a superiority of rhythm control over rate control strategies. This is in part due to the difficulty in restoring and maintaining sinus rhythm in these patients with the drugs currently available for this purpose, the side effects/toxicities of these currently available antiarrhythmic drugs, and the significant patient crossover that has occurred in these studies (i.e. many patients in the rate control arm of the study inadvertently ending up in sinus rhythm for the majority of the study, but still analysed in their original cohort).

There may be prognostic benefits to restoring and maintaining sinus rhythm by catheter ablation, in terms of reduced stroke risk and less heart failure in certain populations, but this is still under investigation in large prospective clinical trials and, at present, these techniques are only offered on the basis of improving atrial fibrillation symptoms that cannot be managed effectively with medical therapy.

Uncontrolled rapid ventricular rates over a prolonged period can lead to a tachycardia-mediated cardiomyopathy, which to a large degree is reversible with correction (slowing) of ventricular rates.

Treatment and its effectiveness

The treatment of atrial fibrillation involves four considerations: (1) emergency vs non-emergent management, (2) management of symptomatic paroxysmal atrial fibrillation, (3) decisions on a rate control or a rhythm control strategy in recurrent persistent atrial fibrillation, and (4) the requirements for anticoagulation.

Atrial fibrillation can present as an emergency in some settings: a paroxysm of atrial fibrillation can result in a precipitous fall in cardiac output in certain patients (e.g. those with severe aortic stenosis, severe mitral stenosis, severe hypertensive heart disease with diastolic impairment, or outflow tract obstruction). Significant hypotension and shock in the setting of atrial fibrillation should prompt a search for such underlying conditions. Emergency cardioversion to sinus rhythm is often required in these cases.

In the setting of rapidly conducted atrial fibrillation which requires urgent rate control, where cardioversion is not felt necessary, many medications are efficacious; IV beta blockade with 1 mg aliquots of metoprolol or atenolol, or 1 mg aliquots of verapamil, titrated to ventricular rate, are effective in reducing ventricular rates acutely, but these agents are contraindicated in patients in shock or with significant hypotension—in which case, digoxin is a safer alternative, but often lacks potency in acute rate control. Amiodarone is another alternative here, as it does not cause significant hypotension, but there is a risk of acutely restoring sinus rhythm with its use, and this may not be desirable. In addition to medications for rate control, a search for the cause of the rapidly conducted atrial fibrillation should be made (e.g. sepsis, hypovolaemia, anaemia, hypoxia, etc.) and corrected.

Atrial fibrillation can be conducted very rapidly to the ventricles in patients who have accessory A–V connections capable of conduction at fast rates—this is termed 'pre-excited atrial fibrillation'. This can lead to shock, the induction of ventricular fibrillation, and death. Emergency cardioversion is frequently required in these cases also. The key to diagnosing pre-excited atrial fibrillation is the presence of a very fast ventricular rate, which is also irregular, with QRS complexes continuously varying in width (reflecting differing degrees of fusion of ventricular activation, via the AV node and the AV bypass tract). Another clue is gained from previous ECGs performed during sinus rhythm, which will usually reveal evidence of pre-excitation (a delta wave). In this situation of pre-excited atrial fibrillation, alone of all tachyarrhythmias, the administration of AV nodal blocking agents (adenosine, verapamil, diltiazem, and digoxin) can be fatal, as it leads to near-complete ventricular activation via the bypass tract at very fast rates, and the induction of ventricular fibrillation as a consequence.

The next consideration is the management of paroxysmal atrial fibrillation. In addition to addressing predisposing medical conditions and identifying triggers for episodes, the options include conservative management (rest, relaxation) if symptoms are mild, or cardioversion (electrical or pharmacological) if symptoms merit this. Medications commonly used for chemical cardioversion include Class I and III antiarrhythmic drugs; in the ambulatory setting, patients often self-treat with 'pill-in-the-pocket' therapy, using flecainide or propafenone, primarily. The absence of significant coronary disease and myocardial scar is considered a prerequisite for the safe use of these drugs, as they can be pro-arrhythmic in such patients. In the emergency room, flecainide, propafenone, ibutilide, sotalol, and amiodarone are all available for acute cardioversion. A newer agent, vernakalant, is promising and demonstrates high acute cardioversion rates, but is not yet widely available.

For patients experiencing frequent paroxysms that require termination, regular daily medication with antiarrhythmic drug therapy is often used, and potential medications include flecainide, propafenone, sotalol, and dronedarone. Amiodarone is still used in this setting, but concerns regarding the drug's multiple toxicities limit its use. In some countries dofetilide and ibutilide are available. Regular antiarrhythmic medication use is effective in a large number of patients for controlling symptoms of atrial fibrillation.

For those who fail to respond to drug therapy or who tolerate it poorly, the next option is percutaneous catheter ablation (left atrial ablation, consisting of pulmonary venous antral electrical isolation and sometimes additional linear and focal ablation). This technique can eliminate atrial fibrillation in 70%–80% of patients, but may require more than one procedure, and carries with it some risks, including vascular trauma, cardiac tamponade, stroke, pulmonary vein stenosis, atrio-oesophageal fistula formation, gastroparesis from oesophageal nerve injury, post-procedure iatrogenic atrial arrhythmias, and even death. Nevertheless, it is an effective treatment in highly symptomatic patients for whom drug therapy has been ineffective or poorly tolerated.

For those patients requiring cardiac surgical treatment for another reason (e.g. coronary bypass grafting, valve surgery), consideration should be given to performing an intra-operative atrial ablation procedure (termed the 'maze' procedure) as a part of the surgery. Some centres also offer surgical maze procedures as stand-alone procedures, but the added risks of an open surgical procedure compared to those of a percutaneous transcatheter approach limit this to a small proportion of patients only.

In patients with long-lasting recurrent persistent or permanent atrial fibrillation, where the restoration of sinus rhythm has been unsuccessful by definition, management options include catheter ablation, as previously described, if a rhythm control strategy is desired, or rate control of the atrial fibrillation. In the case of rate control, AV nodal blocking medications are used in the first instance, consisting of beta blockade, calcium-channel blockade, and digoxin. Occasionally, these medications can result in episodes of symptomatic bradycardia, and a ventricular pacemaker is required. In some cases, drugs alone are insufficient to slow AV nodal conduction, or are poorly tolerated—in these cases, ventricular pacing is implemented, followed by AV nodal ablation. In this case, a patient becomes completely dependent on the pacemaker for the generation of a cardiac rhythm.

As previously mentioned, some patients with atrial fibrillation remain asymptomatic for many years, but eventually present with symptoms of bradycardia. The finding is usually one of AV nodal and/or conduction system disease, and permanent ventricular pacing is usually indicated.

Anticoagulation

Anticoagulation and cardioversion

In the setting of acute cardioversion, thromboembolic risk depends on the duration of the current atrial fibrillation episode, and patient-specific risk factors for stroke. As they presently stand, European Society of Cardiology (ESC) guidelines recommend at least 3 weeks of warfarin (international normalized ratio (INR) 2–3) or uninterrupted DOAC administration prior to and 4 weeks after cardioversion (electrical **or** pharmacological), if atrial fibrillation has been present for ≥48 hours. If the duration of atrial fibrillation is definitely less than 48 hours, but the patient is at high stroke risk, heparin or low molecular weight heparin is recommended pericardioversion, and warfarin/DOAC post cardioversion, in the long term. Finally, if the duration is definitely less than 48 hours, and patient is at low risk for stroke, then pericardioversion anticoagulation is optional, and post-procedure anticoagulation is unnecessary.

An alternative to 3 weeks of pretreatment with warfarin/DOAC is precardioversion transoesophageal echocardiography, which can be used to exclude the presence of a left atrial appendage thrombus—if a thrombus is present, then, obviously, cardioversion is deferred (at least 3 weeks, during which time anticoagulation is administered, followed by repeat transoesophageal echocardiography) but, if there is no thrombus, cardioversion can take place with pericardioversion anticoagulation and with at least 4 weeks of warfarin/DOAC post cardioversion.

Long-term anticoagulation

The decision to anticoagulate in the long term depends on the presence of stroke risk factors (Table 116.1), namely, patient age, sex, history of prior stroke, diabetes, heart failure, vascular disease, and hypertension. Currently, these risk factors are weighted and summed according to the CHA$_2$DS$_2$-VASc algorithm, and the score used to determine the merits of aspirin, vitamin K antagonist/DOAC, or no anticoagulation. The greater the number of risk factors, the higher is the yearly stroke risk—one risk factor gives a 1.3% yearly risk of stroke, whereas all nine give a risk of 15.2% per annum. Consideration must always be made of the risk of bleeding on anticoagulation therapy, and the HASBLED score can help in this respect (see Table 116.2 and Figure 116.2); while it is not used to

Table 116.2 Application of CHA$_2$DS$_2$-VASc score, and HASBLED calculation of bleeding risk on anticoagulation therapy

Clinical characteristics comprising the HAS-BLED bleeding risk score		
Letter	Clinical characteristic	Points awarded
H	Hypertension	1
A	Abnormal renal and liver function (1 point each)	1 or 2
S	Stroke	1
B	Bleeding tendency or predisposition	1
L	Labile INRs (if taking VKA)	1
E	Elderly (e.g., age >65, frail condition)	1
D	Drugs (concomitant aspirin, NSAID) or alcohol (1 point each)	1 or 2
		Maximum 9 points

Abbreviations: INR, international normalized ratio; NSAID, non-steroidal anti-inflammatory drug; VKA, vitamin K antagonist.

Reproduced from Corrigendum to: 'Guidelines: 2012 focused update of the ESC Guidelines for the management of atrial fibrillation: an update of the 2010 ESC Guidelines for the management of atrial fibrillation, European Heart Journal, Volume 34, Issue 36, With permission of Oxford University Press (UK) © European Society of Cardiology, www.escardio.org/guidelines.

preclude a patient from anticoagulation, it helps in making decision regarding frequency of follow-up, and consideration of alternatives to anticoagulation, where available.

For those patients at high risk of stroke, but who are intolerant of or unfit for anticoagulation, another technology is available, namely the left atrial appendage occlusion device. This device is placed percutaneously into the left atrial appendage, and deployed, thus excluding the appendage from the left atrial blood, and thereby reducing the risk of cardiac thromboembolic events. Although still being investigated, preliminary data suggest that this technique reduces stroke in these patients to a degree similar to that obtained via anticoagulation.

These guidelines are revised periodically, and it is important to be familiar with the latest recommendations.

Normally, once a decision has been made to anticoagulate, this is continued throughout the patient's life, as there is still no technique which can definitively cure atrial fibrillation and be sufficient to eliminate ongoing stroke risk and so enable the discontinuation of anticoagulation.

Key points

The key points concerning atrial fibrillation are as follows:

- Atrial fibrillation is defined by rapid and chaotic atrial activity, usually with an irregular ventricular response rate, which may be fast, slow, or of normal speed.
- The clinical significance of atrial fibrillation relates to the risk of thromboembolism and stroke, the risk of uncontrolled rapid ventricular rates (which can lead to a cardiomyopathy), and the risk of excessively slow ventricular rates (and possible syncope).
- Atrial fibrillation requires an ECG for diagnosis in all cases. The absence of uniform P waves is diagnostic of atrial fibrillation.
- The use of **adenosine** or **carotid sinus massage** results in a transient slowing of the ventricular rate, but has no effect on atrial activity.
- Differentials in the diagnosis for atrial fibrillation include atrial tachycardia, atrial flutter, AV nodal re-entrant tachycardia, and atrioventricular re-entrant tachycardia.
- Atrial fibrillation almost never terminates with a closely coupled sinus beat following the termination of atrial fibrillation; if this is seen, then question whether atrial fibrillation is the correct diagnosis (i.e. ventricular tachycardia or another supraventricular tachycardia may be the correct explanation).
- Ventricular pacing may obscure the underlying presence of atrial fibrillation; in any case of pacing on an ECG, look carefully for evidence of atrial activity.
- The need for anticoagulation depends upon the setting (emergent vs long term), and patient-specific risk factors, which are currently

Table 116.1 The CHA$_2$DS$_2$-VASc scoring system for determining risk for stroke in atrial fibrillation patients

a) The risk factor based approach expressed as a point based scoring system, with the acronym CHA$_2$DS$_2$-VASc
(Note: maximum score is 9 since age may contribute 0, 1 or 2 points)

Risk factor	Score
Congestive heart failure/LV dysfunction	1
Hypertension	1
Age ≥75	**2**
Diabetes mellitus	1
Stroke/TIA/TE	**2**
Vascular disease[a]	1
Age 65–74	**1**
Sex category (i.e., female gender)	1
Maximum score	**9**

b) Adjusted stroke rate according to CHA$_2$DS$_2$-VASc score

CHA$_2$DS$_2$-VASc score	Patients (n = 73538)	Stroke and thromboembolism event rate at 1 year follow-up (%)
0	6369	0.78
1	8203	2.01
2	12771	3.71
3	17371	5.92
4	13887	9.27
5	8942	15.26
6	4244	19.74
7	1420	21.50
8	285	22.38
9	46	23.64

Abbreviations: LV, left ventricular; TE, thromboembolism; TIA, transient ischaemic attack.
Note: Actual rates of stroke in contemporary cohorts may vary from these estimates. Stroke, TIA, or systemic embolism and age ≥75 years are regarded as major risk factors, and others are described as clinically relevant non-major risk factors.
[a]Prior myocardial infarction, peripheral artery disease, aortic plaque.
Reproduced from Corrigendum to: 'Guidelines: 2012 focused update of the ESC Guidelines for the management of atrial fibrillation: an update of the 2010 ESC Guidelines for the management of atrial fibrillation, European Heart Journal, Volume 34, Issue 36, With permission of Oxford University Press (UK) © European Society of Cardiology, www.escardio.org/guidelines.

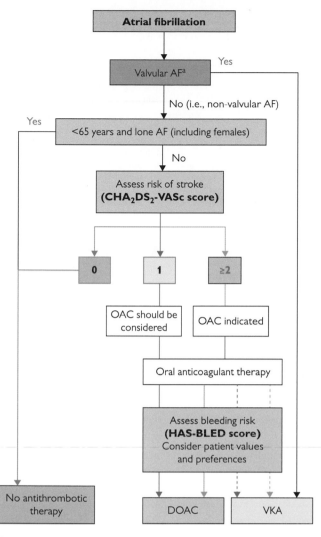

Antiplatelet therapy with aspirin plus clopidogrel, or—less effectively—aspirin only, should be considered in patients who refuse any OAC, or cannot tolerate anticoagulants for reasons unrelated to bleeding. If there are contraindications to OAC or antiplatelet therapy, left atrial appendage occlusion, closure or excision may be considered.

Colour: CHA_2DS_2-VASc; green = 0, blue = 1, red ≥ 2.

Line: solid = best option; dashed = alternative option.

AF = atrial fibrillation; CHA_2DS_2-VASc = see text; HAS-BLED = see text; DOAC = direct-acting oral anticoagulant; OAC = oral anticoagulant; VKA = vitamin K antagonist.

[a]Includes rheumatic valvular disease and prosthetic valves.

Figure 116.2 Choice of anticoagulant: antiplatelet therapy with aspirin plus clopidogrel, or—less effectively—aspirin only, should be considered in patients who refuse any oral anticoagulant or cannot tolerate anticoagulants for reasons unrelated to bleeding. If there are contraindications to oral anticoagulant or antiplatelet therapy, then left atrial appendage occlusion, closure, or excision may be considered. Solid lines indicate the best options; dashed lines indicate alternative options; * includes rheumatic valvular disease and prosthetic valves; AF, atrial fibrillation; NOAC, novel DOAC, direct-acting oral anticoagulant; VKA, vitamin K antagonist.

assessed by the CHA_2DS_2-VASc score. The decision to anticoagulate is individualized to the patient in every case, and involves the family physician and outpatient services significantly.

- Currently, the main indication for catheter ablation is in drug refractory, symptomatic patients.

Further Reading

Freedman B, Potpara TS, and Lip GYH. Stroke prevention in atrial fibrillation. *Lancet* 2016; 388: 806–17.

Piccini JP and Laurent Fauchie L. Rhythm control in atrial fibrillation. *Lancet* 2016; 388: 829–40.

Van Gelder IC, Rienstra M, Crijns HJGM, and Olshansky O. Rate control in atrial fibrillation. *Lancet* 2016; 388: 818–28.

The Task Force for the management of atrial fibrillation of the European Society of Cardiology (ESC). 2016 ESC Guidelines for the management of atrial fibrillation developed in collaboration with EACTS. *Eur Heart J* 2016; 37: 2893–962.

117 Atrial flutter

Michael Jones, Norman Qureshi, and Kim Rajappan

Definition of the disease

Atrial flutter is the term given to one of the four types of supraventricular tachycardia (SVT); in it, atrial activation occurs as a consequence of a continuous 'short circuit': a defined and fixed anatomical route, resulting in a fairly uniform atrial rate, and uniform atrial flutter waves on the ECG.

The ventricles are not a part of this arrhythmia circuit, and ventricular activation is variable, dependent on atrioventricular (AV) nodal conduction. Given that the atrial rate is essentially uniform (e.g. 300 min⁻¹), ventricular activation tends to be regular (i.e. 150 min⁻¹, 100 min⁻¹, 75 min⁻¹, etc. if the atrial rate is 300 mins⁻¹), or regularly irregular if changes are occurring in the fraction of conducted impulses to the ventricles. When AV nodal conduction permits only 4:1 conduction or less, atrial flutter is usually obvious but, when ventricular rates are higher (150 min⁻¹ or more), the flutter waves can be obscured by the QRS complexes, making diagnosis more difficult.

Atrial flutter is of two types: typical and atypical (Figure 117.1). Typical atrial flutter is a right atrial tachycardia, with electrical activation proceeding around the tricuspid valve annulus. This arrhythmia is dependent on a zone of slow electrical conduction through the cavotricuspid isthmus (the tissue lying between the origin of the inferior vena cava and the posterior tricuspid valve). The resulting circuit can be either **anticlockwise** (activation proceeds up the inter-atrial septum, across the atrial roof, down the free wall, and then through the cavotricuspid isthmus to the basal septum) or **clockwise** (down the inter-atrial septum and around the circuit in the opposite direction). Anticlockwise typical atrial flutter is more common.

Atypical atrial flutter refers to all other atrial flutters, and this includes other right atrial flutters (e.g. pericristal flutter), left atrial flutters, post-ablation or post-surgical flutters, and pulmonary vein flutters.

The feature common to all types of flutter and which differentiates flutter from other types of SVT is the presence of a macro-re-entrant anatomical circuit around which the electrical impulse travels continuously and repeatedly, thereby generating the flutter. Even though typical atrial flutter has a fairly obvious and specific appearance on the ECG, atypical flutters do not, and often it is only possible to differentiate atypical flutter from atrial tachycardias by invasive electrophysiology studies, as the ECG alone may be insufficient.

Aetiology of the disease

The cellular change that predisposes to the development of atrial flutter is the presence of regions of atriopathy (scarring, and the presence of tissue with disordered electrical conduction properties), which provide the substrate for re-entry (short circuiting). The underlying etiologies include long-standing hypertension, chronic lung disease, valvular heart disease, left ventricular hypertrophy, coronary disease, pericarditis, prior cardiac surgery, pulmonary embolism, hyperthyroidism, diabetes, and congestive heart failure. Atypical atrial flutter occurs more commonly in patients with prior cardiac surgery or ablation procedures, and is rare in structurally normal hearts.

Typical symptoms of the disease, and less common symptoms

Atrial flutter can be paroxysmal (occurring in self-limiting bursts) or persistent, and can be an asymptomatic and incidental finding on a 12-lead ECG. Symptoms include palpitations, presyncope, syncope, dyspnoea, exertional intolerance, fatigue, and chest discomfort. Symptoms are more common when ventricular rates are fast, or when AV nodal conduction is poor (and significant ventricular pauses occur).

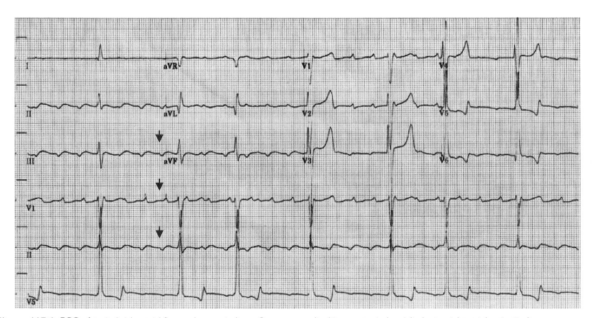

Figure 117.1 ECG of typical right atrial flutter. Arrows indicate flutter waves (in this case, typical anticlockwise right atrial activation).

As there is the potential during flutter for blood to pool in the left atrium and in particular, the left atrial appendage, thrombosis and embolization can occur.

Demographics of atrial flutter

The incidence of atrial flutter is around 88 per 100 000 per year, although the epidemiology is still not fully explored. It makes up 10% of all SVT presentations to the emergency room. The male to female ratio is 2:1, and prevalence increases significantly with age.

Natural history, and complications

Atrial flutter can occur paroxysmally, remain persistent and stable for prolonged periods, or alternate with a closely related but distinct arrhythmia, atrial fibrillation. If ventricular response rates to atrial flutter remain elevated for prolonged periods, a tachycardia-mediated cardiomyopathy can result, which can usually be reversed with ventricular rate control (slowing). The risk of intra-cardiac thrombus formation parallels that of atrial fibrillation, and can lead to arterial embolic complications and stroke.

As with atrial fibrillation, some patients can present late in life with atrial flutter and high-grade conduction block, requiring a permanent ventricular pacemaker.

Approach to diagnosing the arrhythmia, including clinical clues, through concentrating on the ECG diagnosis

The ECG appearance is classic in the majority of cases of atrial flutter, and consists of sawtooth flutter waves, of a uniform morphology, usually with an isoelectric segment between individual waves (in the case of typical flutter). Given that atrial septal activation is the major determinant of the P wave vector, anticlockwise flutter is associated with negative flutter waves in the inferior leads and V6, and positive waves in V1, with the reverse seen for clockwise flutter. The atrial rate is usually 300 min^{-1}, but this can vary considerably, depending on the presence of atrial scarring or distension, and drug therapy (slowing conduction velocity).

If ventricular rates are too fast to clearly see the flutter waves, then, by increasing AV nodal block briefly (with vagal manoeuvres (carotid sinus massage) or with IV adenosine) the flutter waves will become apparent. Adenosine must be avoided if the presence of an antegradely conducting accessory pathway is suspected (due to the possibility of precipitating 1:1 conduction down the pathway, leading to shock and possible ventricular fibrillation).

Other diagnoses that should be considered

Atrial flutter leads to symptoms which are very similar to those of other tachyarrhythmias, and so an ECG diagnosis is imperative to make a definitive diagnosis of atrial flutter. If the ECG is still inconclusive, then dynamic manoeuvres such as carotid sinus massage, or the acute administration of adenosine, can be helpful.

'Gold-standard' diagnostic test

Despite the ECG often appearing highly suggestive of atrial flutter, in some cases, only an invasive electrophysiology study can differentiate atrial flutter from atrial tachycardia, or other SVTs. This is especially the case when the flutter appears atypical, and the patient has a history of prior cardiac surgery or ablation therapy. Whether invasive electrophysiology is warranted in any particular situation depends upon the precise mechanism of the SVT in that particular case.

Acceptable diagnostic alternatives to the gold standard

Atrial flutter can only be diagnosed from the ECG, or at invasive electrophysiology study.

Other relevant investigations

Echocardiography should be routinely performed, to look for structural heart disease and to quantify left ventricular size and function. Blood tests (full blood count, thyroid function tests, renal function, and electrolytes) should be directed at revealing any underlying aetiology and, where clinically appropriate, chest radiography and an assessment for coronary ischemia should be performed. Baseline coagulation studies should be performed prior to commencing anticoagulation.

Prognosis

Atrial flutter can be well tolerated for years, and is often an incidental finding on an ECG. On the other hand, it can have disabling symptoms as previously described. For patients with poor ventricular rate control, a tachycardia-mediated cardiomyopathy can result, which is generally reversible with treatment. The risk of stroke/arterial embolization differs between patients and, generally speaking, the decision to anticoagulate is based on the same algorithms as are used for atrial fibrillation.

Treatment and its effectiveness

Treatment of atrial flutter involves management of the arrhythmia, and management of thromboembolic risk (i.e. requirement for anticoagulation).

The decision to commence long-term anticoagulation is based upon an assessment of individual patient risk, using the CHA_2DS_2-VASc risk calculator, in the same manner as for atrial fibrillation, and taking into account the patient's bleeding risk. Management of the arrhythmia is directed towards either a rhythm-control strategy (the restoration and maintenance of sinus rhythm), or a rate-control strategy (permitting flutter to continue, but ensuring ventricular rates are controlled).

If atrial flutter is persistent, sinus rhythm can be restored acutely by external electrical cardioversion. The risk of thromboembolism associated with cardioversion depends on the duration of the episode of flutter, and the patient's own specific risk of stroke, which is calculated according to the CHA_2DS_2-VASc risk calculator. For low-risk patients who have been in flutter for less than 48 hours, cardioversion may be attempted without anticoagulation, and there is no requirement for post-cardioversion anticoagulation. If the flutter has been present for >48 hours, then cardioversion should be deferred until at least 3 weeks of therapeutic anticoagulation have passed (international normalized ratio (INR) 2–3 for warfarin, or compliant with a direct-acting oral anticoagulant (DOAC) for the same period), and anticoagulation should be continued for at least 4 weeks post-cardioversion; alternatively, a transoesophageal echocardiogram can be performed to exclude the presence of left atrial thrombus, and the cardioversion performed on heparin periprocedure, with warfarin administered for at least 4 weeks post-cardioversion. For high-risk patients, heparin should be administered periprocedurally, and warfarin/DOAC should be continued indefinitely, in the absence of a major contraindication. In an emergency situation, cardioversion may be performed without anticoagulation beforehand and without a transoesophageal echocardiogram, if the benefit (restoring haemodynamic stability) is believed to outweigh the risk of stroke; but this should be performed with periprocedural heparinization, and warfarin/DOAC should be administered for at least 4 weeks post procedure. These guidelines are revised periodically, and it is important to be familiar with the latest recommendations.

Cardioversion can also be achieved pharmacologically, using the same agents as are used for the cardioversion of atrial fibrillation. Care must be taken to avoid merely slowing the atrial flutter rate, as AV nodal conduction can increase to 1:1, leading to syncope (from sudden rapid ventricular rates). As such, pharmacological cardioversion of atrial flutter should be performed with an AV nodal blocking medication co-administered.

While there is no study that clearly establishes the superiority of long-term rhythm control over long-term rate control, rhythm control by ablation does have certain advantages—namely, typical atrial flutter is readily amenable to percutaneous catheter ablation, which is curative in 91%, with a fairly low rate of periprocedural complications (an overall 0.5% risk of adverse outcomes, including bleeding, pericardial effusion and tamponade, stroke, and complete heart block). This is different from the case with catheter ablation of atrial fibrillation, where the risks are higher, and procedural success rates lower. Atypical atrial flutter is also amenable to catheter ablation, in selected cases.

Despite atrial flutter ablation being highly effective, and recurrence rates low, a successful ablation does not necessarily imply that anticoagulation is no longer indicated, and this should be explained to any patient contemplating an invasive treatment strategy.

Long-term rhythm control may also be attempted with antiarrhythmic drugs, but caution needs to be exercised in this case; Class III agents may prolong the QT interval, and can precipitate polymorphic ventricular tachycardia (torsades de pointes) and sudden death, and Class I agents slow conduction velocity and, by slowing the flutter rate, can lead to 1:1 conduction through the AV node, as previously described. The risks and benefits of antiarrhythmic drug therapy in patients with atrial flutter need to be carefully weighed in each case.

Rate control of persistent and permanent atrial flutter is a reasonable management option, and the same medications as are used for atrial fibrillation are used in atrial flutter. Nevertheless, rate control in atrial flutter can often prove difficult, owing to the unpredictable nature of the ventricular response in the setting of additional AV nodal blocking medications; unlike the case of atrial fibrillation, where doses and drugs can be titrated fairly accurately to average ventricular response rates, in atrial flutter, sudden unpredictable increases in AV nodal block can occur with the addition of more medications. In such cases, where flutter ablation is not desired, is not feasible, or is unsuccessful, a permanent ventricular pacemaker may be required to provide rate support, in the setting of multiple AV nodal blocking medications. Quite commonly, an AV node ablation by percutaneous transvenous catheter technique is performed in these cases, to eliminate the need for ongoing pharmacological AV nodal blockade.

Key points

The key points regarding atrial flutter are as follows:

- Atrial flutter is defined by rapid, regular, and uniform atrial activity, manifesting on the ECG as continuous flutter waves.
- Atrial flutter results from a macro-re-entrant atrial circuit, which is a fixed anatomical route for ongoing electrical re-entry to occur.
- Typical atrial flutter is a right-atrial arrhythmia, dependent on slow conduction through the cavotricuspid isthmus, and is either anticlockwise or clockwise in direction of conduction around the circuit.
- Atypical atrial flutter refers to all other atrial flutter (i.e. not right-atrial-isthmus dependent), and is therefore a heterogeneous group, including peripulmonary venous atrial flutter, perimitral atrial flutter, pericristal atrial flutter, peri-coronary-sinus atrial flutter, peri-scar atrial flutter, and pericardiotomy atrial flutter.
- The clinical significance of atrial flutter is the same as for atrial fibrillation—the risk of thromboembolism and stroke, and the need to control the ventricular rate.
- Anticoagulation requirements are treated in the same manner as for atrial fibrillation—that is, a risk score is calculated according to the CHA_2DS_2-VASc scoring algorithm, and a decision regarding the need for anticoagulation, aspirin, or neither of these is made on this basis. As for atrial fibrillation, additional considerations regarding anticoagulation apply in the setting of planned cardioversion to sinus rhythm.
- Both rhythm control and rate control are acceptable management options for recurrent persistent atrial flutter; however, unlike the case for atrial fibrillation, percutaneous ablation techniques are of low risk and very high efficacy, and are associated with a very low long-term arrhythmia recurrence rate.

Further Reading

Bun S-S, Latcu DG, Marchlinski F, and Nadir Saoudi N. Atrial flutter: more than just one of a kind. *Eur Heart J* 2015; 36: 2356–2363.

118 Ventricular tachyarrhythmias: Ventricular tachycardia and ventricular fibrillation

Michael Jones, Norman Qureshi, and Kim Rajappan

Definition of the disease

Ventricular tachycardia

Ventricular tachyarrhythmias are abnormal patterns of electrical activity arising from the ventricular tissue (myocardium and conduction tissue). Ventricular tachycardia (VT) is an abnormal rapid heart rhythm originating from the ventricles. The rhythm may arise from the ventricular myocardium and/or from the distal conduction system. The normal heart rate is usually regular, between 60 and 100 bpm, and there is synchronized atrial and ventricular contraction. In VT, the ventricles contract at a rate greater than 120 bpm and typically from 150 to 300 bpm, and are no longer coordinated with the atria. There is still organized contraction of the ventricles in VT, with discrete QRS complexes. It is a potentially life-threatening arrhythmia, with the risk of degenerating into ventricular fibrillation (VF) and resulting in sudden cardiac death. It is characterized by a broad-complex tachycardia (BCT) on ECG. VT can be classified according to morphology, duration of episodes, and haemodynamic status; it can also be classified as idiopathic.

Classification of VT according to morphology

Monomorphic VT occurs when the shape of the QRS complexes repeats itself in each and every lead of a 12-lead ECG, usually originating from the same focus (or ventricular exit site) and representing either increased automaticity or re-entry as underlying mechanisms. An example is right ventricular outflow tract (RVOT) VT, which has a characteristic pattern on 12-lead ECG, with QRS complexes of left bundle branch block (LBBB) morphology, and an inferior axis. Polymorphic VT refers to VT with beat-to-beat variations in the contours of the QRS complexes. Torsades de pointes (TdP) is a term reserved for polymorphic VT occurring in the context of a prolonged resting QT interval (prolonged repolarization) and early after-depolarizations. The variation in the QRS morphology and axis in TdP takes the form of a progressive, sinusoidal, cyclic alteration of the QRS axis. The peaks of the QRS complexes appear to 'twist' around the isoelectric line of the recording, hence the term TdP, or 'twisting of points'. Bidirectional VT is classically seen in catecholamine polymorphic VT (CPVT), where there is beat-to-beat alternation of the QRS axis.

Classification of VT according to duration of episodes

Sustained VT is usually defined either as that which lasts longer than 30 seconds, or which requires an intervention for termination. A group of three to five beats of non-sustained ventricular tachycardia (NSVT) are often termed a 'salvo'. NSVT in the setting of ischaemic heart disease has been well described and is used as a prognostic marker in risk stratification of sudden cardiac death (SCD). Haemodynamically stable VT that may last for hours is termed 'incessant', and very frequent episodes of VT requiring cardioversion or multiple therapies from an implantable cardioverter defibrillator (ICD) in situ is termed a 'VT storm'.

Classification of VT according to haemodynamic status

Pulseless VT is VT leading to haemodynamic collapse, without sufficient cardiac output to maintain vital organ function, including consciousness, and often leads to cardiac arrest. It is recognized as one of the shockable rhythms on the Advanced Life Support algorithm. Some VT is associated with a good cardiac output, and may even be asymptomatic—termed 'pulsed VT'. However, such patients' clinical course may still be complicated by pulseless VT or VF in the medium-to-long term.

Classification of VT as idiopathic

VT can occur in patients with structurally normal hearts, and this is often termed 'idiopathic VT'. A significant proportion of patients with idiopathic VT have an underlying 'electrical disorder' as part of the inherited arrhythmogenic syndromes.

VF and ventricular flutter

VF is a grossly disorganized, rapid ventricular rhythm condition which results in uncoordinated contraction of the ventricles, with subsequent loss of cardiac output, and haemodynamic collapse. It has been described as 'chaotic asynchronous activity of the heart' (Figure 118.1). It was originally thought to be as a result of simultaneous independent multiple wavelets that follow random, continuously changing pathways through the myocardium. However, experimental evidence now supports the model of organized centres of 'rotors' representing unstable cardiac excitation as the underlying mechanism of sustaining VF. It usually terminates fatally within 3 to 5 minutes unless

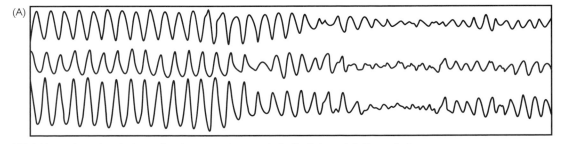

(A)

Figure 118.1 Ventricular tachyarrhythmia often deteriorates into ventricular fibrillation, a lethal heart rhythm.

Reproduced with permission from Roderick Tung, Noel G. Boyle, Kalyanam Shivkumar Catheter Ablation of Ventricular Tachycardia, *Circulation*, Volume 122, Issue 3, pp. e389-e391, Copyright © 2010 Wolters Kluwer Health, Inc.

corrective interventions are undertaken. It is the most common arrhythmia noted in patients with out-of-hospital cardiac arrest (up to 75%). It can occur as a primary arrhythmia or, more frequently, as a result of degeneration of VT. The characteristic ECG finding of VF is that of irregular undulations of varying contour and amplitude, with an absence of distinct QRS complexes, ST segments, and T waves. Fibrillatory waves of low amplitude (termed fine ventricular fibrillation) are present when VF is prolonged, and then all electrical activity ceases (asystole) as an agonal event. Ventricular flutter looks like a sine wave with large regular oscillations at a rate of between 150 and 300 bpm (often 200 bpm); it can be difficult to distinguish between ventricular flutter and rapid VT but the difference between the two is often academic.

Aetiology of the disease

More than 50% of those with symptomatic VT have ischaemic heart disease (either acute ischaemia or scar-related VT). The next-largest group has an underlying cardiomyopathy (dilated cardiomyopathy (DCM), hypertrophic cardiomyopathy (HCM), arrhythmogenic right ventricular cardiomyopathy (ARVC), or infiltrative cardiomyopathies, such as sarcoidosis). The others fall into the following groups: inherited arrhythmogenic syndromes (channelopathies), congenital heart disease (tetralogy of Fallot), idiopathic VT/VF, and VT due to drugs (sympathomimetic agents, antiarrhythmics, QT-prolonging agents) or electrolyte imbalances.

The exact electro-anatomical substrates of ventricular tachyarrhythmias in the conditions associated with SCD are discussed in detail in Chapter 120. They are largely a consequence of structural heart disease, with breakdown of normal conduction patterns, both within the myocardium and within the specialized conduction system of the heart. The general principles of cardiac arrhythmia mechanisms prevail, with abnormal automaticity as a result of hypoxia and increased sympathetic nervous system stimulation, and activation of re-entrant pathways as a result of scarring (which provides a slowly conducting substrate) and differential conduction properties in both myocardial and conduction tissue. A re-entry mechanism accounts for the majority of monomorphic VT. Triggered activity occurs by a non-re-entrant mechanism that appears to be due to after-depolarizations (early and delayed) and is thought to arise from abnormal ionic currents (e.g. long-QT syndrome and Brugada syndrome) and calcium handling (CPVT).

In this section, we will discuss the aetiology and pathophysiology of idiopathic VT and VF, and bundle branch re-entry VT, which is a specific kind of VT that can be seen in those with structural heart disease, as these have not been covered in other sections of the book.

Idiopathic VT

Idiopathic VT, defined as monomorphic VT in patients with no underlying structural heart disease, can have characteristic ECG morphologies based on the foci of the VT: outflow tract tachycardias, annular tachycardias, and fascicular tachycardias (Figure 118.2). These types of VT often respond well to drug therapy, and are amenable to ablative therapy when medical therapy fails. In outflow tract tachycardias (responsible for 75%–90% of idiopathic VT), the monomorphic VT originates from either the left ventricular outflow tract (LVOT) or the RVOT or, more infrequently, above the pulmonary valve or in the aortic cusps. RVOT VT has a typical LBBB appearance in V1 and an inferior axis in the frontal plane. When multiple VT morphologies are present, the possibility of other disease processes (e.g. ARVC) should be considered. The mechanism responsible is cyclic-AMP-triggered activity resulting in early depolarizations or after-depolarizations. A similar tachycardia mimicking RVOT VT can be identified in the LVOT, but with a right bundle branch block (RBBB) morphology (see Figure 118.2). VTs arising from the mitral and the

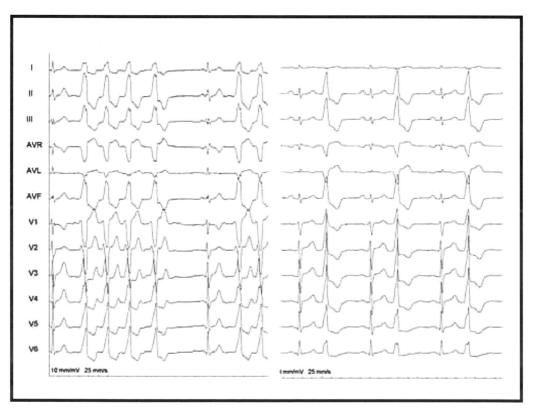

Figure 118.2 (Left) Right ventricular outflow-tract, non-sustained, monomorphic ventricular tachyarrhythmia with left bundle branch block and inferior axis; (Right) left ventricular outflow-tract bigeminy, with right bundle branch block morphology.

Reproduced with permission from Brugada and Diez, How to recognise and manage idiopathic ventricular tachycardia, An article from the e-journal of the ESC Council for Cardiology Practice, Volume 8, Issue 26, 2010 ESC copyright. All rights reserved. https://www.escardio.org/Guidelines-&-Education/Journals-and-publications/ESC-journals-family/E-journal-of-Cardiology-Practice/Volume-8/How-to-recognise-and-manage-idiopathic-ventricular-tachycardia

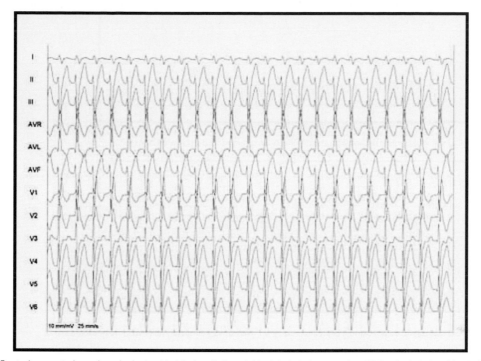

Figure 118.3 Fascicular ventricular tachyarrhythmia with right bundle branch block (relatively narrow) and left-axis deviation (classical 'straight-up' axis with isoelectric in I, and negative in aVF).

Reproduced with permission from Brugada and Diez, How to recognise and manage idiopathic ventricular tachycardia, An article from the e-journal of the ESC Council for Cardiology Practice, Volume 8, Issue 26, 2010 ESC copyright. All rights reserved. https://www.escardio.org/Guidelines-&-Education/Journals-and-publications/ESC-journals-family/E-journal-of-Cardiology Practice/Volume-8/How-to-recognise-and-manage-idiopathic-ventricular-tachycardia

tricuspid valve annuli account for approximately 4%–7% of idiopathic VTs. When the VTs arise from the mitral valve, they have, typically, an RBBB morphology; when they arise from the tricuspid valve, they have a typical LBBB morphology.

Fascicular tachycardia (also known as fascicular VT or idiopathic left VT) arises from the left posterior septum, close to the left posterior fascicle, and is characterized by a RBBB morphology on ECG, with a leftward axis (left anterior fascicular block) and a relatively narrow QRS. This VT is often verapamil sensitive, suggesting that the relevant mechanism relates to the slow inward current in either a small re-entrant circuit (see Figure 118.3) or delayed after-depolarizations. Fascicular tachycardias may be a heterogeneous group, with several mechanisms responsible, and are relatively uncommon.

Bundle branch re-entry VT

Bundle branch re-entry VT is a form of monomorphic, sustained VT which occurs in those with structural heart disease. It is more common in non-ischaemic DCM than in ischaemic DCM. In it, there is conduction delay in the His–Purkinje system, thus creating a substrate for a macro-re-entry involving the bundle branches (see Figure 118.4). This is usually manifest as interventricular delay on ECG during sinus rhythm (LBBB), with or without atrioventricular (AV) nodal disease. Conduction retrogradely over the left bundle system, and antegradely over the right bundle, constitute the most common form, resulting in an LBBB morphology during VT (similar to sinus rhythm; see Figure 118.5). It is important to recognize this as it responds poorly to medical therapy but may be eliminated by catheter ablation. Myocardial VT may concomitantly exist. It is very uncommon in the absence of myocardial disease. The patient profile may still warrant ICD therapy, depending on the presence of underlying DCM, and symptoms.

Idiopathic VF

Idiopathic VF is defined as VF occurring on a background of a structurally normal heart. It has an incidence of 1% of all out-of-hospital cardiac arrests, and 14% of all VF cardiac arrests in those >40 years old. It has been associated with early repolarization, and has been

considered to be part of a spectrum of J-point elevation disorders, including Brugada syndrome. The mechanism of arrhythmogenesis with early repolarization is unclear in this patient group. In a few patients, VF has been triggered by short-coupled premature

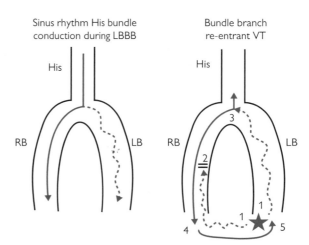

Figure 118.4 Substrate for macro-re-entry in bundle branch re-entry ventricular tachycardia. The His bundle (His), right bundle (RB), and left bundle (LB) are shown, on the left with sinus rhythm with left bundle branch block (LBBB), and on the right with bundle branch re-entrant ventricular tachyarrhythmia (VT). On the right, a ventricular ectopic (indicated by the star) initiates slow retrograde conduction in the LB, and across retrogradely in the RB (indicated by '1'). The retrograde conduction in the RB blocks (indicated by '2'). The slowly conducting retrograde LB wavefront reaches the RB and conducts antegradely (indicated by '3'), and further distally (indicated by '4'); by this time, the LB is able to conduct retrogradely once again, and a re-entrant circuit is completed.

Reproduced with permission from Bashir, Betts, and Rajappan, *Cardiac Electrophysiology and Catheter Ablation*, Oxford University Press, Oxford, UK, Copyright © 2010

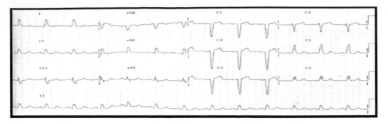

ECG showing sinus rhythm with borderline AV block and LBBB (QRSd 120ms)

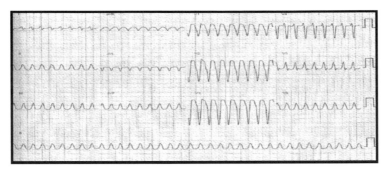

ECG demonstrating a bundle branch re-entry VT with a very similar QRS morphology to sinus rhythm

Reproduced from Cardiac Electrophysiology and Catheter Ablation (Oxford Specialist Handbooks in Cardiology)

Figure 118.5 (*Top panel*) ECG showing sinus rhythm with borderline atrioventricular block and left bundle branch block (QRSd 120 ms) (*Bottom panel*) ECG demonstrating a bundle branch re-entry ventricular tachycardia with a QRS morphology very similar to that of sinus rhythm.
Reproduced with permission from Bashir, Betts, and Rajappan, *Cardiac Electrophysiology and Catheter Ablation*, Oxford University Press, Oxford, UK, Copyright © 2010

ventricular complexes (PVCs), which are often from Purkinje fibres, which can be targeted in ablative therapy.

Typical symptoms of the disease, and less common symptoms

Symptoms occurring during VT depend on the haemodynamic consequences produced by the VT, and several factors influence this: the ventricular rate; the time spent in tachycardia; the presence and severity of any underlying heart disease; and autonomic factors. The localization and the direction of spread of ventricular depolarization can also be important. Patients may present with palpitations, breathlessness (increased pulmonary venous pressures and pulmonary congestion), presyncope/syncope (diminished cerebral perfusion), or cardiac arrest. Some patients may experience chest pain, which may reflect underlying ischaemia as the precipitant of VT, or due to the rhythm itself (rate-related ischaemia). In some instances, patients may tolerate their VT well with adequate haemodynamics, but may drift into heart failure over time. In addition, an incessant VT which is haemodynamically tolerated may itself cause a DCM. This may develop over weeks and months, and resolves with management of the VT. Likewise, those with frequent ventricular ectopy/bigeminy in the absence of high rates can also develop a reversible form of dilated cardiomyopathy. Should there be independence of atrial activity from the ventricular contractions (AV dissociation occurs in some 60% of VTs), patients may report neck fullness (corresponding to cannon A waves, when ventricular and atrial contractions occur synchronously, resulting in raised central venous pressures). Physical examination when AV dissociation is present in a patient in VT may reveal, in addition to cannon A waves in the jugular venous pressure, variable first heart sound, and blood pressure. VF presents with syncope, seizures, apnoea, and, eventually, if left untreated, cardiac arrest and death.

Demographics of the disease

Fifty per cent of all cardiac deaths are sudden, and the majority of SCDs are as a result of ventricular tachyarrhythmias. As previously mentioned, VF is the most common arrhythmia in patients with out-of-hospital cardiac arrest.

Approach to diagnosing the disease

The diagnosis of VT is made on electrocardiography, on a 12-lead ECG, telemetry rhythm strip, or other forms of ambulatory ECG monitoring. VT is a differential diagnosis of a BCT. The other differential diagnoses of a BCT (Figure 118.6) are:

- supraventricular tachycardia (SVT) with aberrancy (preexisting or functional bundle branch block)
- SVT with pre-excitation, including pre-excited atrial fibrillation (see Figure 118.7)
- antidromic Atrioventricular reciprocating tachycardia (AVRT)
- pacemaker-mediated tachycardia (PMT)
- accelerated idioventricular rhythm
- ECG-lead motion artefact

Despite the numerous established criteria in the differentiation of VT from SVT with aberrant conduction, the correct diagnosis of a BCT remains a challenge, but is crucial in acute as well as long-term management (e.g. the administration of verapamil to treat BCT misdiagnosed as SVT with aberrancy may result in severe hypotension and haemodynamic collapse). The commonest cause of a BCT is VT, which represents up to 80% of BCTs presenting in the emergency department. Hence, a BCT should be treated as VT unless proven otherwise. The likelihood of a particular diagnosis is significantly affected by a number of factors, including features on the ECG, and the presence or absence of structural heart disease. A history of

CHAPTER 118 **Ventricular tachyarrhythmias: Ventricular tachycardia and ventricular fibrillation**

372 at bottom left.

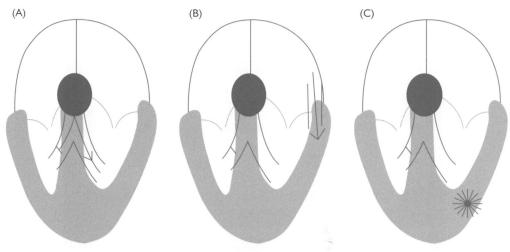

SVT with BBB:
• atrial tachy
• atrial flutter
• atrial fibrillation
• AV nodal tachy
• CMT with AV conduction over AV node and VA conduction over Acc pathway

SVT with AV conduction over Acc pathway:
• atrial tachy
• atrial flutter
• atrial fibrillation
• AV nodal tachy
• CMT with AV conduction over Acc pathway and VA conduction over AV node or second Acc pathway

VT

Figure 118.6 Different types of supraventricular tachycardia: (A) supraventricular tachycardia with bundle branch block; (B) supraventricular tachycardia with atrioventricular conduction over an accessory pathway; (C) ventricular tachycardia resulting in a broad QRS tachycardia; Acc, accessory; AV, atrioventricular; BBB, bundle branch block; CMT, circus movement tachycardia; SVT, supraventricular tachycardia; tachy, tachycardia; VA, ventriculo-atrial; VT, ventricular tachycardia.

Reproduced from Heart, Hein JJ Wellens, ELECTROPHYSIOLOGY: Ventricular tachycardia: diagnosis of broad QRS complex tachycardia, volume 86, issue 5, pp. 579–585, copyright 2001 with permission from BMJ Publishing Group Ltd.

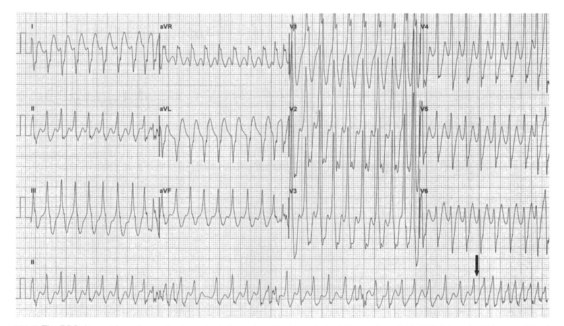

Figure 118.7 The ECG shows a broad, complex irregular tachycardia with right-axis deviation and a variable R–R interval which is consistently <250 ms. No discernible P waves are seen but inspection of the QRS complexes show pre-excitation. The terminal portion of the rhythm strip (not recorded simultaneously with the rest of the 12-lead ECG) shows degeneration of the pre-excited atrial fibrillation into ventricular fibrillation (onset denoted by black arrow) and therefore records the exact moment and cause of cardiac arrest.

Reproduced with permission from Fakhar Z. Khan, David Paul Dutka, Simon Patrick Fynn, Recorded spontaneous sudden cardiac arrest in a patient with pre-excited atrial fibrillation, Europace, Volume 11, Issue 1, p. 124, Copyright © 2009 Oxford University Press.

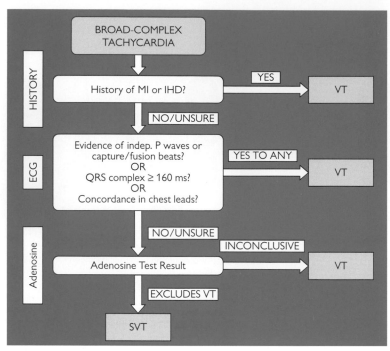

Figure 118.8 A proposed algorithm for the differential diagnosis of ventricular tachycardia versus supraventricular tachycardia; IHD, ischaemic heart disease; indep, independent; MI, myocardial infarction; SVT supraventricular tachycardia; VT, ventricular tachycardia.
Courtesy of Dr Y Bashir, John Radcliffe Hospital, Oxford.

ischaemic heart disease with previous myocardial infarction or heart failure has a positive predictive accuracy of 95% for VT, and can serve as a good discriminator as to the cause of a BCT. The response of the BCT to vagal manoeuvres and/or adenosine is also useful. With VT, there is no response to vagal manoeuvres or adenosine. Termination of the tachycardia with vagal manoeuvres or adenosine strongly suggests a supraventricular origin. Adenosine may not terminate the BCT, but can result in sufficient AV nodal blockade, unmasking the underlying atrial rhythm (e.g. atrial flutter or atrial tachycardia with aberrancy). As with narrow-complex tachycardias, adequate doses of adenosine must be given to achieve AV node blockade. However, unlike the case with narrow-complex tachycardias, an eventual lack of response to increasing doses of adenosine must indicate a VT as opposed to a SVT mechanism.

There are well-described ECG findings that are of value in differentiating the causes of a BCT, but most of these are not 100% specific or sensitive. The following are ECG features of a BCT favouring VT:

- QRS complexes >140 ms for a RBBB tachycardia (a predominantly positive QRS complex in Lead V1)
- QRS complexes >160 ms for a LBBB tachycardia (a predominantly negative deflection in Lead V1)
- a superior frontal plane axis in RBBB tachycardia, and a right inferior axis in LBBB tachycardia
- evidence of AV dissociation
- capture/fusion beats
- negative/positive concordance

In addition, the 12-lead ECG in sinus rhythm may also be helpful. Pre-excitation indicates an antegradely conducting accessory pathway and may suggest an SVT with pre-excitation (antidromic AVRT or pre-excited AF), although the accessory pathway could be a bystander in terms of the BCT. The presence of Q waves in a territory consistent with coronary artery disease (i.e. a QR (Coumel) complex) may indicate myocardial infarction and consequent scarring as a substrate for VT, and the presence of an identical QRS morphology during tachycardia is very suggestive of VT involving this area of scarring.

In summary, the diagnostic approach to VT involves the clinical history, ECG analysis, and the incorporation of adenosine testing

(see 'PMT'). These depend on the clinical predicament of the patient. Always consider whether the apparent tachycardia is artefactual (Figure 118.8).

Other diagnoses that should be considered

Accelerated idioventricular ventricular rhythm

The term 'accelerated idioventricular rhythm' (AVIR) describes an ectopic ventricular rhythm with three or more consecutive ventricular premature beats with a rate faster than the normal ventricular intrinsic escape of 30–40 bpm but slower than that of VT (usually between 100 and 120 bpm). It differs from VT by its mode of onset, which is with a long coupling interval, and its offset, which is by a gradual decrease of the ventricular rate or increase of the sinus rate. Frequently, the mechanism seems to be related to enhanced automaticity in the His–Purkinje fibres and/or myocardium and associated with vagal excess and decreased sympathetic activity. When the enhanced automaticity in the His–Purkinje system or myocardium exceeds the sinus rate, accelerated idioventricular rhythm (AIVR) manifests as the dominant rhythm. There is some overlap between AIVR and some slow VT. It is generally a transient rhythm, rarely of haemodynamic consequence and requiring treatment. It has a good prognosis, and can occur in any form of structural heart disease and, occasionally, in those with no structural heart disease. Rarely, AIVR can degenerate into VT or VF. In patients with poor left ventricular systolic dysfunction, AIVR can lead to haemodynamic compromise due to the loss of AV synchrony, or a relatively rapid heart rate. It is most commonly seen in those with coronary artery disease and occurs in up to 25% of patients during an acute myocardial infarction, as a marker of successful reperfusion. It is also seen in digoxin toxicity.

PMT

PMT in patients with a dual-chamber pacemaker can result in a BCT. It may be obvious if clear ventricular pacing spikes are observed on an ECG of a BCT. However, with the use of bipolar pacemaker leads, the pacing spike may be subtle and difficult to observe on an

ECG. There are two mechanisms that underlie PMT. One involves the 'tracking' of an atrial tachyarrhythmia and normally occurs in a patient with a dual-chamber pacemaker in the setting of complete heart block. Should these patients develop any atrial tachyarrhythmias (atrial fibrillation/atrial flutter/atrial tachycardia), the atrial lead will sense the atrial activity and trigger ventricular pacing at the pacemaker's maximal preprogrammed rate (upper tracking rate), which is usually between 120 and 140 bpm in older patients. If a programmer is no available, a magnet placed over the pacemaker generator deactivates the sensing facility on the pacemaker leads, and induces asynchronous pacing at the preset demand rate, thus allowing diagnosis of the atrial tachyarrhythmia. If a programmer is available, the pacemaker can be reset to the VVI mode, and this will prevent the 'tracking' of the atrial tachyarrhythmia. In most pacemakers now, there is a mode-switch facility, and the pacemaker switches from the DDD to the VVI mode once it detects a high atrial rate (at a preprogrammed setting). The second mechanism occurs when a premature ventricular beat is conducted retrogradely via the AV node, resulting in atrial depolarization (occurring after the atrial refractory period). The atrial lead senses this, and the pacemaker initiates ventricular pacing, which continues as an endless-loop tachycardia. This once again results in a BCT (see Figure 118.9); placing a magnet over the pacemaker generator will terminate this loop, as it will disable the atrial lead sensing facility. Adenosine or Valsalva manoeuvres may or may not terminate this tachycardia, depending on whether the ventriculo-atrial block is sensitive to them. This problem is overcome by altering the post-ventricular atrial refractory period.

Other relevant investigations

Once the diagnosis of VT has been made, the following investigations may be performed to guide further management: resting 12-lead ECG, assessment of left ventricular systolic function, and assessment of cardiac ischaemia.

Resting 12-lead ECG

The 12-lead ECG, once the patient has been successfully cardioverted to sinus rhythm (or, in some cases, atrial fibrillation), is important for elucidating the potential cause of the VT.

Evidence of myocardial ischaemia/infarction

The presence of an ST-segment shift (elevation or depression) suggests myocardial ischaemia or infarction may be the cause of the VT/VF, although cardiac ischaemia may be a representation of a patient's compromised haemodynamics as a result of the VT. Urgent coronary angiography should be considered in such instances. In addition, the presence of Q waves in a territory consistent with coronary artery disease (i.e. a QR (Coumel) complex) may indicate myocardial infarction and scarring as a substrate for VT, and the presence of an identical QRS morphology during tachycardia is very suggestive of VT involving this area of scarring.

Presence of ventricular pre-excitation

As previously mentioned, ventricular pre-excitation indicates an antegradely conducting accessory pathway and may suggest an SVT with pre-excitation (antidromic AVRT or pre-excited AF), although the accessory pathway could be a bystander in terms of the BCT.

Evidence of underlying inherited arrhythmogenic syndrome

As previously discussed, there are particular ECG changes which might prompt the consideration of the diagnosis of an inherited arrhythmogenic syndrome. A prolonged or shortened QT interval may suggest a diagnosis of long-QT syndrome or short-QT syndrome, respectively. The characteristic ECG changes associated with Brugada syndrome (e.g. coved ST elevation with T-wave inversion) may be present and may be helpful in achieving the diagnosis. ARVC should be considered as an underlying diagnosis if an epsilon wave is detected.

Assessment of left ventricular systolic function

Transthoracic echocardiography

In a patient presenting with VT, in addition to the symptoms of presentation, the other crucial information required is whether the patient has a structurally normal heart. Apart from the implications this has for the type of VT, if a patient has a severely impaired left ventricular systolic function, they may be a candidate for ICD implantation. This information can be provided by transthoracic echocardiography.

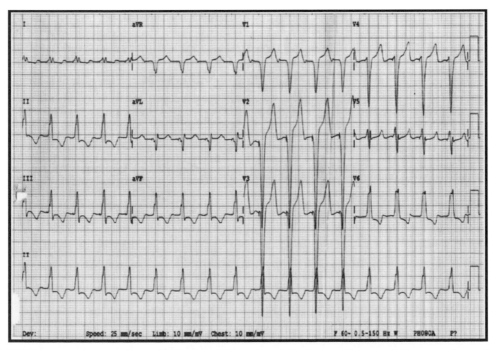

Figure 118.9 ECG demonstrating a pacemaker-mediated tachycardia (paced ventricular rhythm with retrograde P waves at the terminal portion or just after the T wave on Leads II, III, aVF, and V1 (note the QRS morphology of the left bundle branch block, and the superior axis, consistent with right ventricular apical pacing).

Cardiac MRI

Like transthoracic echocardiography, cardiac MRI (CMRI) is primarily used to assess cardiac structure and function. However, CMRI allows for a more detailed assessment of the myocardial structure than transthoracic echocardiography does, particularly via late gadolinium enhancement imaging. This gives information on myocardial composition (i.e. areas of scarring, fibrosis, oedema, and infiltration), which is helpful not only in demonstrating the substrate for VT (e.g. in re-entrant VT), but also in achieving the diagnosis (e.g. in ARVC).

Assessment of cardiac ischaemia

It is important to exclude underlying cardiac ischaemia as the cause or precipitant of ventricular tachyarrhythmias, as it may need to be treated primarily.

Coronary angiography

Coronary angiography is inevitably performed in patients presenting with ventricular tachyarrhythmias, especially if features of the history or other investigations suggest underlying coronary artery disease (e.g. ST-segment shift on ECG, or regional wall motion abnormality on transthoracic echocardiography). The presence of coronary artery disease, if demonstrated on coronary angiography, will need to be interpreted in the context of the clinical predicament before any revascularization is contemplated. Other functional investigations, such as myocardial perfusion scanning, stress echocardiography, or stress CMRI, may be useful in such instances.

Prognosis, and how to estimate it

Numerous approaches have been used to assess the prognosis of those with ventricular tachyarrhythmias, depending on the underlying disease process. Prognostication largely involves risk stratification for SCD and decision on ICD implantation, and may involve invasive and non-invasive assessments, as well as genotyping. These are discussed in greater detail in Chapter 120. Except in patients with inherited arrhythmogenic syndromes (channelopathies), HCM, or ARVC, left ventricular function is the strongest predictor of outcome. In patients with an ischaemic cardiomyopathy and NSVT, the sudden-death mortality rate is almost 30% at 2 years. In general, the prognosis for patients with idiopathic VT, in the absence of either a long QT or structural heart disease, is excellent, and therapy is often directed against symptoms. Their major risk is due to poorly timed syncopal spells.

Treatment and its effectiveness

The management of VT/VF and aborted SCD have dramatically changed over the past decade as the evidence base has expanded. Management decisions can be divided into those for immediate action (i.e. termination of VT), and those for long-term management (i.e. prevention of recurrence and SCD).

Acute management of sustained VT

Treatment of VT may either be directed towards ending an episode of VT or preventing any future episodes from occurring, and subsequent consideration for an ICD to prevent SCD. The severity of the clinical symptoms dictates the urgency with which VT must be treated, regardless of the arrhythmia mechanism. VT associated with cardiac arrest (pulseless VT) should be treated in accordance to the Advanced Life Support algorithm, with immediate electrical cardioversion. It also suggests IV amiodarone as a first-line adjunctive antidysrhythmic in shock-resistant pulseless VT.

In pulsed VT, immediate assessment of the patient's haemodynamic state and end-organ perfusion is a priority. Their level of consciousness (cerebral perfusion), symptoms of chest pains (which may reflect underlying cardiac ischaemia and coronary hypoperfusion), and presence of pulmonary congestion are important indices. VT which leads to angina, left heart failure, right heart failure, low blood pressure, shock, or symptoms of hypoperfusion of the brain (leading to a lowered Glasgow Coma Score and/or confusion) should be treated with prompt electrical cardioversion. If the haemodynamic

status is stable, rhythm conversion may be achieved via either electrical cardioversion or medical therapy with IV antiarrhythmic agents. Figure 118.10 shows an algorithm for the management of tachycardias, including BCT and VT, as produced by the Resuscitation Council (UK). Electrical cardioversion (synchronized) is simple and safe, with close to 100% efficacy and with no risk of haemodynamic depression and the proarrhythmia associated with antiarrhythmic drug therapy. It is ideally performed under general anaesthesia (GA), but can be done with benzodiazepines and opiates if necessary. It may be delayed if a patient has not been fasting, or other contraindications to GA are present. Acute termination of VT can also be achieved with IV antiarrhythmic agents such as amiodarone, lidocaine, and procainamide (not available in the UK), although they are generally ineffective, and many patients end up requiring electrical cardioversion. If left ventricular systolic function is impaired, using amiodarone and then lidocaine is better than using procainamide, due to its potential to exacerbate congestive cardiac failure. With associated ongoing myocardial ischaemia, it is recommended that lidocaine be used as the primary antiarrhythmic drug, as the mechanism in this case rather than being re-entry is thought to be abnormal automaticity. In TdP-type VT, magnesium sulfate may be effective if the QT is found to be pathologically lengthened. Magnesium is rarely effective in those with a normal QT interval. Amiodarone is suggested as the first-line antiarrhythmic agent by the Resuscitation Council (UK).

In cases of VT associated with a background of a previous myocardial infarction (i.e. the mechanism is likely to be that of re-entry), overdrive pacing (pacing of the ventricle by using a temporary pacing lead inserted into the right ventricle at a rate higher than that of the VT) can end the episode of tachycardia. This is especially useful in recurrent VT, where multiple electrical cardioversions have been attempted, and allows time for antiarrhythmic drug therapy to take its effect (e.g. even IV preparations of amiodarone may take 12–48 hours to work). However, a risk of this overdrive pacing approach is that the VT may increase its rate to that of ventricular flutter or even VF. In the treatment of recurrent appropriate ICD discharges or a VT storm, sedation and intubation may be helpful when IV antiarrhythmic agents and beta blockade have failed to control the ventricular tachyarrhythmias. Neuroaxial modulations via thoracic epidural anaesthesia and surgical left-cardiac sympathetic denervation have been also shown to be effective. Emergency VT ablation ('primary VT ablation') can also be considered when other treatment modalities have failed.

Once the VT is terminated, remediable factors contributing to VT initiation and maintenance should be sought and corrected. VT can be triggered by cardiac ischaemia (acute myocardial infarction is found in 20% of patients with a VF arrest), electrolyte imbalances, decompensation of congestive cardiac failure (likely as a result of myocardial stretch), relative bradycardias (as sinus bradycardia or AV block may promote the occurrence of PVCs and ventricular tachyarrhythmias), and drugs.

Long-term therapy for the prevention of recurrence

The aim of long-term therapy is to prevent the recurrence of symptomatic VT, and SCD. The key factors influencing treatment include comorbidity, symptom severity, and the extent of structural heart disease, and they determine whether medical therapy (antiarrhythmic drug therapy, and drugs to treat underlying disease), ICD implantation, and catheter ablation should be considered. Often, combinations of these treatments are implemented when structural heart disease is present.

Antiarrhythmic drug trials have been largely ineffective, especially in those with left ventricular systolic dysfunction, and some antiarrhythmic drugs have been shown to paradoxically increase sudden-death mortality in such patients. Beta blockers can diminish the incidence of ventricular tachyarrhythmias and improve survival in those with VF and symptomatic VT. In patients with VF which is refractory to beta blockers, other antiarrhythmic agents should be considered. Class I Vaughn-Williams antiarrhythmic agents may paradoxically increase mortality in such patients via proarrhythmia, especially in patients with underlying coronary artery disease. Current clinical practice favours the use of Class III antiarrhythmic agents

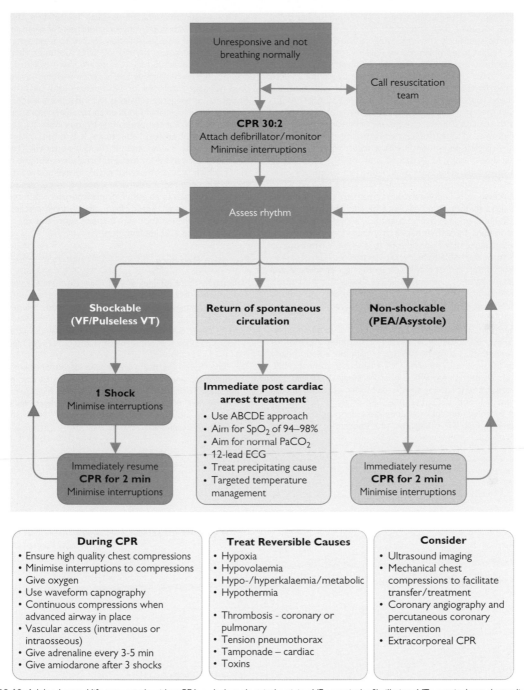

Figure 118.10 Adult advanced life support algorithm; PEA, pulseless electrical activity; VF, ventricular fibrillation; VT, ventricular tachycardia.
Reproduced with the kind permission of the Resuscitation Council (UK).

(sotalol and amiodarone), which prolong myocardial depolarization through potassium-channel blockade and are preferred in those with reduced left ventricular systolic function. Amiodarone is a complex antiarrhythmic agent and is categorized as a Class III antiarrhythmic but has measurable Class I, II, and IV effects. Unlike the Class I antiarrhythmic agents, it seems to be safe for use in those with impaired left ventricular systolic function. The ACC/AHA/ESC guidelines state that, when used together with beta blockers, amiodarone is helpful for those with decreased left ventricular systolic function due to prior myocardial infarction, and with VT symptoms not responding to beta-adrenergic-blocking agents. In those with heart failure, the best proven, but non-specific, antiarrhythmic medical therapy includes, in addition to beta blockade, the use of angiotensin-converting enzyme inhibitors and aldosterone antagonists. The idiopathic VTs often respond well to drug therapy, including calcium-channels blockers (verapamil) and beta blockers. Other specific drug therapies are recommended, each with its own evidence base, in the varying etiologies of ventricular tachyarrhythmias and are discussed in Chapter 120 (e.g. the use of quinidine in Brugada syndrome).

The use of ICDs has had a significant impact on the management of ventricular tachyarrhythmias, especially in the context of an aborted SCD (secondary prevention) and in patients with underlying cardiomyopathy/structural heart disease. ICDs may be indicated on prognostic grounds in many patients, irrespective of any other treatment for their VT. The indications are discussed in further detail in Chapter 121, including their role in primary prevention of SCD, and these may be specific to the underlying cardiac disease process (see Chapter 120). Once implanted, an ICD can be used to diagnose ventricular tachyarrhythmias, and end them with defibrillation/ cardioversion shocks or anti-tachycardia pacing algorithms. These devices can also function as pacemakers in patients with bradyarrhythmias. There have been several large trials (e.g. CASH/AVID) comparing ICD therapy to conventional antiarrhythmic dug therapy in patients with structural heart disease with a history of ventricular tachyarrhythmias. These studies demonstrated the superiority of ICD therapy (reduction in mortality by a reduction in SCD) over antiarrhythmic dug therapy (amiodarone and sotalol), especially in patients with severe left ventricular dysfunction (left ventricular ejection fraction <35%) and haemodynamically unstable sustained VT. In patients who refuse an ICD, the next best treatment may be that of amiodarone, although there is no evidence base for this. For patients with ICDs in situ and who receive frequent ICD shocks due to recurrent VT, concomitant antiarrhythmic drug therapy may be indicated to reduce the incidence of VT episodes or to slow the VT rate and so allow it to be more amenable to being pace terminated. On occasion, multiple antiarrhythmic agents may be required (e.g. amiodarone and flecainide concomitantly). Catheter ablation should also be considered in such circumstances. In a proportion of patients considered for ICD implantation, cardiac resynchronization therapy may also be indicated.

A key treatment in those with recurrent VT is catheter ablation. The EHRA/HRS Expert Consensus on Catheter Ablation of Ventricular Arrhythmias suggests the use of catheter ablation early in the therapy of those with recurrent VT. Previously, catheter ablation was often contemplated when pharmacological options had been exhausted, often following significant morbidity to the patient from recurrent VT and ICD therapies. Advances in technology with the use of three-dimensional activation mapping techniques and understanding of VT substrates (incorporating endocardial and epicardial approaches) now allow for ablation of multiple and unstable VTs with good outcomes and safety, even in those with advanced heart disease. Ablation is used to treat symptomatic VT rather than to reduce the risk of SCD. Catheter ablation of certain types of idiopathic VT (i.e. where there is a structurally normal heart) is very effective and is recommended in those who are drug resistant/intolerant or who refuse long-term drug therapy. Abnormal or triggered activity is the most likely mechanism, and in these patients focal ablation is often curative, with success rates of greater than 90% if the presenting rhythm disturbance is inducible in the electrophysiology laboratory. It is often important to give consideration to haemodynamic stability of the VT. The use of percutaneous left ventricular assist devices allows for the maintenance of VT which would otherwise result in haemodynamic instability, and thus enable more extensive mapping to be performed. There are also strategies to ablate VF or polymorphic VT in certain patient groups where focal triggers from the Purkinje system and RVOT play a role in the initiation of VF. Once again, this approach is used as an adjunct to ICD implantation.

Further Reading

National Institute for Health and Care Excellence. Implantable cardioverter defibrillators and cardiac resynchronisation therapy for arrhythmias and heart failure. Technology appraisal guidance [TA314] 2014. https://www.nice.org.uk/guidance/ta314.

Sapp JL, Wells GA, Parkash R, et al. Ventricular tachycardia ablation versus escalation of antiarrhythmic drugs. N Engl J Med 2016; 375: 111–21.

The Task Force for the management of patients with ventricular arrhythmias and the prevention of sudden cardiac death of the European Society of Cardiology (ESC). 2015 ESC Guidelines for the management of patients with ventricular arrhythmias and the prevention of sudden cardiac death. Eur Heart J 2015; 36: 2793–867. doi: 10.1093/eurheartj/ehv316.

Definition of bradyarrhythmia

A bradyarrhythmia is defined as a rhythm disturbance which results in a heart rate of less than 60 bpm, although it is important to note that many healthy people have a resting heart rate that is less than 60 bpm. The forms of bradyarrhythmia that need to be considered are sinus bradycardia, sinus node disease, sick sinus syndrome, and atrioventricular (AV) block.

Definition of sinus bradycardia

Sinus bradycardia is a rhythm which arises from the sinus node but has a ventricular rate less than 60 bpm (see Figure 119.1).

Definition of sinus node disease

Sinus node disease may also manifest itself as a sinus bradycardia, but is often accompanied by other aspects of abnormal sinus node function. The most common of these is sinus arrest. This is defined as a longer-than-normal pause between two consecutive cardiac cycles (>3 seconds), with an absence of sinus node activity between the two cycles; that is, no P waves are seen (unlike the case in AV block, where the sinus node continues to fire, so P waves are seen but there is no ventricular activity).

Definition of sick sinus syndrome

Sick sinus syndrome is a collection of heart rhythm disorders; it includes sinus bradycardia, sinus tachycardia, and alternating brady-cardia and tachycardia.

Definition of AV block

First-degree AV block

In first-degree AV block, the PR interval is fixed and prolonged. The normal PR interval is 0.12–0.2 seconds; in first-degree AV block, there is a fixed PR interval >0.2 seconds. (Note that the upper limit of the PR interval in children is age dependent and often abnormal if >160 ms in very young children.) Every atrial impulse is conducted to the ventricles in first-degree AV block; however, conduction is delayed within the AV node.

Second-degree AV block

Second-degree AV block is characterized by atrial impulses (generally occurring at a regular rate) which fail to conduct to the ventricles. **Möbitz type I** second-degree AV block, also known as the **Wenckebach** phenomenon, is defined by progressive prolongation of the PR interval with dropped beats (i.e. the PR interval gets longer and longer until finally one beat drops; see Figure 119.2A). **Möbitz type II** second-degree AV block is defined as a PR interval that remains unchanged and is not normally prolonged but where the P wave suddenly fails to conduct to the ventricles, often in a regular fashion (e.g. every second P wave has a dropped beat (in 2:1 second-degree AV block), every third P wave has a dropped beat (in 3:1 second-degree AV block), etc.; see Figure 119.2B) Another, less-recognized, form of second-degree AV block consists of multiple P waves occurring in a row and which should conduct, but do not. The conduction ratio can be three P waves to one conducted beat, or higher, but the PR interval of each of the conducted beats remains

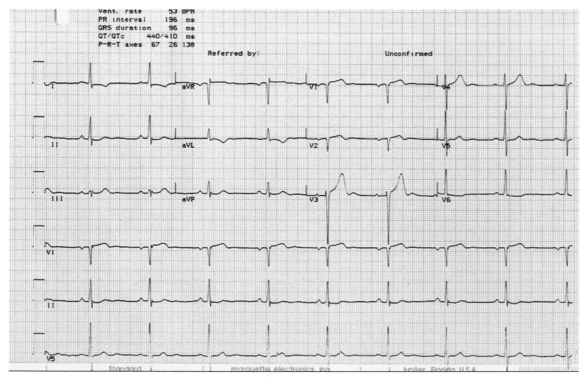

Figure 119.1 12-lead ECG showing sinus bradycardia.

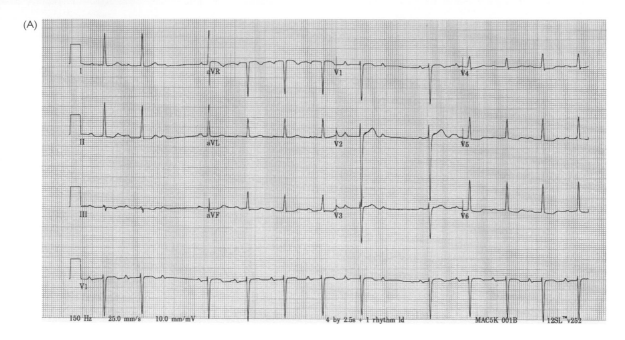

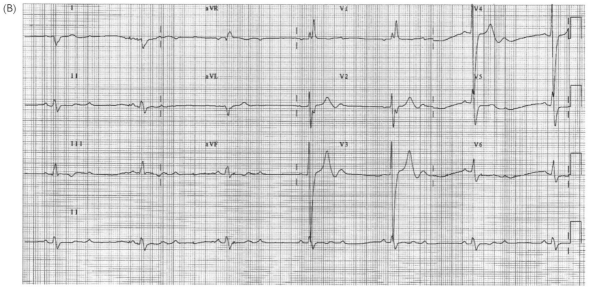

Figure 119.2 12-lead ECGs showing (A) Mobitz type I (Wenckebach) and (B) Mobitz type II second-degree atrioventricular block.

constant. This form of second-degree AV block is clinically distinct from complete heart block in that, in this form, the P waves that conduct to the QRS complexes occur at fixed intervals, unlike the case in third-degree AV block (see 'Third-degree AV block').

Third-degree AV block

Third-degree AV block, also known as complete heart block, is diagnosed when no supraventricular impulses are conducted to the ventricles. In individuals with this, the P waves can normally be identified and seen to demonstrate sinus rhythm, dissociated from the QRS complexes (see Figure 119.3). Ventricular contraction is driven by a pacemaker in junctional (bordering the AV node) or ventricular myocardium. A junctional escape rhythm is typically at a rate of 40–50/min, with a narrow QRS complex, while a ventricular escape rhythm is 30–40/min or slower, with a broad QRS complex. A ventricular escape rhythm is less reliable, with a higher probability of prolonged pauses.

Aetiology of bradyarrhythmia

Aetiology of sinus bradycardia

Sinus bradycardia is often caused by the administration of drugs which depress impulse generation by the sinus node (e.g. beta blockers, calcium-channel blockers, and ivabradine). In addition, athletes often have sinus bradycardia as a physiological response. Other causes of sinus bradycardia include increased vagal tone, hypothermia, hypothyroidism, epileptic seizures (during the postictal state), increased intracranial pressure, and, rarely, infections such as diphtheria, acute rheumatic fever, and viral myocarditis.

Aetiology of sinus node disease

Sinus node disease is a condition that often occurs as people age. However, it is may be seen in patients at a younger age.

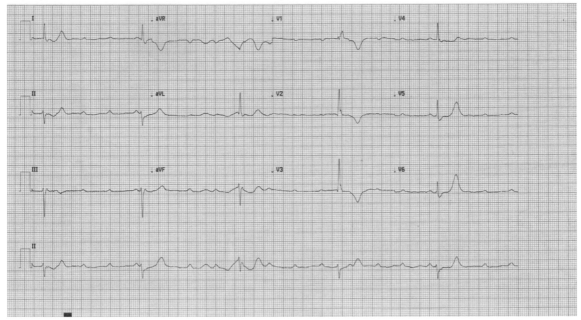

Figure 119.3 12-lead ECG showing third-degree atrioventricular block (complete heart block).

Aetiology of sick sinus syndrome

Sick sinus syndrome is relatively uncommon. It tends to occur in people older than 50. The most common mechanism is thought to be a non-specific, scar-like degeneration of the heart's conduction system, predominantly affecting the atria. In children, sick sinus syndrome is most commonly seen after cardiac surgery, especially where this involves the atria. Coronary artery disease, hypertension, and aortic and mitral valve diseases may be associated with sick sinus syndrome, which is probably related to associated fibrosis within the conduction system.

Aetiology of AV block

AV block can occur at the level of the AV node or at the level of the His–Purkinje system. The AV node (AVN), which lies in the floor of the right atrium, allows electrical impulses to be transmitted from the sinus node to the ventricles with 1:1 conduction., The AVN consists of three parts: the atrionodal region (which is a transitional zone), the nodal region (which is quite compact), and the nodal-His region (which contains the penetrating His bundle). Conduction is slowest through the nodal region. The AVN is supplied by the right coronary artery (in 90% of individuals) or the left circumflex artery (in 10% of individuals), and is innervated by both sympathetic and parasympathetic fibres. The His–Purkinje system comprises the bundle of His, the right and left bundle branches, and the Purkinje fibres, which travel subendocardially to connect with ventricular myocytes; the conduction system enables synchronous ventricular activation.

First-degree AV block and Möbitz type I second-degree AV block usually reflect conduction delay within the AVN, while Möbitz type II second-degree AV block typically reflects conduction delay in the His–Purkinje system. Third-degree AV block may be due to conduction block in the AV node and/or His–Purkinje system.

High vagal tone (e.g. during sleep) may cause first-degree or Möbitz I second-degree AV block in healthy people. Möbitz I second-degree AV block may also occur physiologically at high heart rates (e.g. with rapid atrial pacing).

Causes of AV block may be classed as congenital or acquired, and, if acquired, acute or chronic.

Congenital AV block is rare, occurring in 1:22 000 births. This form of heart block, in the absence of major structural abnormalities, is often associated with maternal antibodies to Ro/SSA) and La/SSB, secondary to maternal SLE. It is most commonly diagnosed between 18 and 24 weeks' gestation and may be first degree, second degree, or third degree. Mortality approaches approximately 20%, with most surviving children requiring pacemakers.

Acquired acute causes of AV block include ischaemia of the AV node and conduction system in the setting of acute coronary syndrome, adenosine administration, drug toxicity (beta blockers, digoxin, verapamil) and hyperkalaemia. Acute injury of the AV node and conduction system may occur in Lyme disease, other causes of acute myocarditis, and infective endocarditis with aortic root abscess. Surgical aortic valve replacement, percutaneous transcatheter aortic valve implantation, repair of congenital cardiac defects, and cardiac trauma may also result in injury of the conduction system. Catheter ablation of the AV node is a therapeutic procedure (combined with pacemaker implantation) used to treat selected patients with atrial fibrillation associated with rapid ventricular rates.

Acquired chronic AV block is most often due to idiopathic conduction system fibrosis (Lenegre–Lev syndrome), or in association with extensive calcification of the mitral annulus or aortic valve. Chronic ischaemic heart disease, infiltrative disorders such as sarcoidosis or haemochromatosis, and cardiomyopathies may involve the conduction system and result in AV block. AV block may be seen in association with neuromuscular disorders (e.g. myotonic dystrophy) and spondyloarthropathies.

Typical symptoms of bradyarrhythmia

Symptoms of sinus bradycardia

Bradycardia is not necessarily symptomatic. However, the slow heart rate arising from any of the bradyarrhythmias can reduce cardiac output, causing symptoms such as presyncope, dizziness, chest pain, hypotension, vertigo, confusion, fatigue, dyspnoea, and syncope. The slow heart rate may also lead to other escape rhythms, including junctional, ectopic atrial, or ectopic ventricular rhythms. Profound bradycardia may predispose the affected individual to R-on-T ectopy and potentially life-threatening torsades de pointes.

Symptoms of sinus node disease

As previously mentioned, sinus node disease may manifest as a sinus bradycardia, but is often accompanied by other abnormal sinus node functions, the most common of which is sinus arrest (see 'Definition of sinus node disease').

Symptoms of sick sinus syndrome

In sick sinus syndrome, symptoms may include palpitations, because of the associated tachycardia component.

Symptoms of AV block

First-degree AV block is usually asymptomatic and an incidental finding on ECG; examination may reveal a soft first heart sound. Second-degree AV block can be asymptomatic or may cause palpitation and effort intolerance; presyncope/syncope may result from intermittent higher degrees of AV block. Acquired third-degree AV block typically causes effort intolerance, and may result in presyncope/syncope from bradycardia or prolonged pauses. Syncope related to AV block (Stokes–Adams attack) is characteristically of abrupt onset; secondary anoxic seizures may occur.

Demographics/natural history of the arrhythmia

Sinus bradycardia

Studies have found that 50%–85% of highly trained athletes have benign sinus bradycardia, as compared to 20%–30% of the general population studied.

Sinus node disease

Sinus node disease often occurs as people age, although it is may be seen in patients at a younger age. It is often accompanied by other aspects of abnormal sinus node function, most commonly sinus arrest.

Sick sinus syndrome

In sick sinus syndrome, the patient's heart rate may be very slow at any time, but can also be very variable. Blood pressure may be affected but not consistently. The presence of sick sinus syndrome may cause heart failure symptoms to occur or worsen.

AV block

The incidence of AV block increases with age, and is more common in patients with underlying coronary or structural heart disease. There is a 60% female preponderance in congenital third-degree AV block, but a 60% male preponderance with acquired AV block. No clear racial trends exist for any bradyarrhythmias including AV block, although some systemic conditions associated with AV conduction demonstrate racial variation and therefore may affect prevalence (e.g. sarcoidosis).

First-degree AV block is seen in 0.5%–2.0% of healthy 20-year-olds, and 5% of healthy 60-year-olds. Möbitz type I second-degree AV block is seen in 1%–2% of healthy young people during sleep.

Approach to diagnosing the arrhythmia

Diagnosing sinus bradycardia

The diagnosis of sinus bradycardia is definitively confirmed by ECG, with a rate <60 bpm and which is normally regular, with P waves that are normal in morphology, and a normal PR interval.

Diagnosing sinus node disease

Sinus node disease is often accompanied by other aspects of abnormal sinus node function. The most common of these is sinus arrest, which is defined as a longer-than-normal pause between two consecutive cardiac cycles (>3 seconds), with an absence of sinus node activity between the two cycles.

Diagnosing sick sinus syndrome

Sick sinus syndrome is diagnosed when the symptoms occur only during episodes of arrhythmia. However, this often can be difficult to prove. An ECG may show various abnormal heart rhythms related to this syndrome. Holter monitoring is can be useful to diagnose sick sinus syndrome because of the episodic nature of the disorder.

Extremely slow heart rate and prolonged pauses may be seen during monitoring, along with episodes of atrial tachycardias. An intra-cardiac electrophysiology study is a very specific test for this disorder, although it is often unable to confirm the diagnosis and is usually not needed in current clinical practice. Exercise testing has been used to assess sinus node function but has not proven effective as a screening tool for this syndrome.

Diagnosis of AV block

AV block is diagnosed on the ECG, on the basis of the features described in 'Definition of AV block'. The hallmark feature of third-degree AV block is that no relationship exists between the P waves and the QRS complexes (i.e. they are completely dissociated). The frequency of the P waves (atrial rate) is normally, but not always, higher than the frequency of the QRS complexes (ventricular rate). In atrial fibrillation, this can be difficult to diagnose, or differentiate from just a slow ventricular response to the atrial fibrillation itself, but it is normally characterized by a very regular slow ventricular rhythm, as opposed to the slight irregularity of slowly conducted atrial fibrillation.

Other relevant investigations

Ambulatory ECG monitoring is indicated in symptomatic patients with first-degree or Möbitz type I second-degree AV block, to detect higher degrees of AV block or associated sinus node disease that may warrant pacemaker implantation. In patients with presyncope/syncope suspected of being due to AV block (e.g. because of the finding of a bundle branch block on ECG or the presence of relevant structural heart disease), ambulatory ECG monitoring is indicated. The type of monitoring chosen depends on the frequency of symptoms and, in some patients, an implantable ECG loop recorder will be used.

In 2:1 AV block, which can be due to Möbitz I or II second-degree AV block, exercise ECG may be used to differentiate these: in Möbitz I, the conduction rate increases (due to adrenergically mediated enhanced conduction through the AV node) while in Möbitz II, it decreases, and so may result in a fall in heart rate.

In general, imaging studies do not provide a significant role in investigating bradyarrhythmias. However, they are needed to exclude underlying structural heart disease and assess left ventricular function, as this may determine the type of pacemaker used if required. Apart from a thorough clinical examination, a transthoracic echocardiogram is the initial investigation of choice to exclude structural heart disease. Where there is a suspicion of coronary heart disease, further investigation of this, with tests including coronary angiography, may be appropriate. Cardiac MRI may be used in patients where a suspicion of a myocardial infiltrative problem exists (e.g. younger patients), with or without other features of a condition that predisposes to heart block (e.g. sarcoidosis).

Intra-cardiac electrophysiological studies may be indicated in a patient with suspected AV block as the cause of syncope. Block that is below the AV node in the His–Purkinje system (so called infra-Hisian block) is more commonly associated with slower heart rates and greater risk of prolonged pauses/asystole. Invasive recording of AH (atrium–His) and HV (His–ventricle) intervals can be used to determine the degree of conduction abnormality and its location and to guide decision-making for pacemaker therapy. However, this is rarely necessary with the current availability of non-invasive monitoring techniques.

Electrolyte imbalance may also cause a variety of arrhythmias, including various forms of bradycardia, so these will normally be checked, and toxicology screening may be performed where there is sufficient suspicion. Where a systemic disorder is suspected, appropriate investigations may be performed.

Prognosis and how to estimate it

Patients with Möbitz II second-degree or third-degree AV block are at risk of syncope (which may result in major injury) and sudden cardiac death. Pacemaker implantation substantially reduces these risks and thus improves their prognosis.

For patients with sinus node disease first-degree AV block, or Möbitz I second-degree AV block, the prognosis for life expectancy largely depends on the presence and type of underlying cardiac disease. Progression of the degree of AV block may occur over time. First-degree AV block is associated with an increased incidence of atrial fibrillation.

Treatment and its effectiveness

Long-term medical therapy is not useful or indicated in bradyarrhythmias. Permanent pacing is the therapy of choice in advanced AV block, and/or symptomatic bradycardia (see Chapter 121). AV nodal blocking medications, such as beta blockers, may exacerbate the symptoms, and therefore need to be discontinued, if possible. Where the patient is symptomatic, and this has been proven to be due to the bradycardia drugs that may be causing the problem, it is common to implant a permanent pacemaker, so the drugs can be continued. Tachycardia associated with sick sinus syndrome may be treated with medication, but again, such treatment may exacerbate the bradycardia component, thus requiring pacemaker insertion. If tachycardia is the predominant problem, then catheter ablation may help.

Temporary transcutaneous or transvenous pacing is the treatment of choice in the emergency setting when there is a slow heart rate (and for asystole) caused by bradyarrhythmia, although transvenous pacing is associated with significant morbidity and mortality. Atropine administration (0.5–1.0 mg) or isoprenaline infusion may improve AV conduction in emergencies with bradycardia but is not a long-term strategy, and normally these measures are only used as a bridge to permanent pacemaker implantation as soon as possible.

Consultation with a cardiologist or cardiac electrophysiologist is indicated in the case of advanced heart block or unexplained syncope. An electrophysiologist will be best placed to decide when invasive electrophysiology testing is needed to determine the level and/or magnitude of conduction disturbance.

Patients with first-degree or benign Möbitz I second-degree AV block do not require hospitalization. Patients with symptomatic second- or third-degree AV block may need hospitalization with monitoring. Transcutaneous or transvenous pacing may need to be used but, where there is an indication for permanent pacing, this needs to be expedited.

Patients with implanted pacemakers require routine follow-up to monitor pacemaker function and assessment for the occurrence of other arrhythmias such as atrial fibrillation.

Further Reading

The Task Force on cardiac pacing and resynchronization therapy of the European Society of Cardiology (ESC). 2013 ESC Guidelines on cardiac pacing and cardiac resynchronization therapy. *Eur Heart J* 2013; 34: 2281–29.

120 Sudden cardiac death

Norman Qureshi and Kim Rajappan

Definition and demographics of sudden cardiac death

Sudden cardiac death (SCD) is defined as **unexpected** death due to a cardiac disease, in a patient with or without known cardiac disease, which occurs **within 1 hour** from the appearance of the **first** clinical symptoms. The sudden cessation of cardiac activity leads to haemodynamic collapse, typically due to sustained ventricular tachyarrhythmias. The event is described as an aborted SCD (or sudden cardiac arrest (SCA)) when an intervention (e.g. defibrillation) or spontaneous reversion restores circulation. The lack of uniformity with this definition complicates SCD statistics. By convention, the use of SCD to describe both fatal and non-fatal cardiac arrests persists.

SCD continues to be a leading cause of death in Western countries, and underlies 15%–20% of all deaths in adults in the developed world, and about half of all cardiovascular deaths. In the US, estimates of SCDs from retrospective death certificate analyses range from 300 000 to 350 000 annually, giving an incidence of 0.1%–0.2% per year amongst the population above the age of 35 years. Event rates are said to be similar in Europe, although worldwide incidence is difficult to estimate and varies in accordance with the prevalence of coronary heart disease (CHD). The incidence of SCD increases with age and underlying cardiac disease. There is also a male preponderance, with men 2–3 times more likely to experience SCD than women, and this reflects the higher incidence of CHD in men.

Aetiology of SCD

SCD usually occurs in the presence of underlying structural heart disease, although the specific causes vary with the age of the population studied. The overwhelming majority of SCD (up to 80%) in adults is attributable to CHD. Accordingly, the risks for SCD are predominantly the same as those of CHD, such as age, male gender, hypertension, dyslipidaemia, smoking, and diabetes mellitus. The frequency of CHD is, however, much lower in SCD in younger populations. Other structural heart disease, both acquired and inherited, account for about 10% of SCD. Many have been covered in other chapters in this book (see Part 3) but, in this chapter, we will discuss specific conditions where risk stratification of SCD is an important aspect of the management of the condition. These conditions include hypertrophic cardiomyopathy (HCM) and arrhythmogenic right ventricular cardiomyopathy (ARVC). There are instances of SCD in the absence of structural heart disease (primary electrical disorder), and these account for approximately 10%–12% of cases amongst populations under the age of 45, with a significantly lower proportion when older subjects are included. There have been significant developments made in the understanding of the genetic, molecular, and electrophysiological basis of SCD in this group of patients, in particular with respect to the inherited arrhythmia syndromes, and this will be discussed further.

Superimposed triggers seem to play a role in SCD in the presence of underlying anatomical and functional substrates. Ischaemia, electrolyte imbalance, drugs (especially antiarrhythmic agents), autonomic nervous system activation, and psychosocial factors can act in concert to disturb cardiovascular function and coalesce together to lead to fatal ventricular tachyarrhythmias. However, only a small percentage of patients with structural heart disease and inherited arrhythmogenic syndromes develop SCD, and the challenge is in the risk stratification of SCD in these patient groups. The most powerful predictor of SCD is significant left ventricular impairment from any cause.

CHD

SCD is the mechanism of death in over 60% of patients with known CHD, and accounts for up to 80% of all SCDs. The incidence of SCD is influenced by the clinical manifestations of CHD, with patients with previous myocardial infarction (MI) being most at risk, and intermediate risk for patients with angina but no previous MI. However, it has been estimated that, in 15%–25% of patients, the initial presentation of CHD is SCD. SCD can occur in the context of an acute coronary syndrome (ACS) or the setting of stable CHD in a patient with a previous MI with the myocardial scar serving as a substrate for ventricular tachyarrhythmias and SCD. An important distinction has to be made with the arrhythmic mechanisms, as the implications for those with an aborted SCD in either setting are different.

In the acute phase of an MI, SCD is usually as a result of acute ischaemia triggering lethal ventricular tachyarrhythmias, and the peak incidence of ventricular fibrillation (VF) within the first 48 hours. The degree of coronary artery stenosis required and the roles of 'vulnerable' atherosclerotic plaques and coronary artery thrombi are debated, but all can result in acute physiological derangements, destabilizing the electrical activity of the heart. Studies have suggested that, before reperfusion therapy, early VF in acute MI is independently associated with anterior MIs and the absence of preinfarction angina (preconditioning). Mechanical complications resulting in acute haemodynamic collapse (e.g. myocardial rupture with pericardial tamponade and septal defects; papillary muscle rupture; and ischaemic valvular dysfunction) may mimic sudden arrhythmic death. Extensive myocardial necrosis with cardiogenic shock may result in a similar consequence.

Following acute MI, the mechanism of SCD evolves as a result of adverse left ventricular remodelling. Myocardial scarring is the substrate for ventricular tachyarrhythmias as a result of regional and intramural re-entry circuits that incorporate areas of diseased myocardium and unexcitable scar tissue. Sustained ventricular tachycardia (VT) can accelerate and subsequently degenerate into VF. The development of heart failure as a result of adverse left ventricular remodelling, with progressive ventricular dilatation and worsening left ventricular systolic function, corresponds to progressive loss of cardiac output, and congestive cardiac failure is the second process underlying the risk of SCD post-MI. Neurohormonal pathways are activated, and this underlies progressive vasculopathy, left ventricular dysfunction, fibrosis, and progression of the disease. Dilatation of the left ventricle predisposes to electrical heterogeneity characterized by a temporal dispersion of repolarization predisposing to re-entrant tachyarrhythmias. It has been suggested that progressive pump failure, sudden arrhythmic death, and sudden death during episodes of clinical deterioration each account for a third of deaths in patients with heart failure. VT degenerating into VF is the most common cause of SCD, and a bradyarrhythmia or pulseless electrical activity (PEA) is responsible in 5%–33% of cases. Pump failure is an additional mechanism; in it, chronic ischaemia causes global hypoxia, giving rise to electrical instability and ectopy and thus leading to the generation of lethal ventricular tachyarrhythmias. An ACS can also be the precipitating factor in some patients with heart failure.

Other structural heart disease

Other structural heart diseases account for up to 10% of all SCDs, and these can be categorized into non-ischaemic cardiomyopathies, valvular heart disease, and congenital heart disease.

Dilated cardiomyopathy

Dilated cardiomyopathy (DCM) is increasingly common and has both primary and secondary forms. The causes are uncertain, and include viral, autoimmune, genetic, and environmental (alcohol and drugs) causes. SCD accounts for approximately a third of deaths in this group of patients, and the predominant mechanism seem to be ventricular tachyarrhythmia, although bradyarrhythmia and PEA have also been seen, especially in those with severe heart failure. Extensive subendocardial scarring resulting in left ventricular dilatation underlies the substrate for re-entrant tachyarrhythmias. As with ischaemic cardiomyopathy, the risk of SCD increases with the decline in left ventricular systolic function, which probably serves as a function of other risk factors such as sympathetic tone, neurohormonal activation, and electrolyte disturbances. Drugs used to treat heart failure, such as antiarrhythmic agents, inotropes, and diuretics (potentially causing electrolyte disturbances), can act as triggers to ventricular tachyarrhythmias.

Hypertrophic cardiomyopathy

Hypertrophic cardiomyopathy (HCM) is an inherited heart muscle disorder caused by mutations (>45) in sarcomeric proteins, resulting in myocyte disarray and myocardial hypertrophy. The commonest form of inheritance is autosomal dominant with incomplete penetrance. Most cases are accounted for by mutations in genes encoding beta-myosin heavy chains and cardiac troponin T. SCD is the most important threat in this population, with 50%–60% of deaths being sudden; the incidence of SCD in patients with HCM is 2%–4% per year in adults, and 4%–6% in children and adolescents. In addition, HCM is the commonest cause of SCD in those under the age of 30; in the vast majority of those cases, the patients had been asymptomatic prior to SCD occurring. In a significant number of patients with HCM, SCD occurs during or after strenuous exercise. HCM is also the single most common cause of SCD in young athletes, and autopsy series have suggested it accounts for up to 36% of cases. Hence, it is an important disease to screen for in athletes.

The mechanism of SCD in HCM is not well understood, and was initially thought to be a result of obstruction of the left ventricular outflow tract as a result of catecholamine activity, but subsequent studies have suggested that patients with non-obstructive HCM are at high risk of SCD as well, primarily via ventricular tachyarrhythmias. The mechanism of arrhythmia is unclear. Myocyte disarray and fibrosis may provide the arrhythmogenic substrate, with the triggers being ischaemia, left ventricular outflow-tract obstruction, vascular instability, and cellular energy depletion. Non-sustained VT is common and is seen in up to 20% of this population. Sustained VT is, however, rare and may suggest the presence of a left ventricular apical aneurysm. Current guidelines advise a primary-prevention implantable cardioverter defibrillator (ICD) in high-risk patients, who are defined as patients having two or more risk factors (severe left ventricular hypertrophy with a septal thickness of 3 cm or greater; family history of SCD; syncope; abnormal blood-pressure response to exercise; and non-sustained VT on ambulatory monitoring). Recent studies have suggested a potential for mutation analysis as part of the risk stratification for SCD in HCM, as there appear to be high-risk genotypes for SCD, particularly related to troponin T. In addition, the extent of late gadolinium enhancement, which reflects fibrosis, on cardiac MRI (CMRI) is currently being studied as an independent prognostic factor in SCD. At this time, there is no definitive evidence to support the use of pharmacological therapy in reducing the risk of malignant arrhythmias in HCM patients, and its use is mainly adjunctive in patients with ICDs.

ARVC/dysplasia

ARVC/dysplasia (ARVC/D) is a rare but increasingly recognized inherited cardiomyopathy. It is characterized by the progressive replacement of cardiac myocytes by adipose and fibrous tissue and leads to electrical instability and ventricular arrhythmias in the early stages, and reduced contractility and heart failure in the later stages. The tissue replacement can also affect the left ventricle, with relative sparing of the septum. The prevalence in the general adult population has been estimated at 1 in 1000, with men being affected more often in a ratio of 3:1. It is an important cause of SCD in young adults and, in some series, it accounts for up to 11% of cases overall and 22% of cases in athletes. There appears to be some discordance to the geographical prevalence of ARVC; this is more likely a result of under-recognition of the disease rather than a true difference in genetic prevalence. In up to 50% of patients with ARVC, a positive family history can be elicited. ARVC is predominantly inherited as an autosomal dominant disease but with incomplete and age-related penetrance, and variable forms of clinical expression. Autosomal recessive inheritance has also been described, often in association with a cutaneous phenotype (Navos disease). Gene identification studies helped the elucidation of the pathophysiology of the disease and have defined ARVC as a disease of the desmosome, an adhesive junction between cells. Mutations in key components of the desmosome, including plakoglobin (most common desmosomal mutation), desmoplakin, and plakophilin, have been reported to result in the phenotype of ARVC.

The diagnosis of ARVC is challenging. Definitive diagnosis requires histologic confirmation of transmural fibrofatty replacement of the right ventricle at post-mortem or surgery. This is clearly not practical in the clinical setting and, due to the patchy nature of the disease, endomyocardial biopsy is not highly sensitive. In 1994, an international task force proposed criteria for the clinical diagnosis of ARVC, to facilitate recognition and interpretation of the frequently non-specific clinical features of ARVC. Structural, histological, electrocardiographic, arrhythmic, and familial features of the disease were incorporated into the criteria and subdivided into major and minor categories according to the specificity of their association with ARVC. There has since been a modification, and the 2010 revised task force criteria incorporates new knowledge and technology to improve diagnostic sensitivity while maintaining diagnostic specificity. Both the original and revised criteria are divided into major and minor criteria, and are subdivided into the following six categories:

- global and/or regional dysfunction and structural alterations
- tissue characterization of wall
- repolarization abnormalities on the ECG
- depolarization/conduction abnormalities on ECG
- arrhythmias
- family history

Definitive diagnosis requires the presence of two major criteria, one major plus two minor criteria, or four minor criteria from different categories. A comparison of original and revised task force criteria is given in Table 120.1.

Approximately half of patients with ARVC have a normal ECG at presentation but, within 6 years of presentation, almost all patients will have one of the characteristic ECG findings (ECG evolution). The characteristic ECG changes seen in ARVC patients include:

- prolonged QRS duration, particularly in V1 and V6, consistent with the delayed right ventricular (RV) activation (>110 ms)
- a pattern of incomplete or complete right bundle branch block
- a prolonged S-wave upstroke (interval from the nadir of the S wave to the isoelectric baseline is >55 ms)
- an epsilon wave (a reproducible distinct wave between the end of the QRS complex and the onset of the T wave) in the right precordial leads, particularly in V1 (major criterion in the 2010 revised task Force Criteria); this represents the low-amplitude signals caused by delayed activation of parts of the RV
- T-wave inversion (TWI) in the right precordial leads, with the extent of TWI correlated with the degree of RV enlargement

In addition, abnormalities in signal-averaged ECGs (SAECG) are also frequently detected in patients with ARVC, and have been proposed as a minor criterion on the 2010 revised task force criteria. Arrhythmias most frequently seen in ARVC include sustained or non-sustained VT with left bundle branch block morphology and frequent ventricular extrasystoles (>500/24-hour period).

The role of non-invasive imaging in the diagnosis of ARVC incorporates the use of echocardiography and CMRI. RV dilatation with

Table 120.1 Comparison of original and revised task force criteria

Original task force criteria	Revised task force a criteria
I. Global or regional dysfunction and structural alterations* Major • Severe dilatation and reduction of RV ejection fraction with no (or only mild) LV impairment • Localized RV aneurysms (akinetic or dyskinetic areas with diastolic bulging) • Severe segmental dilatation of the RV	**By 2D echo:** • Regional RV akinesia, dyskinesia, or aneurysm • and 1 of the following (end diastole): — PLAX RVOT ≥32 mm (corrected for body size [PLAX/BSA] ≥19 mm/m²) — PSAX RVOT ≥36 mm (corrected for body size [PSAX/BSA] ≥21 mm/m²) — *or* fractional area change ≤33% **By MRI:** • Regional RV akinesia or dyskinesia or dyssynchronous RV contraction • *and* 1 of the following: — Ratio of RV end-diastolic volume to BSA ≥110 mL/m² (male) or ≥100 mL/m² (female) — *or* RV ejection fraction ≤40% **By RV angiography:** • Regional RV akinesia, dyskinesia, or aneurysm
Minor • Mild global RV dilation and/or ejection fraction reduction with normal LV • Mild segmental dilation of the RV • Regional RV hypokinesia	**By 2D echo:** • Regional RV akinesia or dyskinesia • *and* 1 of the following (end diastole): — PLAX RVOT ≥29 to <32 mm (corrected for body size [PLAX/BSA] ≥16 to <19 mm/m²) — PSAX RVOT ≥32 to <36 mm (corrected for body size [PSAX/BSA] ≥18 to <21 mm/m²) — *or* fractional area change >33% to ≤40% **By MRI:** • Regional RV akinesia or dyskinesia or dyssynchronous RV contraction • *and* 1 of the following: — Ratio of RV end-diastolic volume to BSA ≥100 to <110 mL/m² (male) or ≥90 to <100 mL/m² (female) — *or* RV ejection fraction >40% to ≤45%
II. Tissue characterization of wall Major • Fibrofatty replacement of myocardium on endomyocardial biopsy Minor	• Residual myocytes <60% by morphometric analysis (or <50% if estimated), with fibrous replacement of the RV free wall myocardium in ≥1 sample, with or without fatty replacement of tissue on endomyocardal biopsy • Residual myocytes 60% to 75% by morphometric analysis (or 50% to 65% if estimated), with fibrous replacement of the RV free wall myocardium in ≥1 sample, with or without fatty replacement of tissue on endomyocardial biopsy
III. Repolarization abnormalities Major Minor • Inverted T waves in right precondal leads (V₂ and V₃) (people age >12 years, in absence of right bundle branch block)	• Inverted T waves in right precordial leads (V₁, V₂, and V₃) or beyond in individuals >14 years of age (in the absence of complete right bundle branch block QRS ≥120 ms) • Inverted T waves in leads V₁ and V₂ in individuals >14 years of age (in the absence of complete right bundle branch block) or in V₄, V₅, or V₆ • Inverted T waves in leads V₁, V₂, V₃, and V₄ in individuals >14 years of age in the presence of complete right bundle branch block
IV. Depolarization/conduction abnormalities Major • Epsilon waves or localized prolongation (>110 ms) of the QRS complex in right precordial leads (V₁ to V₃) Minor • Late potentials (SAECG)	• Epsilon wave (reproducible low-amplitude signals between end of QRS complex to onset of the T wave) in the right precordial leads (V₁ to V₃) • Late potentials by SAECG in ≥ 1 of 3 parameters in the absence of a QRS duration of ≥110 ms on the standard ECG • Filtered QRS duration (fQRS) ≥114 ms • Duration of terminal QRS <40 µV (low-amplitude signal duration) ≥38 ms • Root-mean-square voltage of terminal 40 ms ≤20 µV • Terminal activation duration of QRS ≥55 ms measured from the nadir of the S wave to the end of the QRS, inducing R′, in V₁, V₂, or V₃, in the absence of complete right bundle-branch block
V. Arrhythmias Major Minor • Left bundle-branch block-type ventricular tachycardia (sustained and non-sustained) (ECG, Holter, exercise) • Frequent ventricular (>1000 per 24 hours) (Holter)	 • Nonsustained or sustained ventricular tachycardia of left bundle-branch morphology with superior axis (negative or indeterminate QRS in leads I, III, and aVF and positive in lead aVL) • Non-sustained or sustained ventricular tachycardia of RV outflow configuration, left bundle-branch block morphology with inferior axis (positive QRS in leads II, III, and aVF and negative in lead aVL) or of unknown axis • >500 ventricular per 24 hours (Holter)

Table 120.1 (Continued)

Original task force criteria	Revised task force a criteria
VI. Family history	
Major	
• Familial disease confirmed at necropsy or surgery	• ARVC/D confirmed in a first-degree relative who meets current Task Force criteria • ARVC/D confirmed pathologically at autopsy or surgery in a first-degree relative • Identification of a pathogenic mutation† categorized as associated or probably associated with ARVC/D in the patient under evaluation
Minor	
• Family history of premature sudden death (<35 years of age) due to suspected ARVC/D • Familial history (clinical diagnosis based on present criteria)	• History of ARVC/D in a first-degree relative in whom it is not passible or practical to determine whether the family member meets current Task Force criteria • Premature sudden death (<35 years of age) due to suspected ARVC/D in a first-degree relative • ARVC/D confirmed pathologically or by current Task Force Criteria in second-degree relative

Abbreviations: ARVC/D, arrhythmogenic right ventricular cardiomyopathy/dysplasia; aVF, augmented voltage unipolar left foot lead; aVL, augmented voltage unipolar left arm lead; BSA, body surface area; LV, left ventricular; PLAX, parasternal long-axis view; PSAX, parasternal short-axis view; RV, right ventricular; RVOT, right ventricular outflow tract; SAECG, signal-averaged ECG.

Note: Diagnostic terminology for original criteria: this diagnosis is fulfilled by the presence of two major, or one major plus two minor criteria, or four minor criteria from different groups. Diagnostic terminology for revised criteria: definite diagnosis: two major or one major and two minor criteria, or four minor criteria from different categories; borderline: one major and one minor, or three minor criteria from different categories; possible: one major or two minor criteria from different categories. Hypokinesis is not included in this or subsequent definitions of RV regional wall motion abnormalities for the proposed modified criteria. A pathogenic mutation is a DNA alteration with ARVC/D that alters or is expected to alter the encoded protein, is unobserved or rare in a large non-ARVC/D control population, and either alters or is predicted to alter the structure or function of the protein or has demonstrated linkage to the disease phenotype in a conclusive pedigree.

Reproduced with permission from Marcus, McKenna, Sherrill et al., Diagnosis of arrhythmogenic right ventricular cardiomyopathy/dysplasia, *European Heart Journal*, volume 31, pp806-814, © 2010 American Heart Association, Inc. and European Society of Cardiology.

reduction in systolic function, and widespread regional wall motion abnormality, corresponds to disease severity. CMRI enables the identification of intra-myocardial fat and late gadolinium enhancement, and may be sensitive in identifying early changes leading to the diagnosis of ARVC, although they also have a high rate of CMRI false-positive diagnosis of ARVC. Standardized imaging protocols are available on http://www.arvd.org. Right ventriculography is included as a major criterion in the presence of regional RV akinesis, dyskinesis, or aneurysm.

With greater understanding and recognition of the familial basis of ARVC, and identification of disease-causing genes, the clinical identification of relatives at risk has become central to management. Mutations are frequently detected in patients with ARVC, with greater than 70% of living probands in some series. However, the role of genetic testing remains to be fully established, limited by the uncertainty of the prognostic implications of genetically affected individuals, since penetrance is low, with marked intrafamilial phenotypic diversity. Variable age-related expression of the disease is common, with an unpredictable minority suffering arrhythmic events without overt clinical disease. On the contrary, the majority of patients will not develop clinically significant disease, and those with clinical disease expression have a benign course. There is also the issue of detecting gene sequence variations with uncertain significance.

The prevention of SCD is the major role of therapy in patients with ARVC. In addition, since SCD is the first clinical manifestation of the disease in up to 50% of index cases, surveillance of family members is a crucial part of the management of this disease. Ventricular arrhythmias in patients with ARVC range from ventricular premature beats to sustained VT, and the frequency varies with the severity of the disease. The most common arrhythmia is sustained or non-sustained monomorphic VT which originates from the RV (inflow tract, apex, or outflow tract) and thus have a left bundle branch block morphology. VT from the outflow tract can be indistinguishable from that seen in idiopathic RV outflow-tract tachycardia.

The optimal strategies for preventing SCD, and indications for ICD therapy, are not well defined and, hence, risk stratification is challenging. The evidence available is based on small studies (non-randomized controlled studies) and the opinion of experts due to the relatively low prevalence of ARVC. Current guidelines recommend ICD implantation for secondary prevention of SCD in patients with sustained VT or VF, and aborted SCD. Primary-prevention ICD implantation is suggested in selected high-risk patients such as those with extensive disease, adverse family history, or unexplained syncope. Other putative risk factors that may predict an adverse prognosis include early onset structurally severe disease, and increased QRS dispersion (a difference of >40 ms between maximum and minimum QRS values, occurring in any of the 12 ECG leads). Electrophysiological testing by programmed ventricular stimulation is currently not useful in the risk stratification of patients with ARVC, with conflicting results. Genotyping may help in the assessment of SCD, and certain recessive forms of ARVC have been suggested to be more malignant. It is crucial to note that the potential prognostic benefits offered by ICD therapy may be tempered by the significant risk of complications with some unique to patients with ARVC. Areas of RV myocardium can be perforated during placement of RV leads, and fibrofatty changes in the RV may interfere with adequate lead positioning and compromise sensing of arrhythmias. Hence, indiscriminate ICD implantation may not be beneficial to the majority of patients.

Antiarrhythmic drugs and radiofrequency ablation have not been shown to reduce the risk of SCD in ARVC, but are often used as adjuncts to ICD implantation in patients with frequent ventricular arrhythmias and ICD therapies. In addition, strenuous activity is discouraged in patients with ARVC, due to the proarrhythmic effect of sympathetic stimulation and the risk of disease progression with increased mechanical stress.

Absence of structural heart disease

SCD most commonly occurs in patients with structural heart disease. However, SCD may occur in patients with an 'apparently' normal heart. Failure to detect structural abnormalities may depend on the unknown or concealed nature of the underlying pathological processes along with the limits of our diagnostic tools. This accounts for approximately 10%–12% of cases amongst populations under the age of 45, with a significantly lower proportion when older subjects are included. Previously, these have been termed 'idiopathic', but more complete evaluation has identified the cause of death or SCA as being a primary electrical disorder in many of these patients. Over the last decade, molecular genetic research has established a link between a number of inherited lethal cardiac arrhythmias and their genetic basis, involving mutations in genes encoding for ion channels or other membrane components. These account for the majority of the inherited arrhythmogenic syndromes, and they will be reviewed here.

Long-QT syndrome

Long-QT syndrome (LQTS) is a disease of abnormal myocardial ventricular repolarization and is characterized by a prolonged QTc interval on the ECG; syncope; and SCD due to ventricular arrhythmias, typically torsades de pointes (TdP). The syndrome can be congenital or acquired. Acquired LQTS is largely due to drug therapy (see Box 120.1)

Box 120.1 Commonly prescribed agents that prolong QT interval and should be avoided in patients with congenital long-QT syndrome

Antiarrhythmics
- Amiodarone
- Sotalol

Antibiotics
- Erythromycin
- Clarithromycin
- Ciprofloxacin

Antihistamines
- Terfenadine

Antidepressants
- Fluoxetine
- Sertraline
- Amitryptiline

Reproduced from the BMJ, Dominic J Abrams, Malcolm A Perkin, Jonathan R Skinner, Long QT syndrome, volume 340, copyright © 2010 with permission from BMJ Publishing Group Ltd

and which are located on chromosomes 3, 4, 7, 11, 12, 17, and 21. In all genetic forms, decreases in the outward potassium currents or increases in the inward sodium or calcium current prolong the action-potential duration, resulting in the common phenotype in LQTS, prolongation of the QT interval. The LQT1 and LQT2 syndromes are the two commonest genetic variants, each accounting for approximately 40% of genotyped patients. The LQT3 syndrome accounts for about 10% of genotyped patients. In LQT1, a mutation in KCNQ1, which encodes the alpha subunit of the potassium channel gene, is responsible for a defect (loss of function) in the slowly activating component of the delayed rectifier potassium channel. In LQT2, a mutation in KCNH2 causes a defect in the rapidly activating component of the delayed rectifier potassium current. In LQT3, a mutation in SCN5A, the gene which encodes the alpha subunit of the sodium channel, results in an increase (gain of function) in the late sodium current (I_{Na}). At present, 65%–70% of affected individuals will have an identifiable mutation one of the genes known to cause LQTS. In many families, LQTS exhibits incomplete penetrance and variable expressivity; this observation suggests that factors other than the primary mutation can modify the probability of symptoms.

The genetic basis for congenital LQTS is given in Table 120.2.

The diagnosis of LQTS is clinical and relates to the ECG, clinical findings (syncope), and family history (unexplained SCD). Measurement of the QT interval in the ECG is the primary investigation, with intervals of >450 ms in men, and >460 ms in women, being suggestive of QT prolongation. The QT interval is frequently automatically calculated and printed on the 12-lead ECG but, unfortunately, errors occur frequently, largely due to incorrect determination of the end of the T wave, and incorporation of the U wave into the measurement. The QT interval has to be corrected for the heart rate, and the most common correction used is the Bazett's formula. Incorrect calculation of the QT interval may lead to a false-negative or a false-positive diagnosis. Due to the differential modification of the ionic currents in each cell type by mutations in each LQTS gene, there is a variety of QT-interval and T-wave morphology. Broad-based prolonged T waves are more commonly seen in the LQT1 syndrome, whereas low-amplitude T waves with a notched or bifid configuration are observed more frequently in the LQT2 syndrome. LQT3 patients have late-appearing T waves with a prolonged isoelectric ST segment. However, there are exceptions for all three genotypes, and the T-wave pattern may vary with time in the same patient with a specific mutation. Measurement of the QT interval following exercise testing or at time of relative bradycardia on 24-hour ambulatory ECG monitoring may be useful in

or electrolyte imbalances (e.g. hypokalaemia and hypomagnesaemia), although it may also be secondary to cerebral injury, myocardial disease, and hypothermia. These factors may also unmask the congenital syndrome in a previously asymptomatic individual. LQTS is a potential cause of avoidable SCD, and is thought to be responsible for a significant percentage of all SCD.

The exact prevalence of congenital LQTS is unknown, due to its highly variable disease expression, but current estimates range from 1 in 2000 to 1 in 3000. LQTS is certainly the most common of the inherited arrhythmogenic syndromes. Two phenotypic variants have been described—an autosomal dominant form (Romano–Ward syndrome), which accounts for 90% of LQTS cases, and an autosomal recessive form in association with sensorineural deafness (Jervell and Lange-Nielsen syndrome). Molecular genetic studies have revealed a total of at least 12 forms of congenital LQTS, and the 'family' concept of syndromes has been applied to the multiple LQTS genotypes (LQT1–12). They result from mutations which occur in genes of the potassium, sodium, and calcium channels, or the membrane adaptor,

Table 120.2 Genetic basis for congenital long-QT syndrome

Type	Locus	Gene	Protein	Function	Frequency
LQT1	11p15.5	KCNQ1	KV7.1 α	I_{Ks} ↓	30%–35%
LQT2	7q35	KCNH2	KV11.1 α	I_{Kr} ↓	25%–30%
LQT3	3p21	SCN5A	NaV1.5 α	I_{Na} ↑	5%–10%
LQT4	4q25	ANK2	Ankyrin-B	$I_{Na,K}$ ↓ I_{NCX} ↓	1%–2%
LQT5	21q22.1	KCNE1	mink β	I_{Ks} ↓	1%
LQT6	21q22.1	KCNE2	MiRP1 β	I_{Kr} ↓	Rare
LQT7*	17q23	KCNJ2	Kir2.1 α	I_{K1} ↓	Rare
LQT8†	12p13.3	CACNA1C	CaV 1.2 α1c	$I_{Ca,L}$ ↑	Rare
LQT9	3p25	CAV3	Caveolin-3	I_{Na} ↑	Rare
LQT10	11q23	SCN4B	NaV1.5 β4	I_{Na} ↑	Rare
LQT11	7q21	AKAP9	Yotiao	I_{Ks} ↓	Rare
LQT12	20q11.2	SNTA1	A1-syntrophin	I_{Na} ↑	Rare

*Andersen–Tawil syndrome.
†Timothy syndrome.

Abbreviations: $I_{Ca,L}$, L-type calcium current; I_{K1}, inward rectifier potassium current; I_{Ks}, slowly activating component of the delayed rectifier potassium channel; I_{Kr}, rapidly activating component of the delayed rectifier potassium current; I_{Na}, sodium current; $I_{Na,K}$, sodium–potassium pump current; I_{NCX}, sodium-calcium exchanger current.

Reprinted from *Heart Rhythm*, volume 6, issue 8, Elizabeth S. Kaufman, Mechanisms and clinical management of inherited channelopathies: Long QT syndrome, Brugada syndrome, catecholaminergic polymorphic ventricular tachycardia, and short QT syndrome, pp.s51-s55 Copyright 2009, with permission from Elsevier.

Table 120.3 1993 long-QT syndrome diagnostic criteria

		Points
ECG findings*		
A.	QT_c†	
	≥480 msec¹⸍²	3
	460–470 msec¹⸍²	2
	450 msec¹⸍² (in males)	1
B.	Torsade de pointes‡	2
C.	T-Wave alternans	1
D.	Notched T wave in three leads	1
E.	Low heart rate for age§	0.5
Clinical history		
A.	Syncope‡	
	With stress	2
	Without stress	1
B.	Congenital deafness	0.5
Family history‖		
A.	Family members with definite LQTS#	1
B.	Unexplained sudden cardiac death below age 30 among immediate family members	0.5

LQTS, long QT syndrome.

* In the absence of medications or disorders known to affect these electrocardiographic features.

†QT_c calculated by Bazett's formula, where $QT_c = QT/\sqrt{RR}$.

‡Mutually exclusive.

§Resting heart rate below the second percentile for age.[25]

‖The same family member cannot be counted in A and B.

#Definite LQTS is defined by an LQTS score ≥4.

Scoring: ≤1 point, low probability of LQTS; 2 to 3 points, intermediate probability of LQTS; ≥4 points, high probability of LQTS.

Reproduced with permission from PJ Schwartz, AJ Moss, GM Vincent and RS Crampton, Diagnostic criteria for the long QT syndrome, *Circulation*, Volume 88, pp. 782-784, Copyright © 1993 Wolters Kluwer Health, Inc.

ECG, clinical, and familial findings, and the score ranges from a minimum value of 0 to a maximum value of 9. The point score is arbitrarily divided into three probability categories: (1) ≤1, low probability of LQTS; (2) 2 or 3 points, intermediate probability of LQTS; and (3) ≥4 points, high probability of LQTS.

The risk of SCD in LQTS is attributed to the underlying risk of developing ventricular tachyarrhythmias. In LQTS, the long QT interval and an appropriately timed ventricular ectopic (R on T phenomenon) may lead to the occurrence of TdP, a form of polymorphic VT. The variation in the QRS morphology and axis in TdP takes the form of a progressive, sinusoidal, cyclic alteration of the QRS axis. The peaks of the QRS complexes appear to 'twist' around the isoelectric line of the recording, hence the term TdP, or 'twisting of points'. TdP is usually short-lived and spontaneously terminates, but episodes can occur in rapid succession and may degenerate into VF leading to cardiac arrest and potentially SCD.

The clinical course, triggers, and risk stratification of patients with LQTS are variable, with a significant genotype–phenotype correlation, which has been demonstrated in clinical and experimental studies. This is especially evident in the LQT1, LQT2, and LQT3 syndromes.

In LQT1 patients, cardiac events were most frequent during exercise, with swimming a common trigger. In contrast, in LQT3 patients, cardiac events principally occurred during sleep and rest, and exercise-related events are rare. In LQT2, there was no predilection to cardiac events during exercise or at rest, but a sudden startle in the form of an auditory stimulus is a specific trigger (see Figure 120.1). Exercise should be limited more strictly in LQT1 patients, especially swimming and diving.

The overall population-based risk of patients with expressed phenotypic evidence is low when the patients receive appropriate treatment, most usually with beta blockers. The international LQTS registry indicates an approximately 4% risk of mortality over 40 years (i.e. 0.1%/year). There are statistically significant differences in the incidence of cardiac events and SCD, correlated to the genotype, with those with LQT2 and LQT3 having a greater risk than those with LQT1. Other indicators of high relative risk of SCD include a personal history of aborted SCD; syncope; or QTc >500 ms. Gender and age also play significant roles in influencing the clinical course of LQTS.

With regards to SCD, absolute rates in the respective genotype groups are as follows: LQT1, 0.3%/year; LQT2, 0.6%/year; and LQT3, 0.56%/year (Priori et al., 2003). Based on published data, the risk in LQTS may be determined as high (presence of aborted SCD +/− ECG documented episodes of TdP), intermediate

identifying those who carry an LQTS mutation but have a normal QT interval on a 12 lead ECG at rest.

Commonly prescribed agents that prolong QT interval and should be avoided in patients with congenital LQTS are given in Box 120.1.

The criterion for the diagnosis of LQTS was upgraded in 1993, and is detailed in Table 120.3. Relative points are assigned to various

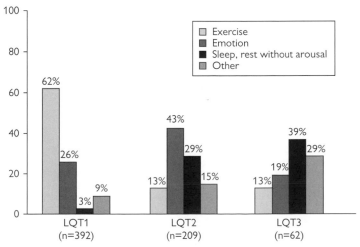

Figure 120.1 Triggers for cardiac events, according to three genotypes.

Reproduced with permission from Schwartz et al., Genotype-Phenotype Correlation in the Long-QT Syndrome: Gene-Specific Triggers for Life-Threatening Arrhythmias, *Circulation*, Volume 103, Issue 1, pp.89-95, Copyright © 2001 Wolters Kluwer Health, Inc.

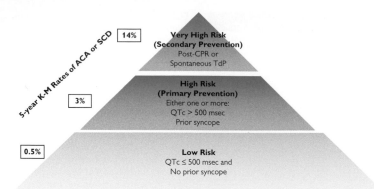

Figure 120.2 Suggested risk-stratification scheme for aborted cardiac arrest or sudden cardiac death in LQTS patients; ACA, aborted cardiac arrest; K–M, Kaplan–Meier; QTc, corrected QT interval; SCD, sudden cardiac death; TdP, torsades de pointes.

Reprinted from *Current Problems in Cardiology*, Volume 33, issue 11, Ian Goldenberg, Wojciech Zareba, Arthur J. Moss, Long QT Syndrome, pp.629-694, Copyright (2008), with permission from Elsevier

(time-dependent syncopal history +/− QTC >500 ms), and low (those free of previous syncope, and QTC <500 ms) (see Figure 120.2). However, as mentioned, risk factors in LQTS are also time dependent and age specific and these features need to be incorporated in any risk-stratification process. Cardiac events probably occur more commonly in children, with boys having a higher risk of events during preadolescence and girls having higher event rates in adolescence and thereafter. Recent data indicate that a family history of premature SCD is not an independent risk factor for subsequent lethal events in an affected individual. Invasive electrophysiological study (EPS) is not helpful in risk stratification of SCD in patients with LQTS.

Beta blockers are the mainstay of the treatment of LQTS. Nadolol and propanolol, agents that block both beta-1 and beta-2 adrenergic receptors, are often preferred, based on long-term experience with their usage. They are most effective in LQT1 patients, in whom the prognosis is excellent if patients avoid QT-prolonging drugs, and specific triggers such as competitive exercise. Although beta blockers are least effective in LQT3 patients, these drugs may still be beneficial. The mechanism of action is likely due to the decrease of adrenergic-mediated triggers in this condition. Patients should continue beta blockade, including during pregnancy and peripartum. However, despite the beneficial effects of beta blockade, high rates of cardiac events have been reported in those receiving this therapy, although data from numerous studies suggest that non-compliance and the use of QT-prolonging drugs underlie most life-threatening 'beta-blocker failures'. Therefore, patients who remain symptomatic despite beta blockade should be considered for more invasive therapies.

Potentially useful but unproven pharmacological options such as calcium-channel blockers, flecainide, and mexiletine are used in those with continuing symptoms with ICDs in situ. Surgical left cervico-thoracic sympathetic denervation (LCSD) should be considered in patients with recurrent syncope despite beta blockade, in patients with a contraindication or intolerance to beta blockade, and in patients with arrhythmia storms with an ICD. LCSD leads to a significant reduction in the frequency of aborted SCD and syncope in high-risk groups, although it does not produce complete protection. It does provide a reasonable alternative to ICD implantation, particularly in children, where the ICD-therapy-associated comorbidity can be high. An ICD is indicated in LQTS patients who have survived an aborted SCD (as secondary prevention) and/or who have repetitive episodes of syncope in the presence of pharmacological and non-pharmacological therapy, regardless of genotype (primary prevention).

Although antibradycardic pacing has been used in selected LQTS patients with sinus bradycardia, long-term follow-up data show that the incidence of SCD in these patients is still unacceptably high. Pacemakers are thought to be beneficial in preventing TdP by suppressing pause-dependent QT prolongation, which is recognized more frequently in LQT2 patients. Focal radiofrequency ablation of ventricular premature beats which trigger VT/VF in LQTS has been reported. Preventative measures are crucial in LQTS, and adrenergic

and auditory stimuli, and QT-prolonging drugs, should be avoided. Further prospective and comprehensive study on genotype–phenotype correlation is needed to improve the management and treatment of patients with LQTS.

Short-QT syndrome

Congenital short-QT syndrome (SQTS) is a relatively recently described, novel inherited disorder characterized by a very short QT interval and by susceptibility to atrial fibrillation and VF, and hence SCD. Although the link between a short QT interval and SCD had been previously suspected, only in the last decade has SQTS been defined as a clinical syndrome. The definitive link between short QT interval and familial SCD was described by Gaita et al. (2003), with a clinical report of two families with SQTS and a high incidence of SCD. The prevalence of SQTS is not known and it appears to be extremely rare. At present, only a few families and some sporadic individuals have been reported to exhibit SQTS. The following features characterize the syndrome:

- an autosomal dominant pattern of inheritance
- a corrected QT interval of ≤320 ms
- an increased risk of SCD due to VF
- atrial fibrillation which occurs at a young age
- short atrial and ventricular refractory periods at EPS
- structurally normal heart

Although the penetrance of SQTS is high, its clinical manifestations can be quite variable, even amongst members of the same family. However, in the largest SQTS study (Giustetto et al., 2006), the most frequent symptom of SQTS is cardiac arrest, which is also the most frequent clinical presentation of this syndrome. First presentation can occur at any age, from a few months old to 60 years old, with the median age of presentation being 30 years. Atrial fibrillation is also common in SQTS, and occurs in some 80% of patients with SQTS, even if they are young. Therefore, in young patients presenting with lone atrial fibrillation, SQTS should be considered as a possible cause of the arrhythmia.

The diagnosis of SQTS is based on the patient's symptoms (syncope and palpitations), family history (syncope, SCD, or atrial fibrillation occurring at <30 years of age), and 12-lead ECG. Secondary causes of a short QT, such as hyperthermia, hyperkalaemia, hypercalcaemia, acidosis, and alterations of autonomic tone, must be excluded. The ECG is characterized by a strikingly short QT interval (typically <320 ms) with a virtual absence of the ST segment, with tall, peaked, narrow-based, symmetrical T waves. In addition, as SQTS is often diagnosed in childhood, the criteria for diagnosing SQTS sometimes includes an age- and gender-adjusted cut-off for the QT interval (a QT interval that is less than 80% of the predicted value is accepted to be consistent with SQTS).

The clinical significance of an incidentally short QT interval is uncertain; however, some have suggested that patients with a QTc

<330 ms (in the case of men) or <340 ms (in the case of women) should be considered to have SQTS even if they have no symptoms, as such short intervals are very rare in the general population. In addition, whereas, in healthy individuals, the QT interval shortens as the heart rate increases, those with SQTS exhibit a paradoxical shortening of QT intervals during slow heart rates, and little shortening with higher heart rates. Hence, frequent ECGs, 24-hour ECG monitoring, and exercise ECG testing can be used to diagnose SQTS in patients with a relative tachycardia at baseline. Invasive EPS in patients with SQTS reveals extremely short atrial and ventricular effective refractory periods. Additionally, in >90% of patients, ventricular tachyarrhythmias (predominantly, VF and ventricular flutter) were inducible.

SQTS is an autosomal dominant syndrome which, in some cases, is caused by mutations in cardiac ion channels. These mutations can lead to either hyperfunction of the delayed rectifier potassium current (KCNQ1, KCNH2, and KCNJ2), or hypofunction of the calcium current (CACNA1C and CACNB2B). As a result, the repolarization period is extended and there is an increase in the transmural dispersion of repolarization, with consequent short atrial and ventricular effective refractory periods, causing susceptibility to atrial fibrillation and VF. (Curiously, four of the five genes associated with SQTS have also been implicated in LQTS; in that case, the mutations lead to hypofunction of the potassium current.) However, these mutations do not occur in all cases of SQTS. In addition, there is no genotype–phenotype correlation for SQTS, due to the relatively few cases described. Nonetheless, genetic testing may assist in the diagnosis of SQTS in symptomatic patients with an abnormal but non-diagnostic ECG.

Although SQTS is characterized by high lethality due to an increased risk of SCD from fatal arrhythmias, there is, at present, insufficient data for risk stratification; therefore, it can be difficult to assess the extent of the risk in asymptomatic patients, especially when there is no family history of SQTS. Although ICD therapy is the only effective treatment for SQTS, it can be associated with T-wave oversensing. Thus, pharmacological therapy may be indicated, to prevent inappropriate ICD discharges or as an alternative to ICD therapy in the young. It has been shown that quinidine and disopyramide can prolong the QT interval; however, further clinical trials are needed before these drugs can be recommended for routine use in SQTS treatment.

Brugada syndrome

Brugada syndrome (BrS) is a clinical entity characterized by the triad of right bundle branch block, coved ST elevation, and risk of SCD as a result of ventricular tachyarrhythmias in an apparently normal heart. It is thought to be responsible for up to 4% of all SCD, and up to 20% of SCD in people under the age of 50 with structurally normal hearts. The prevalence of BrS is estimated at 1–5 in 10 000 worldwide, and studies in hetergenous populations suggest that the majority of affected individuals are Asian. It has a significant male preponderance, being as much as nine times higher in one analysis, with men also having a higher rate of syncope and SCD in a large prospective registry study.

BrS is inherited in an autosomal dominant fashion with incomplete penetrance. Genetic analyses have led to the identification of causative mutations in the SCN5A gene, which encodes the alpha subunit of a cardiac sodium channel, resulting in a functional reduction in the availability of the sodium current (and hence the use of sodium channels blockers in unmasking the Brugada pattern ECG). Of note, other mutations in SCN5A have been found in a number of other cardiac conditions, including LQTS. However, sodium-channel mutations only account for a maximum of 30% of cases, and underlying structural myocardial abnormalities have now been described in what was initially thought to be a purely functional disorder, with a number of studies demonstrating fibrosis in the Brugada right ventricle, suggesting a degenerative process.

Abnormalities in repolarization and depolarization in the RV outflow tract, and heterogeneities of conduction within the epicardium and between the epicardium and endocardium, have been proposed to be responsible for the ECG abnormalities and predisposition to ventricular tachyarrhythmias. Ventricular arrhythmias in BrS take the form of VT, most originating from the RV outflow tract, or VF. BrS is usually diagnosed in adulthood, with the average age of presentation being 41. It is rarely diagnosed in children. Symptoms at presentation are syncope, nocturnal agonal respiration, ventricular tachyarrhythmias, and SCD.

A number of ambiguities surround the diagnosis of BrS, with the characteristic ECG pattern being only one component of the diagnostic criteria of BrS. Patients with ECG changes typical of BrS but with no other clinical criteria are said to have the Brugada pattern but not BrS. Further, the characteristic ECG changes are also

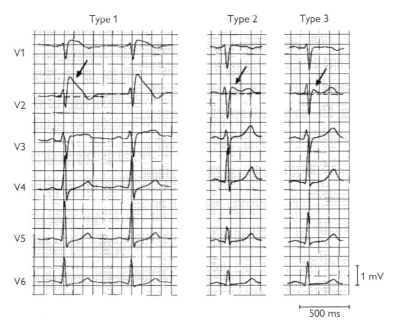

Figure 120.3 Three different types of Brugada ECG pattern.

Reproduced with permission from Wilde et al., Proposed Diagnostic Criteria for the Brugada Syndrome: Consensus Report, *Circulation*, Volume 106, Issue 19, pp. 2514-2519, Copyright © 2002 Wolters Kluwer Health, Inc.

dynamic, and often concealed. Three types of repolarization patterns (recorded in right precordial leads V1–V3) are recognized, either occurring spontaneously or following pharmacological provocation. The type 1 Brugada pattern, initially described by the Brugada brothers (1992), is characterized by a prominent, coved ST elevation which is >2 mm (0.2 mV) and followed by a negative T wave (Figure 120.3). The type 2 pattern is characterized by a saddleback ST elevation which is >2 mm and followed by a trough of >1 mm ST elevation and then a positive or biphasic T wave; it may represent a less severe phenotype. The type 3 pattern is characterized by a saddleback or coved appearance, with an ST elevation of <1 mm. There can be significant variation in the ECG patterns seen in a patient over time. The Arrhythmia Working Group of the European Society of Cardiology published a consensus statement in 2002 based on the available clinical date and molecular basis of BrS. The diagnosis of BrS should be strongly considered in the following two cases:

- the appearance of a type 1 ST elevation in more than one right precordial lead, in the presence or absence of a sodium-channel blocker (with no other factors that can account for the ECG abnormality) and one of the following:
  - documented VF
  - self-terminating, polymorphic VT
  - a family history of SCD (<45 years)
  - a type 1 ECG pattern in family members
  - inducibility of VT on electrophysiologic testing
  - syncope
  - nocturnal agonal respiration
- the appearance of type 2 or 3 ST elevation ('saddleback type') in more than one precordial lead under baseline conditions, with conversion to type 1 ST elevation following a challenge with a sodium-channel blocker, and one of the following features:
  - documented VF
  - self-terminating, polymorphic VT
  - a family history of SCD (<45 years)
  - a type 1 ECG pattern in family members
  - inducibility of VT on electrophysiologic testing
  - syncope
  - nocturnal agonal respiration

Drug-induced conversion of type 3 to type 2 ST elevation is considered inconclusive.

Clinical diagnostic evaluation to exclude other causes is crucial, as there are numerous factors that may contribute to ST-segment elevation. Distinguishing between BrS and ARVC may be challenging, and any structural abnormalities may be found only at the time of autopsy. BrS should also be distinguished from early repolarization syndromes (with eventual J-wave elevation in the left precordial leads), and drug challenges might provide the clue for a proper diagnosis.

The role of genetic testing in diagnosing BrS is limited by the fact that only 18%–30% of BrS patients have mutations in the SCN5A gene, and not all patients with documented Brugada SCN5A mutations have BrS. The use of genetic testing is probably most useful in the context of screening of relatives with BrS patients who have documented specific SCN5A mutations.

The management of patients with BrS largely involves the prevention of SCD. SCD or an aborted SCD (SCA) may be the first and only clinical event in BrS, occurring in as many as a third of BrS patients. Arrhythmic events tend to occur between the ages of 22 and 65, with a nocturnal predilection. SCA is not usually related to exercise, with frequent nocturnal ventricular premature beats preceding an arrhythmia. Risk stratification usually begins with eliciting a history of associated symptoms (previous SCA or syncope).

The role of ICD implantation in secondary prevention in BrS is established, with previous SCA having the highest risk, and a Class I indication. Risk stratification for implantation of primary-prevention ICD (which is the only effective therapy for preventing SCD in BrS) remains controversial, particularly in entirely asymptomatic patients. The benefits of ICD therapy have to be balanced against the potential complications, especially in a younger population of patients, with the need for recurrent generator box changes, and the presence of endocardial leads which might be in situ for many decades. The use of a subcutaneous ICD, which would negate the need for an endovascular lead, may be an attractive alternative. There is a strong evidence base for the prognostic impact of syncope in BrS, and this is a Class IIa indication for ICD implantation. Data from published registries also suggest that a spontaneous (rather than drug-induced) type 1 Brugada ECG and male gender were predictors of arrhythmic events. Of note, familial history of SCD was not predictive of arrhythmic events.

The significance of the inducibility of ventricular arrhythmias during programmed electrical stimulation is not entirely clear. Although this investigation is recommended in the second consensus statement on BrS (endorsed by both the Heart Rhythm Society and European Heart Rhythm Association), several studies published since have shown no prognostic impact from the inducibility of ventricular

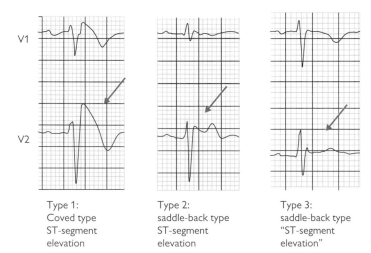

V1		
V2		
Type 1: Coved type ST-segment elevation	Type 2: saddle-back type ST-segment elevation	Type 3: saddle-back type "ST-segment elevation"

Figure 120.4 ECG abnormalities which are diagnostic or suspect of Brugada syndrome. Type 1 (coved-type ST-segment elevation) is the only diagnostic ECG in Brugada syndrome and is defined as a J-wave amplitude or an ST-segment elevation of ≥2 mm or 0.2 mV at its peak (followed by a negative T wave with little or no isoelectric separation). Type 2 (saddle-back-type ST-segment elevation), defined as a J-wave amplitude of ≥2 mm, gives rise to a gradually descending ST-segment elevation (remaining ≥1 mm above the baseline) followed by a positive or biphasic T wave that results in a saddle-back configuration. Type 3 is a right precordial ST-segment elevation (saddle-back type, coved type, or both) without meeting the aforementioned criteria.

Reproduced with permission from Mizusawa and Wilde, Arrhythmogenic Disorders of Genetic Origin: Brugada Syndrome, *Circulation*, volume 5, pp.606-616, Copyright © 2012 Wolters Kluwer Health, Inc.

arrhythmias. The current tools used for risk stratification are not precise, but careful individual patient assessment can yield an estimate of the risk of SCD, and this can be balanced against risks of ICD therapy.

There are pharmacological agents that have been proven to reduce the risk of SCD, including beta blockers and amiodarone. There is some data suggesting the beneficial effects of quinidine, although its use is limited by significant gastrointestinal side effects and prolongation of the QT interval. A multicentre trial of quinidine therapy in asymptomatic patients is currently in progress. Invasive ablative approaches (mapping and ablation of triggers of VF) have also been reported.

As with LQTS, a number of drugs are contraindicated in patients with BrS, as they can provoke the development of type 1 ECG changes. A comprehensive and up-to-date list is available on the website http://www.brugadadrugs.org. Fever can also provoke type 1 ECG changes and should be treated aggressively (Figure 120.4).

Catecholaminergic polymorphic VT

Catecholaminergic polymorphic VT (CPVT) is an inherited arrythmogenic syndrome that is characterized by adrenergically mediated ventricular tachyarrhythmias manifesting in syncope, cardiac arrest, and SCD in young individuals in the absence of structural heart disease. Characteristically, CPVT-associated arrhythmic events are triggered by catecholaminergic stimulation. Thus, they occur under conditions of physical and also mental stress. Sudden noises, physical pain, fear, or sudden movements are all associated with catecholamine release, and can trigger arrhythmias in the setting of CPVT. It was first described by Coumel et al. (1978), but its genetic bases were only discovered in 2001. The prevalence of CPVT in Europe is 1 in 10 000, and it is an important cause of SCD in the young, with some reports suggesting that it may account for 1 in 7 cases of sudden unexplained death. The mean onset of symptoms is between 7 and 9 years of age, with no gender difference. However, it may also manifest in adulthood. SCD can be the manifestation of the disease in a subset of patients (10%–20%). In untreated patients, 8-year overall arrhythmic event rates of 58% and fatal or near-fatal rates of 25% have been reported, and these are higher in patients with aborted SCD.

Most cases of CPVT are caused by autosomal dominant mutations in RYR2, which encodes the cardiac isoform of the ryanodine receptor, which is a calcium channel. CPVT can also be caused by recessive mutations in CASQ2, which encodes the cardiac isoform of calsequestrin, a calcium-binding protein found in the sarcoplasmic reticulum; however, only ~2% of CPVT cases are due to CASQ2 mutations. Both RYR2 and CASQ2 are involved in the control of calcium release from the sarcoplasmic reticulum. Consequently, mutations in these genes lead to an inappropriate release of calcium from the sarcoplasmic reticulum, causing cytosolic calcium overload and thus delayed after-depolarization, triggered activity, and ventricular arrhythmias, especially when beta-adrenergic tone is increased. As with LQTS, CPVT is characterized by variable penetrance, although patients with CASQ2 mutations are thought to carry a greater risk of arrhythmia. In addition, silent mutation carriers (i.e. patients who have a mutation in RYR2 or CASQ2 but do not exhibit ventricular arrhythmia on exercise testing) are also at increased risk of arrhythmia.

The clinical diagnosis of CPVT is made on the basis of symptoms, a family history, and response to exercise or catecholamine infusion. Clinical symptoms can vary from mere palpitations to syncope and SCD. Unfortunately, individuals with CPVT often have normal resting ECGs, so diagnosis is difficult and, not infrequently, these patients are given a diagnosis of 'LQTS with normal QT'. Treadmill ECG or IV catecholamine infusions are the key investigation in terms of the clinical diagnosis, as the arrhythmias are usually reproducible. The 'textbook' arrhythmia with exercise is that of polymorphic or bidirectional VT (beat-to-beat alternation of the QRS axis), but patients may only develop increasing polymorphic ventricular extrasystoles. Although bidirectional VT has been thought to be the hallmark of this condition, this arrhythmia can sometimes occur in other channelopathies, for example LQTS, although this is usually associated with an abnormal resting ECG. Holter monitoring is indicated in the rarer cases where acute emotion represents a more powerful trigger. The

sensitivity (diagnostic yield) from genetic testing is reasonably high; it is approximately 80% in those with typical features, although a negative test does not remove the diagnosis. A positive test has important prognostic implications for the individual patient, and for screening of family members. There is no role for EPS in determining prognosis, as it has poor specificity and sensitivity for 'clinical' arrhythmias with and without catecholamine stimulation.

The risk stratification of SCD in various subgroups in CPVT is much less well defined than that of other inherited arrhythmogenic syndromes such as LQTS and BrS, due to the recent characterization and relative rarity of CPVT, and the current evidence is based on considerably fewer patients. Consequently, it can be difficult to determine whether a CPVT patient is at such low risk of serious arrhythmias that treatment is not required.

Beta blockers (nadolol and propranolol) are the most effective drugs for treating ventricular arrhythmias and preventing arrhythmic events. The use of beta blockade is suggested for all mutation carriers, even those without symptoms. This is due to the possibility of these mutations being highly penetrant, with fatal or near-fatal event rates being as high in family members as in probands. Some reports have suggested that beta blockade should be increased to such a dose as to ensure a maximum exercise heart rate of 110 bpm, based on its effectiveness in suppressing ventricular arrhythmias. As CPVT patients tend to be relatively young, fatigue and other side effects of beta blockers may cause significant limitations to daily life and influence therapeutic compliance. The outcome of exercise stress tests during monitoring are significantly associated with subsequent clinical events, including mortality. The use of calcium-channel antagonists of the verapamil type (L-type calcium-channel blocker) has not been proven to be efficacious in patients who have contraindications to beta blockade, or those who continue to have symptoms on beta blockade and so require additional treatment. An important new development is the discovery that flecainide (a Class Ic antiarrhythmic agent) has RYR2-blocking properties and so directly targets the molecular defect in CPVT. Flecainide greatly reduced the incidence of ventricular arrhythmia during treadmill ECG testing in patients with CPVT. It is unclear whether it is effective in genotype-negative CPVT, and whether it should be used as first-line therapy, either in concert with beta blockers or on its own; however, there is an ongoing randomized clinical trial addressing these questions prospectively.

LCSD may be useful in patients with uncontrolled ventricular arrhythmias on medical therapy, and in patients with ICD, to reduce appropriate ICD therapies. CPVT patients presenting with VF or an aborted SCD without a reversible cause should have an ICD implanted in addition to beta blockade and/or flecainide/LCSD. Patients experiencing exercise-induced ventricular arrhythmias syncope (when VT/VF has not been excluded as the cause) despite medical therapy and/or LCSD should be considered for ICD therapy also. It should, however, be noted that ICD use may have harmful effects in CPVT patients. Both appropriate and inappropriate therapies can trigger catecholamine release, subsequently triggering further VT/VF and resulting in multiple shocks, arrhythmic storms, and death. As such, ICD therapy does have a proarrhythmic potential. Thus, the prevention of VT is crucial even in ICD recipients.

As previously mentioned, CPVT patients are young, and so ICD therapy may produce significant problems. Due to the increased incidence of supraventricular tachyarrhythmias in CPVT patients, they are at an increased risk of receiving inappropriate therapies. This can be prevented with careful ICD programming. Although CPVT is a severe and often lethal disease, early diagnosis and proper treatment can greatly increase life expectancy. Exercise restriction along with medical therapy (and emphasis on importance of drug compliance) and ICD implantation in patients with recurrent symptoms have resulted in a favourable prognosis. The use of sympathomimetic agents is contraindicated in patients with CPVT.

Further Reading

Al-Khatib SM, Stevenson WG, Ackerman MJ, et al. 2017 AHA/ACC/HRS guideline for management of patients with ventricular arrhythmias and the prevention of sudden cardiac death: a report of the American College of Cardiology Foundation/

American Heart Association Task Force on Clinical Practice Guidelines and the Heart Rhythm Society. *Circulation* 2017. http://circ.ahajournals.org/content/early/2017/10/30/CIR.0000000000000548

Gatzoulis M, Webb G, Daubeney P. Diagnosis and Management of Adult Congenital Heart Disease, 3rd ed. Elsevier, 2017.

The Task Force for the management of patients with ventricular arrhythmias and the prevention of sudden cardiac death of the European Society of Cardiology (ESC). 2015 ESC Guidelines for the management of patients with ventricular arrhythmias and the prevention of sudden cardiac death. *Eur Heart J* 2015; 36: 2793–67. doi: 10.1093/eurheartj/ehv316

National Institute for Health and Care Excellence (NICE). Implantable cardioverter defibrillators and cardiac resynchronisation therapy for arrhythmias and heart failure. Technology appraisal guidance [TA314] 2014. https://www.nice.org.uk/guidance/ta314

121 Cardiac device therapy

Kim Rajappan

The term 'device therapy' is used in cardiology to refer to three different types of implantable cardiac-rhythm-management devices: pacemakers, implantable cardioverter defibrillators (ICDs), and cardiac resynchronization therapy (CRT) devices. There has been a steady increase in the number of patients receiving these cardiac devices; in relation to CRT devices, the increase has been almost exponential.

Pacemakers

Background information for pacemakers

Permanent pacemakers (PPMs) are implanted devices that sense intrinsic cardiac electric activity and, if this falls below a given rate, generate impulses to stimulate atrial and/or ventricular contraction.

How PPMs work

PPM systems consist of an implantable pulse generator (IPG) and pacing leads, placed transvenously in the myocardium of the right atrium and/or ventricle. Current leads are almost always bipolar (i.e. they have anode and cathode rings at the tip of the lead), so pacing and sensing only occurs at the tip, unlike unipolar leads, in which the cathode is at the tip, and the IPG acts as the anode. The main advantage of a bipolar lead is that there is much less chance of interference from extrinsic factors such as muscle artefact. The IPG is placed subcutaneously or submuscularly in the chest wall, most commonly in the left infra-clavicular position.

The pulse generator contains electronic sensing, timing, and output circuitry, and a battery (typically lithium–iodide, with a battery life of 7–10 years), housed in a steel case. The sensing circuitry detects intrinsic activity in the cardiac chamber in which the lead is placed. If no activity is detected over a specified interval, an impulse is generated (and may be visible on the ECG as a pacing artefact preceding the P wave or QRS complex). Depolarization of the cardiac chamber occurs by muscle-to-muscle spread of the impulse; with right ventricular pacing, this results in a broad QRS complex on the ECG, of left bundle branch block (LBBB) morphology.

There are three types of pacemakers:

- a single-lead atrial pacing system
- a single-lead ventricular pacing system
- a dual-lead atrial and ventricular pacing system

Single-lead atrial pacing system

In a single-lead atrial pacing system (which can be used with the pacing modes AAI or AAIR), the pacemaker senses and paces the right atrium. If no intrinsic activity is sensed (i.e. no P wave detected), the pacemaker paces the right atrium at its programmed rate. Use of the AAIR mode provides the capability to increase the atrial pacing rate in response to stimuli such as movement, conferring an increase in heart rate with exercise.

Single-lead ventricular pacing system

In a single-lead ventricular pacing system (which can be used with the pacing modes VVI or VVIR), the pacemaker senses and paces the right ventricle. If atrial activity is conducted through the conduction system and depolarizes the ventricles, the pacemaker is inhibited. If no intrinsic activity is sensed (i.e. no R wave detected), the pacemaker paces the right ventricle at its programmed rate. Use of the VVIR mode provides the capability to increase the ventricular pacing rate in response to stimuli such as movement, conferring an increase in heart rate with exercise.

Dual-lead atrial and ventricular pacing system

In a dual-lead atrial and ventricular pacing system (which can be used with the pacing modes DDD or DDDR), the pacemaker senses and paces both the right atrium and right ventricle. If no intrinsic activity is sensed in the right atrium, the pacemaker paces the right atrium at its programmed rate. If the intrinsic or paced atrial activity is not conducted to the ventricles within a preset interval, the pacemaker paces the right ventricle. Use of the DDDR mode provides a rate-adaptive capability.

Pacemaker programming

Programming the mode of a pacemaker can be performed non-invasively by an appropriately trained individual using the appropriate programmer for that device. As there are many pacemaker types, patients should carry with them a card providing information about their particular make and model. Most pacemaker generators have an X-ray code that can be seen on a chest radiograph; however, the chest radiograph may need to be zoomed onto the pacemaker generator for better resolution.

Indications for pacing

Indications for pacing (either temporary or permanent) can be divided into those where pacing can be used to prevent symptoms related to bradycardia, and those where pacing can be used to prevent asystolic arrest. International and national guidelines have been written about the indications for pacing; the following constitute a summary of these indications:

- complete atrioventricular (AV) block (third-degree block; whether symptomatic or asymptomatic)
- second-degree AV block Möbitz type II (whether symptomatic or asymptomatic)
- alternating left and right bundle branch block
- sick sinus syndrome
- symptomatic sinus bradycardia
- tachy brady syndrome
- atrial fibrillation with sinus node dysfunction (Figure 121.1)
- chronotropic incompetence (inability to increase the heart rate appropriately during exercise)

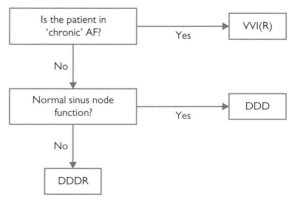

Figure 121.1 Choice of type of permanent pacemaker; AF, atrial fibrillations.

Note that first-degree AV block or Möbitz type I second-degree AV block (Wenckebach) are not clear indications for pacing. Neither is bundle branch block per se, even in the presence of axis deviation and prolonged PR interval, unless it is associated with presyncope/syncope.

Temporary emergency pacing is indicated for the treatment of significant and haemodynamically unstable bradyarrhythmias; for the prevention of bradycardia-dependent malignant arrhythmias when permanent pacing cannot be immediately performed (however, ideally, a permanent system should be implanted as soon as possible to minimize the risk of complications from having a temporary pacing lead); and, very occasionally, where there is a significant chance of recovery of normal conduction (e.g. transient AV block after an inferior myocardial infarction (MI)).

How to implant pacemakers

Pacemaker implantation is typically a day-case procedure. Most pacemakers are implanted in the prepectoral region, just below the clavicle. The most common access route for the pacemaker leads is via the axillary or subclavian vein. This may be through a direct puncture into the vein, or through the cephalic vein, which drains into the axillary vein.

There are a number of different types of pacemaker leads. Lead design has been a major area of development; however, at present the majority of leads consist of conducting coils that are surrounded by insulating material. The outer coating is predominantly made of polyurethane. The lead tips are held in place by one of two methods. The first method is 'passive' fixation, which uses small anchoring tips, or 'tines', which hook into the trabeculation of the tissue. Over a short period, these tips cause fibrotic tissue to form, which helps keep them in place. The second method, known as 'active' fixation, uses a small helical screw that extends out of the tip of the lead and holds the lead in position. The advantage of the active fixation method is that the lead can be inserted into any tissue, not just those areas that have trabeculation. This is often useful when it is necessary to place a lead on the right ventricular septum rather than on the right ventricular apex. The active fixation leads are also normally easier to extract if necessary. However, the passive fixation leads are easier to implant.

During pacemaker placement, the lead parameters are measured and checked to make sure they are optimal. The threshold for the pacing voltage is the minimal voltage (at a given pulse duration) required for depolarization ('capture') of the myocardium that a lead requires to capture myocardium, and the aim is to get readings as low as possible. The signal amplitude (i.e. the size of the intrinsic P or R wave) is also measured. The sensing on the lead is important, as it determines whether the pacemaker will or will not pace. The output and sensing are set high enough to reliably achieve myocardial capture, yet low enough to maximize battery life. Once the leads are in place, they are secured, the IPG is connected, and the entire system is inserted into a pocket which is fashioned in the prepectoral region. Programming of the pacemaker can then be performed remotely.

Temporary systems use an external pulse generator with skin pads or with transvenous leads. Transcutaneous temporary pacing can be instituted quickly, and is the preferred method for use cardiopulmonary resuscitation. Transcutaneous pacing may be uncomfortable, and the patient may require sedation (e.g. benzodiazepine). Once the patient is stabilized and central venous access is gained, transvenous temporary pacing provides a more reliable and comfortable method and is a good bridge to permanent pacing.

Complications of pacemakers

Pacemaker complications include lead displacement, with consequent pacemaker malfunction; cardiac perforation; complications associated with venous access; bleeding; and infection. The administration of antibiotics prior to and around the time of the procedure (including injection of antibiotics into the pocket) may reduce infection risk. However, only preprocedure antibiotics have clear evidence of benefit.

Pneumothoraces may require medical observation, needle aspiration, or even chest-drain placement. Erosion of the PPM through the skin, while rare, normally requires extraction of the entire system and replacement after systemic antibiotics. Haematomas may be treated with direct pressure and observation, but occasionally require surgical drainage, carrying a risk of introducing infection. If lead displacement occurs, it typically does so within 2 days of implantation, and may be visible on chest radiography. Fluctuating lead impedance may also indicate lead displacement, lead impedance is normal when it is in contact with the endocardium, but infinite (or very high) when not. Free-floating ventricular leads may trigger malignant arrhythmias due to mechanical stimulation of the myocardium.

Device-associated deep vein thrombosis is rare. It typically presents with ipsilateral swelling of the arm. Treatment includes elevation of the arm, and anticoagulation.

Advanced Life Support protocols, including defibrillation, may safely be performed for patients with pacemakers. It is recommended that sternal pads are placed at a safe distance (10–15 cm) from the IPG—for a left-sided device, normal pad positions to the right of the sternum and at the apex should be fine. Anterior and posterior positions tend to be acceptable as well, particularly when used for elective cardioversion of atrial fibrillation in a patient with a cardiac device. Temporary pacing may very occasionally become necessary in cases of MI, as the programmed pacemaker output settings may be insufficient to stimulate ventricular contraction if the lead is close to or within the infarcted tissue. If a suitable programmer is available, the output from the permanent pacemaker can be increased and may overcome this.

Pacemaker malfunction may be suspected when a patient with a pacemaker reports presyncope or syncope, or the ECG does not show normal pacemaker function. With new algorithms to preserve intrinsic conduction, the ECG may suggest pacemaker malfunction, whereas, in fact, the appearances reflect normal programmed function. Types of pacemaker malfunction and their causes are summarized in Table 121.1. In suspected pacemaker malfunction, the details of the pacemaker should be checked (to determine if it is a single- or dual-chamber system, and the pacing mode), and a 12-lead ECG, with a long rhythm strip recorded. Chest radiography will establish the position of the leads and may provide evidence of lead fracture; lead fracture most commonly occurs from compression of the lead between the clavicle and the first rib, or entrapment in the subclavius muscle or the costoclavicular ligament, so the segment of the lead in these areas should be carefully examined.

Table 121.1 Types of pacemaker malfunction and their causes

Type of malfunction	Causes
No pacing stimulus when appropriate	Lead displacement
	Complete lead fracture
	Output failure due to complete battery depletion or component failure
	Oversensing
Oversensing (i.e. no pacing stimulus when appropriate, but pacing stimuli seen with fixed-rate pacing)	Inhibition of pacing due to inappropriate sensing of cardiac or non-cardiac electrical activity, with sensing of: • P wave or T wave by the ventricular lead • pectoral muscle or diaphragm contraction • electromagnetic interference (e.g. diathermy) • electrical noise created by partial lead fracture
Failure to capture (i.e. pacing stimulus present but not followed by P wave or QRS complex)	Poor connection between lead and pulse generator (loose set screw)
	Lead displacement
	Partial lead fracture or insulation break
	Myocardial perforation
	Inflammation or fibrosis at lead–myocardium interface
	Increase in pacing threshold due to effect of drugs (e.g. flecainide) or metabolic disorder (e.g. hyperkalaemia)
	Pacing stimulus delivered in ventricular refractory period because of undersensing
Undersensing (i.e. pacing stimulus seen when not appropriate)	Lead displacement
	Myocardial perforation
	Inflammation or fibrosis at lead–myocardium interface
	Low-amplitude P/R wave not sensed
	Sensing threshold too high

CHAPTER 121 **Cardiac device therapy**

Full interrogation of the pacemaker should be done as soon as possible. Application of a magnet over the pulse generator closes a reed switch and turns off the sensing function. This results in fixed-rate pacing, and so can be used to distinguish between output failure and oversensing as causes of inappropriate pacing. Abnormal or changed lead impedance may indicate lead failure. A break in the lead insulation results in a very low impedance, while a complete lead fracture results in a very high impedance. Reprogramming of the pacemaker may be able to address the cause of pacemaker malfunction (e.g. achieve a correct sensing threshold), or provide a temporary solution pending revision of the pacing system. f pacemaker malfunction is confirmed, and the patient is at risk of presyncope/syncope, temporary pacing should be instituted prior to definitive management.

Pacemaker syndrome is the occurrence of dizziness or exertional breathlessness due to loss of AV synchrony, when a single-chamber ventricular pacemaker is inserted in the presence of sinus rhythm, and is treated by upgrading the system to dual-chamber pacing.

Twiddler's syndrome is caused by the (usually subconscious) manipulation of the pulse generator in its subcutaneous pocket, with twisting or coiling of the leads, resultant lead displacement or fracture, and pacemaker malfunction. This is managed by revision of the pacing system, with lead repositioning or replacement, suturing of the pulse generator to subjacent tissues, or placement of the generator in a submuscular pocket, together with counselling of the patient.

In a patient with a dual-chamber pacemaker, and intact retrograde conduction through the AV node, a ventricular extrasystole may result in atrial depolarization, which is sensed by the atrial lead and triggers ventricular pacing, initiating a self-sustaining re-entry circuit. The result is a regular broad-complex tachycardia, at the upper tracking rate of the pacemaker. Application of a magnet disables sensing by the pacemaker and terminates this arrhythmia (pacemaker-mediated tachycardia). Current pacemakers have algorithms to prevent this occurring.

Impact of PPMs on life expectancy and quality of life

In some patients (e.g. those with third-degree (complete) heart block), death is prevented by the insertion of a PPM. In others (e.g. those with tachy brady syndrome), the indication for PPM insertion is mainly to deal with symptoms and improve quality of life.

ICDs

Background information for ICDs

An ICD is designed to directly treat ventricular tachyarrhythmias. If the device senses a ventricular rate that exceeds the programmed threshold, the device may observe with no action, perform anti-tachycardia pacing, deliver a low-energy, synchronized shock, or deliver a high-energy unsynchronized shock (defibrillation). With anti-tachycardia pacing, the device fires a preset number of rapid pulses in succession, in an attempt to terminate the ventricular arrhythmia. This is usually painless. If unsuccessful or if the rate falls above the preprogrammed cut-off rate, the device will perform a cardioversion/defibrillation. Transvenous ICDs (TV-ICDs) are also equipped with a demand pacing system and so can act as a pacemaker as well. Subcutaneous ICDs (S-ICDs) can currently effectively only provide defibrillation, but do not have a lead in the venous system, avoiding all of the associated complications.

How ICDs work

The main difference between a pacemaker and a TV-ICD in terms of components is the presence of a capacitor in the latter. This is needed to store charge before delivering defibrillation and can be used on a chest radiograph as one of the means of distinguishing an ICD from a pacemaker (the others being that fact that ICDs are normally larger than pacemakers and that the ICD lead in the ventricle has one or more coils on it to deliver energy to the tissue). The S-ICD generator sits under the left arm near the mid-axillary line, with the lead running subcutaneously to the xiphisternum and up along the sternum towards the manubrium.

The pacemaker function and coding in a TV-ICD is the same as in a standard pacemaker. The tachycardia therapy delivered by the TV-ICD can be programmed in a variety of ways. Normally, one or more 'zones' are defined. For a defined range of ventricular rates, the ICD is programmed to behave in one of three ways: (1) do nothing and record the rhythm (a monitor zone); (2) deliver anti-tachycardia pacing; or (3) deliver a shock (possibly having delivered anti-tachycardia pacing already). The way in which the device is programmed depends upon a number of factors, including the original reason for the implant, whether or not ventricular tachycardia (VT) or VF has been seen before, and the age of the patient. The S-ICD has simpler programming as it only provides defibrillation.

Indications for an ICD

ICDs were first used for secondary prevention in patients who had had life-threatening ventricular arrhythmias and were survivors of cardiac arrest. Recent trials have shown that for selected patients, ICDs are beneficial for the primary prevention of sudden cardiac death as well. Trials have demonstrated that, in post-MI patients with reduced ejection fraction primary prevention with ICD over conventional medical therapy saved lives. Further studies have shown that primary prevention using ICDs in other patient groups (e.g. hypertrophic cardiomyopathy with high-risk features) is also beneficial.

In the case of post-MI patients, no mortality benefit was observed from placing ICDs in those with reduced ejection fraction until after 40 days post-MI, probably because death in this early period is more likely to be due to non-arrhythmic causes.

International guidelines exist regarding the indications for ICDs, but in different countries this may be determined by local policies/economic constraints; however, broadly speaking, the indications include the following:

- survival of cardiac arrest due to VF or haemodynamically unstable sustained VT, after evaluation to define the cause of the event and to exclude any completely reversible causes
- structural heart disease and spontaneous sustained VT (stable or unstable)
- syncope of undetermined origin with clinically relevant, haemodynamically significant sustained VT or VF induced at electrophysiological study
- left ventricular ejection fraction (LVEF) <35% due to prior MI, in patients who are at least 40 days post-MI and who are in New York Heart Association (NYHA) Functional Classes I–III
- non-ischaemic dilated cardiomyopathy with LVEF ≤35%, in NYHA Functional Class I–III patients
- non-sustained VT due to prior MI, LVEF < 40%, and inducible VF or sustained VT at electrophysiological study
- hypertrophic cardiomyopathy in patients who have a greater than 1% per annum risk for sudden cardiac death as assessed by the European Society for Cardiology risk calculator or similar risk scores
- specific individuals with inherited cardiac conditions such as long-QT syndrome or Brugada syndrome, who have an increased risk of sudden cardiac death

How to implant ICDs

Implantation of a TV-ICD is similar to that of a pacemaker. The main differences are as follows: first, a larger pocket is normally required for an ICD than for a pacemaker, as an ICD is larger than a pacemaker; second, because patients requiring ICDs will often have structurally abnormal hearts (e.g. scarring in the right ventricle, in a patient with arrhythmogenic right ventricular cardiomyopathy), placing the leads in positions with optimal pacing and sensing parameters may be more difficult for an ICD than for a pacemaker; and third, unlike the case with pacemaker implantation, after implanting the ICD, it is sometimes necessary to test its detection and treatment of VF by inducing VF and letting the ICD treat it. However, this test is being performed much less frequently, particularly with primary prevention devices, as ICDs have become very reliable, and the VF induction does carry a small risk of death.

An S-ICD is normally implanted under general anaesthetic and in a very different position to that for the TV-ICD. The generator is inserted into a pocket between serratus anterior and latissimus dorsi on the left and the defibrillator lead is tunnelled from there to the midline at the xiphisternum and up along the sternal edge towards the head. Currently, it is necessary to always induce VF and test these devices.

Complications of ICDs

All of the complications that occur with pacemakers can also occur with TV-ICDs. In addition, because the hearts that these devices are implanted into often have structural abnormalities, it is more common to see problems with sensing and pacing (not only at implantation, as previously mentioned, but also later on). An S-ICD does not carry any of the risks that are associated with vascular access though.

The generators still remain larger for ICDs than for pacemakers, so erosion is slightly more common.

Inappropriate shocks, and shocks while the patient is conscious, are ICD-specific problems. If the ICD detects tachycardia that fulfils all programmed parameters requiring treatment with a shock, then it will deliver that therapy. The most common inappropriate shock comes from atrial fibrillation with a raid ventricular response, as this condition is incorrectly detected and treated as either VT or VF by the ICD. There are a number of algorithms on ICDs that can be used to try and minimize this problem but none are completely fail-safe.

The ICD also cannot determine if the patient is conscious. Therefore, if an arrhythmia which the ICD deems should be treated with a shock occurs when the patient is conscious, then the patient will receive a shock while still conscious. Most patients describe this experience as being very painful, and receiving such shocks can cause significant psychological disturbance.

Failure of an ICD to deliver an appropriate shock may be caused by similar problems to a pacemaker if the sensing is incorrect (see Table 121.1). This could be caused by lead fracture, electromagnetic interference, or inadvertent ICD deactivation. Management includes external defibrillation, and antiarrhythmic medications. Ineffective cardioversion may result from an inadequate energy output from the device. This is much less common with modern devices, which produce higher energy shocks than older devices do. A rise in the defibrillation threshold may occur for a variety of reasons, including:

- the use of antiarrhythmic medications such as amiodarone, flecainide, or phenytoin
- infarction of the subjacent myocardium
- fracture of the lead insulation
- scarring at the lead implantation site
- lead displacement.

Many ICDs deliver a programmed set of therapies per arrhythmic episode, and the number of therapies per episode is program specific. If a delivered therapy does not terminate the arrhythmia, the device proceeds to the next programmed therapy. For example, say that a total of six attempts at defibrillation are attempted per episode of VF. The device attempts defibrillation with the first programmed therapy and then re-evaluates the cardiac rhythm. If the arrhythmia persists, the device will deliver the second programmed therapy, and so on, until all six attempts have been delivered. Once the final attempt has been delivered, the device will not deliver any further therapy until a new episode is recognized. Therefore, theoretically, the therapies may be exhausted before the arrhythmia is terminated. As a result, ICDs do not prevent all sudden deaths, and it is important to understand that cardiac arrest in a patient with an ICD is not necessarily a sign that the ICD malfunctioned: the device may have properly delivered the required shocks for the triggering rhythm but the shocks themselves may have been ineffective in resolving the arrhythmia. This highlights the very important point that the use of an ICD is not a guarantee that a patient will not die from VT/VF.

Impact of ICDs on life expectancy and quality of life

The main reason for implanting an ICD is to increase life expectancy. This may be for primary prevention or for secondary prevention (see 'Indications for an ICD'). Where there is also a pacing indication, or when a combined CRT defibrillator is implanted (see 'CRT devices'), there may be improvement in quality of life. However, many patients

will not see any change in quality of life at all and, owing to the risk of inappropriate or conscious shocks, quality of life may actually be reduced for some patients. End-of-life management is an increasingly important aspect of ICD patient care. Decisions need to be made around the time of a patient's end of life about what to do with the ICD programming to allow a dignified and comfortable death.

CRT devices

Background information for CRT devices

Heart failure is a complex condition caused by structural or functional cardiac disorders which impair the heart's ability to function efficiently as a pump to support physiological circulation. In a healthy heart, the ventricles contract synchronously (i.e. the walls contract almost simultaneously). In some people with heart failure caused by left ventricular (LV) systolic dysfunction, the left ventricle contracts dyssynchronously, either because of dyssynchrony within the ventricle itself (intraventricular dyssynchrony), or because of dyssynchrony with the right ventricle (interventricular dyssynchrony). If the contractions lack synchrony, the heart becomes less efficient as a pump. People with heart failure, who have a reduced LVEF, and, on an ECG have characteristic changes due to abnormal electrical conductivity (normally LBBB, with a QRS duration >150 ms) can be considered for CRT. Echocardiographic assessment, which measures aspects of mechanical dyssynchrony, can also be used to identify patients whose condition is likely to respond to CRT, although it has not proven to be very reliable or reproducible.

How CRT devices work

A conventional pacemaker may have either one or two leads normally. A dual-chamber pacemaker maintains AV synchrony. In contrast, a CRT device aims to restore ventricular synchrony. To do this, it is necessary to pace the left ventricle at two distinctly different sites, generally with the aim of forcing the two walls of the ventricle to actually contract almost simultaneously. The most common way to do this is to first implant a right ventricular lead (and an atrial lead if the patient is in sinus rhythm) in the standard way. This effectively paces the septal wall of the left ventricle. A lead is then implanted on the lateral wall of the left ventricle; when connected to the CRT generator, this can then force contraction of both walls to occur with minimal delay. An ICD component can also be added simply by using a right ventricular ICD lead and a CRT defibrillator generator (CRT-D) instead of a standard CRT pacemaker (CRT-P).

Indications for CRT devices

As with ICD implantation, national and international guidelines vary slightly on the indications for CRT. However, there is broad agreement that, in patients with a diagnosis of heart failure associated with LV systolic dysfunction (symptomatic heart failure at NYHA Functional Classes II–IV and an LVEF >35%), the use of CRT is based primarily on a diagnosis of electrical dyssynchrony, indicated by a widened QRS complex of more than 150 ms on a standard ECG (normally, an LBBB pattern). The confirmation of the presence of mechanical dyssynchrony by echocardiography may be used in patients with electrical dyssynchrony indicated by bundle branch block and a shorter QRS duration (between 120 and 149 ms) but has not been shown to be very useful outside of clinical research. This approach was the same as that provided by the inclusion criteria for the CARE-HF trial, one of the first multicentre studies looking at CRT implantation. Since then, numerous studies have reported a variety of criteria to apply; however, ultimately, the most consensus guidance is that response to CRT is best predicted simply by the LVEF and the QRS duration at implant. Increasing evidence suggests that both patients in sinus rhythm and those in atrial fibrillation benefit from CRT; however, in the latter group, it may be necessary to ablate the AV node to ensure biventricular pacing occurs most of the time. More recent trial data suggest that patients with less severe symptoms of heart failure but severe LV dysfunction and dyssynchrony may also benefit from CRT in terms of mortality and morbidity; however, only some of the guidelines have changed to recognize these findings. It is important to note that many of these patients do not need a pacemaker for conventional bradycardia indications. The decision as to whether to implant a CRT-P or a CRT-D is normally based on whether or not the patient fulfils criteria for both, or just one. In some patients, when an indication for a pacemaker exists but LV function is known to be impaired, then use of a CRT device should be considered, in order to reduce the risk of progressive LV deterioration.

How to implant CRT devices

The implantation of the right atrial and right ventricular leads of a CRT is exactly the same as for a standard pacemaker or ICD. The LV lead is most commonly implanted via the coronary sinus (CS). This is accessed in exactly the same way as the right atrial and the right ventricular leads: via the subclavian vein. The CS os is posterior to the tricuspid valve in the right atrium and allows venous blood from the heart to drain into the right atrium. By entering the CS, a lead can then be passed retrogradely though it and into lateral branches that run along the lateral margin of the left ventricle (i.e. pacing the lateral wall of the left ventricle epicardially). The anatomy of the CS is somewhat variable. This, along with the presence of scarring in the left ventricle, may make implantation difficult or even impossible. Furthermore, the proximity of the left phrenic nerve means that electrical stimulation in this region may cause diaphragmatic twitching, thus rendering the device useless. If it proves impossible to implant the LV lead via the CS, then the lead may be implanted surgically on the epicardial surface, or endocardially using a different approach through the interventricular septum or a direct ventricular puncture. Modern technology, such as multipolar pacing leads, has meant that a number of the challenges that would have made CRT impossible in some patients in the past have now been addressed. Once all of the leads are in place, they are connected to a CRT generator and implanted into a pocket, as with a pacemaker or TV-ICD.

Complications of CRT devices

With CRT, the same complications at implantation are seen as with any pacemaker or TV-ICD implant. In addition, there is a small risk of damage to the CS but this rarely results in a serious complication, although it may mean that the LV lead cannot be inserted. In fact, implant failure related to the placement of the LV lead, together with post-operative lead dislodgement, are the most common problems seen in CRT.

The response to CRT is variable. Estimates of the proportion of patients who have a CRT device implanted successfully but do not experience an improvement in their condition range from approximately 10% to 50%. In some patients, non-response may be due to loss of biventricular stimulation, because of atrial arrhythmias or frequent ventricular extrasystoles, and suppression of these arrhythmias may be beneficial. Recognition of who will and will not respond remains a challenge and there is no difference between CRT-D and CRT-P devices with respect to the number of patients whose condition does not improve. However, the response rate is improving, due to ongoing research, particularly in the field of advanced cardiac imaging.

Impact of CRT devices on life expectancy and quality of life

CRT, via either a pacemaker device or a pacemaker–defibrillator device, improves life expectancy and the quality of life in patients who have heart failure due to LV) systolic dysfunction in NYHA Functional Classes II, III, and IV and who are in sinus rhythm with a broad QRS complex (>130 ms). For example, in the COMPANION study, all-cause mortality was reduced by 24% during a mean follow-up period of 16 months and, in the CARE-HF study, it was reduced by 36% over 29 months. On average, CRT results in an increase in functional capacity by one NYHA class, and reduces hospitalizations for heart failure.

Current European Society of Cardiology guidelines recommend CRT (Class I indication) for symptomatic patients with heart failure in sinus rhythm with a QRS duration >130 ms, and LBBB morphology, and a LVEF <35% despite optimum medical therapy; CRT should be considered (Class IIa) for those with QRS duration >150 ms and non-LBBB morphology.

Most patients for whom CRT is indicated also qualify for an ICD. However, the additional benefit of CRT-D over CRT-P is uncertain, and CRT-D is more expensive. Determining which device will be better for the individual patient is the subject of current research.

CRT can result in reverse remodelling, with reductions in LV volumes and functional mitral regurgitation, and improvement in LVEFs. While the occurrence of reverse remodelling is associated with a favourable effect on prognosis, symptomatic benefit from CRT can be seen in patients who do not demonstrate it.

Other device-related issues

Magnet inhibition

For most PPMs, placing a specific type of magnet over the device does not turn it off but instead temporarily 'reprograms' it into an asynchronous mode. Each pacemaker type has unique asynchronous rates (specific to the device's manufacturer and model) which indicate battery status: BOL (for **b**eginning **o**f **l**ife), ERI (for **e**lective **r**eplacement **i**ndicator), and EOL (for **e**nd **o**f **l**ife). Therefore, if the device parameters are known, a magnet can be used to determine whether the PPM's battery should be replaced. Further interrogation or manipulation of the device should only be performed by an individual competent to do so. A magnet can also be used to temporarily treat oversensing with a PPM.

When a magnet is applied to an ICD, it can temporarily turn off defibrillation and anti-tachycardia pacing therapy without altering the ICD's pacing ability. However, some devices can be programmed to not respond to magnet application and thus will need a device programmer to change the parameters. Indications for ICD deactivation are as follows:

- end-of-life care (after a discussion with the patient and family)
- inappropriate shocks
- during resuscitation
- during transcutaneous pacing (external pacing can cause an ICD to fire)
- during surgical procedures involving electrocautery

Resuscitation

If a patient enters a life-threatening cardiac arrhythmia, Advanced Life Support protocols should be initiated immediately. Although an ICD will attempt defibrillation, chest compressions should be continued. Note that some of the current may enter the rescuer; however, there has never been a reported case of rescuer injury from this, other than mild discomfort. VT and VF refractory to ICD defibrillation will require external defibrillation and/or antiarrhythmic medications, as dictated by Advanced Cardiac Life Support/Advanced Life Support protocols. If external defibrillation is required in a patient with a device, whether a pacemaker, an ICD, or a CRT, placing the electrode pads at least 10–15 cm away, and out of the shockwave reduces the risk of causing device failure. However, it is not appropriate to withhold therapy for fear of damaging the device in this emergency setting.

If rescuers are uncomfortable with ICD discharge during resuscitations, it is appropriate to deactivate the ICD with a magnet; the magnet can be removed to allow the ICD to again treat VF/VT if desired.

Central venous catheter placement

Pacemaker or ICD leads placed in the venous system often lead to surrounding thrombosis, with 20% of patients having complete occlusion at 2 years. This can make subsequent venous access difficult. Furthermore, during central line placement, if the metal guidewire contacts the lead system, there may be sufficient artefacts to trigger an inappropriate shock or inhibit pacing. Therefore, when placing central venous catheters either avoid the use of a metal guidewire or reprogram the device accordingly. Although the contralateral subclavian or internal jugular vein can be cannulated with care, femoral vein access is a much safer option in this circumstance.

**Issues related to driving in patients
with cardiac devices**

In the UK, for driving advice for patients with cardiac devices, specifically refer to the DVLA guidelines on fitness to drive. For a standard driving licence (Group 1) in the UK, in general, any device procedure is associated legally with at least 1 week of driving restriction. With ICDs (TV-ICDs, S-ICDs, or CRT-Ds), a primary prevention implant carries a 1-month restriction, and a secondary prevention implant carries a 6-month restriction. If the patient receives an appropriate shock from an ICD, driving may be restricted for up to 2 years after the event, although, in many cases, the patient will be permitted to drive after 6 months. The restrictions on professional driving licences (Group 2) are much stricter: an ICD implant results in an immediate and permanent ban.

Further Reading

The Task Force on cardiac pacing and resynchronization therapy of the European Society of Cardiology (ESC). 2013 ESC Guidelines on cardiac pacing and cardiac resynchronization therapy. *Eur Heart J* 2013; 34: 2281–329.

National Institute for Health and Care Excellence (NICE). Implantable cardioverter defibrillators and cardiac resynchronisation therapy for arrhythmias and heart failure. Technology appraisal guidance [TA314] 2014. Available at: https://www.nice.org.uk/guidance/ta314

Report of a joint Working Party project on behalf of the British Society for Antimicrobial Chemotherapy (BSAC, host organization), British Heart Rhythm Society (BHRS), British Cardiovascular Society (BCS), British Heart Valve Society (BHVS) and British Society for Echocardiography (BSE). Guidelines for the diagnosis, prevention and management of implantable cardiac electronic device infection. *J Antimicrob Chemother* 2015; 70: 325–59.

122 Drug-induced cardiovascular disease

Yoon Loke

Introduction

Many drugs can cause or exacerbate cardiovascular disease, and clinicians should be vigilant when prescribing potentially cardiotoxic medication to patients at risk, so that preventive measures and close monitoring can be implemented. Conversely, the possibility of drug-related disease should always be considered in patients with cardiovascular symptoms, so that culprit drugs can be identified and alternative therapies considered.

Congestive cardiac failure/oedema

Drugs can typically cause or worsen cardiac failure, either through a direct negative effect on the myocardium or by causing fluid retention via the renal–endocrine axis. Myocardial damage is a particular problem with cancer chemotherapy. Anthracyclines such as doxorubicin have a cumulative, dose-related toxic effect leading to cardiomyopathy and congestive cardiac failure which persists in the long term. Treatment with trastuzumab, a monoclonal antibody against the human epidermal growth factor receptor-2 (HER-2) in breast carcinoma can cause a decline in left ventricular function, and heart failure that may be reversible on cessation of therapy. Echocardiographic monitoring for left ventricular dysfunction is recommended for all patients receiving trastuzumab. Protein kinase inhibitors (such as imatinib and sunitinib) used in the treatment of malignant disease have also been reported to cause oedema and congestive cardiac failure.

While negatively inotropic drugs such as beta blockers and calcium-channel blockers (e.g. verapamil) are not directly toxic to the myocardium, they can lead to symptomatic deterioration in those with preexisting left ventricular dysfunction. Low doses should be used initially, with gradual upward titration as needed.

Some drugs can precipitate cardiac failure and symptomatic oedema in susceptible patients by causing fluid retention. This can be mediated by a negative effect on renal function (e.g. by NSAIDs) or through mineralocorticoid properties (e.g. via high doses of corticosteroids). Other drugs such as the thiazolidinediones (rosiglitazone, pioglitazone) appear to cause cardiac failure and peripheral oedema through increased intravascular volume via an unknown mechanism.

Ischaemic heart disease

Drugs can increase the risk of myocardial ischemia through coronary artery constriction, through prothrombotic effects on blood components, or by increasing cardiac workload and oxygen requirements. The fluoropyrimidines (fluorouracil, capecitabine) have been associated with ischaemic electrocardiographic findings in patients being treated for cancer. The triptans (such as sumatriptan), which are serotonin-receptor (5-HT-1B/1D) agonists used in the acute treatment of migraine, appear to have a marked vasoconstrictive effect due to stimulation of the serotonin receptors in the smooth muscle of the coronary arteries, thus leading to ischaemic symptoms.

Prothrombotic drugs include some selective cyclooxygenase-2 (COX-2) inhibitors (such as rofecoxib) which may have deleterious effects on platelet and endothelial function; these effects are mediated through decreased vasodilatory prostaglandins in the face of continued production of thromboxane. While cardiovascular toxicity may be a common threat amongst conventional and COX-2-selective NSAIDs, the magnitude of risk may vary depending on agent (e.g. diclofenac is thought to carry high risk, while naproxen is thought to carry less risk).

Erythropoetin-stimulating agents (such as epoetin, darbepoetin) have been associated with myocardial infarction, particularly with higher target haemoglobin levels in cancer patients and those with chronic kidney disease. This prothrombotic risk may arise from a more rapid or greater overall increase in haemoglobin, or through a dose-dependent drug toxic effect that has yet to be clarified.

Drugs that increase the cardiac workload and the myocardial oxygen requirement may precipitate ischaemia, especially in those with preexisting atherosclerosis. Short-acting calcium-channel blockers such as nifedipine are associated with myocardial infarction in those with coronary disease, possibly through vasodilation causing reflex tachycardia. Sympathomimetic drugs such as amphetamines, ephedrine, and cocaine have also been associated with myocardial infarction in younger patients. Historically, excessive use of short-acting beta-2 agonists in asthma has been linked to increased cardiovascular mortality, although there is no definite evidence of risk with newer bronchodilators.

Cardiac arrhythmias

By nature of their widespread effect on cardiac conduction, antiarrhythmic drugs themselves are major culprits in the genesis of many forms of cardiac arrhythmias. Digoxin, for instance, can induce both bradyarrhythmias and tachyarrhythmias. In patients who have known heart disease and who present with arrhythmia, the search for a culprit should start with the patient's list of medications, as a variety of factors (such as drug interactions and electrolyte disturbances) can tip the balance over from beneficial cardiac drug to dangerous arrhythmogenic agent. Toxicity from antidepressants and antipsychotics can also cause a diverse range of arrhythmias.

Bradyarrhythmias

Bradycardias commonly arise from drugs that block sympathetic activity or the atrioventricular (AV) node. Beta blockers are widely used in the community and are common associated with dose-dependent bradycardia, as are AV nodal blocking agents such as verapamil and digoxin. Amiodarone, sotalol, and flecainide are the other antiarrhythmic drugs which are highly likely to lead to bradycardias. This risk of bradycardia is heightened by the common practice of prescribing two agents to obtain satisfactory control of atrial fibrillation.

Tachyarrhythmias

Ventricular arrhythmias are a particular concern in patients receiving antiarrhythmic drugs, with agents such as flecainide now being restricted to patients who do not have underlying ischaemic or structural heart disease. However, the discovery of a relationship between the drug quinidine and QT interval prolongation and polymorphic tachycardia (torsades des points) has led to the realization that many other drugs, both cardiac and non-cardiac, are linked to tachyarrhythmia (see Table 122.1). While the incidence of torsades is very much lower with non-cardiac drugs, many of the implicated agents are widely used in the community, thus contributing to a potentially large burden of exposure in the population.

The underlying mechanism behind torsades appears to stem from blockade in transmission of a particular potassium current which is involved in myocardial repolarization and which known as the rapid component of the delayed rectifier, IKr. Drugs that block IKr can increase the duration of the action potential, manifesting in QT prolongation. However, QT prolongation itself has limited predictive value for torsades, as many patients have QT prolongation without serious harm, while some have dangerous arrhythmias despite minimal changes in their QT interval. Other mediating factors

Table 122.1 Drugs that are likely to be associated with prolongation of the QT interval

Clinical application	Class	Specific drug
Antiarrhythmic	Ia	Disopyramide
		Procainamide
		Quinidine
	III	Amiodarone
		Sotalol
		Dofetilide/ibutilide
Antibiotic	Macrolide	Erythromycin
		Clarithromycin
	Fluroquinolone	Sparfloxacin
Antimicrobial	Antimalarial aminoquinolone	Chloroquine
	Antimalarial phenanthrene-methanol	Halofantrine
	Antiprotozoal aromatic diamine	Pentamidine
Antihistamine	Second-generation H1-receptor blockers	Astemizole
		Terfenadine
Antipyschotic	Phenothiazine	Chlorpromazine
		Thioridazine
	Butyrophenones	Haloperidol
	Diphenylbutylpiperidines	Pimozide
Gastrointestinal	Prokinetic	Cisapride
	Dopamine antagonist	Domperidone
		Droperidol
Analgesic	Opioid agonist	Methadone

include hypokalaemia, drug interactions leading to toxic levels (usually through CYP3A4), genetic susceptibility, and the presence of structural heart disease. Indeed, while there is a long list of medications that are implicated in QT prolongation (see Table 122.1), only a relatively small proportion of patients experience serious harm. Preventive measures should focus on correction of electrolyte abnormalities, avoidance of polypharmacy with other drugs that can affect the QT interval or the p450 metabolic pathways, and optimization of the patient's cardiac condition.

Hypertension

Drug-induced elevation in blood pressure can stem from increased sympathetic activity or from interference with the renal–endocrine regulatory axis. Hypertension can occur with sympathomimetic agents such as the amphetamines and ephedrine. Similarly, serotonin–noradrenaline reuptake inhibitors (such as venlafaxine) used in treating depression can cause a dose-related rise of blood pressure by increasing sympathomimetic amines. Sibutramine, an obesity drug which blocks reuptake of serotonin, noradrenaline, and dopamine, is associated with clinically relevant elevation of blood pressure, and

the drug had to be withdrawn from the market after excess cardiovascular risk was detected in a large trial.

Inhibition of protective prostaglandins in the renal and endothelial systems can cause blood pressure elevation in patients exposed to NSAIDs, with a potential relationship to the increased risk of oedema and myocardial infarction discussed elsewhere in this chapter. The increase in blood pressure appears to be more prominent with agents such as rofecoxib, and affects susceptible patients with preexisting hypertension.

Valvular heart disease

Both regurgitant and stenotic lesions can arise as a complication of drug therapy. The implicated drugs are thought to have some effect on 5-HT-2B serotonin receptors or serotonin transporters in heart valves, thereby having an impact on fibroblast proliferation. In the past, drugs used in the treatment of migraine (ergotamine, methysergide) were the most prominent culprits, but these agents are seldom prescribed nowadays. Appetite suppressants (dexfenfluramine and fenfluramine, used alone or in combination with phentermine) were then linked with valvular heart disease, leading subsequently to the withdrawal of dexfenfluramine from the market. However, the threat of valvular complications from the fenfluramines has not been completely eliminated as a multitude of illicit slimming remedies containing fenfluramine and phentermine can be obtained from unlicensed sources. Pulmonary hypertension has also been reported with these drugs, which may arise as a direct toxic effect, or secondary to valvular disease.

Valvular heart disease has recently been noted in patients receiving pergolide and cabergoline, which are ergot-related dopamine agonists used in the treatment of Parkinson's disease. Based on their structural similarity to ergotamine, it is thought that these drugs have an agonist effect at the 5-HT-2B receptor, thus triggering valvular pathology. Patients should have cardiac assessments and echocardiography prior to treatment initiation, and will need regular monitoring clinically and with echocardiography while they remain on these agents (pergolide has been withdrawn in the United States, but is still available elsewhere). It is not yet clear if valvular lesions regress fully after treatment cessation.

Further Reading

Andrejak M and Tribouilloy C. Drug-induced valvular heart disease: An update. *Arch Cardiovasc Dis* 2013; 106: 333–9.

Heist EK and Ruskin JN. Drug-induced arrhythmia. *Circulation* 2010; 122: 1426–35.

Isbister GK and Page CB. Drug-induced QT prolongation: The measurement and assessment of the QT interval in clinical practice. *Br J Clin Pharmacol* 2013; 76: 48–57.

Varga ZV, Ferdinandy P, Liaudet L, and Pacher P. Drug-induced mitochondrial dysfunction and cardiotoxicity. *Am J Physiol Heart Circ Physiol* 2015; 309: H1453–H1467.

2016 ESC Position Paper on cancer treatments and cardiovascular toxicity developed under the auspices of the ESC Committee for Practice Guidelines: The Task Force for cancer treatments and cardiovascular toxicity of the European Society of Cardiology (ESC). *Eur Heart J* 2016; 37: 2768–801.

123 Psychological management of coronary heart disease

Rhiain Morris

Risk factors associated with coronary heart disease outcomes

Both anxiety and depression have been found to increase the risk of developing coronary heart disease (CHD) and lead to exacerbation of cardiac symptoms, with the latter subsequently impacting recovery/rehabilitation (e.g. leading to an increased number of readmissions to hospital, and an increased mortality risk following myocardial infarction (MI)). This may be due to pathophysiologic effects, such as vascular inflammation and autonomic dysfunction, and poor lifestyle/behavioural patterns, including non-attendance at cardiac rehabilitation classes and/or poor treatment adherence. Psychosocial factors such as stress, hostility, social isolation, socio-economic status, and psychological defensiveness can also affect the course of cardiac illness.

Psychological responses to MI

Depression is commonly associated with CHD but anxiety is often the first psychological response in the acute phase of MI, with the anxiety level bearing little relation to the severity of the infarct. Therefore, depression may initially mask anxiety. A study found that 31% of MI patients had elevated depression scores while in hospital, increasing to 38% at 4 months, and 37% at the 12-month follow-up. Similarly, prevalence for depression immediately following MI was 20%, with another 21% becoming depressed over the following year. A high anxiety rate has also been reported, with 26% of MI patients showing elevated anxiety in hospital, increasing to 42% after 4 months, and 40% at 1 year post MI. Women have also been found to be more anxious than men.

Following the cardiac event, some patients find the transition from a healthy self-perception to confronting their own mortality/fragility very stressful. Studies demonstrate that there are parallels between this transition and loss and bereavement: following an MI, patients often experience denial, anger, guilt, depression, and loneliness before acceptance. Indeed, individuals can also suffer loss of functioning, status, role, and identity. Psychological interventions can help this process considerably.

Associations between psychological distress and cardiac outcomes have therapeutic implications, highlighting the need for routine screening at regular intervals, ensuring early detection of psychosocial difficulties and appropriate service referral. Two standardized screening tools, the Hospital Anxiety and Depression Scale, and the Beck Depression Inventory, can be used at all stages in the care of cardiac patients.

Using a psychological approach in acute settings

During the acute phase of treatment, the volume of clinical interventions undertaken may hinder patient engagement in psychological treatment and the amount of information processing that is required. Uncertainty regarding future health may also further impede acceptance. However, interventions can be adapted to take such limitations into account. The majority of patients will not request or need focused psychological intervention during or following hospital stays, only time to adjust.

Recommendations, beneficial to all patients, exist; they outline the most helpful aspects of care at the acute stage of CHD and are defined by 'communication-based care', encouraging staff to develop positive/friendly relationships with patients by displaying empathy and warmth and by using active listening.

There are two basic areas of focus:

- informational care:
  - exploration of what the patient knows and wishes to know
  - memory facilitation through language, diagrams, and information aids
  - checking the patient's understanding of imparted information
- emotional care:
  - allowing the expression of emotional distress to help patients come to terms with their illness
  - facilitating safe feelings
  - share emotional responses

The enhancement of 'control and personal responsibility' is important in rehabilitation. In order for patients to feel involved in their treatment and empowered, an attitude of collaboration and respect needs to be conveyed, whereby staff work 'with' the patient, rather than doing treatment 'to' the patient.

As most of this care is delivered by nursing staff, it highlights the need for skills in both the identification of psychological distress and use of basic strategies to help the patient cope (e.g. stress management). This is particularly important during the transition from hospital to home, when psycho-educational input can help the patient and their family prepare.

Psychological and psychosocial interventions for CHD

The efficacy of psychological interventions in cardiac rehabilitation has been assessed in relation to a variety of outcome criteria, making any comparison between studies complicated. Nevertheless, the main studies are summarized in this section.

Cardiac rehabilitation, which incorporates psychosocial methods of intervention, has been demonstrated to reduce mortality. The main studies include an investigation of lifestyle changes and CHD; the Recurrent Coronary Prevention Project; the Ischemic Heart Disease Life Stress Monitoring Program; and the M-HART Study Group. These and consequent studies show psychosocial intervention is directly linked to reducing mortality and further cardiac events.

An initial study in 1983 investigated the effects of cardiac rehabilitation, utilizing a three-and-a-half-week rehabilitation program of diet, relaxation, and exercise in an attempt to reduce mortality in post-infarction participants, with good effect. Later studies such as the Recurrent Coronary Prevention Project looked at risk factors for Type A behaviour, yielding very positive results, even at a six-and-a-half-year follow-up, where participant mortality was greatly reduced. Most early psychosocial intervention studies predominantly targeted lifestyle and behavioural factors, whereas recent studies focus more on cognitive aspects (e.g. stress/anxiety management) relating to an increased risk of CHD.

As part of the Enhancing Recovery in Coronary Heart Disease Patients study, researchers investigated whether cognitive behavioural therapy (CBT) delivered in individual and/or group formats could reduce high mortality and recurrent infarction levels associated with depression and low perceived social support. Although intervention improved depression and low perceived social support, it did not increase event-free survival. However, the findings from this study have recently been reanalysed. This showed group **plus** individual therapy was associated with a 33% reduction in death or further infarction, compared to usual care or individual therapy alone.

In a review of nine psychological interventions conducted with patients after surgery for an implantable cardioverter defibrillator (ICD), researchers concluded that the most notable effects were reductions in anxiety, and improved exercise capacity. Although some studies found a decrease in depression and quality of life gains, this was a less robust finding. The review supports another study, which found that a brief cognitive-behavioural intervention for ICD patients improved quality of life, reduced incidences of anxiety/depression, and reduced the number of unplanned admissions at 6 months post surgery.

CBT has yet to be explored in relation to congestive heart failure (CHF) patients. However, research has demonstrated that basic relaxation skills can help reduce stress in CHF patients. More recently, there has been interest in the application of mindfulness-based cognitive therapy (MBCT) with CHD patients. Mindfulness encourages recipients to find distance from anxious/negative thinking and is an adjunct to cognitive techniques such as negative-thought identification. A review of an MBCT group for cardiac rehabilitation found favourable outcomes for awareness, acceptance, and within-group experiences. Lastly, CBT combined with antidepressants may be the most effective treatment for patients with cardiovascular disease and depression.

Psychology also has an important role in behaviour change. People are most likely to change when they believe they have the necessary resources to do so. Known as self-efficacy, this has important implications for cardiac rehabilitation. A problem-solving approach can be used to help individuals explore and resolve practical barriers to change. Furthermore, motivational interviewing, developed to help increase an individual's motivation to change, has relevance to many cardiac rehabilitation programmes, being widely used in populations requiring diet/exercise modification and, more recently, with CHF patients to improve self-care.

Overall, there is a paucity of research investigating the efficacy of psychological approaches with cardiac patients. Existing research has tended to focus on medical outcomes, rather than on the reduction of psychological distress per se. Although emerging evidence suggests CBT can be beneficial for cardiac patients suffering from anxiety and/or depression, a need exists for research to address the efficacy of a variety of psychological interventions in reducing psychological distress as a primary goal.

Benign cardiac symptoms

The characteristics of patients presenting with non-cardiac chest pain and benign palpitations have been investigated. This non-cardiac group is more likely than others to be made up of young women reporting other physical symptoms and previous psychiatric problems. At the 6-month follow-up, they continued to report limited activities, concern about the cause of their symptoms (despite reassurance), and dissatisfaction with medical care. Importantly, a common feature of health anxiety is to seek frequent medical reassurance, which serves to maintain the person's preoccupation with their health. Health anxiety also has overlapping features with panic disorder. In another study, patients with benign palpitations were more likely to be female, with a higher prevalence of panic disorder and fear of bodily sensations.

Subsequently, a brief nurse-led psycho-educational intervention (based on CBT principles) was conducted, aiming to reduce disability in patients with benign palpitations. Patients completing the intervention showed significant increases in activity levels at the 3-month follow-up. In general, though, limited research has been conducted to investigate the efficacy of psychological interventions with this patient group.

There is, however, an existing body of literature which can be drawn from and applied to cardiology. The current evidence base supports treatment of health anxiety and panic disorder with specific cognitive-behavioural techniques. Lastly, the role of cardiologists in addressing these problems has been highlighted. It is recommended that cardiologists routinely address psychological factors (particularly anxiety) relevant to the aetiology and management of palpitations and/or chest pain. Such timely identification and explanation may help patients to resolve their uncertainty regarding their symptoms and ultimately reduce anxiety.

Summary

Psychological issues linked to health problems are varied and can be experienced briefly or chronically. Patients differ greatly in their responses to medical conditions; many use their own existing coping styles successfully, but a significant proportion struggle to cope with accepting their condition. Psychological support from the cardiac event and beyond is therefore an important aspect of care with this patient group.

Further Reading

Chambers JB, Marks EM, and Hunter MS. The head says yes but the heart says no: what is non-cardiac chest pain and how is it managed? *Heart* 2015; 101: 1240–49.

Richards SH, Anderson L, Jenkinson CE, et al. Psychological interventions for coronary heart disease. *Cochrane Database Syst Rev* 2017; 4: CD002902.

124 Treatment of terminal cardiovascular disease

Dave Riley

Definition of the disease

This chapter is an introduction to the key components of the palliative treatment of terminal cardiovascular disease; more in-depth resources are listed in 'Further Reading' at the end of this chapter.

While definitions may vary, a person who may die within 6–12 months could be considered to be approaching the terminal stage of their illness, while those expected to die within a number of days or hours would be considered to be at the terminal stage. Either situation is a valid time to implement palliative treatment, but considering end-of-life care earlier provides opportunities that may otherwise be missed.

Aetiology of the disease

All serious cardiovascular disease can end with the patient dying, sometimes quickly, and sometimes, more distressingly, slowly. This is particularly so with heart failure, but can also be the case with profound coronary disease, extensive cerebrovascular disease, and peripheral vascular disease, and often these diseases interact with others, such as COPD, diabetes, and so on, all of which are made worse by increasing age, immobility, and possibly dementia.

Typical symptoms of the disease, and less common symptoms

The patient typically experiences a progressive worsening of exercise tolerance, culminating in symptoms at rest or on minimal exertion. This leads on to limited functional ability, with failing independence and interrupted sleep. A full palliative assessment incorporates a holistic approach to patient needs, including physical, social, and psychospiritual aspects.

Physical aspects include:

- breathlessness
- fatigue
- pain
- constipation
- nausea
- insomnia

Social aspects include:

- financial difficulties
- relationship difficulties
- personal care needs, including carers and equipment

Psychospiritual aspects include:

- anxiety
- depression
- fear
- existential distress, which may be religious, spiritual, or non-specific

Demographics of the disease

The incidence of heart failure has been estimated at 63 000 new cases annually in the UK. In 2001, just over 11 500 deaths due to heart failure were officially recorded in the UK.

However, the number of deaths attributed to heart failure in national mortality statistics is likely to be a huge underestimate.

Combining data on incidence and survival, the British Heart Foundation has estimated that, in 2001, the true number of deaths from heart failure in the UK was at least 24 000. This means at least 4% of all deaths in the UK are due to heart failure.

Natural history, and complications of the disease

The last several months of life are characterized by recurrent episodes of deterioration, either as a result of decompensated cardiac function or concomitant illnesses, and may lead to patients being admitted to the acute hospital setting more frequently. The last hours to days of life are characterized by a bed-bound patient with an altered level of consciousness, difficulty managing oral medication, and a poor oral intake. Sudden, relatively unpredicted death is also a risk.

Complications include:

- uncontrolled symptoms
- hospital admissions, with the associated burden of travelling, time away from home and family, investigations, and invasive treatment
- failing to die in the place of one's choosing
- ICD activation

Deteriorating renal function, low blood pressure, and hyponatraemia are common sequelae of poor cardiac output. However, quality of life takes precedent for those in the terminal stage; efforts to preserve renal function, blood pressure, and serum sodium levels may be at the expense of symptom control and quality of life.

Approach to diagnosing the disease

Recognizing a patient who is approaching the terminal stage can be challenging and uncertain; it should be a team-based decision. It requires a shift of mindset away from active treatments and to moving towards patient-centred care encompassing quality of life and the acceptance of the inevitability of death. This can be difficult for patients, family, friends, and healthcare professionals alike. The process of acceptance opens the way to preparing both patients and their loved ones for the impending death and helping patients with making an advance care plan.

The advance care plan should address:

- symptom control and comfort measures
- anticipatory prescribing of medication to manage exacerbations
- discontinuing inappropriate interventions
- needs for psychological and spiritual care
- care of the family (before and after the person's death)
- when, who, and how to call for help when there is a crisis or acute exacerbation, and what the options are for management

The plan should also include the person's preferences regarding:

- where they wish to be cared for at the end of life
- deactivation of an ICD
- documentation of a do not attempt resuscitation decision

Anticipatory prescribing for end-of-life medication is detailed in 'Treatment and its effectiveness'.

It is essential that the outcome of consultation be disseminated amongst each relevant member of the multidisciplinary team (e.g. GP, district nurse, out-of-hours GP service, ambulance service).

Other diagnoses that should be considered

Optimal management of cardiac failure must be ensured, including any reasons for poor concordance. That aside, a full assessment with a history and examination, plus investigations if appropriate, is required to identify any reversible cause of deterioration of symptoms. The differential diagnosis is large, but includes:

- suboptimal management or acute exacerbation of comorbidities, e.g.:
  - progressive renal impairment
  - anaemia
  - COPD
  - diabetes mellitus
- acute infection

'Gold-standard' diagnostic test and acceptable diagnostic alternatives to the gold standard

There is no tool or test available to accurately ascertain the terminal stage or the prognosis of patients with terminal cardiovascular disease. However, the Gold Standards Framework describes three triggers to aid in identifying the terminal stage:

- Would you be surprised if the patient were to die in the next 6–12 months?
- The patient makes a choice for comfort care only, not 'curative' care.
- Clinical indicators suggest advanced disease.

Other relevant investigations

Investigations should be driven first by the need (or indeed, necessity) to further define the underlying disease process (often no further investigations are needed) and, second, to clarify whether specific treatments designed to relieve symptoms have a role, for example, a chest X-ray may define how much of the symptoms are due to heart failure, and how much to pneumonia—this may be relevant if active treatment with antibiotics is appropriate, but clearly is not if such therapies are not under consideration. The underlying philosophy determining whether any investigations are appropriate is whether the results would lead to specific interventions that would improve the quality of death. If investigations will not lead to such an outcome, they should not be performed.

Prognosis and how to estimate it

Prognosis from heart failure is poor. Comparing 1-year survival rates for heart failure with those for a number of common cancers show that prognosis from heart failure is relatively poor. The 1-year survival rate for heart failure is worse than those for breast, prostate, or bladder cancer, better than those for lung or stomach cancer, and very similar to that for cancer of the colon.

Those patients with Stage III or IV heart failure and who have repeated hospital admissions and difficult-to-control physical or psychological symptoms are likely to die within 6–12 months.

Predicting prognosis becomes more accurate the nearer a person is to death.

Treatment and its effectiveness

Symptoms can be effectively managed in the majority of patients following an assessment of the cause, its impact on the patient, and the initiation of appropriate treatments. However, some symptoms cannot be resolved and supportive measures alone are required. If a patient has ongoing symptoms, intolerable side effects, or complex needs, the specialist palliative care team should be contacted for advice or review of a patient.

Anticipatory prescribing for end-of-life medication is given in Table 124.1. These are suggestions only; all prescribing must be on an individual patient basis.

Table 124.1 Anticipatory prescribing for end-of-life medication

Symptom	Drug	Dose	Route
Pain and breathlessness	Morphine	1.25–2.50 mg	Subcutaneous
Nausea	Haloperidol	500 µg–1.5 mg	Subcutaneous
Anxiety and agitation	Midazolam	2.5–5.0 mg	Subcutaneous
Respiratory secretions	Glycopyrronium	200–400 µg	Subcutaneous

Fatigue

Non-pharmacological management of fatigue includes:

- explanation and reassurance
- cardiac or palliative rehabilitation
- occupational therapist review re home adaptations, equipment, and mobility aids
- support and advice for carers, including a care package

The following is recommended for pharmacological management of fatigue:

- review medication which may contribute to fatigue and reduce, stop, or change to alternatives
- psychostimulant medication is not recommended

Dyspnoea

Non-pharmacological management of dyspnoea includes:

- explanation, reassurance
- cardiac or palliative rehabilitation
- occupational therapist review re home adaptations, equipment, and mobility aids
- use of a handheld fan
- psychological support
- complementary therapies
- support and advice for carers, including a care package

Recommendations for the pharmacological management of dyspnoea are as follows:

- nebulized saline 0.9% 5 ml, when necessary
- low-dose opiates: morphine sulfate solution 2.5 mg, 4 hourly
- lorazepam 0.5–1.0 mg sublingual when necessary (max 2 mg in 24 hours) for acute anxiety
- trial of oxygen via nasal cannulae

Pain

Non-pharmacological management of pain includes:

- explanation, and reassurance
- physiotherapy review
- occupational therapist review re home adaptations, equipment, and mobility aids
- complementary therapies

The following is recommended for the pharmacological management:

- the WHO Pain Relief Ladder (see Table 124.2)

Table 124.2 Pharmacological management

STEP 1	STEP 2	STEP 3
Regular Paracetamol 1g qds	Regular Paracetamol 1g qds	Regular Paracetamol 1g qds
(Avoid NSAIDs as they can cause fluid retention & worsening renal function)	Plus a weak opioid, e.g.: codeine 30mg–60mg qds	Plus a strong opioid, e.g.: Morphine 2.5–5mg qds & prn

Reprinted from WHO, WHO Pain Relief Ladder, Copyright (2009). http://www.who.int/cancer/palliative/painladder/en/.

- all patients started on an opioid need a laxative co-prescribing (e.g. sodium picosulfate 5–10 ml, at night)

Constipation

Non-pharmacological management of constipation includes the following:

- encourage fluid intake and review the diet
- optimize mobility
- optimize privacy for toileting

The following may be used for pharmacological management of constipation:

- stimulant laxative (e.g. sodium picosulfate 5–10 ml, at night)
- softener laxative (e.g. sodium docusate 200 mg, once or twice per day), if stool is hard

Nausea

Non-pharmacological management of nausea includes:

- eating small meals
- avoiding preparing food

Pharmacological management of nausea includes the following:

- review medication that may contribute to nausea and reduce, stop, or change to alternatives
- for a systemic cause, haloperidol 500 μg–1.5 mg, once per day and as necessary (up to 5 mg/day)
- for gastric stasis, metoclopramide 10 mg, three times per day and as necessary

Anxiety

Non-pharmacological management of anxiety includes:

- full exploration of underlying cause and perpetuating factors
- explanation and reassurance to family and carers
- appropriate psychospiritual support; refer to specialists if needed

The following may be used for pharmacological management of anxiety:

- diazepam 2 mg as necessary, up to a maximum of three times per day
- lorazepam 500 μg–1.0 mg sublingual, for acute anxiety

Depression

Non-pharmacological management of depression includes:

- full exploration of underlying cause and perpetuating factors
- explanation and reassurance to family and carers
- appropriate psychospiritual support; refer to specialists if needed

The following is recommended for pharmacological management of depression:

- sertraline

Insomnia

Non-pharmacological management of insomnia includes:

- full exploration of underlying cause and perpetuating factors
- explanation and reassurance to family and carers
- appropriate psychospiritual support; refer to specialists if needed

The following is recommended for pharmacological management of insomnia:

- zopiclone 3.75–7.50 mg, at night

Further Reading

Kavalieratos D, Gelfman LP, Tycon LE, et al. Palliative care in heart failure: rationale, evidence, and future priorities. *J Am Coll Cardiol* 2017; 70: 1919–30

McIlvennan CK and Allen LA. Palliative care in patients with heart failure. *BMJ* 2016; 353: i1010

Steiner JM, Cooper S, and Kirkpatrick JN. Palliative care in end-stage valvular heart disease. *Heart* 2017; 103: 1233–37

PART 4

Respiratory disorders

Abdul Nasimudeen

Introduction

Respiration has two components: external respiration, which enables the absorption of O_2 and the removal of CO_2, and internal respiration, which enables the utilization of O_2 and production of CO_2 and mediates gas exchange between the cells and their fluid medium. This chapter addresses the mechanics of respiration; gas exchange in the lungs; the pulmonary circulation; lung defence mechanisms; and the metabolic and endocrine functions of the lungs.

Mechanics of respiration

Inspiration and expiration

The lungs and chest wall are elastic structures that slide easily against each other but resist being pulled away. The pressure in the intra-pleural space (the space between the lungs and the chest wall) is normally subatmospheric. The contraction of inspiratory muscles during the active inspiratory process results in an increase in intra-thoracic volume and a decrease in intra-pleural pressure. Lungs go into an expanded position, and negative pressure inside the airways aids airflow to the lungs. In end inspiration, lung recoil pulls the chest back to expiratory position, where recoil pressures of the chest wall and lung balance. Airway pressures are now slightly positive and this aids airflow out of lungs. Expiration is a relatively passive event, compared to inspiration.

Respiratory muscles

The diaphragm is the main muscle for inspiration and accounts for 75% of the change in the intra-thoracic volume during inspiration. It has three parts: the costal portion, the crural portion, and the central tendon into which the costal and crural fibres insert. External intercostal muscles are also important for inspiration, and the scalene and sternocleidomastoid muscles act as accessory muscles of respiration. Dilatation of bronchi during inspiration is controlled by the sympathetic system, and constriction during expiration is under parasympathetic control. The work of breathing performed by respiratory muscles involves both elastic work (e.g. stretching the lungs and the chest wall), which accounts for around 65% of the workload, and non-elastic work, such as viscous resistance (which accounts for 7% of the workload) and airway resistance (which accounts for 28% of the workload).

Lung volumes

The amount of air that moves into lungs with each inspiration is called the **tidal volume**. The **minute volume** is the tidal volume times the number of respirations per minute. The air inspired with a maximal inspiratory effort in excess of tidal volume is the **inspiratory reserve volume**. The volume expelled by an active expiratory effort after a passive expiration is the **expiratory reserve volume**, and the volume left in the lungs after a maximal expiratory effort is the **residual volume. Vital capacity** is the largest amount of air that can be expired after a maximal inspiratory effort and this is useful routinely as a measure of pulmonary function; **FEV₁** is the fraction of this vital capacity during the first second and is useful in diagnosing obstructive airways diseases.

Positional variation in ventilation

Both blood flow and ventilation per unit lung volume is greater at the base of the lung than at the apex in the upright position. The ventilation:perfusion (V/Q) ratio is low at the base and high at the apex, as the relative change in blood flow from the apex to the base is greater than the relative change in ventilation. These differences are mainly due to gravity and tend to disappear in the supine position.

Compliance

The change in lung volume per unit change in airway pressure indicates the compliance of the lungs and the chest wall, and its normal value is approximately 0.2 l/cm H_2O. Compliance also depends on the lung volume. Compliance is decreased in conditions such as pulmonary fibrosis and pulmonary oedema, whereas it is increased in conditions such as emphysema. **Surfactant**, a lipid surface-tension-lowering agent produced by type II alveolar epithelial cells, lines the alveoli and is also an important factor affecting the compliance of the lungs.

Dead space

Gas exchange normally takes place in the terminal airways and hence the gas that occupies the rest of the respiratory system is not available for gas exchange. This area is called the **anatomical dead space**, and its volume is around 150 ml. The **physiological dead space** is the volume of gas not equilibrating with blood and, in healthy individuals, the two dead spaces are identical. The physiological dead space can be calculated from the **Bohr equation**:

$$\frac{V_D}{V_T} = \frac{PaCO_2 - PeCO_2}{PaCO_2},$$

where $PeCO_2$ is the partial pressure of CO_2 in expired air, $PaCO_2$ is the partial pressure of CO_2 in arterial blood, and V_T and V_D represent the tidal volume and the dead space volume, respectively. This equation can also be used to calculate the anatomical dead space by replacing $PaCO_2$ with the partial pressure of CO_2 in the alveoli ($PACO_2$).

Gas exchange in the lungs

Alveolar ventilation

Alveolar ventilation is the rate at which a volume of air participates in gas exchange in the alveoli, where the volume of air is equal to the difference between V_T and V_D and is normally around 350 ml. The partial pressure of alveolar oxygen (PAO_2) can be calculated via the alveolar gas equation:

$$PAO_2 = FIO_2(PATM - PH_2O) - \frac{PaCO_2}{R},$$

where FIO_2 is the fraction of inhaled air that is oxygen, PATM is the prevailing atmospheric pressure, PH_2O is the saturated vapour pressure of water at body temperature and the prevailing atmospheric pressure, $PaCO_2$ is the arterial partial pressure of carbon dioxide, and R is the respiratory exchange ratio, assumed to be 0.8.

Alveolocapillary membrane diffusion

The diffusion of alveolar oxygen into capillaries completes gas exchange. The alveolar–arterial O_2 gradient reflects the effectiveness of this diffusion process and is equal to $PAO_2 - PaO_2$. This is normally less than 10–15 mm Hg.

Gases diffuse across the alveolocapillary membrane and achieve equilibrium at various times. Nitrous oxide (N_2O) is not bound to blood with a high partial pressure, and hence its uptake is mainly **flow limited**, whereas carbon monoxide (CO) has a high affinity to haemoglobin with low partial pressure, and its uptake is **diffusion**

limited. Oxygen has an intermediate affinity to haemoglobin, and its uptake is **perfusion limited**.

The diffusing capacity of the lung for a given gas is directly proportionate to the surface area of the capillary membrane and inversely proportionate to its thickness. The diffusion capacity of the lung for carbon monoxide is $\dfrac{V_{CO}}{PACO}$, where V_{co} is the volume of carbon monoxide entering the blood, and PACO is the partial pressure of alveolar carbon monoxide.

Pulmonary circulation

Pulmonary blood vessels

The walls of the main pulmonary arteries are 30% thicker than the aortic wall, but smaller arteries have relatively thin muscles. Each alveolus sits in a pulmonary capillary basket with multiple anastomoses. The pulmonary vasculature is able to accommodate a blood flow equal to that of all other organs of the body. At any one time, pulmonary vessels carry 1 l of blood, of which less than 100 ml is in the capillaries. The pressure gradient in the pulmonary system is about 7 mm Hg and it takes a red blood cell about 0.75 s to traverse the pulmonary capillaries at rest. The normal pulmonary capillary pressure is about 10 mm Hg.

Positional variation in blood flow

Gravity plays an important effect on pulmonary circulation. In the upright position, the pulmonary capillary pressure of the upper lobes is close to the alveolar pressure; in the middle part of lungs, the pulmonary arterial and capillary pressures are greater than the alveolar pressure; and, in lower lobes, the alveolar pressure in lower than that in the pulmonary artery, capillaries, or venules. The V/Q ratio for the whole lung is about 0.8 (4.2 l/min of ventilation divided by 5.5 l/min of blood flow).

Regulation of pulmonary blood flow

Pulmonary blood flow is also affected by both active and passive factors. There is extensive autonomic innervation of the pulmonary vessels; in addition, the pulmonary vessels respond to several circulating humoral agents, such as adenosine, bradykinin, and so on. Stimulation of the cervical sympathetic ganglia reduces pulmonary blood flow by 30%. Exercise increases cardiac output and pulmonary arterial pressure, and the net effect is a marked increase in pulmonary blood flow.

Alveolar hypoxia resulting from bronchial obstruction causes pulmonary vasoconstriction, shunting blood away from the area of hypoxia. A rise in pH from a rising PCO_2 also produces pulmonary vasoconstriction, as opposed to the vasodilatation it produces in other tissues. Consequently, further bronchoconstriction occurs with further shift of ventilation away from the poorly perfused lung.

Lung defence mechanism

Lungs have a variety of defence mechanisms, which include anatomic defences to defend against particle deposition in upper airways, and functional defences, such as the clearance of particles through cough, mucociliary action, and cellular metabolism.

Anatomic defence mechanisms include nostril hairs, and mucus membranes in the nose and pharynx. Coughing is another defence against particles falling on the walls of the trachea and the bronchi. Cilia situated from the anterior third of the nose to the beginning of the bronchioles are instrumental in removing these particles as well. These cilia can beat at a rate of around 1000 cycles/min. Most particles >2 μm are removed by these defences; particles <2 μm are ingested by macrophages upon reaching the alveoli. Pulmonary alveolar macrophages are phagocytic, ingesting bacteria and other particles. They also help in processing inhaled antigens and play a role in inflammation due to cigarette smoke inhalation, by releasing lysosomal products.

Cellular and humoral immune responses play a vital part in lung defence. Lymphokines are produced by T-lymphocytes and regulate immunoglobulin synthesis. B-lymphocytes produce antibodies by transforming into plasma cells. Natural killer cells are lymphocytes that can kill bacteria without prior sensitization. IgAs in the nasopharynx bind to viruses and bacteria and facilitate microorganism agglutination. Protease-activated receptors in the pulmonary epithelium help release prostaglandin E2, which protects epithelial cells. Alpha-1 antitrypsin inactivates proteolytic enzymes from bacteria and necrotic cells. Interferon produced by macrophages and lymphocytes has antiviral activity.

Metabolic and endocrine functions of the lungs

Surfactant produced by type 2 alveolar cells is important at birth and prevents the lungs from collapsing. As well as removing prostaglandins from circulation, the lungs also synthesize and release prostaglandins, histamine, and kallikrein into blood. Angiotensin-converting enzyme located on the pulmonary capillary endothelial cells is responsible for converting inactive angiotensin I to the active hormone angiotensin II in the pulmonary circulation. Lungs also play a role in removing vasoactive substances such as serotonin and norepinephrine.

Further Reading

Scientific Principles of Respiratory Medicine, in *Murray & Nadel's Textbook of Respiratory Medicine*, 6th edition 2016. Elsevier
West JB. *Lectures in Respiratory Physiology.* https://meded.ucsd.edu/ifp/jwest/resp_phys/

126 Diagnosis in suspected respiratory disease

James Bonnington

Introduction

When there is suspicion of respiratory pathology, the clinician's role is to obtain a diagnosis accurately and, where possible, swiftly while subjecting the patient to the minimum of anxiety and invasive or potentially harmful tests. It is not only in rapidly progressive disease and malignancy where speed is of the essence. Potentially reversible airways disease often becomes irreversible once established and conditions that erode into lung reserve lead to increasing levels of disability if unchecked. Furthermore, in the case of respiratory-borne infections, there may be a public health risk.

A pertinent question always to be asked is whether the patient's respiratory symptoms are a consequence of lung pathology or whether the problem lies elsewhere. Shortness of breath is a common presenting symptom in left ventricular failure. Chronic cough may be the sole presenting symptom in a number of extra-pulmonary conditions, in particular postnasal drip syndrome (41%) and gastroesophageal reflux (21%). If the patient's history and examination findings continue to point towards a problem within the respiratory system, this should be considered in some detail. Successful ventilation requires a number of factors. The thoracic cage should be intact and appropriately shaped and orientated. In turn, it must be moved by muscles of adequate strength and assisted by a competent diaphragm. Airways, both large and small, should be of appropriate calibre and elasticity and supported by the lung interstitum without compression from abnormal lymphatics or masses. If ventilation is successful, it needs to be paired with adequate perfusion, requiring the flow of blood laden with functional haemoglobin through pulmonary vessels free of thrombus and unimpeded by increased vascular resistance. The innocuously simple complaint of dyspnoea may be caused by a problem in any one of these! It is the physician's challenge to identify which component is compromised. This can only be achieved by taking a full clinical history, performing a thorough physical examination, and following this with targeted investigations.

The respiratory history

It is widely accepted that roughly 80% of diagnoses are made on reading of a referral letter and taking a clinical history, a further 10% on performing a physical exam, and the final 10% when presented with the results of appropriate investigations. This is nowhere more true than in respiratory medicine, where, although a panoply of investigations are available to the physician, most are hampered by a wide range of normal values, and few have significant positive predictive value unless accompanied by an appropriate pretest probability.

The patient typically presents with one or two major symptoms. The nature of these should be established along with the time for which they have been present and any change in their severity. While many congenital anomalies of the lung are usually noted in the first few weeks of life, others may not be identified until later in childhood while some, such as bronchogenic cysts, may not become problematic until early adulthood. Diagnoses of asthma in young adults are five times more likely in those who experienced symptoms of bronchial hyper-responsiveness in childhood. A range of respiratory disease may first present in middle age, including bronchiectasis as a consequence of childhood infection, pulmonary manifestations of systemic disease, fibrotic lung disease, and malignancy. From the sixth decade onwards, the effects of chronic smoking often manifest themselves,

and patients with indolent forms of usual interstitial pneumonitis may first seek medical attention.

Associated symptoms should be identified and any constitutional symptoms noted. Weight loss may accompany malignancy, but may also be seen in chronic inflammatory conditions, where the work of breathing exceeds calorific intake and where breathlessness precludes good dietary intake.

Wherever possible, a trigger for symptom worsening should be identified which may be either a patient factor or an environmental factor. Patient factors could be a change in smoking habit or an insidious increase in weight. Environmental factors hint at allergen-related disease and may include changes to home life: moving near an active farm, or the acquisition of a new pet. Changes to the working environment need to be elicited (and documented) if a diagnosis of occupational asthma is suspected. A diurnal variation in cough or wheeze hints at a diagnosis of asthma, while profuse early morning expectoration is common in bronchiectasis.

Without quantifying symptom severity, it may be difficult to identify disease progression or response to treatment. For the dyspnoeic patient, the MRC breathlessness scale correlates well with lung function measurements and is useful for stratifying interventions in COPD (Table 126.1). Few will measure their exercise tolerance in absolute terms so a guide to their functional impairment can be sought. Many hospitals provide an exercise load in terms of a remote car park or a sloped corridor: although non-standard, such tests are at least reproducible on a visit-by-visit basis! Patients should be encouraged to describe their sputum production in terms of volume, colour, and viscosity. Cough can be hard to quantify, as patient perception and reporting varies, but validated questionnaires are available.

A synopsis of the patient's past medical history and drugs prescribed may identify an atopic individual, one with multisystem disease, or a patient at risk from pulmonary fibrosis (as a consequence of previous chemotherapy, radiotherapy where the lung was included in the radiation field, or other drugs with recognized pulmonary toxicity). Up to 15% of patients commencing ACE-inhibitor therapy develop dry cough, which is normally relieved by cessation of treatment but may take several months to resolve fully (and may persist in a small minority).

A smoking history, quantified in pack years, should be documented along with any recreational drug abuse. Inhalation of freebase

Grade	Degree of breathlessness related to activities
1	Not troubled by breathlessness except on strenuous exercise
2	Short of breath when hurrying or walking up a slight hill
3	Walks slower than contemporaries on level ground because of breathlessness, or has to stop for breath when walking at own pace
4	Stops for breath after walking 100 m or after a few minutes on level ground
5	Too breathless to leave the house, or breathless when dressing or undressing

Table 126.1 The MRC scale of breathlessness

Reproduced with permission from Chris Stenton, The MRC breathlessness scale, Occupational Medicine, Volume 58, Issue 3, pp.226-227, Copyright © 2008 by permission of Oxford University Press.

Adapted from: Fletcher CM, The clinical diagnosis of pulmonary emphysema—an experimental study. Proc R Soc Med, volume 45, pp 577-584, copyright (c) 1952 SAGE Publications.

cocaine, particularly when mixed with impurities, is associated with significant respiratory pathology ('crack lung'). A family history of respiratory disease may identify inherited disease or shared exposure to an environmental factor such as asbestos in prefabricated housing. It is important to be familiar with local disease patterns and associated socio-economic factors. The UK incidence of TB is modest (12/100 000 in 2014) and the clinician should be aware of the local situation: immigration patterns, uptake of BCG vaccination, and any local resistance patterns. Local industry, current and past, has a profound effect on the patterns of respiratory disease seen, including the incidence of occupational asthma and pneumoconioses.

The respiratory examination

Although much of the diagnosis will have been made from the clinical history, a thorough physical examination is essential. It may seem contrary to note that the most useful information is to be gained away from the chest. On arrival at clinic, all patients should have a height and weight recorded and a BMI calculated. Any significant deviation away from the normal range (19.0–24.9 kg/m2) is to be discussed with the patient to identify rapid or relentless changes. This should be accompanied by measurements of heart rate, blood pressure, and arterial oxygen saturation. Patients noted to be hypoxic should be questioned as to whether this represents arterial oxygen saturation at rest or after exercise (e.g. walking to the clinic) An increased respiratory rate is a non-specific sign, although the clinician should be alert to the presence of Cheyne–Stokes breathing, which is seen in encephalopathy, severe congestive heart failure, and CNS damage at the cerebral level.

Examination of the hands may reveal evidence of cyanosis, anaemia, or occult cigarette smoking, but also signs of systemic disease such as rheumatoid arthritis or scleroderma. Finger clubbing is a non-specific sign and may be found in cases of malignancy, lung abscess, bronchiectasis, and lung fibrosis, along with various extra-pulmonary diseases. Palpation of the peripheral lymph nodes is essential and may provide evidence of an on-going inflammatory process, TB, or disseminated malignancy. Inspection of the chest wall identifies mechanical factors likely to impede ventilation, including central obesity and deformities of the spine, such as kyphosis and scoliosis. Percussion may reveal areas of dullness as a consequence of either fluid accumulation or consolidation (which can be differentiated by vocal resonance, tactile vocal fremitus, or whispering pectoriloquy). Auscultation will detect areas of reduced air entry and the presence or absence of any crackles or wheeze.

Respiratory investigations

Having taken a full history and performed a thorough examination, the clinician should be in a position to offer a diagnosis or, at the least, a short differential. This leaves the role of respiratory investigations as:

- narrowing the differential to a definitive diagnosis
- excluding important diagnoses
- staging disease
- guiding therapy

In a minority of cases, the diagnosis remains uncertain even after extensive investigation and then a trial of therapy may be appropriate. A range of investigations is available and so, by asking which question is being tackled, the clinician can identify which investigations are most suitable.

Lung function tests can be both a source of revelation and consternation and, as such, need to be interpreted with caution. Seldom diagnostic, the patterns of abnormality often fit with a fairly small group of diseases. Patients may be referred following grossly abnormal spirometry results in a number of situations. A typical scenario is the patient who was predicted to have an obstructive defect but not to the extent of that revealed by spirometry. In this instance, it can be educational to simply repeat the test in the clinic room. This often reveals a patient who lacks enthusiasm in expiration and can be encouraged towards a normal FEV1/FVC ratio. Likewise, patients who stop expiring prematurely before reaching FVC may be erroneously found to have a restrictive defect. This is particularly a problem

with computerized spirometers, which terminate the test after a few seconds. A volume–time trace that is still sloping upwards at the end of the test hints towards this scenario. Caution should also be exercised when faced with the presumption that a restrictive spirometry pattern in the presence of breathlessness must indicate fibrotic lung disease. Increasingly, the restriction (and cause of the breathlessness) is found to be extra-thoracic in origin: a consequence of central obesity. Sensitive questioning, calculation of the BMI, and advice may be all that is required in such situations but, if further reassurance is necessary, lung volumes and gas transfer may be established. In intra-thoracic restriction, both the transfer factor for carbon monoxide and the carbon monoxide transfer coefficient may be reduced; when the restriction is extra-thoracic, the latter will be preserved or elevated.

Gas transfer is a sensitive test of lung function and often one of the first abnormalities when pathology develops in the alveoli. In patients with a history suggestive of a dynamic airway problem, a single spirometry recording is largely unhelpful, and thought should be given to peak flow diaries, tests of reversibility, and provocation tests. Where a diagnosis of airway obstruction is considered, the possibility of a reversible element to the disease must be pursued thoroughly. As understanding of asthma improves, it becomes apparent that patients labelled as having 'irreversible' airway obstruction may in fact have 'poorly characterized' or even 'significantly under-treated' disease. This presents the potential opportunity to render patients virtually symptom-free, or at least significantly improve their quality of life. Asthma can be associated with the progression of symptoms and the development of irreversible airflow obstruction. Such airway remodelling may be limited with appropriate treatment.

Cardiopulmonary exercise testing allows the response of the cardiovascular and respiratory systems to a known exercise stress to be measured concomitantly. This is particularly useful where a patient is thought to have elements of both respiratory and cardiac disease and the relative contributions to their symptoms are difficult to quantify. In the area of sleep medicine, many centres will have access to overnight oximetry recording. In conjunction with the clinical scoring systems, this provides a reasonable screening tool, facilitating referral to more specialist units.

A standard chest radiograph is indicated in most patients, if only to guide the choice of more definitive imaging. The effective radiation dose of a posterior–anterior projection is 0.1 mSv. Other views (lateral, oblique, lateral decubitus, etc.) have largely fallen from favour with the increasing availability of CT. Improvements in CT have considerably increased its usefulness in respiratory medicine, and a number of imaging protocols have been developed. In order to perform the most appropriate investigation, it is imperative that the radiologist is provided with thorough clinical details along with the diagnostic thought processes.

Direct examination of the airways by bronchoscopy should only follow appropriate imaging, as a targeted examination has considerably higher yield, both for infection and for identifying malignancy.

Sputum culture is of relatively little value in the diagnosis of community-acquired pneumonia, but may be helpful in those chronically colonized. When considering tuberculosis, the yield is higher when early morning samples are examined (patients should be instructed to provide these via a deep cough shortly after waking). The yield of any single specimen is low (36%–63%) and is insufficient to exclude a diagnosis of active tuberculosis. Sputum cultures positive for *Haemophilus influenzae*, *Streptococcus pneumoniae*, and *Pseudomonas aeruginosa* raise the possibility of bronchiectasis, although the pathogens may also be found in patients with chronic bronchitis. Sputum may be induced safely by inhaling 3% saline, and the yield is improved. Characterizing the inflammatory profile of induced sputum is becoming an increasingly useful step in the management of a variety of airway diseases, including asthma, COPD, and chronic cough.

The choice of venous blood tests should be guided by the likely underlying pathology. Both anaemia and marked polycythaemia may cause breathlessness. Renal and liver dysfunction may suggest systemic disease. Total immunoglobulin levels can be appropriate; raised IgE is suggestive of an allergic process, while depressed IgG levels may be seen in bronchiectasis. Raised IgE against *Aspergillus fumigatus* is required for a diagnosis of allergic bronchopulmonary aspergillosis, while low IgG titres against encapsulated organisms provide a treatment target in bronchiectasis.

Although not always necessary, tissue diagnosis remains the gold standard for a number of conditions where treatment is potentially long or likely to put the patient at significant risk of complications or side effects (e.g. sarcoidosis). While there remains a limited role for blind pleural biopsy in cases of suspected tuberculosis, in all other cases prior imaging should be considered essential. Available sampling techniques include CT-guided needle biopsy, advanced bronchoscopic techniques, thoracoscopy, and open lung biopsy. In general, the choice of technique should be decided in discussion with the reporting radiologist or, where appropriate, in a multidisciplinary meeting. Physical examination and imaging may reveal involvement of peripheral lymph nodes or other organs (e.g. liver) that may provide safer biopsy targets than the lung tissue itself. Note also that, with recent advance in tissue-sampling techniques, some patients may have been empirically initiated on long-term treatment many years ago for conditions that are now amenable to more rigorous investigation.

Diagnosis is continually reviewed against expected clinical progress and response to treatment. If these are not as predicted, thought must be given to both unusual presentations of disease and the presence of uncommon disease.

Conclusion

Faced with a patient with suspected respiratory disease, the problem is far from a lack of diagnostic tools; rather, it is choosing those most fit for purpose. Any investigation is only as good as its interpretation and this in turn will depend upon the context in which it is used. Perform a thorough clinical history and physical examination; being alert to the cardinal symptoms and signs should lead to a logical route of investigation. Together, these approaches should culminate in an appropriate diagnosis and a way forwards for physician and patient.

Further Reading

Bohadana A, Izbicki G, and Kraman SS. Fundamentals of lung auscultation. *N Engl J Med* 2014; 370: 744–51.

Diagnosis and Evaluation of Respiratory Disease. In Murray & Nadel's Textbook of Respiratory Medicine, 6th edition 2016. Elsevier

127 Investigation in respiratory disease

Pranabashis Haldar

Introduction

Investigation in respiratory disease may be broadly classified as:

- tests that aid diagnosis
- tests that assess disease severity; these are usually measures of respiratory function and inform prognosis
- tests that assess disease activity; these are usually non-invasive biomarkers, enabling serial measurement, and may inform therapy

One of the challenges of respiratory medicine is the limited spectrum of clinical expression associated with a diverse spectrum of pathologies. Clinical symptoms in respiratory medicine are often of poor specificity for securing a diagnosis or assessing disease severity. Investigations, therefore, necessarily form a critical part of assessment.

The most appropriate choice of investigation is an important component of clinical decision-making that affects patient care and may be influenced by a number of different questions that the clinician will need to consider. These include:

- what am I trying to find out?
- how will this affect my patient's management?
- what are the investigations available to me?
- which investigation is most likely to give me the information I need with the least discomfort or risk to my patient?
- is my patient in agreement with my assessment and are they aware of the alternatives that may exist?

Of course, more than one investigation may be appropriate and, in such circumstances, the decision may ultimately depend on cost and availability. In practice, investigations are guided by clinical suspicion (from history and examination) and undertaken in a stepwise manner. Easily accessible, low-cost, non-invasive tests are usually performed first and most often serve a screening function, directing further, more specific tests.

This chapter will provide a systematic overview of important tests commonly performed in the investigation of respiratory illness, and the clinical principles that govern their use in practice. More detailed discussion of specific investigations will be presented in Chapters 128–145, which address particular conditions.

Principles of investigating the respiratory system

The respiratory system may be viewed as comprising several related anatomical compartments:

- extra-pulmonary tissues, including the pleural space, the chest wall, and the diaphragm
- pulmonary parenchyma, including terminal airways, alveoli, and the interstitium
- lower airways
- pulmonary vasculature

The relationship of structure with function is shown in Figure 127.1.

The alveolar membrane is the interface for gas exchange between the atmosphere and circulation, and comprises several layers (Figure 127.1). Gas exchange occurs by simple diffusion along a concentration gradient across this membrane. The two principle factors affecting diffusion, and therefore partial pressure of gases in the pulmonary capillaries are:

- the concentration gradient for diffusion; this is primarily determined by the partial pressure of gases in the alveoli; these pressures, in turn, are determined by alveolar ventilation
- the diffusion capacity of the alveolar membrane; this is related directly to the total surface area for exchange and inversely to the thickness of the membrane; it should be noted that the surface

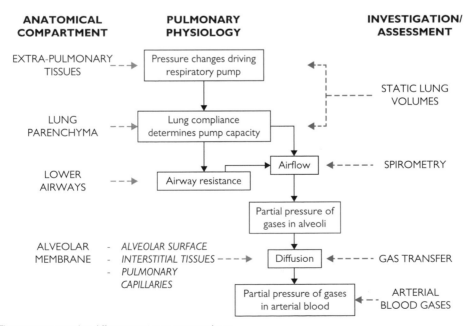

Figure 127.1 The anatomic sites that different respiratory tests evaluate.

area available for gas exchange is not the same as the anatomical surface area provided by the alveoli, but includes only the proportion of this area that is accompanied by blood flow (ventilation–perfusion matching)

Information about each component of these processes can be obtained from specific investigations of pulmonary function (see Figure 127.1), as will be discussed in this chapter.

Arterial blood gases and respiratory failure

Failure of the respiratory system is defined by abnormalities identified in the arterial blood gases (ABGs), that is, the partial pressures of O_2 (PaO_2) and CO_2 ($PaCO_2$) in arterial blood. These represent the final common pathway in respiratory function (Figure 127.1). Resting tachypnoea is often the first sign of respiratory failure, and respiratory rate should always be noted in the assessment of respiratory disease. Respiratory failure is divided into two types:

- type 1 respiratory failure, defined by a low PaO_2 and a low or normal $PaCO_2$
- type 2 respiratory failure, defined by a low PaO_2 and a raised $PaCO_2$.

This distinction has an important physiological basis. The solubility and therefore diffusion capacity of $PaCO_2$ is 20-fold greater than for O_2. This has two implications. First, pathology affecting gas exchange rarely disturbs CO_2 homeostasis; second, pathology leading to a raised $PaCO_2$ will always be associated with hypoxia. The only determinant of arterial $PaCO_2$ is the alveolar $PaCO_2$, which is a function of alveolar ventilation. Thus, type 1 respiratory failure indicates a problem of gas exchange, while type 2 respiratory failure implies insufficient ventilation.

The interpretation of ABGs and, in particular, type 1 respiratory failure is entirely dependent upon the inspired fraction of oxygen (FiO_2). The FiO_2 of room air at atmospheric pressure is 0.21, and this defines the normal range for PaO_2. For this reason, ABG sampling at room air is always preferred, when possible.

Interpreting the PaO_2 at higher FiO_2 requires knowledge of the alveolar PaO_2 (PAO_2), which is calculated from the alveolar gas equation. A simplified form of the equation at sea level is

$$PAO_2 = (95 \times FiO_2) - (1.2 \times PaCO_2),$$

where PAO_2 is in kilopascals. To determine whether a problem of gas exchange exists, the difference between PAO_2 and measured PaO_2 is calculated. This is known as the alveolar–arterial gradient and is normally less than 2 kPa.

ABG is an unusual example of a test that is both an easily accessible screening tool (to determine that a problem of respiratory function exists) and a clinical gold standard (for identifying and characterizing respiratory failure). It should be remembered that ABG sampling has important limitations. First, it is invasive and may be associated with complications (haematoma, infection, distal ischaemia, damage to adjacent structures such as the median nerve in the wrist), particularly when the procedure is technically challenging (low volume pulse, joint deformity, anomalous vascular anatomy, obesity) or performed by inexperienced operators. It is also of limited value prior to the onset of frank respiratory failure and unnecessary for monitoring type 1 respiratory failure. For the latter, measurement of arterial oxygen saturation (SaO_2) with a finger probe provides sufficient information to monitor progress and guide therapy. Subclinical type 1 respiratory failure may be precipitated with controlled exercise.

Investigations of pulmonary function

There are three types of pulmonary function tests:

- spirometry, which is used to measure airflow
- static lung volume, which determines pump capacity
- diffusing capacity, which measures gas transfer across the alveolar membrane

Of these, spirometry is routinely available and easily performed at the bedside. Although primarily used to test airway function, spirometry is also frequently used as a screening test of pulmonary function to guide further investigation.

Spirometry and testing airway function

The lower airways refer to the trachea and all divisions that follow. The primary role of the airways is the conduction of air to and from the gas exchange surface of the lungs. Pathology affecting the airways, therefore, manifests in disordered airflow that is measurable with spirometry. Differences exist in the effects of pathology on airflow at different levels of the bronchial tree and in the different phases of the respiratory cycle (Table 127.1). A basic understanding of these factors will help with interpretation of spirometry.

Airway anatomy

Structurally, large bronchi repeatedly divide into progressively smaller bronchioles that end in terminal respiratory bronchioles and alveoli. Approximately 23 divisions of the bronchial tree (airway generations) are recognized. It is useful to think of the smaller and larger airways as two separate compartments. Larger airways constitute the first four to six generations and are structurally characterized by the presence of supporting cartilage to maintain airway patency. In contrast, smooth muscle that encircles the entire bronchial tree alone maintains structural integrity of smaller airways. The basic anatomy of the airways is dynamic and propagated by changes in pressure and volume during inspiration and expiration. The effects are greatest in the smaller, floppier airways that lack cartilaginous support.

Effects of the respiratory cycle

During inspiration, intra-thoracic pressure falls below atmospheric pressure as the chest wall and the diaphragm expand. This negative pressure applies a force to the airways and pulls them open. Outside the thoracic cavity, a pressure gradient between the atmosphere, and negative pressure within the airway (i.e. the larynx and the trachea), will promote airway collapse, but this is normally prevented by the existing cartilaginous support. Inspiration, therefore, improves airflow in the intra-thoracic airways, but has the opposite effect on the extra-thoracic portion of the lower airway.

During expiration, positive pressure has a compressive effect on intra-thoracic airways, promoting narrowing proximally and closure distally in the smaller airways with no supporting cartilage. In contrast, positive pressure within the extra-thoracic airway acts as a pneumatic splint to improve patency.

Pathology affecting the intra-thoracic airway is, therefore, more apparent in expiration and, for the extra-thoracic airway, is more apparent during inspiration. Clinically, the contrast is usefully made in the distinction between expiratory wheeze (implies narrowing of proximal intra-thoracic airways) and inspiratory stridor (implies pathology affecting either the larynx or the trachea). Despite their size, the smaller airways collectively contribute only a small proportion of total airway resistance because of their large number and arrangement in parallel. Pathology of the small airways will lead to premature closure during expiration, and gas trapping that will be clinically evident as hyperinflation and reduced air entry (Table 127.2).

Interpreting outputs of spirometry

Spirometry provides both quantitative and graphical information. Graphically, there are two outputs that provide related but complementary information:

The volume–time (V–T) curve: This displays the cumulative volume of air that is expired as a function of time (see Figure 127.2A1), and examines expiration only.

The flow–volume (F–V) loop: This displays the flow of air as a function of lung volume during both inspiration and expiration (see Figure 127.2B). The F–V loop is therefore needed to investigate pathology affecting the extra-thoracic airway; most often, the pathology will be evident as flattening of the inspiratory limb.

Basic spirometry requires the patient to take a maximal breath in followed by a forced and complete expiration into the spirometer. The most common indices recorded are:

Table 127.1 Suggested investigations to further evaluate respiratory symptoms

Clinical symptoms		Extra-pulmonary pathology				Airways pathology		Pulmonary tissues pathology	Pulmonary vasculature pathology
		Chest wall	Pleural space	Diaphragm	Mediastinum	Proximal/larger airways	Distal/small airways		
		Chest pain Breathlessness Orthopnoea	Pleuritic pain Breathlessness	Breathlessness Orthopnoea	Usually asymptomatic	Wheeze Productive cough Breathlessness	Dry cough Breathlessness	Dry cough Breathlessness	Breathlessness Chest discomfort Presyncope or syncope
Investigations	Screening and further investigation	CXR CT/MRI (for detailed characterization of soft tissues)	CXR USS CT	CXR	CXR CT/MRI	CXR Spirometry Static lung volumes	CXR Spirometry Static lung volumes	CXR Spirometry Static lung volumes	SaO2 and ABG CXR, spirometry, and static lung volumes (normal) Gas transfer ECG
	Diagnostic	Biopsy EMG/nerve conduction studies	Diagnostic aspiration Pleural biopsy (CT guided or thoracoscopy)	USS	EBUS-TBNA Surgical mediastinoscopy	CT (for diagnosing bronchiectasis) Methacholine PC20 (for diagnosing asthma) Sputum induction Bronchoscopy/BAL	CT Bronchoscopy/BAL Transbronchial biopsy	CT Transbronchial biopsy Lung biopsy (CT guided or surgical)	Echo CTPA MRA

Abbreviations: ABG, arterial blood gas; BAL, bronchoalveolar lavage; CT, computed tomography; CTPA, CT pulmonary angiography; CXR, chest radiography; EBUS-TBNA, endobronchial ultrasound-guided transbronchial needle aspiration; ECG, electrocardiography; Echo, echocardiography; EMG, electromyography; MRA, magnetic resonance angiography; MRI, magnetic resonance imaging; SaO2, arterial oxygen saturation; USS, ultrasound scan.

Table 127.2 Simple lung function tests in respiratory disease

Investigation	Description	Use	Positives	Negatives
Spirometry	Straightforward test to measure FEV1, and FVC	Quick assessment on ward or GP surgery to distinguish between obstructive and restrictive pathologies Determine severity of COPD (GOLD criteria) Serial measurements can track decline in COPD/asthma	Simple Quick Inexpensive Rapidly narrows differential diagnosis	Technique cannot always be mastered; this limits usefulness of results
Pulmonary function test	A 45-minute test to measure FEV1, FVC, TLC, residual volume, KCO, and TLCO	To diagnose and quantify severity of restrictive pathology Serial measurements can monitor decline of interstitial lung disease	Narrows differential diagnosis Reasonably simple to perform	Technique cannot always be mastered Measuring TLCO and KCO requires a 10-second breath hold Requires some sophisticated apparatus not routinely available. Tests cannot be performed in Primary Care
Reversibility	Spirometry is carried out before and after 200 μg (two puffs) salbutamol is administered via inhaler	Improvement in FEV1 by 20% **and** >200 ml is indicative of reversible airways disease	Asthma can be diagnosed COPD/asthma can be characterized as reversible or fixed Effectiveness of inhaled bronchodilator therapy can be assessed	Lack of significant reversibility does not always correlate with a lack of improvement in patient's symptoms
Methacholine PC$_{20}$ challenge	Nebulized methacholine, which causes bronchospasm in hyper-reactive airways, is given in incremental doses; the amount required to cause FEV1 to fall by >20% is called the 'PC$_{20}$'	A positive test (<8 mg/ml) indicates airway hyper-responsiveness and probable asthma or reactive airway dysfunction syndrome; normal values are >16 mg/ml	Helpful confirmatory test for the diagnosis of asthma	Not widely available Causes bronchoconstriction Contraindicated in patients with baseline FEV1 <50% Specificity falls with reducing baseline FEV1 False-negative tests commonly occur in patients who have continued with regular asthma medication or antihistamine therapy prior to testing
Exhaled nitric oxide	Nitric oxide, which is released by inflamed bronchial cells, is measured via a breath test; an elevated result indicates airway inflammation	Assessing treatment effectiveness in asthma May help with assessment of compliance with inhaled corticosteroids	Equipment is inexpensive and can easily be used in smaller hospitals/peripheral clinics	Not widely available Elevated result is not specific to asthma
Induced sputum	Sputum is induced by nebulized hypertonic saline after the teeth are cleaned and inhaled salbutamol is given; it is then mixed with 0.1% dithiothreitol and saline, and the cells in it are filtered out and centrifuged	Characterizing inflammation as neutrophilic or eosinophilic, to target corticosteroid treatment Assessing treatment effectiveness in asthma Serial measurement is used to titrate corticosteroid and immunosuppressive therapy in specialist centres Diagnosing TB and PCP	May make it possible to avoid the need for bronchoscopy in suspected TB and PCP	Available in specialized laboratories only Care required with pulmonary infections
Plethysmography	The patient sits in an air-tight chamber and undergoes pulmonary function tests; a sensitive method of determining absolute lung volumes	Helpful in assessing whether lung volume reduction surgery will be beneficial	True volume of lung and gas trapping can be calculated	Not widely available

Abbreviations: FEV1, forced expiratory volume in 1 second; FVC, forced vital capacity; GOLD, Global Initiative for Chronic Obstructive Lung Disease; GP, general practitioner; KCO, carbon monoxide transfer coefficient; PCP, pneumocystis pneumonia; TB, tuberculosis; TLC, total lung capacity; TLCO, transfer factor for carbon monoxide.

- forced expiratory volume in 1 second (FEV1); this is the volume of air forcefully exhaled in the first second
- forced vital capacity (FVC); this is the maximum volume of air forcefully exhaled from the point of maximum inspiration

Between 75% and 80% of the total expired volume is normally expelled in the first second during forced expiration. Airflow obstruction is defined by an FEV1/FVC ratio of <70% or 0.7. If airflow obstruction is identified, reversibility testing should be performed. This involves inhalation of 200–400 μg salbutamol through a spacer, followed by repeated spirometry after 20 minutes. Severity of obstruction is defined by the reduction in post-bronchodilator FEV1 (as per cent predicted) and not by the ratio. There are a number of common pitfalls to be aware of:

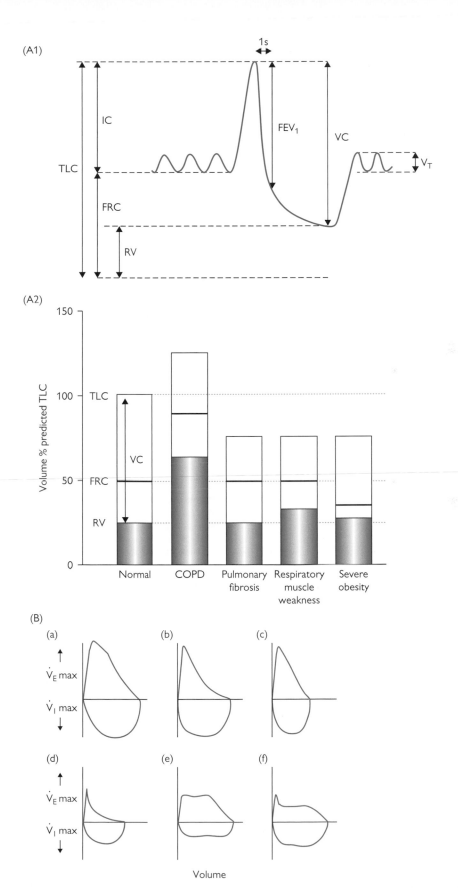

Figure 127.2 (A1) Volume–time curve; (A2) lung volumes in respiratory disease; (B) flow–volume loop; FEV_1, forced expiratory volume in 1 second; FRC, functional residual capacity; IC, inspiratory capacity; RV, residual volume; TLC, total lung capacity; VC, vital capacity; V_T, tidal volume; $\dot{V}_E$ max, maximum airflow on expiration; $\dot{V}_I$ max, maximum airflow on inhalation.

Reproduced with permission from Warrell, Cox and Firth, *Oxford Textbook of Medicine*, Oxford University Press, Oxford, UK, Copyright © 2010

(A)

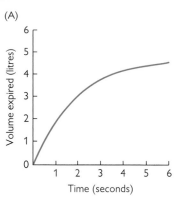

(B)

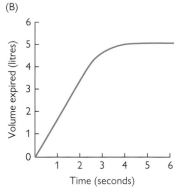

Figure 127.3 (A) An algorithm for interpreting spirometry; (B) an algorithm for interpreting static lung volume measurements; EP, extra-pulmonary; FEV_1, forced expiratory volume in 1 second; FVC, forced vital capacity; RV, residual volume; TLC, total lung capacity.

- The FEV1/FVC ratio falls in the ageing lung. This is physiological senescence, and caution must be exercised when interpreting spirometry in people beyond the age of 70 years, as normal values are not well validated for this group.
- A low FEV1/FVC ratio may be accompanied by a 'normal' FEV1 in young and fit individuals, as defined by the reference range. However, the true FEV1 may be considerably higher in this group, and the measured FEV1 may therefore represent a significant fall from baseline and can be difficult to quantify.
- The FEV1/FVC ratio may improve and even normalize with increasing severity of airflow obstruction, due to a fall in the FVC. This occurs as increasing involvement of the smaller airways leads to air trapping that is exacerbated by forced expiration. For advanced airways disease, a more accurate measure of FVC (and therefore underlying obstruction) may be obtained by performing a slow vital capacity test. In this test, the patient exhales slowly from peak inspiration for as long as possible. The lower intra-thoracic pressures generated reduce the extent of small airway collapse and gas trapping that occurs.

An algorithm for interpreting spirometry is presented in Figure 127.3A.

Measuring static lung volumes

The measurement of static lung volume involves calculation of the residual volume. This is the volume of air that remains in the lungs at the end of a full expiration. This measurement cannot be performed with spirometry and is essential to calculate total lung capacity (TLC; TLC = vital capacity + residual volume). Static lung volume measurements provide information that helps with the assessment of disordered physiology at two levels:

To determine and assess the severity of a restrictive lung deficit: A restrictive deficit is diagnosed by a demonstration of TLC <80% predicted. The severity of the restriction is determined by the size of the reduction in TLC. However, the presence of a reduction does not indicate whether the restriction is due to pulmonary pathology or extra-pulmonary pathology. Determining this requires further investigation (Figure 127.4), which is often done by examining the carbon monoxide- transferring ability of the lung.

To identify gas trapping as evidence for small airways disease: This is determined by measuring the ratio of the residual volume to the TLC ratio. This should be below 40% but is increased with gas trapping seen in small airways disease (increased residual volume, normal TLC) or emphysema (increased residual volume and increased TLC). A raised ratio is not diagnostic of gas trapping as it may also be increased with thoracic neuromuscular weakness (increased residual volume and reduced TLC).

There are two principal techniques used for the measurement of static lung volumes:

Helium dilution: This is the simpler technique and requires patients to gently breathe air containing a known volume of helium (which does not diffuse across the alveolar membrane) until the partial pressure of the gas reaches equilibrium. Total lung volume can

be calculated by knowing the change in partial pressure of helium from baseline. This technique is limited by the assumption that the helium distributes evenly and completely in both lungs. For patients with airways disease, the distribution of gas may be inhomogeneous and incomplete, leading to significant underestimation of the total lung volume.

Body plethysmography: This is considered the gold-standard diagnostic test for respiratory disease, but is limited by technical difficulty and limited availability. Patients also find this investigation less tolerable. The patient is required to sit in a sealed chamber and breathe through a mouthpiece. At the end of a normal breath, a shutter occludes the mouthpiece, and the patient is asked to continue making gentle respiratory efforts against the shutter. By measuring the pressure changes at the mouthpiece (alveolar pressure) and within the chamber, it is possible to derive the volume of gas in the lungs.

An algorithm for interpreting static lung volume measurements is presented in Figure 127.3B.

Measuring diffusion capacity

The diffusion capacity of the alveolar membrane is investigated by measuring the rate of diffusion of a known volume of inspired CO. CO is highly soluble and diffuses rapidly into the blood stream, and is retained there after binding with haemoglobin. Therefore, no back diffusion occurs and the rate at which the measured partial pressure of CO falls with time can be used to determine diffusion.

Diffusion across the alveolar membrane is influenced by numerous factors. Processes leading to thickening of the membrane reduce the rate of gas transfer. These include alveolitis; alveolar disruption as seen with emphysema; interstitial thickening due to pulmonary oedema, mitral stenosis, or lymphangitis; and thickening of the pulmonary capillaries due to vasculitis or primary pulmonary hypertension. In addition, as CO transfer is in part regulated by binding with haemoglobin, it is reduced with anaemia and increased with polycythaemia. Lung function reports can provide a correction for this, but the laboratory needs to be informed of an abnormal haemoglobin level. Finally, the rate of delivery of blood to ventilated lung will also influence gas transfer. Diffusion will be accelerated in high-output states and reduced when blood flow is sluggish (e.g. during cardiac failure or hypovolaemia) or absent (e.g. during ventilation–perfusion mismatching).

Gas transfer is expressed in two variables:

- TLCO, the transfer factor for CO, quantifies the diffusion capacity of the respiratory system
- KCO, the diffusion coefficient for CO, quantifies the diffusion capacity per unit volume of lung

KCO corrects for lung volume changes that may confound the interpretation of TLCO. An important example of when KCO is used is when distinguishing between pulmonary and extra-pulmonary restriction. In both types of restriction, a reduction in lung volume leads to a fall in TLCO. However, with pulmonary restriction, which will be associated with impaired gas transfer across a thickened alveolar membrane, KCO will be reduced as well; in contrast, KCO remains normal with extra-pulmonary restriction.

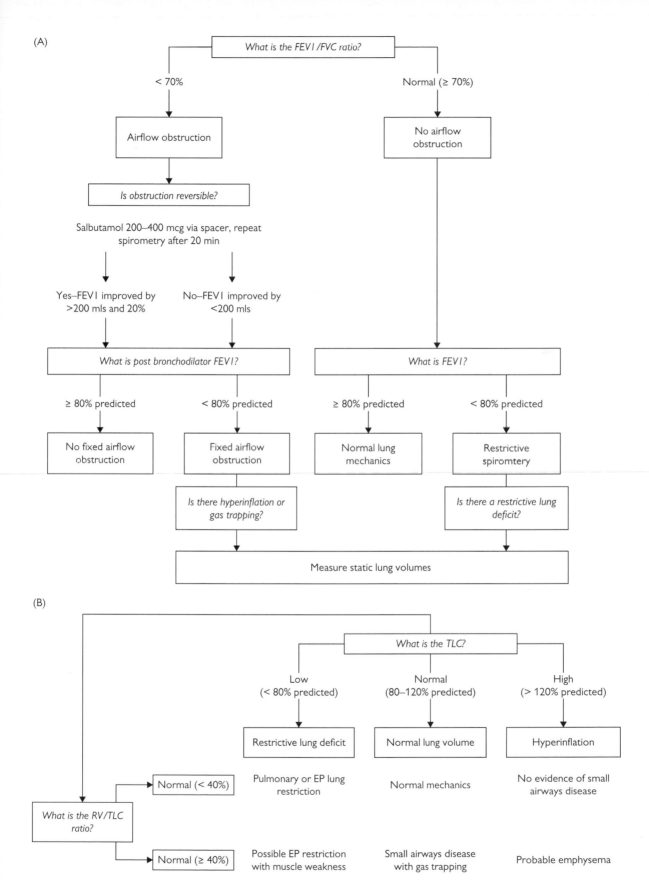

(A)

What is the FEV1 /FVC ratio?

< 70%

Airflow obstruction

Is obstruction reversible?

Salbutamol 200–400 mcg via spacer, repeat spirometry after 20 min

Yes–FEV1 improved by >200 mls and 20%

No–FEV1 improved by <200 mls

What is post bronchodilator FEV1?

≥ 80% predicted

No fixed airflow obstruction

< 80% predicted

Fixed airflow obstruction

Is there hyperinflation or gas trapping?

Normal (≥ 70%)

No airflow obstruction

What is FEV1?

≥ 80% predicted

Normal lung mechanics

< 80% predicted

Restrictive spiromtery

Is there a restrictive lung deficit?

Measure static lung volumes

(B)

What is the TLC?

Low (< 80% predicted)

Restrictive lung deficit

Pulmonary or EP lung restriction

Normal (80–120% predicted)

Normal lung volume

Normal mechanics

High (> 120% predicted)

Hyperinflation

No evidence of small airways disease

Normal (< 40%)

What is the RV/TLC ratio?

Possible EP restriction with muscle weakness

Small airways disease with gas trapping

Probable emphysema

Normal (≥ 40%)

CHAPTER 127 Investigation in respiratory disease

Figure 127.4 Schematic spirograms of two patients with airway obstruction and similar values for the forced expiratory volume in 1 second (FEV₁). (A) Diffuse intra-thoracic airway narrowing (COPD or asthma). Note that forced expiration is continuing after 6 s. (B) Upper airway narrowing with a 'straight' spirogram which corresponds to the plateau of flow in the earlier part of the expiration.

Reproduced with permission from Warrell, Cox and Firth, *Oxford Textbook of Medicine*, fifth edition, Oxford University Press, Oxford, UK, Copyright © 2010

Table 127.3 Radiological investigations in respiratory disease

Investigation	Description	Use	Positives	Negatives
Staging CT	CT scan of the lower neck, chest, and abdomen, usually with contrast; 5 mm slices taken at 5 mm intervals, with image reconstruction, so the whole lung is scanned	Staging of cancer	Whole lung is scanned	High radiation dose (equivalent to 150 chest X-rays) Poorer resolution than ordinary CT
High-resolution CT	CT of 1.25 mm slices at 10 mm intervals of the lung, usually with contrast	Visualization of lung parenchyma and nodules	Diagnosis of most lung diseases Monitor progression of interstitial lung disease Can provide limited information without contrast	Radiation dose Scanning protocol skips segments of lung and therefore small nodules can be missed
CT pulmonary angiogram	CT of 2 mm slices at 2 mm intervals, with contrast timed to visualize pulmonary arteries	Diagnosis of acute and chronic pulmonary embolism Diagnosis of arteriovenous malformations	High sensitivity and specificity, particularly for clots in the proximal third of the vascular tree	Cannot be performed if there is renal impairment or contrast/iodine allergy Loses sensitivity for small, subsegmental emboli (but the clinical importance of these is unknown)
Ventilation/perfusion scan	IV radiolabelled albumin is injected and cannot be filtered by the lungs; areas where there are perfusion defects show as a mismatch in perfusion/ventilation scans; results are divided into low/intermediate/high probability	Diagnosis of pulmonary embolism in patients who have a normal chest X-ray	Lower dose of radiation than with CT pulmonary angiogram Can be used in people who are allergic to the contrast agent	Alternative diagnosis for the symptoms cannot be made if the scan is negative Loses specificity and therefore is of limited value in persons with other chronic or acute lung pathology Patients remain radioactive after the scan (difficult in nursing mothers) Patients with intermediate probability require a CT pulmonary angiogram
Ultrasound thorax	Fluid is a good acoustic window, and ultrasound is a non-invasive method for identifying the site and size of pleural effusions	Can differentiate amongst consolidation, air, and fluid Accurate marking of a safe site for pleural aspiration and biopsy Loculated effusions can be diagnosed	No radiation involved Safe site for pleural aspiration can be marked by the bedside Improved rate of successful pleural aspiration without complications	Users are required to be Level 1 competent
PET–CT	Radiolabelled glucose is administered, and areas with high metabolic activity have high uptake and show up strongly on the image	Accurate cancer staging	Cancer staging is more accurate than with CT alone	Cannot differentiate between infections (particularly TB) and cancer Malignant areas under 10 mm can be missed, so of limited value for assessment of small nodules Bowel has a lot of physiological uptake and there are a high number of false positives in this area
CT-guided biopsy	The site of the tumour is identified on CT, and a fine needle is passed to obtain a cellular aspirate; usual sites of investigation include the lungs, cervical nodes, and the chest wall	Diagnosis, usually in suspected cancer when histology for biomarkers is not required	Diagnosis can be made with safe sampling without general anaesthetic Well tolerated	Fin- needle aspirates provide small samples, so sufficient material for measuring biomarkers such as EGFR may not be obtained Cannot be used for suspected lymphoma, as it provide insufficient material for immunohistochemistry 10% risk of pneumothorax

An isolated reduction in KCO and TLCO in patients that have normal lung volumes and spirometry is seen with pulmonary vascular disease and may also be seen with early interstitial lung disease.

Approach to utilizing investigations in respiratory diagnosis

Pathological processes affecting the respiratory system may be broadly divided into three groups:

- primary diseases of the lung

- diseases that are part of a multisystem disease process (e.g. connective tissue disorders, other immunopathological syndromes)
- secondary physiological manifestations of disease in another organ system; most commonly, pulmonary manifestations of cardiac disease (e.g. pulmonary oedema) or neurological disease (e.g. weakness of the thoracic muscles)

Whatever the cause, the pathway to diagnosis is systematic and seeks to address three questions (see Figure 127.1):

- What is the physiological disturbance causing symptoms?
- What is the site of this disturbance?
- What is the underlying pathology?

Table 127.4 Endoscopic investigations in respiratory disease

Investigation	Description	Use	Positives	Negatives
Bronchoscopic procedures				
Bronchoscopy	A fibre-optic camera is passed into the lungs via the nose or mouth, under local anaesthetic and sometimes sedation; images are then seen on a screen	Visualization of obstructing lesions Targeted wash when infection suspected Bronchoscopy of bronchial and lung tissues can diagnose sarcoidosis	Quick Usually well tolerated Tissue diagnosis usually possible	Possible failure to get a diagnosis Typical complications include sore throat, sore nose, and haemoptysis; large-volume haemoptysis can be settled with ice-cold water and a 1:10 000 adrenaline solution
Bronchoalveolar lavage	The broncoscope is wedged into an airway of the affected area; 50–100 ml saline is used to wash the area and is then aspirated back; the fluid is then sent to specialized laboratories for analysis	Diagnosis of pulmonary infections and parenchymal diseases such as ILD	Can allow the diagnosis of parenchymal lung diseases based on the cell population that predominates; infection can also be diagnosed, although a wash alone is usually insufficient for this	Hypoxia proportional to the volume of fluid used can occur
Transbronchial biopsy	Parenchymal tissue sampled by pushing the biopsy forceps down a bronchiole until resistance is met; clopidogrel should be omitted for 7 days preprocedure	Diagnosis of parenchymal lung diseases, particularly sarcoidosis	Usually well tolerated	There is a 10% risk of pneumothorax Surgical-wedge biopsy is preferable in ILD, suspected bronchoalveolar carcinoma, and organizing pneumonia
TBNA	Blind biopsy of large lymph nodes around the carina at the time of a bronchoscopy; a CT scan is required to determine the site of the nodes.	Diagnosis and staging of cancer (sensitivity 78%, specificity 99%) Diagnosing TB Diagnosing sarcoidosis	Diagnosis and staging possible in centres without EBUS-TBNA so delays to treatment are avoided Cheaper than EBUS-TBNA	Success is operator dependant Diagnostic rate less than EBUS-TBNA Complications include pneumothorax, pneumomediastinum, perforation of adjacent structures, and bleeding
EBUS-TBNA	An ultrasound probe is incorporated into a bronchoscope to allow for detection of enlarged lymph nodes and fine-needle aspiration biopsy under vision	The procedure of choice for investigation of mediastinal lymphadenopathy Diagnosis and staging of cancer (sensitivity 82%–94%, specificity close to 100%) Diagnosing TB Diagnosing sarcoidosis (diagnostic in 88%–93%)	Makes it possible to avoid the need for a mediastinoscopy under general anaesthetic Can be used to stage cancer	Risks include bleeding, puncture of adjacent structures, infection, and pneumomediastinum Not widely available Mediastinoscopy for histology may still be required for non-diagnostic samples and for lymphoma
Autofluorescent bronchoscopy	Blue light is used during bronchoscopy; when viewed through a specialized bronchoscope, normal and abnormal tissues appear to be different colours	Diagnosis of carcinoma in situ and dysplasia Allows for targeted biopsies	Cancer can be detected and treated at a very early stage Clearance at surgical resection sites can be checked	Progression from dysplasia and tumours in situ to invasive cancer is unclear, so the usefulness of the procedure in improving prognosis is unknown Only available in a few centres around the country
Pleural procedures				
LAVAT	Procedure performed under local anaesthetic and conscious sedation by physicians to diagnose the cause of a pleural effusion; the pleural cavity is visualized, and targeted biopsies taken; the effusion can be drained and pleurodesis carried out	Investigation of choice for exudative effusions where aspiration is inconclusive and malignancy is suspected Diagnostic sensitivity for malignancy is 92.6%	Greater yield for TB pleuritis than blind biopsy Pleurodesis is successful in 80%–90%	Complications (2.3%) include pneumonia, empyema, and bleeding Not available at every centre
Diagnostic pleural aspiration	Removal of 50 ml of pleural fluid, under ultrasound guidance, using a green needle and local anaesthetic, in order to diagnose the cause of the effusion; fluid should be sent for pH, protein, LDH, MC&S, AAFB, and cytology	The effusion can quickly be categorized into transudate or exudate Empyema and malignancy can be diagnosed	Quick and simple to perform Well tolerated	Ultrasound guidance should be used to confirm effusion and reduce the complication rate from iatrogenic pneumothorax and organ puncture
Abram's needle pleural biopsy	Blind biopsy of the pleura performed under local anaesthetic and ultrasound guidance	Diagnosis of TB pleural effusions (however, 47% sensitivity vs 87% in CT-guided group); the use of Abram's needle is now limited to investigation of suspected TB only	Can be used in centres where CT-guided pleural biopsy is not available	Risk of pneumothorax and progression to chest drain Risk of bleeding High non-diagnostic rate

Abbreviations: AAFB, acid- and alcohol-fast bacteria; CT, computed tomography; EBUS-TBNA, endobronchial ultrasound-guided transbronchial needle aspiration; ILD, interstitial lung disease; LAVAT, local anaesthetic video-assisted thoracoscopy; LDH, lactate dehydrogenase; MC&S, microscopy, culture, and sensitivities; TB, tuberculosis; TBNA, transbronchial needle aspiration.

CHAPTER 127 **Investigation in respiratory disease**

Clinical assessment

Investigations are always preceded by clinical history and examination. Although respiratory symptoms are non-specific, they provide clues to the underlying site of pathology. A detailed respiratory history should elicit the rapidity of symptom onset, whether additional associated symptoms exist, whether symptoms are progressive or intermittent, and, if intermittent, whether there are identifiable triggers (Table 127.1).

Cough and wheeze indicate disorders of the airways. Cough that is productive of sputum indicates airway inflammation and usually involvement of larger airways. Breathlessness indicates increased work of breathing and is a ubiquitous indicator of respiratory compromise. Chest pain associated with the respiratory system is usually sharp and localized and indicates either injury to the chest wall or, if pleuritic in character, inflammation of the pleural surface.

Screening tests

Three screening tests, providing complementary information, are most often performed in an outpatient setting:

- SaO_2 (screening of respiratory failure)
- spirometry (screening of respiratory physiology)
- chest radiography (CXR; screening of respiratory anatomy)

In combination with detailed clinical assessment, these tests usually provide sufficient information to formulate a short differential diagnosis and direct further investigation.

What is the physiological disturbance causing symptoms?

The principles of investigating respiratory physiology have already been discussed and should inform the likely site of pathology.

What is the site of pathology?
CXR

The site of pathology is frequently evident on the screening CXR, which is useful for revealing structural abnormalities in extra-pulmonary tissues (e.g. skeletal deformities of the thoracic cage, rib fractures, diaphragmatic weakness), pleural pathology (pneumothorax, effusion), and gross changes of the pulmonary parenchyma (interstitial lung disease, consolidation, pulmonary oedema, soft tissue growth).

The CXR is often not helpful for characterizing pathology of the airways, subtle pathology of the lung parenchyma, and pathology of the pulmonary vasculature. Although pathology at these sites may be suspected from the clinical assessment and other screening investigations, the absence of abnormal findings on the CXR can also help alert the clinician to consider these sites more carefully.

CT scan

Continuing advances in scanning technology and computer analysis has put CT scanning at the forefront of detailed imaging for the respiratory system. A number of different scanning protocols are used to optimize imaging of different sites (Table 127.3). Not just a screening test, CT scanning should be regarded as a tool for detailed characterization of suspected pathology. Furthermore, 'low-dose' protocols of targeted imaging are available that significantly lower the radiation dose to patients and permit longitudinal evaluation of abnormalities, most notably pulmonary nodules.

PET–CT

CT scanning combined with positron emission tomography (PET–CT) is now performed routinely for staging of lung cancer (Table 127.3). An expanded future clinical role for PET–CT is likely, as research is presently being undertaken to evaluate its utility in the characterization of interstitial lung diseases, sarcoidosis, and pulmonary infections.

Ultrasound scan

Ultrasound scanning is useful for investigating pleural pathology. It is used routinely to guide appropriate and safe insertion of needles for thoracocentesis or for insertion of intercostal drains. Indeed, recently updated British Thoracic Society guidelines recommend all such pleural interventions should be performed with ultrasound guidance.

MRI

The role of MRI is presently limited for respiratory disease, although this is likely to change. MRI is useful for characterizing abnormalities of the mediastinum and can provide detailed images of the pulmonary vasculature (via magnetic resonance angiography), using software for 3D reconstruction. It is used for the evaluation of pulmonary vascular disease and assessment of the mediastinum in women of childbearing age, when radiation to the breasts is avoided, if possible.

What is the underlying pathology?

A definitive diagnosis may be achieved in a number of different ways. Structural abnormalities may be diagnosed with imaging alone. These include musculoskeletal deformity, bronchiectasis, and pulmonary embolism. Detailed characterization of interstitial lung disease with CT scanning can be diagnostic for subgroups with usual interstitial pneumonitis and asbestosis.

COPD and asthma are diagnosed using physiological criteria. For most other conditions, a sample of tissue is required for cytological, histological, or microbiological analysis. Different strategies exist for obtaining samples from the different anatomical compartments. These are summarized in Table 127.4.

Finally, investigation beyond the respiratory system will be needed for diagnosing systemic pathology that presents with respiratory manifestations. These will be guided by clinical suspicion and from results of preliminary investigations.

Conclusions

In summary, the breadth and scope of investigation of the respiratory system is considerable. The challenge to clinicians is to understand the choices available and organize a strategy for investigation that delivers the necessary information in a patient-centred and cost-effective way.

Further Reading

Diagnosis and Evaluation of Respiratory Disease. In Murray & Nadel's Textbook of Respiratory Medicine, 6th edition 2016. Elsevier

128 Upper respiratory tract infections, including influenza

Pippa Newton

Definition of the disease

Infections of the nasal cavity, sinuses, pharynx, epiglottis, and larynx are termed upper respiratory tract infections (URTIs). These include acute coryza, pertussis, sinusitis, pharyngitis, tonsillitis, epiglottitis, laryngitis, laryngotracheobronchitis, and influenza.

Aetiology of the disease

Rhinoviruses and coronaviruses account for the majority of acute coryzal illnesses. Other causes include human parainfluenza viruses (HPIVs), respiratory syncytial virus (RSV), enteroviruses, adenoviruses, and influenza. Acute coryzal symptoms may be an early manifestation of pertussis.

Acute sinusitis (<4 weeks duration) is usually viral in origin, with rhinoviruses, HPIVs, and influenza responsible for most cases. Approximately 2% of cases are complicated by bacterial infections such as *Haemophilus influenzae*, *Streptococcus pyogenes* (Group A streptococcus; GAS), *Streptococcus pneumoniae*, *Moraxella catarrhalis*, *Staphylococcal aureus*, Gram negative bacteria, and anaerobic bacteria. Chronic sinusitis (>12 weeks duration) can also be caused by *Pseudomonas aeruginosa*, *Bacteroides* spp., and fungal infections.

About 70% of pharyngitis and tonsillitis cases are viral in aetiology. The viruses involved include rhinoviruses, coronaviruses, adenoviruses, enteroviruses, HPIVs, influenza, herpes simplex virus (HSV), EBV, CMV, and HIV. GAS is the commonest bacterial cause, with Group C and G Streptococci, *Corynebacterium diphtheriae*, *Borrelia vincentii* (Vincent's angina), *Neisseria gonorrhoea*, *Treponema pallidum*, and *Fusobacterium* spp. less frequent causes.

Haemophilus influenzae type B is responsible for most cases of epiglottitis. Other causes include *Streptococcus pneumoniae*, other Streptococci, and *Staphylococcus aureus*.

Acute laryngitis and laryngotracheobronchitis are usually caused by HPIVs. Other causes include RSV, adenoviruses, influenza, GAS, *Corynebacterium diphtheriae*, *Mycoplasma pneumoniae*, *Chlamydia pneumoniae*, and *Haemophilus influenzae*.

Typical symptoms of the disease and less common symptoms

Acute coryza has prominent nasal symptoms associated with mild systemic symptoms. Clinical features include sneezing, nasal congestion, a profuse watery nasal discharge, sore throat, conjunctivitis, earache, sinus discomfort, and a cough. Systemic features include a mild fever, headache, myalgia, lethargy, and anorexia.

Pertussis has an insidious onset with an initial catarrhal stage followed by a paroxysmal cough. Initial symptoms last about 2 weeks and include sneezing, rhinorrhoea, conjunctivitis, and a mild dry cough. The cough worsens and becomes productive and paroxysmal in nature. It can be triggered by several stimuli, including laughing, yawning, and eating. Towards the end of the paroxysm, there is an inspiratory gasp of air, termed the inspiratory whoop. This may be absent in young infants. Paroxysms can be associated with cyanosis, subconjunctival haemorrhages, and vomiting. This stage lasts several weeks.

In young children, acute sinusitis often presents with persistent rhinorrhoea, a cough, and fever. Less commonly, facial swelling and tenderness occur. Older children and adults usually present with nasal blockage, purulent rhinorrhoea, facial pressure/pain over the involved sinus (if frontal or maxillary), and headaches. The headache is often unilateral and severe. Fevers are usually absent. Chronic sinusitis presents with a persistent cough, nasal blockage, purulent rhinorrhoea, facial pain/tenderness, and headaches. Both forms of sinusitis may be associated with nausea, lethargy, and a reduced sense of smell and taste.

Pharyngitis and tonsillitis are often associated with a prodromal illness including fever, malaise, headache, and myalgia. Acute coryzal symptoms often accompany the onset of a sore throat. Other clinical features may include gingivostomatitis (HSV), mouth ulcers (enteroviruses, HSV), soft palate petechiae (EBV), conjunctivitis (adenoviruses), cervical lymphadenopathy (HSV, EBV, CMV, HIV), a maculopapular rash (HIV), jaundice (EBV, CMV), lymphocytosis/atypical lymphocytes (EBV, CMV), and splenomegaly (EBV). Bacterial pharyngitis and tonsillitis are often present with a high fever, painful cervical lymphadenopathy, and soft palate/tonsillar exudates. In children, abdominal pain secondary to mesenteric adenitis may occur. The presence of an erythematous rash and a strawberry tongue suggests a diagnosis of scarlet fever (GAS). A greyish pseudomembrane at the back of the throat raises the possibility of diphtheria (*Corynebacterium diphtheriae*). Ulcerative tonsillitis with associated tissue necrosis is suggestive of Vincent's angina (*Borrelia vincentii*).

Epiglottitis typically presents with a fever, sore throat, difficulty swallowing, and breathing. Stridor may be present. Laryngitis and laryngotracheobronchitis may mimic epiglottitis in young children. Other features include a hoarse voice and barking cough. Older children and adults present with a fever, sore throat, and hoarse voice. Cervical lymphadenopathy may be present.

Influenza has an abrupt onset. Clinical features include high fever, headache, myalgia, arthralgia, anorexia, nasal congestion, rhinorrhoea, a sore throat, dry cough, and diarrhoea. The systemic features last a few days, but the cough, sore throat, and lethargy may persist several weeks. In children, influenza often presents with fever, cervical lymphadenopathy, nausea, and vomiting.

Demographics of the disease

URTIs are the commonest infections seen in the general population. Their incidence decreases with age. In temperate and cold climates, the majority of viral infections occur in the winter/spring months and some tend to occur in mini-epidemics (RSV, HPIVs, influenza). Influenza A and B may cause epidemics, and influenza A has caused several pandemics.

Pertussis, epiglottitis, and GAS infections primarily affect young children. Pertussis is endemic in most populations, with epidemics occurring every 2–5 years in late winter/early spring. GAS infections are commoner during the winter.

Natural history and complications of the disease

The majority of URTIs are short-lived illnesses that resolve spontaneously.

Acute coryzal illnesses usually last less than 10 days but can persist for several weeks. Their complications include otitis media, sinusitis, and secondary bacterial infections. They cause exacerbations of asthma and COPD.

Pertussis tends to last several weeks. It complications include cerebral anoxia, seizures, encephalopathy, pneumonia, otitis media, and bronchiectiasis.

Acute sinusitis of viral aetiology usually settles spontaneously. If symptoms persist over a week or there is an associated purulent rhinorrhoea with facial tenderness and a fever, then bacterial infection should be considered. Periorbital oedema, orbital cellulitis, intra-orbital abscess, cavernous sinus thrombosis, meningitis, osteomyelitis, and a cerebral abscess are known complications.

The majority of cases of viral pharyngitis and tonsillitis last a few days. Complications include secondary bacterial infections, thrombocytopenia, haemolytic anaemia, pneumonitis, encephalitis, and myocarditis. GAS pharyngitis and tonsillitis may be complicated by a peritonsillar abscess, otitis media, sinusitis, and scarlet fever. Late complications (several weeks later) include rheumatic fever and acute glomerulonephritis. Tonsillitis secondary to *Fusobacterium* infection can result in thrombophlebitis of the internal jugular vein, causing carotid thrombosis (Lemierre's syndrome). Complications of diphtheria include respiratory obstruction, myocarditis, and cranial/peripheral nerve paralysis.

Epiglottitis may be complicated by a bacteraemia and severe airflow obstruction. Examination of the epiglottis should not be performed until the airway is secured. Most cases of laryngitis settle spontaneously. Complications include respiratory obstruction and bacterial tracheitis.

Influenza is usually a self-limiting illness which lasts a few days. The associated malaise may persist for longer. Complications include pneumonia (viral, secondary bacterial), sinusitis, otitis media, myocarditis, encephalitis, and rhabdomyolysis. In children, Reye's syndrome may occur.

Approach to diagnosing the disease

History and examination play an important role in determining the likely diagnosis and differential diagnosis. The age, vaccination history, prominent clinical features, and associated clinical manifestations all provide important clues. Unusual clinical symptoms, signs, or laboratory results often provide additional information. For example, a young child presenting with coryzal symptoms, a cough, and a very high peripheral lymphocyte count is likely to have pertussis.

As most URTIs are viral in origin, it is important to assess whether the patient is likely to have a bacterial infection (primary or secondary). Knowledge of the usual pathogens and the proportion of infections that they cause often aids the assessment; for example, pharyngitis and tonsillitis in young children are most frequently caused by GAS infections, whilst in adults GAS accounts for only about 10% of cases. Bacterial infections should be suspected in patients with tachycardia, hypotension, a neutrophilia, and a high C-reactive protein result.

Other diagnoses that should be considered

These include otitis media, allergic rhinitis/sinusitis, vasculitis, retropharyngeal abscess, meningitis, and lower respiratory tract infections.

'Gold-standard' diagnostic test

For bacterial infections, the gold-standard diagnostic test remains culture. This also enables antibiotic sensitivities to be determined. Viral culture is now rarely used and viral polymerase chain reaction technologies are often now the preferred diagnostic test. The collection of appropriate clinical specimens for microbiological testing remains of paramount importance.

Acceptable diagnostic alternatives to the gold standard

These include immunofluorescence to detect viral antigens (RSV), the Paul–Bunnell test (EBV), and specific antibody responses.

Other relevant investigations

Routine bloods including a full blood count, renal and liver function tests, and inflammatory markers. CT imaging of sinuses may be required for suspected sinusitis.

Prognosis and how to estimate it

Most URTIs settle spontaneously without complications. The mortality associated with pertussis, diphtheria, and *Haemophilus influenzae* infections has greatly reduced following the introduction of vaccination programmes.

Treatment and its effectiveness

The majority of URTIs are viral in origin and require no specific treatment apart from symptomatic relief. Oseltamivir and zanamivir can reduce the duration of influenza symptoms and have a role in prophylaxis. Specific CMV treatment (ganciclovir, foscarnet) is primarily used in immunocompromised individuals. Antibiotic therapy should be directed against the likely causative bacterial pathogen.

Bacterial sinusitis may require antibiotics, although studies have shown limited benefit in uncomplicated cases. Typically, a 2-week course of amoxycillin, co-amoxyclav, cefixime, or macrolides is given and failure to respond to therapy necessitates ENT referral.

Bacterial pharyngitis and tonsillitis due to GAS is treated with a 10-day course of amoxicillin, erythromycin, or clindamycin to prevent complications and reduce carriage.

Diphtheria and epiglottitis require urgent airway protection. Antitoxin is given in suspected diphtheria cases and antibiotics including penicillin or erythromycin are used. For epiglottis parenteral ceftriaxone or amoxicillin for 10 days is recommended.

Pertussis is treated with erythromycin for at least two weeks. It reduces infectivity and may also reduce the severity and duration of the illness. Erythromycin is also used in prophylaxis.

Summary

URTIs are common and usually self-limiting illnesses. The clinical history, examination, and associated clinical manifestations often provide important clues as to the likely diagnosis and differential diagnosis. Assessment of the likelihood of a bacterial infection should help to determine whether antibiotic therapy is indicated.

Further Reading

Paules C, Subbarao K. Influenza. *Lancet* 2017; 390: 697–708.

129 Pneumonia

Pippa Newton

Definition of the disease

Pneumonia is defined as acute infection of the pulmonary parenchyma, presenting with consistent symptoms and signs and associated with new radiographic shadowing. It may be acute or chronic in onset and involve either one area of a lung (e.g. lobar pneumonia) or be multifocal in nature. It may be community-acquired or hospital-acquired.

Community-acquired pneumonia (CAP) is defined as pneumonia occurring in an individual with no recent contact with a healthcare setting, or in a patient admitted to hospital with development of symptoms and/or signs of pneumonia within 48 hours of admission. Hospital-acquired pneumonia (HAP) or nosocomial pneumonia (NP) occurs when a patient develops symptoms or signs of pneumonia after 48 hours of admission to a healthcare setting or in the context of a long-term nursing home resident. A subtype of NP is ventilator-associated pneumonia (VAP), defined as pneumonia occurring at least 48–72 hours post intubation.

Aetiology of the disease

The majority of cases of CAP are bacterial in origin and include both typical (e.g. *Streptococcal pneumoniae, Haemophilus influenzae, Klebsiella pneumoniae*, and *Staphylococcus aureus*) and atypical (e.g. *Mycoplasma pneumoniae, Legionella pneumophila, Chlamydia pneumoniae/psittaci*, and *Coxiella burnetii*) organisms. The latter are classified as atypical because they replicate within cells and respond to agents that are concentrated intracellularly, such as macrolides, tetracyclines, and quinolones. They are characteristically resistant to beta-lactams.

Viruses such as influenza, parainfluenza, respiratory syncytial virus (RSV), and adenovirus account for almost all of the remaining cases where an etiological agent is found. In some studies, the causative agent remains unclear in up to a third of cases. Rarer viral causes of CAP include metapneumovirus, measles, and varicella zoster. Primary viral pneumonias may be complicated by bacterial infections such as *Streptococcus pneumoniae, Haemophilus influenzae*, and *Staphylococcus aureus*. Rare causes of CAP include other bacterial infections (e.g. Salmonella typhoid/paratyphoid infections; *Bordetella pertussis, Leptospira* spp., and *Brucella* spp., and *Listeria monocytogenes*) fungal infections (e.g. Histoplasmosis, *Aspergillus fumigatus* infection), and parasitic infections (e.g. with migrating helminths).

Viral infections are the commonest cause of CAP in children under the age of 2. RSV, parainfluenza, influenza, and adenoviruses are the commonest pathogens. Mixed viral and bacterial infections also frequently occur. The predominant bacterial cause in neonates is Group B Streptococci, with other causes including *Chlamydia trachomatis* and *Listeria monocytogenes*. In slightly older infants, *Streptococcus pneumoniae* and *Haemophilus influenzae* are more common causes. In children over 2 years old, the frequency of viral, bacterial, and mixed bacterial and viral infections is similar. The viral pathogens seen are similar to those described in younger infants. The main bacterial pathogens in this age group include *Streptococcus pneumoniae, Haemophilus influenzae, Mycoplasma pneumoniae*, and *Staphylococcus aureus*.

In adults, the commonest bacterial causes for CAP are *Streptococcus pneumoniae, Haemophilus influenzae*, and *Mycoplasma pneumoniae*. In patients with underlying lung disease such as bronchiectasis and COPD, *Streptococcus pneumoniae, Haemophilus influenzae, Pseudomonas aeruginosa*, and *Moraxella catarrhalis* are common pathogens. About 20% of cases of CAP in adults are viral in aetiology. Influenza, parainfluenza, RSV, and adenovirus are the most frequent causes.

Immunocompromised individuals may develop CAP with the same organisms as seen in immunocompetent individuals. However, CAP tends to be more severe in these patients. Some immunocompromised patients have an increased susceptibility to *Streptococcus pneumoniae* infections (e.g. HIV infection and hyposplenism/splenectomy). Immunocompromised patients are also susceptible to opportunistic infections with microbes of low pathogenicity that rarely cause significant disease in immunocompetent individuals. These pathogens include *Pneumocystis jirovecii* (formerly *Pneumocystis carinii*), cytomegalovirus (CMV), *Cryptococcus neoformans, Aspergillus fumigatus, Nocardia* spp., and atypical mycobacteria.

The pathogens that cause HAP are usually different from those that cause CAP, except when HAP occurs within 5 days of admission. In that instance, the most commonly isolated organisms are *Streptococcus pneumoniae, Haemophilus influenzae*, and *Staphylococcus aureus*. As the length of inpatient stay increases, enteric Gram-negative bacteria such as *Escherichia coli, Enterobacter* spp., *Proteus* spp., *Klebsiella* spp., and *Serratia marcescens* become more prominent. In late-onset HAP (after 5 days of admission) other pathogens, including MRSA and multidrug-resistant (MDR) strains such *Pseudomonas aeruginosa, Enterobacter* spp, *Klebsiella* spp, and *Acinetobacter* spp., should be considered, and polymicrobial infection may occur. VAP is most frequently caused by enteric Gram-negative bacteria, including MDR strains, followed by *Streptococcus pneumoniae* and *Staphylococcus aureus*. Less common causes of HAP include anaerobes, *Legionella* spp., and viral causes such as influenza, parainfluenza, RSV, and adenovirus.

Typical symptoms of the disease, and less common symptoms

The clinical presentation of pneumonia may be acute or insidious in onset and will vary depending upon the causative organism and the immune status of the individual. It may follow an upper respiratory tract infection. Both constitutional and respiratory symptoms may be present and, in some cases, the constitutional symptoms may be more prominent. The constitutional symptoms include lethargy and fatigue, fever and rigors, anorexia, myalgia, arthralgia, and headache. Respiratory symptoms include cough (dry or productive), haemoptysis, breathlessness, and pleuritic chest pain. In some cases, where lower lobe pneumonia is present, the patient may describe abdominal pain.

Historically, CAP was divided into typical and atypical presentations, but studies have failed to accurately match the etiological agent to clinical presentation and these terms are no longer advocated.

Extra-pulmonary manifestations are less common and include rashes (e.g. erythema multiforme or nodosum), gastrointestinal symptoms (e.g. vomiting and diarrhoea), jaundice, meningitis, meningoencephalitis, encephalitis, myocarditis, pericarditis and delirium.

Elderly patients more frequently present with non-specific symptoms, especially delirium, and are less likely to have fever than younger patients.

Immunocompromised patients are susceptible to the commonly implicated organisms as well to opportunistic pathogens, and presentation will depend on aetiology. For example, Pneumocystis jirovecii pneumonia has an insidious onset, typically of several weeks duration. It often presents with a high fever and night sweats, weight loss, a dry cough, and increasing breathlessness associated with a progressive exertional dyspnoea and chest discomfort. Haemoptysis and extra-pulmonary manifestations, such as lymphadenopathy, are rare.

HAP can be difficult to detect. Patients may present with typical features of pneumonia, but more often their illness is non-specific. Sometimes, the only new feature is a fever. It should be suspected in any patient with a fever who has a recent history of reduced consciousness or known swallowing difficulties. In this instance, aspiration pneumonia should be suspected. VAP tends to occur in the intensive care setting, often in unconscious patients, but can occur in patients invasively ventilated via a tracheostomy. Such patients may develop increased respiratory secretions and worsening breathlessness in addition to fever and chest pain.

Demographics of the disease

CAP occurs worldwide with various incidence rates reported. These range from 1 to 36 cases per 1000 of the population. The highest incidence rates tend to be seen in small children (<5 years old) and in the elderly. The majority of cases of CAP occur during the winter/spring months in temperate and cold climates. This is when some of the causative agents, such as influenza, parainfluenza (type 1 and 2), and RSV, are most prevalent and may also occur in mini-epidemics. As *Streptococcus pneumoniae*, *Haemophilus influenzae*, and *Staphylococcus aureus* may complicate influenza, it is not surprising that these bacterial pathogens cause the majority of CAPs during the winter months.

There are several respiratory pathogens that are more prevalent during later spring or summer. These include *Coxiella burnetii*, enteroviruses, and parainfluenza type 3 infections. *Mycoplasma pneumoniae* most frequently occurs in later summer and autumn in the northern hemisphere and typically affects young adults. Every few years there is a worldwide epidemic. Infections with *Legionella* spp. also tend to occur in the summer months and, as these bacteria are spread by contaminated aerosols, cases may be sporadic in nature or be part of a localized outbreak.

Several potential opportunistic pathogens have a variable worldwide distribution (e.g. *Histoplasma* spp., *Cryptococcus gattii*, and atypical mycobacterial species). Others, such as *Pneumocystis jirovecii*, are often under-reported in some developing countries due to a lack of specific diagnostic tests.

HAP is the second commonest nosocomial infection and is most commonly seen in elderly patients. It is estimated that it extends an inpatient stay of a survivor by between 5 and 9 days on average, resulting in a huge cost burden to the healthcare provider. VAP is very common in the intensive care setting; the risk of a patient developing a VAP is of the order of 1%–3% for each day on a ventilator.

The few studies that have looked into age predilection have found that most pathogens affect the young and old in similar frequency. Having said that, *Mycoplasma pneumoniae* and *Legionella* spp. were isolated less frequently in the elderly, who were more prone to have aspiration pneumonia and infections of unknown aetiology.

Natural history, and complications of the disease

As most cases of pneumonia are bacterial in origin, the patient is at risk of clinical deterioration without appropriate treatment. Immunocompromised patients often present with more severe illness and have a higher risk of deterioration. For viral causes of pneumonia, the majority will settle spontaneously without specific treatment, provided the pneumonia is not complicated by a secondary bacterial infection.

The common complications of pneumonia include severe sepsis/septicaemia in cases of associated bacteraemia (e.g. *Streptococcus pneumoniae*) and pleural collections, which can be either parapneumonic effusion or empyema. Others include bradycardia (e.g. in infection with *Coxiella burnetii*, *Legionella* spp., *Leptospira* spp., *Salmonella typhi/paratyphi*), lung abscess, metastatic infection (e.g. infection with *Staphylococcus aureus*, *Streptococcus pneumoniae*, *Klebsiella* spp., anaerobes), necrotizing pneumonia (e.g. Panton–Valentine leukocidin *Staphylococcus aureus*), respiratory failure, acute respiratory distress syndrome, and death. In cases of pneumonia due to atypical pathogens, in addition to pulmonary complications, there may be complications associated with the extra-pulmonary manifestations of the disease, such as neurological complications from meningitis, or bleeding from an associated thrombocytopenia. *Pneumocystis jirovecii* pneumonia can be associated with the development of a pneumatocele, which may rupture, causing a pneumothorax. As opportunistic infections are often associated with disseminated disease, there may also be complications related to the systemic infection. For example, disseminated CMV infection may cause a hepatitis, oesophageal ulceration, colitis, adrenal failure, and a retinitis. Additional complications may arise for patients with VAP. They may be difficult to wean off a ventilator and, after prolonged ventilation, have an increased risk of herpes simplex virus pneumonitis and Candida infections.

Recurrent episodes of pneumonia may be associated with underlying bronchiectasis or an obstructing bronchial lesion. They should also alert the physician to the possibility of underlying lung disease, malignancy, or immunosuppression.

Approach to diagnosing the disease

The history, examination, and initial investigations, including the radiological findings, play an important role in determining the diagnosis and differential diagnosis. The age of the patient, the vaccination history (e.g. Pneumococcal and *Haemophilus influenzae* vaccines), underlying respiratory diseases (e.g. COPD, bronchiectasis, bronchial obstruction secondary to a tumour), smoking history (increases risk of invasive Streptococcal pneumonia), alcohol excess (e.g. *Klebsiella* spp., *Mycobacterium tuberculosis*), immune status (e.g. immunodeficiency, transplant, immunomodulatory drugs), any neurological illness (e.g. risk of aspiration), travel history, pets (especially birds) and animal contacts, and their clinical presentation all provide useful clues as to the likely diagnosis. Questions relating to recent contact with healthcare settings will help differentiate CAP from HAP.

For CAP, additional questions relating to the prominence of both systemic symptoms and extra-pulmonary manifestations may help to differentiate between typical and atypical pathogens. In the case of immunosuppressed individuals, the nature of the immune defect and the severity may make it easier to ascertain the likely cause. For example, HIV-positive patients are at risk of *Pneumocystis jirovecii* pneumonia once their CD4 count is less than 200 per cubic millimetre or 11% of their total lymphocytes. In the transplant setting, the timing of the infection post transplant often gives a clue to the likely pathogen. The presence of latent infections (e.g. CMV infection) may also be relevant.

Table 129.1 summarizes the different clinical features that may provide important clues to the likely pathogen in CAP. It also describes some of the clinical presentations that may occur in immunocompromised patients with opportunistic infections. For HAPs, the likely pathogens isolated depend upon the timing of the infection. In early onset HAP (between 48 and 120 hours post admission), the pathogen isolated is often similar to that found in CAP (e.g. *Streptococcus pneumoniae*, *Haemophilus influenzae*, and *Staphylococcus aureus*) but, as the inpatient stay lengthens, enteric Gram-negative bacteria become the predominant pathogens, and the risk of developing an infection with a multidrug-resistant pathogen increases, especially following repeated courses of antibiotics. A high index of clinical suspicion is needed to consider this infection, as often patients have limited clinical symptoms and signs. This is particularly important in the setting of VAPs.

Other diagnoses that should be considered

These include mycobacterial infections, cryptogenic organizing pneumonia, pulmonary emboli, alveolitis, pulmonary oedema, primary and metastatic lung malignancies, vasculitis, and pulmonary eosinophilia. Other infections such as typhoid, paratyphoid, brucellosis, and leptospirosis may present with symptoms and signs of pneumonia, often as a minor feature of the overall systemic illness.

Several illnesses such as ischaemic heart disease, peptic ulcer disease, pancreatitis, and liver or subphrenic abscesses can mimic the clinical presentation of pneumonia and must be considered in the differential diagnosis.

'Gold-standard' diagnostic test

As pneumonia is defined as inflammation of the lower respiratory tract, in association with radiological evidence of lung parenchymal involvement, the gold-standard diagnostic test for pneumonia is really

Table 129.1 Clinical features that may provide clues to the underlying causative pathogen in different types of pneumonia

Clinical feature	Likely pathogen
History	
Rusty sputum	*Streptococcus pneumoniae*
Exertional dyspnoea	*Pneumocystis jirovecii*
Prodromal flu-like illness or initial upper respiratory tract infection then lower respiratory tract symptoms	*Mycoplasma pneumoniae*, *Chlamydia* spp., *Legionella* spp., *Coxiella burnetii*, influenza, parainfluenza, RSV, adenovirus
Extra-pulmonary manifestations e.g. diarrhoea	*Legionella* spp., *Streptococcus pneumoniae*, *Mycoplasma pneumoniae*, *Coxiella burnetii*, influenza, adenovirus, CMV
COPD or bronchiectasis	*Streptococcus pneumoniae*, *Haemophilus influenzae*, *Pseudomonas aeruginosa*, *Moraxella catarrhalis*
Alcoholism	*Streptococcus pneumoniae*, *Klebsiella pneumoniae*, *Staphylococcus aureus*, anaerobes, *Mycobacterium tuberculosis*
Immunocompromise	*Pneumocystis jirovecii*, mycobacteria, CMV, *Aspergillus fumigatus*, *Cryptococcus neoformans*, *Norcardia* spp., mycobacteria
Animal exposure	*Chlamydia* spp. (birds), *Leptospira* spp. (rats), *Coxiella burnetii* (cattle)
Examination findings	
Bullous myringitis	*Mycoplasma pneumoniae*
Rash Erythema multiforme Eythema nodosum	*Chlamydia pneumoniae*, *Mycoplasma pneumoniae*
Vesicular rash	Varicella zoster virus
Maculopapular or macular rash	Measles virus, *Chlamydia* spp.
Lymphadenopathy	*Mycoplasma pneumoniae*
Meningitis/encephalitis	*Legionella* spp., *Mycoplasma pneumoniae*
Myocarditis/pericarditis	*Coxiella burnetii*, *Mycoplasma pneumoniae*
Limited chest signs	*Pneumocystis jirovecii*
Radiological findings	
Lobar pneumonia	*Streptococcus pneumoniae*, *Haemophilus influenzae*
Multilobar pneumonia	*Legionella* spp., *Mycoplasma pneumoniae*
Multiple pulmonary abscesses	*Staphylococcus aureus* (including PVL strains), *Streptococcus pneumoniae*, *Klebsiella pneumoniae*
Interstitial shadowing	*Pneumocystis jirovecii* (often perihilar), CMV
Nodular lesions	*Aspergillus fumigatus*, Mycobacteria
Laboratory findings	
Normal white blood cell count	*Mycoplasma pneumoniae*
Lymphopenia	*Legionella* spp.; *Pneumocystis jirovecii* and other opportunistic agents
Atypical lymphocytes	CMV
Hepatitis	*Legionella* spp., *Leptospira* spp., CMV
Renal failure	*Legionella* spp., *Leptospira* spp.
Haemolytic anaemia	*Mycoplasma pneumoniae*, CMV
Thrombocytopenia	*Mycoplasma pneumoniae*, CMV
Hyponatraemia	*Legionella* spp.

Abbreviations: CMV, cytomegalovirus; PVL, Panton–Valentine leukocidin; RSV, respiratory syncytial virus.

a combination of clinical features of pneumonia in the presence of appropriate radiological findings. However, it is important to note that the radiological features of pneumonia can lag behind the clinical presentation, and therefore it is possible that patients with symptoms of lower respiratory tract infections may not initially have radiological evidence of lung parenchymal involvement, but may develop it a few days later.

The gold-standard diagnostic test for bacterial and fungal infections remains culture. This enables antimicrobial sensitivities to be determined. For *Pneumocystis jirovecii* pneumonia, the demonstration of cysts or trophozoites in bronchoalveolar lavage (BAL) or lung tissue by methenamine silver staining is the standard diagnostic test, although polymerase chain reaction (PCR) is often now the preferred diagnostic test. Viral culture is now rarely used, and PCR is the usual diagnostic tool to determine the viral pathogen.

The appropriate collection of microbiological samples for culture, prior to commencement of antimicrobial therapy, remains very important, as the culture yield decreases significantly following antimicrobial therapy.

Acceptable diagnostic alternative to the gold standard

These include urinary antigens (for *Streptococcus pneumoniae*, *Legionella* spp.), blood cultures (in cases of bacteraemia), direct immunofluorescence on respiratory samples (e.g. *Pneumocystis jirovecii*, *Chlamydia* spp.), fungal antigens in blood (e.g. Beta D glucan for *Pneumocystis jirovecii*, galactomannan for *Aspergillus* spp.) or sputum (e.g. for *Aspergillus* spp.), cold agglutinins (e.g. for *Mycoplasma pneumoniae*), and the presence of a specific antibody response (e.g. to *Mycoplasma pneumoniae*, *Coxiella burnetii*, *Chlamydia* spp.).

Other relevant investigations

BAL samples are collected in cases of suspected VAP and may be required in some patients presenting with a non-productive cough. All patients should have routine blood tests, including a full blood count and differential white cell count, renal and liver function tests, and tests for inflammatory markers. Although CT imaging of the chest may provide useful information regarding the likely aetiology, it has no routine role in the investigation of pneumonia. It would be useful when diagnosis is in doubt or to investigate possible complications, such as lung abscess. Patients with associated pleural effusion should have diagnostic thoracocentesis under ultrasound guidance with pH testing to exclude an empyema and samples sent for culture.

Prognosis and how to estimate it

CAP tends to have a better prognosis than HAP. In CAP there are several different methods to assess clinical severity and prognosis. For example, the British Thoracic Society (BTS) guidelines use the CURB-65 score, which uses several clinical parameters (new onset **confusion**, a **urea** above 7 mmol/l, a **respiratory** rate of 30 or more breaths per minute, a systolic **blood pressure** less than 90 mm Hg, or a diastolic blood pressure less than 60 mm Hg and an age of **65** or over) to estimate mortality. Each factor scores 1, and combining the scores gives an overall estimate of mortality. A total score of 1 or less is associated with a mortality of less than 3%, while a score of 3–5 has an estimated mortality of 15–40% (see Figure 129.1).

The prognosis of early early-onset onset HAP is better than that of late-onset disease, presumably due to the reduced prevalence of multidrug-resistant organisms causing the illness. The crude mortality rate for HAP has been estimated to be as high as 70% in some studies, although this is likely to be an overestimate, as several factors may have contributed to death. It is probably responsible for between a third and a half of deaths in patients with HAP. Severity scores for HAP are less well developed than in CAP. Several factors known to increase mortality have been identified. These include evidence of sepsis (systolic blood pressure less than 90 mm Hg or diastolic blood pressure less than 60 mm Hg; greater than 4 hours of vasopressor usage; poor urine output (less than 80 ml in 4 hours), or need for renal support), respiratory failure (mechanical ventilation; requirement of over 35% oxygen to keep oxygen saturations over 90%), multifocal disease, and admission to intensive care.

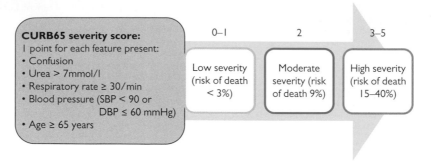

Figure 129.1 CURB-65 severity score; DBP, diastolic blood pressure; SBP, systolic blood pressure.

Reproduced from Lim WS et al. Defining community acquired pneumonia severity on presentation to hospital: an international derivation and validation study, Thorax, volume 58, pp 377, copyright 2003 with permission from BMJ Publishing Group Ltd.

Other factors associated with a higher mortality include underlying pulmonary disease, cardiac disease, immunosuppression, multifocal disease, and treatment delay.

Treatment and its effectiveness

As the majority of cases of pneumonia are bacterial in origin, it is important to start prompt antibiotic therapy for suspected bacterial cases. Treatment is aimed at reducing the severity of the illness, and potential complications. Empirical treatment is usually started, as the causative organism is often unknown at presentation, but treatment should be modified when microbiological results become available. Reviewing previously isolated organisms in the sputum of chronic respiratory patients may also provide useful information on any colonizing organisms and their susceptibility. Viral pneumonias may not require specific treatment but, for infections such as influenza, specific antiviral agents (zanamivir, oseltamivir) may reduce the duration of the illness.

In order to start appropriate empirical treatment, it is important to ascertain whether the patient has a CAP or HAP and whether they are immunosuppressed. Several treatment guidelines are available for the management of CAP, including the BTS guidelines, which provide advice of when, on clinical judgement, it should be safe to manage the patient in the community (CURB65 score of 0) and when admission to hospital may be needed (CURB65 score of 1 to 2) or advised (CURB65 score of 3 and above). For patients treated at home, the preferred antibiotic regimen is amoxicillin 500 mg to 1 g three times per day orally or, in penicillin-allergic individuals, erythromycin 500 mg four times per day or clarithromycin 500 mg twice per day orally. The same treatment regimen can used in hospital for non-severe cases of CAP when treatment was not started in the community. More commonly, these cases are treated with a combination of amoxicillin and macrolide, either IV or oral, and, for penicillin-allergic individuals, levofloxacin 500 mg once daily or doxycycline, with a 200 mg loading dose and then 100 mg once daily. For patients presenting with severe CAP, the guidelines recommend IV co-amoxiclav 1.2 g three times per day or cefuroxime 1.5 g three times per day plus an IV macrolide (plus rifampicin if suspected *Legionella* infection); in penicillin-allergic individuals, IV levofloxacin 500 mg twice per day is advised. The exact duration of treatment is dependent upon the clinic response, but it is usually around 7–10 days in duration for the more severe forms of the illness. The treatment of specific respiratory pathogens, once identified, is also discussed in the BTS guidelines.

Each opportunistic infection requires specific treatment. It is advisable to obtain specialist advice on the most appropriate treatment. For example, *Pneumocystis jirovecii* pneumonia is treated with high-dose co-trimoxazole (120 mg/kg day^{-1} IV in two to four divided doses) for 21 days, and steroids (methylprednisolone, followed by a reducing course of prednisolone) given to patients with moderate to severe disease. Following treatment, secondary prophylaxis with daily co-trimoxazole is given. For CMV infection, ganciclovir or foscarnet may be indicated.

The empirical treatment of HAP is dependent upon whether the infection is of early or late onset, whether there are features of disease severity, and whether there are risk factors for multidrug resistance. If the HAP is of early onset with no other associated features, then IV co-amoxiclav 1.2 g three times per day or IV ceftriaxone 2 g per day would be appropriate; in penicillin-allergic, individuals, levofloxacin 500 mg twice per day would be recommended. In late-onset disease, where the risk of multidrug resistance is higher, empirical dual antimicrobial therapy is often indicated. Treatment regimens may include IV ceftazidime 2 g three times per day, IV meropenem 1 g three times per day, or IV tazobactam with piperacillin 4.5 g three times per day plus an aminoglycoside such as gentamicin or tobramycin. For penicillin-allergic individuals, IV levofloxacin and/or an aminoglycoside may be indicated.

Summary

Both CAP and HAP pneumonia are common medical presentations, and the majority are bacterial in origin. The clinical history, examination findings, and initial investigations often provide useful clues to the likely pathogen. Clinical severity scores help guide the initial empirical treatment of suspected bacterial infections, and treatment should be modified once appropriate microbiology results are available.

Further Reading

National Institute for Health and Care Excellence. Pneumonia in adults: diagnosis and management. Clinical guideline [CG191] 2014. https://www.nice.org.uk/guidance/cg191

Prina E, Ranzani OT, and Torres A. Community-acquired pneumonia. *Lancet* 2015; 386: 1097–108.

Management of adults with hospital-acquired and ventilator-associated pneumonia: 2016 Clinical Practice Guidelines by the Infectious Diseases Society of America and the American Thoracic Society. *Clinical Infectious Diseases* 2016; 63: e61–e111. http://cid.oxfordjournals.org/content/63/5/e61.long.

130 Tuberculosis

Pranabashis Haldar

Definition

Tuberculosis (TB) is an infectious disease caused by the bacterial organism *Mycobacterium tuberculosis*. In this context, reference to the word **disease** is important, as TB implies *Mycobacterium tuberculosis* infection that is associated with symptoms. Approximately 10% of *Mycobacterium tuberculosis* infection is manifest as disease. In the large majority, *Mycobacterium tuberculosis* infection is latent and defined by evidence of a measurable and significant cell-mediated immune response to mycobacterial antigens in the absence of clinical or radiological evidence of disease. TB may be clinically classified further according to the site of disease. Miliary TB refers to systemic disease that may affect multiple organs.

Aetiology

Mycobacterium tuberculosis is one of four species (*Mycobacterium bovis*, *Mycobacterium africanum*, and *Mycobacterium microti* are the others) belonging to the *Mycobacterium* genus of the Mycobacteriaceae family. Collectively, these species share a close genotypic relationship and comprise the *Mycobacterium tuberculosis* complex. The microbiological properties of these organisms are unusual and of clinicopathological relevance. *Mycobacterium tuberculosis* is an obligate aerobe that resides intracellularly within cells of the monocyte–macrophage lineage in vivo. This adaptation is a form of immune sequestration. Structurally, the bacillus has a cell wall with a high lipid content that provides an effective barrier to immune and drug-mediated cytolytic processes. One consequence of the lipid cell wall is a comparatively slow rate of bacterial replication. In vitro, *Mycobacterium tuberculosis* can only be cultured using special media, and this may take up to 6 weeks. 'Acid-fastness' refers to the high retention of dye in the mycobacterial cell wall after washing with dilute acid during staining procedures and is a further consequence of its high lipid content. However, this is not unique to mycobacteria, and therefore identification of acid-fast bacilli at microscopy should not be considered synonymous with mycobacterial infection.

A number of other species from the Mycobacteriaceae family may infect humans and cause disease that may clinically resemble TB. Typically, infections with so-called non-tuberculous mycobacteria are more frequently seen in patients that are immunosuppressed or have chronic lung disease.

Typical symptoms of the disease, and less common symptoms

Symptoms in TB may be broadly categorized as systemic or organ specific (Box 130.1). The lungs are involved most frequently and comprise 75% of all TB cases. Extra-pulmonary TB may include any organ system, but most commonly involves intra- or extra-thoracic lymph nodes, bones, the gastrointestinal tract, and the genitourinary tract. Involvement of the CNS is uncommon (approximately 5% of non-pulmonary TB) but of disproportionate importance due to significant associated morbidity and mortality. Extra-pulmonary TB occurs more frequently in ethnic minorities and the immunocompromised. For the latter, miliary TB is significantly more common, and involvement of multiple extra-pulmonary sites should be considered.

Primary TB (see 'Natural history, and complications') is associated with some specific clinical presentations arising from hypersensitivity reactions. These include:

- erythema nodosum: reddish and painful raised lesions, most frequently seen on the anterior surface of the lower legs

Box 130.1 Symptoms of TB

Systemic
- fever
- night sweats
- weight loss
- anorexia

Organ/system specific

Pulmonary
- cough
- haemoptysis
- chest pain
- breathlessness

Lymphatic
- lymph node enlargement (cold abscess)*

Gastrointestinal
- non-specific abdominal pain
- ascites
- terminal ileitis†

Genitourinary
- haematuria
- dysuria with sterile pyuria
- prostatitis
- infertility

Musculoskeletal
- chronic osteomyelitis with focal bone pain
- chronic back pain (vertebral osteomyelitis)
- chronic discharging sinus
- psoas abscess, presenting with hip and buttock pain

CNS
- non-specific headache
- symptoms of meningitis
- cranial nerve palsies (single or multiple)
- hemiparesis (tuberculoma)

* Lymphadenopathy is most commonly cervical and confined to a single anatomical group. Enlargement is commonly painless to begin with but may become uncomfortable with increasing size.
† Involvement of the terminal ileum may clinically resemble Crohn's disease or appendicitis.

- dactylitis: pain and swelling of fingers and/or toes
- phlyctenular conjunctivitis: characterized by itching and soreness of the eye, with excessive tear production; usually, symptoms are monocular, and small grey nodules may be visualized at the conjunctival periphery; the condition most often affects young girls and is self-limiting

Systemic symptoms may accompany any form of TB and include intermittent fever, night sweats, weight loss, anorexia, and cachexia. Systemic symptoms can often dominate presentation and this raises diagnostic challenges; TB should be high on the differential diagnosis of all patients with an unexplained fever or weight loss, particularly if they are foreign-born and from ethnic minorities with a high TB prevalence in their country of origin (see 'Demographics of the disease').

Box 130.2 Risk factors for TB

Prior latent infection
- previous TB
- recent TB contact
- residence in country with high TB prevalence
- increasing age

Immunodeficiency
- HIV infection
- alcoholism
- chronic malnutrition*
- chronic kidney disease†
- diabetes mellitus
- immunosuppressant therapies‡
- haematological disease

* Malabsorption syndromes are considered to be in this category; jejunoileal bypass is associated with a higher risk of TB.

† Increasing TB risk with Stages 4 and 5 of chronic kidney disease; patients requiring dialysis are at the highest risk in this group.

‡ Notably, anti-tumour necrosis factor agents; consider increased TB risk in patients requiring this therapy for comorbid conditions; profound immunosuppression following organ transplant.

Demographics of the disease

The risk of TB is a function of two factors that reflect demographic characteristics of the disease (see Box 130.2):

- probability of prior latent *Mycobacterium tuberculosis* infection
- level of immunocompetence

There were 5,664 notified cases of TB in England in 2016 (10 per 100,000 population). The rising trend in this figure over the past 20 years is primarily attributable to immigration. Foreign-born UK residents comprise 80% of all cases, and limited data suggest that approximately half of these occur within 5 years of UK entry. Amongst foreign-born persons, the case rate is comparable with the reported rate for their country of origin, suggesting that TB in this setting is due to reactivation of imported latent infection (see 'Natural history, and complications'). Amongst UK-born Caucasians, the case rate is 4 per 100 000. Immunodeficiency is the single most important risk factor for disease in this population (see Box 130.2).

Worldwide, there are approximately 9 million new cases of TB and 1.5 million deaths due to TB each year. Co-infection with HIV is seen in approximately 15% of all cases for which testing has been performed and recorded. HIV co-infection is most prevalent in countries of sub-Saharan Africa (50%–90%), where the incidence of TB is also highest.

Natural history, and complications

Mycobacterium tuberculosis is transmitted almost exclusively by aerosol. Individuals acquire infection by inhaling droplets which are released by pulmonary TB patients when they cough, sneeze, or talk. Infectious droplets are typically 1–5 μm in diameter. Within this range, droplets are small enough to allow suspension in the air for several hours, increasing the likelihood of inhalation, and large enough to deposit in the small airways and alveoli.

Once deposited in the alveoli, *Mycobacterium tuberculosis* is internalized by resident alveolar macrophages. However, the development of infection and disease progression thereafter is variable and determined by a complex interaction between the organism and host immune response; this interaction is poorly understood (see Figure 130.1). The organism replicates within alveolar macrophages, leading to the death of the infected macrophages, and recruitment of further macrophages. An adaptive immune response develops in response to antigen presentation by dendritic cells at regional lymph nodes. Adaptive immunity is a Th1-driven, cell-mediated response that is measurable clinically 6 weeks after infection. Adaptive immunity may prevent disease progression in two ways:

- by *clearance* of the infection, via cytotoxic responses that effectively destroy infecting bacilli
- by *containment* of the infection, via a chronic inflammatory response that ensues after a failed cytotoxic response and leads to the formation of granulomas that localize the infection

In most cases, this 'primary' phase of infection is subclinical and leads to the production of Ghon foci, which are small, rounded, calcified lesions visible at chest radiography in the peripheral lung fields. They represent old granulomas and indicate previous primary *Mycobacterium tuberculosis* infection. The term 'Ghon complex' refers to a Ghon focus associated with ipsilateral hilar adenopathy.

Between 5% and 10% of primary *Mycobacterium tuberculosis* infection is associated with disease. Primary TB occurs most often in young children with immature immune systems that are unable to clear or contain the organism effectively. The tubercle bacillus may spread within the body by passing through the lymphatic system or the bloodstream. Dissemination of the infection via the lymphatic system most common and is typically associated with local or more generalized lymphadenopathy. Passage of *Mycobacterium tuberculosis* in the bloodstream likely occurs by direct invasion of the alveolar

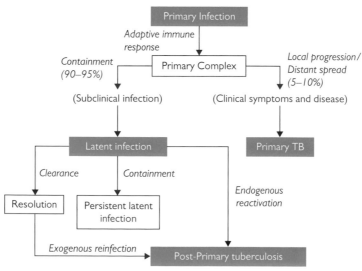

Figure 130.1 Natural history of infection with *Mycobacterium tuberculosis*.

Table 130.1 Disease-related complications of TB		
Body system		**Complication**
Respiratory	Lung	Pulmonary fibrosis, bronchiectasis, extensive cavitation with bullous disease, aspergilloma, accelerated lung function decline, COPD
	Pleura	Secondary pneumothorax arising from bronchopleural fistula, chronic tuberculous empyema with pleural calcification and pulmonary restriction
Cardiovascular	Pericardium	Constrictive pericarditis
	Myocardium	Conduction defects, risk of ventricular arrhythmia
Abdominal	Gastrointestinal system	Bowel strictures, peritoneal adhesions, protein-losing enteropathy with intestinal lymphangiectasia secondary to mesenteric TB lymphadenitis
	Renal system	Hypercalcaemia and secondary nephrolithiasis, renal papillary necrosis, tubulointerstitial nephritis, ureteric strictures
	Adrenal system	Primary adrenal insufficiency
Pelvic	Female reproductive tract	Infertility, ectopic pregnancy
	Male reproductive tract	Infertility
Musculoskeletal	Spine	Pronounced kyphoscoliosis (Pott's disease)
	Other bones and joints	Destructive arthropathy, pathological fractures
CNS	Meninges	Multiple cranial nerve palsies, neurological disability
	Tuberculoma	Secondary epilepsy, neurological disability
	Retina	Visual loss

microvasculature and implies miliary TB; in this form of the disease, lymphadenopathy may be absent. Primary pulmonary TB is notable for involving more often the mid and lower zones of the lungs; involvement of the upper lobes and apical segments of the lower lobes is typical of post-primary TB.

The term 'post-primary TB' (or 'secondary TB') refers to disease in individuals with previous *Mycobacterium tuberculosis* infection. In these cases, the duration of infection that is latent or subclinical is undefined and may be a few weeks or many years. Progression to disease in this setting is uncertain but likely to be heterogeneous. In some cases, disease will occur with disruption of the equilibrium between host immunity and viable bacilli (reactivation); in others, particularly older adults, disease may represent new infection (reinfection).

The complications of TB may be broadly categorized as those arising from specific organ involvement, and those arising from treatment (see 'Treatment and its effectiveness' and Table 130.1). Organ-specific complications are a consequence of chronic granulomatous inflammation that leads to tissue destruction, space-occupying effects, and fibrotic tissue repair (Table 130.1).

Approach to diagnosis

The diagnosis of TB can be challenging, particularly in cases of extra-pulmonary disease. The diagnosis is **suspected** from the history (see 'Typical symptoms of the disease, and less common symptoms' and Box 130.1). Appropriate radiological imaging may identify abnormalities that **support** this suspicion. The diagnosis is ideally **confirmed** by demonstration of tubercle bacilli in tissue samples obtained from the affected organ at microscopy (smear positive) or after culture.

Smear-positive TB is most common with pulmonary disease that is radiologically extensive and cavitating. For suspected pulmonary TB, three or more sputum samples are collected, preferably on waking. It is recommended that the samples are collected prior to or within 7 days of starting antituberculous chemotherapy. In patients unable to provide spontaneous sputum, samples may be induced with nebulized saline or bronchoscopy and washings performed to obtain samples. Children are likely to swallow sputum, and gastric lavage is often useful in this age group and often performed prior to considering bronchoscopy.

Culture confirmation is achieved in approximately 80% of cases with pulmonary TB. However, the yield from other sites may be considerably lower; for example, a positive culture is obtained in less than 50% of samples taken from extra-thoracic lymph nodes. For culture-negative TB, a hierarchy of other findings are considered appropriate for arriving at the diagnosis (see 'Other diagnoses that should be considered').

PCR-based molecular methods have been developed that offer more rapid microbiological confirmation of the diagnosis. Molecular methods are increasingly used in routine practice, and in some low resource settings, replacing culture based methods for the diagnosis of TB. The most well known commercial platform GeneXpert MTB/RIF (Cepheid Inc.) has near 100% specificity for Mtb. While not as sensitive as culture, a recent enhancement of the assay (Xpert ULTRA) offers sensitivity that is approaching culture and more robust detection of drug resistance genes. Results from molecular testing are available within hours, facilitating rapid diagnosis to guide immediate management.

Interferon gamma release assays (IGRAs) are enzyme-linked immunosorbent assays (ELISAs) that detect the production and release of interferon gamma by T-cells reacting to specific *Mycobacterium tuberculosis* antigens. Studies indicate that, while these assays are useful for informing *Mycobacterium tuberculosis* specific cell-mediated immunity, they are unable to distinguish between latent infection and active disease. IGRAs may therefore provide useful supporting evidence in the diagnostic evaluation of TB.

Other diagnoses that should be considered

The differential diagnosis in TB is broad and will depend upon the organ system that is affected. Most commonly, the differential diagnosis includes lymphoproliferative disease, other malignant disease, and granulomatous disorders, such as sarcoidosis and the granulomatous vasculitides.

'Gold-standard' diagnostic test

The gold-standard diagnostic test for TB is microbiological confirmation, with culture of *Mycobacterium tuberculosis*.

Acceptable diagnostic alternatives to the gold standard

A hierarchy exists for grades of evidence used in the diagnosis of TB. For patients that are culture negative with a clinical suspicion of TB, the hierarchy, in order of credibility, is:

- tissue microscopy revealing acid fast bacilli. Note that subjects with partially or completely treated TB may expel dead organisms that are visible at microscopy and in some instances the microscopic appearances are not sufficiently specific to be diagnostic. In treatment naive subjects, positive smear microscopy that is supported by positive rapid PCR testing is equivalent to positive culture for a diagnosis of TB
- histological evidence of tissue necrosis, lymphocytosis, and granulomatous inflammation
- radiological features of TB, with evidence of clinical and radiological improvement after treatment

Other relevant investigations

Chest X-ray

While routinely performed for suspected pulmonary TB, a chest X-ray should also be performed for patients with extra-pulmonary TB, as concomitant pulmonary TB often exists.

Bronchoscopy

Bronchoscopy is useful for obtaining samples from the lower airways in patients who are suspected of having pulmonary TB but do not have a productive cough. In patients with suspected miliary disease, a bronchoscopy with transbronchial biopsy may be performed to obtain samples of lung parenchyma that may reveal acid-fast bacilli at microscopy.

Evaluation of CNS involvement

While uncommon, CNS involvement should be considered in all TB patients, as this will determine the duration of antituberculous therapy. High-risk groups are those with miliary disease, children, and patients with concomitant immunodeficiency. For all patients with miliary TB, a CT or MRI scan of the brain is recommended and should be followed by lumbar puncture if appearances are not diagnostic but there is clinical concern.

HIV testing

UK policy recommends screening for HIV infection in all patients diagnosed with TB.

Vitamin D levels in plasma

There is in vitro evidence that supports a role for vitamin D in cell-mediated immunity to TB. In practice, TB patients identified with vitamin D deficiency may benefit from replacement therapy, although this remains to be clinically proven.

Contact screening

Recent close contacts of a patient with TB (usually other household members) should be screened for disease (via direct questioning about symptoms, and a chest X-ray). In the absence of evidence for active TB, current UK guidelines recommend screening of contacts under 35 years for latent infection with *Mycobacterium tuberculosis* (LTBI). This is diagnosed by demonstrating a positive reaction with tuberculin skin testing and/or a positive IGRA. Recent contacts under 35 years with LTBI are offered a prophylactic regimen of antituberculous chemotherapy that reduces the risk of TB for 2 years after contact by up to 90%.

Treatment and its effectiveness

Overview

In common with other chronic diseases, the care of patients with TB is best managed in a specialist, multidisciplinary TB clinic.

Current UK guidance recommends routine treatment of TB for 6 months. Treatment is divided into an early phase (Months 1 and 2) and continuation phase (Months 3 to 6). Early phase treatment is with four antibiotics: rifampicin, isoniazid, pyrazinamide, and ethambutol. In the continuation phase, rifampicin and isoniazid are continued. Dosing is weight dependent, and medication is available as combination tablets that may help to minimize prescription errors and improve treatment adherence.

Patient information

All of the drugs used for treating TB have significant side effects, and information about these should be provided to all patients before commencing therapy (Table 130.2). Ideally, this should be in the form of an information leaflet that is kept for reference. Although uncommon, side effects carry a risk of significant morbidity and may be potentially life-threatening. Patients are advised to report possible drug-related symptoms early to minimize risk.

Adherence to therapy

A crucial component of patient education is the importance of being adherent to therapy. This can be difficult for a regimen of many tablets over a long period, and the message may require reinforcement at multiple time points during the treatment course. Poor adherence is associated with an incomplete treatment response, and risks development of drug resistance.

Directly observed therapy (DOT) refers to observation of the patient to confirm that treatment is being taken, by a health professional or designated member of family. DOT is recommended for

Table 130.2 Antituberculous chemotherapy in clinical practice

Drug	Mechanism of action	Treatment independent and adverse effects	Monitoring	Patient information and other comments
Rifampicin	Inhibits mRNA transcription and translation Both bactericidal and bacteriostatic function	Hepatitis Rash Nausea, vomiting, diarrhoea, abdominal cramps Flu-like symptoms Inducer of cytochrome P450 enzymes	Liver function tests every 6–8 weeks	Patient should be alert to RUQ pain, pruritus, or jaundice Red/orange colouration of body fluids, particularly urine; this is harmless Accelerated metabolism of drugs may require altered dosing for warfarin and glucocorticoids Accelerated metabolism of OCP; additional contraception should be used Reduced absorption by up to 50% when taken with food; treatment should be taken at least 30 minutes before food
Isoniazid	Inhibits cell-wall formation by blocking fatty acid synthesis Both bactericidal and bacteriostatic function	Hepatitis Rash Peripheral neuropathy Metabolic acidosis (high anion gap) Sideroblastic anaemia Drug interactions may elevate drug levels of some drugs Epilepsy	Liver function tests every 6 to 8 weeks	Patient should be alert to RUQ pain, pruritus, or jaundice Patient should be alert to peripheral paraesthesiae or numbness, which can occur due to vitamin B6 depletion, which is the basis for pyridoxine supplementation Care with use in patients with epilepsy
Pyrazinamide	Inhibits cell-wall formation by blocking fatty acid synthesis Both bactericidal and bacteriostatic function	Hepatitis Rash Arthralgia Nausea, vomiting, diarrhoea, and abdominal cramps Hyperuricaemia Sideroblastic anaemia	Liver function tests every 6 to 8 weeks	Patient should be alert to RUQ pain, pruritus, or jaundice Arthralgia is the commonest side effect and is managed with simple analgesia; it is rarely of clinical concern May exacerbate gout
Ethambutol	Impaired cell-wall synthesis Primarily bacteriostatic	Optic neuritis Red–green colour blindness Peripheral neuropathy Arthralgia Hyperuricaemia	Visual acuity testing performed prior to commencement of therapy; repeated if visual symptoms are reported	Patient should be alert to any visual symptoms May exacerbate gout

Abbreviations: OCP, oral contraceptive pill; RUQ, right upper quadrant.

patients at high risk of treatment non-adherence (e.g. patients with no fixed abode); patients with serious mental illness; for disease with multiple drug resistance; and also for patients with disease recurrence after completing a course of therapy. For convenience, DOT regimens are intermittent (usually three times per week).

Drug-resistant TB

Fortunately, most cases of TB in the UK are fully sensitive to the standard regimen. Drug resistance may be to a single or multiple agents. Single drug resistance is most commonly to isoniazid and is covered by the quadruple regimen described. Multidrug-resistant TB (MDR-TB) is encountered most often in Eastern Europe and South Africa. Treatment for MDR-TB is usually prolonged and should be managed by a doctor with specialist experience. In the UK, a national internet-based forum exists for clinical discussion and advice of MDR-TB cases.

Extended treatment regimens

Antituberculous therapy should be continued beyond 6 months in:

- patients with a slow but continued response to therapy
- patients with CNS disease (treatment should be continued for 12–24 months)
- patients with MDR-TB

Additional treatments

Pyridoxine

Pyridoxine is usually prescribed with antituberculous chemotherapy to minimize the risk of peripheral neuropathy with isoniazid. A dose of 10 mg/day is routinely prescribed, but may be escalated in groups at higher risk of neuropathy. These include patients with malnutrition (who are likely to be vitamin deficient), alcohol dependence, diabetes mellitus, and HIV.

Glucocorticoids

Glucocorticoids have a dual role in TB therapy: as anti-inflammatory agents, and for cortisol replacement. Specific indications for the use of glucocorticoids are:

- TB adrenalitis with adrenal insufficiency
- gross cachexia
- TB meningitis (as glucocorticoid use reduces the risk of long-term neurological sequelae)

- TB pericarditis (as glucocorticoid use reduces the risk of constrictive pericarditis)

Prognosis and how to estimate it

The majority of TB cases are treated successfully with antibiotic chemotherapy. Prognosis is determined by the effectiveness of the treatment; the site and type of disease; coexistent illness; and the age of the patient.

Treatment effectiveness is a function of both the drug sensitivity of the infecting organism, and the site of disease. Sequestration of the organism in immune-privileged sites, such as the CNS and within cavities, will impair drug efficacy. In practice, a common cause for a slow or partial treatment response is poor adherence to the medication regimen.

In the pre-chemotherapy era, untreated tuberculosis had a mortality rate of 50%. While debated, it is likely that both effective chemotherapy and advances in social well-being have contributed to the decline in mortality and TB prevalence over the past 50 years. In the UK, current TB-related mortality is estimated to be 3%; however, this figure is age dependent and increases rapidly with age above 65 years.

Long-term TB-related morbidity is more likely in patients with prolonged disease, due to a significant delay in commencing treatment (either through delayed presentation or diagnosis), leading to extensive tissue destruction.

Further Reading

Alimuddin Zumla A, Raviglione M, Hafner R, et al. Tuberculosis. *N Engl J Med* 2013; 368: 745–55.

National Institute for Health and Care Excellence (NICE) guideline [NG33]. Tuberculosis. 2016. Available at: https://www.nice.org.uk/guidance/ng33.

PHE report for TB in England, accessible from https://www.gov.uk/government/uploads/system/uploads/attachment_data/file/654152/TB_Annual_Report_2017.pdf

WHO global report: http://www.who.int/tb/publications/global_report/en/

131 Pneumothorax

Saifudin Khalid, Rowland J. Bright-Thomas, and Seamus Grundy

Definition of the disease

Pneumothorax is defined as the presence of air within the pleural space. Pneumothoraces are divided into spontaneous and traumatic categories, depending on the presence or absence of preceding trauma. Spontaneous pneumothoraces are subclassified as primary or secondary: a primary spontaneous pneumothorax (PSP) occurs in a person without underlying lung disease, whereas a secondary spontaneous pneumothorax (SSP) takes place in a person who has an underlying lung condition, such as COPD or asthma. Tension pneumothorax is a medical emergency where air entering the pleural space on inspiration is unable to escape on expiration, causing mediastinal shift and cardiovascular compromise.

Aetiology of the disease

The aetiology of spontaneous pneumothoraces depends on their subtype. PSPs are believed to arise from the rupture of an apical sub-pleural bleb, which can often be seen during thoracoscopy. The exact pathogenesis of these blebs is unclear but smoking increases the risk of developing PSP, in a dose-dependent manner (the risk of pneumothorax is 12% in smokers compared with 0.1% in non-smokers), while cannabis use further increases the risk. Taller subjects appear to be at greater risk of developing PSP and this may be because the fall in intra-pleural pressure with the increase in vertical height contributes to the formation of apical blebs.

Many underlying ling diseases are associated with SSP, the commonest being COPD, which is responsible for over 50% of cases. Other common underlying diagnoses are asthma, interstitial lung disease, bronchial carcinoma, pulmonary infection (especially *Pneumocystis jiroveci* infection), tuberculosis, cystic fibrosis, and Langerhans cell histiocytosis. Catamenial pneumothorax is pneumothorax occurring at the time of menstruation.

Iatrogenic pneumothorax may occur during central line insertion, pleural procedures, or transbronchial lung biopsy, or in ventilated patients in the ICU.

Typical symptoms of the disease, and less common symptoms

A high proportion of patients with PSP with normal pulmonary reserve may be relatively asymptomatic initially and may not seek immediate medical attention. Symptoms tend to be more severe in patients with SSP, due to reduced respiratory reserve.

Common symptoms at presentation are chest pain and dyspnoea. The chest pain is usually sudden in onset and ipsilateral. Patients with SSP usually complain of worsening of their breathlessness.

On physical examination, signs of pneumothorax include tachycardia and, on the affected side, there may be reduced movement of the chest wall; a hyper-resonant percussion note; reduced breath sounds; and vocal resonance. In large pneumothoraces, tachycardia may be marked, and a pulse rate of more than 140, together with hypotension, may suggest the presence of tension pneumothorax. Cyanosis may be present in large primary pneumothoraces or in patients with underlying lung disease.

Clinical examination findings are often unreliable in indicating the size of the pneumothorax—many patients with PSP appear well even when they have a large underlying pneumothorax. Patients with SSP can be extremely unwell with relatively small pneumothoraces and it may be more difficult to interpret clinical signs due to the presence of underlying disease.

Demographics of the disease

The incidence of PSP is estimated to be around 18–28/100 000 in males, and 1.2–6/100 000 in females. The peak age of PSP is in the 20s, and the condition becomes rare after the age of 40. Patients with SSP tend to be older, with a peak age of 75 years. It tends to be more common in tall, thin males.

Natural history, and complications of the disease

A pneumothorax without a persistent air leak will resolve at a rate of approximately 2% of the volume of the hemithorax each day. Thus, a small apical pneumothorax can resolve completely within a few days, whereas a large pneumothorax may take many weeks. The likelihood of recurrence after a first PSP is approximately 30%, with most recurrences occurring within 2 years. After a second or third event, the risk of recurrence increases to 62% or 83%, respectively. The risk of recurrence for SSP is higher, with independent risk factors including age, ongoing smoking, and height.

Approach to diagnosing the disease

The diagnosis in cases of both PSP and SSP is often suggested by the clinical history and the physical examination and is confirmed by a chest radiograph demonstrating a pleural line. A standard postero-anterior chest X-ray is normally adequate to diagnose a pneumothorax. However, CT imaging is much more accurate at estimating the volume of pneumothorax and can clearly discern between large emphysematous bullae and pneumothorax, a distinction which isn't always possible with a plain X-ray. The absence of lung sliding on ultrasound is sensitive for diagnosing pneumothorax, although its use is primarily limited to trauma cases.

Pneumothorax size is usually estimated as either 'small' or 'large', depending on whether the rim of air around the lung is <2 cm or >2 cm, respectively. This approach is preferred by the British Thoracic Society and helps in formulating a management plan. Another method of estimating the size of pneumothorax is based an equation known as the Light index, where the size of the pneumothorax is expressed as a percentage: $Pneumothorax = 100(1 - Lung^3/Hemithorax^3)$.

Other diagnoses that should be considered

Moderate-to-large pneumothoraces are normally easy recognized with an X-ray. However, in the presence of large emphysematous bullae, pneumothorax can be misdiagnosed. It can be catastrophic to insert a drain into a bulla and so, if there is any doubt, a CT scan must be performed prior to any intervention.

'Gold-standard' diagnostic test

Although, in most cases, the diagnosis can be made on a postero-anterior chest X-ray, in cases of doubt, a lateral decubitus X-ray may be performed, as its sensitivity is superior to that of a standard chest X-ray. A CT scan is rarely necessary but is regarded as highly accurate. Where there is confusion about the presence of a pneumothorax or a bulla, the two can be differentiated by the shape of the pleural line—a convex-outward line suggests pneumothorax, and a concave-outward appearance suggests a bulla.

Acceptable diagnostic alternatives to the gold standard

If the diagnosis is unclear or if there is complex underlying lung disease, a CT thorax may be requested to delineate the pneumothorax and extent of underlying lung disease.

Prognosis and how to estimate it

In making decisions regarding the management of pneumothorax, it is important to consider the likelihood of spontaneous resolution and the risk and potential consequences of future recurrence. Hence, an asymptomatic, small, first, primary spontaneous pneumothorax can be managed on an outpatient basis, with simple observation, whereas a recurrent, secondary spontaneous pneumothorax causing significant symptoms will require early intervention and consideration of how to prevent future recurrences.

After a first presentation with a PSP, around 30% of patients will have an ipsilateral recurrence within a year, and the risk of a contralateral pneumothorax in such patients is 15%. The risk is greatest within the first year and is increased if smoking is continued. After a recurrence, the risk of a subsequent pneumothorax goes up to 50%. The risk of recurrence in SSP is greater and, after first presentation, around 45% of patients have a recurrence within 3–5 years.

Treatment and its effectiveness

The treatment of spontaneous pneumothorax differs depending on whether it is primary or secondary, the size of the pneumothorax, and the presence or severity of symptoms (see Figure 131.1). Management options available include observation alone, simple aspiration, chest drain insertion, and chemical and surgical pleurodesis.

Management

Observation alone

In the absence of an ongoing air leak, air within the pleural space gradually gets reabsorbed and, for patients with PSP who have a small (<2 cm) pneumothorax and are asymptomatic, it is sufficient to simply observe and repeat a chest X-ray at early outpatient follow-up. It must, however, be explained to these patients that, if they develop worsening breathlessness, they must immediately return to the hospital. Patients with SSP should be admitted to hospital. If such patients have a very small (<1 cm) or isolated apical pneumothorax and few symptoms, observation alone may be considered, if the patient is stable, with close chest X-ray monitoring.

Supplemental oxygen

Supplemental high-flow oxygen should be given to all patients, except those who have a history of CO_2 retention, as these should be admitted to hospital. Supplemental oxygen accelerates the resolution of pneumothorax fourfold by reducing the partial pressure of nitrogen in the blood, encouraging air removal from the pleural space.

Simple aspiration

Simple aspiration in PSP

Simple aspiration in PSP is relatively painless and is successful in up to 60% of patients. While opinion differs among chest physicians, simple aspiration is currently the recommended first procedure in

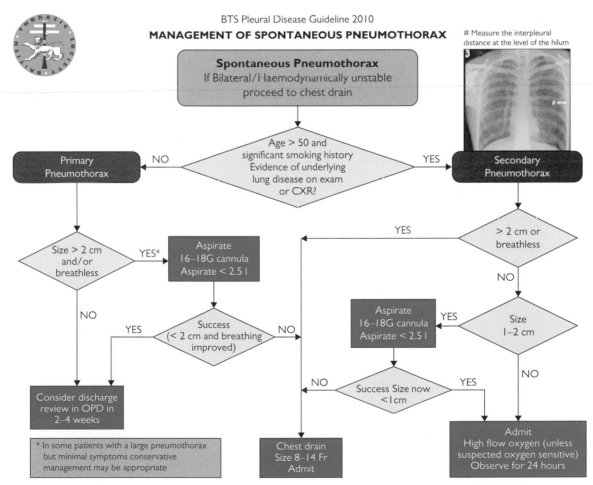

Figure 131.1 Management of spontaneous pneumothorax; BTS, British Thoracic Society; CXR, chest X-ray; OPD, outpatient department.

Management of spontaneous pneumothorax: British Thoracic Society pleural disease guideline 2010. Thorax 2010;65(Suppl 2):ii18-ii31. Available online at: http://www.brit-thoracic.org.uk/clinical-information/pleural-disease.aspx

PSP patients if they are symptomatic or have a pneumothorax >2 cm in size. The risk of recurrence after simple aspiration appears to be similar to that after chest drain insertion. Simple aspiration can be repeated once if there is unsatisfactory improvement after the first attempt but, if a repeat attempt is also unsuccessful, then the next procedure should be the insertion of a chest drain.

Simple aspiration in SSP

Simple aspiration in SSP is much less likely to be successful than simple aspiration in PSP and should only be carried out if the patient has minimal dyspnoea, is less than 50 years old, and has a pneumothorax <2 cm. If aspiration fails, a chest drain should be inserted before clinical deterioration takes place.

Intercostal chest tube drainage

Intercostal chest tube drainage is indicated for PSP patients who have failed simple aspiration, and for all SSP patients who have a large (>2 cm) pneumothorax, are symptomatic, or are more than 50 years old. Patients with tension pneumothorax require urgent insertion of a large-bore cannula into the appropriate intercostal space and, immediately afterwards, insertion of a chest drain. While traditional practice has been to place the cannula in the second intercostal space in the case of tension pneumothorax, a standard cannula may be of insufficient length to reach the pleural space, due to the thickness of the chest wall in this area. Consequently, if this first approach fails, the cannula or chest drain may be inserted in the safe triangle laterally. Most patients with traumatic pneumothorax require an intercostal drain.

In most cases, the initial chest drain should be a small-calibre drain, which is usually as effective as a large-bore chest drain and is more comfortable for the patient. Drains should be attached to an underwater-seal bottle. A swinging drain indicates that the drain is in the pleural space, while bubbling indicates an ongoing air leak. If the drain does not swing, it is blocked, clamped, or not in the correct position. A bubbling chest drain should never be clamped, as this can result in tension pneumothorax.

When a chest drain produces cessation of air leak and full re-expansion of the lung, it is usually removed after a further 24 hours. If the chest drain insertion fails to improve the pneumothorax, after around 48 hours, then low-pressure, high-volume suction should be considered. If this does not resolve the pneumothorax, a surgical opinion should be sought.

Chemical pleurodesis

Chemical pleurodesis with talc or other sclerosing agents such as tetracycline can be employed in patients who are not suitable to undergo surgery, due to their comorbid conditions, or are unwilling to undergo the procedure. Although the risk of recurrence with this technique is reduced, it is still higher than the risk after surgery.

Indications for surgical intervention

The common indications for surgical intervention include failure of re-expansion of lung 5 days after chest drain insertion; second ipsilateral or first contralateral pneumothorax; spontaneous haemopneumothorax; bilateral spontaneous pneumothoraces; and patients working in professions at risk (e.g. scuba divers, pilots). It can also be considered in patients with a first episode of SSP and who are at risk of serious complications from a recurrence.

Video-assisted thoracoscopic surgery (VATS) has generally replaced open thoracotomy, as it is less invasive. In PSP patients, VATS allows apical bullectomy, stapling, and pleurectomy. If pleurodesis is to be performed, this is usually achieved by mechanical pleural abrasion. In SSP with significant underlying lung disease, trauma to the lung may cause a persistent air leak, and simple pleurodesis with talc poudrage is most commonly used.

Further Reading

Bintcliff AJ, Hallifax RJ, Edey A, et al. Spontaneous pneumothorax: time to rethink management? *Lancet Respir Med* 2015; 3: 578–88.

MacDuff A, Arnold A, and Harvey J. Management of spontaneous pneumothorax: British Thoracic Society pleural disease guideline 2010. *Thorax* 2010; 65: ii18–ii31.

Pasquier M, Hugli O, and Carron PN. Videos in clinical medicine. Needle aspiration of primary spontaneous pneumothorax. *N Engl J Med* 2013; 368: e24. http://www.nejm.org/doi/full/10.1056/NEJMvcm1111468

Tschopp J-M, Bintcliffe O, Astoul P, et al. European Respiratory Society task force statement: diagnosis and treatment of primary spontaneous pneumothorax. *Eur Respir J* 2015; 46: 321–35.

132 Cystic fibrosis

Rowland J. Bright-Thomas and Andrew M. Jones

Definition of the disease

Cystic fibrosis is the most common lethal autosomal recessive disorder in Caucasians. There is no known survival advantage of the heterozygote carrier state. Chronic progressive pulmonary infection and bronchiectasis are the major causes of morbidity and mortality. The disease affects all ductal systems where the basic defect is manifest, including the pancreas, gastrointestinal tract, sinuses, hepatobiliary system, and male reproductive system, and has significant effects on nutrition and growth.

Aetiology of the disease

The abnormal gene responsible for cystic fibrosis is found on the long arm of Chromosome 7 and encodes a protein called the cystic fibrosis transmembrane conductance regulator (CFTR). CFTR is a cAMP-regulated anion channel responsible for chloride transport in the apical membranes of epithelial cells. To date, more than 2000 mutations affecting the CFTR gene have been detected, although only about 200 have been shown to be disease-causing, with the commonest one in the UK being Phe508del, found in 70% of patients with cystic fibrosis. Defects in CFTR affect ion and water transport properties across epithelia throughout the body. In the airway epithelium, the CFTR defect gives rise to viscid secretions which promote airway obstruction, bacterial infection, and chronic inflammation. The inflammatory process is characterized by infiltration of massive numbers of neutrophils into the airways. These release an arsenal of oxidants and proteases which damage the architecture of the lung and further enhance bacterial adhesion. The main bacterial pathogens in early childhood are *Staphylococcus aureus* and *Haemophilus influenza*. In late childhood and adult life, *Pseudomonas aeruginosa* predominates.

Typical symptoms of the disease, and less common symptoms

Although cystic fibrosis is a multisystem disorder, it is respiratory disease that accounts for the majority of the associated morbidity and mortality. Classically, patients have upper lobe bronchiectasis initially, which later becomes widespread. Typical symptoms are dyspnoea, malaise, chronic cough, haemoptysis, and excess purulent sputum production, although sputum retention may occur. The clinical course is punctuated by repeated infective exacerbations.

Demographics of the disease

In the UK Caucasian population, approximately 1 in 25 individuals is a carrier of a cystic fibrosis gene, and the disease frequency is about 1 in 2500 live births. There are currently >10 000 patients in the UK with cystic fibrosis, and adult patients now outnumber paediatric patients. Cystic fibrosis cases occur in all races, and cystic fibrosis genes are present worldwide but incidence estimates are not available for most non-Caucasian populations.

Natural history, and complications of the disease

The natural history of untreated cystic fibrosis lung disease is one of inexorable decline until death or double-lung transplantation. With expert care delivered at cystic fibrosis centres, this decline is extremely attenuated, albeit often with a high treatment burden.

Non-pulmonary complications relate to CFTR-mediated epithelial dysfunction (e.g. pancreatic, gastrointestinal, hepatobiliary, and sweat gland manifestations), systemic consequences of chronic infection (e.g. vasculitis and arthropathy), or a combination of these processes (e.g. poor nutrition and growth, and osteoporosis).

Pancreatic and gastrointestinal disease

Approximately 90% of cystic fibrosis patients have exocrine pancreatic insufficiency (PI), with clinical effects including malabsorption, steatorrhoea, malnutrition, deficiencies of fat soluble vitamins, and growth failure. PI patients need lifelong oral pancreatic enzyme supplementation. Exocrine pancreatic sufficient patients have an improved nutritional status and prognosis but a high incidence of acute and chronic pancreatitis.

Gastrointestinal dysmotility is common and may manifest as gastro-oesophageal reflux disease, delayed gastric emptying, reduced small intestinal transit, and reduced large bowel motility. Constipation is a frequent occurrence and may become chronic. Meconium ileus in infancy, and distal intestinal obstruction syndrome in older patients, are characteristic of cystic fibrosis presenting as small bowel obstruction secondary to the build-up of abnormally viscid material.

Hepatobiliary disease in cystic fibrosis

CFTR is present on the apical membrane of intra-hepatic bile duct cells. Abnormal bile salt composition causes cholelithiasis, which is present in approximately 15% of the adult population. Plugging of intra-hepatic bile ducts, with subsequent cirrhosis, portal hypertension, hypersplenism, and risk of variceal bleeding occurs in 2%–5% of patients.

Nutrition, growth, and bones

The poor nutritional state of many cystic fibrosis patients reflects intestinal malabsorption, the increased energy demands resulting from continual respiratory infection, and other factors such as cystic fibrosis-related diabetes and liver disease. Although growth has historically been poor in cystic fibrosis patients, with modern standards of care there is the expectation for normal growth in the vast majority of cystic fibrosis patients. The prevalence of low bone-mineral density is high.

Cystic fibrosis-related diabetes

Loss of beta cell mass, due to pancreatic destruction, end-organ insulin resistance and delayed absorption causes postprandial hypoglycaemia, impaired glucose tolerance, and overt diabetes mellitus. Approximately 25% of patients over 10 years have cystic fibrosis-related diabetes, and the incidence rises with age.

Sinus disease

The sinuses are affected in more than 90% of patients, and nasal polyps and nasal obstruction are extremely common. Medical treatment usually meets with limited success, and surgery is often required.

Arthropathy and vasculitis

Vasculitic rashes and polyarthropathy occur in cystic fibrosis adults with chronic bronchial infection and have been linked with circulating immune complexes.

Fertility in cystic fibrosis

Males with cystic fibrosis are infertile due to the absence or maldevelopment of the vas deferens. Assisted reproduction techniques such as sperm retrieval and intra-cytoplasmic sperm injection now allow males to father their own genetic offspring. Females with cystic fibrosis probably have near normal fertility but pregnancy can risk a deterioration in clinical status.

Approach to diagnosing the disease

Cystic fibrosis can present at any age but is usually diagnosed in infancy. Newborns may present with meconium ileus. In early life, failure to thrive, often with malabsorptive symptoms and recurrent chest infections, is common. Some patients are diagnosed in adulthood, with features including bronchiectasis, pancreatitis, nasal polyps, and male infertility, or on screening following the identification of a family member with cystic fibrosis.

Newborn screening programmes have been introduced in the UK and are estimated to identify >90% of newborn patients with cystic fibrosis. The test measures immunoreactive trypsin on a blood spot from newborns—those with a positive result go on to have a second test and genetic screening.

Other diagnoses that should be considered

In children who present with failure to thrive and pancreatic insufficiency, the diagnosis, once considered, is usually clear. Shwachman–Diamond syndrome, a rare autosomal recessive disorder characterized by exocrine pancreatic insufficiency, bone marrow dysfunction, and skeletal and growth abnormalities, needs to be considered. In adults presenting with bronchiectasis or chronic respiratory infection, the differential includes tuberculosis, non-tuberculous mycobacterial infection, primary ciliary dyskinesia, allergic bronchopulmonary aspergillosis, and immune deficiency states.

'Gold-standard' diagnostic test

Cystic fibrosis is a clinical diagnosis requiring appropriate clinical features. The sweat test is the gold-standard diagnostic test: a sweat chloride of >60 mmol/l is consistent with a diagnosis of cystic fibrosis. However, sweat chlorides as low as 30 mmol/l are seen in some patients, results can be unreliable in adulthood, expertise is required to accurately perform the test, and contamination can occur.

Acceptable diagnostic alternatives to the gold standard

With the advent of genetic screening, cystic fibrosis is often diagnosed on the basis of two disease-causing mutations. However, >2000 cystic fibrosis mutations have been described but not all are disease causing and the presence of two mutations does not signify clinical cystic fibrosis; the diagnosis requires characteristic phenotypic features and/or an abnormal sweat test. Whether healthy men with a congenital bilateral absence of the vas deferens, and two CFTR gene mutations, should be classified as having cystic fibrosis is an ethical dilemma.

Other relevant investigations

Nasal potential difference recordings may be useful in patients with a high clinical suspicion but with a non-diagnostic sweat test or without two identified cystic fibrosis -causing gene mutations.

Prognosis and how to estimate it

With aggressive modern treatment regimens and the multidisciplinary care afforded to cystic fibrosis patients, survival of cystic fibrosis cohorts continues to improve. The current median survival of cystic fibrosis patients is 40 years but extrapolation of the survival curve for babies born in 2000 suggests median survival may be >50 years.

Treatment and its effectiveness

Many cystic fibrosis patients have an enormous treatment burden, and care is best delivered at cystic fibrosis centres, where multidisciplinary teams of staff, including physicians, nurses, physiotherapists, dieticians, pharmacists, social workers, and psychologists, work together to manage the multisystem nature of the disease and achieve best outcomes. The cystic fibrosis team should also have close links with other specialist services such as interventional radiology, diabetes, ENT, obstetric and gastroenterology teams.

Pulmonary treatment

Chest treatment aimed at controlling airway infection, reducing airway obstruction, and improving nutritional status is the cornerstone of successful management of cystic fibrosis. Chest physiotherapy combined with adjuncts providing positive expiratory pressure and/or oscillation forms the major airway clearance strategy. Nebulized mucolytics and expectorants such as dornase alfa and hypertonic (7%) sodium chloride help clear respiratory secretions. Exercise improves prognosis and quality of life.

Oral antibiotics are used continuously, to control the burden of infection, or intermittently, to treat pulmonary exacerbations. A combination of a beta-lactam and an aminoglycoside are usually given intravenously to treat *Pseudomonas aeruginosa* infection. Patients with cystic fibrosis bronchiectasis typically require high doses and a long duration of antibiotic therapy. Nebulized antibiotics are predominantly used in patients infected with *Pseudomonas aeruginosa* to eradicate early infection, and to reduce the number of pulmonary exacerbations and improve lung function in those patients with chronic infection. Inhaled and oral corticosteroids are frequently prescribed in cystic fibrosis but evidence is lacking on their long-term benefit.

Double-lung transplantation offers patients with end-stage lung disease prolonged survival with an improved quality of life. However, lifelong immunosuppressive therapy is required post-transplantation and the incidence of early complications and later graft rejection is high, with a median post-transplant survival of 5–10 years.

Non-pulmonary treatment

Nutritional support is essential, and improved nutritional status is associated with a better prognosis. CFRD needs to be managed closely in conjunction between cystic fibrosis and diabetic teams. PI patients require lifelong supplementation with pancreatic enzymes and the fat soluble vitamins A, D, E, and K. Low bone mineral density is treated with exercise, calcium and vitamin D supplementation. Gastro-oesophageal reflux disease is usually treated with proton-pump inhibitors, and constipation with laxatives. Liver disease and gallstones are usually treated with ursodeoxycholic acid. In severe cases, liver transplantation may be needed.

CFTR-mutation-specific therapies

Restoring CFTR function is the ultimate goal of cystic fibrosis treatment. Patients with CFTR gating mutations have shown remarkable clinical improvements following treatment with ivacaftor, a small-molecule potentiator for CFTR. Another small molecule, lumacaftor, augments the transport of CFTR to the cell surface and, combined with ivacaftor, has been approved as a treatment for patients homozygous for the Phe508del mutation.

Gene therapy and future treatments

The CFTR gene was cloned in 1989 but initial expectations that gene therapy was just around the corner have been tempered by the complex genetics of cystic fibrosis, and difficulties finding safe, effective, non-immunogenic vectors. Despite this, survival continues to improve via the use of aggressive treatment; on the horizon are new inhaled antimicrobials and CFTR-mutation-specific therapies.

Further Reading

Elborn JS. Cystic fibrosis. *Lancet* 2016; 388: 2519–31.

Horsley A, S Cunningham S, and Innes A (eds). *Cystic Fibrosis*, 2015. Oxford University Press.

Plant BJ, Goss CH, Plant WD, et al. Management of comorbidities in older patients with cystic fibrosis. *Lancet Respir Med* 2013; 1: 164–74.

Stoltz DA, Meyerholz DK, and Welsh MJ. Origins of cystic fibrosis lung disease. *N Engl J Med* 2015; 372: 351–62.

133 Asthma

Andrew Jeffrey, Abdul Nasimudeen, and Joshua Agbetile

Definition of the disease

Asthma is a disorder of airway smooth muscle and airway inflammation, manifested by variable airflow limitation. This definition continues to be refined in light of developments in our understanding of asthma's pathophysiology, immunology, and treatment.

Aetiology of the disease

Asthma is genetically heterogeneous. While many genetic wide-association studies have identified common alleles associated with disease risk at all ages, its interaction with environmental factors remains very important. Identifying triggers, which include common environmental aeroallergens, exercise, and emotional factors, consequently play key roles in patient-focused management. Its presentation is correspondingly variable:

- early onset is associated with family history of atopy
- non-allergic late-onset with aspirin sensitivity (when with nasal polyposis, this is known as Samter's triad)
- occupational asthma; it is particularly important to seek occupational triggers in those presenting in adult life, as early removal from a sensitizer may lead to resolution of the asthma

Typical symptoms of the disease, and less common symptoms

Episodic breathlessness, cough, and wheeze, often with associated chest tightness, are regarded as the cardinal symptoms of asthma. Importantly, these symptoms occur at rest as well as on exertion in the vast majority. It is well recognized also that cough alone maybe the sole presenting feature, known otherwise as cough variant asthma, due to airways hyper-responsiveness, the absence of which, in the presence of eosinophilic airway inflammation, is the diagnostic criterion for non-asthmatic eosinophilic bronchitis.

The inflammation in asthma is described as being present from the tip of the nose to the terminal bronchi. It is debatable if this is always true, but rhinitis is frequently found in patients with asthma. This can be diagnosed by the presence of rhinorrhoea, frequent sneezing, post-nasal drip, and an impaired sense of smell. These symptoms should be actively sought in all patients presenting with possible asthma.

Demographics of the disease

Current estimates are that around 300 million people worldwide have asthma, with a projected increase by 100 million persons in the next two decades. Asthma contributes to significant morbidity. with disability-adjusted life years lost due to asthma worldwide similar to that for diabetes, and cirrhosis of the liver. Asthma is most prevalent in Westernized societies, affecting approximately 1 in 8 children, and 1 in 20 adults in Europe.

Difficult or therapy-resistant asthma is estimated at 5%–10% of those with asthma. Clinical trials aimed at escalating treatment until control is achieved in patients with asthma have shown that less than 60% achieve total symptomatic control. The reasons for this are not clear but are almost certainly multifactorial, including behavioural as well as disease factors.

Natural history and complications of the disease

Most patients with asthma are able to achieve adequate control of their symptoms with minimal therapy. Most continue to experience symptoms but not sufficiently to interfere with normal daily activities at a troublesome level.

Asthma does not actuarially reduce life expectancy, and the vast majority of sufferers will remain in employment until the normal retirement age. Many can undertake physically active work and athletic pursuits.

Many 'asthma scores' have been proposed to assess asthma control, but it is perhaps most easily assessed using three questions:

- In the last month/week, have you had difficulty sleeping due to your asthma (including cough symptoms)?
- Have you had your usual asthma symptoms (e.g. cough, wheeze, chest tightness, shortness of breath) during the day?
- Has your asthma interfered with your usual daily activities (e.g. school, work, housework)?

One 'yes' indicates medium morbidity, and two or three 'yes' answers indicate high morbidity.

The consequences of poor symptomatic control can lead to significant additional morbidity. Symptoms frequently unappreciated include:

- urinary stress incontinence
- disturbed sleep
- symptoms interfering with work, sports, or recreation
- side effects of therapy
- consequences of fixed airflow obstruction/airway remodelling, with frequent exacerbations requiring hospital visits

Approach to diagnosing the disease

Traditionally, the diagnosis and management of asthma has been based on patient-reported symptoms, with objective measures of airflow obstruction. More importantly, assessing the 'A to E of airway disease', that is, the factors responsible for morbidity in patients with airway disease—**A**irway hyper-responsiveness, **B**ronchitis, **C**ough reflex hypersensitivity, **D**amage to the airway and surrounding lung, and **E**xtra-pulmonary factors—both utilizes pathophysiological mechanisms and offers a more patient centred approach, particularly in difficult cases (see Table 133.1).

Other diagnoses that should be considered

Other diagnoses that should be considered include:

- dysfunctional breathing
- vocal cord dysfunction
- Churg–Strauss syndrome
- emphysema
- bronchiectasis
- left ventricular failure (in the older patient)
- allergic bronchopulmonary aspergillosis

'Gold-standard' diagnostic test

Asthma has traditionally been regarded as a reversible airway disease with a 20% and 400 ml improvement in FEV_1 following bronchodilation with salbutamol. More advanced techniques, such as airway inflammometry using induced sputum differentials, are helpful in both the diagnosis and management of difficult cases. Direct and indirect airway challenges are becoming more readily available and give useful information to airway hyper-responsiveness, which is itself often mediated through airway inflammation.

Table 133.1 The A to E of airway disease

	Clinical features	Definition	Physiology	Pathology	Mechanism	Existing treatments	Potential new treatments
Airway hyperresponsiveness	Short-term variable breathless, wheeze and chest tightness (i.e. over minutes or hours) Often exercise-induced and nocturnal	One or more of: methacholine PC20 <8 mg/mL; >12% improvement in FEV1 after inhaled bronchodilator; >20% within day variability in peak expiratory flow	Bronchodilator responsive airflow obstruction Exaggerated bronchoconstrictor response to constrictor stimuli Deep breath-induced bronchodilatation	Mast cell infiltration of airway smooth muscle Increased airway smooth muscle mass	Direct interaction between mast cells and airway smooth muscle involving multiple mediators, including histamine, cysteinyl-LT, PGD2 Increased airway smooth muscle contractility Altered airway smooth muscle phenotype	Short- and long-acting β2-agonists Anti-muscarinic agents Inhaled corticosteroids	Bronchial thermoplasty TNF-α antagonists
Bronchitis	Exacerbations, particularly when co-existing with an acute inflammatory stimulus and if A and/or D are present Cough with morning sputum May be clinically silent	Raised induced sputum eosinophil (>2%) or neutrophil (>61%) count Raised neutrophil and total inflammatory cell count may suggest infection Raised exhaled nitric oxide concentration suggests eosinophilic airway inflammation	Bronchodilator resistant corticosteroid responsive airflow obstruction (eosinophilic) Deep breath-induced bronchoconstriction	Eosinophilic or neutrophilic infiltration of mucosa Goblet cell hyperplasia	Allergic, Th2 cytokine driven (eosinophilic) or infection/innate immune response driven (neutrophilic) Airflow obstruction as a result of mucosal oedema and intraluminal impaction with mucus and cellular debris	Inhaled and oral corticosteroids for eosinophilic bronchitis; latter may be more effective for small airway disease Anti-leukotrienes Antibiotics for infective neutrophilic bronchitis	Eosinophilic: • Omalizumab • Mepolizumab Neutrophilic: long-term macrolide antibiotics
Cough reflex hypersensitivity	Excess dry cough with changes in temperature, fumes, talking, laughing	Capsaicin cough reflex hypersensitivity	Heightened cough response to inhaled tussive stimuli such as capsaicin and citric acid	Increased sputum neutrophil numbers BAL lymphocytosis in some Sputum and airway mucosal eosinophilia in 10–15%	Sensitization of sensory nerve endings by pro-tussive mediators such as histamine and PGE2	Removal of aggravating factors (smoking, angiotensin converting enzyme inhibitor therapy, gastrooesophageal reflux, rhinitis) Inhaled and oral corticosteroids helpful in eosinophilic disease	None
Damage	Non-variable breathlessness, wheeze and chest tightness Chest deformity	Post-bronchodilator and oral corticosteroid FEV1/FVC <70% Impaired gas transfer CT criteria for emphysema and bronchiectasis	Bronchodilator resistant corticosteroid unresponsive airflow obstruction Impaired gas transfer Increased lung volumes	Emphysema Small airway fibrosis Thickening of basement membrane Increased lymphoid follicles Bronchiectasis	Likely a result of chronic airway inflammation, particularly if multiple inflammatory hits Airflow obstruction as a result of progressive small airway constriction and loss of airway support Reduction of area for gas exchange Damage induced by aspergillus sensitization and colonization	Smoking cessation	Lung volume reduction for emphysema
Extrapulmonary factors	Episodic dyspnoea and chest tightness Weight loss or gain Rhinitis Premature vascular disease	Specific to individual extrapulmonary factor	Altered vascular reactivity Muscle weakness	Increased systemic inflammation	Hyperventilation Upper airway obstruction and hypersensitivity Vocal cord dysfunction Insulin resistance Muscle wasting Loss of confidence Effect of obesity on lung function Poor adherence with therapy	Breathing retraining Nasal corticosteroids Modification of vascular risk factors Weight loss or dietary support Pulmonary rehabilitation	Anabolic agents

Factors potentially responsible for symptoms and morbidity in a patient with airway disease.

Abbreviations: BAL, bronchoalveolar lavage; FEV1, forced expiratory volume in 1 second; FVC, forced vital capacity; LT, leukotriene; PC20, the provocative concentration required to cause a 20% fall in FEV1; PG, prostaglandin; Th2, T-helper type 2.

Reproduced with permission from D. Pavord and A. J. Wardlaw, The A to E of airway disease, *Clinical & Experimental Allergy*, Volume 40, pp.62–67 Copyright © 2010 John Wiley and Sons.

Acceptable diagnostic alternatives to the gold standard

Home peak flow monitoring, if carried out twice or three times daily, can demonstrate the classical diurnal variation of asthma. Variation should be more than 20%, with a repeated pattern each day: most commonly, the lowest reading being seen first thing in the morning. A therapeutic trial is sometimes required in cases of diagnostic uncertainty of reversible airflow obstruction with either oral prednisolone 30 mg daily for two weeks, or an inhaled corticosteroid for a month.

Other relevant investigations

Other relevant investigations include:

- historical blood eosinophil counts (>4%)
- allergy testing with skin-prick measurements against common aeroallergens such as house dust mite, cat, dog, grass, and fungi, or other specific IgE
- total IgE
- aspergillus IgE and aspergillus IgG
- CT chest
- antineutrophil cytoplasmic antibodies (ANCAs)
- CT nose and sinuses (if symptoms of rhinitis are present)
- FeNO-Fractional expired Nitric Oxide as a measure of eosinophilic inflammation

Prognosis and how to estimate it

The prognosis for patients with asthma is one of ongoing symptoms with significant variability. Many, when they are between the ages of 14 and 25, experience an improvement in symptoms, with this improvement perhaps related to adolescence with its hormonal changes and the growth spurt. In later life, patients can experience periods of up to several years during which symptoms become worse or settle, apparently spontaneously.

Asthmatic patients who are likely to develop treatment-resistant disease and so are at high risk of dying include those who demonstrate:

- non-compliance with treatment or monitoring
- failure to attend appointments
- fewer GP contacts
- frequent home visits
- self-discharge from hospital
- psychosis, depression, other psychiatric illness, or deliberate self-harm
- current or recent major tranquillizer use
- denial
- alcohol or drug abuse
- obesity
- learning difficulties
- employment problems
- income problems
- social isolation
- childhood abuse
- severe domestic, marital, or legal stress

Persistent airflow obstruction has been defined as a post-bronchodilator FEV_1:FVC ratio <0.70, or FEV_1 <80%. This is a frequent observation in therapy-resistant asthma and is thought to arise from factors including smoking, duration of disease, and fungal sensitization. Other risk factors include female gender and genetic factors (e.g. *ADAM33* polymorphisms).

Treatment and its effectiveness

Treatment is summarized in Table 133.1. It can be divided into non-pharmacological of chronic asthma, pharmacological treatment of chronic asthma, and the treatment of acute exacerbations.

Non-pharmacological treatment of chronic asthma

Self-management plans

Most exacerbations of asthma have a preceding history of poor control, a fact often underappreciated by patients. Utilizing peak-flow measurements combined with an action plan allows patients to take more control of their care as well as aborting early exacerbations.

Allergen avoidance

Specific allergic triggers are more readily identified in children with asthma than in most adults. Where present, suitable avoidance strategies should be developed with the patient. Simple domestic measures such as keeping humidity levels low to discourage house dust mite proliferation, and barrier covers for bedding, can be effective. Desensitization is rarely practical, as most patients have multiple allergies but, where dominant allergens are identified, this approach can sometimes be effective in reducing overall symptoms. Similarly, removal of domestic animals to which the patient is allergic can be helpful. There is emerging data suggesting significant improvements in asthma quality of life when nocturnal temperature-controlled laminar airflow treatment, which reduces levels of inhaled allergens and other particles, is used in atopic patients.

Pulmonary rehabilitation

Pulmonary rehabilitation schemes have consistently been shown to be of significant benefit to patients with chronic pulmonary disease, most often COPD. In patients with severe asthma, similar benefits have been found, particularly in deconditioned patients.

Psychological interventions

When psychological issues (predominantly anxiety and depression) are recognized, appropriate interventions—relaxation, counselling, cognitive behavioural therapy, or more complex psychological therapies—should be considered. There is insufficient evidence to indicate routine psychological interventions for most patients.

Pharmacological treatment of chronic asthma

Upper and lower airways

If there is evidence of nasal involvement, this must be treated actively, if overall good control is to be achieved. The choice of inhaler device can be critical in ensuring that the medication reaches the appropriate part of the airway. As well as the ability of the patient to use the relevant device, device flow characteristics and particle size and mass are important in achieving this end. Systemic therapies ensure that the whole airway is treated but, in general, produce more side effects than topical treatments; hence, the latter represent the preferred option for achieving long-term control.

Stepwise incremental management

All national and international guidelines advocate a stepwise approach to the pharmacological treatment of asthma, generally having five steps, with Step 5 including oral steroids. If the patient's first presentation is with a significant episode, then treatment should be started on at least Step 3 and titrated down with improvement in symptoms. Only the mildest symptoms should be treated with the lowest dose therapy (usually bronchodilators alone) in the first instance. The key therapy at all but Step 1 is an inhaled steroid whose dose is increased before introducing long-acting bronchodilators, as separate- or single-inhaler combinations, and subsequently systemic therapies, such as leukotriene antagonists and/or theophyllines. Increasing inhaled steroid doses beyond the equivalent of 1000 µg/day is of doubtful benefit in the majority of patients.

Single-inhaler therapy

Single-inhaler, or combination inhaler, therapy is appropriate for those who do not achieve adequate control on low-dose inhaled steroids and, as required, short-acting bronchodilators. The usual combination is of an inhaled steroid and a long-acting beta agonist. Several different preparations are available and, in general, produce similar overall benefit, the choice being made on the convenience of the device, the need for targeting specific parts of the airway (see 'Small airways targeted treatment'), and patient response to the therapy. If response is poor, an alternative combination should be tried before moving up to the next therapeutic step.

Although normally prescribed in a fixed-dosage regimen, there is evidence that single-inhaler therapies can be used in a more flexible manner during exacerbations. The data are best for the combination of formoterol and budesonide in a dry powder preparation which has been shown to be effective when taken up to six times in a day. Similar effects may exist for other combinations, but there is little published evidence to support this.

Small airways targeted treatment

The small particle size found in two beclomethasone preparations has been shown to result in a higher deposition in the smallest airways. Although there is little or no smooth muscle in these airways, symptoms resulting from their inflammation benefit from direct topical treatment. It is also believed that inflammation in one part of the airway exacerbates inflammation found at other levels (the one airway hypothesis). Although the evidence for overall better symptom control through specifically targeting small airways in all patients is not robust, it is worth considering when control is not easily achieved with large-particle drugs.

Anti-IgE therapy

Omalizumab, an anti-IgE monoclonal antibody therapy, is available for the treatment of resistant asthma. It is given as a once fortnightly or once weekly subcutaneous injection and is indicated when asthma control is poor, exacerbations frequent and potentially life-threatening, and blood IgE levels are elevated. The long-term side effects are not yet clear, but the majority of patients tolerate the injections with only minor discomfort at the injection site. Cost and the logistics of administering the drug are significant barriers to its widespread use at present, although the benefits in some individuals can be quite dramatic.

Antifungal therapy

While steroids have traditionally been the mainstay of therapy in those with allergic bronchopulmonary aspergillosis, antifungal therapy has been shown to offer additional benefits in steroid reduction. Patients with severe asthma and sensitization to fungal allergens but not fulfilling the criteria for allergic bronchopulmonary aspergillosis have also been shown to benefit from antifungal therapy, with improvements in quality of life.

Treatment of premenstrual/menstrual asthma

Most women with asthma will experience variation of their symptoms with the phase of their menstrual cycle. For the vast majority, this difference will be small and not pose an issue. For the minority in whom it is a dominant feature, treatment is indicated. These women present with monthly variations on symptoms, most commonly worst in the week before the and during the onset of their menstrual bleed. The administration of a single-depot contraceptive injection is a useful diagnostic step, as it will substantially relieve the problem with immediate effect. If shown to be helpful, either depot injections or tricycling (taking 3 months of tablets without a monthly break) oral contraceptives can be helpful.

Treatment of acute exacerbations

Exacerbations of asthma can be life-threatening and are always debilitating and frightening for the patient. Severe exacerbations resulting in hospital admission most often occur on a background of ongoing symptomatic disease. Occasionally, severe episodes can have a very rapid onset in a normally asymptomatic patient (so-called type 1 brittle asthma). More often, the exacerbation is mild to moderate and results from an identifiable trigger such as an intercurrent viral infection, or exposure to a known allergic trigger.

Initial assessment includes confirmation of the diagnosis and early physiological assessment. This should include peak expiratory flow and oxygen saturation measurements. The history may be hard to get at presentation. Inability to complete sentences due to breathlessness, poor air entry, or any element of confusion is an indicator of a severe attack.

For mild (peak expiratory flow rate (PEFR) fall of less than 20% from usual levels) to moderate (PEFR fall of 20%–40%) attacks, nebulized bronchodilators may be required. In a mild exacerbation in a patient on Step 1 or 2, the dose of inhaled corticosteroids may be increased but, in all others in these groups, a course of oral corticosteroids should be prescribed at approximately 0.5 mg/kg. There is little good evidence to determine the ideal length of the course, but the dose should not be reduced until the symptoms have settled and the PEFR returned to normal. The dose need not be tailed off unless the course exceeds 2 weeks or there have been previous courses of oral steroids within the preceding 3 months.

In severe exacerbations, after initial therapy with nebulized bronchodilators, preferably delivered by an oxygen-driven nebulizer, intravenous steroids should be given. Close monitoring is needed and should be undertaken in a hospital setting where full resuscitation, including access to mechanical ventilation, is available. The monitoring should include close personal observation of the patient to check for signs of exhaustion. This can in itself be an indication for intubation and mechanical ventilation.

Arterial blood gas sampling is indicated only if the oxygen saturation falls below 94%, as carbon dioxide does not rise in asthma until hypoxia is established. If there is doubt about the diagnosis, particularly in an older patient, the blood gases should be measured at presentation.

Substantial improvement is often delayed for several hours, although some improvement should be noted within 10–15 minutes of use of the nebulized bronchodilator. If it is not, use of the nebulizer can be repeated several times. If no improvement occurs, other measures should be taken. Intravenous magnesium is regularly used in these circumstances, although the evidence for benefit is small. Failure to improve at all within 1 hour is an indication to consider intubation.

Labile peak flows are a normal feature in the recovery phase of acute severe asthma and do not necessarily indicate the need to increase therapy, so long as there is a good response to bronchodilators. For this reason, pre- and post-nebulizer peak flows should be measured while the patient is in the hospital.

Prior to discharge, the trigger for the exacerbation should be identified whenever possible and a self-management plan for the recovery period negotiated with the patient. Clear communication of the follow-up arrangements must occur and include appropriate use of both specialist and community services.

Further Reading

Healthcare Improvement Scotland. *British Guideline on the Management of Asthma: A National Clinical Guideline.* Available at https://www.brit-thoracic.org.uk/document-library/clinical-information/asthma/btssign-asthma-guideline-2014/ (accessed 6 Apr 2017).

Israel E and Reddel HK. Severe and difficult-to-treat asthma in adults. *N Engl J Med* 2017; 377: 965–76.

Tarlo SM and Lemiere C. Occupational asthma. *N Engl J Med* 2014; 370: 640–9.

134 Chronic obstructive pulmonary disease

Patrick Davey, Sherif Gonem, Salman Siddiqui, and David Sprigings

Definition of the disease

The Global Initiative for Chronic Obstructive Lung Disease (GOLD) states that 'chronic obstructive pulmonary disease (COPD), a common preventable and treatable disease, is characterised by persistent airflow limitation that is usually progressive and is associated with an enhanced chronic inflammatory response in the airways and the lung to noxious particles and gases. Exacerbations and comorbidities contribute to the overall severity in individual patients.'

Aetiology of the disease

The majority of cases of COPD worldwide are caused by tobacco smoking. However, a variety of other environmental and occupational exposures may also contribute to the condition, including passive exposure to cigarette smoke, marijuana smoking, exposure to inorganic dusts, and exposure to smoke from biomass fuels used for cooking or heating. Chronic asthma is an underappreciated cause of COPD, with a significant proportion of asthmatic patients developing fixed airflow obstruction in middle age. The most well-characterized genetic abnormality causing COPD is alpha-1 antitrypsin deficiency, although this accounts for only a small proportion of cases. Nevertheless, family studies suggest a significant genetic component to COPD in the general population, and a number of candidate genes have been identified.

Airflow obstruction in COPD is caused by two distinct processes, either of which may be more prominent in a given patient. The first is small airway disease (bronchiolitis), which results in airway wall thickening and luminal obstruction. The second is lung parenchymal destruction (emphysema), which results in both loss of lung elastic recoil and disruption of the alveolar attachments that anchor the airways to the lung parenchyma, thus causing dynamic expiratory airway collapse.

Typical symptoms of the disease, and less common symptoms

The main symptoms of COPD are:

- shortness of breath; this characteristically occurs on exertion and is progressive over a number of years, eventually culminating in shortness of breath at rest in end-stage disease; orthopnoea is relatively common, even in the absence of coexistent congestive cardiac failure
- chronic cough; this is usually dry, or productive of small to moderate quantities of sputum; copious sputum production should raise the suspicion of coexistent bronchiectasis
- wheeze or chest tightness

Other common symptoms of COPD are related to its systemic manifestations. These include:

- oedema; this is a sign of right heart failure (cor pulmonale) or coexistent congestive cardiac failure
- weight loss and muscle wasting; this is not completely understood, but is a poor prognostic indicator
- low mood; depression commonly coexists with COPD and should be actively screened for

Demographics of the disease

COPD is the fourth leading cause of death worldwide and imposes a significant burden in terms of individual morbidity and disability.

The prevalence is difficult to estimate due to variations in diagnostic criteria used in different studies. Most national surveys report prevalence rates of approximately 6%, although it is likely that a significant proportion of patients remain undiagnosed. COPD increases in prevalence with age, being uncommon under the age of 40 years, and most common among those over the age of 60. Although previously more common in men, changing patterns of cigarette smoking have resulted in an approximately equal female prevalence. Some studies have suggested that women may be more susceptible than men to the effects of cigarette smoke, and COPD mortality among women has now surpassed that of men.

Natural history, and complications of the disease

In normal individuals, lung function, measured using the forced expiratory volume in 1 second (FEV_1), increases during childhood and peaks in early adulthood, before gradually declining. The natural history of COPD mirrors this, except that, at a certain point, usually during middle age, a level of lung function is reached that causes functional limitation and symptoms. This can occur either because the expected peak lung function is not achieved, due to early life events, or because the decline in lung function after the peak is accelerated. It has been shown that lung function measured shortly after birth tracks through to young adulthood and that maternal smoking is an important determinant of postnatal lung function. Moreover, a positive correlation has been found between birth weight and FEV_1 in middle age. Childhood asthma and lower respiratory tract infections are associated with lower lung function in adult life, but it is not known whether these events cause loss of lung function, or are themselves a consequence of preexisting diminished lung function during childhood. The most important factor causing accelerated lung function decline during adulthood is tobacco smoking. Moreover, it has been shown that cessation of smoking may result in a return to non-smoking rates of lung function decline, albeit starting from a lower baseline.

In many patients, the natural history of COPD is punctuated by periodic exacerbations of the condition, characterized by an acute onset of worsening shortness of breath and cough, often with increasing sputum quantity or purulence. It is thought that most acute exacerbations of COPD are caused by viral or bacterial infections. Exacerbations of COPD are a major cause of morbidity, mortality, and healthcare utilization associated with the condition. Moreover, there is evidence that patients with frequent exacerbations have a faster rate of lung function decline than those who do not. Other than acute exacerbations of the condition, respiratory complications of COPD include pneumonia, pneumothorax, and respiratory failure. Moreover, it is increasingly recognized that COPD is a systemic disease and that attention should be directed to its extra-pulmonary manifestations. Chief among these are the cardiovascular effects of COPD: It has been shown that reduced FEV_1 is an independent risk factor for cardiovascular disease, including ischaemic heart disease and stroke, even after controlling for smoking history, and much of the morbidity and mortality associated with COPD is due to cardiovascular rather than respiratory complications. Chronic hypoxaemia may also result in pulmonary hypertension and right heart failure. Other important extra-pulmonary manifestations of COPD include skeletal muscle atrophy, weight loss, depression, and osteoporosis.

Approach to diagnosing the disease

The diagnosis of COPD should be considered in people over the age of 40 years who present with progressive exertional dyspnoea or chronic cough, with or without sputum production, in the presence of one or more risk factors for the condition, such as tobacco smoking.

Important features of the clinical assessment

History

Important features to note when taking the history are:

- time course of symptoms: this is usually insidious, often with a lag period of months or years between the onset of symptoms and presentation to medical services
- smoking history: current smoking status and pack year history should be noted
- occupation and other relevant exposures: this includes exposure to inorganic dusts, biomass fuel smoke, and tobacco smoke

Examination

General inspection

Signs of severe COPD include dyspnoea at rest or on minimal exertion, use of accessory muscles of respiration, pursed lip breathing, cyanosis, and muscle wasting. Nicotine staining of the fingers indicates continued cigarette smoking. Clubbing is not a sign of COPD, and suggests an alternative diagnosis.

Examination of the chest

Hyperinflation may be evidenced by a 'barrel-shaped' chest, with an increased postero-anterior diameter. Quiet breath sounds on auscultation are suggestive of emphysema, while wheeze is an indication

of expiratory airflow limitation. Crackles are not a usual feature of COPD, and suggest an alternative or additional diagnosis, such as bronchiectasis or interstitial lung disease.

Other diagnoses that should be considered

A number of conditions should be considered in the differential diagnosis of stable COPD, or may occur in conjunction with it, thus altering the required management. These are shown in Table 134.1, together with the clinical features and investigation results that may suggest these alternative diagnoses. Similarly, acute exacerbation of COPD is a diagnosis of exclusion, and a number of other pathologies should be considered in a patient with COPD who presents with worsening shortness of breath or cough, as listed in Table 134.2.

'Gold-standard' diagnostic test and acceptable diagnostic alternatives

Spirometry is the gold standard for the diagnosis of COPD, as well as its classification into categories of severity. Diagnosis is made on the basis of a compatible clinical picture in conjunction with an FEV_1 to forced vital capacity (FVC) ratio of less than 70% following administration of a bronchodilator. However, there is some concern that this spirometric criterion may result in over-diagnosis of COPD in the elderly, and it may be preferable to define the lower limit of normal in terms of the lower fifth percentile value in an age, sex, and height-matched population. The spirometric classification of COPD is shown in Table 134.3. While the gold-standard diagnostic test is spirometry performed in an accredited pulmonary function laboratory by a qualified respiratory physiologist, it is acceptable and indeed encouraged for spirometry to be available in a community setting. Training is available to enable a wide variety of practitioners to perform spirometry, including practice nurses, general practitioners, and hospital doctors. However, in order to ensure accurate and consistent results across centres, it is important that spirometers are calibrated regularly, that personnel performing spirometry are trained to an appropriate standard, and that spirometry is performed according to

Table 134.1 Differential diagnoses of stable COPD

Condition	Supportive clinical features
Asthma	Young age of onset
	Minimal or no smoking history
	History of atopy/allergy
	Family history of asthma
	Mainly episodic or nocturnal symptoms
	Diurnal variability in peak expiratory flow
	Normal spirometry in the stable state
	Significant bronchodilator reversibility
	Reduced methacholine PC_{20}
Bronchiectasis	Copious daily sputum production
	Coarse crackles audible on auscultation
	Chronic bacterial colonization in sputum (esp. with *Pseudomonas aeruginosa*)
	Bronchial dilatation visible on chest radiograph or CT scan
Interstitial lung disease	Fine crackles audible on auscultation
	Restrictive pattern on spirometry
	Reduced lung volumes
	Interstitial shadowing visible on chest radiograph or CT scan
Bronchiolitis	History of connective tissue disease, toxic fume inhalation, or previous lung or bone marrow transplant (obliterative bronchiolitis)
	History of sinusitis, and East Asian origin (diffuse panbronchiolitis)
Obesity hypoventilation syndrome	Obesity
	Restrictive pattern on spirometry and reduced lung volumes, but with normal or supra-normal carbon monoxide transfer coefficient
Congestive cardiac failure	History of ischaemic heart disease
	Peripheral oedema and orthopnoea out of proportion to other symptoms; paroxysmal nocturnal dyspnoea
	Fine basal crackles on auscultation; gallop rhythm
	Cardiomegaly and evidence of pulmonary oedema on chest radiograph
	Left ventricular failure on echocardiogram

Table 134.2 Differential diagnosis of acute exacerbation of COPD

Condition	Supportive clinical features
Pneumonia	History of pleuritic chest pain
	Fever and other features of the systemic inflammatory response syndrome (e.g. shock)
	Bronchial breathing or localized coarse crackles on auscultation
	Pulmonary infiltrate or lobar collapse on chest radiograph
Pneumothorax	History of pleuritic chest pain
	Sudden onset of symptoms
	Pneumothorax visible on chest radiograph
Pulmonary embolism	History of pleuritic chest pain or haemoptysis
	Personal or family history of venous thromboembolism
	Recent surgery or immobility
	Absence of wheeze or other abnormalities on auscultation
	Shortness of breath out of proportion to clinical signs
	Lack of response to COPD treatment
	New right-heart strain pattern on electrocardiogram
	Raised D-dimers
Silent myocardial infarction	History of ischaemic heart disease
	Absence of hypoxia or abnormalities on chest auscultation
	Ischaemic changes on electrocardiogram
	Raised cardiac enzymes
Congestive cardiac failure	History of ischaemic heart disease
	Peripheral oedema and orthopnoea out of proportion to other symptoms; paroxysmal nocturnal dyspnoea
	Fine basal crackles on auscultation; gallop rhythm
	Cardiomegaly and evidence of pulmonary oedema on chest radiograph
	Left ventricular failure on echocardiogram

Table 134.3 Spirometric classification of COPD

Severity	Postbronchodilator FEV$_1$/FVC	FEV$_1$ % pred.
At risk#	>0.7	≥80
Mild COPD	≤0.7	≥80
Moderate COPD	≤0.7	50–80
Severe COPD	≤0.7	30–50
Very severe COPD	≤0.7	<30

#Patients who smoke or have exposure to pollutants and have cough, sputum, or dyspnoea.
Abbreviations: FEV$_1$, forced expiratory volume in 1 second; FVC, forced vital capacity; pred., predicted.
Reproduced with permission of the European Respiratory Society ©: European Respiratory Journal Jun 2004, 23 (6) 932–946; DOI: 10.1183/09031936.04.00014304.

standard guidelines, such as those published jointly by the American Thoracic Society and the European Respiratory Society.

Other relevant investigations

Further investigations that may be required for the investigation of stable COPD include the following:

Pulmonary function tests: Carbon monoxide uptake in the lung is often reduced, and body plethysmography may show evidence of air trapping, with a raised residual volume/total lung capacity ratio.

Exercise testing: Validated exercise tests include the 6-minute walk test and the incremental shuttle walk test. These may be used to assess the level of disability, as well as providing an objective measure of the effectiveness of interventions such as pulmonary rehabilitation or lung volume reduction surgery.

Pulse oximetry: This, with or without arterial blood gas, is used to assess suitability for long-term oxygen therapy.

Chest radiograph: This may show evidence of hyperinflation or emphysematous bullae.

CT scan: This shows the extent and distribution of emphysema, as well as the presence of bullae. Associated bronchiectasis or interstitial lung disease may be visualized.

Echocardiogram: This allows right-heart function and pulmonary artery pressures to be assessed non-invasively.

Alpha-1 antitrypsin levels: Levels below 15%–20% of normal are suggestive of homozygous alpha-1 antitrypsin deficiency.

Appropriate investigations in patients presenting acutely with exacerbations of COPD may include the following:

Full blood count, and C-reactive protein level: Raised inflammatory markers could indicate bacterial infection.

Chest radiograph: Complications of COPD that may be visualized on a chest radiograph include pneumonia and pneumothorax.

Arterial blood gas: This is used to distinguish between type I and type II respiratory failure, and hence guide oxygen therapy and respiratory support.

ECG: This may show evidence of right-heart strain or right atrial hypertrophy.

Prognosis and how to estimate it

Characteristics associated with a worse prognosis in patients with COPD include severely diminished FEV$_1$, weight loss, poor exercise tolerance, and hypoxaemia at rest. The BODE index is a composite score that is used to estimate prognosis in patients with COPD. It comprises four components:

- **B**ody mass index
- **O**bstruction (FEV$_1$ (% predicted))
- **D**yspnoea (modified Medical Research Council dyspnoea scale)
- **E**xercise capacity (6-minute walk test distance)

Each component is given a score ranging from 0 (best) to 3 (worst), except for body mass index, which is scored as 0 (BMI > 21 kg/m²) or 1 (BMI ≤ 21 kg/m²). The BODE index can therefore range from 0 (best prognosis) to 10 (worst prognosis).

Treatment and its effectiveness

Treatment of stable COPD

The optimal management of stable COPD requires a holistic approach in which interventions are directed not only at improving the function of the lungs, but also at addressing the systemic manifestations of the condition, in addition to psychological and social factors. The treatments available may be divided into general, pharmacological, and interventional categories.

General management

Smoking cessation

Smoking cessation is the only intervention that has been proven to favourably alter the natural history of COPD. All patients with COPD who still smoke should be advised to quit, and those who are motivated to do so should be referred to a smoking cessation service which can provide access to pharmacotherapy in combination with regular follow-up and support. The most commonly used pharmacological treatment is nicotine replacement therapy, which can be administered in the form of gums, lozenges, patches, nasal sprays, and inhalers. Bupropion and varenicline are alternative smoking cessation agents.

Pulmonary rehabilitation

Pulmonary rehabilitation is a comprehensive intervention that has at its core an exercise training programme specifically designed to improve muscle strength and physical endurance. Allied to this may be a number of complementary components, including self-management education, dietary advice, counselling, and occupational therapy.

Long-term oxygen therapy

Long-term oxygen therapy, administered for more than 15 hours per day, has been shown to improve mortality in patients who are chronically hypoxic. It is indicated for patients with a resting arterial oxygen tension ≤7.3 kPa, or between 7.3 kPa and 8.0 kPa with concomitant evidence of cor pulmonale or polycythaemia. Continued smoking is a relative contraindication due to the risk of facial burns, and patients should be warned not to smoke near the oxygen supply or to allow others to do so.

Nocturnal non-invasive ventilation

Nocturnal non-invasive ventilation is used in occasional patients with severe COPD and chronic hypercapnia, particularly those who manifest recurrent admissions with decompensated type II respiratory failure.

Vaccination

Vaccination against influenza and *Pneumococcus* is recommended for all patients with COPD.

Pharmacological therapy

Inhaled bronchodilators

Short-acting beta-2 agonists such as salbutamol are administered via an inhaler or a nebulizer on an as-required basis for relief of symptoms, while inhaled, long-acting beta-2 agonists such as salmeterol and formoterol are used regularly to prevent or reduce chronic symptoms. Anticholinergic agents include the short-acting ipratropium and the long-acting tiotropium.

Inhaled corticosteroids

Inhaled corticosteroids such as beclometasone, budesonide, and fluticasone may be administered singly, but combination inhalers with long-acting beta-2 agonists are preferred. Regular treatment with inhaled corticosteroids has been shown to improve symptoms, lung function, and exacerbation frequency in patients with an FEV$_1$ (% predicted) <60%.

Theophylline

Theophylline is not a first-line treatment for COPD but may provide some benefit as an additional therapy in some patients with poorly controlled disease. Similarly, mucolytics such as carbocisteine may benefit selected patients, particularly those who complain of difficulty expectorating tenacious sputum.

CHAPTER 134 **Chronic obstructive pulmonary disease**

Roflumilast

Roflumilast, a phosphodiesterase-type-4 inhibitor, appears to reduce exacerbations in patients with severe or very severe COPD in combination with chronic bronchitis and a history of exacerbations. It may be considered as an add-on therapy in selected patients.

Surgical and bronchoscopic therapies

Bullectomy

Bullectomy is the surgical removal of a large (i.e. occupying at least one-third of the hemithorax) bulla which is causing compression of the adjacent lung. The procedure may be indicated in patients with severe functional limitation despite maximal medical therapy, and its primary purpose is to reduce dyspnoea.

Lung volume reduction surgery

Lung volume reduction surgery (LVRS) is the removal of emphysematous areas of the lung that are not participating in gas exchange, in order to alleviate hyperinflation and thus allow the respiratory muscles to act at a mechanical advantage. It may be performed via open surgery or video-assisted thoracoscopic surgery. A recent large trial of LVRS has emphasized the importance of careful patient selection. Patients undergoing LVRS should have upper-lobe-predominant emphysema, with significant functional limitation due to their COPD, despite undergoing pulmonary rehabilitation. The FEV_1 and the carbon monoxide transfer factor should both be greater than 20% predicted. Contraindications include age greater than 70 years (with some exceptions); continued smoking; comorbidities which may increase surgical risk; diffuse emphysema; significant hypercapnia (i.e. the partial pressure of carbon dioxide in arterial blood (P_aCO_2) >7.3 kPa); and pulmonary hypertension. LVRS has been shown to improve lung function and symptoms in patients who fit these criteria, but with a perioperative mortality of approximately 5%.

Bronchoscopic alternatives to LVRS have recently been developed. The insertion of one-way endobronchial valves causes collapse of the distal lung segments, thus ameliorating hyperinflation. Extrapulmonary bypass, which is the insertion of stents through the bronchial wall in order to bypass the site of flow limitation, allows trapped gas to escape and reduces the resistance to airflow. Both of these techniques are still under development and not yet widely available except in a research setting.

Lung transplantation

Lung transplantation is suitable for a small proportion of patients with COPD, but carries a 1-year mortality of up to 15%. Factors favouring lung transplantation over LVRS include diffuse emphysema, hypercapnia, pulmonary hypertension, and FEV_1 <20% predicted. Patients should be relatively young (under 65 years) with an absence of cardiac or renal disease, osteoporosis, or malignancy. Bilateral lung transplantation is the preferred option, but organ availability is a limiting factor.

Treatment of acute exacerbations of COPD

Many acute exacerbations of COPD can be managed successfully in the community. However, admission is required for patients who are hypoxic, those who manifest abnormal vital signs, and those who do not have adequate social support at home. Supported early discharge schemes may allow some patients to be discharged home 24–48 hours after admission, with treatment and follow-up provided in the community by specialist nurses. Long-term therapy should be reviewed and optimized before discharge.

The treatment of acute exacerbations of COPD incorporates the following components:

Oxygen: Oxygen should initially be administered via a Venturi mask and titrated to target saturations of 88%–92%, since excessive oxygen administration may result in hypercapnic respiratory failure in susceptible patients. If the P_aCO_2 is found to be normal and there are no other risk factors for hypercapnic respiratory failure, such as previously documented episodes requiring ventilatory support, then the target range may be increased to 94%–98%. Any increase in administered oxygen concentration should be followed by an arterial blood gas 30–45 minutes later to rule out worsening hypercapnia.

Nebulized short-acting bronchodilators: Nebulized short-acting bronchodilators such as salbutamol and ipratropium should be given regularly during the acute phase of the exacerbation.

Oral corticosteroids: Short courses (5–7 days) of oral corticosteroids are routinely given, and antibiotics are appropriate in most cases, particularly if there is an increase in sputum quantity or purulence.

Aminophylline: Intravenous aminophylline may be considered in severe exacerbations which are refractory to nebulized bronchodilator treatment. However, side effects, including cardiac arrhythmias, are not uncommon, and the evidence for benefit is inconsistent. Serum levels should be monitored regularly, and cardiac monitoring is advisable.

Ventilatory support: Invasive or non-invasive ventilatory support is indicated in patients with refractory hypoxaemia or hypercapnic respiratory failure despite maximal medical therapy, including appropriate titration of oxygen. Acute non-invasive ventilation has transformed the management of type II respiratory failure in COPD, and has been shown to reduce the need for invasive ventilation, as well as reducing mortality and length of hospital stay.

Further Reading

National Institute for Health and Care Excellence. *Chronic Obstructive Pulmonary Disease in Over 16s: Diagnosis and Management.* 2010. Available at http://www.nice.org.uk/guidance/cg101/resources/guidance-chronic-obstructive-pulmonary-disease-pdf (accessed 4 Apr 2017).

Rabe KF and Watz H. Chronic obstructive pulmonary disease. *Lancet* 2017; 389: 1931–40

Vogelmeier CF, Criner GJ, Martinez FJ, et al. Global Strategy for the Diagnosis, Management, and Prevention of Chronic Obstructive Lung Disease 2017 Report. GOLD Executive Summary. *Am J Respir Crit Care Med* 2017; 195: 557–82. doi: 10.1164/rccm.201701-0218PP

135 Respiratory failure

Matt Wise and Simon Barry

Definition of the disease

Respiratory failure is a syndrome characterized by defective gas exchange due to inadequate function of the respiratory system. There is a failure to oxygenate blood (hypoxaemia) and/or eliminate carbon dioxide (hypercapnia). Hypoxaemia is defined as an arterial blood partial pressure of oxygen (PaO_2) of <8 kPa, and hypercapnia as an arterial blood partial pressure of carbon dioxide ($PaCO_2$) of >6 kPa.

Respiratory failure is divided into two different types, conventionally referred to as type 1 and type 2. The distinction between these two is important because it emphasizes not only their different pathophysiological mechanisms and etiologies, but also different treatments. The preferred terminology and definitions are:

- oxygenation failure (type I respiratory failure): PaO_2 of <8 kPa
- ventilation failure (type 2 respiratory failure): $PaCO_2$ >6 kPa

Respiratory failure may be **acute** (onset over hours to days), or **chronic** (developing over months to years); alternatively, there may be an acute deterioration of a chronic state.

Physiology and aetiology of respiratory failure

There are only five causes of a low PaO_2 on arterial blood gas sampling:

- low inspired oxygen (altitude)
- ventilation–perfusion (VQ) mismatch
- right-to-left shunt
- diffusion limitation
- alveolar hypoventilation

The first four of these cause failure of oxygenation, while the last results in ventilation failure, as the name suggests. The alveolar gas equation is crucial to understanding why hypoventilation causes hypoxaemia. PAO_2, the partial pressure of alveolar oxygen, is calculated as follows:

$$PAO_2 = PiO_2 - (PCO_2 / 0.8).$$

The partial pressure of inspired oxygen is calculated as follows:

$$PiO_2 = FiO_2 \times (Pb - PH_2O),$$

where

FiO_2 = fraction of inspired oxygen (0.21 if breathing room air)
Pb = barometric pressure (101 kPa at sea level)
PH_2O = water vapour pressure (6.3 kPa)

PiO_2 = breathing room air at sea level = 0.21 x (101 − 6.3)
= 19.9 kPa.

This value, 19.9 kPa, is similar for practical clinical purposes to the percentage of oxygen inspired while breathing air, 21%. If the patient is on oxygen, then the FiO_2 is adjusted to reflect this.

Therefore, to simplify:

$$PAO_2 \sim FiO_2 (\%) - (PaCO_2 / 0.8).$$

From this equation, it is apparent that any rise in $PaCO_2$ results in a fall in PAO_2 and, consequently, also a reduction in PaO_2, since there must be a gradient from the alveolus to the artery. Thus, hypoventilation causes hypoxaemia.

Knowledge of the PAO_2 also enables the difference between the alveolar and the arterial oxygen partial pressures, that is, the A–a gradient to be calculated. This describes the severity of oxygenation failure. By contrast, hypoventilation will cause hypoxaemia with a normal A–a gradient. The lungs are not perfect, and there is a degree of VQ mismatch, with normal values of the A–a gradient up to 2 kPa in most and up to 3 kPa in the elderly.

Apart from causing hypoxaemia, another important result of acute hypoventilation is the development of an acidosis. The acid–base balance is described by the Henderson–Hasselbalch equation. A simplification of this is

$$pH \sim (base / acid),$$

where HCO_3 is the base, and $PaCO_2$ is the acid.

From this equation, a rise in $PaCO_2$ results in a reduction in pH and thus leads to a respiratory acidosis. This can be corrected either by improving ventilation, perhaps with invasive or non-invasive methods, or through renal conservation of bicarbonate (compensation).

Causes of oxygenation failure

The causes of oxygenation failure are ventilation perfusion mismatch, right-to-left shunt, and diffusion limitation.

Ventilation perfusion mismatch

Ventilation perfusion mismatch is by far the most common cause of oxygenation failure. Causes of ventilation perfusion mismatch include:

- pneumonia
- pulmonary embolism
- lobar collapse
- COPD or acute severe asthma

Right-to-left shunt

A right-to-left shunt is caused by either an intra-cardiac shunt, or shunting through a pulmonary arteriovenous malformation. This can be associated with hepatic disease (hepatopulmonary syndrome).

Diffusion limitation

Diffusion limitation is caused by

- pulmonary oedema
- pulmonary fibrosis

Causes of ventilation failure

The common causes of ventilation failure are:

- COPD
- obesity
- chest wall disease
- neuromuscular disease
- depressed respiratory drive

The most helpful way to understand the mechanisms of ventilation failure is to describe the balance between the respiratory drive, the load imposed by the disease process, and the respiratory muscle capacity (see Figure 135.1). Imbalances of any of these three components can result in ventilatory failure. Impaired respiratory drive may be caused by overdoses of opiates, alcohol, or recreational drugs such as gamma-hydroxybutryric acid; alternatively, it may be caused by brainstem disease. Drive may also be reduced as a compensatory mechanism for metabolic acidosis. Increased load is commonly caused by obesity, but COPD can also impose an increased

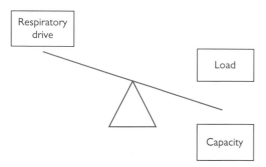

Figure 135.1 Diagram representing the balance between the respiratory drive, the load imposed on respiratory muscles, and the respiratory muscle capacity, as causes of ventilatory failure.

load due to dynamic hyperinflation. Pulmonary fibrosis increases load by impairing lung compliance, and kyphoscoliosis impairs chest wall compliance. The main causes of reduced capacity are neuromuscular diseases encompassing a number of different conditions. These are best considered as diseases affecting nerves, the neuromuscular junction, or muscle (Box 135.1).

Typical and less common symptoms, and signs of respiratory failure

Symptoms of oxygenation failure

The clinical presentation of oxygenation failure strongly suggests the underlying cause. For example, symptoms of fever, productive cough, and dyspnoea, developing over days, with coarse lung crepitations on chest auscultation and hypoxaemia suggests pneumonia. Dyspnoea is the cardinal symptom of oxygenation failure, and careful history taking is paramount, with a particular emphasis on determining the speed of onset of dyspnoea and the severity of change when compared to the baseline. Frequently, patients have a previous history of cardiac or respiratory illness, for example pulmonary fibrosis or COPD, and significant worsening of dyspnoea may represent infection, pulmonary embolism, or another process exacerbating the existing illness.

Important signs in acute oxygenation failure include the following:

- abnormal respiratory rate (>20/min or <8/min)
- low oxygen saturations (<93% on air)
- tachycardia
- hypotension
- confusion
- central cyanosis

Box 135.1 Neuromuscular causes of ventilatory failure

Nerve
- motor neuron disease
- Guillain–Barré
- phrenic nerve palsy
- polio
- high spinal cord lesions (above C3)

Neuromuscular junction
- myasthenia gravis
- botulism

Muscle
- muscular dystrophies (Duchenne, Becker's, myotonic)
- metabolic myopathies (acid maltase deficiency)
- endocrine myopathies (thyroid disease)
- mitochondrial cytopathies
- inflammatory myopathies

In most cases, oxygenation failure is rapidly diagnosed in a dyspnoeic patient with low oxygen saturations, particularly since the widespread adoption of standard nursing assessments such as Early Warning Scoring and its variants, which record observations including respiratory rate and oxygen saturations.

A cause of oxygenation failure that is less commonly identified is that due to obstructive sleep apnoea (OSA), since it occurs at night and is usually associated with normal daytime oxygen saturations. A history of sleep apnoea is easy to obtain once the diagnosis is considered, and an overnight sleep study can readily diagnose the condition.

Symptoms of ventilation failure

While oxygenation failure is rapidly recognized, the converse is true in ventilatory failure, which is frequently missed. The symptoms of ventilation failure are due to the effects of hypercapnia and include increasing drowsiness, confusion, and, eventually, coma. Usually these symptoms occur in a patient at risk of ventilatory failure, such as those with obesity or with chest wall or neuromuscular disease. In addition, COPD patients placed on high-flow oxygen, usually during transport to hospital in an ambulance, constitute another group that frequently presents with ventilation failure.

It cannot be overemphasized that oximetry gives no information about the state of ventilation, and a blood gas is necessary to make the diagnosis. Clinical signs that support ventilatory failure include:

- confusion, drowsiness, and an altered conscious state
- bounding pulse
- vasodilation
- flapping tremor
- papilloedema

Demographics of the disease

There are numerous causes of respiratory failure, and addressing the demographics of all these is impractical and beyond the scope of this chapter. Nevertheless, both acute and chronic respiratory failure are major causes of morbidity and mortality. Data from intensive care units in the UK have demonstrated that 3%–4% of admissions are due to COPD, and 5.9% are due to pneumonia. When chronic ventilatory failure is considered, the UK prevalence of home mechanical ventilation (including tracheostomy ventilation) is 4.1 per 100 000 and, of the 2842 users in 2002, approximately one-third were ventilated for lung/airways disease, one-third for chest wall disease, including obesity, and one-third for neuromuscular disease. There are likely to be significant changes in these proportions over time. If current trends continue, 60% of adults in the UK will be obese by 2050. Studies have demonstrated that 31% of hospital patients with a BMI >35 without lung or neuromuscular disease have daytime hypercapnoea, rising to a staggering 50% of those with a BMI >50.

Natural history, and complications of the disease

Respiratory failure has many causes. Therefore, the natural history, the complications, and the outcomes reflect the underlying disease and patient comorbidities.

Approach to diagnosing respiratory failure

Diagnosing oxygenation failure

As previously discussed, the diagnosis of oxygenation failure is strongly suggested by low oxygen saturations. Pulse oximeters are dependent on good pulsatile flow. Pitfalls include poor oximetry traces in states of poor peripheral perfusion or when nail varnish is present; such traces will lead to an inaccurate or inadequate signal for analysis. Different types of haemoglobin are not distinguished by pulse oximeters. In carbon monoxide poisoning (carboxyhaemoglobin), oxygen saturations will be falsely elevated, while, in methaemoglobinaemia, they may be erroneously low or high, depending on the level of methaemoglobin. Arterial blood gas analysis should be performed in those with oxygen saturations of <93% on air. In addition, modern point-of-care gas analysers measure carboxy- and methaemoglobin directly. Many A & E departments or critical care units have point-of-care blood gas analysers. If the sample is being transported to a laboratory, it should be on ice, and any air bubbles should be expelled, to avoid spurious values. If arterial blood gas tests are performed while the patient is on oxygen, it is crucial that this fact be recorded in the notes and on the request form, so that a correct assessment of oxygenation can be made. Ideally, in patients on oxygen, the A–a gradient should be recorded, as this gives an indication of the extent of oxygenation failure.

Diagnosing ventilation failure

In patients with ventilatory failure, the key approach is to recognize those at risk and then perform blood gas analysis. While there are some symptoms and signs of ventilatory failure, these are often not present, and the patient may appear well with preserved oxygen saturations.

The following patient groups should be considered for blood gas analysis:

- those with severe obesity (BMI >40)
- those with kyphoscoliosis or other significant chest wall deformities
- those with moderate-to-severe COPD
- those with neuromuscular diseases, such as motor neuron disease; muscular dystrophies; or diaphragm palsy of any cause
- those with severe bronchiectasis or cystic fibrosis

Bicarbonate and $PaCO_2$ levels are not clinically significantly different, whether a venous, capillary (ear lobe), or arterial sample is taken, a fact that is frequently not appreciated.

Other diagnosis that should be considered

Patients with acute or acute-on-chronic respiratory failure are critically ill, and this syndrome should be considered in all critically ill patients. There are very few instances where it is not appropriate to obtain a blood gas in a critically ill patient, and this will establish a diagnosis of respiratory failure. Since the symptoms and signs of critical illness are non-specific, there are many instances where the patient may be thought on first inspection to be in respiratory failure. Thus, a patient with diabetic ketoacidosis may complain of dyspnoea and be extremely tachypnoeic (as a consequence of metabolic acidosis and increased work of breathing), and a similar presentation may be observed in severe sepsis. Potential pitfalls in the diagnosis of respiratory failure are due to misinterpretation of arterial blood gas samples. It is easy to establish if the patient is hypoxic or a large A–a gradient exists. If there is evidence of hypercapnia, one must remember to first look at the pH. Rarely, patients have a metabolic alkalosis (diuretics, nasogastric losses, or vomiting) which is partially corrected by alveolar hypoventilation (hypercapnia), but the primary abnormality will be an alkalosis.

'Gold-standard' diagnostic test

Arterial blood gas analysis remains the best method for diagnosing acute respiratory failure.

Acceptable diagnostic alternatives to the gold standard

Pulse oximetry may be used to detect hypoxaemia non-invasively. However, this method gives no information about ventilation ($PaCO_2$), and several factors can adversely affect readings, as previously discussed. Nevertheless, overnight oximetry is very helpful in the diagnosis of OSA. Transcutaneous CO_2 can also be measured, which is helpful during overnight studies in patients who hypoventilate. However, the readings should be anchored with a blood $PaCO_2$ level.

Other relevant investigations

Tests should be chosen in order to support or refute the clinical diagnosis. However, in general, these can be grouped into five main categories: blood tests, imaging, lung function tests, cardiology tests, and sleep tests.

Blood tests

Blood tests relevant to respiratory failure include:

- a full blood count; for leucocytosis or neutropenia (infection), polycythaemia (chronic hypoxia), anaemia (cause of breathlessness)
- blood biochemistry; for electrolyte disturbance (which may precipitate arrhythmias or muscle weakness); amylase levels (pancreatitis); thyroid function (cardiac disease, muscle weakness); creatinine kinase (cardiac or muscle disease); and troponin (ischaemic heart disease, myocarditis)
- toxicology (overdose)

Imaging

Imaging relevant to respiratory failure includes:

- chest radiograph
- ultrasonography (to detect pleural effusions, pneumothorax, consolidation, lung water)
- CT scan (CT pulmonary angiogram, to exclude pulmonary emboli; high-resolution CT, to exclude fibrosis, bronchiectasis, or other structural abnormalities)

Lung function tests

Lung function tests relevant to respiratory failure include:

- spirometry, lung volumes (to determine obstructive and restrictive defects)
- gas diffusion
- tests of diaphragm function (sniff nasal inspiratory pressure, lying and sitting vital capacity); useful in neurological disease
- cardiopulmonary exercise tests (a powerful tool for determining the cause of breathlessness)

Cardiology tests

Cardiology tests relevant to respiratory failure include:

- ECG (ischaemia, arrhythmias)
- echocardiography (for estimates of left ventricular function, diastolic dysfunction, regional wall abnormality, valve function, pericardial disease, pulmonary hypertension, pulmonary emboli)

Sleep tests

Sleep tests relevant to respiratory failure include:

- simple oximetry (screening test for obstructive sleep apnea)
- limited channel sleep study (to differentiate obstructive and central apnoeas, paradoxical breathing)
- transcutaneous CO_2 measurement (helpful in determining nocturnal hypercapnoea in obesity hypoventilation)

Prognosis and how to estimate it

Respiratory failure is a syndrome with a wide aetiology and it is difficult to prognosticate. Clinical scoring systems exist for several of the clinical conditions, including pneumonia (e.g. CURB-65, or pneumonia severity index), which help identify those at high risk of death; however, for many conditions, such tools are not available. Once patients are admitted to a high-dependency or intensive care unit, a number of scoring systems such as the Acute Physiology and Chronic Health Evaluation (APACHE), the Simplified Acute Physiology Score (SAPS), and the Sequential Organ Failure Assessment (SOFA) help to define patient outcome. These scoring systems are similar in their predictive accuracy but describe outcome in groups of patients rather than individuals; therefore, prognosis is often determined by expert opinion.

For acute ventilatory failure, there is good evidence that increasing acidosis results in higher mortality and increased rates of endotracheal intubation and mechanical ventilation.

Treatment and its effectiveness

The differentiation of respiratory failure into oxygenation failure and ventilation failure is particularly important when considering treatment. Simplistically, oxygenation failure requires oxygen, and ventilation failure requires ventilation. Conversely, giving oxygen to patients with ventilation failure may, on occasion, be dangerous.

Treatment of acute respiratory failure

Treatment of patients in acute respiratory failure requires a stepwise approach, addressing the key essentials first.

Resuscitation and Advanced Life Support

Resuscitation must be initiated as soon as respiratory failure is recognized and should follow the standard Airway, Breathing, Circulation (ABC) approach such that immediate threats to life such as airway compromise or tension pneumothorax are addressed first. The patient should be managed in an appropriate area with trained staff and monitoring (respiratory rate, continuous ECG, oximetry, arterial line (blood pressure, arterial blood gas analysis), and use of the Glasgow Coma Scale).

Maintaining oxygen saturations

Patients who are critically ill (peri-arrest, septic shock, multiple trauma) should have high-flow oxygen delivered via a non-rebreathing reservoir mask. However, after a blood gas has been taken and the patient is more stable, the target oxygen saturations for most people should be 94%–98%. There is increasing evidence that maintaining saturations above this level produces adverse outcomes in a variety of condition such as COPD, severe asthma, and cardiac arrest. In patients with known ventilatory failure (i.e. a raised $PaCO_2$ on this admission, or in the past), the target oxygen saturation range should be 88%–92%. For practical purposes, patients with moderate-to-severe COPD should be assumed to have ventilatory failure and given target saturations of 88%–92%, pending a blood gas result. Oxygen, if required at this stage, is best provided through a 24% or 28% Venturi mask, to achieve this range.

Physiotherapy

Sputum retention can lead to acute respiratory failure and may occur when there is an increased sputum load, tenacious sputum, and poor cough. This may be in the context of an acute respiratory infection, but also may occur in post-operative or trauma patients, particularly when pain prevents adequate coughing and sputum clearance. This is a frequent problem in patients who have been mechanically ventilated for a period of time and then extubated. Reintubation for respiratory failure secondary to sputum retention is common and again related to factors such as increased load and tenacity of sputum, poor cough, and physiological reserve. These individuals often require tracheostomy to liberate them from the ventilator and provide ongoing bronchopulmonary toilet.

Sputum retention is also important in those with chronic lung disease such as COPD, bronchiectasis, or cystic fibrosis, as well as those with neuromuscular disease, as the latter commonly have impaired cough reflexes. Physiotherapy, aided by mucolytics such as carbocisteine or dornase alfa, is often effective, but in patients in the high-dependency unit/intensive therapy unit setting, bronchial toilet via a nasopharyngeal airway, bronchoscopy, or even tracheostomy may be required.

Continuous positive airways pressure

Continuous positive airways pressure (CPAP) is an important intervention to improve oxygenation. CPAP is not a ventilatory mode per se, as it provides a constant pressure throughout the respiratory cycle; however, it improves oxygenation by increasing functional residual capacity, improving ventilation perfusion mismatch, and preventing upper airways obstruction.

Ventilatory support: Correcting a respiratory acidosis

Ventilatory support may either be provided non-invasively, via a mask applied to the nose, nose and mouth, or full face, or invasively, via a tracheostomy or endotracheal tube. In the acute setting, patients with a pH <7.25 are more likely to fail with non-invasive ventilation (NIV), and this should be attempted, if appropriate, in a high-dependency setting. Patients more profoundly

acidotic or with other organ instability may require immediate intubation.

The principles behind ventilation are simple. In a conscious patient given NIV, the patient initiates a breath and this triggers the machine to deliver a pressure, or volume, over a set period of time. This augmented breath is then terminated and the cycle repeats. In the UK and Europe, most ventilators are pressure driven. The inspiratory positive airway pressure (IPAP) is set and, at the end of the augmented breath, the machine usually returns not to the baseline, but a set expiratory positive airway pressure (EPAP), which functions like CPAP. It is the difference between the IPAP and EPAP, the pressure support, which determines ventilation and hence effective PCO_2 reduction. In practice, the keys to successful NIV are good communication with the patient, ensuring optimum mask fit, and adjusting the pressures to correct the ventilatory abnormality.

NIV is highly effective, reducing mortality by 50% when compared to standard medical treatment and reducing the need for invasive ventilation.

Treating the underlying pathology

Needless to say, the disease process which has led to the respiratory failure needs to be treated. In some cases, this may be an illness in which there will be complete resolution, such as a pneumonia treated with antibiotics. However, this may not always be possible, as in the case of progressive neuromuscular disease.

Treatment of chronic respiratory failure

Treatment of oxygenation failure

Two landmark studies from the 1980s demonstrated that giving oxygen to COPD patients who were hypoxaemic improved survival. Based on these studies, long-term oxygen therapy is recommended in the stable state if the PaO_2 <7.3 kPa, or less than 8 kPa in the presence of cor pulmonale, polycythaemia, or pulmonary hypertension. Oxygen is generally not recommended in those who continue to smoke.

Treatment of ventilation failure

Evidence for the benefit of long-term ventilation in neuromuscular and airways disease is evolving. Long-term ventilation provides definite survival and quality-of-life advantages in motor neuron disease patients developing ventilatory failure without predominant bulbar features, compared to controls. In addition, NIV is largely responsible for an increase in life expectancy of approximately 10 years in patients with Duchenne muscular dystrophy.

By contrast, it is surprising that only a single recent randomized trial has shown a survival benefit of long-term NIV in COPD patients with ventilatory failure. The likely explanation is that, historically, low ventilatory pressures have been used, and the current vogue is to try more aggressively to correct the abnormal physiology with a greater acceptance for using higher pressures.

Obesity is a growing indication for long-term ventilatory support. The umbrella term 'obesity-related respiratory failure' encompasses those with OSA, OSA and obesity hypoventilation syndrome (OHS), or lone OHS. Only a minority of OSA patients develop ventilatory failure and, even then, most can be managed with CPAP. OSA/OHS overlap or lone OHS requires NIV.

Lastly, severe bronchiectasis and cystic fibrosis can result in ventilatory failure. Usually, the disease is severe, and chronic sputum production may make tolerance more difficult. The evidence base, particularly in cystic fibrosis, is poor.

Invasive ventilation, and end-of-life care

Patients with respiratory failure may not respond to simple measures or NIV and it may be appropriate to escalate to invasive mechanical ventilation in critical care—this is discussed further in Chapter 149.

Escalation of treatment may not be in the patient's best interests or indeed desired by them. In chronic respiratory failure patients in whom the inevitable trajectory of illness is towards ventilator dependence, these issues are best discussed, well in advance of an acute deterioration, with the individuals concerned and their family.

End-of-life care in the context of more acute respiratory failure is discussed in Chapter 153.

Further Reading

Davidson AC, Banham S, Elliott M, et al. British Thoracic Society/ Intensive Care Society Acute Hypercapnic Respiratory Failure Guideline Development Group. BTS/ICS Guidelines for the ventilatory management of acute hypercapnic respiratory failure in adults. *Thorax* 2016; 71: ii1–ii35.

O'Driscoll BR, Howard L, Earis J, et al. British Thoracic Society Emergency Oxygen Guideline Development Group. BTS guideline for oxygen use in adults in healthcare and emergency settings. *Thorax* 2017; 72: i1–i90.

Pepin JL, Timsit JF, Tamisier R, et al. Prevention and care of respiratory failure in obese patients. *Lancet Respir Med* 2016; 4: 407–18.

136 Obstructive sleep apnoea

Sonya Craig and Sophie West

Definition of the disease

Obstructive sleep apnoea (OSA) is caused by the repetitive closure of the pharynx during sleep, leading to sleep fragmentation and, often, daytime somnolence. Traditionally, it is defined as either the number of apnoeas (complete cessation of breathing for longer than 10 seconds) or hyponoeas (reduction in air flow by >30% for more than 10 seconds with >3% oxygen dip) per hour in an overnight sleep study. However, it must be remembered that this definition is arbitrary, and OSA is better viewed as a spectrum with trivial snoring at one end and severe, almost continuous obstruction at the other. In addition to the sleep study findings, if the patient is sleepy during the day, as defined by the Epworth Sleepiness Scale, then this condition is termed 'obstructive sleep apnoea syndrome'. This distinction is important, as patients with this syndrome usually warrant treatment.

Aetiology of the disease

The majority of patients with OSA are overweight, and weight loss can certainly cure OSA. The evidence suggests that most OSA in adults is due to loading of the upper airway, with the loading being caused by obesity and fat deposits in the neck area. This external loading can be fended off during wakefulness but not during sleep, when the withdrawal of postural muscle tone allows the pharyngeal dilators to be overwhelmed, leading to excessive narrowing or collapse of the airway, with consequent apnoea and arousal.

Major risk factors

The major risk factors for developing OSA are:

- being a middle-aged male
- being overweight
- being a snorer
- having a collar size >17 inches
- having craniofacial abnormalities (e.g. retrognathia (may be genetic or acquired))

Less common/minor risk factors

The less common/minor risk factors for developing OSA are:

- having large tonsils
- hypothyroidism (leading to an increase in submucosal tissue)
- neuromuscular diseases with pharyngeal involvement (e.g. stroke, myotonic dystrophy, motor neurone disease)

Rare causes

Rare causes of OSA are:

- mucopolysaccharidoses
- acromegaly
- Marfan syndrome

Typical symptoms of the disease, and less common symptoms

The main symptom of OSA is excessive daytime somnolence, and this correlates broadly with the degree of sleep disruption. Initially, while occupied, there is little difficulty in concentrating and staying awake but, once activities become more boring, unwanted sleepiness intervenes. Driving, especially on motorways, is a particular problem, and accidents are more common in patients with OSA.

Common symptoms of OSA are:

- excessive sleepiness, as determined by the Epworth Sleepiness Score (>9 is abnormal; >15 is severely abnormal)
- loud snoring, witnessed apnoeas, and choking noises
- feeling unrefreshed on waking
- poor concentration
- mood swings, personality changes, or depression
- nocturia

Less common symptoms of OSA are:

- nocturnal sweating
- reduced libido
- oesophageal reflux

Demographics of the disease

OSA affects mainly men with upper body obesity, but the male preponderance is reduced once women have undergone menopause, as postmenopausal women have a threefold increased risk of developing OSA, compared to premenopausal women. The incidence of OSA is estimated to be 1%–2% of middle-aged men, but OSA may be much under-diagnosed, and its incidence has been estimated to be as much as 4% in some studies. Ethnicity also affects the risk of OSA; this is usually due to face shape and mandibular size, so non-obese Asians have a higher prevalence of OSA than Caucasians of similar weight. OSA prevalence generally increases with age, with a 2–3 times greater prevalence in those >65 compared to those aged 30–64.

Natural history, and complications of the disease

Most patients attending a sleep clinic have had symptoms of OSA for many years. It is usually some specific event that prompts initial consultation, such as falling asleep while driving or during a meeting. There will be a long history of gradually worsening snoring with apnoeas, possibly witnessed by the spouse. There is often weight gain over the previous few years, with a BMI >30 kg/m² and a collar size of 17 inches or more (see 'Approach to diagnosing the disease').

Complications from the syndrome are usually due to daytime somnolence and relate to sleep deprivation so that there is poor concentration, forgetfulness, depression, mood swings, and often marital and work problems related to these symptoms. There are also complications due to recurrent arousals and consequent blood pressure rises which can last into the waking hours, leading to hypertension which reduces with continuous positive airways pressure (CPAP) treatment. There may also be an increased incidence of atrial fibrillation and failure of cardioversion in OSA patients, possibly due to increased heart rate and sympathetic activation with OSA.

Approach to diagnosing the disease

In addition to finding apnoeic events on a sleep study, it is important to try to assess the degree of somnolence and how this is impacting on the patient's life. This can be done using the Epworth Sleepiness Score. However, this score should not necessarily be taken at face value: patients may under-report their level of sleepiness, due to concerns regarding driving, or over-report it to 'get something done'. It is also important to differentiate 'sleepiness' from 'tiredness', which has many other causes which are not necessarily related to sleep problems, as these terms are often interchanged by patients.

Examination findings are mostly non-contributory but the following may be helpful:

- neck circumference: collar size >17 inches
- oropharynx: large tonsils and boggy mucosa
- teeth: crowding suggests that the mandible is small
- nasal patency: snoring may be reduced, and CPAP therapy facilitated by improved patency
- respiratory function: signs of cor pulmonale, FEV_1/FVC ratio, oxygen saturation (SaO_2)
- blood pressure: may influence decision to treat with CPAP
- endocrine abnormalities (e.g. acromegaly, hypothyroidism)
- neuromuscular disorders (e.g. recent stroke; motor neuron disease)
- heart failure: can lead to Cheyne–Stokes breathing, or central apnoeas

Other diagnoses that should be considered

OSA should be relatively easy to diagnose in the presence of a patient who snores, has witnessed apnoeas, is sleepy, and has a compatible abnormal sleep study. However, the following alternative diagnoses should also be considered:

- depression: this is often missed and is a cause of daytime somnolence
- periodic leg movements during sleep: this can lead to multiple arousals and daytime somnolence; it is associated with restless legs syndrome during the day
- narcolepsy: excessive daytime somnolence, vivid dreams, and cataplexy should alert one to this diagnosis and lead to a referral to a specialist
- multisystem atrophy: this can present with 'snoring' which is actually due to laryngeal abductor weakness and laryngeal closure during sleep, with stridulous inspiratory obstruction; patients with multisystem atrophy can suddenly die from nocturnal respiratory arrest but can be successfully treated with standard CPAP therapy.
- previous head injury; a head injury can lead to hypothalamic damage and excessive sleepiness
- central sleep apnoea: there may be a few obstructed breaths at the end of the apnoea cycle secondary to the central apnoea
- overlap syndromes: OSA may coexist with COPD or obesity hypoventilation syndrome leading to ventilatory failure

'Gold-standard' diagnostic test

The supposed gold-standard test for OSA is polysomnography, which involves EEG monitoring and multiple 'sleep' channels. This test is not necessary for diagnosing OSA in most cases, but is still used in many sleep centres.

Acceptable diagnostic alternatives to the gold standard

A limited sleep study, with other channels such as snoring, body movement, heart rate, oronasal flow, and chest wall movements, is the usual routine investigation. Oximetry alone can be used, and is often adequate to make a diagnosis, especially in severe cases,

but does have limitations, namely poorly differentiating between Cheyne–Stokes/periodic breathing and OSA. Also, nocturnal hypoventilation in COPD can sometimes look similar to OSA on oximetry alone. Desaturation in COPD will be worse at night, because reduced activity in the intercostal muscles leads to significant desaturation on oximetry. There will be periods of desaturation (especially during REM), interpreted by the computer as 'dips'. If there is a suggestion of an overlap, then limited sleep studies rather than simple oximetry may be needed.

The sleep study report will give information regarding overnight arterial SaO_2, the apnoea hypopnoea index (AHI; the number of such events per hour of sleep), the oxygen desaturation index (ODI; the number of >4% dips in SaO_2 per hour), body movements, pulse, and blood pressure. Generally, the higher the AHI or ODI, the more severe the OSA, but other factors such as daytime symptoms will determine whether treatment is necessary.

Other relevant investigations

Other relevant investigations include:

- blood gas estimation, if respiratory failure is suspected
- thyroid function
- routine haematology and biochemistry
- cholesterol, fasting triglycerides, and glucose, due to the high vascular risk in this population

Prognosis and how to estimate it

OSA patients, once treated, have a normal life expectancy. However, there is evidence from longitudinal studies that untreated OSA patients have reduced life expectancy, due to cardiovascular disease, although it is not clear whether this is an independent effect of OSA or due to obesity-related morbidity.

Treatment and its effectiveness

The most effective treatment for OSA is CPAP, in which pressurized air is blown from a pump, via a mask, into the pharynx to hold it open like a 'pneumatic splint'. There are now numerous types of mask available and the comfort and acceptability of this treatment has increased greatly over recent years. Patients are usually offered a CPAP trial if they have evidence of significant OSA on a sleep study and have daytime symptoms. The patient's health and general well-being is usually helped enormously with CPAP treatment. Patients often describe the abolition of sleepiness together with improvements in mood, concentration levels, and memory, once the effects of the sleep deprivation have been removed. The effects of treatment are mainly within the first few days or weeks, although there is a more gradual improvement in some patients over a few months.

Further Reading

Heinzer R, Vat S, Marques-Vidal P, et al. Prevalence of sleep-disordered breathing in the general population: the HypnoLaus study. *Lancet Respir Med* 2015; 3: 310–18.

Levy P, Kohler M, McNicholas WT, et al. Obstructive sleep apnoea syndrome. *Nat Rev Dis Primers* 2015; 1: 1–20.

137 Bronchiectasis

Andrew M. Jones and Rowland J. Bright-Thomas

Definition of the disease

Bronchiectasis may be defined clinically as the chronic daily production of copious mucopurulent sputum. Pathologically, the disease is characterized by inflamed, thick-walled, dilated bronchi.

Aetiology of the disease

Bronchiectasis has many potential underlying causes and associations with other diseases but, in individual cases, the underlying cause is often unknown.

Possible causes of bronchiectasis include the following:

- infection (e.g. following an episode of severe pneumonia, whooping cough, measles, tuberculosis, or opportunistic mycobacterial infection)
- allergic bronchopulmonary aspergillosis; this leads to a proximal bronchiectasis often with an upper lobe distribution; patients usually have a history of asthma, total serum IgE >1000; raised IgG or IgE to aspergillus; positive skin prick tests; peripheral eosinophilia; and pulmonary infiltrates
- immune deficiencies:
  - congenital (e.g. common variable immunodeficiency)
  - acquired (e.g. due to haematological malignancies, chemotherapy, HIV)
- ciliary disorders:
  - primary ciliary dyskinesia: features include autosomal recessive inheritance; childhood onset of symptoms; otitis media, often leading to hearing loss; sinusitis; middle lobe disease; subfertility; and dextrocardia (Kartagener's syndrome, which occurs in less than 50% of patients with primary ciliary dyskinesia)
  - Young's syndrome: azoospermia, sinusitis, and bronchiectasis
- cystic fibrosis: features include autosomal recessive inheritance, upper lobe distribution, steatorrhoea and malabsorption, male infertility, and *Staphylococcus aureus* and/or *Pseudomonas aeruginosa* as pathogens
- chronic asthma
- aspiration and inhalation injury (e.g. chronic gastric aspiration)
- bronchial obstruction (e.g. tumour or foreign body)
- structural large-airway defects:
  - oesophageal–bronchial fistula
  - Mounier–Kuhn syndrome (tracheobronchomegaly)
  - Williams–Campbell syndrome (cartilage deficiency)
  - tracheomalacia
  - connective tissue disorders (e.g. Marfan syndrome, Ehlers–Danlos syndrome)

Conditions associated with bronchiectasis include:

- inflammatory bowel disease (particularly ulcerative colitis)
- rheumatoid arthritis and other autoimmune arthropathies, including SLE, Sjögren's syndrome, and ankylosing spondylitis
- alpha-1-antitrypsin deficiency
- sickle cell disease
- sarcoidosis
- yellow nail syndrome (comprising bronchiectasis, yellow nails, lymphoedema, and pleural effusions)

Typical symptoms of the disease, and less common symptoms

The typical symptom is cough with sputum. Other common symptoms may include shortness of breath, chest pain, recurrent haemoptysis, malaise, and fatigue. Patients often report a past history of frequent chest infections and may have coexistent symptoms of rhinosinusitis.

Demographics of bronchiectasis

The prevalence of bronchiectasis increases with age. The true prevalence of bronchiectasis remains unclear. It was previously considered to be a relatively rare condition but, with improved diagnostic techniques, it is now known to be much more common than previously thought.

Natural history, and complications of the disease

Bronchiectasis is a chronic condition. Systemic complications are common and include tiredness, malaise, and weight loss. Urinary incontinence is frequently encountered. A common respiratory complication is episodic small-volume haemoptysis. This can usually be managed conservatively with antibiotics and tranexamic acid. Massive haemoptysis is relatively rare, but may be life-threatening and can require urgent bronchial arterial angiography and embolization of the bleeding vessels. Other respiratory complications include pneumothorax and respiratory failure.

Approach to diagnosing the disease (including diagnostic pitfalls)

The diagnosis of bronchiectasis rests upon the clinical history and radiological imaging. Although examination findings may include lung crackles and/or wheeze, it should be noted that clinical signs are often absent. Nail clubbing is present in only a small minority of patients.

Clues to underlying causes for bronchiectasis include:

- a family history of bronchiectasis: consider inherited immune deficiencies, cystic fibrosis, and primary ciliary dyskinesia
- male infertility or subfertility: consider cystic fibrosis, Young's syndrome, and primary ciliary dyskinesia
- upper lobe distribution of disease: consider cystic fibrosis, post-tuberculous bronchiectasis, and allergic bronchopulmonary aspergillosis
- middle lobe distribution of disease: consider primary ciliary dyskinesia and *Mycobacterium avium intracellulare* infection
- malabsorption: consider cystic fibrosis and ulcerative colitis
- *Staphylococcus aureus* or *Pseudomonas aeruginosa* infection: consider cystic fibrosis
- chronic otitis media/hearing problems: consider primary ciliary dyskinesia
- dextrocardia: consider primary ciliary dyskinesia (Kartagener syndrome)
- musculoskeletal problems: consider rheumatoid arthritis, SLE, Sjögren's syndrome, ankylosing spondylitis, and Marfan syndrome

Other diagnoses that should be considered

Other common differential diagnoses include:

- COPD
- asthma
- pulmonary tuberculosis

- lung abscess
- lung cancer
- gastro-oesophageal reflux disease

For patients with obstructive airways disease, the presence of any of the following symptoms should raise the clinical suspicion that bronchiectasis may be the underlying disease:

- chronic purulent sputum production
- bacterial pathogens regularly cultured from sputum (especially if *Pseudomonas aeruginosa*)
- recurrent unexplained haemoptyses
- absence of smoking history
- young age at onset

'Gold-standard' diagnostic test

The gold-standard diagnostic test is a high-resolution CT (HRCT) scan of the chest. Criteria for a radiological diagnosis of bronchiectasis include bronchial dilation with an internal bronchial diameter greater than that of the adjacent artery, bronchi with mucus plugging, non-tapering bronchi, and bronchi visible within 1 cm of the non-mediastinal pleural surface.

Acceptable alternatives to the gold standard

Some patients may be diagnosed on the basis of the clinical history if the chest X-ray has typical features of the condition. However, it should be noted that the chest X-ray can appear normal, particularly in mild cases.

Other relevant investigations

Sputum should be sent for microbiological culture, including myco-bacterial culture, to establish the infecting organism and guide choice of antibiotic therapy. Importantly, it should be noted that failure to culture a pathogen from a sputum sample neither excludes current infection nor contraindicates antibiotic therapy. For patients with symptoms of acute infection, antibiotic treatment should not be delayed; empirical antibiotic therapy can be commenced while awaiting the results of microbiological culture. Spirometry should be measured for all patients to establish if there is an obstructive pattern and the level of impairment. Oxygen saturations and/or arterial blood gas analysis should be recorded.

Tests for underlying causes should include:

- a full blood count
- immunoglobulin (IgG, IgA, and IgM) levels (note that IgG sub-classes are often technically difficult to measure and so are not currently recommended)
- functional antibody levels to tetanus toxoid, pneumococcus, and *Haemophilus influenzae*
- total IgE level and specific IgE and IgG precipitins levels to aspergillus
- HIV test
- rheumatoid factor

Patients with abnormalities of immunoglobulin and/or functional antibody levels, or with a clinical suspicion of underlying immune abnormality, should be referred to an immunologist for more detailed immune-function testing.

Other investigations, as directed by clinical indication, include:

- bronchoscopy (not a standard investigation for bronchiectasis but should be considered for those patients with localized disease)
- cystic fibrosis; a sweat test and genotype screening can be performed; cases where clinical suspicion persists despite negative test results should be referred for an opinion to a specialist cystic fibrosis centre
- ciliary function testing; saccharin tests and nasal nitrogen oxide levels can be used as screening tests where available;

suspected cases should be referred to a specialist ciliary function testing centre
- alpha-1-antitrypsin level (if the patient has features of basal emphysema)

Prognosis and how to estimate it

The prognosis is generally good for the majority of patients, who will have an almost normal life expectancy despite significant morbidity. However, some patients do have progressive deterioration of their lung disease, with eventual risk of respiratory failure and death.

Treatment and its effectiveness

Treatment should be tailored to the individual patient. The aim of therapy should be to control symptoms and prevent complications and disease progression, while minimizing the treatment burden. Patient education should be an integral part of the treatment regimen.

The underlying cause or associated condition should be identified and treated as appropriate. Patients with cystic fibrosis should be under the care of a specialist cystic fibrosis centre. Patients with allergic bronchopulmonary aspergillosis can be treated using a combination of oral prednisolone and/or azole therapy.

Acute infective exacerbations should be treated with antibiotics, usually with at least 2 weeks duration of therapy. The choice of antibiotic should be guided, where possible, by the known pathogen harboured by the individual patient. If this information is not available, empirical antibiotic treatment should be started.

Chronic maintenance therapy involves a combination of regular toilet of the airways and drug therapy. Patients should be assessed by a physiotherapist experienced in the management of patients with chronic lung disease. In addition to physical therapy, pharmacological therapies such as hyperosmolar agents (e.g. nebulized hypertonic (7%) saline), mucolytics (e.g. N–acetylcysteine) and inhaled and nebulized bronchodilators can be used to enhance mucociliary clearance and help ease symptoms of breathlessness. The role of inhaled corticosteroids in bronchiectasis is unresolved, while use of daily, long-term oral corticosteroids should be avoided. Studies are emerging to support chronic maintenance antibiotic therapy using oral and/or inhaled antibiotics, particularly for patients who require frequent oral antibiotic courses or hospital admissions.

Other preventative measures to reduce the frequency and severity of exacerbations include smoking cessation, and influenza and pneumococcal vaccination. Regular cardiovascular exercise should be encouraged. Pulmonary rehabilitation is likely to be beneficial. Surgery is rarely indicated, and only in very localized disease which does not respond to medical management.

Supportive measures for those patients with more advanced disease may include supplemental oxygen and/or non-invasive mechanical ventilation. Lung transplantation is a viable option for some younger patients with end-stage lung disease.

Further Reading

Eva Polverino E, Goeminne PC, McDonnell MJ, et al
European Respiratory Society guidelines for the management of adult bronchiectasis
Eur Respir J 2017; 50: 1700629
McShane PJ, Naureckas ET, Tino G, et al. Non-cystic fibrosis bronchiectasis. *Am J Respir Crit Care Med* 2013; 188: 647–56.
Pasteur MC, Bilton D, and Hill AT. British Thoracic Society guidelines for non-CF bronchiectasis. *Thorax* 2010; 65: i1–i58.
Polverino E, Goeminne PC, McDonnell MJ et al. European Respiratory Society guidelines for the management of adult bronchiectasis. *Eur Respir J* 2017; 50: 1700629.

138 Sarcoidosis and other granulomatous lung disease

Anjali Crawshaw

Definition of the disease

Sarcoidosis is a multisystem disorder characterized by the formation of non-caseating granulomas in many tissues. A granuloma is an organized aggregate of immune cells; it forms in response to an antigenic stimulus. It contains abnormal macrophages (epithelioid histiocytes, which fuse to form multinucleated giant cells), lymphocytes, neutrophils, eosinophils, fibroblasts, and collagen.

Aetiology of the disease

The aetiology of sarcoidosis is unknown, although it is widely believed that the disease occurs following a non-specific trigger in a genetically susceptible host. It is likely that both environmental and genetic factors contribute. The assumption that there is an important genetic component is based on the observations that (i) the prevalence and incidence of sarcoidosis differ between ethnic groups and (ii) the disease tends to cluster in families.

Typical symptoms of the disease, and less common symptoms

The clinical manifestations of sarcoidosis are heterogeneous and overlap with many other multisystem disorders. Pulmonary, cutaneous, and ocular manifestations are most common, but almost any tissue

Table 138.1 Symptoms in sarcoidosis

System	Symptoms	Frequency
Pulmonary	Dyspnoea, non-productive cough, chest discomfort	90%, presenting complaint in 20%–50%
Ocular	Painful red eye, floaters, blurred vision, photophobia	25%–80% Anterior uveitis, posterior uveitis (65% and 30%, respectively, of those with ocular involvement)
Constitutional	Fever, lethargy, malaise	20%–50%
Lymphatic	Palpable, non-tender lymphadenopathy	35%
Cutaneous	Erythema nodosum	10%
	Lupus pernio, hypo-/hyperpigmented areas, macules, papules, and plaques, occurring either in crops or isolation, usually less than 2 cm in diameter	25%–35%
Renal	Hypercalciuria, hypercalcaemia, renal calculi	Hypercalciuria 40% Hypercalcaemia 11% Renal calculi 10%
Cardiac	Palpitations, syncope	5%–25%
Neurological	Cranial nerve palsies, headache, cognitive dysfunction weakness, seizures	10%–25%
Hepatic	Usually silent, cholestatic liver function tests	10%

can be affected; cardiac, neurological, gastrointestinal, and renal involvement are important (see Table 138.1.

Demographics of the disease

Sarcoidosis can present at any age, although there is a bimodal distribution, with the highest incidence at 20–39 years and a second peak (predominantly in women) at 65–69 years. There is geographic variation in the incidence of sarcoidosis. The highest incidence is observed in northern European countries (5–40 cases per 100 000 people).

Natural history, and complications of the disease

At presentation to secondary care with sarcoidosis, it is difficult to predict the clinical course and outcome. A third will resolve spontaneously or with minimal treatment, a third will develop relapsing remitting disease which may intermittently require treatment, and the remainder (up to 40%) may develop progressive pulmonary fibrosis, pulmonary hypertension, and respiratory failure. Cardiac involvement must be actively considered and excluded where relevant; sudden cardiac death and progressive right or left ventricular failure are significant contributors to the overall mortality rate of 1%–5%.

Patients presenting with the combination of erythema nodosum, bilateral hilar lymphadenopathy, and arthritis (Löfgren syndrome) have a good prognosis, with resolution of chest radiograph findings in 64% and clinical remission in 84% at 2 years. The remainder develop chronic sarcoidosis.

Overall, approximately two-thirds of patients with sarcoidosis have improved or have stable clinical features, spirometry, and radiographic changes at the 2-year follow-up. African-Caribbean patients have a worse prognosis than Caucasians presenting with disease of the same stage, as do those from families with lower annual income.

Approach to diagnosing the disease

The diagnosis of sarcoidosis is made on the basis of clinical and radiological findings of granulomatous disease in multiple organs with supporting histology. The findings on chest radiography have been

Box 138.1 Chest X-ray findings and stage of sarcoidosis

- **stage 0:** normal chest radiograph
  - 5-10% of patients at presentation
- **stage I:** hilar or mediastinal nodal enlargement only
  - 45-65% of patients at presentation
  - 60% go onto complete resolution
- **stage II:** nodal enlargement and parenchymal disease
  - 25-30% of patients at presentation
- **stage III:** parenchymal disease only
  - 15% of patients at presentation
- **stage IV:** end-stage lung (pulmonary fibrosis)

Reproduced with permission from Collins and Stern, *Chest radiology: the essentials*, Second Edition, Wolters Kluwer, Copyright © 2008. Original Source: RadioGraphics 1995;15:421-437

Table 138.2 Granulomatous disorders

Infections	Non-infectious diseases
Mycobacteria (*Mycobacterium tuberculosis*, non-tuberculous mycobacteria) Fungi (*Histoplasma, Cryptococcus, Coccidioides, Pneumocystis, Aspergillus*)	Sarcoidosis
	Berylliosis
	Hypersensitivity pneumonitis
	Lymphoid interstitial pneumonia
	Vasculitis (Wegener's, Churg–Strauss)
	Aspiration pneumonia
	Rheumatoid
	Crohn's disease
	Chronic granulomatous disease

historically used to classify the stage of sarcoidosis (see Box 138.1). The increased availability of CT imaging has all but superseded the plain film and gives a better indication of disease-activity level, which can be used to guide treatment. CT is not always required for diagnosis, for example in typical Löfgren syndrome (acute sarcoidosis with erythema nodosum, bilateral hilar lymphadenopathy, migratory polyarthralgia and fever). However, it is important in excluding other causes of granulomatous adenitis. The CT imaging should preferably be reported by a radiologist with a special interest in interstitial lung disease.

In cases where there is no apparent pulmonary involvement, there have been reports that ¹⁸FDG PET scanning may prove useful in identifying biopsy sites, although the sensitivity and specificity of this technique remains uncertain. Cardiac and neurological involvement may be better detected with ¹⁸FDG PET, and MRI with gadolinium.

A biopsy should be obtained from the most accessible site (often the skin) and must demonstrate non-caseating granulomas without evidence of infective organisms or another focus for granuloma formation. In patients who present with Löfgren syndrome, a clinical diagnosis is usually sufficient and a biopsy may not be required. Transbronchial biopsy has a diagnostic yield of 40%–90%. The yield can be increased by performing endobronchial biopsy in conjunction with transbronchial biopsy, giving a rate closer to 90%. The yield can be increased yet further if endobronchial ultrasound is used.

Other diagnoses that should be considered

Lymphoma and TB are important differential diagnoses and should be actively excluded where there is clinical suspicion (dramatic weight loss, night sweats, significant adenopathy, TB exposure; see Table 138.2.

'Gold-standard' diagnostic test

Sarcoidosis is a diagnosis of exclusion. The histological confirmation of non-caseating granulomas and supportive imaging is considered the gold standard. The gold-standard diagnostic test for sarcoidosis is histological confirmation of non-caseating granulomas.

Acceptable diagnostic alternatives to the gold standard

Acceptable diagnostic alternatives to the gold-standard test for sarcoidosis are clinical history and radiological studies consistent with the diagnosis of sarcoidosis.

Other relevant investigations

Serum angiotensin-converting enzyme is an insensitive test (sensitivity, 57%; specificity, 90%; negative predictive value, 60%; positive predictive value, 90%) and is not useful as a diagnostic or therapeutic guide.

ECG, 24h ambulatory ECG and echocardiography should be performed at presentation to screen for cardiac involvement.

Examination of bronchoalveolar lavage fluid for lymphocytes (specifically the CD4/CD8 ratio) can be used as a complementary diagnostic test. If the fluid contains more than 15% lymphocytes, the sensitivity for diagnosing sarcoidosis approaches 90%; the specificity is low.

Prognosis and how to estimate it

The prognosis of pulmonary sarcoidosis can be estimated from the radiographic stage at presentation. In patients with Stage I (bilateral hilar lymphadenopathy only) or Stage II (hilar adenopathy and pulmonary infiltration) disease at presentation, 60%–80% have complete resolution of radiographic changes at 2 years, with a similar, slightly greater proportion showing clinical resolution. Stage III–IV at outset is associated with a poor prognosis; 38% showed radiographic resolution at 2 years.

Lupus pernio, or sarcoidosis in the mucosa of the upper respiratory tract, is associated with chronic fibrotic disease, and intrathoracic resolution is rare.

Ocular involvement is associated with two distinct clinical courses. Those with acute anterior uveitis appear to respond to steroid therapy and have low rates of relapse. In contrast, those with chronic uveitis with insidious onset respond less well to steroid therapy and may progress to glaucoma or cataract formation.

Pulmonary hypertension in sarcoidosis is associated with poor outcomes. Patients with sarcoidosis and high pulmonary artery pressures should undergo aggressive treatment including early referral for transplant.

Cardiac involvement carries a poor prognosis, with a 5-year survival rate of approximately 40%. The increased mortality is attributable to fatal arrhythmia and left ventricular dysfunction.

Treatment and its effectiveness

Oral and inhaled corticosteroids are widely used in the treatment of sarcoidosis, but their use has remained controversial since the 1960s. There is no consensus on when this therapy should be started, in whom, at what dose, and for how long. Indications for steroid therapy include severe pulmonary symptoms; radiographic evidence of active inflammatory disease; cardiac or neurological disease; hypercalcaemia; and sight-threatening ocular involvement.

A meta-analysis of 13 randomized controlled trials of variable quality is included in the Cochrane database. The analysis included 1066 participants on the equivalent of 4–40 mg of prednisolone. Radiographic improvement was reported at 3–24 months, but the authors highlight that this result should be interpreted with caution: differences in methodology and chest X-ray reporting in the different studies may have impacted the results seen. Despite a lack of evidence for steroid treatment, it is difficult to withhold when inflammatory processes seem to predominate or the patient is deteriorating. Patients with more severe disease are more likely to receive steroid treatment and are more likely to relapse.

Hydroxychloroquine is useful in the treatment of hypercalcaemia and skin lesions, but not in the treatment of pulmonary disease. There is some evidence to support the use of steroid-sparing agents such as azathioprine, methotrexate, and cyclophosphamide, but only limited evidence for newer therapies such as anti-tumour necrosis factor alpha.

Further Reading

Patterson KC and Chen ES. The pathogenesis of pulmonary sarcoidosis and implications for treatment. *Chest* 2017 Dec 7. doi: 10.1016/j.chest.2017.11.030. [Epub ahead of print]

Sauer WH, Stern BJ, Baughman RP, Culver DA, and Royal W. High-risk sarcoidosis. Current concepts and research imperatives. *Ann Am Thorac Soc* 2017; 14 (Supplement_6): S437–S444.

139 Interstitial lung disease

Patrick Davey, Sherif Gonem, and David Sprigings

Definition

The interstitial lung diseases (ILDs), also known as the diffuse or diffuse parenchymal lung diseases, represent a broad group of pulmonary disorders which mainly affect the lung parenchyma as opposed to the airways. By convention, infectious and malignant conditions are excluded from this definition. Thus, ILDs comprise a group of conditions characterized by variable degrees of inflammation and fibrosis, centred on the lung interstitium and alveolar airspaces.

Aetiology

ILDs may be brought about by an extraordinary range of extrinsic and intrinsic insults. Extrinsic exposures include inorganic mineral dusts such as asbestos and silica; organic antigens; drugs and toxins; cigarette smoke; and radiation. ILD may also occur in association with a variety of systemic conditions, including connective tissue disorders, pulmonary vasculitis, sarcoidosis, and inflammatory bowel disease. Finally, a large group of ILDs have no identifiable underlying cause.

An etiological classification of ILDs is shown in Table 139.1.

Symptoms

The two main symptoms of ILD are:

Shortness of breath: This is typically exertional and progressive over a period of weeks or months. Less commonly, ILD may have an acute presentation (e.g. acute eosinophilic pneumonia, acute interstitial pneumonia, or lupus pneumonitis). Hypersensitivity pneumonitis may have a relapsing and remitting course due to variable exposure to the causative allergen.

Cough: This is usually dry and non-productive.

Demographics

The epidemiology of ILD varies according to the underlying condition. Among the idiopathic group, the incidence of idiopathic pulmonary fibrosis rises with increasing age, such that most patients present between the ages of 60 and 70, with men affected slightly more commonly than women. The other idiopathic ILDs, namely non-specific interstitial pneumonia (NSIP), acute interstitial pneumonia, and cryptogenic organizing pneumonia, generally have an earlier onset, with an average age of presentation between 50 and 55. The smoking-related ILDs present even earlier, typically between the ages of 20 and 40. Lymphangioleiomyomatosis is unique in that it is confined almost exclusively to premenopausal women.

Natural history, and complications

Among the idiopathic ILDs, idiopathic pulmonary fibrosis (IPF) has the worst prognosis, due to the inexorable nature of the disease. The median survival of this condition is approximately 3 years from diagnosis. The natural history of IPF is of a relentlessly progressive decline in pulmonary function, culminating in hypoxaemic respiratory failure and death. This may be interrupted at any stage by a distinct and catastrophic clinical entity known as 'acute exacerbation of idiopathic pulmonary fibrosis' (AEIPF). AEIPF is characterized by an accelerated decline over a period of weeks with worsening dyspnoea, hypoxaemia, and alveolar infiltrates on chest radiology, in the absence of infection or left ventricular failure. Treatment with pulsed corticosteroids is often attempted but mortality is high. Lung histology during AEIPF shows diffuse alveolar damage, a pattern similar to that seen with adult respiratory distress syndrome and acute interstitial

Table 139.1 The interstitial lung diseases	
Aetiology	**Examples**
Idiopathic	Idiopathic pulmonary fibrosis
	Non-specific interstitial pneumonia
	Acute interstitial pneumonia
	Cryptogenic organizing pneumonia
Smoking	Respiratory bronchiolitis interstitial lung disease
	Desquamative interstitial pneumonia
	Langerhans cell histiocytosis
Inhaled mineral dusts	Asbestosis
	Silicosis
	Berylliosis
	Coal-worker's pneumoconiosis
Inhaled organic antigens	Hypersensitivity pneumonitis
Drugs, toxins, and physical insults	Methotrexate
	Busulfan
	Bleomycin
	Amiodarone
	Nitrofurantoin
	Paraquat
	Radiation pneumonitis
Systemic inflammatory diseases	Rheumatoid arthritis
	SLE
	Mixed connective tissue disease
	Systemic sclerosis
	Polymyositis
	Dermatomyositis
	Sjögren syndrome
	Ankylosing spondylitis
	Ulcerative colitis
	Crohn's disease
Pulmonary vasculitis	Granulomatosis with polyangiitis (Wegener's granulomatosis)[§]
	Eosinophilic granulomatosis with polyangiitis (Churg–Strauss syndrome)[§]
	Microscopic polyangiitis
	Anti-glomerular basement membrane disease (Goodpasture's disease)[§]
Miscellaneous	Sarcoidosis
	Eosinophilic pneumonia
	Lymphocytic interstitial pneumonia
	Obliterative bronchiolitis
	Lymphangioleiomyomatosis
	Pulmonary alveolar proteinosis
	Amyloidosis

[§] Previous name in brackets.

pneumonia. Most other ILDs tend to follow a more benign course than IPF, with some patients remaining clinically stable for many years, and others displaying a slowly progressive decline.

Approach to diagnosis

Diagnostic efforts should be aimed at identifying the precise type of ILD, as this has important prognostic and therapeutic implications. Alternative diagnoses that may mimic ILD should be excluded.

History

The history should focus initially on the patient's symptoms and their time course. As previously described, slowly progressive exertional dyspnoea and dry cough are typical of ILD. Wheeze suggests an airway component to the disease and may occur with hypersensitivity pneumonitis or eosinophilic granulomatosis with polyangiitis (previously known as Churg–Strauss syndrome). Haemoptysis occurs with pulmonary vasculitis, due to associated alveolar haemorrhage. Systemic features such as fever and weight loss are particularly prominent in cryptogenic organizing pneumonia (COP) and hypersensitivity pneumonitis. Arthritis or arthralgia, skin rashes, dry eyes or mouth, and Raynaud's phenomenon are suggestive of associated connective tissue disease.

A meticulous drug history should be taken, including the use of over-the-counter drugs, alternative remedies, and illicit drugs. Recent exposures to drugs known to cause ILD should be elicited, even if these have now been stopped.

The smoking history is particularly important, since a number of ILDs occur mainly or exclusively in smokers, namely respiratory bronchiolitis interstitial lung disease, desquamative interstitial pneumonia, and Langerhans cell histiocytosis. IPF and NSIP occur more commonly in smokers but are reasonably prevalent in non-smokers, while pulmonary sarcoidosis and hypersensitivity pneumonitis are rare in smokers.

The occupational history should include all jobs that the patient has performed since leaving school, with details of the precise nature of the work carried out. Exposure to asbestos at any time in the past should be specifically sought, including secondary exposure; for instance, the wives of plumbers or shipyard workers may have been exposed through washing their husbands' work clothes. There are myriad organic antigens encountered in the workplace or through recreational activities that may cause hypersensitivity pneumonitis. While many of these exposures can be ruled out by a full occupational history, the following additional factors should be enquired about:

- exposure to birds or other animals
- swimming in an indoor pool or hot tub
- the presence of a humidifier or ventilator system at home or at work
- exposure to damp or mouldy environments
- gardening or DIY

Examination

General examination may reveal tachypnoea and cyanosis in advanced disease. Finger clubbing occurs most commonly in IPF and asbestosis. Evidence of an inflammatory arthritis is suggestive of connective tissue disease, and specific features of systemic sclerosis may be elicited, such as Raynaud's phenomenon, sclerodactyly, microstomia, telangiectasia, and calcinosis. Various skin rashes may be seen, including erythema nodosum (sarcoidosis), a purpuric or petechial rash (systemic vasculitis), or facial erythema in a 'butterfly' distribution (SLE). The hallmark of ILD on physical examination is the presence of fine inspiratory crackles on auscultation of the chest, although these are not present in all cases. Hypersensitivity pneumonitis may also cause characteristic inspiratory squeaks due to small airway inflammation (bronchiolitis).

Investigations

Blood tests

The following blood tests may be performed:

- antinuclear antibody, extractable nuclear antigens, and rheumatoid factor levels should be checked to screen for associated connective tissue disease
- antineutrophil cytoplasmic antibody (ANCA) may be positive in pulmonary vasculitis; in particular, cytoplasmic ANCA (cANCA) is associated with granulomatosis with polyangiitis (previously known as Wegener's granulomatosis), and perinuclear ANCA (pANCA) with eosinophilic granulomatosis with polyangiitis; however, a negative ANCA does not completely rule out vasculitis
- Serum angiotensin-converting enzyme is often raised in sarcoidosis; while it is not sensitive or specific enough to act as a definitive diagnostic test, it is a useful marker of disease activity once the diagnosis has been made

- avian and other precipitins should be checked as appropriate if hypersensitivity pneumonitis is suspected

Pulmonary function tests

ILD typically produces a restrictive pattern on spirometry, with a reduction in both forced vital capacity (FVC) and forced expiratory volume in 1 second (FEV_1), but with a normal or high FEV_1/FVC ratio. Measures of lung volume such as the residual volume and total lung capacity are low, whether measured by helium dilution or whole-body plethysmography. Carbon monoxide transfer factor (TLco) levels are also low, even after correcting for reduced lung volumes.

Chest radiograph

The plain chest radiograph (CXR) may reveal interstitial shadowing with a reticular, nodular or reticulonodular pattern. Single or multiple areas of consolidation are suggestive of pulmonary vasculitis with alveolar haemorrhage, COP, or eosinophilic pneumonia. Bilateral hilar lymphadenopathy occurs commonly with sarcoidosis. In a significant minority of cases, the CXR is normal in patients with ILD.

High-resolution CT

High resolution CT (HRCT) is an important diagnostic modality in patients with ILD. The extent and distribution of fibrosis, honeycombing, nodular opacities, consolidation, ground-glass opacification, and cyst formation are used to produce a radiological differential diagnosis. It has been shown that, in the presence of typical HRCT appearances consisting of fibrosis and honeycombing with basal and subpleural predominance, and compatible history and examination findings, a diagnosis of IPF can be confidently made. In such cases, lung biopsy is not usually necessary as it is unlikely to alter the final diagnosis. However, many other cases are less clear-cut and thus histological examination of lung tissue is required to make the diagnosis. In particular, the distinction between atypical IPF and NSIP can be difficult to make radiologically.

Bronchoscopy

Bronchoalveolar lavage (BAL) generally has a minor role in the diagnosis of suspected ILD, although it may be helpful in selected cases. IPF is generally associated with BAL neutrophilia, while sarcoidosis and hypersensitivity pneumonitis cause BAL lymphocytosis. Eosinophilic pneumonia results in a high BAL eosinophil count.

Bronchoscopy is most helpful in patients with suspected sarcoidosis, since the disease process often has a bronchocentric distribution. Transbronchial biopsy may reveal characteristic non-caseating granulomas and, in some cases, visible endobronchial nodularity can be visualized and bronchial biopsies taken. Enlarged mediastinal lymph nodes may also be sampled either via blind transbronchial needle aspiration, or with the use of endobronchial ultrasound.

Surgical lung biopsy

Most ILDs cannot be sampled satisfactorily via the transbronchial route and thus surgical lung biopsy is frequently required. This is often performed using video-assisted thoracoscopic surgery. Multiple samples are taken from different segments of the lung, with the sampling sites chosen according to the areas of florid disease activity on HRCT.

Table 139.2 Conditions that may simulate interstitial lung disease

Category	Examples
Malignant	Lymphangitis carcinomatosa
	Bronchoalveolar cell carcinoma
	Pulmonary lymphoma
Infectious	Viral pneumonitis
	Bacterial pneumonia
	Fungal pneumonia
	Miliary tuberculosis
	Pneumocystis jiroveci pneumonia
Miscellaneous	Pulmonary oedema
	Acute respiratory distress syndrome
	Aspiration pneumonitis

Other diagnoses that should be considered

A number of conditions can simulate the clinical and radiographic features of ILD and therefore need to be considered in the differential diagnosis. These are listed in Table 139.2.

'Gold-standard' diagnostic test

Surgical lung biopsy is the single investigation with the greatest claim for being the gold-standard test for ILD diagnosis. However, the diagnosis of ILD is often challenging, since many patients present with radiological or histological features that are not completely typical of any one condition. Indeed, studies have shown only moderate inter-observer agreement between expert radiologists and between expert pathologists in cases of ILD. This means that neither a HRCT scan nor a surgical lung biopsy can be considered a true gold-standard diagnostic test.

It is now recognized that diagnostic accuracy is maximized by integrating clinical, radiological, and pathological information, and that this is best achieved through a multidisciplinary meeting (MDM). Thus, the gold standard for the diagnosis of ILD is currently considered to be an MDM consensus of expert clinicians, radiologists, and pathologists, with access to good quality clinical information, an HRCT scan, and a surgical lung biopsy, as well as the results of any of the previously mentioned ancillary tests which may be required.

Acceptable diagnostic alternatives to the gold standard

It is accepted that a surgical lung biopsy is not necessary if a HRCT scan shows the so-called usual interstitial pneumonia pattern, which consists of fibrosis and honeycombing with basal and subpleural predominance. In such cases, IPF can be confidently diagnosed on the basis of the clinical features and HRCT appearances alone. Furthermore, many patients will be too frail or elderly to undergo a surgical lung biopsy and, in other cases, this invasive procedure may be deemed unlikely to alter patient management and thus unnecessary. In such cases, a clinicoradiological diagnosis is an acceptable alternative to surgical lung biopsy.

Other relevant investigations

Other investigations should be focused on diagnosing or excluding the differential diagnoses of ILD (see Table 139.2), as well as assessing disease severity and prognosis. Such investigations include:

- bronchoscopy and washings; these may be indicated to exclude infectious or malignant conditions that can simulate ILD; washings should be sent for microscopy and culture, including staining for acid-fast bacilli and *Pneumocystis jiroveci*, as well as cytology
- HIV testing; this should be considered in high-risk groups, since a number of pulmonary complications of HIV can present as an ILD-like illness; these include *Pneumocystis jiroveci* pneumonia, miliary tuberculosis, cytomegalovirus pneumonitis, NSIP, lymphocytic interstitial pneumonia, and obliterative bronchiolitis
- echocardiography; this may show pulmonary hypertension and right ventricular failure in advanced ILD; referral to a tertiary pulmonary hypertension centre should be considered if patients exhibit pulmonary hypertension that is out of proportion to the severity of lung disease, and certainly in the case of pulmonary hypertension associated with a connective tissue disease such as systemic sclerosis

Prognosis and how to estimate it

The prognosis of the idiopathic ILDs varies according to the histological diagnosis. Patients with IPF have the worst prognosis, with a median survival of approximately 3 years from diagnosis. Prognosis is better in patients with NSIP, particularly those with the cellular rather than the fibrotic subtype. NSIP is characterized by more inflammation and less fibrosis than IPF, and is thus more responsive to corticosteroids and other immunosuppressive therapy. COP responds

extremely well to corticosteroids and treated cases have an excellent prognosis. Secondary ILDs have a varied prognosis according to whether the underlying cause can be identified and removed or treated. The best physiological parameter for predicting survival in patients with ILD is the percentage drop in FVC over a 6-month period, with a greater-than-10% drop indicating a poor prognosis.

Treatment and its effectiveness

General measures

The management of ILD may be divided into general supportive measures and specific treatments. General supportive measures include the appropriate provision of oxygen, pulmonary rehabilitation, and palliative care, including the use of opiates for distressing symptoms of shortness of breath.

Environmental exposures that may be contributing to the disease should be eliminated. Most notably, strenuous efforts must be made to achieve smoking cessation through a combination of specialist counselling and pharmacological therapy. In some conditions, namely respiratory bronchiolitis interstitial lung disease, desquamative interstitial pneumonia, and Langerhans cell histiocytosis, smoking cessation may alone result in resolution of the disease process. Drugs that may cause ILD, such as nitrofurantoin, should be withdrawn if possible. In proven hypersensitivity pneumonitis, patients should be strongly encouraged to cease any exposure to the causative antigen, although there is often strong resistance to giving up a much loved hobby or activity, such as keeping pigeons.

Corticosteroids and other immunosuppressants

The response of ILD to corticosteroids and other immunosuppressive treatment depends on whether the underlying pathology is mainly inflammatory or fibrotic. Inflammatory conditions such as COP respond extremely well to steroids, while fibrotic conditions such as IPF respond poorly. Table 139.3 shows examples of ILDs and their responsiveness to steroids.

When corticosteroids are used, they are usually started at moderate or high doses (e.g. prednisolone 30–40 mg daily) and, after an initial treatment period, slowly tapered down over a period of months. In some cases, relapse can occur after withdrawal of treatment, necessitating temporary reintroduction. High-dose steroids (more than 10 mg prednisolone per day) should be avoided in ILD associated with systemic sclerosis, due to the risk of scleroderma renal crisis. The addition of other immunosuppressive agents such as cyclophosphamide or azathioprine to corticosteroid therapy is essential in systemic vasculitis and is often required in connective tissue disease-related ILD.

Treatment of IPF

The treatment of IPF has previously been problematic due to the lack of effective disease-modifying therapies. IPF is predominantly a fibrotic condition and conventional anti-inflammatory treatments do not appear to affect its course. Thus, steroid monotherapy is not recommended in current guidelines.

Table 139.3 Steroid-responsiveness amongst the interstitial lung diseases

Good or moderate response to corticosteroids	Poor response to corticosteroids
Cryptogenic organizing pneumonia	Idiopathic pulmonary fibrosis
Cellular non-specific interstitial pneumonia	Fibrotic non-specific interstitial pneumonia
Hypersensitivity pneumonitis	Langerhans cell histiocytosis
Amiodarone-induced pneumonitis	Asbestosis
Methotrexate-induced pneumonitis	Coal worker's pneumoconiosis
Connective tissue disease-related interstitial lung disease	Lymphangioleiomyomatosis
Sarcoidosis	
Eosinophilic pneumonia	

A recent randomized controlled trial showed that the combination of acetylcysteine, azathioprine, and prednisolone actually increased mortality compared to placebo. However, there are now two new therapies available that appear to slow the progression of IPF, namely pirfenidone and nintedanib.

Lung transplantation is the only treatment that has been shown to improve survival in patients with IPF. Current British Thoracic Society guidelines suggest that patients should be referred for transplantation if the disease is severe (TLco less than 40% predicted) or rapidly progressive (greater than 10% decline in FVC over 6 months). However, patients with significant comorbidities or of age greater than 65 are generally excluded. Similar referral criteria are used for other ILDs, such as fibrotic NSIP and sarcoidosis.

Treatment of acute ILD

The management of acute or rapidly progressive ILD is challenging due to a combination of diagnostic uncertainty and the urgency of initiating definitive treatment. Acute ILD may occur on a background of established ILD, the most common scenario, or de novo.

It is well recognized that IPF patients who were relatively stable previously may manifest a period of rapid decline over a number of weeks, associated with worsening pulmonary infiltrates and type 1 respiratory failure, the distinctive clinical entity AEIPF. The differential diagnosis in such cases includes infection, pulmonary oedema, and pulmonary embolism. Echocardiography and CT pulmonary angiography may be obtained to rule out left ventricular dysfunction and pulmonary embolism, respectively. Empirical antibiotics are often provided, although obtaining a specific microbiological diagnosis is difficult since most patients are too hypoxic to tolerate a bronchoscopy and lavage. Pulsed high-dose IV methylprednisolone may be attempted if infection is thought to be unlikely, although this is supported only by anecdotal evidence. A more pragmatic approach is to prescribe moderate doses of corticosteroids, for example, oral prednisolone 30 mg daily. The mortality of AEIPF is high, and invasive ventilation is almost always inappropriate. It is important to effectively communicate the prognosis to patients and their families, and to switch the focus of care to palliative when appropriate.

Genuine de novo presentations of acute ILD are uncommon. In many cases, a careful history and inspection of old chest radiographs reveals evidence of previously unrecognized chronic ILD. In patients with apparent de novo ILD, a more aggressive approach to diagnosis and treatment is warranted. The ILDs most likely to present in this way are acute interstitial pneumonia, fulminant COP, drug-induced pneumonitis, acute eosinophilic pneumonia, and pulmonary vasculitis. Patients often require admission to the intensive care unit for invasive ventilation. It is vital that any possible drug precipitants are withdrawn unless they are absolutely necessary. Infection should be diagnosed or excluded using BAL, often in an intubated patient. Transbronchial biopsy or surgical lung biopsy should be considered if the results are likely to alter the management sufficiently to justify the risks. In most cases, once infection has been excluded, the mainstay of therapy in acute ILD is high-dose pulsed IV methylprednisolone. The addition of IV cyclophosphamide is occasionally required.

Treatment of rare ILDs

Two rare ILDs merit special mention since their treatments are unique. Pulmonary alveolar proteinosis is characterized by the progressive accumulation of lipoproteinaceous material within the alveolar spaces. It is treated with bronchoscopic whole-lung lavage under general anaesthetic, with both symptomatic and survival benefits. Both lungs are usually treated a few days apart.

Lymphangioleiomyomatosis occurs almost exclusively in women of child-bearing age and it has thus been hypothesized that oestrogen may play a role in the pathogenesis. Sirolimus has shown some promise as a treatment for this condition. Progressive disease may necessitate lung transplantation.

Further Reading

Belloli EA, Martinez FJ, and Flaherty KR. Update in interstitial lung disease 2014. *Am J Respir Crit Care Med* 2015; 192: 538–43.

Fischer A, Antoniou KM, Brown KK, et al. An official European Respiratory Society/American Thoracic Society research statement: interstitial pneumonia with autoimmune features. *Eur Respir J* 2015; 46: 976–87.

Richeldi L, Collard HR, and Jones MG. Idiopathic pulmonary fibrosis. *Lancet* 2017; 389: 1941–52.

Vij R and Strek ME. Diagnosis and treatment of connective tissue disease-associated interstitial lung disease. *Chest* 2013; 143: 814–24.

Rajini Sudhir

Definition of the disease

Pulmonary vasculitis comprises a heterogeneous group of disorders characterized by an inflammatory process damaging the vessel wall, leading to ischaemia and tissue necrosis. Granulomatosis with polyangiitis (Wegener's granulomatosis) Churg–Strauss syndrome (eosinophilic granulomatosis with polyangiitis, EGPA), and microscopic polyangiitis are primary, small-vessel, necrotizing vasculitides linked by an overlapping clinicopathological picture and are collectively referred to as ANCA-associated systemic vasculitis (AASV). The European Vasculitis Study Group has proposed a clinical staging system based on disease activity, to guide treatment (see Table 140.1).

Aetiology of the disease

The exact aetiology of pulmonary vasculitis is unclear, although the disease is associated with exposure to silica, quartz, occupational solvents, or livestock. Drugs such as propylthiouracil, carbimazole, allopurinol, and minocycline have been associated with AASV.

Specific disorders

Granulomatosis with polyangiitis

Definition

Granulomatosis with polyangiitis (abbreviated as GPA, and formerly known as Wegener's granulomatosis) is the most common pulmonary vasculitis. It classically involves the upper and lower respiratory tracts and the kidneys.

Aetiology

The aetiology of GPA is unclear, but the disease is characterized by the histopathological finding of small-vessel necrotizing vasculitis and granulomatous inflammation. Patients with type ZZ alpha-1 antitrypsin deficiency are at a 100-fold increased risk of GPA. *Staphylococcus aureus* nasal carriage is very common with GPA.

Typical symptoms, and less common symptoms

Upper respiratory symptoms

The upper respiratory features of GPA are ENT involvement in 70%–90% of patients, hearing loss in 15%–20%, and nasopharyngeal involvement in 60%, with the latter characterized by nasal crusting, pain, mucosal ulcers, and epistaxis. Septal perforation and saddle nose deformity occur in up to 25% of patients with GPA.

Lower respiratory symptoms

Lower respiratory symptoms of GPA include wheeze, dyspnoea, and stridor. Tracheal stenosis is associated with flattening of both limbs of the flow–volume loop. Subglottic stenosis invariably occurs with nasopharyngeal disease. Lung parenchymal involvement presents as dyspnoea, cough, and haemoptysis with diffuse alveolar haemorrhage (DAH). The chest X-ray is abnormal in up to 70% of patients, showing nodules, cavitation, consolidation, infiltrates, or intra-thoracic lymphadenopathy.

Renal features

Renal features of GPA include glomerulonephritis with hypertension, acute renal failure with casts and proteinuria, and chronic renal impairment.

Optical features

Optical features of GPA include scleritis, episcleritis, and proptosis.

CNS-related features

CNS-related features of GPA include mononeuritis multiplex and cranial nerve palsy.

Demographics

The peak age of onset of GPA is 30–50 years. By the late 1990s, the incidence was around 10.3 per million. The disease is commoner in Northern Europe than elsewhere, with an increased incidence in winter months.

Natural history, and complications

The clinical spectrum of GPA ranges from an asymptomatic form to fulminant respiratory failure with DAH, the latter with a mortality of up to 50%. Subglottic stenosis can cause life-threatening airway compromise. Glomerulonephritis is the most worrying feature, and progressive renal failure can occur in the absence of any other features, needing aggressive immunosuppressive therapy. Even patients with limited GPA and no renal disease can have severe diffuse alveolar haemorrhage or neurological involvement. Consequently, the term 'limited GPA' is defined as necrotizing granulomatous inflammation with (a) no vasculitis component and (b) no disease manifestation that puts the affected organ at risk of irreversible damage. Complications occur in the form of relapse, infections, or drug toxicity and need close monitoring.

Approach to diagnosis

The approach to diagnosing GPA involves identification of the clinical features listed in 'Typical symptoms, and less common symptoms', and exclusion of the differentials listed in 'Other diagnoses that should be considered'.

Other diagnoses that should be considered

The differential diagnosis for granulomatous inflammation is mainly fungal or mycobacterial infection. Ophthalmological features may suggest sarcoidosis. Destructive nasopharyngeal disease should be

Table 140.1 The European Vasculitis Study Group clinical staging system

Class	Localized	Early systemic	Generalized systemic	Severe	Refractory
Constitutional	–	+	+	+	Any
Renal dysfunction	–	–	+	++	Any
Threatened vital organ function	–	–	–	++	+
Induction	Single agent CS, AZA, MTX	CYC/MTX + CS	CYC + CS	CYC + CS + PEX	Investigational drugs

Abbreviations: AZA, azathioprine; CS, corticosteroid; CYC, cyclophosphamide; MTX, methotrexate; PEX, plasma exchange.

Rasmussen N, Jayne DRW, Abraowicz D, et al. European therapeutic trials in ANCA-associated systemic vasculitis: disease scoring, consensus regimes and proposed clinical trials. European Community Study Group on Clinical Trials in Systemic Vasculitis ECSYSVASTRIAL. Clin Exp Immunol. 1995;101(Suppl 1):29-34.

differentiated from cocaine-related disease or lymphoma. Relapsing polychondritis can cause saddle nose deformity or tracheobronchial involvement but ear involvement is the cardinal feature differentiating relapsing polychondritis from GPA. DAH could also be caused by Goodpasture's disease, rheumatoid vasculitis, or SLE.

'Gold-standard' diagnostic test

cANCA (PR3) positivity is a feature of 75%–90% of patients with GPA. The prevalence of this feature increases to 99% if immunofluorescence is used along with target-antigen-specific methods. This is often combined with biopsy of the affected area, showing necrotizing small-vessel vasculitis.

Acceptable diagnostic alternatives to the gold standard

There are no acceptable diagnostic alternatives to the gold standard for Wegener's granulomatosis. The criteria specified in 'Gold-standard' diagnostic test for granulomatosis with polyangiitis must be used for diagnosis.

Other relevant investigations

Chest X-ray abnormalities occur in around 70% of patients sometime during their disease activity. High-resolution CT thorax shows the extent of bronchial or peribronchial involvement. Flow–volume loops are either obstructive or restrictive, with flattening of limbs in tracheal stenosis. With DAH, there is an increase in the diffusing

Table 140.2 Non-Granulomatosis with polyangiitis (GPA) ANCA-associated systemic vasculitis

	Churg–Strauss syndrome (Eosinophilic granulomatosis with polyangiitis)	Microscopic polyangiitis
Definition	Allergic granulomatous angiitis with asthma, small-vessel vasculitis, and hypereosinophilia	Necrotizing small-vessel vasculitis with predominant focal segmental glomerulonephritis
Aetiology	Unclear but similar to GPA	Unclear but similar to GPA
Symptoms	Asthma refractory to most treatments Allergic rhinitis and polyposis Peripheral neuropathy	DAH in 30% Pleurisy, effusion, and lung fibrosis (10%–12%) Focal glomerulonephritis; acute renal failure with casts and proteinuria in around 90% Headache, seizures (cerebral vasculitis) in 30% Abdominal pain, diarrhoea; bowel perforation in 30%–40%
Demographics	40–50 years peak Male = female Commoner in northern Spain	50–55 years peak incidence Male > female Commoner in middle-aged Caucasians
History and complications	First phase with rhinitis and asthma difficult to control, followed by eosinophilia (remitting and relapsing) and then vasculitis Renal involvement is uncommon Main mortality is due to cardiac disease and is a poor prognostic sign	Limited data but upper airway involvement is controversial Occasional acute interstitial pneumonitis or idiopathic pulmonary fibrosis Rapidly progressive glomerulonephritis from renal capillaritis has high mortality Relapses are common
Approach to diagnosis	Asthma with ANCA positivity and high eosinophil count	Renal failure with ANCA positivity
Differential diagnosis	GPA Microscopic polyangiitis Hypereosinophilic syndrome Chronic eosinophilic pneumonia	GPA Polyarteritis nodosa SLE Goodpasture's disease
'Gold-standard' test	Biopsy of peripheral nerve or lung shows eosinophilic exudates, fibrinoid necrosis, and epithelioid/giant cell granuloma	No unique histopathology on biopsy but presence of small-vessel pulmonary or renal capillaritis Pauci-immune glomerulonephritis (minimal or absent immune complex deposit), in contrast to polyarteritis nodosa or Goodpasture's disease
Acceptable alternatives to the gold-standard test; other investigations	PFT ANCA positivity Type of ANCA CXR/HRCT Blood	PFT ANCA positivity Type of ANCA CXR/HRCT Blood
PFT	Obstructive	Obstructive but restrictive with IPF Increased DLCO, with DAH
ANCA positivity	Up to 65%	Up to 90%
Type of ANCA	pANCA (MPO-ANCA)	pANCA (MPO-ANCA)
CXR/HRCT	Transient infiltrates Nodules unusual Ground glass opacities on HRCT	Infiltrates Ground glass opacities on HRCT
Blood	Peripheral eosinophilia	No eosinophilia
Prognosis	Remission in 90%, and relapses in 15%–25% Asthma is often refractory to treatment Mortality is high with cardiac involvement 60%–69% 5-year survival	90% improve, and 75% achieve complete remission; 30% relapse in 1–2 years Mortality high with rapidly progressive renal failure or DAH 45%–53% 5-year survival
Treatment	Glucocorticoids are the mainstay of treatment The role of cytotoxic agents is less well defined, but life-threatening disease is treated with glucocorticoids and cyclophosphamide Recent trials show promising maintenance of remission with IFN-alpha	Treatment similar to that for GPA Single studies are unavailable but mixed studies suggest response to glucocorticoids and cyclophosphamide in renal disease or DAH

Abbreviations: ANCA, antineutrophil cytoplasmic antibody; CXR, chest X-ray; DAH, diffuse alveolar haemorrhage; DLCO, diffusing capacity of the lung for carbon monoxide; GPA, granulomatosis with polyangiitis HRCT, high-resolution CT; IFN-alpha, interferon alpha; IPF, idiopathic pulmonary fibrosis; MPO, myeloperoxidase; pANCA, perinuclear antineutrophil cytoplasmic antibody; PFT, pulmonary function testing; SLE, systemic lupus erythematosus.

capacity of the lung for carbon monoxide (DLCO). Bronchoscopy shows ulcerative tracheobronchitis, subglottic stenosis, or haemorrhagic fluid on bronchoalveolar lavage. Urine dipsticks for blood and protein, and microscopy for casts, are used to indicate renal disease. MRI brain is a sensitive modality for determining neurological involvement.

Prognosis, and how to estimate it

In GPA, there is 30%–93% remission with treatment, 1-year survival is at 80%–85%, and estimated 5-year survival is at 65%–78%. Clinical symptoms, and findings from chest X-ray, lung function, urine dipsticks, microscopy, and the cANCA test are all essential in estimating and monitoring disease activity, although the cANCA tests needs to be interpreted in conjunction with other indicators of disease activity. In addition, 40%–60% of patients will relapse on treatment.

Treatment, and its effectiveness

In the 1950s, glucocorticoid monotherapy was used in the treatment of GPA, since the 1-year mortality of the untreated disease was around 82%. However, an NIH cohort showed that, with steroids along, there was no sustained improvement but instead progressive disease, leading to discontinuation of the monotherapy. Remission is induced with cyclophosphamide at 2 mg/kg day⁻¹, and prednisolone at 1 mg/kg day⁻¹, tapered over 6–12 months.

Significant toxicities from steroids include hypertension, diabetes, intercurrent infections, osteoporosis, psychosis, and Addison's disease. Cyclophosphamide toxicity includes myelosuppression (8%), cystitis (12%), infertility, and solid organ malignancies (5%). This can be reduced by intermittent administration of the drug, although relapse rates are higher on this regime.

Methotrexate (20–25 mg/week) is used with prednisolone for remission induction, and azathioprine (1 mg/kg day⁻¹) is useful in remission maintenance. Pneumocystis prophylaxis with co-trimoxazole is indicated in all patients on immunosuppressive therapy since this carries a mortality of around 35%. Co-trimoxazole at dose of 160/800 mg twice a day is useful in eliminating nasal carriage of *Staphylococcus aureus* and thereby reducing relapse of upper airway disease.

In fulminant disease (DAH; respiratory or renal failure), use pulsed methylprednisolone at 1 g/day for 3 days, with cyclophosphamide at 3–4 mg/day for 3 days and then reduced to 2 mg/day. If this doesn't work, use plasma exchange, with 60 mg/kg exchanged with 5% human albumin solution for 2 weeks.

Rituximab (RTX, a monoclonal antibody directed against the CD20 surface antigen of B lymphocytes) can be given if cyclophosphamide is contraindicated, e.g. because of high risk of infection, or to avoid its effect on fertility in a young patient. RTX is combined with glucocorticoid therapy. The licensed RTX dose is 375 mg/m2 body surface area/week for 4 weeks; an alternative effective regimen is 1 g repeated after 2 weeks.

Sinus disease is treated with local irrigation, local corticosteroids, and antibiotics. Subglottic stenosis is often treated with tracheostomy or a combination of mechanical dilatation of trachea with intra-tracheal glucocorticoid injection.

In addition to GPA, there are two other types of ANCA-associated systemic vasculitis; their features are described in Table 140.2

Goodpasture's disease

Goodpasture's disease is a rare disorder with an incidence of 1–2/million. It is more common in young cigarette smokers who develop pulmonary haemorrhage; 25%–30% of cases have a viral prodrome. It is characterized by an insidious onset of dry cough, dyspnoea, haemoptysis, oligoanuria, uraemia, and respiratory failure.

It is diagnosed by renal biopsy showing crescentic glomerulonephritis with anti-glomerular basement membrane antibodies on immunofluorescence. The antibodies are directed to the alpha-3 chain of type IV collagen. which is present in the basement membrane. In addition, 32% of patients with Goodpasture's disease are ANCA positive. Treatment is by plasmapheresis, with concomitant use of glucocorticoids with cyclophosphamide, and smoking cessation is advised.

Patients who survive the first year with near-normal renal function do well but relapses occur with ANCA positivity.

Secondary pulmonary vasculitis

Secondary pulmonary vasculitis is usually associated with rheumatoid arthritis or SLE, and is often managed in conjunction with rheumatology. It an immune-complex-mediated disease, and haemoptysis and pulmonary infiltrates with systemic upset are common clinical features. Alveolar haemorrhage with SLE has a mortality of over 50%. Survivors may progress to lung fibrosis. Synchronized plasmapheresis with pulsed methylprednisolone and IV cyclophosphamide therapy are useful in treatment.

Respiratory involvement in other vasculitides

Twenty-five per cent of patients with giant cell arteritis have pulmonary involvement. Large- and medium-vessel vasculitis with pulmonary hypertension is seen in up to 50% with Takayasu's disease, and 40% with Behçet's syndrome. Necrotizing sarcoid granuloma occurs with bilateral nodules and is treated with glucocorticoids.

Further Reading

Lally L and Spiera RF. Pulmonary vasculitis. *Rheumatic Disease Clinics* 2015; 41: 315–31.
Ntatsaki E, Carruthers D, Chakravarty K, et al. BSR and BHPR guideline for the management of adults with ANCA-associated vasculitis. *Rheumatology* 2014; 53: 2306–9.

141 Lung cancer (including management of an isolated lung lesion)

Raman Verma and Sarah Deacon

Definition of the disease

Lung cancer is the second most common type of cancer in the UK. It is a disease of uncontrolled cell growth in the lung tissue. It is termed 'primary' if it originates in the lungs, and 'secondary' if it manifests elsewhere in the body but then spreads to the lungs.

There are several types of primary lung cancer. The main types are small cell lung carcinoma (SCLC) and non-small cell lung carcinoma (NSCLC). This distinction is important, because the treatment varies.

SCLCs comprise 20% of lung cancers and are the most aggressive and rapidly growing. They are small cells that are mostly filled with the nucleus and contain dense neurosecretory granules, which give this tumour an endocrine/paraneoplastic syndrome association. They are strongly related to smoking, with only 1% of these tumours occurring in non-smokers. SCLCs metastasize rapidly to many sites within the body and are most often discovered after they have spread extensively.

There are three main types of NSCLC:

Squamous cell carcinoma (25%): Squamous cell carcinoma develops in the cells lining the airways. It usually starts near a central bronchus. A hollow cavity and associated necrosis are commonly found at tumour center.

Adenocarcinoma (40%): Adenocarcinoma develops from cells producing mucus. It usually originates in peripheral lung tissue. A subtype, bronchioloalveolar carcinoma, is more common in females who have never smoked. It occurs in less than 1 in 20 lung cancers.

Large cell carcinoma: In large cell carcinoma, large, rounded cells are seen under the microscope. This type tends to grow quite quickly.

Other types of lung cancers can arise; for example, bronchial carcinoids account for up to 5% of lung cancer. These are generally small when diagnosed and occur most commonly in people under 40 years of age. Unrelated to cigarette smoking, carcinoid tumours can metastasize and a small proportion of these tumours secrete hormone-like substances which may cause specific symptoms related to the hormone being produced. Carcinoids generally grow and spread more slowly than bronchogenic cancers, and many are detected early enough to be amenable to surgical resection.

Mesothelioma is a rare type of cancer that affects the pleura. It is associated with asbestos exposure. It is very different from lung cancer.

Aetiology of the disease

The most common cause of lung cancer is long-term exposure to tobacco smoke. The occurrence of lung cancer in non-smokers, who account for 10% of cases, is often attributed to a combination of genetic factors, radon gas, asbestos, and air pollution (including secondhand smoke).

Tobacco smoke contains carcinogens. The two primary carcinogenic chemicals are nitrosamines and polycyclic aromatic hydrocarbons. Additionally, nicotine appears to depress the immune response to malignant growth. About nine in ten cases are caused by smoking. Among male smokers, the lifetime risk of developing lung cancer is 17.2%; among female smokers, the risk is 11.6%. After about 15 years of smoking cessation, the risk of developing lung cancer is similar to that of a non-smoker. Those who are regularly exposed to passive smoke have a small increased risk.

A family history of lung cancer in a first-degree relative slightly increases the risk of lung cancer. However, most cases of lung cancer do not run in families.

People who have been in prolonged or close contact with asbestos have a higher risk of lung cancer, especially if they smoke. Asbestos and tobacco smoke act synergistically to increase the risk. Asbestos exposure also increases the risk of mesothelioma.

Radon gas is thought to increase risk in high concentrations. This colourless and odourless gas generated by the breakdown of radioactive radium, which in turn is the decay product of uranium, found in the Earth's crust. The decay products ionize genetic material, causing mutations that sometimes turn cancerous. This is more likely in certain parts of the UK where there is a lot of granite, for example in the West Country and the Peak District.

Typical symptoms of the disease, and less common symptoms

Symptoms that suggest lung cancer include:

- dyspnoea
- haemoptysis
- chronic coughing or change in regular coughing pattern
- wheezing
- chest pain (possible rib erosion)
- cachexia, fatigue, and loss of appetite
- hoarse voice (possible recurrent laryngeal nerve involvement)
- clubbing

If the cancer obstructs airflow, it can lead to secretion accumulation behind the blockage, predisposing the patient to pneumonia. A pleural effusion may accumulate which can cause worsening dyspnoea. Facial oedema may develop if a tumour compresses the superior vena cava. Apical lung cancers (Pancoast tumours) may invade the local part of the sympathetic nervous system, leading to Horner's syndrome as well as muscle weakness in the hands due to invasion of the brachial plexus.

Depending on the type of cancer, so-called paraneoplastic phenomena may initially attract attention to the disease (see Table 141.1).

Table 141.1 Paraneoplastic syndromes associated with cancer type

Cancer type	Paraneoplastic symptom
Squamous	Hypercalcaemia (due to parathyroid-like hormone production)
Adenocarcinoma	Hypertrophic pulmonary osteoarthropathy (joint stiffness, gynaecomastia, clubbing)
	Trousseau syndrome of hypercoagulability
Small cell	Syndrome of inappropriate antidiuretic hormone
	Cushing's syndrome (ectopic adrenocorticotropic hormone)

Table 141.2 Complications of the metastatic spread of cancer

Site	Symptom
Brain	Confusion, fits, focal neurological deficit, cerebellar syndrome
Bone	Pain, hypercalcaemia, spinal cord compression
Liver	Pain, hepatomegaly, liver failure
Adrenal	Addison's disease

Demographics of the disease

Lung cancer is the most common cancer in the world, with 1.3 million new cases diagnosed every year. It is the UK's biggest cancer killer, claiming nearly 36 000 lives each year. It is responsible for 23% of all male cancer deaths, and 21% of all female cancer deaths. More than eight in ten lung cancer cases occur in people aged 60 and over. Within the UK, there is a clear north/south divide, with high lung cancer incidence rates in Scotland and northern England, and generally lower incidence in Wales, the Midlands, and southern England. Scottish men and women have amongst the highest rates in the world, reflecting the country's history of high smoking prevalence.

Natural history, and complications of the disease

In many patients, the cancer has already spread beyond the original site by the time they have symptoms and seek medical attention. Primary lung cancers mostly metastasize to the contralateral lung, adrenal glands, liver, brain, and bone. About 7%–10% of patients are asymptomatic at diagnosis, and cancers are often found incidentally on routine chest radiographs (CXRs); 35% of cases present as an emergency. Complications can arise from locoregional or metastatic spread, paraneoplastic syndromes, or treatment regimes (see Tables 141.2 and 141.3).

Approach to diagnosing the disease

Gathering a history and physical examination will reveal the presence of symptoms or signs that are suspicious for lung cancer. Performing a CXR is the most common first diagnostic step. Thereafter, more sophisticated imaging techniques are used to determine the location and extent of the disease. Histological confirmation and staging is the gold standard to enable treatment planning. Further tests may be required to determine the functional and medical baseline of the patient prior to the initiation of treatment.

Other diagnoses that should be considered

The differential diagnoses for those who present with CXR abnormalities include lung cancer and non-malignant diseases. These include infectious causes such as tuberculosis or pneumonia, and inflammatory conditions such as sarcoidosis. These diseases can result in mediastinal lymphadenopathy or lung nodules and sometimes mimic lung cancers.

Table 141.3 Complications of lung cancer therapy

Therapy	Symptom
Chemotherapy	Febrile neutropenia or bleeding from bone marrow suppression
	Renal failure, ototoxicity, hyponatraemia, hypomagnesia from cisplatin nephrotoxicity
	Peripheral neuropathy from cisplatin, paclitaxel, and vinorelbine
Radiotherapy	Lung toxicity
	Bronchial stenosis
Surgery	Mortality:
	6% pneumonectomy
	3% lobectomy
	1% segmentectomy

'Gold-standard' diagnostic test

A number of diagnostic techniques are available for histology and staging:

- thoracentesis (aspiration of a pleural effusion)
- ultrasound-guided fine needle aspiration of enlarged cervical or supraclavicular lymph nodes
- bronchoscopy: examination of the airways may allow diagnostic sampling, including nodes, via transbronchial needle aspiration (TBNA), endobronchial ultrasound, washings, brushings, and direct biopsy
- CT/ultrasound-guided biopsy: 85%–90% sensitivity in lesions >2 cm
- mediastinoscopy: lymph node staging; confirming the presence and location of N2 disease (see Table 141.4) is important for treatment planning

Acceptable diagnostic alternatives to the gold standard

Acceptable diagnostic alternatives to the gold standard are as follows:

- medical thoracoscopy: to determine whether the parietal pleural contains malignant cells
- video-assisted thoracoscopic surgery (VATS): can be used to assess resectability and invasion into mediastinum, and to biopsy the tumour
- FDG-PET scan: while CT and MRI scans look at anatomical structures, PET scans measure metabolic activity and the function of tissues; they can determine whether a tumour tissue is actively growing and can aid in determining the type of cells within a particular tumour; FDG-PET also has a high sensitivity and specificity for metastases

Other relevant investigations

Other relevant investigations include:

- blood tests; these cannot diagnose lung cancer but may reveal the biochemical or metabolic abnormalities that accompany cancer
- spirometry, or pulmonary function tests; for baseline and pre-biopsy/surgery information
- sputum cytology (limited use); reserved for patients who cannot tolerate invasive tests
- MRI (not routinely performed); for assessment of brachial plexus, pericardial involvement, superior sulcus tumours
- bone scans (if metastatic bone disease suspected)

Prognosis and how to estimate it

The most important prognostic indicator is the extent, or stage, of disease. Clinical, laboratory, radiological, and pathological investigations combined aid staging. Severity can be determined using the TNM (for tumour, node, and metastases) staging system. Other major prognostic factors include performance status, serum lactate dehydrogenase, liver function tests, and serum sodium (see Table 141.4).

Staging

Staging (contrast-enhanced) CT scan of the lower neck, thorax and abdomen, including liver and adrenal glands remains the mainstay of radiological clinical staging, providing information about the nature and extent of spread of the tumour, thus guiding therapeutic options and prognosis.

FDG-PET (PET/CT) provides an accurate assessment of mediastinal lymph node involvement, aiding diagnostic sampling and assessment of indeterminate pulmonary nodules and distant metastases (high sensitivity and specificity); in addition, it aids radical radiotherapy planning. Any lymph node greater than 10 mm in diameter is deemed abnormal. If PET/CT of the mediastinum is negative (negative predictive value of 98.4%), biopsy is not required, but a positive study may require tissue sampling (especially N2/3 disease).

Concerning **surgical staging**, mediastinoscopy is recommended for PET-negative nodes measuring over 16 mm. VATS specifically

Table 141.4 International Association for the Study of Lung Cancer International Staging Committee TNM classification of lung cancer (seventh edition; includes non-small cell lung carcinoma, small cell lung carcinoma, and carcinoids)

Stage	Description
T1a	Tumour ≤2 cm
T1b	Tumour 2–3 cm
T2	Main bronchus >2 cm from carina, invades visceral pleura, partial atelectasis
T2a	Tumour 3–5 cm
T2b	Tumour 5–7 cm
T3	Tumour >7 cm **or** local invasion, total atelectasis, additional nodule(s) same lobe
T4	Invasion mediastinum, heart, vessels, carina, vertebrae, vocal nerve, oesophagus, **or** additional nodule(s) different ipsilateral lobe
N0	No lymph node metastasis
N1	Ipsilateral peribronchial, ipsilateral
N2	Ipsilateral mediastinal or subcarinal
N3	Contralateral mediastinal or hilar, scalene **or** supraclavicular
M1a	Intra-thoracic metastasis: additional nodule(s) contralateral lung; pleura nodules **or** malignant pleural or pericardial effusion
M1b	Extra-thoracic metastasis: distant metastases

This article was published in *Thorac Oncol*, Volume 2, Goldstraw et al., International Association for the Study of Lung Cancer International Staging Committee, Participating Institutions. The IASLC Lung Cancer Staging Project: proposals for the revision of the TNM stage groupings in the forthcoming (seventh) edition of the TNM Classification of malignant tumours, pp.706-714, Copyright Elsevier (2007).

assesses pleural and chest wall involvement and nodal stations not accessible by standard mediastinoscopy.

For **assessment of distant metastases** (50% NSCLC, 60%–80% SCLC), CT or MRI brain is used (cerebral metastases are common in SCLC/adenocarcinoma and are silent in only 2%–4% of NSCLC). Bone scintigraphy is used if there is bone pain or local tenderness (only 5% of cases are asymptomatic).

SCLC grows rapidly with early dissemination to regional lymph nodes and distant sites. Approximately two-thirds of patients have extensive metastatic disease at presentation, and only chemotherapy is suitable for these patients. SCLC has a worse prognosis and should be staged by a contrast-enhanced staging CT scan. It is staged as limited (LS; confined to a single hemithorax and regional lymph nodes), extensive (ES; metastatic lesions in the contralateral lung, lymph nodes and/or distant organs, or malignant pericardial/pleural effusion), or recurrent disease.

Performance status

Activity level, measured by a performance status (PS) scale, is an important prognostic factor which helps individualize treatment (see Table 141.5.

Treatment and its effectiveness

Treatment decisions depend on the histological cell type (NSCLC or SCLC); tumour stage; size and location (particularly in NSCLC);

Table 141.5 Performance status scale used in guidelines

WHO (Zubrod/ECOG) Scale	
0	Asymptomatic
1	Symptomatic, but ambulatory (able to carry out light work)
2	In bed <50% of day (unable to work but able to live at home with some assistance)
3	In bed >50% of day (unable to care for self)
4	Bedridden

Abbreviations: ECOG, Eastern Cooperative Oncology Group.

and the patients' general physical condition (performance status). Preoperative assessment of N2 or N3 disease (mediastinal staging) allows appropriate selection for radical treatment. Therapy options (e.g. surgery, chemotherapy, and radiation therapy) should be discussed in a specialist multidisciplinary meeting.

Surgery

Surgical resection is the preferred treatment for early stage (IA, IB, IIA, IIB) NSCLC in patients with adequate lung function (FEV_1 > 1 l) and considered in single zone, non-bulky, non-fixed N2 disease (IIIA). Nodal staging determines suitability for curative surgery and indicates a possible role for neoadjuvant or adjuvant chemotherapy and radiation therapy. Advanced or metastatic disease (Stage IIIB or IV, 60%–80% of all patients) is usually unresectable, the main exceptions being the presence of a solitary adrenal or brain metastasis. Surgery should be considered in early stage SCLC, but is an option in <5%.

Lobectomy is the standard surgical approach. Sleeve lobectomy offers an acceptable alternative for a central tumour, conserving lung function. Sublobar (segmental or wedge) resection is offered in patients with poorer pulmonary reserve. VATS procedures offer lower perioperative morbidity and mortality and less pain and hospitalization. Suitable patients with bronchioloalveolar carcinoma should be offered multiple wedge or anatomical lung resection.

Medical therapy

Chemotherapy and radiation may prolong life or lead to a cure in a small number of patients. SCLC patients should see an oncologist within 1 week of deciding to treat.

Radiation therapy

Radiation therapy is used as emergency treatment for spinal cord compression. **Continuous hyperfractionated accelerated radiotherapy** should be offered to patients with localized SCLS; NSCLC Stage I and II patients who are medically inoperable but suitable for radical radiotherapy (WHO PS 0–1); and Stage IIIA and IIIB NSCLC patients who cannot tolerate chemoradiotherapy. Baseline pulmonary function tests, including lung volumes and transfer factor, should be performed. **Post-operative radiotherapy** is controversial but should be considered in NSCLC, to reduce local recurrence if resection margins show residual microscopic disease.

Chemotherapy

NSCLC

Chemotherapy alone plays no curative role. Chemotherapy can be given as a neoadjuvant (pre-surgery) or as adjuvant (post-surgery) therapy. **Neoadjuvant chemotherapy** can downstage tumours prior to surgery; it can also be used to assess chemotherapy response and control micrometastatic disease. **Adjuvant platinum-based chemotherapy** has survival benefits in patients with good PS 0–1 and Stage II or IIIA NSCLC or if N2 nodes are positive at operation. It can be offered alone for palliative treatment (Stage IIIB or IV and WHO PS 0–1), improving disease control and quality of life.

Combined chemoradiation therapy

NSCLC

Cisplatin-based concurrent chemoradiotherapy improves survival (24.8% 3-year survival) and should be considered for inoperable Stage II and III NSCLC, especially in patients under 75 years of age, WHO PS 0–1, with reasonable lung function, and no major comorbidities. **Platinum-based sequential chemoradiotherapy** may be offered to patients with locally advanced NSCLC but who are not suitable for concurrent chemoradiotherapy.

SCLC

Cisplatin-etoposide concurrent chemoradiotherapy may be considered early in patients with LS-SCLC disease and who are WHO PS 0–1. **Platinum-based combination chemotherapy** should be considered in patients with ES-SCLC and good PS. **Thoracic radiotherapy** is unfit for concurrent chemoradiotherapy in patients with LS-SCLC disease but may be offered to patients with ES-SLCS after chemotherapy, depending on response. **Prophylactic**

cranial irradiation may be offered to patients with SCLC and who are WHO PS <2, following good response to initial chemotherapy.

Molecular-targeted therapies

NSCLC tumours should have specific mutation testing (e.g. for mutations in the epidermal growth factor receptor and anapaestic lymphoma kinase). Monoclonal antibodies and tyrosine kinase inhibitors, which, respectively, block receptors and inhibit the enzyme-mediated activation of cellular signalling pathways, thus preventing cell proliferation, can increase survival.

Palliative treatment

Appropriate skilled palliative care is an important treatment for patients with Stage IV NSCLC, especially non-drug interventions for breathlessness. Participation in clinical trails of radical treatment can be considered.

Other treatment modalities

Radiofrequency ablation may be considered for radical treatment and palliation in non-surgical candidates and for small tumours (≤3 cm). **Radical brachytherapy** (high-dose radiotherapy delivered via a catheter during bronchoscopy) is curative in early mucosal or submucosal disease (tumours ≤4 mm).

Management of solitary pulmonary nodules

British Thoracic Society guidelines outline algorithms for the investigation and management of solid and subsolid pulmonary nodules, including the use of malignancy prediction calculators. Solitary pulmonary nodules, defined as discrete, well-marginated, rounded opacities ≤3 cm in diameter, completely surrounded by lung parenchyma, not touching the hilum or mediastinum, and without associated atelectasis or pleural effusion, are often an incidental finding in asymptomatic patients (0.2% of CXRs, 1% of CTs). Most are benign

(infectious granulomas, 80%: harmatoma, 10%; inflammatory or vascular) but approximately 20%–30% are malignant; 47% of these are adenocarcinomas, 22% are squamous cell carcinomas, and 4% are SCLC or metastases.

Lesions with typical benign features (i.e. lack of change over 2 years, or with a benign pattern of calcification, especially in low-risk patients) require no further investigation. Lesions strongly suggestive of malignancy (>3 cm diameter) or with documented growth should be referred for surgical resection.

Lesions with intermediate probability (8–20 mm) pose a diagnostic challenge, and further imaging is appropriate. Around 95% of patients with a malignant nodule will have an abnormal PET. In selected cases, biopsies are undertaken via CT-guided transthoracic needle aspiration or bronchoscopically performed TBNA; alternatively, for peripheral lesions, a surgical diagnosis can be made thoracoscopically.

Surgical resection (via VATS or a thoracotomy) is indicated for indeterminate nodules with a high probability of malignancy, and especially for PET-positive and biopsy-positive nodules. If frozen sections show evidence of malignancy, lobectomy with mediastinal lymph node sampling or dissection is recommended because of their lower recurrence rates. Resection of nodules greater than 1 cm in diameter has a 5-year survival rate as high as 80%.

Survival

Overall (considering all types and stages of lung cancer), 5-year survival is 16%. Mean survival for extensive inoperable lung cancer is 9 months or less (see Figure 141.1).

SCLC survival

In LS-SCLC, with chemotherapy, the 2-year survival rate is 20%–30%, and the 5-yr survival rate is 10%–15%. In ES-SCLC, the 2-year survival rate is <5%, and median survival time is 8–13 months. In recurrent SCLC, the mean survival time is 2–3 months.

	Persons
Stage I	71.12%
Stage II	48.15%
Stage III	34.59%
Stage IV	14.36%
Stage Not Known	16.61%
All Stages	32.16%

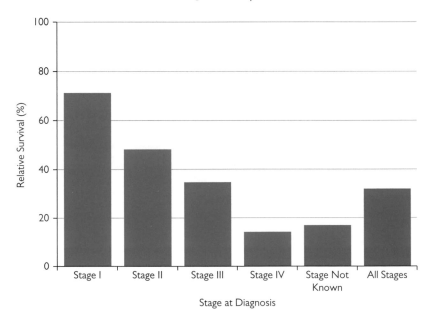

Figure 141.1 One-year relative survival (%) by stage, for adults (age 15–99).
Cancer Research UK, http://www.cancerresearchuk.org/sites/default/files/cstream-node/surv_1yr_bystage_lung.pdf, Accessed March 2016.

Further Reading

Früh M, De Ruysscher D, Popat S, et al. Small-cell lung cancer (SCLC): ESMO Clinical Practice Guidelines for diagnosis, treatment and follow-up. *Ann. Oncol.* 2013; 24 (Supplement 6): vi99–vi105.

Hirsch FR, Scagliotti GV, Mulshine JL, et al. Lung cancer: Current therapies and new targeted treatments. *Lancet* 2017; 389: 299–311.

National Institute for Health and Care Excellence. *Lung cancer: diagnosis and management. Clinical guideline* [CG121] 2011. Available at https://www.nice.org.uk/guidance/CG121 (accessed 11 Apr 2017).

Postmus PE, Kerr KM, Oudkerk M, et al. Early and locally advanced non-small-cell lung cancer (NSCLC): ESMO Clinical Practice Guidelines for diagnosis, treatment and follow-up. *Ann. Oncol.* 2017; 28 (Supplement 4): iv1–iv21.

Reck M and Rabe KF. Precision diagnosis and treatment for advanced non–small-cell lung cancer. *N Engl J Med* 2017; 377: 849–61.

142 Occupational lung disease

Paul Cullinan and Joanna Szram

Definition of the disease

Some occupational lung diseases are defined by their clinical or pathological nature (e.g. occupational asthma or mesothelioma), while others are defined by their specific aetiology (e.g. silicosis, farmer's lung). Most fall into one of three categories:

- airways diseases, including occupational asthma (induced by a workplace agent), work-exacerbated asthma (pre-existing asthma provoked by one or more agents at work), and irritant-induced asthma (initiated by a single, toxic exposure to a respiratory irritant); COPD and obliterative bronchiolitis may arise from workplace exposures, and around 10% of lung cancers have an occupational aetiology
- parenchymal diseases, incorporating the many types of pneumoconiosis, differentiated by the dust that caused them, and extrinsic allergic alveolitis (EAA, or hypersensitivity pneumonitis (HP)) categorised by the occupations and exposures from which they arise
- pleural diseases with an occupational cause comprising pleural plaques, diffuse pleural thickening, and mesothelioma

Aetiology of the disease

Occupational lung diseases arise from the inhalation of toxic dusts, fumes, or gases at work:

- occupational asthma is caused by a specific respiratory hypersensitivity to an airborne allergen; around 300 workplace allergens have been reported but most cases occur in a handful of occupations (see Table 142.1); more comprehensive lists can be found online)
- a wide variety of irritant exposures at work can exacerbate pre-existing asthma; they include dusts or gases, cold or dry air, exertion, or simply an early shift pattern
- obliterative bronchiolitis has been reported in silo, textile, and food-processing workers
- the most common causes of pneumoconiosis are crystalline silica (masons, quarry workers), asbestos, and coal dust (underground mining); many cases are of long latency and reflect past exposures
- rarer causes of occupational lung disease include 'hard metal' (tool grinders) and beryllium (electronics manufacture)

- EAA follows inhalation of (usually) organic, often fungal antigens of small particle size in a very wide variety of occupations (farmers, bird breeders, mushroom pickers, brewers, etc.); in many cases of chronic EAA however, no cause can be identified
- occupational pleural disease is almost always the result of exposure to asbestos, particularly chrysotile ('blue asbestos') or amosite ('brown' asbestos)
- the most common occupational cause of lung cancer is asbestos exposure, which acts in synergy with smoking

Typical (and less common) symptoms of the disease

In most cases, occupational asthma has a short latency with symptoms appearing within 2 years (but rarely sooner than 6 months) of first exposure. Asthma symptoms are often accompanied by nasal and eye symptoms typical of those induced by an airborne, protein allergen such as grass pollen. Symptoms tend to improve away from work, especially during holidays. Less commonly, differences in day-to-day exposures within a job or isolated 'late phase' reactions (felt **after** rather than **at** work) can make a work relationship less clear. Patients with established disease may have persistent bronchial hyper-reactivity with symptoms provoked by exposure to a variety of non-specific respiratory irritants, both at and away from work.

In contrast, patients who have developed irritant-induced asthma generally do so within 48 hours of a clearly identifiable irritant exposure in the workplace.

Simple pneumoconiosis is often asymptomatic, but more advanced 'complicated' disease (progressive massive fibrosis), is characterized by the gradual onset of cough and increasing breathlessness. Some forms of pneumoconiosis (e.g. stannosis) produce only radiographic changes. Chronic beryllium disease is clinically and radiographically indistinguishable from pulmonary sarcoidosis.

EAA has both acute and chronic forms. Acute attacks are characterized by cough, breathlessness, and flu-like symptoms within 12 hours of high antigen exposure and, provided there is no further exposure, resolution within a day or two. Weight loss is common and characteristic. Chronic EAA may be asymptomatic but more usually causes breathlessness of gradual onset after years of exposure.

Table 142.1 Common, high-risk occupations (and relevant exposures) for occupational asthma

Protein allergens		Chemical allergens	
Occupation(s)	Agent(s)	Occupation	Agent
Baking, milling, pastry, and pizza making	Flour(s), alpha-amylase, other enzymes, egg white	Spray painters, French polishers	Diisocyanates
Laboratory animal researchers and technicians; veterinary workers	Mouse, rat, and other animal proteins; egg proteins (embryological research)	Plastics and foam manufacturers and assemblers, chemical processors	Diisocyanates, acid anhydrides, epoxy resins, complex platinum salts, chrome, cyanoacrylates
Seafood processors	Prawn, crab, other fish proteins	Electronic solderers	Colophony fume
Tea packers, coffee processors	Herbal teas, green coffee bean	Healthcare workers	Glutaraldehyde, methyl/butyl methacrylate
Other food processors	Egg, enzymes, flours, legumes, spices	Pharmaceutical manufacturers, healthcare workers	Penicillins, morphine, cimetidine, other drugs
Healthcare workers	Latex	Woodworkers	Red cedar, iroko, other tropical sawdusts
Detergent enzyme manufacturers	Detergent protease, amylase, lipase, cellulase	Textile workers	Reactive dyes
Flower and vegetable farmers	Pollens	Hairdressers, manufacturers of circuit boards	Persulphates

Pleural plaques do not give rise to either symptoms or lung function abnormalities. In contrast, diffuse pleural thickening may be sufficiently restrictive to cause breathlessness. Patients with mesothelioma generally present with chest pain and/or symptoms of a (large) pleural effusion.

Demographics of the disease

The age, sex, and geographic distributions of occupational lung diseases reflect those of current and/or past industrial activities. Overall, there is little doubt the diseases are under-recognized. Population-based surveys suggest that 10% of all new or recurrent asthma in working-age adults is attributable to occupational exposures. Rates of true occupational asthma are high in some groups such as bakers, vehicle spray painters, and those who work with animals.

In most developed economies, new cases of pneumoconiosis are rare and, given the long latency of much disease, may first be recognized in those who have retired, reflecting historic exposures; some types of 'accelerated' silicosis are an exception. EAA that is readily attributable to occupational exposures is uncommon in most settings.

In (post-)industrial communities, pleural plaques are identifiable on CT chest scan in 25% of men aged 50 years or more. Similarly, rates of mesothelioma closely reflect exposures to asbestos 30–40 years previously and are not expected to decline until 2015–2020.

Natural history, and complications of the disease

With continuing allergen exposure, the symptoms of occupational asthma persist, usually deteriorate, are increasingly difficult to treat pharmacologically, and may become irreversible; the natural history of EAA is probably similar.

The fibrosis induced by asbestos or silica tends to progress even after exposure has ceased. Abrupt clinical deterioration is usually a reflection of secondary pulmonary hypertension. Patients with asbestosis, especially those who smoke, have an increased risk of lung cancer.

Pleural plaques frequently calcify but are not premalignant. Given equivalent exposures to asbestos, patients with pleural plaques have the same risk of subsequent mesothelioma as those without.

Approach to diagnosing the disease

All patients of working age with respiratory disease should be asked about their occupation(s), since therein may lie an etiological explanation and the potential for cure or prevention of progression. For diseases of long latency such as pneumoconiosis, a comprehensive and detailed lifetime occupational history is required in order to identify the cause of the disease. Patients with non-occupational respiratory diseases often have difficulties with finding and maintaining productive employment.

Other diagnoses that should be considered

Many occupational lung diseases—especially the pneumoconioses and pleural diseases—are clinically and/or radiologically specific. In the context of an appropriate history of exposure, alternative diagnoses do not need to be considered.

Others are non-specific and have important non-occupational etiologies. Occupational asthma can be demonstrated at an individual level but it is rarely possible to make a firm occupational attribution for a patient with COPD or lung cancer, as most of these patients have a history of heavy smoking.

The distinction between occupational asthma and pre-existing (or coincidental) asthma which is simply exacerbated by one or more exposures at work can be difficult. Injury and repair due to a single, heavy ('toxic') occupational exposure to a respiratory irritant can result in a non-immunologically mediated irritant-induced asthma; fortunately, most 'inhalation incidents' cause temporary symptoms only.

Box 142.1 Criteria for a diagnosis of irritant-induced asthma ('reactive airways dysfunction syndrome')

- onset after a single exposure at very high concentration to a gas, smoke, fume, or vapour with irritant qualities
- onset within 24 hours of the exposure and persistence for at least 3 weeks
- symptoms consistent with asthma (cough, wheezing, dyspnoea)
- evidence of subsequent airflow obstruction
- evidence of subsequent non-specific bronchial hyper-reactivity (methacholine or histamine challenge test)
- absence of prior respiratory symptoms
- other pulmonary disease excluded

'Gold-standard' diagnostic approach

Occupational asthma should be suspected in any working adult with new, recurrent, or difficult asthma. The gold-standard diagnostic test is specific inhalation challenge as an inpatient, a procedure offered at very few hospitals. For occupational asthma arising from protein allergens, evidence of specific IgE sensitization has a very high sensitivity, and a negative result effectively rules out the diagnosis. Immunological testing is generally less helpful with chemical agents and expert advice should be sought.

Criteria for the diagnosis of irritant-induced asthma ('reactive airways dysfunction syndrome') are outlined in Box 142.1.

Acute EAA induces an inflammatory blood picture with peripheral and bronchoalveolar lymphocytosis, pulmonary infiltration on chest X-ray, a reversible fall in gas transfer, and a specific IgG response.

A full occupational history should be taken from all patients with pulmonary fibrosis. Pulmonary function testing reveals a loss of lung volumes, restrictive spirometry, and a reduction in gas transfer. The radiographic changes of many types of pneumoconiosis are characteristic but those of asbestosis are often indistinguishable from idiopathic pulmonary fibrosis. While the co-presence of pleural plaques is confirmatory of asbestos exposure they may develop from far lower levels than the prolonged, heavy exposures required to induce asbestosis.

Mesothelioma is diagnosed using immunohistological techniques from lung tissue obtained at open or video-assisted biopsy.

In chronic beryllium disease, there is a positive response to a specific lymphocyte proliferation test using fresh blood; this assay is performed in very few laboratories.

In cases of suspected pneumoconiosis, a full semi-quantitative occupational history is required; high-resolution CT of the chest is far more sensitive than simple radiology for the detection of fibrosis and pleural disease.

Acceptable diagnostic alternatives to the gold standard

For occupational asthma, the most widely available and best-validated investigative tool is serial measurement of peak flow, which in expert hands has a sensitivity and specificity of approximately 80%. Measurements need to be made both at home and at work, at least four times a day over a period of several weeks; interpretation requires experienced personnel. Cross-shift monitoring of FEV_1 and bronchial reactivity is sometimes used in place of specific inhalation challenge but is logistically complex.

Other relevant investigations

Spirometry in the clinical setting is an insensitive indicator of both occupational asthma and work-exacerbated asthma.

Prognosis and how to estimate it

Once occupational asthma has developed, further exposure to the causative workplace allergen leads, in most cases, to persistent disease which is increasingly difficult to manage, and the risk of irreversible disease is increased by prolonged exposure after onset.

Conversely, avoidance of further exposure is often curative. The prognosis of acute EAA is similar.

The prognosis of the fibrosing pneumoconioses (asbestosis, silicosis) is directly related to the extent of disease but is usually better than that for idiopathic pulmonary fibrosis. The development of secondary pulmonary hypertension carries a very poor prognosis.

Mesothelioma is currently universally fatal, with a median life expectancy of about 12 months.

Treatment and its effectiveness

There are no specific treatments for the occupational lung diseases. In occupational asthma, avoidance of exposure is the most successful intervention and is frequently curative. It may, however, lead to employment difficulties, and successful management requires appropriate support, including, where it is available, occupational health input. Likewise, the cornerstone of treatment for EAA is the avoidance of further exposure; in this disease, respiratory protection may be sufficient. Conventional pharmacological treatment of asthma and rhinitis is rarely effective in occupational asthma when there is continuing allergen exposure but it is often successful in the management of work-exacerbated asthma.

Further Reading

Nicholson PJ, Cullinan P, Burge PS, and Boyle C. *Occupational Asthma: Prevention, Identification and Management: Systematic Review and Recommendations*. 2010. Available at http://www.bohrf.org.uk/downloads/OccupationalAsthmaEvidenceReview-Mar2010.pdf (accessed 12 Apr 2017).

Tarlo S, Cullinan P, and Nemery B. *Occupational and Environmental Lung Diseases: Diseases from Work, Home, Outdoor and Other Exposures*, 2010. Wiley-Blackwell.

Pleural infection

Definition of pleural infection

Pleural infection transitions from simple parapneumonic effusion, to complex parapneumonic effusion, to empyema. Primary empyema occurs without an underlying pneumonic process.

Aetiology of pleural infection

Forty per cent of pleural infections are culture negative. When culture positive, the bacteriology of empyema differs between community-acquired and hospital-acquired empyema (see Table 143.1).

Anaerobes commonly co-infect the pleural space and are not always cultured in the laboratory.

Typical symptoms of pleural infection

Pleural infection commonly presents identically to pneumonia with dyspnoea, purulent sputum, and fevers. It may be associated with pleuritic chest pain. Empyema can cause systemic sepsis leading to cardiovascular instability and multi-organ failure.

Demographics of pleural infection

Often patients will have no known risk factor. However, there is increased risk in the presence of alcohol abuse, immunosuppression, diabetes, and chronic aspiration.

Natural history, and complications of pleural infection

A parapneumonic effusion, if left untreated, will progress through three stages:

Stage 1: Simple parapneumonic effusion
- clear fluid, exudate, sterile, pH >7.20
- normally responds to antibiotics

Stage 2: Complicated parapneumonic effusion
- cloudy fluid, exudate, pH<7.20, culture sometimes positive, septae form
- requires drainage and antibiotics

Stage 3: Empyema
  purulent fluid, pH<7.20, culture sometimes positive, if left untreated pleural thickening develops
  requires drainage and antibiotics and may require surgical intervention

This disease progression emphasizes the importance of early appropriate management of patients with parapneumonic effusions.

Rarely, empyema can drain spontaneously through the chest wall (empyema necessitatis) or can lead to a bronchopleural fistula.

Approach to the diagnosis of pleural infection

All patients with a suspected pleural infection should have a diagnostic pleural aspiration. This should be done under ultrasound guidance,

Table 143.1 Microbiology of pleural infection	
Community acquired	**Hospital acquired**
Streptococcus milleri (28%)	MRSA (27%)
Anaerobes (19%)	Staphyloccoci (22%)
Streptococcus pneumoniae (14%)	Enterobacteria (20%)
Staphylococci (12%)	Enterococci (12%)

which will also allow for evaluation of the presence of septae, which would suggest a complicated parapneumonic effusion which will require drainage.

The following tests should be carried out on the pleural fluid:

- biochemistry: pH (measured accurately with a blood gas analyser), protein, and lactate dehydrogenase
- microbiology: Gram stain and culture; acid/alcohol fast bacilli should be stained for, although pleural fluid culture alone is only positive in 25% of tuberculous effusions; pleural fluid should be sent in blood culture bottles as this increases the pick-up rate for anaerobes

Other diagnoses that should be considered aside from pleural infection

The differential diagnosis of pleural infection includes other causes of exudative effusion, such as malignancy and autoimmune diseases.

'Gold-standard' diagnostic test for pleural infection

The gold-standard diagnostic test for pleural infection is microbiological culture of the pleural fluid. However, this is only positive in 60% of cases and, as such, clinical judgement is always required.

Other relevant investigations for pleural infection

Thoracic ultrasound should be used both to guide any diagnostic aspiration and also to assess for the presence of septae/locules. Contrast-enhanced CT of the thorax may be useful in empyema in order to assess the distribution of the disease and evaluate for the presence of an underlying pulmonary abscess or obstructing bronchial lesion.

If a tuberculous effusion is suspected, pleural biopsy should be undertaken. Tuberculous effusions lead to diffuse infiltration of the pleura with granulomas and, as such, this is the one indication for a blind pleural biopsy. When combined with pleural fluid staining/culture, it has a sensitivity of 90%.

Prognosis of pleural infection, and how to estimate it

The 1-year mortality rate for patients who require intercostal drainage for pleural infection is approximately 20%. Approximately 15% will require surgical intervention within 3 months of the initial drain. Risk factors for a poor outcome include old age, hospital-acquired infection, and markers of associated systemic sepsis, such as hypotension, renal dysfunction, and hypoalbuminaemia.

Treatment of pleural infection, and its effectiveness

Pleural infection should be treated with antibiotics according to local guidelines. Given that the organisms which give rise to hospital-acquired infections are different from those which give rise to community-acquired infections, it is important to differentiate between these two sources of infection when making empirical prescribing decisions. Antibiotics should be rationalized according to microbiology results. It is important to remember, however, that anaerobes commonly co-infect with other bacteria and may not always be identified in the culture. As with pneumonia, early administration of the first dose of antibiotics is essential.

Malignant pleural effusion and mesothelioma

Definition of malignant pleural effusion and mesothelioma

A malignant pleural effusion arises when malignant cells infiltrate the pleura, resulting in increased production and decreased lymphatic

Table 143.2 Primary site of malignant pleural effusion

Primary site	Frequency (%)
Lung	37
Breast	16
Lymphoma	11
Mesothelioma	10
Gastrointestinal	9
Genito-urinary	7
Unknown	10

drainage of pleural fluid (see Table 143.2). Malignant pleural effusions are either metastatic or primary mesothelioma.

Aetiology of malignant pleural effusion and mesothelioma

Malignancy is the commonest cause of an exudative effusion in patients over the age of 60. Mesothelioma is almost always associated with previous asbestos exposure. There is no dose–response relationship between asbestos exposure and the risk of developing mesothelioma. A single exposure may be etiological.

Typical symptoms of malignant pleural effusion and mesothelioma

Malignant pleural effusions may be detected incidentally when a chest X-ray is performed for other reasons. The commonest associated symptoms are breathlessness, chest pain, weight loss, and cough.

Demographics of malignant pleural effusion and mesothelioma

As with malignancy in general, malignant pleural effusion is more common with advancing age and in smokers. The average lag time between asbestos exposure and developing mesothelioma is approximately 35 years. It is rare for mesothelioma to occur within 15 years of asbestos exposure.

Natural history, and complications, of malignant pleural effusion and mesothelioma

When any malignancy presents with a pleural effusion, it is suggestive of advanced disease and a poor prognosis. The major complication associated with malignant pleural effusion is 'trapped lung'. The encasement of the lung by the visceral pleura means that, despite complete drainage of all pleural fluid, the lung will not re-expand and the effusion rapidly recurs.

Approach to diagnosing malignant pleural effusion and mesothelioma

The diagnostic algorithm for determining the cause of any pleural effusion should be systematic and logical (see Chapter 19). Pleural fluid aspiration is the mainstay of diagnosis. If the initial pleural aspirate is non-diagnostic, a second aspiration increases the diagnostic sensitivity, but further samples are unlikely to be beneficial.

Pleural fluid cytology will reveal the diagnosis in approximately 60% of malignant pleural effusions. In cytology-negative cases, a biopsy of the pleura is the next step. This can be performed either with a cutting needle under radiological guidance or with thoracoscopy. The benefit of carrying out thoracoscopy is that the procedure can be both diagnostic, with a sensitivity of >90%, and therapeutic, as talc poudrage can be carried out at the same time.

There is a risk of introducing seeding metastases after therapeutic/diagnostic pleural intervention of mesothelioma. The usefulness of prophylactic radiotherapy to the intervention site is a debated issue, with different studies obtaining conflicting results.

Other diagnoses that should be considered aside from malignant pleural effusion and mesothelioma

The major differential of an exudative effusion is infection. Rarer causes include pulmonary embolism, autoimmune disease, pancreatitis, and drugs. The histological diagnosis of malignant mesothelioma can be challenging, as its appearance can be very similar to that of adenocarcinoma. If the histology is inconclusive, a multidisciplinary team must review the case and come to a consensus diagnosis.

'Gold-standard' diagnostic test for malignant pleural effusion and mesothelioma

There is no single 'gold-standard' test for the diagnosis of a malignant effusion. The gold standard is to make a diagnosis in a timely fashion and in a way that is as minimally invasive as possible. The first test in that algorithm is always a diagnostic pleural aspiration.

Prognosis of malignant pleural effusion and mesothelioma, and how to estimate it

The median survival after diagnosis of a malignant effusion is between 3 and 12 months. This varies according to the primary site of malignancy, with lung cancer having the worst prognosis. As well as tumour staging, pleural fluid pH can be used as a tool for estimating prognosis, with a low pH being associated with a worse outcome.

The prognosis of mesothelioma is poor, with a median survival of less than 1 year. Worse prognosis is associated with the sarcomatoid subtype compared with the epithelioid subtype.

Treatment of malignant pleural effusion and mesothelioma, and its effectiveness

The management of patients with malignant pleural effusion involves symptom control, with drainage of pleural fluid and prevention of its recurrence with pleurodesis, alongside treatment of the underlying condition.

A pleural effusion should not be completely drained until a diagnosis has been obtained, as it may mean that thoracoscopy or radiologically guided biopsy is not possible until the fluid reaccumulates.

Pleurodesis aims to seal the pleural space by causing a fibrinous reaction between the parietal and visceral pleura. The most effective sclerosing agent is talc. There have been previous reports of acute respiratory distress syndrome being caused by talc, but a recent study showed that graded talc is safe to use for pleurodesis. Although less effective, other options include bleomycin, tetracycline, or autologous blood. Pleurodesis can be achieved either with talc slurry via an intercostal drain or with talc poudrage at thoracoscopy. Talc poudrage has a better long-term success rate but is more invasive.

If the effusion is recurrent despite attempts at pleurodesis or if trapped lung is present, a long-term indwelling pleural catheter can be sited which allows the patient to drain the pleural fluid intermittently.

The treatment of mesothelioma is palliative in all cases. Radiotherapy can be used to control chest wall pain or painful nodules. Palliative chemotherapy has been shown to improve survival by 2–3 months, but is associated with significant side effects.

Further Reading

Corcoran JP, Wrightson JM, Belcher E, DeCamp MM, Feller-Kopman D, and Rahman NM. Pleural infection: past, present, and future directions. *Lancet Respir Med* 2015; 3: 563–77.

Debiane LG and Ost ED. Advances in the management of malignant pleural effusion. *Curr Opin Pulm Med* 2017, 23:317–22.

Psallidas I, Kalomenidis I, Porcel JM, Robinson BW, and Stathopoulos GT. Malignant pleural effusion: from bench to bedside. *Eur Respir Rev* 2016; 25: 189–98. doi: 10.1183/16000617.0019-2016.

144 Drug-induced lung disease

Salman Siddiqui and Dhananjay Desai

Background

Pulmonary drug toxicity is being increasingly recognized as a cause of various forms of lung disease. The spectrum of disease can range from transient, minor reactions to rapidly progressive disease with fatal consequences. A large number of drugs are linked to pulmonary disease; however, causality is often difficult to establish, because the length of the latency period between exposure and the onset of disease can vary and because there can be discordance between symptom development and the appearance of radiological changes, which may not be present at all (e.g. angiotensin-converting enzyme (ACE) inhibitors can cause cough-related airways disease in the absence of radiological change).

Pathophysiology and patterns of involvement

Although the lung is often undervalued as a metabolic organ (compared to the kidneys and the liver), it plays an important role in drug metabolism. The total alveolar area available for gas transfer is in the region of 70 m². This allows inhaled agents to be deposited over a very large area and, consequently, they may induce diffuse and heterogeneous damage. Drugs administered systemically can undergo both Phase I and Phase II metabolism in the lungs, albeit to a very minor degree compared to the extent of drug metabolism in the liver. Nonetheless, there is scope for local toxicity due to this metabolism; in addition, drugs metabolized elsewhere in the body may exert their effects by being deposited in the lungs. Overall, however, most drug-induced lung disease (DILD) is idiosyncratic.

A diverse range of structural sites may be involved in DILD. Involvement of bronchial epithelium and pneumocytes may cause central airways disease, such as cough-related syndromes and bronchospasm, as well as peripheral airways disease related to airway narrowing, such as obliterative bronchiolitis, which causes airflow limitation and pulmonary fibrosis. Involvement of the pulmonary vasculature may induce vasculitis or pulmonary hypertension. The pleura and thoracic lymph nodes can also be involved, leading to pleural effusion and lymphadenopathy, respectively. Neuromuscular involvement may lead to ventilatory failure. Allergic drug reactions may involve any of these pulmonary components.

Risk factors for developing DILD

Dose-related drug toxicity is linked with amiodarone and bleomycin (as well as radiation). However, DILD may occur at unpredictably low doses and, therefore, cumulative accrued dose may not be clinically important in some cases (e.g. those due to NSAIDs or eosinophilic pneumonia). In other cases, a combination of several pneumotoxins may result in lung injury, suggesting that multiple hits are necessary for the induction of lung disease. The website http://www.pneumotox.com lists all drugs implicated in lung injury and provides an estimate of the frequency of toxicity. Oral and parenteral routes seem to be associated with the highest incidence of DILD.

Risk factors for developing DILD include low hepatic enzyme activity (e.g. isoniazid acetylation), which can be due to a genetic mutation. Drugs such as geftinib and erlotinib, which inhibit the EGF receptor, also inhibit other tyrosine kinases and are causally linked to pulmonary toxicity. Overall, patients with a history of previous chemotherapy, those with rheumatoid disease, or those with existing underlying fibrosis appear to be at a higher risk of DILD.

Diagnosis of DILD

Diagnosing DILD can be challenging, as previously discussed; the mechanisms of drug toxicity are often unclear and there may be a variable latency period between exposure and disease. Similarly, laboratory studies are often unhelpful and radiographic or even histopathological findings may be non-specific. A detailed history outlining prescription drugs, over-the-counter remedies, herbal remedies, and illicit drugs is necessary to try and identify potential causative agents. Involvement of a dedicated pharmacist with access to primary-care repeat prescription records may be useful.

Physical examination is necessary in order to rule out other diseases that may manifest with interstitial lung disease (ILD). Finger clubbing is not seen in DILD but crackles may be present if the process involves fibrosis. Wheeze may indicate a bronchospastic disorder (e.g. aspirin-induced asthma), and the presence of a pleural effusion is often associated with drug exposure, which is often overlooked.

Pulmonary function tests, on the other hand, are a useful guide to diagnosis. For example, early pulmonary vascular disease may be indicated by a reduced gas transfer coefficient before the onset of established radiological changes of pulmonary hypertension. Furthermore, serial monitoring of static lung volumes and gas transfer may allow determination of disease progression (currently defined by guidelines as a >10% fall in forced vital capacity, and a 15% fall in DLCO (the diffusing capacity of the lung for carbon monoxide) between serial tests). This is especially useful where the causative drug may have been stopped, so the disease process would be expected to improve or remain static.

Radiology involves a high-resolution CT chest scan (HRCT), which may offer some guide to distinguishing disease and response to therapy. For example, the presence of honeycombing and traction bronchiectasis indicates a fibrotic process, whereas the presence of ground-glass opacity (GGO) changes is indicative of active alveolar inflammation that may be steroid responsive. In addition, the HRCT may help to identify the pattern of ILD, for example, hypersensitivity pneumonitis may present with upper lobe predominant centrilobular nodules and GGO change, whereas eosinophilic pneumonia has a characteristic appearance that is the radiographic negative of pulmonary oedema.

Bronchoalveolar lavage, when used in conjunction with HRCT imaging, may be diagnostic. For example, the presence of haemosiderin-laden macrophages in the setting of diffuse pulmonary infiltrates and a fall in haemoglobin would favour diffuse alveolar haemorrhage. Other examples where the lavage may be diagnostic are listed in Table 144.1. Invasive measures such as surgical lung biopsy have low

Table 144.1 Scenarios in which bronchoalveolar lavage may be diagnostic of drug-induced lung disease

Drug-induced lung disease	Typical bronchoalveolar lavage findings
Eosinophilic pneumonia	Eosinophils >25% (preferably >40%)
Amiodarone lung	Foamy macrophages; there may be an increase in neutrophils, lymphocytes, or both; alternatively, neutrophil and lymphocyte counts may be normal (20%)
Lipoid pneumonia	Alveolar macrophages with empty vacuoles; positive result from Oil Red O stain
Hypersensitivity pneumonitis	Bronchoalveolar lavage lymphocytosis
Diffuse alveolar haemorrhage	Progressively bloody lavage return; haemosiderin-laden macrophages

diagnostic yield. Up to 20% of patients who had diffuse infiltrates and who underwent surgical lung biopsy have pathologic findings that can be attributed to a drug reaction.

DILD should remain a diagnosis of exclusion. Rechallenge with the causative agent may be the only way of proving causality but, if these reactions are severe, the consequences may be fatal.

Drugs implicated in DILD

Medications most commonly responsible for lung toxicity include methotrexate, amiodarone, NSAIDs, nitrofurantoin, and ACE inhibitors. These appear in Figure 144.1, with their patterns of involvement.

Amiodarone

With this commonly used antiarrhythmic drug, there appears to be a dose-related toxicity, with a far higher incidence of lung disease in those taking >500 mg per day, and length of treatment is also proportional to the risk of developing DILD. Due to its high lipophilicity and tissue storage, patients taking amiodarone may present with DILD after cessation of therapy (usually within 3 months). The disease spectrum is most commonly in the form of an acute presentation, with cough, fever, and infiltrates on X-ray, with pathological changes that are in keeping with acute interstitial pneumonitis. A more insidious onset with dyspnoea and chronic cough, crackles, and pleural effusions may be seen. An increase in serum lactate dehydrogenase may be seen. HRCT is usually helpful in diagnosis, showing migrating opacities and infiltrates, as well as nodules which may mimic tumours. Some cases may have fibrosis and interlobular septal thickening. Corticosteroid treatment is indicated if no improvement is seen in imaging or lung function after stopping the drug for 1–2 months; the treatment needs to be given over typically 6 months and gradually tapered, as there is a risk of relapse if it is withdrawn too early. The vast majority of cases will improve with this therapy but amiodarone pneumonitis may progress to acute respiratory distress syndrome (ARDS), with poor outcomes. Therefore, a pragmatic step may be to perform pulmonary function tests at the baseline before offering amiodarone therapy to those with no history of underlying lung disease.

Methotrexate

This is the most commonly prescribed disease-modifying anti-rheumatic drug and is estimated to cause DILD in 1% of treated patients. The incidence of rheumatoid ILD is estimated to be 10%–50%, with a higher incidence seen with increasing severity of rheumatoid disease. Therefore, the causality may be very difficult to attribute to drugs unless the temporal association is narrow, and clear evidence of reversibility is demonstrated on withdrawal of the drug. Unlike amiodarone, toxicity is not dose dependent, but the maximal incidence is seen within 1 year of commencing therapy. Clinical symptoms are fever, progressive breathlessness, and cough. HRCT may show reticulation, nodules, or GGO. There may be an accelerated

phase, with worsening dyspnoea and hypoxaemia; at such times, a careful exclusion of atypical lung infection may become necessary. High-dose corticosteroid therapy and ventilatory support if appropriate is the only other management apart from withdrawing the drug. Mortality at these times is estimated in the region of 10%.

Nitrofurantoin

Use of the drug nitrofurantoin for the treatment of chronic urinary tract infection carries the risk of pneumotoxicity leading to 'nitrofurantoin lung'. The acute form may occur within a few days of starting therapy and may cause an ARDS type of picture. The chronic form may cause interstitial pneumonitis or fibrosis. Steroid therapy may be useful.

ACE inhibitors

These drugs are used extensively and well tolerated in a large majority of patients, and the adverse effects are largely manifest as dry cough or airways disease. The potential mechanism of this adverse effect is known but cannot explain why some patient subsets are more prone than others. ACE inhibition causes an accumulation of airway 'irritant' molecules like bradykinin and leukotrienes, resulting mainly in cough (particularly in females) and, to a lesser extent, bronchospasm. Therefore, caution is advised when prescribing these drugs in airways disease patients who have bronchial hyper-reactivity. Up to 20% of patients using an ACE inhibitor may develop a dry cough; however, in only a minority will this be so severe as to cause discontinuation of the drug. In patients that had a 'chronic' cough before commencing therapy, an ACE inhibitor may be proven to be the exacerbating cause, but this may only come to light after discontinuing the drugs for 4–6 weeks. Current national guidelines advocate stopping ACE inhibitors in all patients with chronic cough. Angiotensin II receptor blockers are the logical choice for patients that are intolerant of ACE inhibitors.

NSAIDs

NSAIDs are well tolerated but are associated with a wide variety of airways disease manifestations as a result of their pulmonary adverse effects. Increased levels of leukotrienes from selective cyclooxygenase-1 enzyme inhibition results in cough, bronchospasm, and exacerbations of underlying airways disease and there is a subset of patients that clearly are prone to these effects but why specifically is still unclear. Hypersensitivity pneumonitis-like reactions are also described with fever, cough, eosinophilia, and pulmonary infiltrates. Corticosteroids cause rapid resolution of these effects.

Biological agents

Over the past decade, both the production and the use of biological agents have increased significantly. Pulmonary toxicity has been notably reported with tumour necrosis factor alpha (TNFα) blockers, interferons (IFNs), and anti-CD20 antibodies (rituximab).

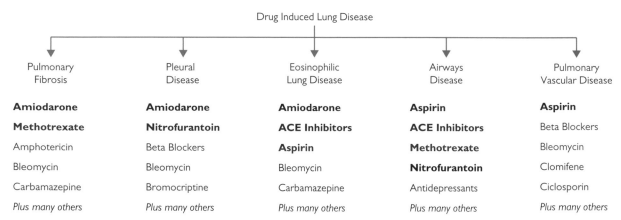

Drug Induced Lung Disease				
Pulmonary Fibrosis	Pleural Disease	Eosinophilic Lung Disease	Airways Disease	Pulmonary Vascular Disease
Amiodarone	**Amiodarone**	**Amiodarone**	**Aspirin**	**Aspirin**
Methotrexate	**Nitrofurantoin**	**ACE Inhibitors**	**ACE Inhibitors**	Beta Blockers
Amphotericin	Beta Blockers	**Aspirin**	**Methotrexate**	Bleomycin
Bleomycin	Bleomycin	Bleomycin	**Nitrofurantoin**	Clomifene
Carbamazepine	Bromocriptine	Carbamazepine	Antidepressants	Ciclosporin
Plus many others	*Plus many others*	*Plus many others*	*Plus many others*	*Plus many others*

Figure 144.1 Drugs implicated in lung disease, classified by the nature of the lung injury; the drugs most commonly implicated in each disease are indicated in bold; ACE, angiotensin-converting enzyme.

Anti-TNFα agents are usually administered to patients with rheumatoid arthritis, who concurrently use or had used methotrexate; hence these drugs have the potential to potentiate lung adverse effects, but cases have also been seen in patients that were never exposed to methotrexate. Agents such as infliximab and etanercept most commonly cause interstitial fibrosis or pulmonary sarcoid-like reactions (estimated incidence 0.5%). Whether these are class effects is unclear, as some case reports suggest an alternative anti-TNFα agent may be safe, but others have reported relapse with this strategy.

Rituximab is an anti-CD20 B-cell antibody widely used in non-Hodgkin's lymphoma and in rheumatoid arthritis. The most common lung toxicity presents typically with an insidious onset. HRCT may reveal GGO in addition to focal alveolar infiltrates. More severe reactions with pulmonary haemorrhage causing acute respiratory failure, and others with pneumonitis, have also been reported. Treatment with corticosteroids and stopping the drug appears to be of benefit.

The interferons interferon alfa-2a and interferon alfa-2b are used for the treatment of hepatitis C viral infection. Pulmonary toxicity from these has been implicated in airways disease exacerbations (asthma), interstitial pneumonitis, OP, and pleural effusions. As earlier, prompt withdrawal is of most benefit but corticosteroids may be administered concomitantly if continuing IFN therapy is indicated, as they may have a protective effect.

Statins

The widespread use of statins, compounded by the fact that the association between statins and DILD has only recently been recognized, means there are relatively few case reports; therefore, there may be a large number of patients who are using statins and who are consequently at risk of DILD. The mechanism of injury with statins is unknown, and the time to the onset of symptoms, which are non-specific, can vary from months to years after initiation of statin therapy. HRCT findings may include reticular opacities or GGOs. The use of steroids together with the discontinuation of statins results in resolution. At this point, it is still contentious if statins do cause ILD, and the only way to improve our understanding is to increase awareness of this association and 'yellow-card' report any suspected cases.

Recommendations and practical management of DILD

DILD remains largely under-recognized and under-reported. Risk factors include cumulative dose for some drugs and concomitant administration of pneumotoxic drugs. Basic investigations are lung function tests and HRCT. Withdrawal of the offending agent, in combination with supportive management, is the only treatment. The only way of definitely establishing causality is to rechallenge with the drug, but this method cannot be recommended.

Further Reading

Camus P. *The Drug-Induced Respiratory Disease Website*. http://www.pneumotox.com/

Schwaiblmair M, Behr W, Haeckel T, et al. Drug-induced interstitial lung disease. *Open Respir Med J* 2012; 6, 63–74.

CHAPTER 144 **Drug-induced lung disease**

145 Psychology in respiratory disease, including dysfunctional breathing

Andrew Jeffrey

Introduction

The real burden to any sufferer of respiratory disease is shown in the human suffering of the individual. It is increasingly understood that there is a link between the psychological aspects of respiratory disease and morbidity and that patients' attitudes to illness can affect their ways of coping and, indeed, impact upon their compliance with treatment. Breathlessness is a symptom of many psychological states, both positive and negative; indeed, it is embedded within the English language—'It took my breath away! I was breathless with anticipation!' An understanding of the links between psychological factors and physical symptoms and behaviours is essential to achieve the best possible outcomes for many patients.

Dysfunctional breathing

Dysfunctional breathing is an umbrella term that refers to the disordered breathing that results from psychological distress. It can occur in the absence of physical lung or cardiovascular disease (usually referred to as hyperventilation), although it is commonly found in association with a physical cause of breathlessness such as asthma, COPD, or heart failure.

Hyperventilation in the absence of physical cardiopulmonary disease can occur at any age after infancy but the onset is usually between the ages of 15 and 55 years, with a female preponderance of around 7:1. Acute hyperventilation comes on suddenly during panic attacks, causing dizziness, breathlessness, and pins-and-needles in the fingers. Chronic hyperventilation is more difficult to diagnose because the body compensates for the chemical changes, so symptoms are less clear. Common complaints are light-headedness, breathlessness, difficulty in taking a deep breath, and even chest pain. These usually occur at rest or when talking rather than during exercise, which is the opposite of significant lung or heart conditions.

Hyperventilation, particularly in its chronic form, can be very debilitating and life-limiting. It is important to acknowledge with the patient that, although not dangerous, it is nonetheless a serious condition that requires appropriate treatment and can be greatly improved by appropriate interventions. This chronic form of dysfunctional breathing is particularly common in association with asthma and COPD (see 'Asthma' and 'COPD').

Precipitation of specific symptoms through voluntary hyperventilation can be a very effective technique for confirming a diagnosis of hyperventilation. This can have the extra beneficial effect of demonstrating to the patient that the symptom and the excess breathing are linked.

Combinations of breath-control training and interventions to target underlying psychological problems are the most effective treatments.

Anxiety and depression

It has been well documented that there is a substantial similarity in symptoms of anxiety and those of respiratory diseases. Individuals often confuse symptoms of anxiety (breathlessness, chest pain, depersonalization, hyperventilation, fainting, etc.) with a worsening of their physical condition. When symptoms seem confusing, patients catastrophize their body sensations; this can lead to inappropriate treatment for respiratory disease. Indeed, the side effects of drugs used to control physical symptoms of respiratory disease, such as salbutamol, can increase anxiety. Symptoms of anxiety can affect the production of cytokines, leading to inflammation of the airways and potentially exacerbating any physical inflammatory-based airways disease.

Indeed, patients with COPD or other lung conditions may also suffer neuropsychological functioning problems due to chronic hypoxemia, which results in memory difficulties, attention deficits, and difficulty with verbal tasks and motor processing.

Psychological factors have a large role to play in the perception of breathlessness. In terms of self-management, it has been shown that anxiety, depression, and alcohol abuse strongly influence how a person self-manages their illness. Self-management plans that better equip and educate patients to make their own decisions improve confidence as well as knowledge. This confidence is believed to be an important element in the improved self-management observed in patients with such plans.

Dyspnoea

Dyspnoea, or breathlessness, is often a strong feature of respiratory disease. It causes a reduction in the quality of life by imposing limitations on functionality and is frequently experienced as life-threatening and terrifying. Emotional perception of breathlessness can contribute to poor outcome. Asthma patients with high negative emotionality were found to be more likely to show breathlessness symptoms than patients who showed low negative emotionality. Generally, these patients also demonstrated a higher degree of asthma-related complaints, a finding which may indicate that this group of patients is less accurate in their perception of breathlessness than groups of patients are.

Asthma

Coexistence of asthma and panic disorder is believed to produce greater morbidity than either alone, as the two disorders essentially overlap, with similar symptoms of breathlessness, chest pain, and tightness, thus leading to symptom confusion. It is accepted that beta-sympathetic agonists used in the treatment of asthma can trigger feelings of panic, as patients catastrophize the bodily sensations produced by this close analogue of adrenaline.

Such has been the confusion for some patients regarding their symptomology that this has resulted in inappropriate treatment and near-deaths, and has even been shown to be implicated in deaths from asthma. Patients who panic may overreact to their asthma symptomology and consequently overuse medication, which can increase anxiety. Evidence that panic disorder and asthma can coexist and lead to misperceptions of symptoms has led to a combined treatment approach using cognitive behaviour therapy (CBT) and education, and improvements were reported in a group of patients using this approach. Patients taught how to differentiate between asthma and panic symptoms reported a significant decrease of more than 50% in panic symptoms alongside a decrease in asthma symptoms, improvement in quality of life, and clinical stability.

Current patient education does not always fulfil the needs of good asthma management, as it frequently does not address the ability to cope. Poor coping skills can interfere with disease management.

Psychological help needs to be culturally appropriate and community based; particularly, it needs to take into account empowerment in minority communities. Social norms help shape attitudes and behaviour. An empowering approach based on active learning rather than didactic teaching in the management of respiratory disease is therefore most likely to be effective. This has significant implications for the manner in which patient education should be undertaken to be effective.

A recent study attempted to determine if a self-management programme could improve psychological outcome by using problem-solving approaches, social support, behaviour modification, and discussion, as determined by measuring peak flow, medication adherence, and other lifestyle behaviours. Improvements in outcome of quality of life, depression, and self-efficacy were demonstrated.

A Cochrane review (Gibson et al., 2002) indicated that teaching adult asthma sufferers self-management skills does have a positive impact on outcome. However, learner-centred self-management programmes that use a facilitator approach rather than a didactic teaching approach may have a better long-term outcome. This is arguably because sufferers manage their physical, emotional, and cognitive aspects of their disease to enhance their quality of life.

COPD

The emotional consequence of disease is often seen in a high prevalence of depression. Depression is frequently unrecognized in COPD patients and may manifest in decreased libido, decreased energy, social withdrawal, and general feelings of hopelessness, with anxiety and panic attacks also being common in this group. COPD sufferers also suffer a decrease in their recreational abilities, domestic management, activities of daily living, and possible reduction in employment opportunities. The impact this has on relationships are problems with social isolation, sexual dysfunction, and general levels of loneliness.

One large-scale study has indicated that, in COPD patients, the prevalence of depression was approximately 42%, and that of anxiousness was around 50%; thus, patients with COPD are 2–3 times more likely to be suffering from anxiety and depression, compared to members of the general population. Depression worsens the outcome and mortality of many physical conditions. Routine screening of COPD patients for anxiety and depression has shown that undetected and untreated depression in COPD patients was a common occurrence and associated with increased disability, increased healthcare usage, and impaired quality of life.

Treatment of patients with COPD has increasingly become focused upon quality of life, assessing the patient's subjective experience of the disease and general satisfaction with their life. The construct of quality of life is, however, very difficult to measure, and what gives this quality differs between individuals and societies. A suggested definition of quality of life is the gap between what is desired and what is achievable in life. A comprehensive measure of quality of life will assess subjective experience of the illness in three dimensions: emotional functioning, physical functioning, and social functioning. Psychological health is clearly a key element in all three domains.

Role of clinical psychology

Much of the evidence for psychological interventions comes from studies of COPD patients, although there is no reason to assume that it does not apply to patients with other chronic respiratory diseases. There are five potential areas of psychological intervention:

- understanding basic personality traits and characteristics
- neuropsychological consequences of the disease, such as memory difficulties and concentration problems
- quality-of-life improvement, facilitating self-efficacy, medical adherence, and the ability to cope
- rehabilitation for patients, encompassing psychological, social, and/or behavioural issues
- CBT interventions to help to modify negative cognitive and behavioural responses

It has been found that clinical psychologists have a great deal to contribute to the management of respiratory disease, with respect to facilitating quality of life, expectations, adjustment difficulties, neuropsychological problems, and so on. At the same time, they have much to offer in terms of the development of rehabilitation

programmes, effective smoking cessation and prevention programmes, and improving the quality of care for patients with respiratory disease. Psychological and behavioural interventions need to be embedded within rehabilitation programmes, delivering education, discussion, and relaxation, with a target of improving the patient's quality of life with respect to anxiety, depression, breathlessness, self-efficacy, and motivation.

While education in physical self-management can be useful, some argue that patients need to know less about the pathophysiology of the disease and more about how to integrate and modify their behaviour to accommodate their disease. This is an area in which the skills and knowledge of the clinical psychologist can be useful.

Significantly, CBT group treatments for both anxiety and depression have been shown to improve mental well-being, quality of life, and education. Antidepressants have often been the treatment of choice for depressed patients and do significantly help in terms of improving mood and symptom management. However, they do not reliably affect self-management skills in chronically ill patients, while this can be achieved with CBT. The effects of relaxation and guided imagery with COPD patients are being explored but further studies are needed to identify the efficacy of these approaches as coping strategies for breathlessness.

Many of these approaches can, with suitable training and support, be integrated into the work of other health professionals.

A holistic approach to care

Holistic approaches take account of the complex mind–body experience, interpreting physical symptoms and taking account of the psychological distress caused to sufferers of respiratory disease. A holistic approach to healthcare can be defined as the appreciation that the impact of physical disease processes extend beyond the usual appreciation of physical health. This includes the emotional challenge that long-term chronic sickness imposes, includes the patient's ways of coping, as well as considering social support that can impact upon a patient's progress.

The management of respiratory disease, like any chronic illness, relies heavily on the patient's perception of their illness. They often have to adapt to their physical limitations, cope with dietary and lifestyle changes, and learn how to deal with difficult life-changing circumstances while taking on the responsibility for monitoring their condition and administering their medication. This may encompass the need to become more dependent on family, carers, and the medical profession. Indeed, this can be in itself very stressful, along with the additional issue of dealing with societal expectations that can lead to anxiety and distortions in their perceptions of their sensations.

In summary, respiratory disease is common across the UK; the direct costs to the NHS include medication, presentations at emergency admissions, treatment, inpatient stays, and outpatient appointments, as well as staffing costs. However, the less obvious costs are to the economy in working days lost, travel, and equipment and also have financial and social implications for the individual. The cost to the individual is, however, far greater as they grieve for their lost healthy self and strive to make the necessary adjustments to chronic respiratory disease and the impact such disease has upon them, their partners, family, and social network.

Further Reading

Gibson PG, Powell H, Wilson A, et al. Self-management education and regular practitioner review for adults with asthma. *Cochrane Database Syst Rev* 2002; 3: CD001117.

Pumar MI, Gray CR, Walsh JR, et al. Anxiety and depression: Important psychological comorbidities of COPD. *J Thorac Dis* 2014; 6: 1615–31.

Sardinha A, Freire RC, Zin WA, et al. Respiratory manifestations of panic disorder: Causes, consequences and therapeutic implications. *J Bras Pneumol* 2009; 35: 698–708.

Wuyts WA, Peccatori FA, and Russell AM. Patient-centred management in idiopathic pulmonary fibrosis: Similar themes in three communication models. *Eur Respir Rev* 2014; 23: 231–8.

146 Terminal care in respiratory illness

Alys Scadding

Introduction

The terminal phase is the period of time between living with a reasonable quality of life, and the process of dying. While lung cancer and pulmonary fibrosis have the potential to deteriorate rapidly, the majority of lung diseases worsen over years. Every exacerbation of the condition leads to a decline in both lung function and performance status, and often the pre-exacerbation level of functioning is never regained. There is not a defining point to indicate whether a patient is entering the terminal stages of their illness but practice shows that the following signs are suggestive:

- increasing breathlessness and thus becoming increasingly housebound
- increasing oxygen requirements
- declining pulmonary function test results
- increasingly frequent exacerbations requiring hospital admission and/or non-invasive ventilation
- developing cor pulmonale
- weight loss and difficulty maintaining weight
- anxiety and depression
- if the death of the patient within the next year would not be a surprise

Symptom control

The symptoms suffered by patients with terminal respiratory disease are often indistinguishable from those experienced by patients with terminal cancer. Recently, the focus has moved towards advance care planning and symptom control. Most commonly, a patient with lung cancer will be cared for by a multidisciplinary team often consisting of respiratory doctors, oncologists, a specialist lung cancer nurse, and palliative care teams, whereas it is the 'Hospital at Home' teams who mainly support patients with chronic respiratory conditions in the community. For the final phases of life, many hospitals have adopted a protocol such as the Liverpool Care Pathway in order to standardize the care received by the dying patient, with a primary aim of reducing any unnecessary interventions, such as routine observations or blood tests, and focusing on improving patient comfort at a time when death is inevitable. Good symptom control benefits both the patient and their loved ones and the management of the most common symptoms is as follows:

Anxiety and dyspnoea: Cochrane reviews have suggested a three-step approach. Non-pharmacokinetic therapies such as relaxation techniques, diaphragmatic breathing, and the use of handheld fans are the first-line treatments. Second-line therapies involve the use of small doses of opiates, such as 1–10 mg morphine sulfate solution, as required. Third-line agents include the use of short-acting benzodiazepines, such as 0.5–1 mg sublingual or oral lorazepam, 5 mg diazepam, or 1–3 mg subcutaneous midazolam, as required. The risk of opiate- or benzodiazepine-related respiratory depression in breathless or hypoxic patients is a concern for many doctors, yet the situation rarely occurs in practice, provided small doses of the medication are used.

Respiratory tract secretions: Subcutaneous hyoscine hydrobromide 400–600 μg every 4–8 hours can help settle this distressing symptom. A dry mouth is a potential side effect; if this occurs, glycopyrronium 200 μg subcutaneously every 4 hours is a good alternative.

Pain: Aim to work up the WHO pain ladder. Once opiates are required, morphine sulfate solution and then subcutaneous morphine or diamorphine are the first-line analgesics. The medication can be given via a syringe driver if multiple doses are required. Pain from bony metastases can be treated with localized radiotherapy and bisphosphonates.

Agitation: Haloperidol 1–3 mg or lorazepam 0.5–1 mg, subcutaneous or oral, can be given as needed.

Nausea: Increasing doses of opiates, particularly in an opiate-naive patient, can cause nausea and vomiting. Good anti-emetics include cyclizine 50 mg three times daily, metoclopramide 10 mg three times daily, and haloperidol starting at 1.5 mg twice daily. If first-line therapies fail, levomepromazine via a syringe driver at a dose of 5–25 mg per 24 hours can be tried.

Loss of appetite: This is very common and can lead to respiratory muscle weakness and exacerbate preexisting breathlessness. This may be due to the cachexia–anorexia syndrome or it could be due to related problems such as oral candidiasis, nausea, or depression. The underlying cause should be treated. Nutritional supplements should be considered in addition to usual meals. In the short term, 20 mg prednisolone for several weeks can help improve the appetite.

Common symptoms in respiratory disease

Haemoptysis

Haemoptysis is a very distressing symptom, particularly when profuse. The usual approach of intubation and bronchoscopy in massive haemoptysis is unlikely to be appropriate in a patient who, for example, has end-stage lung cancer with a tumour adjacent to a large vessel. In this instance, haemoptysis should be anticipated and treated palliatively with anxiolytics and opiates. Less severe haemoptysis can be controlled using tranexamic acid 500 mg orally three times a day.

Pleural effusion

The main causes of pleural effusion are primary lung cancer and pleural metastases. Drainage of the effusion is a palliative measure and should only be performed if the patient is breathless, able to tolerate a chest drain, and likely to survive for sufficient time to feel any benefit. Talc pleurodesis is recommended if the effusion is likely to recur; however, the pleural inflammatory reaction can result in flu-like symptoms, chest pain, and, uncommonly, pulmonary infiltrates.

Fluid retention

Fluid retention forms part of the cor pulmonale syndrome as a result of renal hypoxia, and patients frequently find the leg oedema distressing. Oxygen and diuretics comprise the mainstay of treatment but a balance between mobility, trips to the bathroom, renal function, and control of the oedema needs to be struck.

Intractable cough

For intractable cough, nebulized 0.9% saline and simple cough linctus can be tried. An opiate, such as codeine 30 mg four times daily or morphine sulfate solution 5–10 mg when required, is the preferred choice.

Hypercalcaemia

Hypercalcaemia is often secondary to squamous cell cancers and bone metastases and causes dehydration, confusion, and abdominal pain. Treatment involves IV rehydration with around 4 l of saline over 24 hours, with the concurrent administration of a bisphosphonate. Good choices are disodium pamidronate 30–90 mg IV, zoledronic acid 4 mg IV, or sodium clodronate 300 mg IV daily for 7–10 days or 1.5 g as a single dose.

Advance care planning

Involving the patient and their loved ones in the decision-making regarding future treatment and care in terminal respiratory illness can help alleviate distressing symptoms such as anxiety and fear. Ideally, this is best done when the patient is in a stable condition, in quiet room, and when there is plenty of time to address any concerns. The acute management of poorly inpatients prompts a similar discussion, although, ideally, these topics should be covered early in the admission rather than at the moment when the patient's condition deteriorates. The most important areas to cover are:

- whether the patient wishes to be admitted to hospital if their health deteriorates for any reason
- whether the patient would agree to try non-invasive ventilation should it be required
- whether intensive care treatment, ventilation, and resuscitation would be appropriate based on spirometry results, baseline level of function, quality of life, and underlying diagnosis
- whether the patient has a desired place of care for the end of their life

Discussing the practical issues surrounding dying can help patients regain a sense of control over their future, and approaching the following areas can be helpful:

Making a will and planning a funeral: This enables a nominated executor to follow the patient's wishes regarding the division of their estate, and their desired funeral.

Lasting power of attorney: The nomination of one of the next of kin to hold the lasting power of attorney allows that person to make decisions regarding the patient's welfare and finances in the patient's best interests. The process requires a solicitor and the patient to demonstrate capacity.

Advance directive ('living will'): This document allows a patient to express their wishes regarding future treatment within specific situations. It can include information about cardiorespiratory resuscitation and assisted ventilation. It is wise to involve a solicitor in this process.

Specific respiratory situations

Chronic respiratory failure

The main causes of chronic respiratory failure are COPD, bronchiectasis, pulmonary fibrosis, and neuromuscular disease. The management of these conditions in the terminal phases are outlined in 'Symptom control'; however, patients with neuromuscular disease managed on nasal intermittent positive pressure ventilation (NIPPV) may experience an increasing reliance on ventilatory support requiring nocturnal then daytime NIPPV. Handheld mouthpieces can allow the patient to 'sip' the NIPPV whenever they wish and can alleviate

breathless. Advance care planning is important, and this group of patients in particular are often known to the palliative care services. Hospice admissions are common as their condition deteriorates. During the patient's final hours or days, the decision to switch off the NIPPV machine is often made and the end-of-life medications are given as required.

Acute respiratory failure

All pulmonary conditions can cause acute respiratory failure. In these situations, the ceiling of treatment depends upon the underlying diagnosis and the premorbid function of the patient. If the patient is extremely unwell and previously had a good quality of life, consideration should be given to invasive ventilation. However, if ward care is felt to be more appropriate, the patient can be trialled on non-invasive ventilation such as continuous positive airway pressure or NIPPV. In all these scenarios, the deterioration of the patient's condition should prompt a discussion with the relatives regarding removing the ventilatory support. Once the decision for palliative treatment is made, the end-of-life medications are administered.

Lung cancer

The prognosis and progression to the terminal phase is largely dependent upon the staging of the cancer. Best supportive care and symptom control measures in lung cancer can involve interventions such as stenting in superior vena cava obstruction, low dose radiotherapy in chest wall pain and low grade haemoptysis from invasive tumours. However, these interventions would not be appropriate for a person entering the final phase of life and the symptom control measures discussed previously would be more appropriate.

Further Reading

Ford DW, Koch KA, Ray DE, Selecky PA. Palliative and end-of-life care in lung cancer. Diagnosis and management of lung cancer, (3rd edition). American College of Chest Physicians Evidence-Based Clinical Practice Guidelines. *Chest* 2013; 143(5)(Suppl): e498S–e512S.

Maddocks M, Lovell N, Booth S, Man W D-C, and Higginson IJ. Palliative care and management of troublesome symptoms for people with chronic obstructive pulmonary disease. *Lancet* 2017; 390: 988–1002.

National Institute for Health and Care Excellence. *End of Life Care for Adults.* 2011. Available at http://www.nice.org.uk/guidance/cmg43 (accessed 26 Apr 2017).

National Institute for Health and Care Excellence. *Improving Supportive and Palliative Care for Adults with Cancer.* 2004. Available at http://guidance.nice.org.uk/CSGSP/Guidance/pdf/English (accessed 26 Apr 2017).

PART 5

Intensive care medicine

147 Critical illness

Matt Wise and Paul Frost

Defining critical illness

Critical illness can be considered to be any disease process which causes physiological instability that leads to disability or death within minutes or hours. Fortunately, physiological instability associated with critical illness is easily detected by perturbations of simple clinical observations such as blood pressure, heart rate, respiratory rate, oxygen saturations, level of consciousness, and urine output. Individual abnormalities in these observations are sensitive for the presence of critical illness but non-specific. Unfortunately, poor specificity may contribute to their importance in an individual patient being overlooked. Specificity for critical illness improves as the number of abnormal clinical observations increases. Indeed, the risk of death at 30 days for ward patients can be calculated by the number of these observations that are abnormal, being 0.7% for none, 4.4% for one, 9.2% for two, and 21.3% for three or more.

Over recent years, a greater appreciation of the importance of deviations in simple clinical observations as a method of detecting critical illness has led to the development of a number of 'early warning' or 'track and trigger' systems. These systems attribute a score according to the magnitude and number of abnormal observations that are present, and a high score prompts immediate medical review. Although intuitively sensible, the evidence that these systems are effective in ameliorating or preventing critical illness is currently lacking.

Many routine observations that track physiological instability, particularly respiratory rate, are not reliably recorded either by omission or inter-observer error. Moreover, in the UK there has been no standardized rapid response system with hospitals deploying different early warning scores. In an attempt to address these shortcomings, the Royal College of Physicians has produced the National Early Warning Score (NEWS), which provides for a graded response strategy to acute illness (see Table 147.1 and go to http://www.rcplondon.ac.uk/national-early-warning-score for the full details of NEWS, as well as a detailed observational chart).

Approach to diagnosing critical illness

It remains a common problem that healthcare professionals fail to recognize when a patient is critically ill, and this leads to excess morbidity and mortality. As with any illness, it is impossible to make a diagnosis unless it is specifically considered. One can think of two groups of patients with critical illness: in the first, the aetiology of their critical illness is already known (e.g. a pneumonia); in the second, it remains to be established. The approach to diagnosing critical illness differs from the routine clerking and management of patients in whom critical illness is not present, as it involves a focused examination combined with treatment.

The referral route of potentially critically ill patients may be diverse and include another doctor, a nurse, a physiotherapist, a dietician, or even a visitor. The referral needs be taken seriously and not dismissed because of the role of the referrer. Outcomes in the critically ill are time dependent, and lengthy interrogation of the referrer is inappropriate. However, it is important to ascertain the patient's name, age, location, diagnosis (if known), and resuscitation status. Assessment of the patient begins with an introduction to the patient by the examiner. This immediately provides information about the patient's level of consciousness. Lengthy history taking is inappropriate, but the patient should be briefly questioned about any key symptoms, such as pain or breathlessness. In many cases, the patient will be too ill to provide any direct information and this will be obtained later from other sources, such as notes, charts, other healthcare workers, or visitors.

A brief structured examination should be performed which follows the Airway, Breathing, Circulation, Disability (conscious state), and Exposure (ABCDE) approach. Critically ill patients have little physiological reserve and tolerate prolonged examination and changes in body position poorly. This structure of examining for critical illness is fundamentally different to the standard approach to examination because it focuses on key clinical observations which are abnormal in critical illness, but it also combines treatment with examination. Thus, if a patient has an obstructed airway, further examination is futile unless airway patency is restored, as this is a prerequisite for survival. The ABCDE approach is more than a simple mnemonic but represents a hierarchy to patient survival. For example, a reduced level of consciousness (D) may be the consequence of hypotension (C) caused by haemorrhage; similarly, hypotension (C) may be the result of hypoxia (B) caused by airway obstruction (A). As soon as critical illness is recognized, help should be sought; in some cases, this might require a medical emergency or cardiac arrest team.

Airway

The airway must be patent and this can be assumed if the patient can speak to the individual performing the examination. Partial

---

Table 147.1 Clinical response to National Early Warning Score (NEWS) triggers

NEWS score	Frequency of monitoring	Clinical response
0	Minimum 12 hourly	Continue routine NEWS monitoring with every set of observations
Total: 1–4	Minimum 4–6 hourly	Inform registered nurse who must assess the patient; Registered nurse to decide if increased frequency of monitoring and/or escalation of clinical care is required;
Total: 5 or more or 3 in one parameter	Increased frequency to a minimum of 1 hourly	Registered nurse to urgently inform the medical team caring for the patient; Urgent assessment by a clinician with core competencies to assess acutely ill patients; Clinical care in an environment with monitoring facilities;
Total: 7 or more	Continuous monitoring of vital signs	Registered nurse to immediately inform the medical team caring for the patient—this should be at least at Specialist Registrar level; Emergency assessment by a clinical team with critical care competencies, which also includes a practitioner/s with advanced airway skills; Consider transfer of Clinical care to a level 2 or 3 care facility, i.e. higher dependency or ITU;

Reproduced with permission from National Early Warning Score (NEWS): Standardising the assessment of acute-illness severity in the NHS, Working party report, July 2012, Royal College of Physicians (www.rcplondon.ac.uk/national-early-warning-score).

airway obstruction leads to noisy breathing and is common if consciousness is impaired. Partial obstruction may occur at several levels within the airway and lead to characteristic sounds, such as snoring (tongue obstructing the oropharynx), stridor (obstruction at larynx by oedema, a foreign body, or a tumour), and wheeze (bronchospasm of small airways). Obstruction of the oropharynx by the tongue in an unconscious patient can be relieved by simple airway manoeuvres, such as a chin lift or jaw thrust. The oropharynx should be inspected and any foreign body such as dentures, food, vomit, or blood removed. If airway patency cannot be restored by these simple measures, then experienced help should be sought. The inappropriate insertion of airway adjuncts or suction catheters into semiconscious patients can precipitate laryngospasm and complete airway obstruction. Endotracheal intubation or surgical airway placement should only be performed by appropriately trained staff.

Complete airway obstruction is uncommon; there is no movement of air at the mouth, and paradoxical movement of the chest and abdomen. It requires immediate intervention by an individual trained in airway management, as cardiac arrest and death will occur within minutes.

High-flow oxygen should be applied to all patients to avoid hypoxia.

Breathing

Observation is the most rewarding aspect of examining the breathing system. The respiratory rate should be recorded. Tachypnoea (>20 breaths/min) is the most frequent physiological abnormality amongst patients admitted to the ICU. Patient may also have a reduced respiratory rate (<8 breaths/min) as a consequence of drugs or CNS infection or trauma. The respiratory pattern should be noted and brief auscultation performed. Reduced chest expansion always occurs on the side of disease (pneumonia, pneumothorax, haemothorax, collapse). A pulse oximeter must be applied and the oxygen saturations recorded.

Hypoxaemia can precipitate cardiac arrest, and oxygen must be applied with the aim of maintaining saturations >90%. Oxygen is administered by using a mask with a reservoir bag and a non-rebreathing valve and at high flow (15 l/min), as this will achieve an inspired oxygen of >80%. An arterial blood gas should be performed on oxygen to assess the adequacy of oxygenation (as determined by the oxygen saturation (SaO_2), the partial pressure of oxygen (PaO_2), and the alveolar–arterial oxygen gradient) and ventilation (as determined by the partial pressure of carbon dioxide ($PaCO_2$) and by pH). It may also provide information about the acid–base balance and the circulation (via the base deficit, pH, and lactate level). Lactate is frequently raised in critical illness often long before other indices, usually reflecting an inadequate circulation and a switch to anaerobic metabolism. Removal of oxygen to perform an arterial blood gas is dangerous, as it may precipitate cardiorespiratory arrest, and is therefore avoided. In patients with COPD and type II respiratory failure, a small proportion of individuals retain carbon dioxide on oxygen. In these patients, it is acceptable to initiate a fixed-performance oxygen mask delivering inspired oxygen of 40%. The amount of oxygen delivered can be titrated upwards if oxygen saturations fall to <90%, and downwards if SaO_2 is >93% or consciousness decreases. Oxygen saturations <90%, a rising $PaCO_2$, and a falling Glasgow Coma Scale (GCS) score indicate ventilatory support is needed.

Diagnosis of a tension pneumothorax requires immediate intercostal tube drainage before proceeding to examination of the circulation system.

Circulation

Circulatory dysfunction is characterized by hypotension (systolic blood pressure <90 mm Hg or showing a drop of 30 mm Hg), tachycardia, bradycardia, prolonged capillary refill, low urine output (<0.5 ml/kg hour^{-1}), a falling GCS, raised arterial lactate, and acidosis. It is useful to know the patient's usual blood pressure, as an apparently normal value may represent hypotension in an individual who is normally hypertensive. Circulatory shock can exist in the absence of hypotension, especially in young individuals who have a large physiological reserve. IV access should be set up, and continuous ECG and blood-pressure monitoring established. Invasive blood-pressure monitoring has an advantage in that it is continuous and that

it allows arterial samples to be drawn easily for blood gas analysis. A rapid infusion of fluid is a prerequisite when circulatory failure exists (fluid challenge). The fluid should be given as a bolus of 250–500 ml over a period of 10–15 min. Response to treatment is judged against improvements in blood pressure, pulse, capillary refill, urine output, GCS score, lactate levels, and cardiac output, if this is being measured. Further aliquots may be given if there is a response to therapy. Even in cardiogenic shock, fluid may result in improved tissue perfusion; however, it should be avoided if there is evidence of pulmonary oedema.

Disability

The patient's conscious state should be assessed by recording a response to verbal or painful stimuli. Either a GCS score or the simpler AVPU (**a**lert, **v**oice, **p**ain, **u**nresponsive) score may be used. The response of pupils to light should also be recorded, and a blood sugar taken. Hypoglycaemia must be corrected immediately and the patient's conscious state reassessed. If the GCS score is <8, the patient is unlikely to protect their airway and may aspirate. Endotracheal intubation is indicated under these circumstances, and not only protects the airway but may also facilitate further investigations (such as CT) or treatment (such as surgery).

Exposure

The patient should be fully exposed. Pay particular attention to details such as drains, wounds, deformities, bruising or haematomas, and rashes.

Response to treatment

At each stage of the ABCDE approach, response to any treatment should be assessed. Following resuscitation, outcome depends on establishing the cause of critical illness and having a definitive management plan. A thorough review of notes, charts, investigations, and a corroborative history is appropriate at this stage. Extensive needless history and examination may precipitate further decline. Emphasis should be placed on key findings that will define the management plan, such as a history of abdominal pain, and signs of peritonitis. Definitive treatment and investigation, such as echocardiography for acute mitral regurgitation, CT for suspected subdural haematoma, removal of an infected central line in sepsis, surgical drainage of abscesses, coronary reperfusion in myocardial infarction, and repair of a ruptured abdominal aortic aneurism, should not be delayed, as this increases mortality.

It is always important to consider in critically ill patients, if treatment is futile and the patient is already destined to die, whether any advanced directives or resuscitation orders are in place. These decisions should ideally be made with the involvement of the consultant in charge.

Pitfalls in diagnosing critical illness

Failure of critically ill patients to improve with the plan of treatment should always prompt one to consider if the diagnosis is correct or whether a new complication has arisen.

Young, previously fit individuals have a large physiological reserve and often initially tolerate a catastrophic insult with little physiological instability prior to cardiac arrest. For example, following a road traffic accident, a young patient with impact to the chest but without any fractures may have little complaints other than pain. The only abnormal findings might be tachycardia, hypertension, and a raised lactate. This should prompt investigations for causes of shock, such as a ruptured spleen or acute aortic valve rupture.

Further Reading

Royal College of Physicians. National Early Warning Score (NEWS): Standardising the assessment of acute illness severity in the NHS. Report of a working party. London: RCP, 2012. https://www.rcplondon.ac.uk/projects/outputs/national-early-warning-score-news.

Smith ME, Chiovaro JC, O'Neil M, et al. Early warning system scores for clinical deterioration in hospitalized patients: a systematic review. *Ann Am Thorac Soc* 2014; 11: 1454–65.

148 Role of the intensive care unit

Matt Wise and Paul Frost

Organization

The intensive care unit (ICU) can be defined as an area reserved for patients with potential or established organ failure and has the facilities for the diagnosis, prevention, and treatment of multi-organ failure. Usually, the ICU is located in close proximity to the emergency department the radiology department, and the operating theatres, as it is between these areas that patient flows are greatest.

In large urban hospitals, there may be more than one ICU, some of which serve specific patient populations, such as paediatrics, neurosurgery, cardiothoracic surgery, liver failure, and burns. Many hospitals also have high-dependency units (HDUs) that offer higher nurse-to-patient ratios and more advanced monitoring than a general ward does, as well as limited organ support,

In the UK, the distinction between ICU, HDU, and general ward has been abandoned in favour of a classification based on the patient's needs rather than their location (Table 148.1).

One advantage of this classification is that it increases capacity when compared to the same number of fixed HDU and ICU beds, because there can be flexing between Level 2 and Level 3 beds, depending on patient demand. Despite a recent large investment in critical care services and an expansion in the number of Level 2 and Level 3 beds, the UK still has less capacity than many other European countries.

The ICU may function as either a 'closed' unit or an 'open' unit. This nomenclature refers to how care is undertaken by medical staff. In a closed unit, trained resident intensivists direct all patient care, while, in an open unit, the intensivist is consulted at the discretion of the admitting physician. The closed model of care is associated with a reduction in both morbidity and mortality.

In the UK, many ICUs have developed outreach services with the aim of improving the care of general ward patients at risk or recovering from critical illness. The three main aims of outreach are (1) to identify which ward patients are at risk of critical illness and either avert or facilitate admission, as appropriate, (2) to ensure safe discharge, and (3) to improve critical care skills outside the ICU.

Case mix

Admissions to the critical care unit may be either elective following complex planned surgery or as an emergency in a patient who has become critically ill. The latter tends to form the majority of cases in the ICU, although there are exceptions, such as cardiothoracic ICUs where patients are admitted following elective surgery. It has been recognized for several years that many patients who are admitted to ICU, as emergencies or who sustain a cardiorespiratory arrest on a ward, have a prolonged physiological deterioration that has often gone unrecognized. This has led to greater emphasis on training healthcare workers to recognize critical illness, and a number of specialist postgraduate courses on this topic are available (e.g. Acute Life-threatening Events Recognition and Treatment

(ALERT), Ill Medical Patients' Acute Care and Treatment (IMPACT), Care of the Critically Ill Surgical Patient (CCrISP)).

It does not follow that all critically ill patients require admission to ICU, as many patients will be dying from irreversible end-stage disease. These decisions, and the recognition that further treatment may be futile, are complex. It is for these reasons that potential admissions to critical care should be discussed between the consultant from the referring team, and the consultant intensivist. Generally, patients deemed suitable for ICU admission should have one or more organ failures but a reasonable prospect of recovery to a level of function that is acceptable to the patient. Clearly, there is great variability amongst patients as to what represents a reasonable level of function, and this should be discussed directly with patients or relatives when the opportunity arises.

Management

Referring physicians may have patients admitted infrequently to ICU and therefore have limited contact with this service. Consequently, physicians without previous exposure to ICU may be unfamiliar with what happens to patients in this area and what might be expected when visiting ICU. However, in practice, intensive care medicine should be considered as an extension of general medicine, albeit with more sophisticated monitoring and organ support. The cornerstone of managing any patient in ICU is to establish the correct diagnosis so that an appropriate management plan can be embarked upon. For example, two identical patients may be admitted with respiratory failure: in one, caused by acute asthma; in the other, due to community-acquired pneumonia. Although both patients may require similar support (i.e. endotracheal intubation, mechanical ventilation, sedation, fluid therapy, and enteral feeding), the treatment and expected course of recovery between the two are very different. It is, therefore, insufficient to monitor and 'correct' physiological abnormalities without a diagnosis or plan of treatment.

History and examination

As is the case for patients without critical illness, a detailed history is essential in making a diagnosis. However, little of this may be available from the patient and instead must be obtained from notes, charts, other healthcare workers, or relatives. Examination of the patient remains an important facet of diagnosis but is generally more difficult than in patients who are not critically ill. In particular, sedation, analgesia, and ambient noise may confound aspects of the clinical examination, for example, limiting neurological examination and making auscultation impossible. Moreover, critically ill patients have limited physiological reserves and tolerate changes in body position for clinical examination poorly. Great care must be taken to avoid the accidental removal of medical devices such as the endotracheal tube, IV lines, and monitoring leads. The bedside nurse can be of

Level	Description
Table 148.1 Needs-based classification of high-dependency areas in hospital	
0	Patients whose needs are met by normal ward care in acute hospitals
1	Patients at risk of deterioration, or recently moved from higher levels of care and whose needs can be met on a ward with additional support from intensive care
2	Patients requiring single-organ support or post-operative care, or stepping down from Level 3
3	Patients requiring advanced respiratory support (intubation) alone, or the support of two other organ systems

great help in assisting with these issues so that the examination can be performed safely. Many important aspects of the clinical examination can be accomplished by careful inspection alone of, for example, line sites and wounds for evidence of infection.

Investigation

The majority of hospital investigations are available to the critically ill patient and, given the difficulties of clinical examination, imaging is particularly important. However, transfer of a physiologically unstable patient, for example, for CT, requires careful consideration of the risks and benefits of the investigation being undertaken.

Treatment

Most patients in the ICU will be suffering from one or more organ failures. Although no therapies can reverse this process, most organ failures can be monitored and supported while the underlying disease is treated, as follows:

- respiratory organ failure:
  - monitoring: pulse oximetry, arterial blood gases, capnography, flow-volume loops, respiratory mechanics, chest radiograph, pleural ultrasound, CT chest, bronchoalveolar lavage
  - support: invasive or non-invasive ventilation, continuous positive airway pressure, inhaled nitric oxide or prostacyclin
- cardiovascular organ failure:
  - monitoring: ECG, arterial pressure, central venous pressure, echocardiography, cardiac output measurement, lactate, central mixed venous oxygen saturations
  - support: vasopressors, cardiac pacing, antiarrhythmic drugs, intra-aortic balloon pump, ventricular assist device
- renal organ failure:
  - monitoring: urine analysis, urine output, ultrasound
  - support: intermittent or continuous renal replacement therapy
- gastrointestinal organ failure:
  - monitoring: abdominal radiographs, ultrasound, CT, gastric aspirate volumes, gastric tonometry, intra-abdominal pressure
  - support: enteral or parenteral nutrition, laparostomy, prokinetic drugs
- liver failure:
  - monitoring: liver function tests, ultrasound, indocyanine green dye clearance
  - support: molecular absorbents recirculation system
- neurological organ failure:
  - monitoring: CT, MRI, PET, CT angiography, intracranial pressure monitoring, jugulovenous bulb oximetry, CSF sampling, EEG, microdialysis
  - support: sedation, osmotherapy, cooling, barbiturate coma, CSF drainage

Visiting

Good communication is essential when attending the ICU, and visiting physicians should introduce themselves and their reason for seeing the patient. Any opinions regarding the patient should be discussed with the intensivist and clearly documented in the notes. Critically ill patients are particularly susceptible to nosocomial infection, which is an important attributor to morbidity and mortality. Care must be given to preventing horizontal cross infection, which can be greatly reduced by the use of alcoholic hand gel prior to patient contact. White coats may also be a vector for infection and should be left outside.

Discharges

Discharge from the ICU at night is associated with higher mortality and should be avoided if possible, particularly as many hospitals have reduced medical cover during this period compared to daytime levels. There should be handover of the patient to the receiving physician, outlining the diagnosis, treatment, and any outstanding issues such as pending investigations. A plan should also be in place as to what will happen if the patient subsequently deteriorates, as readmission to ICU may not be appropriate. Ideally, this handover should be performed at the bedside rather than over the telephone, so that both parties have a visual record of the patient. This information should also be clearly documented in the notes.

Outcomes

Mortality varies depending on the case mix of patients; however, a figure of 20%–30% in a general ICU would not be unrepresentative. A number of scoring systems such as the Acute Physiology, Age, Chronic Health Evaluation (APACHE) system or the Simplified Acute Physiology Score (SAPS) have been developed to predict patient outcome. However, these scoring systems describe outcome in groups of patients, not in individuals, and expert opinion is important in estimating outcome. Unfortunately, many patients do not survive ICU. Following death, the referring physician and general practitioner should be informed and hospital records should be amended so that any outstanding appointments can be cancelled. Many ICU now offer a bereavement follow-up service for relatives.

Further Reading

Faculty of Intensive Care Medicine/Intensive Care Society (2013). Core Standards for Intensive Care Units. Available at: https://www.ficm.ac.uk/sites/default/files/Core%20Standards%20for%20ICUs%20Ed.1%20(2013).pdf.

Webb A, Angus D, Finfer S, Gattinoni L, and Singer M (eds). *Oxford Textbook of Critical Care* 2016. Oxford University Press.

149 ICU treatment of respiratory failure

Matt Wise and Paul Frost

Definition of the disease

Respiratory failure is a syndrome characterized by defective gas exchange due to inadequate function of the respiratory system. There is a failure to oxygenate blood (hypoxaemia) and/or eliminate carbon dioxide (hypercapnoea). Generally, hypoxaemia is defined as a value for the partial pressure of oxygen in arterial blood (PaO_2) of <8 kPa, and hypercapnoea as a value for the partial pressure of carbon dioxide in arterial blood ($PaCO_2$) of >6 kPa. Type I respiratory failure describes hypoxaemic respiratory failure with a low or normal $PaCO_2$, while type II respiratory failure is characterized by an elevated $PaCO_2$. Type II failure frequently follows type I as the 'respiratory pump' fatigues.

Respiratory failure can develop over years when it is due to conditions such as kyphoscoliosis or motor neuron disease, or minutes in the case of an acute asthma attack or pneumothorax. In this context, respiratory failure is often called acute (e.g. asthma), chronic (e.g. kyphoscoliosis), or acute on chronic (kyphoscoliosis complicated by pneumonia). Chronic respiratory failure is characterized by compensatory mechanisms which aim to adjust the pH of the blood back to the normal physiological range and involve the retention of bicarbonate by the kidney.

Aetiology of respiratory failure

Hypoxia may be caused by:

- low inspired oxygen (altitude)
- a right-to-left shunt
- diffusion limitation
- alveolar hypoventilation
- ventilation–perfusion mismatch

Ventilation–perfusion mismatch is by far the commonest cause of hypoxic respiratory failure.

Hypercapnoea results from alveolar hypoventilation and may be caused by:

- abnormalities of the chest wall
- depressed respiratory drive
- neuromuscular disease
- increased dead space ventilation

Conditions causing respiratory failure in intensive care include:

- pneumonia (community-acquired pneumonia, healthcare-associated pneumonia, hospital-acquired pneumonia, or ventilator-associated pneumonia (VAP))
- COPD
- asthma
- pulmonary oedema (cardiogenic pulmonary oedema, drug-induced pulmonary oedema, or negative pressure pulmonary oedema)
- pleural disease (pneumothorax, pleural effusions, haemothorax, empyema, chylothorax)
- pulmonary embolus
- adult respiratory distress syndrome (ARDS)
- sputum retention
- drug overdose (opiates, barbiturates, benzodiazepines, gamma-hydroxybutyric acid (GHB))
- central nervous system disease (subarachnoid haemorrhage, traumatic brain injury, stroke, tumour, meningitis, encephalitis)
- aspiration pneumonia
- chest wall deformity (flail chest/rib fractures, kyphoscoliosis, obesity)
- neuromuscular diseases (Guillain–Barré syndrome, spinal injury, myasthenia gravis, motor neuron disease, muscular dystrophy, poliomyelitis)
- hypothyroidism
- tetanus
- obesity hypoventilation syndrome
- pulmonary hypertension
- interstitial lung disease

This list is large but not exhaustive: although some conditions are rare, all (with the exception of polio) have been encountered by the authors in UK intensive care patients. Respiratory failure is often multifactorial in critically ill patients, for example, in an obese, narcotized patient with sputum retention following a laparotomy.

Typical and less common symptoms and signs of respiratory failure

The patient symptoms vary depending on the disease that is leading to respiratory failure; however, dyspnoea, chest pain, cough, snoring, haemoptysis, or headaches may be present. The signs of acute respiratory failure are non-specific and include:

- abnormal respiratory rate (>20 (? >30) or <8 breaths/min)
- tachycardia initially, proceeding to bradycardia and cardiac arrest
- hypotension
- vasoconstriction (hypoxia) or vasodilation (hypercapnoea)
- central cyanosis
- confusion, agitation, drowsiness, seizures, coma

Significant respiratory failure may be present with few symptoms or signs. Therefore, following assessment of the patient, if there is a suspicion that the patient is in respiratory failure, an arterial blood gas should be rapidly obtained.

Demographics of the disease

Respiratory failure is one of the commonest causes of admission to ICU.

Natural history and complications of the disease

Respiratory failure has many causes. Therefore, the natural history of the disease, as well as its complications, and outcome, reflects the underlying disease and patient comorbidities.

Approach to diagnosing respiratory failure

The cornerstone of managing patients with respiratory failure is to establish that they are, in fact, in respiratory failure and then define the underlying aetiology. The diagnosis may be suspected if the patient is known to have a disease (e.g. motor neuron disease or asthma) which may progress or be complicated by respiratory failure. Individuals in whom the onset is acute or acute on chronic are critically ill and may rapidly progress to coma and death. Hypoxaemia and hypercapnoea define respiratory failure but the symptoms and signs attributable to these abnormalities are non-specific and largely cause perturbations of the respiratory, cardiovascular, and neurological systems. An approach to the diagnosis and management of these patients requires a brief history and a clinical examination focused on simple, physiological variables along the lines of the Airway, Breathing, Circulation, Disability, and Environment (ABCDE) approach. It is essential to remember that 'ABCDE' is more than a simple mnemonic but represents a hierarchy of abnormalities which determine patient survival. If the airway is obstructed, attempts to correct hypoxia and the subsequent hypotension and bradycardia will prove unsuccessful unless airway patency is restored. This approach involves both examination and treatment of the patient.

An arterial blood gas sample should be obtained to confirm the diagnosis of respiratory failure. Many emergency departments and critical care units have point-of-care blood gas analysers. If the sample is being transported to a laboratory, it should be on ice, with any air bubbles expelled to avoid spurious values. Respiratory failure is present when the PaO_2 is <8 kPa and/or the $PaCO_2$ is >6 kPa. However, in acutely ill patients, oxygen should not be removed to perform an arterial blood gas, as this may precipitate cardiorespiratory arrest due to hypoxia. Adequate oxygenation should be maintained by delivering sufficient inspired oxygen to maintain oxygen saturations >90% on pulse oximetry. The extent to which oxygenation is impaired may instead be established by using the alveolar gas equation to calculate the alveolar-to-arterial (A–a) gradient. The normal range of the A–a gradient is 2–4 kPa (but increases with age and at inspired oxygen concentrations above 28%) and is a reflection of imperfect ventilation–perfusion matching in normal lungs. The A–a gradient will be normal in hypoxia due to pure hypoventilation and no intrinsic lung disease, and elevated in respiratory failure due to lung pathology:

$$A-a \; gradient = PAO_2 - PaO_2,$$

where PAO_2 is the partial pressure of alveolar oxygen, which can be determined from the alveolar gas equation

$$PAO_2 = FIO_2 \left(atmospheric \; pressure - water \; vapour \; pressure \right)$$
$$-1.25 \left(PaCO_2 \right),$$

where FIO_2 is the percentage inspired oxygen. Thus, the A–a gradient can be calculated as

$$A-a \; gradient = [FIO_2 \left(atmospheric \; pressure - water \; vapour \; pressure \right)$$
$$-1.25 (PaCO_2)] - PaO_2$$

This equation can be used to evaluate the A–a gradient under various circumstances, as in the following two scenarios (both at sea level, where the atmospheric pressure is 101 kPa, and the water vapour pressure is 6.3 kPa):

1. Morphine overdose (pure hypoventilation), with the patient on air (which is 21% oxygen); $PaO_2 = 7$ kPa, and $PaCO_2 = 8.8$ kPa:

$$A-a \; gradient = \left[0.21(101 \; kPa - 6.3 \; kPa) - 1.25 \left(PaCO_2 \right) \right] - PaO_2$$
$$= (19.9 \; kPa - 11 \; kPa) - 7 \; kPa$$
$$= 1.9 \; kPa \; (normal \; A-a \; gradient)$$

2. Acute pulmonary oedema, with the patient on an inspired oxygen concentration of 40%; $PaO_2 = 15$ kPa, and $PaCO_2 = 5.6$ kPa:

$$A-a \; gradient = \left[0.40(101 \; kPa - 6.3 \; kPa) - 1.25 \left(PaCO_2 \right) \right] - PaO_2$$
$$= (37.9 \; kPa - 7 \; kPa) - 15 \; kPa$$
$$= 15.9 \; kPa \; (elevated \; A-a \; gradient)$$

A rough guide to estimating what the PAO_2 should be for a patient on oxygen if there is no lung pathology is to subtract 10 from FIO_2. In the second scenario, where the inspired oxygen concentration is 40%, this would give a PAO_2 of 40 − 10 = 30 kPa for normal lungs; as the measured PaO_2 was 15 kPa, the 'guesstimated' A–a gradient would be 15 kPa (i.e. 30 kPa − 15 kPa).

The arterial blood gas should be scrutinized to see if hypercapnoea is acute or chronic. Hypoventilation that occurs over a long period of time, such as in some neuromuscular disease, is accompanied by the retention of plasma bicarbonate and a shift of arterial pH back to the normal range. Acute rises in the $PaCO_2$ result in a respiratory acidosis and only small changes in plasma bicarbonate. A change in the $PaCO_2$ of 1 kPa causes a change of 0.06 pH units in the opposite direction.

Other diagnosis that should be considered

Patients with acute or acute on chronic respiratory failure are critically ill, and this syndrome should be considered in all critically ill patients. There are very few instances where it is not appropriate to obtain a blood gas in a critically ill patient, and this will establish a diagnosis of respiratory failure. Since the symptoms and signs of critical illness are non-specific, there many instances where the patient may be thought on first inspection to be in respiratory failure. Thus, a patient with diabetic ketoacidosis may complain of dyspnoea and be extremely tachypnoeic (as a consequence of metabolic acidosis and increased work of breathing), and a similar presentation may be observed in severe sepsis. Potential pitfalls in the diagnosis of respiratory failure are due to misinterpretation of arterial blood gas samples. It is easy to establish if the patient is hypoxic or if a large A–a gradient exists. If there is evidence of hypercapnoea, one must remember to first look at the pH. Rarely, patients have a metabolic alkalosis (due to diuretics, nasogastric losses, or vomiting), which is partially corrected by alveolar hypoventilation (hypercapnoea), but the primary abnormality will be an alkalosis.

'Gold-standard' diagnostic test

Arterial blood gas analysis remains the best method for diagnosing acute respiratory failure.

Acceptable diagnostic alternatives to the gold standard

Pulse oximetry may be used to detect hypoxaemia non-invasively. However, this method gives no information about ventilation ($PaCO_2$); furthermore, several factors can adversely affect readings. These include poor peripheral perfusion; motion artefact; fluorescent lights; nail polish (causes falsely low or undetectable readings); carboxyhaemoglobin; and methaemoglobin (causes high readings).

Other relevant investigations

Investigations largely centre on establishing the disease that is causing respiratory failure and this will be determined by the history and examination. A focused clinical approach, rather than merely performing a panel of tests, is essential. However, the following investigations are commonly used and may be useful:

- full blood count (to determine leucocytosis or neutropenia (infection), polycythaemia (chronic hypoxia))
- blood biochemistry:
  - electrolytes (electrolyte disturbances may precipitate arrhythmias and muscle weakness)
  - amylase (to exclude pancreatitis)
  - thyroid function (thyroid disease can contribute to cardiac disease, muscle weakness)
  - creatinine kinase (to exclude cardiac or muscle disease)
  - troponin (to exclude ischaemic heart disease, myocarditis)
  - toxicology (to exclude overdose)
- samples for infectious causes (bacteria, viruses, mycobacteria):
  - blood cultures
  - sputum
  - bronchoalveolar lavage
  - nasopharyngeal swabs (influenza)
  - pleural fluid
  - CSF
- pleural fluid analysis:
  - protein
  - pH
  - lactate dehydrogenase
  - cytology
  - TB
  - amylase
- peak flow rate
- lung biopsy

- imaging:
  - chest radiography
  - ultrasound (to detect pleural disease)
  - CT chest (high resolution and/or volume, angiography); CT head (to exclude subarachnoid haemorrhage, which can lead to neurogenic pulmonary oedema); CT abdomen (to exclude peritonitis, pancreatitis)
  - ECG (to exclude ischaemia, arrhythmias)
  - echocardiography (for left ventricular function, diastolic dysfunction, regional wall abnormality, valve function, pericardial disease, pulmonary hypertension, pulmonary emboli)

Prognosis and how to estimate it

Respiratory failure is a syndrome with a wide aetiology and it is difficult to prognosticate. Even when looking at respiratory failure from a single cause such as pneumonia or ARDS, there is a wide variation in survival rates or hospital discharge between studies. Outcome is dependent on many variables, which include the age of the patient, comorbidities, and the degree of physiological deterioration before diagnosis and commencement of appropriate treatment. A number of scoring systems are used in intensive care, such as the Acute Physiology and Chronic Health Evaluation (APACHE), the Simplified Acute Physiology Score (SAPS), and the Sequential Organ Failure Assessment (SOFA), to define patient outcome. These scoring systems are similar in their predictive accuracy but describe outcome in groups of patients rather than in individuals, and therefore prognosis is often determined by expert opinion.

Treatment and its effectiveness

The cornerstone of managing respiratory failure is to provide organ support, establish the diagnosis, and treat the underlying disease. Resuscitation must be initiated as soon as respiratory failure is recognized and should follow the standard Airway, Breathing, Circulation (ABC) approach, so that immediate threats to life, such as airway compromise or tension pneumothorax, are addressed first. The patient should be managed in an appropriate area with trained staff and monitoring (e.g. respiratory rate, continuous ECG, oximetry, arterial line (blood pressure, arterial blood gas analysis), and Glasgow Coma Scale scoring).

Acute hypoxia is poorly tolerated and, if left untreated, may precipitate cardiorespiratory arrest. Oxygen should be administered. This may be by a fixed device (e.g. a Venturi mask) or via a variable-performance device (e.g. nasal prongs, Hudson mask, or non-rebreathing mask and reservoir bag). In most patients with respiratory failure, a non-rebreathing mask and reservoir bag should be used with high-flow oxygen (15 l/min) and will deliver inspired oxygen in excess of 60% (often approaching 100%). Oxygen saturations >90% represent adequate oxygenation, as most oxygen is carried bound to haemoglobin. Caution should be exercised in COPD patients who are hypercapnic, as approximately 5% of such patients retain more carbon dioxide when the hypoxic respiratory drive is removed. This can be managed with controlled oxygen therapy and repeat blood gas analysis.

Oxygen therapy alone is insufficient in many patients who require ventilatory support to improve oxygenation and eliminate carbon dioxide. This support may be administered as non-invasive positive pressure ventilation or as invasive ventilation via an endotracheal tube.

Non-invasive ventilation (NIV) is suitable for a proportion of critical care patients with respiratory failure. Although both volume- and pressure-cycled ventilators exist, the commonest modes of delivering non-invasive support are pressure-support ventilation, bi-level positive airway pressure (BIPAP) ventilation, and continuous positive airway pressure (CPAP). NIV is delivered to the airway via an interface, which may be a face mask, a nasal mask, a full-face mask, or a helmet. The advantages of NIV over invasive mechanical ventilation are that less sedation is needed, the patient retains the ability to talk, eat, and drink, and airway trauma and VAP are avoided.

CPAP is not a ventilatory mode per se, as it provides a constant pressure throughout the respiratory cycle; however, it improves oxygenation by increasing functional residual capacity and reduces the work of breathing and left ventricular afterload. It is commonly used in type I respiratory failure due to pulmonary oedema and pneumonia. In the pressure-support mode of CPAP, patients initiate, terminate, and control the size of breaths, while the ventilator delivers to a preset inspiratory

pressure. The BIPAP mode alternates between two levels of CPAP, with the switch between levels providing inspiratory drive. Both modes eliminate CO_2 as well as improve oxygenation. NIV is suitable for cooperative patients who have a rapidly reversible cause of respiratory failure and are haemodynamically stable, without severe acidosis. Excessive pulmonary secretions are a relative contraindication. Most frequently used in exacerbations of COPD, NIV has also been used in the treatment of pneumonia, ARDS, asthma, and pulmonary oedema.

Invasive mechanical ventilation is indicated in patients with a Glasgow Coma Scale score <8, apnoea, increasing acidosis, refractory hypoxia, an inability to clear secretions, or who are tiring and have a dyskinetic respiratory pattern and tachycardia. Following endotracheal intubation, the cuff pressure should be maintained <25 mm Hg to avoid tracheal necrosis. Patients in whom long-term ventilation (>7 days) is required may have the endotracheal tube replaced with a tracheostomy. The majority of tracheostomies are performed at the bedside using a percutaneous dilatational technique.

The terminology concerning modes of ventilation is often confusing, and explaining it is outside the scope of this text. Modern ventilators are complex devices allowing a change from mandatory to partial support modes that minimize sedation requirements and allow patients to be conscious but comfortable. Positive end-expiratory pressure (PEEP) is applied to all modes of invasive mechanical ventilation. The principles of ventilation in respiratory failure are:

- treat the underlying cause of respiratory failure
- avoid excessive fluid (which is associated with worse outcome in ARDS)
- set optimal PEEP and minimize FIO_2
- limit plateau pressures to <30 cm H_2O and avoid tidal volumes >6 ml/kg ideal body weight; both of these measures are associated with a reduction in ventilator-induced lung injury (e.g. barotrauma, atelectrauma, volutrauma, biotrauma) in ARDS but will often result in patients having a respiratory acidosis known as permissive hypercapnoea, in which the arterial pH will frequently be 7.2 or lower
- interrupt sedation at least daily (this reduces length of stay on ventilation, and VAP incidence)
- elevate the head of the bed to 30° (this reduces VAP incidence)
- perform microbiological surveillance for VAP
- maintain bronchopulmonary toilet (secretion clearance)
- provide stress ulcer prophylaxis (H2 blocker or proton-pump inhibitor) and thromboprophylaxis
- provide enteral nutrition at an early stage
- ensure that blood glucose levels are controlled in the range 3.8–8.3 mmol/l
- extubate the patient and discontinue ventilation when the cause of respiratory failure has resolved

Note that some of these elements (i.e. sedation break, bed elevation, and DVT and stress ulcer prophylaxis) are grouped together and referred to as 'ventilator care bundles' because, when they are instituted together, there is a reduction in VAP.

Further Reading

Davidson AC, Banham S, Elliott M, et al. British Thoracic Society/Intensive Care Society Acute Hypercapnic Respiratory Failure Guideline Development Group. BTS/ICS Guidelines for the ventilatory management of acute hypercapnic respiratory failure in adults. *Thorax* 2016; 71: ii1–ii35. https://www.brit-thoracic.org.uk/document-library/clinical-information/acute-hypercapnic-respiratory-failure/bts-guidelines-for-ventilatory-management-of-ahrf/.

Goligher EC, Ferguson ND, and Brochard LJ. Clinical challenges in mechanical ventilation. *Lancet* 2016; 387: 1856–866.

Kelly CR, Higgins AR, Chandra SN. Videos in clinical medicine. Non-invasive positive-pressure ventilation. *N Engl J Med* 2015; 372: e30. http://www.nejm.org/doi/full/10.1056/NEJMvcm1313336.

O'Driscoll BR, Howard L, Earis J, et al. British Thoracic Society Emergency Oxygen Guideline Development Group. BTS guideline for oxygen use in adults in healthcare and emergency settings. *Thorax* 2017; 72: i1–i90. https://www.brit-thoracic.org.uk/document-library/clinical-information/oxygen/2017-emergency-oxygen-guideline/bts-guideline-for-oxygen-use-in-adults-in-healthcare-and-emergency-settings/

150 ICU treatment of cardiovascular failure

Matt Wise and Paul Frost

Definition of the cardiovascular failure

Cardiovascular failure or shock is best defined as inadequate delivery or utilization of oxygen for cellular metabolic needs. The majority of shock states are characterized by limitations in perfusion rather than extraction of oxygen by tissues. It is important to recognize that ineffectual tissue perfusion may occur in the absence of hypotension and, therefore, a normal blood pressure does not exclude shock.

Aetiology of shock

Shock can be classified as cardiogenic, obstructive, hypovolaemic, or distributive according to the predominant underlying mechanism.

Cardiogenic shock

In cardiogenic shock, there is inadequate forward flow of blood from the heart. This most frequently occurs following acute myocardial infarction (MI) and complicates between 3% and 10% of infarcts. The incidence of cardiogenic shock following MI increases with failure to establish coronary reperfusion. Less frequent causes of cardiogenic shock include:

- acute valve dysfunction or rupture, most often due to infective endocarditis
- acute ventricular septal rupture complicating acute MI
- myocarditis
- myocardial contusion
- myocardial depression during septic shock (relatively common because of the high prevalence of septic shock)

Obstructive shock

Obstructive shock is defined by pathologies which restrict the outflow of blood from the heart:

- pulmonary embolus
- cardiac tamponade
- tension pneumothorax
- severe asthma

Hypovolaemic shock

Hypovolaemic shock is defined by a pathological reduction in circulating blood volume and is caused by:

- blood loss
- plasma loss

Distributive shock

Distributive shock is characterized by loss of peripheral vascular tone and maldistribution of blood flow:

- septic shock (cardiac output may be increased or decreased)
- spinal shock (disruption of the spinal cord above the sympathetic outflow T1–L2 leads to reduced sympathetic activity resulting in vasodilatation, hypotension, and bradycardia)
- Addisonian crisis
- fulminant hepatic failure
- anaphylactic shock (release of vasoactive histamine and prostaglandins; also accompanied by hypovolaemia due to increased vascular permeability)

It is important to remember that there may be considerable overlap between shock states. Distributive shock, which characterizes sepsis, is compounded by relative hypovolaemia and myocardial depression. Moreover, sepsis with positive blood cultures may occur in up to a fifth of patients with cardiogenic shock. Cardiogenic shock is the common final pathway to death in most severe shock states, particularly when there is severe acidosis.

Typical symptoms of the disease, and less common symptoms

The majority of symptoms associated with shock are attributable to the underlying cause. Diagnoses may be suggested by characteristic pain (MI, pulmonary embolus, or pancreatitis); breathlessness and purulent sputum (pneumonia); and haematemesis and melaena (gastrointestinal haemorrhage). Symptoms attributable to the shock state per se include breathlessness, syncope, and a feeling of impending death.

The presentation of shock is greatly influenced by age, comorbidities, and the time of presentation. At one extreme, an individual may be obtunded while, in another case, they may be sitting up talking with a normal blood pressure and few symptoms. The latter is particularly true in young, previously healthy individuals, who have a large physiological reserve and can compensate during the early stages of shock.

Natural history, and complications of the disease

Untreated shock progresses to multi-organ failure and death. Mortality rises as the number of failing organ systems increases and typically exceeds 50% when four or more organs have failed, whatever the underlying aetiology.

In individuals who survive, the sequelae depend on the underlying cause. Patients with cardiogenic shock due to MI may be left severely limited due to the development of heart failure, while there may be no long-term consequences if cardiogenic shock was the consequence of an overdose of beta blockers. Individuals with shock due to anaphylaxis or pancreatitis may make a full recovery but have recurrent episodes. Survivors of septic shock have a 50% reduction in survival over the following 5 years.

Approach to diagnosing the disease

The diagnosis of shock may be self-evident when there is a corroborating history and clinical findings. There would be little doubt that a patient with known portal hypertension and oesophageal varices who presents with massive haematemesis, hypotension, tachycardia, and oliguria has hypovolaemic shock. However, in clinical practice, the situation is often less clear, as there may be limited history at the time of presentation, and confounding comorbidities, such as hypertension, which may obscure the diagnosis. It is important to appreciate that patients with shock are critically ill; therefore, although the clinical history is crucial in reaching a diagnosis, it is important not to needlessly exhaust the patient with questions that can be answered from other sources, such as staff, and relatives, and medical notes,. Following a brief targeted history, clinical examination should focus on the cardiorespiratory and neurological systems. Observations consistent with a diagnosis of shock would be hypotension (systolic blood pressure <90 mm Hg), tachycardia (pulse >100 bpm), tachypnoea (respiratory rate >20 breaths/min), cold peripheries, cyanosis, prolonged capillary refill, oliguria (<0.5 ml/kg hour^{-1}) or anuria, and altered mental status. These observations are non-specific but nevertheless sensitive for more shock states and are more useful diagnostically when they are considered together, particularly in the context of any history (e.g. haematemesis or ischaemic chest pain) or investigations (e.g. low haemoglobin levels, raised lactate levels, ST elevation on ECG).

The aetiology of the shock state may be suggested by specific features of the history and examination:

- a history of bee sting or ingestion of nuts: anaphylaxis
- chest trauma: tension pneumothorax, myocardial contusion, aortic arch dissection, or traumatic aortic valve rupture
- bronchial breath sounds: pneumonia
- Beck's triad of hypotension, muffled heart sounds, and raised jugular venous pressure: cardiac tamponade
- subcutaneous emphysema: tension pneumothorax
- new murmur: mitral valve rupture, ventricular septal defect, or infective endocarditis
- splinter haemorrhages: infective endocarditis
- purpuric rash: meningococcaemia
- Grey Turner's or Cullen's sign: pancreatitis

The underlying aetiology may not be immediately obvious; however, the classification of shock into cardiogenic, obstructive, hypovolaemic, and distributive is a useful clinical sieve which can be used to plan further investigations which may elucidate the cause. The following investigations may be diagnostic:

- full blood count: to detect low haemoglobin (haemorrhage), raised white-cell count (sepsis), low platelets (haemorrhage)
- amylase: to exclude pancreatitis
- urea and electrolytes: to detect raised urea (Addison's disease, gastrointestinal haemorrhage, vomiting, diarrhoea, polyuria, pericarditis/tamponade) and/or abnormal electrolytes (fluid losses, Addison's disease)
- mast cell tryptase: to exclude anaphylaxis
- blood cultures: to exclude septic shock
- arterial blood gas analysis: lactate levels are frequently abnormal before hypotension, oliguria, and altered mental status are present and is elevated as a consequence of inadequate oxygen delivery and a switch to anaerobic metabolism
- ECG: to exclude MI (indicated by ST elevation), cardiac tamponade (indicated by concave ST elevation and low voltage or electrical alternans), pulmonary embolism (indicated by an S1Q3T3 pattern, right bundle branch block, right-axis deviation), arrhythmias (e.g. ventricular tachycardia)
- chest radiograph: to detect pulmonary oedema (suggests MI), enlarged cardiac silhouette (suggests pulmonary embolism, cardiac tamponade), pneumothorax, consolidation (suggests sepsis)
- echocardiogram: this is an extremely useful investigation because it can be performed at the bedside and can quickly confirm and exclude some major causes of shock; it can be used to detect impaired contractility (suggests MI, contusion, myocarditis), valve lesions (via colour-flow Doppler), hypovolaemia (suggested by small left ventricle chamber size), pulmonary embolism (e.g. clot in transit; pulmonary hypertension; right ventricular dysfunction), pericardial tamponade (indicated by right ventricular collapse in systole, or a large effusion)

In addition, other specialized investigations may be required, such as CT pulmonary angiography (in pulmonary embolism), ultrasonography (in abdominal trauma), CT (in trauma), and angiography (in trauma, gastrointestinal haemorrhage).

Other diagnosis that should be considered

Most often, shock is associated with a single diagnosis, such as MI. Occasionally, other shock-associated diseases may complicate the primary diagnosis. Examples of this include MI precipitating diabetic ketoacidosis, sepsis precipitating an Addisonian crisis, or acute valvular regurgitation complicating endocarditis. Thus, the possibility of dual or even multiple pathologies must always be considered in the shocked patient. Whatever the initial pathology, cardiogenic shock is generally a feature of most advanced shock states as multi-organ failure, severe acidosis, and metabolic mayhem develop.

'Gold-standard' diagnostic test

There is no gold-standard diagnostic test for the presence of shock. Shock is invariably accompanied by abnormalities in cardiac output and blood pressure, and measuring these parameters is important in management; however, there is no number which is diagnostic. Although most shock states have a low cardiac index (<2.2 l/min m^{-2}), this index is elevated in some patients with septic shock. Furthermore, critically ill patients are catabolic, with higher metabolic demands, and so what might be considered an acceptable cardiac output in a healthy individual might be insufficient to meet metabolic demands. Hypotension (systolic blood pressure <90 mm Hg, or a drop in systolic pressure >30 mm Hg from normal) is usually present; however, systolic blood pressure may be preserved or even elevated during the early stages of shock, due to compensatory vasoconstriction. This is particularly true of young, otherwise fit, individuals (e.g. with traumatic blood loss) who maintain blood pressure despite a low cardiac output and poor tissue perfusion up to the point of cardiac arrest. Arterial increments of lactate often precede changes in other parameters such as cardiac output, blood pressure, or urine output, while this may be abnormal in other conditions, so a raised lactate level should raise the possibility the patient is shocked.

Prognosis and how to estimate it

A number of scoring systems, such as the Acute Physiology and Chronic Health Evaluation (APACHE), the Simplified Acute Physiology Score (SAPS), and the Sequential Organ Failure Assessment (SOFA), are used in intensive care to define patient outcome. These scoring systems are similar in their predictive accuracy and are best at describing outcome in groups of patients rather than in individuals.

Treatment and its effectiveness

The treatment of septic shock is discussed in detail in Chapter 152 and therefore will not be considered further here.

General measures

Patients diagnosed with shock are critically ill, and the first stage in the management of these individuals is the recognition of this fact. Resuscitation should follow the standard Airway, Breathing, Circulation (ABC) approach. Treatment within the ICU consists largely of preventing or supporting organ failures, while the underlying condition that precipitated the shock state is treated definitively.

It should be ensured that the airway is patent, high-flow oxygen is applied, and adequate venous access is secured. Intubation and mechanical ventilation protects the airway when consciousness is reduced but also optimizes oxygen delivery and reduces oxygen demand. Even in circumstances where the airway is patent, the patient may require intubation and mechanical ventilation because, in shock states, a high proportion of cardiac output may be consumed by the work of breathing. Moreover, once the patient is intubated, it can be easier and safer to facilitate further investigations (e.g. CT, angiography) or treatments (e.g. surgery, cardiac catheterization).

Monitoring

The patient should be managed in an area with appropriate nursing and medical staff, and monitoring. According to circumstances, this may be the A & E resuscitation room, the CT scanner room, the angiography suite, the surgical theatre, or the ICU. The minimal requirements for monitoring are continuous ECG; blood pressure; pulse oximetry; respiratory rate; hourly urine output; Glasgow Coma Scale score; and blood glucose. If shock does not rapidly resolve with simple measures, additional haemodynamic monitoring, such as arterial line monitoring, central venous access monitoring, or continuous cardiac output monitoring, is required.

Arterial line monitoring

Arterial line monitoring allows continuous display of arterial pressure, and serial measurement of arterial blood gas samples. The latter provides information on oxygenation (e.g. the partial pressure of arterial oxygen; arterial oxygen saturation), ventilation (e.g. the partial pressure of arterial carbon dioxide) and acid–base balance (e.g. pH, base deficit, and lactate levels). Failure of the acid–base balance to improve should lead the physician to reconsider whether the diagnosis and treatment are correct.

Central venous access monitoring

Central venous access monitoring allows continuous measurement of central venous pressure (CVP) and central venous oxygen saturation (ScvO$_2$). Although the CVP is considered a measure of cardiac preload, a specific value does not predict preload responsiveness. Thus, a CVP of 12 mm Hg may represent hypovolaemia, normovolaemia, or hypervolaemia in three different patients. The CVP may be used to guide fluid therapy, with a rise of 2–3 mm Hg following a rapid bolus of fluid representing an adequate change in preload. Ideally, the response to a fluid bolus should be measured against a change in cardiac output; however, when this is unavailable, improvement in heart rate, blood pressure, urine output, or lactate levels may be used instead. ScvO$_2$, which is a measure of the balance between oxygen delivery and extraction by the tissues, can be measured continuously or intermittently and can be a useful guide to the effectiveness of therapy such as fluids and inotropes. In broad terms, the aim is to restore ScvO$_2$ to a value of >70%.

Cardiac output monitoring

There are a number of monitors available which measure cardiac output; generally, familiarity with a device is more important than a specific choice of monitor.

Although the use of pulmonary artery catheters has diminished in Europe, they are capable of measuring cardiac output continuously using a thermodilution technique. They can also measure right atrial, pulmonary artery, and pulmonary wedge (left atrial) pressures. Newer devices such as PiCCO or LiDCO use an injectate dilution step for calibration (cold saline and lithium, respectively) and analysis of the arterial waveform (pulse contour analysis) for continuous cardiac output measurements. Oesophageal Doppler uses a probe which detects blood flow in the descending aorta and calculates cardiac output continuously.

Fluid therapy

Fluid therapy is mandatory in all shock states, with the exception of cardiogenic shock, for restoring tissue perfusion. There is no evidence to support the use of colloid over crystalloid. Fluid should be administered as a rapid bolus; if cardiac output or stroke volume increases by >10%, further fluid is indicated. If no cardiac output monitor is in situ, fluid responsiveness may be titrated against other parameters such as blood pressure, heart rate, urine output, and lactate levels. Additional fluid therapy should be avoided if there is no increase in cardiac output, as this will result in deleterious effects such as oedema, coagulopathy, and hypoxia.

Aside from specific treatment measures, outcomes from shock are equally dependent on the provision of good general intensive care, as outlined in Chapter 152.

Specific measures

Cardiogenic shock

When cardiogenic shock is due to MI, definitive treatment is aimed at the restoration of coronary perfusion, ideally with percutaneous coronary intervention or surgery when available. Early revascularization reduces mortality at 6 months. An intra-aortic balloon pump may be used as a bridge to definitive treatment or recovery of hibernating myocardium by improving coronary perfusion and reducing afterload and myocardial oxygen demand. Inotropic support with vasoactive drugs such as dobutamine, dopamine, adrenaline, milrinone, or levosimendan may be required to achieve adequate perfusion. As is the case with cardiac output monitors, familiarity of use is more important than the specific choice of drug. Patients in the recovery phase (inotropes discontinued) should be treated with normal medical therapy, including angiotensin-converting enzyme inhibitors.

Surgery is also required for acute valve leaks or ventricular septal defect complicating MI; delayed surgery merely hastens the onset of multi-organ failure and death.

Obstructive shock

Specific measures for obstructive shock are as follows:

- for tension pneumothorax: intercostal tube drainage
- for cardiac tamponade: pericardial drain, pericardial window
- for pulmonary embolus: thrombolysis in massive pulmonary embolism is followed by anticoagulation

Hypovolaemic shock

Hypovolaemic shock requires fluid therapy given in rapid boluses, according to improvements in haemodynamic variables. In the case of haemorrhage, fluid is usually given as blood and fresh frozen plasma. In haemorrhage due to trauma fluid, therapy is given sparingly until a definitive surgical approach to bleeding is undertaken. This so-called permissive hypotension involves resuscitation until a radial pulse is palpable. In a trauma setting, aggressive fluid therapy to conventional endpoints leads to clot instability, increased blood loss, and higher mortality.

Distributive shock

Specific measures for distributive shock are as follows:

- for Addisonian crisis: steroids, fluid, treatment of underlying infection
- for anaphylaxis: steroids, adrenaline, antihistamines, fluid
- for septic shock: see Chapter 152

Further Reading

Francis GS, Bartos JA, and Adatya S. Inotropes. *J Am Coll Cardiol* 2014; 63: 2069–078.

Task force of the European Society of Intensive Care Medicine. Consensus on circulatory shock and hemodynamic monitoring. *Intensive Care Med* 2014; 40: 1795–1815. doi:10.1007/s00134-014-3525-z

Van Diepen S, Katz JN, Albert NM, et al. Contemporary management of cardiogenic shock. A scientific statement from the American Heart Association. *Circulation* 2017; 136:00–00. doi:10.1161/CIR.0000000000000525.

Matt Wise and Paul Frost

Definition of acute kidney injury

The Kidney Disease: Improving Global Outcomes (KDIGO) clinical practice guideline for acute kidney injury (AKI) defines AKI as any of the following:

- increase in serum creatinine ≥0.3 mg/dl (≥26.5 μmol/l) within 48 hours
- increase in serum creatinine to ≥1.5 times baseline within the previous 7 days
- urine volume <0.5 ml/kg hour^{-1} for 6 hours

Etiology of AKI

Traditionally, the etiology of AKI is considered in terms of prerenal, renal, and obstructive causes. However, this categorization is less useful in the ICU, where the etiology of AKI is usually multifactorial and often occurs in the context of multi-organ failure (MOF). Hypotension, nephrotoxic drugs, and sepsis or septic shock are the most important identifiable factors. Less frequently encountered causes include pancreatitis, abdominal compartment syndrome, and rhabdomyolysis. Primary intrinsic renal disease such as glomerulonephritis is extremely uncommon.

A previous history of cirrhosis, cardiac failure, or haematological malignancy, and age >65 years, are important risk factors.

Typical symptoms of AKI

The patient may complain of dyspnoea as a consequence of metabolic acidosis or fluid overload. A reduction in urine output may have been noticed or lower abdominal pain may be a complaint if bladder outflow obstruction is present. Occasionally, cardiac arrest (hyperkalaemia, hypoxia due to pulmonary oedema, metabolic acidosis) may be the first manifestation of AKI.

Demographics of AKI

AKI occurs in up to two-thirds of ICU patients; its incidence is increasing, reflecting an ageing population with multiple comorbidities (cardiac failure, cirrhosis, diabetes, malignancy) and a rising prevalence of sepsis.

Natural history of AKI, and its complications

Patients with any form of AKI have increased mortality, as compared to non-AKI patients. Approximately 4%–5% of critically ill patients with AKI require renal replacement therapy. Sequelae of AKI include hyperkalaemia, acidosis, fluid overload, electrolyte disequilibrium, accumulation of waste products of metabolism, and sepsis. Profoundly uraemic patients can become encephalopathic and develop pericarditis and impaired platelet function. Non-resolution of AKI results in chronic renal failure.

Approach to diagnosing AKI

The diagnosis of AKI has been greatly simplified by the development of the KDIGO criteria, which only require a baseline comparison of serum creatinine and hourly urine output measurements. It is important to remember that, occasionally, renal failure may be non-oliguric.

History and examination should focus on known causes of AKI, such as nephrotoxic drugs and poisons; cardiac failure; diabetes; hypertension; urinary tract obstruction; myeloproliferative disease; autoimmune and connective tissue diseases; trauma or excessive exercise; fluid loss; recent abdominal surgery; and symptoms relating to possible sources of sepsis.

Hypotension and sepsis are important causes of AKI in critically ill patients and so assessment of intra-vascular volume status, together with inspection of possible sites of sepsis, is mandatory. It is important to remember that shock can exist without hypotension and that an apparently 'normal' blood pressure may represent hypotension in a previously hypertensive patient.

Other diagnosis that should be considered

Diagnostic pitfalls in the ICU are inadequate recognition and treatment of hypovolaemia and hypotension, overlooking sepsis, poisoning, nephrotoxic drugs, rhabdomyolysis, an obstructed/infected renal tract, and abdominal compartment syndrome.

Diagnostic investigations

Diagnostic investigations can be simply thought of as those required for the diagnosis of AKI (serum creatinine and hourly urine output) and those to establish the cause:

- serum urea and creatinine (high urea:creatinine ratios favour a prerenal cause)
- serum electrolytes, including calcium; to exclude dehydration, multiple myeloma
- urinary sodium (usually <20 mmol/l in prerenal causes)
- liver function tests; to exclude hepatorenal syndrome
- amylase; to exclude pancreatitis
- paracetamol; ethylene glycol levels
- creatinine kinase; to exclude rhabdomyolysis
- ultrasound; to exclude obstruction of renal tract, and determine whether kidneys are of normal size
- urinary dipstick; to detect proteinuria (glomerular or interstitial disease), leukocytes and nitrites (infection), and haemoglobinuria or myoglobinuria (rhabdomyolysis)
- urinary microscopy; to detect red blood cells (bleeding within renal tract); dysmorphic red cells or casts (glomerulonephritis); granular casts (tubular necrosis); leukocytes or white-cell casts (urosepsis, pyelonephritis, interstitial nephritis); eosinophils (allergic interstitial nephritis, embolic disease); crystals (uric acid; calcium oxalate indicates ethylene glycol poisoning)
- intra-abdominal pressure (IAP); to exclude abdominal compartment syndrome
- blood film; to exclude haemolytic–uraemic syndrome, thrombotic thrombocytopenic purpura, malaria
- serology (for anti-glomerular basement membrane antibodies, antineutrophil cytoplasmic antibodies, and immune complexes) and renal biopsy have low yield in critically ill patients
- ECG; early changes of hyperkalaemia (K^+ >5.5 mmol/l) include peaked T waves, shortened QT intervals, and ST depression; later changes include widening of the QRS, increased PR intervals, and bundle branch block; ultimately, the P wave disappears and ventricular tachycardia or fibrillation occurs

Prognosis and how to estimate it

AKI is an independent factor for increased mortality in ICU patients, even if renal replacement therapy is not required. Mortality increases with increasing severity; where renal replacement therapy is required, mortality approaches 50%–60%. More than 85% of survivors are free of renal replacement therapy at 1 year and this approaches 100% by 5 years.

Treatment and its effectiveness

AKI frequently occurs in the setting of multiple organ failure; such patients are critically ill and at risk of imminent death. The first step is to instigate resuscitation using the standard Airway, Breathing, Circulation, Disability, and Exposure (ABCDE) approach. In parallel with resuscitation, the underlying diagnosis should be investigated and managed. During this process, reversible factors contributing to the AKI, such as hypoxaemia, hypovolaemia, and, less commonly, urinary tract obstruction, can be corrected.

Hyperkalaemia is definitively managed by renal replacement therapy (RRT). However, temporizing measures include the administration of IV calcium chloride to stabilize the myocardium, along with IV insulin and glucose, sodium bicarbonate, and nebulized beta-2 adrenergic agonists to promote the movement of K^+ from the extracellular to the intracellular space.

During resuscitation, it is crucial that renal perfusion pressure is optimized. If the AKI is volume responsive, it is possible to restore renal function and avert the need for RRT. Typically, a mean arterial pressure (MAP) of ~70 mm Hg is required. Abdominal perfusion pressure (MAP − IAP) less than 60 mm Hg is associated with increased mortality.

Fluid resuscitation is the cornerstone of haemodynamic manipulation; currently, crystalloids are preferred over colloids, and it does not matter whether normal saline (0.9% NaCl) or balanced electrolyte solutions are selected.

If the patient is volume replete but still hypotensive, vasoactive agents such as noradrenaline may be required. Although low-dose dopamine (< 5 μg/kg min^{-1}) can increase urine flow, it does not confer protection from AKI and is no longer recommended.

Furosemide is often used in the setting of AKI but there is no evidence to suggest that mortality or the eventual need for renal replacement is affected by its use. Moreover, Furosemide may cause irreversible deafness and worsen acute tubular necrosis.

Patients with AKI, particularly in the context of MOF, are invariably catabolic; moreover, RRT contributes to nutrient loss, with up to 30 g/day of amino acids being lost in the dialysate. Therefore, nutritional supplementation should be always be given and titrated to the presence or absence of RRT. Nutritional goals include a total energy requirement of 20–25 kcal/kg day^{-1}. Protein intake should be around 0.6–1.0 g/kg day^{-1} (no RRT) and up to 2.5 g/kg day^{-1} (on RRT).

Potentially nephrotoxic drugs must be avoided, while the doses of essential drugs may require modification to avoid toxicity. Contrast-induced nephropathy is a particular concern because diagnostic imaging and other radiological procedures are frequently required. Generally, analysis of the risk–benefit ratio in ICU patients favours the radiological procedure, and prophylactic measures such as adequate volume resuscitation and the administration of acetylcysteine should occur.

Over recent years, intra-abdominal hypertension (IAH) has been increasingly recognized as an important cause of AKI. Measurement of bladder pressure provides an indirect measure of IAP and this can easily be accomplished using a simple manometer. IAH can usually be managed with medical treatments alone, such as, for example, nasogastric and colonic decompression, fluid restriction, or body positioning. Laparostomy may be required for abdominal compartment syndrome when medical treatment has failed (IAP > 20 mm Hg, and new organ failure).

Despite general supportive measures, AKI may fail to improve or may even deteriorate; in these circumstances, RRT may be required. Currently, there is controversy as to the timing and type of RRT that should be used.

Conventional indications for RRT include refractory hyperkalaemia, fluid overload, severe metabolic acidosis, and overt uraemic symptoms such as encephalopathy or pericarditis.

Broadly, there are two types of RRT: continuous RRT (CRRT) and intermittent RRT (IRRT). Currently, there is no data to support the superiority of either of these modalities, and both are commonly used for AKI in the ICU. Doses of RRT that have been associated with increased survival in ICU patients are at least 35 ml/kg $hour^{-1}$ of haemofiltration or haemodiafiltration, and daily IRRT (dialysis).

Further Reading

Hertzberg D, Ryde L, Pickering JW, et al. Acute kidney injury—an overview of diagnostic methods and clinical management. *Clin Kidney J* 2017; 10: 323–31. doi:10.1093/ckj/sfx003

Kidney Disease: Improving Global Outcomes (KDIGO) Acute Kidney Injury Work Group. KDIGO clinical practice guideline for acute kidney injury. *Kidney Inter Suppl* 2012; 2: 1–138.

National Institute for Health and Care Excellence. *Acute Kidney Injury: Prevention, Detection and Management*. 2013. Available at https://www.nice.org.uk/guidance/cg169?unlid=8859070520174952738 (accessed 28 Apr 2017).

152 ICU treatment of sepsis and septic shock

Matt Wise and Paul Frost

Definition of the disease

The Third International Consensus definitions for sepsis and septic shock (Sepsis-3) were published in 2016; sepsis is defined as 'life-threatening organ dysfunction caused by a dysregulated host response to infection' (Singer et al., 2016, p. 801). Organ dysfunction can be assessed using the Sequential Organ Failure Assessment (SOFA) score (see Table 152.1). SOFA utilizes clinical findings, laboratory data, and therapeutic interventions to quantify organ dysfunction in six organ systems (Table 152.1).

Organ dysfunction is indicated by an acute change in the SOFA score of ≥2 points consequent to the infection. (The SOFA score is assumed to be 0 in patients without preexisting organ dysfunction.) Patients with suspected infection who are at risk of poor outcomes can be promptly identified at the bedside by the quick SOFA score (qSOFA). The criteria for qSOFA are a respiratory rate of >22 breaths/min; altered mentation; and a systolic blood pressure of ≥100 mm Hg. Patients with suspected infection and any two of these three variables are at high risk of death or prolonged intensive care stay.

Septic shock, which is a subset of sepsis, is defined by the presence of particularly profound circulatory, cellular, and metabolic abnormalities and is associated with a greater risk of mortality than sepsis alone. Clinically, septic shock patients are sepsis patients who require vasopressors to maintain a mean arterial pressure (MAP) ≥ 65 mm Hg and have a serum lactate level >2 mmol/l despite adequate volume resuscitation.

Aetiology of sepsis

Bacteria are the most frequent causes of sepsis and septic shock, while viruses, fungi, and parasites are implicated less often. Positive cultures are found in only 60% of cases; this may be the result of previous antibiotic therapy or of inadequate sampling or testing. The aetiology of sepsis is constantly changing; whereas Gram-negative organisms used to make up the majority of cases, Gram-positive bacteria now predominate. Sepsis due to fungal disease has also seen a dramatic rise. These changes may be explained by alterations in patient demographics, such as an increasingly elderly population with multiple comorbidities; an increased frequency of indwelling catheters or devices; and greater numbers of patients with immunosuppression as a result of disease or drug therapy.

The causative organisms depend on the patient population in question; for example, patients with a haematological malignancy and who have prolonged neutropenia following chemotherapy have a high prevalence of invasive fungal disease. The organism type will also depend on whether the infection is acquired in the community or the hospital setting, where antimicrobial resistance is more common.

In European ICUs, one-third of all patients either present with or develop sepsis; in two-thirds of these cases, the sepsis is present on admission. The commonest sites of infection are lung (68%), abdomen (22%), blood (20%), and urinary tract (14%). The most common microorganisms are *Staphylococcus aureus* (30%), *Pseudomonas species* (14%), and *Escherichia coli* (13%). Roughly half of the *Staphylococcus aureus* organisms identified were methicillin resistant (i.e. MRSA).

Typical symptoms of the disease, and less common symptoms

Symptoms of sepsis and septic shock are protean and depend on the site of infection as well as patient factors such as age, immune status, and presence of comorbidity. Altered mental status, such as anxiety or confusion, is a consistent feature while constitutional symptoms such as malaise, loss of appetite, fatigue, and fever are common. The site of infection may be localized by symptoms such as dysuria and frequency for the urinary tract; cough and purulent sputum for the lung; and diarrhoea and vomiting for bowel infection. Localized symptoms may diminish and constitutional symptoms predominate at extremes of age or if the patient is immunosuppressed.

Table 152.1 The Sequential Organ Failure Assessment (SOFA) score

System	0	1	2	3	4
Respiration PaO$_2$/FiO$_2$ mm Hg	>400	<400	<300	<200 with respiratory support	<100 with respiratory support
Coagulation Platelet × 10^3/µL	≥150	<150	<100	<50	<20
Liver Bilirubin µmol/L	<20	20–32	33–101	102–204	>204
Cardiovascular (mm Hg)	MAP ≥70	MAP <70	Dopamine <5 or Dobutamine (any dose)*	Dopamine 5.1–15 or adrenaline ≥ 0.1 or noradrenaline ≥ 0.1*	Dopamine > 15 or adrenaline > 0.1 or noradrenaline > 0.1*
Central nervous System Glasgow Coma Score	15	13–14	10–12	6–9	<6
Renal Creatinine µmol/L Urine output ml/day	<110	110–170	171–299	300–440 <500	>440 <200

Abbreviations: FiO$_2$, fraction of inspired oxygen; MAP, mean arterial pressure; PaO$_2$, partial pressure of oxygen.

*Catecholamine doses are given as micrograms per kilogram per min for at least 1 hour.

Reproduced with permission from J.-L. Vincent, The SOFA (Sepsis-related Organ Failure Assessment) score to describe organ dysfunction/failure, *Intensive Care Medicine*, Volume 22, Issue 7, pp. 707–710, Copyright © 1996 Springer.

Demographics of the disease

One large epidemiological study in the United States analysed hospital discharge data from 1979 to 2000; approximately ten million cases of sepsis were identified from 750 million hospitalizations. During the period of the study, the average age of the patient with sepsis increased; being male and non-white were also relative risk factors. Comorbidities such as cancer, immunosuppression, cirrhosis, renal failure, cardiac failure, and chronic lung disease are also important risk factors for the development of sepsis. Although mortality rates fell during this study, the number of deaths trebled because of an 8.7% annual increase in the incidence of sepsis.

Natural history, and complications of the disease

In a general hospital population, the mortality risk for patients with sepsis is >10%, which increases to >40% for those with septic shock. In European ICUs, the incidence of organ failure in patients with severe sepsis, defined using SOFA, is as follows: cardiovascular, 62.6%; renal, 51.2%; respiratory, 49.8%; CNS, 41.3%; coagulation, 20.1%; and hepatic, 12.2%. Dependence on renal replacement therapy at 1 year can be as high as 20% in survivors. Individuals discharged from hospital have a 50% reduction in life expectancy over the subsequent 5 years, compared to non-septic ICU patients.

Approach to diagnosing the disease

The diagnosis of sepsis requires a documented or suspected infection in association with signs of organ dysfunction (see Table 152.1). Septic shock can be diagnosed when sepsis-induced hypotension persists despite adequate fluid resuscitation. The starting point then is to establish the diagnosis of infection by utilizing a careful history, thorough examination, and appropriate investigations. Clinical examination should be comprehensive and rigorous, as infection may occur in any organ system (Table 152.2). Moreover, some clinical findings are pathognomonic, such as, for example, the petechial rash seen in meningococcal disease.

Clinical signs suggestive of septic shock include a flushed appearance, fever, confusion, tachycardia, a bounding pulse, and hypotension. These signs are consistent with an increased cardiac output. However, if treatment is delayed, then cardiac output may decline and the clinical signs then resemble cardiogenic shock, with cool peripheries, mottled skin, and marked hypotension.

Other diagnosis that should be considered

The differential diagnosis includes:

- hypovolaemic shock: haemorrhagic fluid loss (e.g. gastrointestinal, trauma, retroperitoneal), from diarrhoea, burns, pancreatitis, polyuria, diabetic ketoacidosis, vomiting, or pancreatitis

Table 152.2 Possible signs of infection in each organ system

Organ system	Possible signs of infection
Skin, and soft tissue	Cellulitis, abscess erysipelas, desquamation, necrosis
Locomotor system	Local abscess, draining sinus, pain, pseudoparalysis, bone deformity, swollen joints
Respiratory system	Clubbing, red ear drum, cervical lymphadenopathy, tonsillitis, pharyngitis, stridor, increased respiratory rate, pseudomembranes, cyanosis, bronchial breath sounds, purulent sputum
Cardiovascular system	Pericardial rub, murmurs, dysrhythmia, heart failure, splinter haemorrhages, Osler's nodes, Roth's spots
CNS	Neck stiffness, Kernig's sign, depressed consciousness, confusion, localizing neurological signs
Gastrointestinal system	Bloody diarrhoea, vomiting, abdominal pain, jaundice, hepatosplenomegaly
Genitourinary system	Tenderness in renal angle, rigours, urethral discharge

- cardiogenic shock due to myocardial infarct, myocarditis, acute valve leak, acute ventricular septal defect, or arrhythmia
- obstructive shock due to pulmonary embolus, tension pneumothorax, or cardiac tamponade
- distributive shock: neurogenic, or due to anaphylaxis or Addisonian crisis

It should be remembered that overlap exists between shock states. Infection may precipitate or complicate Addisonian crisis, diabetic ketoacidosis, acute aortic or mitral valve regurgitation, cardiogenic shock, and pancreatitis.

'Gold-standard' diagnostic test

The variables used to diagnose sepsis and septic shock are non-specific (see Table 152.1); accordingly no gold-standard diagnostic test exists for sepsis and septic shock. This fact was recognized by the International Sepsis Definitions Conference (Sepsis-3).

Acceptable diagnostic alternatives to the gold standard

As there is no gold-standard diagnostic test for sepsis and septic shock, there are also no acceptable diagnostic alternatives for a gold-standard test.

Other relevant investigations

Investigations in sepsis and septic shock largely focus on looking for potential sites of sepsis and obtaining microbiological samples or excluding other diagnosis. Blood cultures should be taken in all suspected cases; other samples will be determined by the clinical situation and include urine; sputum or bronchoalveolar lavage; cerebrospinal fluid; pleural fluid; pericardial fluid; ascites; faeces; drain sites; joint effusions; surgically debrided tissue; and abscess fluid.

Imaging is important when looking for occult sources of sepsis and, while plain radiographs of the chest, abdomen, or spine may be diagnostic, other modalities are often required. Ultrasonography has the advantage that it can be performed at the bedside and is particularly useful in identifying collections such as empyema, liver abscesses, abdominal collections, subcutaneous abscesses, and obstruction to the kidneys or biliary tract. CT is employed when other investigations fail to identify a source.

Additional investigations may be helpful with alternative diagnoses and include an ECG; echocardiogram; arterial blood gas, including lactate levels; serum amylase; mast cell tryptase; and CT pulmonary angiography.

Prognosis and how to estimate it

A number of scoring systems are used in intensive care, such as the Acute Physiology and Chronic Health Evaluation (APACHE), the Simplified Acute Physiology Score (SAPS), and SOFA, to define patient outcome. These scoring systems are similar in their predictive accuracy and are best at describing outcome in groups of patients rather than in individuals. For mortality rates for sepsis and septic shock, see 'Natural history, and complications of the disease'.

Treatment and its effectiveness

Resuscitation must be initiated as soon as sepsis or septic shock conditions are recognized and should follow the standard Airway, Breathing, Circulation (ABC) approach, so that immediate threats to life, such as airway compromise or severe respiratory failure, are addressed first.

In a seminal single-centre study published in 2001, early goal-directed therapy (EGDT) aimed at improving tissue oxygenation parameters within the first 6 hours of presentation was shown to increase survival. Resuscitation endpoints of EGDT include a central venous pressure (CVP) of 8–12 mm Hg, an MAP of >65 mm Hg, urine output of >0.5 ml/kg hour^{-1}, and a central venous (superior vena cava) or mixed venous oxygen saturation of >70% or >65%, respectively. IV fluid, red cells, vasopressors, and inotropes were used to attain these goals. However, subsequent large multicentre trials from the USA, UK, and Australasia were unable to replicate the survival benefits of EGDT, and this approach is no longer recommended. Current therapy for sepsis and septic shock emphasizes source control; early, empirical, broad-spectrum antibiotics; judicious IV fluids (typically 2–3 l for an adult), and vasopressors to maintain an MAP ≥ 65 mm Hg. Initially, either a colloid or a crystalloid solution may be given, as there is no evidence to support the selection of one over the other. Balanced electrolyte solutions such as Hartmann's (Ringer's lactate) solution are preferred to normal saline, as the latter can contribute to an undesirable metabolic acidosis.

The quantity of fluid required varies according to the intra-vascular deficit and the severity of the ongoing capillary leak. Fluid requirements are best assessed using a fluid-challenge technique whereby 500 ml of crystalloid is administered over 15 minutes, and its effectiveness assessed against improvements in blood pressure, pulse, and cardiac output. Broadly, fluid administration should continue as long as there is haemodynamic improvement and should be curtailed if filling pressures such as the CVP increase with no concurrent increase in cardiac output. Once resuscitation is completed, IV fluid should be given more sparingly, as cumulative positive fluid balance is associated with increased mortality.

The ability of organs such as the kidneys to autoregulate blood flow is lost below a certain MAP; thus, uncorrected hypotension can lead to ischaemia and organ failure. Vasopressors may be needed to maintain the MAP at around 65 mm Hg. A higher MAP may be required in cases of preexisting hypertension, and a lower MAP may suffice in younger patients without comorbidity. Noradrenaline has predominantly alpha-adrenergic effects and is effective at reversing sepsis-induced vasodilatation. Dopamine has both beta- and alpha-adrenergic effects and increases cardiac output as well as MAP. Before starting either of these agents, it is important that the patient be adequately volume resuscitated.

Catecholamines may have undesirable effects, such as tachyarrhythmias and reduced oxygen delivery. In this context, vasopressin, which can restore vascular tone and blood pressure, has been used as a catecholamine-sparing drug. However, as yet no survival benefits have been demonstrated by this approach.

If, despite restoration of a suitable perfusion pressure and adequate volume resuscitation, there remains evidence of tissue ischaemia, for example, a central venous oxygen saturation ($ScvO_2$) of <70%, then a dobutamine infusion should be introduced. Dobutamine has predominantly beta-adrenergic effects and increases cardiac output.

Source control, such as surgical debridement, abscess drainage, or removal of infected intra-vascular devices, is mandatory and should not be delayed. Early appropriate antimicrobial therapy is crucially important to survival. The risk of death increases by 7.6% for every hour hypotensive septic patients are without antibiotics. Initial, empiric antibiotic therapy should be broad spectrum, as the causative organism is frequently unknown. After 48–72 hours, antibiotic therapy can be de-escalated and refined according to microbiological results and the patient's response.

IV hydrocortisone (<300 mg/day) may improve blood pressure in patients who remain hypotensive despite fluid and vasopressors. However, this therapy does not translate into a survival benefit, even in those patients who had a reduced response to corticotrophin.

Aside from specific treatment measures, outcomes from sepsis and septic shock are equally dependent on the provision of good general intensive care. Patients should be ventilated using a lung-protective strategy aimed at limiting ventilator-induced lung injury, and sedation should be interrupted daily to minimize the duration of ventilation. Enteral nutrition should be established, and blood glucose levels should be controlled in the range 3.8–8.3 mmol/l. Renal replacement therapy may be required to facilitate the management of fluid balance and metabolic derangements. Thromboprophylaxis

with unfractionated or low-molecular-weight heparin should be instigated unless there are contraindications such as bleeding. Stress-ulcer prophylaxis should be provided, using either an H2 blocker or a proton-pump inhibitor.

Despite improvements in the provision of evidence-based care, the mortality rates of sepsis and septic shock remain unacceptably high. A consortium of international intensive care societies spearheaded by the European Society for Intensive Care Medicine has launched the Surviving Sepsis Campaign in an attempt to reduce mortality from these conditions. A central element in this campaign is the promotion of care bundles, which are defined as groups of disease-process-related interventions that, when implemented together, result in better outcomes than when implemented individually (see Box 152.1).

Box 152.1 Surviving sepsis campaign bundles

To be completed within 3 hours
1. Measure lactate level
2. Obtain blood cultures prior to administration of antibiotics
3. Administer broad spectrum antibiotics
4. Administer 30 ml/kg crystalloid for hypotension or lactate > 4 mmol/L

To be completed within 6 hours
5. Apply vasopressors (for hypotension that does not respond to initial fluid resuscitation) to maintain a mean arterial pressure (MAP) ≥ 65 mm Hg
6. In the event of persistent hypotension after initial fluid administration (MAP > 65 mm Hg) or if initial lactate was ≥4 mmol/L, re-assess volume status and tissue perfusion and document findings according to 'Reassessment of volume status and perfusion'.
7. Re-measure lactate if initial lactate elevated.

Reassessment of volume status and perfusion
Document reassessment of volume status and tissue perfusion with:

Either:

Repeat focused exam (after initial fluid resuscitation) including vital signs, cardiopulmonary, capillary refill, pulse and skin findings.

Or two of the following:

* Measure CVP
* Measure $ScvO_2$
* Bedside cardiovascular ultrasound
* Dynamic assessment of fluid responsiveness with passive leg raise or fluid challenge.

Abbreviations: CVP, central venous pressure; $ScvO_2$, central venous oxygen saturation. Reproduced with permission Dellinger RP, Levy MM, Rhodes A, et al. Surviving Sepsis Campaign:
International Guidelines for Management of Severe Sepsis and Septic Shock: 2012. Crit Care Med. 2013; 41(2):580–637. Copyright © 2013 the Society of Critical Care Medicine and Lippincott Williams & Wilkins.

Further Reading

Angus DC and van der Poll T. Severe sepsis and septic shock. *N Engl J Med* 2013; 369: 840–51.

Singer M, Deutschman CS, Seymour CW, et al. The Third International Consensus definitions for sepsis and septic shock (Sepsis-3). *JAMA* 2016; 315: 801–10.

Society of Critical Care Medicine: *Surviving Sepsis Campaign* (http://www.survivingsepsis.org/Bundles/Pages/default.aspx)

Vincent J-L, Mira J-P, and Antonelli M. Sepsis: older and newer concepts. *Lancet Respir Med* 2016; 4: 237–40.

153 Terminal care in the intensive care unit

Matt Wise and Paul Frost

Introduction

In the UK, around 10%–20% of all patients admitted to the intensive care unit (ICU) do not survive, while in the United States, it has been estimated that 22% of all deaths occur in an ICU. Therefore, terminal or palliative care is as important as any of the life-saving interventions that occur in the ICU. The goal of palliative care is to achieve a good death, described by the US Institute of Medicine as one that is 'free from avoidable distress and suffering for patients, families, and caregivers; in general accord with patients' and families' wishes; and reasonably consistent with clinical, cultural, and ethical standards' (Field et al., 1997, p. 95).

Initiation of palliative care

In the ICU, the switch from care with curative intent to palliation occurs when it becomes obvious that the patient is not responding to treatment. Typically, this is manifest by deteriorating physiology and escalating organ support in the setting of overwhelming disease or injury. Although prognostic models such as the Acute Physiology And Chronic Health Evaluation (APACHE) and the Riyadh Intensive Care Programme (RIP) are available, these can never be 100% accurate and are most appropriately used to assess population risk rather than individual risk. Therefore, it is predominantly expert opinion (consensus amongst treating medical and nursing teams) that determines the point at which the patient is recognized as not responding to treatment and, in fact, dying.

Ethical considerations

The decision to start palliative care is framed by the ethical principles of autonomy (the right of patients to make their own decisions), beneficence (treatment should benefit the patient), non-maleficence (treatment should do no harm), and social justice (treatment resources should be used equitably). Although patient autonomy is of paramount importance, understanding the patient's wishes in the ICU is difficult because only around 5% of critically ill patients retain decision-making capacity. In the UK, ultimate responsibility for the decision to discontinue intensive therapies resides with the medical team. However, these doctors will always strive to act in accordance with the patient's wishes. When the patient cannot express their own wishes, then decision-making occurs with surrogates such as the family. In these circumstances, decisions can be made by the 'substituted-judgement standard', if the patient's relatives' wishes are known or by the 'best-interests standard' if their relatives wishes are unknown. Advance directives (living wills), which are legally binding, can inform this discussion but, as these documents rarely cover every eventuality, their usefulness is limited. In the UK, if there is no family, then the Mental Capacity Act allows for the provision of court-appointed deputies who may make proxy decisions about medical treatment in the patients' best interests.

Where the patient retains capacity, then prognostic information should be carefully communicated so that he or she can make informed choices about treatment. Occasionally, contrary to medical advice, patients may refuse continued life-sustaining treatment; in these circumstances, their autonomy must be respected.

Communication

Good communication is essential for effective palliative care and can reduce subsequent psychological morbidity amongst family members. Generally, more time should be spent listening and addressing the families concerns during meetings than talking. End-of-life discussions should occur in private, designated interview rooms and be conducted by a senior clinician accompanied by a senior nurse. No external interruptions should be allowed during the meeting, and pagers and mobile telephones should be switched off. Discussion should be sensitive and appropriate to cultural and religious needs, and interpreters may be required. Language should be clear and unequivocal; care should be taken to avoid medical jargon and euphemisms. The family should be told that the patient is dying and that, in the opinion of the medical team, the emphasis of care should shift to palliation rather than persevering with organ support. The transition from full treatment to a palliative approach should not be hurried; the family often need time to digest the prognosis as well as arrange for other family members to be in attendance. It is always reasonable to enquire whether spiritual or religious support is wanted and to offer to arrange this if necessary.

Family disagreement

Occasionally, the family may disagree with the suggested approach and ask that intensive therapies continue. Even though doctors are not legally obliged to continue treatments which they believe to be ineffectual, it is always appropriate to seek consensus with the family before proceeding to a palliative approach. Therefore, every effort should be made to understand and address the family's concerns. An offer of a second opinion or recourse to a hospital ethics committee may be useful. Usually, with the passage of time, agreement with the family can be reached; as a last resort, a court order may be sought.

Organ donation

The issue of organ donation should not be raised, unless by the family, at the initial end-of-life interview. However, in subsequent family meetings, it is appropriate to seek their views on this. It needs to be established whether the family believe that the patient would wish to be an organ donor. The patient may, in fact, be on the donor register. If the family wish that this option be explored, then the transplant coordinator should be contacted to liaise with the family.

Palliative care practicalities

Environment

Once a palliative approach is embarked upon, it is usually unreasonable to move the patient out of the ICU. Such a move is potentially distressing for the patient and the family, who would then have to acquaint themselves with a new environment and staff (although, in some countries, such as New Zealand, patients have been taken to their home to die, for family and cultural reasons). However, the patient may be moved within the ICU in order to optimize privacy and minimize noise.

Symptom control

Symptom control is a defining feature of palliation, and all care should be directed towards ensuring that the patient remains comfortable. Common distressing symptoms include pain, dyspnoea, and delirium.

Over 50% of seriously ill hospital patients report some level of pain and it is important to be vigilant for evidence of this. Usually, the existence and intensity of pain is self-reported but, in the majority of ICU patients, due to varying degrees of unconsciousness, this is not possible. In the unconscious ICU patient, features suggestive of pain include autonomic responses, such as tears or diaphoresis; facial grimacing, or wincing; and increased muscle tone, particularly on movement.

Care should be taken to avoid iatrogenic causes of pain, such as positioning and turning the patient, tracheal suctioning, and wound, drain, and catheter care. Morphine is the drug of choice for the treatment of pain. In addition to its analgesic effects, it also has additive sedative and potentially beneficial euphoric effects. Undesirable side effects such as pruritus, nausea, and vomiting can be treated with antihistamines and anti-emetics.

Dyspnoea (self-awareness of uncomfortable breathing) in a ventilated patient may be manifest as tachycardia, tachypnoea, accessory muscle activity, nasal flaring, sweating, and agitation. Most commonly, this distressing symptom is dealt with by administering benzodiazepines and morphine. Although these drugs may hasten death, it is ethically acceptable to administer them when the intention is to alleviate distress rather than cause death (the doctrine of 'double effect').

Delirium may be defined as an acute alteration in consciousness with a fluctuating cause, associated with impaired attention, impaired cognition, and increased or decreased psychomotor activity. In a dying ICU patient, the causes of delirium include the underlying illness; sleep deprivation; drug or alcohol withdrawal; medication; pain; and dyspnoea. Delirium can be managed by treating the underlying cause(s), providing a quiet environment, calming nurses and relatives, and using specific drug therapies such as benzodiazepines or neuroleptic drugs (e.g. haloperidol).

Withdrawal of intensive therapies

Symptom control is a prerequisite for withdrawal of intensive therapies; once this is achieved, then organ support can be discontinued. It is important to appreciate that, in these circumstances, there is no legal or philosophical distinction between withholding and withdrawal of treatment. Therefore, inotropes are switched off, renal replacement therapy is stopped, and ventilation and inspired oxygen are reduced. Any exacerbation of distressing symptoms is immediately addressed by titration of sedation and morphine. Monitors are generally switched off, as families can be distracted and distressed by the display of terminal physiological variables. Routine interventions such as blood tests, drug administration, IV fluid, and nasogastric feed are discontinued. If the patient is extubated, then the family are warned that this may be associated with retention of respiratory secretions and noisy breathing. This can be distressing for the family but can usually be addressed by simple airway-opening manoeuvres, positioning, and suction. Where possible, the family should be warned about the likely duration of the dying process, although this can be difficult to predict.

The conscious patient

In the vast majority of cases, the terminally ill ICU patient is deeply unconscious as a consequence of their illness and sedative and analgesic drugs prescribed for their comfort. Rarely, the patient may be wakeful and wish to remain conscious, when therapies such as ventilation are withdrawn, so that they can communicate with their family. This can be accommodated by careful titration of sedation and analgesic drugs to ensure comfort in the very final stages of the illness.

Diagnosing death

Death may be diagnosed after 5 minutes of observed asystole. The absence of the pupillary responses to light, of the corneal reflexes, and of any motor response to supraorbital pressure should be confirmed. The time of death is recorded as the time at which these criteria are fulfilled. Alternatively, where the patient is mechanically ventilated, death may be diagnosed following irreversible cessation of brainstem function. If it accords with the patient's wishes, at this point, organ donation might occur.

Care after death

Following the death, an appointment should be made for the family with the hospital bereavement service. Bereavement advisers not only provide all of the necessary documentation to register the death but can also provide practical information on all aspects of bereavement, including liaison with grief counselling services. Other administrative tasks that should be completed at this time include informing the patient's GP of the death, entering the death into the hospital database and other relevant databases, and following the hospital policy for the property of the deceased.

Many ICUs now offer bereavement follow-up services so that lingering concerns that the family may have about the death can be addressed. Finally, it is important to remember that dealing with death can have a traumatic impact on ICU staff, and appropriate counselling should be readily available.

Further Reading

Aslakson RA, Curtis JR, and Nelson JE. Concise definitive review: the changing role of palliative care in the ICU. *Crit Care Med* 2014; 42: 2418–28.

Cook D and Rocker G. Dying with dignity in the intensive care unit. *N Engl J Med* 2014; 370: 2506–14.

National Institute for Health and Care Excellence. Care of dying adults in the last days of life NICE guideline [NG31] 2015. https://www.nice.org.uk/guidance/ng31?unlid=976936892016102725548

154 Brain death

Matt Wise and Paul Frost

Definitions

Mechanical ventilation has made it possible for the heart to continue to beat and perfuse other organs even when the brain is dead. This means that death can be diagnosed in two distinct ways: first, in the traditional manner, as permanent cessation of cardiorespiratory function; and, second, while the patient is ventilated, as brain death (BD).

In 1976 the Conference of Medical Royal Colleges and their Faculties in the United Kingdom, in a statement on the diagnosis of BD, recognized the brainstem as the centre of brain activity, without which life was not possible. Brainstem death (BSD) occurs when there is complete, irreversible loss of brainstem function, that is, irreversible loss of the capacity for consciousness, coupled with irreversible loss of the capacity to breathe. In the UK, the terms BD and BSD are used interchangeably and are legally synonymous with somatic death.

Aetiology of the disease

In adults, severe head injury accounts for 50% of cases of BSD; 30% occur following subarachnoid or intra-cerebral haemorrhage, and 20% occur as a result of cerebral anoxia, for example, following cardiorespiratory arrest, hanging, or strangulation.

Natural history, and complications of the disease

Cerebral injury following trauma, haemorrhage, or infection causes the brain to swell (cerebral oedema). Usually, deleterious rises in intracranial pressure are prevented by compensatory reductions in CSF and intracranial blood volumes. However, following severe injury, these mechanisms are exhausted, and intracranial pressure rises, often exponentially. This causes a deteriorating cycle of further cerebral ischaemia, neuronal injury, and oedema. In these circumstances, brain tissue is displaced downwards towards the foramen magnum. Ultimately, the cerebellar tonsils may be forced through the foramen magnum (tonsillar coning), compressing the brainstem and causing BSD.

Crucial functions of the brainstem include control of consciousness via the reticular activating system, and control of cardiorespiratory homeostasis. Additionally, all sensory and motor tracts pass through the brainstem and cranial nerves 3–12 emerge from it. Therefore, clinical signs of coning include coma; apnoea; cardiovascular instability and absence of receptivity; movement; and brainstem reflexes.

Following BSD, characteristic pathophysiological changes arise. These include hypotension; cardiac arrhythmias; pulmonary oedema; diabetes insipidus (DI) and other endocrine disturbances; disseminated intra-vascular coagulopathy (DIC); and hypothermia.

Cardiovascular instability occurs in around 80% of brain dead patients; its causes are multifactorial and include loss of sympathetic tone; vasodilatation; and myocardial depression.

The mechanism of myocardial depression is uncertain but is characterized by evidence of myocardial ischaemia and even infarction.

Pulmonary oedema may arise as a result of myocardial dysfunction secondary to massive sympathetic over activity, occasionally seen at the onset of BSD (neurogenic pulmonary oedema).

Following BSD, production of antidiuretic hormone is low to non-existent; consequently, DI occurs in up to 65% of affected patients. DI is characterized by a high urinary output, hypernatraemia (serum sodium >150 mmol/l), plasma hyperosmolality (typically >310 mOsm/kg), and urinary hyposmolality (typically <300 mOsm/kg). Pituitary failure also leads to reductions in circulating thyroid hormones, and these reductions may contribute to myocardial dysfunction.

DIC is common and may be related to the release of tissue thromboplastin from dead brain tissue.

Finally, hypothermia arises as a result of hypothalamic failure; increased heat loss related to vasodilatation; and decreased heat production associated with a reduced metabolic rate.

BSD is always followed by asystolic cardiac arrest; typically, this happens after a few days. Rarely, in countries where the concept of BSD is not recognized and intensive care is continued, cardiac arrest has taken weeks to occur. There has never been a verified report of recovery of brainstem function in these circumstances.

Approach to diagnosing the disease

Before clinical examination for BSD can proceed, the following preconditions must be met. The aetiology of the coma must be established and be irreversible, all reversible causes of coma must be excluded, and the patient must be apnoeic on mechanical ventilation.

Often, the aetiology of the brain damage is immediately self-evident and irreversibility is easy to establish, for example, following a massive intra-cerebral bleed or severe head injury. However, for other conditions, such as cerebral hypoxic ischaemic injury following cardiac arrest, a longer period of observation may be required to increase diagnostic and prognostic certainty.

A number of conditions can confound the clinical examination for BSD and have first to be ruled out. These include hypothermia, drugs, and circulatory, metabolic, and endocrine disturbances.

At the time of BSD, death testing the core temperature must be >34°C as, occasionally, impaired consciousness has been associated with core temperatures of 32°C–34°C.

Anaesthetic drugs such as barbiturates, benzodiazepines, and opiates are routinely used in the management of severely head-injured patients. These drugs and their active metabolites can have persistent effects, particularly if their elimination is reduced because of hepatic or renal failure. Therefore, sufficient time needs to be given to allow clearance of these agents so that they do not confound the clinical examination for signs of BSD. Occasionally, it is helpful to measure drug concentrations, for example, of thiopental, or administer antagonists, for example, to opiates and benzodiazepines, so that confounding influences of these agents can be excluded.

BSD testing should not proceed if thiopental levels are >5 mg/l or if midazolam levels are >10 μg/l.

Neuromuscular blocking agents can mimic coma and respiratory failure and it is important to exclude their presence. This can be done by demonstrating the presence of deep tendon reflexes or by using a nerve stimulator.

Metabolic disturbances and circulatory instability that arise as a direct consequence of brainstem injury should be distinguished from similar, primary disturbances that may cause coma. Hypernatraemia may occur as a consequence of DI complicating BSD or be due to gross dehydration, unrelated to BSD. It is important to emphasize that the establishment of an unequivocal, irreversible cause of the coma outweighs any contribution that minor deviations from normal homeostasis might theoretically make to the comatose state.

Nonetheless, as far as it is possible, metabolic, endocrine, and circulatory contributions to the internal milieu must be normalized prior to BSD testing. So, profoundly abnormal electrolyte levels, for example, sodium <115 mmol/l or >160 mmol/l, potassium <2 mmol/l, and hypoglycaemia (<3 mmol/l) and hyperglycaemia (>20 mmol/l) should be corrected. Additionally, the mean arterial pressure should be >60 mm Hg, and blood gases should be normal.

Rarely, myxoedema, thyroid storm, and Addisonian crisis can present with coma, and appropriate hormone assays should be requested if there is any suspicion that these conditions are present.

Several neurological disorders, for example, acute inflammatory polyneuritis, cause profound neuromuscular weakness resembling loss of brainstem reflexes. Although it would be extremely unlikely for such conditions to coexist with the primary, known cause of irreversible brain damage, nonetheless, these conditions should be considered and excluded. Finally, in the context of traumatic coma, it is essential to exclude a high cervical spinal injury, as this could cause quadriparesis and invalidate the apnoea test.

Once the preconditions have been fulfilled, BSD can be confirmed by clinical examination. In the UK, this examination is undertaken by two doctors, experienced in the procedure, who have been registered for at least 5 years, one being a consultant. These clinicians must confirm the absence of all brainstem reflexes as follows:

- pupils are fixed in diameter and do not respond to light
- no response (i.e. eyelid movement) to direct stimulation of the corneas (corneal reflex)
- no eye movements following direct stimulation of the tympanic membranes with iced water (vestibulo-ocular reflex)
- there should be no motor response in the cranial or somatic distribution to supraorbital pressure
- no contraction of the soft palate when the uvula is stimulated (gag reflex)
- no response to tracheal suctioning as far as the carina (cough reflex)
- no respiratory response to an apnoea test; this means that no breathing movements should be seen following disconnection of the patient from the ventilator; when the partial pressure of carbon dioxide ($PaCO_2$) is above the threshold for maximal stimulation of the respiratory centres in the medulla oblongata (i.e. $PaCO_2 > 6.65$ kPa); during this time, hypoxaemia is prevented by the provision of oxygen at 5 l/min via a catheter placed down the endotracheal tube

In order to reassure the family and remove the risk of observer error, the BSD tests are carried out twice. In the UK, there is no prescribed interval between tests.

Other diagnoses that should be considered

The 'locked-in' syndrome usually arises as a result of destruction of the base of the pons, for example, following haemorrhage, infarction, or trauma. Characteristically, these patients are cognitively intact, retain vertical eye movements, but are otherwise totally paralysed.

Guillain–Barré syndrome involving all of the peripheral and cranial nerves could mimic BSD.

It is vitally important to appreciate that adherence to the preconditions prior to clinical examination will always protect against the misdiagnosis of BSD.

'Gold-standard' diagnostic test

Clinical neurological examination remains the gold-standard method for diagnosing BD.

Other relevant investigations

Various neurophysiological and imaging tests are available that can be helpful in the diagnosis of BSD. EEG shows electrocerebral silence, and somatosensory evoked potentials show loss of all cortically generated components. Imaging, such as magnetic resonance angiography, four-vessel angiography, and CT angiography will all demonstrate absence of intracranial blood flow. All of these tests require further validation studies before they can be recommended as a routine part of the diagnosis of BSD. Until that time, the diagnosis remains a clinical one.

Treatment and its effectiveness

Following the diagnosis of BSD, the grim news is imparted to the family. During this time, it is always reasonable to consider whether the patient is eligible to be an organ donor. In addition to the benefits for organ recipients, grieving families often report some comfort resulting from this act of altruism. If organ donation is not an option, then the patient should be disconnected from the ventilator.

Further Reading

Lewis A and Greer D. Current controversies in brain death determination. *Nature Reviews Neurology* 2017; 13: 505–9.

Magnus DC, Wilfond BS, and Caplan AL. Accepting brain death. *N Engl J Med* 2014; 370: 891–4.

Simpson P, Bates D, Bonner S, et al. *A Code of Practice for the Diagnosis and Confirmation of Death*, 2008. Academy of Medical Royal Colleges. Available at: http://aomrc.org.uk/wp-content/uploads/2016/04/Code_Practice_Confirmation_Diagnosis_Death_1008-4.pdf

PART 6

Disorders of the kidney and urinary tract, and electrolyte and metabolic disorders

155 Normal renal function

Aron Chakera, William G. Herrington, and Christopher A. O'Callaghan

Introduction

The kidney is a vital organ with multiple functions. Without kidney function, death will occur in a matter of days. Fortunately, several forms of effective renal replacement therapy are available.

Urinary tract structure

There are normally two kidneys that are 9–11 cm in length, and each weigh about 150 g. They lie in the retroperitoneum below the levels of the liver and spleen, respectively (see Figure 155.1) The blood supply to the kidneys comes from the renal arteries, which are branches of the aorta. The kidneys receive 20% of cardiac output (approximately 1100 ml/min), and blood is first delivered to the glomeruli in the outer part of the kidney. Inflow to the glomerulus is via the afferent arteriole, with outflow through the efferent arteriole, which then supplies blood to the tubules. Blood then returns to the renal veins, which drain into the inferior vena cava. The glomerulus, tubules, and collecting ducts make up the functional unit of the kidney: the nephron (see Figure 155.2). Each kidney contains approximately 1 million nephrons. Urine is formed by a process of filtration,

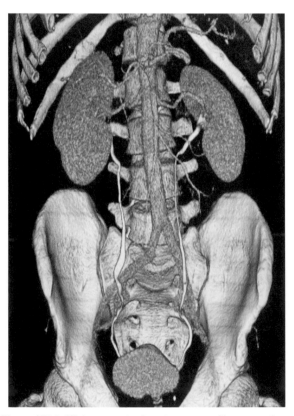

Figure 155.1 CT demonstrating the urinary system. Please see colour plate section.
image courtesy of Nigel Cowan.

as blood passes through the glomerulus. The filtrate (urine) is modified along the course of the tubules, where substances may be reabsorbed or secreted. Urine present at the end of the nephron drains into the renal pelvis and from there passes down the ureters to the bladder, leaving through the urethra.

Kidney function

The kidneys have several important functions:

- they are organs of **excretion**: they remove metabolic products such as urea, organic acids, and unwanted electrolytes
- they are critical to **homeostasis**: they regulate body water content, as well as blood electrolyte and acid–base balance
- they have **endocrine** functions: they sense hypoxia and produce **erythropoietin** in response, promoting red blood cell formation; they are also responsible for **vitamin D** activation by hydroxylation and thus have a central role in calcium, phosphate, and bone metabolism; lastly, they secrete **renin** in response to decreased blood flow, thus activating the renin–angiotensin system, which regulates the salt and water balance; the kidneys are thus central to blood pressure control

The kidneys do not act in isolation. A careful balance of hormones released from other organs act on the kidneys to maintain the body's fluid and electrolyte balance. These include aldosterone, vasopressin, parathyroid hormone, and atrial natriuretic peptide.

Glomerulus function

Each glomerulus is composed of a network of capillaries, supplied by muscular arterioles. The amount of vasoconstriction in the afferent and efferent arterioles determines the pressure within the glomerulus. This intra-glomerular pressure drives filtration of water and solutes through the glomerular filtration barrier, which is composed of three layers: the fenestrated capillary endothelial cells, the basement membrane, and a layer of epithelial cells with foot processes (podocytes) (see Figure 155.3). The epithelium makes up the Bowman's capsule and continues as the tubules. The three layers of the filtration barrier act to limit the passage of large proteins, but allow water and solutes to pass freely. Blood leaves the glomerular capillaries through the efferent arteriole. By modifying tone in the afferent and efferent arterioles, intra-glomerular pressure and, therefore, glomerular filtration rate and the production of urine are regulated. Angiotensin II acts predominantly on the efferent arterioles to cause vasoconstriction, which increases intra-glomerular pressure and filtrate formation.

Tubular function

The tubular system can be divided into four main parts on the basis of function: the proximal tubes, the loop of Henle, the distal tubules, and the collecting ducts.

Proximal tubules

The proximal tubules perform the bulk of the reabsorption. Significant amounts of water and solutes are returned to the blood from the filtrate. This is the main site of glucose and amino acid reabsorption. These cells are highly metabolically active and are thus susceptible to hypoxic damage (acute tubular necrosis).

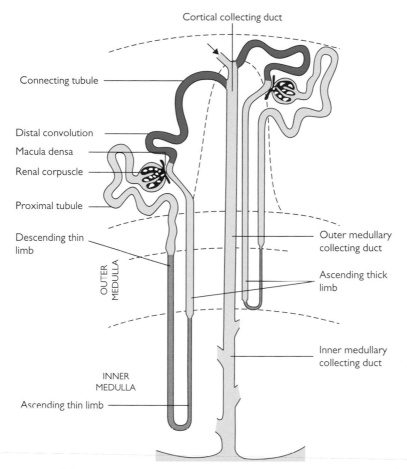

Figure 155.2 The basic organization of short-looped (cortical) and long-looped (juxtamedullary) nephrons; note that the early distal tubule of each type of nephron is in contact with the afferent arterioles of its own glomerulus.

Reproduced with permission from Pocock G et al., *Human Physiology*, Third Edition, Oxford University Press, Oxford, UK, Copyright © 2006.

Loop of Henle

The loop of Henle plays a critical role in concentrating urine through the countercurrent system, which depends on the differing permeability of parts of the loop to water and electrolytes.

Distal tubules

The distal tubules fine tune the urinary acid and electrolyte composition, influenced by the actions of aldosterone.

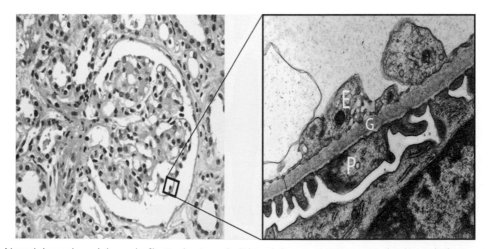

Figure 155.3 Normal glomerulus and glomerular filtration barrier under light and electron microscopy; note the glomerular basement membrane (G), with endothelial cells (E) at its upper edge, and the foot processes of the podocytes (P) abutting its lower edge. Please see colour plate section.

image courtesy of Ian Roberts

Collecting ducts

Collecting ducts modify urinary water content (and therefore osmolality) in response to vasopressin.

Assessment of kidney function

The main assessment of kidney function is by measurement of the serum creatinine. This can be used to provide an estimate of the glomerular filtration rate. This is discussed in detail in Chapter 157.

Natural history of kidney function

Kidney function may deteriorate with age. On average, there is a fall of 1 ml/min year^{-1}. However, this is extremely variable. A mild degree of renal impairment in the elderly is, thus, very common and may not require investigation. However, associated cardiovascular risk factors should still be addressed.

Further Reading

Elger M and Kriz, W. 'The renal glomerulus: The structural basis of ultrafiltration', in Davison A, Cameron JS, Grünfeld JP, et al., eds, *Oxford Textbook of Nephrology* (3rd edition). Oxford University Press.

156 Diagnosis in suspected renal disease

William G. Herrington, Aron Chakera, and Christopher A. O'Callaghan

Introduction

Renal dysfunction can be easily and, in most cases, unambiguously diagnosed from an elevation in serum creatinine and/or abnormal urinalysis. The clinical challenges lie in first suspecting that renal dysfunction is present and therefore requesting the appropriate test (e.g. serum creatinine/urine analysis), and then identifying the underlying aetiology. A major clue to renal dysfunction in the hospitalized patient can be a reduction in urine output. Therefore, urine output should be carefully monitored in those patients who are at risk, which includes most significantly ill hospitalized patients.

Aetiology

The likely causes of renal dysfunction arising de novo in the hospital and community settings are quite distinct. Renal dysfunction arising in hospital is often predictable and caused by a combination of underlying comorbidities, the current illness, and treatment or interventions, such as drugs. For example, septic or post-operative patients are at high risk of hypotensive acute renal failure. In contrast, renal dysfunction arising in the community has a much wider differential diagnosis, which ranges from common causes such as diabetes and hypertension, to rarer primary renal diseases such as glomerulonephritis.

Traditionally, renal dysfunction is arbitrarily divided into acute kidney injury (AKI) and chronic kidney disease (CKD). The key difference is that, in AKI, there is a rapid and potentially reversible fall in kidney function, characterized by a reduction in glomerular filtration rate (GFR). CKD is characterized by long-standing (>3 months) loss of kidney function, which is often, but not always, progressive and is often irreversible due to the presence of fibrotic change within the kidneys.

AKI in hospital is usually divided into:

- prerenal causes, which account for about 60% of hospital-acquired AKI; often, there are multiple contributory factors which may act synergistically, for example, sepsis; with some hypotension during surgery; volume depletion; older age; and diabetes
- intrinsic renal causes, which account for about 20% of hospital AKI and can be further divided into interstitial nephritis, vasomotor nephropathy, toxic tubular injury, and glomerulonephritis
- post-renal causes, which account for about 10% of hospital AKI

In the community setting, obstruction is surprisingly a more common cause of AKI, largely due to prostatic disease (see Figure 156.1).

Box 156.1 Pulmonary renal syndromes

Without alveolar haemorrhage
- acute or chronic kidney disease with pulmonary oedema, due to fluid overload
- pneumonia with renal failure (e.g. legionella)
- heart failure with pulmonary oedema and secondary renal impairment
- poisoning (e.g. with organic solvents or paraquat)

With alveolar haemorrhage
- anti-glomerular basement membrane disease (Goodpasture's disease)
- systemic vasculitis
  - microscopic polyangiitis
  - Wegener's granulomatosis (granulomatosis with polyangiitis)
  - Churg–Strauss syndrome

There are many different causes for CKD, as outlined in Chapter 163.

Often kidney failure occurs in conjunction with failure of other organs. Various autoimmune conditions cause a pulmonary–renal syndrome (see Box 156.1)

Symptoms

Renal impairment *per se* is typically asymptomatic until very near to end-stage renal disease. Presenting symptoms may relate to an underling predisposing condition (see Table 156.1). For example, shortness of breath in cardiac disease, and rashes in autoimmune diseases, such as SLE. Rarely, renal disease presents directly, as, for example, peripheral oedema in nephrotic syndrome, frank haematuria and loin masses in renal malignancy, or uraemic symptoms in end-stage renal disease, such as fatigue, itching, poor appetite, malaise, and nausea.

Importantly, in the hospitalized patient, it is often difficult to tell the non-specific symptoms of kidney failure apart from the underlying illness. Often, kidney failure in this setting is picked up early with frequent blood tests, and managed effectively before the symptoms of advanced AKI can be manifest. However, this is not always the case, and such symptoms may be manifest (see Box 156.2).

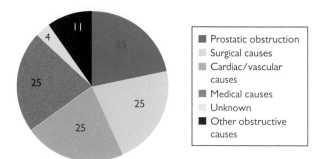

Figure 156.1 Causes of acute kidney injury in a community-based survey.

Reproduced with permission from Barratt, Harris & Topham, *Oxford Desk Reference Nephrology*, Oxford University Press, Oxford, UK, Copyright © 2008.

Pie chart legend:
- Prostatic obstruction
- Surgical causes
- Cardiac/vascular causes
- Medical causes
- Unknown
- Other obstructive causes

Table 156.1 Presentations of renal diseases

Prerenal	Renal	Post-renal
Diarrhoea/ vomiting	Haematuria (GN)	Anuria
Sepsis	Rash (SLE/vasculitis/interstitial nephritis)	Obstructive lower urinary symptoms
Hypotension	Arthralgia (SLE/vasculitis)	Dysuria
Haemorrhage	Myalgia (rhabdomyolysis/GN)	Renal colic
Severe heart failure	Neuropathies (amyloid/ cryoglobulinaemia)	Frank haematuria
Liver failure	ENT symptoms (Wegener's)	Renal mass
	Eye symptoms (vasculitis/SLE/ TINU/others)	Palpable bladder
	Oedema (GN/NS)	
	Frothy urine (NS)	

Abbreviations: ENT, ear, nose, and throat; GN, glomerulonephritis; NS, nephrotic syndrome; SLE, systemic lupus erythematosus; TINU, tubulointerstitial disease with uveitis.

> **Box 156.2 Features of uraemia and an estimated glomerular filtration rate <15 ml/min per 1.73 m² body surface area**
>
> - Anorexia and malnutrition
> - Nausea and vomiting
> - Tiredness
> - Fluid overload with oedema, breathlessness, and orthopnoea
> - Anaemia
> - Pruritus
> - Mental apathy and depression
> - Muscle twitching, restless legs, and cramps
> - Bleeding tendency; haematemesis, epistaxis
> - Sexual dysfunction, loss of libido, and impotence
> - Cardiac-pericarditis
>
> Reproduced with permission from the Oxford Textbook of Medicine (5th edition), Warrell, Cox and Firth (Eds), Published by Oxford University Press 2012)

Demographics

CKD guidelines have been designed to highlight patients at risk of developing renal dysfunction. Renal disease may affect any age group. However certain primary renal diseases do have sex, age, and racial predilections. Myeloma, amyloidosis, and vasculitis are more common in older patients. Lupus is more common in younger women, and patients of black African ethnicity. Minimal change disease is more common in younger patients. Membranous nephropathy is more common in older patients. Renal impairment from obstructive uropathy, secondary to prostatic disease, should always be considered in older men.

In the community setting, the older the patient, the greater the chance of CKD. In the hospital setting, this holds true and, in addition, the more unwell the patient is, the higher the probability is that AKI will be superimposed. It is sensible to consider all hospitalized patients as being at risk of renal dysfunction and to check renal function regularly in patients whose specific illnesses or treatments might increase this risk (e.g. drugs, fluid loss, and sepsis).

Natural history, and complications

Most intrinsic renal diseases are progressive without appropriate treatment. However, some conditions, such as membranous nephropathy, can relapse and remit over time.

Prompt and appropriate management of AKI minimizes both the absolute loss of renal function, and the time period over which this loss occurs. Such intervention lessens the need for renal replacement therapy (dialysis) in the short term, and improves prognosis. Many (but not all) patients with AKI return to their baseline kidney function following treatment.

Renal failure due to obstruction is one of the more benign forms of kidney injury and, once treated successfully, many patients return to a good level of kidney function. Even if renal function does not improve after the relief of obstruction, there is much less chance of progression to end-stage renal failure than there is with intrinsic renal diseases.

Approach to diagnosing the disease

Patients with suspected renal disease should be assessed in the usual manner, with a full history, examination, and appropriate renal investigations. Specific issues to address with suspected renal disease include the following:

- predisposing factors: age is probably the most important predisposing factor, followed by past medical/surgical history (e.g. hypertension, diabetes mellitus, evidence of microvascular complications, or kidney stones)
- family history of heritable kidney diseases (e.g. Alport syndrome, or polycystic kidney disease)
- smoking (a risk factor for renal arterial disease)

- drugs, including analgesics, over-the-counter medications, and herbal/traditional medicines (causes of renal damage)
- symptoms of prostatic disease (which can cause urinary tract obstruction)
- rashes (which may signify a systemic disease, such as SLE, or an allergic response, indicating an interstitial nephritis)
- joint problems (which may signify a systemic disease, such as SLE)
- sinus symptoms (which may indicate granulomatosis with polyangiitis)
- weight loss, or fatigue (indicating a systemic disease; fatigue may indicate anaemia due to erythropoietin deficiency in advanced kidney disease)
- urine (look for blood, discolouration, frothiness, dysuria; see Chapter 157); frank haematuria occurring with upper respiratory infections can indicate IgA nephropathy
- nocturia (which can indicate prostatic disease or poor urine-concentrating capacity, which can arise with advanced renal disease)
- shortness of breath (indicating fluid retention with pulmonary oedema, or lung involvement in a systemic disease)
- swelling/oedema (indicating fluid retention)

The examination should be thorough. Do not forget to check weight, and assess fluid status. This is particularly important in AKI, as volume depletion and heart failure are both common causes. Always measure heart rate (tachycardia may indicate severe dehydration), check blood pressure, and look for a postural drop (indicating either dehydration or autonomic neuropathy, which is common in diabetes). It is important to examine for peripheral oedema and to assess the heart, paying particular attention to the jugular venous pressure, the heart size (clinically and radiologically), and the presence of any murmurs or a third heart sound.

Careful inspection of the skin can be informative (e.g. livedo reticularis, purpura, photosensitive rash, digital infarcts). Palpate for the kidneys, bladder, and masses. Perform a rectal exam for prostate disease. Assess the peripheral vasculature for signs of insufficiency, such as bruits or absent pulses (suggesting renovascular causes for kidney injury). Fundoscopy may reveal changes consistent with hypertension or diabetes mellitus. Always perform dipstick urinalysis.

Standard investigations that may be helpful in suspected renal disease are given in Table 156.2.

Differential diagnosis

There are several standard presentations of renal disease; these can be considered under the following headings:

- asymptomatic haematuria (see Chapter 55)
- asymptomatic proteinuria (see Chapters 55, 161, 164, and 163)
- chronic slowly progressive renal damage (see Chapter 163)
- nephritic syndrome (see Chapter 159)
- acute rapidly progressive renal damage (see Chapter 162)
- nephrotic syndrome (see Chapter 161)

Table 156.2 Standard investigations that may be helpful in suspected renal disease

Prerenal	Renal	Post-renal
Creatinine and urea	CRP	Urine tract ultrasound
Liver function	Myeloma screen	PSA
ECG	ANCA/ANA/complement/ anti-GBM	+/– Urine cytology
Bone chemistry	Urine microscopy	IgG4 levels (IgG4-related disease such as retroperitoneal fibrosis)
CRP	albumin: creatinine ratio or protein: creatinine ratio	
Septic screen	TSH	
Full blood count and clotting	Blood film (particularly looking for haemolytic–uraemic syndromes)	
	Albumin	

Abbreviations: ANCA, antineutrophil cytoplasmic antibody; ANA, antinuclear antibody; ECG, electrocardiography; GBM, glomerular basement membrane; PSA, prostate-specific antigen; TSH, thyroid-stimulating hormone.

Asymptomatic low-grade proteinuria can be caused by many different diseases. These include all the causes of nephrotic syndrome, as well as benign causes. In the absence of other features, proteinuria is not usually investigated with a renal biopsy if it is less than 1 g/day.

'Gold-standard' diagnostic test

The gold-standard diagnostic test for renal dysfunction is the measurement of the GFR by clearance of radioisotopes (e.g. ^{51}Cr-labelled EDTA). However, in routine clinical practice, the diagnosis of renal dysfunction is made on the basis of urinalysis for protein content, and a standardized serum creatinine assay, which is used to calculate an estimated GFR (eGFR). The eGFR is calculated from serum creatinine on the basis of age, gender, and ethnicity.

Other relevant investigations

A small number of patients have structural renal diseases (e.g. horseshoe kidney) that may only be evident on radiological investigation. The clinical context of a patient in whom renal disease is suspected may invoke a number of laboratory or radiological tests (see Chapter 157). The final common test in many cases is a renal biopsy.

Prognosis and how to estimate it

This depends on the nature of the underlying disease. As a generalization, AKI is reversible, whereas CKD, due to intrinsic disease, is slowly but inexorably progressive.

Treatment and effectiveness

Both treatment and its effectiveness will depend on the nature of the underlying disease.

Further Reading

Kidney Disease: Improving Global Outcomes (KDIGO) CKD Work Group. KDIGO 2012 clinical practice guideline for the evaluation and management of chronic kidney disease. *Kidney Inter Suppl* 2013; 3: 1–150.

Kidney Disease: Improving Global Outcomes (KDIGO) Acute Kidney Injury Work Group. KDIGO clinical practice guideline for acute kidney injury. *Kidney Inter Suppl* 2012; 2: 1–138.

Steddon S, et al. *Oxford Handbook of Nephrology and Hypertension* 2nd ed. Oxford University Press, 2014.

Introduction

Renal physicians use a combination of tests to diagnose and monitor renal disease. These include urine, blood, and imaging investigations.

Urine

Appearance

Normal urine is clear to yellow in colour. Conjugated jaundice causes dark yellow urine. Cloudy urine suggests leucocytes. An offensive odour suggests bacterial infection. Frothy urine suggests heavy proteinuria. Frank haematuria causes red- or cola-coloured urine.

Urinalysis

Urine dipstick analysis is an indispensable bedside test. It can be used to detect proteinuria, haematuria, leucocyte levels, nitrate levels, glycosuria, and ketone levels; it is also used to measure specific gravity and pH.

Proteinuria

Proteinuria analysis via a dipstick measures predominately albumin. It does not detect all tubular secreted protein or immunoglobulins/light chains. Urine albumin secretion is <20 mg/day in normal kidneys. Dipsticks cannot reliably detect <300 mg/day of albuminuria (microalbuminuria). A dipstick is semi-quantitative (if concentrated); however, formal quantification is done via the albumin–creatinine ratio (ACR) or the protein–creatinine ratio (PCR).

Haematuria

Haematuria is reliably excluded by a negative dipstick. False positives can occur with myoglobinuria or haemoglobinuria. Microscopy is required to differentiate myoglobinuria, glomerular bleeding, and urinary tract bleeding.

Leucocyte levels

Dipsticks detect an enzyme (leucocyte esterase) produced by leucocytes. A positive result usually indicates bacterial urinary tract infection. If the culture is negative, a cause of sterile pyuria should be sought. This includes infection with a fastidious organism (e.g. *Chlamydia* spp.), prostatitis, tubulointerstitial nephritis (eosinophiluria), renal stone disease, renal tract tumours, papillary necrosis, or renal tract tuberculosis (requires three early morning urine samples).

Nitrite levels

Nitrites are an indicator of nitrate-reducing bacteria, and are best detected after a 4-hour bladder dwell. Nitrites are 98% specific but only 53% sensitive, as many bacteria, including *Pseudomonas* spp. and *Streptococcus faecalis*, do not reduce nitrates. Leucocytes and nitrites are good predictors of infection, if both are positive. Urine culture remains the 'gold-standard' test to exclude an infection.

Glycosuria

Glycosuria is detectable in the urine in hyperglycaemia when reabsorption is overwhelmed, and in proximal tubular disease when reabsorption is impaired. There is large inter-individual variation in the threshold for glycosuria, so it is an insensitive screening test for diabetes.

Ketone levels

Ketones are readily detectable, and useful in diagnosis of diabetic and alcoholic ketoacidosis. They may also be positive in starvation, volume depletion, and isopropyl alcohol poisoning (hand rubs and de-icers).

Specific gravity

The term 'specific gravity' refers to the density of urine compared to distilled water and is a measure of solute content. Concentrated urine has a high specific gravity. Specific gravity normally ranges between 1.005 and 1.035. It is useful to know the specific gravity when trying to estimate degree of proteinuria from a dipstick. Recurrent stone formers can use a dipstick specific gravity, to ensure they are maintaining dilute urine.

pH

The pH of urine ranges from 4.5 to 8.0. Measuring urine pH is useful in the workup for metabolic acidosis. Failure to decrease urine pH below 5.5 in the face of acidosis, suggests renal tubular acidosis. A low urine pH predisposes to uric acid stones. Alkaline urine predisposes to calcium phosphate stones.

Urinary chemical analysis

Urinary chemical analysis can be used to determine osmolality.

Osmolality

Osmolality is more accurate than specific gravity and is used to assess polyuric states, and disorders of sodium balance (see Chapter 174).

Protein–creatinine ratio

The protein–creatinine ratio has replaced 24-hour urinary collections. These collections are inconvenient for patients and are often inaccurate due to timing mistakes. The validity of the ratio relies on the assumption that creatinine excretion remains roughly constant at 10 mmol/day. The test is best performed on concentrated early morning urine. The protein–creatinine ratio detects albumin and tubular secreted protein. The albumin–creatinine ratio is a more sensitive test of glomerular proteinuria. It is preferred for detecting early glomerular renal disease, especially in diabetes mellitus. Thus, although often almost equivalent in practice, the protein–creatinine ratio and the albumin–creatinine ratio are not strictly interchangeable. (see Table 157.1).

Bence Jones proteins

Bence Jones proteins are urinary free light chains secreted by a plasma cell dyscrasia. They are not detected by a standard urine dipstick. They precipitate on heating to 60°C, and redissolve at 90°C. The test for them should be requested in parallel with a serum protein electrophoresis, and serum free light chains as part of a paraprotein screen.

Urinary catecholamines

Urinary catecholamines are indicated when screening for a phaeochromocytoma. Three 24-hour collections of acidified urine are required to reliably exclude the diagnosis.

Urine microscopy

Urine microscopy can be used to detect crystals, cells, and casts.

Crystals

Crystals can be seen by light microscopy, and may display birefringence under polarized light. They aid stone diagnosis, and occasionally indicate a cause for acute renal failure kidney injury (e.g. calcium oxalate crystals in ethylene glycol poisoning, and uric acid crystals in tumour lysis syndrome (see Chapter 166)).

Table 157.1 Converting dipstick albumin–creatinine ratios to 24-hour proteinuria

Dipstick	ACR (mg/mmol) (UK units)	ACR (mg/g) (US units)	24-Hour proteinuria (g/day)	Diagnosis
Negative	<2.5	<30	<0.03	Normal
Trace	3.0–30.0	30–300	0.03–0.30	Microalbuminuria
+	30.0	300	0.30	Overt proteinuria
++	100.0		1.00	
+++	350.0		3.50	Nephrotic range proteinuria
++++	1000.0		10.00	

Abbreviations: ACR, albumin–creatinine ratio.

Cells

Microscopy can identify red cells, white cells, renal tubular epithelium, urothelium, urethral squamous epithelium, and organisms in urine. Finding more than two red cells per high-powered field is significant. Glomerular bleeding damages red cells through the stress they undergo when passing through the filtration barrier and the highly osmotic environment of the tubules. The red cells become dysmorphic with blebs and buds (see Figure 157.1). Red cells from elsewhere in the urinary tract retain normal morphology. Neutrophils usually represent bacterial infection. The number of large, oval renal tubular epithelial cells increases in acute tubular damage but these cells are not diagnostically useful. Urothelial cells are examined by cytologists to screen for malignancy.

Casts

Casts can be cellular or non-cellular. Hyaline casts (Figure 157.2A) are plugs of Tamm–Horsfall mucoprotein from renal tubules and are abundant in concentrated urine. They are not thought to be pathological. Granular casts (see Figure 157.2B) are cellular remnants embedded in hyaline material, and are non-specific for glomerular and tubular disease. Cellular casts are much more useful (Table 157.2). Red cell casts are virtually diagnostic of a glomerulonephritis (confirming the

presence of blood from within the nephron). White-cell casts occur in urinary tract infection and tubulointerstitial nephritis. Epithelial cell casts contain sloughed tubular cells and, like granular casts, are non-specific, occurring in glomerular disease and tubular disease (Figure 157.3). When these epithelial cells are heavily lipid laden, they have a Maltese cross appearance and denote nephrotic syndrome.

Urine culture

The urine culture is deemed significant if there is a pure growth of a single type of organism, at a concentration of 10^5 colony-forming units per millilitre.

Glomerular filtration rate

The normal range of the glomerular filtration rate (GFR) is 90–125 ml/min, depending on the age of the patient. GFR is used to direct renally excreted drug dosing. Serial measurements enable progression of kidney disease to be monitored. GFR can be determined by administering a purely filtered exogenous molecule and then measuring its clearance, or by measuring levels of endogenously produced and filtered molecules such as creatinine and cystatin C.

(A)

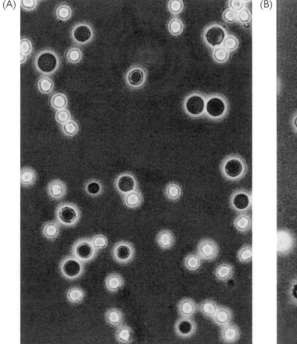

(B)

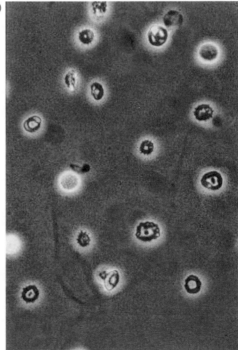

Figure 157.1 Microscopic haematuria. (A) Isomorphic red cells. Isomorphic red cells are seen in non-glomerular haematuria. (B) Dysmorphic red cells. Dysmorphic red cells are seen in glomerular haematuria, but may also be found in non-glomerular and tubulointerstitial disease. Please see colour plate section.

Reproduced with permission from Davidson et al, *Oxford Textbook of Clinical Nephrology*, Third Edition, Oxford University Press, Oxford, UK, Copyright © 2005.

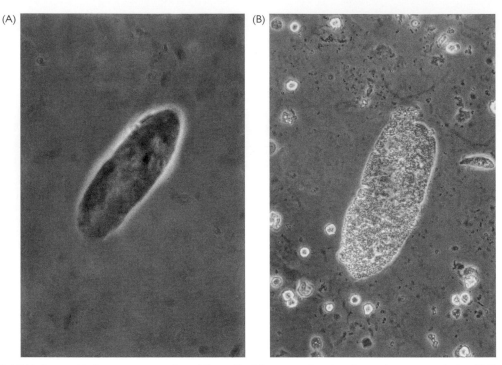

Figure 157.2 (A) Hyaline cast. Hyaline casts are concretions of Tamm–Horsfall mucoprotein and may be seen in concentrated urine. (B) Granular cast. Granular casts are cellular remnants embedded in hyaline material and are non-specific for glomerular and tubular disease. Please see colour plate section.
Reproduced with permission from Davidson et al, Oxford Textbook of Clinical Nephrology, Third Edition, Oxford University Press, Oxford, UK, Copyright © 2005.

Estimated GFR

Creatinine is convenient and cheap to measure. When it is in steady state, renal excretion is balanced with production from skeletal muscle. The steady-state concentration for a given GFR will thus vary with an individual's creatinine production. Factors determining production include sex, age, and size. Equations utilizing these variables are used to convert serum creatinine into an estimation of GFR (eGFR). The conventional units for GFR are millilitres per minute; however, eGFR reports the GFR as a function of body surface area. The units for eGFR are thus millilitres per minute per 1.73 m². eGFR is now routinely reported together with serum creatinine; although it requires four variables for calculation (serum creatinine, age, gender, and ethnicity: the four-variable MDRD formula), it has superseded the Cockcroft–Gault equation, as it does not require a patient's weight. The MDRD formula is based on data derived from a population with chronic kidney disease. Above a GFR of 60 ml/min, the eGFR is less reliable. More recently, an updated formula, the CKD-EPI equation, has been used for reporting eGFR; this equation is more accurate than the MDRD formula, particularly at higher levels of renal function. Like the MDRD formula, it uses creatinine, age, gender, and ethnicity to produce an eGFR.

Creatinine clearance

Creatinine clearance can be measured directly by a timed urine (or peritoneal dialysate) collection (see Box 157.1). It is a reasonable measurement of GFR if collection is accurate (usually over 24 hours).

However, it is seldom used in practice, as it is frequently not possible to obtain an accurate collection of urine samples.

Urea

Urea is a less reliable as a marker of renal function. It is synthesized by the liver as a means of ammonium excretion and undergoes variable tubular reabsorption. However, these facts can be useful diagnostically. Urea can be increased by a gastrointestinal bleed, high dietary protein intake, or a catabolic state. Conversely, liver disease or a low-protein diet reduces urea production. In hypovolaemia, renal perfusion falls, reducing GFR. Creatinine and urea levels thus rise. However, urea reabsorption is increased from the tubules, to increase the peak urine osmolality in the loop of Henle to preserve water. Urea thus rises disproportionately compared to creatinine, in prerenal renal failure.

Isotopic GFR

Isotopic GFR is expensive and thus rarely performed. The radiolabelled marker ^{51}Cr-EDTA is injected and serial venous measurements taken over time.

Renal imaging

Ultrasonography

A renal ultrasound should be performed in acute kidney injury within 24 hours to exclude obstruction and measure kidney size; 10–11 cm is

Table 157.2 Typical urinary findings in acute kidney injury						
	Prerenal	**Acute tubular necrosis**	**Glomerular nephritis**	**Post-renal**	**Acute interstitial nephritis**	**Nephrotic syndrome**
Specific gravity	High: >1.020	Iso-osmotic: 1.010	Normal: 1.010–1.020	Iso-osmotic: 1.010	Iso-osmotic: 1.010	Normal: 1.010–1.020
Protein on dipstick	–	–	+	+/–	+/–	+++
Blood on dipstick	–	–	+	+/–	+/–	+/–
Microscopy	Hyaline casts	Renal tubular epithelial cells Granular casts	Dysmorphic red cells Red cell casts	Normal red cells	Eosinophils White-cell casts	Fatty casts

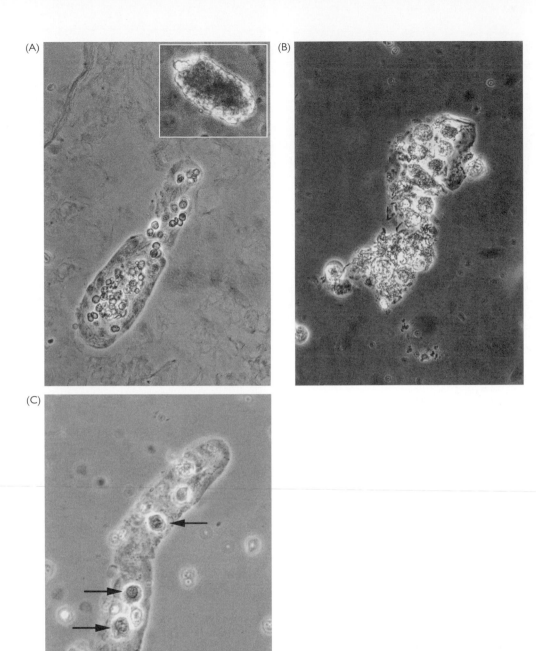

(A)

(B)

(C)

Figure 157.3 (A) Red cell cast; inset: haemoglobin cast. Red cell casts are typically seen in glomerulonephritis. (B) Epithelial cell cast. Epithelial cell casts may be seen in glomerular and tubular disease. (C) White cell cast; individual white cells (arrows) are clearly seen. White cell casts may be seen in pyelonephritis and tubulointerstitial disease. Please see colour plate section.

Reproduced with permission from Davidson et al, Oxford Textbook of Clinical Nephrology, Third Edition, Oxford University Press, Oxford, UK, Copyright © 2005.

normal and suggests an acute cause. An 8–9 cm kidney (+/− acquired cysts) suggests chronic kidney disease. Remember, hydronephrosis may not develop for 48 hours after acute obstruction or in partial obstruction.

Kidney–ureter–bladder imaging

A kidney–ureter–bladder CT scan is a very useful investigation. It does not require IV contrast. It will identify stones, confirm hydronephrosis, and delineate the site and cause of obstruction.

The use of contrast is indicated if a plain scan does not delineate obstruction, or to assess suspicious cysts or renal masses. Performing further CT images after a delay allows time for contrast to be excreted. The ureters can then be imaged. This is called a CT urogram. The presence of fat suggests a benign angiomyolipoma. Enhancing masses greater than 3 cm in diameter, with thick irregular walls, and areas of necrosis are suspicious of malignancy.

Box 157.1 Formula for the calculation of creatinine clearance from a urine collection

Creatine clearance (in millilitres per minute) may be calculated from the following formula:

$$\text{creatine clearance} = \frac{[\text{creatinine}]_{\text{urine}} \times \text{urine volume}}{[\text{creatinine}]_{\text{plasma}} \times \text{collection time}},$$

where urine volume is in millilitres, and collection time is in minutes.

Nuclear medicine

^{99m}Tc-DMSA imaging can be used for assessment of split kidney function. An MAG3 scan with furosemide excretion is useful for the assessment of obstruction and reflux.

Magnetic resonance angiography and CT angiography

Magnetic resonance angiography and CT angiography are used to assess the renal arteries. In expert hands, duplex ultrasound with Doppler and nuclear scans can identify reduced perfusion, but CT angiography or magnetic resonance angiograms are the best screening investigations. However, they may overestimate the degree of stenosis or miss distal stenosis and thus digital subtraction angiography remains the gold-standard investigation for assessment of renal artery disease.

Immunology in renal practice

Immunology is used to assess both chronic and acute renal failure. The standard screen for immunological renal disease includes tests for antinuclear antibody (ANA), complement proteins, and antineutrophil cytoplasmic antibody (ANCA). Additional tests may also be indicated.

Immunoglobulin testing and serum protein electrophoresis

Immunoglobulin testing and serum protein electrophoresis are very commonly requested. In people over 50 years of age with renal disease, a serum and urinary electrophoresis (Bence Jones proteins) should be considered. A free light chain assay is now available to detect light chains in the serum. The interpretations of these tests are summarized in Table 157.3.

Table 157.3 Immunoglobulins/protein electrophoresis interpretation

Test	Diagnosis
Positive serum IgG, IgA, or IgD monoclonal band +/− immunoparesis	Plasma cell dyscrasia (MGUS or myeloma)
Positive serum IgM monoclonal band	Waldenström's macroglobulinaemia
Urinary free light chains (Bence Jones proteins)	Plasma cell dyscrasia (MGUS or myeloma)
	Waldenström's macroglobulinaemia
	B-cell lymphomas and leukaemias
	AL amyloidosis
Raised serum IgA	Associated in 50% of IgA nephropathy cases
Polyclonal gammaglobulinaemia	Very non-specific: connective tissue disorders (including lupus)
	Vasculitis
	HIV infection
	Tubulointerstitial nephritis +/− uveitis
Hypogammaglobulinaemia	Multiple causes, including nephrotic syndrome

Abbreviations: AL, amyloid light chain; MGUS, monoclonal gammopathy of unknown significance.

ANCA

ANCA is requested urgently when a rapidly progressive glomerulonephritis is suspected. ANCA is associated with small vessel vasculitides. There are two different ANCA appearances on immunofluorescence: cytoplasmic (cANCA) and perinuclear (pANCA). The target antigen for cANCA is proteinase 3 (PR3), and for pANCA is myeloperoxidase (MPO). PR3 specificity is associated with granulomatosis with polyangiitis (Wegener's granulomatosis), and MPO specificity with microscopic polyangiitis. Both can cause a focal segmental necrotizing (pauci-immune) glomerulonephritis.

Anti-glomerular basement membrane antibody

An anti-glomerular basement membrane antibody (anti-GBM) test is also requested urgently in rapidly progressive glomerulonephritis. It is highly specific for anti-GBM disease.

ANA

ANA is non-specifically associated with many autoimmune conditions. Elderly patients often have a weakly positive ANA titre. A positive result in the young, however, is more significant. Specific nuclear antigen assays that are useful in nephrology practice include anti-double-stranded DNA (lupus); anti-Scl70 and anti-RNA polymerase (systemic sclerosis); and anti-Ro and anti-La (Sjögren's syndrome).

Complement

Complement proteins are reduced in certain renal diseases where there are high levels of circulating immune complexes (and in other diseases as well). Complement proteins are useful diagnostic pointers, but rarely diagnostic in themselves (see Table 157.4).

Virology

Hepatitis B/C and HIV status are required for haemodialysis patients for infection control purposes. These viruses are associated with several renal diseases (see Chapter 170).

Rheumatoid factor and cryoglobulins

Rheumatoid factor and cryoglobulins are not routinely screened for, but may be indicated where there is a low C4 level, a hepatitis C infection, or a history of rash and peripheral neuropathy. Cryoglobulins precipitate at <37°C and so need to be kept warm after sampling. Type 1 cryoglobulins are monoclonal IgMs or IgGs and are associated with lymphoproliferative diseases. Type 2 mixed essential cryoglobulinaemia is characterized by the presence of a monoclonal IgM with rheumatoid factor function, and polyclonal IgG. It is strongly associated with hepatitis C.

Antiphospholipid antibodies

Antiphospholipid antibodies are indicated with a history of recurrent venous or arterial thrombosis, recurrent miscarriage, livedo reticularis, or a prolonged activated partial thromboplastin time that does not correct. Tests for lupus anticoagulant and anti-cardiolipin antibodies should be requested.

Table 157.4 Complement proteins C3 and C4 in renal diseases

	C3	C4
Lupus nephritis	↓	↓
Post-infective glomerulonephritis	↓	↓/↔
Infective endocarditis	↓	↓
Mesangiocapillary glomerulonephritis type 1 without cryoglobulins	↓	↓
Mesangiocapillary glomerulonephritis type 1 With mixed essential cryoglobulinaemia	↔	↓
Mesangiocapillary glomerulonephritis type 2 (dense deposit disease)	↓	↔

Renal biopsy

Renal biopsy is essential for the diagnosis and estimation of prognosis in many kidney diseases.

Indications

Indications for a biopsy include unexplained acute kidney injury, chronic kidney disease with normal sized kidneys, heavy proteinuria (in adults), assessment of disease cause, assessment of disease activity (e.g. in SLE), and an acute deterioration in renal transplant function. A risk of bleeding is associated with a biopsy, and this should be balanced against the possible diagnostic and prognostic benefit.

Contraindications

Contraindications need to be included in the risk–benefit assessment (see Table 157.5).

Technique

Renal biopsy is now routinely performed as a day case, with real-time ultrasound guidance. CT guidance is reserved for the obese. Local anaesthetic is required. Either kidney can be biopsied, but the left is preferred. In native kidneys, the lower pole is biopsied. The upper part (usually still the lower pole) is biopsied in a transplant, due to the position of the transplant in the pelvis. The mid pole is avoided because of the presence of large vessels. Two cores are taken, usually with a spring-loaded gun. Patients are required to lie flat for 6 hours afterwards. The risk of bleeding falls after 48 hours. Biopsies are processed for light microscopy, immunofluorescence, and electron microscopy.

Complications

Bleeding is the most concerning complication: about 2% of renal biopsy patients experience macroscopic haematuria or a capsular haematoma. Angiography and embolization is indicated for rapid blood loss or persistent bleeding. Rarely, a nephrectomy is required (0.1%) and hence dialysis should be part of informed consent, particularly in a solitary kidney or advance renal failure.

Table 157.5 Renal biopsy contraindications

Relative contraindications	Caution
Hypertension (>160/90 mm Hg)	Small kidneys
Abnormal clotting (INR/APTTr >1.3)	Multiple cysts
Thrombocytopaenia (platlet count < 100)	Uncooperative patient
Hydronephrosis	Single kidney
Urinary tract infection	Antiplatelet therapy within 5 days
Suspected renal tumour	Morbid obesity

Abbreviations: APTTr, activated partial thromboplastin time ratio; INR, international normalized ratio.

Genes and the kidney

Polycystic kidney disease is the commonest inherited kidney disorder. There are a number of other inherited diseases with characterized genes (see Chapter 169). However, genetic analysis is rarely requested in clinical nephrology, as the diagnosis is often confirmed by clinical findings and imaging. This may change when treatments to alter the course of these diseases are found and early treatment is necessary. Research is also ongoing into susceptibility genes for chronic kidney diseases.

Further Reading

Fogazzi GB. 'Urinalysis and microscopy', in Davison A, Cameron JS, Grünfeld JP, et al., eds, *Oxford Textbook of Clinical Nephrology* (3rd edition), 2010. Oxford University Press.

158 Urinary tract infection

William G. Herrington, Aron Chakera, and Christopher A. O'Callaghan

Definition of the disease

A urinary tract infection (UTI) is defined as present when urine culture results in the growth of a single organism at greater than 10^5 colony-forming units/ml of urine.

Etiology

Organisms causing UTI are listed in Table 158.1. Bowel flora are the commonest cause. *Escherichia coli* accounts for 80% of infections. *Klebsiella* spp., *Proteus mirabilis, Enterococcus faecalis,* and *Staphylococcal saprophyticus* account for most of the remaining 20%. *Staphylococcus aureus* culture is usually catheter related or secondary to haematogenous spread.

Host vulnerability factors include urinary tract obstruction, urinary stasis (e.g. incomplete bladder emptying), foreign bodies (e.g. stones or stents), sexual intercourse, diabetes mellitus, and immunosuppression.

Lower UTIs are more common. They represent superficial uncomplicated infection and will respond to a short course of treatment. Upper tract involvement is more serious as it represents deep tissue infection.

Symptoms

Symptoms classically correlate to the site of infection (see Box 158.1). Urethritis causes dysuria. Cystitis irritates the bladder trigone, resulting in suprapubic discomfort, urinary frequency, and urgency. Pyelonephritis may not have associated lower urinary tract symptoms. The usual presentation is a young female with a high fever and renal angle discomfort or tenderness. Renal capsular stretch results in vagal stimulus and can induce nausea and vomiting. Septicaemia is suggested by high fever,

Box 158.1 Common symptoms of lower urinary tract infection

- Severe dysuria, often described as 'scorching' or 'like peeing barbed wire', worse towards the end of or immediately after micturition
- Increased urinary frequency
- Urgency—the sensation of a strong desire to pass urine
- Strangury—the feeling of needing to pass urine despite just having done so
- Offensive-smelling urine, often described as 'strong' or 'fishy'
- Macroscopic haematuria
- Urge incontinence—leakage of urine associated with the desire to pass urine
- Constant lower abdominal aching, not just in the genital area but also in the back, flanks, and lower abdomen
- Nonspecific malaise, aching all over, nausea, tiredness, irritability, and cold sweats

Reproduced with permission from Warrell, Cox and Firth, Oxford Textbook of Medicine, Fifth Edition Oxford University Press, Oxford, UK, Copyright © 2010

rigours, and hypotension and can be life-threatening. In the elderly, the presentation of a UTI may be non-specific, with pyrexia, loss of mobility, and confusion. Prostatitis can give pain on defaecation and a tender prostate on digital rectal examination.

Demographics

Females have a 50% lifetime risk of UTI, and 5% will have recurrent infections. The peak incidence is in sexually active females. Elderly females are also at increased risk, due to a rise in vaginal pH. Males are at low risk of UTI due to a longer urethra and distance of the meatus from the anus. The incidence of UTI in males increases with age, probably as a result of prostatic disease. A UTI in a male should always prompt investigation for an underlying urological cause.

Natural history, and complications

Most UTIs are uncomplicated and can be treated with a short course of antibiotic appropriate for the likely causative organisms (Box 158.2). Asymptomatic bacteriuria can lead to symptomatic infection, but can usually be safely left untreated. The exception to this is in pregnancy and in patients with anatomical abnormalities of their renal tract or renal transplants. Pregnancy is associated with a 5% incidence of bacteriuria. Because of progestogen-mediated ureteric smooth muscle relaxation, the risk of upper UTI is increased, and asymptomatic infections are treated.

Table 158.1 Bacterial etiology of urinary tract infection

Organism	Urinary tract infection (%)	
	Uncomplicated	Complicated
Gram-negative organisms		
Escherichia coli	70–95	21–54
Proteus mirabilis	1–2	1–10
Klebsiella pneumoniae	1–2	2–17
Citrobacter spp.	<1	5
Enterobacter spp.	<1	2–10
Pseudomonas aeruginosa	<1	2–19
Other	<1	6–20
Gram-positive organisms		
Coagulase-negative staphylococci (*S. saprophyticus*)	5–20 or more	1–4
Enterococci	1–2	1–23
Group B streptococci	<1	1–4
Staphylococcus aureus	<1	1–2
Other	<1	2

Reproduced with permission from J Barratt, K Harris and P Topham, *Oxford Desk Reference: Nephrology,* Oxford University Press, Oxford, UK, Copyright © 2008.

This article was adapted from Urinary tract infections in adults, Hooton T. in *Comprehensive clinical nephrology,* Johnson RJ, Feehally J (eds), Table 53.1, p. 695 Copyright Elsevier 2003.

Complicated infections data from: Nicolle LE. A practical guide to the management of complicated urinary tract infection. *Drugs* 1997; 53: 583–592.

Box 158.2 Organisms commonly causing uncomplicated urinary tract infection

- *Escherichia coli*
- *Klebsiella pneumoniae*
- *Proteus*
- *Pseudomonas*
- *Enterococcus*
- *Staphylococcus saprophyticus* (in sexually active females)

Reproduced with permission from Warrell, Cox and Firth, Oxford Textbook of Medicine, Fifth Edition Oxford University Press, Oxford, UK, Copyright © 2010

An adult with appropriately treated acute pyelonephritis will usually have an uncomplicated recovery. However, an obstructed and infected urinary system is an emergency that requires urological drainage.

Recurrent cystitis can eventually result in a sterile inflammation and ulceration of the bladder, termed 'interstitial cystitis'. Treatment of the resultant chronic pain can be difficult but may respond to tricyclic antidepressants.

UTI in children was believed to cause renal scarring. However, it is unclear to what extent the infections contribute to the loss of renal function. The infection itself may simply be an indicator of underlying vesicoureteric reflux, which may itself be injurious. Vesicoureteric reflux affects 1% of newborns, but is present in 50% of children presenting with a UTI. Reflux usually stops at puberty, when the bladder base thickens. After the age of 7, the kidney seems to be resistant to new scarring. The resultant scarred kidney from reflux is termed 'reflux nephropathy' or 'chronic pyelonephritis'. Reflux nephropathy is still responsible for 7% of new dialysis patients.

Approach to diagnosing the disease

Diagnosis is from the history and urinary findings. Urinalysis, plus urine and blood cultures, is a routine screening test in sepsis. Dipstick detection of leucocytes and nitrites is highly sensitive. Blood and protein may also be present. On microscopy of a fresh urine specimen, the presence of >10 white cells per high-power field, or of any bacteria, is significant (Box 158.1 and Figure 158.1). A white-cell count and C-reactive protein and procalcitonin levels may be useful indicators of infection severity. Pitfalls include missing the diagnosis in the elderly, where the presentation may be non-specific, and missing associated urinary tract obstruction or stones.

Differential diagnosis

The differential of renal angle pain is renal stones, renal malignancy, or infection. A renal ultrasound is indicated if there is doubt about the diagnosis (marked loin pain/deterioration in creatinine/history of stones or renal colic/male/elderly/atypical urinalysis).

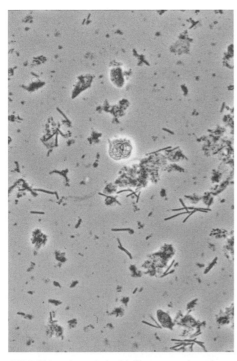

Figure 158.1 Urinary bacteria (rods). Please see colour plate section.

Reproduced with permission from Davidson et al, *Oxford Textbook of Clinical Nephrology*, Third Edition, Oxford University Press, Oxford, UK, Copyright © 2005.

The differential of dysuria includes a *Chlamydia trachomatis* or *Neisseria gonorrhoeae* urethritis. These infections are usually accompanied by a urethral discharge.

'Gold-standard' diagnostic test

The gold-standard diagnostic test for UTI is urine culture, with a finding of $\geq 10^5$ colony-forming units/ml. However, this threshold may miss up to 30% of infections, and a threshold of 10^4 colony-forming units/ml is suggested in the context of symptoms of pyelonephritis or in children, while 10^3 colony-forming units/ml may be significant in men.

Other relevant investigations

An ultrasound is indicated in a second attack of pyelonephritis or in suspected obstruction. Early morning urines are indicated in sterile pyuria with risk factors for tuberculosis.

In older males, an assessment of the prostate, together with cystoscopy and an ultrasound to assess bladder emptying, may be necessary to identify predisposing prostate or bladder disease.

CT scans are useful in severe cases of pyelonephritis or where there is associated stone/obstructive disease.

Children with a UTI may need a renal ultrasound scan to look for anatomical abnormalities. A ^{99m}Tc-DMSA nuclear scan can be used to detect renal scarring. Micturating cystograms are not routinely used but may be helpful under certain circumstances.

Prognosis and how to estimate it

Most UTIs resolve with simple antibiotic treatment.

Treatment and effectiveness

Increased fluid intake is advised. Antibiotics are usually indicated. Empirical choice of antibiotic is directed by local microbiological sensitivities. Treatment duration is an important consideration (Table 158.2).

There are several special situations. A UTI in combination with obstruction can cause rapid renal scarring and is a urological emergency. Decompression is achieved by percutaneous nephrostomy or retrograde stenting.

In children with reflux or recurrent infection, long-term prophylactic antibiotics were previously advocated. However, there is a shift away from this, as there is little evidence that such treatment alters prognosis. Surgery probably offers no long-term benefit over prophylactic antibiotics.

Catheter-related infection is common. Treatment is rarely effective without catheter removal or exchange. Treatment is thus reserved for local symptoms or systemic upset.

Table 158.2 A typical protocol for empirical treatment of a single urinary tract infection; protocols will vary with local patterns of antibiotic sensitivity

Diagnosis	Treatment
Asymptomatic bacteriuria	Well: No treatment
	Pregnant: 7–10 days oral
Uncomplicated lower urinary tract infection	3–7 days oral nitrofurantoin 50 mg four times per day
	3–7 days of co-amoxiclav 375 mg three times per day, or cefalexin 500 mg three times per day in renal impairment
Complicated urinary tract infection	Acute pyelonephritis: 14-day course of oral ciprofloxacin 500 mg twice per day, or co-amoxiclav 625 mg three times per day
	Septicaemia: Inpatient management with IV co-amoxiclav 1.2 g three times per day +/− stat dose of gentamicin +/− IV fluids
	Male: 4–6 weeks oral ciprofloxacin 500 mg twice per day, to clear deep prostate infection
	Recent urinary instrumentation: consider adding vancomycin 1 g IV

Recurrent UTIs are defined by greater than four proven infections within a year. Treatment advice includes increasing fluid intake, double voiding, and avoiding nylon underwear. Prophylactic use of cranberry juice is supported by randomized trials. Cranberry juice contains proanthocyanidins that appear to inhibit the attachment of pathogens to uroepithelium. Between 200 and 750 ml per day of cranberry (or lingonberry) juice can reduce recurrent infection by 12%–20%. Refractory cases may benefit from a year of monthly rotating, low-single-dose antibiotic prophylaxis. In postmenopausal females, oestrogen creams may improve associated atrophic vaginitis. In sexually active women, post-coital voiding and a post-coital dose of antibiotic can be helpful.

Further Reading

Hooton TM. Uncomplicated urinary tract infection. *N Engl J Med* 2012; 366: 1028–37.

Johnson JR, and Russo TA. Acute pyelonephritis in adults. *N Engl J Med* 2018; 378: 48–59.

Shaeffer AJ, Nicolle LE. Urinary tract infections in older men. *N Engl J Med* 2016; 374: 562–71.

159 Glomerulonephritis

William G. Herrington, Aron Chakera, and Christopher A. O'Callaghan

Definition of the disease

Glomerulonephritis (GN) is inflammation of the glomerulus. It can be caused by many different underlying conditions and can present in a range of ways. The key features, however, are evidence of renal dysfunction (clinical and investigative) with associated glomerular disease—the latter is often initially suspected from urine dipstick examination (Chapter 157), and may then be confirmed by a renal biopsy.

Etiology

There are many causes of GN (Table 159.1). Immunological damage to the glomerulus can arise from direct binding of an antibody to the glomerular basement membrane (anti-GBM disease; also known as Goodpasture's disease). In a number of other glomerular diseases, immune mechanisms are implicated, but the exact pathogenesis is not clear.

Symptoms and clinical features

Acute nephritis is characterized by hypertension, fluid retention causing peripheral oedema, and microscopic haematuria and proteinuria. There may also be non-specific systemic features such as fevers, weight loss, anorexia, malaise, myalgias, or arthralgias. Other symptoms may indicate a specific underlying diagnosis (see 'Approach to diagnosing the disease' and 'Other diagnoses that should be considered'). Rapidly progressive GN (RPGN) is an acute destructive GN with renal failure developing over days; typically, features of nephritic syndrome are present. Nephrotic syndrome is defined by the presence of heavy proteinuria (>3.5 g/day), resulting in hypoalbuminaemia and peripheral oedema and is discussed in Chapter 161 (also see Table 159.2). GN may be asymptomatic and detected by abnormal urinalysis on incidental testing.

Some common symptoms of different GNs

Antineutrophil cytoplasmic antibody-positive vasculitis

Antineutrophil cytoplasmic antibody (ANCA)-positive vasculitis affects small vessels. It can be asymptomatic (until uraemia develops) or associated with non-specific systemic upset (fevers, weight loss, anorexia, malaise, myalgias, arthralgias). There may be a vasculitic rash, ocular, or ENT involvement. Granulomatosis with polyangiitis (Wegener's granulomatosis) is characteristically associated with upper respiratory tract involvement, with nasal crusting, epistaxis, sinusitis, or otitis media.

Nephritis in SLE

Nephritis can occur with SLE. There may be features of systemic lupus such as Raynaud's phenomenon, serositis, skin changes including a butterfly rash, alopecia, CNS involvement, or haematological derangements (thrombocytopaenia, haemolysis, leucopenia). It may be associated with antiphospholipid syndrome.

Henoch–Schönlein purpura and IgA nephropathy

Henoch–Schönlein purpura (HSP) and IgA nephropathy share similarities. IgA nephropathy classically presents with macroscopic haematuria, often associated with upper respiratory tract infections. HSP is characterized by systemic symptoms that include palpable purpura, diffuse abdominal pain which may be worse after meals (bowel ischaemia), and symmetrical polyarthralgia. In adults, HSP predominately affects the kidney.

Rarer causes of GN

Anti-GBM disease (Goodpasture's disease)

Anti-GBM disease (Goodpasture's disease) can be asymptomatic. Renal failure often occurs very rapidly. Macroscopic haematuria or 'cola' urine may be reported. A cough, dyspnoea, and haemoptysis suggest pulmonary haemorrhage.

Mesangiocapillary GN

Mesangiocapillary GN can present in a variety of ways ranging from asymptomatic urine abnormalities to a rapidly progressive GN. It can be associated with cryoglobulinaemia or with partial lipodystrophy.

Postinfectious GN

Postinfectious GN can follow any infection, including streptococcal sore throat, infective endocarditis, abscesses, and tropical infections.

Demographics

IgA nephropathy is the commonest cause of GN worldwide. In the Far East, it is responsible for almost half of all cases of glomerular

Table 159.1 Etiology of glomerulonephritis

	Rapidly progressive glomerulonephritis	Acute nephritis	Nephrotic syndrome	Asymptomatic microscopic haematuria +/− proteinuria*
Immune complex	Henoch–Schönlein purpura (IgA nephropathy) Mesangiocapillary glomerulonephritis	IgA nephropathy Lupus nephritis Postinfectious GN Mesangiocapillary glomerulonephritis	Membranous nephropathy	IgA nephropathy Mesangiocapillary glomerulonephritis
Antibody dependent	Anti-glomerular basement membrane disease			
Pauci-immune	ANCA-positive vasculitis (granulomatosis with polyangiitis (Wegener's) and microscopic polyangiitis) Polyarteritis nodosa: does not typically cause glomerulonephritis, but arterial inflammation can cause renal ischaemia and necrosis Churg–Strauss syndrome	Thrombotic microangiopathy†	Minimal-change disease Focal segmental glomerulosclerosis	

* With normal urological investigations.
† Thrombotic microangiopathy is often considered to be a disparate group of systemic disorders rather than a glomerulonephritis.

Table 159.2 Histology of nephrotic syndrome

Histology	Number of children[a] (%)	Number of adults[b] (%)
Minimal-change nephrotic syndrome	76	17
Mesangiocapillary glomerulonephritis	8	3
Focal segmental glomerulosclerosis	7	17
Proliferative (including diffuse mesangial proliferation)	2	0
Membranous	2	30
Other	5	9
Systemic lupus erythematosus	–	8
Amyloid	–	7
Diabetes	–	9

Reproduced with permission from Warrell, Cox and Firth, Oxford Textbook of Medicine, Fifth Edition Oxford University Press, Oxford, UK, Copyright © 2010.

disease. It is also common in Europe. Black and Asian people have a higher prevalence of lupus nephritis.

Vasculitis is rare in all populations. The prevalence of ANCA-positive vasculitis and anti-GBM disease are 20 and 0.5 per million population, respectively.

Mesangiocapillary GN, lupus nephritis, and Henoch–Schönlein purpura tend to affect the young (10–40 years of age). ANCA-positive vasculitis peaks between the ages of 55– 70. Anti-GBM disease can affect any age, but the full syndrome with pulmonary haemorrhage is more common in younger patients. The younger patients are more commonly male, and older patients are more commonly female. Lupus nephritis affects ten times as many women as men.

Natural history, and complications

The progression rate varies with disease. For example, renal survival is 80% at 20 years in IgA nephropathy, while untreated ANCA-positive vasculitis carries a 90% 2-year mortality. Pulmonary haemorrhage is a serious complication of ANCA-positive vasculitides and anti-GBM

disease. The risk is increased by pulmonary oedema and cigarette smoking.

Complications of treatment are largely related to immuno-suppression.

Approach to diagnosing the disease

GN is easily missed. A thorough history may elicit suspicion. Non-specific systemic upset with a combination of fevers, weight loss, anorexia, malaise, myalgias, or arthralgias is common with autoimmune and infective diseases and should prompt further assessment. In any patient with hypertension, peripheral oedema, or impaired renal function urine dipstick testing should be performed.

Urinary abnormalities or abnormal renal function should initiate further investigations to identify the cause and, when indicated, to prepare for a renal biopsy. Often, knowledge of the demographics of the relevant diseases and a thorough history and examination will narrow the diagnosis.

Other diagnoses that should be considered

Microscopic haematuria can be caused by urinary tract stones or tumours and sometimes infections. Alport's syndrome and thin basement membrane disease also present with microscopic haematuria alone and thus resemble IgA nephropathy. They are hereditary nephropathies with urine abnormalities but no inflammation and are thus not strictly GNs. Thin basement membrane disease has a good prognosis and rarely causes renal impairment. Alport's causes a progressive decline in renal function and high-tone sensorineural deafness. End-stage renal failure usually occurs around 20 to 30 years of age. Staining for type IV collagen is negative on biopsy. It is most important to differentiate the conditions causing benign abnormalities on urinalysis from RPGN, which requires urgent investigation and treatment.

'Gold-standard' diagnostic test

The gold-standard diagnostic test is renal biopsy (see Table 159.3 and Figures 159.1 and 159.2). In benign disorders, it may not be indicated.

Table 159.3 Renal biopsy findings in glomerulonephritis

Disease	Light microscopy	Immunofluorescence	Electron microscopy
ANCA-positive vasculitis	Focal and segmental necrotizing glomerular lesions +/– arteritis +/– crescents	Pauci-immune (negative)	
Anti-glomerular basement membrane disease	Diffuse global necrotizing lesions +/– Bowman's capsule rupture with crescents	Linear IgG+ C3+	
Mesangiocapillary glomerulonephritis	Basement membrane duplication + mesangial hypercellularity	Type 1: C3+ IgG+	Sub-endothelial immune complex deposits
Lupus nephritis	I: Normal II: Mesangial hypercellularity III: Focal endocapillary proliferation (<50% glomeruli) IV: Diffuse endocapillary proliferation (>50% glomeruli); can be segmental or global V: Glomerular basement membrane thickening with sub-epithelial 'spikes' on silver staining VI: Advanced sclerosis	IgA/IgG/IgM+ C3/C1q+ (Full house)	All: mesangial electron-dense deposits +/– sub-endothelial (Class III/IV) +/– sub-epithelial (Class V)
Postinfectious GN	Acute proliferative glomerulonephritis Intra-capillary neutrophils	C3+ IgG+/–	Sub-epithelial electron-dense deposits ('humps') Endocapillary swelling with widening of endothelial spaces
Thrombotic microangiopathy	Glomerular capillary fibrin thrombi and sub-endothelial oedema Ischaemic changes	Negative	Capillary fibrin thrombi Endocapillary swelling + injury
Henoch–Schönlein purpura/IgA nephropathy	Mesangial hypercellularity +/– increased mesangial matrix +/– endocapillary proliferation +/– segmental sclerosis +/– tubular atrophy +/– crescents	IgA +	Mesangial electron-dense deposits +/– sub-endothelial deposits

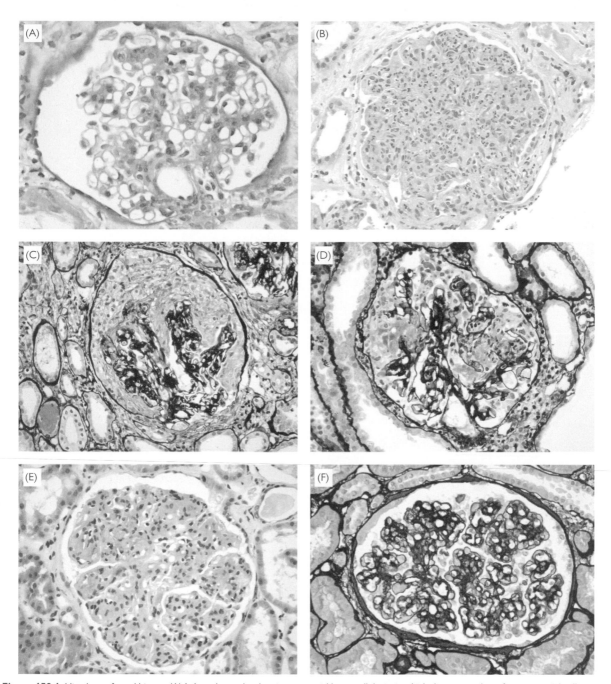

Figure 159.1 Histology of renal biopsy. (A) IgA nephropathy showing mesangial hypercellularity in which there are at least four mesangial cells in a peripheral mesangial area (periodic acid-Schiff stain). (B) Postinfectious glomerulonephritis showing endocapillary hypercellularity, in which the capillary lumina are filled with infiltrating leucocytes (hematoxylin and eosin stain (H&E)). (C) Antiglomerular basement membrane disease, showing extracapillary proliferation (a cellular crescent), in which there is partial tuft collapse and proliferation of cells within Bowman's space (H&E and silver). (D) ANCA-associated vasculitis, showing necrosis with capillary wall rupture and fibrin exudation (H&E and silver). (E, F) Membranoproliferative pattern, showing a lobular appearance of the glomerular tuft, with mesangial hypercellularity and thickened capillary walls, with glomerular basement membrane duplication evident on the silver stain (H&E and silver). Please see colour plate section.

Reproduced with permission from Turner, Oxford Textbook of Clinical Nephrology, Fourth Edition Oxford University Press, Oxford, UK, Copyright © 2015.

Acceptable diagnostic alternatives to the gold standard

Other investigations in GN are adjuncts to diagnostic biopsy material. If RPGN is suspected, a rapid ELISA test can demonstrate anti-PR3, anti-myeloperoxidase, and anti-GBM antibodies within hours.

Other relevant investigations

With GN, urine microscopy may demonstrate dysmorphic red cells with or without red-cell casts—a sign of glomerular bleeding. Other standard investigations include renal function, liver function, bone chemistry, and a nephritic screen (antinuclear antibody (ANA), complement, ANCA, anti-GBM, immunoglobulins, serum, and urine electrophoresis, hepatitis virus serology, and C-reactive protein). Tests for infection such as anti-streptolysin O and anti-DNase B titres are requested if postinfectious GN is suspected. Diarrhoea and thrombocytopaenia should prompt a request for a blood film, haemolysis screen, and stool culture to assess for a thrombotic microangiopathy (see Chapter 170). In vasculitis, a chest X-ray and test to determine the diffusion constant for carbon monoxide (as this constant is elevated with pulmonary haemorrhage) are usually requested.

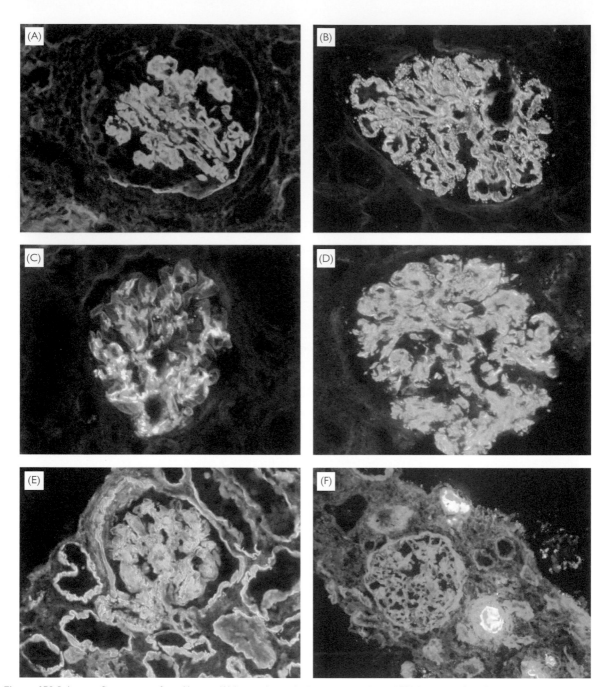

Figure 159.2 Immunofluorescence of renal biopsy. (A) Linear glomerular basement membrane (GBM) positivity for IgG in anti-GBM disease. (B) Granular capillary wall positivity for IgG in membranous nephropathy. (C) Mesangial positivity for IgA in IgA nephropathy. (D) Mesangial and capillary wall positivity for C3 in C3 glomerulonephritis. (E) Mesangial and tubular basement membrane positivity for kappa light chains in light chain deposition disease. (F) Positivity for lambda light chains in tubular casts in light chain cast nephropathy. Please see colour plate section.
Reproduced with permission from Turner, Oxford Textbook of Clinical Nephrology, Fourth Edition Oxford University Press, Oxford, UK, Copyright © 2015.

Membranous nephropathy, which often presents as nephrotic syndrome, is secondary to systemic diseases, drugs, or malignancy in only a minority of cases. There are geographical differences in the prevalence of secondary causes, and these should be considered carefully for each patient. Important secondary causes are SLE in younger women, and chronic hepatitis B infection, especially in East Asia (Box 159.1). It has recently been shown that the majority of patients with idiopathic membranous nephropathy have circulating antibodies against the M-type phospholipase A2 receptor, but such antibodies are typically absent in secondary membranous nephropathy.

Renal biopsy requires a full blood count, a coagulation screen, a negative urine culture, and a renal ultrasound. If polyarteritis nodosa is suspected (because of prominent myalgias, neuropathy, hepatitis B infection, or livedo reticularis), a formal renal angiogram should be performed to exclude microaneursyms before biopsy (see Chapter 170).

Clues in screening investigations are as follows:

Clues indicating ANCA-positive vasculitis: Granulomatosis with polyangiitis (Wegener's granulomatosis) is typically associated with a positive cANCA titre and an elevated PR3 titre. Microscopic polyangitis typically has a positive pANCA titre and an elevated myeloperoxidase titre.

Clues indicating anti-GBM disease: Anti-GBM disease is indicated by a positive anti-GBM antibody titre.

Box 159.1 Conditions associated with membranous nephropathy

Autoimmune diseases
- Systemic lupus erythematosus
- Rheumatoid arthritis

Drugs
- Gold
- Penicillamine
- Captopril

Malignancy
- Carcinoma (bronchus, colon, stomach, prostate, breast)

Infections
- Hepatitis B
- Syphilis
- Filariasis
- Leprosy

Miscellaneous
- Autoimmune thyroid disease
- Diabetes mellitus

Reproduced with permission from Warrell, Cox and Firth, *Oxford Textbook of Medicine*, Fifth Edition Oxford University Press, Oxford, UK, Copyright © 2010

Clues indicating Churg–Strauss syndrome: The patient may be pANCA positive and has an associated eosinophilia.

Clues indicating mesangiocapillary GN: Type 1 mesangiocapillary GN with essential mixed cryoglobulinaemia is indicated by low C4 with positive rheumatoid factor and cryoglobulin. Look for hepatitis C co-infection. Type 2 mesangiocapillary GN (characterized by dense deposits in the glomerular basement membrane on electron microscopy) is indicated by low C3. Look for a C3 nephritic factor.

Clues indicating lupus nephritis: Lupus nephritis is associated with positive ANA and anti-double-stranded DNA antibody titres with low complement titres. Look for antiphospholipid antibodies.

Clues indicating postinfectious GN: Postinfectious GN has a low C3 with normal C4 and evidence of recent or ongoing infection.

Clues indicating Henoch–Schönlein purpura/IgA nephropathy: In Henoch–Schönlein purpura and IgA nephropathy, 50% of cases have a raised IgA, and skin biopsy demonstrates IgA.

Prognosis and how to estimate it

Prognosis is difficult to individually predict. Renal and patient survival is affected by age and the degree of renal impairment at diagnosis. Patients who are dialysis dependent at presentation have a high mortality rate. Progression in those with renal survival can be predicted by extrapolation a plot of the eGFR over time. Anti-GBM disease does not typically relapse, but most other GNs can have a relapsing–remitting pattern over time. Each active phase of GN can leave behind significant chronic damage. Chronic damage with fibrosis and atrophy of the renal tubules on a renal biopsy is a marker for progression, as is significant proteinuria.

Treatment and effectiveness

Treatment can be divided into general measures and disease-specific immunosuppression.

General measures

Fluid overload is treated with salt and water restriction, and diuretic therapy or dialysis. Hypertension should be treated.

Immunosuppression

Immunosuppression is often given as a short, intense course of high-dose immunosuppression (induction) followed by low-dose, long-term therapy (maintenance). The aim is to balance toxicity with efficacy. All drugs predispose to infection as well as other drug-specific toxicities. Specific regimes have been designed for each disease. As many of the diseases are rare, the evidence base for treatment is often weak. This and the potential toxicity of any therapy should be explained to the patient.

Commonly used immunosuppression and drug-specific side effects are given in Table 159.4.

Induction therapy for ANCA-positive vasculitis and anti-GBM disease involves high-dose immunosuppression, typically with cyclophosphamide and steroids. If the creatinine is over 500 µmol/l or there is pulmonary haemorrhage, plasma exchange may be helpful. Maintenance therapy after 3 months of induction is usually with azathioprine.

Lupus nephritis is treated if there is histological evidence of risk of progression (International Society of Nephrology Grades III and IV). Steroids, in combination with high-dose oral mycophenolate

Table 159.4 Commonly used immunosuppression and drug-specific side effects

Drug/treatment	Uses	Toxicity	Prophylaxis	Monitoring
Corticosteroids	Induction (high dose) Maintenance (low dose)	Weight gain and glucose intolerance Osteoporosis Gastric toxicity Insomnia Cataracts	Bone Gastric	Blood sugars
Cyclophosphamide	Induction	Leucopaenia Infertility Premature menopause Haemorrhagic cystitis Urothelial cancer	PJP (TB if at risk) Mesna (if IV)	White-cell count
Azathioprine	Maintenance	Leucopaenia Hepatic toxicity Skin tumour		White-cell count Liver function
Mycophenolate mofetil	Induction (high dose) Maintenance (low dose)	Leucopaenia Diarrhoea Teratogenicity		White-cell count
Rituximab	Induction/maintenance	Rare: anaphylaxis PML Autoimmunity: ITP, and thyroid disease		
Plasma exchange	Induction	Line-related infection		

Abbreviations: ITP, immune thrombocytopenia; PJP, pneumocystis jiroveci pneumonia; PML, progressive multifocal leukoencephalopathy; TB, tuberculosis.

mofetil or cyclophosphamide, have been shown to be useful in inducing remission. Maintenance therapies include mycophenolate and azathioprine. Trials are also underway to assess the effectiveness of new biological agents, such as rituximab, for these conditions.

Some GNs do not require immunosuppression. Postinfectious GN tends to resolve spontaneously with clearance of the infection. There is no convincing evidence that immunosuppression is helpful with IgA nephropathy or mesangiocapillary GN. However, mesangiocapillary GN, in conjunction with hepatitis C infection, may respond to interferon alfa and ribavirin to reduce viral load.

Further Reading

Floege J and Amann K. Primary glomerulonephritides. *Lancet* 2016; 387: 2036–48.

KDIGO Glomerulonephritis Work Group. KDIGO clinical practice guideline for glomerulonephritis. Kidney Inter Suppl 2012; 2: 139– 274.

Pani A, Porta C, Cosmai L, et al. Glomerular diseases and cancer: evaluation of underlying malignancy. *J Nephrol* 2016. 29: 143–52.

160 Interstitial renal disease

William G. Herrington, Aron Chakera, and Christopher A. O'Callaghan

Definition of the disease

Tubulointerstitial renal diseases affect the renal tubules and/or the supporting interstitial tissue around them. The glomeruli are typically spared in early disease. Acute interstitial nephritis is characterized by an inflammatory infiltrate (often containing eosinophils). Chronic tubulointerstitial nephritis (TIN) is characterized by extensive tubular atrophy and interstitial fibrosis. The processes are clinically distinct but a prolonged acute interstitial nephritis will develop into chronic disease.

Etiology

There are many different causes of tubulointerstitial renal damage. Acute interstitial nephritis is an important cause of acute kidney injury. In 90% of cases, it is caused by drugs. It is rarely caused by infections (including leptospirosis, legionella, or TB).

Chronic TIN is a slower fibrotic process. An untreated, drug-associated interstitial nephritis may develop into tubulointerstitial fibrosis. There are many other specific causes (see Table 160.1). Tubulointerstitial fibrosis is the end result of tissue ischaemia and is, therefore, a non-specific finding in nearly all causes of chronic kidney disease.

Causes of tubulointerstitial damage include drugs and toxic substances; multiple myeloma; renal infiltration; kidney cysts; renal ischaemia; autoimmune disease; and crystal formation.

Drugs and toxic substances

Drugs commonly associated with interstitial renal disease include proton-pump inhibitors, NSAIDs, antibiotics (e.g. trimethoprim, penicillins, cephalosporins, and rifampicin), and allopurinol. Analgesic nephropathy was previously reported with phenacetin (a prodrug of paracetamol), but is not seen now. Long-term lithium use can cause renal damage, but most patients with renal damage can safely be managed with a lithium alternative. If lithium must be used, levels should be kept below 1 mmol/l and continued only if necessary. Lithium also causes a nephrogenic diabetes insipidus. Chinese herb nephropathy and Balkan nephropathy are caused by ingestion of aristolochic acid and are associated with rapidly progressive disease and late urothelial tumours. Endemic Balkan nephropathy is very similar and probably also caused by aristolochic acid ingestion.

Multiple myeloma

Multiple myeloma can cause renal impairment via several mechanisms. These include cast nephropathy (30%–60%), light chain amyloidosis (20%), light chain deposition disease (10%), hyperuricaemia, and hypercalcaemia. Cast nephropathy is caused by tubular blockage and inflammation caused by casts consisting of urinary light chains and tubular Tamm–Horsfall protein. On renal biopsy, these casts can

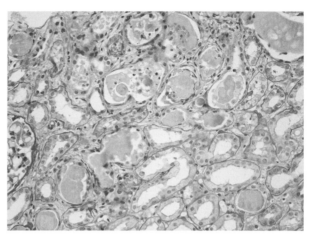

Figure 160.1 Cast nephropathy. Please see colour plate section.
Reproduced with permission from Turner et al, *Oxford Textbook of Clinical Nephrology*, Fourth Edition, Oxford University Press, Oxford, UK, Copyright © 2015.

be characteristically fractured and may be surrounded by multinucleate giant cells (see Figure 160.1).

Renal infiltration

Lymphoma and leukaemia can infiltrate the kidney and can be typed by immunohistochemistry on biopsy. Tuberculosis can infiltrate the kidney and causes granulomas. The differential of granulomatous interstitial nephritis includes tuberculosis, sarcoidosis, Sjögren's syndrome, and drugs.

Kidney cysts

Kidney cysts can be macroscopic (polycystic kidney disease) or microscopic (nephronophthis and medullary cystic kidney disease). These are discussed in Chapter 169.

Renal ischaemia

Sickle cell erythrocytes may obstruct flow in the relatively hypoxic medullary capillaries. Recurrent ischaemic damage results in tubulointerstitial fibrosis. Papillary necrosis can occur and cause loin pain and macroscopic haematuria.

Autoimmune disease

In the autoimmune disease tubulointerstitial nephritis with uveitis syndrome (TINU), tubulointerstitial damage is associated with anterior uveitis, but the eye and kidney inflammation do not necessarily occur at the same time. There is often evidence of systemic upset, with

---

Table 160.1 Causes of chronic tubulointerstitial disease

Vascular/ischaemic	Drug related	Occupational	Neoplastic	Immunological	Infectious	Metabolic	Disease related	Other causes
Hypertensive nephrosclerosis	NSAIDs	Lead	Myeloma	Sjögren's syndrome	Chronic pyelonephritis	Hypercalcaemia	Polycystic kidney disease	Obstructive uropathy
Atheroembolic disease	Analgesic nephropathy	Mercury	Lymphoma	Sarcoidosis	Tuberculosis	Hypokalaemia	Nephronophthisis	Balkan nephropathy
Sickle cell anaemia	Lithium	Cadmium	Leukaemia	Tubulointerstitial nephritis with uveitis syndrome		Oxalosis	Medullary cystic kidney disease	
	Ciclosporin					Hyperuricaemia	Medullary sponge kidney	
	Chinese herb nephropathy					Cystinosis		

weight loss, a raised erythrocyte sedimentation rate (ESR), abnormal liver function, and anaemia.

Crystal formation

Hypercalcaemia and oxalosis are examples of crystals that can precipitate in the tubules and interstitium. Oxalosis is most commonly caused by small bowel resection, which affects gut oxalate absorption. It is also seen in hereditary hyperoxalosis. Hyperoxalosis also occurs acutely with ethylene glycol poisoning.

Symptoms

An acute interstitial nephritis can present with rash, arthralgias, and systemic upset. Renal function is abnormal and there may be an eosinophilia. These features, however, can be entirely absent.

In contrast, chronic TIN is often asymptomatic. Polyuria and nocturia can occur due to loss of urine concentrating ability or due to salt wasting. There may be symptoms from the underlying condition causing the TIN. Proximal tubular disease can lead to excess urinary loss of bicarbonate, sodium, potassium, phosphate, and glucose. The patient has a normal anion gap acidosis, with hypokalaemia, hypouricaemia, and hypophosphataemia. Disease of the more distal nephron can cause distal renal tubular acidosis. Late disease is associated with glomerular fibrosis and the usual manifestations of chronic kidney disease.

Demographics

Acute interstitial nephritis peaks in the late middle age and has no sex predilection. Tubulointerstitial disease demographics are dictated by the underlying etiology. TINU predominately affects young females.

Natural history, and complications

Most cases of acute interstitial nephritis resolve spontaneously with withdrawal of the causative drug. Between 10% and 20% of patients entering dialysis in the developed world have end-stage renal disease due to one or another of the tubulointerstitial diseases. However, the rate of renal progression is very variable. There is an increased risk of urothelial malignancy with analgesic nephropathy, Chinese herb nephropathy, and Balkan endemic nephropathy. Annual urine dipstick testing and cytology is recommended.

Approach to diagnosing the disease

The diagnosis is usually made on the basis of history, examination, and a series of screening tests. The classic triad of rash, eosinophilia, and arthralgias are present in only 10% of acute interstitial nephritis. Acute interstitial nephritis may occur more than a year after the first prescription of the offending drug.

Urinalysis can be normal or exhibit a sterile pyuria, glycosuria, or low-grade proteinuria. The urinary protein:creatinine ratio is generally less than 100 mg/mmol. If there is salt wasting due to an impairment of tubular function, then hypertension is typically absent. The key blood tests include electrolytes, creatinine, and bone and liver chemistry. Urine microscopy may find eosinophils.

Depending on the clinical context, specific investigations may be indicated. These may include a paraprotein screen (urinary free light chains, and serum protein electrophoresis) and an autoimmune screen, which may include an ESR test; tests for rheumatoid factor and antinuclear, anti-Ro, and anti-La antibodies; a test to measure serum angiotensin-converting enzyme; and collection of early morning urine samples (x3) to look for acid-fast bacilli.

Ultrasound scanning in chronic tubulointerstitial disease usually demonstrates small kidneys. Multiple small simple cysts in small

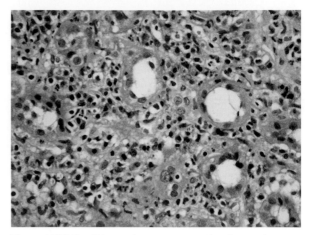

Figure 160.2 Renal biopsy of an acute interstitial nephritis with oedema and a prominent inflammatory infiltrate of lymphocytes and eosinophils separating the tubules (image courtesy of Ian Roberts). Please see colour plate section.

Reproduced with permission from Turner et al, *Oxford Textbook of Clinical Nephrology*, Fourth Edition, Oxford University Press, Oxford, UK, Copyright © 2015.

kidneys are common. Large encysted kidneys suggest polycystic kidney disease. Kidneys that are of normal size despite evidence of significant chronic renal impairment may suggest infiltrative disease or myeloma.

'Gold-standard' diagnostic test

The diagnosis of tubulointerstitial disease is confirmed on renal biopsy. The biopsy may indicate the underlying cause (see Figure 160.2).

Acceptable diagnostic alternatives

A biopsy is also not always necessary in the presence of a suitable clinical finding. However, it is usually performed in the acute setting. It is also recommended in a suspected chronic TIN if there is diagnostic doubt or a course of potentially toxic treatment is to be recommended (e.g. corticosteroids).

Prognosis and how to estimate it

Inflammation is reversible and, hence, acute interstitial nephritis often exhibits some recovery on removal of the causative insult. Progression of chronic TIN can be predicted from a plot of 1/creatinine or the estimated glomerular filtration rate against time, once the cause has been treated.

Treatment and effectiveness

The aim is to identify the causative agent and remove further exposure. Drug-associated acute interstitial nephritis may recover more quickly with steroids, and many nephrologists will prescribe a course. There is no reliably designed randomized control trial. Specific causes should be treated appropriately.

Further Reading

Wise GJ and Schlegel PN. Sterile pyuria. *N Engl J Med* 2015; 372: 1048–54.

161 Nephrotic syndrome

William G. Herrington, Aron Chakera, and Christopher A. O'Callaghan

Definition of the disease

Nephrotic syndrome is a clinical syndrome of heavy proteinuria (greater than 3.5 g per 24 hours), oedema, and hypoalbuminaemia, which is associated with hyperlipidaemia and a procoagulant state.

Etiology of nephrotic syndrome

The glomerular filtration barrier restricts proteinuria to around 30 mg/day (of which albumin is around 10 mg). The barrier consists of fenestrated endothelium (negatively charged), glomerular basement membrane, and a slit diaphragm of interdigitating podocyte foot processes. Loss of normal podocyte function and morphology is associated with albumin leakage through the barrier. Various factors contribute to sodium retention. For example, plasminogen is amongst the proteins lost in the urine and is cleaved by urokinase in the distal tubule to plasmin. Plasmin activates the epithelial sodium channel, driving salt and water retention, and oedema. In addition, there is activation of the renin–angiotensin–aldosterone system, which drives sodium and water retention. Lipids, smaller immunoglobulin molecules (IgG mainly), and anticoagulant clotting factors are also lost in the urine.

Causes of nephrotic syndrome are traditionally classified by their histopathological descriptions. In most cases, the histological picture can have a primary (idiopathic) or secondary cause. Minimal change, membranous nephropathy, and focal segmental glomerulosclerosis account for over 60% of cases.

Primary causes of nephrotic syndrome

Minimal change disease

The pathogenesis of minimal change disease remains unclear. The disease may be triggered by viral infections, NSAIDs, and, rarely, malignancy. Oedema is often massive, with periorbital swelling, pleural effusions, and ascites.

Membranous nephropathy

Membranous nephropathy (see Chapter 159) is associated with autoantibodies directed against the M-type phospholipase A2 receptor (PLA2R) in ~70% of cases. Secondary causes include malignancies (breast, lung, colon, renal cell, and lymphoma), particularly in the >65 age group, and drugs such as gold, D-penicillamine, and captopril. Infective causes include hepatitis B and C and other chronic infections. Lupus nephritis (type V) can have histological features of membranous nephropathy.

Focal segmental glomerulosclerosis

A circulating factor is implicated in idiopathic focal segmental glomerulosclerosis. Focal segmental glomerulosclerosis can also be secondary. Causes include HIV, hyperfiltration induced by reduced nephron numbers (e.g. renal dysplasia, reflux nephropathy, renovascular disease), and morbid obesity.

Mesangiocapillary glomerulonephritis

Mesangiocapillary glomerulonephritis is also known as membranoproliferative glomerulonephritis. Type 1 mesangiocapillary glomerulonephritis is characterized by immune complex deposition, and activation of the classical complement pathway. It is more common in the developing world, where it is associated with recurrent infections. It can be associated with cryoglobulins and a hepatitis C infection. Type 2 mesangiocapillary glomerulonephritis is now referred to as 'dense deposit disease' and is caused by abnormal activation of the alternative complement pathway.

Secondary causes of nephrotic syndrome

Glomerulosclerosis

Glomerulosclerosis caused by diabetes can sometimes result in proteinuria severe enough to cause nephrotic syndrome, but symptoms are usually not marked. (see Chapter 164).

Renal amyloidosis

Renal amyloidosis usually occurs as part of systemic amyloid deposition. Ninety per cent of patients with amyloid have kidney involvement; 60% have nephrotic-range proteinuria (see Chapter 170).

Monoclonal deposition diseases

Monoclonal deposition diseases are a heterogeneous group of conditions caused by plasma cell dyscrasias where the deposits are fibrils that do not organize into discrete fibrils and are therefore Congo red negative. Only 30% will have a detectable monoclonal paraprotein. Assessment of serum free light chains may assist in monitoring the underlying disease.

Symptoms

Patients present with progressive weight gain with peripheral oedema and often orthopnoea. Urine may be frothy. Creatinine is often normal (at least initially).

Demographics

Minimal change disease is the dominant cause of childhood nephrotic syndrome. It also represents 25% of adult nephrosis. Membranous nephropathy and focal segmental glomerulosclerosis are the commonest causes of nephrotic syndrome in the developed world. Nephrotic syndrome is rare before 35 years of age and peaks in the fifth and sixth decades. Black patients with nephrotic syndrome have focal segmental glomerulosclerosis in two-thirds of cases.

Complications of the disease

Large fluid shifts associated with hypoalbuminaemia or treatment can cause acute kidney injury with acute tubular necrosis. There is an increased risk of thrombosis. Loin pain, haematuria, and increasing creatinine may herald renal vein thrombosis (screen with a magnetic resonance venogram) (see Figure 161.1). Infections with capsulated organisms are increased due to low immunoglobulin levels. Longstanding proteinuria predisposes to progressive loss of renal function.

Approach to diagnosing the disease

Diagnosis can be delayed if a patient with oedema does not have a urine dipstick analysis performed. Nephrotic-range proteinuria will show up as at least 3+ protein on urinalysis. The diagnosis is confirmed by a protein–creatinine ratio over 300 mg/mmol, and hypoalbuminaemia. In adults, renal biopsy is the diagnostic test. Minimal change disease classically presents with rapid onset gross peripheral and facial oedema, and haematuria is usually absent. Demographics and associated findings may be pointers. A peripheral neuropathy may be associated with amyloidosis or a cryoglobulinaemia.

Standard investigations are used to help with diagnosis, assess severity, and prepare for a renal biopsy. A urinary PCR, renal function,

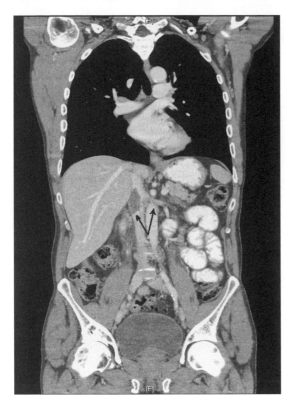

Figure 161.1 CT scan demonstrating renal vein and inferior vena cava thrombus.
Image courtesy of Nigel Cowan.

fasting lipids, and albumin confirm nephrotic syndrome. A renal biopsy requires a full blood count, coagulation screen, renal ultrasound, urine microscopy, and culture. Tests to aid the diagnosis of the etiology include a liver function test; a bone chemistry blood test; tests for antinuclear antibody, complement proteins C3 and C4, and

antineutrophil cytoplasmic antibody, as well as an immunoglobulins test; serum and urine electrophoresis; anti-PLA2R antibodies; hepatitis virus serology; and a C-reactive protein test. In mesangiocapillary glomerulonephritis, an isolated low C4 may indicate the presence of cryoglobulins. An isolated low C3 may indicate the presence of C3 nephritic factor.

Differential diagnosis

Causes of hypoalbuminaemia without nephrotic-range proteinuria are frequently confused with nephrotic syndrome. These include liver failure, acute and chronic inflammatory states, malnutrition, and malabsorption.

'Gold-standard' diagnostic test

Histological findings in nephrotic syndrome are given in Table 161.1; also see Figure 161.2.

Acceptable diagnostic alternatives

In children, a renal biopsy is rarely performed, as minimal change disease dominates the cause. Instead, children are given a trial of corticosteroid.

Treatment

Treatment is divided into general supportive measures applicable to all nephrotic syndrome causes, and disease-specific measures.

General measures

General measures are as follows:

Salt and water restriction: Aim for 0.5 to 1.0 kg weight loss a day until oedema is controlled. This is partially achieved by restricting salt (3 g a day if possible) and fluid (as low as 500 ml a day, if required).

Diuretics: Large doses of diuretics are often required. If 250 mg of furosemide is insufficient, metolozone (a thiazide diuretic) is added. Amiloride may have a specific role in treatment through blockade of the epithelial sodium channel. Close monitoring of

Table 161.1 Histological findings in nephrotic syndrome			
Disease	**Light microscopy**	**Immunofluorescence**	**Electron microscopy**
Minimal change disease	Normal	Negative	Podocyte foot-process effacement
Membranous nephropathy	Glomerular basement membrane thickening with sub-epithelial 'spikes' on silver staining	IgG positive C3 positive	Sub-epithelial electron-dense deposits (often with foot-process effacement)
Lupus nephritis (type V)	Glomerular basement membrane thickening	IgA/IgG/IgM positive C1q/C3/C4 positive (full house)	Sub-epithelial and mesangial electron-dense deposits (often with foot-process effacement)
Focal segmental glomerulosclerosis	Focal (some glomeruli are spared) segmental (only some parts of glomeruli are affected) mesangial matrix expansion with sclerosis Collapsing glomerular tufts suggest HIV	IgM positive C3 positive	
Mesangiocapillary glomerulonephritis	Capillary-wall thickening with basement membrane duplication +/− mesangial hypercellularity	Type 1: granular IgG positive C3 positive Type 2: C3 positive only	Type 1: Sub-endothelial immune complex deposits Type 2: Linear, dense deposits with glomerular basement membrane +/− mesangial hypercellularity
Diabetic glomerulosclerosis	Mesangial expansion Nodular glomerulosclerosis (Kimmelstiel–Wilson disease)	Negative	Glomerular basement membrane thickening
Renal amyloidosis	Amorphous pale hyaline deposits in glomeruli and arteries with positive Congo red stain	AL: Light chain positive (75% lambda) AA: −S-AA +	8–10 nm amyloid fibrils
Light chain deposition disease	Nodular glomerulosclerosis; negative for Congo red	AL: light chain positive (65% kappa)	Electron-dense material along glomerular and tubular basement membranes

Abbreviations: AA, AA protein-related renal amyloidosis; AL, amyloid light chain amyloidosis.
Note: Renal biopsy is the 'gold-standard' investigation in adults.

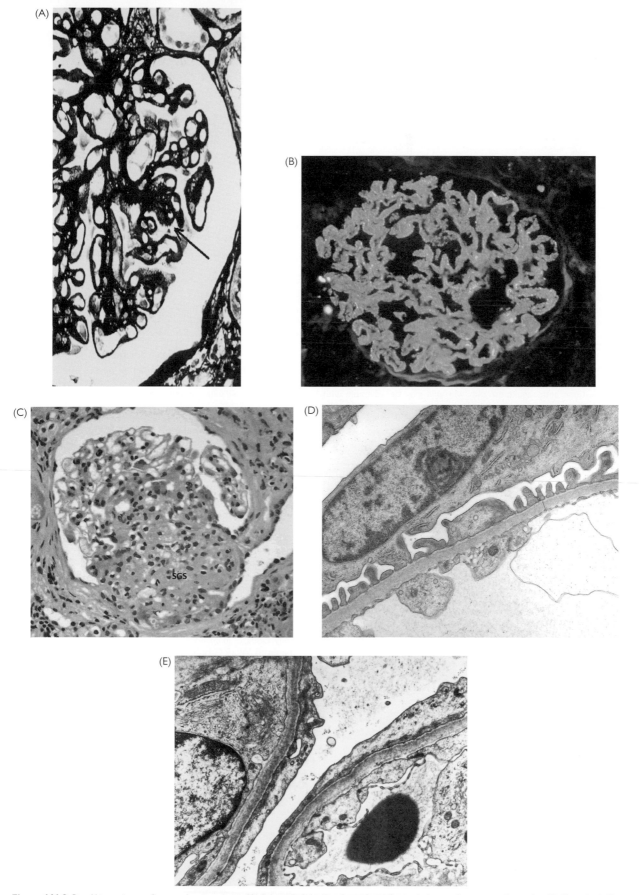

Figure 161.2 Renal biopsy images from nephrotic patients. (A) Sub-epithelial spikes (arrow) on silver stain in membranous nephropathy. (B) Granular IgG on immunofluorescence in membranous nephropathy. (C) Focal segmental glomerulosclerosis (indicated by SGS). (D) Normal podocytes. (E) Podocyte effacement on electron microscopy. Please see colour plate section.

images courtesy of Ian Roberts Reproduced with permission from Turner et al, Oxford Textbook of Clinical Nephrology, Fourth Edition, Oxford University Press, Oxford, UK, Copyright © 2015.

Table 161.2 Commonly used immunosuppression, and drug-specific side effects

Drug/treatment	Uses	Toxicity	Prophylaxis	Monitoring
Corticosteroids	Induction (high dose) Maintenance (low dose)	Weight gain and glucose Intolerance Osteoporosis Gastric toxicity Insomnia Cataracts	Bone Gastric	Blood glucose
Cyclophosphamide	Induction	Leucopenia Infertility Premature menopause Haemorrhagic cystitis Urothelial cancers	PJP (TB if at risk) Mesna (if IV)	White-cell count
Ciclosporin	Induction Maintenance	Nephrotoxicity Tremor/hirsutism/gum hypertrophy Dyslipidaemia Hypertension		Drug levels Renal function

Abbreviations: IV, intravenous; PJP, *Pneumocystis jiroveci* pneumonia; TB, tuberculosis.

fluid balance and electrolytes is required, as the response can be profound.

Angiotensin-converting enzyme inhibition: Angiotensin-converting enzyme inhibitors should be used; alternatively, angiotensin II receptor blockers can be used in the long term.

Blood pressure control: The current recommended target for blood pressure in the presence of heavy proteinuria is ≤130/80 mm Hg.

Anticoagulation: Inpatients should receive prophylactic heparin; long-term anticoagulation with warfarin may be advisable with severe nephrotic syndrome and when the albumin is consistently below 20 g/dl.

Lipid-lowering therapy: Dietary modification, together with a statin-based regimen, should be used.

Specific treatments

Treatment of a secondary cause often successfully treats the nephrotic syndrome. This is, however, not usually the case in diabetic nephrosclerosis. Primary causes also have specific treatments.

Treatment of minimal change disease

Minimal change disease will remit within 3 months in 90% of cases with a course of high-dose corticosteroids. Treatment-resistant cases may be focal segmental glomerulosclerosis that was not detected on biopsy due to a sampling error. Relapse is common. Frequent relapsing, and steroid-dependent disease, can be treated with ciclosporin or a course of cyclophosphamide (see Table 161.2).

Treatment of membranous nephropathy

Membranous nephropathy treatment is reserved for disease associated with a poor prognosis. Up to a third of cases spontaneously improve. Indications of poor prognosis include persistent nephrosis for a year, proteinuria greater than 10 g per day, and falling renal function. The modified 'Ponticelli regime' is a 6-month course of alternating corticosteroid with oral cyclophosphamide and may be preferable

to the traditional alternative ciclosporin. Rituximab, and tacrolimus are sometimes used. A suggested screen for associated malignancy includes a chest X-ray, mammogram, a prostate-specific antigen test, and endoscopy if faecal occult blood tests are positive.

Treatment of focal segmental glomerulosclerosis

Focal segmental glomerulosclerosis can be treated with a 6-month course of high-dose corticosteroids. HIV-associated nephropathy is effectively treated with antiretroviral agents.

Treatment of mesangiocapillary glomerulonephritis

Mesangiocapillary glomerulonephritis has a poor prognosis, as there is no proven therapy other than general measures. End-stage renal disease occurs in 50% at 10 years and it frequently recurs following transplantation.

Treatment of diabetic glomerulosclerosis

Diabetic glomerulosclerosis is treated with intensive blood pressure and glycaemic control.

Treatment of renal amyloidosis and monoclonal deposition diseases

Renal amyloidosis and monoclonal deposition diseases are managed by treatment of the underlying chronic disease or plasma cell dyscrasia.

Further Reading

Kidney Disease: Improving Global Outcomes (KDIGO) Glomerulonephritis Work Group. KDIGO clinical practice guideline for glomerulonephritis. *Kidney Inter Suppl* 2012; 2: 139–274.

Königshausen E and Sellin L. Recent treatment advances and new trials in adult nephrotic syndrome. *BioMed Res. Int.* (2017), Article ID 7689254. https://doi.org/10.1155/2017/7689254

162 Acute kidney injury

Aron Chakera, William G. Herrington, and Christopher A. O'Callaghan

Definition of the disease

Acute kidney injury (also referred to as acute renal failure) refers to a rapid decrease in renal function; it is reflected by an increase in blood urea and creatinine and is often associated with oliguria (a urine volume of less than 400 ml/24 hours). It usually develops over days to weeks. Acute kidney injury has been variously classified, but the current classifications are based on the glomerular filtration rate (or creatinine), looking at changes from baseline, and the presence of oliguria or anuria. The KDIGO (Kidney Disease: Improving Global Outcomes) staging system is shown in Table 162.1. In this classification system, acute kidney injury is indicated by one or more of the following:

- an increase in creatinine by ≥26.5 µmol/l within 48 hours
- an increase in creatinine to ≥1.5 times baseline, known or presumed to have occurred within the prior 7 days
- urine volume <0.5 ml/kg h^{-1} for 6 hours

Etiology of the disease

The potential etiologies of acute kidney injury are usually considered anatomically under the headings prerenal, renal (intrinsic), and postrenal (Table 162.2). Relative frequencies of the major causes of acute kidney injury in hospitalized patients are given in Figure 162.1.

Typical symptoms of the disease, and less common symptoms

Due to the large physiological reserve of the kidneys, many cases of acute kidney injury are initially asymptomatic. Oliguria often precedes significant increases in urea and creatinine. Prerenal causes can be associated with low blood pressure, postural hypotension, and signs of sepsis or cardiac failure, whereas intrinsic renal diseases may cause haematuria or proteinuria (which may be noted as frothy urine) or there may be an associated rash or respiratory tract involvement, as can occur with vasculitis (see Chapters 140 and 247). Postrenal

Table 162.2 Causes of acute kidney injury

Prerenal	Hypotension
	Sepsis
	Medications
	Cardiac failure
	Hypovolaemia
	Haemorrhage
	Dehydration
	Impaired glomerular haemodynamics
	Angiotensin-converting enzyme inhibitors
	NSAIDs
	Vascular disease
	Renal artery stenosis
	Embolization
	Renal arteriole obstruction in haemolytic–uraemic syndrome
	Renal vein thrombosis
	Small vessel obstruction from accelerated phase hypertension
Prerenal/renal	Hepatorenal syndromes
	Pulmonary-renal syndromes
Renal (intrinsic)	Glomeruli
	Antiglomerular antibodies
	Antibody–antigen complex deposition
	Tubules
	Drug-induced tubulitis
	Antibiotics
	Contrast agents
	Chemotherapy agents
	Acute tubular necrosis (usually provoked by prerenal causes)
	Acute cortical necrosis (usually provoked by prerenal causes)
	Obstruction with casts, stones
	Interstitium
	Infection
	Granulomatous diseases
Postrenal	Ureteral obstruction
	Stones
	Tumours
	Sloughed papillae
	Clots
	Bladder outflow obstruction
	Benign prostatic hypertrophy
	Gynaecological malignancy
	Neurogenic bladder
	Urethral obstruction
	Strictures
	Intra-renal crystalluria

Table 162.1 KDIGO (Kidney Disease: Improving Global Outcomes) classification of acute kidney injury in adults

	Serum creatinine	Urine output
1	1.5–1.9 times baseline Or ≥26.5 umol/l increase	<0.5 ml/kg/h for 6–12 hours
2	2.0–2.9 times baseline	<0.5 ml/kg/h for ≥ 12 hours
3	3.0 times baseline Or Increase to ≥ 353.6 umol/l Or Initiation of renal replacement therapy	<0.3 ml/kg/h for ≥ 12 hours Anuria for ≥ 12 hours
Loss	Persistent ARF (complete loss of kidney function) >4 weeks	
ESRD	ESRD >3 months	

Abbreviations: ARF, acute renal failure; ESRD, end-stage renal disease.

Reprinted by permission from Macmillan Publishers Ltd: *Kidney International Supplements*. Kidney Disease: Improving Global Outcomes (KDIGO) Acute Kidney Injury Work Group. KDIGO clinical practice guideline for acute kidney injury. 2(1):1-138, copyright 2012. http://www.nature.com/ki/index.html.

causes may present with abdominal or loin pain and, in males, there is often a history of prostatic symptoms. Late presentations may be associated with electrolyte disturbances, especially hyperkalaemia (see Chapter 173), as well as confusion, a metallic taste, or pericardial and pleural effusions from uraemia.

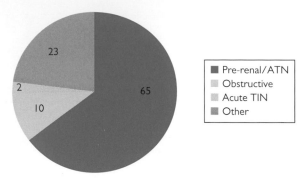

Figure 162.1 Relative frequencies of the major causes of acute kidney injury in hospitalized patients; ATN, acute tubular necrosis; TIN, tubulointerstitial nephritis.

Demographics of the disease

Acute kidney injury occurs in up to 10% of patients admitted to hospital, with an increased incidence in the elderly and patients in critical care settings. Patients with preexisting renal impairment or cardiovascular disease are particularly vulnerable. There is no racial or gender bias. The demographics follow the causes (Table 162.3)

Natural history, and complications of the disease

In hospitalized patients, the development of acute kidney injury is associated with a mortality of up to 50% in some series. Early diagnosis and correction of significant electrolyte abnormalities, together with optimization of fluid balance, are essential to minimize the incidence of complications. Death is usually from cardiac arrhythmias or pulmonary oedema. As acute kidney injury in hospital is usually the consequence of the conditions leading to hospitalization (rather than the cause), the natural history is highly dependent on the management of these condition (e.g. sepsis, cardiac failure). If treated early, many prerenal causes may be rapidly reversible; however, if treatment is delayed, and acute tubular necrosis results, a period of established renal failure lasting weeks may occur. If the renal insult is more profound, acute cortical necrosis may occur which may not be reversible.

Approach to diagnosing the disease

Unless there are prior results available, all elevations in urea and creatinine should be assumed to represent acute kidney injury. Potential causes can be considered anatomically and divided into prerenal, renal, and postrenal (see Chapter 156 for further details). A thorough medication history (including documentation of any herbal remedies and over-the-counter preparations taken) as well as a detailed family history should be elicited. Males should be directly questioned regarding symptoms of prostatic disease.

As many systemic diseases affect the kidneys, a complete examination should be performed, including fundoscopy (hypertensive changes, Roth's spots, and cholesterol emboli), inspection of the skin for rashes (SLE, IgA nephropathy, vasculitis, sepsis), palpation of the bladder and, where indicated, digital rectal examination in males. Dipstick urinalysis, ideally from a non-catheter specimen, is an essential part of the workup, with active urinary sediment (containing blood, protein, and/or leukocytes) being consistent with intrinsic renal disease. As patients with acute kidney injury may be unwell and unable to give a full history or cooperate with examination, it is essential to review any available notes. This includes operation and anaesthetic records, as the majority of cases of acute kidney injury developing in hospital have an easily recognizable cause, such as a period of perioperative hypotension or the prescription of a nephrotoxic drug.

Table 162.3 Causes of development of acute impairment of renal function in 2216 consecutive medical and surgical admissions

Cause	Number of patients
Acute tubular necrosis	
• Hypovolaemia	22
• Congestive cardiac failure	10
• Sepsis	10
• Nephrotoxins	25
• Postsurgical	23
• Other	12
Hepatorenal syndrome	5
Obstruction	3
Vasculitis	2
Other/multifactorial/unknown	17
Total	129 (5.8% of admissions)

Reproduced with permission from Warrell, Cox and Firth, Oxford Textbook of Medicine, Fifth Edition Oxford University Press, Oxford, UK, Copyright © 2010.

Other diagnoses that should be considered

Acute renal impairment in hospitalized patients is usually prerenal in aetiology, so particular attention should be given to assessing cardiac function and fluid balance. A rough heuristic is that the ratio of the creatinine (μmol/l) to urea (μmol/l) should be ~20:1 (i.e. someone with a urea of 20 μmol/l would be expected to have a creatinine of ~400 μmol/l). Significant elevations of this ratio (e.g. urea of 35 μmol/l with a creatinine of 400 μmol/l) should raise the suspicion of dehydration (necessitating optimization of fluid balance) or gut haemorrhage. Syndromes associated with acute kidney injury are given in Table 162.4.

'Gold-standard' diagnostic test

The gold-standard diagnostic test is measurement of the serum urea and creatinine, demonstrating an acute deterioration in renal function. Oliguria often precedes changes in creatinine and urea.

Acceptable diagnostic alternatives to the gold standard

A variety of biomarkers are under investigation to improve the early identification of acute kidney injury (e.g. cystatin C, neutrophil gelatinase-associated lipocalin, and kidney injury molecule-1). Currently, these are not generally available for clinical use.

Other relevant investigations

It is essential to ensure that the patient is not dangerously hyperkalaemic. An ECG should be performed and the patient placed onto cardiac monitoring. If there are diagnostic ECG changes, initial treatment should be commenced while awaiting laboratory results (see Chapter 173).

Renal tract ultrasonography can provide information on renal size and morphology (which may support the presence of some preexisting renal impairment), identify obstruction, and, in most cases, comment on renal blood flow and perfusion. If there is rhabdomyolysis, serum creatinine kinase is usually substantially elevated.

Where intrinsic renal disease is suspected from systemic causes, immunological tests, including tests to detect anti-double-stranded DNA antibodies, antinuclear antibodies, antineutrophil cytoplasmic antibodies, anti-glomerular basement membrane antibodies, and complement proteins C3 and C4, may be indicated, as may viral serology, and assessment for a paraprotein with urine and plasma electrophoresis or free light chain quantification. Often, a definitive diagnosis of the underlying cause requires a renal biopsy.

Table 162.4 Syndromes associated with acute kidney injury

Acute kidney injury and a rash	Vasculitis
	Infective endocarditis
	Cryoglobulinaemia
	Sepsis
	SLE
	Henoch–Schönlein purpura/thrombotic thrombocytopenic purpura
Acute kidney injury and jaundice	Hepatorenal syndrome
	Infections (e.g. leptospirosis, EBV, CMV)
	Drugs (e.g. anaesthetic agents)
	Sickle cell disease
	Severe sepsis
Acute kidney injury and hypercalcaemia	Myeloma
	Malignancy
	Milk-alkali syndrome
	Sarcoid
Acute kidney injury and lung involvement	Pneumonia with ATN (or TIN)
	Systemic vasculitis
	SLE
	Goodpasture's disease
Acute kidney injury and joint involvement	Systemic vasculitis
	SLE
	Amyloidosis
Acute kidney injury and haemolysis	Haemolytic–uraemic syndrome/thrombotic thrombocytopenic purpura
	Accelerated hypertension
	Scleroderma
	Pre-eclampsia

Abbreviations: ATN, acute tubulointerstitial nephritis; CMV, cytomegalovirus; EBV, Epstein–Barr virus; SLE, systemic lupus erythematosus; TIN, tubulointerstitial nephritis.

Particularly in older patients, routine testing of thyroid function may be worthwhile, as subclinical hypothyroidism can cause significant elevations in creatinine.

Prognosis and how to estimate it

The prognosis of acute kidney injury is largely dependent on the underlying aetiology. The poor outcome of acute kidney injury in hospitalized patients largely reflects significant comorbidities in this population, with these having led to the renal impairment. When the inciting agent(s) are removed or the underlying cause treated, many patients with acute kidney injury due to prerenal causes can be expected to recover to their baseline level of renal function, even should they reach the point of temporarily requiring renal replacement therapy. Where intrinsic renal disease is suspected, a renal biopsy may provide some information regarding prognosis (e.g. percentage of sclerosed glomeruli and degree of tubular atrophy).

Treatment and its effectiveness

Therapy in acute kidney injury is initially directed at managing any immediate life threats (e.g. hyperkalaemia or pulmonary oedema) before identifying and treating any underlying causes.

Management of prerenal renal impairment aims to improve renal perfusion, by optimizing fluid balance and blood pressure and stopping any offending medications, such as angiotensin-converting enzyme inhibitors, angiotensin receptor blockers, or NSAIDs. When assessment of intravascular fluid status is difficult, insertion of a central line for central venous pressure monitoring and/or an arterial line for accurate measurement of blood pressure, and considering the use of inotropic agents to improve renal perfusion, may be indicated.

Postrenal causes are managed by relieving the obstruction, by catheterization or insertion of a nephrostomy tube. (Note that unilateral obstruction should not cause an elevation in the urea or creatinine, provided the unaffected kidney is normal.)

Management of intrinsic kidney injury is directed at the underlying abnormality where possible, for example, cessation of medications that may be responsible for interstitial nephritis, or commencement of immunosuppression in autoimmune diseases. Where appropriate, dialysis may be instituted (either haemodialysis or, less commonly, peritoneal dialysis) to support patients through the acute illness, with the hope of eventual renal recovery. For patients who are haemodynamically unstable, haemofiltration is often preferred to haemodialysis. This is a slower therapy that minimizes rapid fluid and electrolyte shifts; it is used by most intensive care units. Up to 10% of patients will remain dialysis dependent following the development of acute kidney injury.

Further Reading

Kidney Disease: Improving Global Outcomes (KDIGO) Acute Kidney Injury Work Group. KDIGO clinical practice guideline for acute kidney injury. *Kidney Inter Suppl* 2012; 2: 1–138.

National Institute for Health and Care Excellence. Acute kidney injury: prevention, detection and management. Clinical guideline [CG169] 2013. https://www.nice.org.uk/guidance/cg169?unlid=42993108620169292525215.

Rosner MH and Perazella MA. Acute kidney injury in patients with cancer. *N Engl J Med* 2017; 376: 1770–81.

163 Chronic kidney disease

William G. Herrington, Aron Chakera, and Christopher A. O'Callaghan

Definition of the disease

Chronic kidney disease (CKD) is defined as abnormalities of kidney structure or function, where the abnormalities have been present for >3 months and have implications for health. It is characterized by a reduced estimated glomerular filtration rate (eGFR) or other renal abnormalities. CKD is staged according to the eGFR (see Table 163.1) or the degree of albuminuria (see Table 163.2). The KDIGO (Kidney Disease: Improving Global Outcomes) criteria for CKD is either an eGFR that is <60 ml/min 1.73 m^{-2} and has been present for >3 months, or one or more markers of kidney damage, when these have been present for >3 months. The accepted markers of kidney damage are:

- albuminuria (albumin excretion rate ≥30 mg/24 hours; albumin–creatinine ratio ≥3 mg/mmol)
- urine sediment abnormalities
- electrolyte and other abnormalities due to tubular disorders
- abnormalities detected by histology
- structural abnormalities detected by imaging
- history of kidney transplantation

The staging uses the eGFR to produce a 'G' stage (Table 163.1), and albuminuria to produce an 'A' stage (Table 163.2). These are combined so that a patient will have both a 'G' and an 'A' stage (e.g. G4, A3). Stage G5 is often referred to as end-stage renal disease. This staging does not incorporate information on the precise diagnosis, on comorbidities, or on the historical rate of renal decline, all of which may be important in assessing the significance of CKD for an individual patient.

Etiology of CKD

There are many causes of CKD, but the most common are diabetes, hypertension, and renovascular disease. Diabetes mellitus is the commonest cause of end-stage renal disease in developed countries and accounts about a quarter of new dialysis patients in the UK (see Figure 163.1).

Symptoms

The biochemical and physiological derangements of CKD occur much earlier than the clinical manifestations (Table 163.3). Therefore, most patients with CKD are asymptomatic. The subtle and late

Table 163.2 KDIGO (Kidney Disease: Improving Global Outcomes) albuminuria, or 'A', staging system for chronic kidney disease

Albuminuria or A stage	AER (albumin excretion rate)	ACR (albumin–creatinine ratio)
A1	<30 mg/24 hours	<3 mg/mmol
A2	30–300 mg/24 hours	30–30 mg/mmol
A3	>300 mg/24 hours	>30 mg/mmol

Reproduced with permission from Kidney Disease: Improving Global Outcomes (KDIGO) Acute Kidney Injury Work Group. KDIGO clinical practice guideline for acute kidney injury. Kidney Int Suppl. 2012 Mar;2(1):1–138.

symptomatology of CKD accounts for late presentations and a large untreated population with early disease. Unfortunately, it is not uncommon for a patient's first contact with renal services to be for the initiation of dialysis.

Polyuria and nocturia can arise if there is a loss of renal tubular concentrating ability. Oedema and hypertension present later and can reflect either a defect in the regulation of body salt and water content associated with raised renin levels or, in the later stages, a loss of ability to excrete salt and water. Renal anaemia causes tiredness. The classic 'uraemic' symptoms, including persistent nausea and vomiting, anorexia, malaise, and itching, are uncommon until there is severe renal impairment with an eGFR usually well below 15 ml/min 1.73 m^{-2}. Renal replacement therapy is often started on the basis of these 'uraemic' symptoms before there is an absolute biochemical need.

Demographics of CKD

The prevalence of CKD depends on the definition used. The prevalence of CKD Stages 3–5 as defined in Table 163.1 may be as high as 10% in Western developed populations. Renal function declines with age, so most CKD occurs in the elderly. However, in the elderly, progression of CKD Stage 3 and non-proteinuric CKD Stage 4 to end-stage renal disease is rare. A fatal cardiovascular event is much more common. Consequently, the prevalence of CKD Stage 5 is perhaps as low as 0.2%. The rising prevalence of obesity and diabetes, and the growing elderly population, are, however, increasing the numbers of patients on renal replacement therapy by up to 6% per annum.

Table 163.1 KDIGO (Kidney Disease: Improving Global Outcomes) estimated glomerular function rate, or 'G', staging system for chronic kidney disease

GFR or G stage	Description
G1	eGFR >90 ml/min 1.73 m^{-2} with markers of kidney damage
G2	eGFR 60–89 ml/min 1.73 m^{-2} with markers of kidney damage
G3A	eGFR 45–59 ml/min 1.73 m^{-2}
G3B	eGFR 30–44 ml/min 1.73 m^{-2}
G4	eGFR 15–29 ml/min 1.73 m^{-2}
G5	eGFR <15 ml/min 1.73 m^{-2} or on dialysis

Abbreviations: eGFR, estimated glomerular function rate.

Reproduced with permission from Kidney Disease: Improving Global Outcomes (KDIGO) Acute Kidney Injury Work Group. KDIGO clinical practice guideline for acute kidney injury. Kidney Int Suppl. 2012 Mar;2(1):1–138.

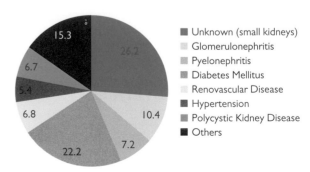

Figure 163.1 Causes of kidney disease in new maintenance renal replacement therapy patients.

data from United Kingdom Renal Registry 2007.

Table 163.3 Physical features indicating the etiology and chronicity of chronic kidney disease

System	Feature	Comment
General	Pallor	Anaemia is a common feature of advanced CKD
	Pigmentation, scratch marks, brown nails	Indicate long-standing CKD
Cardiovascular/ respiratory	Blood pressure	Hypertension is a common association (but uncommon cause) of CKD
	Elevated jugular venous pressure, enlarged heart, gallop rhythm, mitral regurgitant murmur, pulmonary crackles, peripheral oedema	Manifestations of fluid overload caused by CKD and/or cardiac failure associated with hypertension or 'uraemia'
	Aortic systolic murmur	Valvular calcification is more common in CKD
	Peripheral pulses, vascular bruits	Absence of pulses and/or presence of bruits increase the likelihood of renovascular disease as the cause of CKD
Abdominal	Palpable kidneys	Likely to indicate adult polycystic kidney disease in this context
	Palpable bladder, malignant-feeling prostate on digital examination	Consider urinary obstruction as cause of CKD
	Hernias	Require repair if peritoneal dialysis otherwise preferred as RRT
Neurological	Peripheral neuropathy	Indicates long-standing CKD
	Proximal myopathy	Indicates long-standing CKD
Rheumatological	Arthritis	Gout and pseudogout are associated with CKD
	Carpal tunnel syndrome	
Ocular fundi	Features of hypertension	

Abbreviations: CKD, chronic kidney disease; RRT, renal replacement therapy.

Reproduced with permission from the Oxford Textbook of Medicine (5th edition), Warrell, Cox and Firth (Eds), Published by Oxford University Press 2012.

Natural history and complications of CKD

CKD progresses at a different rate in different patients. Factors associated with accelerated decline are listed in Box 163.1. Some of these factors are modifiable and provide the basis for current treatment.

Proteinuria is one of the most important factors associated with chronic kidney damage. It can arise with glomerular damage and raised intra-glomerular pressures. Large amounts of proteinuria are thought to be toxic to the tubules, inducing interstitial inflammation that progresses to fibrosis. With each gram increase in daily proteinuria, there is a significant increase in risk of progression (see Figure 163.2). Proteinuria is an independent marker of cardiovascular risk. It is readily quantifiable on a spot urine protein–creatinine ratio or spot albumin–creatinine ratio and can often be reduced by controlling hypertension and inhibiting the renin–angiotensin system.

CKD is remarkable in that usually more than 90% of renal function is lost before renal replacement therapy is required. However, significant complications begin earlier.

Cardiovascular risk

A reduced eGFR is associated with an increased risk of cardiovascular events (see Figure 163.3). This continues on dialysis, where cardiovascular disease is the leading cause of death. A 20-year-old on dialysis has the same cardiovascular risk as an 80-year-old in the general population. An elderly patient with an eGFR less than 60 ml/min 1.73 m^{-2} has a 1% annual chance of progression to end-stage renal disease but a 10% risk of death.

Box 163.1 Factors that have been associated with the rapid progression of chronic kidney disease

- raised blood pressure
- poor glycaemic control
- persistent primary renal disease activity
- persistent proteinuria
- family history of progression
- recurrent urinary tract infections
- obesity
- smoking
- hyperfiltration states
- dyslipidaemia

The increased cardiovascular risk with CKD arises largely because key risk factors such as age, hypertension, and diabetes mellitus predispose to both CKD and cardiovascular disease. However, CKD does increase cardiovascular risk directly through left ventricular hypertrophy (secondary to renal-induced hypertension, chronic fluid overload, and anaemia), proteinuria, dyslipidaemia, accelerated atherosclerosis, accelerated vascular calcification, oxidative stress, inflammation, and endothelial dysfunction. Management of cardiovascular risk in CKD thus involves more than the control of blood pressure and lipids.

Mineral and bone disorders

The term 'renal osteodystrophy' has now been replaced by the term 'chronic kidney disease–mineral and bone disorders' (CKD-MBD). The kidney excretes phosphate and activates vitamin D, so renal impairment can cause hyperphosphataemia and

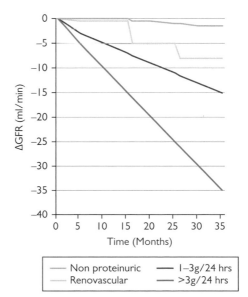

Figure 163.2 Examples of rate of glomerular filtration rate decline, stratified by degree of proteinuria or disease; ΔGFR, change in glomerular filtration rate.

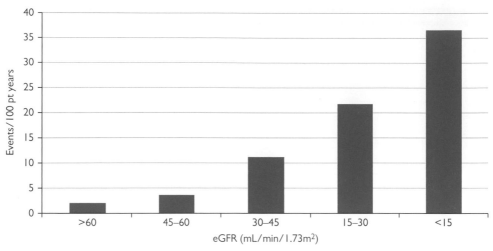

Figure 163.3 Age-standardized risk of cardiovascular events by estimated glomerular filtration rate; eGFR, estimated glomerular filtration rate. Adapted from data by Go et al. 2004.

lead to insufficient levels of active vitamin D. As a consequence, parathyroid hormone levels rise to maintain plasma ionized calcium. This hyperparathyroidism can become autonomous (tertiary hyperparathyroidism) and result in abnormal turnover of bone. In extreme cases, cystic resorption of bone (osteitis fibrosa cystica) occurs. Abnormalities of bone in renal disease can also include the changes of osteomalacia and osteoporosis. Low-turnover bone disease can arise with overzealous suppression of parathyroid hormone with vitamin D treatment and may be linked to accelerated vascular calcification. CKD patients are at higher risk of fracture from all these bony abnormalities.

Biochemical markers of bone turnover are used to direct treatment. A raised alkaline phosphatase and parathyroid hormone level indicate high bone turnover. A low parathyroid hormone level indicates possible low turnover.

Overt bone disease is, however, infrequent in renal practice. Vascular calcification, however, is two to five times greater in CKD patients than age-matched controls with coronary artery disease. Vascular smooth muscle cells can transform to osteoblast-like cells, which lay down a bone-like matrix in blood vessel media. This then calcifies in the setting of a high calcium–phosphate product. The result is increased arterial stiffness. This may explain part of the increased vascular risk in renal patients.

Renal anaemia

Deficiency of erythropoietin secretion results from the atrophy of peritubular interstitial fibroblasts. It typically can occur below an eGFR of 30 ml/min 1.73 m^{-2} (<45 in diabetics). Other causes of anaemia, especially iron deficiency, should be excluded and, occasionally, it is helpful to measure erythropoietin levels. Uraemia reduces dietary intake of iron, impairs intestinal absorption, and increases capillary fragility/platelet dysfunction, promoting gastrointestinal blood loss.

Hyperkalaemia

The kidney excretes potassium. A decreased eGFR reduces delivery of sodium to the aldosterone-mediated distal tubular Na^+/K^+ exchanger, causing potassium retention. Drugs targeting the renin–angiotensin system exacerbate this effect. Extracellular shifts of potassium are encouraged by concomitant acidosis and poor glycaemic control. Refractory hyperkalaemia is an indication for dialysis.

Acidosis

The kidneys regulate acid excretion. The accumulation of organic acids in CKD impairs bone turnover, promotes hyperkalaemia and protein catabolism, and exacerbates uraemic symptoms. Refractory acidosis is an indication for dialysis.

Fluid overload

The kidney excretes salt and water, so salt and water retention is common with renal impairment. This can cause hypertension and oedema and should be managed with diuretics and salt restriction. Occasionally, predominant tubulointerstitial disease can cause tubular salt wasting with hypotension, but this is uncommon.

Nutrition

Dietary modification is important to avoid electrolyte disorders. Potassium, phosphate, and sodium intake must be reduced. With severe disease, fluid intake may needs to be reduced. However, it is important to maintain good nutrition in CKD despite dietary restrictions.

Uraemic pericarditis and encephalopathy

These are very rare and only occur with severe uraemia. They are both indications for urgent dialysis. Pericarditis requires careful heparin-free dialysis. Encephalopathy requires careful short and slow dialysis to allow re-equilibration of uraemic small molecules across the blood brain barrier.

Approach to diagnosing the disease

A raised creatinine should be considered to be acute kidney injury unless there are grounds for believing otherwise. CKD is confirmed by longitudinal follow-up of creatinine results. It is also suggested by the finding of small kidneys on an ultrasound scan (bipolar length of less than 8 cm). Exceptions include polycystic kidneys, infiltrative diseases such as amyloid or lymphoma, and occasionally diabetes mellitus.

'Gold-standard' diagnostic test

The gold-standard' diagnostic test for CKD is longitudinal follow-up of creatinine and eGFR (see Table 163.1). Although total proteinuria is often measured, measurement of albuminuria is now regarded as the gold-standard test for assessing urinary protein loss.

Other relevant investigations

Dipstick urinalysis is important in the assessment of CKD. The absence of proteinuria or microscopic haematuria reduces the likelihood of a significant glomerular disease. Microscopic haematuria or proteinuria greater than 0.5 g/day suggests glomerular disease. Diagnosis relies on an autoimmune screen and renal biopsy. In patients above 50, isolated microscopic haematuria could arise from a urinary tract tumour, and this should be excluded in this age group.

Causes of non-proteinuric CKD include renovascular disease, ischaemic/hypertensive nephropathy, structural kidney diseases, obstructive kidney disease, and tubulointerstitial disease. Patients older than 45 years could be screened for paraproteinaemia by serum protein electrophoresis and free light chain analysis. Additional investigations include ultrasonography, magnetic resonance angiography, and, occasionally, renal biopsy. The renal biopsy is the best test to establish the cause of acute kidney injury. It is seldom of use in advanced CKD, as the biopsy is likely to show non-specific fibrotic changes. Biopsy is also often unnecessary if the diagnosis is obvious from the history, examination, or investigations.

Prognosis and how to estimate it

The progression of CKD can be predicted from a plot of 1/creatinine or eGFR against time. These graphs are commonly a straight line, and the time to dialysis can therefore be estimated by extrapolation. A change in the rate of decline may indicate a new renal insult, such as prostatic obstruction. Renovascular disease may progress in a stepwise fashion with long intervening periods of stability (see Figure 163.2).

Baseline proteinuria is a strong predictor of future progression, with >1 g/day associated with progression.

Treatment and its effectiveness

Treatment is divided into prevention of progression, modification of cardiovascular risk, and management of complications. In practice, many of the interventions used to reduce progression of CKD also reduce cardiovascular risk. Later in the disease, preparations for renal replacement therapy are made.

Prevention of progression

Specific renal diseases may require specialist treatment of the underlying condition. However, regardless of the underlying condition, it is important to control modifiable risk factors for progression (Box 163.1).

Blood pressure control is critical. An accepted target is 130/80 mm Hg, although some guidelines recommend higher or lower targets. For example, if proteinuria is greater than 1 g/day, the target may be lowered further (AASK/MDRD trials). Angiotensin-converting-enzyme (ACE) inhibitors are the first-line antihypertensives, but renal function should be checked within 2 weeks of introduction or a dose change. Commonly used second-line agents include furosemide, beta blockers, alpha-blockers, and calcium-channel blockers. The choice may be dictated by coexisting medical problems.

Proteinuria is minimized by blood pressure control. ACE inhibitors have an additional benefit beyond that of blood pressure control (REIN study). The dose should be titrated against proteinuria. Angiotensin II receptor blockade is similarly efficacious but adds no further benefit (IDN/RENALL trials).

Glycaemic control should be optimized (DCCT/UKPDS trials).

The SHARP study demonstrated that intensive lowering of LDL cholesterol reduces risk of major atherosclerotic events in CKD patients, but does not have any meaningful effect on renal progression.

Dietary protein restriction does not significantly improve progression (MDRD trial). Obesity and smoking are associated with progression and are important causes of mortality. Salt restriction and a diet high in fruit and vegetables reduce blood pressure (DASH study). Exercise 3–5 times a week is advocated.

Hyperuricaemia is independently associated with progression and can be reduced with allopurinol. However, no trial has demonstrated it slows renal progression.

Correction of acidosis with oral sodium bicarbonate may have beneficial effects, including slowing renal progression.

Acute renal insults should be minimized. Physicians should consider renal dose reduction and renal toxicity for any new medications. Patients should be advised that NSAIDs are contraindicated. It is also helpful to ask patients to stop ACE inhibitors in acute illnesses associated with hypovolaemia. Radio-opaque contrast agents should be used where there is no alternative.

Table 163.4 Suggested target ranges for CKD patients

	Target
Haemoglobin or erythropoietin (g/dl)	10–12 g/dl
Phosphate	0.9–1.5 mmol/l
Calcium–phosphate product	<4.8 mmol²/l²
Parathyroid hormone	1–2 times normal range, for Stage 4 CKD
	2–9 times normal range, for Stage 5 CKD
Bicarbonate	22–26 mmol/l

Abbreviations: CKD, chronic kidney disease.

Management of complications

There is no hard clinical endpoint trials which show that correcting anaemia, acidosis, and calcium–phosphate balance slows CKD progression, but these factors are considered important in their own right.

Renal anaemia is corrected by optimizing iron stores, often with IV iron, before administering subcutaneous erythropoietin. Reversing anaemia reduces left ventricular hypertrophy, improves quality of life, and reduces the requirement for blood transfusion. The target haemoglobin is generally between 10 and 12 g/dl (see Table 163.4). Overcorrection is associated with possible increased cardiovascular events (CHOIR/CREATE/TREAT trials). Some IV iron preparations have been associated with allergic reactions. Erythropoietin can increase blood pressure.

Parathyroid hormone levels are controlled by optimizing phosphate levels and using vitamin D replacement therapy. Phosphate levels are controlled by dietary restriction and, if necessary, with phosphate binders. These agents (e.g. calcium carbonate, calcium acetate, sevelamer, and lanthanum) are taken with food and bind dietary phosphate, preventing absorption. Vitamin D suppresses parathyroid hormone secretion, and preparations include alfacalcidol and calcitriol. With tertiary hyperparathyroidism, parathyroidectomy may be necessary. Cinacalcet is a 'calcimimetic' drug and is an alternative for patients unfit for parathyroidectomy. It binds the calcium-sensing receptor on the parathyroid gland and so inhibits parathyroid hormone secretion.

Acidosis is controlled with oral sodium bicarbonate.

Modification of cardiovascular risk

Applying evidence from the general population, all patients with CKD with a history of myocardial infarction, stroke, or peripheral vascular disease should be prescribed aspirin, an ACE inhibitor, a beta blocker, and a statin-based regimen (unless contraindicated).

Preparation for renal replacement therapy

Preparation for dialysis or transplantation requires multiple timely interventions to deal with both medical and psychosocial aspects of care. All progressing patients should be vaccinated against hepatitis B and helped to make an informed decision on dialysis modality in time to arrange formation of an arteriovenous fistula or insertion of a peritoneal dialysis catheter. Referral for transplant assessment should occur within 6 months of estimated date of dialysis. Ideal renal replacement therapy in those fit for surgery is a pre-emptive, live-related transplant.

Further Reading

Kalantar-Zadeh K and Fouque D. Nutritional management of chronic kidney disease. *N Engl J Med* 2017; 377: 1765–76.

Kidney Disease: Improving Global Outcomes (KDIGO) CKD Work Group. KDIGO 2012 clinical practice guideline for the evaluation and management of chronic kidney disease. *Kidney Inter Suppl* 2013; 3: 1–150.

Webster AC, Nagler EV, Morton RL, and Masson P. Chronic kidney disease. *Lancet* 2017; 389: 1238–52.

164 Diabetic renal disease

William G. Herrington, Aron Chakera, and Christopher A. O'Callaghan

Definition of the disease

Diabetic nephropathy is kidney damage occurring as a result of diabetes mellitus. Overt diabetic nephropathy is defined as proteinuria greater than 0.5 g/day.

Etiology of diabetic nephropathy

Diabetic nephropathy has a complicated pathogenesis including glomerular hypertension with hyperfiltration and advanced glycation end products. Poor glycaemic control is associated with progression to microalbuminuria and overt diabetic nephropathy. The lifetime risk is fairly equivalent for type 1 and type 2 diabetes mellitus.

Symptoms

Early disease is usually asymptomatic. Hyperglycaemia causes an osmotic diuresis and, thus, diabetes can present with polyuria. Hypertension develops with microalbuminuria; oedema indicates abnormal sodium and water retention and, occasionally, the development of nephrotic syndrome. Patients with diabetes, perhaps due to accompanying cardiac disease, are particularly susceptible to fluid overload and uraemic symptoms. End-stage renal disease can occur as early as when the estimated glomerular filtration rate (eGFR) is 15 ml/min 1.73 m^{-2}.

Demographics of diabetic nephropathy

Diabetes mellitus affects 6%–9% of the UK population, and the incidence of type 2 diabetes is increasingly annually affecting > 30% of over 60 year olds where obesity is common, such as North America. The peak age of diagnosis of type 2 diabetes mellitus is between 60 and 65 years of age; 25% of these patients will develop overt diabetic nephropathy over 20 years. Only a proportion of patients will, thus, live long enough to develop end-stage renal disease. However, type 2 diabetes mellitus is still the commonest cause of end-stage renal disease in the developed world, with type 2 diabetics representing over 20% of the dialysis population. Type 1 diabetes now accounts for as little as 3% of all cases of diabetes mellitus. After 20 years, type 1 diabetics have a 40% incidence of overt diabetic nephropathy. Susceptibility to diabetic nephropathy differs between populations and individuals and may have a genetic basis. Pima Indians are particularly at risk, with a 40% progression to end-stage renal disease 10 years after developing microalbuminuria.

Natural history of diabetic nephropathy

The degree of hyperglycaemia correlates with the development of microalbuminuria and overt nephropathy (UKPDS/DCCT trials). Hyperglycaemia is also more likely with hypertension or a genetic predilection. Very strict glycaemic control reduces progression to nephropathy, but once overt proteinuria is established, it does not greatly alter prognosis.

The natural history of nephropathy in type 1 diabetes has been divided into five stages (see Figure 164.1):

- Stage 1 is transitory functional kidney changes, which decrease with correction of hyperglycaemia
- Stage 2 is hyperfiltration and increased glomerular filtration rate (GFR) due to activation of the renin–angiotensin system
- Stage 3 is the development of microalbuminuria (30–300 mg/day), which is often accompanied by hypertension; this amount of proteinuria is below the threshold for a standard urinary dipstick, is detected by elevations of the albumin–creatinine ratio (ACR), and is a powerful predictor of future overt nephropathy
- Stage 4 is overt diabetic nephropathy with dipstick-positive proteinuria and an accompanying progressive fall in GFR
- Stage 5 is end-stage renal disease

Complications of the disease

Diabetic nephropathy usually progresses to end-stage renal disease if the patient does not die from the associated vascular disease.

Approach to diagnosing the disease

Diagnosis is usually on clinical grounds and on exclusion of other diagnoses. It requires at least a 5-year history of diabetes mellitus

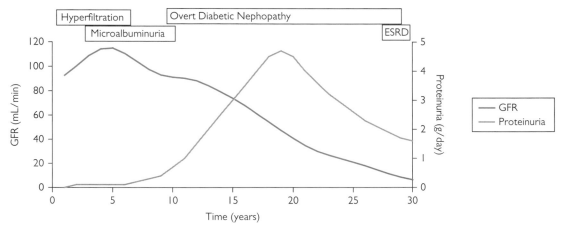

Figure 164.1 The stages of diabetic nephropathy; GFR, glomerular filtration rate.
Adapted from www.EdRen.org with permission from Professor Neil Turner.

(although, in type 2 disease, the onset of hyperglycaemia is difficult to date and typically precedes the formal diagnosis of diabetes by many years). The commonest first presentation is microalbuminuria detected on routine screening during diabetic follow-up. Diabetic neuropathy and retinopathy support the diagnosis, but nephropathy can occur in their absence.

Gold-standard diagnostic test

A renal biopsy is the gold-standard diagnostic test for diabetic renal disease. It is useful where there is diagnostic doubt but, in practice, is infrequently performed because the chance of finding anything other than diabetes is very small. A biopsy might be considered in:

- rapidly increasing proteinuria, particularly with a preserved GFR
- rapidly falling GFR
- microscopic haematuria with microscopic evidence of dysmorphic red cells or red-cell casts
- absence of retinopathy (approximately one-third of biopsied diabetic patients without retinopathy have an alternative glomerular disease)
- short history of diabetes (particularly in type 1 diabetics)
- symptoms of a multisystem disorder
- a positive paraprotein or autoimmune screen

Early histology reveals glomerular basement membrane thickening. Mesangial expansion begins about 5 years after disease onset. This expansion enlarges into intercapillary nodules with glomerulosclerosis (Kimmelstiel–Wilson disease; see Figure 164.2).

Other relevant investigations and differential diagnosis

A dipstick revealing microscopic haematuria in a patient over 50 should prompt a urological referral to exclude urinary tract malignancy, but haematuria can occur in late diabetic nephropathy. Ultrasonography excludes obstructive renal disease. Diabetic kidneys are frequently enlarged, and so asymmetrical or small kidneys may suggest concomitant renovascular disease. This can be confirmed by magnetic resonance angiography.

Diabetics are also predisposed to other renal diseases. These include urinary tract infections and autonomic bladder dysfunction. They also have increased susceptibility to acute insults like radio-opaque contrast nephropathy.

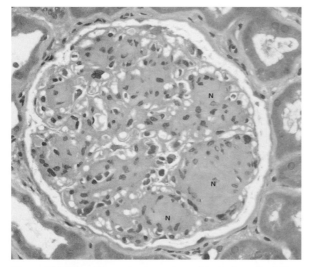

Figure 164.2 Renal biopsy demonstrating nodular (indicated by 'N') glomerulosclerosis. Please see colour plate section.

Reproduced with permission from Turner et al, *Oxford Textbook of Clinical Nephrology*, Forth Edition, Oxford University Press, Oxford, UK, Copyright © 2015.

Prognosis and how to estimate it

As with other cases of chronic kidney disease, prognosis is predicted by extrapolation from a plot of 1/creatinine or eGFR against time. However, once diabetic nephropathy has developed, there is usually a continuous steady decline in GFR, despite treatment. People with diabetes also have significantly increased risk of vascular disease. Mortality in those with nephropathy is 25-fold greater, compared to that in other diabetics. Diabetics are also high-risk dialysis patients and transplant recipients. On average, those with diabetes on dialysis have a 30% 2-year mortality (twice the rate of the non-diabetic dialysis population).

Treatment and its effectiveness

Treatment can be divided into prevention of nephropathy, slowing progression of nephropathy, and preparation for renal replacement therapy.

Prevention of nephropathy

Diabetic patients should have their urine screened for microalbuminuria at least once a year. A spot urine (preferably early morning) ACR can be used to estimate daily albuminuria. Multiplying the ACR by 10 gives an approximation of daily albumin excretion (Table 164.1).

Primary prevention measures include controlling glycaemia and blood pressure. Intensive glycaemic control reduces the onset of nephropathy. Newer agents slow nephropathy in type 2 diabetes. For example, sodium-glucose co-transporter-2 inhibitors offer renoprotection, probably through a non-glycaemic mechanism. Glucagon-like peptide receptor antagonists may also be renoprotective. Patients should not smoke and should ideally adhere to a healthy lifestyle.

Management of microalbuminuria/overt nephropathy

Blood pressure should ideally be maintained below 130/80 mm Hg, and even lower blood pressure may have cardiovascular benefits. It is, unknown if intensive blood pressure lowering is more renoprotective than standard blood pressure control.

Angiotensin-converting enzyme (ACE) inhibitors are the first-choice antihypertensive. They reduce progression to dialysis and death, compared to other antihypertensives. Angiotensin blockade similarly reduces dialysis and death, compared to other antihypertensives. Halving proteinuria with these agent nearly halves the kidney risk (IDNT/RENAAL trials).

Angiotensin blockers, however, afford no added renoprotection above ACE inhibitors. A combination of ACE inhibitor and angiotensin blockade may modestly reduce proteinuria further, but increases the risk of hyperkalaemia and acute kidney injury, and trials have not shown improved renal outcomes.

It is thought that strict glycaemic control may not affect the rate of progression once overt nephropathy has developed. However, biopsy studies from pancreatic transplant recipients have shown resorption of glomerular nodules and normalization of basement membrane thickness after 10 years of true euglycaemia.

If metformin is used for diabetic control, the dose should be dose reduced at eGFR of 60 ml/min 1.73 m^{-2} and probably stopped at an eGFR of 20 ml/min 1.73 m^{-2}. Short-acting sulfonylureas (e.g. gliclazide) are preferred to long-acting versions. Pioglitazone is an option if fluid overload is not a problem. Dipeptidyl peptidase 4 inhibitors are increasingly being used for glycaemic control in patients with advanced renal failure, and linagliptin does not need dose adjustment with renal impairment and might delay the need for insulin. Insulin is partially excreted by the kidney, and insulin doses may need to be reduced as GFR falls. CREDENCE is a large ongoing diabetic kidney disease trial testing if sodium-glucose co-transporter-2 inhibition reduces cardiovascular mortality or kidney disease progression.

Salt restriction improves blood pressure control and may also reduce proteinuria and improve oedema.

Hypercholesterolaemia is associated with progressive nephropathy. There is no evidence that reducing it alters the rate of renal

Table 164.1 Interpretation of albumin–creatinine ratio

albumin–creatinine (mg/mmol)	24-hour albuminuria	Standard dipstick for protein	Stage
<2.5	<30 mg/day	Negative	1 + 2
2.5–300	30–300 mg/day	Negative/trace	3 (Microalbuminuria)
>300	>300 mg/day	Positive	4 + 5 (Overt diabetic nephropathy)

deterioration. However, lipid control is an important in its own right to reduce the risk of cardiovascular disease.

Renal replacement therapy

Preparation for renal replacement therapy should begin early in diabetics. Uraemia occurs earlier, and preparation for transplantation often requires cardiac and peripheral vascular investigations. There is no difference between peritoneal and haemodialysis in terms of survival. Type 1 diabetics can be temporarily 'cured' by a combined pancreas and kidney transplant.

Further Reading

Chan GC and Tang SC. Diabetic nephropathy: landmark clinical trials and tribulations. *Nephrol Dial Transplant* 2016; 31: 359–68.

Wanner C, Inzucchi SE, Lachin JM, et al. Empagliflozin and progression of kidney disease in type 2 diabetes. *N Engl J Med* 2016; 375: 323–34.

165 Urinary tract obstruction

William G. Herrington, Aron Chakera, and Christopher A. O'Callaghan

Definition of the disease

The urinary tract can become obstructed by various disease processes, including tumours. Obstruction at any level of the urinary tract can impair the free flow of urine and may be partial or complete, and unilateral or bilateral.

Etiology

There are many causes of obstruction. Bilateral obstruction usually occurs at the level of the bladder or lower. Retroperitoneal fibrosis and extrinsic compression of both ureters by a malignancy are exceptions. The probability of a specific cause typically varies with the anatomical location of the obstruction and the age of the patient (see Table 165.1). Children are affected by congenital vesicoureteric junction (VUJ) or pelvic–ureteric junction (PUJ) obstruction. Young adults suffer stone disease. The elderly are prone to urothelial cancers, and older men to bladder outflow obstruction. Retroperitoneal fibrosis is an inflammatory condition that typically affects men over 50 years of age. Diagnosis should be confirmed by biopsy to exclude a lymphoma or malignancy.

Symptoms

Bilateral obstruction is more likely to cause easily detectable renal impairment. Complete bilateral obstruction causes anuria. Acute obstruction is often very painful, with colicky pain and sometimes nausea and sweating (see Chapter 166). Chronic obstruction is more subtle. PUJ obstruction may be asymptomatic apart for loin pain, which is worse after drinking a large volume or consuming alcohol, which can trigger a diuresis. Bladder outflow obstruction usually progresses slowly and the bladder capacity may increase to over 2 l. Bladder outflow obstruction is often accompanied by characteristic obstructive and irritative lower urinary tract symptoms. Obstructive prostatic disease can cause hesitancy, poor flow, and terminal dribbling. Bladder distension induces detrusor instability characterized by urgency and frequency. A significant residual volume after voiding predisposes to infection. Obstruction can also cause reflex activation of the renin–angiotensin system resulting in hypertension.

Demographics

Table 165.1 summarizes how age predicts likely cause of obstruction.

Natural history, and complications

Renal recovery in complete obstruction will usually occur if the obstruction is relieved promptly. However, recovery seldom occurs after more than 3 months of obstruction. Chronic partial obstruction is less predictable with the majority of any recovery occurring within 7 to 10 days of treatment. An infected obstructed renal tract is a urological emergency. It can cause rapid irreversible loss of renal function and severe septicaemia.

Approach to diagnosing the disease

Obstruction is often suggested by a history of obstructive lower urinary symptoms or loin pain. Examination of a patient with renal impairment must always include palpation for an enlarged bladder. A renal tract ultrasound is an important screening tool and should be included in the assessment of all cases of acute and chronic renal failure. It should be performed promptly with any acute deterioration in renal function.

Differential diagnosis

If obstruction is detected, a cause must be identified and treated. Ultrasound will demonstrate hydronephrosis in 90% of cases of obstruction. The remaining cases may develop hydronephrosis over the next 72 hours. Partial obstruction can cause a rise in creatinine without obvious hydronephrosis. Anuric obstructed kidneys will not develop hydronephrosis. Chronic hydronephrosis may persist after the cause is removed, due to prolonged stretch of the renal pelvis (a 'baggy system'). Similarly, chronic reflux may leave a large dilated 'megaureter'. Delayed excretion on a MAG3 renogram or intravenous pyelogram/computed tomography urography can help define any ongoing functional obstruction. In some cases, a trial of decompression by nephrostomy or stenting is necessary to establish whether this improves renal function.

'Gold-standard' diagnostic test

The gold-standard for diagnosing obstructive urinary tract disease is CT scanning. Most hydronephrosis is detected by ultrasound examination (see Figure 165.1A, B), but an unenhanced CT kidney–ureter–bladder can confirm hydronephrosis and identify the level and cause of obstruction (Figure 165.1C).

Table 165.1 Common causes of obstruction			
Level of obstruction	**Infants/children**	**Adult**	**Middle aged/elderly**
Kidney	Pelvi-ureteric junction obstruction	Late-presenting pelvi-ureteric junction obstruction Stones (staghorn)	Urothelial tumours Stones
Ureter	Vesicoureteric junction obstruction	Stones	Urothelial tumour Retroperitoneal fibrosis Malignant extrinsic compression (e.g. lymphadenopathy/pelvic tumours)
Bladder		Neuropathic bladder (e.g. from diabetes, or spinal cord damage)	Bladder tumour Clot retention
Bladder neck, or urethra	Congenital urethral valves	Urethral stricture	Prostate disease

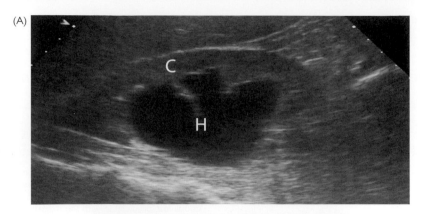

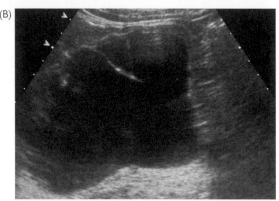

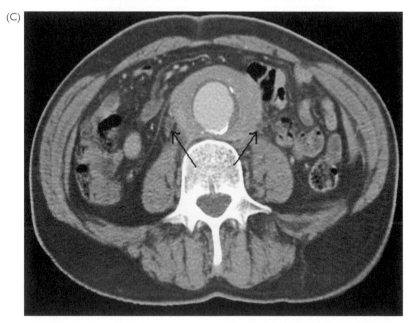

Figure 165.1 (A) Moderate hydronephrosis on ultrasound; C, cortex; H, hydronephrosis. (B) Severe hydronephrosis with loss of cortical thickness. (C) CT scan showing bilateral ureteric stenosis (arrow) due to retroperitoneal fibrosis on CT.

Other relevant investigations

A DMSA/MAG3 with diuretic can help confirm obstruction when in doubt.

A nephrostogram (dye instilled down a nephrostomy tube) or retrograde pyelogram (dye instilled into the ureter during cystoscopy) are alternatives to a urogram to assess ureteric obstruction (see Figure 165.2A).

Digital rectal examination and a prostate specific antigen (PSA) test should be undertaken in men with haematuria or obstruction.

A prostate biopsy may be indicated if the PSA and examination findings are unable to differentiate between benign prostatic hypertrophy and cancer.

Prognosis and how to estimate it

If obstruction is treated early, any associated renal impairment will usually improve. A creatinine taken 10 days after treatment is likely to represent the new baseline kidney function.

(A) 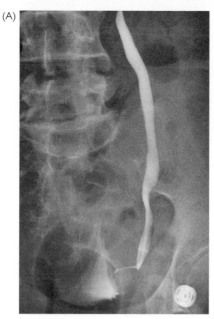 (B)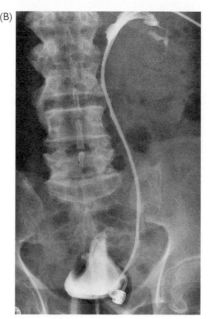

Figure 165.2 (A) Vesicoureteric junction obstruction. (B) Successful treatment of vesicoureteric junction obstruction with a JJ stent.

Treatment and effectiveness

Ureteric obstruction is often treated initially with a percutaneous nephrostomy followed by a ureteric stent inserted percutaneously at the same time as the nephrostomy or placed retrogradely per urethra (see Figure 165.2B). PUJ obstruction (often detected in utero or perinatally) can be managed by pyeloplasty. Stones may require lithotripsy or operative intervention.

Treatment of retroperitoneal fibrosis requires relief of the initial obstruction (often with JJ stents) and cessation of any suspected medications. Medical therapies include corticosteroids and immunosuppressant medications such as azathioprine and tamoxifen. Definitive surgery involves ureterolysis and omental wrapping.

Bladder outflow obstruction is initially treated by urinary catheterization. The collapse of a distended bladder and the rapid refilling of veins can result in bleeding with frank haematuria. Some advocate clamping a catheter after drainage of a litre of urine. Prostate cancer is treated surgically, hormonally, or with radiotherapy. Benign prostatic hypertrophy can be treated with alpha blockade. Tamsulosin has the least orthostatic hypotensive effect. A 5-alpha reductase inhibitor such as finasteride is an alternative. A transurethral resection of prostate is the definitive treatment for failed medical therapy, and long-term catheterization is required in those unfit for surgery.

A diuresis is common following the relief of any obstruction. This occurs because the previously obstructed kidney has a reduced capacity to concentrate urine. If there is renal impairment, it may reflect an osmotic diuresis from retained osmotically active metabolites (e.g. urea). Careful attention to fluid balance is important—it may be necessary to provide fluid replacement at half the urinary volume to prevent dehydration without driving a diuresis.

Further Reading

Fiuk J, Bao Y, Calleary JG, et al. The use of internal stents in chronic ureteral obstruction. *J Urol* 2015; 193: 1092–100.

Yaqoob MM, Bennett-Richards K, and Junaid I. The patient with urinary tract obstruction. 'The patient with urinary tract obstruction', in Turner N, Lameire N, Goldsmith DJ, et al., eds, *Oxford Textbook of Clinical Nephrology* (4th edition), 2015. Oxford University Press.

166 Renal calculi

William G. Herrington, Aron Chakera, and Christopher A. O'Callaghan

Definition of the disease

Nephrolithiasis is the presence of kidney stones, which are also known as 'renal calculi'.

Etiology of the disease

Renal calculi arise when urine becomes supersaturated with insoluble components. This may occur when there is excessive production of these components, a decrease in factors maintaining their solubility (e.g. citrate), or a reduction in urine volume (leading to increased concentration). Infection may play a significant role in the initiation of renal calculus formation, by creating a nidus for further crystal growth (see Figure 166.1). Renal calculi are usually classified into two categories: those containing calcium (80%), and non-calcareous calculi (20%; see Table 166.1).

Typical symptoms of the disease, and less common symptoms

Passage of renal calculi into the ureter causes severe, often colicky pain which is often described as 'worse than childbirth' and classically radiates from loin to groin. Calculi in the renal pelvis cause loin pain, due to obstruction and dilatation of the renal capsule. Calculi that remain within the renal parenchyma or that are too large to pass through the ureter may be asymptomatic. There is usually no fever, and the presence of an increased temperature should raise the suspicion of infection. Calculi that pass into the bladder are usually asymptomatic, but can cause complete anuria if they obstruct the urethra at the bladder outlet. This may be positional, occurring on standing. Patients with calculi anywhere in the urinary tract occasionally present with haematuria.

Demographics of the disease

The lifetime incidence of renal calculi is ~10% for men, and 5% for women, but varies greatly between countries, and is increased in hot climates. Peak incidence occurs between the third and fifth decades, and the overall incidence appears to be increasing. Up to half of all people with a renal calculus will suffer from a recurrence.

Natural history, and complications of the disease

The majority of renal calculi are relatively small (<5 mm), and pass spontaneously. Approximately 20% of patients fail to pass the calculus, or develop infections that necessitate hospitalization. The major complications are urinary system obstruction, which can occur anywhere between the kidney and urethra, leading to hydronephrosis and impaired renal function (note that, if only one kidney is affected, the urea and creatinine may not increase), and infection. Infections, particular those proximal to an obstruction, can be serious and necessitate surgical intervention to prevent urosepsis, abscess formation, and permanent loss of kidney function.

Once renal calculi have formed, they tend to increase in size with time, potentially leading to obstruction

Approach to diagnosing the disease

The diagnosis is often suspected from the history (many patients will have had previous renal calculi), and examination, especially when the classic loin-to-groin colicky pattern of pain is present. A urine dipstick should be performed to assess for any evidence of infection (note that, if the infection is above an obstructing calculus, the urinalysis may be normal), and serum electrolytes and chemistry should be checked to determine renal function, and to identify secondary causes. Imaging of the urinary tract should be performed, to identify the location, number, and size of any calculi.

Other diagnoses that should be considered

Differential diagnoses that should be considered include abdominal aortic aneurysms, ectopic pregnancies, appendicitis, and testicular torsion in males.

The classical pain and radiological appearance of renal calculi may be mimicked by sloughed papillae or clots.

'Gold-standard' diagnostic test

Non-contrast CT KUB (kidneys, ureter, and bladder) (see Chapter 157) is currently the diagnostic test of choice. This technique provides excellent visualization of the kidneys and urinary tract; it may identify anatomical abnormalities that can predispose to calculus formation (medullary sponge kidney, horseshoe kidneys) and reveal other pathologies (see 'Other diagnoses that should be considered') that may be part of the differential diagnosis.

Acceptable diagnostic alternatives to the gold standard

An IV urogram is an acceptable alternative to CT KUB. As contrast is routinely given, some assessment of renal function may be made at the same time. Plain-film KUB X-ray should not be done if non-contrast CT KUB is available for diagnosis, but is useful for follow-up (see Figure 166.2).

Ultrasonography may be used in pregnant patients to avoid radiation exposure, as may MRI. Both techniques are less sensitive than CT. Ultrasonography is highly user dependent.

Other relevant investigations

Urinalysis should be performed to identify any coexisting infection. Renal function should be assessed, particularly if there is a concern that obstruction may be present. If any calculi are passed, they should be collected, and sent for analysis.

As increasing fluid intake and reducing dietary sodium significantly reduces the likelihood of further calculus formation (by reducing the concentration of calculus-promoting factors), many units will not perform further investigations, unless there are atypical features present, or there have been recurrent calculi. In these cases, serum calcium, phosphate, urate, and parathyroid hormone levels should be measured, as well as urinary pH (ideally, on a pH meter in the clinic; otherwise, samples should be collected under oil), calcium, citrate, cysteine, urate, phosphate, and oxalate levels (24-hour collection).

Prognosis and how to estimate it

The prognosis after an isolated renal calculus is good, although the risk of further calculi is high. Where large calculi have caused prolonged obstruction, there can be significant permanent loss of renal function.

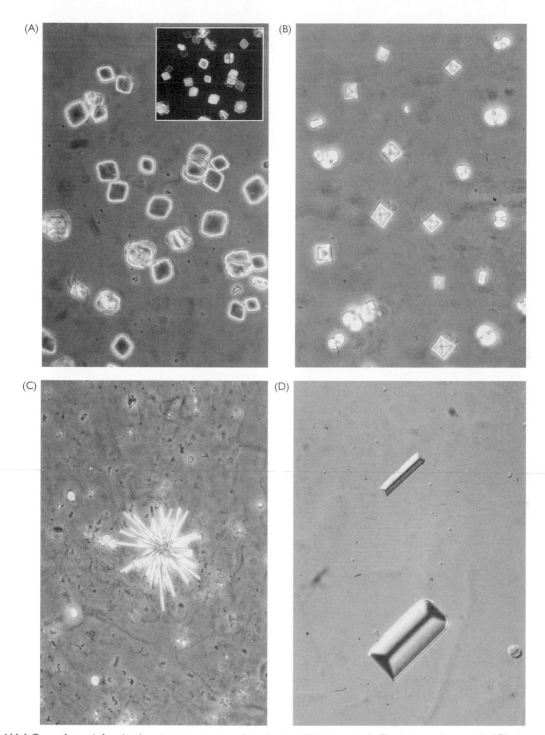

Figure 166.1 Types of crystals found in the urine in association with renal stones: (A) urate crystals, (B) calcium oxalate crystals, (C) calcium phosphate crystals, and (D) triple phosphate (struvite) crystals.

Images by Giovanni B. Fogazzi reproduced with permission from the Oxford Textbook of Clinical Nephrology, edited by Davison et al, Published by Oxford University Press 2005.

Treatment and its effectiveness

Management of calculi depends primarily on their size and location. Calculi that are likely to pass spontaneously can be managed conservatively with analgesia, and by encouraging fluids. Where there is obstruction or infection present, intervention may be required. Conservative treatments include:

- analgesia: as pain is primarily mediated by prostaglandin, NSAIDs are particularly effective; opioids may be used for additional pain relief, or if NSAIDs are contraindicated

- encouraging calculus expulsion: calcium-channel blockers and adrenergic blockers decrease ureteric spasm, and encourage passage of the calculus down the ureter; an oral steroid is often added for several days to decrease inflammation

- antibiotics: should be commenced if there is evidence of infection; usually, a broad-spectrum penicillin (e.g. amoxicillin or fluoroquinolone) is appropriate

Obstructed patients, or those with ongoing pain, should be referred to the urology service. Options for calculus removal include extracorporeal shock wave lithotripsy, percutaneous

Table 166.1 Major types of renal calculi			
Type	**Major constituents**	**Risk factors for formation**	**Shape of crystals**
Calcium containing	Calcium oxalate, calcium phosphate, and calcium urate	Hyperuricosuria Primary hyperparathyroidism Distal renal tubular acidosis Phosphate-losing nephropathies	Dumbbell or envelope shaped
Non-calcium containing	Struvite (magnesium ammonium phosphate)	Proteus infection High urinary pH	Coffin lid
	Uric acid	Gout Myeloproliferative disorders Inflammatory bowel disease	Rhomboid
	Cystine calculi	Cystinuria	Hexagonal
	Medications	Antiretrovirals Aciclovir Sulpha-containing drugs	

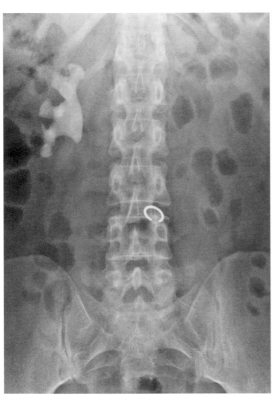

Figure 166.2 Plain-film X-ray showing a right staghorn calculus.

nephrolithotomy, and ureteroscopy or, less commonly, open nephrostomy.

Once the calculus has passed or been removed, all patients should be encouraged to increase their fluid intake to prevent urine supersaturation and crystal formation. Specific treatments where the cause of calculus formation is known are:

- hypercalciuria
  - potassium citrate
  - thiazide diuretics
- hyperoxaluria:
  - calcium supplements to decrease enteric oxalate absorption
  - *Oxalobacter formigenes* probiotic treatment is under investigation
- hypocitraturia:
  - potassium citrate
- hyperuricaemia:
  - allopurinol
  - potassium citrate
- cystine calculi:
  - potassium citrate
  - captopril
  - penicillamine
  - tiopronin

Further Reading

Türk C, Knoll T, Petrik A, et al. *Guidelines on Urolithiasis*. 2014. Available at https://uroweb.org/wp-content/uploads/22-Urolithiasis_LR.pdf (accessed 03 May 2017).

Turner N, Lameire N, Goldsmith DJ, et al., eds, The patient with urinary stone disease. In *Oxford Textbook of Clinical Nephrology* (4th edition), 2015. Oxford University Press.

Hannah Chapman and Christine Elwell

Bladder cancer

Definition of bladder cancer

Bladder cancer is the fourth most common cancer in men, and the eighth most common cancer in women. There were 10 335 new cases and 5 002 deaths from bladder cancer in the UK in 2008. Bladder cancer arises from the bladder urothelium. In the UK, 90% of bladder cancers are transitional cell carcinomas. Of those, 90% are papillary type. Other types of bladder cancer include:

- squamous cell carcinoma
- adenocarcinoma
- small cell carcinoma
- sarcoma

Aetiology of bladder cancer

Smoking is associated with a fourfold increased risk of bladder cancer. Carcinogens present in tobacco are excreted in the urine (e.g. 4-aminobiphenyl and nitrosamine). Occupational exposure to aromatic amines and aniline dyes (e.g. in the textile industry) has been an important risk factor. With improvements in health and safety, this factor is becoming less significant. Radiotherapy to the pelvis, and cyclophosphamide use, are other risk factors.

Chronic urinary stasis (e.g. due to neuropathic bladder) can lead to squamous metaplasia, a precursor for squamous cell carcinoma. Chronic infection with the parasite *Schistosoma haematobium* is associated with squamous cell carcinoma of the bladder. It is most prevalent in Egypt and sub-Saharan Africa.

Typical symptoms of bladder cancer, and less common symptoms

Symptoms of bladder cancer include:

- painless macroscopic haematuria (80%–90%)
- dysuria, urinary frequency, urinary urgency (20%–30%)
- flank pain and symptoms of uraemia (due to ureteric obstruction)
- bony pain (due to metastases)
- leg oedema (due to compression of iliac vessels by tumour)

Demographics of bladder cancer

The peak incidence of bladder cancer is at 69–71 years. Transitional cell carcinoma is four times more common in men than in women. However, squamous cell carcinoma is twice as common in women as in men. Bladder cancer is more common in Caucasians.

Natural history of bladder cancer, and complications of the disease

Eighty per cent of patients have non-muscle-invasive disease. Although the prognosis is good, in around 70% of cases, the cancer recurs. However, progression to muscle-invasive disease is uncommon.

Twenty per cent of patients have muscle-invasive disease. The natural history is one of local spread to surrounding organs, such as prostate, seminal vesicles, rectum, uterus, and vagina. Metastasis to lymph nodes, lung, liver, and bone is also common.

Carcinoma in situ (CIS) is a precursor to cancer, and 80% of patients will develop muscle-invasive cancer if untreated.

Approach to diagnosis of bladder cancer

The presence of microscopic or macroscopic haematuria should raise the suspicion of bladder cancer. Haematuria can be intermittent, so a negative repeat urinalysis does not exclude cancer. Diagnosis requires histopathological evidence, ideally corroborated by evidence from imaging, and/or examination under anaesthetic.

Other diagnoses that should be considered aside from bladder cancer

Other diagnoses that should be considered aside from bladder cancer include:

- urinary tract infection (may coexist with cancer; if treatment with antibiotics fails to resolve symptoms and/or haematuria, consider further evaluation)
- nephrolithiasis
- renal cancer
- haemorrhagic cystitis

'Gold-standard' diagnostic test for bladder cancer

Flexible cystoscopy and trans-urethral resection of bladder tumour (TURBT) is the gold-standard investigation for bladder cancer. Muscle should be included in the resection specimen. TURBT provides information on tumour grade and depth of invasion, which will influence management. It can also reveal the presence of coexisting CIS.

Acceptable diagnostic alternatives to the gold-standard test for bladder cancer

Urine cytology is the standard non-invasive test for bladder cancer. It is particularly useful if a patient is not fit enough for cystoscopy. It has an 80% sensitivity, and specificity for Grade 3 tumours. It is less reliable for lower-grade tumours. Bladder washings are sensitive, but the false-positive rate is high. Urinary cytology is affected by instrumentation, such as catheterization.

Other relevant investigations for bladder cancer

Other relevant investigations for bladder cancer include:

- a full blood count and renal function and liver function tests
- an IV urogram (may reveal a filling defect)
- ultrasound renal tract
- CT of the chest, abdomen, and pelvis (to assess local disease, and identify lymph-node and distant metastases)

Prognosis of bladder cancer and how to estimate it

Prognostic factors for bladder cancer include tumour grade, depth of invasion (T stage), multifocality, and the presence of CIS.

The 5-year survival rates for bladder cancer are:

- non-muscle-invasive disease: 80%–100%
- muscle-invasive disease: 40%–50%
- metastatic disease: <5% (median survival 3–6 months)

For squamous cell carcinoma of the bladder, the 5-year survival rate for T3/4 disease is 19%. Small cell carcinoma of the bladder usually presents in the advanced stage, and has a poor prognosis.

Treatment for bladder cancer, and its effectiveness

Treatment of non-muscle-invasive bladder cancer

TURBT is the standard treatment for non-muscle-invasive bladder cancer. If the risk of progression is low, a single dose of adjuvant intravesical mitomycin is given. For high-risk patients, a course of adjuvant BCG halves the recurrence rate. Patients require cystoscopy surveillance, due to the high recurrence rate. Cystectomy can be considered for patients who develop recurrence despite BCG and for patients with multifocal disease or with multiple high-grade recurrences.

Treatment of muscle-invasive bladder cancer

Radical cystectomy and pelvic nodal clearance is associated with a 3% mortality rate. It requires the formation of either an ileal conduit or an orthotopic neobladder. The 5-year survival rate with cystectomy is 40%–50%. Radical radiotherapy is the alternative, with similar outcomes but bladder preservation. The decision between cystectomy and radiotherapy depends upon a patient's preference, and their fitness for surgery.

Neoadjuvant chemotherapy (prior to either definitive treatment) adds a 5% survival benefit.

Palliative treatment for bladder cancer

If a patient is not fit enough for cystectomy or radical radiotherapy, palliative radiotherapy to the bladder can alleviate pain and haematuria. There is also a role for palliative chemotherapy in metastatic or locally advanced disease.

Renal cancer

Definition of renal cancer

Renal cancer accounts for 3% of cancers in adults in the UK. There are approximately 6000 new cases in England and Wales each year. Renal cell carcinoma is the most common type (80%), and arises from the proximal renal tubule epithelium. A further 5%–10% are transitional cell (urothelial) carcinomas of the renal pelvis. Renal cell carcinomas are subdivided histologically into clear cell (70%), papillary, chromophobic, and collecting duct carcinomas. Benign kidney tumours, such as cysts, are also common.

Etiology of renal cancer

Risk factors for renal cancer include:

- smoking (doubles the risk)
- obesity
- hypertension
- phenacetin analgesics in large quantities
- acquired cystic kidney disease (associated with dialysis)
- asbestos exposure
- von Hippel–Lindau syndrome (an autosomal dominant condition associated with disordered angiogenesis; due to a mutation in the VHL gene on Chromosome 3)
- tuberous sclerosis
- adult polycystic kidney disease

Typical symptoms of renal cancer, and less common symptoms

Renal cancer is frequently asymptomatic and detected incidentally on CT or ultrasound. Symptoms related to the primary tumour may occur, such as:

- painless haematuria (40%)
- flank pain
- flank mass
- left varicocele in males (due to obstruction of the left testicular vein)

Patients might also have pain secondary to bone metastases. Paraneoplastic syndromes are common in renal cell cancer, and 10% present with related symptoms.

Demographics for renal cancer

The mean age at diagnosis for renal cancer is 70 years. Renal cell carcinoma is twice as common in men as in women.

Natural history and complications of renal cancer

Renal cancers spread locally to the adrenal gland, renal vein, inferior vena cava, and perinephric fat. Metastases at presentation are common (30%). The most common sites are lung, bone, liver, and brain. The following complications might also arise due to a paraneoplastic syndrome:

- hypercalcaemia (due to secretion of parathyroid hormone-related peptide, causing confusion, constipation, abdominal pain, and renal impairment)
- polycythaemia (due to secretion of an erythropoietin-like molecule, causing hyperviscosity)
- hypertension (due to secretion of renin)
- hepatic dysfunction (Stauffer syndrome; uncertain mechanism)

Urothelial tumours are often multifocal, and are bilateral in up to 10% of patients.

Approach to diagnosing renal cancer

The main challenge in the diagnosis of renal cancer is distinguishing a benign from a malignant tumour. Renal biopsy is avoided where possible, due to the risk of haemorrhage and tumour seeding.

Other diagnoses that should be considered aside from renal cancer

If a renal mass is discovered on imaging, consider the following differential diagnoses:

- renal cyst
- renal abscess
- renal infarction
- adenoma
- oncocytoma
- metastasis

'Gold-standard' diagnostic test for renal cancer

Contrast-enhanced CT is the diagnostic test of choice for renal cancer. It can differentiate cystic from solid masses. It also permits assessment of lymph node spread and renal vein involvement.

Acceptable diagnostic alternatives to the gold-standard test for renal cancer

Renal ultrasound is useful for diagnosing renal cancer if CT is inconclusive or if a patient cannot be given IV contrast. Cystoscopy with retrograde pyelography can identify filling defects caused by renal pelvis tumours. Ureteroscopy allows direct visualization and biopsy.

Other relevant investigations for renal cancer

Other relevant investigations for renal cancer include a full blood count, a renal function test, a corrected calcium level, an alkaline phosphatase level test, erythrocyte sedimentation rate, and a coagulation profile, as these might identify a paraneoplastic syndrome or suggest metastasis.

If there is doubt about involvement of the inferior vena cava, MRI can be useful. A bone scan is indicated if a patient has bony pain or raised alkaline phosphatase.

Prognosis for renal cancer and how to estimate it

The overall 5-year survival in renal cancer is 44%. Advanced stage and high-grade tumours are associated with a poor prognosis. The 5-year survival for Stage IV disease is only 0%–2%. Other poor prognostic features include:

- poor performance status
- low haemoglobin
- raised lactate dehydrogenase
- raised corrected calcium

In metastatic disease, the prognosis is better when there is a long disease-free interval between nephrectomy and the development of metastases.

Treatment for renal cancer, and its effectiveness

Nephrectomy is the only potentially curative treatment for renal cancer. Radical nephrectomy is associated with a 65% 5-year survival rate. Partial nephrectomy is possible for tumours less than 4 cm in diameter. Compared with open nephrectomy, laparoscopic surgery is less invasive and requires less post-operative analgesic and a shorter recovery time.

In advanced disease, palliative nephrectomy can relieve pain and haematuria. Spontaneous regression of metastases following nephrectomy is a recognized, but rare, phenomenon. Arterial embolization and radiofrequency ablation are alternative palliative treatments for the primary tumour.

Metastastectomy of an isolated metastasis can improve survival in renal cancer. Palliative radiotherapy reduces pain related to bone metastases. Radiotherapy can also be used to treat intractable haematuria.

Renal cell cancers are chemoresistant. However, there now are several promising targeted treatments in use:

- sunitinib (multikinase inhibitor)
- sorafenib (multikinase inhibitor)
- temsirolimus (mTOR inhibitor)

- bevacizumab (recombinant humanized anti-vascular endothelial growth factor monoclonal antibody)

Further Reading

Capitanio U and Montorsi F. Renal cancer. *Lancet* 2016; 387: 894–906.

Choueiri TK and Motzer RJ. Systemic therapy for metastatic renal-cell carcinoma. *N Engl J Med* 2017; 376: 354–66.

Kamat AM, Hahn NM, and Efstathiou JA, et al. Bladder cancer. *Lancet* 2016; 388: 2796–810.

National Institute for Health and Care Excellence. *Bladder Cancer: Diagnosis and Management*. 2015. Available at https://www.nice.org.uk/guidance/ng2?unlid=9874814692015129115552,1759956462017219171532 (accessed 4 May 2017).

168 Renal replacement therapy

William G. Herrington, Aron Chakera, and Christopher A. O'Callaghan

Definition

Renal replacement therapy (RRT) provides a substitute for the function of normal kidneys. Options for RRT include haemofiltration, haemodialysis, peritoneal dialysis, and renal transplantation. Haemofiltration is only used in the acute setting (see Chapter 162). Endocrine functions of the kidney are replaced with erythropoietin and vitamin D therapy.

Etiology

The most common cause of end-stage renal disease (ESRD) in the developed world is diabetes mellitus. Other common causes include renovascular disease, hypertension, chronic glomerulonephritis, adult polycystic kidney disease, and chronic pyelonephritis (see Chapter 163). In about a quarter of cases, the cause remains unknown.

Symptoms

Classic 'uraemic' symptoms include persistent nausea and vomiting, anorexia, malaise, and itching, and usually only occur when the estimated glomerular filtration rate (eGFR) is <15 ml/min 1.73 m^{-2}.

Demographics

The prevalence of ESRD in the UK is approximately 0.1%. This number is growing by 6% a year, due to the rising prevalence of obesity, diabetes mellitus, and an increasingly elderly population. In the UK, around 40% of patients on RRT are on haemodialysis, 10% are on peritoneal dialysis, and 50% have a functioning transplant. Haemodialysis costs can be approximately £20 000–23 000 a year. RRT accounts for 2% of the NHS budget.

Natural history, and complications

Patients with chronic kidney disease who commence dialysis usually remain dependent on RRT, and progressively lose any residual renal function. Patients with acute kidney injury may recover renal function (depending on the cause), although recovery can take several months. In addition to the complications associated with chronic kidney disease (see Chapter 163), there are also dialysis- and transplantation-specific problems. These include infections; hypo- and hypertension related to fluid shifts; access difficulties; and dialysis modality failures.

Approach to diagnosing the disease

Indications for RRT include acidosis, hyperkalaemia, volume overload, or symptomatic uraemia. Uraemic encephalopathy and pericarditis are rare phenomena.

Differential diagnosis

Where there is a steady decline in the glomerular filtration rate (GFR), it is often possible to predict the timing of ESRD. Occasionally, acute illnesses can precipitate acute on chronic kidney disease. If there is a sudden decline in GFR, an alternative renal insult should be sought (e.g. dehydration, urinary tract infection, drug toxicity (see Table 168.1).

Table 168.1 Percentage distribution of primary renal diagnosis in patients starting on renal replacement therapy

Diagnosis	UKRR	ANZDATA	USRDS
Uncertain	26.2	5	4
Diabetes	22.2	32	44.8
Glomerulonephritis	10.4	23	8.5
Chronic pyelonephritis	7.2	4	0.5
Renal vascular disease	6.8	Not specified	1.9
Adult polycystic kidney disease	6.7	6	2.2
Hypertension	5.4	15	25.2
Other	15.3	15	13.3

Abbreviations: ANZDATA, Australia and New Zealand Dialysis and Transplant Registry; UKRR, UK Research Reserve; USRDS, United States Renal Data System.

Reproduced with permission from Warrell, Cox and Firth, *Oxford Textbook of Medicine*, Fifth Edition Oxford University Press, Oxford, UK, Copyright © 2010.

'Gold-standard' investigation

The gold-standard investigation for RRT is serial serum creatinine measurement, which can be converted into eGFR.

Other relevant investigations

The main investigations for a patient heading for RRT are focused on the mode of RRT. For example, this might include imaging of blood vessels in the arm if an arteriovenous fistula is to be created for haemodialysis.

Prognosis and how to estimate it

There is no difference in the mortality for haemodialysis and that for peritoneal dialysis. Transplantation, however, has lower mortality and lifestyle benefits, if the patient is fit for surgery; the 5-year mortality on dialysis is strongly predicted by age (see Table 168.2).

Treatment (effectiveness and complications)

Patients with progressive renal disease should be referred to renal services at least 6 months before the expected requirement for RRT. This allows time for education and discussion about RRT modalities, optimization of medical therapies, and workup for renal transplantation to be completed. If patients choose haemodialysis, an

Table 168.2 Approximate unadjusted 5-year survival in UK incident dialysis patients 1997–2010

Age (years)	Five-year survival (%)
18–34	90
35–44	80
45–54	70
55–64	55
65–74	35
>75	20

Data from www.renalreg.org.

arteriovenous fistula is created where possible as it can take several weeks to mature sufficiently for use. Following insertion of a peritoneal dialysis catheter (e.g. Tenckhoff), there is usually at least a 2-week delay before it is used.

Patients should be given enough information about each dialysis modality to allow an informed choice to be made. Not all patients wish to undergo dialysis. In particular, patients with other terminal conditions or are very elderly may opt for conservative therapy (see Chapter 172).

Haemodialysis

Haemodialysis is the process of blood being exposed to dialysate fluid across a semipermeable membrane. Waste products pass into the dialysis fluid from the blood and are removed. Most dialysis machines can also remove fluid by ultrafiltration. Vascular access is achieved through centrally inserted catheters (see Figure 168.1A),

or more preferably through arteriovenous fistulae or grafts. A large-bore dual lumen venous catheter is used for temporary haemodialysis. Usual access sites are the internal jugular or femoral veins. Tunnelling a line allows a cuff to form and protects from ascending infection (Figure 168.1B). Most patients attend three times per week, with each session lasting 4 hours. Patients on home haemodialysis may choose to dialyse for shorter periods 5–6 times per week.

Arteriovenous fistulae are the preferred form of access, as they provide the best blood flow and lowest infection risk. They are fashioned surgically by anastomosing the radial or brachial artery to the cephalic or basilic veins (see Figure 168.1B). Dialysis access is precious. Forearm and antecubital veins in renal patients should be protected. IV cannulae should only be placed on the dorsum of the hand (wherever possible).

If veins are damaged, a synthetic graft can be used to join an artery to a distant patent vein.

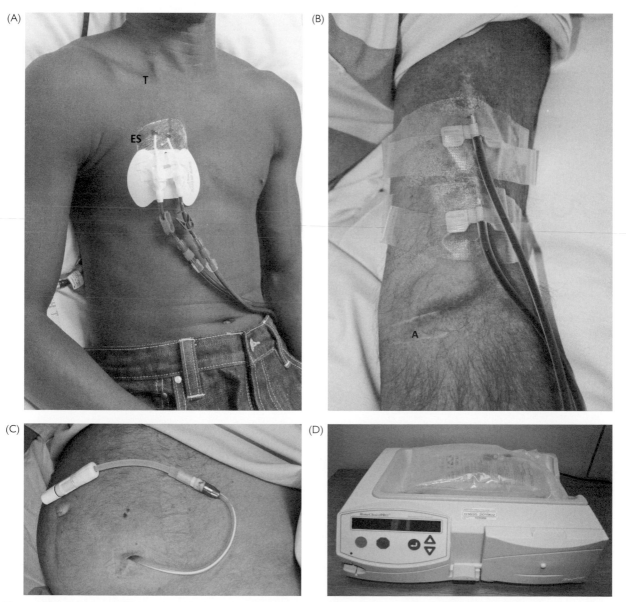

Figure 168.1 (A) A tunnelled, dual-lumen dialysis catheter. (B) A left brachiocephalic arteriovenous fistula, showing arterial and venous needles in situ. (C) A Tenckhoff catheter. (D) An automated peritoneal dialysis machine and a dialysate bag; A, area of arteriovenous anastomosis; ES, exit site; T, subcutaneous tunnel from point of insertion in internal jugular vein. Please see colour plate section.

Dialysis catheters and grafts carry a high risk of infection. Transmission of hepatitis B and C between patients is now rare due to screening for blood-borne viruses, and segregation of infected patients. Despite the introduction of high-flux dialysers, removal of beta-2 microglobulin is still poor, and dialysis-related amyloidosis causing joint degeneration can be problematic after several years of dialysis.

Peritoneal dialysis

Peritoneal dialysis uses the peritoneal membrane as a dialysis membrane. Peritoneal dialysis requires a catheter to be inserted into the peritoneal cavity (Tenckhoff catheter; see Figure 168.1C). The catheter tip coils in the pelvis. Dialysate is infused into the abdominal cavity, where it dwells, allowing the blood to equilibrate with the dialysate. Ultrafiltration is primarily achieved through the presence of hypertonic glucose in the dialysate, driving the movement of water into the abdomen. Patients can perform peritoneal dialysis at home or at work, and usually do four exchanges per day. This is called continuous ambulatory peritoneal dialysis. Alternatively, patients can set up dialysis on a machine next to the bed, and do dialysis overnight. This is termed automated peritoneal dialysis (see Figure 168.1D). Survival rates on haemodialysis and peritoneal dialysis are similar.

Contraindications

It may not always be possible to offer a patient peritoneal dialysis, due to concomitant medical or social problems. Peritoneal dialysis requires space at home to store dialysate, and sufficient visual acuity, manual dexterity, and cognitive function to perform exchanges. Abdominal herniae will usually need repair. Dialysate drainage may not be possible in patients with multiple adhesions from previous surgery. However, in general, peritoneal dialysis is a well-tolerated and popular RRT.

Complications

The most common complication of peritoneal dialysis is peritonitis. It is heralded by cloudy bags with or without abdominal pain. It is usually treated with intra-peritoneal antibiotics and does not always necessitate removal of the catheter. The most common cause is contamination during an exchange, so patients undergo a strict education process to reduce infection rates. Peritoneal dialysis peritonitis, however, must be differentiated from an unrelated intra-abdominal cause of peritonitis (e.g. perforation).

Renal transplantation

Renal transplantation involves the implantation of a kidney from either a deceased donor or a living donor. Transplanted kidneys are usually implanted extra-peritoneally into either iliac fossa, with the transplant renal artery and vein attached to the internal or external iliac artery and vein, respectively (see Figure 168.2).

Table 168.3 NHS Blood and Transplant annual activity report 2010/2011

Type of transplant	One-year graft survival (%)	Five-year graft survival (%)	One-year patient survival (%)	Five-year patient survival (%)
Living donor	97	92	99	96
Donation after brain death	94	84	96	89
Donation after cardiac death	92	86	95	88

Data from NHS Blood and Transplant annual activity report 2010/2011 www.nhsbt.nhs.uk.

As the immune system recognizes the transplant as foreign tissue, immunosuppressive therapies are required to prevent rejection. Often, this involves monoclonal or polyclonal antibodies as part of induction therapy to block lymphocyte activation or cause lymphocyte depletion, with maintenance therapy including a calcineurin inhibitor (e.g. ciclosporin or tacrolimus), an antimetabolite (e.g. mycophenolate or azathioprine), and, often, a steroid.

Over 2000 renal transplants are performed each year in the UK, with increasing numbers coming from living donors. The short-term outcomes following transplantation are very good (see Table 168.3); however, overall graft survival still only averages approximately 10 years.

The average waiting time for cadaveric transplantation is over 2 years in the UK, but difficulties finding a good match can make the wait much longer for patients from some ethnic groups, those with rarer blood groups, or those who have previously received a transplant (prior sensitization).

Complications of renal transplantation include those related to the operation or, more commonly, are the result of the immunosuppression.

Complications are divided into early onset (within 3 months) and late-onset groups, although, in reality, these exist on a continuum (see Table 168.4).

For eligible patients, transplantation is regarded as the renal replacement modality of choice, as it is usually associated with improved quality of life, and reduced mortality and morbidity when compared with age- and comorbidity-matched controls on dialysis.

Where renal disease is secondary to dysfunction of other organs, for example Factor H deficiency (which causes MPGN/TMA and has a high risk of recurrence in the transplanted kidney) or type 1 diabetes, combined organ transplantations, (e.g. liver–kidney or kidney–pancreas) may be offered at specialized centres.

Advantages and disadvantages of transplantation are given in Table 168.5.

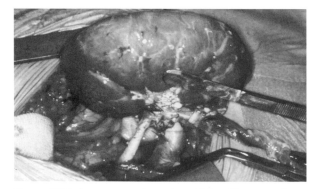

Figure 168.2 An anastomosed transplanted kidney. Please see colour plate section.

Table 168.4 Complications of transplantation

Early complications of transplantation	Late complications of transplantation
Wound dehiscence	Chronic allograft nephropathy
DVT/pulmonary embolism	Chronic rejection
Delayed graft infection	Calcineurin toxicity
Acute rejection	Graft dysfunction from calcineurin toxicity
Viral infections	
CMV infection in non-exposed recipients of organs from positive donors	Skin cancers
	Hypertension
	Accelerated atherosclerosis
Post-transplant lymphoproliferative disorder	Osteoporosis (steroid-containing regimes)
EBV infection/reactivation	Diabetes (often calcineurin induced)
Diabetes	

Table 168.5 Advantages and disadvantages of transplantation

Advantages	Disadvantages
No need for dialysis	Operation
Continuous therapy	Need for immunosuppression
Performs all the functions of a normal kidney	Regular clinic visits initially

Further Reading

Jha V, Martin DE, and Bargman JM, et al. Ethical issues in dialysis therapy. *Lancet* 2017; 389; 1851–56.

Kidney Disease: Improving Global Outcomes (KDIGO) Transplant Work Group. KDIGO clinical practice guideline for the care of kidney transplant recipients. *Am J Transplant* 2009; 9: S1–S157.

Turner N, Lameire N, Goldsmith DJ, et al., eds, In The patient on dialysis. *Oxford Textbook of Clinical Nephrology* (4th edition), 2015. Oxford University Press.

169 Inherited renal diseases

William G. Herrington, Aron Chakera, and Christopher A. O'Callaghan

Definition of the disease

There are many hereditary diseases that affect kidney function. By far, the most common of these in clinical practice is autosomal dominant polycystic kidney disease (PKD).

Etiology

The causes of inherited kidney diseases can be divided into cystic, glomerular, tubular, and systemic diseases (see Table 169.1).

Autosomal dominant PKD is the main focus of this chapter. The majority of cases are caused by mutations in the PKD1 gene, which is located on Chromosome 16 and encodes the polycystin-1 protein. A minority of cases are caused by mutations in the PKD2 gene, which is located on Chromosome 4 and encodes the polycystin-2 protein. PKD2 mutations tend to cause a slower decline in renal function than PKD1 mutations. Both polycystin-1 and polycystin-2 co-localize to a calcium channel that regulates cilia function in the renal tubule collecting ducts, but it is unclear exactly how this leads to the development of the cysts. Most cysts are in the renal cortex and can grow to several centimetres in size, occluding normal renal tissue as they expand and so leading to renal impairment.

Nephronophthisis and medullary cystic kidney disease are rare inherited causes of medullary cysts and feature prominent tubulointerstitial fibrosis. The affected genes in these diseases are all also believed to be involved in cilia function. Cysts are not usually big enough to be seen on ultrasound.

Symptoms

PKD can be asymptomatic, but can also cause haematuria, loin pain, urinary stone formation, urinary tract infection, abnormal urinalysis, or renal impairment. Cyst bleeds, infection, or associated stones may present as loin pain or haematuria. Complications are more common late in the disease and when the kidneys are over 15 cm in length. Hypertension is common. Occasionally, the first presentation is an intracranial bleed due to a ruptured berry aneurysm.

Failure to thrive or anaemia is a common presentation in children with autosomal recessive polycystic kidney disease (ARPKD) and nephronophthisis.

Demographics

The prevalence of PKD in Europe is approximately 1 in 800.

Natural history and complications

Polycystic kidney diseases typically progress to end-stage renal disease over many years. Risk factors for progressive renal failure include male sex, hypertension, PKD1 mutations, and large kidneys (>750 ml for each kidney). Complications of cysts include infection, bleeding, and stones (20%). Polycystin proteins also regulate tubular and vascular development in other organs. PKD is associated with liver cysts (80%), pancreatic cysts, other biliary diseases, and intracranial aneurysms (8%). Screening for a berry aneurysm with a magnetic resonance angiogram is indicated if there is a family history or personal history of intracranial haemorrhage or suggestive headaches. PKD is also associated with diverticular disease, inguinal herniae, and mitral valve prolapse.

ARPKD and nephronophthisis cause end-stage renal disease in childhood. ARPKD is associated with liver fibrosis and portal hypertension. Medullary sponge kidney does not usually impair renal function, but may cause recurrent stone formation and urinary stasis, which predisposes to infections.

Approach to diagnosing the disease

PKD is a major differential diagnosis in any patient with renal impairment. A family history may not be present. Diagnosis is more challenging when it is a first presentation of the disease. Large polycystic kidneys may be ballottable but the diagnosis is usually made first with an ultrasound scan. Screening of young people is usually delayed until after they are 20. However, the absence of cysts does not exclude the disease until at least the late 20s.

Other diagnoses to be considered

Cortical cysts can arise with age, or with chronic kidney disease (acquired cystic disease). These cysts are usually less than 3 cm in diameter and are associated with a reduced kidney size. They have no functional significance.

'Gold-standard' diagnostic test

The gold standard for diagnosis of PKD is ultrasound examination (see Table 169.2).

Without a family history of cysts, criteria have to be correlated to the clinical situation.

Acceptable diagnostic alternatives

Other imaging techniques such as CT or MRI scanning can also be used to diagnose polycystic kidney disease. Genotyping is not routinely performed, due to the large number of mutations and large size of the PKD genes. Nephronophthisis and medullary cystic kidney disease cysts are not seen on ultrasonography, but may be identifiable on fine-cut CT or renal biopsy, and there are genetic tests for some variants.

Prognosis and how to estimate it

A reciprocal creatinine or estimated glomerular filtration rate plot against time can be useful in predicting the rate of decline. Sudden changes in renal function may represent obstruction from a stone or a clot.

Treatment and effectiveness

Genetic screening for children is not routinely advocated, as there are currently no proven disease-modifying treatments.

Management is similar to that for most chronic kidney disease (see Chapter 163); however, patients with PKD often have high haemoglobin levels, and do not develop renal anaemia. This may in part reflect increased erythropoietin secretion by cystic kidneys.

Treatments to prevent cyst growth and renal decline are under investigation. Increasing water intake to >3 l per day to reduce vasopressin levels is advocated by some nephrologists. Alternatively, for selected patients, vasopressin-2 antagonists like tolvaptan slow cyst growth and probably modify the rate of renal progression. Patients on tolvaptan need to drink large volumes of water each day and have their liver function monitored.

Table 169.1 Causes of inherited renal diseases

Cystic diseases

Disease	Gene product	Clinical features
Adult polycystic kidney disease	Polycystin	Polycystic kidneys Polycystic livers Intracranial aneurysms
Autosomal recessive kidney disease	Fibrocystin	Polycystic kidneys Liver fibrosis
Tuberous sclerosis	Hamartin Tuberin	Renal angiomyolipomas Epilepsy/developmental delay Angiofibromas
Nephronophthisis	Nephrocystin	Progressive renal impairment Cerebellar vermis aplasia (Joubert syndrome) Retinitis pigmentosa (Senior–Løken syndrome)
Medullary cystic kidney disease	Tamm–Horsfall protein?	Progressive renal impairment

Glomerular diseases

Disease	Gene/gene product	Clinical features
Alport syndrome	Type IV collagen	Sensorineural deafness
Thin basement membrane	Type IV collagen	Haematuria (benign course)
Congenital nephrotic syndromes	Nephrin Podocin Laminin	Steroid resistant
Focal Segmental Glomerulosclerosis	APOL1	Proteinuria and progressive renal impairment

Tubular diseases

Disease	Gene/gene product	Association
Bartter syndrome	Na-K-Cl co-transporter Luminal potassium channel Basolateral Cl channel	Growth and mental retardation
Gitelman syndrome	Na-Cl co-transporter	Salt craving Cramps
Dent's disease	CLCN5	Nephrocalcinosis Rickets Renal stones
Renal tubular acidosis: • type 1 (distal) • type 2 (proximal)	Multiple	Exclude underlying autoimmune disease Most cases in adults are secondary to myeloma or drugs
Hereditary nephrogenic diabetes insipidus	Vasopressin-2 receptors	Polyuria
Cystinuria	SLC3A1 SLC7A9	Renal stones

Systemic diseases

Disease	Gene/gene product	Association
Fabry's disease	Alpha-galactosidase	Angiokeratomas Atherosclerosis
Thin basement membrane	Type IV collagen	Benign course
Cystinosis	CTNS	Renal failure Growth retardation Corneal deposits
Hereditary renal amyloidosis	Transthyretin Lysozyme Apolipoprotein A	Renal failure
Nail–patella syndrome	LMX1B	Absent patella Dystrophic toenails and fingernails

Table 169.2 Ultrasound criteria for the diagnosis of adult polycystic kidney disease in patients with a family history

Age (years)	No. of cysts required for diagnosis
<30	≥2 in a single kidney, or bilateral cysts
30–59	≥2 in both kidneys
>60	≥4 in both kidneys

Data from Pei et al., Unified Criteria for Ultrasonographic Diagnosis of ADPKD, volume 20, issue 1, pp. 205-212. *Journal of the American Society of Nephrology* (2009).

Further Reading

Devuyst O, Knooers NVAM, Remuzzi G, et al. Rare inherited kidney diseases: Challenges, opportunities, and perspectives. *Lancet* 2014; 383: 1844–59.

Harris PC and Torres VE. Genetic mechanisms and signaling pathways in autosomal dominant polycystic kidney disease. *J Clin Invest* 2014; 12: 2315–24.

Muller R-U, Haas CS, and Sayer JA. Practical approaches to the management of autosomal dominant polycystic kidney disease patients in the era of tolvaptan. *Clin Kidney J* 2017: 1–8. doi: 10.1093/ckj/sfx071

170 The kidney in systemic disease

William G. Herrington, Aron Chakera, and Christopher A. O'Callaghan

Definition of the disease

Many systemic diseases can affect the kidney (see Box 170.1). The main categories are autoimmune conditions, haematological malignancies, and infections. Many details of these conditions are covered in other chapters.

Etiology

Systemic conditions can affect the kidney in a variety of ways:

(a) Malignancy can cause infiltration of normal renal tissue; immunoglobulin deposition in the renal vessels, glomeruli, or tubules; and paraneoplastic renal dysfunction as occurs in secondary focal segmental glomerulosclerosis.

(b) Autoimmune conditions can cause inflammation of the glomeruli or tubules, or deposition of inflammatory proteins (AA amyloidosis).

(c) Infections can cause inflammation in glomeruli in association with immune complex deposition.

(d) Vascular disease and vasculitis reduce kidney blood supply and cause renal ischaemia.

(e) Multiple myeloma: Myeloma can cause renal impairment by multiple mechanisms. These include cast nephropathy (30%–60%; see Chapter 160), amyloid light-chain (AL) amyloidosis (20%), light chain deposition disease (10%; see Chapter 161), hyperuricaemia, and hypercalcaemia. Renal disease can occur with a paraprotein, before myeloma bone disease and immunoparesis develop.

(f) Amyloidosis: Deposition of amyloid protein in the kidney causes renal impairment. AA amyloid fibrils contain serum amyloid A, an acute phase protein that arises with chronic inflammation. AL amyloid fibrils contain immunoglobulin light chains secreted by a plasma cell dyscrasia. With AL amyloidosis, there is a detectable monoclonal paraprotein in 90% of cases; 75% have detectable urinary free light chains; and 15% will meet the diagnostic criteria for multiple myeloma (see Table 170.1). Patients with amyloidosis can present with oedema due to nephrotic syndrome. They may also have coexisting cardiac failure, orthostatic hypotension, or peripheral neuropathy. AL amyloidosis and multiple myeloma carry a poor prognosis, particularly if there is cardiac involvement. Survival at 1 year in dialysis patients has been quoted at 50%, but recent improvements in haematological management may improve this. Kidney involvement in AA amyloidosis is arrested by aggressive treatment of the underlying cause. This may include antibiotics for infections, or intensive immune modulation for autoimmune conditions. The target is a significant reduction in C-reactive protein levels. Treatment of AL amyloidosis with myeloma is with chemotherapy with or without a stem cell transplant.

(g) Vasculitis is autoimmune inflammation of blood vessels. The size of the vessel affected characterizes kidney involvement. Small vessel vasculitides, including ANCA-positive vasculitis, Henoch–Schönlein purpura, and cryoglobulinaemia, cause a glomerulonephritis. Polyarteritis nodosa is a medium vessel vasculitis which can cause renal impairment secondary to ischaemic damage. Vasculitis is treated with high-dose

---

Box 170.1 Multisystem diseases that affect the kidney

Neoplastic
- multiple myeloma*
- amyloid light-chain amyloidosis†
- lymphoma/leukaemia*

Autoimmune
- vasculitis‡
- SLE‡
- antiphospholipid syndrome
- scleroderma
- sarcoidosis*
- rheumatoid arthritis
- AA amyloidosis†

Infective
- hepatitis B†‡
- hepatitis C†‡
- HIV†
- infective endocarditis‡
- tuberculosis*
- AA amyloidosis†

Vascular
- hypertension
- renovascular disease

Metabolic
- diabetes mellitus§
- Gaucher's disease

Others
- thrombotic microangiopathy
- sickle cell anaemia*

* See Chapter 169.
† See Chapter 161.
‡ See Chapter 159.
§ See Chapter 164.

Table 170.1 The differences between amyloid light-chain amyloidosis and AA amyloidosis

	Amyloid light-chain amyloidosis	AA amyloidosis
Sites of amyloid deposition	Gut Liver Spleen Peripheral nerves Autonomic nerves Adrenals Heart Tongue	Gut Liver Spleen Peripheral nerves Autonomic nerves Adrenals
Cause	Plasma cell dyscrasia	Chronic infection (e.g. bronchiectasis) Osteomyelitis Autoimmune disease (e.g. rheumatoid arthritis) Ankylosing spondylitis
Prognosis	20% 5-year survival	Dependent on cause

steroids, and immunosuppression with cyclophosphamide or rituximab.

(h) SLE can cause several different patterns of glomerulonephritis. Antiphospholipid antibodies can activate the clotting cascade, causing recurrent arterial and venous thrombosis. Antiphospholipid syndrome can be primary or associated with lupus (see Warrell et al., 2010, Table 21.10.3.1). Antiphospholipid syndrome is associated with the lupus anticoagulant, and antibodies against cardiolipin and beta-2 glycoprotein 1. Lupus anticoagulant may cause a raised activated partial thromboplastin time that does not correct on mixing with normal plasma.

(i) Scleroderma affects the renal vasculature and can cause a hypertensive renal crisis with a microangiopathy. These crises can usually be prevented by early control of hypertension using angiotensin-converting enzyme (ACE) inhibitors. Scleroderma is often associated with serological abnormalities such as anti-ribonucleoprotein and anti-Scl-70 antibodies. Scleroderma is treated with ACE inhibition. Early therapy and control of blood pressure has almost eliminated severe acute renal failure in patients with scleroderma.

(j) Rheumatoid arthritis is mainly associated with renal dysfunction as an adverse effect of therapy, especially NSAIDs. Rarely, it can be associated with a small vessel vasculitis, or AA amyloidosis. Gold and penicillamine treatment are associated with membranous nephropathy.

(k) Sarcoidosis can cause a granulomatous tubulointerstitial nephritis and can also cause renal impairment through hypercalcaemia, which can develop into diffuse nephrocalcinosis.

(l) Thrombotic microangiopathy results from platelet aggregation and thrombosis in small vessels. It is characterized by thrombocytopaenia, haemolysis, and tissue ischaemia. The causes include pre-eclampsia, haemolytic–uraemic syndrome (HUS) (usually accompanied by diarrhoea, typically caused by *Escherichia coli* serotype 0157 or *Shigella* spp.), and thrombotic thrombocytopenic purpura (TTP) (usually accompanied by central nervous system involvement). Thrombotic microangiopathy often presents with a fever, hypertension, purpura, and acute kidney injury. The clinical context usually suggests the cause. HUS is usually associated with bloody diarrhoea. TTP can cause fits and confusion. Thrombotic microangiopathy is suggested by thrombocytopenia and anaemia, with evidence of haemolysis (a raised bilirubin and lactate dehydrogenase, low haptoglobins, red-cell fragments on blood film, and a negative Coomb's test). Culture of stool and blood is indicated in HUS associated with diarrhoea. In classical HUS, ADAMTS13 activity is normal. Plasma exchange (with fresh frozen plasma) may improve outcomes and the complement inhibitor Eculizumab is now also recommended for selected cases.

(m) Hepatitis B is associated with membranous nephropathy (see Chapter 161).

(n) Hepatitis C can cause a mixed essential cryoglobulinaemia which may inflame small and medium sized vessels. Renal disease associated with hepatitis C often responds well to antiviral therapy.

(o) HIV infection is classically associated with a collapsing variant of focal segmental glomerulosclerosis, HIV-associated nephropathy. HIV infection can also cause a diffuse proliferative glomerulonephritis or a thrombotic microangiopathy. Treatment can have renal side effects. Indinavir is associated with crystalluria, tubular stones, and interstitial nephritis. Cidofovir and adefovir can cause proximal tubular toxicity. HIV-associated nephropathy may respond to antiviral therapy.

(p) Infective endocarditis is associated with renal impairment, which can be an immune-complex-mediated glomerulonephritis. Aminoglycosides and septicaemia can cause acute tubular necrosis, and penicillin antibiotics may induce a tubulointerstitial nephritis. Valvular vegetations may break off and deposit as septic emboli in the kidney.

Symptoms

A systemic illness may be present if there are symptoms, signs, or abnormal investigations that indicate the involvement of other organ systems. For this reason, a careful and full history and examination are necessary in all patients with suspected kidney disease, to help determine whether the renal condition is secondary to a systemic illness (which may or may not be known about) or is a primary illness restricted to the kidneys. Renal disease may be the presenting feature for some multisystem diseases but sometimes a systemic disease has already diagnosed. Renal complications can occur with many chronic multisystem diseases, and renal function and urinalysis should be monitored routinely in conditions such as SLE, scleroderma, and sarcoidosis.

Demographics

Diabetic and ischaemic nephropathy are the most common. By contrast, thrombotic microangiopathies, polyarteritis nodosa, and antiphospholipid syndrome are very rare. However, they often affect the young (10–40 years of age). Better rheumatological and antibiotic treatments mean AA amyloidosis is becoming rarer. Amyloidosis and plasma cell dyscrasias are diseases of late middle age (>50 years).

Natural history, and complications

The natural history of renal complications of systemic disease is very variable. If the underlying cause can be treated, prognosis is often good. Delay in treatment may be associated with permanent renal impairment.

Approach to diagnosing the disease

A good clinical history with a thorough systems review will normally give clues to diagnosis. In nephrotic syndrome, suspected glomerulonephritis, or acute kidney injury, the standard immunological and paraprotein screens will often highlight plasma cell dyscrasias and viral infections (see Chapter 157). Finding anaemia, a raised bilirubin, and thrombocytopenia will usually trigger a clinician to perform a haemolysis screen.

Differential diagnosis

When considering a vasculitis, always exclude systemic infection (especially infective endocarditis) or paraneoplastic states.

'Gold-standard' diagnostic test

A renal biopsy is usually the best investigation for diagnosing a disease affecting the kidneys, when other investigations do not indicate the cause. However, it is not always diagnostic, depending on the underlying disease process. Biopsy findings in vasculitis, myeloma, and glomerulonephritides are discussed in Chapters 159 and 161. Biopsies in scleroderma, thrombotic microangiopathy, polyarteritis nodosum, and antiphospholipid syndrome usually demonstrate ischaemic glomerular collapse, as the disease occurs in the vessels leading to the glomeruli.

Other relevant investigations

Other investigations offer important diagnostic clues and may direct treatment (see 'Aetiology' for specific details).

Prognosis and how to estimate it

If the underlying cause can be treated, prognosis is often good. Delay in treatment may be associated with permanent renal impairment.

Treatment and effectiveness

The general supportive measures for nephrotic syndrome, glomerulonephritis, and acute kidney injury are employed as usual. However, additional treatment is also directed to the systemic disorder that has involved the kidneys.

Further Reading

Fakhouri F, Zuber J, Frémeaux-Bacchi V, and Loirat C. Haemolytic uraemic syndrome. *Lancet* 2017; 390: 681–96.

Georg JN and Nester CM. Syndromes of thrombotic microangiopathy. *N Engl J Med* 2014; 371: 654–66.

Shwartz N, Goilav B, and Putterman C. The pathogenesis, diagnosis and treatment of lupus nephritis. *Curr Opin Rheumatol* 2014; 26: 502–9.

Remuzzi G (ed). Section 6: The patient with another primary diagnosis. In Oxford Textbook of *Clinical Nephrology*, eds Turner NN et al. (4th edition), 2015. Oxford University Press

171 Renal vascular disease

William G. Herrington, Aron Chakera, and Christopher A. O'Callaghan

Definition of the disease

Renal vascular disease typically occurs with progressive narrowing of the main renal artery or smaller arterial vessels. Often, both patterns of disease coexist and result in 'ischaemic nephropathy' with damage to renal tissue. Much less commonly, inflammatory vasculitis can affect small or medium vessels.

Aetiology of renal vascular disease

Ninety per cent of renal vascular disease is caused by atherosclerosis. It is associated with the usual cardiovascular risk factors of smoking, diabetes mellitus, hypertension, and dyslipidaemia. Patients with renal vascular disease have an increased risk of cardiovascular death from associated cerebrovascular and coronary heart disease.

Less than 10% of renal vascular disease is caused by fibromuscular dysplasia. The cause is unknown, but smoking is a risk factor. The disease is often bilateral and multifocal. It tends to affect the mid-portion of the renal artery, while atherosclerosis tends to occur at points of stress, especially at the junction of renal arteries with the aorta.

Symptoms

Renal artery stenosis in itself is usually asymptomatic. Renal vascular disease reduces renal perfusion. This activates the renin–angiotensin system, increasing angiotensin II levels. The elevated angiotensin II level causes hypertension through vasoconstriction and increased aldosterone secretion, which promotes sodium and water retention.

Patients with salt and water retention present with peripheral oedema and orthopnoea. Secondary hyperaldosteronism can also cause a hypokalaemic metabolic alkalosis.

Demographics

Atherosclerosis is increasingly prevalent with age. Renal vascular disease has a prevalence of 7% in those over 65 years old. Fibromuscular dysplasia, in contrast, occurs predominately in females under the age of 30 years.

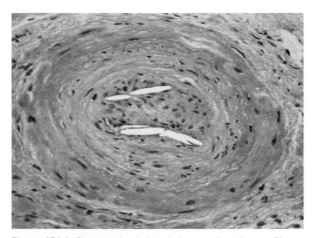

Figure 171.1 Cholesterol emboli occluding a small renal artery. Please see colour plate section.
image courtesy of Ian Roberts.

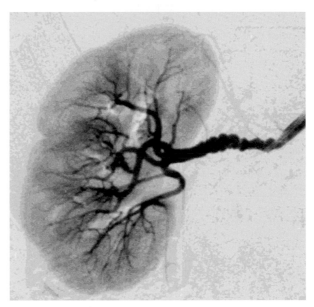

Figure 171.2 Angiogram demonstrating fibromuscular dysplasia ('string of beads').

This article was published in *Grainger & Allison's Diagnostic Radiology* 5e, Adam & Dixon, Copyright Elsevier 2007.

Complications of the disease

Chronic fluid overload can episodically and rapidly decompensate, causing flash pulmonary oedema even when cardiac function is normal. The concept is that reduced renal perfusion, perhaps caused by a dip in blood pressure, results in a sudden activation of the renin–angiotensin system. In practice, however, patients with renal vascular disease often have concomitant coronary artery disease or hypertensive heart disease.

Acute deterioration in renal function can occur due to renal infarction (associated loin pain and raised lactate dehydrogenase) or due to cholesterol emboli. Cholesterol emboli can result from instrumentation or aortic surgery (usually angiography) or thrombolysis/anticoagulation. A shower of cholesterol crystals can occlude small renal vessels (see Figure 171.1). There may be concomitant evidence of digital infarction or livedo reticularis. There is often associated

Table 171.1 Medical treatment of renal vascular disease

	Treatment	Suggested minimum targets
Blood-pressure control	Furosemide Calcium blocker/beta blocker Trial of angiotensin-converting enzyme inhibitor	<130/80 mm Hg
Antiplatelet therapy	Low-dose aspirin	
Lipid-lowering therapy	Statin +/− ezetimibe	As low as possible
Lifestyle advice	Stop smoking Low-salt diet	

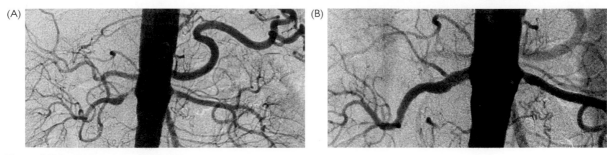

Figure 171.3 (A) Proximal left renal artery stenosis. (B) Angiographic appearance after angioplasty and stent insertion.
This article was published in *Grainger & Allison's Diagnostic Radiology* 5e, Adam & Dixon, Copyright Elsevier 2007.

inflammation with a raised C-reactive protein level and eosinophil count. Complement levels may be reduced. Therapy is supportive.

Approach to diagnosing the disease

Renal artery disease is suspected in a patient with known vascular disease with hypertension that is difficult to control (hypertensive despite full dose of three antihypertensive agents). Fluid overload and renal dysfunction are common. Supporting examination findings including bruits and absent peripheral pulses. An abdominal bruit is useful but not a specific sign because it may or may not localize to the renal artery. Dipstick is bland or may show low-grade proteinuria. Ultrasonography may show renal asymmetry (>1.5 cm is suspicious) in unilateral disease; however, disease is frequently bilateral.

The only reliable indicator of functional stenosis is a significant (>15%) rise in creatinine on starting an angiotensin-converting enzyme (ACE) inhibitor or angiotensin blocker. If there is sufficient clinical suspicion of the diagnosis, imaging is the key to diagnosis.

A pitfall to avoid is not checking plasma creatinine about a week after initiating or changing an ACE inhibitor or angiotensin II receptor blocker dose.

Differential diagnosis

Any cause of chronic kidney disease can cause renal impairment and hypertension. Alternative diagnoses to consider in resistant hypertension with or without renal impairment include high alcohol or salt intake, obesity, obstructive sleep apnoea, concomitant NSAID use, and primary hyperaldosteronism.

'Gold-standard' diagnostic test

The digital subtraction angiogram is the gold-standard diagnostic test (see Figure 171.2). Magnetic resonance angiography (MRA) is, however, the most common first screening test. It visualizes ostial lesions well, but has the propensity to overestimate a stenosis.

Invasive angiography has the benefit of accurate assessment of stenosis, better visualization of distal arteries and the opportunity for angioplasty and stent placement. The procedure is associated with a 7% complication rate. Complications include bleeding, contrast-induced nephropathy, and cholesterol emboli. Formal angiography is thus reserved for equivocal cases or when angioplasty is under consideration.

Acceptable alternative investigations

The best screening test is MRA or CT angiography. A duplex ultrasound with Doppler can demonstrate reduced perfusion in experienced hands, but is a not a standard screening investigation.

Prognosis and how to estimate it

Renal vascular disease may progress in a stepwise fashion with long intervening periods of stability making it difficult to predict prognosis. Mortality is 8%–16% per year, due to associated vascular disease.

Treatment and its effectiveness

Treatment is medical or interventional. Medical therapy should be universal to prevent progression of vascular disease (Table 171.1). An ACE inhibitor can still be used, providing there is no serious increase in creatinine after starting.

Angioplasty is used for fibromuscular dysplasia, but is seldom indicated for atherosclerotic renal arterial disease. Angioplasty seldom sees benefit compared to medical treatment in terms of recovery of renal function or blood pressure. Anecdotal evidence may still support angioplasty in less common clinical situations, such as rapidly deteriorating renal function (acute occlusion) and flash pulmonary oedema (see Figure 171.3). The lack of benefit from angioplasty may be due to concomitant small vessel atherosclerosis downstream of the proximal lesion (ischaemic nephropathy). Angioplasty can also do harm, and a shower of cholesterol emboli may precipitate the need for dialysis.

Further Reading

Cooper CJ, Murphy TP, Cutlip DE, et al. Stenting and medical therapy for atherosclerotic renal-artery stenosis. *N Engl J Med* 2014; 370: 13–22.

Persu A, Giavarini A, Touzé E, et al. European consensus on the diagnosis and management of fibromuscular dysplasia. *J Hypertens* 2014; 32: 1367–78.

172 Management of terminal care in renal disease

William G. Herrington, Aron Chakera, and Christopher A. O'Callaghan

Definition of the disease

The World Health Organization defines palliative care as an approach that improves the quality of life of patients and their families facing the problem(s) associated with life-threatening illness, through the prevention and relief of suffering by means of early identification and impeccable assessment and treatment of pain and other problems—physical, psychosocial, and spiritual.

Aetiology of the disease

With the increasing age and burden of comorbidities experienced by patients with significant renal impairment in developed countries, many patients are deciding that they do not want renal replacement therapy or elect to withdraw from dialysis. In some countries, over 30% of deaths in dialysis-dependent patients are reported as being due to withdrawal from treatment. For these patients and patients who opt for conservative (supportive) management, rather than renal replacement therapy, symptom control and maintenance of quality of life are the primary goals.

Several aspects of terminal care are unique in the context of renal impairment. These include the management of symptoms caused by the loss of normal kidney function, such as anaemia, oedema, and hyperphosphataemia, and also altered pharmacokinetics of medications that are renally cleared.

Typical symptoms of the disease, and less common symptoms

The metabolic derangements caused by end-stage renal disease can lead to a variety of distressing symptoms. Table 172.1 lists some of these symptoms and potential treatment options. In addition to the physical manifestations of renal impairment, significant psychological symptoms related to the decision to withdraw from dialysis (or to opt for conservative management) may occur, and these should be addressed.

Demographics of the disease

With the ageing of the population, there are an increasing number of elderly patients, who often have multiple comorbidities, reaching end-stage renal disease. Recent UK renal registry data show that over 50% of dialysis patients have one or more significant comorbid conditions in addition to their renal disease, with the highest incidence occurring in the 65–74-year age group. Although elderly patients dominate the group receiving supportive care, patients of all ages are represented, and the needs and issues may be very different, particularly in younger patients. A proportion of patients will have another terminal disease, which causes their death, and also have end-stage renal disease.

Natural history, and complications of the disease

The terminal course is highly dependent on the degree of renal impairment, which influences the ability to maintain fluid balance and control acidosis. Patients who were previously dialysis

Table 172.1 Common symptoms and treatment options in terminal renal failure

Symptom	Potential treatments
Nausea and vomiting	Haloperidol
	Metoclopramide
	Levomepromazine
Pruritus	Optimize magnesium and calcium concentrations
	UVB
	Thalidomide
	Capsaicin cream
	Mirtazapine
Bone pain	Paracetamol
	NSAIDs
	Opioids: reduced dose, as these can accumulate; in some units, methadone and fentanyl are preferred for use, as their metabolites are less likely to accumulate with renal impairment
	Bisphosphonates
Neuropathic pain	Paracetamol
	Opioids
	Amitriptyline
	Gabapentin
Restless legs	Optimize iron status
	Pramipexole
	Clonazepam
Oedema and dyspnoea	Non-pharmacological: reassurance, having the patient sit upright, use of fans
	Pharmacological: diuretics, oxygen, opioids, benzodiazepines, antisecretory agents (e.g. glycopyrrolate)
Delirium	Benzodiazepines
	Levomepromazine

dependent have a mean survival on withdrawal of 8–10 days, but some may live for several weeks. Major complications relate to fluid balance, which can cause distressing dyspnoea and uncertainty regarding the duration of survival. With conservative management of end-stage renal disease becoming an increasingly chosen option for patients (over 10% of patients with end-stage renal disease in some centres), progression to death may be very slow. This creates significant opportunities to improve symptom control and optimize quality of life.

Approach to diagnosing the disease

Advanced care planning should be an integral component of the management of all patients with end-stage renal disease. Patients' wishes should be documented, and patients should be supported through their decision-making.

Although patients may have elected for conservative management, if there are sudden declines in clinical state, it may be appropriate for reversible factors to be sought and treated, depending on the patient's wishes and advanced directives. Patients and their families should be fully informed of their prognosis (as far as possible) and made aware of the treatment options available to them.

The UK's National Service Framework for renal services defined six markers of good practice for terminal care in renal disease:

1. Access to communication skills and knowledge of symptom control
2. Offering prognostic assessment
3. Timely information and joint palliative care plan
4. Ongoing medical care for patients opting not to dialyse
5. Dying with dignity
6. Culturally appropriate bereavement support

Importantly, all members of the renal multidisciplinary team, including pre-dialysis counsellors, nurses, pharmacists, dieticians, social workers, and doctors, can make important contributions to the terminal management of patients with renal diseases and should be involved in their care.

Other relevant investigations

If reversible causes for a sudden deterioration in clinical state are suspected, and the patient wishes treatment, appropriate investigations should be performed, as they would for any other patient group. These may include blood tests, chest X-ray, or other imaging.

Prognosis and how to estimate it

Serial measurements of renal function and electrolytes may help gauge the rate of decline.

Treatment and its effectiveness

A variety of treatments are available for symptom control in patients with end-stage renal disease (see Table 172.1). It is essential to remember that many of the commonly used medications and their metabolites are cleared by the kidneys, and appropriate dose adjustments should be made.

As maintenance of quality of life is important and the time course can be long (particularly in patients with slowly progressive renal diseases), it is important that these patients are not denied therapies that can maintain or improve quality of life, including erythropoietin, for the treatment of anaemia; vitamin D preparation, to prevent bone pain and reduce the risk of fractures; and bicarbonate tablets, to reduce acidosis. Specialist palliative care advice should be sought early or if symptom control is proving difficult.

Further Reading

Kane PM, Vinen K and Murtagh FEM. Palliative care for advanced renal disease: A summary of the evidence and future direction. *Palliative Med* 2013; 27: 817–21.

Pinkhasov A, Germain MJ, and Cohen LM. Chapter 261: Dialysis withdrawal and palliative care. In *Oxford Textbook of Clinical Nephrology*, eds Turner NN et al. (4th edition), 2015. Oxford University Press

NHS Scotland. Scottish Palliative Care Guidelines: Renal disease in the last days of life. Available at: http://www.palliativecareguidelines.scot.nhs.uk/guidelines/end-of-life-care/renal-disease-in-the-last-days-of-life.aspx

173 Disorders of plasma potassium

Aron Chakera, William G. Herrington, and Christopher A. O'Callaghan

Definition of the disease

Potassium is the major intracellular cation, and maintenance of potassium homeostasis is critical for normal cellular function. Serum potassium levels usually range from 3.5–4.5 mmol/l (compared with intracellular levels of ~150 mmol/l). Hypokalaemia is defined as a serum potassium level <3.5 mmol/l, and hyperkalaemia as a serum potassium level > 4.5 mmol/l. Serum potassium levels between 3 and 6 mmol/l are usually well tolerated without adverse signs or symptoms; the only exception to this is in those with established severe heart disease (e.g. heart failure with significant left ventricular systolic dysfunction). In these patients, hypokalaemia quite significantly increases the risk of lethal ventricular arrhythmias, in part possibly through QT-interval prolongation. Part of the mechanism of benefit for drugs such as spironolactone and eplerenone is that they help maintain potassium in the normal range and so lessen arrhythmia risk.

Aetiology of the disease

The major cause of hypokalaemia is loss of potassium through either the gut or the kidneys (see Table 173.1); however, it may also be seen transiently with medications that move potassium into cells

Given the high intracellular potassium concentration, hyperkalaemia may be caused by tissue damage, or by impaired renal secretion of potassium. Hyperkalaemia also occurs with acidaemia, as the decrease in pH leads to intracellular buffering of hydrogen ions, which are exchanged with potassium to maintain electrical neutrality (see Table 173.2).

Typical symptoms of the disease, and less common symptoms

Maintenance of the normal intracellular–extracellular potassium gradient determines the resting membrane potential. Both hypo- and hyperkalaemia affect cellular depolarization, leading to neuromuscular symptoms which can rapidly become life-threatening, primarily from cardiac arrhythmias (see Table 173.3).

Table 173.1 Causes of hypokalaemia

Gastrointestinal losses	Vomiting
	Chronic diarrhoea
Renal losses	Medications
	• Diuretics
	• Antimicrobials
	• Penicillins
	• Aminoglycosides
	• Amphotericin
	Endocrine disorders
	• Steroid excess
	• Conn's syndrome
	Tubular disorders
	• Renal tubular acidosis
	• Channelopathies
	• Gitelman syndrome
	• Bartter syndromes
Redistribution into cells	Glucose administration
	Bicarbonate administration
	Beta agonists

Table 173.2 Causes of hyperkalaemia

Release from cells	Haemolysis
	Large haematomas
	Severe tissue damage
	Acidaemia
Decreased renal potassium losses	Hyperaldosteronism
	Medications
	• Antibiotics (e.g. trimethoprim)
	• Potassium-sparing diuretics
	• NSAIDs
	• Angiotensin-converting enzyme inhibitors and angiotensin receptor blockers
	Acute renal failure

Demographics of the disease

Hyperkalaemia occurs in over 5% of hospitalized patients and is most common in older age groups, where it is associated with renal impairment and medication use. Medications that block the renin–angiotensin system, such as angiotensin-converting-enzyme inhibitors (ACE-Is) and angiotensin receptor blockers (ARBs) are often responsible. This is mainly because they lower aldosterone levels, and aldosterone promotes renal potassium excretion.

Hypokalaemia is also common, affecting over 15% of hospitalized patients, and is usually related to diuretic use, gastrointestinal losses, or inadequate potassium in the diet. It is often first noted as an incidental laboratory finding.

Natural history, and complications of the disease

There are no pathognomonic features of hypo- or hyperkalaemia on history or examination, and the presence of clinical signs can depend on the duration of the abnormality. Some patients with significant chronic kidney disease may maintain stable potassium levels of 6.5–7.0 mmol/l, with no symptoms. Where abnormal serum potassium levels are noted, the rate of change is also important. Rapid shifts are associated with worse outcomes. When significant abnormalities in potassium levels are noted before the onset of cardiac or neurological symptoms and treatment is instituted, the prognosis is generally good.

Table 173.3 Symptoms of hypo- and hyperkalaemia

Hypokalaemia	Hyperkalaemia
Weakness (usually severe hypokalaemia)	Fatigue
Cramps	Weakness
Nausea and vomiting	Paraesthesia
Palpitations (reflecting supraventricular and ventricular arrhythmias, especially with underlying cardiac disease)	Paralysis
	Palpitations
	Cardiac arrest (due to ventricular arrhythmias and cardiac standstill)
Constipation	
Polyuria (uncommon and typically reflecting chronicity)	
Psychosis (uncommon)	
Depression (uncommon)	

Approach to diagnosing the disease

Most cases of mild–moderate hypo- or hyperkalaemia are identified as incidental findings on routine laboratory tests and do not necessitate extensive investigation. As the presence of clinical signs and symptoms are a late manifestation, a high index of suspicion is often necessary to diagnose the condition. Hyperkalaemia, in particular, should be suspected in any patient with decreased urine output or significant renal impairment, especially if they are on ACE-I/ARB. The priority in any patient with acute kidney injury is to determine whether their potassium level is high, because this can cause imminent cardiac arrest if undiagnosed and untreated. If there is a concern that significant hyper- or hypokalaemia may be present, potassium levels should be assessed urgently on a blood gas machine (using venous or arterial blood taken through a needle that is 22 gauge or larger, to minimize haemolysis), an ECG performed, and a concurrent serum sample sent to the laboratory for formal reporting. A thorough review of the patient's medications and diet should be undertaken, and any causative medications stopped. Examination should focus on cardiovascular status and fluid balance to assess potential causes of renal dysfunction, and any tissue damage or large haematomas noted.

Other diagnoses that should be considered

Hypokalaemia and hypomagnesaemia often coexist, and correction of hypokalaemia can be difficult if there is ongoing hypomagnesaemia. The presence of an abdominal bruit on examination should raise the suspicion of renal artery stenosis, particular if the onset of hyperkalaemia follows the introduction of medications that affect the renin–angiotensin system. Hypokalaemia is an important feature of hyperaldosteronism (e.g. Conn's syndrome) and can also occur with the use of exogenous steroid agents that have mineralocorticoid activity.

If significant unexplained hypokalaemia is noted, the serum bicarbonate level should be measured, as hypokalaemia with acidosis in the presence of normal renal function is suggestive of renal tubular acidosis (which will be hyperchloraemic), whereas hypokalaemia with normal or elevated bicarbonate is consistent with a channelopathy.

'Gold-standard' diagnostic test

The gold-standard test used to detect disorders of plasma potassium is the laboratory serum potassium level.

Acceptable diagnostic alternatives to the gold standard

Accurate potassium levels can be obtained from blood gas machines and, when clinically worrying hypo- or hyperkalaemia is suspected, this test should be performed first, as the results will be available immediately.

Other relevant investigations

As the major cause of mortality from hypo- or hyperkalaemia is cardiac arrhythmia, an ECG should be performed early, whenever these abnormalities are suspected. ECG findings of hyperkalaemia include tall, tented T-waves, increased PR intervals, and broadening of the QRS complex, with loss of P waves and presence of sine wave morphology when severe (see Figure 173.1).

Hypokalaemia is associated with the development of U waves. Assessment of urinary pH, urinary potassium, and other electrolytes may be performed if a primary tubular disorder is suspected. Investigation of hyperaldosteronism includes plasma renin levels, aldosterone levels, and abdominal imaging to differentiate between adrenal adenomas and bilateral adrenal hyperplasia (although small adenomas may be difficult to detect). If needed, direct sampling of blood from each adrenal vein can be performed (see Chapter 188).

Prognosis and how to estimate it

The prognosis depends on the severity of the derangement and how rapidly it has occurred. In some series, the mortality is over 50% when there are significant delays in treatment. The presence of ECG abnormalities due to hypo- or hyperkalaemia is indicative of a poor prognosis, unless urgent treatment is instituted.

Treatment and its effectiveness

The management of hypokalaemia relies on replacement with oral or IV potassium, depending on the patient's status. As most potassium is intracellular, a decrease in serum potassium of 1 mmol/l equates to a total body potassium loss of 100–300 mmol. IV potassium should not usually be given faster than 20 mmol/hour, unless the patient is on a cardiac monitor. Patients on long-term diuretic therapy (e.g. patients with congestive cardiac failure, particularly if not receiving a potassium-sparing diuretic) are at high risk and should have serum potassium levels assessed regularly.

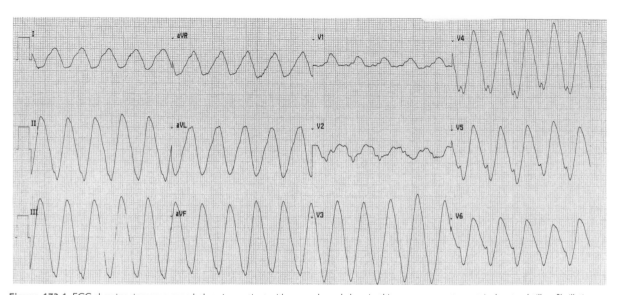

Figure 173.1 ECG showing sine wave morphology in a patient with severe hyperkalaemia; this may progress to ventricular standstill or fibrillation.

Table 173.4 Treatment of severe hyperkalaemia

Action	Medication	Time to effect	Duration of effect
Stabilize the myocardium	Calcium gluconate, calcium chloride	1–2 minutes	20–30 minutes
Intracellular redistribution of potassium	Glucose + insulin	10 minutes	2–4 hours
	Sodium bicarbonate	10 minutes	2–4 hours
	Beta agonists (e.g. salbutamol)	5–10 minutes	2–4 hours
Removal of potassium	Diuretics (e.g. furosemide)	30–60 minutes	2–3 hours ≥6–12 hours Continues while on machine
	calcium polystyrene sulfonate, sodium polystyrene sulfonate*	4–6 hours orally, 1–2 hours rectally	
	Dialysis	1–2 minutes	

Note: Calcium gluconate/chloride should be used with caution in cases where digitalis toxicity is suspected, as it may potentiate arrhythmias. IV magnesium sulfate can be given as an alternative.
*New oral potassium binders are being developed, including patiromer and sodium zirconium cyclosilicate.

The treatment of hyperkalaemia also depends on the severity of the elevation and the rate of increase (see Table 173.4). In general, a serum potassium in the range of 5.0–6.0 can be considered mild elevation; 6–6.5, moderate elevation; and >6.5 should be considered severe elevation in most cases, particularly if it is unclear whether the levels may still be increasing. Management of severe hyperkalaemia involves:

- stabilization of the myocardium (where there are ECG changes or neuromuscular signs or symptoms)
- temporizing measures to redistribute potassium to the intracellular space
- definitive treatment to remove potassium from the body

Further Reading

McDonald TJ, Oral RA, Vaidya B. Investigating hyperkalaemia in adults. *BMJ* 2015; 351: h4762 doi: 10.1136/bmj.h4762
UK Renal Association Clinical Practice Guidelines. Treatment of acute hyperkalaemia in adults 2014. https://renal.org/wp-content/uploads/2017/06/hyperkalaemia-guideline-1.pdf
Unwin RJ, Luft FC, and Shirley DG. Pathophysiology and management of hypokalemia: A clinical perspective. *Nat Rev Nephrol* 2011; 7: 75–84.

174 Disorders of plasma sodium

Aron Chakera, William G. Herrington, and Christopher A. O'Callaghan

Definition of the disease

The normal range for serum sodium levels in most laboratories is 135–145 mmol/l. Hyponatraemia is defined as a serum sodium concentration of < 135 mmol/l (<120 mmol/l is severe), and hypernatraemia as a concentration >145 mmol/l. As sodium is the major extracellular electrolyte, and freely diffuses throughout the extracellular space, it plays a key role in regulating osmolarity. Hyponatraemia is almost always associated with a hyposmolar state, except for the rare circumstances when there are other osmotically active substances present at high levels (e.g. glucose).

Aetiology of the disease

As sodium freely diffuses through the extracellular spaces, abnormalities in serum sodium reflect changes in the total amount of sodium and/or (more commonly) the total amount of fluid present. (In healthy individuals, regulation of serum sodium levels is tightly controlled by osmoreceptors.)

Given the relationship between sodium and water, accurate assessment of fluid balance is an integral part of determining the causes of hypo- or hypernatraemia (see Table 174.1).

An important cause of hyponatraemia in clinical practice is the syndrome of inappropriate diuresis (SIAD). Table 174.2 lists the major etiologies of SIAD.

Hypernatraemia, in contrast, almost always indicates dehydration, due to excessive free water loss (see Table 174.3 for other symptoms). This may be due to gastrointestinal losses, sweating, or renal losses, as occur in diabetes insipidus or with severe hyperglycaemia in diabetes mellitus. Iatrogenic causes of hypernatraemia include excessive infusions of normal saline, sodium bicarbonate, or Gelofusine which contain ~150 mmol/l sodium. As dehydration causes a hyperosmolar state, in normal circumstance this triggers thirst; for hypernatraemia to develop, there must also be inadequate access to water. This is a particular problem with elderly and hospitalized patients, who may be unable to regular their own water intake.

Typical symptoms of the disease, and less common symptoms

The typical and less common symptoms of the disease are stated in Table 174.3.

Demographics of the disease

Hypo- or hypernatraemia occurs in 5% of patients in general hospital wards, and at higher levels in high-dependency and intensive care

Table 174.2 Major causes of syndrome of inappropriate diuresis

Causes	Common examples
Tumours	Small cell carcinoma of bronchus, mesothelioma
	Head and neck cancers
	Gastrointestinal malignancies
	Lymphomas
Lung diseases	Pulmonary infections
	Severe asthma
Neurological conditions	Bleeds (e.g. subarachnoid haemorrhage)
	Trauma
	Infections
	Tumours
	Other: Guillain–Barré syndrome, multiple sclerosis
Endocrine disorders	Hypothyroidism
	Addison's disease
Medications	Amiodarone
	Chlorpropamide
	NSAIDs
	Carbamazepine
	Selective serotonin reuptake inhibitors
	Tricyclic antidepressants
	Ecstasy (MDMA)
Miscellaneous	Surgery
	Pain
	Stress
	Severe nausea

Table 174.1 Mechanisms and causes of hyponatraemia

Mechanism	Cause
Reduced water excretion (hypervolaemic hyponatraemia)	CCF
	Cirrhosis
	Nephrotic syndrome
	Renal failure
	SIAD
	• drugs
	• cancers
	• CNS and pulmonary diseases
	• pain
Increased water intake (hypervolaemic hyponatraemia)	Polydipsia
	Hypotonic IV infusions
Increased sodium loss (euvolaemic or hypovolaemic hyponatraemia)	Diuretics
	Salt-wasting tubular diseases
Miscellaneous	Pseudohyponatraemia
	Spurious (drip arm)
	Hypothyroidism
	Adrenal insufficiency

Abbreviations: CCF, congestive cardiac failure; CNS, central nervous system; IV, intravenous; SIAD, syndrome of inappropriate diuresis.

Table 174.3 Symptoms of hypo- and hypernatraemia

Hyponatraemia	Hypernatraemia
Attention deficits	Irritability
Impaired gait	Muscle twitches
Confusion	Confusion
Hyporeflexia	Hyperreflexia
Muscle cramps	Spasticity
Seizures	Seizures
Lethargy→ coma	Lethargy→ coma
Dysgeusia (uncommon)	

units. Elderly patients and patients with renal disease or head injuries that affect their ability to regulate sodium excretion or fluid intake are particularly at risk.

Natural history, and complications of the disease

Hyponatraemia has been shown to be an independent predictor of mortality in unselected general medical patients (whereas mortality from hypernatraemia generally reflects the presence of multiple comorbidities). Although relatively uncommon, rapid correction of hyponatraemia (especially if chronic) can cause an osmotic demyelination syndrome (central pontine myelinolysis), characterized by altered sensorium, cranial nerve, and long-motor tract dysfunction which can progress to loss of consciousness and death. The risk of this is increased when the initial serum sodium level is <120 mmol/l and if correction to normal is too rapid. As a guide, sodium levels should not be increased by more than 12 mmol/l in the first 24 hours (0.5 mmol/l hr^{-1}) of treatment.

Approach to diagnosing the disease

As the symptoms of hypo- or hypernatraemia are non-specific, these diagnoses will be missed, unless there is a high index of suspicion in hospitalized patients, and regular assessment of serum sodium levels in at risk groups. An awareness of the common medications and diseases associated with abnormalities of sodium homeostasis is important. Given the relationship between sodium and fluid balance, a thorough clinical assessment of volume status is essential. Once a diagnosis is made, ongoing clinical and laboratory assessment is crucial to determine the response to treatment and to tailor further treatment.

The following drugs are associated with hyponatraemia:

- diuretics
- antidepressants (e.g. selective serotonin reuptake inhibitors, monoamine oxidase inhibitors)
- antipsychotics
- anticonvulsants (e.g. chlorpromazine)
- chemotherapy agents (e.g. cyclophosphamide, cisplatin)
- ecstasy (MDMA)
- arginine vasopressin analogues (e.g. desmopressin, oxytocin)
- sulfonylureas (e.g. glipizide, glibenclamide, chlorpropamide)
- NSAIDs

Other diagnoses that should be considered

Hypervolaemic hyponatraemia, with evidence of fluid overload, such as a raised jugular venous pressure, and peripheral or pulmonary oedema, should prompt assessment of cardiac, hepatic, and renal function. Hyponatraemia in hospital may be secondary to SIAD, and assessment for potential CNS or respiratory diseases should be considered.

Most laboratories now analyse sodium with ion-specific electrodes on whole-blood specimens (without dilution) whereas, previously, measurements were made on prediluted serum or plasma. These prediluted samples could result in pseudohyponatraemia in the presence of hyperlipidaemia or hyperproteinaemia, due to an increase in the non-aqueous phase of plasma (which does not contain sodium).

'Gold-standard' diagnostic test

The gold-standard diagnostic test is laboratory assessment of serum sodium levels.

Acceptable diagnostic alternatives to the gold standard

Venous or arterial blood gas measurements, or measurements with portable devices such as the iSTAT® are useful alternatives, particularly when repeated assessment is needed, for example in the treatment of hyponatraemia.

Other relevant investigations

Abnormalities of other electrolytes often occur at the same time and it is important that these are assessed. Measurement of serum and urine osmolarity may be useful in determining the cause. For example, an inappropriately high urine osmolarity, in the presence of low plasma osmolality with hyponatraemia and fluid overload, suggests SIAD. As thyroid and adrenal insufficiency may be subclinical, biochemical assessment of these endocrine axes, with a serum thyroid-stimulating hormone and short tetracosactide test should be considered, if no other diagnoses are evident.

When diabetes insipidus is suspected as the cause of hypernatraemia, a water-deprivation test has high sensitivity and specificity for distinguishing central and nephrogenic diabetes insipidus, but should only be performed in a supervised inpatient setting. This test involves repeated measurements of simultaneously collected urine and serum electrolytes and osmolarity, body weight, and urine output, while all fluid intake is prevented.

Prognosis and how to estimate it

Prognosis is dependent on the degree of hypo- or hypernatraemia, and the presence of comorbid conditions. The increased mortality in hospitalized patients with hypo- or hypernatraemia should be appreciated and prompt regular review.

Treatment and its effectiveness

Where possible, the underlying cause of the hypo- or hypernatraemia should be treated. A euvolaemic state should be aimed for, with appropriate prescription of IV fluids when necessary. In general, hypertonic saline solutions are not necessary for the correction of hyponatraemia and can produce a correction that is too rapid. A new class of medications, the vaptans (non-peptide arginine vasopressin antagonists), which inhibit the action of vasopressin, have been trialled for euvolaemic and hypervolaemic hyponatraemia with good effect, and conivaptan (IV preparation) is now approved for this use in the USA. Demeclocycline 300–600 mg twice per day is now seldom used in the treatment of hyponatraemia, due to its adverse side effect profile, which includes renal impairment.

Hypernatraemia should be treated by careful clinical estimation of fluid deficit, and its correction with appropriate fluids, usually a combination of glucose and saline. Fluid deficit can be estimated using the following equation:

$$\text{Fluid deficit} = \text{TBW} \times (\text{current Na level} - 140)/140,$$

where TBW is total body water; in males, TBW = 0.6 × lean weight; in females, TBW = 0.5 × lean weight.

Further Reading

Spasovski G, Allolio B, Annane D, et al. Clinical practice guideline on diagnosis and treatment of hyponatraemia. *Eur J Endocrinol* 2014; 170: G1–G47.

Sterns RH. Disorders of plasma sodium: Causes, consequences, and correction. *N Engl J Med* 2015; 372: 55–65.

175 Disorders of plasma calcium

Aron Chakera, William G. Herrington, and Christopher A. O'Callaghant

Hypercalcaemia

Definition of hypercalcaemia

The extracellular calcium ion concentration is tightly regulated through the actions of parathyroid hormone (PTH) and vitamin D (1,25-dihydroxyvitamin D) on bone, kidney, and intestines. Abnormalities in these homeostatic mechanisms may lead to increased serum calcium concentrations, resulting in hypercalcaemia. Hypercalcaemic disorders may be divided into those associated with a high/high-normal serum PTH level, and those associated with a low serum PTH concentration.

Aetiology of hypercalcaemia

The aetiology of hypercalcaemia is given in Box 175.1

Primary hyperparathyroidism is the most common cause of hypercalcaemia in ambulant patients, with 85% of cases being due to a single adenoma, and the remainder being parathyroid hyperplasia; <1% are parathyroid carcinomas. Hyperparathyroidism is commonly found in patients with multiple endocrine neoplasia (MEN; types I and II). Chronically low vitamin D levels and chronic renal failure with persistently low calcium levels may stimulate the autonomous increased production of PTH, resulting in tertiary hyperparathyroidism, which in turn causes hypercalcaemia. Malignancy-induced hypercalcaemia is the more common cause in hospitalized patients. Familial hypocalciuric hypercalcaemia (FHH) accounts for 2% of all asymptomatic hypercalcaemia.

Typical symptoms of hypercalcaemia, and less common symptoms

With mild hypercalcaemia (<3.0 mmol/l), many patients are asymptomatic. As calcium levels rise, symptoms develop secondary to increased calcium concentrations and end-organ damage.

Typical symptoms include malaise, depression, confusion, lethargy, polyuria, polydipsia, constipation, abdominal or flank pain, musculoskeletal vague aches, and nausea or vomiting. Patients may have band keratopathy or show signs of proximal myopathy, dehydration, underlying malignancy, or hypertension. Some may present with coma.

Demographics of hypercalcaemia

The average age of diagnosis of primary hyperparathyroidism is 50–60 years, with an approximate incidence of 30–40 per 100 000

in the general population. It is two to three times more common in women than in men. The condition is rare in children. In MEN I, it is found in virtually all gene carriers by the age of 40 years, while it is seen in 10%–30% of families with MEN IIa. Hypercalcaemia secondary to malignancy increases with age and there is no sex preponderance. FHH is caused by mutations in the calcium-sensing receptor and is an autosomal dominant disorder with virtually complete penetrance.

Natural history of hypercalcaemia, and complications of the disease

Patients with primary hyperparathyroidism frequently present without symptoms and are detected after routine laboratory screening reveals hypercalcaemia. Although asymptomatic, these patients commonly develop bone disease, such as osteoporosis. Most sites are affected, but bone loss occurs predominantly in peripheral cortical bone such as the distal radius, with minimal involvement of the lumbar spine, although 15% of patients present with vertebral osteopaenia. With advanced disease, osteolytic lesions may result in bone cysts and, rarely, the condition osteitis fibrosa cystica; the latter is mainly found in tertiary hyperparathyroidism. As calcium levels increase, patients are predisposed to develop renal stones, which are present in 10%–20% of patients. Other renal complications include hypercalciuria and nephrocalcinosis. Both renal and skeletal complications are progressive. Peptic ulcer disease related to hypercalcaemia-induced gastrin release may be found, especially in patients with MEN I. Pancreatitis is rarely found. More commonly, patients develop neuropsychiatric and cognitive complaints with features of depression and anxiety. Cardiovascular complications may be related to hypertension.

Patients with chronic hypercalcaemia may present with other complications associated with long-standing high calcium levels, such as calcification of the basal ganglia, resulting in extrapyramidal symptoms and seizures, or epidermal changes with dry skin and brittle nails.

Hypercalcaemia of malignancy mainly presents with non-specific symptoms which overlap with the clinical features of the underlying disease and may lack many features associated with hyperparathyroidism.

Approach to diagnosing hypercalcaemia

The following approaches should be used to diagnose hypercalcaemia:

- check for hypercalcaemia-related symptoms, which may be vague and long-standing, and for complications related to end-organ damage
- identify symptoms and signs of hyperthyroidism and malignancy, especially of the breast, thyroid, lung, kidney, and prostate, as well as any squamous cell tumours and haematological malignancies (e.g. myeloma, lymphoma)
- confirm corrected hypercalcaemia
- identify drugs causing hypercalcaemia
- check serum PTH and, if high or normal, perform a fractional urine calcium excretion test, where
- if PTH is high or normal, and urine calcium excretion > 0.01 mmol/l, this indicates primary hyperparathyroidism; if, in addition, the renal function is abnormal, consider tertiary hyperparathyroidism
- if PTH is high or normal, and urine calcium excretion < 0.01 mmol/l, this indicates FHH
- if PTH is low or suppressed, exclude malignancy, hyperthyroidism, Addison's disease, sarcoidosis, and other granulomatous disorders

---

Box 175.1 The aetiology of hypercalcaemia

Common (>90% of cases)
- hyperparathyroidism (primary, tertiary)
- malignancy (PTH-rP (parathyroid-hormone related peptide) secreting tumours, bony metastases, multiple myeloma)

Uncommon
- vitamin D intoxication
- familial hypocalciuric hypercalcaemia
- thyrotoxicosis
- sarcoidosis and other granulomatous disorders
- milk-alkali syndrome

Rare
- thiazides, lithium
- Addison's disease
- vitamin A poisoning
- immobilization

Other diagnoses that should be considered aside from hypercalcaemia

Primary hyperparathyroidism may be associated with MEN types I and II.

'Gold-standard' diagnostic test for hypercalcaemia

Confirm hypercalcaemia, and then take a morning blood sample of PTH together with a corrected serum calcium level. Measure urinary calcium excretion if PTH is normal or high.

Acceptable diagnostic alternatives to the gold-standard test for hypercalcaemia

If PTH is high-normal or high, investigate for primary and tertiary hyperparathyroidism and FHH. If PTH is low, investigate for other causes, via the following tests:

- serum phosphate: this is low or normal in primary hyperparathyroidism and malignancy, and high in vitamin D-related disorders
- fasting urine calcium excretion
- serum alkaline phosphatase; this is high in primary hyperparathyroidism and malignancy
- thyroid function tests (to exclude hyperthyroidism)
- renal profile and liver function tests, including albumin
- plasma and urine protein electrophoresis (to exclude myeloma)
- a short tetracosactide test (to exclude adrenal insufficiency)
- skeletal X-rays (of hands, knees, and the lateral thoracolumbar spine)

Other relevant investigations for hypercalcaemia

Other relevant investigations for hypercalcaemia include:

- PTHrp (parathyroid hormone-related peptide); this peptide mediates hypercalcaemia associated with some malignancies
- vitamin D levels (calcitriol); this is useful in diagnosing hypercalcaemia secondary to granulomatous disorders (serum angiotensin-converting enzyme may be elevated in sarcoidosis)
- creatinine clearance; to exclude tertiary hyperparathyroidism and screen for hypercalcaemia-induced kidney disease
- 24-hour urine calcium, with or without biochemical stone analysis
- renal tract ultrasound, X-ray, and CT; to exclude calculi, nephrocalcinosis
- bone mineral density and bone turnover markers; for PTH-induced osteoporosis

In addition, consider chest radiographs and bone scintigraphy, to investigate for malignancy.

Prognosis for hypercalcaemia, and how to estimate it

The prognosis for malignancy-induced hypercalcaemia is poor, with the 1-year survival being 10%–30%. The prognosis for other hypercalcaemia-related disorders is excellent once the disease is treated.

Treatment for hypercalcaemia, and its effectiveness

Treatment of acute hypercalcaemia

If serum calcium >3.0 mmol/l or the patient is symptomatic or dehydrated, prompt IV infusions of large quantities of 0.9% normal saline, around 3–6 l over the first 24 hours. Loop diuretic may be added **only** if there is a risk of salt or fluid overload. Dialysis may be required in severe renal failure.

When the patient is well hydrated, IV bisphosphonates may be used to treat the cause of hypercalcaemia. These drugs are usually effective for conditions with increased PTH and PTHrp inhibiting bone resorption and tubular reabsorption of calcium, and are mainly used in malignancy and primary hyperparathyroidism, but are less effective in the latter. Pamidronate is given as a single IV infusion of between 30 mg and 90 mg, and plasma calcium usually falls by about 72 hours. The drug is usually well tolerated but patients may develop bone pains or a flu-like illness. The dose must be reduced with a glomerular filtration rate <30 ml/min. IV zoledronic acid 4 mg is more effective in achieving normocalcaemia than pamidronate and provides a longer median time to relapse of approximately 4 weeks vs 2.5 weeks. Zoledronic acid is mainly indicated in malignancy-induced hypercalcaemia. Denosumab can be used if malignancy-induced hypercalcaemia does not respond to zolendronic acid.

Salmon calcitonin may need to be given in patients resistant to bisphosphonates. In addition, some resistant cases respond to corticosteroid therapy such as prednisolone 40 mg/day. High-dose steroids are also used as first-line treatment of hypercalcaemia from vitamin D intoxication and granulomatous disorders (e.g. sarcoidosis).

Treatment of primary hyperparathyroidism

For a discussion of the treatment of primary hyperparathyroidism, see Chapter 187.

Hypocalcaemia

Definition of hypocalcaemia

Hypocalcaemia occurs when there are abnormalities in the physiological regulation of PTH, and vitamin D results in calcium levels are lower than the desired normal range. Failure of release of calcium from bone, and increased binding of calcium in the circulation, are other factors causing hypocalcaemia.

Aetiology of hypocalcaemia

The aetiology of hypocalcaemia is given in Box 175.2

Typical symptoms of hypocalcaemia, and less common symptoms

With mild hypocalcaemia, patients are usually asymptomatic. As calcium levels decrease, individuals may develop fatigue; tingling and numbness of toes, fingers, or lips; tetany; carpopedal spasm; cramps; confusion; bone pain; proximal myopathy; or prolonged QT interval on the ECG. Some patients may complain of dry skin, alopecia, or brittle nails. Less common features are cataracts, dental hypoplasia, papilloedema, psychoneuroses, seizures, and subnormal intelligence. Two important signs for diagnosis are Chvostek's sign (twitching of the corner of the mouth with tapping of facial nerve) and Trousseau's sign (carpopedal spasm by inflation of sphygmomanometer cuff above arterial pressure for 3 minutes).

Demographics of hypocalcaemia

Hypocalcaemia is found in all ages, with the differential diagnosis depending on patient age. It is found in males and females equally.

Box 175.2 The aetiology of hypocalcaemia

- hypoparathyroidism, due to
  - autoimmunity
  - surgery
  - infiltration
  - radiation
  - poor development
  - pseudohypoparathyroidism (a receptor defect resulting in high parathyroid hormone and low calcium)
- vitamin D deficiency
- phosphate administration
- tumour lysis syndrome
- hungry bone syndrome
- renal failure
- rhabdomyolysis
- pancreatitis
- drugs (e.g. phenytoin, cisplatin, calcitonin)
- malabsorption syndromes
- respiratory alkalosis (normal total calcium but low ionized calcium)
- hypomagnesaemia (functional hypocalcaemia due to an inhibition of PTH release)
- apparent hypocalcaemia (may be an artefact of low albumin levels)

The incidence will depend on the cause. It is found in around 20% of hospitalized patients.

Natural history and complications of hypocalcaemia

The hallmark of acute hypocalcaemia is neuromuscular irritability. Patients often complain of paraesthesia of the extremities, along with fatigue and anxiety. As calcium levels decrease, painful muscle cramps develop and may progress to tetany and spasms. In extreme cases, bronchial or laryngeal spasms may occur. Patients may also develop cardiovascular complications, including ECG changes such as prolonged QT or T-wave abnormalities, and reversible cardiomyopathy.

Dental abnormalities may be present if hypocalcaemia started in young age. Subcapsular cataracts may develop with chronic disease, as well as psychotic or neurotic disorders.

Patients with pseudohypoparathyroidism (type 1a) display short stature, obesity, short metacarpals, and a round face. This condition is known as Albright's hereditary osteodystrophy.

Approach to diagnosing hypocalcaemia

Symptoms and signs of hypocalcaemia should be elicited from the patient. Questions should be directed towards establishing the possible cause for low calcium levels, and appropriate laboratory tests performed. Patients with acute hypocalcaemia require immediate resuscitation.

Other diagnoses that should be considered aside from hypocalcaemia

In patients with vitamin D deficiency, besides acquired disorders (renal, liver disease, malabsorption, decreased sunlight), inherited disorders such as vitamin D-dependent rickets types I and II and X-linked hypophosphataemic rickets should be considered. Hypoparathyroidism may be part of DiGeorge syndrome, Kearns–Sayre syndrome, Kenny–Caffey syndrome, HDR (hypoparathyroidism, sensory neural deafness, renal dysplasia) syndrome, and autoimmune polyendocrine syndrome type I.

'Gold-standard' diagnostic test for hypocalcaemia

The gold-standard test for hypocalcaemia is a corrected serum calcium level, taken concurrently with a morning serum PTH.

Acceptable diagnostic alternatives to the gold-standard test for hypocalcaemia

Acceptable diagnostic alternatives to the gold-standard test for hypocalcaemia include tests for:

- vitamin D levels
- magnesium levels (abnormal levels are found with prolonged diarrhoea, diuretics, cisplatin, and alcohol abuse)
- phosphate levels (these are high in PTH deficiency, and low in non-parathyroid disease)

- renal and liver function, including tests for albumin (raised serum alkaline phosphatase suggests osteomalacia; renal failure causes vitamin D deficiency)

In addition, consider a coeliac screen.

Other relevant investigations for hypocalcaemia

Other relevant investigations for hypocalcaemia include:

- ECG
- imaging studies (e.g. chest X-ray if infiltrative disorders are suspected)
- thyroid function test, fasting glucose (random if symptomatic); Synacthen test if autoimmune polyglandular syndrome type 1 is suspected
- thyroid function test and gonadal status in pseudohypoparathyroidism (G-protein abnormalities)

Prognosis of hypocalcaemia, and how to estimate it

Severe, symptomatic hypocalcaemia may result in cardiovascular instability with hypotension, arrhythmias, and syncope, and may rarely progress to death. The disease causing the hypocalcaemia influences prognosis and varies accordingly.

Treatment of hypocalcaemia, and its effectiveness

In chronic hypocalcaemia secondary to parathyroid dysfunction, the aim is to raise calcium levels at or just below the normal limit. This may be done initially with large doses of calcium supplements, and if disease is not controlled vitamin D analogues, such as calcitriol or alfacalcidol, should be added. Plasma calcium levels should be checked frequently after each change in dose, and three monthly while on maintenance. In vitamin D deficiency, patients are usually treated with ergocalciferol or cholecalciferol.

Acute asymptomatic hypocalcaemia (<1.9 mmol/l), or symptomatic hypocalcaemia (with tetany or seizures) requiring control over a short time period, should be treated urgently with an infusion of 10 ml of 10% calcium gluconate diluted in 50–100 ml of 5% glucose infusion over about 10 minutes. This should be repeated until symptoms resolve. A maintenance infusion over 24 hours may be required, with careful monitoring of calcium levels and ECG. Concurrent oral calcium should be given, as well as calcitriol if the patient is PTH deficient.

Further Reading

Goldner W. Cancer-related hypercalcemia. *J Oncol Pract* 2016; 12: 426–32. doi: 10.1200/JOP.2016.011155.

Turner J, Gittoes N, Selby P, et al. Society for Endocrinology endocrine emergency guidance: Emergency management of acute hypocalcaemia in adult patients. *Endocr Connect* 2016; 5: G7–G8.

Walsh J, Gittoes N, Selby P, et al. Society for Endocrinology emergency endocrine guidance: Emergency management of acute hypercalcaemia in adult patients. *Endocr Connect* 2016; 5: G9–G11.

Disorders of plasma phosphate

Aron Chakera, William G. Herrington, and Christopher A. O'Callaghan

Definition of the disease

The normal serum level of phosphate is between 0.8 and 1.4 mmol/l.

Aetiology of the disease

Hyperphosphataemia

The commonest cause of sustained hyperphosphataemia is renal impairment, because the kidney normally excretes phosphate (note that phosphate levels normally rise following meals and that there is significant diurnal variation). A considerable phosphate load may also be provided by some medications, in particular, those used for bowel preparation.

Hypophosphataemia

Hypophosphataemia (see Table 176.1) may arise from reduced intake or absorption, increased renal excretion, or intracellular redistribution, particularly in response to carbohydrate loads with refeeding after starvation. Excessive renal phosphate loss can reflect tubular damage or inherited phosphate-wasting nephropathies.

Typical symptoms of the disease, and less common symptoms

As serum levels of calcium and phosphate are reciprocally related, high serum phosphate levels produce the same symptoms as hypocalcaemia. Hypophosphataemia is usually asymptomatic unless severe (serum phosphate <0.3 mmol/l), when it may cause generalized muscle weakness, rhabdomyolysis, and neurological symptoms, including dysaesthesia, confusion, and, eventually, coma.

Demographics of the disease

Hyperphosphataemia is common amongst patients with chronic kidney disease, with phosphate levels generally rising as the glomerular filtration rate falls below 30. Hypophosphataemia is usually encountered in malnourished patients and patients receiving total parenteral nutrition.

Natural history, and complications of the disease

Mild derangements in calcium or phosphate are usually asymptomatic and are not associated with any complications. Increased serum phosphate levels and a high calcium–phosphate product are associated with increased cardiovascular mortality and can promote dystrophic calcification (see Figure 176.1).

Approach to diagnosing the disease

As the laboratory tests for calcium and phosphate have high sensitivity and specificity, false-positive or false-negative results are unusual. Therefore, the key issue is to establish the underlying cause of the disorder.

'Gold-standard' diagnostic test

The gold-standard diagnostic test for disorders of plasma phosphate is the ionized serum phosphate level.

Acceptable diagnostic alternatives to the gold standard

There are no acceptable alternatives to the ionized serum phosphate level for diagnosing disorders of plasma phosphate.

Other relevant investigations

Calcium levels should always be measured, given the reciprocal nature of its relationship with phosphate. Ionized calcium levels are usually between 1.1 and 1.3 mmol/l (NB serum albumin levels must

Table 176.1 Causes of hypophosphataemia	
Reduced phosphate intake/absorption	Alcoholism
	Malnutrition
	Chronic diarrhoea
	Phosphate-binding medications
Renal phosphate loss	Hyperparathyroidism
	Diuretics
	X-linked and autosomal dominant hypophosphataemic syndromes
	Fanconi syndrome
Intracellular phosphate redistribution	Refeeding syndrome
	Glucose infusions
	Malignancies
	Growth hormone excess
	Adrenergic agents

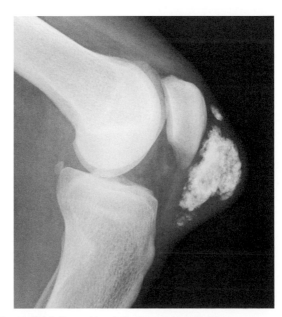

Figure 176.1 Dystrophic calcification involving the left pre-patellar bursa.

always be checked to allow for correction for albumin binding if ionized calcium levels are not measured). As hypomagnesaemia impairs the release of parathyroid hormone, assessment of serum magnesium levels should also be performed. If a renal cause of a phosphate abnormality is suspected, a 24-hour urine collection for calcium, phosphate, magnesium, and other electrolytes is indicated.

Prognosis and how to estimate it

Prognosis is dependent on the underlying condition.

Treatment and its effectiveness

Hyperphosphataemia in managed by dietary phosphate restriction; avoidance of high phosphate foods such as dairy products, sardines, chocolate, and nuts; prescription of phosphate-binding medications (to be taken with meals); and/or commencement of renal replacement therapy in patients with severe renal impairment.

Further Reading

Crook MA. Refeeding syndrome: Problems with definition and management. *Nutrition* 2014; 30: 1448–55.

Ketteler M, Elder GJ, Evenepoel P, et al. Revisiting KDIGO clinical practice guideline on chronic kidney disease: Mineral and bone disorder: A commentary from a Kidney Disease: Improving Global Outcomes controversies conference. *Kidney Int* 2015; 87: 502–28.

177 Disorders of plasma magnesium

Aron Chakera, William G. Herrington, and Christopher A. O'Callaghan

Definition

Normal serum magnesium levels are in the range of 0.7–1.0 mmol/l and, as for calcium, most of the total body magnesium is found in bone and soft tissues. Magnesium is essential for normal cell metabolism (as a cofactor for numerous enzymes) and for neuronal function, and regulates parathyroid hormone release. Alterations in serum magnesium levels are usually asymptomatic unless severe.

Aetiology of hypomagnesaemia and hypermagnesaemia

As there are large tissue reserves of magnesium, hypomagnesaemia usually only develops with chronic gastrointestinal or renal losses, or prolonged dietary insufficiency. Hypermagnesaemia is almost always iatrogenic, due to excessive supplementation. The main causes of hypomagnesaemia are listed in Table 177.1.

Typical symptoms of hypomagnesaemia and hypermagnesaemia, and less common symptoms

As magnesium, like calcium, is a divalent cation, the symptoms of magnesium deficiency are similar to those of calcium deficiency. The deficiency is generally characterized by neuromuscular and cardiac excitability, manifesting as cramps, twitching, and palpitations and, in severe cases, confusion and seizures. Vertigo, ataxia, and psychosis are uncommon presenting complaints.

Demographics of hypomagnesaemia and hypermagnesaemia

Hypomagnesaemia is a common finding in hospitalized patients, particular in acute care setting such as the ICU. Diabetic patients are particularly at risk. Hypomagnesaemia in the community is usually secondary to chronic malnutrition. The commonest cause is alcoholism. Hypermagnesaemia is almost always iatrogenic.

Table 177.1 Causes of hypomagnesaemia	
Renal magnesium loss	Inherited diseases
	• Bartter's syndrome
	• Gitelman syndrome
	Medications
	• Diuretics
	• Platinum-containing chemotherapy agents
	• Calcineurin inhibitors
	Osmotic diuresis
	• Diabetes
	• Mannitol
Inadequate intake/ increased gut losses	Malnutrition
	Chronic diarrhoea
	Inflammatory bowel disease
	Prolonged nasogastric suction
	Fistulae
	Proton-pump inhibitors

Natural history, and complications of hypomagnesaemia and hypermagnesaemia

Severe hypomagnesaemia can be life-threatening. It can cause tetany, convulsions, and cardiac arrhythmias. The prognosis is usually related to the underlying disease. Deficiency states due to excessive renal losses often respond to cessation of the offending medication or adequate replacement and, in these cases, the prognosis is good.

Approach to diagnosing hypomagnesaemia and hypermagnesaemia

The history and examination findings in hypomagnesaemia are non-specific, but the diagnosis should be considered in patients who complain of muscle cramps, particularly where there are risk factors present (see Table 177.1). Where increased renal losses are suspected, urinary magnesium levels should be measured, and inherited forms of tubular dysfunction considered. These are often associated with a history of salt craving. If a positive family history is elicited, genetic testing for some inherited disorders is now available. These include inherited channelopathies such as Gitelman syndrome, which causes sodium, potassium, and magnesium loss in the distal tubule, and Bartter's syndrome, which causes similar losses from the loop of Henle.

Other diagnoses that should be considered aside from hypomagnesaemia and hypermagnesaemia

Depending on the cause of the abnormal magnesium level, other electrolyte abnormalities may also be present and should be excluded.

'Gold-standard' diagnostic test of hypomagnesaemia and hypermagnesaemia

A serum magnesium level is the gold-standard test for hypomagnesaemia and hypermagnesaemia.

Acceptable diagnostic alternatives to the gold standard

There are no acceptable diagnostic alternatives to the gold-standard test for of hypomagnesaemia and hypermagnesaemia.

Other relevant investigations for hypomagnesaemia and hypermagnesaemia

As most tests measure total serum magnesium, free and bound (which accounts for ~20%) levels may be falsely low in hypoalbuminaemic states. Therefore, the serum albumin should be measured.

A fractional excretion of magnesium of greater than 3%, with a low serum magnesium and normal kidney function, is diagnostic of renal magnesium wasting. Twenty-four-hour urine collections to calculate renal magnesium excretion may also be performed. The fractional excretion of magnesium ($FEMg^{2+}$) may be calculated as follows:

$$FEMg^{2+} = 100 \times \left([Mg]_{urine} \times [Cr]_{plasma} \big/ [Mg]_{plasma} \times [Cr]_{urine} \right).$$

Intracellular assessment of magnesium in red blood cells, mononuclear cells, or skeletal muscle may provide a better measure of total body magnesium levels, as serum levels do not correlate well with intracellular levels. These tests are only routinely performed in research laboratories.

If a patient with symptoms consistent with hypomagnesaemia has a normal serum magnesium, and other diagnoses have been excluded, a magnesium loading test (IV infusion of magnesium, to see if symptoms resolve) can be performed, but false-positive results are common.

Hypocalcaemia and hypokalaemia frequently coexist with hypomagnesaemia, and serum levels should be measured.

An ECG should be performed if there are palpitations or evidence of cardiac arrhythmias. Findings are usually non-specific, but may include widened QRS complex and a prolonged PR interval. It is associated with ventricular arrhythmias, and evaluation of magnesium levels is, therefore, of particular value in patients with cardiac conditions such as heart failure.

Prognosis of hypomagnesaemia and hypermagnesaemia, and how to estimate it

The prognosis of hypomagnesaemia and hypermagnesaemia is generally good, as many causes are reversible on cessation of the offending agent, or respond well to replacement therapy.

Treatment of hypomagnesaemia and hypermagnesaemia, and its effectiveness

Severe depletion generally requires IV replacement with magnesium sulfate. Mild depletion, or chronic renal losses may be managed with oral magnesium preparations (which usually contain 2–4 mmol of magnesium/tablet), but these are often poorly tolerated due to adverse gastrointestinal side effects.

Further Reading

Ayuk J and Gittoes NJ. Treatment of hypomagnesemia. *Am J Kidney Dis* 2014; 63: 691–95.
Agus ZS. Mechanisms and causes of hypomagnesemia. *Curr Opin Nephrol Hypertens*. 2016; 25: 301–07.

178 Disorders of acid–base balance

Aron Chakera, William G. Herrington, and Christopher A. O'Callaghan

Definition of the disease

A change in the pH of the blood to outside the normal physiological range (pH 7.35–7.45) defines a disorder of acid–base balance. The disorder can be either acidaemia (pH <7.35) or alkalaemia (pH >7.45).

Aetiology of the disease

Normal metabolism results in a net acid production of approximately 1 mmol/kg day^{-1}. Physiological pH is regulated by excretion of this acid load by the kidneys and the lungs (as carbon dioxide). A series of buffers in the body reduces the effects of metabolic acids on body and urine pH. For acid–base disorders to occur, there must be excessive intake, or loss of acid (or base), or, alternatively, an inability to excrete acid. For these changes to result in a substantially abnormal pH, the various buffer systems must been overwhelmed. The pH scale is logarithmic, so relatively small changes in pH signify large differences in hydrogen ion concentration. Causes of acidaemia and alkalaemia are outlined in Tables 178.1 and 178.2, respectively.

Typical symptoms of the disease, and less common symptoms

Most minor perturbations in acid–base balance are asymptomatic, as small changes in acid or base levels are rapidly controlled through consumption of buffers, or through changes in respiratory rate. Alterations in renal acid excretion take some time to occur. Only when these compensatory mechanisms are overwhelmed do symptoms related to changes in pH develop (Table 178.3). Patients may be symptomatic from the underlying cause of the acid–base disturbance earlier.

Demographics of the disease

Acidaemia and alkalaemia are common in hospitalized patients, and typically reflect the severity of the underlying disease process. Over 50% of patients in critical care areas may have pH levels outside the normal range. Patients with renal or respiratory disease are

Table 178.1 Causes of acidaemia

Cause	Mechanism	Examples
Acid gain	Exogenous intake	Ethylene glycol
		Methanol
		Salicylate
	Endogenous production	Lactic acidosis • ischaemic tissue • metabolic syndromes (e.g. metformin related) Ketoacidosis • diabetes • starvation Renal failure Hypoventilation
Alkali loss	Gastrointestinal	Diarrhoea
		Large bowel fistulae
	Renal	Renal tubular acidosis

Table 178.2 Causes of alkalaemia

Cause	Mechanism	Examples
Acid loss	Gastrointestinal	Vomiting
		Prolonged nasogastric suctioning
		Villous adenomas
	Renal	Medications (e.g. diuretics)
		Channelopathies (e.g. Gitelman syndrome)
		Hyperaldosteronism
		Cushing's syndrome
	Respiratory	Hyperventilation
Alkali gain	Excessive intake	IV bicarbonate solutions
		Medications (e.g. antacids)

particularly at risk, because of the key roles played by the renal and respiratory systems in excreting excess acid.

Natural history, and complications of the disease

The natural history of acid–base disturbances primarily depends on the underlying cause. When the cause is reversible, for example, acidosis due to acute renal failure from obstruction, the prognosis is good. The presence of underlying chronic renal or respiratory disease is associated with a worse prognosis.

Alkalaemia with a pH >7.55 is associated with a high risk of mortality. As a general rule, alkalaemia is tolerated less well than acidaemia. Alkalaemia causes hypocalcaemia by increasing the affinity of calcium for proteins, and hypokalaemia by driving intracellular potassium redistribution. It also results in vasoconstriction, which in combination with hypoventilation (to retain carbon dioxide) leads to hypoxaemia and promotes tissue ischaemia and organ dysfunction. The consequence is neuromuscular irritability, cardiac arrhythmias, seizures, and, eventually, coma and death.

Acidaemia with pH levels less than 7.2 also increases the risk of cardiac arrhythmias and has negative inotropic effects, impairing cardiac output. Chronic acidaemia results in bone buffering of excess acid, which can lead to significant bone loss and fractures.

Approach to diagnosing the disease

A history should be taken to determine the presence of any preexisting diseases, particularly renal, respiratory, or gastrointestinal disorders that may explain impaired acid–base balance. The possibility of toxin ingestion should be considered, and a list of all current

Table 178.3 Symptoms of alkalaemia and acidaemia

Symptoms of alkalaemia	Symptoms of acidaemia
Hypoventilation (which can lead to hypoxia)	Nausea and vomiting
Muscle spasms	Hyperventilation (Kussmaul respiration)
Tetany	Confusion
Palpitations (from cardiac arrhythmias)	Palpitations
Seizures	
Renal stones (chronic)	

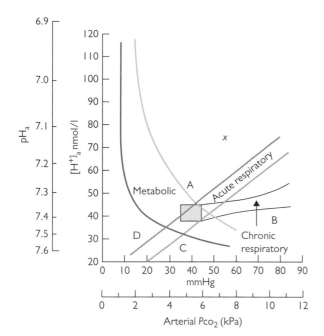

Figure 178.1 A practical acid–base diagram. The band marked 'acute respiratory' is the 95% confidence range of values obtained in normal individuals voluntarily hyperventilating or breathing air or carbon dioxide mixtures for short periods. After a few days of carbon dioxide retention, an increase in plasma bicarbonate produces substantial or complete compensation for the respiratory acidosis; the band in chronic respiratory acidosis is, therefore, different from that for the acute response, as the presence of the extra bicarbonate means that the arterial pH (pH$_a$) decreases to a lesser extent than would be expected for a given rise in the partial pressure of carbon dioxide in arterial blood (Arterial P$_{CO2}$).

medications and over-the-counter preparations reviewed. If the patient is clinically stable a family history should be taken to determine whether inherited renal (or other) diseases may be contributing to the impaired homeostasis.

Initial clinical assessment should focus on 'ABCs' and the identification of any imminent life threats (e.g. an impaired conscious state, cardiac arrhythmias, or evidence of ischaemic tissue (e.g. raised lactate)) before a complete examination is performed. Hyperventilation with a low carbon dioxide level is the normal response to severe acidaemia; therefore, a normal respiratory rate (or normal carbon dioxide level) suggests imminent respiratory collapse. An arterial blood gas should be performed early on, to identify whether there is a primary respiratory or metabolic disorder (based on the carbon dioxide and bicarbonate levels; see Figure 178.1), to provide an estimate of the base excess or base deficit, and to allow calculation of the anion gap. In the presence of acidosis, a high carbon dioxide level suggests a respiratory acidosis, whereas a low carbon dioxide level suggests a metabolic acidosis with respiratory compensation. Conversely, in the presence of alkalosis, a low carbon dioxide level suggests a respiratory alkalosis, whereas a high carbon dioxide level suggests a metabolic alkalosis with respiratory compensation.

If a chloride level is available, the anion gap can be calculated by using the following equation:

$$\text{anion gap} = \left(K^+ + Na^+\right) - \left(Cl^- + HCO_3^-\right).$$

The normal range of the anion gap is 12–20 mmol/l. An elevated anion gap should prompt review of the plasma lactate (lactate is

produced by anaerobic metabolism (e.g. in ischaemic tissue)), assessment for ketones (particularly in diabetics), and increase suspicion of poisoning with alcohols, including methanol and ethylene glycol or salicylates.

Further workup should be guided by results from the blood gases and initial blood tests and will usually include a chest radiograph to assess for respiratory disease. Abdominal imaging should be performed if there is evidence of renal dysfunction, or suspicion of intra-abdominal pathology.

Excess aldosterone can cause a metabolic alkalosis by promoting renal acid excretion. Therefore, plasma renin and aldosterone levels should be measured if derangements in adrenal hormones are suspected with alkalaemia. Adrenal imaging may then be indicated.

Other diagnoses that should be considered

Unexplained metabolic alkalosis, particularly if associated with hypokalaemia and hypomagnesaemia, may reflect diuretic abuse. A urine screen for diuretics can be performed.

'Gold-standard' diagnostic test

Arterial blood gas assessment is the gold-standard test for diagnosing abnormalities of acid–base balance.

Acceptable diagnostic alternatives to the gold standard

A venous blood gas can provide useful information if there is likely to be a delay, or difficulty in obtaining an arterial sample.

Other relevant investigations

If a renal cause of acidosis is suspected, a urinary pH is helpful, as a failure to appropriately acidify the urine is the presence of acidaemia suggests renal tubular acidosis.

Ethylene glycol poisoning causes oxalate crystal formation in the urine, which may be visible on microscopy.

Prognosis and how to estimate it

Alkalaemia is a poor prognostic sign, with mortality approaching 100% when pH levels are >7.6. Acidaemia with a pH <7.2 is also associated with significantly increased mortality, and consideration should be given to escalation of care to a high-dependency or intensive care unit. Regular assessment of pH in response to treatment provides the best marker for estimating prognosis.

Treatment and its effectiveness

The treatment of severe acidosis depends on whether it is primarily respiratory or metabolic in aetiology. Where an underlying cause is identified, specific measures should be employed where available (e.g. fomepizole, for ethylene glycol or methanol poisoning; antibiotics, for sepsis; surgery, for ischaemic bowel). Metabolic acidosis may be also be corrected by IV infusion of base (usually bicarbonate) but, in the presence of multi-organ dysfunction and/or cardiac disease, current evidence suggests it should be used with caution. A significant problem that arises with IV bicarbonate therapy is the sodium and water administration that this entails. The concomitant volume expansion increases the risk of pulmonary oedema. Other concerns include the possibility of worsening intracellular acidosis through the generation of carbon dioxide, and lowering calcium and potassium levels, which could increase cardiac arrhythmias. Haemodialysis or filtration can rapidly correct bicarbonate deficiency.

Treatment of alkalaemia involves correction of chloride deficits if present (renal bicarbonate reabsorption requires adequate chloride levels) and treatment of the underlying cause. Excess mineralocorticoid or renal tubular diseases associated with salt wasting are characterized by hypokalaemia and may respond well to potassium-sparing diuretics. In severe cases, IV infusions of acidic compounds (sodium chloride, hydrogen chloride, or potassium chloride) may be given. Specialist advice should be obtained.

Further Reading

Berend K, de Vries APJ, and Gans ROB. Physiological approach to assessment of acid–base disturbances. *N Engl J Med* 2014; 371: 1434–45.

Seifter JL. Integration of acid-base and electrolyte disorders. *N Engl J Med* 2014; 371: 1821–31.

179 Porphyria

Patrick Deegan

Definition of the disease

This section discusses six diseases caused by inborn errors of metabolism affecting the biosynthesis of haem. Haem is a tetracyclic metal-binding compound involved in oxygen transport (in haemoglobin and myoglobin) and redox reactions (e.g. in the cytochrome P450 system). A few very rare forms are not discussed.

Aetiology of the disease

Each of these conditions is caused by a single gene defect in one of the enzymes involved in the biosynthesis of haem. Inheritance is usually autosomal dominant with incomplete penetrance. The enzyme defect results in disease, not as a result of deficiency of the reaction product, but as a result of accumulation of precursors. Early, soluble precursors, 5-aminolaevulinic acid, and porphobilinogen (not porphyrins as such) are neurotoxic and, when present in great excess, as occurs when flux through the haem synthetic pathway is increased in response to particular medications or hormones, lead to acute neurovisceral crises. Later cyclical precursors (porphyrins) in the pathway are also water soluble and excreted in urine, but are susceptible to activation by electromagnetic radiation in the visible spectrum and are converted to free-radical metabolites that cause pain, inflammation, and tissue damage in the skin. The final haem precursors (also porphyrins) are hydrophobic and excreted in the bile and faeces and are also activated by light to toxic metabolites.

Typical symptoms of the disease, and less common symptoms

There are three main clusters of clinical features:

- neurovisceral crises (acute attacks)
- blistering photosensitive skin rashes with scarring
- photosensitive skin pain

The acute attack presents as severe abdominal pain with constipation; altered mentation and behaviour, including psychosis; autonomic instability with fluctuating heart rate and blood pressure; and peripheral neuropathy, including ascending paralysis and respiratory failure. The urine is typically a dark reddish colour and darkens further on exposure to light. The first attack may be fatal. Acute intermittent pophyria is associated with acute attacks alone. Variegate porphyria and hereditary coproporphyria are associated with both acute attacks and blistering skin rashes. Porphyria cutanea tarda is associated with blistering on sun-exposed areas, but without acute attacks: this condition is more usually sporadic than inherited and the sporadic form is associated with iron overload and chronic liver injury. Congenital erythropoietic porphyria is inherited in an autosomal recessive manner; the condition gives rise to haemolytic anaemia and severe photosensitivity, resulting in facial disfigurement. Erythropoietic protoporphyria is associated with intense pain, sometimes erythema, on light-exposed skin, but without blistering. In a small proportion of patients with erythropoietic protoporphyria, a syndrome of haemolysis and progressive cholestatic liver disease may occur.

Demographics of the disease

Porphyria acute attacks affect women more than men and often have their onset around puberty. Each condition is rare; the prevalence of heterozygosity for mutations causing acute intermittent pophyria, the most frequent porphyria, is around 1 in 10 000, but only around one-tenth of these individuals will develop acute attacks. Porphyria cutanea tarda is more common in middle-aged men. The skin manifestations of congenital erythropoietic porphyria and erythropoietic protoporphyria present in childhood, while the other cutaneous porphyrias may present later. Variegate porphyria is more common in South Africa, as a result of a founder mutation. Acute intermittent pophyria is more common amongst the inhabitants of Northern Sweden.

Natural history, and complications of the disease

As mentioned, only about 10% of individuals heterozygous for acute intermittent pophyria or variegate porphyria develop acute attacks. The remaining 90% are regarded as having 'latent' porphyria and are at risk of development of acute attacks, especially when exposed to certain 'unsafe' medications that upregulate the flux through the haem biosynthetic pathway. Acute attacks may also be precipitated in the few days before the menstrual period. Acute attacks, especially if left untreated, may lead to neuropathy and ascending paralysis with respiratory failure, requiring ventilation and prolonged intensive care support. Death or long-term disability may result from neurologic injury. In the course of an acute attack, the patient may develop a marked hyponatraemia associated with inappropriate antidiuretic hormone secretion: convulsions, cerebral oedema, and death may result. In the case of the cutaneous porphyrias, scarring and extensive photodamage occur on sun-exposed skin. This is particularly evident and disfiguring in congenital erythropoietic porphyria. Patients with erythropoietic protoporphyria complain of sun-induced pain from an early age and avoid light. A small proportion (around 5%) of patients with erythropoietic protoporphyria develop a self-perpetuating syndrome of haemolysis, increasing photosensitivity, and cholestatic liver failure.

Approach to diagnosing the disease

It is critical to make an early diagnosis of an acute porphyric attack. The key to the diagnosis is awareness. A careful family history will often provide the essential clue. Anaesthetists, surgeons, and intensivists should be aware of the association of acute attacks with anaesthetic drugs, particularly barbiturates used in induction. Acute porphyria should be on every physician's list of the medical causes of abdominal pain and on the list of causes of dark or red urine. Blistering porphyrias will be referred to a specialist. Skin pain without signs should not be ignored.

Other diagnoses that should be considered

Other causes of non-surgical abdominal pain include diabetic ketoacidosis, heavy metal poisoning, herpes zoster, sickle cell crises, and familial Mediterranean fever. Neuropathy with ascending paralysis and autonomic instability also suggests Guillain–Barré syndrome. Organic causes of psychosis clearly include the effects of alcohol and drugs.

'Gold-standard' diagnostic test

The definitive diagnosis of porphyria should take place in a specialist laboratory. Samples of urine, blood, and faeces, protected from light and sent to a specialist laboratory, will reveal patterns of excess porphyrins and their precursors and will thus allow the specific defect to be pinpointed in most cases. Difficulty sometimes arises in cases of suspected latent acute intermittent pophyria, where the pattern of metabolite excretion can be normal. Activity of hydroxymethylbilane synthase, the enzyme defective in acute intermittent pophyria, will be reduced by approximately 50% in heterozygotes, but this difference is often not sufficiently robust for diagnosis. For each porphyria, where facilities allow, sequencing of the relevant gene will allow confirmation of a biochemical diagnosis.

Acceptable diagnostic alternatives to the gold standard

In the acute situation, where the clinical question is whether the current signs and symptoms might be due to an acute attack of porphyria, a widely available urine porphobilinogen screening test is very helpful. Most hospital clinical chemistry departments should be able to offer this test and interpret the results. Some patients with acute intermittent pophyria will have a positive porphobilinogen screening test result between attacks, but no patient with a genuine acute attack should have a negative result.

Other relevant investigations

Serum sodium should be estimated at least daily in patients in an acute attack. Patients with erythropoietic protoporphyria should have 6-monthly blood tests looking for evidence of haemolysis and cholestasis. Serum liver-related blood tests are required in the monitoring of patients with porphyria cutanea tarda and erythropoietic protoporphyria. As porphyria cutanea tarda is associated with hepatitis C and HIV, the physician should inquire into these possibilities. Patients with acute intermittent pophyria, variegate porphyria, and hereditary coproporphyria may have an increased risk of hepatoma, and some experts recommend 6-monthly to annual liver ultrasound examinations. Renal impairment may develop in patients with acute intermittent pophyria.

Prognosis and how to estimate it

In women, acute attacks often remit after the menopause. Neuropathy can recover with careful medical support. It is difficult to predict which patients with erythropoietic protoporphyria will develop liver failure, but attention should be paid to coexisting risk factors for liver disease, including alcohol intake, gallstone disease, and hepatic steatosis. Increasing photosensitivity is an early warning symptom.

Treatment and its effectiveness

For patients at risk of acute attacks, patient and physician awareness of provoking factors is essential. Patient support groups and specialist websites are useful sources of information. Medic-alert bracelets and similar patient-held information can be helpful in the acute setting. Lists of safe and unsafe medication are available on websites and national formularies. Prevention of acute attacks can often be achieved through hormonal manipulation gonadotropin-releasing hormone analogues to suspend the menstrual cycle), avoidance of fasting, and institution of high carbohydrate intake during periods of intercurrent illness. An acute neurovisceral attack presents several difficulties in management. The patient is often very distressed, agitated, and behaviourally disturbed. Great care is required in all aspects of prescribing, but morphine is a safe analgesic, and prochlorperazine is a safe antiemetic. Careful fluid balance is required to avoid hyponatraemia; avoid 5% glucose solutions if possible. IV haem arginate is indicated for the acute treatment of moderate, severe, or unremitting acute attacks, and is usually effective in arresting the acute aspects of the attack, although established neuropathy may take months to resolve.

The dermatologic features of porphyria are managed by avoidance of light in the visible spectrum, through the use of clothing and pigmented barrier creams. Porphyria cutanea tarda often responds very well to venesection to control the modest degree of iron overload. The dermatological aspects of erythropoietic protoporphyria are sometimes helped by oral therapy with betacarotene or acetylcysteine. Many patients gain benefit from the use of narrow-band UVB exposure to induce skin pigmentation.

Established liver failure in a number of patients with erythropoietic protoporphyria has been rescued by liver transplantation, but disease can recur in the graft.

Genetic counselling and family-based case finding is recommended, to allow preventative measures to be taken in individuals with latent porphyria.

Further Reading

Puy H, Gouya L, and Deybach J-C. Porphyrias. *Lancet* 2010; 375: 924–37.
Ventura P, Cappellini MD, Biolcati G, et al. A challenging diagnosis for potential fatal diseases: Recommendations for diagnosing acute porphyrias. *Eur J Intern Med* 2014; 25: 497–505.

180 Aminoacidopathies, urea cycle disorders, and organic acidurias

Robin Lachmann and Elaine Murphy

Definition of the diseases

Aminoacidopathies, urea cycle disorders, and organic acidurias, are rare disorders resulting from disturbed protein or intermediary metabolism. Deficiency of an enzyme leads to accumulation of its substrate and deficiency of its product, both of which can contribute to pathogenesis.

Aetiology of the diseases

Aminoacidopathies are caused by deficiencies in enzymes involved in amino acid metabolism and are often characterized by the accumulation of a toxic amino acid. The two diseases most likely to be encountered in adult medicine are phenylketonuria (PKU), which is caused by a deficiency of phenylalanine hydroxylase, and maple syrup urine disease (MSUD), which is due to a branched-chain amino acid decarboxylase deficiency. High levels of phenylalanine progressively damage the developing brain, leading to severe learning difficulties. The high levels of leucine which accumulate in MSUD produce an acute encephalopathy which, if not treated, can be rapidly fatal.

The urea cycle is necessary for the detoxification of ammonia and the elimination of excess nitrogen. Patients in whom the cycle is impaired are at risk of hyperammonaemia, which leads to an acute encephalopathy and cerebral oedema. The commonest urea cycle disorder (UCD), ornithine transcarbamylase (OTC) deficiency, is X-linked and is the only condition discussed here which is not inherited in an autosomal recessive manner.

Organic acidurias are a complex group of disorders involving the metabolism of protein and fat into products which can be used in the general metabolism of the cell. Most present early in life with acute acidosis and encephalopathy, due to the accumulation of toxic metabolites.

For these disorders of protein breakdown, acute decompensations are triggered when the metabolic flux through the affected pathway cannot be supported by the residual enzyme activity. Decompensation can be triggered by a dietary protein load, with the most severe cases presenting in the neonatal period. In older children and adults, a catabolic state (such as intercurrent infection or fasting) with breakdown of endogenous protein for gluconeogenesis, frequently precipitates the acute presentation.

Typical symptoms of the diseases, and less common symptoms

Acute presentations of these disorders generally involve encephalopathy with confusion and an altered level of consciousness. Cerebral oedema then leads to seizures, coma, and death. In adults, hyperammonaemia can present subacutely with personality change, abnormal behaviour, and psychiatric symptoms.

Long-term complications of these disorders may include learning difficulties and behavioural problems. Patients with organic acidurias are particularly prone to basal ganglia damage. Specific features of other diseases include spastic paraparesis (arginase deficiency, a UCD) and certain forms of methylmalonic acidaemia (MMA, an organic aciduria), chronic renal failure (MMA), and eczema (PKU).

Demographics of the diseases

Aminoacidopathies are all rare. PKU has a carrier frequency of 1 in 50 and an incidence of about 1 in 10 000 births in Northern Europe: the other conditions are all less common than this.

Although the classical, severe forms of disease will present in the first few months of life, there are more attenuated forms which can present later in life.

Natural history, and complications of the diseases

The natural history of aminoacidopathies depends on the severity of the metabolic defect. In untreated patients with PKU, the degree of brain damage relates directly to the phenylalanine level. Patients with classical MSUD require continuous dietary therapy to prevent frequent decompensation but people with the milder, intermittent form maintain a normal amino acid profile except under conditions of metabolic stress.

Although mild mutations in the OTC gene can present for the first time in adult men, OTC deficiency in most hemizygous males is untreatable and they die in the neonatal period. Heterozygous female relatives can, however, have extremely variable clinical involvement, ranging from presentation in infancy with hyperammonaemia to adults who only have a slight aversion to high-protein foods. This range of presentation in females is thought to relate to skewed X-inactivation.

Late presentations of organic acidurias are not well recognized, possibly because adults presenting with reduced level of consciousness rarely have a full range of metabolic investigations performed.

Metabolic decompensations at any time in life can result in permanent brain damage. An adult with MSUD, a UCD, or organic aciduria may only have had one or two episodes of encephalopathy in early childhood, but can be left with significant learning difficulties and other features such as epilepsy or a movement disorder.

Approach to diagnosing the disease

There can be raised levels of the substrate of the affected enzyme, decreased levels of its product, or the presence of metabolites which cannot normally be detected at all. While, with modern analytical techniques, most metabolites can be detected in plasma, many substances are concentrated in the urine and are more easily detected there. Detection of a single metabolite can be pathognomic, but more often it is the pattern of metabolites which is important.

Hypoglycaemia or metabolic acidosis should raise the possibility of an inherited metabolic disease (IMD) and trigger the search for abnormal metabolites. Urine should be tested for ketones; the presence of non-ketotic hypoglycaemia implies a problem with intermediary metabolism. Measure plasma lactate and ammonia in the acute stage. A large anion gap implies the presence of an undetected acid which is most likely due to poisoning or metabolic mayhem.

Definitive diagnosis is complicated by the fact that abnormal metabolites may only be detectable during an acute decompensation and by the delay which can occur in obtaining the results of specialist tests. Where the patient presents in crisis, the approach must be to think of metabolic disease, to obtain as much information as possible acutely, and to save plasma and urine for further, directed analysis over the following days and weeks.

Other diagnoses that should be considered

Most physicians will never come across a patient with IMD presenting for the first time. However, improved treatment of these individuals in childhood means that they are now surviving into adulthood and it is increasingly likely that acute metabolic decompensations in patients with known metabolic disease will be seen in the general medical setting. An encephalopathic patient cannot always tell you about a preexisting condition, so it is always important to consider these rare diseases as well as commoner causes such as infection or cerebrovascular events.

'Gold-standard' diagnostic test

Direct demonstration of the enzyme deficiency is not always possible, as the enzymes in question are not always expressed in easily accessible cells such as leukocytes or fibroblasts (e.g. some urea cycle enzymes are only expressed in the liver). It may therefore be sufficient to demonstrate pathological mutations in the relevant gene.

Acceptable diagnostic alternatives to the gold standard

Diagnosis is often based on specialist interpretation of a characteristic pattern of abnormal metabolites in blood and/or urine.

Other relevant investigations

Other relevant investigations are guided by the clinical situation.

Prognosis and how to estimate it

Prognosis is largely determined by whether a patient survives their initial metabolic decompensation. For this to happen, the correct diagnosis has to be made and appropriate treatment initiated in a timely manner. Steps can then be taken to avoid future decompensations and prompt treatment given if they do occur.

Nonetheless, there are still cases where the metabolic block is so severe that current treatment is not effective and children die. For those who survive childhood, the risk of decompensation tends to reduce as they get older and, providing they are compliant with their treatment, their prognosis in adulthood relates to any chronic complications, often more than the risk of acute deterioration.

The danger for those who do have metabolic decompensations in adulthood, either as an initial presentation or where the diagnosis is already made, is that the cause of the acute illness will not be recognized and appropriate treatment not given.

Treatment and its effectiveness

The principles underlying the treatment of these disorders are similar. For detailed protocols see the British Inherited Metabolic Disease Group website (http://www.bimdg.org.uk).

In acute decompensation, first stop catabolism by giving large amounts of carbohydrate as a source of calories. Each patient should have a specific emergency regimen. At home, this includes glucose polymer drinks: in hospital, glucose is given as an IV infusion, usually 10% dextrose running at 2 ml/kg hr^{-1}.

Second, stop protein intake, to minimize the need for protein metabolism. If, however, patients do not recover quickly and require inpatient treatment for more than a few days, a lack of dietary protein will itself trigger endogenous protein breakdown. In MSUD, this is overcome by using a synthetic amino acid supplement free of the branched-chain amino acids, which cannot be catabolized, but, in the UCDs, for example, where the block affects general protein catabolism, specialist metabolic dietetic advice should be sought regarding the gradual reintroduction of dietary protein.

Third, remove toxic metabolites. Continuous haemodiafiltration will effectively remove ammonia, leucine, and other small molecules from the circulation, and has a role in UCDs, MSUD, and organic acidurias. Specific treatments may also be available. In MSUD, use of a synthetic amino acid supplement can reduce plasma leucine levels by stimulating its incorporation into newly synthesized proteins. In hyperammonaemia, arginine is given to stimulate protein synthesis, and the alternative pathway ammonia scavengers sodium benzoate and sodium phenylbutyrate can be given. Carnitine may be used in some organic acidurias.

With appropriate and aggressive treatment, it should be possible to terminate an acute decompensation, but patients can still suffer long-term neurological consequences due to cerebral oedema or metabolic stroke.

Long-term treatment relies on the same principles. In PKU and MSUD, a low-protein diet is combined with an amino acid supplement containing all the vitamins and minerals which are missing from the restricted diet. In UCDs, a low-protein diet is combined with essential amino acid supplements and oral ammonia scavenger treatment to optimize nutrition and prevent hyperammonaemia. Treatment for organic acidurias is specific to the condition but may include a low-protein diet, vitamin B$_{12}$ (in the case of MMA), carnitine, and general vitamin and mineral supplementation.

Further Reading

Blau N, van Spronsen FJ, and Levy HL. Phenylketonuria. *Lancet* 2010; 376: 1417–27.

Lee PJ and Lachmann RH. Acute presentations of inherited metabolic disease in adulthood. *Clin Med* 2008; 8: 621–4.

181 Amyloidosis

Sajjan Mittal

Introduction

Amyloidosis is a systemic disease caused by extracellular deposition of insoluble abnormal fibrils that injure tissues and organs. The fibrils are formed by the aggregation of misfolded, normally soluble proteins.

Systemic amyloid light-chain (AL) amyloidosis (primary) is the commonest type of amyloidosis in the developed world, accounting for 80% of cases. The remainder are due to AA amyloidosis (secondary or reactive), familial amyloidosis, or other rare types of amyloidosis.

Classification of amyloidosis

Amyloidosis is broadly classified in five subgroups which are further described in Table 181.1.

Systemic AL amyloidosis

Aetiology

Systemic AL amyloidosis is associated with a clonal plasma cell dyscrasia, and results from extracellular deposition of monoclonal light chain fragments in an abnormal insoluble fibrillar form. In some cases, this may be associated with myeloma or other B-cell malignancies. However, no definite predisposing factor is known.

Epidemiology

AL amyloidosis occurs in about 1 in 1300 people, and the frequency increases with age. Most patients with AL amyloidosis are aged over 45 years, but it occasionally occurs in young adults. The median age of presentation is 64 years, with a male:female ratio of 2:1.

Clinical features

The most common clinical features at diagnosis are nephrotic syndrome with or without renal impairment, heart failure (typically with predominant right heart failure), sensorimotor and/or autonomic peripheral neuropathy, and hepatosplenomegaly. Carpel tunnel syndrome is seen in approximately one-fifth of patients. Macroglossia is found in 5%–10% of cases but is almost pathognomonic of AL amyloidosis. Purpura, particularly in the periorbital (raccoon eyes) and facial areas, is noted in about one-sixth of patients. Gross bleeding is reported in approximately 3% of cases, as a result of acquired deficiency of Factor X and sometimes also Factor IX or with increased fibrinolysis. Bone pain is a major symptom in only 5% and usually is related to lytic lesions or fractures associated with myeloma. AL amyloidosis can affect most organs except the CNS. Fatigue and weight loss are very common symptoms.

Natural history, and complications of the disease

AL amyloidosis is a progressive disorder which, without treatment, is usually fatal within 5 years. Most of patients die of heart or renal failure.

Diagnostic investigations

Initial investigation should confirm the diagnosis of amyloidosis on tissue biopsy, and this should be followed by investigations to establish the type of amyloid present and the extent of organ involvement. Amyloid deposits stain with Congo red and produce pathognomonic apple-green birefringence under cross-polarized light microscopy, irrespective of type of amyloidosis (Figure 181.1). This is a gold-standard diagnostic test.

Biopsy of an affected organ is usually diagnostic but less invasive alternatives are possible. Screening biopsy of abdominal fat or rectum is diagnostic in 50%–80% of cases. Immunohistochemical staining of tissue sections with a panel of antibodies is used to differentiate AL amyloidosis from AA amyloidosis. DNA analysis is required to exclude hereditary forms.

Serum amyloid protein P (SAP) scintigraphy is a nuclear medicine imaging technique in which radiolabelled protein is injected intravenously to assess the presence and distribution of amyloid deposits. Patients are referred to National Amyloidosis Centre in London for this investigation.

Other investigations to evaluate organ involvement include measurement of plasma brain natriuretic peptide (to detect cardiac involvement), echocardiography (cardiac amyloidosis typically results in a restrictive cardiomyopathy), measurement of 24-hour urine protein excretion, liver function tests, and nerve conduction studies.

Other relevant investigations

Other relevant investigations include full blood count, urea and electrolytes, creatinine, calcium, immunoglobulin electrophoresis, and quantitative serum free light chain assay. Bone marrow aspirate and trephine biopsy, and skeletal survey, are routinely done in amyloidosis patients to confirm or exclude underlying plasma cell dyscrasia.

A coagulation screen is helpful in excluding associated acquired coagulopathy.

Monitoring

Measurement of serum free light chains and immunoglobulins, SAP scintigraphy, and specific functional tests of involved organs are used to assess the response to treatment.

Prognosis

Without treatment, AL amyloidosis has always a progressive course with rapid development of heart or renal failure. Treatment of heart and renal failure is usually ineffective, with median survival of 18–20 months. Outcomes for symptomatic cardiac AL patients remain relatively poor (median overall survival, 10 months).

Treatment and its effectiveness

Treatment of AL amyloidosis is directed at the underlying bone marrow disorder. In principle, chemotherapy in patients with AL amyloidosis is the same as in those with myeloma. The aim of chemotherapy is to decrease the number of abnormal plasma cells, as this will proportionately reduce the production of amyloid-forming protein (light chain protein). As a result, new amyloid formation will decrease and

Table 181.1 Classification of amyloidosis		
Amyloid type	**Classification**	**Amyloidogenic protein involved**
Amyloid light-chain amyloidosis	Primary, including myeloma	Kappa or lambda light chains
AA amyloidosis	Secondary	Protein A
Familial amyloidosis	Familial amyloid polyneuropathy / Cardiopathic	Mutant transthyretin
Senile systemic amyloidosis	Senile cardiac	Normal transthyretin
Dialysis amyloidosis	Dialysis arthropathy	Beta-2 microglobin

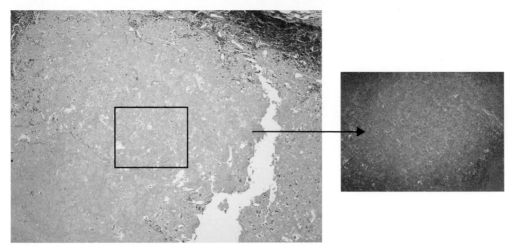

Figure 181.1 Amyloid deposition (amorphous material; boxed area) in a lymph node in amyloid light-chain amyloidosis. Please see colour plate section.

existing amyloid deposits may gradually regress as well. However, regression of amyloid is slow, and often takes 6– 12 months after chemotherapy is completed. A consultant haematologist supervises the treatment of patients with AL amyloidosis. Effective and high-quality care requires a multi-speciality and multidisciplinary team familiar with the range of clinical problems likely to be encountered.

CTD (a combination of cyclophosphamide, thalidomide, and dexamethasone), VCD (bortezomib, cyclophosphamide, and dexamethasone) or VTD (bortezomib, thalidomide, and dexamethasone) are the standard first line treatment options with an estimated 3- year survival of 100% in the responders. However, low- dose treatment, such as a combination of melphalan and prednisolone, is used in elderly patients. Upfront autologous transplant is possible in AL amyloidosis. About two- thirds of patients benefit substantially from this type of treatment. However, given a high rate of treatment- related mortality, autologous transplant is not very popular in the UK. Lenalidomide, pomalidomide, carfilzomib and daratumumab are the newer treatment options.

Localized AL amyloidosis

AL amyloidosis can occur in a localized form that is most often identified in the upper respiratory, urogenital, and gastrointestinal tracts, in the skin, and in the orbits. In such circumstances, the amyloidogenic light chains are produced by a subtle focal infiltrate of clonal plasma cells in proximity to the amyloid deposits. This type of amyloid is frequently nodular in character. Local AL amyloid rarely progresses into a true systemic disease. Systemic chemotherapy is not indicated in localized AL amyloidosis. Local radiotherapy or surgical excision is the treatment of choice.

AA amyloidosis

Reactive systemic AA (secondary) amyloidosis is seen in a small proportion of patients with chronic inflammatory diseases (<5%). AA amyloid fibrils are derived from circulating acute phase reactant (serum amyloid A protein (SAA)). Common associated conditions in the developed world are rheumatoid arthritis and Crohn's disease. Familial Mediterranean fever and chronic infections are the other important causes of AA amyloidosis. Most patients present with nephropathy (proteinuria), although liver and gastrointestinal involvement may occur at a late stage. Clinical cardiac and nerve involvement are extremely rare.

Once the process of AA amyloid deposition has started, excessive amounts of SAA continue to be produced and deposited as amyloid in the organs, as long as the underlying inflammatory disease remains active. The aim of treatment in AA amyloidosis is to control the underlying inflammatory disease and thereby reduce the amount of SAA in the blood. Some underlying inflammatory diseases have very specific and highly effective treatments, for example colchicine in patients with familial Mediterranean fever.

Familial amyloidosis

Hereditary amyloidosis is less common than AL or AA amyloidosis. It is due to the inheritance of an abnormal gene which leads to life-long production of a potentially amyloid-forming protein. Most familial forms of amyloidosis do not cause any symptoms until middle age or later. They are all inherited in an autosomal dominant fashion.

Familial amyloid polyneuropathy (FAP) is the most common type of hereditary amyloidosis in the world. It is characterized by deposition of amyloid in nerves, causing limb weakness, loss of sensation, nerve pain, bowel, bladder, and blood pressure disturbances, and sexual dysfunction. FAP is common in some parts of Portugal, Sweden, and Japan, but occurs throughout the world in very small numbers.

Liver transplantation as a treatment for hereditary amyloidosis has been used most extensively so far in patients with FAP as, in these patients, the abnormal amyloid-forming protein, mutant transthyretin, is made almost exclusively in the liver. Replacement of the liver by a liver that makes normal transthyretin protein is aimed at preventing the formation of further amyloid and can stabilize the disease. Combined liver and heart transplant has been successfully performed in a small number of cases with cardiopathic subtype of familial amyloidosis.

Senile cardiac amyloidosis

This condition occurs as a result of transthyretin deposition in heart in old age, resulting in heart failure. This syndrome is extremely rare before 65 years of age. There is no specific treatment but the patients can survive for many years with reasonable quality of life on diuretics.

Dialysis amyloidosis

Dialysis amyloidosis occurs due to accumulation of beta-2 microglobin in renal failure, and this condition predominantly affects articular and periarticular structures in patients who have end-stage renal failure and who have been on dialysis for at least 7–10 years. Arthralgia may respond to NSAIDs or corticosteroids. However, there is no definite treatment.

Further Reading

Banypersad SM, Moon JC, Whelan C, et al. Updates in cardiac amyloidosis: A review. *J Am Heart Assoc* 2012; 1: 1–14.

Sipe JD, Benson MD, Buxbaum JN, et al. Nomenclature 2014: Amyloid fibril proteins and clinical classification of the amyloidosis. *Amyloid* 2014; 21: 221–4.

PART 7

Diabetes mellitus and endocrine disorders

182 Normal function of the endocrine system

John Newell-Price, Alia Munir, and Miguel Debono

Definition

Endocrinology is the study of hormones (and their glands of origin), their receptors, the intracellular signalling pathways they invoke, and their associated diseases. The clinical specialty of endocrinology focuses specifically on the endocrine organs, that is, the organs whose primary function is hormone secretion, including the hypothalamus, the pituitary, the thyroid, the parathyroid, the adrenal glands, the pancreas, and reproductive organs. An endocrinologist specializes in the diagnosis and management of hormonal conditions.

Hormones

Introduction

Hormones (from the Greek word *harmon*, meaning 'excite') are chemical messengers that are released from cells into the bloodstream to exert their action on target cells. Blood-borne hormones acting at distant sites are 'endocrine' and hormones acting on adjacent cells are 'paracrine', while hormones which feed back on the cell which releases them are 'autocrine'. An 'intracrine' signal is generated by a chemical acting within the same cell. Hormones are crucial mediators of body homeostasis.

Hormone classes

There are five main classes of hormones. These are categorized into the following groups according to structural and/or functional similarities: amine hormones; peptide hormones; cholesterol derivatives and steroids; thyroid hormones; and eicosanoids.

Amine hormones

Amine hormones are hormones that are derived from the modification of amino acids. There are three main amine hormones, which also act as neurotransmitters: **adrenaline**, **noradrenaline**, and **dopamine**. These are phenylalanine derivatives (via the conversion of phenylalanine to tyrosine) and are all secreted by the adrenal medulla; they are also known as **catecholamines**. The synthesis of catecholamines is rate limited by the conversion of tyrosine to dihydroxy-phenylalanine by tyrosine hydroxylase. Subsequently, dopamine, then noradrenaline, and then adrenaline are synthesized. Methylation of adrenaline from noradrenaline is mediated by phenylethonalamine-N-methyltransferase. This reaction is cortisol dependent. Amine hormones are then stored in the adrenal medulla and are secreted in response to either nerve or humoral stimuli. Release is episodic, and catecholamines have a short half-life. They bind to alpha and beta adrenoceptors, while dopamine binds to D1 and D2 receptors to exert their physiological effects. Noradrenaline and adrenaline are broken down via catechol-O-methyl transferase into **normetanephrine** and **metanephrine**, respectively. These products are further degraded to **vanillylmandelic acid**. Catecholamines and nor/metanephrines may be found both in plasma and in urine.

Melatonin is another amine hormone; unlike the catecholamines, it is derived from tryptophan. It is synthesized in and released from the pineal gland at night. It is involved in the resynchronization of sleep and circadian rhythm disturbances.

Peptide hormones

Peptide hormones are composed of amino acids. The number of amino acids may vary from very few—3 in **thyrotropin-releasing hormone (TRH)**—up to 180 or more in pituitary gonadotrophins. Peptide hormones may be linear (e.g. **angiotensin II**) or may contain a ring structure (e.g. **oxytocin** and **vasopressin**). The larger protein hormones like **insulin, thyroid-stimulating hormone (TSH; also known as thyrotropin), follicle-stimulating hormone (FSH)**, and **luteinizing hormone (LH)** are composed of two peptide chains. Intra-chain disulphide bonds, found in some hormones, including **prolactin** and **growth hormone**, help protect from enzyme breakdown and create a tertiary structure necessary to produce an active site. Insulin is made up from both inter- and intra-chain disulphide bonds. Some of the larger proteins may bind to carbohydrate residues and form glycoproteins.

Peptides are mainly stored in secretory granules and are usually released in pulses, which may either be regular or as a response to a stimulus. These hormones, mainly hydrophilic, do not usually diffuse passively through plasma membranes and mainly exert their action by activating receptors at the surface. They have the potential to cause receptor downregulation. Circulating peptides are then broken down either by circulating enzymes or by tissue-bound enzymes.

Cholesterol derivatives and steroids

Cholesterol-derived hormones include **vitamin D** and its metabolites, as well as adrenocortical and gonadal steroids. The adrenal steroidogenic tissue produces glucocorticoids (**cortisol**, corticosterone, and cortisone), mineralocorticoids (**aldosterone**), and sex steroids (androgens), while the gonad steroidogenic tissue produces the sex steroids: **androgens, oestrogens**, and **progestins**.

As steroids are insoluble in water, in circulation they are mainly bound to proteins such as albumin, cortisol-binding globulin (CBG), and sex hormone-binding globulin (SHBG). This gives them longer half-lives. These hormones are lipophilic and may passively diffuse into cells and bind with receptors in the nucleus to induce a response, or bind with receptors in the cytoplasm to form a steroid-receptor complex which is then carried to the nucleus. Some are altered to active metabolites intracellularly. Inactivation and clearance of steroid hormones is not very rapid and occurs mainly in the liver (some in the kidney), although a small amount is secreted unchanged in the kidneys.

Vitamin D is synthesized in the skin and then released into the bloodstream to exert its effects in tissues. Cholecalciferol is synthesized in the skin from cholesterol and 7-dehydrocholesterol (obtained from diet); this is then converted to 25-hydroxycholecalciferol in the liver and is then converted to the active 1,25-hydroxycholecalciferol (calcitriol) in the kidney or the inactive 24,25-hydroxycholecalciferol. The main targets of calcitriol are the kidneys, gut, and bone.

Thyroid hormones

The thyroid gland synthesizes two hormones, **thyroxine (T_4)** and **triiodothyronine (T_3)**, from the precursor tyrosine. Tyrosine is cleaved from thyroglobulin in the colloid. T_4 and T_3 contain iodine, which is extracted from the circulation and incorporated into their structures, as it is required for their biological activity. Initially, T_4 and T_3 are bound to thyroglobulin but, when the thyroid is stimulated by TSH, these are cleaved and pass into the circulation. Most of T_3 in the circulation (80%) comes from peripheral conversion from T_4 through the actions of deiodonase enzymes. Thyroid hormones are not water soluble and are carried by proteins such as albumin, transthyretin, and thyroxine-binding globulin (TBG). There is active uptake in cells. The thyroid hormones, like steroids, exert their actions through receptors in the nuclei, where they bind directly to DNA. T_3 is the main active hormone in the cell, while T_4 is its prohormone.

Eicosanoids

Eicosanoids are chemical messengers that are derived from arachidonic acid or other polyunsaturated fatty acids. Prostaglandins, including prostacyclins and thromboxanes, comprise one class of eicosanoids and mainly act locally (via paracrine or autocrine signalling), although some, like prostacyclins, do have an endocrine effect. Leukotrienes comprise another family of eicosanoids.

Eicosanoids have important roles in uterine contraction, ovulatory cyclicity, inflammation, platelet aggregation, pain sensation, and bronchospasm.

Hormone receptors

Hormone receptors may be found at different sites on cells and play an important role in the effects of hormones on target tissue.

Cell surface receptors

Hormones that do not diffuse across plasma membranes, such as peptide hormones, have receptors at the cell surface. The receptors are commonly coupled with intracellular signalling molecules, and the majority are G-protein-linked receptors. When hormones bind to the receptor, this stimulates either the opening of ion channels in the membrane or the activation of a membrane-bound enzyme that stimulates the production of a secondary messenger. These secondary messengers, such as cyclic AMP, diacylglycerol, and inositol triphosphate, activate protein kinases, which then regulate transcription.

Another common type of cell surface receptor is a transmembrane receptor with either inherent protein tyrosine kinase activity on the intracellular site, or associated molecules with tyrosine kinase activity. Binding of a hormone such as insulin, growth hormone, prolactin, or one of the cytokines to the receptor results in dimerization with another receptor, initiating phosphorylation followed by transcription regulation.

Intracellular receptors

Receptors for steroid and thyroid hormones, which, being lipophilic, readily diffuse across cell membranes, are typically intracellular. All steroid receptors are transcription factors. They bind to DNA and, in conjunction with other transcription factors, initiate, or suppress, RNA synthesis. The receptors predominantly found in the cytoplasm are type 1 receptors and include glucocorticoid, mineralocorticoid, androgen, and progesterone receptors. They are bound to heat-shock proteins. As the steroid binds the receptor, the heat-shock protein is released and the receptor dimerizes with another identical receptor. The hormone–receptor complex then translocates to the nucleus and binds to DNA. The thyroid hormone receptor is a type 2 receptor, which, in contrast, is typically located in the nucleus. The receptors recognize and bind to a base sequence, which known as a hormone response element, on the DNA in order to alter transcription. Steroid hormones may also bind to and activate or repress other transcription factors (e.g. NF-kappa B), either in the nucleus or in the cytoplasm ('non-genomic effect'). Steroid and thyroid hormones may stimulate rapid responses in cells by interacting with poorly characterized receptors at the cell surface.

Hormone receptor regulation

Receptor regulation occurs by up- or downregulation of the number of receptors or by desensitization of the receptors. Interactions between hormones and their receptors depend on the number of receptors, the concentration of circulating hormone, and the affinity of the hormone for the receptor. For example, when receptor numbers are reduced, a higher concentration of hormone is needed to occupy a similar number of receptors and achieve an equal target cell response.

Hormonal regulation

In order to induce a specific action at a required time, hormone action needs to be controlled. Hormones are regulated in a number of ways. They may be secreted constantly or in a pulsatile fashion. Many rhythms for hormone secretion, such as the cortisol circadian rhythm, are regulated by the circadian pacemaker in the suprachiasmatic nucleus, which is mainly influenced by the light–dark cycle through information delivered through retinohypothalamic tracts. Hormones may be released as a response to a nerve stimulus or a hormone (e.g. a releasing hormone). Stimuli may either provoke release from secretory vesicles to produce a rapid effect (in the case of peptide hormones and catecholamines), or enhance hormone synthesis, producing a delayed effect.

Inhibition of hormone release may occur via release-inhibiting factors (e.g. dopamine inhibits prolactin release, and somatostatin inhibits growth hormone release) or by negative feedback inhibition. Feedback loops may involve the hypothalamic–pituitary–adrenal (HPA) axis, which detects changes in the concentration of hormones secreted by peripheral glands (see Figure 182.1A); alternatively, an organ may respond to changes in a variable in the internal environment (see Figure 182.1B).

An important interaction exists between immune and endocrine systems, demonstrating bidirectional communication. Cytokine regulation of the HPA axis during the stress response occurs by stimulation of hypothalamic corticotrophin-releasing hormone (CRH), with resultant release of adrenocorticotropic hormone (ACTH) from the pituitary, and cortisol from the adrenal.

Hormonal physiology

Thyroid

The thyroid gland secretes all T_4 and 20% of T_3. The concentration of T_4 is about 50 times greater than that of T_3. In blood these hormones are almost entirely (>99%) bound to plasma proteins: 70% to TBG, 15% to transthyretin, and 15% to albumin. Only the free hormone is available to the tissues and biologically active; this fraction correlates closely with the metabolic state of the individual but the concentration does not vary directly with the total hormones.

T_3 binds weekly to TBG, compared to T_4, and so has a faster onset of action and is four times more active than T_4. T_4 has a half-life of 6.7 days, while T_3 has a half-life in serum of only 1 day. T_4 is converted peripherally in extra-glandular tissue, especially in liver and muscle, to the active T_3 or the inactive form of T_3, reverse T_3, according to the tissue requirements for cell growth and metabolism. T_4 and T_3 are metabolized in the liver. Free T_3 shows a circadian rhythm with a periodicity that lags behind TSH, suggesting that the periodic rhythm of free T_3 is due to the proportion of T_3 derived from the thyroid.

The levels of thyroid hormones in the blood are regulated by feedback mechanisms from the HPA axis. TRH from the hypothalamus stimulates release of TSH from the pituitary. TSH secretion is pulsatile, with increased amplitude at night. TSH then enhances uptake of iodide, and both synthesis and release of T_3 and T_4. T_4 and T_3 subsequently exert negative feedback on TSH synthesis and secretion

The functions of thyroid hormones are mainly to increase basal metabolic rate, regulate protein, fat, and carbohydrate metabolism, regulate long-bone growth and neuronal maturation, and increase body sensitivity to catecholamines

Adrenal cortex

The major hormones synthesized in the adrenal cortex are cortisol, aldosterone, and the adrenal androgens. The pathways for the synthesis of these hormones are shown in Figure 182.2.

Cortisol

Cortisol is produced in the zona fasciculata of the adrenal cortex from stored cholesterol. It is derived from the hydroxylation of cortisone; 80% of plasma cortisol is bound to CBG, and 10% is bound to albumin; the remaining 10% is free cortisol (unbound fraction), which provides biological activity. The half-life of cortisol is around 90 minutes.

Cortisol has one of the most distinct and interesting circadian rhythms in the body. The circadian clock (pacemaker) in the suprachiasmatic nucleus drives the paraventricular nucleus in the

(A)

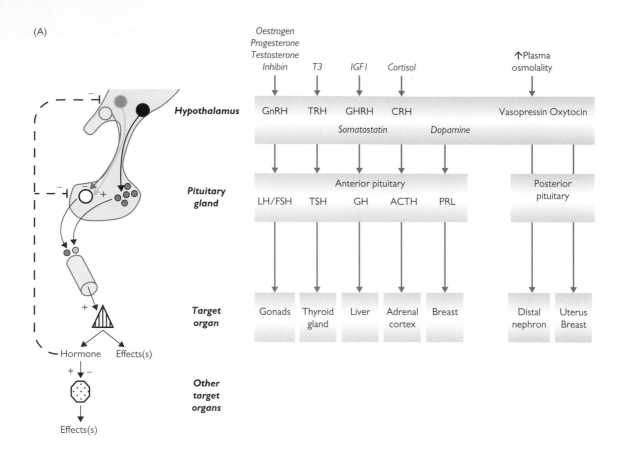

(B)

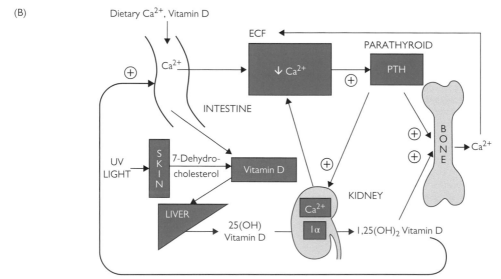

Figure 182.1 (A) Control of hormone production: regulatory pathways integrating the hypothalamus, the pituitary, and various end organs. Hormones shown in italics exert inhibitory effects. Negative feedback regulation occurs at both the hypothalamic and the pituitary level; ACTH, adrenocorticotropic hormone; CRH, corticotropin-releasing hormone; FSH, follicle-stimulating hormone; GH, growth hormone; GHRH, growth hormone-releasing hormone; GnRH, gonadotropin-releasing hormone; IGFI, insulin-like growth factor-1; LH, luteinizing hormone; PRL, prolactin; T3, triiodothyronine; TRH, thyroid-releasing hormone; TSH, thyroid-stimulating hormone. (B) Regulation of extracellular fluid (ECF) calcium (Ca^{2+}) by parathyroid hormone (PTH) action on kidney, bone, and intestine. A decrease in ECF Ca^{2+} is sensed by the calcium-sensing receptor (CaSR), leading to an increase in the secretion of PTH, which predominantly acts directly on the kidneys and bones, as these possess the PTH receptor (PTHR). PTH acts to increase (+) osteoclastic bone reabsorption but, as osteoclasts do not have PTHRs, this action is mediated via the osteoblasts, which do have PTHRs and, in response to PTH, release cytokines and factors that activate osteoclasts. In the kidney, PTH stimulates (+) 1-alpha hydroxylase (1α to increase the conversion of 25-hydroxyvitamin D (25(OH)D) to the active metabolite 1,25-dihydroxyvitamin D (1,25(OH)2D). In addition, PTH increases (+) the reabsorption of Ca^{2+} from the renal distal tubule and inhibits the reabsorption of phosphate from the proximal tubule, thereby leading to hypercalcaemia and hypophosphataemia. PTH also inhibits Na^+–H^+ antiporter activity and bicarbonate reabsorption, thereby causing a mild hyperchloraemic acidosis. The elevated 1,25(OH)2D acts on the intestine to increase (+) absorption of dietary calcium and phosphate, and it is important to note that PTH does not appear to have a direct action on the gut. Thus, in response to hypocalcaemia and the increase in PTH secretion, all of these direct and indirect actions of PTH on the kidney, bone, and intestine will help to increase ECF Ca^{2+}, which, in turn will act via the CaSR to decrease PTH secretion.

Reproduced with permission from Warrell, Cox and Firth, *Oxford Textbook of Medicine*, Fifth Edition Oxford University Press, Oxford, UK, Copyright © 2010.

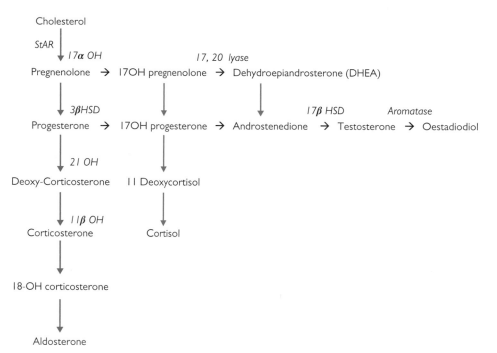

Figure 182.2 Biosynthesis pathways for aldosterone, cortisol, and the adrenal androgens; 3βHSD, 3-beta hydroxysteroid dehydrogenase; 11βOH, 11-beta hydroxylase; 17αOH, 17-alpha hydroxylase; 21 OH, 21 hydroxylase; StAR, steroidogenic autoregulatory protein.
Reproduced with permission from William Jeffcoate, *Lecture Notes on Endocrinology* fifth edition, Wiley-Blackwell, Oxford, UK, Copyright © 1993.

hypothalamus to produce CRH. This stimulates the pituitary to produce pulsatile ACTH in a circadian rhythm rising at 3 am. This drives the adrenal gland to produce cortisol also in a circadian rhythm; hence, cortisol levels are low at the time of sleep onset, rise between 2 a.m. and 4 a.m., peak just after waking, and then fall during the day. Cortisol then exerts a negative feedback on both the hypothalamus and the pituitary.

Around 13–15 cortisol secretory episodes occur during the 24 hours of the day, with a quiescent phase of minimal secretory activity starting prior to sleep and lasting up to after sleep onset. Advances in the measurement of the total amount of cortisol produced in a day shows that this is around 5.7–7.4 mg/m² per day, or 9.5 to 9.9 mg per day. These findings support regimes with lower oral daily hydrocortisone doses of 15–20 mg, allowing for first-pass hepatic metabolism and bioavailability.

In body tissues, interconversion occurs between the active and inactive metabolites, cortisol, and cortisone. Two isoenzymes, 11-beta hydroxysteroid dehydrogenase types 1 and 2, are responsible for this process. The first, expressed mainly in visceral adipose tissue, liver, and gonads, converts exogenous or endogenous cortisone to cortisol. The second converts cortisol to cortisone.

Cortisol stimulates glycogenolysis and gluconeogenesis; causes protein and selective fat breakdown, which is important for skeletal and cardiac muscle function; inhibits bone formation; maintains blood pressure; stimulates free water excretion; and has immunosuppressive and anti-inflammatory functions.

Aldosterone

Aldosterone is produced by the zona glomerulosa of the adrenal cortex and is part of the renin–angiotensin system, which is its main regulator. Aldosterone has a diurnal rhythm which peaks at around 6–7 am and has a nadir at around midnight. Aldosterone secretion is stimulated by plasma angiotensin II, high potassium, acidosis, stretch receptors in the atria, and ACTH. Low renal blood pressure, low sodium, and the sympathetic system will stimulate renin release, which will enhance aldosterone secretion. Aldosterone stimulates potassium and H⁺ secretion into urine, and sodium ions and water into the circulation. It increases blood pressure.

Adrenal androgens

Dehydroepiandrosterone (DHEA) and its metabolite androstenedione are produced in the zona reticularis. These can undergo further conversion to testosterone. In the blood, most DHEA is found as its sulphate, DHEAS. The synthetic pathway is under the control of ACTH. DHEA naturally peaks in the early morning, while serum DHEAS concentrations do not vary throughout the day. The half-life of DHEA is around an hour, and DHEA is secreted episodically.

Gonads

Oestradiol and progesterone

Puberty

The average age of onset of puberty in girls is 10–12 years. Pulsatile secretion of luteinizing hormone-releasing hormone from the hypothalamus at night is the first step in puberty initiation. This results in the pulsatile secretion of LH and FSH from the pituitary. As puberty progresses and sexual characteristics develop, menarche commences.

Menstrual cycle

Through the influence of a rise in FSH during the first days of the cycle, a few ovarian follicles are stimulated and, as they mature, they secrete increasing amounts of oestradiol. The oestrogens initiate the formation of a new layer in the endometrium. One of the follicles becomes dominant and, unlike the other follicles, grows to maturity (this is the 'follicular' or 'proliferative' phase).

As oestrogen levels increase at around day 12, through positive feedback, they trigger release of LH. This LH matures the egg and weakens the wall of the follicle so that ovulation occurs.

The solid body left in the ovary after egg release, the corpus luteum, then produces progesterone and oestrogen. Progesterone makes the endometrium receptive to implantation. The hormones produced by the corpus luteum then suppress LH and FSH, which are essential for the viability of the corpus luteum. After a few days, the corpus luteum atrophies and progesterone levels fall, triggering menstruation and the beginning of the next cycle. This phase usually lasts two weeks and the period is usually consistent (this is the 'luteal' or 'secretory' phase). Menstruation usually lasts for 3–5 days.

Menopause

Menopause is a retrospective diagnosis of 12 months of amenorrhoea. The average age is usually 50 years. Cycles become increasingly anovulatory, even up to 4 years before the menopause, and patients complain of hot flushes, urine symptoms, mood changes, and vaginal dryness. FSH levels start to fluctuate until they remain persistently high. This is followed by low oestradiol levels which correlate with the amenorrhoea.

Oestradiol

Oestradiol is produced from ovarian follicles, by conversion from testosterone, and also by the liver, the adrenals, and the breasts. In males, some oestradiol is produced in the testis but most oestrogens are formed from aromatization of androgens in adipose tissue. Oestradiol is largely bound to SHBG and albumin. Its main function is to promote secondary sexual characteristics in females, increase vaginal lubrication, increase bone formation, decelerate height growth, accelerate metabolism, increase production of binding proteins, increase clotting factors, increase HDL, and decrease LDL.

Progesterone

Progesterone is mainly formed in the ovaries and the brain. It mainly functions to prepare the uterus for implantation, decrease contractility of uterine muscle, and inhibit lactation. Other effects include anti-inflammatory actions, reduction of bronchial spasm, normalization of clotting, and prevention of endometrial cancer.

Testosterone

Leydig cells in the testis produce testosterone. Sertoli cells support spermatogenesis in the seminiferous tubules, in the presence of high testosterone concentration. Gonadotropin-releasing hormone, in a pulsatile manner, stimulates secretion of LH and FSH. LH stimulates synthesis and secretion of testosterone, while FSH stimulates production of seminiferous tubule fluid and substances essential for spermatogenesis. Testosterone exerts negative feedback on both LH and FSH.

The secretion of testosterone has a circadian rhythm, with maximal secretion at around 8 a.m. Spermatogenesis takes approximately 74 days. Testosterone is bound to SHBG and albumin. Around 4% is free and is the active fraction. In target tissues, testosterone is converted to the more potent dihydrotestosterone by 5-alpha reductase. Testosterone is inactivated in liver and excreted in urine. Testosterone functions include promoting increased muscle mass and strength, increased bone density, stimulation of bone growth, maturation of sex organs, and development of secondary sexual characteristics, libido, and erections; it also maintains cardiovascular health.

Adrenal medulla

Catecholamines are produced mainly by the chromaffin cells of the adrenal medulla, as well as by the postganglionic fibres of the sympathetic nervous system. Adrenaline is under the control of the CNS. The most abundant catecholamines are adrenaline, noradrenaline, and dopamine. Adrenaline and noradrenaline are broken down into metanephrines and normetanephrines, respectively. Dopamine acts as a neurotransmitter in the CNS. Noradrenaline is a neuromodulator of the peripheral sympathetic nervous system. During times of stress, adrenaline is released from the medulla; 20% of noradrenaline is released from the medulla, while the rest spills out from the sympathetic nerves supplying blood vessels.

Effects of catecholamines include increased heart rate and inotropy (beta-1 receptor); vasoconstriction in most vessels (alpha-1 and alpha-2 receptors); vasodilatation in skeletal muscle and liver at low concentrations (beta-2 receptor; adrenaline only) and vasoconstriction at high concentrations (alpha-1 receptor); glycogenolysis; and lipolysis. Other agonist effects on alpha receptors result in increased sweating, pupil dilatation, and alertness.

Anterior pituitary

The main hormones produced by the anterior pituitary are growth hormone, LH, FSH, TSH, ACTH, and prolactin. Growth hormone and prolactin will be discussed here.

Growth hormone

Growth hormone is synthesized, stored, and secreted by somatotroph cells in the anterior pituitary. Growth hormone is secreted more commonly at night (five to six 90-minute pulses/24 hours) and in the circulation is bound to growth hormone-binding protein. Growth hormone-releasing hormone released by neurosecretory nuclei in the hypothalamus into the portal circulation surrounding the pituitary stimulates the release of growth hormone. Other stimulating factors are sleep, hypoglycaemia, and exercise. The effects of growth hormone include increasing height in children and adolescents, increasing muscle mass and protein synthesis, promoting lipolysis and gluconeogenesis, and stimulating the immune system. In addition, in the liver, growth hormone stimulates the production of insulin-like growth factor 1 (IGF1), which itself has growth-stimulating effects on a wide variety of tissues. Growth hormone secretion is inhibited by negative feedback from growth hormone itself and from IGF1, as well as by somatostatin and high glucose.

Prolactin

Prolactin is synthesized and secreted by the lactotroph cells in the anterior pituitary; the secretion is pulsatile, with around 14 pulses/24 hours. A nocturnal peak occurs during sleep, and a lesser peak in the evening. Dopamine secreted from neuroendocrine neurons in the hypothalamus causes tonic inhibition of prolactin. Therefore, any mass effect of compression/disconnection of the pituitary stalk will result in an elevated prolactin measurement, as will the use of any dopamine-antagonist medication.

High prolactin levels suppress LH and FSH. Prolactin also stimulates the mammary glands to produce milk, and increased levels of prolactin are found during pregnancy. Levels of prolactin may also rise with stress, meals, nipple stimulation, and minor surgery. In addition, TRH has a stimulating effect on prolactin levels.

Posterior pituitary

The main hormones released by the posterior pituitary are oxytocin and vasopressin (also known as antidiuretic hormone). They both have a short half-life. Both hormones are synthesized in the suprachiasmatic and paraventricular hypothalamic neurons. Oxytocin causes contractions in the pregnant uterus, and breast milk ejection during breast feeding. Vasopressin mainly acts to reduce free water excretion. Its release is stimulated by high osmolality and a low blood volume and it acts in the kidney at the collecting duct and the thick ascending loop of Henle to affect water permeability.

Parathyroid glands

The parathyroid glands secrete parathyroid hormone, which acts to increase the concentration of calcium in the blood. Decreased calcium concentrations, through activation of the calcium sensory receptors on the parathyroid cells, stimulate parathyroid hormone secretion. The release of parathyroid hormone then enhances the release of calcium from the bones through indirect stimulation of osteoclasts, which cause bone resorption. In the kidneys, it enhances the reabsorption of calcium from the distal tubules as well as promoting phosphate excretion. It also increases the intestinal absorption of calcium by stimulating the production of active vitamin D (1,25-hydroxycholecalciferol). Vitamin D also promotes reabsorption of calcium from the kidneys, promotes bone growth and remodelling, and has immunomodulatory effects.

A severe decrease in serum magnesium, or a high calcium concentration, may inhibit parathyroid hormone. In addition, the effects of parathyroid hormone are opposed by calcitonin, which acts to decrease calcium concentrations.

Further Reading

Danks JA, and Richardson SJ. 'Endocrinology and evolution: Lessons from comparative endocrinology', in Wass JAH, Stewart PM, Amiel SA, et al., eds, *Oxford Textbook of Endocrinology and Diabetes* (2nd edition), 2011. Oxford University Press.

Gurnell M, Burrin J, and Chatterjee VK. 'Principles of hormone action', in Warrell DA, Cox TM, and Firth JD, eds, *Oxford Textbook of Medicine* (5th edition), 2010. Oxford University Press.

183 Diagnosis and investigation in endocrine disorders

John Newell-Price, Alia Munir, and Miguel Debono

The aim of this chapter is to introduce the reader to some of the common investigations used in the diagnosis and management of endocrine disorders. Tests used to identify specific disorders will be discussed in Chapters 184–192.

Thyroid disorders

Primary hypothyroidism

Primary hypothyroidism is diagnosed on the basis of an elevated basal level of thyroid-stimulating hormone (TSH), and low free thyroxine (FT4). Anti-thyroid peroxidase (TPO) antibodies are found in patients with autoimmune thyroid disease. In a patient started on thyroxine replacement, TSH should be rechecked 6–10 weeks later. Ideal treatment yields a TSH between the lower limit of the reference range and 2 mU/l. Values between 2 mU/l and the upper limit of the reference range probably imply mild under-treatment, especially if the patient remains symptomatic. There is no place for measuring FT4 in patients who are on replacement thyroxine, as this only proves that the patient took levothyroxine on the morning in question. Patients with persistently elevated TSH levels, despite being on levothyroxine doses of 200 micrograms or more, are frequently non-compliant, and tests often show normal FT4 and elevated TSH. Alternative diagnoses, such as thyroxine malabsorption due to, for example, coeliac disease, should also be considered. There is no place for measuring triiodothyronine levels in suspected hypothyroidism.

Secondary hypothyroidism

Secondary hypothyroidism is diagnosed by a low FT4 and inappropriately normal or low TSH. It is monitored via FT4 levels. TSH values are usually in the normal range or low and are not useful for monitoring.

Hyperthyroidism

The diagnosis of hyperthyroidism is confirmed by a suppressed TSH (i.e. below 0.03 mU/l) with an elevated FT4 or an elevated free triiodothyronine level (FT3). Normally, obtain the FT4 first and, if normal, then measure the FT3 to confirm the diagnosis of triiodothyronine toxicosis. Positive antithyroid antibodies (TPO/thyroglobulin antibodies) or anti-TSH-receptor antibodies favour a diagnosis of Graves' disease. TSH/FT4 levels should be monitored when the patient is treated with antithyroid medication. Detectable TSH and elevated FT4/FT3 are found in TSH-secreting pituitary tumours or in thyroid-hormone resistance. Exclude the presence of heterophile antibodies causing a falsely high TSH level.

Thyroid nodules

All patients with a **dominant nodule** (i.e. larger or different in consistency, compared to other nodules) in a multinodular goitre should be suspected of having a malignancy, as should all patients who have a solitary nodule in their thyroid. The only investigations needed for thyroid nodules are a TSH test and thyroid antibodies, coupled with fine-needle aspiration cytology (FNAC). Ultrasound or radioisotope scans are not routinely indicated. Repeat FNAC at the first return visit if the first sample is clinically suspicious or was non-diagnostic. Other tests include:

Scintiscanning: This is **rarely required** to define areas of increased or decreased function, to detect the presence of a retrosternal goitre or ectopic thyroid tissue, and to detect functioning metastases of thyroid carcinoma; homogenous uptake is increased in Graves' disease and reduced in thyroiditis.

Ultrasound scan: This is used to differentiate between cystic and solid nodules and to follow change in size of a nodule; calcification may suggest malignancy.

Non-contrast CT scan: This is used for evaluation of retrosternal and retrotracheal extension of goitre.

Flow–volume loop: This is rarely indicated: tracheal diameter may be assessed on non-contrast CT.

Pituitary disease

Suspected pituitary tumour

Clinical assessment for a suspected pituitary tumour should include assessment of visual fields; if they are determined to be abnormal with a red pin, formal testing should be considered. Measurements for pituitary function include tests for basal levels of:

- prolactin
- FT4
- TSH
- testosterone or oestradiol
- sex hormone-binding globulin
- luteinizing hormone (LH)
- follicle-stimulating hormone (FSH)
- insulin-like growth factor 1

Cortisol can be measured as a 9 a.m. sample and, if the basal level is >500 nmol/l, no further dynamic tests need to be made. If it is <500 nmol/l, one should consider doing an insulin tolerance test (the gold standard), a glucagon test, or a short tetracosactide test including a basal 9 a.m. adrenocorticotropic hormone (ACTH) test. For all three tests, any oestrogen should be stopped 6 weeks beforehand to allow cortisol-binding globulin levels to return to normal (if a large pituitary tumour is present, the need for urgent clinical management may override the need for assessment, and the patient should be given glucocorticoid cover). Where there is clinical suspicion of a functioning tumour, the appropriate tests should be performed (see Chapters 189 and 192).

Radiological investigations in pituitary disease

The following radiological investigations can be used in pituitary disease:

- MRI: provides optimal imaging; IV gadolinium is used for contrast enhancement (a normal pituitary appears very bright)
- CT scans: this is used for certain tumours (e.g. craniopharyngioma)

Dynamic tests for pituitary disease

Insulin tolerance test

An insulin tolerance test is used to diagnose secondary adrenal failure, or growth hormone (GH) deficiency. In the test, IV insulin is given to induce hypoglycaemia (blood glucose <2.2 mmol/l) and stimulate ACTH and GH secretion. Cortisol levels should rise to >550 nmol/l. A peak GH response of <3 µg/l is associated with severe GH deficiency. This test is contraindicated in ischaemic heart disease, epilepsy, severe long-standing hypoadrenalism, and glycogen storage diseases, or when the patient's age is <2 years, or the cortisol level is <100 nmol/l. In addition, the ECG must be normal.

Glucagon test

A glucagon test is used to diagnose secondary adrenal failure and GH deficiency in patients in whom the insulin tolerance test is contraindicated. This is a routine first-line test for GH deficiency, but is a poor stimulus for ACTH. Glucagon stimulates a glucose rise followed by a drop in sugar, due to insulin secretion. The maximal glucose level is achieved after 90 minutes. Cortisol levels should rise to >550 nmol/l. A peak GH response of <3 μg/l is associated with severe GH deficiency. The test is contraindicated in patients who have not eaten for 48 hours or who have a glycogen storage disease or severe cortisol deficiency (i.e. situations where glycogen stores are low). This test is unreliable in diabetes patients.

Short tetracosactide test

The short tetracosactide test is used for the assessment of primary and secondary adrenal insufficiency (following pituitary surgery, the test should only be utilized after a period of 6 weeks, to avoid false-negative results). In this test, 250 μg tetracosactide is administered intramuscularly, and then cortisol levels are assessed after 30 minutes. In a normal response, cortisol levels rise to >550 nmol/l if the response is normal.

Growth hormone-releasing hormone–arginine test

The growth hormone-releasing hormone (GHRH)–arginine test is used to assess for GH deficiency. The following cut-off levels have been validated for this test: for those with a BMI <25 kg/m², the peak GH is <11 μg/l; for a BMI of 25–30 kg/m², the peak GH is <8 μg/l; and, for a BMI >30 kg/m², the peak GH is <4 μg/l.

Gonadotropin-releasing hormone test

The gonadotropin-releasing hormone test is used to assess LH/FSH reserves. It is rarely used.

Thyrotropin-releasing hormone test

The thyrotropin-releasing hormone (TRH) test is rarely used but may be indicated to distinguish between a TSH-secreting tumour (no change) and thyroid-hormone resistance (increase) or to distinguish between pituitary TSH and hypothalamic TRH deficiency.

Water-deprivation test

The water-deprivation test is extremely difficult to perform properly and is best left to dedicated endocrine units. It is indicated for the diagnosis of diabetes insipidus, and differential diagnosis of thirst, polyuria, and nocturia. Care should be taken in patients with severe clinical diabetes insipidus. Thyroid and adrenal reserve must be normal or adequately replaced, and diabetes mellitus and hypercalcaemia excluded.

For the test, patients are initially allowed fluids overnight. They are then deprived of fluids for 8 hours or until 3% of the body weight is lost. Plasma osmolality and urine volume/osmolality are then measured. A rise in serum osmolality to >305 mOsm/kg confirms diabetes insipidus. If a urine osmolality ≤300 Osm/kg improves with desmopressin, this is suggestive of cranial diabetes insipidus (CDI); no improvement would be suggestive of nephrogenic diabetes insipidus. If urine concentrates with no desmopressin to >800 Osm/kg in a patient with increased thirst and polyuria, and diabetes and hypercalcaemia have been excluded, psychogenic polydipsia may be the cause.

CDI is usually caused by hypothalamic lesions such as craniopharyngiomas; head trauma; cranial surgery; infiltrative disorders; or infections. Alternatively, it may be idiopathic. CDI is virtually never seen as the presenting feature of an anterior pituitary tumour. Familial CDI is rare.

Nephrogenic diabetes insipidus can be caused by chronic renal insufficiency, lithium toxicity, tubulointerstitial disease, hypokalaemia, or hypercalcaemia. Very rarely, it may be familial.

Adrenal gland and sex hormone disorders

Primary hyperaldosteronism

Aldosterone–renin ratio

A random plasma aldosterone–renin ratio is currently the preferred screening test for primary hyperaldosteronism (also known as Conn's syndrome), as it is easy to do and is less affected by drug therapy, day and diurnal variation, and patient position than tests for either aldosterone or renin alone; in primary hyperaldosteronism, the plasma aldosterone–renin ratio is high. During the test, hypokalaemia should be avoided, and patients should be well hydrated and have an adequate intake of sodium. Spironolactone, other aldosterone antagonists, and oestrogens **must** be discontinued 6 weeks before the test. Angiotensin-converting enzyme inhibitors, beta blockers, dihydropyridine calcium-channel blockers, NSAIDs, and diuretics should be stopped 2 weeks before the test, although alpha blockers may be used. Sometimes one may adopt the approach of not stopping any of the drugs; if the test is abnormal, the drugs are then stopped for subsequent confirmatory suppression tests.

Confirmatory suppression tests

The **fludrocortisone suppression test** is considered by some to be the definitive diagnostic procedure for hyperaldosteronism. In this test, plasma aldosterone should initially be measured mid-morning; the subject should be upright for at least 30 minutes prior to venepuncture. Then, for the next 4 days, fludrocortisone 0.1 mg is administered 6 hourly, and slow Na 3 × 10 mmol tabs are administered 8 hourly. In addition, slow K tabs are administered in sufficient quantity to maintain plasma potassium concentration within the reference range. On Day 4, plasma aldosterone is again measured mid-morning. In primary hyperaldosteronism, aldosterone levels will not be suppressed by fludrocortisone (normal response <140 pmol/l). However, if hypokalaemia develops, aldosterone will be suppressed even if primary hyperaldosteronism is present (false-negative result).

The **furosemide posture test**, acute 4-hour IV saline loading, and a postural stimulation test are other confirmatory tests which may be considered.

States of excess mineralocorticoids

In the presence of hypertension and hypokalaemic alkalosis with low renin and normal or low aldosterone, consider (i) apparent mineralocorticoid excess from a deficiency (congenital, or caused by liquorice) in 11-beta hydroxysteroid dehydrogenase type 2; (ii) congenital adrenal hyperplasia, or adrenal tumours with increased secretion of deoxycorticosterone or corticosterone; or (iii) ectopic ACTH. Alternatively, consider Liddle's syndrome (a renal tubular abnormality; autosomal dominant).

In the presence of hypokalaemic alkalosis without hypertension but with increased renin and aldosterone levels, consider:

* Bartter syndrome (presents at a young age, with seizures, tetany, and hypercalciuria; autosomal recessive)
* Gitelman syndrome (hypomagnesaemia, hypocalciuria)

Cushing's syndrome

Circadian rhythm study

To diagnose Cushing's syndrome, a circadian rhythm study may be performed in which a patient is admitted to hospital and, when unstressed on Day 2, has serum cortisol and ACTH levels taken at 9 a.m., 6 p.m., and midnight. The midnight sample should preferably be taken when patient is asleep, within 5 to 10 minutes from waking. Salivary cortisol samples may also be taken, allowing the test to be done on an outpatient basis.

Dexamethasone suppression tests

For initial screening for Cushing's syndrome an overnight dexamethasone suppression test is recommended. In this test, the patient is instructed to take 1 mg dexamethasone tablets at between 11 p.m. and midnight and to return for a blood test at 9 a.m. on the following morning. In normal subjects, the cortisol will fall to <50 nmol/l.

If there is a high index of suspicion of Cushing's syndrome or if the overnight test contradicts other investigations, a low-dose dexamethasone test should be used. The test is started at 9 a.m.; dexamethasone 0.5 mg orally strictly 6 hourly for 48 hours is given. Cortisol and ACTH levels are taken at 9 a.m., before the first dose of dexamethasone, and then again 48 hours later (also at 9 a.m.). In

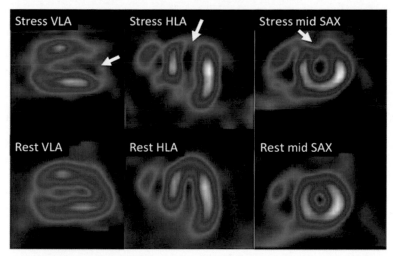

Figure 87.8 Myocardial perfusion imaging with single-photon emission computed tomography (SPECT): An example of inducible hypoperfusion in the anterior wall and apex. Panels, from left to right, show representative vertical long-axis (VLA), horizontal long-axis (HLA), and mid short-axis (SAX) slices, with stress above rest. The white arrows show a perfusion defect which is present on the stress slices but which resolves at rest.
Reproduced with permission from Warrell, Cox and Firth, *Oxford Textbook of Medicine*, fifth edition, Oxford University Press, Oxford, UK, Copyright © 2010

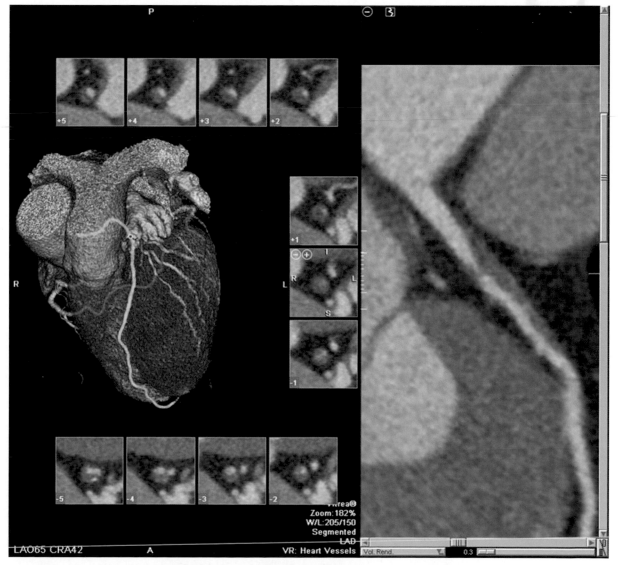

Figure 87.9 CT coronary angiography showing a critical soft plaque stenosis in the left main stem.
Reproduced with permission from Warrell, Cox and Firth, *Oxford Textbook of Medicine*, fifth edition, Oxford University Press, Oxford, UK, Copyright © 2010

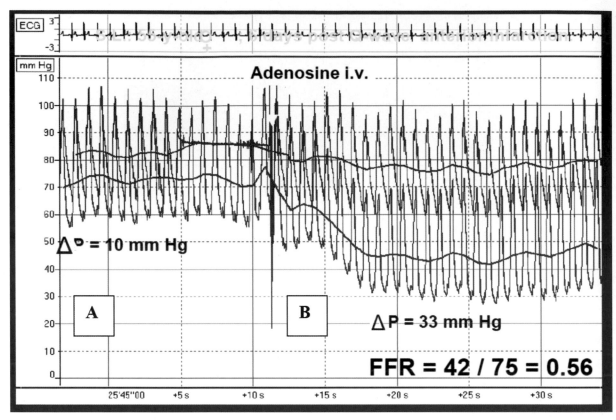

Figure 87.11 To assess the fractional flow reserve, which is the ratio of the pressures distal to and proximal to a stenosis, a small flexible wire with two separate pressure sensors is placed across a candidate coronary artery stenosis. Under resting conditions (A), there is only a 10 mm Hg gradient (ΔP) across the lesion but, under maximal hyperaemia ('adenosine i.v.'; B), the gradient increases markedly to 33 mm Hg, with a mean distal-to-proximal pressure ratio of 0.56. Thus, in this case, the fractional flow reserve indicates the presence of a functionally significant stenosis, and coronary angioplasty is indicated; FFR, fractional flow reserve; i.v., intravenous.

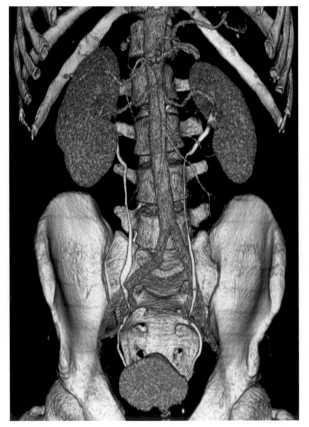

Figure 155.1 CT demonstrating the urinary system.
image courtesy of Nigel Cowan

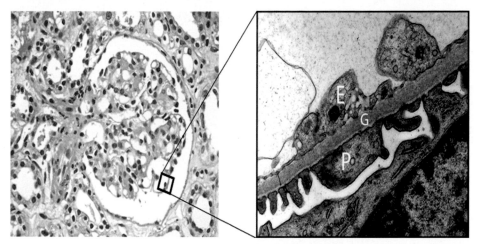

Figure 155.3 Normal glomerulus and glomerular filtration barrier under light and electron microscopy; note the glomerular basement membrane (G), with endothelial cells (E) at its upper edge, and the foot processes of the podocytes (P) abutting its lower edge.
image courtesy of Ian Roberts

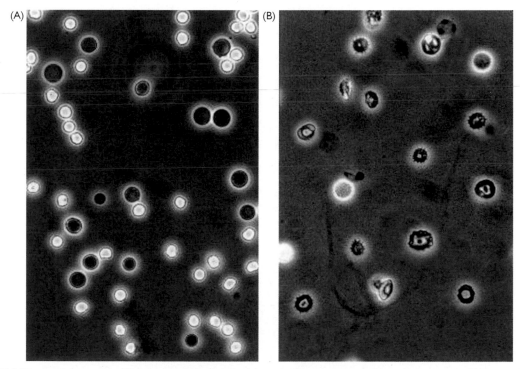

Figure 157.1 Microscopic haematuria. (A) Isomorphic red cells. Isomorphic red cells are seen in non-glomerular haematuria. (B) Dysmorphic red cells. Dysmorphic red cells are seen in glomerular haematuria, but may also be found in non-glomerular and tubulointerstitial disease.
Reproduced with permission from Davidson et al, *Oxford Textbook of Clinical Nephrology*, Third Edition, Oxford University Press, Oxford, UK, Copyright © 2005

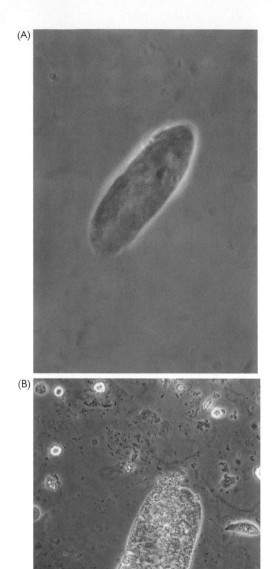

(A)

(B)

Figure 157.2 (A) Hyaline cast. Hyaline casts are concretions of Tamm–Horsfall mucoprotein and may be seen in concentrated urine. (B) Granular cast. Granular casts are cellular remnants embedded in hyaline material and are non-specific for glomerular and tubular disease.
Reproduced with permission from Davidson et al, Oxford Textbook of Clinical Nephrology, Third Edition, Oxford University Press, Oxford, UK, Copyright © 2005

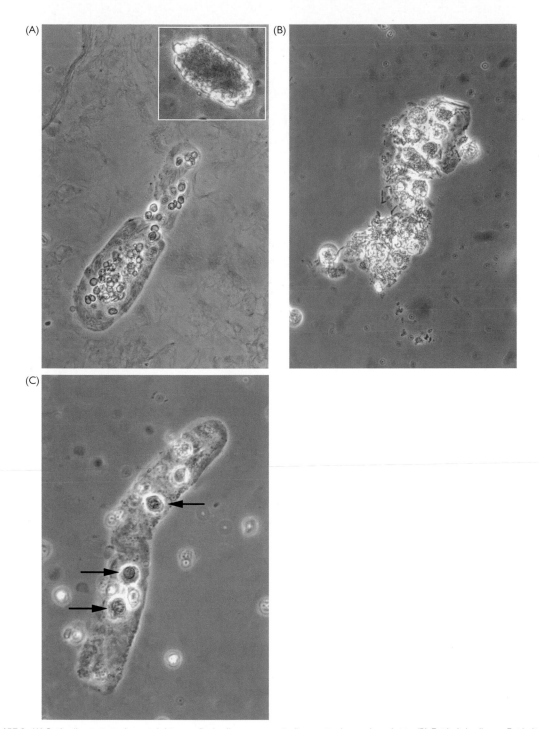

Figure 157.3 (A) Red cell cast; inset: haemoglobin cast. Red cell casts are typically seen in glomerulonephritis. (B) Epithelial cell cast. Epithelial cell casts. may be seen in glomerular and tubular disease. (C) White cell cast; individual white cells (arrows) are clearly seen. White cell casts may be seen in pyelonephritis and tubulointerstitial disease.

Reproduced with permission from Davidson et al, Oxford Textbook of Clinical Nephrology, Third Edition, Oxford University Press, Oxford, UK, Copyright © 2005.

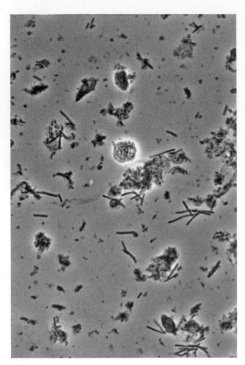

Figure 158.1 Urinary bacteria (rods).
Reproduced with permission from Davidson et al, *Oxford Textbook of Clinical Nephrology*, Third Edition, Oxford University Press, Oxford, UK, Copyright © 2005

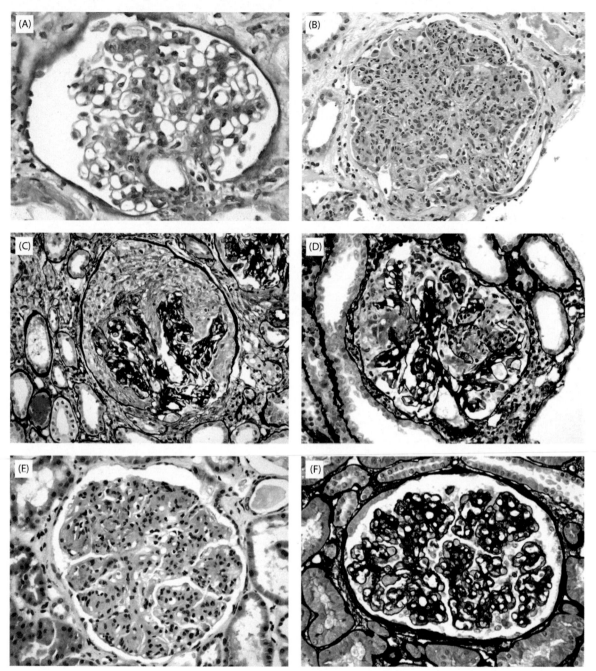

Figure 159.1 Histology of renal biopsy. (A) IgA nephropathy showing mesangial hypercellularity in which there are at least four mesangial cells in a peripheral mesangial area (periodic acid-Schiff stain). (B) Postinfectious glomerulonephritis showing endocapillary hypercellularity, in which the capillary lumina are filled with infiltrating leucocytes (hematoxylin and eosin stain (H&E)). (C) Antiglomerular basement membrane disease, showing extracapillary proliferation (a cellular crescent), in which there is partial tuft collapse and proliferation of cells within Bowman's space (H&E and silver). (D) ANCA-associated vasculitis, showing necrosis with capillary wall rupture and fibrin exudation (H&E and silver). (E, F) Membranoproliferative pattern, showing a lobular appearance of the glomerular tuft, with mesangial hypercellularity and thickened capillary walls, with glomerular basement membrane duplication evident on the silver stain (H&E and silver).

Reproduced with permission from Turner, Oxford Textbook of Clinical Nephrology, Fourth Edition Oxford University Press, Oxford, UK, Copyright © 2015

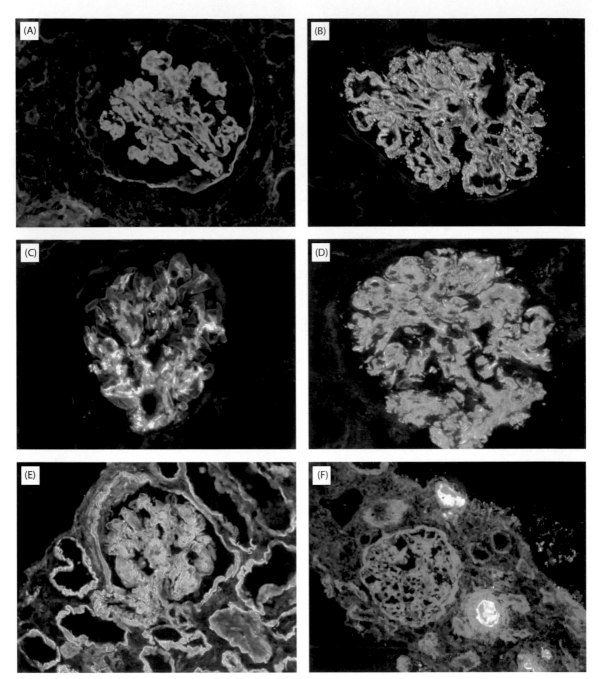

Figure 159.2 Immunofluorescence of renal biopsy. (A) Linear glomerular basement membrane (GBM) positivity for IgG in anti-GBM disease. (B) Granular capillary wall positivity for IgG in membranous nephropathy. (C) Mesangial positivity for IgA in IgA nephropathy. (D) Mesangial and capillary wall positivity for C3 in C3 glomerulonephritis. (E) Mesangial and tubular basement membrane positivity for kappa light chains in light chain deposition disease. (F) Positivity for lambda light chains in tubular casts in light chain cast nephropathy.
Reproduced with permission from Turner, Oxford Textbook of Clinical Nephrology, Fourth Edition Oxford University Press, Oxford, UK, Copyright © 2015

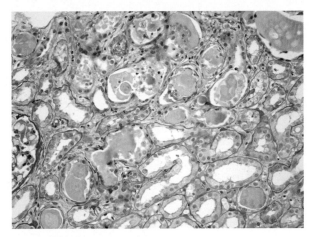

Figure 160.1 Cast nephropathy.
Reproduced with permission from Turner et al, *Oxford Textbook of Clinical Nephrology*,
Fourth Edition, Oxford University Press, Oxford, UK, Copyright © 2015

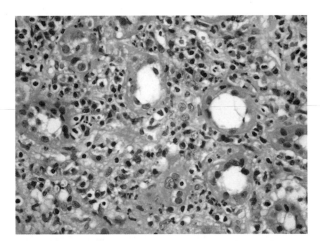

Figure 160.2 Renal biopsy of an acute interstitial nephritis with
oedema and a prominent inflammatory infiltrate of lymphocytes and
eosinophils separating the tubules (image courtesy of Ian Roberts).
Reproduced with permission from Turner et al, *Oxford Textbook of Clinical Nephrology*,
Fourth Edition, Oxford University Press, Oxford, UK, Copyright © 2015

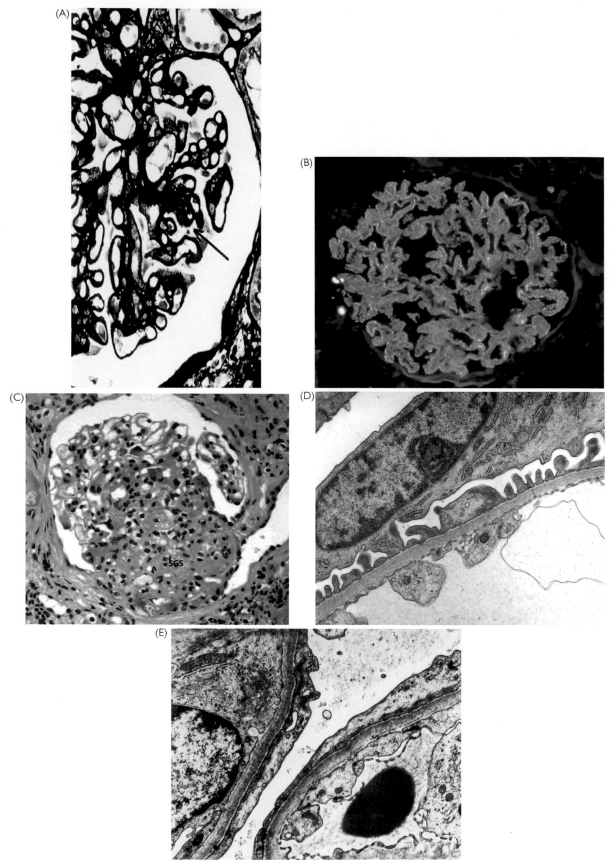

Figure 161.2 Renal biopsy images from nephrotic patients. (A) Sub-epithelial spikes (arrow) on silver stain in membranous nephropathy. (B) Granular IgG on immunofluorescence in membranous nephropathy. (C) Focal segmental glomerulosclerosis (indicated by SGS). (D) Normal podocytes. (E) Podocyte effacement on electron microscopy.

images courtesy of Ian Roberts

Reproduced with permission from Turner et al, Oxford Textbook of Clinical Nephrology, Forth Edition, Oxford University Press, Oxford, UK, Copyright © 2015

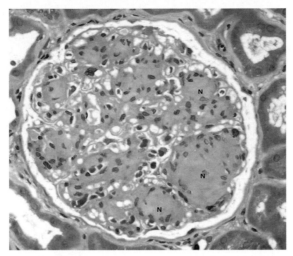

Figure 164.2 Renal biopsy demonstrating nodular (indicated by 'N')
glomerulosclerosis..
Reproduced with permission from Turner et al, *Oxford Textbook of Clinical Nephrology*,
Fourth Edition, Oxford University Press, Oxford, UK, Copyright © 2015

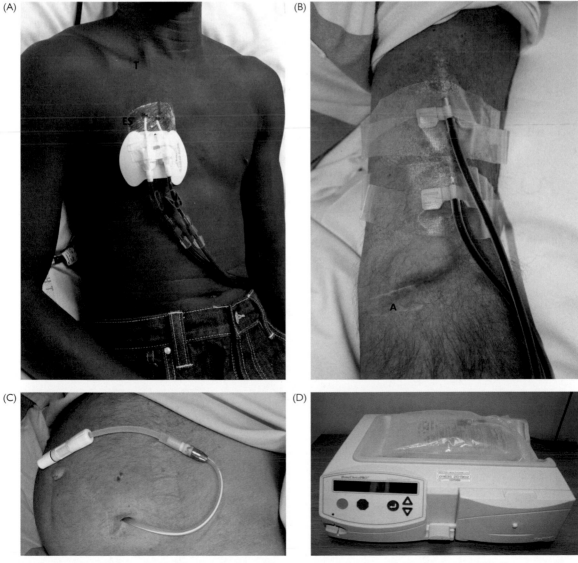

Figure 168.1 (A) A tunnelled, dual-lumen dialysis catheter. (B) A left brachiocephalic arteriovenous fistula, showing arterial and venous needles in situ. (C) A Tenckhoff catheter. (D) An automated peritoneal dialysis machine and a dialysate bag; A, area of arteriovenous anastomosis; ES, exit site; T, subcutaneous tunnel from point of insertion in internal jugular vein.

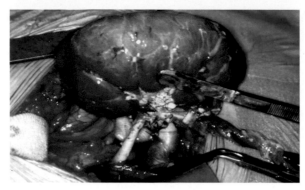

Figure 168.2 An anastomosed transplanted kidney.

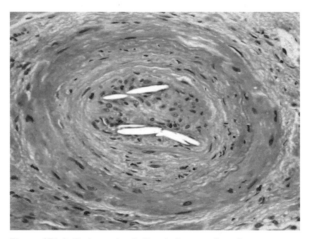

Figure 171.1 Cholesterol emboli occluding a small renal artery.
image courtesy of Ian Roberts

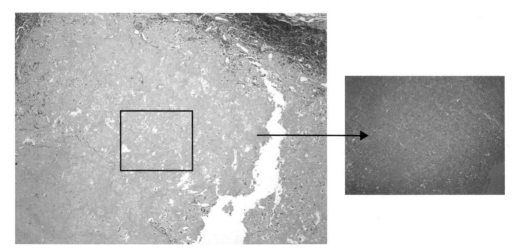

Figure 181.1 Amyloid deposition (amorphous material; boxed area) in a lymph node in amyloid light-chain amyloidosis.

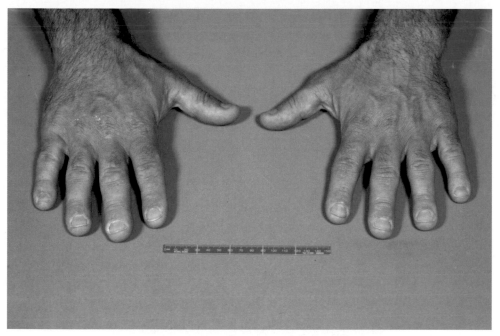

Figure 192.1 Hands of a patient with acromegaly.

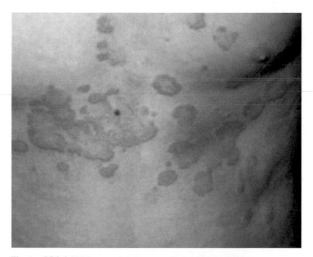

Figure 251.1 Widespread ordinary urticaria; the smooth erythematous papules and plaques may expand into annular shapes.
Reproduced from Burge, S., Wallis, D. Oxford Handbook of Medical Dermatology (Copyright Oxford University Press 2010)

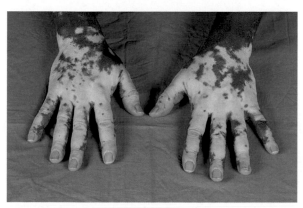

Figure 258.1 Extensive vitiligo of the hands.

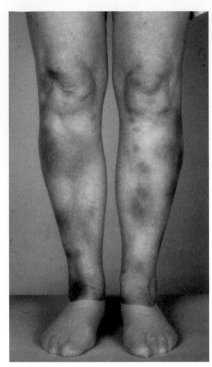

Figure 260.1 Erythema nodosum, with painful bruise-like lesions on the shins.
From: *Ethnic Dermatology: Clinical Problems and Skin Pigmentation*, Archer CB, Copyright 2008, Informa Healthcare, reproduced by permission of Taylor & Francis Books UK

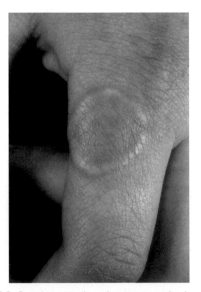

Figure 260.2 Granuloma annulare, showing an annular dermal lesion on the dorsum of the hand.
From: *Ethnic Dermatology: Clinical Problems and Skin Pigmentation*, Archer CB, Copyright 2008, Informa Healthcare, reproduced by permission of Taylor & Francis Books UK

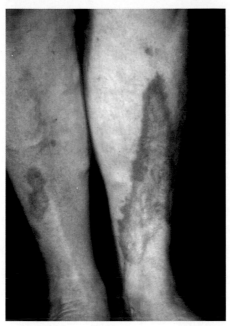

Figure 260.3 Necrobiosis lipoidica, showing atrophic plaques on
the shins.

From: *Ethnic Dermatology: Clinical Problems and Skin Pigmentation*, Archer CB, Copyright
2008, Informa Healthcare, reproduced by permission of Taylor & Francis Books UK

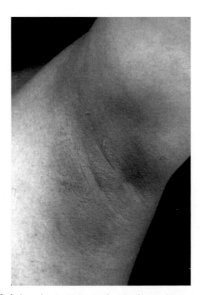

Figure 260.4 Acanthosis nigricans, showing hyperpigmentation and
hyperkeratosis of the axillary skin.

From: *Ethnic Dermatology: Clinical Problems and Skin Pigmentation*, Archer CB, Copyright
2008, Informa Healthcare, reproduced by permission of Taylor & Francis Books UK

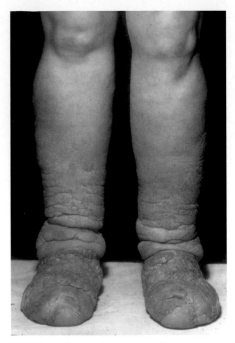

Figure 260.5 Pretibial myxoedema associated with hyperthyroidism.
From: *Ethnic Dermatology: Clinical Problems and Skin Pigmentation*, Archer CB, Copyright
2008, Informa Healthcare, reproduced by permission of Taylor & Francis Books UK

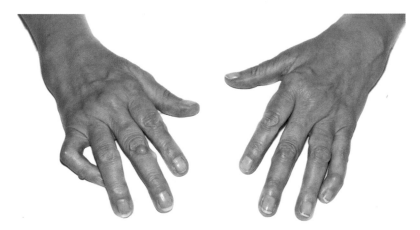

Figure 267.1 Hands of a patient with rheumatoid arthritis. Synovitis of the wrists and metacarpophalangeal joints is apparent. Rheumatoid
nodules (present here over the right middle finger proximal interphalangeal joint) and fixed deformity (present here at the right little finger proximal
interphalangeal joint) are unusual in early disease.

normal subjects, cortisol levels will be <50 nmol/l at 48 hours after the start of the test.

The high-dose dexamethasone test is used in the differential diagnosis of ACTH-dependent Cushing's syndrome, or Cushing's syndrome of unknown aetiology. Like the low-dose test, this test is also started at 9 a.m.; however, dexamethasone 2 mg orally strictly 6 hourly for 48 hours is given. Cortisol and ACTH levels are taken at 9 a.m., before first dose of dexamethasone, and then again 48 hours later (also at 9 a.m.). Suppression of serum cortisol by 50% at the end of the test is consistent with Cushing's disease (ACTH dependent).

For dexamethasone suppression tests, all patients need to be off oestrogens for 6 weeks, and caution is recommended in patients with diabetes and gastric ulceration.

Twenty-four-hour urinary free cortisol test

A 24-hour urinary free cortisol test indicates the level of free cortisol in tissues. However, it has a high false-negative rate and should not be used alone.

Adrenal insufficiency

The tetracosactide test is used in the diagnosis of adrenocortical insufficiency—primary or secondary. The test is started at 9 a.m. Cortisol levels are taken at baseline and at 30 minutes after intramuscular or IV injection of 250 μg tetracosactide. If looking for the cause of the insufficiency, whether primary or secondary, basal ACTH is also taken. With a normal adrenal reserve, the cortisol levels should rise to a peak level of >550 nmol/l. This test is not sensitive for early secondary adrenal insufficiency (<6 weeks post pituitary surgery). In addition, it should be avoided in pregnancy.

Hyperandrogenism

Five-day dexamethasone suppression test of adrenal androgens

The 5-day dexamethasone suppression test of adrenal androgens is used in hyperandrogenism to assess the degree of ACTH regulation. In the test, oral dexamethasone 1.5 mg is given twice per day for 5 days. A baseline sample and a Day 6 sample are taken for cortisol, testosterone, sex hormone-binding globulin, androstenedione, dehydroepiandrosterone sulphate (DHEAS), and 17-hydroxyprogesterone. Androgens are unlikely to suppress in adrenal or ovary adenomas. There may be moderate suppression in polycystic ovary syndrome. In congenital adrenal hyperplasia, good suppression will occur.

Short tetracosactide test for congenital adrenal hyperplasia

The short tetracosactide test is used to diagnose late-onset congenital adrenal hyperplasia. Preferably, the test should be done during the follicular phase of the menstrual cycle. During the test, cortisol and 17-hydroxyprogesterone levels are taken at baseline and at 60 minutes after the administration of 250 μg tetracosactide. A basal 17-hydroxyprogesterone level <6 nmol/l and a peak 17-hydroxyprogesterone level <30 nmol/l are normal.

Adrenal incidentalomas

Approximately 5% of all abdominal CT scans disclose clinically non-suspected adrenal tumours known as incidentalomas. The majority are non-functioning but some may be hormone producing. If adrenal incidentalomas are found, it is necessary to exclude metastases or adrenal cancer, and all patients should be referred to an endocrinologist for investigation. The workup should include renal function tests, fasting glucose, a lipid profile, liver function tests, a full blood count, and the erythrocyte sedimentation rate. In addition, the following tests should be done:

- blood pressure check
- basal DHEAS
- an aldosterone–renin ratio, if the patient is hypertensive
- a 1 mg overnight dexamethasone suppression test
- 2 × 24-hour urine collections for urinary metanephrines

Repeat the CT scan after 6 months to assess for growth if tumours not definitely benign on non-contrast CT scans.

Further Reading

Wallace M. 'Measurement of hormones', in Wass JAH, Stewart PM, Amiel SA, et al., eds, *Oxford Textbook of Endocrinology and Diabetes* (2nd edition), 2011. Oxford University Press.

184 Diabetes mellitus

Kevin Shotliff

Definition

Diabetes mellitus, often referred to simply as diabetes, is a syndrome of disordered metabolism (insulin deficiency and/or insulin resistance) resulting in abnormally high blood glucose levels (hyperglycaemia). The term 'diabetes' relates to passing large volumes of urine (polyuria); 'mellitus' refers to the fact that the urine is sweet (glycosuria). Currently, 2%–6% of the UK population have diabetes but only one-half to one-third are thought to be diagnosed. Worldwide, 189 million people were known to have diabetes in 2003 and this may reach 324 million by 2025.

Symptoms

The symptoms of diabetes are split into acute and chronic problems. Acute symptoms are metabolic abnormalities related to high blood glucose levels, although treatment can also cause acute problems with low blood glucose levels or lactic acidosis. Chronic complications are split into macrovascular (cerebrovascular, cardiovascular, and peripheral vascular disease) and microvascular disease (neuropathy, retinopathy, and nephropathy). As type 2 diabetes is often undiagnosed for some time, chronic complications, such as a myocardial infarct or a foot ulcer, can be the presenting problem.

It is hyperglycaemia which largely causes the acute signs and symptoms of diabetes. About 25% of people with type 1 diabetes have some degree of ketoacidosis at diagnosis. This can be associated with abdominal pain and breathlessness (Kussmaul respiration) in those with significant acidosis.

Polyuria (large amounts of urine) and **polydipsia** (thirst) are caused by renal osmotic diuresis due to hyperglycaemia. The kidneys are typically able to conserve glucose up to a certain level (often blood levels up to 10 mmol/l but less in certain situations, such as pregnancy), and excess glucose is then lost in the urine. This glucose takes water with it, so increasing the volume of urine passed. Symptoms of **nocturia**, **incontinence, and frequency**, due to the dramatic increase in urine production, may be reported.

Blurred vision is caused by osmotic changes in the lens of the eye; these are associated with fluctuations in blood glucose levels. Glucose and water enter the lens of the eye, and the associated swelling of the lens alters its focal length.

People with poorly controlled diabetes often **lose weight** as they are unable to utilize carbohydrates efficiently. Glucose lost in the urine represents unused calories, so other energy stores such as fat or protein must be used instead. Lethargy is also commonly reported.

At very high levels of serum glucose, **confusion** may develop, and may progress further to **coma**. **Mood changes** may also be noted, often by a partner or relative, although both are more common with low blood glucose levels associated with treatments for diabetes.

Recurrent infections (often skin) should alert the physician to screen for diabetes, as hyperglycaemia provides not only high blood levels but also high extracellular tissue fluid levels of glucose.

Diagnosis

Diabetes mellitus is a biochemical diagnosis, indicated when blood glucose levels are over a certain level, as shown in Table 184.1. Investigation and a subsequent diagnosis of type 1 diabetes, and many cases of type 2, is usually prompted by recent-onset symptoms of polyuria and polydipsia, often accompanied by weight loss. These symptoms typically worsen over days to weeks. With type 1 diabetes, diabetic ketoacidosis may be present. Diagnosing other cases of type 2 diabetes is often incidental on routine health screening, during other medical investigations, or when investigating symptoms such as vision changes, recurrent skin infections, or unexplained fatigue. Diabetes is often detected when a person is admitted to hospital for an illness often associated with diabetes (e.g. heart attack, stroke, neuropathy, cellulitis, poor wound healing, foot ulcers, new visual impairment, fungal infections), or after delivering a baby with macrosomia or hypoglycaemia.

Other causes of increased urine production (polyuria) and thirst which should be considered include:

- increased solute load (e.g. with glycosuria or diuretic use)
- water diuresis (e.g. with cranial or nephrogenic diabetes insipidus; hypercalcaemia; or sickle cell disease)
- other causes, such as paroxysmal tachycardias or migraine

Diagnosis in suspected diabetes mellitus

A diagnosis of diabetes is based on blood glucose levels—fasting, postprandial, or both. In a symptomatic person, a random blood glucose >11.1 mmol/l (200 mg/dl) is diagnostic. Asymptomatic patients or those with intercurrent illness require a further abnormal result when well before a diagnosis of diabetes can be made. The timing of a blood glucose test is important, with fasting and 2-hour post-oral glucose-load measurements being the accepted standards.

Impaired fasting glucose and impaired glucose tolerance are sometimes called prediabetes. The latter in particular is a major risk factor for progression to full-blown diabetes mellitus as well as cardiovascular disease.

Type 1 diabetes

Type 1 diabetes often presents with the patient acutely unwell with breathlessness (air hunger or Kussmaul respiration, with deep regular rapid breaths, suggesting acidosis), abdominal pain, muscle cramps, weight loss, polyuria, and polydipsia. Subsequent nausea and vomiting can worsen both the dehydration and electrolyte losses which often precede the onset of coma (occurring in about 10% of cases of ketoacidosis). The duration of symptoms is typically short, over days to weeks. It is more usually diagnosed in people <40 years old, but can occur later; the peak age of onset is 12 years old. Twenty-five per cent of hospital admissions with diabetic ketoacidosis are a first presentation of type 1 diabetes. Diabetic ketoacidosis is precipitated in 30%–50% cases by infection, 25% of cases relate to poor compliance with therapy, and 10%–13% with inappropriate dose adjustments.

Table 184.1 Blood glucose levels for the diagnosis of diabetes mellitus

Condition	Glucose test	Venous plasma glucose (mmol/l)
Normal	Fasting	<6.0
	Two-hour postprandial	<7.8
Diabetes	Fasting	>7.0
	Two-hour postprandial	>11.1
Impaired glucose tolerance	Fasting	<7.0
	Two-hour postprandial	7.8–11.1
Impaired fasting glycaemia	Fasting	6.0–6.9

The presence of ketones in the urine (++ or more on dip testing) and blood (normal <1.0 mmol/l, ketonaemia >3 mmol/l), with or without metabolic acidosis (arterial pH <7.28, or venous pH <7.3) aids the diagnosis. In obese patients and in those of Afro-Caribbean origin, in particular those from sub-Saharan Africa, type 2 diabetes may present with ketoacidosis. The family history and phenotype of the patient are therefore also useful for making an accurate diagnosis. In patients where the diagnosis is equivocal, measurement of anti-glutamic-acid-decarboxylase and anti-islet-cell antibodies can help to clarify this (e.g. antibody-negative, overweight patients may not need insulin once they recover).

Type 2 diabetes

Type 2 diabetes is a common condition affecting 1 in 10 people over 65 years of age in the UK, with many having evidence of end-organ damage at the time of diagnosis. It is a combination of insulin resistance and an insulin secretory defect or pancreatic 'pump' failure.

Other types of diabetes

While type 1 and type 2 diabetes account for the majority of cases seen, other forms to consider include:

- genetic defects of beta-cell function:
  - maturity-onset diabetes of the young (MODY)
  - mutations in: HNF4B (Chromosome 20; MODY 1), GCK (Chromosome 7; MODY 2), HNF1A (Chromosome 12; MODY 3), IPF1 (Chromosome 13; MODY 4)
  - the mitochondrial DNA 3242 mutation
  - mutations associated with neonatal diabetes (KIR6.2, SUR)
- other defects:
  - genetic defects of insulin action
  - type A insulin resistance
  - leprechaunism (type 2 diabetes, intrauterine growth retardation + dysmorphic features)
  - Rabson–Mendenhall syndrome (diabetes mellitus + pineal hyperplasia + acanthosis nigricans)
  - lipoatrophic diabetes
  - diseases of the exocrine pancreas
  - pancreatitis
  - trauma/surgery (pancreatectomy)
  - neoplasia
  - pancreatic destruction (e.g. cystic fibrosis, haemochromatosis)

- endocrinopathies (e.g. Cushing's syndrome, acromegaly, phaeochromocytoma, glucagonoma, hyperthyroidism, somatostatinoma)
- drug- or chemical-induced diabetes mellitus
- infections (e.g. congenital rubella or CMV)
- uncommon forms of immune-mediated diabetes (e.g. anti-insulin-receptor antibodies, stiff man syndrome (type 1 diabetes, rigidity of muscles, painful spasms))
- Wolfram syndrome (or DIDMOAD: **d**iabetes **i**nsipidus, **d**iabetes **m**ellitus, **o**ptic **a**trophy + **d**eafness (sensorineural))
- other genetic syndromes associated with diabetes: these include Down's syndrome, Klinefelter syndrome, Laurence–Moon–Biedl syndrome, myotonic dystrophy, Prader–Willi syndrome and Turner's syndrome
- gestational diabetes

Aetiology

Table 184.2 outlines the different types of diabetes and their frequency, potential mechanisms, and symptoms.

Demographics

The incidence of diabetes mellitus is increasing rapidly. Type 2 diabetes is more common in developed countries, although both types occur throughout the world. One in three Americans born after 2000 will potentially develop diabetes in their lifetime. Asian and African populations are likely to have the greatest increases in prevalence. An increasing incidence of diabetes in developing countries follows the trend of urbanization and lifestyle changes particularly associated with a 'Western' diet and lifestyle. There is a higher prevalence and increasing incidence of diabetes in indigenous populations in first-world countries than in their corresponding non-indigenous populations. In Australia the age-standardized prevalence of self-reported diabetes in Indigenous Australians is almost four times that of non-indigenous Australians. The Centers for Disease Control and Prevention have termed the change an epidemic. The National Diabetes Information Clearinghouse estimates that diabetes costs $132 billion/year in the United States.

Diabetes mellitus prevalence increases with age, and the numbers of older persons with diabetes are expected to grow as the elderly population increases in number. Insulin production decreases because of age-related impairment of pancreatic beta cells. Additionally, insulin resistance increases because of the loss of lean tissue and the accumulation of fat, particularly intra-abdominal fat, and the decreased tissue sensitivity to insulin.

Table 184.2 The aetiology of diabetes

	Type 1 diabetes (previously known as insulin-dependent diabetes mellitus)	Type 2 diabetes (previously known as non-insulin-dependent diabetes mellitus)	Maturity-onset diabetes of the young	Latent autoimmune diabetes in adults	Gestational diabetes (diabetes occurring during or first diagnosed in pregnancy)
Frequency	5%–25% of cases	75%–95%	1%–5%	10% of cases of type 2 diabetes	2%–5% of pregnancies
Potential mechanism	Destruction of insulin-producing beta cells in the pancreas by antibodies, alcohol, cystic fibrosis, surgery, neoplasia, pancreatitis, etc.	Combination of genetic and environmental factors; there are also secondary causes, such as acromegaly and Cushing's syndrome	Autosomal or mitochondrial gene mutations presenting as type 2 diabetes by <30 years of age	GAD antibodies to beta cells	A combination of relatively inadequate insulin secretion and responsiveness during pregnancy
Antibodies	ICA, IA2, GAD65, IAA	None	None	Mostly GAD65	None
Potential effect/problem	Absence or deficiency of insulin	Combined resistance to and relative deficiency of insulin	Defects in beta-cell function	Insulin deficiency	Combined resistance to and relative deficiency of insulin
Symptoms	Rapid onset of symptoms (weeks–months)	Insidious onset over years; may be asymptomatic	May have an insidious onset over years; may be asymptomatic	Onset of symptoms may be rapid (weeks–months)	May be asymptomatic; macrosomia and hypoglycaemia soon after birth in the baby

Abbreviations: GAD65, glutamic acid decarboxylase autoantibody; IA2, islet antigen 2 autoantibody; IAA, insulin autoantibody; ICA, islet cell autoantibody.

Complications

Acute complications (hypoglycaemia, ketoacidosis, or non-ketotic hyperosmolar coma) may occur if the disease is not adequately controlled. Patient education, understanding, and participation is vital since the complications of diabetes are far less common and less severe in people who have well-controlled blood glucose levels. Serious long-term complications include cardiovascular disease (doubled risk), chronic renal failure (commonest reason for dialysis in the UK and the US), retinal damage (which is believed to be the commonest cause of blindness in the working population of the Western world) and nerve damage. Poor healing of wounds, particularly of the feet, can lead to gangrene, and possibly to amputation (diabetes is the leading cause for non-traumatic lower limb amputation in adults). Adequate treatment of diabetes, as well as increased emphasis on lipid and blood pressure control and lifestyle factors (such as not smoking and maintaining a healthy body weight), may improve the risk profile of most chronic complications. Lifestyle modification may also help prevent people predisposed to type 2 diabetes and those at prediabetic stages from developing type 2 diabetes. Although few people actually go into total 'remission' as a result of lifestyle modification, exercise, and weight loss, some with type 2 diabetes may find they need less oral hypoglycaemic agent or insulin therapy since the body tends to have lower insulin requirements during and shortly following exercise.

Other relevant investigations

While not used for diagnosis, an elevated level of glucose irreversibly bound to haemoglobin (termed 'glycosylated haemoglobin', or 'Hb A1c') of 6.0% (42 mmol/mol) or higher (the 2003 revised US standard) is considered abnormal by most labs, and is starting to be considered as a diagnostic tool. The units for Hb A1c are changing from percentage to millimoles of Hb A1c per mole of haemoglobin. Hb A1c is primarily used as a treatment-tracking test reflecting average blood glucose levels over the preceding 90 days (approximately). However, some physicians may order this test at the time of diagnosis to track changes over time. The current recommended goal for Hb A1c in patients with diabetes is 6.5%–7.5% (48–58 mmol/mol) but physicians often aim for <7.0% (53 mmol/mol), which is considered good glycaemic control, although some guidelines are stricter (<6.5% or 48 mmol/mol). People with diabetes with Hb A1c levels within this range have a significantly lower incidence of complications such as retinopathy and nephropathy.

Treatments

After diagnosis, all patients with diabetes need to see a dietitian and a diabetes nurse specialist and have a full medical assessment. The first priority is to decide whether the patient has type 1 or type 2 diabetes, as patients with type 1 diabetes need insulin immediately. Patients with type 2 diabetes need initial dietary advice with or without medication. Typically, metformin was added in after 3 months of diet and exercise alone but is now recommended to be added in at diagnosis. The advice given should always take into account the patient's circumstances and culture and be individually tailored in order to be achievable.

The education of all newly diagnosed patients is intended to provide an incentive for good compliance. A full education package should include:

- an explanation as to what diabetes is and what it means to the patient
- aims of treatment, (e.g. rationale of reducing complications and exact values of blood glucose, Hb A1c, lipids, and blood pressure to aim for)
- types of treatment—not just drugs but also dietary advice and lifestyle modification such as increased physical activity, stopping smoking, and, if needed, reducing alcohol intake
- self-monitoring (e.g. the method(s) of doing this, the reasons for doing it, the target fasting and postprandial levels for that individual (e.g. 4.5–7.0 mmol/l fasting and 4.5–9.0 mmol/l postprandial) and what to do with the results (e.g. whether to alter therapy or not))
- an idea of some chronic complications of diabetes and what to look out for (e.g. a podiatrist's input and review is advised,

especially for those with type 2 diabetes) and reinforcing the need for regular checks (e.g. annual eye screening)
- advice regarding DVLA, insurance companies, and Diabetes UK

While insulin therapy is mandatory from diagnosis in all people with type 1 diabetes, patients with type 2 diabetes should be entered into an educational package with an initial trial of diet, exercise, and weight reduction (if obese, which most will be) with consideration of **metformin** in most patients, especially the overweight, and possibly **sulfonylureas** in the lean, if there are no contraindications. After this initial assessment, all patients should be put into a formal review system, whether by their GP or in a hospital diabetic clinic, for further education, maintenance of good control, and complication screening.

General management and treatment

Dietary advice

In the overweight patient (e.g. BMI >25) a reduction in total calorie intake to aid weight reduction is also required. A standard diabetic diet should aim to have:

- <10% of its energy in the form of saturated fat (<8% if the patient is hyperlipidaemic)
- <30% from all fats
- 50%–60% as carbohydrate, mostly consisting of complex high fibre carbohydrates
- sugar limited to about 25 g/day
- sodium content <6 g/day in most people, or <3 g/day if the patient if hypertensive

Alcohol is a significant source of calories, and reducing alcohol consumption by the overweight or hypertriglyceridaemic patient is advisable. The current 'standard' diet for a person with diabetes is a weight-reducing, low-fat, low-glycaemic-index diet with a reduction in sodium content, as most patients will have type 2 diabetes and are slightly overweight; this needs to be modified according to the individual patient, however.

Oral hypoglycaemic agents

Biguanides

Metformin is the first-line therapy in the obese or in overweight people with type 2 diabetes and is also used in some insulin-treated, insulin-resistant, overweight subjects to reduce insulin requirements. The UK Prospective Diabetes Study (UKPDS) showed significantly better results from metformin for complications and mortality compared to other therapies in the overweight patient with type 2 diabetes. Although a 1–2 kg weight loss is seen initially after the start of metformin usage, UKPDS data suggests metformin does not significantly alter weight over a 10-year period.

Metformin's mode of action

Metformin works by decreasing hepatic gluconeogenesis and increasing muscle glucose uptake/metabolism, so increasing insulin sensitivity. With long-term use a 0.8%–2.0% reduction in Hb A1c occurs.

Side effects/contraindications of metformin

Metformin is contraindicated in patients with renal (suggested as a creatinine >140 nmol/l, although an estimated glomerular filtration rate <30 has also been suggested), hepatic, or cardiac impairment, or who consume significant amounts of alcohol. Gastrointestinal side effects include nausea, epigastric discomfort, and diarrhoea and occur in up to half of patients in the first 1–2 weeks of treatment, but are usually transient. If the starting dose is low (e.g. 500 mg once daily) and it is taken with food, this can be reduced and many people develop a tolerance to these symptoms and are able to take higher doses; <5% are totally intolerant. Rarely, skin rashes and lactic acidosis occur. The latter, when seen, is usually in patients with significant sepsis, hepatic, renal, or cardiac impairment. Using radiological contrast media with metformin is associated with an increased risk of lactic acidosis and therapy should be stopped at the time of or prior to such investigations and restarted 2 days after the test unless renal function has been affected by the procedure, in which case, delay until this has resolved. Lactic acidosis occurs very infrequently (e.g. 0.024–0.15 cases/1000 patient years in a Swedish study). Although it is known to reduce folic acid and vitamin B_{12} absorption, this is not usually a significant problem clinically with metformin.

Sulfonylureas

Sulfonylureas are used as a first-line treatment in non-obese patients with type 2 diabetes. The first-generation agents chlorpropamide, tolbutamide, and tolazamide are rarely used today. Instead, second-generation agents such as glibenclamide, gliclazide, and glipizide are now more commonly used. Third-generation agents, such as glimepiride, are also available.

Mode of action of Sulfonylureas

Sulfonylureas act by stimulating a receptor on the surface of beta cells, closing a potassium channel and opening a calcium channel, with subsequent insulin release. A doubling of glucose-stimulated insulin secretion can be expected, with both first- and second-phase insulin secretion affected. This results in a 1%–2% reduction in Hb A1c long term.

Side effects of Sulfonylureas

The side effects of Sulfonylureas are hypoglycaemia and weight gain. In the UKPDS, the mean weight gain seen after 10 years of sulfonylurea therapy was 2.3 kg, while the incidence of major hypoglycaemic events was 0.4%–0.6%/year. The elderly are particularly at risk of hypoglycaemia with longer-acting agents such as glibenclamide and these should be avoided in that age group. Occasional skin reactions, alterations in liver function tests, and minor gastrointestinal symptoms may occur. Also avoid sulfonylureas in porphyria.

Prandial glucose regulators

Prandial glucose regulators can be used in type 2 patients who have inadequate control on diet or metformin, predominantly targeting postprandial hyperglycaemia due to their short duration of action.

Repaglinide, a carbamoylmethyl benzoic acid derivative, is a non-sulfonylurea oral hypoglycaemic agent which stimulates the secretion of insulin from pancreatic beta cells. It works on separate parts of the beta-cell sulfonylurea receptor from the sulfonylureas. Its use results in an approximate 0.6%–2% reduction in Hb A1c levels. Its very short duration of action reduces the risk of hypoglycaemia, compared to some sulfonylureas. It has an insulinotropic effect within 30 minutes of oral administration and causes a return to normal insulin levels within 4–6 hours (the elimination half-life is around 1 hour). It should not, however, be used in patients with renal or hepatic impairment and may result in hepatic dysfunction, so periodic liver function test monitoring is required.

Nateglinide is a D-phenylalanine derivative with an insulinotropic effect within 15 minutes of oral administration and causes a return to normal insulin levels by 2 hours (the elimination half-life is 1.5 hours), so reducing the risk of subsequent hypoglycaemia. Its efficacy is similar to that of repaglinide.

Alpha-glucosidase inhibitors

Alpha-glucosidase inhibitors are used in type 2 patients who have inadequate control on diet or other oral agent alone. When taken with food, acarbose reduces postprandial glucose peaks by inhibiting the digestive enzyme alpha-glucosidase, which normally breaks carbohydrates into their monosaccharide components, thus retarding glucose uptake from the intestine and reducing postprandial glucose peaks. Some improvement in lipids has also been reported.

These undigested carbohydrates then pass into the large intestine, where bacteria metabolize them, which may explain the common side effects of postprandial fullness/bloating, abdominal pain, flatulence, and diarrhoea. Starting at 50 mg once daily and gradually increasing the dose at 2–3 weekly intervals to a maximum of 200 mg three times per day improves tolerance to this therapy. Less commonly, jaundice and elevated hepatic transaminase levels can also be seen. In the UKPDS, adding acarbose to other therapies resulted in a further 0.5% drop in Hb A1c.

Thiazolidinediones

Thiazolidinediones act as insulin-sensitizing agents by activating the peroxisome proliferator-activated receptor, which stimulates gene transcription for glucose transporter molecules such as GLUT1 and GLUT4. The first of this class was troglitazone, which was withdrawn soon after its UK launch because of reports of hepatotoxicity but was still used in other countries until newer agents were available. Rosiglitazone was withdrawn due to cardiovascular concerns. Pioglitazone gives a 0.6%–2.0% drop in Hb A1c. It does not seem to have the same problem with hepatotoxicity, and there is often an improvement in liver function, especially with non-alcoholic steatohepatitis. Although the risk of hepatic dysfunction is not high with this drug, initial checks of liver function and monitoring of liver function tests are still currently advised. In view of the more common problem with fluid retention, avoidance in heart failure is also strongly suggested. The indication for using these agents varies around the world and in the UK they are used in combination with other oral agents but not with insulin, although the combination with insulin is licensed in the US. Recent studies suggest a possible link with osteoporosis, and side effects also include fluid retention, weight gain, and hepatotoxicity.

The incretin system (glucagon-like polypeptide-1 mimetics and dipeptidyl peptidase-4 inhibitors)

Glucagon-like polypeptide-1 (GLP-1) and gastrointestinal polypeptide are hormones made in the L-cells of the jejunum and ileum in response to a food load entering the gastrointestinal tract. These incretin hormones stimulate glucose-dependent insulin secretion, suppress glucagon secretion, and slow gastric emptying, with an improvement in insulin sensitivity.

Exenatide (Byetta) is a GLP-1 mimetic taken as a twice-daily injection of 5 μg or 10 μg doses or as a once-weekly 2 mg modified-release depot injection with a 0.6%–0.8% reduction in Hb A1c after 30 weeks use and a 1.6–2.8 kg weight loss over the same period. Liraglutide 1.2 mg is a once-daily version.

Dipeptidyl peptidase-4 (DPP-4) breaks down gastric inhibitory polypeptide and GLP-1 and this enzyme can be inhibited by oral drugs such as sitagliptin, vildagliptin, saxagliptin and linagliptin (i.e. DPP-4 inhibitors) with a resultant 0.4%–0.7% reduction in Hb A1c over a 12-month period and are weight neutral, if not helping to reduce weight. Liver monitoring with vildagliptin is currently recommended, and linagliptin needs no dose adjustment in renal impairment.

Side effects of incretin-system drugs

Side effects of incretin-system drugs are as follows:

- sitagliptin: gastrointestinal disturbance, upper respiratory tract infection, nasopharyngitis, and peripheral oedema
- vildagliptin: as for sitagliptin, plus abnormal liver function tests
- exenatide: gastrointestinal upset with nausea, vomiting, abdominal distension, diarrhoea, headache, dizziness, increased sweating, and injection site reactions

Gliflozins (sodium glucose transport protein 2, or SGLT-2 inhibitors)

The SGLT-2 inhibitors block reabsorption of glucose in the kidney, by inhibiting a pathway in the kidney, which normally exchanges sodium for glucose, this can cause people to lose up to 70g of glucose in the urine daily, is independent of insulin action, and whilst reducing circulating glucose, also helps reduce weight in view of the calories lost by this glycosuria. Potential electrolyte loss and an increased risk of lower urinary tract infections need to be monitored.

Insulin

Insulin is required in all patients with type 1 diabetes, and some with type 2, for the preservation of life; in other patients with type 2 diabetes it is needed to achieve better glycaemic/metabolic control or for the relief of hyperglycaemic symptoms. Most insulin is now in a biosynthetic human form (from yeast or bacteria) but there is also a sizable minority of patients still taking bovine or porcine insulin. Bovine insulin is extracted from cattle pancreas and is more antigenic than both human and porcine alternatives and so gives more lipohypertrophy and lipoatrophy.

Insulin can be given by IV or subcutaneous routes; more recently, short-acting insulin was also given as an inhaled formulation, but this was recently withdrawn. Standard insulins come as 10 ml vials for use with a 0.5 ml or 1.0 ml syringe or as 3.0 ml cartridges for use in pen devices. The insulin itself is unmodified/neutral or mixed with agents such as protamine or zinc to alter its onset of action, peak effect, and duration of action. Human insulin analogues that give more rapid onset or greater duration of action are also widely available and used. There are >30 types of insulin preparation available, which should allow full 24-hour cover for a wide variety of lifestyles.

The main problems with all insulin regimens are weight gain and hypoglycaemia. The latter occurring overnight can be troublesome, especially as the patient may not know it has occurred and may just react to the morning hyperglycaemia by increasing their evening insulin dose. Occasional checks of 3 am blood glucose levels may help sort this out. Care with alcohol and adjustments of insulin and pre-bed snacks if nocturnal physical activity such as sex is on the cards will also reduce nocturnal 'hypos'.

Types of insulin

Short-acting (soluble/neutral) insulins

Unmodified or neutral insulins are short-acting but are not identical. Humulin® S has an onset 30 min after injection, with a peak onset at 2–3 hour and a duration of up to 6–8 hours. In contrast, Hypurin® Porcine Neutral has an onset 60 minutes after injection, with a peak at 2–5 hours, and a duration of 6–8 hours. All the soluble human formulations require a 20–30-minute interval between injecting and eating to be maximally effective.

Insulin analogues

Insulin lispro, insulin aspart, and insulin glulisine have been modified to allow injecting and eating to occur simultaneously, as they have a more rapid onset of action and earlier peak effect, with peak blood insulin levels approximately 1.5–2.5 times that from the same dose of standard neutral human insulin. The duration of action is also shorter at 5 hours and this may cause problems if there are long gaps between meals

Long-acting analogues such as insulin glargine and insulin detemir are also available, which give a flatter profile with a duration of action of 22–24 hours. These can be used as part of a basal bolus regimen with short-acting analogues or standard soluble insulins. They appear to be associated with less hypoglycaemia than other background insulins and may reduce the risk of nocturnal hypoglycaemia. Their use as a once-daily insulin alone or in combination with oral agents such as glimepiride or the prandial glucose regulators is also proving popular in the elderly type 2 patient.

While insulin glargine has a slightly longer duration of action, making it a popular once-daily preparation, insulin detemir, because of its albumin-binding properties, is reported to give less between-dose variability in the same individual and, with a duration of action of 20–22 hours, may be used in similar situations, although a significant proportion of people need to use it twice daily.

Intermediate-acting (isophane) insulins

Insulin action can be extended by the addition of protamine to give isophane insulin, with an onset of action 1–2 hours after injection, a peak at 4–6 hours, and a duration of action of 8–14 hours. Different preparations have slightly different profiles when looking at peak effect and maximal insulin concentrations, as with soluble preparations.

Biphasic/mixed insulins

Combinations of soluble/neutral insulins or short-acting insulin analogues with isophane insulins are extremely popular. The amount of soluble insulin present varies from 10%–50%, with 30% being the most popular. Depending on its monocomponents, onset is normally at 30 minutes, the peak effect is at 2–6 hours, and the duration is at 8–12 hours. Insulin analogue biphasic preparations have an onset, peak, and duration all slightly shorter than these.

Insulin regimens

Twice-daily free mixing

Twice-daily free mixing was historically very popular, although now it is used much more rarely. The usual starting regimen was two-thirds isophane insulin and one-third soluble insulin, with two-thirds of the total daily dose given before breakfast, and one-third before the evening meal. The main problems are (1) mixing the two types of insulin, and (2) pre-lunch hypos. If on the same doses twice daily, watch out for pre-evening-meal hyperglycaemia and increase the morning isophane dose to compensate for this, with a reduction in the morning soluble insulin dose often needed to reduce pre-lunch hypoglycaemia.

Twice-daily fixed mixture

Most commonly, a twice-daily fixed mixture consists of 30% soluble insulin and 70% isophane insulin; although this is not ideal for pre-lunch control or alterations in diet and exercise that are not pre-planned, it is indicated in type 2 patients with poor control, those with significant osmotic symptoms, and those in whom there is no room to increase oral agents. A suitable starting regimen is a 30:70 mixture, with two-thirds taken before breakfast, and one-third before the evening meal. The exact doses tend to vary widely depending on insulin sensitivity but a reasonable starting regimen may be 10–15 units before breakfast, and 5–10 units before the evening meal.

Basal bolus regimen

In a basal bolus regimen, soluble insulin or an insulin analogue is given three times per day in pre-meal doses, with a pre-bed dose of isophane insulin or a long-acting insulin analogue; this regimen potentially has more flexibility with meal times, portions, and exercise than the previous regimens. The larger number of injections and the more frequent capillary blood glucose measurements needed makes it less popular with some patients.

If starting with a basal bolus regimen as the first type of insulin regimen, give three equal pre-meal doses and alter as required (e.g. 4–6 units is a reasonable starting dose, with 6–8 units of isophane insulin before bed). If converting to a basal bolus regimen from a twice-daily biphasic regimen, you need to reduce the total daily insulin dose by up to 10%. Initially, give 30%–50% of the total daily insulin needed as a pre-bedtime dose of isophane insulin or a long-acting insulin analogue and split the remaining insulin evenly between the meals as soluble or short-acting insulin analogue. Once the patient is on this regimen, the evening isophane insulin or insulin analogue often needs to be increased to maintain adequate fasting sugars.

In patients using short-acting insulin analogues and, less often, those on standard soluble insulins, a twice-daily dose of isophane insulin or a long-acting insulin analogue is occasionally needed, especially if there is a long gap between lunch and the evening meal.

Continuous subcutaneous insulin infusion

Continuous subcutaneous insulin infusion is used in the US but not as commonly in the UK, possibly because of cost issues as well as potential problems with pump failure, ketoacidosis, and cannula site infections, although, with improvements in technology, these are less common problems now. Soluble insulin or a short-acting insulin analogue is given continuously via a subcutaneous cannula into the anterior abdomen. National Institute of Clinical Excellence guidance on the use of insulin pumps is available and worth reading.

Insulin and oral agent mixtures

In type 2 patients, several combinations are occasionally used. The two most popular are bedtime insulin plus daytime tablets, or more frequent insulin plus metformin. In the first, oral agents continue during the day with a pre-bed dose of isophane insulin or a long-acting insulin analogue used to give acceptable fasting sugars before breakfast. Although often starting at 10 units/night, doses five to six times that are not infrequently needed. This regimen is suitable if someone else such as a district nurse or relative gives the insulin. The second regimen adds up to 2 g/day of metformin to any standard insulin regimen to reduce insulin requirements and improve control without the problem of further weight gain often seen if the insulin is continually increased.

Further Reading

National Institute for Health and Care Excellence diabetes pathways at http://pathways.nice.org.uk/pathways/diabetes#path=view%3A/pathways/diabetes/diabetes-overview.xml&content=view-index

185 Hypoglycaemia

Kevin Shotliff

Introduction

Hypoglycaemia, which is a common complication of the treatment of diabetes, should be excluded in any unconscious or fitting patient, even if diabetes is not known. If prolonged, it can result in death. Most insulin-treated patients can expect to experience hypoglycaemic episodes at some time, with up to one in seven having a more severe episode each year, and 3% suffering recurrent episodes. In addition, 25% of people on long-term insulin lose their hypoglycaemic awareness, and these are of particular concern. Nocturnal hypoglycaemic episodes with a hyperglycaemic response the next morning (due to increased counter-regulatory hormones—the Somogyi phenomenon) tend to occur in younger insulin-treated patients; such episodes should not be forgotten, although it may only present with morning headaches or a 'drunken' feeling.

Definition/diagnosis

Hypoglycaemia is a biochemical diagnosis made when the blood glucose is <2.5 mmol/l and the patient shows symptoms of neuroglycopenia. However, it is often first picked up by the patient, their family, or their doctor from the symptoms listed in 'Clinical features'. In any patient not known to have diabetes, a detailed screen should be undertaken to determine the cause.

Pathogenesis

Hypoglycaemia occurs when there are imbalances between the glucose supply, glucose utilization, and the insulin level so that there is more insulin than is needed at that time. A reduced glucose supply can occur when a meal or snack is missed, or as a late effect of alcohol, which reduces hepatic gluconeogenesis. It can also be due to delayed gastric emptying with autonomic neuropathy, be associated with malabsorptive states such as coeliac disease, Addison's disease, or an acute illness, such as gastroenteritis. Increased utilization of glucose occurs with exercise, and high insulin levels (exogenous or endogenous) occur mostly with sulfonylurea or exogenous insulin therapy and rarely with insulinomas (incidence of 1–2 per million per year). The net result of such imbalances is hypoglycaemia.

Therapies for people with diabetes and hypoglycaemia

Human insulin therapies have a slightly faster onset of action and a shorter duration of action than their animal predecessors, and many patients report alterations in hypoglycaemic awareness when they switch from one to the other. Even so, no definite evidence of specific hypoglycaemic alterations due to human insulin itself has been reported. The shorter-acting insulin analogues may have a similar effect in some patients, compared to standard human insulin therapies, as well.

Sulfonylurea therapy can cause hypoglycaemia due to beta cell stimulation. This is most commonly seen from **glibenclamide (~50% greater risk of hypoglycaemia with this agent than with other secretagogues)**, especially in the elderly and those with reduced renal excreting ability, but can occur in anyone who takes this therapy and fasts.

Other secretagogues can have a similar effect to sulphonylureas, such as the meglitinides (e.g. nateglinide and repaglinide) as can insulin-sensitizing agents such as angiotensin-converting-enzyme inhibitors and thiazolidinediones (e.g. **pioglitazone**). But the biguanide **metformin** and the alpha-glucosidase inhibitor **acarbose** are unlikely to precipitate hypoglycaemia.

Hypoglycaemia in those without known diabetes

In patients without known diabetes who are not taking drugs known to cause hypoglycaemia, other causes need to be sought. These are typically split into either fasting hypoglycaemia (occurring >5 hours after food) or reactive/postprandial hypoglycaemia (typically occurring 2–5 hours after food). The main conditions to consider/exclude in these patients are:

- drug-induced hypoglycaemia resulting from:
  - exogenous insulin or sulfonylurea therapy (either deliberate or accidental)
  - alcohol (impairs gluconeogenesis and alters glycogen stores)
  - salicylates (alters hepatic glucose efflux)
  - quinine (causes hyperinsulinaemia)
- infections:
  - septicaemia (e.g. Gram-negative or meningococcus septicaemia) has high metabolic requirements and causes a reduced energy intake
- tumours:
  - insulinomas (85% benign, 15% malignant)
  - non-islet cell tumours (e.g. large mesenchymal tumours such as fibrosarcomas)
- hormone deficiency:
  - Addison's disease
  - hypopituitarism
  - growth hormone deficiency
- organ failure:
  - acute liver failure
  - chronic renal failure
- starvation:
  - anorexia nervosa
  - kwashiorkor
- autoimmune disorders:
  - the presence of anti-insulin antibodies causing hypoglycaemia; this is a rare condition which is commonest in Japanese patients (insulin autoimmune syndrome, or Hirata's disease; strongly associated with HLA-DR4)
  - the presence of insulin-receptor activating antibodies (again rare but commonest in middle-aged women)
- inborn errors of metabolism:
  - glycogen storage disease
  - hereditary fructose intolerance
  - maple syrup disease
- post-surgery hypoglycaemia:
  - post-gastrectomy hyperglycaemia (e.g. 'dumping'): rapid gastric emptying produces a greater-than-normal insulin response, causing an hypoglycaemic episode 2–3 hours postprandially

Clinical features

Hypoglycaemia should be considered in any patient with an unexplained collapse, loss of consciousness, or 'funny turn'. The features of hypoglycaemia can be divided into two main groups: autonomic symptoms and neuroglycopenic symptoms. The autonomic symptoms usually occur first (when the blood glucose is <3.6 mmol/l), but some drugs, such as alcohol and non-selective beta blockers, may mask these with neuroglycopenia (at a blood glucose <2.6 mmol/l) so that confusion then occurs with no warning. Some patients lose these predominantly autonomic warning symptoms and are therefore at higher risk of injury. Typically, there is a deterioration in neuropsychological performance as the blood glucose falls to 3.0–3.5 mmol/l and there is a subjective perception of hypoglycaemia at 2.7–2.9 mmol/l. EEG changes are evident when the blood glucose falls to 2.0 mmol/l.

Signs and symptoms of hypoglycaemia

Autonomic

The autonomic symptoms of hypoglycaemia are:

* sweating
* pallor
* anxiety
* nausea
* tremor
* shivering
* palpitations
* tachycardia

Neuroglycopenic

The neuroglycopenic symptoms of hypoglycaemia are:

* confusion
* tiredness
* lack of concentration
* headache
* dizziness
* altered speech
* incoordination
* drowsiness
* aggression
* coma

Investigation

Capillary blood glucose testing strips are widely used but are unreliable for low glucose levels, and any symptomatic patient with a capillary testing strip reading <4.0 mmol/l should at least have a laboratory glucose measured. In view of the potential causes for this, any patient with hypoglycaemia and no obvious therapy for this should be investigated fully. Even diabetics who are taking oral or injectable therapies known to cause hypoglycaemia warrant further review. Renal dysfunction and hepatic dysfunction are both well-known causes and so initial tests should include:

* laboratory blood glucose
* urea and electrolytes
* liver function tests

In patients not known to have diabetes with hypoglycaemia, further investigation may be needed and can include:

* laboratory blood glucose
* insulin and C-peptide (if high insulin and no C-peptide consider exogenous insulin)
* beta-hydroxybutyrate (elevated in most cases but suppressed with insulinoma, sulphonylureas, and exogenous insulin)
* sulfonylurea screen
* cortisol ± a short tetracosactide test
* consider insulin-like growth factors 1 (reduced) and 2 (high) if non-islet cell tumour hypoglycaemia suspected
* consider an autoimmune screen for anti-insulin and anti-insulin-receptor antibodies
* chest X-ray for fibrosarcoma, mesothelioma
* consider an overnight or 72-hour fast, to look at glucose/insulin levels

Management

In the conscious patient, oral carbohydrate (high glycaemic index and usually 20 g) is often sufficient to resolve the problem. This 20 g is equivalent to (can be given as):

* seven Dextrosol tablets
* four jelly babies
* 15–20 jelly beans
* 115 ml Lucozade (310 ml Lucozade Sport)
* 180 ml Coca-Cola
* 144 ml of a carton of Ribena
* 200 ml of milk

Having raised the sugar rapidly with a high-glycaemic-index food, then give the patient something to maintain a normal blood glucose level when this quick-acting carbohydrate wears out (e.g. a lower-glycaemic-index food such as a sandwich or two digestive biscuits). In the confused patient, buccal gels (e.g. a 30% glucose gel) are an alternative, although this should not be used in the unconscious patient as there is a risk of aspiration.

In the unconscious patient, once a blood sample has been taken for glucose estimation, treat with 25–50 ml of 50% IV glucose or 1 mg of intramuscular or deep subcutaneous glucagon. However, glucagon mobilizes glycogen from the liver and will not work if given repeatedly or in starved patients with no glycogen stores. In this situation or if prolonged treatment is needed, IV glucose is better (50% initially then 10%). The worry with 50% glucose is tissue necrosis if extravasation occurs; because of this, some units use 20% glucose initially and convert to 5% or 10% glucose for continuation therapy. The potential for larger fluid loads being needed to give the same amount of glucose with the lower concentration does not seem to be a problem in this situation but will need to be tailored to the individual patient.

Subsequent management

Having corrected the acute event, determine why it happened, especially if the patient is not known to have diabetes or to take therapy known to be associated with hypoglycaemic episodes. If possible, then alter treatment or lifestyle to keep the hyperglycaemia from recurring. Extreme exercise may require an alteration in insulin doses for 24 hours afterwards, and alcohol causes not only initial hyperglycaemia but also a degree of hypoglycaemia 3–6 hours after ingestion, and may alter insulin requirements the next morning. Education to avoid precipitating hypoglycaemic episodes in these situations is advisable. A severe hypoglycaemic episode may be associated with a deterioration in the patient's ability to respond, as well as a subsequent hypoglycaemic episode in the next few days, and education regarding care to adjust therapy and lifestyle to avoid this risk is important. During an acute hypoglycaemic event, patients who are on a long-acting sulfonylurea will need careful monitoring, as the drug may last longer than the glucose or glycogen given to correct it, and repeated hypoglycaemic episodes may occur. A continuous IV glucose infusion is therefore often needed for 24 hours, particularly in overdose with these agents. Repeated hypoglycaemic exposure or severe individual episodes can be associated with significant long-term cognitive impairment, although this is a rare end result.

Further Reading

Choudhary P and Amiel SA. 'Hypoglycaemia in the treatment of diabetes mellitus', in Wass JAH, Stewart PM, Amiel SA, et al., eds, *Oxford Textbook of Endocrinology and Diabetes* (2nd edition), 2011. Oxford University Press.

Cryer PE. Mechanisms of hypoglycemia-associated autonomic failure in diabetes. *N Engl J Med* 2013; 369: 362–72.

Frier BM. Hypoglycaemia in diabetes mellitus: Epidemiology and clinical implications. *Nat Rev Endocrinol* 2014; 10: 711–22.

186 Thyroid disease

John Newell-Price, Alia Munir, and Miguel Debono

Hypothyroidism

Definition of hypothyroidism

Hypothyroidism occurs when there is insufficient secretion of thyroid hormones, commonly caused by autoimmune disease. In primary hypothyroidism, the level of thyroid-stimulating hormone (TSH) is elevated, and that of free thyroxine (FT4) is reduced. However, when the origin of the hypothyroidism is pituitary or hypothalamic, FT4 is low and TSH is inappropriately normal or low. Subclinical hypothyroidism is when TSH levels are elevated in the context of an FT4 level in the normal range. Myxoedema is severe hypothyroidism with accumulation of mucopolysaccharides in the dermis and other tissues.

Aetiology of hypothyroidism

In the vast majority of cases, hypothyroidism is caused by autoimmune destruction of the thyroid. The different types of hypothyroidism and their causes are highlighted in Table 186.1

Typical symptoms of hypothyroidism, and less common symptoms

Non-specific onset symptoms include fatigue; lethargy; constipation; cold intolerance; muscle stiffness; cramps; carpal tunnel syndrome; menorrhagia; slowing of movements, deep tendon reflexes, and intellect; decreasing appetite and weight gain; dry skin and hair loss; hoarsening of voice; decreasing visual acuity and hearing; and obstructive sleep apnoea.

In severe hypothyroidism (myxoedema), there may be a dull, expressionless face; sparse hair; periorbital puffiness; macroglossia; and pale, cool skin that feels rough and doughy; but severe hypothyroidism is rare nowadays. Other features of hypothyroidism include an enlarged heart (dilated/pericardial effusion), megacolon/intestinal obstruction, cerebellar ataxia, psychiatric symptoms, peripheral neuropathy, and encephalopathy.

Demographics of hypothyroidism

Hypothyroidism affects 1% of the female population (it is much less common in men). Incidence increases with advancing age. Low dietary iodine and relative iodine deficiency appear to protect against hypothyroidism.

Natural history of hypothyroidism, and complications of the disease

Hypothyroidism is associated with atherosclerosis, hyponatraemia, hypercholesterolaemia, myopathy with raised creatine phosphokinase, and hypochromic microcytic anaemia. Homocysteine and lipoprotein levels may also be raised. Severe complications affect the elderly, and those with myxoedema coma tend to be elderly.

This group is also more likely to have undiagnosed hypothyroidism and thus is at a greater risk of developing perioperative complications.

Patients with subclinical hypothyroidism and positive autoantibodies should be treated, as there is a 5% per year rate of overt hypothyroidism.

Approach to diagnosing hypothyroidism

To diagnose hypothyroidism, measure the TSH level. If this is elevated, check the FT4 level and screen for autoantibodies.

Other diagnoses that should be considered aside from hypothyroidism

If a thyroiditis is suspected, do a full blood count (FBC) and check the erythrocyte sedimentation rate (ESR) and the level of C-reactive protein (CRP).

'Gold-standard' diagnostic test for hypothyroidism

The gold-standard diagnostic tests for hypothyroidism are the tests for TSH and FT4.

Acceptable diagnostic alternatives to the gold-standard tests for hypothyroidism

There are no acceptable diagnostic alternatives to the gold-standard tests for hypothyroidism.

Other relevant investigations for hypothyroidism

Always check the lipid profile and perform an FBC and a test for urea and electrolytes (U&E). In addition, consider investigations to exclude other autoimmune diseases such as type 1 diabetes mellitus, Addison's disease, premature ovarian failure, hypoparathyroidism, myasthenia gravis, and coeliac disease. Vitiligo and alopecia may also exist. Polyglandular autoimmune syndrome type I consists of hypothyroidism, Addison's disease, and mucocutaneous candidiasis.

Prognosis for hypothyroidism, and how to estimate it

Patients who have primary hypothyroidism but are on adequate thyroxine (T4) replacement therapy have a normal life expectancy. The mortality associated with myxoedema coma is very high (>80%).

Treatment of hypothyroidism, and its effectiveness

T4 replacement therapy should be started gradually, to avoid precipitation of arrhythmias. Start with 25–50 µg in the elderly, and 50–100

Table 186.1 The different types of hypothyroidism				
Non-goitrous	**Goitrous**	**Pituitary**	**Hypothalamic**	**Self-limiting**
Post ablative	Chronic thyroiditis	Panhypopituitarism	Neoplasm	Following withdrawal of antithyroid therapy
Congenital defect	Iodine deficiency	Isolated thyroid-stimulating-hormone deficiency	Infiltrative	Subacute thyroiditis and chronic thyroiditis with transient hypothyroidism
Atrophic thyroiditis	Drug elicited		Congenital defect	Post-partum thyroiditis
Post radiation	Heritable biosynthetic defects		Infection	

µg in young patients. Optimize the dosage using TSH measurements approximately 8–10 weeks after any changes. For patients with central or secondary hypothyroidism, FT4 is measured.

Treatment of myxoedema coma

To treat myxoedema coma, treat the precipitating illness. Manage hypothermia by external warming, in the intensive care unit if the patient is comatose. Monitor for cardiac arrhythmias and use central venous pressure for cautious volume expansion.

Check cortisol prior to commencing treatment and replace if low, using hydrocortisone 100 mg IV four times per day. Thyroid replacement can be administered IV or via a nasogastric tube (NGT). Liaise with the pharmacy for preparations. Administer T4 300–500 µg IV or via an NGT; then, 50–100 µg per day until oral medication can be taken. If there is no improvement, give T3 10 µg IV three times per day.

Thyrotoxicosis

Definition of thyrotoxicosis

Thyrotoxicosis results from exposure to excessive thyroid hormone. The term 'hyperthyroidism' denotes only those conditions in which thyroid hyperfunction results in thyrotoxicosis. The most common cause of hyperthyroidism is Graves' disease.

Aetiology of thyrotoxicosis

The aetiology of thyrotoxicosis is outlined in Table 186.2.

Typical symptoms of thyrotoxicosis, and less common symptoms

Patients with thyrotoxicosis may present with hyperactivity; irritability; altered mood; insomnia; heat intolerance; increased sweating; palpitations; fatigue; weakness; dyspnoea; weight loss with increased appetite (weight gain in 10%); pruritus; increased stool frequency; and oligomenorrhoea, amenorrhoea, or loss of libido. Signs include sinus tachycardia; atrial fibrillation; fine tremor; hyperreflexia; warm, moist skin; palmar erythema; hair loss; and muscle weakness. Rarely, patients may develop onycholysis, chorea, high-output heart failure, and periodic paralysis.

Manifestations and conditions associated with Graves' disease

The following manifestations and conditions are associated with Graves' disease:

- diffuse goitre by palpation
- anti-thyroid peroxidase (anti-TPO) or anti-thyroglobulin antibodies (anti-TSH-receptor antibodies are not routinely measured but this test may be of use if the patient is pregnant)

Table 186.2	Aetiology of thyrotoxicosis
Associated with hyperthyroidism	
Excessive thyroid stimulation	**Graves' disease** 80%, Hashitoxicosis
	Pituitary thyrotroph adenoma
	Pituitary thyroid hormone resistance syndrome (excess thyroid-stimulating hormone) (rare)
	Trophoblastic tumours producing Human chorionic gonadotropin with thyrotrophic activity (rare)
Thyroid nodules with autonomous function	**Toxic solitary nodule, toxic multinodular goitre** 20%
	Very rarely, thyroid cancer
Not associated with hyperthyroidism	
Thyroid inflammation	Silent and post-partum thyroiditis, subacute (de Quervain's) thyroiditis
Exogenous thyroid hormones	Overtreatment with thyroid hormone
	Thyrotoxicosis factitia (thyroxine use in non-thyroidal disease)
Ectopic thyroid tissue	Metastatic thyroid carcinoma
	Struma ovarii (a teratoma containing functional thyroid tissue)

- ophthalmopathy, such as:
  - grittiness and discomfort of the eye
  - retrobulbar pressure/pain
  - eyelid lag or retraction
  - periorbital oedema
  - chemosis
  - scleral injection
  - exopthalmos
  - extraocular muscle dysfunction
  - exposure keratitis
  - optic neuritis
- localized dermopathy
- lymphoid hyperplasia
- thyroid acropachy
- associated autoimmune disease in patient or family, such as:
  - type 1 diabetes
  - Addison's disease
  - vitiligo
  - pernicious anaemia
  - alopecia areata
  - myasthenia gravis
  - celiac disease
  - other autoimmune conditions associated with the HLA-DR3 haplotype

Demographics of thyrotoxicosis

Thyrotoxicosis is ten times more common in women than men in the UK. The prevalence in the female population is 2%, with an annual incidence of 3 per 1000 women. Graves' disease accounts for 70% of iodine-sufficient causes.

Natural history and complications of thyrotoxicosis

Graves' disease is caused by an autoimmune reaction to the thyroid, leading to the production of autoantibodies to the TSH receptor; these autoantibodies then mimic the action of TSH. Thirty to forty per cent of patients with Graves' disease have ophthalmopathy.

Toxic multinodular goitre and toxic adenoma, which cause 10% of all cases of thyrotoxicosis, are also common causes of thyrotoxicosis, particularly in iodine-deficient regions. Adenomas are benign, isolated thyroid tumours that independently secrete thyroid hormone. Extranodular tissue may atrophy as the level of endogenous TSH becomes suppressed. Prevalence is thought to be 2.7%, occurring in the older female age group. There is slow growth over many years; eventually, this is enough to produce overt thyrotoxicosis. Twenty to eighty per cent of cases are thought to be due to a somatic mutation in TSH receptor gene. In other cases, the G_s alpha subunit of the TSH-receptor-coupled adenylate cyclase is mutated. Toxic multinodular goitre has a similar natural history; the slow growth and advanced age of patients frequently mean not many symptoms are reported.

Complications of thyrotoxicosis can occur in every system of the body, as follows:

- cardiovascular system: palpitations, atrial fibrillation, heart failure, angina
- respiratory system: decreased lung compliance, respiratory muscle weakness, exercise intolerance
- renal system: mild polyuria, oedema; occasionally, renal tubular acidosis liver and gastrointestinal tract: increased liver enzymes, hepatomegaly, autoimmune hepatitis, weight loss, hunger, diarrhoea
- muscles: weakness and fatigue, myasthenia gravis, hypokalaemic periodic paralysis
- bones: bone loss, osteoporosis, increased risk of fracture, thyroid acropachy
- reproductive system: disturbed menstrual cycle in females; increased libido and testosterone in males
- eyes (if Graves' ophthalmopathy): double vision, blindness

Approach to diagnosing thyrotoxicosis

The following groups should be screened for thyroid disease:

- patients with atrial fibrillation or hyperlipidaemia
- patients on amiodarone or lithium (6-monthly assessments)

- diabetics (annual review)
- women with type 1 diabetes, in the first trimester of pregnancy and in the post-partum period
- women with a history of post-partum thyroiditis
- patients with Down's syndrome, Addison's disease, or Turner's syndrome, in view of the high prevalence of hypothyroidism in these groups (annual review)

In thyrotoxicosis due to Graves' disease, thyroid function tests reveal a raised FT4 and suppressed TSH (alternatively, raised FT3 in T3 toxicosis). The following antithyroid antibodies are typically present: anti-TPO (70%–80% of cases), anti-thyroglobulin (30%–50% of cases), and anti-TSH receptor antibody (70%–100% of cases). A radionuclide scan may be considered if the diagnosis is uncertain; if the result is positive, the scan will show a diffuse high uptake of radioiodine.

Other diagnoses that should be considered aside from thyrotoxicosis

Other diagnoses that should be considered aside from thyrotoxicosis include T3 toxicosis (suppressed TSH with elevated FT3); euthyroid sick syndrome, which occurs in the context of severe illness, and starvation (biochemistry typically reveals a low T4 and T3 with an inappropriately normal/suppressed TSH); phaeochromocytoma; myeloproliferative disease; and diabetes mellitus.

'Gold-standard' diagnostic test for thyrotoxicosis

The gold-standard diagnostic tests for thyrotoxicosis are blood tests to check for:

- TSH suppression (<0.03 mU/l)
- elevation of FT4 and/or FT3 (usually, if TSH is suppressed, the FT4 test is performed automatically by the laboratory; if the FT4 test is normal, the FT3 level should be checked)
- autoantibodies

Acceptable diagnostic alternatives to the gold-standard tests for thyrotoxicosis

There are no acceptable diagnostic alternatives to the gold-standard tests for thyrotoxicosis.

Other relevant investigations for thyrotoxicosis

Other relevant investigations for thyrotoxicosis include:

- FBC
- U&E
- liver function tests
- ECG
- DEXA, if osteoporosis likely
- uptake scan, if the cause of the thyrotoxicosis is uncertain

Prognosis of thyrotoxicosis, and how to estimate it

If thyrotoxicosis is treated medically, there is a 40% remission rate at 5 years. If, at presentation, the FT3 is very high and there is a large goitre, relapse is likely within the first year, and definitive treatment should be considered.

If thyrotoxicosis is treated with radioiodine, 50%–70% of patients have restored thyroid function and goitre shrinkage at 8 weeks post treatment. If hyperthyroidism persists, it may be treated with a maximum of two further treatments. The incidence of hypothyroidism is 50% at 1 year.

If thyrotoxicosis is treated surgically with subtotal thyroidectomy, hypothyroidism occurs in 10%–20% of those treated, after 10 years.

Treatment of thyrotoxicosis, and its effectiveness

Medical treatment of thyrotoxicosis

Manage thyrotoxicosis initially with thionamides (carbimazole (CBZ) or propylthiouracil (PTU)). There are two regimens that can be used: block and replace (not in pregnancy), or dose titration.

There is a 50% chance of remission with medical treatment of thyrotoxicosis.

Block and replace

The procedure for block and replace is as follows:

- start CBZ 20 mg twice or three times per day, but warn of agranulocytosis (0.1%–5% of patients): if patients develop a sore throat or ulcers, they need to stop therapy and go for an FBC (a written warning sheet should be given)
- 3 weeks after starting block and replace, check the FT4 level:
  - if it is within the normal range, reduce CBZ to 40 mg daily and start T4 100 μg once daily
  - if it is 20–25 pmol/l, continue CBZ for a further week, and then add in the T4
  - if it is 25–35 pmol/l, continue the CBZ for a further 2 weeks and then add in the T4
  - if it is >35 pmol/l, review compliance or any other problems
- 4 weeks after starting block and replace, check the FT4 level again and alter T4 to maintain the FT4 level in the middle of the normal range
- review at 4 months
- stop treatment at 6–12 months
- review at 6 weeks after stopping to check for relapse
- if agranulocytosis develops, thionamides are contraindicated

Dose titration

Titrated therapy can be used in the long term; in pregnancy, PTU is used to avoid aplasia cutis. The procedure for the titration method is as follows:

- if the FT3 level is >6 pmol/l, start CBZ at 40 mg/day (or PTU 150 mg twice daily)
- check the FT4 level at 4–6 weeks and reduce the dose of CBZ to keep the TSH level within the normal range
- continue for 18 months

Note that relapses are more likely if the level of FT3 is high and the goitre is large.

Radioiodine therapy for thyrotoxicosis

Radioiodine therapy is the definitive treatment for multinodular goitre, adenoma, and relapsed Graves' disease. The following guidelines should be observed when performing radioiodine therapy:

- the patient should be clinically euthyroid, to avoid post-radioiodine thyroiditis
- the therapy must be performed by a specialist unit; in addition, it must be patient consented and discussed with both a consultant and an ARSAC holder
- technicium scanning may be required
- precautions are required, and written advice should be given
- radioiodine therapy is contraindicated in children, in pregnant or lactating women, and when the safety of others is in question
- care must be taken if the patient has Graves' ophthalmopathy, as radioiodine therapy may worsen eye signs, particularly in smokers; steroid cover may be indicated

Surgery for thyrotoxicosis

Indications for the use of surgery in the treatment of thyrotoxicosis include:

- a suspicious lesion
- pregnancy, when medical treatment has failed
- patients with poor compliance, relapsed Graves' disease, Graves' ophthalmopathy, or radioiodine failures/fears, or when radioiodine is contraindicated

Thyroiditis

Definition of thyroiditis

Thyroiditis is inflammation of the thyroid gland. It often leads to transient thyrotoxicosis followed by hypothyroidism.

Table 186.3 Cause and characteristic features of thyroiditis

Cause	Characteristic features
Autoimmune thyroiditis (Hashimoto's)	Grossly lymphocytic, and fibrotic thyrotoxicosis or hypothyroidism
Subacute de Quervain's	Viral
Pyogenic	Presence of *Staphylococcus aureus*, streptococci, *Escherichia coli*, TB, fungal pathogens
Post-partum thyroiditis	Chronic lymphocytic thyroiditis, transient thyrotoxicosis, or hypothyroidism
Riedel's thyroiditis (very rare)	Extensive fibrosis of the thyroid
Radiation thyroiditis	Transient thyrotoxicosis
Drug induced	Amiodarone use

Aetiology of thyroiditis

The causes and characteristic features of thyroiditis are outlined in Table 186.3.

Typical symptoms of thyroiditis, and less common symptoms

In autoimmune (Hashimoto's with a goitre) or atrophic (without a goitre) thyroiditis, there is usually hypothyroidism. Acute suppurative thyroiditis usually presents with a painful, tender thyroid, and thyroid function is usually normal. In subacute (de Quervain's) thyroiditis, there is malaise, arthralgia, and a recent upper respiratory tract infection with a painful neck; in addition, there is early thyrotoxicosis and late hypothyroidism.

Demographics of thyroiditis

Post-partum thyroiditis has a prevalence of 5%–7% and occurs in 30%–52% of women who are positive for anti-TPO antibodies.

Natural history of thyroiditis, and complications of the disease

In Hashimoto's the goitre is usually non-tender. In de Quervain's thyroiditis, there is an exquisitely tender and nodular thyroid. Symptoms are of malaise and pain. In mild cases, NSAIDs may help; in severe cases, steroids may be of use. Antithyroid drugs are not indicated, but T4 replacement may be required if the patient is rendered hypothyroid.

Post-partum thyroiditis occurs within the first 6 months after delivery; and in most cases, there is complete remission, but progression to hypothyroidism can occur. It is twice as common in patients with type 1 diabetes mellitus.

Riedel's thyroiditis is rare and is characterized by intense fibrosis of the gland and the surrounding region. There may be associated fibrosis of the mediastinum, the retroperitoneum, and the salivary, lacrimal, and parathyroid glands. Sclerosing cholangitis may also occur. Tamoxifen is the first-line treatment in this case, but surgery may be required.

Pyogenic thyroiditis is also rare, and occurs when there is sepsis elsewhere. There is redness and swelling of the thyroid, with systemic upset. Antibiotics, together with incision and drainage, are required.

Approach to diagnosing thyroiditis

After history and examination, the following tests should be used to establish the presence or absence of thyroiditis:

- thyroid function tests (TFTs)
- a screen for antithyroid antibodies
- ESR
- CRP
- FBC

Other diagnoses that should be considered aside from thyroiditis

If there is a dominant nodule, consider fine-needle aspiration biopsy (FNA). There is an association between Hashimoto's thyroiditis and thyroid lymphoma.

'Gold-standard' diagnostic test for thyroiditis

The gold-standard test for thyroiditis is a TSH test.

Acceptable diagnostic alternatives to the gold-standard test for thyroiditis

There are no acceptable diagnostic alternatives to the gold-standard test for thyroiditis.

Other relevant investigations for thyroiditis

Another relevant investigation for thyroiditis is a radionuclide (technicium) uptake scan; in subacute thyroiditis, the uptake is suppressed.

Prognosis of thyroiditis, and how to estimate it

The prognosis for Hashimoto's thyroiditis is good, as it can be optimally treated with T4 replacement. However, Reidel's thyroiditis can prove very difficult to treat, as not all cases respond to tamoxifen, and surgery is challenging due to the intense fibrotic reaction.

Treatment of thyroiditis, and its effectiveness

T4 replacement is very effective in the treatment of thyroiditis. If there is a rapidly increasing goitre in Hashimoto's (very unusual), steroids can sometimes help with pain.

Amiodarone-induced thyroid disease

Definition of amiodarone-induced thyroid disease

Amiodarone is a drug commonly used to treat arrhythmias. Amiodarone-induced thyrotoxicosis type I occurs as a result of iodine excess (due to the amount of iodine in amiodarone; see 'Aetiology of amiodarone-induced thyroid disease') in patients who have latent thyroid disease (usually multinodular goitre). Amiodarone-induced thyrotoxicosis type II is a destructive form of thyroiditis caused directly by amiodarone as a side effect of the drug. Differentiating between amiodarone-induced thyrotoxicosis types I and II is often difficult. Abnormalities of the thyroid occur in up to half of those on amiodarone therapy. Amiodarone-induced hypothyroidism may also occur on long-term amiodarone therapy.

Aetiology of amiodarone-induced thyroid disease

Amiodarone is 30% iodine: while the daily recommended iodine intake is 200 µg, the daily dose of amiodarone contains up to 21 mg of iodine. In addition, amiodarone closely resembles T4. In the euthyroid patient, acutely, there is a protective effect of the iodide concentrations (Wolff–Chaikoff effect), but the thyroid soon escapes this, and T4 production is restored to normal or even elevated. There is inhibition of the 5'-deiodination of T4 to T3 in the peripheral tissues, especially the liver. On treatment the TFTs are usually abnormal, but do not indicate thyrotoxicosis: TSH levels rise early on and then fall to low normal, while FT4 is usually at the upper end of normal or elevated, and FT3 is normal. Conversely, TSH levels may rise but, unless they are >10 mU/l and the FT3 is low, this is not usually indicative of hypothyroidism.

Typical symptoms of amiodarone-induced thyroid disease, and less common symptoms

Patients with amiodarone-induced thyrotoxicosis may present with very few symptoms, due to the inherent beta-blocking action of amiodarone. Amiodarone-induced hypothyroidism is commonly associated with lethargy or worsening heart failure.

Demographics of amiodarone-induced thyroid disease

About 2% of those on amiodarone develop amiodarone-induced thyrotoxicosis, and 6%–13% develop amiodarone-induced hypothyroidism. Those residing in iodine-deficient areas develop amiodarone-induced thyrotoxicosis, and those in high-intake areas develop amiodarone-induced hypothyroidism. Goitre may be associated with amiodarone-induced thyrotoxicosis type I. As the half-life of amiodarone is up to 52 days, amiodarone-induced thyrotoxicosis can occur several months after discontinuing amiodarone. Amiodarone-induced hypothyroidism is more common in women, and those positive for autoantibodies.

Natural history of amiodarone-induced thyroid disease, and complications

Amiodarone-induced hypothyroidism

A significant proportion of amiodarone-induced hypothyroidism cases settle spontaneously. The risk of amiodarone-induced hypothyroidism is higher in elderly and female patients. When such patients are positive for autoantibodies, the relative risk increases to 13.5. The likely explanation is the inhibitory effects of iodine on T4 release and synthesis. A goitre is found in about 20% of cases and usually predates use of the amiodarone. Many patients will eventually become euthyroid on stopping the amiodarone, particularly if there was no preexisting thyroid disease; however, stopping the drug may not be possible, due to the underlying cardiac disease. In amiodarone-induced hypothyroidism, amiodarone may be continued, T4 added, and TSH monitored. In some patients, liothyronine may be needed, due to the inhibitory effects of amiodarone on the conversion of T4 to T3. All patients should be referred to a specialist.

Amiodarone-induced thyrotoxicosis

Amiodarone-induced thyrotoxicosis is less common and more complex than amiodarone-induced hypothyroidism and can be difficult to treat in some cases. Clinically, new arrhythmias may give rise to suspicion, as there may be few clinical signs due to the anti-adrenergic effects of amiodarone. Amiodarone-induced thyrotoxicosis occurs more frequently in men and is often acute in onset, but may spontaneously remit. There are two forms: amiodarone-induced thyrotoxicosis type I and amiodarone induced thyrotoxicosis type II. Amiodarone-induced thyrotoxicosis type I is associated with latent Graves' disease or a multinodular goitre. Here, the iodine load accelerates the thyroid hormone synthesis. Amiodarone-induced thyrotoxicosis type II occurs in a normal thyroid, and the toxic effect of amiodarone causes a subacute thyroiditis. Distinguishing between amiodarone-induced thyrotoxicosis type I and amiodarone-induced thyrotoxicosis type II can be challenging, but Doppler flow ultrasound may show increased flow in amiodarone-induced thyrotoxicosis type I (see Table 186.4). However, in general, there may be a mixture of the two forms.

If amiodarone is withdrawn, the cardiac status may deteriorate, as the beta-blocking effects are lost. In addition, most patients with amiodarone-induced thyrotoxicosis type I still have hyperthyroidism 6–9 months after stopping amiodarone. Long-term follow-up is required, with 6-monthly tests even after remission, as there is a risk of relapse.

Table 186.4 Characteristics of amiodarone-induced thyrotoxicosis types I and II

	Type I	Type II
Underlying thyroid abnormality	Yes	No
Pathogenetic mechanism	Excessive hormone synthesis due to iodine excess	Excessive release of preformed hormones due to thyroid destruction
Goitre	Multinodular or diffuse goitre usually present	Occasionally small, diffuse, firm, sometimes tender
Thyroidal radioiodine uptake	Normal/raised	Low/absent
Serum IL-6	Normal/slightly raised	Profoundly raised
Thyroid USS/Doppler	Nodular, hyperechoeic, increased volume	Decreased

Abbreviations: IL-6, interleukin 6; USS, ultrasound.
Reproduced from Newman et al Heart 1998;79:121–7.

Approach to diagnosing amiodarone-induced thyroid disease

Check TFTs every 6 months in patients on amiodarone. Look for signs of clinical thyroid disease and/or a goitre. If antithyroid antibodies are present, the radionuclide scan is normal, thyroglobulin and interleukin 6 (IL-6) levels are normal, and there is increased vascularity on vascular Doppler, then amiodarone-induced thyrotoxicosis type I (from iodine toxicity) is indicated. In amiodarone-induced thyrotoxicosis type II, there is a destructive thyroiditis, IL-6 and thyroglobulin levels are increased, and there is decreased uptake on radionuclide scan.

Other diagnoses that should be considered aside from amiodarone-induced thyroid disease

Other diagnoses that should be considered aside from amiodarone-induced thyroid disease include other side effects and complications of amiodarone.

'Gold-standard' diagnostic test for amiodarone-induced thyroid disease

The gold-standard tests for amiodarone-induced thyroid disease are baseline TSH and a screen for antithyroid antibodies. In addition, sex hormone-binding globulin is raised in thyrotoxicosis and is a useful marker where TFTs are equivocal and signs few.

Acceptable diagnostic alternatives to the gold-standard test for amiodarone-induced thyroid disease

There are no acceptable diagnostic alternatives to the gold-standard tests for amiodarone-induced thyroid disease.

Other relevant investigations for amiodarone-induced thyroid disease

Other relevant investigations for amiodarone-induced thyroid disease include a radionuclide scan, and a Doppler ultrasound scan of the thyroid. However, although these may be helpful, they are not often used in routine practice.

Prognosis of amiodarone-induced thyroid disease, and how to estimate it

Prolonged monitoring of TFTs is necessary on and after treatment with amiodarone in amiodarone-induced thyrotoxicosis as patients may become hypothyroid, and relapses occur in amiodarone-induced thyrotoxicosis type II. Complications can include thyroid storm; hypothyroidism; aplastic anaemia secondary to perchlorate use; agranulocytosis; and hepatitis from thioamides. The prognosis for amiodarone-induced hypothyroidism is usually good but for amiodarone-induced thyrotoxicosis it may be poor, as there is likely to be an underlying serious cardiac disorder.

Treatment of amiodarone-induced thyroid disease and its effectiveness

The first-line treatment for amiodarone-induced thyrotoxicosis type I is antithyroid medication (CBZ 30–60 mg/day; rarely, in combination with potassium perchlorate (1 g/day)). If possible, withdraw amiodarone, but this should be done on a case-by-case basis. Radioiodine is not usually effective in amiodarone-induced thyrotoxicosis type II, but surgery is successful, and used particularly if medical treatment is unsuccessful and amiodarone cannot be stopped. In amiodarone-induced thyrotoxicosis type II, steroids, such as prednisolone 40 mg once daily, may be required for 8–12 weeks. Practically, many patients are given both prednisolone and CBZ (if they are euthyroid within 2–3 weeks, the diagnosis is amiodarone-induced thyrotoxicosis type II, so CBZ can be discontinued, and prednisolone tapered).

All antithyroid drugs have a marrow suppressant effect, and patients should be warned and given an information leaflet wherever possible.

Thyroid storm

Definition of thyroid storm

Thyroid storm (crisis) occurs as a result of exacerbation of thyrotoxicosis. It is a rare but life-threatening condition.

Aetiology of thyroid storm

Thyroid storm occurs in patients who have hyperthyroidism or a family history of thyroid disease. It may develop in patients with hyperthyroidism during an acute infection or trauma; when they are undergoing surgery or radioiodine treatment; in the post-partum situation; after radiological contrast; or when antithyroid treatment has been withdrawn. Strokes and seizures have also been documented to precipitate thyroid storm.

Typical symptoms of thyroid storm, and less common symptoms

The symptoms of thyroid storm are similar to those found in acute sepsis and are as follows:

- change in cognitive state
- pyrexia >38.5
- tachycardia or tachyarrhythmia
- severe signs of hyperthyroidism
- vomiting, jaundice, and diarrhoea
- multisystem decompensation: cardiac failure, respiratory distress, prerenal failure

Demographics of thyroid storm

Thyroid storm occurs in up to 1%–2% of patients admitted to hospital with thyrotoxicosis. It is becoming significantly less common, due to earlier diagnosis and treatment of thyrotoxicosis.

Natural history of thyroid storm, and complications of the disease

The exact pathogenesis of thyroid storm is unclear. Frequently, TFT levels are those of uncomplicated thyrotoxicosis. It may be caused by high catecholamine levels or high FT4 levels; alternatively, it may be the acute discharge of thyroid hormones in a particular clinical background that causes the storm. Vigorous palpation of thyroid goitres has also been reported to cause thyroid storm. The high mortality associated with the condition is greater the longer the patient remains untreated. If the patient survives the episode, after appropriate treatment, surgery maybe the treatment option of choice.

Approach to diagnosing thyroid storm

Even if the diagnosis of thyroid storm seems unlikely, initiation of treatment for thyroid storm is prudent management, as therapy may always be discontinued when the patient is stable.

Other diagnoses that should be considered aside from thyroid storm

Another diagnosis that should be considered aside from thyroid storm is underlying precipitating illness.

'Gold-standard' diagnostic test for thyroid storm

The gold-standard diagnostic tests for thyroid storm are as follows:

- clinical diagnosis; in particular, the presence of a goitre with a thrill and a bruit, and ophthalmopathy
- TFTs: abnormal but within the range of uncomplicated thyrotoxicosis
- FT3: may even be low/or normal, due to underlying systemic illness
- FT4: an urgent FT4 test should be available as an emergency procedure in most hospitals
- 2-hour radioiodine uptake

Acceptable diagnostic alternatives to the gold-standard tests for thyroid storm

There are no acceptable diagnostic alternatives to the gold-standard tests for thyroid storm.

Other relevant investigations for thyroid storm

Other relevant investigations for thyroid storm are tests to exclude:

- modest hyperglycaemia
- moderate leucocytosis
- increased serum calcium

- hepatic dysfunction
- altered cortisol levels

In addition, search for any underlying precipitating illness.

Prognosis of thyroid storm, and how to estimate it

Thyroid storm has a poor prognosis, but early diagnosis and institution of treatment may reduce its severity. Mortality rates in hospital, even with early diagnosis, are high, ranging from 10% to 75%.

Treatment of thyroid storm, and its effectiveness

The aim of treatment for thyroid storm is to inhibit thyroid hormone synthesis completely, using the following agents:

- PTU blocks T4 to T3 conversion; give 200–300 mg four times per day via an NGT
- potassium iodide 60 mg four times per day via an NGT, started 6 hours after the initial PTU dose, to inhibit thyroid hormone release
- propranolol 160–480 mg/day in divided doses or as an infusion 2–5 mg/hour, for beta blockade (calcium-channel blockers may be used when beta blockade is contraindicated)
- colestyramine, to reduce enterohepatic circulation of thyroid hormones
- prednisolone 60 mg/day, or intramuscular hydrocortisone 40 mg four times per day

In addition, any precipitating illness should be addressed.
    When all pharmacological therapies fail, plasmapheresis and peritoneal dialysis may be effective.

Thyroid adenoma and multinodular goitre

Definitions of thyroid adenoma and multinodular goitre

A thyroid adenoma is a solitary nodule present in the thyroid. In contrast, in a multinodular goitre, multiple nodules are present. These nodules may be palpable or non-palpable, and toxic or non-toxic.

Etiologies of thyroid adenoma and multinodular goitre

Thyroid adenoma

Thyroid adenomas are usually follicular; common types include colloid nodules, cysts, and benign neoplasms (Hürthle cell adenomas). Lymphocytic thyroiditis is a common cause of thyroid adenomas. Uncommon causes include granulomatous thyroiditis, infection, and malignancy (papillary, follicular, medullary, anaplastic, metaplastic; also lymphoma).

Multinodular goitre

Multinodular goitres are most commonly caused by autoimmune thyroid disease; sporadic, endemic iodine deficiency; pregnancy; and thyroiditis syndromes. They may also be drug induced.

Typical symptoms of thyroid adenoma and multinodular goitre, and less common symptoms

The thyroid mass may be discovered by the patient or clinician. Important symptoms to ask about include a rapidly enlarging mass or discrete nodule within the goitre; previous history of radiation to head or neck; family history of thyroid cancer; and hoarse voice, dysphagia, or dyspnoea. Fixation of the mass to adjacent tissue, lymphadenopathy, and a short history of the mass may indicate malignancy, depending on the age of the patient (see 'Demographics of thyroid adenoma and multinodular goitre').

Demographics of thyroid adenoma and multinodular goitre

The prevalence of non-toxic goitre is high (3.2% in the UK); the disease is more common in women (5.3%) than in men (0.8%). Thyroid nodules are common: the prevalence of thyroid nodules is 5%–50% and increases with radiation exposure, iodine deficiency, and increasing age. Ten per cent of the population have clinically apparent nodules; these are four times more common in women than in men. Less than 5% of such nodules are cancerous, but they are more likely to be so if the patient is <20 years old, >60 years old, or male.

Natural history of thyroid adenoma and multinodular goitre, and complications of the disease

The generation of a non-toxic goitre is thought to occur when there is an intense growth stimulus over a short period of time, resulting in a diffuse goitre, whereas a mild stimulation over longer periods results in a nodular goitre. Expansion of thyrocytes may eventually ensue, along with autonomous thyroid function. Patients with multinodular goitre tend to be older and have larger goitres. The goitre size is negatively related to TSH levels; thus, the larger the multinodular goitre, the more suppressed the TSH and the higher the FT4. Solitary nodules without suspicion of malignancy generally change very little. Those that increase in size or are predominantly solid are more likely to be malignant. Those that are cystic may decrease in size or disappear.

Approach to diagnosing thyroid adenoma and multinodular goitre

With a multinodular goitre, thyroid function must be ascertained, as well as the presence of any pressure effects. With a solitary lesion, again check the biochemical thyroid status with TSH, and establish whether the nodule is benign or malignant. FNA should be used for this. Imaging in these lesions is controversial, and radionuclide and ultrasound scanning of the thyroid should be discussed with a specialist. A hot spot on the radioisotope scan makes malignancy less likely, as cancers are generally cold, but the specificity and positive predictive value of scanning is poor.

Other diagnoses that should be considered aside from thyroid adenoma and multinodular goitre

Other diagnoses that should be considered in addition to adenoma and multinodular goitre include multiple endocrine neoplasia, Gardner's syndrome, familial polyposis coli, and Cowden's syndrome.

'Gold-standard' diagnostic tests for thyroid adenoma and multinodular goitre

The gold-standard diagnostic tests for adenoma and multinodular goitre are TSH and FNA (Thy1 - Thy5 classification); these are the best and most cost-effective ways of making the diagnosis.

Acceptable diagnostic alternatives to the gold-standard tests for thyroid adenoma and multinodular goitre

Imaging is an acceptable diagnostic alternative to the gold-standard tests for adenoma and multinodular goitre (U1 to U5 classification).

Other relevant investigations for thyroid adenoma and multinodular goitre

Other relevant investigations for adenoma and multinodular goitre include pulmonary function tests, CT for suspected retrosternal goitre, and follow-up of malignant disease. In cases of medullary thyroid carcinoma, calcitonin may be measured, but this is only recommended in the case of positive family history.

Prognosis of thyroid adenoma and multinodular goitre, and how to estimate it

For benign adenoma and multinodular goitre, the prognosis is good. For tailored-treatment prognoses, see 'Prognosis of thyrotoxicosis, and how to estimate it'.

Treatment of thyroid adenoma and multinodular goitre, and its effectiveness

The optimal therapy for thyroid nodules depends on whether they are functioning or non-functioning, and benign or malignant. If they are functioning, see 'Treatment of thyrotoxicosis, and its effectiveness' for an outline of the medical and radioiodine therapies that may be used.

Surgery for the treatment of thyroid adenoma and multinodular goitre

Surgery for the treatment of adenoma and multinodular goitre is indicated when a lesion is malignant, or when the cytology has suspicious features. The success of surgery is high in specialist centres and, depending on the extent of the thyroidectomy, post-operative, life-long T4 is given.

Further Reading

Caturegla P, De Remigisa A, and Rose NR. Hashimoto thyroiditis: Clinical and diagnostic criteria. *Autoimmun Rev* 2014; 13: 391–7.

Chaker L, Bianco A, Jonklaas J et al. Hypothyroidism. *Lancet* 2017; 390: 1550–62.

Cooper DS and Biondi B. Subclinical thyroid disease. *Lancet* 2012; 379: 1142–54.

De Leo S, Lee, SY, and Braverman LE. Hyperthyroidism. *Lancet* 2016; 388: 906–18.

Fuhrer D and Lazarus JH. 'Management of toxic multinodular goitre and toxic adenoma' in Wass JAH, Stewart PM, Amiel SA, et al., eds, *Oxford Textbook of Endocrinology and Diabetes* (2nd edition), 2011. Oxford University Press.

Klubo-Gwiezdzinska J and Wartofsky L. 'Thyrotoxic storm', in Wass JAH, Stewart PM, Amiel SA, et al., eds, *Oxford Textbook of Endocrinology and Diabetes* (2nd edition), 2011. Oxford University Press.

Ross DS. Radioiodine therapy for hyperthyroidism. *N Engl J Med* 2011; 364: 542–50.

Vaidya B and Pearce SHS. Diagnosis and management of thyrotoxicosis. *BMJ* 2014; 349: g5128.

Zimmermann MB and Boelaert K. Iodine deficiency and thyroid disorders. *Lancet Diabetes Endocrinol* 2015; 3: 286–95.

187 Primary hyperparathyroidism

John Newell-Price, Alia Munir, and Miguel Debono

Definition of the disease

Primary hyperparathyroidism is a disorder of bone mineralization and renal physiology due to excess parathyroid hormone (PTH) secretion.

Aetiology of the disease

PTH is produced and released by the parathyroid chief cells. Its principal actions are stimulation of bone resorption; increased renal calcium reabsorption and phosphate excretion; and stimulation of the conversion of 25-hydroxy vitamin D to the active form 1,25-hydroxy vitamin D. PTH is under the regulation of the G-protein-coupled calcium-sensing receptor (CaSR), and primary hyperparathyroidism occurs when there is a loss of the inhibitory feedback of PTH release by extracellular calcium. The rise in PTH levels is initially associated with a normal serum calcium, and then over time with hypercalcaemia. The most common cause is a benign solitary adenoma (80 %). Other causes include multiple adenomas and hyperplasia. Rare causes include parathyroid carcinoma, lithium therapy, thiazide diuretics, and mutation of the CaSR, such as occurs in familial hypocalciuric hypercalcaemia or as part of the multiple endocrine neoplasia (MEN) type I or II spectrum. Head and neck irradiation maybe a risk factor. PTH levels will rise secondary to hypocalcaemia, vitamin D deficiency, or hyperphosphataemia and are blunted by magnesium deficiency.

Primary hyperparathyroidism is the most common cause of hypercalcaemia in ambulant patients, with 85% of cases being due to a single adenoma, and the remainder to parathyroid hyperplasia. Hyperparathyroidism is commonly found in patients with MEN types I or II. Chronically low vitamin D levels, and chronic renal failure with persistently low calcium levels, may stimulate the autonomous increased production of PTH, resulting in tertiary hyperparathyroidism, causing hypercalcaemia.

Typical symptoms of the disease, and less common symptoms

With the advent of widespread measurement of serum calcium within standard biochemical requests, most patients will be asymptomatic or complain of non-specific fatigue, feelings of weakness, and cognitive blunting. Fewer patients present with symptoms of hypercalcaemia, such as renal tract calculi, abdominal pain, constipation, and low mood.

Demographics of the disease

Primary hyperparathyroidism has a community prevalence of 0.5% to 0.1% but is a common diagnosis in patients presenting with hypercalcaemia. It is three times more common in women, and peaks in the sixth decade.

Natural history and complications of the disease

Approximately 15% of asymptomatic patients with primary hyperparathyroidism progress over years, in terms of increases in serum calcium and PTH. The complications are commonly low bone density, fragility fractures, and renal stones. While commoner in the past, peptic ulcers, myopathy, and pancreatitis are now rare complications. Severe protracted hyperparathyroidism results in multiple bone cysts or brown tumours as part of osteitis fibrosa cystica. These can be a site of bone pain and pathological fracture. In protracted secondary hyperparathyroidism, a small proportion will develop tertiary hyperparathyroidism, where there is autonomous escape from regulation, and extreme hypercalcaemia.

Approach to diagnosing the disease

The key is to establish an inappropriately high or high normal level of circulating PTH with respect to serum calcium. The exclusion of other causes of raised calcium or secondary hyperparathyroidism is usually straightforward. Once a diagnosis of primary hyperparathyroidism is likely, and vitamin D deficiency either excluded or treated, it is essential to request a 24-hour urinary calcium and creatinine collection, with paired serum calcium and creatinine to exclude familial hypocalciuric hypercalcaemia (FHH). A calcium:creatinine clearance ratio ((urine calcium ÷ serum calcium) × (serum creatinine ÷ urine creatinine)) < 0.01 indicates FHH, not primary hyperparathyroidism. Where there is diagnostic uncertainty, family screening for hypercalcaemia is helpful. In cases of primary hyperparathyroidism in young adulthood, it is worth screening for other tumours of MEN type I or II.

Once a diagnosis is established, the most important step is to refer to an experienced endocrine surgeon for a minimally invasive exploration and excision. The surgical team will have a local protocol for then working up patients to identify the site of adenoma. This usually includes functional localization by sestamibi nuclear scan with anatomical localization by MRI, CT, or ultrasound. In cases with concomitant thyroid disease, subtraction-imaging ^{123}I may be needed. Additional diagnostic modalities include SPECT and selective venous sampling.

Other diagnoses that should be considered

Another diagnosis that should be considered is FHH. In addition, secondary hyperparathyroidism may be secondary to hypocalcaemia, vitamin D deficiency, and/or hyperphosphataemia, such as occurs in chronic kidney disease. Patients with primary hyperparathyroidism often have a concomitant vitamin D deficiency that can lower the serum calcium to within the normal range or lower the urine calcium. The diagnostic strategy is to treat the vitamin D deficiency and then remeasure the serum calcium. Even with high-dose replacement of vitamin D, the increment in serum calcium in patients with primary hyperparathyroidism is usually small and asymptomatic. Subsequent unmasking of hypercalcaemia in these patients reveals the diagnosis of primary hyperparathyroidism.

'Gold-standard' diagnostic test

The gold-standard diagnostic test for primary hyperparathyroidism is a blood test to confirm hypercalcaemia with elevated intact PTH. In addition, a technetium-99m sestamibi nuclear scan, with anatomical localization via either MRI or ultrasound, can be used.

Other relevant investigations

Other relevant investigations include blood tests to determine whether there is associated low serum phosphate and/or high alkaline phosphatase. It is also necessary to exclude vitamin D deficiency and renal disease, especially in patients with normocalcaemic hyperparathyroidism. Dual-energy X-ray absorptiometry should be performed, to exclude low bone density and increased fragility fracture risk. In addition, a 24-hour urinary calcium and creatinine collection, with paired serum calcium and creatinine, should be carried out.

In those presenting in young adulthood, a screen to rule out MEN type I/II should be performed.

Prognosis and how to estimate it

Epidemiological studies have confirmed that untreated hyperparathyroidism leads to an excess mortality, reduced quality of life from cardiovascular disease, and bone fragility.

Treatment and its effectiveness

Surgery is the only definitive treatment for this disease. In Guidelines for the Management of Asymptomatic Primary Hyperparathyroidism: Summary statement from the Fourth International Workshop 2013 parathyroidectomy was recommended for patients with 1) serum calcium 0.25mmol/l > upper limit of normal, 2) creatinine clearance <60ml/min and/or 24 hour urine calcium >400mg/day and increased stone risk by biochemical stone analysis and/or nephrolithiasis or nephrocalcinosis on imaging, 3) BMD T-score <-2.5 at any site and/or vertebral fracture, 4) or age <50 years. In patients who do not undergo surgery an annual serum calcium and serum creatinine/eGFR is recommended and bone density every one to two years. If renal stones suspected do 24 hour biochemical stone analysis and imaging. The American Association of Clinical Endocrinologists and the American Association of Endocrine Surgeons also state that operative management should be considered and recommended for all asymptomatic patients with a reasonable life expectancy, and suitable operative and anaesthetic risk factors. When the operation is performed by a qualified surgeon, the disease is cured with low risk in 90%–95% of cases. Radiological imaging is usually performed only as part of the workup for surgery, and may include technetium-99m sestamibi scans, ultrasound scans, CT scans, and MRI scans, depending on tumour location.

If patients do not undergo surgery, they need biannual calcium levels and annual creatinine or creatinine clearance, blood pressure monitoring, and annual bone density scans. If the patient is not suitable for surgery, sex hormone replacement therapy and bisphosphonates should be considered to prevent bone loss. A more targeted approach is the use of calcimimetics, a group of drugs which increase the affinity of the receptor for extracellular calcium, leading to an increase in intracellular calcium. This inhibits the secretion of PTH from the parathyroid cell. Rapid normalization of calcium levels have been achieved with the use of cinacalcet hydrochloride, with maintenance of normal calcium levels, but the drug is expensive.

Minimally invasive parathyroidectomy by an experienced endocrine surgeon is curative. Surgery is indicated in those who have skeletal complications (such as osteoporosis), renal complications (stones or impaired creatinine clearance), a history of parathyroid crisis, or presentation when under 50 years old. In those not meeting these criteria, a comparison of the risks and benefits of the curative procedure needs to be made on a case-by-case basis. Pre-surgical correction of vitamin D deficiency and dietary calcium repletion reduces the incidence of post-operative hungry bone syndrome. It is important to avoid use of potent parenteral anti-resorptive agents prior to surgery to minimize post-operative hypocalcaemia.

In those not eligible for surgery, medical management involves adequate hydration and a moderate dietary calcium intake of 600–800 mg/day. In those with evidence of osteoporosis, anti-resorptive therapy should be considered. In those with parathyroid carcinoma, and even inoperable patients with primary hyperparathyroidism the calcimimetic cinacalcet is indicated. Tests for serum calcium and the estimated glomerular filtration rate should be repeated annually, and bone mineral density should be measured every two years to check for progression.

Where the cause is thought to be lithium or thiazide related, the drug should be stopped for 3 months, and then PTH and calcium levels remeasured.

Further Reading

Kunstman JW, Kirsch JD, Mahajan A, et al. Parathyroid localization and implications for clinical management. *J Clin Endocrinol Metab* 2013; 98: 902–12.

Marcocci C and Cetani F. Primary hyperparathyroidism. *N Engl J Med* 2011; 365: 2389–97.

Silverberg SJ, Walker MD, and Bilezikian JP. Asymptomatic primary hyperparathyroidism. *J Clin Densitom* 2013; 16: 14–21.

188 Adrenal disease

John Newell-Price, Alia Munir, and Miguel Debono

Adrenal insufficiency

Definition of adrenal insufficiency

Adrenal insufficiency (AI) is a disorder characterized by impaired adrenocortical function, with destruction of the adrenal cortex (primary AI (PAI)) resulting in a decreased production of glucocorticoids, mineralocorticoids, and/or androgens. Secondary AI (SAI) is due to disordered pituitary and hypothalamic function resulting in decreased secretion of adrenocorticotropic hormone (ACTH) or corticotrophin-releasing hormone, with consequent reduction in glucocorticoid and/or androgen secretion.

Aetiology of AI

The aetiology of AI is given in Table 188.1.

Typical symptoms of AI, and less common symptoms

Common symptoms of AI include fatigue; loss of energy; abdominal pain; anorexia; weight loss; weakness; hyperpigmentation (primary); myalgia; dizziness secondary to hypotension; and joint pains. Less common symptoms include impaired libido (women), salt craving (primary), axillary or pubic hair loss, and diarrhoea. In SAI, patients may have alabaster-coloured pale skin, and headaches or visual field defects secondary to a pituitary tumour. Hirsutism, acne, and oligomenorrhoea around the onset of puberty may indicate congenital adrenal hyperplasia (CAH).

Demographics of AI

The prevalence of PAI is 93–140 per million, with an incidence of 4.7– 6.2 per million in Caucasian populations, while SAI has a prevalence of 190– 280 per million. Women are affected more often than men in both PAI and SAI. AI may occur at any age but the autoimmune PAI is often discovered in the third to the fifth decade, while SAI peaks in the sixth decade.

Table 188.1 Aetiology of adrenal insufficiency

Primary adrenal insufficiency (Addison's disease)	Secondary adrenal insufficiency
Autoimmune (commonest in UK; isolated or part of autoimmune polyendocrine syndrome type 1, 2, or 4)	Tumours of hypothalamus and pituitary gland (rare; granulomatous disease in these regions)
Malignancy (metastatic (lung, breast, kidney), infiltration, or lymphoma)	
Infiltration (amyloid, sarcoidosis)	
Infection (tuberculosis (commonest worldwide), histoplasmosis, AIDS, CMV, *Mycobacterium intracellulare*)	Long-term steroid-induced suppression of hypothalamic–pituitary–adrenal axis
Vascular haemorrhage (meningococcaemia, anticoagulants, trauma)	Following cure of Cushing's syndrome
Congenital adrenal hyperplasia	High-dose opioid analgesia
Congenital adrenal hypoplasia	
Adrenoleucodystrophy	
Bilateral adrenalectomy/drugs (steroid-synthesis inhibitors)	
Congenital unresponsiveness to adrenocorticotropic hormone	

Natural history of AI, and complications of the disease

The onset of AI is usually gradual and insidious, and may go undetected until an illness or stress precipitates an adrenal crisis. Patients with acute AI usually present unwell with hypotension, collapse, abdominal pain, fever, and a history or signs of a condition precipitating the event. Typically, these patients do not respond fully to fluid resuscitation unless glucocorticoids are given. If the condition is not treated, it may result in confusion, coma, and death.

As symptoms are non-specific in chronic AI, late diagnosis is common. In PAI, besides glucocorticoid deficiency, patients develop mineralocorticoid deficiency, with resultant electrolyte abnormalities and postural hypotension (may also occur with cortisol deficiency), and androgen deficiency with loss of axillary and pubic hair and loss of libido. Patients with AI may have poor quality of life despite being on conventional hydrocortisone treatment.

Approach to diagnosing AI

A thorough history and examination for symptoms and signs directly related to AI are mandatory. Further, history taking should also be directed to identifying a possible cause for AI, such as a history of autoimmune conditions or malignancy; a family history of endocrine disorders; use of drugs affecting cortisol production; or the use of long-term steroids. Social history should be directed towards the identification of risk factors, including risks for sexually transmitted disorders. Clinical examination should also focus on identifying signs of pituitary disease, such as visual field defects or signs of other hormone deficiencies. Signs of autoimmune disorders, such as vitiligo, or signs of underlying malignancy may also be useful in suggesting the diagnosis.

Other diagnoses that should be considered aside from AI

Autoimmune PAI may be associated with autoimmune polyendocrine syndrome 1 (rare; mainly hypoparathyroidism, chronic mucocutaneous candidiasis) or autoimmune polyendocrine syndrome 2 (mainly primary hypothyroidism, type 1 diabetes mellitus).

'Gold-standard' diagnostic test for AI

The gold-standard diagnostic test for AI is the short tetracosactide test: 250 µg of tetracosactide administered intramuscularly or IV. A serum cortisol level >550 nmol/l at 30 minutes afterwards indicates an adequate response—a 'negative result' (recent onset (<6 weeks) SAI may result in a false negative test).

Acceptable diagnostic alternatives to the gold-standard test for AI

The following tests are acceptable diagnostic alternatives to the gold-standard test for AI:

- 9 a.m. cortisol/ACTH:
  - a single 9 a.m. or random serum cortisol level >500 nmol/l almost always indicates adequate adrenal function
  - an inappropriately low cortisol with high ACTH is indicative of PAI
  - an inappropriately low cortisol with low or normal ACTH is indicative of secondary AI; high ACTH also present in uncontrolled CAH
- insulin tolerance test: rarely indicated unless pituitary disease known (a test for ACTH reserve; avoid if basal cortisol <100 nmol/l)

Other relevant investigations for AI

Other relevant investigations for AI include:

- plasma renin activity (elevated in aldosterone deficiency)
- dehydroepiandrosterone sulphate levels
- calcium levels (hypercalcaemia in PAI)
- electrolytes (hyponatraemia, hyperkalaemia—especially in PAI)
- urea (elevated)
- full blood count (FBC; normochromic, normocytic anaemia, eosinophilia)
- glucose (hypoglycaemia may occur)
- adrenal antibodies
- CT scan of adrenal glands (if adrenal antibodies negative)
- MRI pituitary (if SAI confirmed biochemically)
- thyroid function tests (cortisol deficiency may result in abnormal results that resolve on treating AI)
- very long chain fatty acids (adrenoleucodystrophy)
- other endocrine tests for associated pituitary hormone deficiencies or autoimmune endocrine disorders
- tests for 17-hydroxyprogesterone (at 9 a.m. and then 60 minutes after ACTH administration (diagnostic)), testosterone, and androstenedione (best for disease control monitoring in CAH)

Prognosis of AI, and how to estimate it

Patients with PAI, even if on full replacement therapy, have a mortality rate which is twofold greater than that of the background population, with the greatest number of deaths occurring from cardiovascular, malignant, endocrine, respiratory, and infectious diseases. It is possible that a major contributor to cardiovascular mortality is relative overdosing with hydrocortisone. The mortality rate for patients with secondary AI is up to seven times that of the normal population.

Treatment of AI, and its effectiveness

Glucocorticoid replacement in AI

For glucocorticoid replacement in AI, oral hydrocortisone is usually given three times per day: 10 mg on waking, 5 mg at midday, and 5 mg at 6 p.m. No definite method for monitoring treatment is available at present. Clinical assessment may be as effective as repeated day serum cortisol levels, the latter having particular benefit when patients are also on inducers or inhibitors of cytochrome P450 3A4, as these may result in lower or higher levels of circulating cortisol. Achieving physiological replacement is impossible with conventional glucocorticoid replacement. Oral formulations providing circadian cortisol profiles are being introduced.

Mineralocorticoid replacement in AI

For mineralocorticoid replacement in AI, fludrocortisone is given at a dose of 0.05–0.2 mg/day, with dose adjustment according to clinical status and plasma renin and electrolytes.

Androgen replacement in AI

Dehydroepiandrosterone replacement in patients with PAI may have beneficial effects on well-being.

Sick-day rules

- patient education
- double dose of glucocorticoids during febrile illness; in addition, a vial of 100 mg hydrocortisone is required if parenteral treatment is needed
- major illness should be covered with 50–100 mg hydrocortisone intramuscularly every 6 hours until the patient has recovered
- major surgery should be covered with 100 mg hydrocortisone intramuscularly every 6 hours for the first 3 days, and longer if prolonged post-op complications develop

Treatment of acute AI

Acute AI is a medical emergency and, if suspected, should be treated before biochemical confirmation of low serum cortisol. After a blood sample for serum cortisol and, if possible, plasma ACTH for later analysis is taken, large volumes of 0.9% saline are needed and hydrocortisone 100 mg should be given as an IV bolus, followed by 100 mg intramuscularly every 6 hours. On recovery, double-replacement oral doses are given until the patient is well. Glucose supplementation may be necessary if hypoglycaemia develops. The precipitant should be identified and treated.

Treatment of CAH

In CAH, glucocorticoid therapy is used to replace low cortisol and control androgen excess. Hydrocortisone, prednisolone, and dexamethasone have been used. Androstenedione may be used to monitor disease.

Primary hyperaldosteronism (primary aldosteronism)

Definition of primary hyperaldosteronism

Aldosterone is produced in the zona glomerulosa of the adrenal cortex. Abnormal overproduction of aldosterone results in autonomous primary hyperaldosteronism, leading to hypertension and hypokalaemia.

Aetiology of primary hyperaldosteronism

The aetiology of primary hyperaldosteronism is shown in Box 188.1.

Typical symptoms of primary hyperaldosteronism, and less common symptoms

Common features of primary hyperaldosteronism are hypertension and hypokalaemia (9%–37%). Less commonly, myopathy, tetany, polyuria, abdominal distension, and cardiac arrhythmias may be evident.

Demographics of primary hyperaldosteronism

Primary aldosteronism is found in around 10% of resistant hypertensive patients. Studies report rates of between 0.05% and 14.4% in all patients with hypertension, the variability being due to differences in biochemical definitions. Conn's adenomas and adrenal carcinomas are more common in women than men, and adenomas usually present between the third to the sixth decade. Idiopathic adrenal hyperplasia is found in older people. Previous studies have shown that aldosteronomas are responsible for 70% of cases of primary aldosteronism but the incidence of bilateral adrenal hyperplasia is growing. Less than one per cent of cases are caused by the autosomal dominant condition, glucocorticoid-responsive aldosteronism (GRA).

Natural history of primary hyperaldosteronism, and complications of the disease

The clinical presentation of primary hyperaldosteronism is not distinctive, and a high index of suspicion is necessary. Hypertension is common amongst patients with primary hyperaldosteronism, and may be severe or refractory to therapy. Spontaneous hypokalaemia should warrant consideration of hyperaldosteronism, especially in patients who develop severe or persistent hypokalaemia in the setting of low to moderate doses of potassium-wasting diuretics. In view of resistant hypertension, patients may develop related complications, including cardiac failure, stroke, hypertensive encephalopathy, and retinal changes. Direct actions of aldosterone result in cardiac fibrosis and vascular smooth muscle hypertrophy, while persistent hypokalaemia causes neuromuscular symptoms and nephrogenic diabetes insipidus.

Box 188.1 Aetiology of primary hyperaldosteronism

- aldosterone-secreting adenoma of the adrenal cortex (Conn's adenoma)
- bilateral idiopathic adrenal hyperplasia
- primary adrenal hyperplasia
- adrenal carcinoma
- glucocorticoid-responsive aldosteronism

CHAPTER 188 **Adrenal disease**

Approach to diagnosing primary hyperaldosteronism

The following patients should be screened for primary hyperaldosteronism:

- patients with a blood pressure >160–179/100–109 mm Hg or drug-resistant hypertension
- patients with hypertension and spontaneous or diuretic-induced hypokalaemia
- patients with hypertension with adrenal incidentaloma
- patients with hypertension and a family history of early onset hypertension or a cerebrovascular accident at a young age (<40 years old)

All hypertensive first-degree relatives of patients with primary aldosteronism should also be screened.

Other diagnoses that should be considered aside from primary hyperaldosteronism

Other diagnoses that should be considered aside from primary hyperaldosteronism are:

- secondary hyperaldosteronism: aldosterone hypersecretion occurs secondary to elevated renin levels (e.g. from cirrhosis of the liver, congestive heart failure, nephrotic syndrome, renal artery stenosis, or, very rarely, a renin-secreting tumour)
- other mineralocorticoid excess syndromes (e.g. low renin, aldosterone not high (apparent mineralocorticoid excess), liquorice ingestion, ectopic ACTH)

'Gold-standard' diagnostic tests for primary hyperaldosteronism

The following are gold-standard diagnostic tests for primary hyperaldosteronism:

- for screening: plasma aldosterone:renin activity ratio (ARR; hypokalaemia should be normalized prior to the test as this may impair circulating levels of aldosterone)
- for confirmation:
  - oral sodium loading test
  - saline infusion test
  - fludrocortisone suppression test
  - captopril challenge

NB: alpha antagonists and non-dihydropyridine calcium-channel blockers have minimal effects on ARR; other antihypertensives may need to be stopped 4 or 2 weeks prior to testing.

Acceptable diagnostic alternatives to the gold-standard tests for primary hyperaldosteronism

The following tests may be performed if primary aldosteronism is confirmed:

- adrenal CT (for subtype classification and to exclude carcinoma)
- adrenal vein sampling (when surgical treatment is considered and it is desirable to distinguish between unilateral and bilateral disease)
- genetic screening for GRA in those with a family history of strokes or hypertension at age <40 years or in those developing hypertension at age <20 years

Other relevant investigations for primary hyperaldosteronism

Other relevant investigations for primary hyperaldosteronism are:

- serum potassium levels
- bicarbonate levels (to exclude metabolic alkalosis)
- urine potassium excretion (to determine if >30 mmol/24 hours)
- sodium levels (to exclude reset osmostat with hypernatraemia)

Prognosis of primary hyperaldosteronism, and how to estimate it

In unilateral disease, surgical removal of the tumour results in improvement in hypertension and hypokalaemia, with cure of hypertension

in 50%. In patients with bilateral disease, the use of spironolactone results in a mean reduction in blood pressure of approximately 25%. The prognosis of adrenal carcinoma is extremely poor.

Treatment of primary hyperaldosteronism, and its effectiveness

For patients with unilateral primary aldosteronism, laparoscopic adrenalectomy is recommended. Blood pressure typically normalizes within 1–6 months.

For patients with bilateral disease, spironolactone (starting dose 12.5–25 mg/day) or eplerinone (25 mg once or twice daily) should be used and titrated against blood pressure levels

In patients with GRA, the lowest dose of glucocorticoid that can normalize blood pressure and potassium levels should be used. The aim is to suppress pituitary ACTH secretion. Prednisolone or dexamethasone may be used.

For adrenal carcinoma, surgery and post-operative use of mitotane is usually required.

Phaeochromocytoma

Definition of phaeochromocytoma

Phaeochromocytomas are rare tumours of the adrenal medulla, arising from chromaffin cells, and produce catecholamines. Tumours arising from extra-adrenal ganglia, both sympathetic and parasympathetic, are called paragangliomas. As the majority of sympathetic paragangliomas secrete catecholamines, they are also called extra-adrenal phaeochromocytomas.

Aetiology of phaeochromocytoma

The aetiology of phaeochromocytoma is shown in Box 188.2.

Typical symptoms of phaeochromocytoma, and less common symptoms

Common symptoms of phaeochromocytoma include headache (80%), sweating (>80%), palpitations (65%), nervousness, abdominal/chest pain, and constipation. Hypertension may be paroxysmal or persistent, while pallor and fever may also be present. Nausea, fatigue, dizziness, heat intolerance, anxiety, and postural hypotension are less common.

Demographics of phaeochromocytoma

Overall, phaeochromocytoma is rare (~1 per million per year) and usually benign. It has equal incidence in both sexes, and usually occurs between the third and the fourth decades. The 25% caused by inherited syndromes are much more frequently bilateral in the adrenal glands, extra-adrenal, or malignant, especially if caused by SDHB mutations. They account for <0.1% of cases of hypertension.

Natural history of phaeochromocytoma, and complications of the disease

Although the presence of symptoms and signs may raise suspicion of a phaeochromocytoma, many tumours go undiagnosed and are identified incidentally (incidentalomas) during investigation of other non-related complaints. The classic history of a phaeochromocytoma is characterized by headaches, palpitations, and sweating, together with persistent or episodic hypertension, and constipation.

Box 188.2 Aetiology of phaeochromocytoma

- 75% of cases are sporadic
- 25% of cases are inherited:
  - multiple endocrine neoplasia type IIa and type IIb
  - paraganglioma syndrome (mutations of subunits B–D of succinate dehydrogenase (SDHB, SDHC, SDHD))
  - von Hippel–Lindau syndrome
  - neurofibromatosis
  - Carney's triad

Episodes may vary in time, usually lasting less than an hour, but, rarely, may last for days. Some may occur weekly, several times daily, or sometimes every few months. Episodes increase in number as the tumour grows. Diverse symptoms may be related to the type of catecholamines secreted (e.g. postural hypotension secondary to adrenaline) or to co-secretion of other peptides (e.g. diarrhoea from vasoactive intestinal peptide). Although rare, the condition may be fatal if not diagnosed. Complications are mainly cardiovascular (arrhythmias, cardiomyopathy, myocardial infarction) and neurological (hypertensive encephalopathy, stroke); hyperglycaemia and hypercalcaemia can also occur.

Approach to diagnosing phaechromocytoma

The following patients should be screened for phaechromocytoma:

- patients with paroxysmal symptoms, especially palpitations, headaches, sweating, and hypertension
- patients who are well but with hypertension and tachycardia at rest
- patients with hypertensive crises induced by specific precipitants (e.g. tumour palpation; postural changes; exertion; trauma; drugs, including beta blockers, opiates, and tricyclic antidepressants; anaesthesia; tyramine-containing foods)
- patients with a family history of related syndromes
- young patients with hypertension
- patients with unexplained heart failure

Other diagnoses that should be considered aside from phaechromocytoma

Other diagnoses that should be considered aside from phaechromocytoma are associated syndromes, including multiple endocrine neoplasia (MEN) type IIa (hyperparathyroidism, medullary thyroid cancer), MEN type IIb (similar to MEN type IIa but with marfanoid habitus and mucosal and intestinal ganglioneuromas), von Hippel–Lindau syndrome (retinal and cerebellar haemangioblastomas; renal cysts and carcinoma; pancreatic cysts), and neurofibromatosis (café au lait spots, neurofibromas).

'Gold-standard' diagnostic tests for phaechromocytoma

The following are gold-standard diagnostic tests for phaechromocytoma:

- 24-hour urine metanephrines × 2 (specificity 99.7%)
- plasma metanephrines (sensitivity 96%)

Acceptable diagnostic alternatives to the gold-standard tests for phaechromocytoma

An acceptable diagnostic alternative to the gold-standard tests for phaechromocytoma is the chromogranin A test. The following tests may be performed **after** diagnosis has been confirmed biochemically:

- MRI adrenal; if a phaechromocytoma is not detected, then body imaging (a phaechromocytoma appears hyperintense on T2-weighted images)
- CT adrenal
- ^{123}I-MIBG scan (ideal for multiple tumours, extra-adrenal tumours)
- venous sampling
- if phaechromocytoma is non-sporadic or extra-adrenal, consider FDG-PET scan (or DOPA PET, if available) or octreotide scan

Other relevant investigations for phaechromocytoma

Patients with phaechromocytoma and presenting <40 years of age or with multifocal disease should be screened for:

- MEN type II (via serum calcium, serum calcitonin, RET mutation analysis)
- von Hippel–Lindau syndrome (via ophthalmoscopy, MRI posterior fossa, ultrasound kidneys, VHL mutation analysis)
- paraganglioma syndrome (mutations in SDHB, SDHC, and SDHD)

Prognosis of phaechromocytoma, and how to estimate it

The 5-year survival rate for patients with non-malignant phaechromocytoma is >95%, with a low recurrence rate. For malignant phaeochromocytoma, the 5-year survival rate is <50%.

Treatment of phaechromocytoma, and its effectiveness

As soon as diagnosis of phaechromocytoma is made, alpha blockade should be started, using phenoxybenzamine orally 10 mg two times daily, and then titrated against blood pressure. This may then be followed 72 hours later by beta blockade using beta blockers especially if palpitations are problematic.

The definitive treatment for phaechromocytoma is surgical excision. This may be open or laparoscopic. Careful control of blood pressure is essential. IV phenoxybenzamine may be used before surgery. Prognosis after surgery is excellent, although 25%–50% of cases may remain hypertensive. Repeat urine/plasma metanephrines 14–28 days post-operatively. Long-term follow-up is essential.

Hypertensive crisis

Endocrine causes of malignant hypertension are uncommon, but may be suggested by features in the history that indicate catecholamine excess or by biochemical abnormalities. Any patient with hypertension and tachycardia should be screened for phaeochromocytoma. Look out for clinical features of Cushing's syndrome or acromegaly.

Features of hypertensive crisis

Features of hypertensive crisis are as follows:

- usually, very high BP ≥ 200/120
- encephalopathy and coma may be present
- angina, with or without myocardial infarction, left ventricular dysfunction, and aortic dissection
- eclampsia
- renal failure, with proteinuria
- retinopathy, with or without papilloedema

Management of hypertensive crisis

In hypertensive crisis, secure IV access, ECG monitoring, and high-dose oxygen. Take blood for an FBC, to measure urea and electrolytes, and to assess calcium, glucose, and creatine kinase levels. Order a chest X-ray and get a 12-lead ECG. Also get a dipstick urine test and send a midstream specimen of urine for microscopy. In addition, check pulse symmetry, radiofemoral delay, and blood pressure in both arms and examine for renal bruits.

Reducing arterial pressure very rapidly can endanger watershed areas of the brain; aim for a smooth reduction over a few hours. In general, use oral therapy, unless there is encephalopathy or congestive heart failure. Usually prescribe bed rest with amlodipine 2.5 mg once daily to begin with.

Parenteral treatment should really only be attempted in an intensive care (or at least high-dependency unit) setting, with senior involvement. Appropriate parenteral agents include sodium nitroprusside, labetalol, and hydralazine, but are rarely needed.

Avoid beta-blocker treatment if phaeochromocytoma is suspected: such patients should always receive adequate alpha blockade first with phenoxybenzamine. In addition, if a phaeochromocytoma is suspected, at least two 24-hour urinary samples (preferably off all treatment) for metanephrines should be the routine screening test and should be collected in acid. A number of drugs may interfere with catecholamine or metanephrine concentrations. Tests for hyperaldosteronism should also be taken. Any patient with an abnormal screening test should be referred to an endocrinologist.

For all tests for phaeochromocytoma or hyperaldosteronism, patients should preferably be only on an alpha blocker, as this causes little interference with investigations of phaeochromocytoma and/or hyperaldosteronism.

Further Reading

Aronova A, Fahey TJ III, and Zarnegar R. Management of hypertension in primary aldosteronism. *World J Cardiol* 2014; 6: 227–33.

Charmandari E, Nicolaides NC, and Chrousos GP. Adrenal insufficiency. *Lancet 2014*; 383: 2152–67.

Hellman P (ed.). *Primary Aldosteronism: Molecular Genetics, Endocrinology, and Translational Medicine*, 2014. Springer.

Lenders JWM, Duh Q-Y, Eisenhofer G, et al. Pheochromocytoma and paraganglioma: An Endocrine Society clinical practice guideline. *J Clin Endocrinol Metab* 2014; 99: 1915–42.

189 Cushing syndrome

John Newell-Price, Alia Munir, and Miguel Debono

Definition of the disease

Endogenous Cushing's syndrome results from chronic, excessive, and inappropriately high cortisol exposure. It comprises a large group of signs and symptoms.

Pseudo-Cushing's syndrome is a state of hypercortisolaemia that may have some of the clinical features of Cushing's syndrome, but the clinical and biochemical features resolve when the underlying condition is treated: causes include alcohol dependence and depression.

Aetiology of the disease

By far, the most common cause of Cushing's syndrome is iatrogenic, from medically prescribed glucocorticoids.

Endogenous Cushing's syndrome may be caused by either:

- adrenocorticotropic hormone (ACTH)-dependent Cushing's syndrome (80%); from pituitary adenoma (70%; termed 'Cushing's disease') or ectopic ACTH secretion (10%)
- ACTH-independent Cushing's syndrome (20%); from adrenal causes (adrenal adenoma; rarely, carcinoma or nodular hyperplasia)

Typical symptoms of the disease, and less common symptoms

Cyclical Cushing's syndrome may be particularly challenging to diagnose, as its features and biochemistry vary over time.

Demographics of the disease

Cushing's syndrome is uncommon, with an incidence of 2–3 per million per year. It is more common in women (3–15:1) and presents between 20 and 40 years of age.

Natural history, and complications of the disease

Glucocorticoid receptors are present in virtually all cells, reflecting the diverse actions of cortisol. Many of the symptoms are common and non-specific, such as obesity, lethargy, weakness, menstrual abnormalities, loss of libido, hirsutism, acne, depression, and psychosis. Those of greater specificity include proximal myopathy, easy bruising, purple striae, and thin skin. Development of diabetes mellitus, osteoporosis, and hypertension is common; 2%–5% of poorly controlled hypertensive patients with type 2 diabetes may have Cushing's syndrome. Seventy per cent of patients with Cushing's syndrome will have some form of psychiatric symptoms (often agitated depression).

Approach to diagnosing the disease

The following patients should be tested for Cushing's syndrome:

- patients who exhibit symptoms that are unusual for their age (e.g. osteoporosis)
- patients with multiple and progressive features that are predictive of Cushing's syndrome
- patients with adrenal incidentaloma compatible with adenoma
- children with a low height percentile and a high weight

Diagnosis is a two-step process: hypercortisolaemia must first be confirmed and **then** the cause can be searched for. Reliance is placed initially on biochemistry rather than imaging.

A biochemical hallmark of Cushing's syndrome is inappropriate cortisol secretion, with a loss of negative feedback and circadian rhythm.

For unknown reasons, some patients with Cushing's syndrome exhibit cyclical cortisol secretions that may fluctuate and remit spontaneously, sometimes over many years. This can cause considerable diagnostic difficulty; reinvestigation at intervals, and on several occasions, may be required.

Oral oestrogens increase cortisol-binding globulin and therefore lead to falsely elevated serum cortisol levels, and should be stopped for 6 weeks before investigation.

Other diagnoses that should be considered

Another diagnosis that should be considered aside from Cushing's syndrome is pseudo-Cushing's syndrome.

'Gold-standard' diagnostic tests

Step 1: Confirming Cushing's syndrome

For initial testing to confirm the presence of Cushing's syndrome, one of the following tests, based on the suitability for the patient, is used:

- urinary free cortisol (at least twice; NB: this is reduced in renal impairment)
- late-night salivary cortisol or plasma level (at least twice)
- 1 mg overnight dexamethasone suppression test (DST; in this test, dexamethasone 1 mg is given at 11:00 pm and serum cortisol is measured at 9:00 a.m. the next day)
- longer low-dose DST (2 mg/day for 48 hours; dexamethasone 0.5 mg is given at 9:00 a.m., 3:00 p.m., 9:00 p.m., and 3:00 a.m. and serum cortisol is measured at 9:00 a.m. at the start and end of the test)

For individuals with normal tests but progressive symptoms, re-evaluate in 6 months. For those with one or more abnormal test, further evaluation by an endocrinologist is recommended.

In healthy subjects, the serum cortisol level is less than 50 nmol/l (1.8 μg/dl) following any test; however, 5% of patients with Cushing's disease will show serum cortisol suppression <50 nmol/l. Thus, if the clinical index of suspicion is high, retest.

Both types of DST may give false-positive results if patients are taking drugs that increase the hepatic clearance of dexamethasone, including carbamazepine, phenytoin, phenobarbital, and rifampicin.

Midnight plasma cortisol

The normal circadian rhythm of cortisol level is lost in Cushing's syndrome. Following admission of the patient to hospital for 48 hours, a single, sleeping, midnight plasma cortisol level of >50 mmol/l is the most sensitive indicator of Cushing's syndrome, but this test is best left to dedicated endocrine centres.

Step 2: Isolating the cause of Cushing's syndrome

Once Cushing's syndrome is confirmed, the next step is to measure plasma ACTH. The sample needs careful handling, since ACTH is labile and, unless the sample is immediately processed and stored at −40°C, a falsely low level of ACTH may be recorded. A plasma ACTH level <5 pg/ml indicates a primary adrenal cause of Cushing's syndrome, and the adrenals should be imaged by CT or MRI. Levels of ACTH persistently more than 15 pg/ml can confidently be ascribed to ACTH-dependent pathologies and require investigation as discussed in 'Plasma potassium'. Levels of 5–15 pg/ml require cautious interpretation, because individuals with Cushing's disease may have a plasma ACTH level <10 pg/ml. At least two or three estimations are made, to avoid inappropriate classification.

Plasma potassium

Ectopic ACTH secretion is usually associated with higher circulating levels of cortisol in Cushing's disease. These high levels overwhelm the 11-beta hydroxysteroid dehydrogenase type II enzyme, allowing cortisol to act as a mineralocorticoid in the kidney. Hypokalaemia is consequently more common in ectopic ACTH secretion, but it is also present in 10% of patients with Cushing's disease.

ACTH-dependent Cushing's syndrome

ACTH-secreting non-pituitary neuroendocrine tumours (carcinoid tumours) may mimic many of the clinical features of ACTH-dependent Cushing's disease caused by pituitary tumours. Biochemical evaluation, rather than imaging, should be relied on to differentiate pituitary from non-pituitary sources of ACTH, and it is strongly recommended that this is performed in major referral centres.

High-dose DST

In the high-dose DST, dexamethasone 2 mg is administered orally, strictly 6-hourly, and the plasma cortisol level is measured basally and at 48 hours. In about 80% of patients with Cushing's disease, cortisol is reduced to >50% of the basal level. This is, however, **lower** than the pretest likelihood of Cushing's disease in women (90%); thus, this test is no longer be recommended where there is access to **bilateral inferior petrosal sinus sampling** (BIPSS; see 'Corticotrophin-releasing hormone test').

Corticotrophin-releasing hormone test

Corticotrophin-releasing hormone (CRH) stimulates the release of ACTH from the corticotrophs of the anterior pituitary. Patients with Cushing's disease typically exhibit an excessive increase in plasma cortisol, whereas those with ectopic ACTH secretion usually do not.

BIPSS is a highly specialized, invasive investigation, but is the most reliable test for differentiating between pituitary and non-pituitary sources of ACTH. A basal central:peripheral ACTH ratio of more than 2:1, or a CRH-stimulated ratio of more than 3:1, is indicative of Cushing's disease.

Imaging

Pituitary MRI

Most corticotroph adenomas are <1 cm in diameter and, on MRI, give a hypo-intense signal that fails to enhance with gadolinium. When standard MRI protocols are used, 40% of corticotroph microadenomas are not visualized and incidentalomas are found in 10% of the healthy population; this emphasizes the importance of biochemical assessment.

Adrenal CT

Adrenal CT provides the greatest spatial resolution for the assessment of adrenal anatomy.

Imaging in ectopic ACTH secretion

The most common sites of ectopic ACTH secretion are small cell lung cancers and bronchial carcinoid tumours, but tumours may be in any tissue. High-definition multislice CT is required. Carcinoid tumours may be visualized on radiolabelled octreotide scintigraphy

Acceptable diagnostic alternatives to the gold standard

There are no acceptable diagnostic alternatives to the gold-standard tests for Cushing's syndrome.

Other relevant investigations

Other investigations that are relevant for Cushing's syndrome are tests for glucose and glycated haemoglobin, DEXA bone scan, and

investigations for associated conditions, such as multiple endocrine neoplasia.

Prognosis and how to estimate it

Untreated Cushing's syndrome (severe hypercortisolism) has a 5-year survival of 50%. If hypercortisolism persists, the SMR is increased 3.8–5.0-fold, compared with the population. Most deaths are caused by vascular (myocardial infarction, cerebrovascular accident) or infective complications.

Treatment and its effectiveness

Successful treatment reverses but may not normalize features of Cushing's syndrome. Bone mineral density and cognitive function improve. Quality of life improves (but remains below that of age- and gender-matched subjects).

Trans-sphenoidal surgery

Selective microadenomectomy by an experienced surgeon is the treatment of choice in most patients with Cushing's disease. Long-lasting remission without other pituitary hormonal deficiency is achieved in 50%–60% of cases.

Adrenal surgery

Laparoscopic unilateral adrenalectomy is the treatment of choice in patients with an isolated adrenal adenoma. The prognosis following removal of adrenocortical cortisol-secreting adenomas is good. In contrast, the prognosis is almost always very poor in patients with adrenocortical carcinoma.

In ACTH-dependent Cushing's syndrome of any cause, bilateral adrenalectomy may be required to control cortisol levels. Nelson's syndrome (development of a locally aggressive pituitary tumour secreting high levels of ACTH, resulting in pigmentation) is a major concern following bilateral adrenalectomy in patients with refractory Cushing's syndrome. The tumour may be treated with further surgery and radiotherapy, but these seldom cure the disease.

When the syndrome is due to ectopic ACTH, complete excision of an ACTH-secreting tumour usually results in long-lasting remission.

Medical therapy

Medical therapy to lower cortisol may be used in preparation for surgery or after unsuccessful surgery. It is seldom a long-term solution, and is mainly used as an adjunctive treatment with other modalities such as pituitary radiotherapy. There is no **established** treatment to lower ACTH directly in Cushing's disease, and this is needed.

Metyrapone 500–1000 mg three or four times daily, increasing every 72 hours, and ketoconazole, 200–400 mg three times daily, increasing at 2–3-weekly intervals, are often used to inhibit cortisol synthesis, aiming for a mean plasma cortisol level of 150–300 mmol/l, or normalization of elevated urinary free cortisol levels. Metyrapone causes an increase in steroid androgenic precursors, and hirsutism is a major adverse effect in women; this does not occur with ketoconazole. In the UK, o,p′DDD (mitotane) is usually reserved for the treatment of adrenocortical carcinoma.

Pituitary radiotherapy

Following trans-sphenoidal surgery, persisting hypercortisolaemia may be treated with pituitary radiotherapy or gamma knife radiosurgery. Progressive anterior pituitary failure is the major side effect; growth hormone deficiency is present in almost all patients 10 years after treatment, and gonadotrophin deficiency in about 15%. About 4 years after treatment, 80% of patients are in remission with respect to circulating plasma cortisol levels.

Further Reading

Newell-Price J, Bertagna X, Grossman AB, et al. Cushing's syndrome. *Lancet* 2006; 367: 1605–17.

Nieman LK, Biller BM, Findling JW, et al. The diagnosis of Cushing's syndrome: An Endocrine Society clinical practice guideline. *J Clin Endocrinol Metab* 2008; 93: 1526–40.

190 Short stature

John Newell-Price, Alia Munir, and Miguel Debono

Definition of the disease

Short stature is defined as a height less than those in the second centile for age and sex on the appropriate growth chart. Abnormalities of growth may be detected earlier by assessing growth velocity. Specialists refer to an absolute height for which the z score is <-2 SDs for age, or a linear growth velocity with a z score <-1 SDs for age.

Aetiology of the disease

The aetiology of short stature is given in Box 190.1.

Typical symptoms of the disease, and less common symptoms

Features of the different causes of short stature are given in Table 190.1. The child or the child's parent(s) may complain of short stature; commonly, this may be in relation to peers or siblings. Ideally, collection of data from school, GP, health visitor, or home height and weight records can be used to help with calculating growth velocity. Notably, auxology is performed poorly by non-specialists.

Demographics of the disease

Organic disease is increasingly found as a cause of short stature; it is found in approximately 50% of cases. Twenty to thirty per cent of non-organic short stature has been attributed to social or environmental factors. Studies have shown that 80% of cases are due to familial short stature, constitutional delay, or both. Only 5% of cases are attributable to growth hormone (GH) deficiency, Turner syndrome, or hypothyroidism.

The prevalence of adult-onset GH deficiency is approximately 1 in 10 000. If adults who had childhood onset of GH deficiency are included, the prevalence of GH deficiency amongst adults is increased to 3 in 10 000. In children, GH deficiency has a prevalence of 1 in 3480, with a male:female ratio of 3:1.

Natural history, and complications of the disease

The nature history of short stature, as well as the complications associated with it, depends on the cause of the short stature. Untreated systemic disease will result in failure to thrive in the paediatric group, and ongoing chronic disease in the older age group. In GH deficiency, untreated short stature and delayed puberty will result.

Approach to diagnosing the disease

Consistently slow-growing children require full systemic and endocrine assessment. If the growth velocity (measure in centimetres per year) is normal, there is unlikely to be a significant endocrine disease. If the growth velocity is low, without an underlying systemic cause, further investigation is warranted. Sudden cessation of growth suggests major physical disease. If there is no gastrointestinal, respiratory, renal, or skeletal abnormality, a cerebral tumour and hypothyroidism must be excluded. The diagnosis is guided by history, clinical signs, and growth performance.

History

When taking the history, assess the birthweight and the length of gestation, calculate the mid-parental height and the weight for height, and take note of any maternal illnesses, childhood illnesses, medication, and milestones. Also note any family history of short stature or delayed puberty.

Examination

For the examination, assess height and height velocity over at least 4–6 months. Low weight for height suggests a nutritional or gastrointestinal cause.

In addition, stage puberty, using Tanner staging. Also, observe for features of dysmorphism or chronic disease states.

Growth

The persistence of a poor growth rate (below the 25th percentile on a velocity chart over 12 months) would be indicative of the need for investigation. However, if the presentation includes signs or symptoms suggestive of intracranial pathology, urgent investigation is indicated.

Other diagnoses that should be considered

See 'Aetiology of the disease' and 'Approach to diagnosing the disease'.

'Gold-standard' diagnostic tests

Many tests are used in the assessment of short stature, depending on the clinical history and signs.

Basal tests

The following basal tests should be performed:

- full blood count
- erythrocyte sedimentation rate

Box 190.1 Aetiology of short stature

- familial short stature and constitutional delay in growth and puberty (40%)
- growth hormone deficiency: primary (idiopathic; accounts for 50%–70% of cases of growth hormone deficiency) or secondary (pituitary/hypothalamic) from malformation, brain tumours, cranial irradiation, or psychosocial deprivation (8%)
- intrauterine growth retardation (7.5%)
- skeletal dysplasia (e.g. achondroplasia, hypochodroplasia)
- dysmorphic syndromes (e.g. Turner syndrome, Noonan syndrome, Down's syndrome)
- chronic illness (e.g. coeliac disease, Crohn's disease, chronic renal failure, chronic respiratory conditions (cystic fibrosis, severe asthma); chronic infection (HIV, TB); haematological diseases, such as chronic anaemias (thalassaemia, Fanconi syndrome); congenital heart disease)
- malnutrition (anorexia nervosa; marasmus; kwashiorkor; rickets due to vitamin D deficiency)
- endocrine disorders (hypothyroidism, hypoparathyroidism, pseudohypoparathyroidism, Cushing's syndrome)
- metabolic bone disease (hypophosphataemic rickets)
- growth hormone resistance (rare)

Table 190.1 Features of the different causes of short stature

	Constitutional delay	Familial short stature	Growth hormone insufficiency	Primary hypothyroidism	Small bowel disease
Family history	Often present	Positive	Rare	Rare	Sometimes
Growth/clinical feature/puberty	Slow from birth/immature but appropriate, with late but spontaneous puberty	Slow from birth Clinically normal, with normal puberty	Slow growth Immature Often overweight Delayed puberty	Slow growth Immature Delayed puberty	Slow Immature Usually thin for height Delayed puberty
Bone age	Moderate delay	Normal	Moderate delay increasing with time	Marked delay	Delay
Comments	Often difficult to differentiate from growth hormone deficiency Growth velocity vital	Need family member heights	Early investigation vital, especially if plump child	Measure thyroid-stimulating hormone and free thyroxine in all cases of short stature Clear clinical signs may not be obvious in all cases	Diarrhoea Anaemia Macrocytosis

- urea and electrolytes
- thyroid function test
- bone profile
- coeliac serology
- insulin-like growth factor 1 (IGF-1), and insulin-like growth-factor-binding protein 3
- karyotype (in girls), for chromosomal anomalies
- urinalysis

Dynamic tests

There may be indication for anterior pituitary function testing, GH provocation testing (insulin tolerance test (ITT); clonidine or glucagon testing) and IGF-1 generation testing. The **gold standard for assessment of GH deficiency is an ITT**, but it should only be requested in specialist centres.

Imaging

Skeletal survey

A skeletal survey will enable the assessment of bone age: non-dominant hand and wrist X-rays allow comparisons that can be used to set standards (this may indicate that sex-steroid priming is required).

MRI pituitary

In a child, a GH peak <20 mU/l, on an ITT or another stimulatory test, is a classic sign of GH deficiency, and other pituitary deficiencies should be excluded. GH treatment is indicated.

If the basal GH is elevated or the level of growth hormone-binding protein is >2 SDs below the mean, the patient has GH insensitivity syndrome, which is a group of disorders including Laron syndrome and its variants; malnutrition; and chronic disease. In this case, IGF-1 treatment is effective.

Acceptable diagnostic alternatives to the gold standard

If ITT is contraindicated (e.g. in the case of epilepsy or ischaemic heart disease, or in children) to assess the GH axis, then tests for growth hormone-releasing hormone, arginine, or glucagon (if the patient is on steroids) may be used.

Other relevant investigations

A DEXA scan may be useful for investigation in short stature.

Prognosis and how to estimate it

If the short stature is due to a systemic disease, treatment of the systemic disease, such a gluten-free diet for coeliac disease, results in complete recovery, and catch-up of lost height will occur.

If the short stature is due to GH deficiency, then, in general, growth rates are improved in children on GH replacement, although the effectiveness of GH replacement may decrease with prolonged treatment. If short stature due to GH deficiency is left untreated, extreme short stature and delayed puberty will result. If the diagnosis of GH deficiency is certain, normal height may be achieved in childhood and adolescence. A reduction in BMI, together with an improved body composition, will occur.

Treatment and its effectiveness

Any underlying systemic illness should be treated. In the case of primary hypothyroidism, replace levothyroxine at 50–200 µg/day.

In the case of GH insufficiency, injections of recombinant GH (this is synthetic GH, so there is no infection risk) should be given but only by specialists. Evidence suggests that this treatment leads to an improvement in quality of life, cardiac risk profile, body composition, and bone density. GH treatment in disorders such as Turner syndrome, Prader–Willi syndrome, and chronic renal insufficiency should also be done by specialists. A dose of 0.025–0.05 mg/kg per day for children, and 0.15–0.3 mg/day (or 0.6–0.9 IU/day) for adults may be used.

The aim of treatment for short stature is to correct growth failure and improve body composition. Data has shown an increase in growth velocity in response to treatment but there is some debate over whether there is also an increase in final height.

Further Reading

Allen DB and Cuttler L. Short stature in childhood: Challenges and choices. *N Engl J Med* 2013; 368: 1220–8.
Wass J and Shalet S. *Oxford Textbook of Endocrinology and Diabetes*, 2002. Oxford University Press.

191 Infertility

John Newell-Price, Alia Munir, and Miguel Debono

Causes of female infertility

Polycystic ovary syndrome

Definition of polycystic ovary syndrome

Polycystic ovary syndrome (PCOS) is a disorder characterized by two of the following three characteristics: (1) chronic anovulation; (2) chronic hyperandrogenism; (3) and polycystic-appearing ovaries on ultrasound. A diagnosis should be made after exclusion of conditions which cause irregular menstrual cycles and androgen excess.

Aetiology of PCOS

PCOS is commonly polygenic but rarely may be monogenic. Genes involved with insulin and gonadotropin secretion and action and those involved with androgen biosynthesis, secretion, transport, and metabolism are responsible. Ethnic origin, race, and environmental factors also have an influence on the phenotype.

Typical symptoms of PCOS, and less common symptoms

Common features of PCOS are oligo/amenorrhoea (70%), hirsutism (60%), obesity (35%–70%), infertility (30%), and acne (25%). Male pattern hair loss and acanthosis nigricans are less common.

Demographics of PCOS

PCOS is one of the most common endocrine disorders of women in the reproductive age group, with a prevalence of around 5%–10%.

Natural history of PCOS, and complications of the disease

The symptoms of PCOS usually begin around menarche/puberty, but onset after puberty may occur in someone who gains weight, indicating both genetic and environmental influences. Menstrual irregularities occur mainly as oligomenorrhoea or amenorrhoea. Chronic anovulation results in infertility. The majority of women with PCOS have ovarian hyperandrogenism, with hypersecretion of luteinizing hormone (LH) occurring in about 70% of patients. This is thought to occur by an increased frequency of hypothalamic gonadotropin-releasing hormone (GnRH) pulses, which stimulate an increased frequency of LH pulses, which act on the ovarian theca cells to produce increasing amounts of androgens. Women with PCOS are hyperinsulinaemic and insulin resistant, probably because of defects in insulin-signalling pathways. Approximately 10% of patients with PCOS have type 2 diabetes, and 30%–40% have abnormal glucose tolerance. A significant number of patients are obese, and the incidence of the condition in different populations parallels the incidence of obesity. Hypertriglyceridaemia, high very-low-density lipoprotein, high LDL, low HDL, vascular endothelial dysfunction, and reduced vascular compliance increase the risk for cardiovascular disease and hypertension. There is a 43% prevalence of metabolic syndrome in patients with PCOS. In view of persistent unopposed oestrogen stimulation of the endometrium, endometrial hyperplasia or endometrial carcinoma may occur. Obstructive sleep apnoea is another complication of the disease.

Approach to diagnosing PCOS

To diagnose PCOS, a thorough menstrual history should be taken, including time of menarche, frequency of periods, onset of irregularities, and presence of inter-menstrual bleeding. Difficulties with conception should be elicited.

Cutaneous features such as hirsutism, acne, acanthosis nigricans, male pattern hair loss, and obesity are all suggestive of PCOS.

Hirsutism that is rapidly progressive and associated with virilization (deep voice, increased muscle size, clitoromegaly, frontal balding) are associated with ovarian and adrenal tumours. Include an external genitalia examination. In addition, patients may have a family history of PCOS.

Features of associated complications should be recorded, including chest pain, polyuria, polydipsia, high blood pressure, retinopathy, peripheral neuropathy, daytime somnolence, or frequent snoring. Enquire about risk factors for glucose intolerance (e.g. elevated BMI, race, family history of diabetes, gestational diabetes).

Other diagnoses that should be considered aside from PCOS

Other diagnoses that should be considered aside from PCOS are:

- non-classic congenital adrenal hyperplasia
- Cushing's syndrome
- hyperprolactinaemia
- premature ovarian failure (POF)
- virilizing adrenal or ovarian tumour
- drug-related causes

'Gold-standard' diagnostic test for PCOS

The best diagnostic test for PCOS is the serum testosterone level (no gold-standard test available).

Acceptable diagnostic alternatives to the gold-standard test for PCOS

Acceptable diagnostic alternatives are:

- the ratio of LH to follicle-stimulating hormone (FSH)
- sex hormone-binding globulin (SHBG) level (low in 50%)
- transvaginal ultrasound of ovaries and endometrium (>12 follicular cysts of <10 mm in diameter in at least one ovary; or increased ovarian volume (>10 ml); also exclusion of endometrial hyperplasia and ovarian tumours)

Other relevant investigations for PCOS

Other relevant investigations for PCOS are:

- prolactin (to exclude hyperprolactinaemia)
- 9 a.m. 17-hydroxyprogesterone ± response to Synacthen test (to exclude non-classical congenital adrenal hyperplasia)
- androstenedione, dehydroepiandrosterone sulphate (DHEAS; both may be raised in PCOS; DHEAS is a marker for adrenal hyperandrogenism)
- overnight dexamethasone suppression test (if signs of Cushing's only)
- serum lipids and fasting glucose ± an oral glucose tolerance test (OGTT)

Prognosis for PCOS, and how to estimate it

In obese patients with PCOS, endocrine–metabolic markers improve after 4–12 weeks of dietary restriction. With loss of 5% of their starting weight, women with PCOS show a 40% improvement in their hirsutism. In a meta-analysis, metformin therapy resulted in ovulation in 46% of patients compared with 24% who received placebo. Approximately three-quarters of women with PCOS ovulate on clomiphene citrate alone. In women who are resistant to clomiphene citrate alone, addition of metformin may increase ovulation.

Treatment of PCOS, and its effectiveness

Patients may be concerned about cosmetic issues, infertility, or menstrual irregularities. These should all be discussed in detail with the patient, as will all influence the decisions regarding management. In view of long-term risks, all patients should be treated.

Weight loss

Diet and exercise should be recommended, as they may improve frequency of ovulation and fertility and lower diabetes risk and androgen levels.

Fertility

If fertility is the primary goal, consider clomiphene, metformin and, if these are unsuccessful, gonadotrophins. IVF or laparoscopic ovarian diathermy may also be considered.

Hirsutism

Treatment for hirsutism includes:

- short-term non-pharmacologic approaches, such as shaving and use of chemical depilatories and/or bleaching cream
- suppression of androgens (ovarian: oral contraceptive pills (OCPs), commonly co-cyprindiol; GnRH analogues for severe cases)
- androgen receptor blockers (e.g. cyproterone acetate, spironolactone, flutamide)
- 5-alpha reductase inhibitors (e.g. finasteride)
- eflornithine (Vaniqa; an ornithine decarboxylase inhibitor; available as a topical cream that can be used to slow the hair growth)

Amenorrhoea

It is important that women achieve a withdrawal bleed at least once every three months, to reduce the risk of endometrial hyperplasia. Use OCPs or metformin for this.

Premature ovarian insufficiency

Definition of premature ovarian insufficiency

Premature ovarian insufficiency (POI) is a disorder characterized by amenorrhoea, low oestradiol levels, and elevated gonadotropins, developing in women <40 years. As the natural history of POI may begin with infertility but still have persistent follicular development at later stages, the name POI is more accurate than the commonly used POF.

Aetiology of POI

The aetiology of primary ovarian insufficiency is given in Box 191.1

Typical symptoms of POI, and less common symptoms

Patients with POI typically present with amenorrhoea (primary or secondary) and menopausal symptoms (flushes, night sweats, mood changes, low sex drive, sleeping problems).

Demographics of POI

Estimates of the prevalence of POI range between 0.3% and 1%. Age of onset may be as early as the teenage years but varies widely.

Natural history of POI, and complications of the disease

POI at any stage could result from a decrease in the initial primordial follicle number, an increase in follicle destruction, or a failure of the follicle to respond to gonadotrophin stimulation. The disease develops insidiously and the first sign of the disease may be unexplained

---

Box 191.1 Aetiology of primary ovarian insufficiency

- idiopathic causes (common)
- genetic associations: mutations in X-chromosomal or autosomal genes (e.g. Turner syndrome, fragile X syndrome, mutations in the receptors for follicle-stimulating hormone or luteinizing hormone)
- enzyme defects (galactosaemia, 17 alpha-hydroxylase deficiency (congenital adrenal hyperplasia))
- autoimmune causes (e.g. autoimmune polyendocrine syndrome types I and II, isolated; 20%)
- iatrogenic causes (e.g. chemotherapy, radiotherapy, pelvic surgery)
- infective causes (e.g. viral)

---

infertility in a patient failing to respond to gonadotrophin stimulation, although basal FSH levels may be normal (occult POI). As the disease progresses, FSH levels increase (biochemical POI). Following this stage, patients develop menstrual irregularities (overt POI) and, finally, amenorrhoea, permanent infertility, and elevated gonadotrophins (POF). Most patients who develop POI do so after undergoing normal puberty and establishing regular menses. Some do not develop regular periods, and progress to POI years later. Ten per cent of patients present with primary amenorrhoea. Menopausal symptoms may precede menstrual irregularities. Health concerns for patients with POI include osteoporosis, osteopenia, and heart disease.

Approach to diagnosing POI

When diagnosing POI, a thorough menstrual history should be taken, including time of menarche, frequency of periods, onset of irregularities, and presence of inter-menstrual bleeding. Difficulties with conception should be elicited. In addition, enquire about menopausal symptoms.

A history of chemotherapy, radiotherapy, pelvic surgery, or recent infections should be recorded. A family history of overt POI is an important clue to the diagnosis.

A review of systems and a full physical examination should be performed, to uncover other autoimmune disorders or genetic causes. In addition, examine external genitalia.

Other diagnoses that should be considered aside from POI

Other diagnoses that should be considered aside from POI are:

- Turner syndrome (short stature, webbing of the neck, a highly arched palate, short fourth metacarpals, widely spaced nipples)
- autoimmune polyendocrine syndrome types I (hypoparathyroidism, chronic mucocutaneous candidiasis, primary adrenal insufficiency, primary hypothyroidism) and II (adrenal insufficiency, primary hypothyroidism, type 1 diabetes mellitus, vitiligo)
- hyperandrogenic states

'Gold-standard' diagnostic test for POI

The gold-standard diagnostic test for POI is the basal serum FSH level (measured at two occasions at least 1 month apart; may fluctuate; a high level indicates POI).

Acceptable diagnostic alternatives to the gold-standard test for POI

Acceptable diagnostic alternatives to the gold-standard test for POI are tests to measure:

- LH (high in POI)
- oestradiol (low in POI)

Other relevant investigations for POI

Other relevant investigations for POI include:

- a pelvic ultrasound (for uterine and ovarian anatomy assessment)
- karyotype analysis
- a screen for autoimmune disease (thyroid and adrenal antibodies, thyroid function test, fasting glucose test)

Consider a tetracosactide test or other tests for autoimmune diseases, if they are clinically indicated. Also consider a bone density test, for osteoporosis.

Prognosis of POI, and how to estimate it

About 6%–8% of women with POF will become pregnant spontaneously. Sometimes this may occur years after diagnosis. Spontaneous remission may occur.

Treatment of POI

The following may be used in the treatment of POI:

- patient education and counselling
- sex hormone replacement therapy: conjugated oestrogens and oestradiol (add on progestogen for 12–14 days a month in a non-hysterectomized patient)
- oocyte donation and IVF

Causes of male infertility

Male hypogonadism

Definition of male hypogonadism

Male hypogonadism is the failure of testes to produce adequate amounts of testosterone, spermatozoa, or both. The term primary (hypergonadotrophic) hypogonadism refers to testicular disorders characterized by low serum testosterone despite high levels of FSH and LH. Secondary (hypogoadotrophic) hypogonadism is the deficient release of GnRH, characterized by low normal or low levels of LH, FSH, and testosterone.

Aetiology of male hypogonadism

The aetiology of male hypogonadism is given in Box 191.2.

Typical symptoms of male hypogonadism, and less common symptoms

Common features of male hypogonadism are absence and loss of secondary sexual characteristics; reduced libido; erectile dysfunction; low energy; depressed mood; increased irritability; hot flushes; and decreased muscle strength.

Demographics of male hypogonadism

In men with hypergonadotrophic hypogonadism, the more common cause is Klinefelter syndrome, which has an incidence of 1 per 500–1000 live births. Hypogonadism may occur at any age, and hypergonadotrophic hypogonadism is commoner in males.

Natural history of male hypogonadism, and complications of the disease

Hypogonadism will manifest differently depending on the time of onset, duration, and severity. If the onset is in prepubertal males, the patient will present with long arms, long legs, sparse body hair (eunuchoidism), and failure to progress through puberty, while, post puberty, erectile dysfunction and infertility are the chief concerning issues, together with non-specific symptoms of lethargy, irritability, and mood changes. Post puberty penile length and skeleton are of normal proportions, hair is of normal distribution but reduced in amount, and patients progressively claim to be shaving less frequently. Complications of low testosterone levels are loss of libido; decreased physical strength; increase in visceral fat; anaemia; and reduced bone density or osteoporosis. In addition, there is an important association with type 2 diabetes mellitus and the metabolic syndrome.

Numerous studies have established a close relationship between obesity and low serum free or total testosterone levels in healthy males. An inverse relationship exists between testosterone levels and insulin concentrations in healthy men. Importantly, free testosterone levels, independently of SHBG (also low in insulin resistance), are low in one-third of diabetic men, while obesity and visceral adiposity, as assessed by both BMI and waist circumference, are negatively associated with low levels of testosterone.

After the age of 50, mean serum testosterone levels decrease progressively. Associated with advancing age, there is an increase in the levels of SHBG, translating into a decrease in the bioavailable testosterone (both albumin-bound and free fractions). A combination of primary and secondary hypogonadism may be seen with ageing.

Approach to diagnosing male hypogonadism

When diagnosing male hypogonadism, enquire about the presence of developmental anomalies associated with the genital tract and elicit features of delayed puberty. If the hypogonadism is post pubertal, establish symptoms of testosterone deficiency. In addition, record:

- events leading to hypogonadism (trauma, infections, chemotherapy, radiotherapy)
- a drug history, including over the counter drugs and drugs of abuse
- a general medical history for systemic illnesses
- any family history of genetic disorders
- a thorough sexual history, for erectile function and frequency of intercourse

Also, perform an external examination for body hair distribution, muscle mass, sense of smell, visual fields, and gynaecomastia. In addition, examine external genitalia for reduced testicular volume or anomalies.

Other diagnoses that should be considered aside from male hypogonadism

Other diagnoses that should be considered aside from male hypogonadism are Klinefelter syndrome (small testis, gynaecomastia, eunuchoidism), Kallmann syndrome (anosmia, cleft lip or palate, sensorineural deafness), type 2 diabetes mellitus, and metabolic syndrome.

'Gold-standard' diagnostic test for male hypogonadism

The gold-standard diagnostic test for male hypogonadism is a fasting 9 a.m. serum total testosterone test (if the level is low, the test should be repeated).

Acceptable diagnostic alternatives to the gold-standard test for male hypogonadism

Acceptable diagnostic alternatives to the gold-standard test for male hypogonadism are:

- free testosterone levels (especially in patients with diabetes or who are obese)
- SHBG levels (high in elderly; low in type 2 diabetes and in obese patients)
- LH, FSH (high in primary hypogonadism; inappropriately low in pituitary or hypothalamic hypogonadism)
- prolactin levels

Other relevant investigations for male hypogonadism

Other relevant investigations for male hypogonadism are:

- oestradiol levels (especially if gynaecomastia is present or an adrenal or testicular tumour is suspected)
- human chorionic gonadotropin stimulation test (to examine for Leydig cell function)
- clomifene test (examining integrity of hypothalamic–pituitary–testicular axis)
- prostate-specific antigen (PSA), full blood count (FBC), and lipids, if considering testosterone replacement
- fasting glucose ± OGTT

Also consider bone density assessment.

Box 191.2 Aetiology of male hypogonadism

Primary hypogonadism
- genetic (Klinefelter syndrome)
- anatomic defects (cryptorchidism)
- orchitis (infection, autoimmune causes)
- tumour
- trauma/torsion
- iatrogenic causes (e.g. chemotherapy, surgery, radiotherapy, trauma)
- chronic illness
- alcohol abuse
- varicocele
- systemic illness (e.g. cirrhosis, anaemia, chronic renal failure)

Secondary hypogonadism
- hyperprolactinaemia
- gonadotropin-releasing hormone deficiency (Kallmann syndrome; associated with anosmia)
- hypothalamic lesions or disorders
- pituitary lesions or disorders
- systemic illness (e.g. haemochromatosis, stress, myocardial infarction)

Prognosis of male hypogonadism, and how to estimate it

Men with hypogonadism may live a normal life if on hormone replacement.

Treatment for male hypogonadism, and its effectiveness

Testosterone replacement therapy is used as treatment for male hypogonadism, as intramuscular, buccal, and transdermal formulations, as well as gels and implants. It improves well-being, libido, virilization, and sexual function, increases muscle mass, and prevents osteoporosis. Testosterone replacement therapy may also reduce cardiovascular risk by possibly improving markers of insulin resistance in patients with hypogonadism and type 2 diabetes. However, it is contraindicated in prostate or breast cancer and should be avoided in sleep apnoea.

During the course of the therapy, monitor PSA levels, FBCs (for polycythaemia), lipids, liver function tests (if on oral testosterone), and testosterone levels.

Androgen replacement therapy does not restore fertility. In secondary hypogonadism, if fertility is desired, this may be stimulated by pulsatile luteinizing hormone-releasing hormone or gonadotropins.

Further Reading

Basaria S. Male hypogonadism. *Lancet* 2014; 383: 1250–63.

Ehrmann DA. Polycystic ovary syndrome. *N Engl J Med* 2005; 352: 1223–36.

Legro RS, Arslanian SA, Ehrmann DA, et al. Diagnosis and treatment of polycystic ovary syndrome: An Endocrine Society clinical practice guideline. *J Clin Endocrinol Metab* 2013; 98: 4565–92.

John Newell-Price, Alia Munir, and Miguel Debono

Prolactinoma

Definition of prolactinoma

A prolactinoma (a prolactin-secreting pituitary tumour) is defined as a macroprolactinoma when it is >1 cm in diameter, and as a micro-prolactinoma when it is <1 cm in diameter.

Aetiology of prolactinoma

The causes of hyperprolactinaemia are listed in Box 192.1. The pathogenesis of prolactinoma is unknown, but the rare malignant prolactinomas may harbour the Ras mutation.

Typical symptoms of prolactinoma, and less common symptoms

Patients with micro- or macroprolactinomas may develop galactor-rhoea (up to 90% in women, and 10%–20% in men) and gonadal dysfunction (in women, menstrual disturbance in up to 95%; in men, loss of libido and erectile dysfunction). They also have a long-term risk of reduced bone mineral density. Further, patients with macro-prolactinomas may develop mass effects such as headaches, visual field defects, hypopituitarism, and invasion of the cavernous sinus; the latter may lead to cranial nerve palsies and, occasionally, erosion of bone, CSF leakage, and meningitis.

Demographics of prolactinoma

Prolactinomas are the commonest functioning pituitary tumour. Microprolactinomas are more common in females and are more common than macroprolactinomas.

Natural history of prolactinoma, and complications of the disease

Microprolactinomas are common post-mortem, and less than <17% show an increase in size. In one-third of women with hyperpro-lactinaemia, the condition resolves after pregnancy or menopause. Dopamine-agonist treatment can be titrated down after 2–5 years of treatment and withdrawn to assess whether resolution of hyperpro-lactinaemia has occurred.

For macroprolactinomas, dopamine-agonist dose reduction should only be considered >5 years of treatment, as tumour enlarge-ment may occur and definitive treatment may be required (radio-therapy or surgery).

Approach to diagnosing prolactinoma

Hyperprolactinaemia is indicated by prolactin levels above the sex-specific normal range. Since stress can cause an elevation in prolactin levels, two to three cannulated prolactin measurements over 30–60 minutes can be used to confirm abnormal prolactin elevation.

In the context of a pituitary macroadenoma on MRI, a prol-actin level >6000 mIU/l is diagnostic of a macroprolactinoma as opposed to a non-functioning tumour with stalk compression.

If history and biochemistry are consistent with disease, proceed to pituitary MRI with gadolinium contrast. Microadenomas appear hypodense on T1-weighted images. Macroadenomas are space-occupying lesions and are sometimes associated with invasion.

Other diagnoses that should be considered aside from prolactinoma

The following should be considered in the differential diagnosis of prolactinoma:

- rule out hypothyroidism and chronic renal failure, as these also cause elevations in serum prolactin
- the Hook effect: in some assays, a very high level of prolactin may be incorrectly reported as a low level, as the antibodies used in the assay may fail to bind all prolactin molecules
- macroprolactinaemia: macroprolactin ('big prolactin') is a non-bioactive isoform of prolactin that binds to the antibodies used in the prolactin assay and can cause the prolactin level to appear elevated; macroprolactinaemia presents biochemically as hyper-prolactinaemia, but ovulatory cycles are normal
- idiopathic hyperprolactinaemia: this may be due to alterations in hypothalamic function, as MRI does not demonstrate a pitui-tary lesion in these patients; in one-third of cases, prolactin levels return to normal; in 10%–15% of cases, prolactin levels increase; in the remaining cases, prolactin levels remain stable

'Gold-standard' diagnostic test for prolactinoma

The gold-standard diagnostic test for prolactinoma is a cannulated prolactin measurement.

Box 192.1 Aetiology of hyperprolactinaemia

Physiological causes
- pregnancy
- sexual intercourse
- nipple stimulation/suckling
- neonatal
- stress

Pituitary tumours
- prolactinoma
- mixed growth hormone-secreting and prolactin-secreting tumour
- stalk compression (non-functioning pituitary tumour)
- empty sella
- hypothalamic disease
- infiltration
- stalk section
- cranial irradiation

Drugs
- dopamine-receptor antagonists
- neuroleptics
- antidepressants
- cardiovascular drugs
- opiates
- protease inhibitors
- others

Metabolic causes
- hypothyroidism
- chronic renal failure (reduced clearance)
- severe liver disease

Other causes
- polycystic ovary syndrome
- chest wall lesions (zoster, burns, trauma)

Acceptable diagnostic alternatives to the gold-standard test for prolactinoma

There are no acceptable diagnostic alternatives to the gold-standard test for prolactinoma.

Other relevant investigations for prolactinoma

Another relevant investigation for prolactinoma is a full anterior pituitary function tests (to rule out hypopituitarism and to check for co-secretion), including tests for:

- adrenocorticotropic hormone (ACTH)
- luteinizing hormone (LH)
- follicle-stimulating hormone (FSH)
- testosterone
- growth hormone (GH)
- insulin-like growth factor 1 (IGF-1)
- oestradiol
- urea and electrolytes

In addition, liver function tests and a short Synacthen test should be carried out.

Prognosis for prolactinoma, and how to estimate it

Most prolactinomas are treated successfully with medical therapy, with minimal morbidity. Lack of normalization of prolactin levels can be found in 25%–50% of patients taking bromocriptine, and 5%–18% taking cabergoline. Regarding failure to achieve at least a 50% decrease in tumour size, resistance can be expected in about one-third of those taking bromocriptine, and 5%–10% of those taking cabergoline. Prolactinomas in multiple endocrine neoplasia (MEN) type 1 may act more aggressively. Dopamine-agonist resistance is commoner in macroprolactinomas, especially in men.

Treatment of prolactinoma, and its effectiveness

The aim of treatment for prolactinoma is to restore gonadal function (for both microprolactinomas and macroprolactinomas) and reduce tumour size and prevent expansion (in macroprolactinomas). Thus, definitive tumour treatment is necessary.

Medical therapy for the treatment of prolactinoma

Dopamine-agonist treatment is the mainstay of treatment for all types of prolactinomas and leads to suppression of prolactin in most patients, so that galactorrhoea ceases and gonadal function returns to normal. Tumour shrinkage is the norm and must be carefully monitored. Cabergoline is more effective than bromocriptine. If prolactin levels fall but no shrinkage of a macroadenoma is seen on an MRI scan, the diagnosis is likely to be that of a non-functioning pituitary adenoma, and surgery may be indicated. Dopamine-agonist resistance may occur.

Surgery for the treatment of prolactinoma

Trans-sphenoidal hypophysectomy for the treatment of microprolactinoma is only indicated in patients who are intolerant to or resistant to dopamine agonists. The surgical cure rate for macroprolactinoma is poor (<30%); therefore, drug treatment should be trialled for all tumours. For microprolactinoma, the surgical cure rate is high (>80%) but the risk of subsequent hypopituitarism is also high (25%), and recurrence occurs at a rate of 4% at 5 years.

Radiotherapy for the treatment of prolactinoma

Pituitary irradiation leads to a slow reduction of prolactin levels in the majority of patients with prolactinoma. It is useful in the treatment of macroprolactinoma, provided the optic chiasm is not involved. Stereotactic radiosurgery may be used in selected cases.

Acromegaly

Definition of acromegaly

Acromegaly occurs as a result of excessive secretion of GH and, consequently, insulin-like growth factor 1 (IGF-1) in adults. It is termed 'pituitary gigantism' in the paediatric setting when excessive GH secretion occurs prior to epiphyseal plate fusion.

> **Box 192.2 Aetiology of acromegaly**
>
> - pituitary adenoma, in the majority of cases (>99%)
> - growth hormone-releasing hormone secretion (hypothalamic or ectopic; rare)
> - ectopic growth hormone secretion (very rare)

Aetiology of acromegaly

The aetiology of acromegaly is given in Box 192.2.

Typical symptoms of acromegaly, and less common symptoms

Symptoms of acromegaly include increased sweating (>80%), headaches, tiredness and lethargy, joint pains, and change in ring size or shoe size. Signs of acromegaly include coarsening of facial features; oily skin; frontal bossing; an enlarged nose; prognathism; interdental separation; a deep voice; macroglossia; musculoskeletal changes such as degenerative joint disease (osteoarthritis; 70%) and generalized myopathy; and soft tissue swelling, such as carpal tunnel syndrome (40%), goitre, and organomegaly (see Figure 192.1).

Demographics of acromegaly

Acromegaly is rare, with a prevalence of 40–60 cases/million population and a new case incidence of 4/million per year. There is an equal sex distribution. Most cases are insidious in onset and diagnosed in middle age.

Natural history of acromegaly, and complications of the disease

Acromegaly is a chronic debilitating disease. Often there is a delay in diagnosis for up to 7–10 years. The clinical manifestation of acromegaly depends on the chronicity and severity of disease. Patients frequently experience hyperhydrosis and fatigue. Acral enlargement may also be an early feature. Thickening of the soft tissue of the hands and feet results in enlargement of ring and shoe sizes. Coarsening of the facial features has a deleterious effect on self-image, markedly affecting self-confidence and quality of life. Local pituitary tumour enlargement may cause headaches and cranial nerve defects; in particular, optic chiasm compression may cause visual field defects (typically, bitemporal hemianopia).

There is a two- to threefold increase in mortality in patients with acromegaly, with cardiovascular, cerebrovascular, and respiratory disease contributing to the reduced life expectancy. It has been shown that disease duration and GH levels are independent predictors of overall mortality. Excess GH and IGF-1 have major detrimental effects on the heart and vasculature. At diagnosis, 60% of patients have hypertension, arrhythmias, valvular heart disease, and, consequently, diastolic heart failure. In terms of respiratory disorders, upper airways obstruction caused by pharyngeal hypertrophy and macroglossia, with obstructive sleep apnoea, occurs in over 50% of patients. Mortality returns to normal when GH and IGF-1 levels are in their normal ranges.

Up to 70% of patients with acromegaly develop large-joint and axial arthropathy due to bone and cartilage overgrowth and periarticular calcification. Clearly, these problems represent the most significant functional disability associated with acromegaly. Another serious consequence is the development of type 2 diabetes mellitus. GH blocks the action of insulin, inhibiting phosphorylation of the insulin receptor and the signalling molecule insulin receptor substrate 1. This results in impaired glucose tolerance and insulin resistance. Both peripheral glucose uptake and suppression of gluconeogenesis are reduced.

Twenty-five per cent of GH-producing adenomas co-secrete prolactin. This may contribute to the 40%–80% of menstrual irregularities seen in women with acromegaly. Tumour compression effects may also cause hypopituitarism in some patients, who may therefore require replacement hormonal therapy.

Patients with acromegaly have a twofold increased risk of developing colonic polyps; this is attributed to the effects of IGF-1 on proliferating epithelial cells. Interestingly, the incidence rate of colon

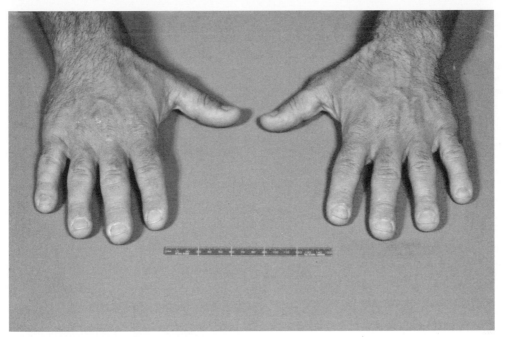

Figure 192.1 Hands of a patient with acromegaly. Please see colour plate section.

cancer is lower but the rate of death from colon cancer is higher in this patient group compared to the normal population.

Complications of acromegaly include:

- hypertension (60%)
- impaired glucose tolerance (40%)
- insulin resistance and diabetes mellitus (20%)
- obstructive sleep apnoea (50%)
- increased risk of colonic polyps
- ischaemic heart disease
- cerebrovascular disease
- congestive cardiac failure
- visual field defects
- hypopituitarism

Approach to diagnosing acromegaly

A high index of suspicion is required to consider a diagnosis of acromegaly. Key questions in the history and careful examination are essential. It is useful to ask about changes in appearance; often, patients do not notice, so asking for an old photograph of the patient for comparison and, in particular, asking about changes in ring, shoe, or hat size may be helpful. Biochemical confirmation of the disease should be the initial investigative approach.

Other diagnoses that should be considered aside from acromegaly

Acromegaly is associated with the following rare syndromes: MEN type 1, Carney complex, and isolated familial somatotrophinomas.

'Gold-standard' diagnostic test for acromegaly

The gold-standard diagnostic test for acromegaly is failure to suppress GH levels to <1 µg/l in response to a 75 mg oral glucose tolerance test with at least five measures (normally, GH suppresses to undetectable levels); in addition, 30% of patients show a paradoxical rise. This test may diagnose glucose intolerance as well. However, note that failure to suppress GH may also be seen in advanced liver disease, anorexia nervosa, and opiate abuse; in addition, a paradoxical rise in GH levels may be seen in diabetes mellitus and renal failure.

After the biochemical test, it is essential to proceed to an MRI (with gadolinium) of the pituitary to demonstrate a tumour.

Acceptable diagnostic alternatives to the gold-standard test for acromegaly

An IGF-1 test alongside GH measurements during the oral glucose tolerance test can be useful, as a normal IGF-1 level with a GH level <1 µg/l excludes acromegaly. It is also useful in disease monitoring.

Note that a random GH test will be unhelpful, as GH is secreted in a pulsatile fashion.

Other relevant investigations for acromegaly

Other relevant investigations for acromegaly are:

- serum prolactin; this is essential, as some tumours co-secrete
- serum calcium: some patients are hypercalcaemic due to increased levels of 1,25-dihydroxycholecalciferol, as GH stimulates renal 1-alpha hydroxylase
- full anterior pituitary function (i.e. ACTH, GH, prolactin, testosterone, LH, FSH), to exclude hypopituitarism
- a short tetracosactide test

In the absence of a pituitary lesion, a serum growth hormone-releasing hormone measure may be useful. Imaging the thorax and abdomen will also help demonstrate a carcinoid tumour (rare; <1% of cases).

Prognosis of acromegaly, and how to estimate it

If acromegaly is untreated, its mortality is double that of the normal population, with the cause of death usually being cardiovascular, cerebrovascular, or respiratory in origin.

Treatment of acromegaly, and its effectiveness

Treatment for acromegaly is tailored to the patient.

Surgical treatment of acromegaly

The first-line management of acromegaly is surgical resection of the pituitary tumour, usually through trans-sphenoidal surgery, although a transfrontal approach may be necessary, depending upon the tumour. More recently, endoscopic endonasal trans-sphenoidal surgery has been shown to be less invasive. Optimal surgical outcome depends on the surgeon. Cure is defined as a mean GH <1 µg/l. Surgery achieves biochemical control in 80% of acromegalics with microadenomas (<1 cm), and 50% of those with macroadenomas. As over

70% of acromegalics have macroadenomas, adjunctive medical treatment is required in about half of all cases.

Medical treatment of acromegaly

Dopamine agonists

Cabergoline has been shown to be more effective than bromocriptine at reducing IGF-1 levels. Levels of GH and IGF-1 are reduced but not usually to the normal range. Tumour shrinkage may occur if prolactin is co-secreted. ECG is recommended prior to and as monitoring with this class of drugs.

Somatostatin analogues

Somatostatin analogues lead to GH suppression in 60% of patients with acromegaly. Up to 40% of patients are complete responders, with normalization of GH and IGF-1 levels.

GH receptor antagonists

Pegvisamont is a new drug that has been shown to reduce IGF-1 levels in >90% of patients.

Radiotherapy for the treatment of acromegaly

Radiotherapy is used following unsuccessful surgery, or, very occasionally, as a primary therapy. The greatest reduction in GH levels following radiotherapy usually occurs in the first 2 years but GH levels may continue to fall for many years after therapy. Selected patients may also undergo stereotactic radiosurgery but this procedure is only performed at a few centres.

Pituitary apoplexy

Definition of pituitary apoplexy

Pituitary apoplexy is infarction of the pituitary gland, via haemorrhage or ischaemia, with resulting hypopituitarism. The clinical syndrome is characterized by sudden-onset headache, vomiting, visual impairment, and decreased consciousness. This may be accompanied by neurological symptoms involving the second, third, fourth, and sixth cranial nerves. Classical pituitary apoplexy is a medical emergency. Prompt diagnosis and hydrocortisone administration may be life-saving. Referral should be made to a multidisciplinary team consisting of (amongst others) a neurosurgeon and an endocrinologist.

Aetiology of pituitary apoplexy

Apoplexy may occur in patients with pituitary adenomas, most commonly with macroadenomas. It occurs when bleeding into a necrotic area of a pituitary tumour which has outgrown its blood supply causes infarction. Other factors which predispose to pituitary apoplexy include radiation therapy, diabetes mellitus, anticoagulant therapy, reduced intracranial pressure, major surgery, and post-partum haemorrhage (Sheehan's syndrome, where the enlarged post-partum pituitary gland is infarcted following severe hypotension from blood loss).

Typical symptoms of pituitary apoplexy, and less common symptoms

Consider pituitary apoplexy in all patients who have severe headache and:

- subarachnoid haemorrhage and meningitis have been excluded
- the headache is of sudden onset (may be retro-orbital), with vomiting and meningism
- visual disturbance and cranial nerve palsies (neuro-ophthalmic symptoms) are present; most commonly, bitemporal hemianopia; at worst, blindness
- there are preexisting pituitary tumours
- hypopituitarism is present, with symptoms similar to those of target organ insufficiency; this may be clinically apparent

If blood bursts through the sellar diaphragm, subarachnoid haemorrhage will develop.

Demographics of pituitary apoplexy

Pituitary apoplexy is rare. In preexisting pituitary tumours, the risk is higher in macroadenomas and it has been reported that 0.6%–10.0% of such cases experience apoplexy. The average age of onset is 50 years. Men are more affected than women. The majority of the tumours involved in pituitary apoplexy are non-functioning adenomas. In most cases, the pituitary tumour was previously undiagnosed.

Natural history of pituitary apoplexy, and complications of the disease

After pituitary apoplexy, 80% of patients develop hypopituitarism; 60%–80% require hydrocortisone replacement, either permanently or when unwell; 50%–60% require thyroid hormone replacement; and 60%–80% of men require testosterone replacement therapy. GH deficiency is, however, a common problem in these patients and, if left untreated, may cause decreased muscle mass, obesity, and fatigue; in addition, 10%–25% of patients develop diabetes insipidus. Hypopituitarism should be identified, and patients informed, as glucocorticoid deficiency is a life-threatening complication.

Approach to diagnosing pituitary apoplexy

There must be a high index of suspicion to consider a diagnosis of pituitary apoplexy. Consider this diagnosis in patients with known pituitary tumours; patients who have had major surgery, such as a coronary artery bypass; patients who are on anticoagulation; patients who have undergone radiation therapy to the pituitary; patients with a traumatic brain injury; and patients who are pregnant or on oestrogen treatment. In addition, hormone stimulation tests have been reported to provoke apoplexy.

In the acute situation with sudden-onset headache, haemodynamic stability must be maintained through supportive means (fluids and steroids), and urgent tests for urea, creatinine, renal function, liver function, clotting, random serum cortisol, thyroid-stimulating hormone (TSH), free thyroxine (FT4), prolactin, IGF-1, LH, FSH, testosterone (men), and oestradiol (women), as well as a full blood count, are to be sent. MRI pituitary are the imaging of choice. Subarachnoid haemorrhage and meningitis must be excluded. Depending on the severity of illness, admission to a high-dependency unit may be indicated.

Other diagnoses that should be considered aside from pituitary apoplexy

Other diagnoses that should be considered aside from pituitary apoplexy are:

- subarachnoid haemorrhage
- bacterial/viral meningitis
- brainstem infarction
- cavernous sinus thrombosis

'Gold-standard' diagnostic tests for pituitary apoplexy

'Gold-standard' diagnostic tests for apoplexy in the anterior pituitary

The following are the gold-standard diagnostic tests for apoplexy in the anterior pituitary:

- basal hormones:
  - LH
  - FSH
  - 9 a.m. testosterone
  - oestradiol
  - TSH
  - FT4
  - 9 a.m. cortisol
  - prolactin
  - IGF-1
  - ACTH; deficiency leads to a low glomerular filtration rate (an inability to excrete water load will mask diabetes insipidus); replace corticotropic function first and then TSH
- further dynamic testing if indicated (e.g. insulin tolerance test (ITT))
- MRI pituitary

'Gold-standard' diagnostic tests for apoplexy in the posterior pituitary

The gold-standard diagnostic tests for apoplexy in the posterior pituitary are paired urine and plasma osmolalities at baseline (usually enough).

Acceptable diagnostic alternatives to the gold-standard tests for pituitary apoplexy

The following are acceptable diagnostic alternatives to the gold-standard diagnostic tests for pituitary apoplexy:

- a glucagon test (if ITT is contraindicated)
- CT (if MRI pituitary is contraindicated)

Other relevant investigations for pituitary apoplexy

The following tests may be used if infiltration of the pituitary is suspected and further investigation is needed:

- angiotensin-converting enzyme levels (serum and CSF; to exclude sarcoidosis)
- ferritin level (to exclude haemochromatosis)
- pituitary biopsy

Prognosis of pituitary apoplexy, and how to estimate it

In a large case series, mortality in pituitary apoplexy was thought to be 1.6% overall, and 1.9% in those requiring pituitary surgery. If pituitary apoplexy is untreated, there is an increased mortality from hypopituitarism. Before the introduction of steroid replacement, mortality was 50%.

Treatment of pituitary apoplexy, and its effectiveness

Empirical steroids are indicated in the treatment of pituitary apoplexy if there is haemodynamic instability, altered consciousness, reduced visual acuity, and severe visual field defects. In adults administer a 100 mg intramuscular bolus of hydrocortisone and then 50–100 mg 6 hourly intramuscular injections; alternatively, administer a 100–200 mg IV bolus and then an IV infusion of 2–4 mg/hour. Ideally, blood samples for basal anterior pituitary blood tests should be taken urgently for analysis; the tests should include random serum cortisol, TSH, FT4, prolactin, IGF-1, LH, FSH, testosterone (men), and oestradiol (women).

A bedside assessment of visual acuity and fields should be made, with further neuro-ophthalmic assessment when the patient is stable. CT brain (+/− lumbar puncture) to exclude subarachnoid haemorrhage and meningitis should be undertaken, if not done already. The imaging of choice is an MRI of the pituitary and will confirm diagnosis in 90%. After emergency care, refer to a joint neurosurgical/endocrine team for definitive management and arrange a formal visual field assessment when the patient is stable, preferably within 24 hours. Where visual acuity and field defects occur, early surgery (trans-sphenoidal hypophysectomy) significantly improves the neuro-ophthalmic outcome.

Consider surgery if any of the following is present:

- severely reduced visual acuity
- severe, persistent visual field defects
- a deteriorating level of consciousness

If urgent empirical steroids are not indicated, consider treatment if the 9 a.m. serum cortisol is <400–500nmol/L (depending on assay).

Repeat pituitary and visual assessments are required at 4–6 weeks post apoplexy. Long-term follow-up 6–12 monthly is required to optimize hormone replacement and monitor tumour progression or recurrence.

Further Reading

Baldeweg SE, Vanderpump M, Drake W, et al. Society for Endocrinology Endocrine Emergency Guidance: Emergency management of pituitary apoplexy in adult patients. *Endocr Connect* 2016; 5: G12–G15.

Katznelson L, Laws ER Jr, Melmed S, et al. Acromegaly: An Endocrine Society clinical practice guideline. *J Clin Endocrinol Metab* 2014; 99: 3933–51.

Wong A, Eloy JA, Couldwell WT, et al. Update on prolactinomas. Part 1: Clinical manifestations and diagnostic challenges. *J Clin Neurosci* 2015; 22: 1562–7.

Wong A, Eloy JA, Couldwell WT, et al. Update on prolactinomas. Part 2: Treatment and management strategies. *J Clin Neurosci* 2015; 22: 1568–74.

PART 8

Gastrointestinal disorders

Introduction

The gastrointestinal (GI) system accomplishes the tasks of digestion, absorption of nutritional compounds, and removal of waste products. This is a complex process that involves the hollow GI tract and the hepatic, pancreatic, and biliary systems. Symptoms and signs of disease relate directly to the digestive and/or absorptive processes they interrupt.

In this section, we will follow the progress of food through the GI tract.

Swallowing

There is first an oral and then a pharyngeal phase of swallowing. When food enters the mouth, mastication helps break down the bolus while mixing liquids, solids, and saliva, which helps lubricate and dissolve solid boluses. Taste sensation is carried by afferent fibres from the anterior two-thirds of the tongue (Cranial nerve (CN) VII), the posterior third of the tongue (CN IX), and the epiglottis (CN X); these fibres terminate in the nucleus tractus solitarius. When the bolus is a suitable size for swallowing, it is voluntarily moved to the back of the oral cavity by the tongue. The tongue then presses its anterior, superior aspect against the hard palate to prevent the bolus from entering the anterior part of the oral cavity, and creates a pressure wave which propels the bolus into the oropharynx as the soft palate raises. The posterior dorsum of the tongue then presses against the soft palate, thus preventing the bolus from re-entering the oral cavity.

The pharyngeal phase of swallowing transports the bolus through the pharynx and upper oesophageal sphincter, while protecting the airway. The soft palate raises to seal off the nasopharynx; the vocal cords and arytenoids adduct; and the epiglottis swings down to protect the laryngeal vestibule. In addition, the larynx and hyoid bone move forwards and upwards to move the larynx under the tongue and out of the path of the bolus. Overall, the bolus moves through the oropharynx at a velocity of 20–40 cm/s, and usually ~15 ml of air is swallowed with the bolus. At rest, the upper oesophageal sphincter is naturally closed, and prevents air from entering the oesophagus during respiration. However, the pressure reduces during sleep and anaesthesia. The upper oesophageal sphincter opens due to a reduction in tone plus traction from associated muscles, allowing the bolus to pass through.

The muscles involved in the initiation of swallowing are all striated, while the lower oesophageal muscles are non-striated. CN V and VII are required for mastication, while movement of the tongue requires CN XII, and the overall swallowing process requires further input from CN IX, X, XI, and XII. Acetylcholine is the major neurotransmitter.

Oesophagus

The oesophagus lies behind the trachea and enters the abdominal cavity through an opening in the diaphragm, the oesophageal hiatus. The upper third is composed of striated muscle, and peristalsis is controlled by parasympathetic nerves originating from the vagus nerve. The lower two-thirds is composed of smooth muscle and is innervated by the myenteric plexus, which lies between the inner circular and outer longitudinal muscle layers. There is also input from Meissner's plexus within the submucosa.

Peristalsis within the oesophagus, alongside the natural effect of gravity, transports boluses from the upper oesophagus into the stomach, through the lower oesophageal sphincter. Peristalsis involves lumen-occluding contractions that travel the oesophagus at ~4 cm/s,

caused by alternating, vagally controlled inhibition and excitation. Secondary peristalsis (peristalsis without the swallowing reflex, pharyngeal contractions, or relaxation of the upper oesophageal sphincter) clears food debris from the oesophagus. Tertiary contractions are simultaneous (non-propagated) contractions, of which the relevance is not known. The basal resting tone of the lower oesophageal sphincter is high, and on manometry is seen as a high-pressure zone, which relaxes within 2 s of swallowing, to allow the bolus into the stomach.

Belching

During belching, gas passes from the stomach into the oesophagus, causing oesophageal distension. This distension causes neurally mediated reflex relaxation, which, along with the pressure of the gas, causes relaxation of the upper oesophageal sphincter and release of the gas.

Reflux events

Transient relaxations of the lower oesophageal sphincter are often seen and, although not all are associated with reflux events, most reflux episodes occur during these relaxations. Distension of the oesophagus from liquid occurs much more slowly than in belching, resulting in contraction of the upper oesophageal sphincter and thus preventing fluid from entering the pharynx and causing aspiration.

Vomiting

During vomiting, the upper oesophageal sphincter relaxes and is pulled open by suprahyoid muscles, and the vocal cords actively close to prevent aspiration.

Stomach

The stomach is divided into four sections: the cardia, the fundus, the body, and the antrum. The oesophageal and pyloric sphincters keep the contents of the stomach contained. The stomach receives its blood supply from several sources:

- the right gastric artery (supplies the inferior part of the lesser curvature)
- the left gastric artery (supplies the superior part of the lesser curvature, and the cardia)
- the right gastroepiploic artery (supplies the inferior part of the greater curvature)
- the left gastroepiploic artery (supplies the superior part of the greater curvature)
- the short gastric artery (supplies the fundus and the upper portion of the greater curvature)

The layers of the stomach are found throughout all luminal surfaces of the GI tract, and are shown in Table 193.1.

The stomach has three main functions:

- to store food and release it into the duodenum at a slow steady rate
- to 'churn' food, aiding its breakdown by gastric acid and enzymes
- to kill ingested pathogens

As digestive products enter the stomach and cause distension of the antrum, G-cells release gastrin, which stimulates the release of hydrochloric acid. This acid aids in killing bacteria, and initiates protein digestion by catalysing the conversion of pepsinogen to pepsin, which is a protease. Gastrin stimulates the release of pepsinogen from chief cells. Intrinsic factor is produced by parietal cells, and binds to dietary hydroxocobalamin (vitamin B_{12}), preventing its degradation, and aiding its absorption in the ileum. The production of gut hormones is controlled by the autonomic nervous system; details of

Table 193.1 Layers of the gastrointestinal tract

Mucosa	This layer is exposed to luminal contents; there are three layers within the mucosa: • epithelium • lamina propria (contains connective tissue and glands) • muscularis mucosa
Submucosa	This contains fibrous connective tissue, and Meissner's plexus
Muscularis externa	This muscular layer has two layers throughout the gastrointestinal tract: the inner circular layer and the outer longitudinal layer; Auerbach's plexus lies between these layers; the stomach has an additional inner oblique layer, which helps create motion and churn food
Serosa	This is a connective tissue layer, continuous with the peritoneum

this are listed in Table 193.2. Absorption is not one of the major roles of the stomach, although the stomach does absorb some lipid-soluble compounds, such as caffeine, alcohol, and aspirin.

Duodenum

The duodenum is the first part of the small intestine. It is approximately 25 cm long, and connects the stomach to the jejunum, ending at the ligament of Treitz. It is largely retroperitoneal. The duodenum is C-shaped, and is divided into four parts:

• the first part is the duodenal bulb, which passes laterally, superiorly, and posteriorly, before making a sharp downward turn into the second part
• the second part passes downwards, and contains the ampulla of Vater, where the pancreatic duct and common bile duct connect to the GI tract
• the third part passes transversely to the left, crossing the aorta and vertebrae
• the fourth part terminates at the duodenojejunal flexure, which is surrounded by a peritoneal fold called the ligament of Treitz

The duodenum represents the join between the embryological foregut and midgut, with the transition point at the level of the ampulla of Vater. As such, it has two blood supplies: the foregut is supplied by the gastroduodenal artery and its branch, the superior pancreaticoduodenal artery, and the midgut is supplied by the superior mesenteric artery and its branch, the inferior pancreaticoduodenal artery.

The duodenum is responsible for digestion and controls the rate of emptying food from the stomach. As food enters the duodenum, fat and acid stimulate the release of secretin and cholecystokinin from duodenal epithelial cells. These hormones stimulate the gallbladder and liver to release bile, and the pancreas to release bicarbonate and digestive enzymes. These digestive enzymes include trypsin (breaks down proteins), lipase (breaks down fat), and amylase (breaks down carbohydrates). The bicarbonate neutralizes gastric acid, and Brunner's glands release mucus.

Jejunum and ileum

The jejunum is approximately 2.5 m long, and the ileum is 3–4 m long; overall, the small intestine is approximately 5–7 m long. The mucosal layer of the small intestine is permanently folded (plicae circulares), with further finger-like projections of the mucosa, and microvilli projections on the epithelial cells. Overall, this increases the absorptive surface area of the small intestine by 500-fold, to approximately 250 m². Each villus has a blood supply which transports nutrients to appropriate sites throughout the body. Most of the nutrients are absorbed in the jejunum, with the following exceptions:

• vitamin B_{12} and bile salts are absorbed in the terminal ileum
• water and lipids are absorbed throughout the ileum
• iron is absorbed in the duodenum

The GI tract secretes approximately 8 l of fluid per day: 1–1.5 l of saliva, 2–3 l of stomach secretions, 2 l of pancreaticobiliary secretions, and 2 l of small intestinal secretions. However, the small intestine reabsorbs the majority of this fluid, so only ~1 l enters the colon. Any pathological process that affects this absorptive process (e.g. cholera) can lead to excess fluid loss. Water absorption is passive, but other electrolytes (e.g. sodium, chloride) have both active and passive transport mechanisms. The nutritional role of the small intestine is clearly affected by conditions affecting the small bowel (e.g. coeliac disease, Crohn's disease), and these can lead to malnutrition.

Pancreas

The pancreas is an organ that lies beneath the stomach, and secretes hormones and enzymes into the GI tract via the pancreatic duct. It is divided into the head (from which extends the uncinate process), neck, tail, and body and sits in the retroperitoneum. The blood supply is from the superior and inferior pancreaticoduodenal arteries and the splenic artery. The pancreas is both an endocrine gland and an exocrine gland. Islets of Langerhans produce hormones: alpha cells secrete glucagon, beta cells produce insulin, delta cells secrete somatostatin, and PP cells secrete pancreatic polypeptide. Table 193.2 provides information about these hormones. Acinar cells produce

Table 193.2 Gut hormones

Hormone	Site of production	Stimulus for secretion	Mode of action
Gastrin	G-cells in the stomach	Distension of the antrum and duodenum; pancreas	Increases secretion of gastric acid, pepsinogen, and intrinsic factor
Cholecystokinin	Duodenum	Acid and fat entering the duodenum	Release of bile; decreases gastric emptying; increases release of pancreatic juice; mediates satiety
Secretin	Duodenum	Low pH from acid entering the duodenum	Stimulates release of pancreatic enzymes, bile, insulin, pepsin, glucagon, pancreatic polypeptide, and somatostatin; stimulates water and bicarbonate release from Brunner's glands; inhibits gastrin release
Gastric inhibitory peptide	Duodenum and jejunum	Glucose in the duodenum	Decreases gastric acid and motility; increases insulin secretion
Somatostatin	Delta cells, islets of Langerhans, stomach, intestine		Inhibitory hormone; inhibits release of gastrin, cholecystokinin, secretin, motilin, vasoactive intestinal polypeptide, gastric inhibitory peptide, enteroglucagon, insulin, glucagon, and pancreatic enzymes; decreases gastric emptying
Pancreatic polypeptide	PP cells, islets of Langerhans	Protein meal; fasting; exercise; hypoglycaemia	Stimulates release of pancreatic hormones and enzymes
Glucagon	Alpha cells, islets of Langerhans	Hypoglycaemia, catecholamines, cholecystokinin	Stimulates liver to convert glycogen into glucose
Insulin	Beta cells, islets of Langerhans	Protein and glucose ingestion	Stimulates glucose absorption, and conversion into glycogen
Vasoactive intestinal polypeptide	Brain, gut, pancreas		Causes smooth muscle relaxation; stimulates water and electrolyte secretion; inhibits gastric acid secretion

digestive enzymes; these cells are regulated by hormones and via the sympathetic and parasympathetic innervation.

Biliary tree

The biliary tree provides the pathway by which bile secreted by the liver reaches the duodenum. The bile first travels from the bile canaliculi to the canals of Hering and then to the bile ductules (in portal tracts). From there, it goes to the intra-hepatic bile ducts and then to the left and right hepatic ducts, which join to form the common hepatic duct. This joins the cystic duct to form the common bile duct, which then joins the pancreatic duct. From there, the bile travels to the ampulla of Vater and then to the duodenum. The gallbladder is connected to the common bile duct via the cystic duct, and acts as a reservoir for bile when the bile does not need to be delivered into the duodenum.

Bile has three main functions:

- to increase the solubility of cholesterol, fats, and fat-soluble vitamins and aid in their absorption
- to stimulate the secretion of water, to help move the contents along
- to aid the excretion of drugs and other waste products

The term 'enterohepatic circulation' refers to the way bile salts are reabsorbed in the terminal ileum, extracted by the liver, and then resecreted into bile. Bile salts are recirculated about 10–12 times per day.

Colon

The colon is the most caudal part of the GI tract. It starts at the caecum and can be divided into the following regions: ascending, transverse, descending, and sigmoid. The ascending colon and the proximal two-thirds of the transverse colon are supplied by the superior mesenteric artery, and the rest of the transverse colon, the descending colon, and the sigmoid colon are supplied by the inferior mesenteric artery. The main functions of the colon are:

- absorbing water
- storing waste
- absorbing some vitamins (e.g. vitamin K)

As chyme passes into the colon, most of the water is removed, and the chyme is mixed with bacteria and mucus to become faeces. Some fibre is broken down by bacteria to create butyrate, acetate, and propionate, which provide some nourishment for the mucosal lining.

Rectum and anus

The rectum acts as a reservoir for faeces. As the rectum becomes full, stretch receptors initiate the desire to defaecate; the increase in intra-rectal pressure forces the faecal matter into the anal canal, and peristaltic waves propel the faeces out of the body. The anus has an internal and external sphincter, with the external sphincter remaining in a constant state of tonic contraction. The rectum receives a blood supply from the rectal arteries.

Further Reading

Guyton AC and Hall J. *Textbook of Physiology*, 2010. Saunders Elsevier.
Johnson, LR. *Gastrointestinal Physiology* (8th edition), 2013. Elsevier Mosby.

194 Diagnosis in suspected gastrointestinal disease

Satish Keshav and Alexandra Kent

Symptoms of suspected gastrointestinal disease

The most frequent presenting complaints suggesting gastrointestinal disease are diarrhoea, constipation, nausea, vomiting, anorexia, and abdominal pain, which can localize to any of the quadrants of the abdomen observed from the front. Loss of weight is a feature of some gastrointestinal disease, and general symptoms such as fever, malaise, and arthralgia may also occur. According to the National Institute for Health and Care Excellence (NICE), alarm symptoms include unintentional weight loss, dysphagia, chronic gastrointestinal bleeding, iron deficiency anaemia, an abdominal mass, and/or persistent vomiting.

The characteristics of diarrhoea and vomiting are important: for instance, is the stool loose, liquid, fatty, or blood stained? Urgency in the need to defaecate is characteristic of pathological bowel movements. Steatorrhoea, with the passage of pale, floating, malodorous stool suggests malabsorption, which can arise from pancreatic insufficiency and coeliac disease, amongst other causes. Watery diarrhoea is usually due to hypersecretion, and can be caused by viral, parasitic, or bacterial infection; toxins; laxatives ingested deliberately or inadvertently; and hormonal excess, for example, from thyrotoxicosis or neuroendocrine tumours. Bloody stools usually indicate inflammatory, vascular, or neoplastic disease such as bacterial dysentery, inflammatory bowel disease, neoplasia, and so on. Haematemesis or vomiting of coffee grounds is a feature of peptic ulcer disease and oesophageal varices, which are major causes for emergency presentation in gastroenterology.

Abdominal pain is a common symptom and, when it is chronic, associated with bloating of the abdomen, and altered bowel habit; it is a diagnostic criterion for irritable bowel syndrome. Typically, abdominal pain is relieved by defaecation in irritable bowel syndrome. Pain felt in the epigastrium or left upper quadrant may indicate gastric or duodenal disease. Pain in the right upper quadrant may be associated with hepatobiliary disease. Epigastric pain that radiates through to the back may indicate a penetrating peptic ulcer or pancreatic disease. Periumbilical pain may indicate disease in any part of the midgut, that is, any structure from the duodenum to the splenic flexure of the colon. Pain in the right lower quadrant may arise from structures such as the appendix or the caecum, and pain in the left lower quadrant suggests pathology in the sigmoid colon, such as diverticulitis.

Other important symptoms include dysphagia and odynophagia, acid reflux, dyspepsia, rectal bleeding, and difficulties with defaecation. Conversely, many serious gastrointestinal diseases can remain asymptomatic, and are only suspected because of abnormal tests indicating, for example, anaemia or elevated inflammatory markers, or when complications occur.

Family history is important because many gastrointestinal conditions have genetic or familial associations. These include colorectal cancer, inflammatory bowel disease, and coeliac disease.

Reassurance is the key to the management of most benign conditions. However, patients have access to the internet and often attend the outpatient clinic with preconceived ideas about their underlying diagnosis. Identifying a patient's specific concern is vital to preventing recurrent hospital attendances. Discussing these concerns with the patient will often lead to a more honest portrayal of their symptoms, and prevents the patient purely presenting the symptoms that they feel will lead to what they consider to be the necessary investigation.

Signs of suspected gastrointestinal disease

General examination is as important in gastroenterology as in all specialities. Particular attention must be paid to:

Colour: Pallor and jaundice are important.
Weight: Is the patient underweight for height? Has their weight changed?
Evidence of being systemically unwell: Tachycardia, fever, and hypotension occur in varying combinations in intra-abdominal sepsis, inflammation, and haemorrhage.
Stigmata of chronic liver disease: clubbing, Dupuytren's contracture, loss of body hair, gynaecomastia, and spider naevi.
Finger clubbing: Finger clubbing is also a feature of inflammatory bowel disease.

Various unusual rashes, such as acanthosis nigricans, are associated with gastrointestinal malignancy. Carcinoid syndrome is characterized by flushing and sclerosis of the skin.

Abdominal examination is used to detect an enlarged liver or spleen, ascites, tumours, and inflammatory masses. Nausea, vomiting, and constipation may arise from an incarcerated hernia, and examination for herniae is part of the gastroenterological assessment. Examination of the perineum may show signs of perineal Crohn's disease, or excoriation of the anal skin from chronic diarrhoea. Digital rectal examination is used to detect distal rectal masses, and proctoscopy and sigmoidoscopy, performed at the bedside, can be used to detect haemorrhoids, fissures, and rectal inflammation. Mucosal biopsies of the rectum can be obtained at the same time.

Examination of the stool is frequently helpful—it is an essential part of the evaluation when the patient presents with reported melaena or haematemesis, and blood-stained faeces can indicate the presence of neoplasia or inflammation in the colon and rectum.

Tests for suspected gastrointestinal disease

Blood tests

Routine test results will usually be available to the physician in secondary care, and are easily obtained in primary care. These are frequently very helpful.

Haematology

Anaemia may be the earliest and only indicator of gastrointestinal disease, particularly in non-menstruating individuals with no other comorbidity. Iron deficiency can be caused by reduced absorption in coeliac disease and inflammatory bowel disease, or by intestinal bleeding in peptic ulcer disease, excessive use of NSAIDs, and intestinal neoplasia. For these reasons, unexplained iron deficiency should prompt further gastrointestinal investigation. Iron deficiency should be suspected in patients with microcytosis, and the most helpful further test is to determine the ferritin level. Hypoferritaemia indicates iron deficiency. The ferritin may, however, be normal or even slightly elevated in iron-deficient patients with an inflammatory condition, because increased ferritin production is a feature of the hepatic acute phase response. In these cases, more careful examination of the full blood count, the transferrin level, and the clinical context is necessary.

In acute gastrointestinal haemorrhage, of course, the haemoglobin level will not be reduced immediately while bleeding is occurring.

Rather, the initially normal haemoglobin level is seen to fall in the subsequent hours as the circulating volume is replenished. Therefore, in such cases, the best guide to the extent of blood loss is the haemodynamic assessment of pulse and blood pressure rather than the full blood count.

Vitamin B$_{12}$ and folate levels are easily checked. Low vitamin B$_{12}$ may indicate atrophic gastritis (pernicious anaemia) or ileal disease such as Crohn's ileitis. Low folate levels may be due to dietary insufficiency or malabsorption, caused by, for instance, coeliac disease.

Biochemistry

Inflammatory markers such as C-reactive protein (CRP) and the erythrocyte sedimentation rate (ESR) are useful to detect inflammatory bowel disease, infection, pancreatitis, and so on. In ulcerative colitis, the CRP level and the ESR are typically normal or only slightly elevated whereas, in Crohn's disease, the CRP level is usually moderately elevated. Very high levels of CRP, usually accompanied by leucocytosis, typically indicate infection or severe systemic inflammation associated with, for example, acute pancreatitis, cholecystitis, or appendicitis. An elevated platelet count should make the clinician suspicious of intra-abdominal septic collections or an abscess.

Electrolyte disturbances may be seen in diarrhoeal diseases and vomiting, especially when severe or prolonged. Typical changes include hypokalaemia and hyponatraemia. Diarrhoea may cause a metabolic acidosis, while persistent vomiting of gastric contents may cause a metabolic alkalosis. In coeliac disease, there may be malabsorption of calcium and magnesium with hypocalcaemia, and hypophosphataemia due to secondary hyperparathyroidism. In upper gastrointestinal haemorrhage, the urea level may be elevated because of increased digestion, absorption, and degradation of blood protein, resulting in increased production of urea.

Liver dysfunction and disease produce characteristic alterations in the levels of circulating transaminases, indicating hepatocellular damage, and the alkaline phosphatase and gamma-glutamyl transferase enzymes, indicating biliary tract damage. Hyperbilirubinaemia may indicate hepatic or post-hepatic cholestasis. Reduced liver function is best demonstrated by a prolonged prothrombin time, provided that the patient is not deficient in vitamin K (vitamin K deficiency is an important cause of coagulopathy), or by a reduced serum albumin level, provided that this is not caused by poor nutrition, an exaggerated acute phase response, or loss of albumin from the intestine or kidneys (e.g. via protein-losing enteropathy or nephritic syndrome). In hepatic encephalopathy, serum ammonia levels may be elevated. However, ammonia levels only approximately relate to clinical severity and, in chronic liver disease, can be totally misleading.

Stool samples can be tested for excessive fat, indicating malabsorption, and for levels of pancreatic elastase, which are reduced in cases of pancreatic insufficiency.

Serology

Specific blood tests can be used to provide near-diagnostic information. These include antibodies to tissue transglutaminase, which indicate coeliac disease, anti-mitochondrial antibodies, which indicate primary biliary cholangitis, and antibody tests for viral hepatitis. The tumour markers carcinoembryonic antigen, alpha-fetoprotein, and CA-19-9 are associated, respectively, with colon, liver, and pancreatic cancer, although they are not diagnostic and can only be used to monitor progress.

Endoscopy

Endoscopy of the upper and lower gastrointestinal tract is a direct and highly accurate means of diagnosing gastrointestinal disease. Biopsies taken at the time of endoscopy can be used to detect helicobacter infection, coeliac disease, various gastrointestinal infections, cancer, and inflammatory bowel disease. Endoscopy is usually performed by gastroenterologists, and the specific test should be discussed in advance. Endoscopy can also be used therapeutically, for example to control bleeding from a peptic ulcer or to remove a colonic polyp. The reach of endoscopy is increasing, for example, with the development of enteroscopy, biliary endoscopy, and wireless capsule endoscopy.

Radiology

Radiological examination of the gastrointestinal tract, liver, and pancreas is also expanding rapidly. Barium swallow is an important modality used to study the function of the oesophagus, although upper endoscopy has almost completely replaced barium meals. Small bowel enema and small bowel follow-through allow visualization of the small intestine, and are used particularly for detection of strictures and diverticula rather than for evaluation of the mucosal surface. Colonic polyps and cancer can be detected without the need for colonoscopy, using CT scanning with or without tagging of faeces with radio-opaque material, and gas distention of the lumen. Ultrasound scanning of the liver is highly sensitive to gallstones and fatty infiltration of the liver. The liver and the biliary tract are also well visualized with MRI.

Histopathology

Liver biopsy, and biopsy and histological examination of tumours, are critically important diagnostic tests. A liver biopsy can be performed percutaneously, using ultrasound guidance, or via the jugular vein (transjugular liver biopsy).

Microbiology

Examination of stool and urine may also help the diagnosis. Diarrhoea is frequently due to microorganisms such as viruses, parasites, and bacteria that can be detected by microscopy and culture, for instance. Antibiotic-associated diarrhoea may be caused by toxin-expressing *Clostridium difficile* strains, and the toxin can be detected in the stool by ELISA. Porphyria is a rare cause of recurrent abdominal pain, and a urine sample is used to detect excessive porphyrin excretion.

Summary

Diagnosis in gastroenterology should still proceed along standard lines, with an emphasis on history and examination, and attention to simple tests such as the full blood count. Specific diagnoses can be reliably established by more specialized tests, including serology, endoscopy, radiology, histopathology, and microbiology. However, it is critically important that clinical judgement is used in deciding which tests to perform, and when and how to interpret the results in the context of the patient's presentation.

Further Reading

Emmanuel A and Inns S (eds). *Lecture Notes: Gastroenterology and Hepatology*. 2010. Wiley Blackwell.

Warrell DA, Cox TM, and Firth JD. *Oxford Textbook of Medicine* (5th edition). 2010. Oxford University Press.

195 Investigation in gastrointestinal disease

Satish Keshav and Alexandra Kent

Blood tests

Blood tests used for investigation in gastrointestinal disease include a full blood count, haematinics tests, and tests for biochemistry, immunology, and microbiology.

Full blood count

Haemoglobin

Haemoglobin is reduced in occult blood loss and malabsorption. However, it may remain normal for some time even in iron, vitamin B_{12}, or folate deficiency and in acute haemorrhage.

White-cell count

The white-cell count is raised in infection. It is also raised in patients taking steroids (e.g. for inflammatory bowel disease (IBD)).

Platelets

The platelet level is raised in inflammatory disorders (e.g. IBD).

Mean corpuscular volume

The mean corpuscular volume is a measure of the average red blood cell volume; it differentiates between microcytic (iron deficiency) and macrocytic (B_{12} and folate deficiency) anaemia and is normal in acute blood loss.

Haematinics tests

Serum iron

Serum iron measures circulating iron bound to transferrin; iron is predominantly absorbed in the duodenum and upper jejunum. The results of this test are highly variable diurnally and in relation to meals and so of little clinical use.

Transferrin

Transferrin is a circulating protein that transports iron around the body. It is high in iron-deficiency anaemia due to the liver producing more in order to maximize use of available iron. It is low in anaemia of chronic disease.

Transferrin saturation is the ratio of serum iron and total iron-binding capacity (TIBC). It is low in iron-deficiency anaemia, and normal in anaemia of chronic disease. TIBC measures the bloods capacity to bind iron and transferrin. It is high in iron-deficiency anaemia, and low in anaemia of chronic disease.

Vitamin B_{12}

Vitamin B_{12} levels indicate the status of the stomach, the pancreas, and the ileum. First, proteases released by the exocrine pancreas digest R-proteins to release vitamin B_{12}. In order to be absorbed, vitamin B_{12} must first bind intrinsic factor, which is produced by parietal cells in the stomach. This complex is then absorbed in the terminal ileum. Therefore, B_{12} absorption requires that the stomach, exocrine pancreas, and terminal ileum be intact.

Folate

Folate is absorbed in the proximal jejunum and its status can be indicated by folate levels. Folate deficiency can also occur in small bowel disease such as coeliac disease, and in diets deficient in green leafy vegetables. Conversely, small bowel bacterial overgrowth may result in elevated folate concentrations, because bacteria produce folic acid.

Biochemistry

Calcium

Calcium absorption occurs mainly in the proximal small intestine. Calcium levels are reduced in vitamin D deficiency and coeliac disease.

Magnesium

Magnesium is absorbed from the upper small intestine. Its absorption is hindered by the presence of calcium, alcohol, protein, phosphates, or fats. Magnesium levels are also low in short-bowel syndrome.

Albumin

Albumin levels can be reduced via protein-losing enteropathy, due to an increase in its loss from the gastrointestinal tract. It can also be reduced in inflammatory states, as it is a negative acute phase protein and so is downregulated during inflammation, and in nutritional deficiency. It is produced by the liver; therefore, in severe liver failure, albumin levels fall.

Glucose

Hypoglycaemia can be a feature of acute liver failure. Chronic pancreatitis may be associated with diabetes mellitus and hyperglycaemia. In addition, diabetes mellitus is associated with autonomic neuropathy, which can manifest as gastroparesis and chronic diarrhoea; however, these usually occur in patients with a long-standing history of diabetes and associated complications.

Zinc and selenium

Zinc and selenium are trace elements absorbed by the small intestine (jejunum). They are usually only reduced in malnutrition/malabsorption.

Thyroid function

Thyroid dysfunction can be associated with diarrhoea (hyperthyroidism) and constipation (hypothyroidism).
Cortisol levels and the Synacthen test
Addison's disease can present with weight loss and diarrhoea.

Immunology

Antibodies positive in coeliac disease include anti-gliadin antibody, anti-endomysial antibody, anti-reticulin antibody, and anti-tissue transglutaminase. IgA levels should also be checked, as 2% of patients with coeliac disease have IgA deficiency.

Microbiology

Blood serum can be used for specific bacterial serology (e.g. salmonella, brucella, proteus, giardia, and campylobacter). *Helicobacter pylori* serology confirms exposure to the bacteria, and titres will reduce following eradication therapy. Table 195.1 lists available tests for helicobacter.

Stool investigations

Stool samples for microscopy and culture are the most important investigation for acute diarrhoea. It is important to state on the request form details regarding risk factors, as different bacteria require selective culture medium. Furthermore it is important to specify if testing for *Clostridium difficile* is required. If the patient has travelled abroad it is also important to send stool samples for ova, cysts, and parasites. If the stool sample is not received by the microbiologist within 2 hours it should be refrigerated at below 4°C.

Stool samples are also useful when assessing fat malabsorption. Previously, the laboratory required a 3-day collection to assess abnormal faecal fat content, but nowadays most laboratories can perform this test on a single sample. Faecal elastase is a simple and non-invasive method for detecting pancreatic exocrine insufficiency and is performed on a single stool sample.

Radiology

Abdominal plain X-ray

Normally, an abdominal plain X-ray (AXR) is taken in a supine position, although an erect AXR gives the added benefit of visualizing air–fluid levels. Normally, the gastric gas bubble is seen in the left upper quadrant, and air is seen through the large bowel. The large bowel is normally in the periphery of the film, has a diameter ≤5 cm, and has haustra that only partially cross the bowel wall. The small bowel sits centrally and should have a diameter ≤3 cm, with valvulae conniventes that traverse the whole bowel wall. The caecum may have a greater diameter (up to 9 cm). There should not be air in the biliary tree unless the patient has recently undergone endoscopic retrograde cholangiopancreatography (ERCP). Gas outside the bowel is invariably abnormal, and is best seen under the right diaphragm on a supine film. Faecal matter has a mottled appearance. Colitis can have a characteristic appearance on the AXR, with narrowing, loss of haustrations, and thumbprinting. Calcium is radiolucent and may be identified in blood vessels (in calcified vessels), the pancreas (in chronic pancreatitis), gallstones, the kidneys (renal calculi or nephrocalcinosis), and the pelvis. Usually, you can see the outline of soft tissues and organs.

The AXR is an excellent tool for rapid diagnosis in support of clinical findings, including emergency conditions such as bowel perforation, chronic pancreatitis, and colitis, as well as benign conditions such as constipation.

Barium studies

Barium studies utilize barium, which is radiolucent and coats the bowel lining. The integrity of the bowel wall can then be seen on plain AXR. It can be used to look at the oesophagus (via a barium swallow), the stomach (via a barium meal), the small bowel (via barium follow-through or enteroclysis), or the colon (via a barium enema). Contrast studies permit the detection of mucosal abnormalities, including diverticulosis, dilation, polyps, and cancers. Air can be instilled into the colon along with the barium contrast medium to enhance and further define structures of the large bowel and rectum. Polyps and small cancers are more readily found using this method, which is called a double-contrast barium enema. A barium study may also provide information about gastrointestinal motility (e.g. delayed transit, nutcracker oesophagus, etc.). Barium enemas are used far less commonly now, given the greater availability of colonoscopy and CT pneumocolon, which are invariably more detailed. Barium is an irritant to the mediastinum and the peritoneum so, in cases of possible perforation, alternative contrast media (e.g. Gastrografin®, Omnipaque®) are used.

Ultrasound

Ultrasound uses reflected sound waves to produce a picture of abdominal structures via a non-invasive and risk-free procedure. It can gain an image of all abdominal structures (unless prevented due to body habitus) and is particularly good at assessing:

- gallstones
- biliary dilatation +/− cause
- organ (liver, spleen, pancreas, kidneys) size, shape, and texture
- the presence of masses
- hepatic fatty infiltration
- blood flow (e.g. through the portal vein)
- renal stones
- cysts
- aortic aneurysms

It is also used for guiding biopsies and aspirations.

CT

CT combines multiple X-rays with a computer to generate three-dimensional images of the body. CT can provide far more information than plain X-rays, contrast radiography, or ultrasound can. There are multiple reasons to perform CT scans, but the commonest indications include:

- diagnosing or staging cancer
- infections (e.g. appendicitis, abscesses, or fluid collections)
- inflammatory processes (e.g. pancreatitis or pyelonephritis)
- kidney and bladder stones
- abdominal aortic aneurysms
- when combined with angiography, assessing for blood vessel diseases such as thrombosis and stenosis
- rapidly identifying trauma
- guiding therapeutic procedures such as biopsies and drain insertion

CT colonoscopy (CT pneumocolon) is widely used, especially in patients in whom a colonoscopy is felt to be high risk (e.g. patients with heart disease). Patients require bowel preparation beforehand with purgatives, and have carbon dioxide passed into the colon via a rectal tube. They then undergo a CT scan, which can be used to create three-dimensional endoluminal views of the colon. CT colonoscopies are generally less uncomfortable than conventional colonoscopy, and do not require sedation. However, they are less accurate for polyps <5 mm, and do not allow mucosal biopsies. Patients in whom it is not necessary to identify polyps and in whom a CT is being performed to purely exclude colorectal cancer (e.g. the elderly, who would not benefit from polyp surveillance) are usually offered a CT colon with oral contrast alone. This is referred to as 'faecal tagging', and aids the radiologist in excluding faecal residue as pathology.

MRI

MRI utilizes magnets and radio waves to create three-dimensional images, and has the added benefit of not requiring ionizing radiation to produce images. Gadolinium is routinely used as a contract agent and is usually well tolerated, with less risk of renal dysfunction, compared to the contrast agents used for CT scans.

The high-contrast resolution of MRI allows discrimination between two adjacent tissue types as well as between normal and abnormal structures, to a greater degree than in CT. This accounts for the common practice of performing an MRI in patients with equivocal CT findings. MRI is more sensitive and specific for the detection and characterization of small disease processes such as hepatocellular carcinoma and liver metastases. Phases of contrast enhancement allow hepatic lesions to be assessed when contrast is in the arterial, venous, and intermediate stages, aiding differentiation amongst vascular, benign, and malignant lesions in the liver. In much the same way, small pancreatic cancer is much better shown on MRI.

MR cholangiopancreatography allows clear images of the biliary system and is often used to clearly assess for biliary obstruction prior to referral for therapeutic ERCP. The uses of MRI are expanding rapidly, and MRI small bowel is often used to assess young people for small bowel Crohn's, while reducing their radiation exposure.

MRI can also combine images with physiological responses. For example, secretin-enhanced MRI pancreas involves the exocrine pancreas being stimulated to produce a fluid containing digestive enzymes which are released into the pancreatic duct.

Nuclear medicine

SeHCAT scan

In a SeHCAT scan, the patient takes, orally, a capsule containing radiolabelled bile salts (23-seleno-25-homo-tauro-cholate) and then undergoes a baseline scan. The scan is then repeated after 7 days. Normally, bile salts are reabsorbed as part of the enterohepatic circulation; a retention value less than 15% signifies bile salt malabsorption. This scan is not routinely used, as treatment with colestyramine (a bile acid sequestrant) is quicker and simpler. If patients have bile salt malabsorption, they will respond rapidly to colestyramine.

HIDA scan

A HIDA scan involves injection of a radioactive tracer (hydroxy-iminodiacetic acid (HIDA)) into the bloodstream, from which it is preferentially taken up by the liver and excreted into the bile. The HIDA then enters the biliary tree and the gallbladder and then exits into the small intestine. A HIDA scan is used to identify biliary obstruction; if the gallbladder is not filled, this suggests blockage of the cystic duct +/− cholecystitis. When used in conjunction with an injection of cholecystokinin, a gallbladder ejection fraction (the percent of bile expelled) can be calculated. When this ejection fraction is very low, gallbladder disease may be present.

Gastric emptying study

A gastric emptying study is used to calculate the rate at which the stomach empties, and can be used to diagnose gastroparesis. This study requires the ingestion of a meal containing a radioactive tracer. The test is completed in approximately 1–2 hours and is painless.

Endoscopy

Endoscopy is a minimally invasive procedure which uses a fibre-optic telescope passed into the body via the mouth or anus. It provides a video image, allowing direct inspection of the mucosal surface. The instrument also has additional channels and equipment, to allow passage of the following instruments:

- biopsy forceps: for mucosal biopsies
- snares: for removal of polyps, either alone ('cold') or with electro-diathermy ('hot')
- injection needles: a needle is passed through the endoscopic channel and attached to a syringe held by an assistant; it can be used to inject bleeding points with adrenaline, inject gastric varices with glue or thrombin, mark colonic cancers with dye (tattoo) to aid surgeons to identify cancer sites at the time of surgery, or inject beneath flat polyps ('lifting') to aid their removal and reduce the risk of perforation
- cauterization instruments: heat probes or argon plasma coagulation probes can be passed through the biopsy channel to apply heat to bleeding lesions
- endoscopic basket: used to pick up and remove objects (e.g. polyps, foreign objects) from the lumen
- endoloops: these are ligatures that can be placed on long polyp stalks to reduce bleeding from any vessels within the stalk

Oesophagogastroduodenoscopy

Oesophagogastroduodenoscopy (OGD) can be performed with local anaesthetic sprayed into the throat, or under conscious sedation with a short-acting benzodiazepine. In this procedure, the endoscope passes into the second part of the duodenum. There are many indications for OGD. The main side effects and risks include a sore throat, bleeding, and perforation, although the latter two are rare in diagnostic OGD and usually only seen when the OGD is accompanied by therapeutic procedures.

Lower GI endoscopy

A flexible sigmoidoscopy can pass as far as 60 cm, which is enough to reach the transverse colon, although usually it is only used to view as far as the descending colon. A colonoscopy can view the entire colon and pass into the terminal ileum. Sigmoidoscopies are usually performed with the patient unsedated whereas a colonoscopy usually requires conscious sedation with a short-acting benzodiazepine with or without an opiate (usually pethidine or fentanyl). Prior to the procedure, the patient requires bowel preparation, which, for sigmoidoscopy, involves an enema and, for colonoscopy, requires a full bowel purge. Lower GI endoscopies are often accompanied with simple procedures such as polypectomy, especially in patients >50, when polyps are common. Perforations occur in ~1 in 1000 diagnostic colonoscopies and ~1 in 500 therapeutic colonoscopies (e.g. polyp removal), and are rare in sigmoidoscopies. Bleeding occurs in 0.001%–0.240% of colonoscopies, is usually related to polypectomy, and settles with conservative measures in the majority.

Endoscopic retrograde cholangiopancreatography

Endoscopic retrograde cholangiopancreatography (ERCP) is now only used as a therapeutic procedure, as radiology is able to give clear visualization of the biliary tree. However, an ERCP is performed with radiological guidance. Initially, an endoscope is passed into the duodenum in a similar way as in an oesophagogastroduodenoscopy. However, an ERCP utilizes a side-viewing endoscope, allowing clearer visualization of the ampulla of Vater. Initially, the ampulla is cannulated so that radiolucent dye can be injected into the biliary tree, which is visualized via radiological images so that any obstruction to biliary flow can be identified. Operators can then treat the biliary obstruction according to the underlying pathology. Treatment can include sphincterotomy (cutting the sphincter of Oddi to open the exit into the duodenum and allow passage of gallstones), clearing of the bile ducts, dilatation of strictures, and placement of biliary stents. Samples can also be taken to aid diagnosis. ERCP usually requires heavier sedation with benzodiazepines and opiates.

Therapeutic endoscopy

There are several procedures that can be performed endoscopically:

Endoscopic mucosal resection: This is the removal of large polyps, by injecting saline underneath the polyp to lift, snare, and retrieve it. More recently, endoscopic submucosal dissection has been introduced, allowing lesions to be removed in one section.

Dilatation: This is most often used for oesophageal strictures, whether benign or malignant, although it is occasionally used for colonic fibrotic strictures. Balloon dilatation is most commonly used, allowing direct visualization of the mucosa as it is stretched. Bougie dilatation involves passing bougies of increasing size over an endoscopically placed guidewire. The risk of perforation should be clearly explained to the patient, at approximately 1%–2% for benign strictures and 4%–6% for malignant strictures.

Stent insertion: Self-expanding metal stents can be endoscopically placed within GI tumours to prevent obstruction and provide some palliation to symptoms. These can also be placed on a temporary basis in benign recurrent strictures in an attempt to prevent strictures reforming. Furthermore, stents are occasionally used to cover small mucosal tears (usually oesophageal) to prevent leakage as the perforation heals.

Laser therapy: This can be used for oesophageal cancers to reduce obstruction.

Radiofrequency ablation: This is used for Barrett's oesophagus associated with high grade dysplasia or early cancer in specialist centres. A balloon-mounted coil is passed into the oesophagus, and a controlled emission of radiofrequency energy is delivered. This ablates the abnormal tissue to good effect.

Photodynamic therapy: This is used in some specialist centres for oesophageal and gastric cancers. The basis behind photodynamic therapy is that a photosensitive drug is given to the patient, which is attracted to cancer cells. When the light is directed at the cancer, the drug is activated.

Capsule endoscopy

In capsule endoscopy, a capsule containing a camera, a light source, batteries, and a transmitter is swallowed. The capsule is approximately 1.5–2.0 cm long, and images are taken every 2 seconds and relayed to a data recorder worn by the patient. The commonest indications for this procedure include:

- iron-deficiency anaemia with normal OGD and colonoscopy, for suspected obscure gastrointestinal bleeding
- diagnosis of early or suspected small bowel Crohn's disease
- diagnosis of benign and malignant small intestinal lesions
- diagnosis of small bowel abnormalities identified via other investigations (e.g. CT, MRI, or barium X-rays)

Side effects are rare, and capsule retention occurs in <0.75% of cases.

Breath tests

Lactulose/glucose-hydrogen breath test for small bowel bacterial overgrowth

In a lactulose/glucose-hydrogen breath test for small bowel bacterial overgrowth, baseline expired air samples are taken to assess the patient's basal hydrogen concentrations, prior to consuming 75 g lactulose or 50 g glucose. Repeat expired air samples are taken every 15 minutes for 3 hours following this. A positive test is defined as a rise in hydrogen concentration >10 ppm over basal values within the first 2 hours, suggesting bacterial colonization of the small intestine. This initial peak will be followed by a much larger peak signifying the colonic response. Glucose (unlikely lactulose) is absorbed and so is less accurate for determining distal end bacterial overgrowth.

Lactose/hydrogen breath test for lactose intolerance

In a lactose/hydrogen breath test for lactose intolerance, following baseline samples, the patient consumes ~20 g lactose.

If the expired hydrogen concentration rises >20 ppm over the baseline value, the patient is typically diagnosed as having lactose intolerance.

Urea breath test for *H. pylori*

In a urea breath test for *H. pylori*, following baseline samples, patient consume a solution containing ^{13}C- or ^{14}C-labelled urea, which is broken down by the *H. pylori* bacteria to release CO_2. This is absorbed into the bloodstream and excreted in the breath, which is measured for the radiolabelled carbon 10–20 minutes later. This test is >90% accurate for the presence of *H. pylori*.

Further Reading

Aktas H and Mensink PB. Small bowel diagnostics: Current place of small bowel endoscopy. *Best Pract Res Clin Gastroenterol* 2012; 26: 209–20.

Warrell DA, Cox TM, and Firth JD. *Oxford Textbook of Medicine* (5th edition), 2010. Oxford University Press.

196 Immunology and genetics in gastrointestinal and hepatic medicine

Satish Keshav and Alexandra Kent

Introduction

Immunology

The gut has a pivotal role in immune homeostasis. It is constantly exposed to a wide array of antigens in food, and resident and consumed microorganisms. It is estimated that the number of bacterial cells in the gastrointestinal tract is tenfold greater than the number of cells in the human body. The gut needs to recognize harmful bacteria and, consequently, contains the largest number of immune cells in the body. However, it must remain tolerant to commensal bacteria. Bacteria express antigens that stimulate an immunological response via the gut-associated lymphoid tissue (GALT). The GALT includes the appendix, tonsils, Peyer's patches, and mesenteric lymph nodes. Therefore, the intestinal immune system is finely balanced between tolerance and reactivity. An example of an abnormal response that generally the individual should be tolerant to is gliadin peptides in coeliac disease. An example of excessive tolerance to an otherwise controllable infection is cryptosporidiosis, which causes diarrhoea in patients with HIV infection.

Genetics

The understanding of genetics in disease has progressed rapidly with the introduction of genome-wide association studies. The Welcome Trust Case Control Consortium has performed extensive research on the genetics of many illnesses, including Crohn's disease, ulcerative colitis, Barrett's oesophagus, oesophageal adenocarcinoma, and primary biliary cholangitis. Although these studies have increased our understanding of the molecular basis of disease, they have had little impact on clinical management. This may change as studies associate genotype and phenotype.

Several gastrointestinal diseases have an aetiology based on immunological or genetic aberrations, and these immunological mechanisms and genetic mutations can be utilized for diagnostic purposes. However, there is no genetic or immunological marker that is 100% specific to a disease and, consequently, the markers are used to support clinical, histological, and/or radiological findings. Immunological and genetic tests that can be done for specific gastrointestinal conditions are listed in Tables 196.1 and 196.2, respectively.

Inflammatory bowel disease

Inflammatory bowel disease (IBD) is caused by an aberrant immune response in genetically susceptible individuals. The genetic component of IBD is confirmed by the increased concordance in monozygotic twins (50%–70%) compared to dizygotic twins (5%–10%); 15%–20% of IBD patients have an affected family member. Genome-wide scanning has identified a number of genes that alter the risk of developing IBD. Some genes, including the one with the strongest effect, NOD2, affect bacterial recognition. The NOD2 gene is on Chromosome 16, and the gene product is expressed in Paneth cells, which are specialized intestinal epithelial cells that have an antibacterial role, and in mononuclear phagocytes, including monocytes. Other genes are the IRGM and ATG16L autophagy-related genes, the interleukin 23 receptor gene, and PTPN2 (protein tyrosine phosphatase, non-receptor type 2) gene, which is also associated with other autoimmune diseases. Certain HLA types affect the exact type of IBD that is manifest, and affect prognosis. Many more genes have been identified, but the results concerning their roles in IBD are less well replicated, although studies are ongoing. Studies are now directed at correlating genotype and phenotype; for example, mutations in the NOD2 gene are associated with small bowel disease.

The underlying mechanism of inflammation in IBD is driven by immunological responses, including macrophage activation, leucocyte trafficking, and production of inflammatory cytokines such as tumour necrosis factor alpha (TNFα). Cytokines are inflammatory mediators which interact with the colonic mucosa and associated immune cells, resulting in colonic inflammation and ulceration. IBD patients have raised TNFα levels in inflamed mucosa, and this has led to the development of anti-TNFα therapy (e.g. infliximab, adalimumab). TNFα levels are not routinely measured. However, studies have suggested measurements of anti-TNFα trough levels or antibodies to anti-TNFα may allow for more accurate dosing, checking for adherence, and provide a rationale for switching to alternative therapies.

Table 196.1 Immunological tests in gastrointestinal disease

Disease	Autoantibodies
Coeliac disease	Anti-tissue transglutaminase IgA Anti-endomysial IgA Anti-reticulin IgA
Autoimmune pancreatitis	Raised IgG4 levels
Autoimmune hepatitis	Type 1: ANA, anti-SMA, anti-actin antibody, anti-SLA, anti-liver–pancreas antigen, pANCA, AMA Type 2: anti-LKM, anti-liver cytosol-1 Raised IgG
Primary biliary cholangitis	AMA (raised in 90%–95%) ANA (raised in 20%) Raised IgM
Primary sclerosing cholangitis	pANCA Anti-biliary epithelial cells (60%) AMA, ANA, anti-SMA

Abbreviations: AMA, anti-mitochondrial antibody; ANA, antinuclear antibody; anti-LKM, anti-liver kidney microsomal type 1 antibody; pANCA, perinuclear antineutrophil cytoplasmic antibody; anti-SLA, anti-soluble liver antigen antibody; anti-SMA, smooth muscle antibody.

Table 196.2 Diagnostic genetic tests in gastrointestinal disease

	Disease	Gene	Chromosome
Colon cancer	Familial adenomatous polyposis	APC	5
	Hereditary non-polyposis colorectal cancer	MLH1 MSH2 MSH6	3 2 2
Liver disease	Haemochromatosis	HFE	6
	Wilson's disease	ATP7B	13
	Alpha-1-antitrypsin deficiency	Alpha-1-antitrypsin	14
Pancreatitis	Cystic fibrosis	CFTR	7
Luminal disease	Coeliac disease	HLA DQ2 HLA DQ8	6 6

641

Coeliac disease

Coeliac disease, also known as gluten-sensitive enteropathy, is due to an immunologically mediated reaction to gliadin, leading to intra-epithelial lymphocyte infiltration, loss of intestinal villi, and lengthening of the intestinal crypts. Loss of the intestinal villi significantly reduces the absorptive capacity of the small bowel, leading to malabsorption. This immunological component is reflected in the presence of autoantibodies, which form part of the diagnostic workup. The most sensitive and specific antibodies are the anti-tissue transglutaminase IgA, anti-endomysial IgA, and anti-reticulin IgA, and these antibodies have been show to correlate with the degree of mucosal damage. It is important to remember that approximately 1 in 500 people are deficient in IgA; therefore, the routine, IgA-based serological tests for coeliac disease will be falsely negative. A routine check on IgA levels will avoid this diagnostic pitfall. In any case, cases of suspected coeliac disease should undergo endoscopic biopsy of the duodenum to confirm the diagnosis.

There is a hereditary component with a prevalence of 10% in first-degree relatives and 75% concordance between monozygotic twins. Coeliac disease is almost never seen without an appropriate, permissive HLA background: DQ2 or DQ8.

Colon cancer

Colorectal cancer is associated with specific genetic mutations which are now well-characterized and which are usually acquired by somatic mutation, although they may also be inherited in the germline. An individual colorectal cancer has an average of nine mutant genes per tumour. These mutations are not tested for routinely, but a strong family history should initiate genetic testing for specific mutations; this testing should be done in specialist centres, alongside genetic counselling. Even without a specific inherited mutation, the risk of colorectal cancer is increased in family members. One first-degree relative with colorectal cancer will increase an individual's risk of colorectal cancer (relative risk (RR) 2.3), with additional first-degree relatives increasing the risk (RR 4.3). Familial conditions associated with a significant increase in colorectal cancer include familial adenomatous polyposis coli, which is very rare, hereditary non-polyposis colorectal cancer, which is less rare, and juvenile polyposis and Peutz–Jeghers syndrome. Genes associated with specific conditions are listed in Table 196.2.

Haemochromatosis

Haemochromatosis is a common autosomal recessive genetic disorder in certain Western European populations, and is caused by two common mutations in the HFE gene. This gene is located within the HLA Class I region on Chromosome 6, and affects iron homeostasis. Identifying the gene responsible has made diagnosing cases easy, by virtue of genetic testing, although clinical and biochemical testing, for instance, for a very high ferritin level, is also reliable. Most cases are caused by mutations C282Y or H63D, which block the normal HFE activities, leading to enhanced iron accumulation. C282Y homozygotes account for 95% of cases, and C282Y/H63D compound heterozygotes account for 3%. More unusual causes of haemochromatosis have been mapped to Chromosome 2 (HFE2; juvenile haemochromatosis) and Chromosome 7 (HFE3).

Wilson's disease

Wilson's disease is an autosomal recessive disease characterized by excessive copper absorption from the small intestine. This abnormality is caused by a mutation in the ATP7B gene, with over 40 different mutations found, including small deletions, insertions, and missense mutations. This variety of mutations means genetic testing is not feasible as a diagnostic test for this disease.

Autoimmune hepatitis

Autoimmune hepatitis (AIH) is more common in women than men, and can cause cirrhosis and liver failure rapidly. It is characterized by the presence of elevated levels of circulating IgG, and autoantibodies. It is likely that liver damage is a consequence, however, of the activation of T-lymphocytes, and consequent release of cytokines in the liver. Histologically, there is interface hepatitis, and a tendency to for rapid progression to cirrhosis. There are two types of AIH, according to serology: type 1 is characterized by the presence of antinuclear antibodies and/or anti-smooth muscle antibodies, whereas type 2 has anti-liver kidney microsomal type 1 antibody. AIH is associated with other autoimmune diseases and usually responds well to corticosteroid and immunosuppressive therapy. There is a genetic component to the disease. In Europe and the USA, susceptibility to AIH type 1 is conferred by the presence of HLA DR3 and DR4, and AIH type 2 by HLA DR7 and DR3. HLA DR7 confers a more aggressive disease.

Primary biliary cholangitis

In primary biliary cholangitis (PBC), increased expression of HLA Class II antigens makes hepatocytes more vulnerable to CD4 and CD8 lymphocyte-mediated attack, leading to the progressive destruction of small and medium bile ducts. It is also characterized by circulating autoantibodies (anti-mitochondrial antibodies), which are directed against the pyruvate dehydrogenase enzyme, raised levels of circulating IgM antibodies, and granuloma formation in the liver and regional lymph nodes. Genetic factors play an etiological role, as there is a significantly increased risk in first-degree relative (500–1000-fold), although no specific gene has been identified as yet. PBC has been associated with haplotype HLA-DR8 and, for some populations, HLA-DPB1.

Primary sclerosing cholangitis

Primary sclerosing cholangitis occurs mainly in the context of ulcerative colitis, although it may also occur in patients with Crohn's colitis, and in some cases with no apparent IBD. It is probably due to immune-mediated damage to large, medium, and, occasionally, small bile ducts. Circulating levels of IgG and IgM may be raised in some patients, and 60%–82% of patients are positive for pANCA (perinuclear antineutrophil cytoplasmic antibody). Studies have suggested a genetic component, with increased incidence in first-degree relatives, and it is strongly associated with HLA-B8 and HLA-DR3.

Viral hepatitis

Hepatitis B virus (HBV) has been classified by the genetic variation in a partial sequence of the HBV genome, with nine genotypes (A, B, C, D, E, F, G, H, J) identified to date. However, only four of these genotypes are tested for in routine clinical practice. These genotypes vary between populations and have been associated with differences in disease progression and response to therapy. Many doctors use genotyping to guide therapy, and educate the patient on the likelihood of a sustained response. However, there is disagreement between major national and international organizations as to whether genotyping should be part of routine management or simply used as a research tool. Further details regarding HBV genotypes can be found in Chapter 212. Eleven hepatitis C virus (HCV) genotypes have been identified throughout the world, designated 1–11, with further subtyping and strains identified according to the genomic sequence heterogeneity. This heterogeneity has hindered the development of vaccines, although this research is ongoing. The genotype may influence response to treatment.

The immune response to viral inoculation allows diagnosis from simple serological tests. An antibody to HCV confirms exposure, with further tests required to confirm ongoing infection. Presence of the hepatitis B surface antigen means HBV infection, with further tests required to assess whether infection is acute or chronic. Chapter 212 gives further information regarding serological testing in viral hepatitis

Variations in the gene for interleukin 28 (interferon lambda) have an apparently profound effect on the outcome of infection and treatment for HCV. This relatively new discovery may also alter our understanding of the pathogenesis of this disease.

Further Reading

Barbosa T and Rescigno M. Host-bacteria interactions in the intestine: Homeostasis to chronic inflammation. *Wiley Interdiscip Rev Syst Biol Med* 2010; 2: 80–97.

Ge D, Fellay J, Thompson A, et al. Genetic variation in IL28B predicts hepatitis C treatment-induced viral clearance. *Nature* 2009; 461: 399–401.

Kinzler KW and Vogelstein B. Lessons from hereditary colon cancer. *Cell* 1996; 87: 159–70.

197 Gastrointestinal infections

Satish Keshav and Alexandra Kent

Definition of the disease

Gastrointestinal infections includes diarrhoeal diseases that are major causes of morbidity and mortality worldwide; viral hepatitis; and infections such as *Helicobacter pylori* infection in the stomach, and intestinal tuberculosis. Here, only luminal gastrointestinal infections causing gastroenteritis, manifested by diarrhoea and/or vomiting, are considered.

Aetiology of the disease

Gastrointestinal infections can be caused by viral, bacterial, or parasitic infections. Risks include contact with infected individuals, travel to areas with endemic infection, poor sanitation, eating uncooked or poorly cooked food, and immunocompromise. Table 197.1 lists the most common pathogens.

Table 197.1 Pathogens causing gastrointestinal disease

Pathogen	Risk factors	Incubation period	Duration	Symptoms	Treatment
Bacteria					
Escherichia coli	Enterotoxigenic *Escherichia coli* is the commonest cause of traveller's diarrhoea *Escherichia coli* O157 is found in undercooked meat (especially beef) and milk	1–7 days	3–5 days	Bloody diarrhoea Severe abdominal cramps	Co-trimoxazole Second or third generation cephalosporin Avoid antibiotics in *Escherichia coli* O157
Campylobacter spp.	Dairy products Undercooked meat, especially poultry	2–5 days	7 days	Abdominal pain Bloody diarrhoea Malaise Myalgia Fever	Erythromycin Ciprofloxacin
Salmonella spp.	Uncooked food Eggs	8–48 hours	10 days	Nausea Vomiting Diarrhoea (watery, +/− blood) Fever	Ciprofloxacin Co-trimoxazole Third generation cephalosporins
Shigella spp.	Shellfish Fruit Vegetables	2–4 days	7 days	Bloody diarrhoea Fever	Ampicillin Co-trimoxazole Ciprofloxacin
Yersinia spp.		3–7 days	1–3 weeks	Fever Watery diarrhoea, Abdominal pain	Ciprofloxacin Tetracycline
Vibrio cholerae	Seafood Contaminated water	6–48 hours	5–7 days	Rice-water diarrhoea	Tetracycline Co-trimoxazole Erythromycin Doxycycline
Listeria monocytogenes	Dairy products, especially soft cheese	3 weeks	48 hours	Fever Myalgia Nausea Diarrhoea	Ampicillin
Staphylococcus aureus	Undercooked meat	1–6 hours	1 day	Vomiting and diarrhoea Mediated by toxin production	
Clostridium perfringens	Inadequately reheated or undercooked meat	6–24 hours	1 day	Watery diarrhoea Abdominal pain Fever Nausea Vomiting Caused by enterotoxin	Supportive
Clostridium difficile	Occurs in hospitals, after antibiotics	Variable	Variable	Fever Profuse watery (green) diarrhoea Abdominal pain Leucocytosis	Stop broad-spectrum antibiotics Vancomycin Metronidazole

Table 197.1 (Continued)

Pathogen	Risk factors	Incubation period	Duration	Symptoms	Treatment
Aeromonas spp.	Fresh water and fish	1–7 days	>10 days	Fever Abdominal cramps Diarrhoea Vomiting	Third and fourth generation cephalosporins
Bacillus cereus	Food, especially rice	1–24 hours	12–24 hours	Vomiting Diarrhoea	Usually self-limiting Vancomycin or clindamycin in severe disease
Viruses					
Rotavirus	Occurs in outbreaks	1–3 days	3–8 days	Vomiting Watery diarrhoea	Supportive
Norovirus	Occurs in outbreaks Commonly in hospitals, nursing homes, and schools	1–3 days	24–48 hours	Diarrhoea Vomiting Myalgia Headaches Spreads rapidly	Supportive
Astrovirus	More common in the winter Affects the extremes of age	1–3 days	3–4 days	Vomiting Diarrhoea	Supportive
Enteric-type adenovirus	Mainly in children <2 years	1 week	3–4 days	Vomiting Diarrhoea	Supportive
Hepatitis A	Water Shellfish Raw vegetables	2–6 weeks	10–30 days	Flu-like illness Myalgia Diarrhoea Vomiting Abdominal pain Jaundice	Supportive
Parasites					
Entamoeba histolytica	Exotic travel	1–2 weeks	1–3 weeks	Amoebic dysentery Can cause liver abscesses	Metronidazole, followed by a luminal agent to prevent colonization (paromomycin, diloxanide furoate)
Giardia	Contaminated food or water	2–12 days	Variable	Abdominal pain Diarrhoea Can cause a chronic illness with malabsorption	Metronidazole Tinidazole
Microsporidia	Immunosuppression	1 week	Variable	Chronic diarrhoea Weight loss Abdominal pain Nausea Vomiting	Albendazole
Cryptosporidia	Untreated water Unpasteurized milk	7 days	5–10 days	Profuse diarrhoea	Nitazoxanide Paromomycin
Schistosomes	Still-water bathing in Africa, the Caribbean, South and Central America (*Schistosoma. mansoni*), or the Far East (*Schistosoma japonicum*)	Variable	Variable	Acute or chronic diarrhoeal illness	Praziquantel

Bacterial

Bacteria exert pathological responses via various mechanisms. Non-invasive bacteria adhere to the luminal wall, causing an inflammatory response, whereas invasive bacteria cause mucosal ulceration and inflammation. Bacteria can also produce toxins that can cause diarrhoea, inflammation, and systemic toxicity. For example, the verotoxin produced by enterohaemorrhagic *Escherichia coli* leads to complications such as haemolytic–uraemic syndrome (HUS).

Viral

Viral gastroenteritis is highly contagious, and is spread by direct contact or via food (contaminated water, shellfish). Norovirus can be spread via droplets.

Parasitic

Entamoeba histolytica is responsible for amoebiasis, and causes 40 000–100 000 deaths worldwide annually. Humans acquire microsporidiosis through ingestion or inhalation of microsporidia spores. Cryptosporidiosis and microsporidiosis rarely cause problems in immunocompetent hosts.

Helminthic

Helminthic infections include ascariasis, trichuriasis, hookworm infection, enterobiasis, strongyloidiasis, filariasis, and trichinosis. Many are prevalent in warm moist climates. Worms can infect humans via ingestion, larval penetration, or the introduction of larvae by a vector (usually mosquitoes or flies).

Typical symptoms of the disease, and less common symptoms

Gastrointestinal infections usually manifest as mild to severe diarrhoeal illness, often with associated nausea, vomiting, and abdominal pain. Infections are often accompanied by non-specific flu-like symptoms, such as myalgia and headaches. Bacterial and viral illnesses are usually self-limiting, but parasitic infections (e.g. giardia or helminth infections) can cause chronic illnesses, leading to malabsorption and/or nutritional deficiencies.

Gastrointestinal parasitic infections, such as schistosomiasis, microsporidiosis, and cryptosporidiosis can cause chronic illness with diarrhoea and weight loss, especially in immunocompromised individuals.

Helminth infections can cause abdominal pain, weight loss, diarrhoea, malaise, or can be asymptomatic. *Trichuris trichiura* can cause bloody diarrhoea when there is a heavy parasite load. *Enterobius vermicularis* infection (pinworm) causes nocturnal perianal pruritus and, occasionally, appendicitis or ulceration in the bowel. Ascariasis can cause small bowel obstruction if a mass of worms obstructs the lumen, although this is usually observed in children with heavy infections. The major manifestations of hookworm disease include iron deficiency anaemia and chronic protein–energy malnutrition. Worm attachment to the small intestine mucosa can cause abdominal pain, diarrhoea, and weight loss. Malabsorption has also been reported in children and, less commonly, in adults. *Strongyloides stercoralis* infection can cause abdominal pain and diarrhoea, nausea, vomiting, weight loss, and a protein-losing enteropathy.

Demographics of the disease

Gastrointestinal infections affect both genders and all ages and races, but certain groups are more susceptible, including returning travellers, children, elderly, and the immunocompromised.

Natural history and complications of the disease

The majority of bacterial and viral infections are self-limiting, without long-term sequelae. Parasitic and helminth infections respond well to specific treatments. The commonest complication is dehydration with or without associated prerenal failure, and is a leading cause of death in developing countries. However, specific complications for infection by the following microorganisms should be kept in mind:

- *Escherichia coli*: HUS, caused by *Escherichia coli* O157:H7; seen in 10% of cases, with an overall mortality of between 1% and 5%
- *Yersinia* spp.: erythema nodosum, reactive polyarthritis
- *Listeria monocytogenes*: septicaemia and meningitis
- *Clostridium difficile*: pseudomembranous colitis, toxic dilatation, and paralytic ileus
- *Campylobacter* spp.: peritonitis, pancreatitis, cholecystitis, bacteraemia, meningitis, Reiter's syndrome, Guillain–Barré syndrome
- *Salmonella* spp.: osteomyelitis, meningitis, bacteraemia, endocarditis, Reiter's syndrome
- *Shigella* spp.: Reiter's syndrome, HUS
- *Entamoeba histolytica*: fulminant colitis, toxic megacolon, cerebral amoebiasis
- schistosomes: disseminated disease
- helminths: anaemia, protein-losing enteropathy

It is important to recognize that salmonella and *Clostridium difficile* can result in asymptomatic carriage and so patients should continue to follow strict hygiene.

Approach to diagnosing the disease

Epidemics in the UK are usually caused by rotavirus, especially in children. However, norovirus is a common cause of 'winter vomiting', and rapidly spreads. It is important to ask about recent travel abroad, as the country of travel may give clues to the causative organism:

- Africa (*Entamoeba histolytica*, *Vibrio cholerae*, *Schistosoma mansoni*, *Strongyloides* spp., *Loa loa*)

- Central and South America (*Entamoeba histolytica*, *Vibrio cholerae*, *Schistosoma mansoni*)
- the Caribbean (*Schistosoma mansoni*, *Strongyloides* spp.)
- the tropics (*Entamoeba histolytica*, *Trichuris trichiura*, *Ascaris* spp.)
- Asia (*Vibrio cholerae*, *Schistosoma japonicum*, *Strongyloides* spp., *Trichinella* spp.)
- India (*Entamoeba histolytica*, *Vibrio cholerae*)
- Mexico (*Aeromonas* spp., *Entamoeba histolytica*, *Plesiomonas shigelloides*, *Yersinia* spp.)
- New Guinea (*Clostridium* spp.)
- Japan (*Vibrio parahaemolyticus*)
- Australia (*Yersinia* spp.)
- Canada (*Yersinia* spp.)
- Europe (*Yersinia* spp., *Giardia* spp.)

If a number of people who ate together are affected, specific foods consumed and the incubation period may give an indication of the responsible organism (see Table 197.1). Bloody diarrhoea should arouse suspicion of bacterial infection, which is commonly caused by *Escherichia coli*, salmonella, campylobacter, or shigella. Fever in adults suggests an invasive organism; children are often febrile irrespective of the underlying pathogen. Notably, campylobacter and salmonella are the commonest causes of bacterial gastroenteritis in the UK. If diarrhoea lasts for more than a fortnight, the aetiology is likely to be different from that of shorter duration.

Other diagnoses that should be considered

Gastrointestinal infections are usually easily identified, characterized by an acute onset, and often associated with systemic signs of infection (e.g. fever). The differential diagnoses include all causes of diarrhoea, including drugs, inflammatory bowel disease, coeliac disease, diverticular disease, microscopic colitis, colorectal cancer, bile acid malabsorption, pancreatic insufficiency, ischaemic colitis, bacterial overgrowth, lactose intolerance, toxin ingestion, vitamin deficiencies, and endocrine disorders.

'Gold-standard' diagnostic test

Stool microscopy and culture are the critical investigations. Light microscopy can identify ova, cysts, and parasites, including *Entamoeba histolytica*, *Cryptosporidium parvum*, microsporidia, and *Giardia lamblia*. One gram of faeces contains >10^{11} bacteria; however, selective media must be used to identify specific pathogens. Blood agar is suitable for *Plesiomonas shigelloides*, *Listeria monocytogenes*, *Staphylococcus aureus*, *Bacillus cereus*, and *Salmonella*, *Shigella*, *Aeromonas*, and *Vibrio* spp. *Campylobacter* spp., *Clostridium difficile*, *Escherichia coli*, and *Yersinia* spp. require selective culture mediums. Unfortunately, stool cultures have a low yield, especially if the sample is not cultured within 2 hours of collection or is refrigerated at below 4°C.

Acceptable diagnostic alternatives to the gold standard

Treatment for gastrointestinal infections is largely supportive, but septic patients are often treated empirically with suitable antibiotics until the organism is identified. Antibiotic choice should be based on risk factors and travel history. Microsporidiosis has the greatest parasitic burden in the proximal jejunum, and diagnosis can be made from biopsies and/or jejunal fluid retrieved at endoscopy.

Other relevant investigations

Leucocytosis and faecal leucocytes are seen in enteroinvasive organisms but are unusual with enterotoxin-producing bacteria. Persistent diarrhoea may require endoscopic evaluation via flexible sigmoidoscopy, and mucosal biopsies may identify organisms and can exclude differential diagnoses. Endoscopic evaluation can also diagnose pseudomembranous colitis as seen in *Clostridium difficile* infection. Serological tests are available for *Entamoeba histolytica*, *Escherichia coli* O157:H7, enteroviruses, rotaviruses, *Salmonella typhi*, *Salmonella paratyphi*, Q fever, and campylobacter, but are usually reserved for patients who fail to respond to treatment and in whom the pathogen has not been identified. *Staphylococcus aureus* enterotoxin and *Clostridium difficile* toxin can be identified in stool samples. *Salmonella typhi* and *Salmonella paratyphi* are found in the blood <10 days after infection, and in urine and bone marrow >10 days after infection. Helminth infections are associated with eosinophilia and elevated serum IgE.

Prognosis and how to estimate it

The prognosis from gastrointestinal infections should be good when medical help is available, as the illness is responsive to supportive and specific therapy. Unfortunately, diarrhoeal illnesses are a massive cause of morbidity and mortality worldwide where medical and supportive care is lacking and where patients live in poverty. In the UK, mortality is rare except in very young, very old, or frail patients and those with significant comorbidities such as compromised immunity and renal, hepatic, cardiac, or respiratory disease.

Treatment and its effectiveness

The mainstay of treatment is the following procedure:

1. Rehydrate.
2. Correct electrolyte disturbances.
3. Isolate infective diarrhoea.
4. Notify the CDC about cases of infective diarrhoea.

The use of antibiotics for bacterial infections is not straightforward. Unnecessary antibiotic use has been seen to prolong symptoms, and may increase the risk of complications (HUS in infection with *Escherichia coli* O157). Furthermore antibiotics may have gastrointestinal side effects and increase the risk of concomitant *Clostridium difficile* infection. Generally, antibiotics should be reserved for the immunocompromised, the elderly, and those with bacteraemia or prolonged symptoms. Patients with severe ischaemic heart disease are also often treated with antibiotics.

Antihelminth treatments include albendazole, mebendazole, ivermectin, piperazine, pyrantel, and diethylcarbamazine citrate.

Further Reading

Kaiser L and Surawicz CM. Infectious causes of chronic diarrhoea. *Best Pract Res Clin Gastroenterol* 2012; 26: 563–71.
Schiller LR and Sellin JH. 'Diarrhea', in Feldman M, Friedman LS, and Brandt LJ, eds, *Sleisenger and Fordtran's Gastrointestinal and Liver Disease* (9th edition), 2010. Saunders Elsevier.

198 Benign oesophageal disease

Satish Keshav and Alexandra Kent

Definition of the disease

Benign oesophageal disease includes several conditions, including:

- gastro-oesophageal reflux disease (GORD), which is reflux of gastric juices into the oesophagus with or without mucosal injury (oesophagitis)
- achalasia, which is an oesophageal dysmotility disorder characterized by aperistalsis in the distal oesophagus, and failure of lower oesophageal sphincter (LOS) relaxation
- motility disorders, such as:
  - oesophageal spasm, which is characterized by simultaneous, non-propagated contractions
  - nutcracker oesophagus, which is diagnosed by high-amplitude (≥180 mm Hg) contractions associated with chest pain
  - ineffective oesophageal motility, which is characterized by low-amplitude contractions (≤30 mm Hg) in the distal oesophagus
- eosinophilic oesophagitis, which is diagnosed on a combination of clinical features and oesophageal biopsies confirming the presence of >15 eosinophils per high-powered film

Aetiology of the disease

GORD has been associated with a hypotensive LOS, or transient relaxations of the LOS. Certain substances increase GORD by either decreasing the LOS pressure (caffeine, alcohol, nitrates, theophyllines, beta blockers, and calcium channel blockers) or increasing gastric acid (citrus fruits, spicy food). Reflux is more likely to occur in the presence of a hiatus hernia as it disrupts the synergistic action of the diaphragmatic crura and LOS. Obesity increases the intra-abdominal pressure, precipitating reflux.

Achalasia is due to degeneration of inhibitory neurons of the myenteric plexus and oesophageal wall. The cause is unknown, although studies have suggested there are associations with HSV-1 infection and HLA-DQw1.

The aetiology of motility disorders is unknown. Similarly, the exact cause of eosinophilic oesophagitis is unknown, although its association with allergic conditions such as asthma and rhinitis suggests it is a response to environmental antigens.

Typical symptoms of the disease, and less common symptoms

Symptoms in benign oesophageal disease have an insidious onset (see Table 198.1).

Table 198.1 Typical and less common symptoms of benign oesophageal disease

Disease	Common symptoms	Less common symptoms
GORD/hiatus hernia	Heartburn Acid reflux Regurgitation	Cough, wheeze, hoarseness, laryngitis, odynophagia, water brash, nausea
Achalasia	Dysphagia Regurgitation/vomiting	Chest pain, heartburn, weight loss
Motility disorders	Heartburn Chest pain Dysphagia	Regurgitation
Eosinophilic disorders	Dysphagia Food impaction	Heartburn, reflux

Abbreviations: GORD, gastro-oesophageal reflux disease.

Demographics of the disease

Symptoms of GORD affect 14%–20% of the population, although only 20%–40% of patients with symptoms have diagnostically proven GORD. It affects all age groups and races, with no gender predilection.

Motility disorders and achalasia have an incidence of ~1–3 in 100 000 population and affect the genders equally. They can affect all age groups but more commonly affect those aged 25–60.

To date, eosinophilic oesophagitis is a disease of the developed world, mainly affecting children and young adults. Its incidence is currently estimated at 10–40 per 100 000 population in the Western world and is increasing, although the increase is likely to be due to increasing recognition of the condition.

Natural history and complications of the disease

Persistent exposure of the lower oesophagus to gastric acid, and the associated mucosal inflammation, can lead to the development of peptic strictures. These usually present with dysphagia and are treated with a soft diet +/− endoscopic balloon dilatation.

Persistent exposure of the oesophagus to gastric acid can lead to oesophagitis, peptic strictures, replacement of the squamous epithelium with columnar epithelium (Barrett's oesophagus), and adenocarcinoma. Barrett's oesophagus and adenocarcinoma are more common in men. Barrett's is found in ~1% of all endoscopies, and ~12% endoscopes performed for symptoms of GORD. Five per cent of these patients will develop low-grade dysplasia, with 10%–50% of these patients progressing to high-grade dysplasia and adenocarcinoma over 4–5 years. For this reason, endoscopic screening is performed for patients with histologically proven Barrett's oesophagus.

Achalasia has a gradual onset, with patients often suffering for years before seeking medical attention. Patients have an increased risk of squamous cell carcinoma of the oesophagus.

Motility disorders have no long-term complications aside from discomfort related to symptoms.

Many patients will suffer with eosinophilic oesophagitis for years prior to presentation. Complications include oesophageal ulceration and strictures.

Approach to diagnosing the disease

The insidious onset of symptoms is compatible with the benign nature of these conditions. It is often difficult to distinguish GORD from functional dyspepsia on symptoms alone, although response to treatment is compatible with true GORD. In patients with typical symptoms of GORD who respond to medication, no further investigations are necessary. Achalasia and motility disorders are usually only considered once endoscopy has ruled out mechanical obstructive lesions or eosinophilic oesophagitis.

Other diagnoses that should be considered

The common symptoms that occur in benign oesophageal disease are associated with all diagnoses: GORD, achalasia, motility disorders, and eosinophilic oesophagitis. Therefore, the initial differential diagnosis will include all of these conditions. Chagas disease, due to infection with *Trypanosoma cruzi*, can cause neuronal degeneration and symptoms consistent with achalasia. Other diseases associated with achalasia-like motor abnormalities include sarcoidosis, amyloidosis, juvenile Sjögren's syndrome, Fabry's disease, and neurofibromatosis. Often, patient demographics and risk factors will clarify the most likely diagnosis. Secondary causes of oesophageal dysmotility include scleroderma, diabetes mellitus, alcohol consumption, psychiatric disorders, and presbyesophagus.

Eosinophilic oesophagitis is diagnosed on a combination of clinical symptoms and histology. Other conditions associated with oesophageal eosinophilia include GORD, parasitic and fungal infections, congenital rings, Crohn's disease, periarteritis, allergic vasculitis, drug injury, connective tissue diseases, and bullous pemphigoid.

'Gold-standard' diagnostic test

Oesophageal physiology tests are the gold-standard diagnostic tests for GORD and motility disorders. GORD is most accurately diagnosed by pH monitoring, which will detect exposure of the lower oesophagus to pH <4. This can be performed using standard pH-monitoring probes or, as is the case more recently, by pH-monitoring capsules which are attached to the oesophageal mucosa at the time of endoscopy. Oesophageal manometry is the gold-standard diagnostic test for motility disorders. Achalasia is characterized by aperistalsis and failure of LOS relaxation. The LOS is often hypertensive with a raised oesophageal-body resting pressure. The diagnostic findings of the other motility disorders are as described in their definitions. Oesophageal impedance testing and high-resolution manometry are not yet in widespread use. Multichannel intra-luminal impedance testing measures electrical resistance and can more accurately monitor bolus transit and gas or fluid reflux. Manometry probes normal contain 4–8 pressure sensors. High-resolution manometry utilizes up to 36 pressure sensors, thereby providing far more information about oesophageal motility.

Eosinophilic oesophagitis is diagnosed histologically from oesophageal biopsies.

Acceptable diagnostic alternatives to the gold-standard tests

A barium swallow can easily diagnose the presence of a hiatus hernia, and may demonstrate reflux of barium into the oesophagus. Endoscopy cannot diagnose GORD unless there are associated complications, such as peptic strictures or Barrett's oesophagus. Therefore, patients should ideally only be referred for endoscopy in the presence of alarm symptoms (unintentional weight loss, chronic gastrointestinal bleeding, dysphagia, persistent vomiting, iron-deficiency anaemia, epigastric mass, suspicious barium meal), or in patients ≥55 years with persistent symptoms.

Achalasia has a virtually diagnostic appearance on barium swallow, with a dilated oesophagus and beak-like narrowing due to the contracted LOS, although a normal appearance does not exclude the diagnosis. Gastroscopy will often confirm the dilated oesophagus with food residue, and a tight LOS.

Motility disorders cannot be diagnosed by alternative methods. Eosinophilic oesophagitis is diagnosed by oesophageal biopsies,

but endoscopic appearances can show characteristic oesophageal mucosal 'rings'

Other relevant investigations

There are no further investigations required to diagnose these symptoms. It is important to state that *Helicobacter pylori* is not associated with oesophageal disease.

Prognosis and how to estimate it

Prognosis in benign oesophageal disorders is dependent on response to treatment and presence of complications. Oesophageal symptoms can significantly impair quality of life, and treatments can result in dramatic improvements. In GORD, 80%–90% patients will respond to medications; however, recurrence is common on discontinuing therapy. Long-term prognosis in eosinophilic oesophagitis is not yet known, but the disease remains confined to the oesophagus, with studies confirming the persistence of oesophageal eosinophilia and symptoms. Hopefully, increasing recognition and implementation of therapy should improve the long-term prognosis.

Treatment and its effectiveness

Lifestyle measures for GORD include weight loss, alcohol reduction, smoking cessation, raising the head of the bed, avoiding tight garments, avoiding large meals, and not consuming meals 3 hours prior to bedtime. Proton-pump inhibitors (PPIs) are more effective at treating oesophagitis (83% response) than H2 antagonists (52% response). Patients with persistent symptoms are commonly offered prokinetics, to increase gastric emptying, although evidence for this approach is lacking. Nissan's fundoplication is equally efficacious as PPIs, but 60% of patients will have recurring symptoms after 10–12 years. The occurrence of Barrett's and adenocarcinoma is equal between medically and surgically treated groups.

Peptic strictures causing dysphagia are treated with endoscopic balloon dilatation and high-dose PPIs. Repeat dilatations are often required, and patients may require a Nissan's fundoplication to reduce acid reflux precipitating the stricture.

Achalasia has three main treatment strategies, which are shown in Table 198.2.

Motility disorders are difficult to treat. Reflux and heartburn are usually controlled with antisecretory agents. In patients with chest pain due to spastic disorders, clinical trials support the use of smooth muscle relaxants (nitrates, calcium channel blockers) and pain modulators (tricyclic antidepressants and selective serotonin reuptake inhibitors). Further treatments, with less evidence, include sildenafil and botulinum toxin.

Eosinophilic oesophagitis can be treated with elimination diets, with a 77% response seen when elimination is guided by skin prick or atopy patch testing. Milk, wheat, soy, and egg are the most common allergens associated with this disorder. Elemental diets have been successfully used in children, with smaller studies in adults showing a 94% symptomatic response and a 78% histological response. Topical steroids have been used widely, using steroid inhalers, but instructing

Table 198.2 Treatment of achalasia

Treatment	Procedure	Short-term response (1 year)	Long-term response (5–10 years)
Medications	Calcium channel blockers/nitrates	10%	Overall poor response; reserved for patients refusing further treatment options
Botulinum toxin	Endoscopic injection into the LOS; response lasts only 6–12 months	30%	N/A
Pneumatic dilatation	Endoscopic dilatation; associated with 5% perforation rate and 25% post-procedure GORD	70%–80%	45%–60%
Surgical myotomy	Post-operative GORD in 10%–15%; reduced by simultaneous partial fundoplication	85%–95%	70%–85%

Abbreviations: GORD, gastro-oesophageal reflux disease; LOS, lower oesophageal sphincter.

the patient to swallow rather than inhale the medication. There is an 80%–100% response to topical steroids, although up to 90% of symptoms recur off therapy. Small preliminary studies have shown a response to the following therapies: montelukast (leukotriene inhibitor), mepolizumab (a monoclonal antibody against interleukin 5), and azathioprine.

Further Reading

Kahrilas PJ. Clinical practice. Gastroesophageal reflux disease. *N Engl J Med* 2008; 359: 1700–7.

Spechler SJ and Castell DO. Classification of oesophageal motility abnormalities. *Gut* 2001; 49: 145–51.

199 Peptic ulcer disease

Satish Keshav and Alexandra Kent

Definition of the disease

Peptic ulcer disease (PUD) describes ulceration limited to the stomach and duodenum and characterized by mucosal damage related to pepsin and gastric acid.

Aetiology of the disease

Helicobacter pylori and NSAIDs are the predominant cause of peptic ulcers. *H. pylori* is associated with >90% of duodenal ulcers (DUs), and >70% of gastric ulcers (GUs); 10%–15% of patients with *H. pylori* develop ulceration. NSAIDs confer an annual risk of 1%–4% in those taking long-term therapy. NSAIDs inhibit prostaglandin synthesis and cyclooxygenase-2, reducing mucus and bicarbonate secretion, mucosal blood flow, and epithelial cell proliferation. Other causes of peptic ulcers include steroids, bisphosphonates, malignancy, critical illness, surgery, or hypovolaemia (due to splanchnic hypoperfusion).

Chronic renal failure, cirrhosis, and sarcoidosis have an increased incidence of PUD. In addition, Zollinger–Ellison syndrome presents with multiple ulcers due to gastrin-producing tumours (gastrinomas).

Typical symptoms of the disease, and less common symptoms

The typical symptom associated with PUD is a gnawing or burning epigastric pain, occurring on an empty stomach or 2–5 hours after meals. Less common symptoms include nausea, vomiting, heartburn, bloating, anorexia, or haematemesis/melaena due to underlying bleeding.

Demographics of the disease

The worldwide incidence rates of PUD are closely related to the presence of *H. pylori* and NSAID-prescribing habits. Approximately 10% of the population have a lifetime risk of PUD. However, incidence and prevalence rates may be underestimated due to many patients self-medicating with antacids. Incidence is equal between genders, with the majority of patients between 25 and 64 years of age. Zollinger–Ellison syndrome is a rare condition, affecting ~1 per million population, but is the cause of peptic ulceration in 0.1%–1% of cases.

Natural history and complications of the disease

Ulcers will heal when the injurious agent is removed, although antacid therapy will accelerate healing. However, significant morbidity and mortality are associated with PUD, with older patients having a significantly higher mortality risk.

Mortality is related to associated perforation and gastrointestinal (GI) bleeding. Approximately 30 in 100 000 patients require hospitalization, with an overall mortality of 1 in 100 000 cases of PUD. Fifteen to twenty per cent of patients with PUD will develop GI bleeding. The mortality rate is higher in older patients, of whom 20% present with asymptomatic ulcers. Two to ten per cent of peptic ulcers will perforate, with 60% duodenal, 20% in the gastric antrum, and 20% on the gastric lesser curve. Recurrent duodenal or pyloric canal ulceration may lead to pyloric stenosis, with resultant gastric outlet obstruction. In addition, 10% of GUs are malignant.

Approach to diagnosing the disease

Symptoms of PUD are difficult to distinguish from those of gastritis and non-ulcer dyspepsia, with only 20%–25% of patients with symptoms consistent with PUD actually having an ulcer. The presence of associated symptoms can provide more information, suggesting the presence of complications, for example persistent vomiting, in gastric outlet obstruction; haematemesis, in bleeding ulcers; and severe abdominal pain radiating through to the back, in gastric or duodenal perforation. In patients <55 years old, with no alarm symptoms, it is standard practice to give a trial of proton-pump inhibitor (PPI) and 'test and treat' for *H. pylori*. Referral for further investigations should be performed on older patients (≥55 years old), in the presence of alarm symptoms (weight loss, anaemia, persistent vomiting, haematemesis) or in patients who have persistent symptoms despite antisecretory therapy.

Other diagnoses that should be considered

The differential diagnosis for patients presenting with right upper quadrant/epigastric pain includes:

- gastric carcinoma
- biliary colic
- cholelithiasis
- cholecystitis
- gastritis/duodenitis
- functional dyspepsia
- gastro-oesophageal reflux disease
- pancreatitis
- pancreatic carcinoma
- mesenteric ischaemia
- Crohn's disease affecting the upper GI tract

'Gold-standard' diagnostic test

The only investigation that can absolutely confirm the present of peptic ulceration is an upper GI endoscopy (oesophagogastroduodenoscopy). This allows accurate recording (including photographs) of ulcer size, depth, features, and stigmata of haemorrhage. It allows for biopsies to be taken, especially from GUs, which have a 10% malignancy risk. Gastric biopsies can also be taken for an *H. pylori* urease test. Endoscopy is fundamental in patients with possible GI bleeding, as bleeding lesions can be treated endoscopically by sclerosant injections, cauterization, and/or application of haemoclips.

Acceptable diagnostic alternatives to the gold standard

In patients in whom endoscopy is considered to be high risk, a barium/Gastrografin meal and follow-through will provide information regarding mucosal integrity. If abnormalities are seen on the barium studies, a more accurate risk–benefit assessment can be applied. CT can be used to identify abnormal, usually thickened, mucosa, which is often found in association with peptic ulcers. However, CT is less accurate than barium or endoscopic investigations and is usually reserved for patients with symptoms or signs suggestive of visceral perforation, when it should be performed immediately.

Other relevant investigations

Young patients without alarm symptoms or suggestion of complications can be treated empirically with antisecretory therapy and tested and treated for *H. pylori*. All patients diagnosed with peptic ulcers should be tested for *H. pylori* and treated as necessary. In patients with bleeding ulcers, when *H. pylori* tests are not available or results are delayed, treatment should be given empirically.

Table 199.1 Diagnostic tests for *Helicobacter pylori*

Diagnostic test	Sensitivity (%)	Specificity (%)
Helicobacter serology	92	83
Helicobacter stool antigen	96	97
Helicobacter/urea breath test	95	96
Urease test	96	96

Hospitals vary in modes of *H. pylori* tests, but available tests are listed in Table 199.1.

In patients with multiple ulcers or in whom ulcer healing is unresponsive to antisecretory therapy, a fasting serum gastrin level should be measured to exclude Zollinger–Ellison syndrome as an underlying cause. PPIs and H2 antagonists should be stopped 3 and 7 days, respectively, prior to this test.

Prognosis and how to estimate it

Peptic ulceration can inflict substantial morbidity and mortality if left untreated. True peptic ulcers response well to treatment and removal of precipitants, but recurrence is not uncommon. In patients with a previous history of PUD, care should be taken when prescribing medications (e.g. aspirin or NSAIDs) associated with peptic ulceration. The benefits and risks of such medications should be balanced, and prophylactic antisecretory medication considered, in the following groups:

- patients with NSAID-induced ulcers but who require chronic, daily NSAID therapy
- patients over the age of 60
- patients with a history of PUD or a complication such as GI bleeding
- patients taking concomitant steroids or anticoagulants
- patients with significant comorbid medical illnesses

Treatment and its effectiveness

H. pylori eradication reduces ulcer recurrence from 69% to 6% in DU and from 59% to 4% in GU, and has been shown to be cost-effective.

Treatment of *H. pylori* infection is more effective than antisecretory therapy in preventing recurrent bleeding from PUD. Consequently, the most important and efficacious treatments for peptic ulcers are *H. pylori* eradication and avoidance of precipitants (e.g. NSAIDs). All patients who have undergone *H. pylori* eradication should be retested to ensure eradication has been effective.

PPIs bind to and inhibit the H^+/K^+-adenosine triphosphatase pump of the parietal cell, resulting in a marked decrease in acid secretion. In those patients who need to remain on NSAIDs, co-treatment with PPIs can reduce ulcer recurrence from 67% to 11%.

H2 antagonists selectively block H2 receptors on parietal cells, resulting in diminished acid secretion and ulcer healing. Both H2 antagonists and PPIs can reduce the incidence of duodenal and gastric ulceration as primary and secondary prophylaxis, in ulcers that are not associated with *H. pylori*.

Misoprostol inhibits gastric mucosal release of endogenous prostaglandin E2 and thromboxane B2, and reduces gastric ulcer recurrence from 7.7% to 1.9%.

Visceral perforation is treated surgically.

All patients with GUs should undergo repeat endoscopy at 8–10 weeks, to ensure healing and obtain biopsies from persistent ulcers, to ensure there is no underlying malignancy.

Further Reading

Gralnek IM, Barkun AN, and Bardou M. Management of acute bleeding from a peptic ulcer. *N Engl J Med* 2008; 359: 928–37.

Lanas A and Chan FKL. Peptic ulcer disease. *Lancet* 2017; 390: 613–24.

Laine L. Clinical Practice. Upper gastrointestinal bleeding due to a peptic ulcer. *N Engl J Med* 2016; 374: 2367–76.

McColl KEL. *Helicobacter pylori* infection. *N Engl J Med* 2010; 362: 1597–604.

Ramakrishnan K and Salinas RC. Peptic ulcer disease. *Am Fam Physician* 2007; 76; 1005–12.

200 Gall bladder disease

Satish Keshav and Alexandra Kent

Definition of gall bladder disease

The gall bladder is a sac which lies underneath the liver and stores and concentrates bile produced by the liver. As food enters the duodenum, it stimulates the release of cholecystokinin, which in turn stimulates the release of bile, which passes via the cystic duct to the common bile duct, which connects to the duodenum at the sphincter of Oddi. Bile is required in digestion, especially for the emulsification and absorption of fat. Biliary disease can take several forms:

- cholelithiasis, which is the presence of gallstones in the gall bladder
- choledocholithiasis, which is the presence of gallstones in the biliary tree
- cholecystitis, which is inflammation and infection of the gall bladder
- cholangitis, which is inflammation and infection of the biliary tree
- sphincter of Oddi dysfunction (SOD), which is characterized by symptoms of biliary obstruction, with no structural cause
- gall bladder polyps
- primary biliary cholangitis (see Chapter 213)
- primary sclerosing cholangitis (see Chapter 218)

Approach to diagnosing gall bladder disease

Gall bladder disease is easily diagnosed on a combination of history and examination, and radiology will clarify the exact underlying condition. SOD is more difficult to diagnose and requires the exclusion of structural causes of symptoms. An ampullary tumour is found in approximately 4% of patients suspected of having SOD, so multiple investigations may be required prior to establishing the diagnosis. The presence of associated functional or psychiatric symptoms may correlate with type III SOD. However, this should not defer the doctor from excluding structural causes, especially given the complications that can occur with a delay in diagnosis.

Other diagnoses that should be considered aside from gall bladder disease

The differential diagnosis of biliary pain includes:

- hepatitis
- pancreatitis
- gastroenteritis
- right lower lobe pneumonia
- mesenteric ischaemia
- myocardial infarction
- small bowel obstruction
- renal calculi
- abdominal aneurysm

'Gold-standard' diagnostic test for gall bladder disease

An ultrasound scan (USS) of the biliary tree is considered to be the gold-standard test for gall bladder disease. A USS can clearly identify the presence of gall bladder polyps and gallstones as small as 1–2 mm and determine whether they are impacted in the biliary tree, as well as detect any associated biliary dilatation. Normally, the common bile duct is <8 mm. Cholecystitis is characterized by gall bladder distension, wall thickening, and pericholecystic fluid, and Murphy's sign is often duplicated when the USS probe is pushed down on the gall bladder. Air in the gall bladder wall indicates gangrenous cholecystitis.

USS is also advantageous in that it can identify complications, for example abscesses, empyemas, and perforations. It can also image other abdominal structures, such as the pancreas and the aorta, helping to exclude differential diagnoses. Sphincter of Oddi manometry is considered the gold standard for diagnosing SOD, although this test is only available at specialized centres. An elevated sphincter pressure of >40 mm Hg is diagnostic and corresponds to the obstruction seen in SOD. Manometry results correlate well with the type of SOD, with raised pressure seen in 60%–85% of patients with type I SOD, 18%–55% of patients with type II SOD, and 7%–28% of patients with type III SOD.

Acceptable diagnostic alternatives to the gold-standard test for gall bladder disease

MRI

Magnetic resonance cholangiopancreatography (MRCP) can give clear information about the biliary tree, including biliary dilatation and choledocholithiasis. It is often more sensitive for biliary sludge and tiny gallstones. The use of MRCP with secretin-stimulating pancreatic flow is being evaluated in diagnosing SOD, but studies are still needed to verify the usefulness of the technique.

Biliary scintigraphy

A HIDA scan is performed in the nuclear medicine department. A radioisotope is injected intravenously and is naturally removed by the liver and excreted into the bile. A two-dimensional image is then produced that shows where the isotope is located. Failure to see the isotope in the liver suggests a diseased liver. Blockages within the biliary system can be clearly seen, as only clear ducts will show up on the image. A gall bladder that is not visualized (i.e. no isotope seen within it) suggests a blockage in the cystic duct, supporting a diagnosis of acute calculus cholecystitis.

HIDA scans will show obstruction to biliary flow in SOD, especially in types I and II. However, reproducibility is uncertain and, therefore, scintigraphy is not yet used consistently.

CT

CT is not usually useful for evaluating biliary disease, and should only be used to identify complications (perforation, empyema) or in patients with failed USS (usually due to body habitus).

Other relevant investigations for gall bladder disease

Liver function tests

Uncomplicated gallstones and biliary colic will have normal blood parameters, and abnormal liver function tests (LFTs) should alert the physician to an alternative diagnosis. LFTs may be raised in cholecystitis, but normal parameters do not exclude the diagnosis. Cholangitis and biliary colic will result in raised LFTs, with the bilirubin and alkaline phosphatase levels rising to a greater extent than the transaminase levels. Type I and type II SOD patients may have raised alkaline phosphatase and transaminases, with levels of up to three times the upper limit of normal.

Full blood count

Cholangitis will cause leucocytosis, whereas only 60% of patients with cholecystitis will have a raised white-cell count.

C-reactive protein

C-reactive protein levels will be raised in inflammatory conditions, such as cholecystitis and cholangitis.

Amylase

Amylase levels may rise in cholecystitis and cholangitis, but usually no higher than three times the upper limit of normal. An amylase level higher than this should alert the physician to the possibility of gallstone pancreatitis.

Blood cultures

All febrile patients should have blood cultures taken to help identify any bacterial pathogens.

Gallstones

Aetiology of gallstones

Gallstones are formed when there is an imbalance in the composition of bile, and can be formed from cholesterol (75%–80%), pigment (15%), or a mixture of both. Cholesterol stones form when there is too much cholesterol in the bile, and pigment stones form when there is too much bilirubin. Biliary stasis and impaired gall bladder motility increase the risk of gallstone formation. Gallstones can range in size from millimetres to centimetres. Cholecystitis and cholangitis invariably occur as a consequence of gallstones obstructing the cystic or common bile duct, respectively, impairing biliary flow. Inflammation of the gall bladder is usually chemically mediated by lysolecithin, although 20% of cases are complicated by bacterial infection: *E. coli* (41%), *Enterococcus* spp. (12%), *Klebsiella* spp. (11%), and *Enterobacter* spp. (9%).

Typical symptoms of gallstones, and less common symptoms

Gallstones are asymptomatic in the majority and are often coincidental findings. Pain related to the gall bladder or biliary tree is usually constant and located in the upper abdomen (right upper quadrant or epigastrium) and is worsened by eating, especially fatty meals. The nature of the pain can vary, being described as a dull, gnawing, aching, band-like burning or tightness. Simple gallstones often cause mild-to-moderate pain, whereas cholecystitis or cholangitis can produce a more severe pain lasting for days. Gallstones impacted in the biliary tree cause biliary colic, which is usually severe, lasting for 1–5 hours on average. Biliary pain can radiate through to the back or be referred to the right shoulder or scapula, and can be associated with nausea and vomiting. Cholangitis is more likely to be accompanied by signs of sepsis, including fever, tachycardia, and hypotension. Fever can occur in cholecystitis, but is less common. Tenderness in the right upper quadrant ('Murphy's sign') is indicative of cholecystitis. Jaundice will only be seen when there is an obstructed biliary tree causing a blockage to the flow of bile.

Demographics of the gallstones

In the UK, approximately 3.5 million people have gallstones, although only 30% will develop symptoms. The highest prevalence is in fair-skinned Northern Europeans, and gallstones are more common in females. It has been proposed that the reason for the female preponderance is oestrogens causing increased cholesterol secretion and progesterone promoting biliary stasis. Pregnancy increases the risk of gallstones. Other risk factors include obesity, rapid weight loss, diabetes mellitus, haemolysis (e.g. sickle cell disease), cirrhosis, exogenous oestrogens, and medications (e.g. octreotide, fibrates). The risk of gallstones increases with age. The classic presentation is with the '3 F's': 'fat, female, and forty'!

Natural history of gallstones, and complications of the disease

Seventy per cent of patients with asymptomatic gallstones will have no complications. The majority of patients with complications related to gallstone will recover with standard therapy. Seventy per cent of patients would have suffered with a recurrence of their symptoms, but laparoscopic cholecystectomy has significantly improved the prognosis for patients.

Complications of gallstones include:

- sepsis
- choledocholithiasis (10%)
- acute cholecystitis
- cholangitis
- gallstone pancreatitis
- gall bladder perforation (10%)
- a gall bladder-enteric fistula caused by a gallstone eroding through the gall bladder wall into the small bowel
- gall bladder ileus: following formation of a gall bladder-enteric fistula, a gallstone ≥2.5 cm can obstruct the ileocaecal valve
- conversion of a laparoscopic cholecystectomy to an open procedure (5%)

Prognosis of gallstones, and how to estimate it

Uncomplicated acute cholecystitis has a low mortality. However, complications significantly increase the mortality: there is 25% mortality in patients with a gangrenous gall bladder or gall bladder empyema, and up to 60% in patients with a gall bladder perforation. Complications are more common in the elderly or immunocompromised.

In patients treated with a cholecystectomy, post-cholecystectomy syndrome affects ~10%–15% of patients. This condition is thought to be due to the continuous passage of bile into the upper gastrointestinal tract, due to the loss of the gall bladder reservoir. This can result in gastritis, duodenitis, abdominal pain, or diarrhoea.

Treatment of gallstones, and its effectiveness

Incidental asymptomatic gallstones do not require treatment.

Laparoscopic cholecystectomy has revolutionized treatment for gallstones, being a procedure with fewer complications and quicker recovery than an open cholecystectomy. It is the commonest treatment strategy, resolving symptoms in approximately 90%.

In patients unable to undergo the operation for medical or personal reasons, medical therapy can be offered. Ursodeoxycholic acid can promote dissolution of cholesterol stones, but requires treatment for a minimum of 6 months, and trials have shown wide-ranging results, achieving complete dissolution of gallstones in 20%–75%. Furthermore, it does not prevent new stone formation once the treatment is stopped.

Lithotripsy utilizes extracorporeal ultrasonic waves to shatter gallstones. It has a reported success rate as high as 90%, although it is more successful in patients with few, small non-calcified gallstones.

Treatment of cholecystitis

When treating cholecystitis, fluid losses should be replaced with IV fluids. Patients normally remain 'nil by mouth' until symptoms are settling and complications are excluded. Analgesia should be given: opiates are often necessary, although morphine should be avoided as it can increase sphincter of Oddi tone. Anticholinergic antispasmodics (dicyclomine, Buscopan) can be useful for biliary colic. Gall bladder distension can be effectively treated with anti-inflammatory drugs (indomethacin). Anti-emetics should be given as required.

Although bacterial infection only complicates 20% of cases, antibiotics are usually given to all patients with cholecystitis. The antibiotic choice should depend on each individual hospital policy. However, commonly used antibiotics include penicillin or cephalosporin plus metronidazole, or piperacillin and tazobactam.

Cholecystectomy should be performed on all patients with complications from gallstones, as gallstones have a high risk of recurrence (~70%). However, it is no longer performed during an acute attack of cholecystitis, unless complications develop (perforation, gall bladder gangrene). If a cholecystectomy is performed for acute cholecystitis, it is preferable for it to be performed immediately once the diagnosis has been established. Following admission, the inflammation will often progress, making a laparoscopic procedure more difficult, and more often requiring conversion to an open procedure. Emergency drainage of a distended gall bladder can be performed using a radiologically placed drain. Cholecystectomy is usually performed when the patient has fully recovered from the cholecystitis, on an elective basis.

Treatment of cholangitis

Cholangitis treatment mirrors that of acute cholecystitis. However, since its aetiology is due to a blockage in the biliary tree, treatment is required to relieve this. Usually, endoscopic retrograde cholangiopancreatography (ERCP) is performed, when a sphincterotomy can be performed; the ducts are trawled to clear stones, and stents placed, if required, to maintain drainage. When ERCP cannot achieve drainage, a percutaneous biliary drain can be placed under radiological guidance and, once inflammation has settled, an ERCP is often more successful.

SOD

Aetiology of SOD

The aetiology of SOD is not entirely known. Biopsies from the ampulla have shown inflammation or fibrosis in ~40%, and this would fit with the papillary obstruction seen in some patients with SOD. Biliary dyskinesia, causing a motor abnormality of the sphincter of Oddi, has been considered, and would correspond with studies that have shown increased frequency of phasic contractions, retrograde propagation of contractions, and a paradoxical response to cholecystokinin. Visceral hyperalgesia has also been proposed as an underlying cause, with increasing incidence of anxiety, depression, and psychiatric problems being seen in patients with type III SOD.

The three types of SOD are defined as follows:

- type I: biliary pain with elevated LFTs and a dilated common bile duct (CBD); thought to be related to sphincter of Oddi stenosis
- type II: biliary pain and either elevated LFTs or dilated CBD; represents an overlap of type I and type III
- type: biliary pain alone; thought to be a functional disorder with sphincter of Oddi dyskinesia

Typical symptoms of SOD, and less common symptoms

SOD has three distinct clinical scenarios: (1) post-cholecystectomy syndrome, (2) acalculus biliary pain, and (3) recurrent pancreatitis. Patients suffer with biliary-type pain, as described, with no structural abnormalities to explain their symptoms.

Demographics of SOD

SOD can affect any age or gender, but classically affects women between the ages of 20 and 50.

Natural history of SOD, and complications of the disease

The main complications of SOD are persistent pain, requiring continuing use of analgesia, and the risk of recurrent pancreatitis. Sphincterotomy in patients with SOD carries a much higher risk of associated pancreatitis, which occurs in over twice as many SOD patients undergoing sphincterotomy as those undergoing sphincterotomy for biliary pathology.

Prognosis of SOD, and how to estimate it

SOD can have a very variable prognosis. Type I SOD patients and many type II SOD patients will respond to a sphincterotomy, although symptoms may recur after time. Type III SOD is far more difficult to treat, with no benefit from a sphincterotomy and medications being poorly tolerated or poorly effective.

Treatment of SOD, and its effectiveness

Medical therapy, including calcium channel blockers (nifedipine) and nitrates, has been used, but studies are often small and therapy is limited by side effects. Studies are ongoing into the use of octreotide and prostaglandin analogues, aimed at reducing sphincter pressures.

Sphincterotomy, performed endoscopically, can relieve symptoms in 85% of patients with type I SOD, and 69% of patients with type II SOD. It is usually only offered to type II SOD patients who have high sphincter pressures. It is far less effective in type III SOD.

Botulinum toxin, injected endoscopically into the sphincter, can give relief of symptoms, and the procedure is relatively easy to perform. However, it is limited by its short duration of action (3–6 months). Response to botox can also be used to predict those who will respond to a sphincterotomy.

Gall bladder polyps

Aetiology of gall bladder polyps

Gall bladder polyps are common, with a prevalence of 4%–9%, but have an unknown aetiology. Cholesterol polyps are the most common (70%), and other types of polyps include inflammatory polyps, hyperplastic polyps, lymphoid polyps, fibrous polyps, granulation tissue, and adenomas.

Typical symptoms of gall bladder polyps, and less common symptoms

The majority of polyps are asymptomatic and diagnosed on a USS incidentally. Large polyps may cause abdominal pain, which is thought to be due to hypercontraction of the gall bladder, or intermittent obstruction of gall bladder emptying. Occasionally, the polyp can break off and cause obstruction of the CBD.

Demographics of gall bladder polyps

Benign gall bladder polyps affects all ages equally. They are slightly more common in men and in patients of Indian origin, with an increased incidence in patients with primary sclerosing cholangitis and hepatitis B.

Natural history gall bladder polyps, and complications of the disease

The main concern with polyps is the adenoma-to-cancer sequence which is seen in colonic adenomas. Polyps <5 mm are unlikely to be malignant, whereas those >15 mm have a much higher risk; for this reason, gall bladder polyps should remain under surveillance.

Prognosis of gall bladder polyps, and how to estimate it

The overall prognosis of gall bladder polyps is unknown, and the benefit of surveillance USS to monitor growth has not yet been established.

Treatment of gall bladder polyps, and its effectiveness

Generally, gall bladder polyps ≥1.0–1.5 cm are removed via a cholecystectomy. Smaller polyps usually are monitored closely for 2 years, with 6–12 monthly USS, to assess the rate of growth. When there is no clear growth, USS can be done yearly; however, it has not yet been established how long these polyps should be monitored for.

Further Reading

Sanders G and Kingsnorth AN. Gallstones. *BMJ* 2007; 305; 295–9.
Strasberg SM. Acute calculous cholecystitis. *N Engl J Med* 2008; 358: 2804–11.
Yamashita Y, Takada T, Kawarada Y, et al. Surgical treatment of patients with acute cholecystitis: Tokyo guidelines. *J Hepatobiliary Pancreat Surg* 2007; 14: 91–7.

201 Pancreatic disease

Satish Keshav and Alexandra Kent

Acute pancreatitis

Acute pancreatitis is an acute inflammatory process of the pancreas and is potentially reversible. It is characterized by oedema and necrosis of peripancreatic fat and may progress to necrosis of glandular and surrounding tissue. Activation of pancreatic enzymes leads to pancreatic autodigestion and systemic effects.

Aetiology of acute pancreatitis

Fifty to fifty-five per cent of cases of acute pancreatitis are caused by gallstones impacted in the common bile duct, and 20%–25% of cases are caused by alcohol. Other causes include drugs (e.g. azathioprine, pentamidine, didanosine), endoscopic retrograde cholangiopancreatography (ERCP), hypercalcaemia, hyperlipidaemia, pancreatic tumours, familial pancreatitis, ischaemia, trauma, vasculitis, pregnancy, viral infection, venom (e.g. scorpion bite), intra-ductal parasites (e.g. ascariasis), mycoplasma, and end-stage renal failure; alternatively, acute pancreatitis may be idiopathic.

Typical symptoms of acute pancreatitis, and less common symptoms

Pancreatic pain is classically described as epigastric in origin, radiating through to the back, and worsened by lying down or eating. The pain can be severe, and be associated with nausea and vomiting. Cullen's sign and Grey Turner's sign, respectively, describe periumbilical and flank bruising seen with haemorrhagic pancreatitis, and are uncommon features. Patients with acute pancreatitis usually have severe pain, which is relieved only by opiates, and are often systemically unwell, with fever, tachycardia, dehydration, and leucocytosis.

Demographics of acute pancreatitis

Acute pancreatitis has an annual incidence of 2 per 100 000 population, with an increasing incidence with age. It affects the genders equally.

Natural history of acute pancreatitis, and complications of the disease

Approximately 10%–30% of patients will develop severe disease, and account for the over 2%–10% mortality associated with acute pancreatitis. Severe inflammation can lead to the systemic inflammatory response syndrome and multi-organ failure. Mortality from acute pancreatitis is almost exclusively due to patients with necrotizing pancreatitis, which has a mortality rate of 20%–40%. Infected pancreatic necrosis has a mortality reaching almost 100% if not debrided.

Approach to diagnosing acute pancreatitis

The differential diagnosis of any patient presenting with acute abdominal pain and with an underlying history of excess alcohol consumption should include acute pancreatitis. A raised amylase level in a patient with typical symptoms is virtually diagnostic, and a CT scan should simply confirm the diagnosis. A history of gallstones or a change in medication may aid in the diagnosis. Infectious causes may have prodromal illness.

Diagnostic tests for acute pancreatitis

A rise in the serum amylase level, which peaks in the first 24 hours of acute pancreatitis, combined with clinical signs and symptoms, is virtually diagnostic of acute pancreatitis. Serum lipase levels also rise in the first 24 hours of acute pancreatitis, and may remain elevated longer than amylase levels, due to the longer half-life

Box 201.1 Balthazar grading system for acute pancreatitis

A: Normal pancreas

B: Heterogeneous attenuation, focal or diffuse glandular enlargement, irregular contour of the gland, no peripancreatic inflammation

C: Grade B plus peripancreatic inflammation

D: Grade C plus a single fluid collection

E: Grade C plus multiple fluid collections or abscess formation

Data from Balthazar EJ, Robinson DL, Megibow AJ, Ranson JH; Robinson; Megibow; Ranson, Acute pancreatitis: value of CT in establishing prognosis, *Radiology*, volume 174, issue 2, pp. 331–336. Copyright © 1990

of lipase in serum. However, the lipase test is less readily available in hospital laboratories. Other pancreatic enzymes have no diagnostic value.

CT can be used to confirm acute pancreatitis and can be evaluated with the Balthazar grading system, which can be correlated with mortality (see Box 201.1). However, the optimal timing of CT is open to discussion. Early scans may confirm the diagnosis, but the use of IV contrast media can worsen necrosis and renal failure, and early scans may be too early to identify developing necrosis. A scan at 4 days will invariably detect necrosis.

MRI has been evaluated as an alternative to CT, but as yet is not in widespread use for diagnosing acute pancreatitis. Ultrasound may show inflammation of the pancreas and is especially good for identifying biliary obstruction or gallstones.

The APACHE scoring system lists the blood parameters that should be checked in patients with acute pancreatitis. These include a full blood count and tests for urea, creatinine, electrolytes, C-reactive protein (CRP), and arterial blood gas. Liver function tests should be checked, as the vast majority of patients have a history of excess alcohol consumption, and these results may confirm concurrent hepatic damage, inflammation, and synthetic function. Calcium and triglyceride levels also should be checked to ensure they are not etiological factors for acute or chronic pancreatitis.

Prognosis of acute pancreatitis, and how to estimate it

Amylase and lipase levels have no prognostic role in pancreatitis. Scoring systems have been developed to predict outcomes. The Ranson and Glasgow scoring systems have been used in the past, but can only be applied at 48 hours. Subsequently, the APACHE II score has come into widespread use, and can be applied from 24 hours. The variables used in the APACHE system are listed in Table 201.1. A score of >8 at initial presentation or 24 hours later is considered in keeping with severe pancreatitis. CRP levels can reflect disease severity, rising with the degree of inflammation. However, there may be no rise for 48 hours, reducing the usefulness of CRP levels in initial assessment.

Treatment of acute pancreatitis, and its effectiveness

The initial approach to acute pancreatitis is to assess severity, using scoring systems (Ranson, APACHE, Glasgow), serum markers (CRP, haematocrit), and clinical assessment (blood pressure, pulse, and dehydration). Fluid resuscitation is integral to restore intravascular volume and third-space losses, with placement of a urinary catheter

Table 201.1 The APACHE II scoring system		
Physiological variables	**Age**	**Pancreatic history**
Rectal temp (°C)	<44	Non-operative patients
Mean arterial pressure (mm Hg)	45–54	Post emergency operation
Heart rate (bpm)	55–64	Post elective operation
Respiratory rate (bpm)	65–74	
Oxygen delivery (ml/min)	>75	
PO_2 (mm Hg)		
Arterial pH		
Sodium (mmol/l)		
Potassium (mmol/l)		
Creatinine (mg/dl)		
Haematocrit (%)		
White-cell count (10^3/ml)		

Reproduced with permission from Knaus WA, Draper EA, Wagner DP, Zimmerman JE, APACHE II: a severity of disease classification system, *Critical Care Medicine*, volume 13, issue 10, pp.818-29, copyright © 1985 Wolters Kluwer Health Inc.

to monitor urine output. Pain should be controlled and usually requires opiate analgesia.

Patients with moderate-to-severe pancreatitis, or any suggestion of organ failure (respiratory, circulatory, renal, etc.), should be monitored in a high-dependency or intensive care unit. Those with milder disease should still have close monitoring in view of the risk of rapid deterioration.

Patients are usually kept 'nil by mouth', as any oral intake further stimulates the pancreas, causing the release of pancreatic enzymes and potentially worsening pain. Nutrition is extremely important, given the hypercatabolic state of the patient; usually, nasojejunal feeding is implemented early via endoscopically placed nasojejunal tubes. Total parenteral nutrition is an alternative, particularly in patients who develop an ileus. However, the higher costs and increased rate of septic complications preclude the routine use of parenteral nutrition.

If patients fail to respond to treatment within 72 hours, a repeat CT scan should be performed to assess for pancreatic necrosis or abscess formation.

The use of antibiotics in acute pancreatitis is contentious, with studies showing variable results, and recognition of the increased risk of developing antibiotic-resistant bacterial strains. However, the general consensus is that pancreatic necrosis requires treatment with prophylactic broad-spectrum antibiotics, with doctors being advised to refer to their hospital's antibiotic policy when it comes to choice. If antibiotics are given, a minimum of 14 days treatment should be advocated. Fine-needle aspiration of the necrotic area can be cultured and used to guide antibiotic therapy.

ERCP has only been shown to be useful when performed early (within 72 hours) in patients with evidence of biliary obstruction, with a sphincterotomy performed to allow biliary drainage. The use of magnetic resonance cholangiopancreatography (MRCP) allows clear views of the biliary system, and has led to the avoidance of unnecessary ERCP. In general, sterile necrosis will be treated conservatively, whereas infected pancreatic necrosis requires surgical debridement by open surgical techniques. However, minimally invasive procedures (laparoscopic or endoscopic) may hold promise for the future.

Chronic pancreatitis

Chronic pancreatitis is characterized by progressive inflammation and fibrosis, leading to the irreversible loss of pancreatic structure and function.

Aetiology of chronic pancreatitis

Sixty to eighty per cent of cases of chronic pancreatitis are related to alcohol and, conversely, 10% of alcoholics develop chronic pancreatitis. Idiopathic chronic pancreatitis is responsible for ~20% of cases; other causes include recurrent acute pancreatitis (and all causes thereof), gallstones, trauma, and autoimmune pancreatitis

(AIP). Chronic pancreatitis has also been associated with primary biliary cholangitis, Sjögren's syndrome, SLE, and renal tubular acidosis. Genetic studies have suggested several genetic mutations may be associated with hereditary and idiopathic chronic pancreatitis.

Typical symptoms of chronic pancreatitis, and less common symptoms

Chronic pancreatitis can present with constant discomfort, or with recurrent episodes of severe pain. Postprandial pain may lead to food avoidance and subsequent weight loss. Persistent pancreatic destruction may lead to the patient presenting with symptoms of exocrine insufficiency (diarrhoea and/or weight loss) or endocrine insufficiency (diabetes).

Demographics of chronic pancreatitis

Chronic pancreatitis affects men twice as often as women and is more common in the fourth to the sixth decades.

Natural history of chronic pancreatitis, and complications of the disease

The natural history of chronic pancreatitis is highly variable, but the overall survival is approximately 70% at 10 years and 45% at 20 years. In the majority, the pain will gradually resolve or reduce over the course of years to decades, although, in alcohol-related disease, abstinence may expedite pain relief. Endocrine dysfunction may lead to a reduction in insulin secretion and subsequent diabetes, with all associated complications.

The exocrine pancreas produces digestive enzymes, including trypsin, chymotrypsin, lipase, and amylase, and lack of these leads to malabsorption and resultant diarrhoea, steatorrhoea, and/or weight loss. However, nutritional deficiencies are not seen until 90% of exocrine function is lost. Chronic pancreatitis is also associated with pseudocyst (10%) and pseudoaneurysm formation, biliary and duodenal obstruction (5%–10%), venous thrombosis, and pancreatic cancers. The cancer risk is 4% after 20 years of disease.

Approach to diagnosing chronic pancreatitis

Chronic pancreatitis is less straightforward, since the pain is often chronic, but an alcohol history may be a clue to the diagnosis. The presence of symptoms of pancreatic insufficiency (diarrhoea or diabetes) may help confirm chronic damage to the organ.

Diagnostic tests for chronic pancreatitis

Amylase is less useful in chronic pancreatitis as there is often no rise in serum levels, due to atrophy and fibrosis, with overall destruction of exocrine cells which normally produce this enzyme. Chronic pancreatitis is often diagnosed on the clinical history of recurrent abdominal pain, commonly in a setting of alcohol excess.

A CT scan of chronic pancreatitis may appear normal in mild disease, but moderate-to-severe disease will produce an atrophic fibrotic gland with dilated ducts and calcifications. CT has an overall sensitivity of 80% and a specificity of 85%.

A plain abdominal X-ray will reveal pancreatic calcification in ~30% of cases. Anterolateral and oblique views should be performed to ensure the vertebral column does not conceal small calcifications.

MRCP can provide clear views and is growing in popularity, as it is safe, fast, and accurate. It can also be combined with a secretin-stimulation test to provide information on pancreatic function (so-called functional MRI).

Criteria have been produced for diagnosing chronic pancreatitis from features seen from endoscopic ultrasound (EUS), including the presence of stones, irregular ducts, lobularity, and cysts. Pancreatic exocrine insufficiency can be assessed by a taking a stool sample to measure faecal pancreatic elastase. This will be reduced in advance pancreatic exocrine insufficiency (loss of ≥90% exocrine function). Other pancreatic function tests have been superseded by the simple faecal elastase test, but previously included the non-invasive para-aminobenzoic acid (commonly known as PABA) and pancreolauryl tests, and the invasive secretin-stimulation test and Lundh test.

As with acute pancreatitis, liver function tests, calcium levels, and triglyceride levels should be checked.

CHAPTER 201 **Pancreatic disease**

Treatment of chronic pancreatitis, and its effectiveness

Patients should be encouraged to stop drinking alcohol and smoking, as this can reduce pain and further pancreatic damage. Analgesics are required for pain relief; often, simple analgesics do not suffice and opiates are required. In extreme cases, a celiac ganglion block can relieve pain in ~50% of patients, but the relief is often short term, and complications (haemorrhage, transverse myelopathy) preclude regular use.

Pancreatic enzyme supplements can reduce symptoms of exocrine insufficiency and may reduce pain in some patients, by allowing the pancreas to 'rest'. Vitamin supplements (especially vitamin B_{12}) should be given where necessary, and low-fat meals may reduce symptoms.

Pancreatic duct strictures can be treated endoscopically by stent insertion and sphincterotomy, with resolution of pain in 65%. Pancreatic pseudocysts can often be treated endoscopically in specialist centres. Surgical procedures include a pancreaticojejunostomy to relieve pancreatic duct obstruction, or a pancreatic resection. However, the operative mortality is 3% and 10%, respectively, so it is reserved for patients who are severely affected but have an otherwise healthy premorbid status.

AIP

AIP is a relatively newly recognized disorder characterized by pancreatitis and biliary and/or pancreatic duct strictures and with autoimmune aetiology.

Aetiology of AIP

AIP has an autoimmune aetiology, and has been associated with other autoimmune conditions, including rheumatoid arthritis, primary biliary cholangitis, primary sclerosing cholangitis, Sjögren's syndrome, and inflammatory bowel disease. Recent studies have suggested that genetic factors related to the HLA complex may play a role in the development of this condition.

Typical symptoms of AIP, and less common symptoms

AIP can present with a variety of features, including mild acute pancreatitis, biliary or pancreatic strictures, and a pancreatic mass. Subsequently, symptoms are in keeping with those of acute pancreatitis, and also include jaundice and weight loss.

Demographics of AIP

AIP is more common in elderly men.

Natural history of AIP, and complications of the disease

Most patients with AIP will respond to either medical treatment, or endoscopic therapy of biliary strictures, and exocrine dysfunction is rarely detected after treatment. The long-term complications, including the potential increased risk of pancreatic cancer, are, as yet, unknown.

Approach to diagnosing AIP

Several criteria have been developed to aid diagnosis of AIP. The Mayo Clinic criteria state diagnosis can be made when ≥1 of the following are present:

- a diagnostic histology consistent with lymphoplasmacytic sclerosing pancreatitis
- response to steroid therapy
- a characteristic appearance on CT, with elevated IgG4 levels

Diagnostic tests for AIP

A diagnosis of AIP usually requires a histological sample and raised IgG4 levels. Increased serum levels of other autoantibodies, including rheumatoid factor, antinuclear antibody, and antibodies against lactoferrin and carbonic anhydrase, are often seen and can aid the diagnosis.

The CT appearance of the pancreas in AIP includes pancreatic enlargement, irregular narrowing of the pancreatic duct, sclerosing cholangitis, and/or stenosis of the intra-pancreatic duct. MRCP and EUS can also be used, but their usefulness is restricted by the limited availability of personnel with the technical skills needed to perform these techniques, and the difficulty of differentiating abnormalities from pancreatic or biliary cancer.

Prognosis of AIP, and how to estimate it

The overall prognosis is difficult to ascertain in AIP, due to it being a relatively new rare condition.

Treatment of AIP, and its effectiveness

The main treatment for AIP is steroid therapy. First, this can confirm the diagnosis, but the treatment also can relieve symptoms, improve structural abnormalities, and improve endocrine function in the short term. Steroids have been shown to help biliary strictures biochemically and structurally, although many patients undergo endoscopic therapy for biliary strictures before the diagnosis is confirmed. The long-term benefit of steroids is, however, not yet known.

Further treatment options require trials before they can be advocated.

Diabetes

Type 1 diabetes mellitus is caused by the autoimmune destruction of pancreatic beta cells, which normally produce insulin. Diabetes mellitus is dealt with in more detail in Chapter 184.

Cystic fibrosis

Cystic fibrosis is a condition caused by abnormalities in exocrine gland function and leads to the production of thick secretions affecting the lungs in 90% of patients with cystic fibrosis. It also leads to pancreatic exocrine insufficiency.

Aetiology of cystic fibrosis

Cystic fibrosis is an autosomal recessive genetic disorder caused by mutations in the cystic fibrosis transmembrane conductance regulator gene and disrupts chloride transport at the cellular level. Chloride ions, and associated sodium ion and water, are not secreted into the lumen, leading to the development of thick secretions in the airways and impaired mucociliary clearance. The pancreatic duct is lined with cells similar to those in the airways and, consequently, there is also a reduction in bicarbonate-related water secretion. As in the airways, this leads to the production of thick secretions which cause obstruction, dilatation, cellular damage, and fibrosis. Cystic fibrosis is the major cause of pancreatic insufficiency in childhood, and 85% of cystic fibrosis patients develop pancreatic insufficiency.

Demographics of cystic fibrosis

In the UK, cystic fibrosis affects over 8000 people, with a current life expectancy of 31 years.

Natural history of cystic fibrosis, and complications of the disease

Most complications and fatalities from cystic fibrosis are related to progressive lung disease. The pancreatic disease in cystic fibrosis can present as acute or chronic pancreatitis or progressive malnutrition due to malabsorption from pancreatic exocrine insufficiency.

Approach to diagnosing cystic fibrosis

Cystic fibrosis is usually diagnosed in childhood in a child with recurrent respiratory illnesses, failure to thrive, or diarrhoea.

Pancreatic cancer

Please see Chapter 204 for details about pancreatic cancer.

Other diagnoses that should be considered aside from pancreatic cancer

Upper abdominal pain has various differential diagnoses, including biliary colic, cholangitis, cholecystitis, gastritis, peptic ulcer disease, intestinal perforation, mesenteric ischaemia, Crohn's disease, and myocardial infarction.

Further Reading

Anand N, Park JH, and Wu BU. Modern management of acute pancreatitis. *Gastroenterol Clin North Am* 2012; 41: 1–8.

Forsmark CE, Vege SS, and Wilcox CM. Acute pancreatitis. *N Engl J Med* 2016; 375: 1972–81.

Majumder S, and Chari ST, Chronic pancreatitis. *Lancet* 2016; 387: 1957–66.

Sugumar A. Diagnosis and management of autoimmune pancreatitis. *Gastroenterol Clin North Am* 2012; 41: 9–22.

Trikudanathan G, Navaneethan U, and Vege SS. Modern treatment of patients with chronic pancreatitis. *Gastroenterol Clin North Am* 2012; 41: 63–76.

CHAPTER 201 **Pancreatic disease**

202 Malabsorption

Satish Keshav and Alexandra Kent

Definition of the disease

Malabsorption is defined as a defect in the digestion and absorption of nutrients by the gastrointestinal tract. It can lead to a specific nutritional deficiency ('selective' malabsorption, such as vitamin B_{12} deficiency) or a general nutritional deficiency (global malabsorption, such as that due to diseases affecting the mucosa diffusely, such as Crohn's disease).

Aetiology of the disease

Causes of malabsorption are listed in Table 202.1, and many of these diseases are dealt with elsewhere in this book. The commonest causes are coeliac disease and pancreatic exocrine insufficiency. Pancreatic insufficiency is dealt with in Chapter 201.

In coeliac disease, also known as gluten-sensitive enteropathy, an immunologically mediated reaction to gliadin peptides in cereals such as wheat, rye, and barley causes damage to the intestinal mucosa. Pathological features of coeliac disease include increased numbers of intra-epithelial lymphocytes, reduced height of intestinal villi, and increased length of the intestinal crypts. Loss of intestinal villi reduces the absorptive capacity of the small bowel, leading to malabsorption. There is a strong association with two HLA haplotypes: HLA-DQ2 and HLA-DQ8. Furthermore there is a hereditary component, with a prevalence of 10% in first-degree relatives, and 75% concordance between monozygotic twins.

There is an increased incidence of coeliac disease in patients with type 1 diabetes mellitus, Down's syndrome, Turner's syndrome, autoimmune thyroid disease, primary sclerosing cholangitis, primary biliary cholangitis, autoimmune cholangitis, autoimmune adrenal disease, Sjögren's syndrome, rheumatoid arthritis, and SLE.

Typical symptoms of the disease, and less common symptoms

Symptoms of malabsorption include diarrhoea, steatorrhoea, weight loss, anaemia, oedema, abdominal pain/bloating, defective bone metabolism, neurological manifestations, and others.

Diarrhoea

Diarrhoea is the most common presenting symptom, and is due to the reduced absorption of nutrients leading to an increased osmotic load reaching the colon, resulting in watery diarrhoea.

Steatorrhoea

Steatorrhoea is caused by fat malabsorption. It is characterized by the passage of pale, bulky, and often malodorous stools which are often difficult to flush. It is usually caused by pancreatic insufficiency, and may also be seen in severe coeliac disease.

Weight loss

Weight loss is more common in conditions affecting a larger surface area of the gastrointestinal tract, such as coeliac disease. Patients may increase their oral intake masking the reduced absorption of nutrients.

Anaemia

Anaemia can be caused by iron deficiency, vitamin B_{12} deficiency, or folate deficiency. Iron is absorbed in the duodenum and upper jejunum, folate is absorbed in the proximal jejunum, and vitamin B_{12} is absorbed in the terminal ileum after it is bound to intrinsic factor

Table 202.1 Causes of malabsorption	
Mechanism	**Cause**
Defects in digestion	
Enzyme deficiency	Pancreatic insufficiency (e.g. chronic pancreatitis, cystic fibrosis)
	Lactase deficiency
	Alpha-glucosidase deficiency
Bile salt deficiency	Cirrhosis
	Cholestasis
	Small bowel bacterial overgrowth
Defects in absorption	
Damage to the intestinal wall	Coeliac disease
	Crohn's disease
	Eosinophilic gastroenteritis
	IgA deficiency
	Radiation enteritis
	Autoimmune enteropathy
	Intestinal lymphangiectasia
	Systemic mastocytosis
	Abetalipoproteinaemia
	Acrodermatitis enteropathica
	Enterokinase deficiency
	Small bowel lymphoma
	Short bowel syndrome
Circulatory defects	Mesenteric ischaemia
	Venous insufficiency (e.g. thrombosis, portal stasis, infiltration, trauma)
	Chronic heart failure ('cardiac cachexia')
	Constrictive pericarditis (due to dilated lymphatics leading to excessive protein loss)
Small bowel overgrowth	Small bowel diverticulosis
	Gastric atrophy
	Fistulae
	Diabetic neuropathy
	Scleroderma
	Obstruction
Microbial agents	Intestinal parasitosis (e.g. giardiasis)
	Tropical sprue
	Whipple's disease
	HIV
Miscellaneous	
	Achlorhydria
	Hyperthyroidism
	Drug related (e.g. orlistat, acarbose, colchicines)
	Amyloidosis
	Autonomic neuropathy
	Zollinger–Ellison syndrome (leads to inactivation of pancreatic enzymes)

produced by gastric parietal cells. Disease processes affecting any of these parts of the bowel can lead to anaemia. Small intestinal bacterial overgrowth can cause impaired B_{12} absorption, but bacteria produce folate, so folate deficiency is rare.

Oedema

Chronic protein malabsorption leads to hypoalbuminaemia, with resultant oedema. This often affects the peripheries initially, but can cause ascites as it progresses. Intestinal lymphangiectasia can cause obstruction of the lymphatic system, with resultant oedema.

Abdominal pain/bloating

Bacterial fermentation of unabsorbed food substances releases gaseous products such as hydrogen and methane and this can cause bloating, abdominal discomfort, and excess flatulence.

Defective bone metabolism

Osteopenia and osteoporosis are caused by vitamin D and calcium malabsorption, and are well-recognized complications of coeliac disease.

Neurological manifestations

The following nutritional deficiencies may lead to the specific neurological manifestations listed, although these are rare:

- hypocalcaemia: tetany
- hypomagnesaemia: tetany
- thiamine deficiency: peripheral neuropathy
- vitamin A deficiency: night blindness
- vitamin D deficiency: hypocalcaemia, hypomagnesaemia, bone pain, and muscle weakness
- vitamin B_{12} deficiency: anaemia, and loss of vibration sense and joint position sense

Other symptoms

Other symptoms recognized in coeliac disease include fatigue, alopecia, mouth ulcers, dyspepsia, headaches, dermatitis herpetiformis, infertility, amenorrhoea, and miscarriage.

Demographics of the disease

Approximately 1% of the UK population has coeliac disease, although it is estimated that only 1 in 8 have their condition diagnosed. Approximately 3 million people in Europe have coeliac disease, and it is more common in temperate climates, with the highest incidence in Ireland, Finland, and North America. However, the incidence is increasing in the Indian and Middle Eastern population. It has a bimodal age distribution, with peaks at 8–12 months and again in the third and fourth decades. It affects women slightly more than men.

Natural history and complications of the disease

Generally, patients respond rapidly to a gluten-free diet, with resolution of symptoms and a return to a normal small bowel mucosa. Complications can arise due to malabsorption, and nutritional deficits should be supplemented. There is a greater incidence of osteoporosis seen in coeliac patients, especially those with a low BMI and poor compliance with a gluten-free diet. Current guidelines advocate performing a DEXA bone densitometry scan in those patients with two or more of the following:

- persisting symptoms on a gluten-free diet for 1 year, or poor adherence to gluten-free diet
- weight loss >10%
- BMI <20
- age >70

Uncontrolled coeliac disease increases the risk of cancer, including enteropathy-associated T-cell lymphoma, as well as adenocarcinoma of the oropharynx, oesophagus, pancreas, small and large bowel, and hepatobiliary tract.

Approach to diagnosing the disease

Initial laboratory investigations in any patient with symptoms of malabsorption should always include coeliac serology. The most sensitive and specific antibodies are the tissue transglutaminase IgA, endomysial IgA, and reticulin IgA, and these antibodies have been show to correlate with the degree of mucosal damage. It is important to remember that a significant number of patients with coeliac disease have IgA deficiency and, as such, the IgA level should be checked in patients with negative serology results.

Supporting laboratory evidence of malabsorption includes iron, folate, and B_{12} deficiencies, anaemia, hypoalbuminaemia, hypoproteinaemia, hypocalcaemia, hypomagnesaemia, hypokalaemia, and secondary hyperparathyroidism.

Other diagnoses that should be considered

Causes of malabsorption are listed in Table 202.1, which also serves as a list of differential diagnoses to consider.

'Gold-standard' diagnostic test

The gold-standard diagnostic test for malabsorption is an upper gastrointestinal endoscopy, with mucosal biopsies taken from the duodenum. This will provide a histological diagnosis of coeliac disease, which is staged using the Marsh classification:

- type I: normal mucosal architecture with an increased number of intra-epithelial lymphocytes
- type II: increase in crypt depth without villous flattening
- type III: villous atrophy; divided into:
  - type IIIa: partial villous atrophy
  - type IIIb: sub-total villous atrophy
  - type IIIc: total villous atrophy

Acceptable diagnostic alternatives to the gold standard

The only reason for employing alternative methods of diagnosis is when patients are unable to tolerate endoscopic investigations and it is impossible to obtain mucosal biopsies. In this instance, most centres would advocate implementing a strict gluten-free diet, and monitoring a serological and clinical response. Genetic testing can be useful to exclude coeliac disease, as >97% of patients are HLA DQ2 and/or HLA DQ8 positive, compared with ~40% of the general population.

Other relevant investigations

Further investigations would be used to diagnose alternative causes of malabsorption, and Table 202.2 provides diagnostic investigations for these differential diagnoses. Investigations to confirm carbohydrate malabsorption (e.g. an oral D-xylose tolerance test) are not generally performed nowadays.

Prognosis and how to estimate it

Apart from the slightly increased risk of malignancy, and the effect on quality of life of having to adhere to a strictly gluten-free diet, coeliac disease has a benign prognosis once the diagnosis has been established.

Treatment and its effectiveness

The only definitive treatment is lifelong adherence to a strictly gluten-free diet. Ancillary assistance that should be offered to patients is summarized in the mnemonic CELIAC:

C: consultation with a skilled dietitian
E: education about the disease
L: lifelong adherence to a gluten-free diet
I: identification and treatment of nutritional deficiencies
A: access to an advocacy group
C: continuous long-term follow-up by a multidisciplinary team

The mainstay of treatment for coeliac disease is compliance with a strict gluten-free diet. This involves close interactions between the physician, the dietician, and the patient. Patients are able to receive gluten-free products on prescription and are encouraged to join Coeliac UK or other appropriate patient organizations. These can

Table 202.2 Treatment of causes of malabsorption

Disease	Diagnostic investigation(s)	Treatment
Pancreatic insufficiency	Faecal elastase	Pancreatic supplements
Lactase deficiency	Hydrogen breath test Intestinal biopsy with measurement of lactase levels	Dairy-free diet Lactase supplements Calcium +/− vitamin D supplements
Alpha-glucosidase deficiency	Acid alpha-glucosidase activity in cultured skin fibroblasts or peripheral blood lymphocytes	Enzyme replacement
Bile salt deficiency	SeHCAT scan	Colestyramine
Eosinophilic gastroenteritis	Intestinal biopsy	Corticosteroids Elimination diet
IgA deficiency	Serum IgA level	Preventative measures to reduce, and early treatment of, infections
Radiation enteritis	Intestinal biopsy/histology	Antidiarrhoeals Bile-sequestering agents Corticosteroids Anti-emetics 5-Aminosalicylic acid Sucralfate Endoscopic therapy (e.g. argon plasma coagulation)
Autoimmune enteropathy	Antienterocyte autoantibodies	Exclusion diet Immunosuppressive therapy
Intestinal lymphangiectasia	Low protein, albumin, and immunoglobulin levels Small bowel endoscopy with jejunal biopsies	Dietary modifications Bulking agents Octreotide Antidiarrhoeals Investigate for secondary causes
Systemic mastocytosis	Total serum tryptase levels ≥ 20 ng/ml Bone marrow aspirate	Symptomatic treatment for anaphylaxis, malabsorption, peptic ulcer, diarrhoea, and pruritus Chemotherapy not seen to be effective
Abetalipoproteinaemia	Low serum cholesterol level No apolipoprotein B (confirmed by immunoelectrophoresis)	Vitamins A and E
Acrodermatitis enteropathica	Low serum zinc	Zinc supplementation
Enterokinase deficiency	Enterokinase activity in duodenal juice and intestinal mucosa	Pancreatic enzyme replacement
Small bowel lymphoma	Radiology Small bowel studies Histology	Surgical resection Chemotherapy
Short bowel syndrome	Previous medical history of bowel resections	Oral or IV replacement of nutrients Total parenteral nutrition
Circulatory defects	Mucosal biopsy/histology	Treat underlying disease
Small bowel overgrowth	Glucose hydrogen breath test	Antibiotics
Microbial agents	Stool culture Mucosal biopsy/histology	Antibiotics

provide support and information regarding the source of appropriate foods, and potential hazards. Patients are advised to avoid all wheat, rye, and barley, but oat is generally considered to be acceptable in the diet. Unfortunately, oat products are often contaminated with other gluten-containing grains. The majority of patients respond to gluten avoidance; should symptoms recur or persist, the first step is to assess compliance. Approximately 5% of patients develop refractory coeliac disease, despite a strict gluten-free diet. Corticosteroids can be effective, usually given as a tapering 6–8 week course.

Treatments for other, less common causes of malabsorption are listed in Table 202.2.

Further Reading

Fasano A and Catassi C. Clinical practice. Celiac disease. *N Engl J Med* 2012; 367: 2419–26.

Montalto M, Santoro L, D'Onofrio F, et al. Classification of malabsorption syndromes. *Dig Dis* 2008; 26: 104–11.

203 Inflammatory bowel disease

Satish Keshav and Alexandra Kent

Definition of the disease

Inflammatory bowel disease (IBD) encompasses ulcerative colitis (UC) and Crohn's disease (CD). Both conditions cause chronic relapsing inflammation in the gastrointestinal (GI) tract, but have different characteristics, as shown in Table 203.1.

UC causes diffuse mucosal inflammation limited to the colon, extending proximally from the anal verge, with the rectum involved in 95% of patients. UC is described in terms of the disease extent: proctitis (confined to the rectum), proctosigmoiditis (disease confined to the recto-sigmoid colon), distal disease (distal to the splenic flexure), and pan-colitis (the entire large intestine). The extent of disease can change, with proximal extension seen in approximately a third of patients with proctitis, although there is great variation between studies.

CD causes inflammation that can affect the entire thickness of the wall of the intestine, and is not confined to the mucosa. CD can affect any part of the GI tract. The terminal ileum is affected in approximately 80% of cases, the colon in approximately 60% of cases, and the rectum and perianal region in approximately 40% of cases. CD is classified by location (ileal, colonic, ileocolonic, upper GI tract), by the presence of stricturing or penetrating disease, and by the age of onset (before or after the age of 40). Penetrating disease refers to the development of fistulae, which can lead to complications such as abscesses or perforations. An earlier age at onset is associated with more complicated disease.

The diagnosis of UC or CD is established through a combination of clinical, endoscopic, radiological, and histological criteria rather than by any single modality. Occasionally, it is not possible to establish an unequivocal diagnosis of CD or UC in IBD, and a third category, accounting for nearly 10% of cases, is used, termed IBD unclassified.

Aetiology of the disease

The pathogenesis of IBD is considered to be due to an aberrant immune response to luminal bacteria in genetically susceptible individuals, although no specific pathogen has been identified. Inflammation is driven by immunological responses, including macrophage activation, leucocyte trafficking, and the production of inflammatory cytokines such as tumour necrosis factor alpha, which seems to be a critically important mediator in IBD. Genome-wide scanning has confirmed multiple genetic loci that confer an increased risk of developing IBD, and many of these have roles in bacterial recognition within the intestinal lumen. The first gene, and the one for which the most results have been replicated, is the NOD2 gene, which is found on Chromosome 16, is associated with ileal disease, and has a role in the innate immune system. Further genes identified include the autophagy gene IRGM, the interleukin 23 receptor gene, the autophagy gene ATG16, and other loci in the region. Many more genes have been identified, but the results for these genes are less well replicated, although studies are ongoing. The importance of genetics in IBD development is confirmed by the greater incidence of IBD in first-degree relatives (5–20-fold increased risk), a 5%–10% concordance in dizygotic twins, and 50% concordance for disease in monozygotic twins.

Typical symptoms of the disease, and less common symptoms

UC is typically characterized by diarrhoea, often with the passage of blood and/or mucus. The extent of symptoms is related to the disease extent and depth of ulceration within the colon. Abdominal pain, or discomfort, is not uncommon. It is important to document the bowel frequency and the need to defaecate at night. More serious signs include tachycardia or fever (>37.5°C); these indicate the need for hospital admission. Criteria developed by Truelove and Witts have been used to indicate the need for inpatient intensive treatment of acute severe colitis, which is a medical emergency.

Symptoms of CD are more varied, and related to the site of disease activity and nature of disease. Colonic inflammation (Crohn's colitis) may present with diarrhoea, with or without the presence of blood, in a fashion similar to that for UC. However, small bowel disease may be less evident, with abdominal pain prevailing. Stricturing disease may be due to active CD or to fibrosis from previous active inflammation. Stricturing can lead to progressive obstructive symptoms, with bloating, abdominal pain, and vomiting if the stricture is high in the GI tract. Penetrating disease most commonly affects the

Table 203.1 Comparison of ulcerative colitis and Crohn's disease		
	Ulcerative colitis	**Crohn's disease**
Depth of inflammation	Mucosal/superficial inflammation	Transmural inflammation
Histology	Diffuse inflammatory infiltrate	Diffuse inflammatory infiltrate
	Goblet cell depletion	Goblet cell depletion
	Cryptitis	Cryptitis
	Crypt abscesses	Crypt abscesses
	No granulomas	Granulomas
		Fibrosis
Location	Colonic	Any part of the gastrointestinal tract
Pattern of inflammation	Continuous; starts at the rectum and progresses proximally	Patchy/segmental
		Cobblestoning
		Skip lesions
Response to immunosuppression	Yes	Yes
Response to 5-aminosalicylic acid medications	Yes	No
Strictures	No	Yes
Fistulae	No	Yes
Smoking history	Associated with non-smokers	Associated with smokers

perianal region, leading to fistulae and abscesses which are at risk of crossing the anal sphincters. Perianal fistulae lead to persistent discharge, and abscesses can be extremely painful. Perianal skin tags and anal fissures are also seen in Crohn's disease.

Fatigue is a common symptom, and IBD is commonly associated with anaemia. This is usually due to iron deficiency from chronic blood loss and the anaemia of chronic disease, which is a consequence of the effect of chronic inflammation on iron absorption and utilization. Small bowel disease can also disrupt absorptive capacity, reducing iron, folate, and B$_{12}$ absorption; this, in turn, can lead to anaemia.

IBD is associated with extra-intestinal manifestations, the commonest of which include oral ulceration, arthralgia, arthritis, erythema nodosum, pyoderma gangrenosum, iritis, uveitis, and mouth ulcers. Therefore, patients should be asked, as a matter of routine, about symptoms associated with these conditions: rashes, skin changes, painful or red eyes, and joint swelling or arthralgia.

Demographics of the disease

In the UK, UC has an annual incidence of 10–20 per 100 000 population, compared to the incidence of CD being 5–10 per 100 000 population. The prevalence rates for IBD are 100–200 per 100 000 population. Overall, IBD affects 1 in 400 people in the UK. The peak incidence is at 10–40 years old, with both genders equally affected. IBD is more common in the Western world, although immigrants have the same incidence as the indigenous population. Studies have also shown IBD to have a higher prevalence in colder climates and in urban areas.

Natural history and complications of the disease

Both UC and CD are relapsing–remitting conditions with an unpredictable course for any individual patient. The average UC patient has a 50% chance of a flare in 2 years, and up to 10% may have only one flare in their lifetime. Up to 80% of CD patients and 30% of UC patients require surgery at some point. However, the overall risk is dependent on the site and extent of the disease, and varies widely between studies. Patients with disease limited to the recto-sigmoid have a 12% risk of colectomy, while those with pan-colitis have a 60% risk. However, up to 50% of patients with proctitis may have some proximal extension during their lives. The prognosis and risk of colectomy in acute severe colitis can be calculated using the Truelove–Witts criteria, which are shown in Table 203.2. If, on Day 3 of admission, patients have a bowel frequency of >8 times per day or a C-reactive protein (CRP) level >45 mg/l combined with a bowel frequency of 3–8 times per day, they have an 85% risk of requiring colectomy on that admission.

There are multiple complications associated with IBD, beyond the nutritional deficiencies related to malabsorption. Extra-intestinal manifestations which physicians should play close attention to include:

- dermatological manifestations such as erythema nodosum, pyoderma gangrenosum, Sweet's syndrome (neutrophilic dermatosis), and vasculitis
- ophthalmological manifestations such as iritis, uveitis, and episcleritis; these require urgent treatment in conjunction with an ophthalmological specialist, to prevent visual loss

- arthritis: axial arthritis, including ankylosing spondylitis and sacroiliitis, affects approximately 5% of IBD patients (usually those with CD) and is usually associated with HLA-B27; peripheral arthritis occurs in up to 10% of IBD patients
- hepatobiliary manifestations: primary sclerosing cholangitis (PSC) is associated with IBD, most commonly UC, and any patient with abnormal liver function should undergo investigations for this condition; there is a high incidence of cholangiocarcinoma in PSC, so establishing the diagnosis is vital
- renal associations: calcium oxalate renal stones are more common in CD
- osteoporosis: can occur due to malabsorption and recurrent steroid use
- thromboembolic phenomena: patients admitted to hospital with flares of IBD should be prescribed prophylactic heparin, as there is an increased risk of deep vein thrombosis and embolic phenomena

Approach to diagnosing the disease

The classic patient with IBD is a young adult (20–40 years) with a 4–8 week history of diarrhoea, often waking at night to defaecate. It is often difficult to differentiate them from patients with other conditions, although raised inflammatory markers and/or anaemia support the diagnosis. Most gastroenterologists would advocate performing a rigid sigmoidoscopy in the outpatient clinic, as the presence of proctitis would support the diagnosis and allow the doctor to initiate treatment in the absence of histological confirmation. Initiating topical (rectal) 5-aminosalicylic acid (5-ASA) therapy can often improve symptoms, and may well reduce the risk of progression prior to biopsy results. However, if infective colitis is a possible diagnosis, it may be necessary to withhold steroids until a histological diagnosis, or until negative stool cultures have excluded an infective cause. An endoscopy is required to accurately assess the extent of disease and obtain serial biopsies.

Other diagnoses that should be considered

The major diagnosis that needs to be excluded, prior to commencing steroid therapy in undiagnosed IBD, is infective colitis. In view of this, known IBD patients presenting with diarrhoea flares should always have stool samples sent to exclude concomitant infectious diarrhoea, particular dysentery caused by organisms such as shigella and campylobacter; amoebiasis; and diarrhoea associated with *Clostridium difficile* toxin. The exact presenting symptom influences differential diagnoses to be excluded, but the commonest include infectious diarrhoea, microscopic colitis, diverticulitis, coeliac disease, eosinophilic gastroenteritis, giardiasis, irritable bowel syndrome, lactose intolerance, bacterial overgrowth, radiation injury, and colorectal cancer.

'Gold-standard' diagnostic test

A colonoscopy, including intubation of the terminal ileum, will diagnose the vast majority of IBD cases. Many patients will have characteristic mucosal appearances, and typical histological changes confirm the diagnosis. Furthermore, in continuous or distal inflammation, histological results will differentiate between UC and CD.

Acceptable diagnostic alternatives to the gold standard

A true diagnosis of IBD requires histological confirmation, and treating patients for IBD without such confirmation requires the expertise of experienced physicians. A flexible sigmoidoscopy is the appropriate first-line investigation, especially in patients with severe inflammation, as these patients have a higher risk of perforation during a total colonoscopy. As UC is characterized by continuous inflammation, a sigmoidoscopy may pass beyond the extent of inflammation. As long as the full extent of inflammation is confirmed macroscopically and histologically, further investigations can be avoided. Patients unable to tolerate bowel purgation or an endoscopic examination may require CT colonography. Although it is not possible to obtain biopsies during a CT scan, characteristic inflammation with bowel wall thickening is easily identified, and can at least confirm the extent of disease. CT

Table 203.2 Truelove and Witts classification for activity of ulcerative colitis

	Mild	Moderate	Severe
Bowel frequency per day	<4	4–6	>6
Temperature	Afebrile	<37.8	≥37.8
Heart rate	Normal	Indeterminate	≥90
Haemoglobin (g/dl)	>11	10.5–11	<10.5
ESR (mm/hour)	<20	20–30	>30

Reproduced from *The BMJ*, S. C. Truelove, L. J. Witts, Cortisone in ulcerative colitis: final report on a therapeutic trial, volume 2, pp. 1041-8, copyright © 1955 with permission from BMJ Publishing Group Ltd.

scanning is also the first-line investigation for patients with an inflammatory mass, and/or possible luminal perforation.

Small bowel CD will require small bowel imaging, by MRI, CT, or barium radiography. CD of the upper GI tract may require an upper GI endoscopy or enteroscopy, with biopsies. In patients with stricturing CD or an inflammatory mass, a histological diagnosis is usually made after surgical resection of the affected bowel. Capsule endoscopy is rarely used for a diagnosis of small bowel CD, although it may be picked up in patients undergoing the procedure to investigate persistent anaemia.

Other relevant investigations

The following investigations should be performed:

- a full blood count: patients may be anaemic due to iron, folate or B_{12} deficiency, or anaemia of chronic disease; a leucocytosis is unusual in IBD, unless the patient is taking steroids, and should direct the physician to exclude infections, especially infectious diarrhoea; thrombocytosis is common in active inflammation
- renal function: persistent diarrhoea can cause dehydration
- electrolytes: persistent diarrhoea causes hypokalaemia, and reduced oral intake and malnutrition or reduced absorptive capacity in IBD patients often leads to hypomagnesaemia and hypocalcaemia
- liver function: abnormal liver function tests can be due to associated PSC or medications (5-ASA, azathioprine, 6-mercaptopurine (6MP)); serum albumin drops in active disease
- inflammatory markers: the most commonly used markers of inflammation are CRP and the erythrocyte sedimentation rate (ESR), both of which correlate with disease activity, although CRP is probably more reliable and preferred
- haematinics: vitamin B_{12}, folate, and iron levels should be checked in all patients, as chronic blood loss, chronic disease, or malabsorption can lead to deficiencies
- coeliac serology: this should be checked to exclude celiac disease as an alternative or concomitant diagnosis
- stool culture: all patients, on initial presentation and in the setting of a flare, should have stool samples sent for microscopy and culture and assessment for *Clostridium difficile* toxin
- plain abdominal X-ray: this should be performed on all patients presenting with a flare of their disease, as it can identify bowel wall thickening or thumbprinting, which are consistent with inflammation; proximal faecal loading (formed stool in the right colon) is not uncommonly seen in distal colitis, and helps delineate disease extent; it is also important to exclude toxic dilatation
- fistulogram: in patients with penetrating disease, a fistulogram can assess the depth, extent, and course of a fistula

Prognosis and how to estimate it

Studies have suggested there is a small, but significant mortality increase in IBD compared to non-IBD populations. However, the mortality rates have reduced dramatically in the last 40–50 years, due to the introduction of anti-inflammatory treatment, particularly hydrocortisone, for acute and severe disease. Earlier and more intensive management of chronically active IBD, and appropriate surgery, also contribute to the generally favourable prognosis in IBD. While the effects of the disease are mitigated by treatment, the major emerging cause of morbidity and mortality is also treatment, especially the use of powerful immunosuppressives such as thiopurines, anti-tumour necrosis factor (anti-TNF) antibodies, and corticosteroids.

Treatment and its effectiveness

Treatment for IBD should be tailored to the individual, and is influenced both by disease distribution, activity, and extent and by drug potency and side effects. There are a number of differences between treatment for UC and that for Crohn's.

5-ASA

5-ASA therapy is appropriate for treating active UC and maintaining remission. It is ineffective for CD. There are several 5-ASA products available, including sulfasalazine, mesalazine, balsalazide, and olsalazine. 5-ASA can be given orally or topically as suppositories or rectal foam or liquid enemas (1 g per day). Proctitis should be initially treated with topical treatment, with suppositories more appropriate for rectal disease, and enemas reaching more proximally. Topical therapy is effective in a median of 67% of patients with active disease. In patients with disease extending beyond the rectum, topical treatment is combined with oral therapy (≥2 g per day). Remission rates vary between 20% and 60% amongst studies, although the response rates are higher. 5-ASA medications are the first-line treatment for maintaining remission, and studies have suggested 5-ASA therapy reduces the risk of colorectal cancer in the long term.

Steroids

If patients with mild-to-moderately active UC fail to respond after 2 weeks of combined oral and topical 5-ASA, or in Crohn's colitis, steroid therapy will be introduced. This is usually with prednisolone 40 mg daily, reducing over the course of 5–8 weeks, and can induce remission in 70%–80% of patients. Patients with severe colitis are usually commenced on steroids from the outset, and the majority, especially those with acute severe colitis, should be admitted to hospital for IV steroid therapy. Acute severe colitis is a potentially life-threatening condition, and treatment should not be delayed. Treatment with hydrocortisone 100 mg four times per day, combined with rectal steroid therapy is advocated, with a response seen in approximately 70%.

Small bowel CD is initially treated with budesonide. This achieves remission in 50%–60% over 8–10 weeks. It is preferred to prednisolone due to the reduced systemic bioavailability. However, if patients fail to respond, prednisolone can induce remission in up to 90%. In severely active disease, IV steroids should be commenced.

Nutrition

All patients with IBD should be carefully monitored for nutritional deficiencies. Enteral nutrition is important, but is less effective as a treatment option than steroids. The exception to this rule is in children, who are equally responsive to steroids or enteral nutrition, with the latter often used due to the reduced side effects.

Antibiotics

Many studies have been performed, assessing the efficacy of antibiotics in IBD. Overall, antibiotics are only suitable in the setting of infection such as, for example, perianal CD, abscess formation, or pouchitis. Treatment is usually instituted with metronidazole or ciprofloxacin.

Thiopurines: Azathioprine/6MP

IBD patients who become steroid dependent, or have early recurrence of disease, are commenced on azathioprine or 6MP. These drugs are associated with a higher rate of remission and mucosal healing than steroids or 5-ASA medications are, and avoid the complications of long-term steroids. These medications take up to 16 weeks to take effect, so patients often require steroid maintenance therapy until the drugs take full effect. The main side effects are bone marrow suppression, deranged liver function, pancreatitis, infections relating to immunosuppression, and GI symptoms. Bone marrow suppression and abnormal liver function may respond to reduced doses, but pancreatitis should prevent further use.

Ciclosporin

Ciclosporin is an effective therapy for IV-steroid-resistant, severe UC, with a response seen in 50%–80% of patients. However, Ciclosporin has a poorer long-term response, with many patients requiring a colectomy within the subsequent year.

Methotrexate

Studies have shown methotrexate to be an effective treatment for IBD, but there is less evidence than for azathioprine or 6MP. As such, it is reserved for patients who are resistant to, or intolerant of, these medications, with clear explanations of the teratogenic potential.

Therapeutic antibodies

Infliximab (a chimeric anti-TNF monoclonal antibody) is an effective therapy in moderate-to-severe UC and CD, where steroids and immunomodulator therapy fail to induce remission. Adalimumab (humanized anti-TNF monoclonal antibody) and certolizumab (an anti-TNF Fab fragment conjugated to poly-ethylene glycol) are alternatives administered subcutaneously that induce remission in CD. The use of these and other therapeutic antibodies and other protein-based therapeutics should be closely supervised by those who are specialists in the field and have a good working knowledge of the risks and benefits of these agents, and of strategies to manage the patient's overall therapy.

Vedolizumab is a humanized antibody that blocks a surface protein found on lymphocytes and which mediates the movement of immune cells form the circulation into the intestine and liver exclusively. It is highly effective in treating UC, and is also effective in CD. Because it interrupts only the movement of immune cells to the intestine, this treatment should not cause global immunosuppression, and therefore may represent a new and more effective treatment strategy.

Subcutaneous heparin

Acute flares of IBD are associated with thromboembolic complications and, as such, all patients admitted to hospital for treatment of active disease should be commenced on heparin prophylaxis.

Surgery

In acute severe colitis, patients should be introduced to the surgical team and stoma nurses early on, as those in whom there is an inadequate response to treatment 3 days may well require colectomy. Even when secondary or 'rescue' treatment is introduced, the risk of needing surgery remains high. Surgery for colitis usually has two stages, with a colectomy and ileostomy formation performed initially. At a later date, an anastomosis can be performed, with the formation of an ileo-anal pouch and pouch–anal anastomosis. The pouch acts as a reservoir, and the intact anus provides continence.

Surgery in CD is more varied, as the disease affects a greater extent of the GI tract. Surgery is kept to a minimum, and resections are planned to be as conservative as possible, to minimize the risk of short bowel syndrome and intestinal failure. Perianal CD requires integrated care from medical and surgical teams, often requiring a combination of surgical debridement, placement of seton sutures, and medical therapy.

Further Reading

Bamias G, Pizarro TT, and Cominelli F. Pathway-based approaches to the treatment of inflammatory bowel disease. *Transl Res* 2016; 167: 104–15.

Baumgart DC and Sandborn WJ. Crohn's disease. *Lancet* 2012; 380: 1590–605.

Ordás I, Eckmann L, Talamini M, et al. Ulcerative colitis. *Lancet* 2012; 380: 1606–19.

Torres J, Mehandru S, Colombei JF, et al. Chrohn's disease. *Lancet* 2017; 389: 1741–55.

Ungaro R, Mehandru S, Allen PB, et al. Ulcerative colitis. *Lancet* 2017; 389: 1756–70.

204 Gastrointestinal tumours

Satish Keshav and Alexandra Kent

Approach to the patient with gastrointestinal cancer

Gastrointestinal (GI) tumours can affect any part of the GI tract, and colorectal cancer is the most common. Throughout the GI tract, chronic inflammation seems to promote the development of neoplasia: for example, chronic reflux oesophagitis is linked to oesophageal adenocarcinoma; chronic *Helicobacter pylori* infection is linked to gastric cancer; chronic pancreatitis is linked to pancreatic cancer; cirrhosis is linked to hepatocellular cancer; chronic biliary inflammation is linked to cholangiocarcinoma; untreated coeliac disease is linked to intestinal lymphoma; and chronic inflammatory bowel disease is linked to colorectal cancer. Symptoms depend on the location of the tumour, and occur as a result of local anatomical disruption, with consequent functional consequences and, less frequently, as a result of hormonal, metabolic, and immune effects. Weight loss is a common symptom seen in the gastroenterology outpatient clinic, given the high overall incidence of GI tumours. Often, the associated symptoms will direct the doctor to the site of a possible underlying cancer. Anaemia is another non-specific finding with a strong association with luminal cancers. Patients with anaemia with or without weight loss will normally undergo upper and lower GI investigations, usually via oesophagogastroduodenoscopy (OGD) and colonoscopy (either CT or endoscopic colonoscopy).

In tumours that are difficult to identify or for which assessing the malignant potential is difficult, PET scanning can provide a large amount of information. PET scanning is a nuclear medicine scanning technique that utilizes 18F-fluorodeoxyglucose (FDG), which is taken up by metabolically active tissue. When combined with CT scanning, it can provide information about both anatomical and metabolic activity. FDG is rapidly taken up by malignant tumours and, as a result, is often used for diagnosing, staging, and monitoring response in cancers.

Oesophageal cancer

Aetiology of oesophageal cancer

Oesophageal cancers are squamous cell carcinomas (SCCs) occurring in the mid- or upper oesophagus, or adenocarcinomas occurring at the gastro-oesophageal junction or associated with Barrett's oesophagus. Barrett's oesophagus is associated with gastro-oesophageal reflux disease (GORD). Etiological factors associated with SCC include tobacco smoking and alcohol (independently and synergistically), riboflavin deficiency (explaining the higher incidence in China), and tylosis.

Typical symptoms of oesophageal cancer, and less common symptoms

Progressive dysphagia is a worrying symptom, alongside odynophagia, oesophageal pain, weight loss, nausea, vomiting, and haematemesis. Aspiration pneumonia is more common due to poor clearance of food from the oesophagus. Invasion of the recurrent laryngeal nerve can lead to hoarseness and makes the cancer unresectable.

Demographics of oesophageal cancer

In 2005, 7823 people were diagnosed with oesophageal cancer, and it is the ninth most common cancer in the UK. It has a male-to-female ratio of 1.8:1, which rises to 4.8:1 for adenocarcinoma. Most patients are over 60 years old, and risk increases with age. It is more common, as the SCC form, in developing countries, with the highest reported area in the Asian 'oesophageal cancer belt': eastern Turkey, north-eastern Iran, northern Afghanistan, and southern Russia to northern China.

Natural history of oesophageal cancer, and complications of the disease

Oesophageal cancer arises from the mucosa and spreads to the submucosa, the muscle layers, and surrounding structures such as the lymph nodes (LN) and the bronchial tree. It eventually metastasizes to the lung and liver. The main complication is progressive dysphagia, which can lead to total obstruction of the oesophagus, with the associated nutritional deficiencies. Delayed clearance of food from the oesophagus can lead to aspiration pneumonia.

Other diagnoses that should be considered aside from oesophageal cancer

The symptoms associated with oesophageal cancer include dysphagia and dyspepsia. The differential diagnosis should include erosive and non-erosive GORD, peptic stricture, Schatski ring, eosinophilic oesophagitis, oesophageal web, oesophageal dysmotility, and achalasia.

'Gold-standard' diagnostic test for oesophageal cancer

Gastroscopy is the gold-standard test for identifying upper GI cancers, allowing direct visualization and mucosal biopsy for a histological diagnosis.

Acceptable diagnostic alternatives to the gold-standard test for oesophageal cancer

In patients unsuitable for OGD, a barium (or alternative contrast agent) swallow can identify strictures and intra-luminal masses. In addition, intra-abdominal malignancies can often be identified on CT scanning, which also allows the detection of metastases, and may be used in patients with non-specific symptoms that do not aid the physician in identifying the likely site. CT scanning is also a safer investigation than interventional procedures, such as endoscopy, and may be used in patients seen to be unsuitable for endoscopic procedures. However, the physician must consider the benefit of diagnosing cancer in patients unable to undergo endoscopic procedures, as endoscopic procedures are far less risky than most cancer treatment strategies.

Other relevant investigations for oesophageal cancer

All patients should undergo the following routine blood tests: a full blood count, renal function tests, liver function tests, and a calcium profile. Haematinics should be done if anaemia is present, and the patient should be treated accordingly. All patients with GI cancers will need to undergo staging investigations, which usually involve a CT scan of the chest and abdomen, mainly to identify lung and liver metastases. If the patient describes bone pain, and/or X-rays or CT scans suggest bone metastases, a nuclear medicine bone scan can confirm this. Bone metastases are often associated with hypercalcaemia, which can worsen symptoms. In the case of upper GI cancers (oesophageal, gastric, duodenal, biliary, or pancreatic), endoscopic ultrasound can be used to assess for depth of invasion and lymphatic spread.

Prognosis of oesophageal cancer, and how to estimate it

Prognosis from oesophageal cancer is invariably poor, with an overall 5-year survival rate of <5%. Overall prognosis (expressed as 5-year survival rate) can be related to the depth of invasion as follows:

- mucosa: 80%
- submucosa: 50%
- muscularis propria: 20%
- invasion into adjacent structures: 7%
- distant metastatic spread: 3%

Treatment of oesophageal cancer, and its effectiveness

Curative treatment is possible with surgery: an oesophagectomy. This is only possible if the cancer is localized (20%–30%) and the patient is able to undergo such a procedure. An oesophagectomy involves pulling up the stomach to replace the oesophagus and is a large, complicated operation with a significant associated mortality (5%–18%). The mortality is associated with cardiorespiratory and septic complications. Even curative surgery only has a 25% 5-year survival rate. Surgery is usually preceded by (neoadjuvant) chemo-radiotherapy to shrink the cancer, and chemotherapy may be given after surgery to reduce metastases. Chemotherapy is usually cisplatin based. Photodynamic therapy can be used in small cancers. Only a small number of patients are suitable for surgical intervention; in the majority of these, treatment is aimed at reducing tumour growth and providing palliation of dysphagia. This can be done with laser therapy, radiotherapy, or insertion of expanding stents. Such treatment strategies are purely palliative, with no improvement in prognosis.

Gastric cancer

Aetiology of gastric cancer

The majority of gastric cancers are adenocarcinomas, with lymphomas, GI stromal tumours (GISTs), carcinoids, adenoacanthomas, and SCCs accounting for the rest. There are several factors which have been implicated in the development of gastric cancer. *H. pylori* is strongly associated with gastric cancer, although <5% of people with *H. pylori* infection develop cancer. However, patients with *H. pylori* infection can develop chronic atrophic gastritis, with a subsequent sixfold increase in the risk of gastric cancer. Previous gastric surgery, in particular partial gastrectomy, is also associated with gastric cancer, probably owing to an associated change in gastric pH. Smoking increases the risk, in proportion to number of cigarettes and length of smoking, with studies showing the risk is increased approximately 1.6-fold. Dietary factors, including salt and smoked meat, are associated with an increased incidence, as is obesity. Genetic factors may play a role, although these are poorly understood. Pernicious anaemia and some hereditary syndromes increase the risk of gastric cancer, including hereditary non-polyposis colorectal cancer, familial adenomatous polyposis, and Peutz–Jeghers syndrome.

Typical symptoms of gastric cancer, and less common symptoms

Indigestion and epigastric pain are common symptoms, alongside nausea, vomiting, early satiety, weight loss, haematemesis, and melaena. Gastric cancers can present as ulcerated lesions; consequently, patients diagnosed with gastric ulcers must have biopsies taken in order to exclude an underlying malignancy, which is found in approximately 10% of cases. Bleeding from the cancer may lead to anaemia with the associated symptoms. Examination may reveal a palpable mass and/or Virchow's (left supraclavicular) node. Persistent vomiting of undigested food, with or without a succussion splash, suggests the patient is suffering from gastric outlet obstruction.

Demographics of gastric cancer

In 2005, 7980 people were diagnosed with gastric cancer in the UK, with 95% of patients over 50 years of age. It is the sixth most common cancer in men, and the eleventh in women and leads to 5250 deaths per annum in the UK. It has a slight predominance for men, and has the highest incidence in the eighth decade. There are far higher rates in Asian countries, particularly Japan, Taiwan, Korea, and China; this has led to the implementation of screening programmes.

Natural history of gastric cancer, and complications of the disease

Forty per cent of gastric cancers arise in the lower part of the stomach, 40% in the middle, and 10%–15% in the upper part. The remainder involve more than one part. At presentation, 25% of patients have localized disease; of the remainder, half have regional disease, and half have metastatic disease. Stomach cancer spreads into surrounding tissue directly, via lymphatics, or haematogenously. Cancers in the lower stomach can obstruct the pyloric sphincter, leading to gastric outlet obstruction.

Other diagnoses that should be considered aside from gastric cancer

Gastric cancer can present with dyspepsia. Gastric ulcers are related to *H. pylori* or drugs (NSAIDs), in the majority of cases.

'Gold-standard' diagnostic test for gastric cancer

As for oesophageal cancer, gastroscopy is the gold-standard test for gastric cancer, allowing direct visualization and mucosal biopsy for a histological diagnosis.

Acceptable diagnostic alternatives to the gold-standard test for gastric cancer

A barium meal will identify gastric mucosal lesions, although it removes the ability to obtain biopsies for a histological diagnosis.

Other relevant investigations for gastric cancer

All patients should undergo the following routine blood tests: a full blood count, renal function tests, liver function tests, and a calcium profile. Haematinics should be done if anaemia is present, and the patient should be treated accordingly. CT scanning will be necessary to stage the disease.

Prognosis of gastric cancer, and how to estimate it

Gastric cancer is staged using the TNM system, which further classifies staging into Stages I–IV, and correlates with prognosis as follows:

- Stage 0: >90% survival
- Stage I: 50%–80% survival
- Stage II: 30%–40% survival
- Stage III: 10%–20% survival
- Stage IV: <5% survival

The overall 5-year survival for gastric cancer has improved over the past 25 years, but is still low at 15%. Linitis plastica, where the stomach becomes rigid and thickened due to infiltration of the gastric wall, occurs in approximately 5% of cases and has an extremely poor prognosis.

Treatment of gastric cancer, and its effectiveness

Curative surgery usually involves LN dissection, with more extensive LN resection gaining popularity. Five-year survival rates following 'curative' surgery are related to tumour stage: 60%–90% in Stage I, 30%–50% in Stage II, and 10%–25% in Stage III. Neoadjuvant chemotherapy may be given to shrink the tumour. Chemoradiotherapy may shrink the tumour, but cannot cure the cancer. Newer biological treatments are currently used in clinical trial settings, but are not in widespread use as yet.

Pancreatic cancer

Aetiology of pancreatic cancer

Ninety-five per cent of pancreatic cancers are adenocarcinomas, of which the majority are ductal adenocarcinomas. Seventy-five per cent occur in the head of the pancreas, 15%–20% in the body of the pancreas, and 5%–10% in the tail of the pancreas. Specific genetic mutations have been associated with pancreatic cancer, although these are not yet applied to clinical practice. Patients known to carry the BRCA2 mutation, which is associated with breast cancer, have a higher incidence of pancreatic cancer. Smoking accounts for 25%–30% of cases of pancreatic cancer and double the risk of it developing. Studies have also associated obesity, high-fat diets, and caffeine with an increased risk. Chronic inflammation (as with many other cancers) has been shown to increase the incidence of dysplastic change (e.g. chronic pancreatitis), but there is no screening programme for patients with chronic pancreatitis. Alcohol consumption has not been directly linked to the development of pancreatic cancer, except when it has led to the development of chronic pancreatitis.

Typical symptoms of pancreatic cancer, and less common symptoms

The classic symptom of pancreatic cancer is painless jaundice, although symptoms are often non-specific, such as weight loss, malaise, and anorexia. Pain is usually epigastric, radiating through to the back, and patients have been known to develop diabetes mellitus. Many patients are diagnosed at a late stage and, consequently, may present with symptoms related to local or distant metastases (e.g. ascites).

Demographics of pancreatic cancer

Pancreatic cancer is the tenth-commonest cancer in the UK, with an incidence of approximately 10 per 100 000 population per year. The incidence rises with age, being rare before the age of 40, with 75% of cases occurring in people aged 65 years or older.

Natural history of pancreatic cancer, and complications of the disease

Pancreatic cancer can spread locally and commonly presents with biliary obstruction, leading to jaundice and the associated complications of cholangitis and sepsis. Invasion into surrounding organs can cause gastric outlet, duodenal, and/or colonic obstruction. Metastatic disease spreads via the lymphatics to the regional LNs, the liver, and the lungs, with peritoneal spread leading to metastasis to any abdominal surface. It can also be associated with painful metastatic skin nodules.

Other diagnoses that should be considered aside from pancreatic cancer

The jaundice associated with pancreatic cancer, cholangiocarcinoma, or gall bladder cancer can also be associated with benign biliary disease (choledocholithiasis, biliary colic) or pancreatic cysts, which in themselves may cause nausea and/or weight loss. Chronic pancreatitis with exocrine insufficiency can imitate pancreatic cancer, presenting with abdominal pain, malabsorption, and weight loss.

'Gold-standard' diagnostic test for pancreatic cancer

CT has become the easiest and most reliable way of diagnosing pancreatic cancer and can also provide the means for percutaneous biopsy. Furthermore, it can identify tumour invasion and metastatic disease.

Acceptable diagnostic alternatives to the goldstandard test for pancreatic cancer

Endoscopic ultrasound is extremely accurate at diagnosis, even with small pancreatic lesions, and can also provide information regarding the staging of the tumour by assessing the depth of spread, and LN and portal vein involvement. Furthermore, fine-needle aspiration can be performed to obtain a histological diagnosis. MRI is also an excellent modality for diagnosing pancreatic cancer and may be more accurate for very small lesions, which are usually found incidentally on CT. Magnetic resonance cholangiopancreatography (MRCP) is usually used to identify the cause of obstructive jaundice when it is not clear from a transabdominal ultrasound scan.

Other relevant investigations for pancreatic cancer

All patients should undergo the following routine blood tests: a full blood count, renal function tests, liver function tests, and a calcium profile. Pancreatic and biliary cancers presenting with obstructive jaundice will reveal a raised conjugated bilirubin level, usually alongside raised alkaline phosphatase and gamma-glutamyltransferase levels. In pancreatic cancer, the amylase level will be raised in 30%–50%

of patients, whereas the level of the tumour marker CA-19-9 will be raised in 75%–85%. CA-19-9 levels are also raised in gall bladder cancer. Ultimately, normal amylase or CA-19-9 levels do not exclude pancreatic cancer, and these levels can also be raised in the setting of gallstones, cholecystitis, pancreatitis, and cirrhosis.

Prognosis of pancreatic cancer, and how to estimate it

Pancreatic cancer has a high mortality rate, as it is difficult to diagnose at an early stage; 52% of patients have distant metastases, and 26% have spread to the regional LNs at the time of diagnosis. The 1-year survival rate is 20%–25%, and the 5-year survival rate is <5%, with a median survival of 4–6 months. Staging also utilizes the TNM system.

Treatment of pancreatic cancer, and its effectiveness

Surgical treatments for resection of pancreatic cancer involve a large and complicated procedure, with patients being monitored on an intensive care unit following the procedure. The position of the cancer will dictate the surgical approach used, and the patient's premorbid status will influence their suitability for this approach. Chemotherapy is used in combination with surgery and for unresectable disease, and fluorouracil, gemcitabine, capecitabine, and erlotinib have been shown to be effective. Palliative treatment can involve surgery (in cases of luminal obstruction), chemotherapy, and endoscopically placed biliary stents to relieve jaundice. Relief of pain is paramount.

Cholangiocarcinoma

Aetiology of cholangiocarcinoma

Cholangiocarcinomas arise from the biliary epithelium, and 90% are adenocarcinomas, with SCC accounting for the remainder. There is a higher incidence of cholangiocarcinomas in Asian populations, due to chronic endemic infestations of parasites such as *Clonorchis sinensis* and *Opisthorchis viverrini*. There is an association with primary sclerosing cholangitis (PSC), with 5%–15% of PSC patients developing cholangiocarcinoma. Inflammatory bowel disease (both ulcerative colitis and Crohn's disease) incurs an increased risk, even in the absence of PSC. In addition, congenital diseases (Caroli disease and choledochal cysts), biliary adenomas, and biliary papillomatosis have been associated with cholangiocarcinoma.

Typical symptoms of cholangiocarcinoma, and less common symptoms

Cholangiocarcinoma classically presents with obstructive jaundice, with associated pale stools, bilirubinuria, and pruritus. Weight loss and abdominal pain are also commonly seen. A palpable mass and/or lymphadenopathy is an uncommon finding.

Demographics of cholangiocarcinoma

Cholangiocarcinoma has an incidence of 1–2 per 100 000 population, with a higher incidence in women. The incidence in South East Asia, Japan, and Israel is higher.

Natural history of cholangiocarcinoma, and complications of the disease

Cholangiocarcinomas grow slowly and insidiously, invading local structures, including the bile ducts, the porta hepatis, the liver, and the regional LNs. Fifty per cent of patients have LN involvement at presentation, and 10%–20% of patients have peritoneal or distant metastases. The main complication is obstruction of the biliary tree and the associated risk of cholangitis and sepsis. These should be treated aggressively with antibiotics and biliary drainage. Secondary biliary cirrhosis occurs in 10%–20% of patients.

Other diagnoses that should be considered aside from cholangiocarcinoma

The differential diagnosis for cholangiocarcinoma includes all conditions that can cause an obstructive jaundice.

'Gold-standard' diagnostic test for cholangiocarcinoma

Endoscopic retrograde cholangiopancreatography (ERCP) will enable the doctor to perform a cholangiography and image the site of obstruction and also obtain brushings or biopsies for a histological diagnosis. Furthermore, therapy can be performed at the same time, with placement of a biliary stent to relieve the obstruction.

Acceptable diagnostic alternatives to the gold-standard test for cholangiocarcinoma

Patients will undergo imaging to identify the probable cause of obstruction prior to therapeutic procedures. Often, a patient will initially undergo an ultrasound scan, which can confirm biliary dilatation and absence of gallstones as the cause. However, this modality has a poor sensitivity for cholangiocarcinomas, and patients will subsequently undergo a CT or MRI for further information. Currently, MRI should be considered the optimal investigation for diagnosing cholangiocarcinoma. Endoscopic ultrasounds can provide further information for diagnosis, provide the ability for obtaining samples of tissue, and stage the cancer.

Other relevant investigations for cholangiocarcinoma

All patients should undergo the following routine blood tests: a full blood count, renal function tests, liver function tests, and a calcium profile. CA-19-9 levels are also raised in 85% of patients with cholangiocarcinoma, and a level >100 U/ml, in the setting of PSC, has a sensitivity of 75% and specificity of 80% for cholangiocarcinoma. Carcinoembryonic antigen and CA-125 are raised in approximately 30% and 40%–50% of patients with cholangiocarcinoma, respectively.

Prognosis of cholangiocarcinoma, and how to estimate it

Cholangiocarcinoma has a poor prognosis. Distal tumours are associated with the greatest survival rate, which is related to these tumours being the most amenable to resection: 40% 5-year survival, with a median survival of 17–27 months. Intra-hepatic tumours carry the worst prognosis. Overall, cholangiocarcinoma has an average survival of 12–18 months and is considered to be an incurable and rapidly lethal disease in the majority of cases.

Treatment of cholangiocarcinoma, and its effectiveness

Relief of obstruction is achieved by placement of biliary stents, either endoscopically or percutaneously under radiographic control. Biliary stents can also become occluded, so it is not unusual for patients to require a repeat procedure. Chemotherapy is usually fluorouracil based, and can provide some survival benefit. Surgical resection offers the only chance of cure, but only 10% of patients present with disease with an early enough stage for this to be a reasonable treatment option. Resection requires a major operative procedure; thus, it is vital to know a patient's premorbid status when deciding on their suitability. The 5-year survival in patients undergoing surgery is 9%–18% in proximal lesions, and 20%–30% in distal lesions. The evidence for adjuvant therapy is yet to be established, and is mainly used in a trial setting. Unfortunately, there is a high rate of recurrence, closely correlated with TNM staging, and so patients require aggressive follow-up.

Gall bladder cancer

Aetiology of gall bladder cancer

Eighty to eighty-five per cent of gall bladder cancers are adenocarcinomas, with the remainder including SCCs, carcinoids, melanomas, sarcomas, and lymphomas. Chronic inflammation is known to be an etiological factor for gall bladder cancer, most commonly associated with gallstones, which increase the risk of cancer four- to fivefold. Obesity is associated with an increased risk, but this may be due to the increased incidence of gallstones in obese people. Other, less common, sources of inflammation which are associated with inflammation include PSC, chronic infections (with *H. pylori, Salmonella*

typhi, S. paratyphi, liver flukes, etc.), and ulcerative colitis. Gall bladder polyps and a calcified gall bladder increase the risk of cancer, and the latter has a 10%–25% risk of associated cancer. Therefore, gall bladder polyps bigger than 5 mm or so should be monitored with annual ultrasound to check there is no increase in size, and are generally removed if they are ≥1 cm.

Hereditary syndromes associated with gall bladder cancer include hereditary non-polyposis colorectal cancer, Gardner's syndrome, and neurofibromatosis type I. Congenital abnormalities, including choledochal cysts and anomalous pancreaticobiliary duct junctions, are also associated with an increased risk of gall bladder cancer. In addition, certain exposures increase the risk of gall bladder cancer, including drugs (methyldopa, oral contraceptives), chemicals (vinyl chloride, pesticides, rubber), heavy metals (lead, chromium, cadmium), and occupational exposures (paper mill, petroleum, textile industries).

Typical symptoms of gall bladder cancer, and less common symptoms

Unfortunately, gall bladder cancer may remain asymptomatic until it has spread to adjacent structures. Symptoms include jaundice, nausea, anorexia, weight loss, weakness, abdominal pain (which can be due to biliary peritonitis in the setting of a perforated gall bladder), palpable right upper quadrant mass (Courvoisier sign), palpable Virchow nodes, and lymphadenopathy.

Demographics of gall bladder cancer

Gall bladder cancer is rare in the UK, with less than 600 cases per year; 70% of cases occur in women. There is considerable variation in incidence, associated with gender, age, and ethnicity. The UK, Norway, and Denmark have the lowest incidence rates, whereas the highest incidence rates are found in Peru, Chile, India, Korea, Japan, Bolivia, Spain, Columbia, Slovakia, the Czech Republic, and Ecuador. Females from India have the highest rate overall.

Natural history of gall bladder cancer, and complications of the disease

At presentation, only 10%–20% of patients have disease confined to the gall bladder wall; in 40%–60%, disease will have breached the gall bladder wall; 20% will have peritoneal spread; and 45%–50% will have disease that has spread to regional LNs. The disease can spread, via direct local invasion, to the liver, the duodenum, the pancreas, the stomach, the colon, and the peritoneum. The main complications are due to invasion of adjacent structures; perforation of the gall bladder, leading to biliary peritonitis; and biliary obstruction, with the associated risk of sepsis and kernicterus.

Other diagnoses that should be considered aside from gall bladder cancer

Gall bladder cancer often presents with non-specific symptoms, making it difficult to provide specific differential diagnoses, although you should consider alternative GI cancers and causes of dyspepsia, weight loss, and right upper quadrant pain.

'Gold-standard' diagnostic test for gall bladder cancer

CT is the most effective investigation and can identify tumour invasion into surrounding structures and metastatic disease.

Acceptable diagnostic alternatives to the gold-standard test for gall bladder cancer

Ultrasound scanning can identify a gall bladder mass in approximately 50%–70% of cases. MRI and/or MRCP may identify a lesion, whereas endoscopic ultrasound provides a means of obtaining bile samples for cytological analysis (sensitivity of 73%) and assessing tumour stage. Other methods of obtaining histology include ERCP and CT-guided biopsies.

Other relevant investigations for gall bladder cancer

All patients should undergo the following routine blood tests: a full blood count, renal function tests, liver function tests, and a calcium profile. Haematinics should be done if anaemia is present, and the patient should be treated accordingly.

Prognosis of gall bladder cancer, and how to estimate it

Prognosis is correlated with the TNM staging; a large number of patients have LN and distant metastases at presentation, leading to an overall 5-year survival rate of 15%–20%. Localized cancer has a 5-year survival of approximately 40%, regional disease 15%, and metastatic disease <10%. Advanced disease has a median survival of 2–4 months.

Treatment of gall bladder cancer, and its effectiveness

Unfortunately, only approximately 25% of patients are suitable for surgical resection, which involves a complicated procedure with a significant associated morbidity and mortality, as with surgery for cholangiocarcinoma. If residual disease remains post-operatively, the survival is approximately 6 months, which can be extended to 12 months with adjuvant radiotherapy. Given the low numbers of patients presenting with potentially resectable disease, the evidence for adjuvant therapy is low, but chemotherapy regimens usually utilize fluorouracil or gemcitabine. There are no defined standards for chemotherapy treatment in gall bladder cancer. Patients with unresectable disease can be offered radiotherapy and/or chemotherapy on a palliative basis, as there is little evidence of any survival benefit. Endoscopic biliary stents may provide palliation by relieving biliary obstruction.

Colorectal cancer

Aetiology of colorectal cancer

Genetic mutations are well recognized to be associated with an increased risk of colorectal cancer. These mutations are not tested for in general practice but, in patients with a strong family history, genetic counselling should be sought in order to assess for inheritable mutations and the need for increased screening. Familial conditions associated with a significant increase in colorectal cancer include familial adenomatous polyposis, hereditary non-polyposis colorectal cancer, juvenile polyposis, and Peutz–Jeghers. These conditions are usually monitored by specialist centres. Other conditions associated with an increased risk of colorectal cancer include inflammatory bowel disease, PSC, acromegaly, and having undergone a ureterosigmoidoscopy. The majority of cancers develop in adenomatous polyps. Consequently, patients who have adenomatous polyps should undergo regular screening, as this has been clearly seen to reduce the development of colorectal cancer. Smoking is associated with an increased risk of colorectal cancer. Dietary factors also have a role, including a diet high in red meat and low in fresh fruit, vegetables, fish, and poultry. Industrialized countries have a higher incidence of colorectal cancer, probably related to the differences in diet. Low physical activity and alcohol have also been associated with an increased risk.

Typical symptoms of colorectal cancer, and less common symptoms

Common symptoms of colorectal cancer include rectal bleeding, a change in bowel habit, anaemia (due to occult blood loss), and abdominal pain, but these symptoms can be associated with many other colonic diseases and, therefore, have a low predictive value. Tenesmus can also occur in rectal tumours. If the tumour grows large enough to fill the colonic lumen, obstruction can occur, with symptoms of distension, constipation, vomiting, and abdominal pain. This can lead to perforation and subsequent peritonitis. Deep vein thrombosis can occur as a paraneoplastic syndrome. Liver metastases can cause jaundice or abdominal pain.

Demographics of colorectal cancer

Colorectal cancer is the third most common cancer in the UK, with 100 new cases diagnosed daily. It accounts for 9% of new cancer cases worldwide. Eighty-three per cent of cases occur in people over 60. The male-to-female ratio is 1.2:1.0, with the lifetime risk being 1 in 18 for men, and 1 in 20 for women. Worldwide, the highest incidence rates are in Europe, North America, and Australasia, and the lowest are in Africa and Asia. There is a rapid increase in colorectal cancer risk in migrants moving from low- to high-risk countries. Incidence rates in the UK have slightly decreased, but colorectal cancer screening is likely to significantly increase the number of cases diagnosed in the next decade.

Natural history of colorectal cancer, and complications of the disease

Regardless of aetiology, most colorectal cancers arise from adenomatous polyps, and this information has led to colonoscopic surveillance in patients with adenomatous polyps (see Chapter 354). The size of polyps is proportional to the risk of cancer, with small polyps (<1 cm) posing less than 1% risk, and large polyps (>2 cm) with a cancer incidence of 50%. The worst complications are bowel obstruction and bowel perforation, both of which entail a worse prognosis. Ulcerative tumours are also associated with a worse prognosis. The cancer can spread locally, invading adjacent structures and the peritoneum, and usually metastasizes to the liver and lungs.

Other diagnoses that should be considered aside from colorectal cancer

Colonic symptoms independently have an overall poor predictive value for colorectal cancer. The strongest combination of symptoms to predict colorectal cancer is a change in bowel habit, with rectal bleeding and no anal symptoms in patients 60 or older. Many patients with classic colonic symptoms such as diarrhoea, constipation, and rectal bleeding have alternative diagnoses such as diverticular disease, irritable bowel syndrome, inflammatory bowel disease, haemorrhoids, microscopic colitis, or slow-transit constipation.

'Gold-standard' diagnostic test for colorectal cancer

Colonoscopy allows direct visualization of the tumour and the ability to obtain mucosal biopsies. Colorectal cancers require a total colonoscopy to exclude synchronous lesions.

Acceptable diagnostic alternatives to the gold-standard test for colorectal cancer

CT scanning is extremely good at identifying colorectal cancers. CT can be performed with oral contrast, which coats any faecal material, or with full bowel purgation and air insufflation (CT colonoscopy). CT colonoscopy has been considered to be safer than endoscopic investigations, due to a reduced risk of perforation. However, if lesions are seen at CT, an endoscopic examination is subsequently required for tissue diagnosis. Double-contrast barium enemas are used less often nowadays, as CT colonoscopy becomes more widely available.

Other relevant investigations for colorectal cancer

All patients should undergo the following routine blood tests: a full blood count, renal function tests, liver function tests, and a calcium profile. Haematinics should be done if anaemia is present, and the patient should be treated accordingly. Carcinoembryonic antigen is often raised in colorectal cancer, but cannot be used as a diagnostic tool, although it is often used to monitor response to treatment.

Prognosis of colorectal cancer, and how to estimate it

Colorectal cancer is the third most common cancer and the second leading cause of cancer-related death in the Western world. Prognosis is related to staging, and three systems can be used to classify tumour stage: the TNM staging system, the AJCC staging system, and the Dukes classification. The Dukes classification is older and simpler, with the following overall 5-year survival rates:

- Dukes A (confined to the intestinal wall): 90%
- Dukes B (invading through intestinal wall): 55%–85%
- Dukes C (LN involvement): 20%–55%
- Dukes D (distant metastases): <5%

Ulcerative cancers and those associated with bowel obstruction or perforation entail a worse prognosis.

Treatment of colorectal cancer, and its effectiveness

Surgery remains the only treatment for curing colorectal cancer and is usually combined with adjuvant chemotherapy to reduce cancer recurrence. Fluorouracil remains the backbone of chemotherapy, but oral fluoropyrimidines (e.g. capecitabine) are increasingly used. Newer chemotherapeutic agents and biological therapies (e.g. bevacizumab) are likely to increase survival, especially in patients with metastatic disease. Radiotherapy is standard therapy in rectal cancer but has limited used in colonic tumours. Palliative therapy includes endoscopically or radiologically placed stents, which can prevent obstruction by tumours which are encroaching the colonic lumen.

Anal cancer

Aetiology of anal cancer

Anal cancer is usually SCC. The human papilloma virus (HPV) is a strong risk factor for the development of anal cancer, with anal cancers being positive for the virus in 100% of homosexual men, 90% of women, and 58% of heterosexual men. The incidence of anal cancer is significantly higher in homosexual men, mainly related to anal intercourse increasing the exposure to HPV. In addition, having multiple sexual partners increases the risk of anal cancer. Smoking, immunosuppression, and benign anal lesions (inflammatory bowel disease, haemorrhoids, fistulae) have also been associated with anal cancer. Overall, the highest incidence is in homosexual HIV patients. Although there is no national screening programme, many HIV specialist centres advocate regular screening with anoscopy in homosexual HIV-positive patients. Anal smears are being studied to assess if they can be used to identify anal intra-epithelial neoplasia (AIN) in the same way that cervical screening is used to identify cervical neoplasia.

Typical symptoms of anal cancer, and less common symptoms

The commonest symptom of anal cancer is rectal bleeding. Other symptoms include lumps, discomfort, rectal mucus, or faecal incontinence. Twenty per cent of patients have no symptoms. Anal cancers may be identified during a rectal examination.

Demographics of anal cancer

Anal cancer is rare, with only 850 new cases annually in the UK. The incidence increases with age, with most patients 50 or older. The incidence is slightly higher in women, although the reason for this is not known.

Natural history of anal cancer, and complications of the disease

Anal cancer usually arises from a dysplastic area (AIN), which can progress to a carcinoma in situ and eventual frank cancer. Initially, it spreads locally, invading surrounding tissue, but can spread more distantly via the lymphatic system. Distant metastases usually occur in the liver and lungs. The main complication is faecal incontinence.

Other diagnoses that should be considered aside from anal cancer

Rectal symptoms are commonly associated with benign conditions such as anal fissures or haemorrhoids.

'Gold-standard' diagnostic test for anal cancer

Anal cancers can be diagnosed at anoscopy or proctoscopy.

Acceptable diagnostic alternatives to the gold-standard test for anal cancer

Pelvic CT or MRI scanning may identify anal cancers. Ideally, an MRI is performed in all patients with anorectal cancers to assess direct invasion into surrounding structures.

Other relevant investigations for anal cancer

Patients with anorectal carcinomas will require a pelvic MRI, to assess the overall local spread of disease.

Prognosis of anal cancer, and how to estimate it

The 5-year survival for patients with anal cancer is approximately 80%, dropping to 60% if it has spread locally and 20% in patients with distant metastases.

Treatment of anal cancer, and its effectiveness

Previously, surgical resection was the mainstay of treatment, involving removal of the anal sphincter; this meant that patients required permanent colostomies, to avoid faecal incontinence. However, combination chemoradiotherapy has been shown to be as effective as surgical resection, and preserves the anal sphincter. The commonest chemotherapy used is fluorouracil in combination with mitomycin or cisplatin.

Hormone-secreting tumours

Aetiology of hormone-secreting tumours

Hormone-secreting tumours found in the GI tract include pancreatic neuroendocrine tumours and carcinoids. These are rare, slow-growing tumours which are often found incidentally. Carcinoid tumours are derived from enterochromaffin cells, of which 55% occur in the GI tract (small intestine 45%, rectum 20%, appendix 16%, colon 11%, stomach 7%). Pancreatic neuroendocrine tumours arise from APUD (for **a**mine **p**recursor **u**ptake **d**ecarboxylase) cells. Approximately 25% appear to be non-secreting; however, it is probably more likely that the secretion of hormones is so low that any effects are subclinical. The commonest tumours are gastrinomas, insulinomas, VIPomas, somatostatinomas, and glucagonomas.

Typical symptoms of hormone-secreting tumours, and less common symptoms

Carcinoid tumours can cause intestinal symptoms related to luminal obstruction or fibrosis. However, they are often more recognized for their hormone-secreting potential, with symptoms related to the specific hormone secreted. Typical symptoms of carcinoid syndrome are flushing, diarrhoea, bronchospasm, and valvular heart disease. Although these symptoms are usually associated with serotonin release, other hormones also play a role. For example, neuropeptide K, histamine, and bradykinin cause flushing, and glucagon, gastrin, prostaglandins, and vasoactive polypeptide cause diarrhoea. Seventy-five to eighty per cent of patients with carcinoid syndrome have small bowel carcinoid, and 90% have metastases.

Pancreatic neuroendocrine tumours are often diagnosed incidentally but can present with a palpable mass, biliary obstruction, or symptoms related to hormone production, as follows:

- gastrinoma: peptic ulcer disease, diarrhoea
- insulinoma: hypoglycaemia
- VIPoma: profuse diarrhoea, achlorhydria, hypokalaemia, hyperglycaemia
- somatostatinoma: gallstones, diarrhoea, steatorrhoea, diabetes mellitus
- glucagonoma: glucose intolerance, diarrhoea, anaemia, thromboembolic phenomena, dermatitis (necrolytic migratory erythema), stomatitis

Demographics of hormone-secreting tumours

Carcinoid tumours are rare, with only 1500–2000 cases per year in the UK. They have an incidence of 1.5 per 100 000 population, although the incidence rises to 650 at post-mortem, confirming the undiagnosed incidence in the majority. Patients are usually over 60 years of age and the tumours are slightly more common in men.

Neuroendocrine tumours are extremely rare, with an incidence of 3–10 per million in the UK. They are solitary and sporadic in those aged 30–50, and only occur in younger patients (aged 10–30) in the setting of multiple endocrine neoplasia type 1 (an autosomal dominant condition associated with hyperparathyroidism and pituitary adenomas).

Natural history of hormone-secreting tumours, and complications of the disease

Carcinoid tumours are slow-growing and often multiple. They are often found incidentally and there are a significant number found at autopsy, with patients dying from other diagnoses. Only 10% of patients will develop carcinoid syndrome, and metastases usually spread to the liver.

Other diagnoses that should be considered aside from hormone-secreting tumours

As hormone-secreting tumours are usually diagnosed incidentally, the main differential includes neoplastic tumours. Consequently, patients with hormone-secreting tumours often undergo various imaging and/or endoscopic techniques prior to a final diagnosis being made, especially when there are pancreatic lesions causing biliary obstruction.

'Gold-standard' diagnostic test for hormone-secreting tumours

A 24-hour urine collection for 5-hydroxyindoleacetic acid, which is a breakdown product of serotonin and is usually raised in carcinoid tumours, is the gold-standard diagnostic test for hormone-secreting tumours, with a sensitivity of 75% and a specificity of 100%. Neuroendocrine tumours can also be diagnosed in the following ways, although usually in combination with an octreotide scan:

- gastrinoma: fasting serum gastrin level (normally <110 pg/ml); any proton-pump inhibitors and H2 antagonists should be stopped 7 days 2 days, respectively, prior to the test
- insulinoma: 72-hour fasting study with insulin, proinsulin, C-peptide, and glucose levels
- VIPoma: fasting VIP levels during symptoms should be 2–10 times the upper limit of normal
- somatostatinoma: fasting somatostatin >160 pg/ml
- glucagonoma: serum glucagon >500 pg/ml

Acceptable diagnostic alternatives to the gold-standard test for hormone-secreting tumours

Octreotide scans can be useful for carcinoid and most neuroendocrine tumours, based on the fact that they usually express somatostatin receptors. Octreotide scans are performed in the nuclear medicine department, utilizing radiolabelled octreotide, a somatostatin analogue. ^{123}I-MIBG scans work in a similar way. The vast majority of hormone-secreting tumours are identified on CT scans performed for unrelated reasons. MRI scans may be used to further image small lesions. Endoscopy may be used for lesions in the upper GI tract or colon, allowing visualization and biopsy. Endoscopic ultrasound is often used for pancreatic neuroendocrine tumours, assessing size, invasion, and LN involvement. Provocation tests are currently rarely used.

Other relevant investigations for hormone-secreting tumours

Several investigations can confirm the diagnosis of a hormone-secreting tumour. Gastrinomas can be confirmed by secretin stimulation tests, with levels rising to >200 pg/ml. Furthermore, a gastric pH of <3 excludes secondary hypergastrinaemia. VIPomas cause hypochlorhydria, and this can also be confirmed by gastric pH. Furthermore, VIPomas cause >700 ml diarrhoea per day in all patients, and >3 l/day in 70%.

Prognosis of hormone-secreting tumours, and how to estimate it

The prognosis for carcinoids tumours, as with all cancers, depends on the degree of spread. The approximate 5-year survival is 78% in localized disease, 72% with regional disease, and 39% in patients with distant metastases. The overall 5-year survival for all stages is 68%. The prognosis for pancreatic neuroendocrine tumours is not dissimilar, dependent on the degree of spread, tumour grade, or age. Unfortunately, they may remain undetected for years, and only become symptomatic when metastases cause symptoms from tumour bulk or increased hormone secretion.

Treatment of hormone-secreting tumours, and its effectiveness

There are several forms of treatment for hormone-secreting tumours:

- surgery
- radiotherapy
- chemotherapy
- chemoembolization: this involves injecting a chemotherapeutic agent into the blood vessel supplying a liver metastasis, and then embolizing the artery and subsequently cutting off the blood supply
- percutaneous ethanol injection
- biological therapy: octreotide, lanreotide, interferon

Further Reading

Ciocirlan M, Gincul R, Lepilliez V, et al. Non-Barrett's esophageal and gastric tumors: Diagnosis and treatment. *Gastrointest Endosc* 2012; 76: 501–5.

Michl P and Gress TM. Current concepts and novel targets in advanced pancreatic cancer. *Gut* 2013; 62: 317–26.

Muniraj T, Vignesh S, Shetty S, et al. Pancreatic neuroendocrine tumors. *Dis Mon* 2013; 59: 5–19.

Patel SG and Ahnen DJ. Familial colon cancer syndromes: An update of a rapidly evolving field. *Curr Gastroenterol Rep* 2012; 14: 428–38.

205 Functional gastrointestinal diseases

Satish Keshav and Alexandra Kent

Definition of the disease

Irritable bowel syndrome (IBS) is a functional bowel disorder characterized by chronic abdominal pain associated with a change in bowel habit or stool consistency in the absence of any definite organic abnormality. It is the commonest functional gastrointestinal syndrome. Many others have been defined clinically, including functional dyspepsia, functional biliary pain, functional abdominal pain, and so on. Functional dyspepsia is dealt with in Chapter 25.

Aetiology of the disease

Mechanisms leading to the development of IBS are thought to include visceral hypersensitivity, altered intestinal motility, altered autonomic function, bacterial flora, and stress. Sixty per cent of patients with IBS show a disproportionate pain response to rectal balloon distension, and imaging has shown increased cerebral blood flow in response to pain. Intestinal mediators such as bradykinin and serotonin induce visceral hypersensitivity and may play a role. A large number of patients develop IBS following on from gastroenteritis, and this may be related to the raised concentration of serotonin-containing enteroendocrine cells which develop after gastrointestinal infections. Psychological factors are thought to play an integral role, with studies showing that up to 50% of IBS patients who seek medical care have concurrent depression or anxiety. Finally, the increased incidence in twins suggests there is a genetic link, although, to date, no specific genetic loci have been identified.

Typical symptoms of the disease, and less common symptoms

International consensus meetings have defined diagnostic criteria for IBS, and the latest is the Rome III criterion, which can be summarized as follows: recurrent abdominal pain or discomfort for 3 days per month for the past 3 months, with onset ≥6 months earlier and associated with two or more of:

- improvement with defaecation
- onset associated with change in appearance of the stool
- onset associated with change in frequency of the stool

IBS can be further subdivided into constipation-predominant IBS, diarrhoea-predominant IBS, or mixed IBS. Other symptoms associated with IBS include bloating, abdominal pain after eating, rapid gastrocolic reflex, passage of rectal mucus, urgency, incomplete evacuation, lethargy, nausea, and food intolerances. Most symptoms are intermittent, with 'flares' lasting an average of 1–4 days. Patients who have IBS-like symptoms but do not meet the Rome III criterion may still have a functional bowel disorder.

Demographics of the disease

IBS is very common, with a prevalence of 10%–20% of the general population and with the majority treated in primary care. The highest incidence is in the 20–30-year-old age group, with women being affected twice as often as men.

Natural history and complications of the disease

IBS symptoms are usually intermittent but protracted, lasting several years. IBS patients attend their general practitioner twice as much as non-IBS patients, incurring huge costs to the NHS. The diagnosis does not need to be re-evaluated unless new symptoms develop. There are no long-term complications of IBS, although it can impact hugely on the patient's quality of life.

Approach to diagnosing the disease

The most important approach to diagnosing IBS is a good history. Many patients will not volunteer symptoms unless specifically asked, especially 'embarrassing' symptoms such as faecal incontinence. It is important to be sensitive to cultural and gender barriers in these patients, and assess how symptoms affect their quality of life, in particular time off work. Although investigations 'just to exclude …' are to be avoided, because negative investigations may reinforce the patient's view that the underlying pathology has simply not yet been uncovered, it is pragmatic to perform some simple tests that make certain common diagnoses that can mimic IBS unlikely. These tests include a full blood count to check for anaemia, C-reactive protein levels as a sign of inflammation, a coeliac antibody test, and *Helicobacter* serology. If these tests are normal, then significant gastrointestinal disease such as peptic ulcer, coeliac disease, inflammatory bowel disease, and colorectal cancer are unlikely. In cases where there is an inadequate response to reassurance and symptomatic treatment, a case could be made for more specialized tests, such as an abdominal ultrasound scan and upper and lower endoscopy.

Other diagnoses that should be considered

Symptoms not compatible with IBS and so requiring further investigation include weight loss, rectal bleeding, abdominal masses, anaemia, and raised inflammatory markers. Furthermore, patients >50 years old with a persistent change in bowel habit should not be diagnosed with IBS until organic pathology, in particular colorectal cancer, is excluded. The main differential diagnoses to be excluded include microscopic colitis, inflammatory bowel disease, colorectal cancer, bacterial overgrowth, and lactose intolerance.

'Gold-standard' diagnostic test

Patients who meet the criteria for IBS, have no additional symptoms or signs, and are <50 years old need no additional investigations. Therefore, the majority of patients can be diagnosed from a history and examination, especially those with constipation-predominant IBS. For patients with diarrhoea-predominant IBS, most centres would advocate screening blood tests with a full blood count, erythrocyte sedimentation rate, C-reactive protein level, coeliac serology, and immunoglobulins. The role of these investigations is to ensure inflammatory and malabsorptive conditions are excluded.

Acceptable diagnostic alternatives to the gold standard

Since IBS is diagnosed on clinical presentation rather than results of investigation, there are no alternative diagnostic tests.

Other relevant investigations

Patient with persistent diarrhoea may require a more extensive workup, including stool microscopy and culture, haematinics, calcium, thyroid function, and a lower gastrointestinal endoscopy with mucosal biopsies. A more detailed description of investigations into chronic diarrhoea is in Chapter 29.

Prognosis and how to estimate it

The overall prognosis is unpredictable, and patients should be warned that there is a variable response to treatment. Some patients suffer intermittent, short-lived symptoms, while others suffer chronic, severe symptoms that seriously affect their quality of life.

Treatment and its effectiveness

Appropriate treatment can be highly effective, particularly when delivered professionally and with empathy and reassurance. Many patients are convinced there is something serious wrong with them; subsequently, reassurance is integral to patient care, as this may address accompanying anxiety and depression. The treatment of IBS aims at reducing symptoms, and includes changes in lifestyle as well as pharmacotherapy.

Dietary modification

Self-help booklets on IBS and the effect of diet on its symptoms can be very useful. In more complex cases, specialist help from a trained dietician may be needed. Those with constipation as a major symptom should be given advice regarding fibre levels, which should be optimized. Fibre intake should neither be inadequate nor excessive, and soluble fibre, such as ispaghula, is better than insoluble fibre, such as bran. Dietary advice can help avoid foods that can cause diarrhoea, such as caffeine, citrus fruits, and sorbitol. Wheat and dairy products are commonly identified as substances that can worsen symptoms.

Exercise and stress

Patients should be advised to take regular exercise and try to reduce stress levels, although the evidence behind these interventions is limited.

Pharmacological therapy

Peppermint oil has been shown to be an effective treatment for abdominal discomfort and bloating. Other antispasmodics that are effective in some patients include hyoscine butylbromide, mebeverine, and alverine.

Diarrhoea and urgency can be controlled with loperamide. Codeine should be avoided because it can cause sedation and other psychotropic effects, and may be addictive. Laxatives such as cracked linseed, syrup of figs, and sodium docusate are used to treat constipation. Lactulose is usually avoided because it aggravates wind and bloating.

Tricyclic antidepressants (TCAs) such as amitriptyline at low doses such as 20–50 mg daily reduce abdominal pain, and have been shown to be most effective in diarrhoea-predominant IBS. Constipation is a recognized side effect, and may help diarrhoea. In patients unresponsive to TCA, selective serotonin reuptake inhibitors (SSRIs) can be tried. With both TCAs and SSRIs, patients should be warned of possible side effects, and doses should be titrated slowly.

Newer preparations that treat constipation and diarrhoea by targeting various serotonin-receptor subtypes are being developed and may radically improve the treatment of these two symptoms. Abdominal pain and bloating, however, remain a therapeutic challenge.

Complementary therapy

In patients with refractory IBS or in whom stress is a major factor, cognitive behavioural therapy, psychological therapy, or hypnotherapy may be effective, although their use is restricted by limited availability. In hypnotherapy, specific 'gut-related' hypnosis is applied, whereby the patient is taught to control gut function while in a hypnotic state.

Biofeedback

Biofeedback is a behavioural technique that teaches a patient to raise awareness and conscious control of their physiological responses.

Probiotics

There have been several controlled trials which have shown that probiotics can help abdominal distension and flatulence, with a reduction in IBS composite scores. However, it is difficult to draw definitive conclusions, as the studies use different bacterial species and doses.

Herbal medicines

Studies have suggested herbal or Chinese medicines can be effective at controlling symptoms. However, evidence for this is limited, so such treatment cannot be recommended at this time.

Further Reading

Camilleri M, Lasch K, and Zhou W. Irritable bowel syndrome: Methods, mechanisms, and pathophysiology. The confluence of increased permeability, inflammation, and pain in irritable bowel syndrome. *Am J Physiol Gastrointest Liver Physiol* 2012; 303: G775–85.

Ford AC and Talley NJ. Irritable bowel syndrome. *BMJ* 2012; 345: e5836.

National Institute for Health and Care Excellence. *Irritable Bowel Syndrome in Adults: Diagnosis and Management.* 2008. Available at https://www.nice.org.uk/Guidance/CG61 (accessed 12 Jun 2017).

Satish Keshav and Alexandra Kent

Psychiatric conditions with gastrointestinal consequences

Eating disorders

Anorexia nervosa is characterized by extreme weight loss, which is maintained by dieting, excessive exercise, fear of weight gain, and a disturbed body image. Bulimia nervosa is characterized by binge eating following by purging, normally by self-induced vomiting. Patients classically develop these disorders in adolescence; the incidence is greater in women. Patients with bulimia may maintain their body weight due to the binge eating, while anorectics have a low BMI and typically appear emaciated.

The mainstay of treatment is provided by specialist psychiatry. However, gastroenterologists are commonly asked for advice for treating severe malnutrition. Electrolyte and nutritional deficiencies should be replaced, including trace elements such as selenium and zinc. As a healthy diet is introduced, the patient is at risk of refeeding syndrome. The increased oral intake causes a shift from metabolizing fat and ketones to carbohydrate metabolism. The result can be rapid and cause profound alterations in the concentration of critical ions, including K^+, Na^+, Mg^{2+}, and phosphate; K^+ and phosphate, particularly, may need to be replenished rapidly to prevent cardiac arrhythmias and seizures. Severe starvation and refeeding syndrome are both life-threatening emergencies, carrying a high risk of death.

Depression

One of the diagnostic criteria of depression is weight loss, related to a reduced appetite and disinterest in eating. Depression should be considered in any patient presenting with weight loss, and can be associated with stressful life events, such as bereavement. This usually responds to treatment of the underlying problem, and weight gain is a common sign of improvement in mood. Studies suggest that up to 70% of patients with irritable bowel syndrome (IBS) meeting the Rome III criteria (see Chapter 205) have underlying depressive disorders. Further studies have confirmed that antidepressants can improve IBS symptoms, a result that is almost certainly related to treating the symptoms of depression.

Psychiatric medications

Medications used to treat psychiatric conditions commonly have gastrointestinal (GI) side effects, and this emphasizes the importance of taking an accurate drug history. The GI side effects associated with each drug group are as follows:

- antidepressants: dry mouth, constipation, diarrhoea (selective serotonin reuptake inhibitors), nausea, weight gain, and abdominal pain
- neuroleptics: dry mouth, constipation
- lithium: at treatment doses, this can cause nausea and weight gain; toxic levels can cause diarrhoea, nausea, and vomiting

GI diseases with psychiatric symptoms

Hepatic encephalopathy

Hepatic encephalopathy is a neuropsychiatric condition that occurs acutely or chronically in the setting of liver failure. Portal hypertension leads to the development of a collateral circulation, with shunting of portal venous blood flow from the intestinal tract directly into the systemic circulation. This shunting, as well as reduced liver function, allows toxins in portal venous blood to enter the cerebral circulation and impair brain function. The severity of hepatic encephalopathy varies from subclinical to frank coma, with decerebration and brain death. Early symptoms include reversal of the sleep–wake pattern, impaired cognition, impaired spatial perception, asterixis, lethargy, apathy, and subtle personality changes. Laxatives that accelerate intestinal transit, and reduce bacterial production of toxins such as ammonia, are the mainstay of treatment. Lactulose is particularly favoured because bacterial metabolism of lactulose acidifies intestinal contents and so inhibits the absorption of ammonia from the intestine.

Acute encephalopathy in patients with stable chronic liver cirrhosis can be precipitated by upper GI haemorrhage, infection, and electrolyte disturbances, which can be caused, for instance, by the use of diuretics to treat ascites. In these cases, an attempt is made to reverse or treat the precipitant. Coma and decerebration are more likely to occur in acute liver failure, such as that caused by paracetamol overdose, than in chronic liver disease.

Coeliac disease

Neuropsychiatric symptoms are well recognized in coeliac disease, and are especially prevalent in the untreated coeliac population. These may be the only presenting symptom, and include cerebellar ataxia, neuropathy, memory impairment, multifocal leucoencephalopathy, dementia, myoclonus, epilepsy, and internuclear ophthalmoplegia, amongst others. GI symptoms may be absent, and this fact accounts for the large undiagnosed population. The pathophysiology behind the neuropsychiatric disturbances is not completely understood, but improvement following a gluten-free diet suggests that nutrient deficiencies may contribute. Nutrients which could be implicated include folic acid, vitamin B_6, and tryptophan. Treatment involves a gluten-free diet and replacement of nutritional deficiencies. Overall, it is important that coeliac testing should be part of the workup in patients presenting with neurological and psychiatric symptoms.

Wilson's disease

Wilson's disease is an autosomal recessive disorder, characterized by copper deposition in the brain, liver, kidney, and cornea. This leads to a widely variable presentation, but neurological and psychiatric symptoms are well described. Neurological symptoms and signs include dysarthria, dysdiadochokinesis, tremor, bradykinesia, ataxia, chorea, seizures, and dystonia. Many of these signs are extremely subtle, and not identified without careful examination. Psychiatric conditions are far less common than neurological ones, and are predominantly found in patients with neurological disease. Conversely, the majority of patients with neuropsychiatric symptoms already have established cirrhosis. Ten to twenty per cent of patients present with psychiatric symptoms, which can be divided into behavioural, affective, schizophrenic, and cognitive categories. Symptoms include emotional lability, belligerence, disinhibition, impaired social judgement, and temper outbursts. Case reports have also identified patients developing these abnormalities after years of treatment with penicillamine.

Acute intermittent porphyria

Acute intermittent porphyria is an autosomal dominant condition involved in defective haem processing. It is characterized by attacks consisting of abdominal pain, mild mental disturbance, and autonomic dysfunction. The autonomic neuropathy can cause neurovisceral symptoms, including constipation, abdominal pain, delirium, seizures, depression, and coma. Encephalopathy can develop, and psychosis has been reported. Most symptoms resolve with the attacks, which are treated conservatively. Anxiety and depression are more common in patients with acute intermittent porphyria and are most likely related to the impact of chronic illness

Functional GI disease

It is well recognized that that there is a strong association of functional disorder (functional dyspepsia, IBS) with psychiatric problems. The pathophysiology underlying functional disorders in not completely understood, but is thought to be due to visceral hypersensitivity, a disrupted hypothalamic–pituitary–adrenal axis and/or an altered brain–gut axis. Overall, it is thought there is a disrupted balance between the neural system, the neuroendocrine system, and the immune system. It is well recognized that stressful life events can exacerbate IBS symptoms. Studies have shown that approximately 25%–40% of patients with panic disorder, 35% of patients with obsessive–compulsive disorder, and 25%–30% of those with major depressive illnesses have IBS. It is important for a GI physician to identify underlying psychiatric disturbances, as treatment of the psychiatric disorder may provide relief of the GI symptoms. This may also explain the benefit seen in some patients for alternative therapies such as hypnotherapy or acupuncture. Given the limited

effective treatment strategies in functional disorders, psychiatric treatment may be a far more efficacious option.

Inflammatory bowel disease

Inflammatory bowel disease, as with many chronic illnesses, has a higher incidence of depressive illness, occurring in 16% in one large study. Children and adolescents have a higher risk of developing depressive illness. Depressive illnesses impact on quality of life, with symptoms increasing with progressive disease severity. There is no evidence that stress or psychiatric illness can initiate disease, but studies have suggested stress may play a role in exacerbating inflammation, although this is not a unanimous opinion.

Further Reading

Jones MP, Crowell MD, Olden KW, et al. Functional gastrointestinal disorders: An update for the psychiatrist. *Psychosomatics* 2007; 48: 93–102.
Sobel RM and Markov D. The impact of anxiety and mood disorders on physical disease: The worried not-so-well. *Curr Psychiatry Rep* 2005; 7: 206–12.

PART 9

Disorders of the liver

207 Normal hepatic function

Satish Keshav and Palak Trivedi

Liver anatomy

Anatomy

The liver is the largest internal organ of the body, weighing about 1.5 kg in an adult. It is a wedge-shaped structure situated under the right hemidiaphragm and is covered by a connective tissue capsule (Glisson's capsule). Morphologically, the liver can be divided into four lobes: right, left, caudate, and quadrate. Three ligaments attach the liver to surrounding structures: the falciform ligament (anteriorly and superiorly) and two posterior triangular ligaments. The falciform ligament separates the larger right lobe from the smaller left lobe. It also attaches the liver to the anterior abdominal wall and diaphragm. A smaller structure called the ligamentum teres attaches the falciform ligament to the umbilicus. The two posterior triangular ligaments enclose the retrohepatic vena cava and the small bare area of the liver.

Inferiorly, Glisson's capsule is attached to the lesser curve of the stomach. At the hepatic hilus, it encases the hepatic pedicle, which consists of the hepatic artery, the portal vein, and the common hepatic bile duct.

Vasculature of the liver

The portal vein is formed by the union of the superior mesenteric vein and the splenic vein and divides into left and right branches to supply each lobe. The left gastric vein also enters the portal vein and is important in the development of varices.

The hepatic artery arises from the coeliac artery. Several anatomical variants of the liver arterial blood supply exist and become important when considering transplantation.

Venous drainage of the liver is through the right, middle, and left hepatic veins. The caudate lobe has a separate drainage system through the spigelian veins directly into the inferior vena cava. In hepatic vein obstruction, as occurs in, for instance, Budd–Chiari syndrome, more hepatic venous blood flows via the spigelian system, with hypertrophy of the caudate lobe.

The liver receives approximately one-quarter of the total cardiac output (one-third from the hepatic artery, and two-thirds from the portal vein). The flow rate at rest varies between 1.6 and 1.8 l/min. The rate depends on physiological states such as feeding (following which the flow rate will be increased), respiration (flow rate increases in the expiratory phase), and posture (hepatic flow is reduced on adoption of an upright position). The portal venous system is passive, without pressure-dependent autoregulation, and the major physiological factors controlling flow are those modulating supply between the intestines and spleen. There is an important relationship between portal venous flow and hepatic arterial flow: a reduction in portal venous input results in a compensatory decrease in hepatic arterial resistance and, hence, an increase in the arterial flow rate.

Biliary anatomy of the liver, and lymphatic drainage

Bile canaliculi drain from the right and left hepatic bile ducts before coalescing to form the common hepatic duct. The cystic duct then joins the common hepatic duct to form the common bile duct. The common bile duct passes behind the first part of the duodenum and joins the pancreatic duct before entering the duodenum through the ampulla of Vater.

The gall bladder lies on the underside of the liver and is connected to the cystic duct via a spiral valve. The gall bladder functions as a storage organ with a capacity of up to 50 ml of bile.

Lymphatic vessels drain via the portal tract, closely applied to the branches of the hepatic artery, up to the hepatic hilum and subsequently via the thoracic duct. In addition, a smaller proportion drain via the hepatic veins, and some interstitial fluid drains through Glisson's capsule directly into the peritoneum. The lymph flow of the liver is approximately 0.5 ml per kilogram of liver per minute.

Innervation of the liver

The liver receives sympathetic and parasympathetic autonomic innervation. Sympathetic stimulation leads to:

- glycogenolysis and subsequent glucose release
- reduced ammonia uptake
- reduced bile formation
- reduced oxygen consumption by the liver
- increased hepatic vascular resistance
- increased portal pressure
- the release of blood from the liver into the systemic circulation; sympathetic nerve stimulation may reduce hepatic blood volume by up to 50%

Functional anatomy of the liver

The central area where the common bile duct, the hepatic portal vein, and the main hepatic artery proper enter is termed the porta hepatis. There, they divide into left and right branches. The portions of the liver supplied by these branches constitute the functional left and right lobes, which are distinct from the anatomical right and left lobes. The right functional lobe is divided into anterior and posterior segments by the right hepatic vein. The left functional lobe is divided into medial and lateral segments by the left hepatic vein. The medial segment corresponds to the quadrate lobe.

In the Couinaud nomenclature system, each functional lobe is divided into eight subsegments, each of which is a complete functional unit with a single portal pedicle and hepatic venous drainage (see Figure 207.1 and Table 207.1). Within each functional segment of the liver, the structural unit is the hepatic lobule.

The hepatic lobule

Although the liver is the largest internal organ, it is only a few cells thick. This is because hepatocytes form hepatic plates that are one to two cells thick and are separated from each other by large capillary spaces called liver sinusoids. The plates are assembled in hexagonally shaped lobules (see Figure 207.2). In each lobule, there is a central vein, a peripheral portal triad (containing a bile duct and the respective branches of the portal vein and the hepatic artery), and the hepatic plates, which lie between the two. In venous congestion (as occurs in right heart failure), the zone around the central vein sustains injury while, in hepatitis/cirrhosis, damage begins at the portal triads and spreads outwards in ripples. The components of the hepatic lobule and their roles are discussed in Table 207.2.

Basic physiology of the liver

The liver is critical to the maintenance of homeostasis, and life cannot be supported in the anhepatic state.

Bile formation

Each day, the liver produces 600 ml of bile via osmotic filtration and active transport across the canalicular membrane. The principle bile salt conjugates are cholic acid and chenodeoxycholic acid. Once in bile ductules, the bile is modified as the duct cells absorb glucose

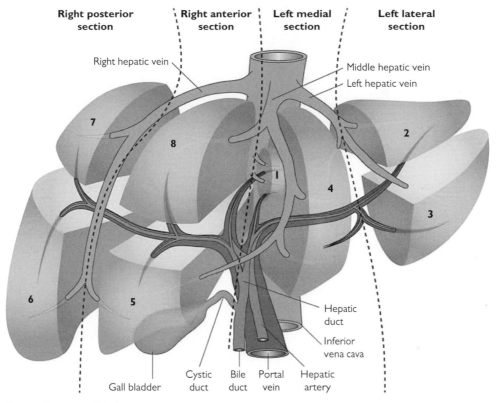

Right posterior section | Right anterior section | Left medial section | Left lateral section

Right hepatic vein

Middle hepatic vein
Left hepatic vein

7

8

2

1

4

3

6

5

Hepatic duct

Inferior vena cava

Gall bladder | Cystic duct | Bile duct | Portal vein | Hepatic artery

Figure 207.1 Functional segments of the liver.
Reprinted by permission from Macmillan Publishers Ltd: *Nature Reviews Clinical Oncology*, Siriwardena et al., volume 11, issue 8, pp. 446–459, copyright 2014.

from the bile and actively secrete amino acids and additional bile salts. Active secretion of bicarbonate and chloride also occur via the cystic fibrosis transmembrane regulator protein.

Bile salt conjugates secreted from hepatocytes into bile are deconjugated in the jejeunum and ileum with reabsorption and reuptake by the liver. This is termed the enterohepatic circulation. This mechanism is responsible for conserving bile acids and hence maintains the high concentration of bile. Five per cent of bile acids will pass through the ileocecal valve and undergo deconjugation by colonic bacteria. They will then be reabsorbed as the secondary bile acids deoxycholic acid and lithocholic acid.

There are many digestive functions of bile, including the neutralization of duodenal pH, emulsifying fat (hence making fat and fat-soluble molecules absorbable), and activating lipase enzymes. In addition to their role in digestion, bile acids are the principal mechanism for the biliary secretion and clearance of cholesterol.

Bilirubin metabolism and transport

Bilirubin is transported within plasma, bound to albumin. A few substances can displace bilirubin from albumin (e.g. antibiotics from the sulfonamide group). Unbound bilirubin is insoluble in water. Fortunately, unbound bilirubin is only present in miniscule amounts in normal circumstances. Levels of insoluble bilirubin rise in the absence of the hepatic enzyme UDP-glucuronyl transferase. This is

an enzyme of the glucuronidation pathway and transforms bilirubin into a water-soluble metabolite. This enzyme is undetectable in the rare disorder Crigler–Najjar syndrome. Two main forms of this disorder exist:

- type I: absence of any recognizable forms of the enzyme
- type II: <10% of normal UDP-glucuronyl transferase; phenobarbital can be used as a therapeutic measure as it is an enzyme inducer and thus will increase levels of UDP-glucuronyl transferase

Coagulation

The liver produces Factors I (fibrinogen), II (prothrombin), V, VII, IX, X, and XI, as well as protein C, protein S, and antithrombin. The liver also produces the glycoprotein thrombopoietin, which regulates the production of platelets by the bone marrow.

Hepatic metabolic processes

Hepatic metabolic processes have a central role in protein, carbohydrate, and lipid metabolism. Adverse alteration to these processes results in the major metabolic consequences of acute and chronic liver disease.

Carbohydrates

During fasting, hepatic glucose release via glycogenolysis, and more so by gluconeogenesis (from lactate, pyruvate, glycerol, and glucogenic amino acids), takes place. This process is regulated by hormonal control through glucagon (accounting for fasting glucose output), cortisol, growth hormone, and catecholamines. After a carbohydrate load, insulin will suppress hepatic glucose release and promote the storage of glucose as glycogen.

Proteins and amino acids

Most circulating proteins are produced by hepatocytes (the exceptions being immunoglobulins produced by lymphocytes, and von Willebrand factor, which is produced by platelets). Acute-phase

Table 207.1 Correspondence between anatomical lobes and functional segments

Anatomical lobe/segment	Couinaud segments
Caudate	1
Lateral	2, 3
Medial	4a, 4b
Right	5, 6, 7, 8

(A)

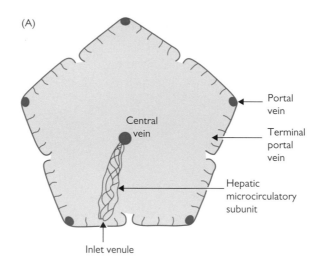

Central vein

Portal vein

Terminal portal vein

Hepatic microcirculatory subunit

Inlet venule

(B)

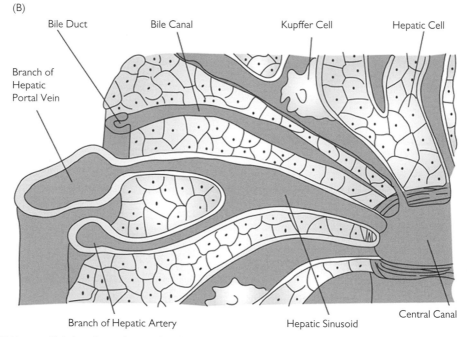

Bile Duct

Bile Canal

Kupffer Cell

Hepatic Cell

Branch of Hepatic Portal Vein

Branch of Hepatic Artery

Hepatic Sinusoid

Central Canal

Figure 207.2 (A) Hexagonal lobule with portal venous branches and a hepatic microcirculatory subunit: the sinusoid. (B) Liver lobule and portal triad.
(A) Reproduced with permission from Warrell, Cox and Firth, *Oxford Textbook of Medicine*, Fifth Edition, Oxford, UK, Copyright © 2010. (B) Reproduced with permission from Mark Harrison, *Revision Notes for MCEM Part A*, Oxford University Press, Oxford, UK, Copyright © 2011.

proteins (e.g. C-reactive protein (CRP)) have a reciprocal relationship to albumin synthesis and other carrier proteins. This is demonstrated in acute inflammatory conditions when CRP rises and albumin levels fall.

The liver is also the most important organ in controlling plasma concentrations of amino acids. During prolonged starvation, glucagon stimulates hepatic proteolysis whereas, during the post-prandial absorptive state, amino acid uptake is increased. The liver has a critical role in clearing portal venous ammonia generated within the gut lumen.

Lipids

During carbohydrate intake, free fatty acids (FFAs) formed within the liver are exported as components of very-low-density lipoproteins (VLDLs) and taken up by muscle and adipose tissue, with extraction of FFAs via the degradation of VLDLs. This leaves intermediate-density lipoproteins (IDLs) and, subsequently, low-density lipoproteins (LDLs). Hepatocytes bear specific LDL receptors and remove LDL from the circulation so that the associated cholesterol may be utilized

for bile salt metabolism or excreted into bile (there are also peripheral LDL receptors, present in extra-hepatic tissues, that extract cholesterol). High-density lipoproteins (HDLs) transport cholesterol from peripheral tissues (including the blood vessel lumen) to the liver, where it can be used in bile synthesis.

Vitamin D

Whether it is made in the skin or ingested, vitamin D_3 (cholecalciferol) is hydroxylated by hepatocytes to 25-hydroxycholecalciferol (25(OH) D_3, or calcidiol) and stored until it is needed. 25-Hydroxycholecalciferol is further hydroxylated in the kidneys into the biologically active hormone 1,25-dihydroxycholecalciferol (1,25(OH)$_2$D$_3$, or calcitriol) and 24R,25(OH)$_2$D$_3$.

Other functions

Production of insulin-like growth factor 1

The liver produces insulin-like growth factor 1, which plays an important role in childhood growth and has anabolic effects in adults.

Table 207.2 The components of the hepatic lobule

Component	Main functions	Additional points
Sinusoids	Specialized capillaries Allow low-molecular-weight proteins to permeate into the space of Disse (the space between sinusoids and hepatocytes) Postulated to be a major site of portal venous resistance	Lack basement membrane Lined with endothelial lining cells The sinusoidal membranes of hepatocytes surrounding the sinusoids contain microvilli that increase the surface area sixfold
Bile canaliculi	Collect bile secreted by the hepatocytes and pass it into the bile ductile	The volume of bile passing into the duodenum is small and has a low flow rate Secretion is controlled by gall bladder tone and sphincter of Oddi tone
Hepatocytes	Protein synthesis and storage Carbohydrate synthesis and metabolism Synthesis of cholesterol, bile salts, and phospholipids Detoxification, modification, and excretion of exogenous and endogenous substances Synthesis and secretion of bile Vitamin D metabolism	Make up 70%–80% of liver parenchyma Possess specialized cell membranes: • sinusoidal membrane (70% of surface area); for exchange of material between the space of Disse and the intracellular compartments (via endo- and exocytosis) • canalicular membrane (15%); for exchange with the smallest of biliary canaliculi or hemicanals • lateral membrane (15%); connected to the canalicular membrane by tight junctions and involved in intercellular transport between hepatocytes
Endothelial lining cells	Control entry and exit of molecules from the sinusoidal flow into the space of Disse Express a range of surface adhesion molecules that enhance leucocyte adherence, activation, and migration towards sites of inflammation	Possess numerous specialized endocytotic mechanisms, some of which are linked to known receptors
Kupffer cells	Specialized macrophages; part of the mononuclear phagocyte system	Found in a periportal distribution, adherent to the sinusoidal surface
Hepatic stellate cells	Control sinusoidal perfusion Contain most of the body's vitamin A stores	Located within the space of Disse Morphologically very similar to fibroblasts but contain fat droplets Central to the process of hepatic fibrogenesis; mediators released by parenchymal and Kupffer cells cause hepatic stellate cells to transform into myofibroblasts
Pit cells	Act as natural killer cells	Located between endothelial cells

Erythrocyte production in the fetus

In the first-trimester fetus, the liver is the main site of erythrocyte production. By the thirty-second week of gestation, the bone marrow has almost completely taken over that task.

Nutrient storage

The liver is involved in the storage of vitamin A (which can be stored up to 4 years), vitamin B_{12}, iron, and copper.

Drug and toxin metabolism

The liver metabolizes virtually every drug or toxin introduced in the body. Many drugs are capable of inducing liver enzymes (e.g. cytochrome P450 enzymes) and so can decrease the effectiveness of other drugs by causing them to be more rapidly metabolized. The induction of microsomal enzymes (so called because they are found in microsomes) takes place over days because it requires transcription and translation of genetic material. The drugs that induce cytochrome P450 enzymes are as follows:

• phenobarbital
• phenytoin
• carbamazepine
• ethanol
• glucocorticoids
• rifampin
• griseofulvin
• quinine
• omeprazole

Similarly, many drugs are capable of inhibiting microsomal enzymes; this reduces the metabolism of many drugs, hence increasing their concentrations and the risks of side effects. Unlike induction, inhibition occurs immediately following drug ingestion. Agents that cause inhibition include:

• amiodarone
• cimetidine

• erythromycin
• grapefruit juice
• isoniazid
• metronidazole
• sulfonamides
• omeprazole

An introduction to liver dysfunction

Most insults to the liver bring the threat of necrosis and liver failure—a series of functional changes which can lead to the following features of hepatic decompensation:

• jaundice
• encephalopathy
• portal hypertension
• bleeding
• ascites

Jaundice

The yellowish discolouration of jaundice (also known as icterus) is caused by increased levels of bilirubin in the blood, as the bilirubin subsequently accumulates in extravascular spaces, particularly those high in protein (the skin, the conjunctiva, etc.). In order for jaundice to be picked up clinically, the bilirubin in plasma must exceed ~40 μmol/l.

Jaundice is discussed further in Chapter 31. A brief summary of the biochemical anomalies observed in the classes of jaundice is provided in Table 207.3.

Encephalopathy

Hepatic encephalopathy is a potentially reversible situation occurring in severe liver impairment. Toxic substances normally cleared by the liver accumulate in the blood and, due to portal hypertension and subsequent bypassing of the hepatic filtration system, travel directly to the brain without being purified or modified. This is discussed further in Chapter 209.

CHAPTER 207 **Normal hepatic function**

683

Table 207.3 Biochemical anomalies in jaundice

	Pre-hepatic jaundice	Hepatic jaundice	Post-hepatic jaundice
Total bilirubin	Normal/increased	Increased	Increased
Conjugated bilirubin	Increased	Normal/increased	Increased
Unconjugated bilirubin	Increased	Normal/increased	Normal
Urobilinogen*	Increased	Normal/increased	Decreased/negative
Urine colour	Dark	Light	Dark
Stool colour	Dark	Normal	Pale
Alkaline phosphatase levels	Normal	Increased	Increased
Alanine transferase and aspartate transferase levels	Normal	Increased	Increased
Conjugated bilirubin in urine	Not present	Present	Present

*In pre-hepatic jaundice, no bilirubin will be present in urine but urobilinogen may be increased more than twofold. However, in neonates who have yet to develop gut flora, this trend will be absent.

Portal hypertension

The portal vein enters the liver at the porta hepatitis and sends a branch to each lobe. When portal flow is obstructed (from outwith or within the liver), a collateral circulation develops to carry blood into the systemic veins. This causes two main problems:

- the liver's metabolic function is bypassed
- increasing pressure in collaterals (known as varices) causes bleeding

Varices are commonly oesophageal, derived from the left gastric vein (usually from deep intrinsic layer of oesophagus). Other sites include the stomach, the colon, and the rectum.

A hyperdynamic circulation accompanies portal hypertension and may, in part, develop to maintain portal flow (collaterals will lower portal pressure). Causes of portal hypertension may be:

- presinusoidal (e.g. from splenic or portal vein thrombosis, schistosomiasis, or extrinsic compression)
- intra-hepatic (sinusoidal; e.g. from cirrhosis, acute hepatitis, or congenital hepatic fibrosis)
- post sinusoidal (e.g. from hepatic venous obstruction or constrictive pericarditis)

The clinical consequences of portal hypertension are:

- gastrointestinal haemorrhage; this can often be the first indication of varices; in addition, there may be mucosal congestion and bleeding from the stomach, the small bowel, or the colon; this is termed port-systemic enteropathy
- development of caput medusae
- an audible venous hum
- splenomegaly
- secondary hypersplenism (causing peripheral blood cytopenias)
- ascites

The diagnosis of portal hypertension can be made through imaging. Doppler-duplex ultrasound demonstrates portal flow, portal vein cavernous transformation, and portal vein or splenic vein thrombosis. The finding of splenomegaly and a collateral circulation may be seen. The disadvantages of this technique include a lack of data reproducibility, and inter-observer variability.

Spiral CT and CT angiography may allow more accurate demonstration of liver vasculature and collateral circulations. Dilatation of the inferior vena cava is also suggestive of portal hypertension and may be seen. Magetic resonance angiography has the additional advantage of providing quantitative data regarding portal vein and azygous vein flow. Direct portal pressure measurements (assessing the hepatic venous pressure gradient) are not routinely performed due to the invasive nature and risk of complications.

Treatment is directed at the cause of portal hypertension. Gastroesophageal variceal haemorrhage is the most dangerous complication of portal hypertension. Most of the treatment focuses on the prevention and treatment of variceal haemorrhage. This is discussed in Chapters 22 and 210.

Bleeding

Bleeding is consequent upon a number of problems:

- prolonged prothrombin time (consequent upon depletion of coagulation factors) due to impaired synthetic hepatic function
- thrombocytopenia: splenomegaly and hypersplenism; alcohol as an etiological factor is directly marrow toxic and will further affect platelet count; liver dysfunction also impairs the release of thrombopoietin
- portal hypertension leading to the development of variceal shunt vessels (very friable; bleeding can be profuse)
- gastritis and peptic ulceration associated with alcohol-induced liver disease

Ascites

Ascites is caused by the accumulation of fluid in the peritoneal cavity. In general, ascites may occur because of three main mechanisms:

- raised portal pressure
- reduced oncotic pressure
- direct peritoneal irritation

It is not unusual for more than one mechanism to be in play at any one time.

In liver cirrhosis, ascites can occur in up to 50% of patients during the 10 years following the diagnosis (Cardenas and Gines, 2005). The median 2-year survival is reduced from 90% (compensated cirrhosis) to 50% in those who develop ascites. Ascites usually develops gradually and continuously, with onset over weeks to months, and is relatively painless. When ascites becomes massive, there may be vague discomfort caused by stretching of the abdominal wall and parietal peritoneum. If ascites is painful, one should always consider the presence of infected peritoneal fluid or the presence of a hepatoma. In gross ascites, there may be respiratory embarrassment or the development of a leak of fluid through diaphragmatic lymphatics causing pleural effusions.

The mechanisms thought to be in play in cirrhotic ascites are as follows. First, there is peripheral vasodilatation due to an impaired metabolism of vasodilator substances; increased endothelial nitric oxide and prostacyclin may play a role. As a consequence, renal blood flow is reduced, stimulating the renin–angiotensin–aldosterone system. Salt and water retention occurs.

Portal venous (sinusoidal) hypertension then encourages fluid transudation into the peritoneal cavity. Ascites is rare in those with a hepatic-wedge pressure gradient of <12 mm Hg. Interestingly, those individuals with presinusoidal portal hypertension without cirrhosis rarely develop ascites.

The salt retention is followed by worsening water retention through the action of vasopressin. This will cause hyponatraemia (but increased total body sodium) and reduced renal blood flow predisposing to hepatorenal failure. Reduced oncotic pressure (due to hypoalbuminaemia) also contributes to the process.

The examination of ascitic fluid content, and other causes of ascites, are explained in Chapter 208. The management of ascites is discussed in Chapter 210.

Further Reading

Cardenas A and Gines P. Management of refractory ascites. *Clin Gastroenterol Hepatol* 2005; 3: 1187–91.

Hall JE. *Guyton and Hall Textbook of Medical Physiology* (13th edition), 2015. Saunders.

Longo DL and Fauci AS. *Harrison's Gastroenterology and Hepatology*, 2010. McGraw-Hill Medical.

208 Investigation in liver disease

Satish Keshav and Palak Trivedi

Blood tests

Liver chemistry

Liver chemistry tests are frequently abbreviated as LFTs, for liver function tests. In reality, they comprise mainly markers of liver injury rather than true measures of liver function, although a number of other blood tests, such as the prothrombin time and albumin level, offer a reliable measure of liver function. Routine liver chemistry includes tests to determine the levels of serum bilirubin, transaminases, alkaline phosphatase, gamma-glutamyl transpeptidase, and lactate dehydrogenase.

Bilirubin

Bilirubin (normal reference range: 3–17 μmol/l) is a breakdown product of haem, which is metabolized in the liver. Bilirubin is taken up by hepatocytes, conjugated, and secreted into bile before being released into the intestine. Bilirubin metabolism is discussed further in Chapters 31 and 207. Jaundice does not necessarily reflect hepatic dysfunction, as bilirubin levels reflect production, hepatic uptake, conjugation, and secretion. Conjugated bilirubin is highest in cholestatic disease whereas unconjugated bilirubin may reflect a pre-hepatic cause such as haemolysis (total bilirubin levels rarely >50–90 μmol/l) or genetic causes such as Gilbert's syndrome (a relatively benign condition where there is deficient glucuronyl transferase activity and hence reduced conjugation of bilirubin; individuals with Gilbert's syndrome become jaundiced at times of physical stress or fasting. In addition, certain drugs metabolized by the liver are more likely to cause side effects, given the reduced activity of the glucuronyl transferase enzyme). Rising levels of (conjugated) bilirubin reflect approaching end-stage disease in many chronic liver conditions, and in secondary malignancy often signal a preterminal event.

Transaminases

Transaminase levels do not reflect the functional capacity of the liver as such, but are more so tests of liver injury. They are produced following cytosol burgeoning, which leads to plasma membrane leak and hepatocyte lysis. Marked elevations (>1000 IU/l) are unusual in alcoholic liver disease, wherein levels rarely exceed 350 IU/l. Massive elevations are usually seen in paracetamol overdose, untreated autoimmune hepatitis, and acute viral hepatitis. Persistent elevation should arouse suspicion of significant chronic liver disease (e.g. chronic viral hepatitis, autoimmune disease, or haemochromatosis).

Transferases include:

- aspartate aminotransferase (AST; normal reference range: 5–45 IU/l); this is also known as serum glutamic oxaloacetic transaminase and occurs in two isoforms:
  - glutamic oxaloacetic transaminase 1, which is located in the cytoplasm and is found mainly in cardiac muscle and erythrocytes
  - glutamic oxaloacetic transaminase 2, which is located in the mitochondria and is expressed mainly in the liver
- alanine aminotransferase (ALT; normal reference range: 5–45 IU/l); this is also known as serum glutamic pyruvate transaminase and is a more liver specific transaminase enzyme

AST is also found in skeletal muscle, the pancreas, and the kidneys. AST is usually more markedly raised than ALT (alanine transaminases) in alcoholic liver disease, whereas the ratio is reversed in non-alcoholic fatty liver disease unless advanced fibrosis is present.

Alkaline phosphatase

Alkaline phosphatase (the normal reference range is centre specific) is located in the biliary membrane of hepatocytes lining the bile ducts. This enzyme is associated with cholestasis (where it can reach three or more times the upper limit of normal). Milder elevations can also be seen in hepatocellular injury. Other sources of this enzyme include bone, the small bowel, placental tissue, and the kidneys. In cases where elevated alkaline phosphatase level is observed in isolation, consider an extra-hepatic cause.

Gamma-glutamyl transferase

Gamma-glutamyl transferase (normal reference range: 5–40 IU/l) is a membrane-bound enzyme found in all cells but with particularly high concentrations in the liver, the bile ducts, and the kidney. It is elevated in even minor, subclinical levels of hepatic dysfunction. It is particularly useful when attempting to attribute the origin of a raised alkaline phosphatase level. Elevated levels may also be associated with pancreatitis, obesity, hyperlipidaemia, anorexia nervosa, hyperthyroidism, diabetes mellitus, and certain enzyme inducers such as anticonvulsants.

Lactate dehydrogenase

Lactate dehydrogenase (normal reference range: 105–330 IU/l) is another enzyme present in all cells, with a variety of isoenzymes. The test for lactate dehydrogenase becomes particularly useful when the enzyme level is raised out of proportion to other LFTs, whereby its presence points toward ischaemic liver injury (see Chapter 217). It is also raised in the presence of secondary malignancy.

Tests of liver synthetic function

Serum albumin

Serum albumin (normal reference range: 39–50 g/l) is the most abundant plasma protein and is produced by the liver. Its concentration is dependent upon nutrition, hepatic synthesis, and losses. In chronic liver disease, low albumin is a major prognostic indicator representing diminishing hepatocyte function. Albumin has a half-life of 17–26 days. Reduced levels of albumin may also occur with malnutrition and increased losses (e.g. nephrotic syndrome).

Prothrombin time and internationalized normalized ratio

Vitamin K-dependent clotting factors are synthesized by the liver. The prothrombin time (PT; normal reference range: 11–14 seconds) assesses the activity of these clotting factors and is a surrogate marker for the extrinsic clotting pathway. The internationalized normalized ratio (INR; 0.9–1.2) is the ratio of a patient's plasma PT divided by that of a laboratory control. By logic, one can deduce that, in significant liver disease, vitamin K-dependent clotting factors will fail to be synthesized; hence, the PT (the time it takes for blood to clot) will increase. A raised INR or PT may also reflect poor intake of vitamin K or malabsorption; parenteral administration of vitamin K may correct the abnormality in these circumstances, provided the intrinsic hepatocellular function is intact. (NB: in cases of large-volume transfusion, one should recall that stored blood contains anticoagulant but no clotting factors, which may also need replacing.)

Alpha-fetoprotein

Alpha-fetoprotein is normally produced by the yolk sac of the embryo during pregnancy, and by the liver. Pathologically raised levels are observed in two-thirds of patients with hepatocellular carcinoma, but levels may be mildly elevated in acute and chronic liver disease without malignancy. For this reason, alpha-fetoprotein is no longer recommended as part of hepatocellular carcinoma surveillance

Table 208.1 Viral hepatitis: Serology testing

Test positive	Interpretation	Additional points
HAV		
Anti-HAV IgM	Recently infected with HAV	Confirms acute HAV illness
Anti-HAV IgG	Previous infection with HAV **or** immunity to HAV through vaccination	
HBV		
Anti-HBc IgM	Recent infection of HBV	Confirms acute HBV illness
HBsAg	Present or chronic HBV infection	
HBeAg (e antigen)	Active viral replication present	Highly infectious
HBV DNA*	Presence of complete virus†	Highly infectious
Anti-HBe	No active viral replication	No longer infectious
Anti-HBs	Previous infection or vaccination	
HCV		
Anti-HCV	Exposure to HCV	
HCV RNA	Confirms the presence of the virus	Useful in monitoring response to treatment
HCV genotype		Helps identify serotype which is important in treatment
Other viral hepatitides		
EBV IgM	Recent EBV infection	Cross reactivity with CMV IgM
Glandular fever test	Recent EBV infection	
EBV IgG	Previous EBV infection	
CMV IgM	Recent CMV infection	Cross reactivity with EBV IgM
CMV IgG	Previous CMV exposure	

Abbreviations: anti-HBe, antibody to the hepatitis B e antigen; anti-HBs, antibody to the hepatitis B surface antigen; EBV, Epstein–Barr virus; HAV, hepatitis A virus; HBc, hepatitis B core protein; HBsAg, hepatitis B surface antigen; HBeAg, hepatitis B e antigen; HBV, hepatitis B virus; HCV, hepatitis C virus.

Note: Acute hepatitis D and E virus infection can be diagnosed with positive IgM serology to the respective viruses.

* This is a quantitative marker.

† This may be used as a surrogate marker for those with active disease in presence of 'precore mutant disease' and who do not produce HBeAg but are still highly infectious.

programmes, although it may be of prognostic significance in monitoring treatment response in those with confirmed liver cancer.

Viral serology

Viral hepatitis has been covered in more detail in Chapter 212. Testing for viral serology is important when investigating the cause of deranged LFTs. A summary of the common tests for viral hepatitis is provided in Table 208.1.

Autoantibodies and immunoglobulins

Autoantibodies and autoimmune liver disease have been covered in more detail in Chapter 213. Despite obtaining positive autoantibody serology in the workup of someone with chronic liver disease, confirmation often requires liver biopsy. Moreover, up to 19% of patients with autoimmune hepatitis, and 5% of patients with primary biliary cholangitis, may lack identifiable autoantibodies (i.e. they are 'seronegative'). A summary of the common tests in autoimmune liver disease is given in Table 208.2.

Other laboratory tests

Other laboratory tests include iron studies for haemochromatosis; copper studies for Wilson's disease; alpha-1-antitrypsin levels for alpha-1-antitrypsin deficiency (see Chapter 214); thyroid function tests; and lipid and glucose tests, for hepatic steatosis (see Chapter 216).

Ascitic fluid analysis

The mechanisms in ascites development are explained in Chapter 207. Examination of ascitic fluid is essential, particularly when ascites is first diagnosed or when the patient's clinical picture changes. Consider non-hepatic causes if LFTs and coagulation studies are normal. Remember, serum albumin levels may be low in protein-losing nephropathies and enteropathies. Ascitic fluid should always be sent for red and white blood cell counts, blood culture, albumin, total protein, glucose, amylase, triglyceride, and cytology. The peritoneal fluid characteristics for common causes of ascites are outlined in Tables 208.3 and 208.4.

Table 208.2 Autoimmune liver disease serology

Test	Association
Antinuclear antibody	Autoimmune hepatitis type I (classical variety; good response to immunosuppression)
Anti-smooth muscle antibody	Autoimmune hepatitis type I
Raised IgG	Autoimmune hepatitis (any type but more so with type I)
Anti-liver kidney microsomal antibody	Autoimmune hepatitis type II (females/teenagers; frequently steroid dependent)
Anti-soluble liver antigen	Autoimmune hepatitis type III (behaves like type I)
Anti-mitochondrial antibodies	Primary biliary cholangitis (95% sensitivity)
Raised IgM (subclass 2)	Primary biliary cholangitis
Raised IgA	Alcoholic liver disease
Anti-endomysial antibody (an IgA antibody)	Coeliac disease: can predispose to liver steatosis (5% of the coeliac population will be total IgA deficient)
Antineutrophil cytoplasmic antibody (p type)	Non-specific; found in up to 92% of patients with autoimmune hepatitis, and 94% of individuals with primary sclerosing cholangitis; may also be detectable in ~>70% of patients with ulcerative colitis alone

Imaging

Hepatobiliary ultrasound

Hepatobiliary ultrasound is usually the first-line approach in terms of imaging when deranged liver biochemistry, jaundice, hepatomegaly, or ascites is present. It is used for assessing gross hepatic architecture, ductal dilatation, stone disease, and tumours. Doppler studies of venous flow can be performed in both hepatic venous and portal venous systems to aid in the diagnosis of certain conditions.

Table 208.3 Causes of ascites

High SAAG	Low SAAG	Other rarer causes
Liver cirrhosis*	Malignancy with peritoneal spread[†]	Vasculitis
Cardiac failure	Tuberculosis	Myxoedema
Hepatic venous occlusion/ Budd–Chiari	Pancreatitis	Peritoneal mesothelioma
Constrictive pericarditis	Serositis	
Portal vein thrombosis	Protein-losing states	
Fatty liver of pregnancy		
Internal malignancy with liver metastasis		

Abbreviations: SAAG, serum–ascites albumin gradient.

Note: A high SAAG (≥11 g/l) indicates that the ascites is due to portal hypertension; a low SAAG (<11 g/l) indicates that the ascites is not due to portal hypertension

* Occurs in 80% of cases of ascites.

[†] Common malignancies which spread to the peritoneum are ovarian cancer, bladder cancer, colon cancer, stomach cancer, breast cancer, pancreatic cancer, lung cancer, and lymphoma (with nodal obstruction).

Ultrasound is also useful in differentiating solid from fluid-filled lesions; this is not always possible on CT scans. Ultrasound is widely accessible and relatively inexpensive. Individuals undergoing hepatobiliary ultrasound should abstain from oral intake for 4 hours prior to the test if the biliary tree and gall bladder are to be looked at in the study. The disadvantages are an inability to depict smaller lesions, and the possibility of inaccuracy when dealing with individuals with a larger body habitus.

CT

CT provides excellent detail of anatomy and has the advantage of picking up smaller lesions that are often missed on ultrasound. It has the advantage in cases where doubt regarding diagnosis persists on ultrasound and in cases where ultrasound is not technically feasible (e.g. when there is a large quantity of intra-abdominal fat). CT is also better at looking at other retroperitoneal structures. The main disadvantage of CT is that it is not as portable as ultrasound and is relatively more expensive. Frequent CT scans also entail the risk of radiation exposure.

MRI

MRI may be needed if it is the only modality that can pick up the lesion in question. For example, MRI is usually indicated for the evaluation of isolated hepatic lesions to distinguish adenomas from focal nodular hyperplasia or tumours. Magnetic resonance cholangiography is indicated for detailed evaluation of the hepatobiliary tree before endoscopic biliary intervention (i.e. endoscopic retrograde cholangiopancreatography), as it can detect smaller ductal stones that are missed on ultrasound.

Endoscopic ultrasound

Endoscopic ultrasound is a procedure in which upper gastrointestinal endoscopy is combined with internal ultrasound in order to obtain images of the internal organs. It is particular useful in the identification of small (<1 cm) lesions in the distal hepatobiliary tree and the pancreas, as well as the identification of gallstones which have migrated into the distal common bile duct.

Liver biopsy

Liver biopsy has been practised for over a century and is still used in establishing the underlying aetiology of many liver diseases. The broad indications for proceeding with a liver biopsy are:

- liver disease in general; to determine the severity and extent of the disease
- persistently elevated LFTs without an underlying cause being identified through laboratory or radiological testing
- serological diagnosis (e.g. of autoimmune liver disease), for confirmation of the diagnosis, and prognostication
- indeterminate hepatic lesions (see Chapter 218) on radiological scanning

Contraindications to percutaneous liver biopsy are:

- elevated PT (>1.5 seconds)
- thrombocytopenia (platelet count <50 × 10⁹)
- large body habitus, or ascites (although a transjugular liver biopsy can be performed in experienced hands)
- echinococcal infection (due to the risk of severe anaphylaxis)
- suspected haemangioma
- hepatic peliosis (i.e. randomly distributed multiple blood-filled cavities throughout the liver; associated with AIDS, the use of synthetic oestrogens, and the use of anabolic steroids)

Complications of a liver biopsy are rare, but can be serious when they occur; 95% of complications occur in the first 24 hours. Possible complications are as follows:

- pain:
  - normally localized in the right upper quadrant or may radiate to the shoulder
  - usually not more than a dull ache
  - relatively short-lived
  - responds to simple analgesia
  - more severe and longer-lasting pain may indicate a biliary leak or intra-peritoneal haemorrhage
- haematoma:
  - occurs either as a parenchymal haematoma or as a subcapular haematoma

Table 208.4 Characteristics of ascitic fluid

Aetiology	Colour	SAAG (g/l)	RBCs (10⁶ cells/l)	WBCs (10⁶ cells/l)	Cytology	Other comments
Cirrhosis	Straw	≥11	Few	≤250		
Infected	Straw Turbid	≥11	Few	≥250 PMN ≥400 total		Culture is essential: any growth is abnormal
Tuberculosis	Turbid Haemorrhagic	<11	Abundant	≥1000 (lymphocytes)	Ziehl/Nielsen stain	Send for AAFB and culture
Neoplasia	Haemorrhagic mucinous	<11 (unless directly due to liver mets)	Variable	Variable	Large volume (50 ml) needed	Malignant cells diagnostic
Cardiac failure	Straw	≥11	Few/nil	<250		Echo should be performed
Pancreatitis	Turbid Haemorrhagic	<11	Variable	Variable		Amylase may be increased
Chylous	Milky	<11	Nil	Nil		Fat globules Triglyceride >5 mmol/l is abnormal
Biliary leak	Yellow	<11	Few	Variable		Ratio of ascitic fluid to serum bilirubin is >1.0

Abbreviations: AAFB, acid- and alcohol-fast bacteria; Echo, echocardiography; PMN, polymorphonuclear; RBC, red blood cell; SAAG, serum–ascites albumin gradient; WBC, white blood cell.

- the majority are asymptomatic
- the few that are painful will respond to simple analgesia (avoid aspirin and NSAIDs)
- haemobilia:
  - although rare, this is one of the most serious complications
  - may present as rapid exsanguination through a gastrointestinal bleed or give rise to a chronic anaemia
  - biliary colic and jaundice are common in cases of gastrointestinal blood loss
  - the interval between onset and presentation of symptoms may be as long as 5 days
  - although conservative treatment usually suffices, consider biliary angiography in severe cases
- intra-peritoneal haemorrhage:
  - the most serious complication

- occurs in the first few hours post procedure (late-onset haemorrhage >24 hours post procedure is associated with a poorer outcome)
- suspect if severe abdominal pain and haemodynamic instability are present
- angiography with embolization is the treatment of choice
- rarer complications include pneumothorax, bacteraemia, surgical emphysema, and biopsy of other organ tissue

Further Reading

Hall JE. *Guyton and Hall Textbook of Medical Physiology* (13th edition), 2015. Saunders.

Longo DL and Fauci AS. *Harrison's Gastroenterology and Hepatology*, 2010. McGraw-Hill Medical.

209 Acute liver failure

Satish Keshav and Palak Trivedi

Definition of the disease

Acute liver failure (ALF) is the term given to a potentially reversible condition characterized by rapid deterioration in hepatocyte function, coagulopathy, and encephalopathy in the absence of preexisting liver disease.

Aetiology of the disease

Ingestion of drugs or toxins, and viral hepatitis, are the most common causes of ALF (Table 209.1), with a large number of other causes accounting for the remaining cases.

Typical symptoms of the disease and less common symptoms

The key features are a rapid deterioration in liver function with nausea, anorexia, malaise, fatigue, altered consciousness, jaundice, and disordered clotting parameters progressing to hepatic encephalopathy (Table 209.2), coma, and death, if uncorrected. Most patients with ALF demonstrate 'warm shock' with profound vasodilatation, intravascular depletion, and low mean arterial pressures. Severe alterations in nearly all clotting parameters are seen in ALF in part due to failure of synthesis as well as factor consumption. The classic interpretation has been that severe bleeding is a likely outcome. Overall, however, there are abnormalities in both the coagulation and fibrinolytic pathways, and recent data suggest that the defects are balanced.

Patients with ALF have an overwhelming susceptibility to the development of infection. Proposed mechanisms include severe complement deficiency and impaired polymorphonuclear cell and Kupffer cell function. The quoted incidence of bacteraemia varies between 22% and 80%, and fungaemia 32%.

The varying etiologies of ALF may harbour phenotypic differences although, in practice, diagnostic tests including liver biopsy may be requested early in order not to miss dual pathology, and also to ensure that a diagnosis is reached quickly.

Table 209.1 Causes of acute liver failure

Type	Cause
Common	Paracetamol/acetaminophen overdose
	Viral hepatitis: HBV, HEV, HSV, CMV, EBV
	Drugs: e.g. isoniazid, halothane, tetracycline, thioglitazones, amphetamines, cocaine, herbal remedies
Uncommon	Autoimmune hepatitis
	Cryptogenic (no cause found)
	Alcoholic hepatitis
Rare	HELPP syndrome and fatty liver of pregnancy
	Budd–Chiari syndrome
	Acute hypotension or vascular catastrophe: e.g. catastrophic antiphospholipid syndrome
	Amanita phalloides mushroom poisoning
	Wilson's disease

Abbreviations: CMV, cytomegalovirus; EBV, Epstein–Barr virus; HBV, hepatitis B virus; HEV, hepatitis E virus; HSV, herpes simplex virus.

Table 209.2 West Haven grading of hepatic encephalopathy

Grade	Features
I	Altered mood or behaviour, shortened attention span, dyspraxia, altered sleep
II	Drowsy, lethargy, or apathy disorientation for time or place
III	Somnolence responsive to verbal stimuli, confusion, asterixis
IV	Coma unresponsive to verbal or noxious stimuli, abnormal plantar reflex
V	Coma unresponsive to painful stimuli, abnormal plantar reflex

This article was published in *Gastroenterology*, Volume 72, issue 4 (pt 1), Conn HO, Leevy CM, Vlahcevic ZR, et al., Comparison of lactulose and neomycin in the treatment of chronic portal-systemic encephalopathy. A double blind controlled trial, pp. 573-583, Copyright Elsevier 1977.

Symptoms of ALF due to acetaminophen/paracetamol overdose

Symptoms of acetaminophen/paracetamol overdose present 1–3 days after the overdose, which may be deliberate or accidental. Clinical features include anorexia, malaise, abdominal discomfort, and altered consciousness. Jaundice occurs early. Therapeutic doses of paracetamol are converted to non-toxic metabolites by conjugation with sulphate and glucuronide. Approximately 5% of paracetamol is oxidized by cytochrome p450 (Cyp450) to a highly reactive intermediary, N-acetyl-p-benzoquinone imine (NAPQI). NAPQI is then detoxified by conjugation with glutathione. In cases of overdose, the sulphate and glucuronide pathways are saturated, resulting in the generation of excessive levels of NAPQI that cause hepatocellular necrosis.

Symptoms of ALF due to acute viral hepatitis

Acute viral hepatitis typically presents acutely or subacutely, with typical viraemic prodromal symptoms, followed by jaundice that progresses rather than resolves. The prognosis after transplantation appears to be better if the presentation is acute, particularly for hepatitis B.

Symptoms of ALF due to drugs or herbal remedies

There may be no clues to the diagnosis of ALF due to drugs or herbal remedies, apart from a history of exposure to potential hepatotoxins.

Symptoms of ALF due to autoimmune hepatitis

Autoimmune hepatitis (AIH) affects females more frequently than males and tends to occur in middle age or later. Classical immunoserological and histological features of AIH may be absent or altered in fulminant disease and, in a recent retrospective review of the US Acute Liver Failure Registry, >50% of patients with acute liver failure of previously indeterminate origin were considered to have probable AIH. The commonest histological finding in fulminant AIH is central perivenulitis or centrilobular (Zone 3) necrosis. In such situations, the severity of necroinflammatory activity can be variable, ranging from mildly active hepatitis to massive hepatic necrosis. It is important not to mistake such changes for cirrhosis.

Symptoms of ALF due to alcoholic hepatitis

Alcoholic hepatitis typically occurs on a background of chronic excessive alcohol use followed by a brief period of abstinence (~4 weeks). The patient may be feverish and have signs of chronic liver disease, although splenomegaly, ascites, and portal hypertension can occur acutely and do not necessarily indicate cirrhosis.

Symptoms of ALF due to pregnancy-associated liver failure

Acute fatty liver in pregnancy typically occurs in the third trimester and is more often associated with pre-eclampsia and twin pregnancy. HELLP (haemolysis, elevated liver enzymes, and low platelets) is a severe complication of pre-eclampsia (10%–15% of cases), with mortality approaching 25% (usually due to cerebral haemorrhage and disseminated intravascular coagulation). Elevations in liver enzymes can be dramatic, and there is a risk of hepatic rupture. True failure of hepatic synthetic function is rare.

Symptoms of ALF due to Wilson's disease

Wilson's disease can present with acute hepatitis and liver failure in young patients and, for unknown reasons, haemolysis is a typical feature. Although liver enzymes may be elevated, serum alkaline phosphatase level is usually normal or disproportionately closer to normal.

Symptoms of ALF due to Budd–Chiari syndrome

Budd–Chiari syndrome presents with ascites and jaundice, and typically occurs in the context of a myeloproliferative syndrome, other malignancy, or prothrombotic diathesis, all of which may be subclinical at the time of liver failure.

Demographics of the disease

ALF is uncommon, affecting ~2000 patients annually in the US; approximately 7% of all US liver transplants are performed for ALF. Paracetamol overdose accounts for over 70% of cases of acute hepatic failure in the UK. Where viral hepatitis is endemic, it accounts for more cases; for instance, in the Indian subcontinent, it accounts for 30% of cases.

Natural history, and complications of the disease

ALF can be divided into three categories according to the time from the onset of jaundice to the onset of hepatic encephalopathy: hyperacute (<7 days), acute (7–28 days), or subacute (>28 days). The outcome after hyperacute failure is often better than that for subacute failure.

Different aetiologies typically have different time frames. For example, paracetamol cases are virtually always hyperacute, while viral hepatitis, idiosyncratic drug reactions, or cases of indeterminate cause demonstrate slower onset and evolution (acute or subacute). The etiologic diagnosis per se appears to be the strongest driver of outcome. Untreated liver failure may progress to death, which may occur from cerebral oedema and coma, metabolic failure including hypoglycaemia, coagulopathy and haemorrhage, autonomic and haemodynamic instability, and/or infection.

Elevated liver enzymes alone give little information about hepatic function. The key tests demonstrating progressive liver failure are elevated bilirubin, prolonged prothrombin time (PT) or international normalized ratio (INR), and reduced serum albumin. The PT can worsen precipitously over a few hours and so it is essential to take repeated measurements. The albumin level falls over a period of days. Elevated bilirubin may persist or even continue to rise even when the liver is recovering. The development of ascites, particularly in cases of subacute failure, indicates worsening disease.

Oliguria and renal dysfunction occur in approximately 50% of cases. Frequently, these are poor prognostic signs and can be associated with worsening liver failure or even hepatorenal syndrome. In other cases, however, they may be independent of the precipitating cause, for instance high doses of paracetamol causing renal damage; alternatively, they may result simply from dehydration, which can be readily corrected.

Potential outcomes from ALF include full recovery; progressive deterioration and death; death from complications such as renal failure and sepsis; and recovery after liver transplantation. Patients with ALF due to autoimmune liver disease or, in some cases, viral hepatitis, may recover but then progress to chronic liver disease.

Differential diagnosis

The full constellation of signs and symptoms of ALF are rarely seen together in any other context. ALF is distinct from decompensation in a patient with chronic liver disease and cirrhosis triggered by intestinal haemorrhage from varices, infection, alcoholic binge drinking, hepatotoxic drugs, hepatocellular carcinoma, and so on.

The differential diagnosis for acute jaundice includes biliary obstruction, haemolysis, and infection such as Weil's disease. The differential diagnosis for an elevated PT includes warfarin poisoning, disseminated intravascular coagulation, and sepsis. The differential diagnosis for coma and encephalopathy includes extremely rare inherited defects of the urea cycle, hyperammonemia, uraemia, and overdose with psychoactive drugs.

Approach to diagnosing the disease

The diagnosis of ALF must be considered in anyone presenting with a quick onset of hepatic illness with prolonged PT/INR and encephalopathy, provided they have had an illness of short duration and do not have cirrhosis. Patients often appear hypotensive and vasodilated with low systemic vascular resistance.

The following laboratory studies should be checked where there is suspicion of ALF:

- coagulation, including PT
- glucose
- electrolytes
- creatinine
- bilirubin
- albumin
- liver enzymes
- amylase
- full blood count
- group and save
- serum lactate

In addition, blood cultures and a chest X-ray should be obtained, as sepsis is a frequent complication.

Causes of acute liver injury that can be readily tested for should be tested. These include viral hepatitis, paracetamol, serum copper and caeruloplasmin, IgG levels, and autoantibodies (although these are often negative in acute fulminant presentations of AIH). An urgent liver ultrasound with Doppler measurement of hepatic venous and portal venous flow should be obtained. If there is ascites, an ascitic tap should be performed to quantify the number of leukocytes, and measure albumin and protein.

'Gold-standard' diagnostic test

The constellation of clinical signs of liver decompensation, with elevated PT, elevated bilirubin, and low serum albumin make the diagnosis of ALF when they occur in the appropriate timescale. However, no single feature distinguishes between acute and acute-on-chronic liver failure.

Other relevant investigations

Transjugular liver biopsy can be performed safely even in the presence of ascites and coagulopathy. Findings may be non-specific, although they may provide clues to the underlying aetiology. In particular, AIH, acute alcoholic hepatitis, and drug-induced liver damage may require biopsy to support the diagnosis. The presence of microvesicular steatosis suggests certain medications (e.g. sodium valproate, salicylates) and is also found in acute fatty liver of pregnancy. Central perivenulitis is the commonest feature in acute, fulminant AIH, which may progress to Zone 3 necrosis, making distinction from drug-induced disease difficult. In such situations, the severity of necroinflammatory activity can be variable, ranging from mildly active hepatitis to massive hepatic necrosis. It is important not to mistake such changes for cirrhosis. Less specific findings include ballooning degeneration, spotty hepatocyte necrosis, apoptotic bodies, and syncytial multinucleated hepatocyte giant cells. Giant cell hepatitis is seen more frequently in children but also in atypical viral infections and idiosyncratic drug injury.

Prognosis and how to estimate it

If the patient survives an episode of ALF and its immediate complications, they usually have an excellent long-term prognosis. Overall survival is approximately 70%. Where recovery with supportive care seems unlikely, orthotopic liver transplantation offers a good chance of recovery, albeit with the long-term implications of living with an allograft and lifelong immunosuppression. Transplantation is performed in ~25%–30% of patients.

Paracetamol-related ALF carries a better prognosis than drug-induced ALF, cryptogenic ALF, and ALF of most other etiologies, largely through the advent of acetylcysteine (NAC) therapy.

Treatment and its effectiveness

ALF is a medical emergency, of which good coma care is the hallmark of management. By establishing timely diagnosis and determining the aetiology and severity, appropriate triage to an intensive care unit or transfer to a transplant centre can be rapidly accomplished. Determining eligibility and listing for transplantation must be an early consideration.

Should the individual progress beyond Grade II encephalopathy, the airway should be protected. Cerebral oedema is a frequent cause of mortality, and occurs secondary to osmotic changes and loss of capillary integrity within the brain. Sedation should be avoided, as this can worsen encephalopathy. Invasive monitoring of intracranial pressure is to be considered in the intensive care setting (preferably in a dedicated liver unit) in cases of higher-grade encephalopathy. Phenytoin can reduce subclinical seizure activity, and mannitol can be given in cases of raised intracranial pressure, provided there is adequate renal output.

Cardiovascular support with fluid resuscitation is essential, and consideration given to central venous pressure monitoring. This will assist in accurate fluid balance and avoid exacerbating encephalopathy. Low systemic vascular resistance and renal artery vasoconstriction is potentially reversible with improvement in liver function.

Patients should have the serum glucose monitored and, if hypoglycaemic, treated as appropriate. In addition, blood tests should be checked regularly, particularly electrolytes, renal function coagulation, full blood count, and albumin. This is essential in the first 48–72 hours. Fresh frozen plasma, cryoprecipitate, or platelets are reserved for active bleeding or if an invasive procedure is planned. Moreover, withholding fresh frozen plasma allows for the use of INR as a continuously available surrogate and reliable measure of hepatic synthetic function and outcome.

Patients with paracetamol poisoning may demonstrate acute kidney injury due to the direct toxic effects of acetaminophen, with oliguria requiring continuous venovenous haemofiltration. The initial aim should be volume resuscitation and, if the mean arterial pressure falls to <80 mm Hg, consideration should be given to inotropic support. Renal failure is also a well-recognized manifestation of fulminant hepatic failure secondary to acute Wilson's disease.

As up to 80% of ALF cases are complicated by sepsis, and meticulous care of lines, catheters, and procedures should be taken. It is essential to take all relevant material for culture prior to the institution of antibiotics. Patients will often be critically ill and, as a result,

recognized signs of sepsis may not manifest. There should be a low threshold for administering IV antibiotics and antifungals, pending further sensitivities.

Osmotic laxatives such as lactulose reduce intestinal bacterial production of ammonia and psychoactive amines, and therefore reduce encephalopathy. Intestinal decontamination such as neomycin may also be used.

Rapid evaluation should be performed, with initiation of specific antidotes where feasible. NAC infusion is an effective antidote to the depletion of hepatic glutathione caused by paracetamol overdose. Historically, clinical practice was to institute therapy based on the serum paracetamol level (in the case of 'single-point' overdose); however, recent guidelines advocate NAC to be commenced immediately for suspected overdose (before serum levels become available) and only discontinued in cases where the time of overdose is certain and serum levels fall below the nomogram treatment line (http://www.mhra.gov.uk/Safetyinformation/DrugSafetyUpdate/CON185624). NAC is to be continued until the PT returns to normal. Paracetamol toxicity is dose dependant but its effects are enhanced by induction of Cyp450 by chronic use of alcohol or drugs such as antiepileptics. Patients receiving NAC within 24 hours of overdose have the best prognosis; however, benefit can be demonstrated even when treatment is provided after 36 hours ingestion. In addition, early consideration should be made to use NAC in non-paracetamol settings, as this may improve transplant-free survival.

In cases of pregnancy-induced ALF, the fetus should be delivered. In idiosyncratic reactions, withdrawal of the causative agent can potentially reverse hepatic injury. Early discussion with a transplant centre is vital. Indications for transfer are highlighted in Table 209.3. Wilson's disease is an indication for early transplantation, as these individuals deteriorate rapidly.

Further Reading

Bernal W and Wendon J. Acute liver failure. *N Engl J Med* 2013; 369: 2525–34.

Lee WM. Recent developments in acute liver failure. *Best Pract Res Clin Gastroenterol* 2012; 26: 3–16.

Table 209.3 Guidelines for referral for liver transplantation

Guidelines for referral for liver transplantation		
Hyperacute	**Acute**	**Subacute**
Encephalopathy	Encephalopathy	Encephalopathy
Renal failure	Renal failure	Renal failure
PT > 30 sec	PT > 30 sec	PT > 20 sec
		Sodium <130 mmol/l
		Shrinking liver volume
Guidelines for referral to a liver unit following paracetamol overdose		
Day 1	**Day 2**	**Day 3**
Acidosis: arterial pH <7.3	Acidosis: arterial pH <7.3	Progressive rise in PT
Oliguria	Oliguria	Oliguria
Creatinine >200 μmol/l	Creatinine >200 μmol/l	Creatinine >300 μmol/l
PT > 50 sec	PT > 60 sec	PT > 75 sec
Hypoglycaemia	Encephalopathy	Encephalopathy

Abbreviations: PT, prothrombin time.

210 Chronic liver failure

Satish Keshav and Palak Trivedi

Definition of the disease

Chronic liver failure is the functional syndrome resulting from cirrhosis. Clinical features of chronic hepatic decompensation include encephalopathy, coagulopathy, and hepatocellular jaundice (also see Chapters 207 and 209). Cirrhosis is the final common pathway for a variety of chronic liver diseases and is characterized by fibrosis and the conversion of normal liver architecture into structurally abnormal nodules.

There often exists a poor correlation between biopsy findings and the clinical presentation. Some individuals with cirrhosis are asymptomatic and have a reasonably good life expectancy, while others have severe symptoms of chronic liver failure and limited life expectancy.

Aetiology of the disease

There are many causes of cirrhosis, the most prevalent being alcohol, viral hepatitis (usually hepatitis C), and, as is increasingly recognized, non-alcoholic fatty liver disease. A list of causes is given in Table 210.1.

Typical symptoms of the disease and less common symptoms

Patients with cirrhosis are often asymptomatic. In fact, up to 80%–90% of liver parenchyma must be destroyed before liver failure can be manifest clinically. Early, well-compensated disease may manifest as weight loss, fatigue, and anorexia. Osteoporotic fracture may result from defective vitamin D and calcium metabolism. In addition, the patient may show heightened sensitivity to a range of drugs normally metabolized by the liver.

Decompensated disease (see also Chapter 207) may manifest as

- jaundice
- pruritus
- ascites, with or without spontaneous bacterial peritonitis
- hepatic encephalopathy (see Chapter 209)
- portal hypertension
- variceal bleeding
- hepatopulmonary syndrome (15% of cirrhotics) due to the overproduction of nitric oxide and overexpression of the endothelin

B receptor, resulting in pulmonary vessel vasodilatation, shunting, and hypoxaemia
- portopulmonary hypertension; this is less common and is probably caused by excess of pulmonary artery vasoconstrictors and profibrogenic factors

Physical signs of decompensated chronic liver disease include:

- signs in the hands, such as:
  - Dupuytren's contracture
  - clubbing
  - palmar erythema
  - asterixis
  - half-and-half nails (chronic disease of any cause)
  - leukonychia
- conjunctival icterus
- gynaecomastia
- spider naevi (also occur in severe malnutrition and pregnancy)
- hepatomegaly
- splenomegaly
- ascites
- caput medusae
- testicular atrophy

Demographics of the disease

The exact prevalence of cirrhosis worldwide is unknown. There are an estimated 30 000 people living with cirrhosis in the UK, and at least 7000 new cases being diagnosed each year. The numbers of people living with both alcoholic cirrhosis and non-alcohol-related cirrhosis seems to be rising. The number in developing countries is higher due to the prevalence of viral hepatitis. Since the disease often goes undetected for extended periods, a reasonable estimate is that up to 1% of the population may have histological evidence of cirrhosis.

Natural history, and complications of the disease

The natural course of cirrhotic liver disease depends on the cause of underlying disease and treatment provided. Decompensation rates with chronic viral hepatitis B and C are 10% and 4%, respectively, per year. Decompensation in alcoholics is even higher with continued alcohol consumption and may be associated with an acute hepatitis on a background of cirrhosis. The complications of cirrhosis are essentially those of hepatic decompensation. This defines chronic liver failure.

Approach to diagnosing the disease

Imaging

Ultrasound, MRI, and CT are not usually sensitive enough to detect the presence of cirrhosis, but may give evidence of hepatic decompensation (e.g. ascites and other features of portal hypertension). They can also be used in the investigation of hepatocellular carcinoma.

Ultrasound is an inexpensive way of providing clues about hepatic architecture and may show increased echogenicity, irregularity, atrophy, and a nodular appearance (some of these feature may also be present in steatosis). The diagnosis of portal hypertension can be made through Doppler/duplex ultrasound by demonstration of portal flow. This can also diagnose portal vein cavernous transformation and portal vein or splenic vein thrombosis. The finding of

Table 210.1 Causes of liver cirrhosis

Common	Less common	Less prevalent causes
Alcohol	Autoimmune hepatitis	Carbohydrate disorders:
Chronic viral (C or B) hepatitis	Drug induced	• galactosaemia
Haemochromatosis	Alpha-1-antitrypsin deficiency	• glycogen storage disease
Non-alcoholic fatty liver disease	Porphyria	Lipid disorders:
Primary biliary cirrhosis	Wilson's disease	• abetalipoproteinaemia
Congenital:	Veno-occlusive diseases	Sarcoidosis
• cystic fibrosis		Vascular:
• congenital biliary cysts		• right-sided heart failure
• biliary atresia (neonatal hepatitis)		• hereditary haemorrhagic telangiectasia
		Polycystic liver disease
		Infections:
		• brucellosis
		• syphilis
		• echinococcus

Table 210.2 Making a diagnosis of specific causes of chronic liver disease

Aetiology	Screening test
Alcohol	AST:ALT >1
	Raised γGT
Autoimmune hepatitis	ANA
	Anti-liver/kidney microsomal antibodies
	Anti-soluble liver antibodies
	Immunoglobulins
Chronic hepatitis B	Hepatitis B surface antigen
Chronic hepatitis C	Hepatitis C antibody
Haemochromatosis	Ferritin or fasting transferring saturation
Non-alcoholic fatty liver disease	ALT:AST >1
	Lipids
	Fasting glucose
	Thyroid function
	Coeliac serology
Primary biliary cirrhosis	AMA (IgM)
Wilson's disease	Serum caeruloplasmin and urinary

Abbreviations: ALT, alanine aminotransferase; AMA, anti-mitochondrial antibody; ANA, antinuclear antibody; AST, aspartate aminotransferase; γGT, gamma-glutamyl transferase.

splenomegaly and a collateral circulation may be seen. The disadvantages include the lack of reproducibility of data due to inter-observer variability.

Spiral CT and CT angiography may allow more accurate demonstrations of liver vasculature and collateral circulations. Dilatation of the inferior vena cava is also suggestive of portal hypertension. Magnetic resonance angiography has the additional advantage of providing quantitative data regarding portal vein and azygous vein flow. MRI can sometimes differentiate between regenerating or dysplastic nodules and hepatocellular carcinoma; it is best used as a follow-up study to determine whether lesions have changed in appearance and size.

Direct portal pressure measurements are not routinely performed due to their invasive nature and the risk of complications.

Blood tests

Although liver function test results may not correlate exactly with degree hepatic dysfunction, interpreting certain patterns from the liver panel in conjunction with the clinical picture may give clues toward certain etiologies (see Table 210.2).

Other diagnoses that should be considered

See Table 210.2 for other diagnoses that should be considered.

'Gold-standard' diagnostic test

Liver biopsy is often considered the 'gold standard' not only for diagnosing cirrhosis but also for sequential histological grading of inflammation and staging of fibrosis. It also becomes important in determining aetiology in about a fifth of patients. Ascites and coagulopathy need correcting prior to percutaneous biopsy but, if correction is needed urgently, a transjugular approach may be attempted. Liver biopsy is subject to a degree of sampling variability regardless of underlying aetiology. Biopsy confirmation of cirrhosis is not needed if clear signs of cirrhosis, such as ascites, coagulopathy, or a nodular, shrunken appearance of the liver, are present.

Acceptable diagnostic alternatives to the gold standard

Non-invasive biomarkers to stage liver fibrosis have been researched extensively (e.g. TIMP1, fibrotest). A problem is the heterogeneity of liver disease, with different stages being present at different parts of the liver during any one time.

A newer imaging technique to determine the 'stiffness' of the liver is based on the velocity of an elastic wave via intercostally located

wave transmitters. Shear wave velocity correlates with liver stiffness. The disadvantage is that the test is less accurate in those who are obese or those with ascites.

Other relevant investigations

Other relevant investigations include liver chemistry, immunoglobulins, and a full blood count (also see Table 210.2).

Liver chemistry

Liver chemistry may be normal in the compensated phase. Marked elevation of levels of alanine aminotransferase or alkaline phosphatase can occur in primary biliary cirrhosis or alcoholic hepatitis (alanine aminotransferase and aspartate aminotransferase levels rarely exceed 350 IU/l if the sole aetiology is alcohol). In terminal disease, these levels may fall. This is due to loss of hepatocyte function, in which case no enzymes can be produced.

Immunoglobulins

Raised IgA is common in alcoholics. IgM is common in primary biliary cirrhosis. IgG is common in other autoimmune conditions.

Full blood count

When performing the full blood count, look for features of hypersplenism (e.g. leucopenia, thrombocytopenia).

Prognosis and how to estimate it

Once decompensation occurs in any type of cirrhosis, mortality can be as high as 85% in 5 years, without transplantation. The Child–Turcotte–Pugh classification is used to gauge disease severity in patients with liver disease (Table 210.3). However, at the turn of the century, the Model for End-Stage Liver Disease (MELD) was developed to provide a more accurate prediction of short-term mortality:

$$MELD = (3.78)(\ln [bilirubin]) + (11.2)(\ln INR)$$
$$+ (9.57)(\ln [creatinine]) + 6.43,$$

where '[bilirubin]' is the serum concentration of bilirubin (in milligrams per decilitre), 'INR' is the international normalized ratio, and '[creatinine]' is the serum concentration of creatinine (in milligrams per decilitre). This equation is used to identify patients who are most likely to die without liver transplantation.

Treatment and its effectiveness

Cirrhosis need not be progressive. Once complications have developed, appropriate patients should be referred to a specialist liver

Table 210.3 Child–Turcotte–Pugh scoring system to assess liver disease severity

Measure	1 point	2 points	3 points
Bilirubin (total) in µmol/l	<34 (<2)	34–50 (2–3)	>50 (>3)
Serum albumin in g/l	>35	28–35	<28
INR	<1.7	1.71–2.20	>2.20
Ascites	None	Suppressed with medication	Refractory
Hepatic encephalopathy	None	Grade I–II (or suppressed with medication)	Grade III–IV (or refractory)

Score 5–6 ≡ Class A: 100% survival from liver cirrhosis at 1 year; 85% survival at 2 years.
Score 7–9 ≡ Class B: 81% survival from liver cirrhosis at 1 year; 57% survival at 2 years.
Score 10< ≡ Class C: 45% survival from liver cirrhosis at 1 year; 35% survival at 2 years.
Abbreviations: INR, international normalized ratio.

Reprinted from *The liver and portal hypertension* Edited by CG Child, Surgery and portal hypertension by Child CG, Turcotte JG, pp50–64, Philadelphia: Saunders 1964 with permission from Elsevier.

unit for management of end-stage liver disease, and consideration for transplantation. This section deals with the features of hepatic decompensation, but treatment of the underlying aetiology (e.g. venesection for haemochromatosis) is also important.

Conservative measures for the treatment of chronic liver failure

Conservative measures for the treatment of chronic liver failure are as follows:

- abstinence from alcohol: this is essential if alcohol is thought to be an etiological factor; for other causes, restriction to <10 units a week should be advised
- salt restriction, in those with ascites
- good nutritional intake, in those with compensated disease

Treatment for ascites

Managing ascites can be difficult, but the aim is a gradual, controlled reduction of ascitic fluid volume, with weight loss of 0.5–1.0 kg per day. Fluid losses at a rate greater then this exceed the capacity of the peritoneum to absorb ascites and can result in hypovolaemia. Medications which can cause fluid retention (e.g. NSAIDs, calcium channel blockers) should be stopped. The mainstays of treatment are:

- dietary sodium restriction (intake not to exceed 2000 mg/day)
- water restriction (1.5 l/day), if the sodium level is below 125 mmol/l
- diuretic therapy

Note that most patients cannot be managed without diuretic therapy. If ascites is present in moderate quantities, then outpatient management is adequate, starting with spironolactone 100 mg daily. Amiloride (up to 15 mg daily) is an alternative if patients cannot tolerate spironolactone. Eplerenone is a newer drug akin to spironolactone; it is licensed for use in cardiac failure but not yet widely used in the management of ascites. It has the advantage of not causing gynaecomastia. Loop diuretics (bumetanide 1–3 mg daily or furosemide 40–120 mg daily) augment the response to spironolactone. Renal function must be monitored closely and should be normal for these medications to work. A weight loss of 2–4 kg per week till the disappearance of clinical ascites is the aim. Spironolactone can be increased by 100 mg every few days to achieve response (maximum 400 mg daily).

Refractory ascites (5%–10% of cases) is defined as an inadequate response to sodium restriction and maximal diuretic treatment (400 mg of spironolactone and 160 mg of furosemide daily). In these cases, one should ensure all appropriate samples have been sent for analysis to exclude treatable causes. If the ascites is tense, and particularly if it is causing respiratory distress or discomfort despite the measures previously mentioned, then therapeutic paracentesis should be instituted. The aim is to drain to dryness; however, one should not leave the drain in situ for greater than 6 hours, in order to prevent the development of iatrogenic bacterial peritonitis. IV colloid replacement should be provided (5–8 g 20% albumin for every 1–2 l of fluid drained). This latter measure is essential to avoid hypotension and hepatorenal syndrome. Diuretics are continued to prevent reaccumulation of ascites. Other measures for refractory ascites include peritoneovenous shunting, use of a transjugular intra-hepatic portosystemic shunt (TIPS), and transplantation.

Peritoneovenous shunting

Peritoneovenous (LeVeen) shunting was introduced in the early 1970s for the treatment of refractory ascites (in patients with cirrhosis). Unfortunately, this procedure has many reported complications, particularly in those with significant hepatocellular insufficiency. Shunt obstruction (particularly at the venous end) is the main problem, necessitating replacement of the shunt. This remains an option in those who are not candidates for TIPS or transplantation.

TIPS

TIPS creates an artificial fistula between the hepatic vein and portal vein via the placement of an expandable metal stent. It can also be used to treat those with persistent variceal haemorrhage, by reducing portal pressure. However, shunt dysfunction is still quite common.

Recent trial data comparing the use of TIPS and medical therapy to large-volume paracentesis and medical therapy demonstrate that the former approach is superior for ascites control but does not improve survival, hospital stay, or subjective quality of life. Hepatic encephalopathy is more common in those who receive TIPS but variceal bleeding and renal impairment have similar rates of occurrence. The recent development of PTFE-coated shunts improves patency and reduces the incidence of TIPS dysfunction and possibly even encephalopathy.

Transplantation

Individuals who develop diuretic resistant ascites have an increasingly worse prognosis. Any individual who develops diuretic resistance should be considered for transplantation, as the 1-year survival rate can be increased to greater than 75%.

Treatment for bacterial peritonitis

Recognition of spontaneous bacterial peritonitis and differentiation of it from bacterial peritonitis due to a secondary cause is important. The latter often warrants surgical intervention, whereas the former is treated medically. Secondary peritonitis should be considered in the following circumstances:

- ascitic total protein >1 g/dl
- ascitic lactate dehydrogenase >225 mU/ml (or higher than the upper limit of normal for sodium)
- ascitic glucose >2.75 mmol
- polymicrobial ascitic fluid

Patients with secondary peritonitis must be evaluated by urgent imaging to exclude viscus perforation.

Cirrhotic patients are at risk of developing spontaneous bacterial peritonitis. This can have a mortality of 40%–70%. Increased risk is present in the following conditions:

- gastrointestinal haemorrhage
- ascitic fluid total protein <10 g/l; this is particularly important if bilirubin is very high and the patient is thrombocytopenic
- a history of previous episodes of spontaneous bacterial peritonitis
- fulminant hepatic failure

Spontaneous bacterial peritonitis is usually caused by *E. coli*, and enteric organisms have been isolated from ascitic fluid in >90% of cases of spontaneous bacterial peritonitis, suggesting that the gastrointestinal tract is the source of bacterial contamination. Because of the predominance of enteric organisms in spontaneous bacterial peritonitis, it was once thought that spontaneous bacterial peritonitis was caused by the direct transmural migration of bacteria from the intestinal lumen, or 'bacterial translocation', although experimental evidence suggests that bacterial translocation might not be the only factor responsible. Nonetheless, a key predisposing factor may be intestinal bacterial overgrowth (attributed to decreased intestinal transit time), combined with impaired phagocytic function, low serum and ascites complement levels, and decreased activity of the reticuloendothelial system; an increased number of microorganisms, combined with a decreased capacity to clear them from the bloodstream, may result in their migration to and proliferation within ascitic fluid.

A diagnosis of spontaneous bacterial peritonitis is made when the ascitic fluid total white-cell count exceeds 400 cells/mm³, or the total polymorph count exceeds 250 cells/mm³. This is the case even if no organisms are identified in the ascitic fluid. In patients with haemorrhagic ascites, when the ascitic fluid red-cell count is >10 000 cells/mm³, 1 neutrophil should be subtracted for every 250 red blood cells, to adjust for the presence of blood.

Following a diagnosis of spontaneous bacterial peritonitis (by diagnostic paracentesis), the following treatment should be started promptly:

- all diuretic treatment should be stopped, and large-volume paracentesis should be avoided (except for diagnostic purposes); this will reduce risk of progression to hepatorenal syndrome
- cefotaxime should be provided at 2 g twice daily for 5 days
- if the patient is systemically unwell but with normal renal function, then a single dose of gentamicin 5 mg/kg should also be given, for rapid bactericidal kill

- 20% human albumin solution should be provided: 1.5 g/kg on Days 1 and 2 of treatment, followed by 1.0 g/kg on Day 3; this may improve mortality and reduce the incidence of developing renal failure
- following treatment, a fluoroquinolone should be prescribed in the long term, to prevent future recurrence

Portal hypertension

Regardless of the aetiology of liver cirrhosis, the development of portal hypertension is usually inevitable and occurs due to an increased resistance to portal flow secondary to scarring, narrowing, and compression of the hepatic sinusoids (see also Chapter 207). Raised portal pressure leads to the development of varices. The British Society of Gastroenterology guidelines recommend that endoscopic surveillance for varices should take place every 3 years in those who have not had an episode of variceal bleeding in the past.

Primary prophylaxis (of varices) is aimed at reducing portal pressure with propranolol 40 mg two or three times per day. This is also the treatment of choice in portosystemic gastropathy. Variceal banding is not usually indicated as a prophylactic measure unless bleeding has occurred, and has to be done repeatedly to be of any value. Isosorbide mononitrate (20 mg twice daily) can be used if propranolol is contraindicated. Acute variceal bleeding is covered in Chapter 22; band ligation is the first treatment of choice in an acute oesophageal, variceal bleed. Injection of Histoacryl glue has been used successfully in managing gastric varices. Vasoconstrictors terlipressin (2 mg bolus followed by 2 mg every 4 hours) and octreotide can be used as a bridge to endoscopy. Varices recur after obliteration in about 40% of cases. In recurrent cases of variceal bleeding, TIPS should be considered. Surgery is another option in refractory cases in the absence of deranged liver function and encephalopathy. Options available include surgical shunting, oesophageal stapling, and transection.

Hepatic encephalopathy

See Chapter 209 for a discussion of hepatic encephalopathy.

Hepatorenal syndrome

The term 'hepatorenal syndrome' (HRS) refers to acute renal failure that occurs in the setting of cirrhosis or fulminant hepatic failure and is sometimes associated with portal hypertension in the absence of intrinsic diseases of the kidney. Type I HRS is characterized by rapidly progressive renal failure with a doubling of serum creatinine to a level greater than 221 μmol/l. This carries a very poor prognosis, usually with less than 50% survival at 1 month. Patients with type I HRS are usually ill, may have low blood pressure, and may require therapy with inotropes or IV drugs to maintain blood pressure. In contrast, type II HRS is characterized by a slowly progressive increase in serum creatinine level to greater than 133 μmol/l. It is typically associated with ascites unresponsive to diuretics and also carries a poor outlook, unless the patient undergoes transplantation.

It can be challenging to distinguish HRS from other entities that cause renal failure in the setting of advanced liver disease. The key to effective treatment is early recognition; once HRS has been recognized, the following steps should be taken:

- diuretics and all nephrotoxic drugs should be stopped
- intravascular albumin (colloidal solution) should be provided, to correct hypovolaemia
- terlipressin should be provided (to vasoconstrict the splanchnic circulation; 0.5 mg twice daily); this is not a definitive treatment, but may lead to short-term improvements in cases of reversible liver disease
- haemodialysis or continuous venovenous haemofiltration may be needed to correct uraemia and electrolyte imbalances, although these procedures have no impact on survival
- it may be too late for liver transplantation once HRS has developed, but it is the only treatment that can affect survival

Other therapies for HRS

Some studies have demonstrated improvements in renal blood flow and glomerular filtration rate in type 1 HRS after 20 days treatment with oral midodrine and parenteral octreotide, compared with treatment with dopamine. These therapies may improve survival rates and act as a bridge to liver transplantation.

Further Reading

El-Serag HB. Hepatocellular carcinoma. *N Engl J Med* 2011; 365: 1118–27.

Ge PS and Runyon BA. Treatment of patients with cirrhosis. *N Engl J Med* 2016; 375: 767–77.

Tsochatzis EA, Bosch J, and Burroughs AK. Liver cirrhosis. *Lancet* 2014; 383: 1749–61.

211 Alcoholic liver disease

Satish Keshav and Alexandra Kent

Definition of the disease

Alcoholic liver disease (ALD) develops in excessive drinkers and can manifest in three forms:

- alcoholic fatty liver (steatosis): >80%
- alcoholic hepatitis: 10%–35%
- cirrhosis: 10%

Aetiology of the disease

The more alcohol consumed, the greater the risk of ALD (the recommended daily intake of alcohol is ≤14 units for women, and ≤21 units for men). However, other important etiological factors are as follows:

- 10%–20% of patients have a genetically inherited susceptibility to the harmful effects of alcohol
- women are more sensitive to the harmful effects of alcohol than men are
- daily drinking is more harmful than binge drinking
- poor nutrition and alcohol work synergistically to cause hepatotoxicity

Typical symptoms of the disease and less common symptoms

Alcohol can cause significant damage without producing any symptoms, and many patients will only have liver dysfunction detected on routine blood tests. Many patients report non-specific symptoms, such as anorexia, morning nausea, diarrhoea, and vague right upper quadrant abdominal pain.

Alcohol withdrawal produces additional symptoms of tremulousness, headache, anxiety, tachycardia, and hypertension. Severe withdrawal ('delirium tremens') can produce profound confusion, disorientation, hallucinations, hyperactivity, and extreme cardiovascular disturbances.

Patients with ALD may present with complications related to alcohol misuse, such as rib fractures, head injuries, pancreatitis, and so on. Alcoholic hepatitis can present with a constellation of symptoms, including rapidly developing jaundice, ascites, and liver failure. ALD symptoms may also reflect complications of liver disease, for example haematemesis from bleeding varices, a distended abdomen from ascites, and/or confusion from encephalopathy.

Demographics of the disease

Since 1950, alcohol consumption in the UK has risen from 3.9 l of pure alcohol per capita per year to a peak of 9.4 l in 2004. In the UK, there are 150 000 hospital admissions per year due to alcohol, with >39 000 due to ALD, and 22 000 alcohol-related deaths. Alcohol misuse costs the NHS £1.7 billion per year.

Of adults in England, aged 16–64, 38% of men and 16% of women have an alcohol use disorder, 21% of men and 9% of women are binge drinkers, 23% (7.1 million) consume alcohol at hazardous or harmful levels (32% of men, 15% of women), and 3.6 % (1.1 million) are alcohol dependent (6% of men, 2% of women). In addition, there is an increasing incidence of women drinking in excess of the recommended daily alcohol intake. However, there is wide variation in alcohol consumption between racial groups: 91% of Caucasian British drink alcohol, but only 52% of British of African descent and 10% of those of Pakistani and Bangladeshi descent. Nonetheless, UK teenagers report more alcohol consumption, more episodes of intoxication, and more adverse effects from drinking than do teenagers in any other European country.

Natural history, and complications of the disease

The underlying pathogenesis of alcohol-induced injury is not fully understood but is thought to involve various mechanisms, including reactive acetaldehyde derivatives; oxygen-derived free radicals; the pro-inflammatory cytokines interleukin 1 beta, interleukin 6, and tumour necrosis factor alpha (TNFα); elevation of hepatocyte and Kupffer cell iron; mitochondrial damage; reduced levels of cellular antioxidants; and alterations in intracellular signalling and hormones.

Minimal change/steatosis

In alcoholic fatty liver, the cytoplasm of affected hepatocytes is occupied by a single large triglyceride occlusion, thought to be due to increased free fatty acid synthesis, diminished triglyceride utilization, decreased fatty acid oxidation, a block in lipoprotein excretion, and enhanced lipolysis, thus increasing delivery and uptake of free fatty acid. Fatty change in the liver is universal 3–7 days after a large amount of alcohol is consumed, and lasts for 2–4 weeks.

Alcoholic hepatitis

In alcoholic hepatitis, hepatocyte ballooning due to water, fat, and protein accumulation occurs, along with inflammation. Mallory's hyaline bodies are seen histologically.

Cirrhosis

Continuing alcohol exposure leads to the development of cirrhosis, which is characterized microscopically by regeneration nodules (containing regenerating hepatocytes) surrounded by fibrous septa. Portal tracts, central veins, and the radial pattern of hepatocytes are absent. Biliary ducts may become damaged, proliferate, or distend, leading to biliary stasis.

Patients who drink excessive volumes of alcohol are at risk of the complications of alcohol toxicity and all complications of chronic liver disease. Box 211.1 lists complications of excessive alcohol consumption. Specific hepatic complications include:

- varices
- ascites
- spontaneous bacterial peritonitis
- encephalopathy
- hepatorenal syndrome

The presence of one or more of these complications significantly worsens prognosis (see Chapter 210 for more information regarding the complications of chronic liver disease).

Approach to diagnosing the disease

Patients may self-present for detoxification or requesting help. Ultimately, a good clinical history and suspicious mind is all that is required to diagnose ALD, and friends and relatives are often useful in providing a collateral history. Questionnaires, such as the Alcohol Use Disorders Identification Test (AUDIT) or CAGE may aid diagnosis. The CAGE questionnaire consists of four questions:

- Have you ever felt you should **c**ut down on your drinking?
- Have people **a**nnoyed you by criticizing your drinking?

Box 211.1 Complications of excess alcohol consumption

- peptic ulcers
- dyspepsia/acid reflux
- throat and mouth cancer
- enteropathy and diarrhoea
- pancreatitis
- malnutrition
- vitamin deficiency
- cardiomyopathy
- peripheral neuropathy
- cerebellar atrophy/syndrome
- Korsakoff's syndrome
- Wernicke's encephalopathy
- depression
- immunosuppression
- coagulopathy
- bone marrow suppression
- reduced libido
- erectile dysfunction
- congenital disorders in babies born to alcoholic mother (fetal alcohol syndrome)

- Have you ever felt **g**uilty about your drinking?
- Have you ever had a drink first thing in the morning (an **e**ye opener) to steady your nerves or get rid of a hangover?

Other diagnoses that should be considered

It is important to ensure the patient has no other underlying liver disease, as alcohol will increase susceptibility to liver damage. Most gastroenterologists would advocate a full liver screen to ensure there is no concomitant diagnosis. In patients presenting with bleeding oesophageal varices, an ultrasound of the liver should be performed to ensure there is no portal vein thrombosis related to turbulence from portal hypertension.

'Gold-standard' diagnostic test

The only investigation which can truly gauge the degree of liver damage is a liver biopsy. This is normally performed under ultrasound guidance but, in patients with coagulopathy or thrombocytopenia, a transjugular approach may be a safer alternative. Histological analysis will help identify features of steatosis, hepatitis, and/or cirrhosis and can exclude pathognomonic features of other liver diseases. The presence of a typical pattern of fine pericellular reticulin fibrosis and Mallory's hyaline are highly suggestive of alcohol-related liver damage.

Acceptable diagnostic alternatives to the gold standard

Various tests are performed to help clarify a diagnosis of ALD, although each test individually has a low sensitivity. The gamma-glutamyltransferase (γGT) test and mean corpuscular volume test each have a sensitivity of 30%–40% in ALD but, in when the tests are taken in combination, the sensitivity increases. However, the γGT level also increases proportionally with BMI. Serum carbohydrate-deficient transferrin is a sensitive and specific test of alcohol excess, but is not widely available. Serum transaminases are often only mildly raised in ALD, and hyperbilirubinaemia is more suggestive of acute alcoholic hepatitis. Hepatic synthetic function is assessed by the albumin level and prothrombin time.

Ultrasound examination can provide information about the liver; fatty infiltration produces a hyperechogenic, bright image, whereas an irregular shrunken liver is in keeping with cirrhosis. An ultrasound can also identify other features of chronic liver disease, such as splenomegaly, ascites, varices (splenic, abdominal wall), and portal vein patency.

Newer investigations assessing the degree of hepatic fibrosis are not in widespread use but include serum fibrosis markers (e.g. procollagen III propeptide, laminin, type IV collagen) and Fibroscan®.

Other relevant investigations

Patients with cirrhosis or evidence of portal hypertension should undergo endoscopic variceal surveillance, at least once every 3 years. Cirrhosis predisposes to hepatocellular carcinoma (HCC); therefore, patients should undergo 6-monthly alpha-fetoprotein measurements and liver ultrasound scans. These guidelines should be adapted for each patient, as patients with severe chronic liver disease will not be eligible for treatment of an underlying HCC, so screening investigations will not be of benefit.

Prognosis and how to estimate it

Prognosis is dependent on patients remaining abstinent from alcohol, as steatosis is reversible. Cirrhosis causes irreversible damage, but abstinence prevents further hepatic damage. Survival for cirrhotic patients is dependent on the degree of liver damage, but overall is 60%–70% at 1 year, and 35%–50% at 5 years. Alcoholic hepatitis has a high mortality rate: 50% in 30 days. Each additional complication (e.g. spontaneous bacterial peritonitis, variceal bleeding) worsens prognosis. The Maddrey discriminant function (DF) was originally used in studies investigating the use of corticosteroids in acute alcoholic hepatitis. The formula used to calculate this index is

$$DF = 4.6\,(\text{prothrombin time} - \text{control prothrombin time}) + [\text{bilirubin}],$$

where the prothrombin time and the control prothrombin time are in seconds, and '[bilirubin]' is the concentration of bilirubin in milligrams per decilitre (NB: if bilirubin is measured in micromoles per litre, then divide the measurement by 17.1). A DF ≥32, with or without encephalopathy, is associated with a 65% 28-day survival, and a DF <32 with a 93% 28-day survival.

Treatment and its effectiveness

Abstinence is integral to prognosis and should be encouraged with help from family, friends, social services, and support groups such as Alcoholics Anonymous. Naltrexone and acamprosate have been shown to reduce alcohol cravings, although their effect on abstinence is not known. Vitamin deficiency is common, particularly for thiamine, folate, pyridoxine, and riboflavin. Patients admitted to hospital usually receive IV vitamins (Pabrinex® I + II ampoules, twice daily for 3 days) and then oral supplements. Patients suffering with withdrawal should receive chlordiazepoxide or clomethiazole in reducing doses, to reduce agitation and withdrawal phenomena.

Nutrition is extremely important; patients should be reviewed by the dietician, and enteral supplements provided. In severely malnourished patients, nasogastric feeding can be given as a supplement.

The use of corticosteroids in ALD has been the subject of much debate. However, a pooled analysis of three large, well-designed studies showed that steroids improved survival (85%), compared to placebo (65%), when used in patients with a DF ≥32 and/or encephalopathy, although the survival benefit only lasted for 1 year post treatment. Furthermore, it suggested that a reduction in bilirubin by Day 7 might be a prognostic factor.

Pentoxifylline is a phosphodiesterase inhibitor with anti-TNFα activity and has been shown to reduce mortality by 40%, mainly due to a reduction in hepatorenal syndrome. Antioxidant therapy has not yet been shown to have a beneficial effect, and the use of anti-TNFα biological therapies is still being investigated.

Liver transplantation is considered in patients who meet the following criteria:

- abstinence from alcohol for 6 months, to allow for spontaneous liver recovery, allow time for other alcohol-related morbidities to recover, and on the theory that preoperative abstinence can

predict a reduced risk of post-operative relapse, although this theory is not substantiated
- advanced liver disease with complications
- no other organ damage
- good social or family support

Propranolol should be given to all patients with Grade 2–4 varices, with doses escalated as tolerated.

Further Reading

Bernstein D. A practical approach to the spectrum of alcoholic liver disease. *Clin Liver Dis* 2012: 16: 659–890.

Lucey MR, Mathurin P and Morgan TR. Alcoholic hepatitis. *N Engl J Med* 2009; 360: 2758–69.

Reuben A. Alcohol and the liver. *Curr Opin Gastroenterol* 2007; 23; 283–91.

Definition of the disease

Hepatitis means 'inflammation of the liver' and is manifest with symptoms that include malaise, anorexia, fever, flu-like symptoms, and pain in the right upper quadrant of the abdomen, with the pain being caused by swelling of the liver and its capsule. Elevations in circulating hepatic enzymes, particularly aspartate transaminase (AST) and alanine transaminase (ALT), are common, with jaundice occurring some time after the onset of other symptoms and signs.

There are five viruses that primarily cause viral hepatitis (see Table 212.1): hepatitis A, B, C, D, and E viruses, abbreviated HAV, HBV, HCV, HDV, and HEV, respectively. These viruses are all hepatotrophic, in that the liver is the primary site of infection. HAV, HBV, and HEV are most often acute, self-limiting infections that may nonetheless cause morbidity and, in the case of HEV, fatality in selected groups of patients. However, HBV and, more so, HCV can cause chronic carriage of the virus over many years, as well as the development of chronic hepatitis. HDV is only pathogenic in conjunction with HBV. There is also emerging evidence of chronic hepatitis E virus infection in patients who are immunosuppressed.

After recovery from acute infection with HAV, individuals have long-lasting immunity against further infection. The same holds true for the majority of individuals with acute HBV infection. There seems to be little natural immunity to HCV infection, and a significant proportion of cases result in chronic hepatitis. Immunity to HEV is not long-lasting, and repeated infections are possible.

Many other viruses can cause hepatitis; of these, cytomegalovirus (CMV), herpes simplex virus (HSV), Epstein–Barr virus (EBV), and flaviviruses such as dengue and yellow fever are the most important. The liver, however, is not their primary site of replication or cellular damage.

Aetiology of the disease

Replication of hepatotrophic viruses in hepatocytes causes cellular damage, resulting in elevations in circulating liver enzymes and compromise of liver function. Activation of the immune system by the infection, and immune-mediated damage to hepatocytes, are also important in causing liver damage. This is demonstrated by the potential for asymptomatic carriage of HBV infection, with overt hepatitis becoming apparent only when the immune system is activated, whereupon the infection may be cleared entirely (seroconversion).

Hepatitis A is transmitted via the faecal–oral route and, hence, has a higher prevalence in areas with poor hygiene and sanitation. Increased incidences are recognized after natural disasters that disrupt sanitation systems that were already marginal at best. Deepwater crustaceans can concentrate the virus and can be a risk if consumed when undercooked or raw.

Hepatitis B is transmitted by infected blood and bodily fluids, percutaneously or through sexual contact. Hepatitis B can also be transmitted vertically from mother to child, and this is one of the most common modes of transmission worldwide. A major mechanism of acquired infection in the UK is IV drug use. Prior to the use of effective methods of blood testing (pre-1990s), blood products also carried a risk of transmission. The majority of observed new cases in the UK arise through immigration from those who resided in endemic countries.

Hepatitis C infection is primarily acquired following contact with infected blood; this can occur through IV drug use, nasal drug use, tattooing, and, less so, skin piercings. Hepatitis C transmission through blood products was particularly an issue in the haemophiliac population prior to the use of heat-treated Factor VIII concentrates, which started in 1985. Fortunately, the proportion of cases due to this route of transmission has fallen greatly. Sexual transmission of hepatitis C through heterosexual relationships is low, but up to 20% of those with hepatitis C infection have no known percutaneous risk factor, and report exposure to sexual contact with a known carrier. However, promiscuous homosexual behaviour amongst men is a risk factor. Vertical transmission of hepatitis C is between 1% and 6%, and does not appear to be affected by the mode of delivery chosen during labour.

Hepatitis D virus infection only occurs with co-transmission of hepatitis B. Its presence should be suspected when an individual with known, stable hepatitis B has an acute deterioration in their clinical condition.

Hepatitis E virus is transmitted through the faecal–oral route and is endemic in countries with poor sanitation, particularly Mexico, Central America, Asia, and Africa. Increasing frequencies have been identified in the Indian subcontinent, with epidemic outbreaks being attributed to contamination of drinking water. Sporadic outbreaks are also recognized in developed countries, usually attributed to travellers returning from endemic countries. Some authorities report a zoonotic source, and pigs are a recognized reservoir. Direct person-to-person transmission is uncommon.

Typical symptoms of the disease, and less common symptoms

Acute infection with HCV is asymptomatic in 50%–90% of cases, although failure to eradicate infection and subsequent progression to chronic disease is the rule rather than the exception (discussed later). HDV suprainfection should be suspected when an individual with previously stable chronic HBV suddenly develops features of an acute hepatitis flare or decompensated liver disease. Acute infection with HAV, HBV, or HEV often presents with the classical symptoms of acute viral hepatitis.

Table 212.1 Hepatitis viruses

	Hepatitis A virus	**Hepatitis B virus**	**Hepatitis C virus**	**Hepatitis D virus**	**Hepatitis E virus**
Transmission	Enteric	Parenteral	Parenteral	Parenteral	Enteric
Classification	Picornavirus	Hepadnavirus	Hepacivirus	Deltavirus	Hepevirus
Genome	ssRNA	dsDNA	ssRNA	ssRNA	ssRNA
Incubation period	15–45 days	45–60 days	15–160 days	30–60 days	15–60 days
Icteric period	Variable	Begins 10 days after the incubation period, lasting up to 4 weeks	Usually occurs in decompensated, chronic infection	N/A	Variable

Abbreviations: dsDNA, double-stranded DNA; ssRNA, single-stranded RNA.

Common symptoms

Infection begins with an incubation period as the virus multiplies and spreads without symptoms. Following the incubation period, a viral prodrome of up to 2 weeks is recognized, including anorexia, malaise, nausea, severe fatigue, myalgia, and fever. Some patients may have a serum-sickness-type presentation including arthralgia, arthritis, and urticarial skin lesions. This is seen more with HBV (up to 20% of infected patients) than with the other hepatitis viruses. It is associated with the formation of immune complexes between antibodies and viral antigens.

When one starts to notice the onset of jaundice, prodromal symptoms will start to resolve and the patient begins to feel much better. Palpable, smooth hepatomegaly may be felt. Jaundice develops within 1–2 weeks and peaks around 4 weeks.

Examination findings often reveal the presence of jaundice and tender hepatomegaly. Other signs of chronic liver disease are rare in acute infection; however, splenomegaly is common in EBV infections.

Resolution of the acute illness is usually spontaneous over the next 4–8 weeks in the majority of patients.

Less common symptoms

Pruritus is unusual with jaundice due to viral hepatitis, although obstructive symptoms (dark urine, pallor to stools) may be noticed.

HBV infection may become chronic in a minority of affected patients, and can lead to features of chronic liver disease as a consequence (discussed later).

Demographics of the disease

Hepatitis A occurs worldwide, with an estimated 1.5 million cases occurring per year. The regions where hepatitis A is endemic include the Indian subcontinent, sub-Saharan and North Africa, the Far East, Middle and Central America, and the Middle East. Interestingly, clinical cases of hepatitis A in adults are uncommon in endemic countries, as most people in those countries are exposed to the virus at a very young age and hence acquire lifelong immunity.

There are over 350 million carriers of hepatitis B worldwide, most of them being concentrated in developing countries. Sub-Saharan Africa, most of Asia, and the Pacific are hit hardest, with 10% of those infected becoming chronic carriers. Five per cent of all people in India and the Middle East are affected. The estimate chronic HBV carrier rate in South East Europe and Central Europe is between 2% and 7%. Australia, New Zealand, Northern Europe, Western Europe, and North America have a prevalence of chronic hepatitis B viral infection of approximately 2%. In the UK, 0.5% of the population is hepatitis B surface antigen (HBsAg) positive, which is representative of chronic infection. Furthermore, up to 2% have prior evidence of hepatitis B virus infection.

Hepatitis C virus is also prevalent worldwide, but epidemiological data is difficult to interpret accurately, as many infections are asymptomatic. It is estimated that 3% (130–210 million) of the world's population are chronically infected with HCV. The highest prevalence rates are found in the African continent, particularly Egypt (up to 50% in some areas), the Eastern Mediterranean, South East Asia, and the Western Pacific. The United Kingdom and Western Europe are considered to be low-prevalence regions; in 2003, the estimated number of individuals with positive hepatitis C antibodies in England and Wales was just over 230 000 (aged 15–59).

Large outbreaks of hepatitis E have been seen in Central and South America, the Indian subcontinent, and bordering nations.

Natural history and complications of the disease

Rarely, acute liver failure may occur with the initial infection. One per cent of symptomatic, acute HBV infections can lead to fulminant liver failure. This complication is more common in the elderly, in whom mortality approaches 15%. Acute liver failure is typical of HEV in pregnancy and elderly men. However, this complication is uncommon outside these settings. Acute liver failure does not usually occur with hepatitis A or C. Complete recovery from the acute

episode can take many weeks to months, with lethargy and anorexia persisting. However, acute HCV inevitably leads to the development of chronic hepatitis. In addition, type III mesangiocapillary glomerulonephritis (immune deposits in sub-endothelial space and mesangium) is associated with HBV or HCV infection.

Viral hepatitis infection typically resolves completely, except in 5% of cases of HBV infection, and in the majority of patients with HCV infection, where disease may persist and become chronic. These viruses represent some of the commonest etiological risk factors worldwide for the development of chronic liver disease and its associated complications.

Chronic HBV infection

Chronic HBV infection has six distinct, dynamic phases of infection: the immune tolerance phase, the immune active phase, the inactive-HBV carrier phase, the HBeAg-negative phase, the HBsAg-negative phase, and HBeAg-negative chronic hepatitis. These do not necessarily occur in a sequential manner.

Immune tolerance phase

The immune tolerance phase of chronic HBV infection is characterized by persistent positivity for the hepatitis B e antigen (HBeAg) following the acute infection (see " 'Gold-standard' diagnostic test for hepatitis B"), high levels of viral replication, and mild or no hepatic necroinflammation with little progression to fibrosis.

Immune active phase

The immune active phase of chronic HBV infection usually occurs after many years of immune tolerance and is characterized by HBeAg positivity, lower levels of HBV DNA and viral replication, increased/fluctuating levels of transaminases, and moderate-to-severe hepatic necroinflammation with rapid progression to fibrosis. The rate of spontaneous HBeAg loss is enhanced. This phase ends with seroconversion to antibodies against HBeAg (anti-HBe).

Inactive carrier phase

The inactive carrier phase (5%–10% of all patients infected) may follow seroconversion to anti-HBe and is characterized by very low/undetectable serum HBV DNA levels and normal serum aminotransferases. ALT levels (usually <40 IU/ml) and serum HBV DNA levels (<2000 IU/ml) should be tested every 3–4 months. HBV DNA levels <2000 IU/ml with elevated ALT values necessitate liver biopsy. The inactive carrier state confers a favourable long-term outcome with a very low risk of cirrhosis or hepatocellular carcinoma (HCC) in the majority of patients. HBsAg loss and seroconversion to antibodies against HBsAg (anti-HBs) may occur spontaneously (in a minority) but, conversely, some individuals progress to develop chronic hepatitis (HBeAg negative). Therefore, inactive carriers should be followed up for life with regular ALT determinations and measurements of HBV DNA levels.

HBeAg-negative chronic hepatitis

HBeAg-negative chronic hepatitis may follow seroconversion from the immune active phase, or develop after years of the inactive carrier state. It is characterized by periodic reactivation with a pattern of fluctuating levels of HBV DNA and aminotransferases, and an active hepatitis. These patients harbour HBV viruses which have developed mutations that render the viruses unable to express HBeAg, and so undergo low rates of prolonged spontaneous disease remission. It is important yet difficult to distinguish true inactive carriers from patients with active HBeAg-negative chronic HBV but who are undergoing spontaneous remission, as the latter have active liver disease with a high risk of progression to advanced hepatic fibrosis, cirrhosis, and subsequent complications such as decompensated cirrhosis and HCC.

HBsAg-negative phase ('occult' HBV disease)

In some patients who achieve loss of HBsAg following HBV infection, low-level viral replication persists, with detectable HBV DNA in the liver. Generally, HBV DNA is not detectable in the serum, while antibodies against the HBV core protein HBcAg (anti-HBc), with or without anti-HBs, are. Immunosuppression for other diseases may lead to HBV reactivation in individuals in this phase, emphasizing the importance of HBV serology testing in all patients for whom immunosuppression is being proposed. Should such an individual show evidence of past infection (e.g. anti-HBc), antiviral therapy is advised prior to starting immunosuppressive therapy.

Long-term impact of chronic HBV infection

The long-term impact of chronic HBV infection on hepatic disease varies greatly, and all grades and stages of hepatitis, including minor changes, chronic hepatitis, fibrosis, and cirrhosis with or without HCC may be observed. Hepatitis B also has a rare association with polyarteritis nodosa, membranous glomerulonephritis, and nephrotic syndrome.

Chronic HCV infection

In most cases, chronic HCV infection usually leads to the development of histologically identifiable hepatitis which may progress to cirrhosis. Cryoglobulinaemia is also a recognized association with hepatitis C leading to type I mesangiocapillary glomerulonephritis.

Approach to diagnosing the disease

History and examination will provide evidence that viral hepatitis is a diagnostic possibility. In acute infection, elevated serum ALT and AST levels signify acute liver damage; levels are typically >10× normal levels. In 10%–15% of those infected with hepatitis A, a characteristic cholestasis with a rise in alkaline phosphatase levels occurs following the acute phase, and an apparent relapse may occur after initial recovery. However, the condition does not become chronic.

As the illness progresses, transaminase levels decline over weeks, and the serum bilirubin level rises. The peak bilirubin level typically occurs weeks after the peak transaminase levels.

With chronic infection, apart from mild-to-moderate elevation in the levels of transaminases, clinical hepatitis may be inapparent. The key to making the diagnosis is to proceed to serological and virological testing for viral hepatitis.

Hepatitis C may not necessarily present as a notable acute, symptomatic hepatitis, and transaminases may not reach the high levels seen in other acute virus infections.

Ultrasound scanning of the liver and the gall bladder is usually indicated to exclude biliary disease, liver abscesses, or mass as a cause of symptoms.

Other diagnoses that should be considered

Other diagnoses that should be considered aside from viral hepatitis include:

- glandular fever (acute EBV infection): a glandular fever test or equivalent (monospot, Paul–Bunnell test) should be performed if hepatitis A and hepatitis B serology are negative, in order to exclude infectious mononucleosis
- acute CMV infection: serology (CMV IgM) may be useful in diagnosing acute CMV infection (does not usually present with posterior cervical lymphadenopathy as seen in acute EBV infection)
- HSV infection
- malaria
- toxoplasmosis infection
- flavivirus/leptospirosis (**always** ask travel history and occupation)
- other causes of hepatitis:
  - alcohol (AST and ALT very rarely rise above 350 IU when solely due to alcohol)
  - mycoplasma pneumonia is an important differential not to miss (often treatable with antibiotics of the macrolide class)
  - drug-induced liver injury
  - autoimmune hepatitis
  - ischaemic hepatitis

'Gold-standard' diagnostic tests

Most viral hepatitis can be readily diagnosed on serological testing.

'Gold-standard' diagnostic test for hepatitis A

Acute infections can be diagnosed on testing hepatitis A IgM. This antibody appears within 8 weeks of the acute illness, may persist for 3–6 months, and clears with the end of jaundice. Hepatitis A IgG indicates immunity either from past infection or through vaccination.

'Gold-standard' diagnostic test for hepatitis B

Hepatitis B testing is complex. To understand the test, it is worth reviewing the structure of the virus and immune response of the host.

HBV is part of the hepadnavirus family, and the complete virus is called the 'Dane particle.' The virus particle consists of an outer lipid envelope and a nucleocapsid core. The nucleocapsid encloses the viral DNA and a viral DNA polymerase bearing reverse transcriptase activity.

There are four known HBV genes: C, X, P, and S. The core protein, HBcAg, is encoded by C. HBcAg cannot be detected in the serum. Upstream to the start codon for the core protein is the coding region for what is known as the 'pre-core' protein. HBeAg is produced by proteolytic processing of the pre-core protein. The DNA polymerase is encoded by P. S is responsible for encoding HBsAg.

About 5–6 weeks following acute hepatitis B infection, the HBsAg titre begins to rise (see Figure 212.1). A level of the HBsAg titre persisting for >6 months indicates chronic infection (see 'Chronic HBV infection'). Once an individual has been identified as HBsAg positive, the HBeAg status should be checked. This begins to rise about 5–6 weeks following infection. HBeAg positivity is a marker of infectivity.

A certain percentage of individuals will not produce HBeAg, due to what is known as pre-core mutant disease. These individuals should have HBV DNA levels assessed as an alternate marker of infectivity. This phenomenon is more common in those who have received prior antiviral therapy (e.g. for coexisting retroviral disease).

IgM antibodies to HBcAg (HBc IgM) generally start to appear 7 weeks after the initial/acute infection. Anti-HBe should appear 15 weeks following infection. Anti-HBs begins to manifest 22 weeks after infection.

During the incubation period of acute infection, the patient will be positive for HBsAg and HBeAg. The acute viral hepatitis is evidenced by derangement of liver function in the presence of HBsAg, HBeAg, anti-HBc IgM, and, later, IgG. Anti-HBe may also be present.

Chronic carriers will bear HBsAg (>6 months after acute infection) and may or may not be HBeAg positive. Anti-HBc IgG should be present, but anti-HBe status is variable.

Recovery is evidenced by anti-HBs, anti-HBe, and anti-HBc (anti-HBc IgM will only remain positive in the acute recovery phase; anti-HBc IgG will remain positive for life). A previously vaccinated individual should only be anti-HBs positive, with anti-HBc and anti-HBe being negative.

A summary of hepatitis B serology is outlined in Table 212.2. **The gold standard for identifying HBV infection (acute or chronic) is an HBsAg test. Following a diagnosis of chronic HBV infection, infectivity should be assessed by determining HBeAg and HBV DNA titres.**

Gold-standard' diagnostic test for hepatitis C

The diagnosis of hepatitis C is rarely made during the acute phase of the disease because the majority of people infected experience no symptoms during this period. The diagnosis of chronic phase hepatitis C is also challenging due to the absence or lack of specificity of symptoms until advanced liver disease develops. This may not occur for many years.

Chronic hepatitis C is usually suspected based on previous medical history and usually begins with serological testing (via an ELISA) to detect antibodies to hepatitis C (anti-HCV). These antibodies usually appear 3–5 months following acute infection in up to 80% of individuals. The pick-up rate approaches 100% at 6 months into the disease. Although anti-HCV antibodies have a strong positive predictive value for exposure to hepatitis C, they cannot determine the presence of ongoing infectivity and tests for these antibodies may fail to identify a significant number of individuals who have not yet undergone, or in the process of undergoing, seroconversion. In addition, the ELISA, although highly sensitive, is not terribly specific and yields many false-positive results. Moreover, the antibody that is detected by the ELISA is non-neutralizing and so does not signal immunity.

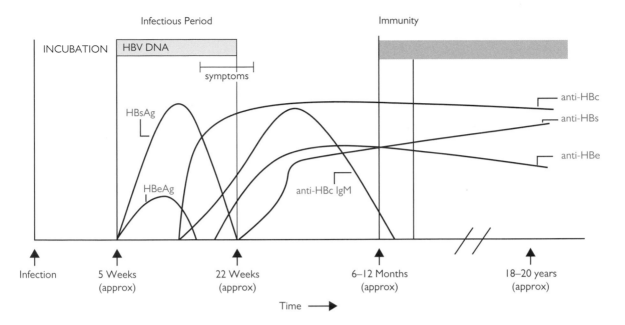

Infectious Period   Immunity

INCUBATION   HBV DNA

symptoms

HBsAg

HBeAg

anti-HBc IgM

anti-HBc
anti-HBs
anti-HBe

Infection   5 Weeks (approx)   22 Weeks (approx)   6–12 Months (approx)   18–20 years (approx)

Time →

HBsAg: hepatitis B surface antigen
HBeAg: hepatitis B e antigen
Anti-HBc IgM: IgM antibody to hepatitis B core antigen
Anti=HBs: antibody to hepatitis B surface antigen
Anti-HBe: antibody to hepatitis e antigen.

Figure 212.1 Hepatitis B antigens and serology in acute infection and recovery; Anti-HBc IgM, IgM antibody to hepatitis B core antigen; Anti-HBe: antibody to hepatitis e antigen; Anti-HBs, antibody to hepatitis B surface antigen; HBeAg, hepatitis B e antigen; HBsAg, hepatitis B surface antigen.

The diagnosis of hepatitis C should be confirmed in cases with positive serology by PCR testing for circulating viral RNA. In acute HCV infection, or in those patients who are profoundly immunosuppressed, anti-HCV antibodies may not be detected; if clinical suspicion remains high, then confirmation should be sought with HCV RNA testing.

Gold-standard' diagnostic test for hepatitis D

As HDV can only be present with the aid of HBV, initial testing in the workup of liver disease is not needed. Hepatitis D should be suspected in any individual who has had long-standing, stable hepatitis B but suddenly deteriorates. Antibodies to hepatitis D can be detected (via an ELISA) in serum or plasma samples; the presence of these antibodies correlates with ongoing viral replication. PCR can also be performed to detect the presence of viral RNA.

Gold-standard' diagnostic test for hepatitis E

There should be a high index of suspicion of hepatitis E for anyone who has travelled to an endemic area and presents with a hepatitis A-like illness that is HAV-IgM negative. Commercial ELISAs are also available in specialist centres for detecting antibodies against HEV.

Acceptable diagnostic alternatives to the gold-standard tests

As most assays for hepatitis A, B, and C are widely available throughout the UK, alternatives to the investigations already mentioned are rarely necessary.

Acceptable diagnostic alternatives to the gold-standard test for hepatitis B

The issue of pre-core mutant disease and HBeAg negativity in the presence of active disease has already been touched upon. In this situation, testing for HBV DNA serves as an alternative for signalling infectivity.

Histological analysis serves as a useful tool to guide treatment and assess the severity of liver damage; however, liver biopsy with staining for HBV is seldom needed to make a diagnosis.

Acceptable diagnostic alternatives to the gold-standard test for hepatitis C

Second-generation serological tests for HCV are more reliable than earlier tests. All individuals who are anti-HCV positive should be referred for specialist hepatology intervention, staging of disease, and suitability for genotype testing and treatment. Treatment must be guided by initial and subsequent estimation of circulating viral RNA levels, and by the specific genotype or subtype of virus causing the infection.

Other relevant investigations

All individuals who test positive for hepatitis B or hepatitis C should have a full assessment detailing travel history, sexual practices, IV drug use, social habits involving needles (e.g. body art, tattoos, piercings), previous transfusions, and any significant family history. Social circumstances should also be discussed (e.g. sharing of razors, cutlery, crockery, and toothbrushes). Once a diagnosis of hepatitis B is made, testing for hepatitis C co-infection is mandatory (and vice versa).

Table 212.2 Hepatitis B serology

	Acute infection	Chronic carrier	Recovered	Vaccination
Anti-HBc	+	+	+	−
HBsAg	+	+	−	−
Anti-HBs	−	−	+	+
HBeAg	+	+/−	−	−
Anti-HBe	+/−	+/−	+	−

Abbreviations: anti-HBc, antibody to the hepatitis B core antigen; anti-HBe, antibody to the hepatitis e antigen; anti-HBs, antibody to the hepatitis B surface antigen; HBeAg, hepatitis B e antigen; HBsAg, hepatitis B surface antigen.

Liver biopsy

Liver biopsy in hepatitis B

Although a liver biopsy is not needed to establish the diagnosis of hepatitis B, it is important for assessing the severity of inflammation, particularly as some treatment modalities can exacerbate hepatic inflammation.

Liver biopsy in hepatitis C

In hepatitis C, assessment of liver disease severity is recommended prior to starting therapy. Identifying patients with cirrhosis is of particular importance, as their likelihood of responding to therapy, and post-treatment prognosis, are altered. Significant fibrosis may be present in patients with repeatedly normal ALT; thus, evaluation of disease severity should be performed, regardless of liver biochemistry. Based on the available evidence, current guidelines advocate using alternative, non-invasive methods (such as transient elastography (Fibroscan®)) of assessing the severity of fibrosis in patients with chronic HCV infection, reserving liver biopsy for difficult or indeterminate cases.

Liver biopsy and cirrhosis

The presence of cirrhosis identifies the subgroup of patients with chronic viral hepatitis most likely to develop complications of chronic liver disease and HCC.

Additional investigations

Additional investigations worth noting once a diagnosis of hepatitis B or C are made include:

- HIV testing (document any reasons why this has not been done)
- sexual health screening, and screening for other sexually transmitted disease, where appropriate
  - investigations to exclude other etiologies of chronic liver disease; perform a liver ultrasound and appropriate follow-up, depending on the results

Prognosis and how to estimate it

Prognosis for hepatitis A

Hepatitis A usually has a self-limiting course with no long-lasting sequelae. As a result, most patients have an excellent prognosis with long-lasting immunity. Acute liver failure is rare, with cases confined to those having underlying chronic liver disease of another aetiology.

Prognosis for hepatitis B

Most adults with acute HBV infection have a self-limiting illness, developing full immunity. Chronicity is commoner in those who acquire infection as newborns (>90% chronicity) as a result of vertical transmission. These individuals do not tend to develop immunity.

Sixty per cent of chronic carriers may not have active inflammation with normal levels of transaminases. Markers of infectivity may be negative. In contrast, those with marked inflammation have a mortality approaching 50% in 5 years and may progress to cirrhosis. Furthermore, 20%–30% of inactive carriers may develop reactivation of HBV.

Morbidity and mortality in chronic HBV are linked to persistence of viral replication and evolution to cirrhosis. Cirrhosis is a cardinal factor leading to the development of HCC, which has an annual incidence of 2.5%–8.0%. Non-cirrhotic patients with chronic HBV infection may also be at risk (0.2% annual incidence of HCC), as HBV is able to integrate into the human genome and is believed to be pro-oncogenic. The incidence rises in the presence of coexisting HCV.

The 5-year cumulative incidence of developing cirrhosis ranges from 8% to 20%. The 5-year cumulative incidence of hepatic decompensation is approximately 20% for untreated patients with compensated cirrhosis. Untreated patients with decompensated cirrhosis have a poor prognosis, with a 14%–35% probability of survival at 5 years.

Prognosis for hepatitis C

Acute hepatitis C is usually an asymptomatic illness; however, progression to chronic infection is frequent. Cirrhosis occurs over 20 years in up to 20% of those with chronic infection; this figure is higher in those with coexisting liver disease of other etiologies (e.g. alcohol). Many factors will enhance this process:

- excessive alcohol
- coexisting fatty liver disease
- HIV co-infection
- hepatitis B co-infection
- coexisting liver disease of any aetiology

HCC develops in 2%–8% of those with cirrhosis each year after an average of 30 years. The worldwide incidence of HCC has increased, mostly due to persistent HBV and/ or HCV infections; presently, it constitutes the fifth-most-common cancer, representing around 5% of all cancers.

Prognosis for hepatitis E

Hepatitis E usually causes an acute, self-limiting illness which does not progress to chronic carrier status. There is, however, a high case fatality rate in pregnant women (mostly those in their second and third trimesters), with death usually resulting from fulminant hepatic failure resulting in encephalopathy and disseminated intravascular coagulation. The overall mortality rate is in the order of 1%–4%.

Treatment and its effectiveness

In discussing the various treatment options of viral hepatitis, one should differentiate between treatment of the acute infection, treatment of the chronic infection (if appropriate), and vaccination. All types of viral hepatitis in the acute setting are notifiable diseases.

Treatment of hepatitis A

Acute HAV infection

No specific treatment of acute HAV infection is necessary, as most individuals settle on their own. Hospital admission is rarely needed unless there are complications of significant hepatic failure (evidenced by encephalopathy, coagulopathy, etc.). Prevention against transmission of contacts is essential (good sanitation and cleanliness is key; avoid contact with bodily fluids). Contact tracing should include all household contacts, sexual partners, and those who share washroom facilities with the patient. Patients should be advised to abstain from alcohol (until liver function returns to a normal level) and other known hepatotoxic substances.

Vaccination for HAV

There are two forms of vaccination for HAV. The first is active immunization with live-attenuated and killed vaccines. This form is offered to those travelling to endemic areas, those in the military, childcare workers, and other high-risk individuals. The second form is passive immunization with human immunoglobulin. With this form, immunity lasts for 3–4 months. This form can be offered to those with acute hepatitis A and those travelling to endemic areas but who not able to complete the full immunization schedule for active vaccination.

Immunoglobulin therapy has not been shown to be of any additional benefit in changing the outcome in immunocompetent patients.

It is thought to be good practice that all individuals with retroviral disease and chronic liver disease should be screened and offered vaccination if they are non-immune, although the evidence and cost-effectiveness of this approach is a topic for academic debate.

Treatment of hepatitis B

Acute HBV infection

Most cases of acute HBV are self-limiting, and individuals should adopt the same measures as for acute HAV infection. Fewer than 1% of patients may develop a severe acute hepatitis (usually those with coexisting liver disease or immunosuppression). These individuals may require antiviral therapy to suppress active viral replication. Interferon (see 'To treat or not to treat') should be avoided in this situation, due to the risk of the patient developing fulminant liver failure.

Chronic HBV infection

Indications for treatment in chronic HBV infection depend on the serum HBV DNA titre, serum transaminase levels, fibrosis stage, presence of coexisting disease (e.g. HIV or HCV), and patient choice. The specific regimen is determined by evolving protocols developed in specialist hepatitis clinics.

To treat or not to treat?

Patients who are chronic carriers (HBeAg positive or not) bearing a high viral load (> 10^5 ml^{-1}) **and** evidence of hepatic damage (elevated transaminases for 6 months, or liver biopsy showing active inflammation) should be considered for therapy. All patients with evidence of chronic HBV infection and cirrhosis mandate treatment. All patients with co-infection (HCV/HIV) also require treatment. All those with HBV/HCV or HBV/HIV co-infection should be considered for anti-HBV treatment.

Carriers with normal liver biochemistry, negative HBeAg, positive anti-HBe, and non-detectable/low-level DNA titres need not receive antiviral therapy, as low levels of hepatitis B DNA are not associated with progressive liver disease. These patients should, however, be followed up in the long term with regular (3–4 monthly) assessment of liver biochemistry and HBV DNA levels.

Patients who are HBeAg negative and have evidence of active disease at lower HBV DNA levels may, under specialist supervision, require therapy if they have elevated liver enzymes or there is histological proof of active disease.

Regular-interval ultrasound screening, together with alpha-fetoprotein tests, is recommended for patients who are cirrhotic and at risk of HCC, although a false-positive raised alpha-fetoprotein level is not uncommon in cirrhotic patients. Regular surveillance for the development of HCC is also recommended for the following categories of non-cirrhotic individuals who have chronic hepatitis B:

- Asian male HBV carriers above the age of 40, and Asian female HBV carriers above the age of 50
- hepatitis B carriers with a family history of HCC
- African or North American blacks with chronic hepatitis B and who are above the age of 20

Effective antiviral therapy must ensure a degree of virological suppression, biochemical remission, histological improvement, and prevention of complications. Although HBsAg seroconversion is extremely rare (<15% of cases), long-lasting immunity and remission are likely if this end point is achieved. Additional target end points of therapy include:

- durable anti-HBe seroconversion in those who are HBeAg positive (serological remission)
- sustained biochemical remission (normal ALT levels)
- maintained virological response, as defined by HBV DNA <2000 IU/ml.

Durable HBV DNA suppression also increases the likelihood of HBe seroconversion in HBeAg-positive patients, and the possibility of HBsAg loss in HBeAg-positive and HBeAg-negative patients.

Drugs for treating chronic HBV infection

At present, there are three main drug classes for the treatment of chronic HBV infection: interferon (IFN), nucleoside analogue reverse transcriptase inhibitors (e.g. lamivudine, entecavir), and nucleotide analogue reverse transcriptase inhibitors (e.g. adefovir, tenofovir). Treatment practice varies and combination regimens of two agents may be given by some.

IFN IInterferon alfa is usually indicated in cases of HBeAg positivity with evidence of significant necroinflammatory activity. IFN enhances clearance of HBV while improving the immune response. Controlled studies of conventional IFN have shown that a 4–6-month course achieves HBeAg loss in 29%–32% of HBeAg-positive patients compared with 12% of controls. Seroconversion is sustained in 80% of cases. The standard IFN formulation used (IFN-α_{2b}) has largely been replaced by pegylated IFN-α_{2a} in routine practice. A recognized side effect of interferon is the emergence of flares of acute disease. This can be seen in 25%–40% of patients with IFN treatment and is due to the stimulatory effect of IFN, which is capable of increasing T-cell cytolytic activity and natural killer cell function. Predictors of flares during IFN treatment include preexisting cirrhosis and initial low levels of ALT.

Nucleoside/nucleotide analogues Lamivudine directly inhibits viral replication (via reverse transcriptase) without stimulating the immune response. Lamivudine significantly reduces viral DNA and normalizes liver function tests. It has few side effects and rarely leads to flares of hepatitis. For this reason, it is particularly useful for those with cirrhotic liver disease but for whom IFN is contraindicated. Lamivudine is effective for a combination virologic and biochemical response, and demonstrates histological improvement in both HBeAg-positive and HBeAg-negative patients. The incidence of lamivudine resistance, however, increases with a greater duration of time spent on therapy, and peaks at 80% after 5 years of treatment. Lamivudine is not recommended as a first-line therapy for this reason.

Adefovir inhibits both reverse transcriptase and DNA polymerase activity. Like lamivudine, adefovir has few side effects, but the resistance rates are relatively low (<2% per year). Adefovir also has the advantage of suppressing lamivudine-resistant disease. The major disadvantage is that the drug is nephrotoxic (this is a dose-dependent effect).

Entecavir is a potent selective inhibitor of HBV polymerase and has shown superiority to lamivudine in pivotal Phase III randomized controlled trials. Resistance rates in treatment-naive patients over 2 years are low. Entecavir is effective in lamivudine-refractory patients, but exhibits higher rates of resistance.

Tenofovir exerts strong and early suppression of infection of HBV with or without lamivudine-associated mutations. It is more potent than adefovir, without the associated renal toxicity: results from multicentre, randomized, adefovir-controlled trials in HBeAg-positive patients showed that tenofovir has better efficacy with respect to histological improvement, viral suppression, ALT normalization, and HBeAg seroconversion, and it achieved a virologic and histological response in a higher proportion of HBeAg-negative patients.

The efficacy of each of the drugs mentioned is variable (see Tables 212.3a–c), and it is not uncommon to use a combination of agents in order to achieve treatment end points. Treatment rationale is largely based the on the presence of HBeAg status, viral load, and the severity of liver injury (inflammatory activity and fibrosis). Predictors of anti-HBe seroconversion include:

- the pretreatment viral load (HBV DNA <2 ×10^8 IU/ml)
- a decrease of HBV DNA levels to <20 000 IU/ml at 12 weeks of treatment with pegylated IFN alpha (PEG-IFNα) regimens, or an undetectable viral load at 24 weeks of treatment with regimens based on nucleoside/nucleotide analogues
- high pretreatment ALT levels (2–5× the upper limit of normal) and/or high inflammatory activity on liver histology
- a decline of HBsAg levels below 1500 IU/ml at 12 weeks of treatment (in contrast, an HBsAg level >20 000 IU/ml or no decline of HBsAg levels at 12 weeks is associated with a very low probability of subsequent anti-HBe seroconversion)

Treatment duration with peg-interferon alfa is finite, usually for 48 weeks, and restricted to well-compensated, non-cirrhotic individuals. Notably, IFN therapy is contraindicated in pregnancy. By contrast, monotherapy with nucleoside/nucleotide analogues (usually entecavir or tenofovir) is often continued indefinitely, with the aim of suppressing viral replication to undetectable levels. Peg-interferon alfa is also the only medication of proven efficacy in treating HDV, although the optimal duration of treatment in this setting is unclear.

Transplantation is an option for HBV-induced cirrhosis and end-stage liver disease, but antiviral cover will be needed to prevent recurrence in the graft. The use of anti-HBV immunoglobulin during and after the transplant period dramatically reduces the recurrence rate of HBV infection.

Vaccination for HBV

Active immunization against HBV has been available since the 1980s and the vaccine has evolved to consist of modified surface antigen proteins. It is a three-course vaccine, given at 0, 1, and 6 months. The efficacy of the vaccine has been quoted to reach up to 90% following the full course. About one-fifth to one-third of those vaccinated will have a drop in antibody titre below critical protective levels within 5 years, necessitating booster therapy at 5–10 yearly intervals.

Active immunization is recommended for:

- contacts of those with acute hepatitis B
- patients undergoing dialysis

Table 212.3a Treatment efficacy in HBeAg-positive patients

	PEG-IFNα	Nucleoside analogues		Nucleotide analogues	
		Lamivudine	Entecavir	Adefovir	Tenofovir
Anti-HBe seroconversion (%)	29–32	16–18	21	12–18	21
HBsAg loss (%)	3–7	0–1	2	0	3
Biochemical remission (%)	32–41	41–72	68	48–54	68
HBV DNA <60–80 IU/ml (%)	7–14	36–44	67	13–21	76

Abbreviations: HBV, hepatitis B virus; PEG-IFNα, pegylated interferon alpha.
Note: Values provided are in per cent of patients.
Data from EASL practice guidelines (see 'Further reading').

Table 212.3b Treatment efficacy in HBeAg-negative patients

	PEG-IFNα	Nucleoside analogues		Nucleotide analogues	
		Lamivudine	Entecavir	Adefovir	Tenofovir
HBsAg loss (%)	4	0	0	0	0
Biochemical remission (%)	59	71–9	78	72–7	76
HBV DNA <60–80 IU/ml (%)	19	72–3	90	51–63	93

Abbreviations: HBV, hepatitis B virus; PEG-IFNα, pegylated interferon alpha.
Data from EASL practice guidelines (see 'Further reading').

Table 212.3c Pegylated interferon alpha versus nucleoside/nucleotide analogues: Advantages and disadvantages

	Pegylated interferon alpha	Nucleoside/nucleotide analogues
Advantages	Finite duration No resistance High rates of anti-HBe and anti-HBs seroconversion	Well tolerated Potent antiviral effect Oral administration route
Disadvantages	Subcutaneous injections Poorly tolerated Risk of adverse events	Usually indefinite duration of treatment Long-term safety issue and risk of resistance

Data from EASL practice guidelines (see 'Further Reading').

- haemophiliacs and those receiving regular blood products
- individuals in high-risk professions (healthcare personnel, those in endemic areas, prisoners and prison staff, and those who work in laboratories)
- sex workers and others at high risk of sexually transmitted diseases
- those with chronic liver disease

Acute HBV exposure in non-vaccinated individuals who are immunocompromised requires passive immunization with anti-HBV immunoglobulin. This may be administered with the first dose of vaccine (given at a separate site). Infants of hepatitis B mothers should receive the immunoglobulin and full active vaccine course, with the first dose given at birth.

Guidelines regarding healthcare professionals and hepatitis B

The goal of assessing a healthcare professional identified as being HBV positive is to determine infectivity and hence risk of transmission to co-workers and patients. Healthcare professionals identified as being HBsAg positive should have their HBeAg titres checked. Should they be positive for HBeAg, then restrictions upon practice will be imposed on them (especially against exposure-prone procedures).

If a healthcare professional is anti-HBe negative or has HBeAg negativity, the HBV DNA level should be checked. If viral DNA titres are >10^3 ml^{-1}, then restrictions should be imposed. Those whose viral DNA load does not exceed 10^3 ml^{-1} **and** who are HBeAg negative need not have restrictions imposed, **but** should have retesting performed every 12 months.

Healthcare workers with chronic HBV infection and who are responsible for undertaking exposure-prone procedures should be treated if they are HBeAg positive or if the HBV DNA load is >10^3 ml^{-1}. Healthcare workers should not perform exposure-prone procedures while on IFN or on antiviral therapy. Individuals having undergone any treatment with IFN or antivirals need to show that they have a viral DNA load not exceeding 10^3 ml^{-1} 1 year after stopping therapy before returning to unrestricted practice.

Treatment of hepatitis C

Acute HCV infection is difficult to detect; however, given the high rates of chronicity, individuals with HCV infection, when identified, should be considered for antiviral treatment. In contrast to the response during chronic infection, response rates during the acute phase can be as high as 90% when treatment is initiated within the first 2–4 months.

In chronic HCV infection, the primary goal of treatment is to eradicate HCV infection in order to prevent the complications of HCV-related chronic liver disease. Extra-hepatic manifestations such as mixed (type III) cryoglobulinemia may also respond to hepatitis C treatment. Specific end points include:

- achievement of a sustained virologic response (SVR), which is defined as viral levels persistently undetectable within 12 weeks (SVR12) or 24 weeks (SVR24) months after the end of therapy; achievement of SVR has shown to be a reliable indicator of viral clearance
- preventing decompensation to cirrhosis, end-stage liver disease, or HCC.

Treatment is indicated for all treatment-naive and treatment-experienced patients with compensated and decompensated liver disease. Priority for treatment is given to:

- patients with significant fibrosis or established cirrhosis, including decompensated disease
- patients with HIV co-infection
- patients with HBV co-infection
- patients with an indication for liver transplantation
- patients with recurrence of HCV infection after liver transplantation
- patients with clinically significant extra-hepatic manifestations
- patients with debilitating fatigue
- individuals at risk of transmitting HCV (active IV drug users; men who have sex with men with high-risk sexual practices; women who are of childbearing age and wish to get pregnant; haemodialysis patients; incarcerated individuals)

Table 212.4 Virological response classification in chronic hepatitis C infection while on treatment

Classification	Description
Rapid virological response	Undetectable HCV RNA at Week 4 of treatment, maintained until the end of therapy
Early virological response	HCV RNA detectable at Week 4 but undetectable at Week 12, maintained up to end of treatment
Delayed virological response	More than 2 $\log_{10}$ drop but detectable HCV RNA at Week 12; HCV RNA undetectable at Week 24, maintained up to end of treatment
Partial non-response	More than 2 $\log_{10}$ IU/ml decrease in HCV RNA level from baseline at 12 weeks of therapy, but detectable HCV RNA at Weeks 12 and 24
Non-response	Less than 2 $\log_{10}$ IU/ml decrease in HCV RNA level from baseline at 12 weeks of therapy
Virological breakthrough	Reappearance of HCV RNA at any time during treatment after virological response
End-of-treatment response	Undetectable HCV RNA at the end of treatment (24 weeks with G2/3 patients, and 48 weeks with G1 patients)
Relapse	Detectable HCV RNA within 6 months of stopping therapy after a previous EOTR
Sustained virological response	Undetectable HCV RNA level till 6 months after treatment course completed

Abbreviations: EOTR, end-of-treatment response; G1, genotype 1; G2, genotype 2; G3, genotype 3; HCV, hepatitis C virus.

Note: Applicable to pegylated-interferon and ribavirin regimens.

Additionally, moderate fibrosis is a justification for treatment, whereas treatment can be deferred in those with no or very mild disease on biopsy, or non-invasive fibrosis and an absence of extra-hepatic manifestations.

Historically, the drugs used to treat chronic HCV infection were restricted to PEG-IFNα and oral ribavirin. The major side effects with ribavirin are haemolysis, rapid development of anaemia, and thrombocytopenia. For anaemia, ribavirin dose reduction and/or the use of erythropoietin is the preferred management approach. Other side effects include rash, glossitis, and nausea. Side effects of IFN can be profound and, for unknown reasons, develop more commonly in patients with HCV than in those with HBV. Commonly recognized side effects include flu-like symptoms, lethargy, headaches (up to 55%), severely altered mood, and depression. In contrast to the case in patients with hepatitis B, cirrhotic liver disease is not a contraindication to IFN therapy in hepatitis C, provided there are no signs of decompensation.

Before initiating treatment, the genotype of the virus with which the patient is infected should be sequenced. This is essential when evaluating an individual's response to treatment, and in determining the duration of therapy. Although six HCV genotypes have been classified, only the first three will be discussed here:

- patients infected with genotype 2 or genotype 3 (commoner in the USA) have a higher chance of achieving SVR (65%–82%) than those infected with genotype 1, and treatment is usually administered for 24 weeks
- genotype 1 (the commonest strain in the UK) is harder to eradicate and generally requires a 48-week course of treatment; moreover, SVR rates were, up until recently, only 40%–46% with standard treatment; however, with the advent of newer agents and advanced translational research, success rates approaching those seen in patients infected with genotype 2 or 3 are now being seen

In addition to HCV genotype, other predictors of SVR, particularly for patients infected with genotype 1, include:

Favourable genetic polymorphisms near the gene IL28B: IL28B encodes for the protein interferon lambda-3 (IFN-λ3). Both IFN-λ and IFN-α activate the same intracellular pathway, which results in expression of many IFN-stimulated genes. Individuals who are infected with genotype 1, are of European ancestry, and carry the favourable CC alleles have been reported to achieve SVR rates as high as 69%, whereas those with CT alleles achieve an SVR rate of 33%, and those with TT alleles achieve a rate of 27%. The CC polymorphism also confers a higher rate of disease response and lower rates of disease relapse in individuals infected by genotypes 2 or 3.

Baseline HCV RNA levels: Lower baseline HCV RNA levels (<400 000–800 000 IU/ml) are associated with higher rates of SVR.

On-treatment virological response: While the patient is on treatment, HCV RNA should be assessed at baseline, Week 4, Week 12, Week 24, and, if continued, Week 48. HCV RNA should also be assessed during the 6 months after the treatment course has been completed, in order to assess SVR. The likelihood of achieving SVR is directly correlated to the time taken to achieve viral negativity

(<50 IU/ml; see Table 212.4), being greatest in those patients who achieve a rapid virological response (i.e. viral negativity at 4 weeks of treatment). Treatment durations may be modified based on the virological response; however, a detailed discussion of this area is beyond the scope of this book.

Body mass index: Body weight reduction prior to therapy is recommended and has been associated with better SVR rates.

Insulin resistance: Insulin resistance is associated with fibrosis progression, and an increased HOMA-IR index is an independent predictor of treatment failure.

Race: Black patients are less likely to respond to therapy; this is explained in part by a lower frequency of the favourable IL28B polymorphism in this population.

Until 2011, the combination of PEG-IFNα and ribavirin for 24 or 48 weeks was the approved treatment for chronic hepatitis C. With this regimen, patients infected with HCV genotype 1 had SVR rates of approximately 40%–50%; higher SVR rates were achieved in patients infected with HCV genotypes 2, 3, 5, or 6 (60%–80%), and intermediate SVR rates were achieved in those with HCV genotype 4. However, treatment algorithms are rapidly evolving and heavily influenced by ongoing clinical trials. To this effect, newer generation protease inhibitors, polymerase inhibitors, and inhibitors of HCV RNA replication (e.g. NS5A inhibitors) have entered clinical practice, and enable SVR rates of 80%–95% as part of durable, IFN-free regimens (see Tables 212.5, 212.6, and 212.7) with a limited side-effect profile.

Orthoptic liver transplantation is the treatment of choice in anyone who has end-stage liver disease and, in fact, is the leading cause for transplantation in the US. Recurrence of hepatitis C is almost universal, with progression to fibrosis or cirrhosis occurring in 10%–30% within 5 years of transplantation. Once cirrhosis develops post transplant, complications tend to occur more rapidly than in the native liver. Viral re-entry inhibitors are currently being evaluated in early phase clinical trials, and it is hoped that they will be of benefit in treating HCV infection of the donor liver.

Vaccination for HCV

There is no effective hepatitis C vaccine at present. IV drug users should be advised to use clean needles if they refuse to abstain from

Table 212.5 Emerging antiviral therapies for chronic hepatitis C virus infection

Drugs	Mechanism of action
Simeprevir Paritaprevir	Inhibits the protease NS3/4A
Daclatasvir Ledipasvir Ombitasvir	Inhibits the non-structural protein NS5A responsible for viral replication
Sofosbuvir Dasabuvir	A pro-drug, the metabolite of which serves as a defective substrate for NS5B; a protein involved in viral replication
Ritonavir	Booster of other proteases (CYP3A4 inhibitor)

Table 212.6 Approved recommendations for chronic hepatitis C virus infection (for treatment-naive patients and those with prior treatment failure with pegylated interferon alfa and ribavirin) **without cirrhosis**

Genotype	PEG-IFNα, RBV, and sofosbuvir	PEG-IFNα, RBV, and simeprevir	Sofosbuvir and RBV	Sofosbuvir and ledipasvir	Ritonavir-boosted paritaprevir, ombitasvir, and dasabuvir	Sofosbuvir and simeprevir	Sofosbuvir and daclatasvir
1a	12 weeks	12 weeks, then PEG-IFNα and RBV only for 12 weeks (for treatment-naive patients or patients with prior relapse); or 36 weeks (for partial or null responders)	No	8–12 weeks	12 weeks with RBV	12 weeks	12 weeks
1b	12 weeks	12 weeks, then PEG-IFNα and RBV only for 12 weeks (for treatment-naive patients or patients with prior relapse); or 36 weeks (for partial or null responders)	No	8–12 weeks	12 weeks without RBV	12 weeks	12 weeks
2	12 weeks	No	12 weeks	No	No	No	12 weeks
3	12 weeks	No	24 weeks	No	No	No	12 weeks

Abbreviations: PEG-IFNα, pegylated interferon alfa; RBV, ribavirin.
Data from EASL Guidelines for Management of Chronic HCV Infection 2015.

Table 212.7 Approved recommendations for chronic hepatitis C virus infection (for treatment-naive patients and those with prior treatment failure with pegylated interferon alfa and ribavirin) **with compensated cirrhosis**

Genotype	PEG-IFNα, RBV, and sofosbuvir	PEG-IFNα, RBV, and simeprevir	Sofosbuvir and RBV	Sofosbuvir and ledipasvir	Ritonavir-boosted paritaprevir, ombitasvir, dasabuvir, and ribavirin	Sofosbuvir and simeprevir	Sofosbuvir and daclatasvir
1a	12 weeks	12 weeks (for treatment-naive patients or patients with prior relapse); or 24 weeks (for partial or null responders)	No	12 weeks with RBV; or 24 weeks without RBV; or 24 weeks with RBV if negative predictors of response	24 weeks	12 weeks with RBV; or 24 weeks without RBV	12 weeks with RBV; or 24 weeks without RBV
1b	12 weeks	12 weeks (for treatment-naive patients or patients with prior relapse); or 24 weeks (for partial or null responders)	No	12 weeks with RBV; or 24 weeks without RBV; or 24 weeks with RBV if negative predictors of response	12 weeks	12 weeks with RBV; or 24 weeks without RBV	12 weeks with RBV; or 24 weeks without RBV
2	12 weeks	No	16–20 weeks	No	No	No	12 weeks
3	12 weeks	No	No	No	No	No	24 weeks with RBV

Abbreviations: PEG-IFNα, pegylated interferon alfa; RBV, ribavirin.
Data from EASL Guidelines for Management of Chronic HCV Infection 2015.

their habit. Vaccination against HAV and HBV is recommended to all those at high risk, to prevent co-transmission.

Treatment of hepatitis B and C co-infection

Most patients in this category have quiescent hepatitis B, and antiviral therapy needs to be directed toward hepatitis C only. If both are active, then the individual should be on the recommended treatment regimens for HBV and HCV, bearing in mind the potential for drug–drug interactions. A flare of clinical hepatitis is not unusual when treating patients with hepatitis B.

Further Reading

European Association for the Study of the Liver. EASL clinical practice guidelines: Management of chronic hepatitis B virus infection. *J Hepatol* 2012; 57: 167–85.
European Association for the Study of the Liver. EASL clinical practice guidelines: Management of hepatitis C virus infection. *J Hepatol* 2011; 55: 245–64.

213 Autoimmune hepatitis

Satish Keshav and Alexandra Kent

Definition of autoimmune hepatitis

Autoimmune hepatitis (AIH) is a condition characterized by hepatic inflammation associated with elevated levels of circulating immunoglobulin and autoantibodies to hepatic antigens.

Aetiology of AIH

In AIH, human leukocyte antigen (HLA) Class II displayed on the surface of hepatocytes facilitates the presentation of normal liver cell membrane constituents to cytotoxic T-lymphocytes, which, in turn, infiltrate liver tissue, release cytokines, and destroy hepatocytes. Subsequently, AIH is characterized by raised transaminases, the presence of autoantibodies, raised IgG and, histologically, interface hepatitis. There are two types of AIH according to serology: Type 1 is characterized by the presence of antinuclear antibodies (ANAs) and/or anti-smooth muscle antibodies (anti-SMAs), whereas type 2 has the anti-liver–kidney microsomal type 1 antibody (anti-LKM). The immunological basis of AIH is further confirmed by its association with other autoimmune diseases (see Box 213.1) and response to steroids and immunosuppressive therapy.

The exact aetiology leading to the immunological response is unknown, although genetic and environmental factors are known to be involved.

Genetic factors in AIH

In Europe and the USA, susceptibility to AIH type 1 is conferred by the presence of HLA-DR3 and HLA-DR4, and AIH type 2 by HLA-DR7 and HLA-DR3. HLA-DR7 confers a more aggressive disease.

Environmental factors in AIH

Studies have suggested the immune response is triggered by viral infections (e.g. EBV, hepatitis A or B) or drug reactions (e.g. nitrofurantoin, interferon).

Typical symptoms of AIH, and less common symptoms

Patients can present with an acute hepatitis, chronic hepatitis, or established cirrhosis. Approximately one-third present with an acute hepatitis, with typical symptoms of jaundice, fever, and right upper quadrant tenderness. Rarely, AIH presents as acute fulminant hepatic

failure. Many patients have cirrhosis at presentation, with up to 20% of patients showing signs of decompensated liver disease. Many patients will present with a chronic hepatitis and be diagnosed following investigations into asymptomatic raised transaminases. Other symptoms associated with chronic hepatitis include fatigue, mild pruritus, anorexia, abdominal discomfort, myalgia, arthralgia, and amenorrhoea.

Demographics of AIH

The incidence of type 1 AIH is between 0.1 and 1.9 per 100 000 population per year, with a higher incidence in Northern Europeans. Type 2 AIH is more common in Southern Europe, the USA, or Japan; 70%–80% of patients are female, with the disease predominantly affecting children and young people. However, AIH can affect all ages and both genders, and therefore should be considered as a differential diagnosis in all patients presenting with deranged transaminases.

Natural history of AIH, and complications of the disease

AIH is a progressive disease and, without treatment, most patients will die within 10 years; 20%–40% of patients will progress to cirrhosis despite treatment with immunosuppression. However, patients who achieve clinical remission have the same life expectancy as that of the general population. Complications of AIH are mainly related to progressive disease and cirrhosis. However, AIH is associated with various other autoimmune conditions, and therefore patients may suffer with complications associated with these conditions (see Box 213.1). Hepatocellular carcinoma is less common in AIH cirrhosis than in other causes of cirrhosis, but is still recognized.

Approach to diagnosing AIH

The symptoms and signs of liver disease can be non-specific. The typical indicator of autoimmune liver disease is the presence of liver dysfunction and, therefore, all patients presenting with liver dysfunction should be tested for the following serological markers of autoimmune disease: ANA, anti-SMA, anti-mitochondrial antibody (AMA), anti-LKM, and perinuclear antineutrophil cytoplasmic antibody (pANCA). A combination of elevated IgG, liver damage, and hepatic autoantibodies (e.g. anti-SMA) is highly indicative of AIH. It is critically important to make the diagnosis of AIH, as early treatment can be life-saving.

Other diagnoses that should be considered aside from AIH

As AIH can be associated with acute or chronic hepatitis, many other causes of liver disease should be considered, as dealt with in Chapters 209 and 210. Histological features are those of acute or chronic hepatitis, with no features specific to the disease.

'Gold-standard' diagnostic test for AIH

The diagnosis of all autoimmune liver diseases is based on characteristic histological, serological, biochemical, and clinical findings. However, generally the gold standard required to diagnose AIH is considered to be a liver biopsy. Although a liver biopsy may not provide direct evidence of AIH, it helps exclude other diagnoses (e.g. viral or drug-induced hepatitis).

Box 213.1 Autoimmune diseases associated with autoimmune liver disease

- haemolytic anaemia
- pernicious anaemia
- Graves' disease
- autoimmune thyroiditis
- inflammatory bowel disease
- coeliac disease
- fibrosing alveolitis
- rheumatoid arthritis
- Sjögren's syndrome
- systemic sclerosis
- proliferative glomerulonephritis
- pericarditis
- myocarditis

Prognosis for AIH, and how to estimate it

Thirteen to twenty per cent of patients will have spontaneous resolution of disease, and it is impossible to predict these patients. However, without treatment most patients will die within 10 years; 20%–40% of patients will progress to cirrhosis despite treatment with immunosuppression. HLA-DR3-positive patients are more likely to have active disease, respond less to therapy, and are more likely to require liver transplantation at some point than patients with other HLA types.

Treatment of AIH, and its effectiveness

Indications for treatment of AIH are listed in Table 213.1. The standard treatment is high-dose prednisolone (60 mg per day), reduced slowly over the course of 6–8 weeks (usually by 5–10 mg per week), while monitoring liver function tests. It should be maintained at the lowest dose possible to reduce side effects. Patients requiring long-term steroid therapy should be commenced on azathioprine as a steroid-sparing agent. Immunosuppression has been shown to improve survival, achieving remission in 65% of patients within 18 months, and 80% of patients by 3 years. It is unknown how long treatment should be continued for before being withdrawn, and most centres would advocate a minimum of 2 years to allow for histological improvement, which lags behind clinical and biochemical improvement by 3–6 months. However, 80% of these patients relapse following drug withdrawal. Drug reinstitution is usually successful. There is limited evidence to support the use of alternative immunosuppressants including ciclosporin, tacrolimus, mycophenolate mofetil, cyclophosphamide, and methotrexate. Patients with decompensated cirrhosis should be referred for consideration of liver transplantation.

Primary biliary cholangitis

Definition of primary biliary cholangitis

Primary biliary cholangitis (PBC) is an autoimmune disease, characterized by destruction of the bile ducts, leading to cholestasis and progressive liver disease.

Aetiology of PBC

CD4 and CD8 lymphocytes mediate progressive destruction of small and medium bile ducts. The disease is autoimmune in nature, as evidenced by circulating autoantibodies (AMA), raised IgM, granulomas found in the liver and regional lymph nodes, and the association with other autoimmune diseases. It has been associated with haplotype HLA-DR8 and, for some populations, HLA-DPB1. There is a significantly increased risk in first-degree relatives (500–1000 fold), suggesting genetic factors play an etiological role, although no specific gene has been identified as yet. Increased expression of HLA Class II antigens makes hepatocytes more vulnerable to T-cell-mediated attack. The bile contains toxic substances (e.g. bile acids and copper), and this means that cholestasis results in further destruction of bile ducts and hepatocytes.

Typical symptoms of PBC, and less common symptoms

Twenty-five to fifty per cent of patients are asymptomatic and will be diagnosed after investigations into abnormal liver function tests. Presenting symptoms and signs include fatigue (30%–65%), pruritus

(20%–55%), hyperpigmentation (40%), right upper quadrant discomfort (10%–15%), hepatomegaly (25%), splenomegaly (15%), jaundice (10%), and sicca syndrome (50%). As the disease progresses, patients may present with signs and symptoms of chronic liver disease. Furthermore, they may have symptoms from associated autoimmune diseases.

Demographics of PBC

Ninety per cent of PBC sufferers are women, and they are commonly affected between the ages of 30 and 60. Epidemiological studies show 1 in 4000 people are affected, with 1 in 1000 women over the age of 40 years affected. The disease is more common in the UK and Scandinavia.

Natural history of PBC, and complications of the disease

PBC patients tend to be diagnosed at an earlier stage than in the past, and this means treatment is instituted earlier, with a resultant improvement in prognosis. However, PBC is a progressive disease, and the extent to which medication can slow progression varies between studies. Complications include osteoporosis, deficiency of fat-soluble vitamins, hypercholesterolaemia, steatorrhoea (related to reduced bile-salt excretion), and asymptomatic bacteriuria (35%). Symptoms from associated autoimmune conditions may occur, including hypothyroidism in 20% and autoimmune thrombocytopenia. Finally, symptoms and signs of chronic liver disease, and the associated complications occur, including hepatocellular carcinoma, which occurs in ~6% of PBC patients.

Approach to diagnosing PBC

Patients with PBC usually present with abnormal liver chemistry, in particular, with an elevated bilirubin. AMA is highly sensitive and specific for PBC. Early diagnosis of PBC allows appropriate monitoring, and prevention of complications of cirrhosis.

Other diagnoses that should be considered aside from PBC

The differential diagnosis of PBC includes causes of cholestasis, for example biliary obstruction (gallstones, pancreatic tumour, cholangiocarcinoma), primary sclerosing cholangitis, or sarcoidosis.

'Gold-standard' diagnostic test for PBC

The gold-standard diagnostic test for PBC is a liver biopsy, and would be advocated prior to commencing therapy. The majority of patients undergo percutaneous liver biopsies, but a transjugular approach can be used in high-risk situations (e.g. coagulopathy). Imaging does not provide diagnostic features of autoimmune liver disease, but is important in the setting of cholestatic liver tests in order to exclude biliary obstruction.

Prognosis of PBC, and how to estimate it

PBC is a progressive disease, and studies have shown the median time from diagnosis to death or liver transplantation is only 9.3 years. Factors associated with decreased survival include raised bilirubin, presence of cirrhosis, presence of associated autoimmune diseases, and loss of bile ducts. Bilirubin level is the most reliable determinant of prognosis:

- serum bilirubin >2 mg/dl (34.2 µmol/l): mean survival rate = 4.1 years
- serum bilirubin >6 mg/dl (102.6 µmol/l): mean survival rate = 2.1 years
- serum bilirubin levels >10 mg/dl (171 µmol/l): mean survival rate = 1.4 years

Treatment of PBC, and its effectiveness

Unfortunately, the treatment options for PBC are still limited. Ursodeoxycholic acid (UDCA) is the major treatment option for patients with PBC, being effective in up to 30% of patients. It has been shown to normalize liver function tests and slow disease progression in trials, reducing the need for liver transplantation or death.

Table 213.1 Indications for treatment in autoimmune hepatitis

Absolute	Relative
AST 10× upper limit of normal	AST or IgG less than absolute criteria
AST 5× upper limit of normal **and** IgG ≥2× upper limit of normal	Symptoms: fatigue, arthralgia, jaundice
Bridging or acinar necrosis on liver biopsy	Interface hepatitis

Abbreviations: AST, aspartate aminotransferase.

There have been many studies investigating the efficacy of immuno-suppressants in PBC (ciclosporin, azathioprine, prednisolone, penicillamine, budesonide, chlorambucil) but, as yet, there is no evidence to support their use in patient care. In patients unresponsive to UDCA, methotrexate or colchicine is occasionally used, as studies have shown that these agents can provide an improvement in liver parameters. However, there is no evidence on survival benefit, and efficacy has not been duplicated in further trials.

Primary sclerosing cholangitis

Definition of sclerosing cholangitis

Primary sclerosing cholangitis (PSC) is a chronic cholestatic liver disease with obliterative inflammatory fibrosis of the bile ducts.

Aetiology of PSC

The exact aetiology of PSC is unknown, although bacteria, toxins, viral infections, and immunologic and genetic factors have all been proposed. Immune-mediated destruction of the hepatobiliary tract is the most likely cause, possibly secondary to transient bacterial infection. Supporting evidence for an immunological cause include an increased number of T-cells in the portal tracts, with a concurrent decrease in the total number of circulating T-cells, although the ratio of CD4 lymphocytes to CD8 lymphocytes in the circulation is increased. Furthermore, there is an increase in IgG and IgM, in 48% and 80% of patients, respectively, and 60%–82% of patients are positive for pANCA. There is a close association between PSC and inflammatory bowel disease (IBD), more specifically ulcerative colitis (UC). Only 3%–4% of patients with ulcerative colitis have PSC, but 75% of patients with PSC have UC. Studies have suggested a genetic component, with increased incidence in first-degree relatives, and it has been associated with HLA-B8 and HLA-DR3.

Typical symptoms of PSC, and less common symptoms

The presentation of PSC is variable, ranging from being asymptomatic, to presenting with non-specific symptoms of lethargy, fatigue, pruritus, abdominal pain, nausea, or fevers, to presenting with cholestasis and associated cholangitis. Many patients are diagnosed following investigations into abnormal liver function tests or hepatomegaly, which is found in ~50% at presentation.

Demographics of PSC

PSC is a rare condition, with an incidence of <1 per 100 000, and is more common in Northern Europe, with a mean age of 40 years and a male predominance (70%).

Natural history of PSC, and complications of the disease

PSC is a progressive disease which will eventually develop into cirrhosis. Many patients will suffer with one or more complications. Many have recurrent episodes of cholestasis and cholangitis related to biliary strictures, which may require endoscopic therapy. Cholangiocarcinoma develops in 10%–15% and there is no infallible method for cancer screening, with limited evidence for the use of the tumour marker CA 19-9, which can also rise during episodes of cholestasis. Furthermore, malignant strictures are often indistinguishable from PSC benign strictures. The risk of colorectal cancer in patients with concurrent UC and PSC is significantly higher, and patients should be entered into a colon surveillance programme (usually annual). Although liver transplantation can give tremendous relief of symptoms, PSC will recur in 10%–20% of patients.

Approach to diagnosing PSC

The diagnosis of PSC is usually made by imaging and predominantly occurs in the context of IBD.

Other diagnoses that should be considered aside from PSC

PSC should be differentiated from any cause of hepatitis or cholestasis.

'Gold-standard' diagnostic test for PSC

Endoscopic retrograde cholangiopancreatography used to be the most effective method for diagnosing PSC, but has now been superseded by MRI of the biliary tree, as this procedure has a much better safety profile. Classically, multiple strictures will be seen, separated by

Table 213.2 Investigations for autoimmune liver disease

	AIH	Primary biliary cholangitis	Primary sclerosing cholangitis
Transaminases	↑↑↑ (200–300 U/l)	Normal/↑	Normal/↑
Alkaline phosphatase	Normal	↑↑	↑↑↑
Bilirubin	Normal	Normal/↑↑	Normal/↑
Immunoglobulins	Raised IgG	Raised IgM	Raised IgG (48%) and IgM (80%)
Autoantibodies	Type 1: ANA, anti-SMA, anti-actin antibody, anti-SLA, anti-LPA, pANCA, AMA Type 2: anti-LKM, anti-liver cytosol-1	AMA (90%–95%) ANA (20%)	pANCA Anti-biliary epithelial cells (60%) AMA, ANA, anti-SMA
Histology	Mononuclear cell infiltrate, piecemeal necrosis, and bridging necrosis Majority will have some evidence of fibrosis Acute-onset AIH has more interface, lobular hepatitis, and necrosis, but less fibrosis and cirrhosis Steatosis is not common	Early damage of the bile duct basement membrane Reactive hyperplasia of the epithelial lining Lymphocytic and plasma cell infiltration, with eosinophilic condensation in the portal tracts Epithelioid aggregates or granulomas may be found Fibrosis and cirrhosis eventually develop	Periductal fibrosis with inflammation, bile duct proliferation, and ductopenia Periductal concentration of mononuclear cells and ductular proliferation Can resemble AIH
Other abnormal blood parameters's	Normochromic anaemia Mild leucopenia Eosinophilia Thrombocytopenia Raised ESR	Raised lipids and cholesterol Raised ESR	
Radiology	No specific diagnostic features	No specific diagnostic features	

Abbreviations: AIH, autoimmune hepatitis; AMA, anti-mitochondrial antibody; ANA, antinuclear antibody; anti-LKM, anti-liver–kidney microsomal type 1 antibody; anti-LPA, anti-liver–pancreas antigen antibody; anti-SLA, anti-soluble liver antigen antibody; anti-SMA, smooth muscle antibody; ESR, erythrocyte sedimentation rate; pANCA, perinuclear antineutrophil cytoplasmic antibody.

dilated segments, giving the biliary tree a beaded appearance. PSC is less well diagnosed on a liver biopsy, with findings often non-specific and non-diagnostic. However, it is useful to exclude other causes of cholestasis and for staging of the disease.

Prognosis of PSC, and how to estimate it

PSC is an insidiously progressive disease, with a median survival of 9–11 years from diagnosis, although in symptomatic patients this may be further reduced.

Treatment of PSC, and its effectiveness

Multiple treatments have been used in trials for the treatment of PSC, but with little success. The only medication currently used is UDCA, which can improve biochemical abnormalities, although the evidence for decreasing overall disease progression or improving survival is limited. More recently, evidence suggests that UDCA reduces the incidence of colorectal cancer, supporting its continuing use. Biliary strictures can be treated endoscopically with balloon dilatation or stent insertion, and associated cholangitis should be treated with antibiotics promptly. Patients often need nutritional and fat-soluble vitamin supplements. Patients should be observed closely for complications of chronic liver disease, and

referred early to tertiary centres for consideration of orthotopic liver transplant, which has been performed successfully in PSC patients.

Other relevant investigations for autoimmune liver disease

See Table 213.2 for a summary of investigations in autoimmune liver disease. As these diseases progress, investigations may reflect progressive liver disease with a reduction in synthetic function (low albumin, prolonged prothrombin time), excretory function (raised bilirubin), or portal hypertension (thrombocytopenia). In such situations, patients should also be screened for complications of chronic liver disease with upper gastrointestinal endoscopy for varices, and alpha-fetoprotein for hepatocellular carcinoma.

Further Reading

Lata J. Diagnosis and treatment of autoimmune hepatitis. *J Dig Dis* 2012; 30: 212–5.
Ponsioen CY. Recent insights in primary sclerosing cholangitis. *J Dig Dis* 2012; 13: 337–41.

Genetic liver disease

Satish Keshav and Palak Trivedi

Introduction

This chapter will discuss three of the major inherited forms of liver disease (all autosomal recessive):

- hereditary haemochromatosis
- Wilson's disease
- alpha-1-antitrypsin deficiency

Hereditary haemochromatosis

Definition of hereditary haemochromatosis

Hereditary haemochromatosis is characterized by excessive absorption of dietary iron, with a pathological increase in total body iron that accumulates in tissues and organs, disrupting their function. The liver, adrenal glands, heart, pituitary, and pancreas are most affected. The disease is usually caused by mutations in the HFE gene, although similar conditions are now recognized, being caused by other genes that regulate iron absorption and distribution. Normal total body iron is approximately 4 g, with 3.5 g in circulating red blood cells, and the rest in the bone marrow, the reticuloendothelial system, including the liver, and other tissues such as muscle and nerves (Figure 214.1). Secondary haemochromatosis may occur, for instance with iron overload as a consequence of multiple transfusions. Excessive deposition of iron in the liver may also occur in liver disease due to alcohol excess and other etiologies; however, levels rarely exceed those found in hereditary haemochromatosis. Circulating ferritin levels generally reflect body iron stores, and a ferritin level consistently and repeatedly greater than 1000 ¼g/l is almost pathognomonic of hereditary haemochromatosis and is rarely observed in any other condition.

Aetiology of hereditary haemochromatosis

Hereditary haemochromatosis is the commonest genetic disorder in the Caucasian population within the UK and the USA. The main gene responsible for the disorder is HFE, on Chromosome 6, which encodes an MHC Class-I related protein responsible for regulating iron absorption. The commonest mutations of the HFE gene in hereditary haemochromatosis are:

- C282Y: cysteine to tyrosine mutation at position 282; this mutation is present in almost 90% of patients with hereditary haemochromatosis

- H63D: histidine to aspartate mutation at position 63
- S65C: serine to cysteine mutation at position 65

The latter two mutations have less of a clinical effect than the first one but can present with first in a compound heterozygote. Genetic mutations in other iron transport proteins such as haemojuvelin and ferroportin may also lead to hepatic iron overload.

Typical symptoms of hereditary haemochromatosis, and less common symptoms

The manifestations of hereditary haemochromatosis are those of chronic iron overload but signs/symptoms may be difficult to differentiate from those for other diagnoses of specific organ systems; symptoms include:

- non-specific fatigue and malaise
- slate-grey pigmentation, or bronzing of the skin
- hepatomegaly
- liver cirrhosis with an increased risk of hepatocellular carcinoma (HCC)
- insulin resistance and type 2 diabetes due to pancreatic iron deposition (suspect in any individual who has diabetes and abnormal liver biochemistry, although non-alcoholic fatty liver disease is more commonly responsible for abnormal liver enzymes in this setting)
- erectile dysfunction, hypogonadism, and testicular atrophy, due to iron deposition in the pituitary gland
- cardiomyopathy, dysrhythmias, and cardiac failure
- arthritis and arthralgia, due to chondrocalcinosis, **not** iron deposition; usually present in the first and second metacarpophalangeal and proximal interphalangeal joints
- adrenal insufficiency due to deposition in the adrenal glands (occasional finding)

Given the increase in iron stores, affected individuals are prone to infections from siderophoric organisms such as *Yersinia enterocolitica* and *Listeria monocytogenes*, as well as salmonella and klebsiella pneumonia. In addition, hereditary haemochromatosis may be asymptomatic, in which case it can be diagnosed either from abnormal iron studies or from family screening. The clinical symptoms tend to manifest later in women than men (given the indirect venesecting effects of menstruation in the former). The age of presentation is between 40 and 50 years but may be much later. Physical findings may not manifest in early disease, and diagnosis may only be suspected on family history and results of investigations.

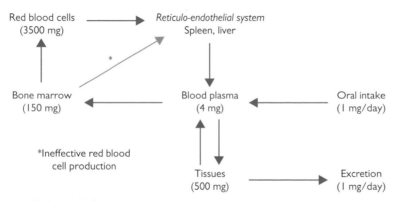

Figure 214.1 Iron distribution in the human body.

Demographics of hereditary haemochromatosis

The reported frequency of homozygosity of the C282Y mutation is 0.4%, although a frequency of up to 1% may be observed in Northern European populations. Due to the variable penetrance of this mutation, not all individuals have features of iron overload.

Penetrance is higher in men than women. Elevated liver enzymes are found in approximately 30% of males homozygous for C282Y; liver fibrosis in 18%; and cirrhosis in 6%. In contrast, 5% of females homozygous for C282Y may have liver fibrosis, and only 2% have cirrhosis. Anywhere between 10% and 33% of C282Y homozygotes eventually develop morbidity associated with hereditary haemochromatosis.

Natural history of hereditary haemochromatosis, and complications of the disease

Survival is normal if diagnosis has been made prior to the onset of irreversible liver damage. However, those who have established cirrhosis are at risk of developing HCC in up to 45% of cases. This is discussed in more detail in Chapter 218.

Approach to diagnosing hereditary haemochromatosis

Suspect hereditary haemochromatosis in any first-degree relative of a known case, or in any individual with abnormal liver function tests (LFTs) and diabetes. Iron studies should be part of the workup of any chronic liver disease screen; the most widely used biochemical surrogate for iron overload is serum ferritin.

Serum ferritin is usually >400 ng/ml in patients with clinical disease. The ferritin may be very high, over 1000 ng/ml, and this makes a presumptive diagnosis of hereditary haemochromatosis in the appropriate clinical setting. Ferritin is an acute phase protein, and values may be elevated in inflammatory states (e.g. Still's disease), sepsis, alcoholic excess, and acute hepatitis unrelated to hereditary haemochromatosis. Values greater than 1000 ng/ml, however, are unusual outside hereditary haemochromatosis.

In hereditary haemochromatosis, serum iron is high, the total iron binding capacity is low, and the transferrin saturation is >45%. However, serum iron concentration and transferrin saturation do not quantitatively reflect body iron stores and should therefore not be used as surrogate markers of tissue iron overload.

Other diagnoses that should be considered aside from hereditary haemochromatosis

Chronic viral hepatitis, certain porphyrias, non-alcoholic fatty liver disease, and excess alcohol intake can be associated with abnormal iron studies and may even have excess iron deposition in the liver. Iron deposition, however, is rarely in the quantities seen in hereditary haemochromatosis.

Non-alcoholic fatty disease is an important differential in an individual with deranged LFTs and diabetes mellitus. Another differential, African iron overload (Bantu haemosiderosis), was initially thought to be caused by excessive amounts of iron being ingested through the consumption of alcoholic beverages brewed in ungalvanized iron drums. However, there may also be a genetic element (not HFE) linked to the iron protein ferroportin.

Transfusion haemosiderosis is the accumulation of iron, mainly in the liver, in patients who receive frequent blood transfusions (e.g. thalassaemia). Another differential is myelodysplastic syndrome, which results in the disordered production of red blood cells. This leads to increased iron recycling from the bone marrow and accumulation in the liver.

'Gold-standard' diagnostic test for hereditary haemochromatosis

Should iron studies be abnormal, genetic studies looking for HFE mutations are the next step. If homozygosity for the C282Y is detected, or an individual is a compound heterozygote (C282Y/H63D) with normal liver chemistry **and** below 40 years, then no further tests are necessary.

Those older than 40 years or with abnormal liver chemistry **and** ferritin >1000 ng/ml should proceed to liver biopsy for determining the extent of fibrosis/cirrhosis. Although the latter holds little prognostic value, it is important to ascertain as advanced histological liver disease warrants surveillance for oesophageal varices and HCC.

Liver biopsy with Perl's stain is diagnostic.

Other relevant investigations for hereditary haemochromatosis

CT scanning can detect excessive iron in massively 'iron-loaded' patients. Other investigations are specific to other organ involvement (e.g. echocardiography or cardiac MRI for myocardial involvement).

Prognosis for hereditary haemochromatosis, and how to estimate it

Most patients feel better after venesection, with marked improvement of constitutional symptoms. Survival can be normal if the diagnosis is made before irreversible liver damage has occurred. Liver enzymes improve typically on depletion of hepatic iron stores. Hepatomegaly may also resolve and a noticeable improvement in histology will be observed. Cardiac function may improve, although the presence of cardiac failure is a poor sign.

The following features may not improve despite venesection:

- advanced, already developed cirrhosis (with complications of decompensated liver disease) and the subsequent risk of HCC; these are the commonest reasons for death
- arthropathy
- hypogonadism
- diabetes mellitus; however, some degree of improvement in glycaemic control may be noticed once regular venesection has been commenced

Treatment for hereditary haemochromatosis, and its effectiveness

The mainstay of medical treatment for hereditary haemochromatosis is venesection, with initially twice-weekly phlebotomy with one whole unit of blood (each unit bearing ~200–250 mg of iron). The aims of treatment are:

- haematocrit <50%
- transferrin saturation <35%–40%
- ferritin <50 ng/ml

Once these targets have been achieved, venesection intervals can be prolonged (e.g. 2–3 monthly). Note that desferrioxamine (an iron-chelating agent) has been used to treat excess iron in the body but is not currently licensed for this use.

Complications from end-organ damage (e.g. heart failure) should be addressed. In addition, the following conservative treatment measures should be instituted:

- limit alcohol intake
- reduce intake of vitamin C (which enhances the gastrointestinal absorption of iron)
- increase intake of substances that inhibit iron absorption (e.g. tea (tannin) and calcium)
- vaccinate against hepatotropic viruses (hepatitis A and B)

Family screening for hereditary haemochromatosis

All first-degree relatives should be offered screening with genetic testing, transferrin saturation, and ferritin. Incomplete penetrance means not everyone with the genetic anomaly will develop iron overload. Venesection is indicated for the indications already outlined. Heterozygotes should only have liver biopsy if hepatic enzymes and iron studies are abnormal.

Wilson's disease

Definition of Wilson's disease

Wilson's disease (hepatolenticular degeneration) is an autosomal recessive genetic disorder in which copper accumulates in tissues. Wilson's may present primarily with neuropsychiatric features or with liver disease, and both typically coexist in patients.

Aetiology of Wilson's disease

The gene responsible for Wilson's disease is ATP7B on Chromosome 13. It encodes a transmembrane copper transport protein. Altered function of this gene impairs excretion of copper into bile and promotes accumulation in the liver and in nerve tissue.

Typical symptoms of Wilson's disease, and less common symptoms

A spectrum of liver diseases may be encountered in patients with Wilson's disease, and clinically evident hepatic involvement may precede neurologic manifestations by >10 years. The majority of individuals with neurological symptoms have some degree of liver disease at presentation.

Symptoms of liver disease at presentation can be highly variable. The commonest presentation is with liver disease or neuropsychiatric disturbance; however, patients may be asymptomatic and only detected by family screening. Wilson's disease typically affects young adults (ages 5–35) but can affect individuals of any age.

Acute hepatitis and fulminant liver failure are often accompanied by a Coombs-negative haemolytic anaemia, acute renal failure, deep jaundice with only mildly elevated transaminases, and an alkaline phosphatase (ALP) level that is normal/lower than expected in the context of other liver test abnormalities. Although preexisting cirrhosis may be present in most cases, the clinical presentation is acute, progressing rapidly to hepatic failure. Acute liver failure (ALF) occurs predominantly in women (4:1) and accounts for 6%–12% of all patients with ALF referred for emergency transplantation.

Many patients present with signs of chronic liver disease and cirrhosis, with a presentation that may be indistinguishable from that observed in other etiologies. Haemolysis may be the only presenting feature in the early stage in up to 12% of patients. This becomes more marked as liver disease progresses due to hepatocyte death and copper release, which exacerbates haemolysis.

Neuropsychiatric symptoms are predominantly those pertaining to a basal ganglia disorder (parkinsonism, ataxia, dystonia, and tremor), although some patients may just present with mild cognitive impairment, behaviour changes, and general clumsiness. Psychiatric problems include depression, anxiety, and psychosis.

Kayser–Fleischer (KF) rings may be visible around the iris. They are due to copper deposition in Descemet's membrane of the cornea and are found in 95% of patients with neurological disease, and in approximately half without. KF rings may only be visible on slit lamp examination, although they are frequently absent in young children with hepatic disease.

Wilson's disease is also associated with sunflower cataracts resulting from the deposition of brown or green pigmentation in the anterior and posterior lens capsules. Significant visual loss is unusual. Type 2 renal tubular acidosis is recognized as leading to nephrocalcinosis and arthropathy.

Demographics of Wilson's disease

The incidence worldwide of Wilson's disease is 1 in 30 000. Most mutations in families are unique or rare and there are no common mutations.

Natural history of Wilson's disease, and complications of the disease

Patients with liver disease tend to come to medical attention earlier, either as children or as teenagers. Those with neurological and psychiatric symptoms tend to present in their twenties or older. Some are identified only because relatives have been diagnosed with Wilson's disease. In the few presenting with fulminant hepatic failure, the condition is inevitably fatal without transplantation.

Approach to diagnosing Wilson's disease

When one presents with symptoms from Wilson's disease, it is highly likely that cirrhosis is already present. Most patients have only mildly abnormal liver chemistry. If liver damage is significant, albumin levels may be decreased and the prothrombin time may be prolonged. ALP may be relatively low in patients with Wilson's-related ALF.

Initial investigations should encompass:

- serum caeruloplasmin (low; <0.1 g/l)
- 24-hour urinary copper (high; >0.64 µmol per 24 hours)

Other diagnoses that should be considered aside from Wilson's disease

The differential diagnoses include conditions with altered mental status or cognition in the presence of deranged liver function, and certain types of haemolytic anaemia. The following diagnosis should also be considered:

- alcohol withdrawal (e.g. delirium tremens, Wernicke–Korsakoff encephalopathy)
- thrombotic thrombocytopenic purpura (by definition, the prothrombin time should not be prolonged)

Screening should be performed for the other causes of acute and chronic liver failure. The acute presentation may mimic many features of viral hepatitis, or an autoimmune hepatitis (AIH), including hypergammaglobulinaemia; positivity for anti-smooth muscle antibodies, antinuclear antibodies, or anti-liver kidney microsomal type 1 antibody (~60%); and an active histological hepatitis or cirrhosis.

'Gold-standard' diagnostic test for Wilson's disease

For many patients, a combination of tests reflecting disturbed copper metabolism is needed, as no single diagnostic modality is specific. Although the combination of KF rings and low serum caeruloplasmin (<0.1 g/l) alone is often sufficient to establish a diagnosis, KF rings may not be present in the absence of neurological involvement. Moreover, caeruloplasmin levels are not always reliable, because they may be low for reasons other than Wilson's disease (e.g. AIH; severe hepatic insufficiency in advanced liver disease, in coeliac disease, or in patients who are heterozygous carriers of ATP7B mutations but do not show copper overload disease). The Leipzig score, based on all available tests assessing copper metabolism, provides good diagnostic accuracy (Table 214.1).

Acceptable diagnostic alternatives to the gold-standard test for Wilson's disease

Total serum copper is usually decreased in proportion to the decreased caeruloplasmin. Non-caeruloplasmin-bound copper ('free copper') in untreated patients is often >200 µg/l, but may be elevated in ALF (due to release from dying hepatocytes) of any aetiology, or in disorders of chronic cholestasis. A 24-hour urinary copper >1.6 µmol per 24 hours (100 µg per 24 hours) is taken as diagnostic but may be lower than this in up to 23% of children and asymptomatic siblings. Lower levels (>0.64 µmol per 24 hours) can be suggestive of Wilson's disease and should prompt further testing if clinical suspicion remains high. In the paediatric population, the penicillamine test may be applied, whereby penicillamine is administered orally and after 12 hours; a subsequent urine protein excretion with >5x the normal urobilinogen level in 24 hours is considered diagnostic. However, this test has not been standardized in adults.

Liver biopsy with staining for copper-associated protein, together with the typical clinical context, can be reliable and diagnostic. Hepatic copper accumulation (>4 µmol/g dry weight) is the hallmark of Wilson's disease; however, the hepatic parenchymal copper concentration can be inhomogeneous in distribution in later stages of Wilson's disease; thus, the concentration can be underestimated due to sampling error.

Linkage analysis has been used in family studies for presymptomatic testing. However, due to the large number of mutations that require screening in individuals without affected family members, such analysis is not practical.

Other relevant investigations for Wilson's disease

CT/MRI brain scanning may be used to detect low attenuation in the basal ganglia. However, abdominal imaging is neither sensitive nor specific for Wilson's disease.

As Wilson's disease is autosomal recessive, all first-degree relatives should be screened for caeruloplasmin and 24-hour urinary copper.

Table 214.1 Leipzig 2001 scoring system for diagnosing Wilson's disease*

Diagnostic parameter	Score
Kayser–Fleischer rings	
• Present	2
• Absent	0
Neurological symptoms/lesions detectable on MRI brain	
• Severe	2
• Mild	1
• Absent	0
Serum caeruloplasmin	
• >0.2 g/l	0
• 0.1–0.2 g/l	1
• <0.1 g/l	2
Coombs-neg. haemolytic anaemia	
• Present	1
• Absent	0
Liver copper (in the absence of cholestasis)	
• >4 µmol/g	2
• 0.8–4.0 µmol/g	1
• <0.8 ¼mol/g	−1
• Rhodanine-positive granules	1
Urinary copper (in the absence of acute hepatitis)	
• Normal	0
• 1–2× ULN	1
• >2× ULN	2
• Normal but >5× ULN after D-pencillamine chelation	2
Mutation analysis	
• Both chromosomes detected	4
• Only one chromosome detected	1
• No mutations detected	0

*Total score >4: diagnosis established; total score = 3: diagnosis possible but more tests needed; total score <2: diagnosis unlikely.

Abbreviations: MRI, magnetic resonance imaging; ULN, upper limit of normal.

Reprinted from *Journal of Hepatology*, volume 56, issue 3, Leipzig 2001 , EASL Clinical Practice Guidelines: Wilson's disease. Pp. 671-85, copyright 2012. With permission from Elsevier.

Prognosis of Wilson's disease, and how to estimate it

Lifelong copper chelation therapy is necessary in all patients with Wilson's disease. Patients are at risk of liver failure even in stable chronic disease. The development of fulminant hepatic failure is inevitably fatal without liver transplantation.

Treatment and its effectiveness

The mainstay of medical treatment is chelation therapy, and an argument can be made for early liver transplantation. D-pencillamine is the drug of choice. However, ALF occurs if this drug is stopped abruptly. Due to the side effects of pencillamine (both drug-induced lupus and drug-induced myasthenia can occur in up to 20% of cases), many individuals are switched to trientine hydrochloride or tetrathiomolybdate.

Zinc may be used to maintain stable copper levels in those whose results have returned to normal or in those parts of the world where primary agents are not available. Zinc monotherapy appears to be effective and safe in neurologic Wilson's disease and in asymptomatic siblings, but caution is needed in patients with advanced or symptomatic hepatic disease. Hepatic deterioration has been reported when zinc was commenced and may relate to less efficient de-coppering.

Liver transplantation is the only cure for Wilson's disease but is used only in particular scenarios because of the numerous risks and complications associated with the procedure. It is reserved mainly in patients with fulminant liver failure.

Alpha-1-antitrypsin deficiency

Definition of alpha-1-antitrypsin deficiency

Reduced circulating levels of alpha-1-antitrypsin, a liver-derived protease inhibitor, and accumulation within the hepatocytes of the abnormal, poorly degraded protein, are the defining features of alpha-1-antitrypsin deficiency. Excessive activity of proteases, such as elastase, in pulmonary alveoli, unopposed by protease inhibitors, leads to emphysema, whereas accumulation of alpha-1-antitrypsin in hepatocytes causes liver dysfunction.

Aetiology of alpha-1-antitrypsin deficiency

Mutations leading to alpha-1-antitrypsin deficiency alter the configuration of the alpha-1-antitrypsin molecule so that it cannot be released efficiently from hepatocytes. As a result, serum levels of the protein are decreased, leading to low concentrations of it in pulmonary alveoli, where it normally would serve as protection against proteases.

The gene for alpha-1-antitrypsin is located on Chromosome 14; over 100 different mutations in this gene have been described in various populations. The alpha-1-antitrypsin genotype of a patient can be determined through protein phenotyping via protein gel electrophoresis; the normal alpha-1-antitrypsin isoform is encoded by the 'M' allele, and common variants are encoded by the 'S' and 'Z' alleles. Circulating levels of alpha-1-antitrypsin depend on the patient's genotype and determine the severity of the condition. Alpha-1-antitrypsin serum levels for various genotypes are as follows, where Pi stands for protease inhibitor:

- PiMM: 100% of normal serum levels
- PiMS: 80% of normal serum levels
- PiSS: 60% of normal serum levels
- PiMZ: 60% of normal serum levels
- PiSZ: 40% of normal serum levels
- PiZZ: 10%–15% of normal serum levels (severe deficiency)

Typical symptoms of alpha-1-antitrypsin deficiency, and less common symptoms

The commonest respiratory effects of alpha-1-antitrypsin deficiency are dyspnoea, cough, wheeze, and premature emphysema localized to the basal lung areas. The disease affects individuals aged 30–35 years, particularly smokers.

The liver is rarely involved, except in severe deficiency. In this situation, disease usually presents in the first two decades of life. Adults with liver involvement may not have any symptoms until the onset of chronic liver disease with decompensation.

Demographics of alpha-1-antitrypsin deficiency

Alpha-1-antitrypsin deficiency is present in 1 in 3000–5000 individuals. The highest-risk populations are those residing in Northern Europe, Liberia, and Saudi Arabia; 5% carry the PiZ allele. Women and men are equally affected. The enzyme deficiency is congenital and has a bimodal distribution with respect to symptoms. It can rarely be seen in neonates as a cause of neonatal jaundice and hepatitis. It can present in infants as cholestatic jaundice and in children as hepatic cirrhosis or liver failure.

Natural history, and complications of alpha-1-antitrypsin deficiency

Patients with alpha-1-antitrypsin deficiency are subject to all the complications characteristic of patients with COPD from cigarette smoking. Chronic liver disease is uncommon but often hastened by excessive alcohol consumption. When present, hepatic involvement usually manifests in the first two decades of life. HCC has also been reported in alpha-1-antitrypsin deficiency.

Approach to diagnosing alpha-1-antitrypsin deficiency

It is useful to consider a diagnosis of alpha-1-antitrypsin deficiency in anyone who is being worked up for chronic liver disease. Early onset emphysema is particularly suggestive of the diagnosis.

Other diagnoses that should be considered aside from alpha-1-antitrypsin deficiency

Respiratory disease with cor pulmonale leading to congestive hepatomegaly is a more common cause for dual lung/liver pathology than alpha-1-antitrypsin deficiency is. Liver cirrhosis is unusual in these circumstances. As respiratory disease tends to dominate the clinical picture in adults, other conditions that may have to be considered include:

- bronchiectasis
- bronchitis
- chronic bronchitis
- COPD
- Kartagener syndrome
- vasculitides

'Gold-standard' diagnostic test for alpha-1-antitrypsin deficiency

The gold-standard test for alpha-1-antitrypsin deficiency is genotype and protein-phenotype assessment.

Acceptable diagnostic alternatives to the gold-standard test for alpha-1-antitrypsin deficiency

Moderately reduced levels of alpha-1-antitrypsin in the circulation may indicate heterozygosity and do not require further investigation, particularly if enzyme levels are only slightly low.

Other relevant investigations for alpha-1-antitrypsin deficiency

Family screening should be performed by measuring alpha-1-antitrypsin levels and by phenotype testing. Chest radiography (plain-film and high-resolution CT scanning) can be useful as, in alpha-1-antitrypsin deficiency, emphysematous areas are distributed uniformly throughout the acinus and, for reasons that are not known, are found more commonly in the basilar portions of the lung. In contrast, centrilobular emphysema is characteristic of cigarette smoking and predominantly affects the respiratory bronchioles in the central portion of the lobule, initially at the apex of the lung. Spirometry is another useful investigation.

Prognosis of alpha-1-antitrypsin deficiency, and how to estimate it

The prognosis of alpha-1-antitrypsin deficiency depends entirely on the severity of underlying lung or liver disease, as well as how patients are identified. Patients found as a result of screening often have a prognosis near that of healthy people. Those identified because of their symptoms face a more limited future. Specific features that confer a poor prognosis include:

- severe airflow obstruction
  - FEV_1 >50%: 5-year mortality rate, 4%
  - FEV_1 35%–49%: 5-year mortality rate, 12%
  - FEV_1 <35: 5-year mortality rate, 50%
- smoking
- male sex
- PiZZ genotype: individuals with this genotype have a 16% likelihood of surviving to age 60, with the most common causes of death being emphysema (~70%) and chronic liver disease (~10%); the latter is often hastened by excessive alcohol consumption

The quoted mortality rate is approximately 3% per year. HCC has also been reported in deficiency.

Treatment of alpha-1-antitrypsin deficiency, and its effectiveness

Conservative treatment of alpha-1-antitrypsin deficiency

Conservative treatment of alpha-1-antitrypsin deficiency involves:

- abstinence from alcohol and tobacco
- standard emphysema treatment (e.g. bronchodilators, inhaled steroids)
- pulmonary rehabilitation
- long-term oxygen, where indicated
- preventing severe respiratory tract infections (e.g. via yearly influenza and pneumococcal vaccinations)

Replacement therapy in alpha-1-antitrypsin deficiency

Individuals who have alpha-1-antitrypsin deficiency and who show signs of developing significant emphysema can be treated with alpha1–proteinase inhibitor (e.g. Prolastin ®), which is a purified human plasma protein concentrate replacement for the missing enzyme. This should be performed only under specialist supervision.

Surgery for treating alpha-1-antitrypsin deficiency

The only definitive treatment for alpha-1-antitrypsin deficiency is transplantation.

Further Reading

European Association for the Study of the Liver. EASL clinical practice guidelines for HFE hemochromatosis. *J Hepatol* 2010; 53: 3–22.

European Association for the Study of the Liver. EASL clinical practice guidelines: Wilson's disease. *J Hepatol* 2012; 56: 671–85.

Köhnlein T and Welte T. Alpha-1 antitrypsin deficiency: Pathogenesis, clinical presentation, diagnosis, and treatment. *Am J Med* 2008; 121: 3–9.

Powell LW, Seckington RC, and Deugnier Y. Haemochromatosis. *Lancet* 2016; 388: 706–16.

215 Drug-induced liver disease

Satish Keshav and Palak Trivedi

Definition of the disease

Drugs are an important and common cause of hepatic injury. This is unsurprising, as the liver is a major site for drug clearance, biotransformation, and excretion.

A careful history of drugs taken (prescribed, over the counter, herbal, or illicit) is vital when assessing anyone with abnormal liver function tests. Although toxic or idiosyncratic adverse reactions may occur with many therapeutic agents, drug-induced jaundice is not so common.

Aetiology of the disease

Abnormalities seen in drug-induced liver disease cover a wide spectrum, from acute inflammation, to cholestasis, to fulminant necrosis. The pattern of the disease depends on the agent.

Intrinsic liver injury can be caused by hepatotoxins (drugs or their respective metabolites) leading to direct damage to the liver by covalently bonding to cellular macromolecules (hydroxyl radicals, hydrogen peroxide, or lipid peroxides). This type of injury is usually dose dependant but occurs infrequently. The classical example is acetaminophen/paracetamol (see Chapter 209).

More commonly, reactions are idiosyncratic and not predictable. Simvastatin, for example, may cause a mild rise in liver enzymes, but occasionally a more severe acute cholestatic hepatitis may occur through changes in mevalonic acid metabolism. Isoniazid and halothane are other well recognized examples of drugs that can cause idiosyncratic drug-induced hepatitis and may produce chronic inflammation if consumption continues. Progressive fibrosis and cirrhosis can develop with methotrexate.

Immune mechanisms (hypersensitivity) are responsible for some drug reactions. Only a few have concomitant evidence of an allergic reaction (rash, eosinophilia, etc.).

Polymorphisms of certain cytochrome p450 and acetylator enzymes may also influence an individual's risk of drug-induced liver injury, by affecting the rate of production of toxic metabolites.

Cholestatic reactions may either be of the inflammatory or non-inflammatory (so-called bland) subtype:

- chlorpromazine, allopurinol, and flucloxacillin may cause an acute periportal necro-inflammatory reaction with biochemical cholestasis and features of inflammation on biopsy
- certain steroids (oral contraceptives) cause relatively pure impairment of bile outflow with no associated inflammatory change; this arises due to the effect of sex hormones on bile canalicular transport

Oral contraceptives may also be associated with the development of hepatic adenomas, focal nodular hyperplasia, gallstones, and veno-occlusive disease.

Typical symptoms of the disease, and less common symptoms

Symptoms of drug-induced liver injury vary, depending on the type of liver injury caused. For example, allergic hepatitis (e.g. in response to phenytoin) may present with systemic symptoms such as pharyngitis, lymphadenopathy, and atypical lymphocytosis. Jaundice, when present, may persist for a limited period after withdrawal of some agents, particularly drugs that cause inflammatory cholestasis. Chronic hepatitis can occur in response to amiodarone, nitrofurantoin, methyldopa, dantrolene, and co-amoxiclav and its individual components.

Demographics of the disease

Over 600 medicines have been reported to cause liver injury. Drug-induced hepatic injury is the one of the most frequent reasons cited for withdrawing a drug from the market. In the US, it accounts for 2%–5% of admitted cases of jaundice and over 50% of cases of acute liver failure, most due to acetaminophen poisoning.

Natural history, and complications of the disease

The natural history and the complications of the disease depend on the drug in question (see Table 215.1).

Approach to diagnosing the disease

The diagnosis is suspected from the history of liver dysfunction or jaundice, which may occur soon after first or early exposure to a drug. Occasionally, liver damage can present many months after starting the drug.

A good drug history assessing aspects of not only prescribed medication but also herbal, over-the-counter, and illicit drug use is vital. It is also important to ascertain a temporal association in cases of acute dysfunction, as most reactions occur within days to weeks of starting a new drug.

Other diagnoses that should be considered

Diagnosis requires exclusion of viral, toxic, cardiovascular, inherited, autoimmune, and malignant causes of liver injury. When drug-induced liver injury is suspected, withdrawal of the offending agent and close observation often provide adequate circumstantial evidence for a diagnosis.

'Gold-standard' diagnostic test

Reliable evidence of exposure, and an expected pattern of injury, are usually sufficient, provided that the injury ceases and liver injury recedes on stopping the drug. Occasionally, it is necessary or worthwhile to reintroduce the drug and monitor for recurrent injury.

Acceptable diagnostic alternatives to the gold standard

Liver biopsy should be reserved for situations when discontinuation of the drug is not followed by prompt improvement, the disease remains in question, and/or the severity necessitates urgent intervention (e.g. immunosuppression, liver transplantation).

Other relevant investigations

The following investigations are largely aimed at assessing liver damage and liver function while excluding the wide range of differential diagnoses:

- full blood count (including differential)
- renal function
- liver enzymes (alanine transaminase and alkaline phosphatase)
- liver synthetic function (bilirubin, albumin, clotting)

Table 215.1 Drugs and hepatotoxicity

Type of liver injury	Features	Drug examples
Deranged LFTs alone		
Microsomal enzyme induction	No clinical features Raised ALP/γGT	Warfarin Phenytoin
Hyperbilirubinaemia	Jaundice (rarely occurs)	Rifampicin
Steatosis		
Acute fatty change	Clinical features of hepatitis, liver failure	Tetracycline NSAIDs Catabolic steroids Valproate
Steatohepatitis	Features of chronic liver disease	Amiodarone Parenteral nutrition
Cholestasis		
Bland cholestasis	Pruritus ALP > 2× normal	COCP Androgens Phenytoin
Inflammatory cholestasis	Systemic symptoms ALT and ALP raised	Erythromycin Flucloxacillin Co-amoxiclav Chlorpromazine Allopurinol Amitriptyline Azathioprine Captopril Carbamazepine
Cholestasis with bile duct injury	Destructive lesions of bile ducts, similar to acute cholangitis	Flucloxacillin Chlorpromazine
Vanishing bile duct syndrome*	Chronic cholestasis > 3 months Resembles primary biliary cholangitis (AMA negative)	Chlorpromazine Flucloxacillin Amitriptyline
Hepatocellular necrosis (variable inflammation). ALT >5 times normal		
Focal necrosis	Can resemble viral hepatitis histologically	Isoniazid Halothane
Bridged necrosis		Isoniazid Methyldopa
Zonal necrosis		Paracetamol Halothane (severe)
Massive necrosis	Fulminant hepatic failure	Halothane (fatal) NSAIDs Valproate
Chronic parenchymal damage (deranged LFTs >3/12)		
Chronic hepatitis	Clinical and biochemical features of chronic liver disease Liver failure may occur	Methyldopa Nitrofurantoin Sodium dantrolene Minocycline can induce autoimmune hepatitis that is indistinguishable from the spontaneous variety
Fibrosis and cirrhosis	Portal hypertension (LFTs may be normal)	Methotrexate Retinoids Hypervitaminosis A
Vascular problems		
Sinusoidal dilatation	Can be an isolated finding Hepatomegaly may be the only feature	COCP
Non-cirrhotic portal hypertension	Splenomegaly Varices (features of portal hypertension)	Azathioprine
Hepatic venous outflow tract obstruction	Budd–Chiari syndrome and related	COCP 6MP
Nodular regenerative hyperplasia	Features of portal hypertension	Azathioprine

(continued)

Table 215.1 (Continued)

Type of liver injury	Features	Drug examples
Hepatic granulomas		
Non-caseating granuloma (usual presentation)	Mixed LFT picture Can present with cholestasis or even cholangitis	Allopurinol Isoniazid Phenytoin Sulfonamides Chlorpromazine Quinidine Penicillins Diltiazem Nitrofurantoin Gold COCP Diazepam Phenytoin
Hepatic tumours		
Focal nodular hyperplasia	Hamartomas	COCP
Hepatic adenoma		Androgens COCP
Hepatic carcinoma		Androgens COCP

*Histology shows chronic portal inflammation and degeneration of the bile duct referred to as progressive ductopenia.

Abbreviations: γGT, gamma-glutamyl transferase; 6MP, 6-mercaptopurine; ALP, alkaline phosphatase; ALT, alanine transaminase; AMA, anti-mitochondrial antibody; COCP, combined oral contraceptive pill; LFT, liver function test; NSAID, non-steroidal anti-inflammatory drug.

- hepatic viral serology
- autoantibody and immunoglobulin screen
- copper and iron studies

Box 215.1 Dose-related and dose-independent side effects

Dose-dependent hepatotoxicity
- halothane:
  - rarely used now
  - partly related to dose (should be avoided for anaesthetics <6 weeks apart)
- methotrexate:
  - varying grades of damage from fibrosis to portal inflammation
  - toxicity is usually associated with excess alcohol use
  - dose-dependent fibrosis (unusual if total dose <2 g)
  - jaundice may occur in terminal stages, with liver function remaining normal earlier on
- paracetamol
  - >10 g per 24 hours
  - >6 g per 24 hours if underlying liver disease (e.g. from alcohol, malnutrition) is present

Dose-independent hepatotoxicity
- isoniazid
- valproate
- rifampicin
- NSAIDs
- azathioprine
- co-amoxiclav
- chlorpromazine
- gliblenclamide
- nitrofurantoin
- dantrolene sodium
- methyldopa
- verapamil
- allopurinol

- alpha-1 antitrypsin (to exclude other causes of liver disease)
- liver ultrasound
- chest X-ray (to look for pulmonary infiltrates associates with certain drug toxicities (e.g. sulphasalazine))

Prognosis and how to estimate it

The prognosis depends on the offending agent, the pattern of distribution, and the presence of coexisting liver disease.

Treatment and its effectiveness

Exclude other causes of hepatic dysfunction and jaundice. Minor elevations in transaminases (2–3 times the normal limit) after starting potentially hepatotoxic drugs (e.g. anti-mycobacterial agents) are not an indication for stopping the drug, as improvement usually occurs. Remember, not all injury is dose dependant. (Box 215.1)

If enzymes continue to deteriorate or the patient develops jaundice, then all potential drugs leading to hepatic dysfunction should be stopped. Monitor liver enzymes until a normal level is reached. Although most hepatotoxic effects resolve completely after withdrawal of the drug, in rare cases persistent loss of small bile ducts can occur. If liver enzymes fail to return to normal after 8 weeks and the history is uncertain, proceed to liver biopsy.

Further Reading

Leise MD, Poterucha JJ, and Talwalkar JA. Drug-induced liver injury. *Mayo Clinic Proc* 2014; 89: 95–106.

LiverTox is a freely available website that provides comprehensive information about drug-induced liver injury. LiverTox is a joint effort of the Liver Disease Research Branch of the National Institute of Diabetes and Digestive and Kidney Diseases, and the Division of Specialized Information Services of the National Library of Medicine, National Institutes of Health. The web address is http://livertox.nih.gov/

216 Miscellaneous liver diseases

Satish Keshav and Palak Trivedi

Non-alcoholic fatty liver disease

Definition of non-alcoholic fatty liver disease

Non-alcoholic fatty liver disease (NAFLD) comprises a spectrum of disorders which are characterized by the deposition of lipid material in hepatocytes in the absence of a history of excess alcohol ingestion.

Aetiology of NAFLD

There are many conditions that can lead to the development of NAFLD (see Table 216.1).

Typical symptoms of NAFLD, and less common symptoms

Most patients with NAFLD remain asymptomatic, with the diagnosis of NAFLD being made incidentally. Occasionally, individuals may present with non-specific symptoms such as malaise or with right upper quadrant discomfort. Hepatomegaly is not an uncommon clinical finding on examination. Individuals with steatohepatitis may eventually progress to cirrhotic liver disease and demonstrate all the symptoms/signs of decompensated liver disease.

Demographics of NAFLD

With the obesity pandemic sweeping across the world, and the rising number of individuals with type 2 diabetes, the incidence of NAFLD has dramatically increased. NAFLD is now the commonest diagnosis in patients with incidental abnormal liver biochemistry, both in secondary care (60%–70%) and in primary care (26%). The true overall prevalence can be difficult to measure, given the large proportion of asymptomatic individuals, but is estimated to affect up to 20%–30% of the adult population and >90% in the morbidly obese. The implications of such rates on the future burden of NAFLD are heightened by a reported prevalence of 3% and 53% in the general and obese paediatric populations, respectively. The reported prevalence is higher in patients of European or Hispanic descent; this is largely a reflection of ethnic differences in lipid metabolism and insulin resistance. The more clinically relevant form of NAFLD, non-alcoholic steatohepatitis (NASH), is less common and affects 2%–3% of the general population, and 37% of the morbidly obese.

Natural history of NAFLD, and complications of the disease

The spectrum of NAFLD ranges from simple steatosis, in which there is a mildly elevated level of serum alanine transaminase (ALT) or aspartate transaminase (AST; ≤100 IU/l or less than 3 × urobilinogen) and/or an isolated rise in gamma-glutamyl transpeptidase (with fatty appearances of the liver detected on ultrasound), through to NASH, which is indistinguishable from alcoholic hepatitis histologically.

Simple steatosis was historically thought to be a benign condition. However, despite progression from simple steatosis to advanced liver fibrosis being rare, patients with simple steatosis have increased mortality, which is largely attributable to cardiovascular causes.

Steatohepatitis may progress to cirrhosis with complications of decompensated liver disease. Individuals who have impaired glucose tolerance or with a raised BMI are at a higher risk of progression to fibrosis. Changes in aminotransferases do not necessarily parallel the changes in fibrosis.

Approach to diagnosing NAFLD

A diagnosis of NAFLD should be suspected in any individual who is overweight (BMI > 25 kg/m²), is diabetic or hyperlipidaemic, and has abnormal liver biochemistry. There is no specific cut-off regarding the quantity of alcohol consumption that is allowable for individuals to be included in the NAFLD group as opposed to the alcoholic hepatitis group; however, an arbitrary limit is set at 24 units/week.

Table 216.1 Causes and associations with non-alcoholic fatty liver disease

Metabolic	Drugs	Surgical	Miscellaneous
Inherited:	Amiodarone	Jejunoileal bypass‡	Inflammatory bowel disease
• lipoproteinemias	Oestrogens	Biliopancreatic diversion	Jejunal diverticuli
• Wilson's disease	Tamoxifen	Extensive bowel	
• tyrosinemia	Glucocorticoids	resection	
• galactosemia	Tetracycline		
• glycogen storage diseases	Valproic acid		
Acquired:			
• metabolic syndrome*			
• obesity†			
• type 2 diabetes			
• hypertriglyceridaemia			
• coeliac disease			
• lipodystrophy			
• severe malnutrition			

*Characterized by insulin resistance, centripetal obesity, dyslipidaemia, and microalbuminuria; this is the disorder most consistently associated with non-alcoholic fatty liver disease.

†Non-alcoholic fatty liver disease may also occur in 2%–3% of lean individuals.

‡The risk of developing steatohepatitis and even subacute hepatic failure has been seen to be high following jejunoileal bypass, with up to 95% patients developing steatosis at the end of the first year. The association of jejunoileal bypass with hepatic dysfunction has prompted proximal gastric bypass as a method of choice for bariatric surgery. The head-to-head comparison of these two surgical modalities has indicated that proximal gastric bypass is more effective and safer than jejunoileal bypass. However, changes suggestive of steatohepatitis were observed following both jejunoileal and proximal gastric bypass surgeries. The predominant mechanism behind the hepatocellular injury is thought to be metabolic stress induced by rapid weight loss in the post-bypass period.

Most individuals diagnosed will be asymptomatic, with deranged liver biochemistry being diagnosed incidentally. The ratio of ALT:AST is usually >1 in NAFLD but this ratio is reversed in the presence of fibrosis or cirrhosis.

Other diagnoses that should be considered aside from NAFLD

Other diagnoses that should be considered aside from NAFLD include:

- alcoholic liver disease
- hereditary haemochromatosis (in a diabetic with deranged biochemistry)
- Wilson's disease (in a young patient with modest elevations in serum liver enzymes, and a fatty liver on ultrasound)
- other causes (see Chapter 210)

Gold-standard diagnostic test for NAFLD

Non-invasive imaging can assess the amount of fatty infiltration within the liver but not the presence of inflammation, fibrosis, or cirrhosis. Liver biopsy is currently the most accurate way of determining the presence of steatosis, degree of fibrosis, and severity of liver injury. However, liver biopsy is invasive and costly, and findings may be indistinguishable from alcoholic hepatitis and prone to sampling error. Common histological changes include:

- balloon degeneration
- Mallory's hyaline (highly eosinophilic cytoplasmic inclusions found in hepatocytes)
- sinusoidal fibrosis

Acceptable diagnostic alternatives to the gold-standard test for NAFLD

Ultrasound in NAFLD

In NAFLD, the liver is hyperechogenic or bright liver (only when >30% of the liver parenchyma has become steatosis). However, ultrasound cannot distinguish a simple fatty liver from steatosis with hepatitis.

Assessment of steatosis in NAFLD

Vibration-controlled transient elastography with a controlled attenuation parameter (recorded in decibels per metre) measures the degree of ultrasound attenuation by hepatic fat at the central frequency of the Fibroscan® probe and can be performed simultaneously with liver stiffness measurement. Median parameter values correlate with the percentage of hepatocytes with lipid droplets and histological steatosis grade:

- Stage 0 steatosis: ~250 dB/m
- Stage 1 steatosis: ~300 dB/m
- Stage 2–4 steatosis: ≥320 dB/m (301–338 dB/m)

Assessment of fibrosis in NAFLD

Transient elastography or Fibroscan® assessing liver stiffness has been validated as a tool in assessing the severity of liver fibrosis in NAFLD. A value <10 kPa excludes the presence of advanced fibrosis, although values may be underestimated with increasing subcutaneous adiposity.

Biomarkers of liver fibrosis in NAFLD

An AST:ALT ratio more than 0.8 or a NAFLD fibrosis score (http://nafldscore.com) less than −1.455 excludes advanced fibrosis (negative predictive value >90%).

Other relevant investigations for NAFLD

Evaluation of cardiovascular risk in NAFLD

The following investigations should be performed to evaluate cardiovascular risk in NAFLD:

- waist circumference
- BMI
- blood pressure

Laboratory tests directed at identifying the underlying cause of NAFLD

The following laboratory tests may be performed to identify the underlying cause of NAFLD:

- fasting glucose and postprandial (post 2 hours) glucose to detect impaired glucose tolerance
- fasting lipid screen
- thyroid function
- coeliac serology
- iron studies (may reveal moderate elevations in ferritin with reduced transferrin saturation; levels are seldom as deranged as in untreated haemochromatosis)
- other laboratory tests to exclude other causes of chronic liver disease

Prognosis of NAFLD and how to estimate it

Liver disease is the third leading cause of death amongst people with NAFLD, behind cardiovascular-related mortality and extra-hepatic malignancy. A greater death rate is seen in those individuals with increasing age at diagnosis, cirrhosis, and diabetes. Liver-related outcomes are dependent upon the degree of hepatic fibrosis, with all-cause mortality being 13% over 7.6 years.

Simple hepatic steatosis does not usually follow a progressive course, although such patients are at risk of adverse cardiovascular events. The rate of progression from steatohepatitis to advanced fibrosis/cirrhosis is the same as that observed in patients with steatohepatitis secondary to alcohol. Longitudinal studies of patients with NASH undergoing repeat biopsies have shown that one-third of these patients progress, one-third remain stable, and one-third improve, as determined by histology, over a 3-year period without pharmacologic intervention. End-stage/decompensated NASH cirrhosis accounts for ~3% of patients undergoing liver transplantation.

The rate of development of primary liver malignancy in NAFLD is thought to be comparable to those with other primary liver diseases. However, there is emerging evidence that non-cirrhotic patients may also be at risk of developing hepatocellular carcinoma (HCC).

Biomarkers for prognostication in NAFLD

The fatty liver index (FLI) is a validated algorithm derived from the serum triglyceride level, the gamma-glutamyl transferase level, BMI, and waist circumference, and was originally designed as a non-invasive marker of hepatic steatosis. However, it has recently been shown that FLI also correlates with 15-year liver-related death as well as all-cause mortality.

Other laboratory scoring systems which assist in predicting liver-related morbidity, death, and need for transplantation include the enhanced liver fibrosis test and the aminotransferase-to-platelet ratio.

Treatment of NAFLD and its effectiveness

The management of NAFLD is complex and requires a multidisciplinary approach encompassing dietetic input, management of cardiovascular risk factors, and diabetes, as well as assessment and targeted therapy directed towards liver disease. The cornerstones of treatment are directed towards weight loss through diet and exercise, and control of comorbidities (e.g. tight glycaemic control, lipid-lowering therapies, and exclusion of gluten exposure in patients with coeliac disease; see Box 216.1).

Box 216.1 Factors increasing the likelihood of fibrosis with non-alcoholic fatty liver disease

- age >45
- BMI > 28 kg/m²
- type 2 diabetes, or insulin resistance
- systemic hypertension
- ALT > 2× normal upper limit
- AST:ALT > 1
- hypertriglyceridaemia

Abbreviations: ALT, alanine transaminase; AST, aspartate transaminase; BMI, body mass index.

Lifestyle changes for the management of NAFLD

Weight reduction by lifestyle modification with diet and exercise should be recommended to all, as this will:

- favourably improve the cardiovascular profile
- improve hepatic steatosis
- ameliorate hepatic inflammation (only with >7%–9% weight loss)

Pharmacological therapies for the management of NAFLD

Multiple pharmacological therapies have been trialled in the management of NAFLD and NASH, although most are used off-label.

Orlistat

Orlistat has been shown to lower aminotransferase levels, total cholesterol, triglycerides, and low-density lipoprotein, with an improvement in insulin resistance. Histologically, improvement is also seen with regard to fatty infiltration and inflammatory indices.

Antiglycaemics

Glitazones improve transaminase levels and steatosis and reduce inflammation (but not fibrosis) in the liver, but only as long as therapy continues. Due to adverse publicity regarding the effect of glitazones on cardiovascular mortality, further trials regarding their safety as therapeutic drugs are underway.

Some studies have shown short-term radiological and biochemical improvement with metformin, although histological changes have yet to be proven. However, there is emerging evidence that metformin has inherent anticancer effects, with >60% reduction of HCC in diabetics.

Glucagon-like peptide-1 analogues reduce serum transaminases and radiological evidence of steatosis, but not independently of weight loss and improvement in glycohemoglobin levels. Their therapeutic potential in non-diabetic individuals with NAFLD is currently the subject of a large, multicentre clinical trial.

Lipid-lowering agents

Fibrates and statins should be considered where indicated in view of their cardiovascular protective effects and are safe in patients with liver disease. Statins may also have inherent chemoprotective effects with respect to HCC.

Antihypertensives

Certain agents targeting the renin–angiotensin system have been shown to improve hepatic steatosis and, through the induction of hepatic-stellate-cell apoptosis, may also possess inherent antifibrotic properties.

Vitamin E

Vitamin E is associated with a reduction in serum transaminases and a significantly higher rate of improvement in steatosis, steatohepatitis, and lobular inflammation but not fibrosis.

Bariatric surgery for the treatment of NAFLD

Bariatric surgery should be considered for severely obese persons (BMI >40, or >35 if comorbidity is present) and for those who clearly wish to lose weight. It induces long-term weight loss and decreases morbidity, the incidence of cancer, and mortality. Compelling data show a sustained decrease in steatosis in >90% of patients, and an improvement of steatohepatitis and fibrosis in >80%.

Liver abscesses

Definition of liver abscess

There are two main types of liver abscess: pyogenic and amoebic. Fungal abscesses are rare and usually caused by *Candida* spp. in immunocompromised individuals. Tubercular abscesses also represent a rare hepatic manifestation of *Mycobacterium tuberculosis* infection.

Aetiology of liver abscesses

Pyogenic abscesses usually arise by portal vein seeding from the following intra-abdominal infections:

- diverticulitis
  - Crohn's disease and ulcerative colitis
- bowel perforation
  - delayed diagnosis of appendicitis
- subphrenic abscess or gall bladder empyema
- haematogenous spread (e.g. endocarditis, pyelonephritis with bacteraemia)

Gram-negative infections are usually the cause, with *Escherichia coli* and *Enterobacter* spp. being the commonest cultured organisms. Anaerobic organisms are a close second. It is not uncommon for a patient with a liver abscess to also have a polymicrobial infection.

Amoebic liver abscesses are usually caused by the organism *Entamoeba histolytica*. Predisposing factors include:

- living in endemic areas
- poor hygiene and overcrowding
- immunosuppression

Liver abscesses can also be caused by biliary tract disease (35%) related to cholangitis or cholecystitis. In addition, parasitic infections by roundworms or liver flukes can be causative. Pancreatobiliary malignancy can account for abscesses **originating** in the biliary tree.

Typical symptoms of liver abscesses, and less common symptoms

Symptoms of pyogenic liver abscesses

The features of pyogenic liver abscesses are relatively non-specific, with fever, rigours, right upper quadrant pain, and, occasionally, weight loss. On examination, there may be right upper quadrant tenderness or features of an underlying condition such as appendicitis. Jaundice may indicate the presence of biliary disease.

Symptoms of amoebic liver abscesses

Coupled with a travel history to an endemic area, there may be an antecedent history of diarrhoea, but 90% of infected people will be asymptomatic in the initial stages of amoebic infection before liver abscesses develop. Once hepatic involvement is present, the majority will present with symptoms that develop quickly over a couple of weeks. These include right upper quadrant pain, fever, and a variety of constitutional symptoms. Involvement of the diaphragm can lead to referred right shoulder pain or symptoms of pleurisy. Pain is more common with point tenderness on examination. Hiccups may herald impending rupture.

Demographics of liver abscesses

The estimated annual incidence for pyogenic liver abscesses is around 2–3 per 100 000 people per year in the UK. Worldwide, 40–50 million people are affected with amoebic liver abscesses annually (with the majority found in the developing world). The right lobe is affected in isolation in 60% of cases.

Natural history of liver abscesses, and complications of the disease

Natural history of pyogenic liver abscesses, and complications

Untreated cases of pyogenic liver abscesses can lead to overwhelming, fulminant sepsis. The abscess may rupture into adjacent areas (e.g. pleural or peritoneal space with development of subphrenic, perihepatic, or subhepatic abscesses). Metastatic septic embolic may occur. One rare association is endophthalmitis (infection of intra-ocular fluid), particularly in the presence of klebsiella infection. Larger abscesses may result in the compression of hepatic venous drainage, causing a Budd–Chiari-type picture. Even with appropriate treatment, this condition can yield mortality rates approaching 30%.

Natural history of amoebic liver abscesses, and complications

Amoebic liver abscesses have a much better prognosis with treatment, with considerably lower mortality rates, compared to pyogenic liver abscesses. Impending rupture may be indicated by the presence of hiccups. Rupture into the lung parenchyma may result in a lung abscess or bronchopleural fistula. Haematogenous spread leading to infected emboli has been reported, but this is comparatively rare. Clinical improvement is usually noted within the first week of therapy, with a marked lag in radiological resolution.

Approach to diagnosing liver abscesses

Ultrasound of the liver is always indicated when a patient is febrile and has a derangement in liver biochemistry. Ultrasound enables distinction between solid and fluid-filled structures, but patient body habitus may cause difficulty leading to diagnostic inaccuracy.

Other diagnoses that should be considered aside from liver abscess

The differential for liver abscess includes the multitude of conditions giving rise to fever, right upper quadrant pain/tenderness, and deranged liver biochemistry, such as:

- cholecystitis
- right lower lobe pneumonia
- pulmonary tuberculosis
- hepatic malignancy
- ascending cholangitis
- acute alcoholic hepatitis
- hepatic infarction
- hepatic adenoma (radiological differential)
- hepatic haemangioma (radiological differential)

Another radiological differential is hydatid cystic disease (caused by *Echinococcus* spp.). Primary hosts are usually dogs, with sheep and cattle acting as secondary hosts. This disease usually causes asymptomatic hepatomegaly and normal liver function tests. Serology is often negative. On ultrasound, one may see multiple daughter cysts. If the patient is asymptomatic, leave them alone, as rupture may cause massive anaphylaxis. If the patient is symptomatic, a suitable alternative to surgery is albendazole. Surgery is indicated for increasing size or pressure symptoms.

Gold-standard diagnostic test for liver abscesses

Gold-standard diagnostic test for pyogenic liver abscesses

Ultrasound-guided aspiration confirms the diagnosis of pyogenic liver abscess in 90% of cases.

Gold-standard diagnostic test for amoebic liver abscesses

Ultrasound, with positive antibodies to *Entamoeba histolytica*, is diagnostic for amoebic liver abscesses in over 90% of cases.

Acceptable diagnostic alternatives to the gold-standard diagnostic tests for liver abscesses

Acceptable diagnostic alternatives to the gold-standard diagnostic test for pyogenic liver abscess

Blood cultures are positive in 50% of cases of pyogenic liver abscesses. Helical CT may aid in the diagnosis of smaller abscesses and perhaps give further clues to the underlying source for the abscess.

Acceptable diagnostic alternatives to the gold-standard diagnostic test for amoebic liver abscess

Aspiration of an amoebic liver abscess will reveal a thick, 'anchovy sauce'-like paste which is odourless (unlike that from a pyogenic abscess). Aspiration is indicated when pyogenic or secondary infection cannot be excluded, the abscess is very large, or the patient is not responding to treatment or is in severe pain. Unfortunately, aspiration does not usually yield diagnostic material in most cases.

Serological tests (e.g. immunoelectrophoresis, complement fixation, haemagglutination assays) are positive in patients with invasive disease only (not asymptomatic carriers). These tests are extremely sensitive (except the complement fixation test). Depending on the test used, the titres may remain positive for some time after the infection (e.g. indirect haemagglutination may remain positive for many years).

The biliary tree is not usually involved in amoebic liver abscesses, as bile is toxic to amoebae. Compression of the biliary system may give rise to jaundice but, in the presence of a cholangitis, suspect ascending secondary bacterial infection.

Other relevant investigations for liver abscesses

Other relevant investigations for liver abscesses include:

- full blood count (to look for neutrophil leucocytosis, or anaemia of sepsis or chronic disease)
- serum liver biochemistry
- blood cultures (essential in any febrile patient)
- hot (fresh) stool (for trophozoites)
- a plain chest film (may show a flat right hemidiaphragm)
- cholangiography (if indicated; to demonstrate the site of biliary obstruction)

Prognosis for liver abscess, and how to estimate it

Prognosis for pyogenic liver abscesses

If untreated, pyogenic liver abscesses are associated with high mortality.

Prognosis for amoebic liver abscesses

With good treatment, the mortality of amoebic liver abscesses falls to 1%–3%.

Treatment of liver abscesses, and its effectiveness

Treatment of pyogenic liver abscesses

Treatment of pyogenic liver abscesses includes the following:

- broad-spectrum antibiotic cover (e.g. IV metronidazole and IV ceftriaxone) while awaiting microbial sensitivities
- urgent percutaneous drainage of a single abscess or the larger abscess in the case of multiplicity
- surgical drainage, if there is evidence of the causative disease process (e.g. peritonitis from viscus perforation), if the abscess is very large (>5 cm), if the location of the abscess makes percutaneous drainage difficult, or if previous treatment via percutaneous drainage and antibiotics has failed

Treatment of amoebic liver abscesses

A 10-day course of IV metronidazole is effective in the majority of cases. This should be followed by a further 10-day course of diloxanide, to prevent recurrence.

Consider aspiration with/without drainage if abscesses are >5 cm or located on the left side of the liver (left-sided liver abscesses have a higher mortality and an increased frequency of leaking into peritoneum and pericardium), or if a response is not detected in the first 5 days.

Amphotericin or fluconazole can be used to treat fungal abscesses (seek specialist microbiology advice).

Nodular regenerative hyperplasia

Definition of nodular regenerative hyperplasia

Nodular regenerative hyperplasia (NRH) is the diffuse transformation of normal hepatic parenchyma into smaller regenerative nodules in the presence of little or no fibrosis. This leads to nodules pressing directly onto one another with small atrophic hepatocytes in between (cf. cirrhosis, which has nodules separated by fibrous tissue).

Aetiology of NRH

NRH is hypothesized to be due to alterations in blood flow, with frequent observations of portal and central vein anomalies. This pathological entity has been explained by uneven microcirculatory perfusion, leading to atrophy of the poorly perfused areas, and compensatory (regenerative) hypertrophy of the areas of maintained perfusion. The nodular areas are thus hypothesized to be hypertrophied areas which develop in response to slightly increased blood flow.

Etiological associations of NRH have been provided in Table 216.2.

Typical symptoms of NRH, and less common symptoms

NRH can remain asymptomatic for many years before incidental deranged liver biochemistry is found in the absence of other identifiable causes. Tests of synthetic function may often be normal. Nonspecific features may be malaise, abdominal pain, and fatigue. In other cases, the features that dominate are fundamentally those of (non-cirrhotic) portal hypertension and decompensated liver disease,

Table 216.2 Associations of nodular regenerative hyperplasia

Rheumatological	Haematological	Hepatobiliary disease (without cirrhosis)	Cardiovascular	Other
Systemic sclerosis Polyarteritis nodosa Polymyalgia rheumatica Rheumatoid arthritis Felty's syndrome SLE	Hodgkin's and non-Hodgkin's lymphoma Chronic lymphocytic leukaemia Waldenström's macroglobulinaemia Multiple myeloma	Primary biliary cholangitis Budd–Chiari syndrome	Congestive cardiac failure Hypertension Severe coronary artery disease Hereditary haemorrhagic telangiectasia	Thiopurines and other drugs (probably the most important cause) Type 2 diabetes mellitus Renal transplantation Coeliac disease Certain anticonvulsants.

although ascites is less common than in cirrhosis. Examination findings may reveal the presence of hepatosplenomegaly.

Demographics of NRH

Older studies of autopsy figures have shown that NRH is present in 5.3% of those over 80, with most patients having systemic disease. Case series reviews point towards NRH being the cause for >25% of cases of non-cirrhotic portal hypertension.

Natural history of NRH, and complications of the disease

There is little documentation regarding the true course of NRH, given the large percentage of asymptomatic disease. The medical literature tends to focus on the symptomatic cases, thus giving a slightly skewed view on the condition. In the same breath, it is not fully known whether NRH is **fully** reversible following treatment of the underlying cause.

Complications, when present, are essentially those of decompensated liver disease. Extra-hepatic portal vein thrombosis has been reported to occur in >70% of cases.

Approach to diagnosing NRH

Although NRH can be suspected based on abnormal liver function tests (usually a cholestatic picture) in the absence of other underlying causes, a significant proportion of patients will have normal biochemistry. Further suspicion raised in the presence of unexplained portal hypertension in the absence of cirrhosis. Ultrasound may demonstrate nodularity in the liver.

Other diagnoses that should be considered aside from NRH

NRH and cirrhotic liver disease can be difficult to distinguish, but differentiation is important, as treatment for the two and consequent prognoses are different. Other nodular disorders of the liver include:

- malignancy (see Chapter 218)
- liver cysts
- hepatic adenoma
- focal nodular hyperplasia

Gold-standard diagnostic test for NRH

The gold-standard diagnostic test for NRH is liver histology with reticulin stain.

Acceptable diagnostic alternatives to the gold-standard test for NRH

Increasingly, advanced MRI and CT techniques are being employed to evaluate nodular liver disease. However, confirmation of NRH can only be reached through tissue diagnosis.

Other relevant investigations for NRH

Other investigations in NRH are directed at excluding other causes of chronic liver disease, identifying possible underlying causes, and assessing portal hypertension (see Chapter 210).

Prognosis of NRH, and how to estimate it

See 'Natural history of NRH, and complications of the disease'.

Treatment of NRH, and its effectiveness

Treatment is guided towards the underlying diagnosis and complications of portal hypertension and should be along standard lines. Antiplatelet and anticoagulant therapy should be managed in a specialist setting, given the risks of variceal bleeding with portal hypertension. The need for liver transplantation is rare.

Further Reading

Dowman JK, Tomlinson JW, and Newsome PN. Systematic review: The diagnosis and staging of non-alcoholic fatty liver disease and non-alcoholic steatohepatitis. *Aliment Pharmacol Ther* 2011; 33: 525–40.

Harleb M, Gutkowski K, and Milkiewics P. Nodular regenerative hyperplasia: Evolving concepts on underdiagnosed cause of portal hypertension. *World J Gastroenterol* 2011; 17: 1400–9.

Pang TCY, Fung T, Samra J, et al. Pyogenic liver abscess: An audit of 10 years' experience. *World J Gastroenterol* 2011; 17: 1622–30.

Schwenger KJP and Allard JP. Clinical approaches to non-alcoholic fatty liver disease. *World J Gastroenterol* 2014; 20: 1712–23.

Introduction

The liver may be involved in systemic diseases that primarily affect other organs. In most cases, the systemic disease should be treated effectively first.

The liver in cardiovascular disease

Definition of cardiovascular-disease-related liver disease

Circulatory disturbances can cause liver dysfunction by ischaemia (due to arterial hypoperfusion) and hepatic venous congestion. Liver congestion usually occurs in the setting of acute or chronic right-sided cardiac failure causing hepatic venous congestion and sinusoidal stasis, and is also termed 'passive congestion of the liver' (cf. Budd–Chiari syndrome). In ischaemic hepatitis, patients develop a dramatic transaminitis, raised bilirubin, and raised lactate dehydrogenase (LDH) after a very short time (e.g. 24–48 hours) following a period of haemodynamic compromise leading to liver hypoperfusion. Hepatic infarction is relatively rare compared to ischaemic hepatitis (due to the fact that the liver has a dual blood supply, which is provided by the hepatic portal vein and the hepatic arteries) and represents focal liver injury, which is usually iatrogenic. In contrast, the bile ducts receive their blood supply solely from the hepatic artery and peribiliary plexus. Any interruption of blood flow to the latter damages the perihilar intra-hepatic and extra-hepatic bile ducts, leading to ischaemic cholangiopathy.

Aetiology of cardiovascular-disease-related liver diseases

Hepatic congestion mainly results from the causes of right-sided heart failure, such as:

- congestive cardiac failure
- tricuspid regurgitation (pressure from the right ventricle is transmitted directly through to the hepatic veins so the degree of congestive hepatopathy can be severe)
- right ventricular failure (and, hence, the causes of pulmonary hypertension (e.g. mitral stenosis, severe respiratory disease))
- pericardial constriction

Many conditions can predispose to hepatic ischaemia; some are provided in Table 217.1.

Typical symptoms of cardiovascular-disease-related liver disease, and less common symptoms

In congestive hepatic disease, individuals may be asymptomatic but with deranged liver function tests (LFTs). There may be pain from stretching of the Glisson's capsule. Look for ascites, peripheral oedema, and signs of hepatosplenomegaly on examination.

In ischaemic hepatitis and hepatic infarction, a haemodynamic insult is usually apparent before the appearance of liver injury. Patients may show features of an acute hepatitis (e.g. fever, right upper quadrant pain, vomiting, and jaundice). Suspect ischaemic hepatitis and hepatic infarction in the post-transplant patient.

In ischaemic cholangiopathy, patients may present with the features of biliary obstruction (pale stools, dark urine, jaundice, and pruritus). There may also be features of a cholangitis with fever, vomiting, and rigours.

Demographics of cardiovascular-disease-related liver disease

No accurate data are available on the demographics of cardiovascular-disease-related liver disease.

Natural history of cardiovascular-disease-related liver disease, and complications of the disease

The natural course of congestive liver disease depends on that of the underlying cardiac disorder. Liver function tends to return to normal within 1 week of improvement in cardiac failure. Long-standing liver congestion and sinusoidal stasis may result in the accumulation of deoxygenated blood; parenchymal atrophy; necrosis; collagen deposition; and, ultimately, fibrosis. This rare eventuality is termed cardiac cirrhosis.

In ischaemic hepatitis, typically, there will be elevation of liver enzymes (transaminitis peaks at 24–72 hours post insult) following the hypoperfusion insult, coupled by a rise in LDH. The transaminase level will settle within a week or so following resolution of haemodynamic compromise. Following the decline in liver enzymes, the

Table 217.1 Causes of hepatic ischaemia

Ischaemic hepatitis	Focal hepatic infarction	Ischaemic cholangiopathy
Any cause of left ventricular dysfunction:	Hepatic artery thrombosis:	Paroxysmal nocturnal haemoglobinuria (hypercoagulability)
• acute myocardial infarction	• atherosclerosis	Iatrogenic:
• cardiac dysrhythmia	• prothrombotic states	• post liver transplantation
• cardiac tamponade	• post liver transplant	• vascular injury post biliary surgery
• restrictive cardiomyopathy	Embolic phenomenon:	• chemoembolization
Causes of shock:	• therapeutic embolization	• radiotherapy
• dehydration	• tumour embolization	AIDS related
• haemorrhage	• infective endocarditis	
• burns	Iatrogenic:	
• dehydration	• hepatic artery ligation during transplantation	
Focal interruption of blood supply to liver:	• chemoembolization	
• sickle cell crisis	Toxaemia of pregnancy	
• portal venous thrombosis	Vasculitides (esp. polyarteritis nodosa)	
• post-transplantation arterial thrombosis	Amphetamine use	
• any cause of left ventricular dysfunction	Dissection of the aorta	

bilirubin rises while synthetic function (clotting and albumin) usually remain unchanged. The liver recovers completely.

Ischaemia-related, non-anastomotic biliary strictures and necrosis of bile ducts are well-described complications of liver transplantation. The natural course and, consequently, prognosis of ischaemic cholangiopathy depends on the location of the blockage and underlying aetiology. In proximal hepatic artery blockade via hepatic artery ligation/embolization (outside the transplant setting), limited consequences are seen due to rapid development of collateral 'shunt' vessels and a retrograde portal supply.

In the transplanted liver, proximal blockade (thrombosis) is generally followed by severe morbidity from biliary damage. The transplanted liver differs from the non-excised liver in that excision interrupts arterial blood supply from transcapsular peripheral arteries, and therefore compromises collateralization through this route. In contrast, distal occlusion of smaller hepatic arteries has been shown (in experimental data) to cause significant ischaemic biliary injury.

Approach to diagnosing cardiovascular-disease-related liver disease

Congestive hepatic disease is more common with right-sided heart failure and should be included in the differential workup of deranged liver function in the presence of underlying cardiopulmonary disease. A clue is provided by Doppler studies of liver vasculature, with loss of the normal triphasic flow in the hepatic veins.

In contrast, suspect ischaemic hepatic injury in those with an acute hepatitis with predominant transaminitis in the presence of left ventricular dysfunction, systemic shock, or sickle cell crisis, or post liver transplant. A haemodynamic insult is usually apparent clinically before the appearance of liver injury, although transient minor reductions of hepatic perfusion may produce ischaemic injury and not be clinically apparent. The precipitating cause is usually evident before focal hepatic infarction ensues.

Ischaemic cholangiopathy should be suspected post transplant in the presence of clinical cholangitis with obstructive LFTs.

Other diagnoses that should be considered aside from cardiovascular-disease-related liver disease

Differential diagnoses of an ischaemic hepatic injury include an acute hepatitis, such as drug-induced liver injury, viral hepatitis (not just from hepatotropic viruses, such as the hepatitis A and B viruses, but also EBV, rubella, CMV, and mumps), and alcohol. These should be screened for in any case of acute hepatitis.

Three features distinguish ischaemic hepatitis from acute viral hepatitis: LDH elevation is more marked in ischaemia; serum aspartate aminotransferase (AST) and alanine aminotransferase (ALT) concentrations rapidly return to normal in ischaemic hepatitis upon correction of the underlying cause; and ischaemic hepatitis is more often complicated by renal dysfunction. It can be sometimes be difficult to differentiate between focal hepatic infarction and pyogenic liver abscess radiologically, in which case, attempt at aspiration may be helpful. Other entities which can mimic the presence of an ischaemic cholangiopathy include the various causes of biliary stricturing disease, biliary obstruction, and cholangitis (e.g. biliary, pancreatic, or duodenal malignancy; biliary stones). Another important diagnosis to consider is primary sclerosing cholangitis, although other coexisting features may also be present (e.g. history of inflammatory bowel disease or other autoimmune disease).

Gold-standard diagnostic test for cardiovascular-disease-related liver disease

Characteristic features of congestive liver disease are present on histological analysis, but biopsy is rarely needed, as other clues point towards the diagnosis. The gross histological appearance of congestive liver disease has earned it the name 'nutmeg liver'. There will be a central red area (sinusoidal congestion, bleeding into atrophic areas surrounding an enlarged hepatic vein) intermixed with a yellow area (representing fatty liver). In the absence of cardiac cirrhosis, there will be no inflammatory change. Chronic cardiac failure will cause the accumulation of collagen, with fibrous bands extending outwards from the central veins. This is the appearance of cardiac sclerosis; eventually, a micronodular cirrhosis will result.

In contrast, no real gold-standard diagnostic test for ischaemic hepatitis is available, so the diagnosis is made from the accumulation of clinical signs, biochemical tests, and, occasionally, histological tissue. Biopsy shows hepatocyte necrosis in Zone 3 (the region most poorly perfused by the hepatic artery), with architectural collapse around the central vein. With a prolonged insult, necrosis may reach the mid-zone of hepatocytes.

Concerning ischaemic cholangiopathy, following a history of the condition, definitive diagnosis can be made on cholangiography.

Other relevant investigations for cardiovascular-disease-related liver disease

In patients with congestive liver disease, echocardiography with right-sided and pulmonary pressures is essential. Doppler hepatic venous studies are also helpful. LFTs show that serum bilirubin is elevated mostly in the unconjugated form. Bilirubin concentrations rapidly (i.e. within days) return to normal following improvement of right-sided heart failure. In those who show a transaminitis, the change in AST is more marked than that in ALT. Elevated serum alkaline phosphatase (ALP) is observed in 10%–20% of patients with right-sided heart failure, but ALP levels return to normal within 1 week after improvement of heart failure. Other investigations focus on diagnosing the cause of cardiac failure. A high LDH favours the diagnosis of ischaemic hepatitis over that of an acute viral hepatitis. In hepatic infarction, an abdominal CT scan may reveal a wedge-shaped low-attenuation area indicating the infarct.

Prognosis for cardiovascular-disease-related liver disease, and how to estimate it

The prognosis for congestive liver disease depends on the aetiology of the underlying cardiac failure, as well as its severity and reversibility. Ischaemic hepatitis usually has a benign prognosis, once resolution of the underlying problem has taken place. However, if it is superimposed on underlying cirrhotic liver disease or cardiac failure, fulminant liver failure may occur. There is limited data on the management of ischaemic cholangiopathy and, thus, outcome after treatment. If it occurs in the first 4 weeks or so post liver transplant, retransplantation is indicated.

Treatment of cardiovascular-disease-related liver disease, and its effectiveness

In congestive liver disease, right upper quadrant discomfort rapidly resolves with **effective** diuretic treatment; the remainder of management rests on cardiac failure therapy. In ischaemic liver disease, treatment rests on that of the underlying condition. Little data are available regarding the effectiveness of treatment of ischaemic cholangiopathy but there is some evidence for endoscopic dilatation and stenting of strictures. Disease occurring in the first month post transplantation warrants urgent retransplantation.

Sepsis-induced liver dysfunction

Definition of sepsis-induced liver dysfunction

The liver is a key organ in sepsis, both as source of inflammatory mediators and as a victim of the inflammatory response. The two main characteristics that illustrate this 'dual' role are:

- the heterogeneous cellular makeup of the liver: Kupffer cells, hepatocytes, and cells lining the sinusoidal endothelium are all involved in the immune response
- the liver's unique blood flow: the portal vein receives blood from the splanchnic circulation; in sepsis there can be marked vasoconstriction and translocation of harmful pathogens across this vascular bed

As an active participant in the response to sepsis, the liver will scavenge, attempt to inactivate bacterial products, and modify its metabolic functions towards amino acid synthesis and increased gluconeogenesis. There will be increased production and release of coagulation factors, complement, and acute phase proteins.

As a victim in sepsis, the liver can suffer primary dysfunction related to shock and hypoperfusion (see discussion of ischaemic hepatitis in 'The liver in cardiovascular disease'), or secondary dysfunction, which is more related to microcirculatory changes in the hepatic circulation. Secondary dysfunction is insidious in its presentation and is characterized by functional and structural hepatic injury, as well as bacterial and endotoxin spillover, with the liver becoming the source of soluble mediators in the systemic inflammatory response syndrome. Cholestasis is also a common complication in patients with extra-hepatic bacterial infections and sepsis and is increasingly recognized as a cause of jaundice in hospitalized patients, as part of the secondary dysfunction triggered by a burst of inflammatory mediators.

As hypoxic liver injury has already been discussed (see 'The liver in cardiovascular disease'), the bulk of the discussion in this section primarily focuses on sepsis-induced jaundice and cholestasis.

Aetiology of sepsis-induced liver dysfunction

Sepsis-induced jaundice occurs most frequently with Gram-negative bacteria. The primary site of infection is usually intra-abdominal (e.g. peritonitis, diverticulitis) but can be from a pneumonia or endocarditis. Other specific extra-hepatic infections known to cause jaundice are pneumococcus, clostridia, legionella, and typhoid infections.

Jaundice can occur in isolation in patients with sepsis, but is frequently associated with other elements of cholestasis. As the principal clinical manifestation of cholestasis is also jaundice, literature to date has primarily focused on the sepsis syndrome of jaundice with cholestasis. Accurate epidemiological documentation regarding the incidence of isolated jaundice (without cholestasis) in sepsis remains unclear. Possible causes of jaundice in sepsis are:

- aberrant processing of bilirubin by hepatocytes
- increased bilirubin load from haemolysis
- hepatocellular injury
- cholestasis (decreased bile acid transport secondary to lipopolysaccharide and various cytokines)
- antibiotics/drugs

Typical symptoms of sepsis-induced liver dysfunction, and less common symptoms

Functional cholestasis with jaundice usually predominates as the liver manifestation in sepsis. Ischaemic hepatitis or progressive sclerosing cholangitis can be found in severe cases, with the presentation varying according to the severity of the infection. Primary hepatic dysfunction can lead to disseminated intravascular coagulation; reduced lactate and amino acid clearance; and reduced gluconeogenesis and glycogenolysis, thus leading to hypoglycaemia. A raised LDH with transaminase leakage can be seen, reflecting hepatocyte injury. Reduced perfusion appears to be the primary initiating event here (caused by reduced cardiac output with the vasoconstriction of hepatic artery and portal veins that is observed in sepsis). Secondary hepatic dysfunction may be silent and involve localized hepatic areas, which become inflamed as a consequence of bacterial detoxification by Kupffer cells. This induces activation of the coagulation, kallikrein, and complement cascades.

Demographics of sepsis-induced liver dysfunction

Sepsis and bacterial infection are responsible for up to 20% of cases of jaundice seen in all patient groups. Sepsis with jaundice is more likely to present in children than in adults.

Natural history of sepsis-induced liver dysfunction, and complications of the disease

Cholestasis usually resolves with the appropriate antibiotics. Persistent/worsening hyperbilirubinemia can indicate ongoing sepsis and is associated with a worse outcome. Persistently high ALP and gamma-glutamyl transpeptidase (γGT) levels should raise suspicion of progressive sclerosing cholangitis due to sepsis. Ischaemic hepatitis usually resolves on correction of haemodynamic instability and hypoxia.

Approach to diagnosing sepsis-induced liver dysfunction

Sepsis-related cholestasis gives rise to a hyperbilirubinemia (mostly conjugated) with a modest rise in ALP and transaminases in the presence of a normal LDH. Resolution should occur with appropriate antibiotic therapy. Ischaemic hepatitis is discussed in 'The liver in cardiovascular-disease-related liver disease'.

Other diagnoses that should be considered aside from sepsis-induced liver dysfunction

Other diagnoses that should be considered aside from sepsis-induced liver dysfunction are:

- antibiotic-induced liver dysfunction (see Chapter 215)
- progressive sclerosing cholangitis: this can occur following severe sepsis, burns, or severe trauma; patients with this disease have rising levels of ALP and γGT, and deep jaundice over several months; as this disease tends to involve the smaller bile ducts, diagnosis is usually confirmed on cholangiography (severe intra-hepatic stenosis); prognosis is usually poor
- cholecystitis
- structural biliary tract obstruction
- parenteral nutrition
- liver abscess

Gold-standard diagnostic test for sepsis-induced liver dysfunction

Biopsy is occasionally needed for diagnosis of sepsis-induced liver dysfunction and demonstrates the following characteristic findings in cholestasis:

- Kupffer cell hyperplasia
- portal mononuclear cell infiltrates
- an increased amount of smooth endoplasmic reticulum as a result of cholestasis; this may lead to hepatocytes having a ground-glass appearance
- focal hepatocyte dropout

Acceptable diagnostic alternatives to the gold-standard test for sepsis-induced liver dysfunction

A thorough history, examination, and investigation of the septic illness, coupled with exclusion of other common causes of jaundice, usually suffice in achieving the diagnosis.

Other relevant investigations for sepsis-induced liver dysfunction

Other relevant investigations for sepsis-induced liver dysfunction include:

- split bilirubin (to help evaluate the cause of jaundice in sepsis)
- hepatobiliary ultrasound
- full septic screen, including
  - blood
  - urine
  - lines and drains
  - recent operation sites
  - lumbar puncture (if appropriate and safe)
  - chest X-ray

Prognosis for sepsis-induced liver dysfunction, and how to estimate it

In the absence of systemic signs of sepsis, the cholestasis that can accompany an extra-hepatic bacterial infection is usually mild and of no prognostic significance. Should sepsis develop (with systemic features), jaundice is associated with a poor prognosis, and most patients with sepsis-associated cholestasis die from extra-hepatic causes associated with sepsis-related multiple organ failure. It is crucial that emphasis is placed on identifying the focus of infection and providing treatment by appropriate antibiotic therapy and other anti-infective strategies (e.g. aspiration or drainage of collections).

Treatment of sepsis-induced liver dysfunction, and its effectiveness

The cornerstone of the treatment of sepsis-induced liver dysfunction rests on appropriate antibiotic therapy and effective management of the complications of sepsis. Ursodeoxycholic acid has been shown to improve parameters in other cholestatic diseases, but its use in sepsis-induced cholestasis is still under investigation.

The liver in malignancy

Definition of malignancy-related liver disease

There are many ways in which an oncological process may affect hepatic function. For example, tumours in and around the liver can affect function by directly reducing the volume of healthy, functioning tissue or by causing biliary obstruction. In addition, portal venous infiltration or hypercoagulability may compromise vascular supply. Paraneoplastic phenomena have been well documented, and humoral and immunological factors related to the primary malignancy are known to contribute to further cholestasis and inflammatory hepatic changes. Underlying malignancy may also affect hepatic drug metabolism (tumour cells release a host of cytokines as part of an inflammatory response which reduce the activity of certain cytochrome enzymes). Other ways that malignancy can affect hepatic function include:

* chemotherapy-induced hepatotoxicity
* graft-versus-host disease
* metastases of cancer cells to the liver

In-depth discussion regarding the latter two points is beyond the scope of this section and will not be discussed further.

Aetiology of malignancy-related liver disease

The chronic myeloproliferative disorders (including polycythaemia rubra vera and essential thrombocythemia) tend to cause damage or blockage to the hepatic circulation and can lead to:

* Budd–Chiari syndrome
* portal vein thrombosis (PVT)
* nodular regenerative hyperplasia (see Chapter 216)

These topics will form the bulk of the discussion in this section.

Other haematological malignancies that lead to liver disease

Acute leukaemia in liver disease

Hepatic involvement is mild in the initial stages of leukaemia, and so patients may initially be asymptomatic. Acute lymphocytic leukaemia (ALL) generally gives rise to portal tract infiltration only, whereas infiltration in acute myeloid leukaemia (AML) involves the sinusoids also.

Chronic leukaemia in liver disease

Mild-to-moderate hepatomegaly, together with extensive infiltration by lymphocytes with consequent impairment of liver function, is observed in chronic lymphoid leukaemia (CLL). Half of all cases of chronic myeloid leukaemia at presentation will show hepatomegaly. During blast crises, infiltration of sinusoids can cause massive liver enlargement.

Myelofibrosis in liver disease

Liver enlargement is present in most patients, in keeping with extramedullary haemopoiesis and increased hepatic blood flow. Nodular regenerative hyperplasia (see Chapter 216: Miscellaneous liver diseases) may accompany intra-hepatic portal vein obstruction.

Lymphoma in liver disease

In lymphoma, infiltration of the liver by malignant cells, leading to hepatomegaly, may be seen. A mild transaminitis and a relatively greater increase in ALP can also occur due to tumour infiltration. These are more common in non-Hodgkin's than in Hodgkin's lymphoma. Cholestasis not due to extra-hepatic duct obstruction or infiltrative disease has also been described. Acute liver failure may also occur.

Myeloma in liver disease

Sinusoidal and portal infiltration occurs in up to 50% of cases. There may also be nodular regenerative hyperplasia. Extramedullary haemopoiesis may also contribute to hepatomegaly and deranged LFTs.

Specific solid tumours in the liver

Stauffer syndrome is a constellation of signs and symptoms of liver dysfunction that arises due to the presence of renal cell carcinoma, but it is not due to tumour infiltration into the liver and/or intrinsic liver disease: it is a true paraneoplastic syndrome. It leads to elevated LFTs, which result from cholestasis (i.e. a cessation of bile flow). The symptoms resolve if the renal cell cancer is successfully treated.

Typical symptoms of malignancy-related liver disease, and less common symptoms

Budd–Chiari syndrome (hepatic venous outflow obstruction, of the hepatic vein, the inferior vena cava (IVC), or both) causes congestion, necrosis, and, eventually, fibrotic change and cirrhosis. Features include abdominal pain, hepatomegaly, jaundice, ascites, and hepatic failure with features of decompensation. PVT (in any part of the portal circulation, including the mesenteric system, the splenic vein, and the intra-hepatic veins) can also present with features of portal hypertension and hepatic decompensation (e.g. variceal bleeding and ascites).

Demographics of malignancy-related liver disease

Hepatomegaly is found in the majority of individuals with ALL or AML, at the time of diagnosis. CLL is largely an incidental finding, with most patients being asymptomatic, so most of the demographics on hepatic involvement in CLL come from post-mortem studies; one study revealed that 98% of patients with CLL had hepatic leukaemic infiltration at autopsy. In myeloma, sinusoidal and portal infiltration occurs in up to 50% of cases and, in 10% of cases, there will be immunoglobulin light chain deposition or amyloid in the space of Disse; there may also be non-specific changes, such as haemosiderosis, in a smaller percentage of patients. Budd–Chiari syndrome is rare in Western countries. The exact frequency of PVT in malignancy is unknown; however, it occurs in approximately 5% of patients with cirrhosis and portal hypertension.

Natural history of malignancy-related liver disease, and complications of the disease

The natural history of malignancy-related, veno-occlusive liver disease is not well known and its manifestation can change from asymptomatic presentation to fulminant liver failure in a matter of days to weeks. A chronic form of Budd–Chiari progresses over a matter of months, and rapid deterioration with encephalopathy, renal failure, coma, and death can occur in untreated disease. In extensive PVT, the patient may present with mesenteric ischaemia. The natural history of hepatic involvement in other haematological malignancies is dependent on the underlying disorder.

Approach to diagnosing malignancy-related liver disease

In Budd–Chiari syndrome, obstruction of hepatic venous drainage leads to elevated sinusoidal pressure, dilatation, and congestion. This leads to portal hypertension. When all three hepatic veins are obstructed, drainage from the caudate lobe (through separate spigelian veins) directly into the IVC becomes the only route of drainage, and this leads to caudate hypertrophy. This can be observed on Doppler ultrasound, CT, or MRI angiography. Absence of flow in the hepatic veins, as well as other features of portal hypertension, may also be seen.

In PVT, simple imaging may identify splenomegaly with or without hepatomegaly and an enlarged azygous vein. Ultrasound may demonstrate a lack of normal portal flow or the presence of a thrombus in the portal vein.

Table 217.2 Predisposing factors for hepatic veno-occlusive disease

Myeloproliferative disorders	Prothrombotic disorders	Other malignancies	Vascular disorders	Infections	Other
Polycythaemia rubra vera	Factor V Leiden	Hepatocellular carcinoma	Behçet's syndrome	Amoebic abscesses	Pregnancy
Essential thrombocythemia	Protein C deficiency	Adrenal cancer	Sjögren's syndrome	Pyogenic abscesses	Oral contraceptives
Myeloid leukaemia	Lupus anticoagulant	Renal cancer		Echinococcus infections	Cirrhotic liver disease
	Paroxysmal nocturnal haemoglobinuria	Leiomyosarcoma			Splenectomy
	Homocystinuria				

Other diagnoses that should be considered aside from malignancy-related liver disease

Other diagnoses that should be considered aside from malignancy-related liver disease include:

- other predisposing factors for hepatic veno-occlusive disease (see Table 217.2)
- congestive cardiac failure
- constrictive pericarditis
- IVC web (a common cause of Budd–Chiari syndrome in the East)

The main cause of PVT in children is sepsis with dehydration and consequent haemoconcentration. In adults, cirrhosis, pancreatic cancer, and hepatomas are other major causes.

Gold-standard diagnostic test for malignancy-related liver disease

Hepatic venography may show the characteristic 'spider-web' appearance of intra-hepatic veins in Budd–Chiari syndrome. This may also demonstrate non-patency of the IVC. Contrast-enhanced CT can identify portal vein patency and any thrombi within.

Acceptable diagnostic alternatives to the gold-standard test for malignancy-related liver disease

A liver biopsy is also crucial in Budd–Chiari syndrome. Pathological findings are a high-grade venous congestion and centrilobular liver cell atrophy. There may be thrombi within the terminal hepatic venules. The presence of necrosis or end-stage fibrosis indicates a need for urgent decompression.

Other relevant investigations for malignancy-related liver disease

Other relevant investigations for malignancy-related liver disease include:

- ascitic fluid analysis (serum ascites: albumin gradient <1.1)
- endoscopy, to identify varices
- other tests as part of a chronic liver disease screen
- investigations for possible underlying malignancy and other possible causes

Prognosis for malignancy-related liver disease, and how to estimate it

The following features have been shown to indicate a favourable prognosis in Budd–Chiari syndrome:

- younger age at diagnosis
- a low Child–Pugh score

- the absence of ascites, or easily controlled ascites
- a low serum creatinine level

The 5-year survival rate for Budd–Chiari syndrome is 38%–87%, following portosystemic shunting. The 5-year survival rate following liver transplantation is 70%. The prognosis is poor in patients who have Budd–Chiari syndrome and remain untreated or have venous occlusion caused by malignancy. There is high mortality in untreated cases of Budd–Chiari syndrome, with death resulting from progressive liver failure at 3 months to 3 years from the time of diagnosis.

In contrast, PVT has a much better prognosis, with 75% of patients alive after 10 years and an overall mortality rate of less than 10%. In the presence of cirrhosis and malignancy, the prognosis is understandably worse and is dependent upon the underlying condition.

Treatment for malignancy-related liver disease, and its effectiveness

The aims of treatment in Budd–Chiari syndrome are threefold:

- to relieve hepatic congestion
- to preserve histology
- to preserve synthetic function

Diuretics are helpful for the management of ascites, and chronic anticoagulation may prevent further clot formation. Thrombolysis is only useful in the acute situation, but is risky. In cases of portal hypertension, decompression of the hepatic vasculature should be offered. Transjugular intra-hepatic portosystemic shunts can be used as a bridge to transplantations, but is not without complication. Surgical decompression is also an option, and transplantation is recommended for those in fulminant liver failure. Medical therapy cannot prevent progression of liver disease or reverse hepatic congestion.

As most patients with PVT present with variceal bleeding, this should be an essential focus of treatment, both during an acute episode and also in prevention of further bleeding events (see Chapters 23, 210, and 206). Mesenteric ischaemia warrants further surgical intervention.

Further Reading

Field KM, Dow C, and Michael M. Part I: Liver function in oncology: Biochemistry and beyond. *Lancet Oncol* 2008; 9: 1092–101.
Malnick S, Melzer E, Sokolowski N, et al. The involvement of the liver in systemic diseases. *J Clin Gastroenterol* 2008; 42: 69–80.

218 Liver cancer

Satish Keshav and Palak Trivedi

Definition of the disease

Primary hepatocellular carcinoma (HCC) arises from hepatocytes and is one of the commonest solid-organ malignancies in the world, particularly in the Far East and in sub-Saharan Africa. Cholangiocarcinoma arises from the biliary epithelium. The incidence is rising in the West, and primary sclerosing cholangitis (PSC) is an important risk factor (15% lifetime risk).

Other forms of liver cancer include metastatic cancer, hepatoblastoma, haemangiosarcoma, and gall bladder cancer. Metastatic cancer is much more common in the West than any primary liver cancer, accounting for 90% of liver cancers, and its common primary sites are the colon, the stomach, the breasts, and the lungs. Hepatoblastoma is an uncommon malignancy in children, originating from immature liver cell precursors. Haemangiosarcomas are also rare; these are malignant tumours arising from the blood vessels in the liver and can be very rapidly growing. Gall bladder cancer arises from the gall bladder epithelium. Gallstones and PSC are risk factors for gall bladder cancer; in particular, PSC confers a risk >160 times that of the control population.

The remainder of this chapter will primarily focus on HCC.

Aetiology of the disease

The great majority of HCC develops in cirrhotic liver, and all causes of cirrhosis are associated with an increased risk of HCC. Secondary metastases are said to be less frequent in cirrhotic liver. Chronic hepatitis C is associated with about one-third of HCC cases worldwide. Chronic hepatitis B is associated with over half of all HCC cases worldwide. Viral integration into the hepatocyte DNA may confer a direct oncogenic effect and, in those infected early in life, HCC may develop in the absence of established cirrhosis.

Other causes of HCC include alcoholic liver cirrhosis (alcohol also confers increased risk in patients with coexisting viral hepatitis), haemochromatosis, which is associated with a 45% lifetime risk in cirrhotic individuals, fatty liver disease, and alpha-1-antitrypsin deficiency. Cirrhosis from autoimmune hepatitis, primary biliary cholangitis (PBC), or PSC also increases the risk of HCC, although the incidence is clearly dwarfed by viral and metabolic liver diseases in particular.

A rare, autosomally recessive glycogen storage disorder, von Gierke disease, may cause hepatic adenomas that can transform to HCC. In contrast, hepatic adenomas associated with the use of the oral contraceptive pill (OCP) rarely or never transform.

Another important etiological factor for the development of HCC is exposure to aflatoxins, which are produced by many species of the fungal genus aspergillus. Aflatoxin-producing aspergillus can colonize and contaminate foods such as cereals, groundnuts, and sunflower seeds during periods of prolonged storage.

Typical symptoms of the disease, and less common symptoms

HCC should be considered in any patient who has established cirrhosis and develops features of hepatic decompensation, ascites, an increased liver size, or jaundice over a very short period of time. Rarely, a hepatic arterial bruit may be audible; however, this can also be heard in acute alcoholic hepatitis.

HCC can have distinct patterns of growth:

- nodular: multiple nodules of varying size throughout the liver (this is the most common form)
- solitary: larger, solitary masses (more common in younger patients; these can be massive)
- diffuse: widespread infiltration of minute tumour foci

Demographics of the disease

HCC accounts for ~80% of primary liver cancers. The incidence is increasing and, at present, is about 2–3 per 100 000 in Europe and the US. Much higher rates of 90 per 100 000 are observed in the Far East. The incidence of HCC increases progressively with advancing age in all populations, reaching a peak at 70 years. The mean age of onset in Chinese and black patients is much earlier. The age differences and higher incidence of HCC in Asia and Africa (85% of all HCC cases worldwide) are largely related to viral hepatitis. In addition, the disease is more prevalent in men than in women (4:1).

Natural history, and complications of the disease

The median survival for those diagnosed with HCC is poor. This is usually because of advanced disease being present at time of symptom presentation. This issue is discussed further in 'Prognosis and how to estimate it'.

Approach to diagnosing the disease

International guidelines advocate that individuals with established liver cirrhosis be surveyed for HCC via ultrasound scanning every 6 months (Table 218.1). Select individuals with chronic hepatitis B infection in the absence of cirrhosis are also at risk of HCC, although the evidence base for offering surveillance to non-cirrhotic individuals with chronic liver disease is contentious.

Finding the following features on initial assessment should always raise suspicion of HCC, particularly in the context of existing cirrhotic liver disease:

- hepatomegaly, with or without bruit
- haemorrhagic ascites
- acute rise in alkaline phosphatase
- secondary polycythaemia (a paraneoplastic phenomenon)
- pyrexia of unknown origin

Table 218.1 Groups in whom surveillance for hepatocellular carcinoma is recommended by international guidelines

Population group	Incidence of hepatocellular carcinoma (%/year)
Non-cirrhotic hepatitis B males >age 40	0.2
Non-cirrhotic hepatitis B females >age 50	0.2
African/North American blacks with hepatitis B	0.2
Cirrhotic hepatitis B carriers or non-cirrhotic carrier with family history of hepatocellular carcinoma	2.5–8.0
Hepatitis C cirrhosis	2.0–8.0
Stage 4 primary biliary cholangitis	3.0–11.0
Genetic haemochromatosis and cirrhosis	3.0–4.0
Alpha-1-antitrypsin deficiency and cirrhosis	Unknown, but probably >1.5

Other diagnoses that should be considered

The differential diagnosis must distinguish between other causes of hepatic decompensation in a patient with previously stable chronic liver disease (see Chapter 210), other tumours of the hepatobiliary system (malignant and benign), and abscesses and anomalies on ultrasound scanning that may simulate a focal liver mass. It includes:

- cholangiocarcinoma
- hepatic adenoma:
  - increased risk with oestrogen use (was rarely seen prior to the use of OCPs)
  - can spontaneously rupture during menstruation or pregnancy
  - can progress to HCC
  - although surgical resection is usually offered, hepatic ademonas have been known to remit once the etiological agent (usually OCP) has been removed
- haemangioma:
  - this is a common benign hepatic tumour (develops in 20% of the normal population), occurring more commonly in women as a single, asymptomatic mass
  - usually located in the right lobe, existing as a blood-filled vascular sinusoid
  - risks of tumour growth or bleeding are minimal
  - intervention is usually not needed
- focal nodular hyperplasia:
  - a round, non-encapsulated mass with a vascular scar and with fibrous septa radiating from the scar like 'bicycle spokes from a central hub', with hepatocytes in-between
  - the second most common benign liver tumour
  - although not thought to cause the anomaly, OCPs have been shown to enhance its growth once the lesion is already present, and should be stopped
  - resection is not usually necessary
- focal fatty infiltration:
  - often seen in alcoholism, obesity, diabetes, retroviral disease, and starvation
  - can look similar to focal liver lesions; once the underlying disease process is corrected, this appearance rapidly disappears
- liver abscesses and cysts (discussed in further detail in Chapter 216).

Gold-standard diagnostic test

A single, universally acceptable diagnostic test for liver cancer does not exist. Ultrasound scanning (USS) has a sensitivity of 58%–89% and a specificity of >90% and is the first imaging modality of choice when suspecting HCC. However, diagnosing HCC radiologically on a background of nodular cirrhosis can be challenging. Once concern of HCC has been raised with USS, additional radiological modalities should be employed in order to confirm the diagnosis (Figure 218.1).

Current guidelines advocate that lesions <1 cm in diameter should be followed up with a repeat USS in 4 months. Lesions 1–2 cm in diameter should be followed up by means of two consecutive radiological tests: a four-phase-contrasted CT and a contrast-enhanced MRI. However, some experienced centres may rely on only one modality if the lesion appears 'bright' during the arterial phase before 'washing out' in the late/venous phase. This radiological finding is characteristic of an HCC lesion, which receives its blood supply from the hepatic artery, and thus helps to differentiate HCC from relatively hypovascular tumours (e.g. metastasis). Lesions >2 cm in diameter require confirmation by only one of the contrast-enhanced investigations.

Acceptable diagnostic alternatives to the gold standard

Liver biopsy, even with expert histopathology, is not as reliable as might be expected because well-differentiated HCC can resemble the surrounding cirrhotic liver parenchyma. Moreover, liver biopsy may lead to 'tumour seeding' along the biopsy tract. Nonetheless, this remains a useful tool in investigating indeterminate lesions or in situations which preclude more advanced imaging techniques (e.g. contrast allergy, pacemaker insertion).

Other relevant investigations

Alpha-fetoprotein (αFP) is the most widely used serum biomarker, although its use as a marker is no longer advocated for surveillance. When combined with USS, αFP provides additional detection of HCC in only 6%–8% of cases. When used as a diagnostic test, αFP values of 20 ng/ml show good sensitivity but poor specificity.

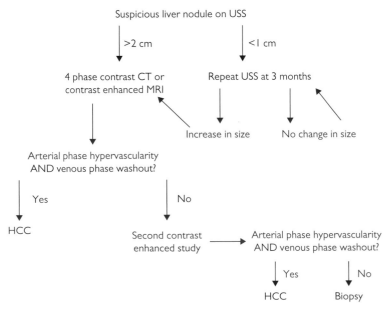

Figure 218.1 Approach to diagnosing hepatocellular carcinoma; HCC, hepatocellular carcinoma; USS, ultrasound.

Conversely, when using a cut-off of 200 ng/ml, the specificity is high but sensitivity falls to 22%. Furthermore, only 10%–20% of small tumours may lead to an elevated serum αFP level.

Efforts to uncover the underlying aetiology (e.g. hepatitis B virus, hepatitis C virus) should be made, as this has implications for further treatment as well as for family screening. Full-body staging CT should also be undertaken as part of the workup to identify distant metastasis.

Prognosis and how to estimate it

Based on data reporting the natural history of the disease, the main clinical prognostic factors in HCC patients are related to tumour number; the size of the nodules; the presence of vascular invasion and/or extra-hepatic spread; liver function (Child–Pugh's score, bilirubin, albumin); portal hypertension; and the premorbid state. Aetiology has not been identified as an independent risk factor. When a HCC is detected due to symptoms, survival can be as little as 12 weeks. However, in broad terms, 5-year survival when picked up through screening programmes can approach 50%.

In untreated disease, death can occur due to liver failure or metastatic disease. Unfortunately, most patients have non-resectable disease with prognosis depending more on the state of the liver rather than on tumour size alone. The tumour size, however, helps predict the likelihood of major venous involvement, whereas the Child–Pugh score is useful in predicting perioperative survival following surgical resection.

Treatment and its effectiveness

The Barcelona Clinic Liver Cancer (BCLC) score is the most widely used staging system in the West. It is very useful in deciding amongst potential treatment options and correlates best with patient outcome. A detailed discussion of the different staging systems is beyond the scope of this chapter, although we turn the reader's attention to the recent European Association for the Study of the Liver guidelines for further reading. Using the BCLC criteria, available treatment options can be stratified depending on the size, number, and location of tumours; the presence or absence of cirrhosis; operative risk factors based on extent of cirrhosis and comorbidity; overall performance status; portal vein pressure/patency; and presence of metastases.

Any decision regarding treatment should take place in a specialist centre with expertise in dealing with HCC, and in a multidisciplinary meeting with radiologists, hepatologists, surgeons, oncologists, specialist nurses, and histopathologists. However, a brief discussion of the different modalities is provided in this section. Up until recently, surgical resection and liver transplantation were the only chances of cure. However, newer treatment modalities show promise in those patients not meeting criteria for surgical intervention. Local ablative therapies in particular can be used either as a bridge to transplant by reducing tumour progression, or as a palliative procedure to extend disease-free survival.

Surgical treatments

Resection

Resection is the operation of choice in patients with tumours <2 cm in diameter and with well-compensated liver disease. Amongst patients who undergo successful resection, long-term survival is possible, with 5-year survival rates of up to 74% in patients without significant decompensation. Unfortunately, less than 5% of candidates are suitable for this procedure at time of diagnosis, and those with cirrhosis tolerate resection less well. Moreover, up to 75% of cirrhotic patients will develop intra-hepatic recurrence within 5 years, due to either de novo HCC or local intra-hepatic metastasis. Clinically evident portal hypertension is a significant predictor of poor outcome with significant resection, and resection of more than two liver segments is thus contraindicated in individuals with Child–Pugh Class B or C. Selection criteria for resection include:

- non-cirrhotics/Child–Pugh Class A
- solitary lesion <2 cm in diameter
- lack of vascular involvement or extra-hepatic spread

A distinctive variant of HCC known as the 'fibrolamellar variant' is a slow-growing tumour occurring in the third decade. Patients seldom have a history of previous liver disease. This most commonly occurs in the left lobe, presenting as pain. Histologically, neoplastic hepatocytes are separated by thin layers of fibrosis. It is important to recognize these variants, as nearly one-half are amenable to resection. Post-transplant survival appears to be equivalent to that of 'classical' HCC.

Transplantation

Transplantation has the potential to not only eliminate the cancer but also cure underlying liver disease; thus, it is often the treatment of choice in patients with cirrhosis. Only about 5% of HCC patients are suitable; however, down-staged disease following embolization or radiofrequency ablation (RFA) may confer suitability for transplantation. This option should be considered in the following cases:

- solitary lesion ≤5 cm in diameter
- nodular disease with <3 nodules, each ≤3 cm in diameter
- no metastatic or regional node involvement
- no vascular invasion

Carefully selected individuals with established cirrhosis and a single HCC lesion ≤5 cm in diameter, or up to three HCC lesions all ≤3 cm in diameter, have a 4-year overall survival rate of 85% and a tumour-free survival rate of 92% with liver transplantation (these are known as the Milan criteria). Survival for patients with much larger tumours is below 50%.

Ablative therapies

Tumour ablation is probably as effective as surgical resection in cirrhotic patients. Possible approaches that can be considered include percutaneous ethanol injection (PEI) and RFA.

PEI into the tumour can lead to complete ablation in up to 70% of lesions ≤3 cm in diameter. This requires several sessions but 3-year survival rates of 40%–79% have been achieved depending on the severity of underlying liver disease. However, PEI can result in tumour seeding, and treated lesions have a high rate of local recurrence (33%–43%). This technique is rarely used nowadays and has largely been superseded by more advanced modalities.

RFA is useful for smaller tumours and, compared with PEI, is associated with an improved recurrence-free survival at 24 months (64% vs 43%). Complication rates are low but may include fever, pain, bleeding, pleural effusion, haematoma, and an intermittent transaminitis.

Embolization

Trans-arterial embolization, or trans-arterial chemo-embolization (TACE), is now the most widely used treatment for non-resectable HCC. The rationale is that intra-arterial infusion of a cytotoxic agent (usually doxorubicin or cisplatin), followed by embolization of the tumour-feeding blood vessels, will result in a strong cytotoxic and ischaemic antitumour effect. Patients require well-preserved liver function and, before instituting definitive therapy, it is best to treat the complications of cirrhosis, using diuretics with or without paracentesis, for ascites; lactulose, for encephalopathy and control of variceal bleeding; and antibiotics, for spontaneous bacterial peritonitis.

The efficacy of TACE appears to be dependent on careful patient selection, although a reduction in tumour burden can be achieved in 16%–61% of treated patients. A 2-year survival rate of 63% has been achieved in patients with Child–Pugh A cirrhosis, an absence of cancer-related symptoms, and large or multinodular HCC with no vascular invasion or extra-hepatic metastasis. However, patients with portal vein invasion achieve 2-year survival rates of only 31%. This is still superior to that of the untreated control group (2-year survival, 11%). TACE has thus been established as the standard of care for patients with multinodular HCC, relatively preserved liver function, an absence of cancer-related symptoms, and no evidence of vascular invasion or extra-hepatic spread.

The tolerability of conventional TACE seems to be affected by the type of regimen and the frequency of the treatment. The most common complication is postembolization syndrome, which is characterized by fever, elevated alanine aminotransferase levels, and abdominal pain; it occurs in 32%–80% of treated patients. TACE is contraindicated in patients with advanced cirrhosis and hepatic decompensation because the ischaemic damage associated with embolization can lead to a rapid decline in liver function with worsening encephalopathy, increased ascites, and, ultimately, death.

Synergistic and combination therapies

Locoregional therapies have long been used in the setting of combined treatment strategies. An accepted indication is the use of interventional treatment in patients awaiting transplantation, to prevent tumour progression when the waiting time exceeds 6 months. Moreover, preliminary data suggests that both RFA and TACE may be able to 'down-stage' patients with larger tumours to the point of patients meeting the Milan transplant criteria.

The combined use of TACE and tumour ablation techniques is very popular in the treatment of HCC tumours of intermediate size (i.e. 3–7 cm in diameter). Despite promising results, no robust randomized controlled trial comparing the efficacy of combined techniques over monotherapy has been completed so far.

Newer modalities

Many patients with advanced HCC are not candidates for surgical resection, liver transplantation, or localized ablation. Unfortunately, HCC is a relatively chemotherapy-resistant tumour. Moreover, chemotherapy is usually not well tolerated and seems to be less efficacious in patients with HCC with underlying hepatic dysfunction. Younger patients with well-compensated cirrhosis have better outcomes with chemotherapy than older patients or those with alcoholic cirrhosis, and may be a candidate for entry into clinical trials.

Sorafenib (a multitargeted oral kinase inhibitor) has recently been shown in a Phase III trial to slightly prolong survival (up to 14.7 months) in select patients with HCC.

Anti-angiogenesis agents (e.g. bevacizumab) work by disrupting the formation of blood vessels that feed tumours. The highly vascular nature of HCC suggests that the use of such agents may be effective in combination with the chemotherapy agents gemcitabine and oxaliplatin. However, bevacizumab is not currently licensed for use in the UK.

Palliative care

For patients with Child Class C cirrhosis and contraindications to transplantation or entry to clinical trials, any further intervention has the potential to result in progressive hepatic decompensation. In these patients, treatment focuses on managing pain, ascites, oedema, and encephalopathy. Patients with large tumours have a short life expectancy, and care should be designed to preserve and enhance quality of life. Early referral to palliative care practitioners should be considered.

Further Reading

El-Serag HB. Hepatocellular carcinoma. *N Engl J Med* 2011; 365: 1118–27.
European Association for the Study of the Liver, European Organization for Research and Treatment of Cancer. EASL-EORTC Clinical Practice Guidelines: Management of hepatocellular carcinoma. *J Hepatol* 2012; 56: 908–43.

PART 10

Neurological disorders

219 Normal neurological function

Dirk Bäumer

Introduction

A basic understanding of the anatomy and physiology of the nervous system is necessary in order to understand and diagnose neurological disease. This chapter will give a brief outline of those aspects of neuroanatomy and neurophysiology which are helpful in daily clinical practice and form the basis of the clinical neurological method outlined in Chapter 220.

Consciousness

A simple operational definition of consciousness includes awareness of the self and the environment, and responsiveness to external stimulation. This implies content (awareness of something) as well as arousal and alertness. Arousal is thought to be mediated by the ascending reticular activating system (RAS), which is located in the upper brainstem and diencephalon (medial thalamus) and has reciprocal connections with wide parts of the cerebral cortex. Localized lesions of the RAS or interruption of its diffuse connections will lead to diminished arousal, which manifests as disturbance of consciousness. This could be a mild reduction of attention; confusion; drowsiness; or coma.

Cognition

Intact arousal and attention are prerequisites for all other cognitive processes, including memory and executive function, which can be secondarily impaired by attentional deficits. Attention, memory, and executive function are examples of functions that are anatomically distributed over different parts and both hemispheres of the brain.

Episodic memory function is dependent upon structures in the diencephalon (mamillary bodies and thalamus), basal forebrain nuclei, and medial temporal lobe structures including the hippocampal formations and their related structures on both sides. These structures are connected in the 'circuit of Papez' of the extended limbic system. Note that the thalamus comprises a group of nuclei with diverse functions not only in cognition but also in the relay of motor, sensory, and visual information.

Executive function—goal-directed behaviour, planning, initiating action, monitoring action, and shifting attention to different tasks—is attributed to the frontal lobes, as are social cognition, inhibitory control, and aspects of emotion.

Other functions are localized and/or lateralized to more specific brain regions, such as, for example:

- language: dominant hemisphere (peri-Sylvian region)
- praxis (i.e. the ability to perform learned skilled motor acts) and calculation: dominant parietal lobe
- visuospatial skills, constructional ability, and prosody (the rhythm and intonation of speech): non-dominant hemisphere

See Table 219.1 for an abbreviated list of the localization of cognitive functions and deficits arising from lesions.

Motor function

Voluntary movements require efficient interplay between higher cortical centres, the basal ganglia and cerebellum, and the descending motor pathways, including the pyramidal tract. The activity of the lower motor neurons, which synapse directly onto the muscle, is further modified at spinal level.

In a simplified scheme, movements are thought to be initiated in the supplementary motor area in the frontal lobes, with access to stored motor programmes in a wider range of the cortex. Before the signals initiating planned movement leave the brain via the corticospinal (pyramidal) tract, they are adjusted and fine-tuned through feedback loops with both the basal ganglia and the cerebellum.

The main basal ganglia input from the cortex is the striatum; its main output is via the medial globus pallidus and thalamus back to the cortex—the cortical–striatal–pallidal–thalamic–cortical motor loop. A number of other loops exist, for example for eye movements (see 'Eye movements'). The function of the basal ganglia as a whole is to facilitate and initiate movement, and a number of basal ganglia (or 'extrapyramidal') disorders lead to either too much or too little movement.

The cerebellum receives cortical inputs from the frontal lobes via the pontocerebellar tracts and the middle cerebral peduncle, as well as information from the vestibular and proprioceptive systems; inputs are continually integrated, and outputs are adjusted, to allow for smooth and coordinated movements. Cerebellar efferents back to the cerebral cortex are mainly via the superior cerebellar peduncle, from where tracts cross the midline to reach the contralateral thalamus. Because the cerebellar outflow paths are crossed, and the descending motor pathways are crossed again, the cerebellar hemispheres control the ipsilateral limbs.

The corticospinal tract is the only descending motor tract directly connecting with the lower motor neurons in the spinal cord. It originates predominantly, but not exclusively, from the motor cortex, where body areas are represented topographically in the 'motor homunculus'. Body parts with the most delicate movements, including the hand and the face, have a proportionally larger representation than proximal muscles. The corticospinal tract descends through the internal capsule into the brainstem, giving off collaterals to the basal ganglia and cerebellum. It then crosses to the other side (decussates) in the lower medulla. In the spinal cord, it runs in the anterior and posterolateral white matter tracts before synapsing with the alpha motor neurons in the anterior horn (grey matter).

Lower motor neuron axons pass through the anterior roots, nerve roots, and peripheral nerves (and plexuses in the cervical and lumbosacral regions) before connecting with muscle fibres at the neuromuscular junction. The neurotransmitter used here is acetylcholine.

The number of muscle fibres innervated by each motor neuron (the motor unit) varies from muscle to muscle and can be high (up to 1000) in the case of proximal muscles, and low (about 20 in the case of extraocular muscles).

The activity of the alpha motor neuron determines muscle tone. This in turn is modulated by a monosynaptic reflex with afferents coming from the muscle spindle—the basis for the tendon reflex. If a muscle is stretched by tapping a tendon, muscle spindle afferent sensory fibres are activated. After passing through the posterior spinal root, these synapse directly onto and activate the alpha motor neuron. The sensitivity of the muscle spindle is set by intra-fusal muscle fibres innervated by gamma motor neurons. Both alpha and gamma motor neurons are under supraspinal control from descending tracts. These are mostly inhibitory, so that a lesion of the descending tracts will lead to an exaggeration of muscle tone and tendon reflexes.

In an analogous fashion, lower motor neurons in the brainstem are under control of the corticobulbar tract. Their cell bodies are located in cranial nerve motor nuclei. Importantly, unlike spinal motor neurons, brainstem motor neurons are often under bilateral cortical control. This is true for the motor neurons innervating the 'bulbar' musculature of pharynx and tongue, as well as motor neurons innervating the upper face and the muscles controlling eye closure (hence, the sparing of the forehead in 'upper motor neuron' facial weakness).

Table 219.1 Abbreviated list of the localization of cognitive functions and deficits arising from lesions

Structure	Function	Deficit
Frontal lobe		
Primary and supplementary motor area	Motor control of contralateral face and limbs	Apraxia Hemiparesis Localized weakness(e.g. the 'cortical hand')
Frontal eye field	Initiation of voluntary gaze	Gaze deviation
Prefrontal cortex (highly connected with wide areas of the cortex, the limbic system, and the basal ganglia)	Executive abilities Social cognition Inhibitory control Emotion	Poor executive function Apathy or disinhibition Personality change
Broca's area (dominant hemisphere)	Speech	Expressive dysphasia
Temporal lobe		
Temporal neocortex	Language (Wernicke's area) Semantic memory (left) Hearing	Receptive dysphasia Poor semantic memory
Temporal optic radiation	Visual pathways	Upper homonymous quadrantanopia
Medial temporal lobes (hippocampi and related structures)	Episodic memory formation (verbal on left, non-verbal on right) Emotions (limbic system)	Memory dysfunction Disinhibition Aggression Placidity
Parietal lobe		
Parietal optic radiation	Visual pathways	Lower homonymous quadrantanopia
Sensory cortex	Sensation	Cortical sensory loss (e.g. two-point discrimination)
	Representation of motor tasks	Apraxia
Inferior parietal lobe/angular gyrus	Calculation	Left-right disorientation Acalculia Finger agnosia
	Integration of complex visual and somatosensory information	Inattention Visuospatial difficulties
Occipital lobe		
Visual cortex	Vision	Hemianopia Cortical blindness

Sensory function

In the peripheral nerves, pain and temperature sensation is conveyed through small nerve fibres, whereas touch, vibration, and joint-position sense tend to be transmitted in large fibres. Sensory nerve cell bodies are located in the dorsal root ganglia. Fibres enter the spinal cord through the dorsal roots. Within the cord, anatomically distinct tracts carry sensory information to the brain. The dorsal columns carry the 'large-fibre' information (touch, vibration, and joint-position sense). These tracts decussate in the medulla and reach the contralateral thalamus as the medial lemniscus. The 'small-fibre' information of pain and temperature is conveyed through the spinothalamic tracts. Axons carrying these impulses cross the midline several segments above the level of root entry; their fibres join the medial lemniscus only in the midbrain before reaching the thalamus. From the thalamus, sensory information of the contralateral side of the body reaches the sensory cortex 'homunculus'.

The different sensory pathways explain the frequent occurrence of dissociated sensory loss, for example loss of pain and temperature but not touch, vibration, or joint-position sense in selective neuropathies or in focal spinal cord and brainstem lesions.

Vision

Vision is one of the special senses. Visual information from the retina is conveyed to the occipital cortex via the optic nerves, optic tracts, and optic radiation. At the optic chiasm (which lies just above the pituitary gland), optic nerve fibres derived from the nasal half of each retina cross the midline and continue in the optic tract, together with the uncrossed temporal fibres of the other eye.

Lesions of the chiasm can therefore cause a deficit in the temporal field of each eye ('bitemporal hemianopia'), while lesions in the visual pathways behind the chiasm cause homonymous defects, for example of the left nasal and right temporal field.

Afferent fibres subserving the pupillary light reflex leave the optic radiation to reach the Edinger–Westphal nucleus of the third cranial nerve in the midbrain. Visual problems arising posterior to his point, that is, in the optic radiation or the visual cortex, therefore do not impact on the light reflex. The efferent, parasympathetic pupilloconstrictor fibres of the light reflex travel in the third nerve.

Eye movements

Eye movements depend on the intact function of the extraocular muscles and their neuromuscular junctions; the cranial nerves III, IV, and VI, and their brainstem nuclei; and internuclear as well as supranuclear pathways. For example, voluntary gaze to the left starts with cortical activation of the right frontal eye field. Impulses from there travel down to the contralateral pontine gaze centre, which activates the adjacent left sixth nerve nucleus, which is the origin of the abducens nerve innervating the left lateral rectus muscle, which turns the left eye to the left (abduction). To maintain conjugate gaze, the right eye also needs to turn left (adduction) at the same time. To achieve this, the left pontine gaze centre activates the contralateral (right) oculomotor nucleus, which is the origin of the third nerve innervating the right medial rectus, which turns the right eye inwards. The connection between the left sixth nerve nucleus in the pons and the right third nerve nucleus in the midbrain is the medial longitudinal fasciculus. Lesions here lead to a failure of the right eye to adduct and left eye nystagmus—this is called internuclear ophthalmoplegia.

Similar considerations apply for voluntary upgaze, which relies on intact midbrain function.

To maintain gaze on an object while moving the head, short-latency conjugate eye movements in the opposite direction are produced by the vestibulo-ocular reflex, which can be examined with the doll's head manoeuvre.

Balance

Balance is maintained by the integration of proprioceptive, visual, and vestibular information in the cerebellum and can therefore be upset by a variety of mechanisms.

Cerebrospinal fluid

Cerebrospinal fluid (CSF) is actively produced by the choroid plexus of the ventricular system at a rate of about 500 ml per day. CSF circulates from the lateral ventricles to the third ventricle, then via the aqueduct into the fourth ventricle, and from there through the foramina of Magendie and Luschka to the subarachnoid CSF spaces around the brain and spinal cord. The CSF is then reabsorbed via the arachnoid villi, which protrude into the sagittal sinus and other venous structures around the brain and cord. CSF pressure is a function of venous pressure; CSF pressure as measured by lumbar puncture in the recumbent position is usually between 6 and 20 cm H_2O, and is considered raised when above 25 cm H_2O.

Obstruction to CSF flow leads to hydrocephalus. The block can occur within the ventricular system or in the subarachnoid space, for example due to a fibrosing meningeal reaction around the base of the brain.

Nervous system function in ageing

Cross-sectional studies of intelligence in the population suggest a steady decline in cognitive function after the age of 30 but, from a practical point of view, only very a mild decline in processing speed, memory, and problem-solving becomes apparent in healthy elderly people after 70 years of age. In this population, the prevalence of mild cognitive impairment, a possible precursor to more specific dementias, is estimated to be between 14% and 18%, but signs might not always be easy to tell apart from a more benign senescent forgetfulness.

Other 'abnormal' neurological signs that may appear in up to 30% of otherwise healthy people over 70 include a glabellar sign, a snout reflex, altered eye movements with limited vertical gaze and abnormal pursuit, and a degree of muscle rigidity. Frequently, there is some thinness and weakness of muscles, seen more in proximal muscles than in distal muscles, and a loss of the ankle jerks. Vibration sense is often impaired, but proprioception is largely maintained. Walking becomes slow and cautious, with short steps and a slightly stooped posture. One might expect progressive hearing loss, a reduced sense of smell, and small pupils with a decreased reaction to light and decreased accommodation.

Further Reading

Baehr M and Frotscher M. *Duus' Topical Diagnosis in Neurology* (5th edition), 2012. Thieme.

Clarke C and Lemon R. 'Nervous system structure and function', in Clarke C, Howard R, Rossor M, et al., eds, *Neurology: A Queen Square Textbook*, 2009. Wiley-Blackwell.

220 Diagnosis in suspected neurological disease

Dirk Bäumer

Introduction

It is not always clear that a symptom is due to a problem in the nervous system. Delirium, generalized weakness, and fatigue are frequently due to systemic illness. Transient loss of consciousness may have a neurological or cardiac cause. It is, therefore, important to keep an open mind before focusing on a primary neurological diagnosis in these presentations.

The principles of the neurological method are described in 'General approach', followed by their application in common clinical presentations.

General approach

Pattern recognition

Experienced neurologists often make a diagnosis on the basis of pattern recognition. For example, a patient with a unilateral tremor, slowness of movement, stiffness, and an expressionless face will be recognized as suffering from Parkinson's disease. However, in many cases, the cause of symptoms is not immediately obvious, and a careful analytical approach is needed to reach a diagnosis. It is helpful to ask where in the nervous system a problem may be located before thinking about the possible aetiology.

What part or parts of the nervous system are affected?

If a neurological problem is suspected, the first key question to be answered is 'where is the lesion?' in neuroanatomical terms. The degree of precision of localization on clinical grounds varies. It can sometimes be very specific (e.g. 'this is a problem in the dorsolateral medulla oblongata'), while at other times it may only be possible to make a general statement like 'this is a problem in the central nervous system'. Localization relies on the patient history as much as on the examination and, in cases of transient symptoms (like suspected seizures (see Chapter 39) or transient ischaemic attacks), it is in the history only. A clear history is, therefore, indispensable, and it is often worthwhile to spend some time on the review of old notes and obtaining a collateral history to clarify facts.

It may not be possible to explain all symptoms and signs on the basis of a single lesion, in which case multifocal pathology needs to be considered. With the help of the anatomical diagnosis, an attempt should be made to group the key features of a presentation into a syndromic classification. For example, if history and examination suggest a lesion affecting both spinothalamic tracts and pyramidal tracts below a certain spinal level, and there is nothing to suggest dorsal column involvement, then a diagnosis of an anterior spinal cord syndrome is made, and this will help to narrow the differential diagnosis. It will also avoid jumping to conclusions by immediately associating this constellation of signs with a spinal cord infarct without considering other possibilities.

What is the likely underlying pathology?

While occasionally the localization of the problem greatly narrows down the differential diagnosis (e.g. the dorsolateral medulla oblongata syndrome is almost always due to an infarct), usually the most important clues about the aetiology of a condition come from the history.

The mode of onset and the temporal evolution of symptoms help to make a judgement about the likely category of pathology:

- sudden onset: vascular cause (infarct, haemorrhage)
- subacute: infectious/inflammatory
- slowly progressive: neoplastic, degenerative
- fluctuating/relapsing–remitting: metabolic, inflammatory

The a priori likelihood of specific diagnoses is further influenced by the demographics of the patient, in particular age, sex, preexisting diseases, and degree of immunosuppression, as well as medication and substance use.

If there is evidence of multifocal pathology, the possibilities are that:

- some signs are old and related to disease not relevant to the current presentation (e.g. an extensor plantar response due to an old stroke in someone now presenting with a myopathy)
- the presentation defies 'Occam's razor' and is due to more than one acute problem rather than a single unifying diagnosis (e.g. pins and needles in both feet and one hand due to a peripheral neuropathy and unilateral carpal tunnel syndrome), this is Hickam's dictum
- the presentation is due a single condition affecting several parts of the nervous system (e.g. mitochondrial disease, HIV infection, sarcoidosis, or vasculitis)

How can the diagnosis be confirmed?

A syndromic diagnosis together with demographic factors will usually lead to a differential diagnosis. To reach a final diagnosis, neurology employs a number of investigations, which are outlined in Chapter 221. The clinician should be reasonably familiar with the limitations of tests, all of which have false positive and negative rates. For example, an interictal EEG cannot be used to rule out epilepsy, and a CT brain scan can be normal in acute ischaemic stroke. If there are many differential diagnoses and, therefore, the list of possible investigations is long, it is important to find a balance between taking a pragmatic approach, limiting tests to looking for what is common, and not missing rare but potentially important diagnoses. In difficult cases, a repeat history and examination, perhaps after an interval, can be extremely helpful, as can be a second opinion from a colleague.

The following paragraphs are intended to give some more specific pointers of how to use the neurological method in common presentations, in particular in relation to the anatomical diagnosis.

The neurological approach to common presentations

The unconscious patient

Is this a neurological problem? The majority of cases of coma are due to metabolic–toxic encephalopathies, including hypoxia–ischaemia and poisoning, in which case the 'lesion' localizes to diffuse dysfunction of the cerebral cortex. This conclusion is often reached by the absence of signs pointing towards a focal lesion of the reticular activating system located in the upper brainstem and thalamus. Perhaps the most useful part of the examination is to look at the eyes and pupils:

- roving eye movements indicate an intact brainstem, implying diffuse cortical dysfunction as the cause of coma

- many spontaneous eye movement abnormalities occur in diffuse hemispheric dysfunction
- intrinsic brainstem lesions (e.g. haemorrhage or infarction) may cause skew deviation of the eyes, small or unequal pupils, and motility disorders like an internuclear ophthalmoplegia or absent oculocephalic reflex in the doll's head manoeuvre
- brainstem compression, for example by herniation, may cause a third nerve palsy with a fixed dilated pupil but otherwise intact brainstem reflexes

The patient with cognitive problems

Where is the lesion? Is this a problem predominantly of maintaining attention (a distributed cognitive function; see Chapter 112) or is it a more localized problem indicative of a focal brain lesion or specific dementia? Tests of attention include 'serial 7s' and digit span, and deficits here will impact on the performance in other domains, including memory, perceptuospatial skills, and executive function. How quickly did the problem develop? An acute or subacute onset of symptoms and fluctuations in performance throughout the day point towards a delirium. An insidious onset and slowly progressive course indicates a degenerative cause.

The patient with weakness

Where is the lesion? The assessment relies on both the distinction between lower and upper motor neuron lesions, and a broad classification of the pattern of weakness. **Lower motor neuron lesions** produce signs related to muscle denervation and are characterized by normal or reduced muscle tone, muscle wasting, fasciculations, and depressed or absent deep tendon reflexes. **Upper motor neuron lesions** always involve problems with a group of muscles, and the pattern is often 'pyramidal', with weakness affecting arm extensors more than flexors, and leg flexors more than extensors. Movements are slow and there is a reduction in control of fine finger movements. Because muscles are still innervated, there is no wasting or fasciculations. Muscle tone is increased due to lack of inhibition of spinal reflexes, resulting in spasticity, exaggerated deep tendon reflexes, clonus, and an extensor plantar response: the big toe 'goes up' after stroking the lateral plantar surface of the foot, a sign first described by Babinski in 1896.

Spasticity is velocity-dependent increase in tone and must be distinguished from extrapyramidal rigidity, in which the resistance to muscle stretch is constant. Slowness of movement in spasticity does not generally lead to true bradykinesia. This is defined as slowness with a progressive decrease of speed and amplitude of repetitive movements.

Distribution of weakness

Global weakness

When global weakness is observed, consider metabolic problems (such as hypokalaemia, disorders of the neuromuscular junction, a myopathy, or polyneuropathy). A brainstem problem, for example from basilar artery thrombosis, can present with weakness of all limbs, the bulbar muscles, and eye movements. Look for impairment of consciousness (upper brainstem), sensory disturbance, altered brainstem reflexes, and brisk reflexes in the limbs. Predominantly distal weakness points to a length-dependent neuropathy, while predominantly proximal weakness is often myopathic. Some diseases affect peripheral nerves and nerve roots in a non-length-dependent fashion and lead to proximal and distal weakness (e.g. Guillain–Barré syndrome).

Quadriparesis

When quadriparesis is observed, consider a cervical spinal cord lesion, a myopathy, or a polyneuropathy. Again, the reflexes will be most helpful in distinguishing a spinal cord lesion (upper motor neuron) from a neuropathy or myopathy (lower motor neuron). Acutely, reflexes may be absent in a spinal cord lesion. In this case, weakness above the neck (e.g. of neck flexion and the facial muscles) favours a neuropathy or myopathy. A sensory level and sphincter involvement favour a cord problem.

Paraparesis and bibrachial paresis

Paraparesis (weakness of both legs) is caused by thoracic or lumbar spinal cord lesions, in which case there is often a sensory level and sphincter impairment. Other possibilities include multiple radiculopathies, which are often asymmetrical, or 'paraparetic' forms of a neuropathy affecting mainly the legs. Finally, bilateral frontal lobe lesions can lead to a paraparesis.

Weakness of both arms (bibrachial paresis) is less common. It can be caused by a lesion located in the central cervical cord, the cervical anterior horn cells, the cervical nerve roots, or brachial plexus.

Hemiparesis

Hemiparesis (weakness on one side of the body) points to a problem in the brain or, less commonly, one side of the cervical cord. Facial weakness shows that the problem is in the brain. The presence of other signs will help to localize this further. Are there cortical signs, for example hemianopia, dysphasia, or neglect? If not, are there symptoms or signs pointing to a brainstem problem, such as vertigo, ataxia, or double vision? Brainstem lesions also frequently produce bilateral signs, or a hemiparesis with 'crossed' signs, for example contralateral ataxia or contralateral cranial nerve palsies. The latter may help to pinpoint the lesions to the brainstem level involved, depending on their site of origin (brainstem nuclei):

- midbrain: Cranial nerves III (oculomotor) and IV (trochlear)
- pons: Cranial nerves V (trigeminal), VI (abducens), and VII (facial)
- medulla: Cranial nerves VIII (vestibulocochlear; also pons), and IX–XII (glossopharyngeal, vagus, accessory, hypoglossal)

Single limb weakness

Single limb weakness can be due to peripheral mononeuropathies, a plexopathy, a radiculopathy, an anterior horn cell problem, or an upper motor neuron lesion in the spinal cord or brain. The pattern of weakness, the general features of upper versus lower motor neuron lesions outlined in 'The patient with weakness', and associated sensory features help to distinguish amongst the different causes.

Reaching a diagnosis in the patient with weakness

After establishing the anatomical diagnosis (or differential diagnosis) on clinical grounds, other features in the history are taken into account to reach a differential diagnosis of the underlying pathology. For example, the occurrence of a paraparesis with brisk reflexes, extensor plantar responses, sphincter disturbance, and a sensory level coming on over weeks in a patient with known prostate cancer would make cord compression by malignancy most likely, while the same syndrome developing acutely in someone admitted with aortic dissection suggests a spinal cord infarct.

The patient with sensory problems

As for the patient with weakness, one should try to localize sensory symptoms to a problem in a peripheral nerve (e.g. numbness of Fingers 1–3 in a median neuropathy), nerve roots (dermatomal distribution), plexus, spinal cord (sensory level), or brain (hemisensory loss and often 'cortical' sensory loss: intact light touch but impaired two-point discrimination and stereognosis). The sensory examination is difficult and can easily lead to spurious results. It is, therefore, often helpful to try and confirm an hypothesis, rather than to do a complete sensory examination of all nerves and dermatomes.

Occasionally, it is difficult to distinguish between sensory loss from a neuropathy and that from a spinal cord lesion. However, the reflexes are absent or depressed in the former case, but are brisk in the latter case.

The unsteady patient

The unsteady patient may have a problem of proprioception (large-fibre neuropathy or dorsal spinal cord disease) and get significantly worse in the dark, displaying a positive Romberg's test and impaired joint position sense. Removal of visual clues also worsens the unsteadiness of vestibular disorders, which, in addition, show an abnormal vestibulo-ocular reflex. Patients with cerebellar disease have problems integrating the visual, proprioceptive, and vestibular inputs with reflex movements, leading to incoordination. This can affect gait and stance in isolation, or be combined with ataxia of the limbs, cerebellar dysarthria, and abnormal eye movements. Romberg's test is usually negative in cerebellar disease, and patients do not report vertigo.

The patient with abnormal movements

For the patient with abnormal movements, the usual approach is to classify abnormal movements into broad categories of tremor (a rhythmic sinusoidal oscillation of a body part), myoclonus (a very brief jerk), chorea (irregular, fidgety, purposeless movements flowing from one body part to another), tics (involuntary, stereotyped movements that can be suppressed briefly), and dystonia (abnormal posture). These movements can occur alone or in combination, and be due to a primary movement disorder, a heredodegenerative disease with other features, or be secondary to lesions or systemic illness. It is important not to equate the phenotype of the movement with a specific disorder, but to reach a syndromic diagnosis first and then think about the possible aetiology. For example, chorea can occur in Huntington's disease, but can also occur in SLE, or as a medication side effect. Chorea affecting only one part of the body can be due to a focal lesion of the basal ganglia.

The patient with a functional disorder

Many patients present with symptoms and signs that are not explicable anatomically, inconsistent over time, distractible, and often associated with dissociative symptoms and other medical complaints. Overt psychiatric features may or may not be present. 'Hard' neurological signs are absent but, of course, functional symptoms can occur in patients with an organic disorder. There are a number of signs supportive of a functional disorder, but the sensitivity and specificity of many is limited or unknown. For example, Hoover's sign is positive when a patient shows weakness of hip extension when tested directly, but strong (involuntary) hip extension when flexion of the contralateral hip is tested. While widely considered the most useful test for functional weakness, it can also be positive in patients with cortical neglect.

Summary

In conclusion, diagnosis in neurology is predominantly guided by the history, with physical examination and investigations used to confirm or refute hypotheses generated by it.

Further Reading

Biousse V and Newman NJ. Diagnosis and clinical features of common optic neuropathies. *Lancet Neurol* 2016. 15: 1355–67.

Fowler T, Losseff N, and Scadding J. 'Symptoms of neurological disease', in Scadding, JW and Losseff, N, eds, *Clinical Neurology* (4th edition), 2012. Hodder Arnold.

Fowler T, Scadding J, and Losseff N. 'Examination of the nervous system', in Scadding, JW and Losseff, N, eds, *Clinical Neurology* (4th edition), 2012. Hodder Arnold.

Ropper A and Samuels M. 'Cardinal manifestations of neurologic disease', in Ropper A and Samuels M, *Adams and Victor's Principles of Neurology* (9th edition), 2009. McGraw-Hill Medical.

221 Investigation in neurological disease

Kannan Nithi and Sarosh Irani

Introduction

This chapter provides a brief overview of the more commonly available neurophysiology and neuroradiology techniques, guidance on how to perform a lumbar puncture, and a summary of biochemical, immunological, and genetic tests relevant to neurological disorders.

EEG

Surface-recorded EEG monitors underlying brain electrical currents generated by synaptic activity in cortical neurones. The actual traces obtained are only a low-resolution summation of this activity. An EEG will normally report the wake background rhythms, which are typically dominated by sinusoidal oscillations at a frequency of 8–12 Hz (alpha wave) activity over the occipital area, as well as any focal slow wave activity, sharp waves, or spike discharges.

EEG is used clinically in the investigation of epilepsy, states of altered consciousness, and in some cases of dementia.

Epilepsy

In adults, EEG still has a role in defining the epilepsy syndrome and directing further investigation and treatment. A baseline 'interictal' recording may reveal an underling potential for idiopathic generalized epilepsy or a focal epilepsy syndrome. It should be noted, however, that a significant percentage of patients with a definite diagnosis of epilepsy have a normal interictal recording. Conversely, recordings in non-epileptic subjects can show abnormalities in 1%–10% of cases. Using a routine EEG to rule in or rule out epilepsy when the history is equivocal is, therefore, not recommended.

A recording during an attack has much higher sensitivity and specificity, first in confirming whether or not a clinical episode does represent an epileptic seizure and, second, in determining whether it is clearly of focal or generalized onset. The EEG may remain abnormal for several hours after an epileptic seizure.

Prolonged EEG recordings can be carried out in a home/work environment with an ambulatory system or in an inpatient setting (video telemetry). The latter may be helpful in patients being considered for epilepsy surgery and in identifying the small number of patients who may have a normal surface EEG during an epileptic seizure.

Altered consciousness

EEG in the context of altered consciousness often shows a non-specific disturbance of cortical rhythms. It can be of particular help in demonstrating the presence of non-convulsive status epilepticus (see Figure 221.1); in this situation, a patient may appear to be confused or unconscious with no clearly identifiable clinical epileptic features. Although certain EEG patterns, most notably triphasic waves, are classically associated with hepatic encephalopathy, even these are not entirely specific and are occasionally seen with other metabolic causes of altered consciousness. Therefore, in this setting, the EEG really only helps confirm the existence of an encephalopathic state, which is usually readily clinically apparent in any case. An EEG is sometimes requested in order to support a diagnosis of herpes simplex encephalitis but, again, it lacks the sensitivity and specificity to either refute or confirm this diagnosis. An EEG may be helpful in providing prognostic information in coma. However, the cause, depth, and duration of the coma, as well as the clinical signs, are of greater importance in this respect. Only one EEG pattern (complete generalized suppression greater than 24 hours after cardiac arrest) has a uniformly poor prognosis.

Dementia

EEG tends to show a progressive non-specific slowing of cortical rhythms in dementia syndromes. It can be of particular use in the diagnosis of sporadic Creutzfeldt–Jakob disease as, during the course of the disease, the EEG often becomes dominated by periodic generalized sharp-wave complexes.

Nerve conduction studies

The basic principle in nerve conduction studies (NCSs) is the application of an electrical stimulus at one point along a nerve (causing depolarization of the underlying nerve fibres) and recording, with surface electrodes, the potentials generated and propagated further along the nerve. Sensory and motor nerve fibres can be studied. The report will normally comment on the amplitudes (measured in microvolts), onset, and peak latencies (measured in milliseconds) of the sensory nerve action potentials; the amplitudes (measured in millivolts) and distal latencies of compound muscle action potentials (CMAPs); and motor conduction velocities (expressed as metres per second).

Some limitations of conventional NCSs should be noted: they do not assess the very smallest sensory nerve fibres, they may not be possible in the context of severe limb oedema, and abnormalities may lag some time behind the onset of clinical symptoms and signs. There is also a wide range of normal values for each of the parameters measured, allowing for age, sex, and skin temperature.

NCSs are used in the investigation of single nerve lesions (mononeuropathies) and more generalized polyneuropathies; when they are used in combination with needle EMG, they can be helpful in the investigation of lesions of the brachial and lumbosacral plexus, nerve root lesions (radiculopathies), and disorders of the neuromuscular junction.

Mononeuropathies

NCSs are often used to confirm the presence of an entrapment neuropathy, which is most commonly located in the median nerve in the carpal tunnel (see Figure 221.2), and the ulnar nerve at the elbow (see Figure 221.3); the degree of abnormality reported will often influence the decision regarding surgical intervention. In acute compressive lesions (e.g. 'Saturday night palsy' of the radial nerve), NCSs and EMG may not demonstrate any abnormality for several weeks following the precipitating event.

Polyneuropathies

NCSs may be used to document the presence and/or severity of peripheral nerve involvement in hereditary and acquired neuropathies. They are particular helpful in identifying whether the underlying pathological process is likely to be due to primary axonal degeneration or to inflammation of the myelin sheath. The latter process, demyelination, is usually manifested by marked slowing of nerve conduction velocities (the report may also comment on prolongation of distal latencies, temporal dispersion, evidence of conduction block, and absence or dispersal of proximal nerve responses (F waves)). In the acute setting, NCSs can be particularly helpful in supporting a diagnosis of Guillain–Barré syndrome. Even here, studies can be normal, especially early on in the disease process.

Neuromuscular junction disorders

Application of repetitive nerve stimulation (RNS) of varying frequencies (usually 3–10 Hz) to motor nerve fibres in muscles at rest and after exercise can be used to identify disorders such as myasthenia

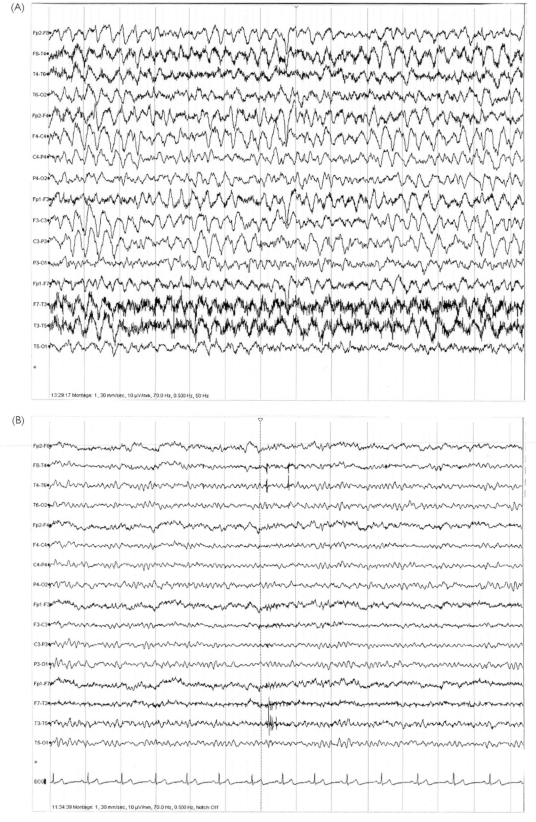

Figure 221.1 Upper non-convulsive status epilepticus; EEG recordings from a patient who had a past history of epilepsy, was no longer on anticonvulsants, and was admitted with an 'acute confusional state'. (A) This trace, taken 48 hours into admission, is dominated by frequent bursts of high-amplitude slow-wave activity. (B) This trace, recorded three days later after reintroduction of anticonvulsants, shows a marked improvement, mirrored by resolution of the confusional state.

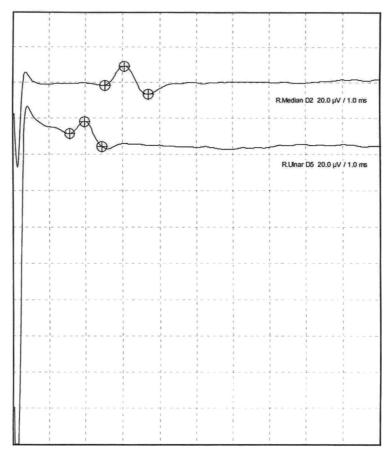

R.Median D2 20.0 µV / 1.0 ms

R.Ulnar D5 20.0 µV / 1.0 ms

Figure 221.2 Sensory nerve conduction study in a patient with carpal tunnel syndrome; the upper trace shows a delayed latency of onset of the sensory nerve action potential from the second digit, which is innervated by the median nerve. The lower trace shows a normal latency response from the fifth digit, which is innervated by the ulnar nerve.

gravis and botulism. Typically, in these disorders, RNS will show a decrement in the amplitudes of successive CMAP responses (the decrement is usually maximal by the fourth response), and this will be accentuated if the muscle to be studied is contracted maximally for a few seconds before stimulation.

Needle EMG

EMG records electrical potentials generated by contracting muscle fibres. Unlike NCSs, this activity is usually studied using needle rather than surface electrodes. A 0.3–0.7 mm concentric needle electrode, consisting of an insulated platinum wire within a steel cannula, is inserted directly into the muscle to be studied. The signal obtained has an auditory as well as visual component.

The EMG report will comment on any activity in the muscle at rest (normally electrically silent) as well as during increasing levels of voluntary muscle contraction. Abnormal spontaneous activity includes fasciculations, fibrillation potentials, and positive sharp-wave discharges, as well as more prolonged activity such as myotonia (see Figure 221.4). The morphology and recruitment pattern of motor units can be analysed qualitatively and quantitatively.

In clinical practice, EMG has, to a large extent, been superseded by histopathology and genetic testing in establishing a precise diagnosis in primary and acquired muscle disease. It does, however, still have a role in narrowing the differential diagnosis in muscle weakness and, in particular, determining whether weakness is due to a neuropathic or myopathic process. Similarly, although neuroimaging is now the modality of choice for the investigation of radiculopathy, EMG may help in the preliminary localization of the site of pathology. EMG remains an important investigation in the assessment of motor

neuron diseases, in particular, in providing objective evidence of denervation in limb muscles in cases of predominantly upper motor neuron/bulbar presentations.

A more specialized EMG recording (single-fibre EMG) is of particular use in the neurophysiological assessment of disorders of the neuromuscular junction, particularly when used in conjunction with RNS.

Evoked potential studies

Evoked potential studies are a way of measuring how sensory information is processed within the CNS. The stimuli applied may be visual, auditory, or somatosensory (see Figure 221.5).

In clinical medicine, the role of these studies is largely restricted to the investigation of multiple sclerosis (MS) and, in particular, demonstrating evidence of a 'clinically silent' demyelinating lesion (i.e. one with no associated clinical deficit).

Neuroradiology

This section will deal primarily with CT and MRI. There are a number of less commonly used, more specialized techniques (including magnetoencephalography, magnetic resonance spectroscopy, functional MRI, and DaT scanning) which may gain more widespread clinical use over the next few years. Imaging of acute stroke is covered in Chapter 227.

CT

CT is an X-ray-based technique which is readily available and remains the first-line radiological investigation in many acute neurological/

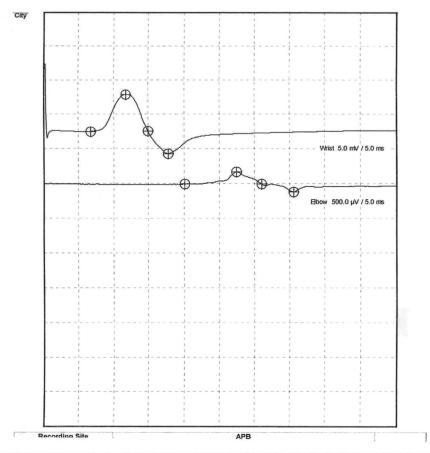

Figure 221.3 Ulnar entrapment neuropathy: recordings of compound muscle action potentials from the abductor digiti minimi. The upper trace shows a normal-amplitude response following stimulation of the ulnar nerve at the wrist. The lower trace shows a marked reduction in amplitude following stimulation in the ulnar groove at the elbow.

neurosurgical situations. CT is particularly helpful in identifying acute bleeding, and remains the imaging modality of choice in the initial workup of subarachnoid haemorrhage. CT is often the first radiological investigation in acute stroke and traumatic brain injury, although it is often followed by MRI. CT (with contrast) will usually identify the presence of significant space-occupying lesions, but subsequent MRI is nearly always needed in such situations, due to its better resolution. In particular, CT may be inadequate if there is a strong clinical suspicion of a posterior fossa abnormality.

MRI

MRI is based on the properties of hydrogen nuclei (protons). In simple terms, an MRI can be regarded as displaying the relative amount of fat and water within the region being studied (see Figures

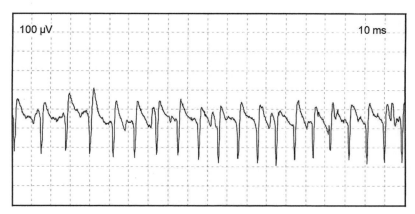

Figure 221.4 Myotonia: a needle recording from the tibialis anterior in a patient with myotonic dystrophy. The trace shows a prolonged burst of myotonia; the sound this produces is often compared to that made by a dive-bomber.

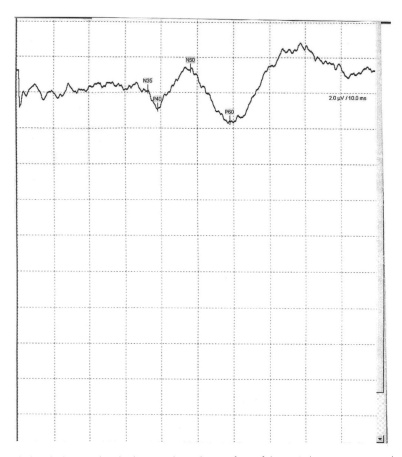

Figure 221.5 A posterior tibial evoked potential study: this trace shows the waveform of the cortical somatosensory evoked potential obtained by stimulation of the posterior tibial wave in a normal subject.

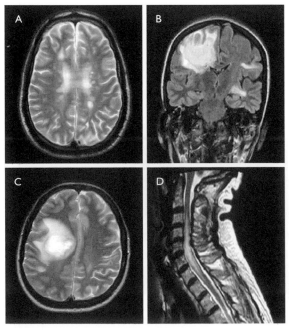

Demyelination in the central nervous system.

A. Multiple small ovoid periventricular hyperintense white matter lesions (T2 weighted axial image) in relapsing-remitting multiple sclerosis.

B. One large and three smaller confluent white matter lesions on coronal FLAIR.

C. Single large right hemispheric white matter lesion on T2 weighted axial image. This is an example of tumefactive multiple sclerosis.

D. Sagittal spinal cord T2-weighted image showing swelling in upper cervical cord with high signal within the central cord, extending over 3 vertebral segments. These features are consistent with the longitudinally extensive transverse myelitis (LETM) of neuromyelitis optica (MMO).

Figure 221.6 MRI findings in multiple sclerosis: demyelination in the CNS. (A) Multiple small, ovoid, periventricular, hyperintense white matter lesions (T2-weighted axial image) in relapsing–remitting multiple sclerosis. (B) One large and three smaller confluent white matter lesions on coronal FLAIR MRI. (C) Single large, right-hemispheric white matter lesion on T2-weighted axial image. This is an example of tumefactive multiple sclerosis. (D) Sagittal spinal cord T2-weighted image showing swelling in the upper cervical cord with high signal within the central cord, extending over three vertebral segments. These features are consistent with the longitudinally extensive transverse myelitis of neuromyelitis optica.

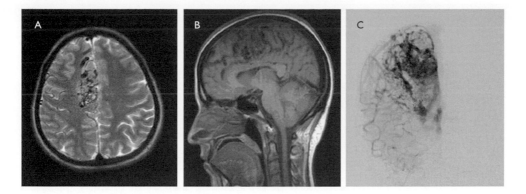

Cerebral angioma.

Tortuous parasagittal vasculature structure within the right hemisphere shown on T2 (A) and T1 (B)-weighted MRI and the angiogram (C).

Figure 221.7 Imaging of cerebral angioma: tortuous parasagittal vasculature structure within the right hemisphere shown on (A) T2- and (B) T1-weighted MRI and (C) an angiogram.

221.6–221.8). Following the application of a radiofrequency pulse in the magnetic field, hydrogen nuclei are perturbed and then relax back to their resting state by two mechanisms—spin–lattice relaxation (T1) and spin–spin relaxation (T2). Each tissue type has a characteristic T1 and T2 time, which are measured in milliseconds. Setting the MRI scanner to emphasize one or other of these produces distinctly different images.

A basic MRI image series will include T1-weighted images (in which fat is designated by a high signal, and water by a low signal) and T2 (in which fat is designated by a low signal, and water by a high signal). T1 images are best for delineating normal anatomy, providing grey/white matter contrast, and differentiating fat from water. T2 sequences are very sensitive to increases in water content (i.e. oedema), and thus are used for detecting pathology. T1 sequences pre- and post-administration of gadolinium contrast are also obtained in certain circumstances, notably to look for breaches in the blood–brain barrier (such breaches are characteristic of active/acute MS lesions), to help radiologically differentiate tumour types and grades, and to look for abnormal enhancement of the meninges. By altering the radiofrequency pulse sequence and other technical aspects of the acquisition protocol, a number of different MRI sequences result, each with their own advantages and disadvantages (Table 221.1). It is often most informative to compare the behaviour of the area of interest across the different sequence types, and the specific set of sequences run will depend on the clinical scenario and the information needed from the MRI (see Table 221.1).

The sensitivity of MRI can lead to diagnostic uncertainty and undue patient anxiety when interpreting a report. Around 10% of MRI brain scans will reveal an incidental abnormality. In particular, the significance of the finding of high-signal lesions in white matter on T2 sequences needs to be interpreted in the clinical context, as it may be supportive of a diagnosis of MS or be purely a reflection of small vessel ischaemic changes.

Although MRI, (unlike CT), does not have the same health concerns with respect to radiation, there are contraindications to MRI scanning with respect to implanted devices/metal such as cardiac pacemakers and cerebral aneurysm clips. The concern with respect to cardiac devices is malfunction due to the magnetic field and heating of the leads whereas, for implanted metal, there may be direct tissue damage due to heating or displacement of the metal. Many currently available cardiac devices and prosthetic heart valves are MRI compatible.

CHAPTER 221 **Investigation in neurological disease**

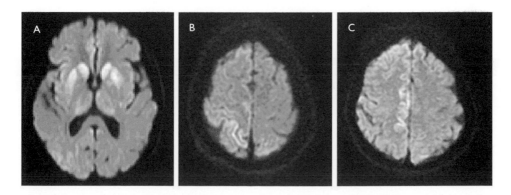

Sporadic Creutzfeld-Jacob disease.

Hyperintensities in the caudate and putamen nuclei and the posterior thalamus in addition to assymetric cortical hyperintensities

Figure 221.8 Imaging in sporadic Creutzfeld–Jacob disease, showing hyperintensities in the caudate and putamen nuclei and the posterior thalamus, as well as asymmetric cortical hyperintensities.

Table 221.1 The advantages and disadvantages of various MRI sequences

Sequence	Advantages/utility	Disadvantages
Spin echo	Higher signal-to-noise ratio Less susceptibility	Longer scan times (much improved with fast spin echo)
Gradient echo	Faster image acquisition More and thinner slices (allows multiplanar reconstructions) More readily reveals blood, calcium, and other metallic deposits (increased susceptibility) Allows flow-related enhancement (MRA and MRV)	Poorer T2 contrast Increased susceptibility to perturbations in the magnetic field also gives more artefact
Echo planar imaging	Rapid image acquisition for uncooperative patients and for fetal or paediatric scanning	Marked susceptibility distorts anatomy at tissue interfaces Much poorer image quality
FLAIR	Suppresses CSF signal Allows detection of more subtle T2 abnormalities (particularly periventricular MS lesions) Incomplete CSF suppression can suggest subarachnoid blood, pus, or malignant meningitis Distinguishes perivascular spaces (black) from ischaemic foci (white)	Flow-related artefact and incomplete CSF suppression (notably in the posterior fossa) can confuse Inferior to fast spin echo for detecting ischaemic lesions in the posterior fossa Old, fluid-filled ischaemic foci will also supress
STIR	Supresses fat signal, including water content Allows detection of pathology in areas of high fat content (orbits and brachial plexus especially)	Fat suppression not absolutely specific, as blood, mucus, and protein-rich fluid may also supress; fat-saturation techniques are better in this regard
DWI/ADC	DWI is highly sensitive in detection of acute infarction ADC differentiates old (high signal) and new (low signal) ischaemic stroke DWI is sensitive and specific for CJD	DWI high signal is not completely specific to infarction; it is also seen with, for example, acute MS demyelination May not be positive with reversible ischaemia (i.e. TIA) Relatively poor delineation of anatomy

Abbreviations: ADC, apparent diffusion coefficient; CJD, Creutzfeldt–Jakob disease; CSF, cerebrospinal fluid; DWI, diffusion-weighted imaging; FLAIR, fluid attenuated inversion recovery; MRA, magnetic resonance angiography; MRV, magnetic resonance venography; MS, multiple sclerosis; STIR, short T1 inversion recovery; TIA, transient ischaemic attack.

Angiography

Radiological visualization of the vasculature can be carried out as part of a CT or an MRI study (see Figure 221.7C). In addition, it can also be carried out by catheter (femoral artery puncture) study under X-ray, whereby it can be analysed on sequential films or by digital subtraction techniques. Over the last few years, catheter angiography has expanded to encompass endovascular treatment of cerebral aneurysms and vascular malformations.

Myelography

MRI is the most commonly used technique for imaging of the spinal cord/column. However, when MRI is contraindicated, then CT or X-ray myelograms can be produced following injection of an iodinated contrast material into the subarachnoid space.

Lumbar puncture

Lumbar puncture is the removal of fluid from around the spinal cord, usually by inserting a needle between two of the higher lumbar vertebrae, through the ligamentum flavum, and into the subarachnoid space, allowing the removal of CSF.

Indications for lumbar puncture

The indications for lumbar puncture are both diagnostic and therapeutic. Table 221.2 highlights typical test results in the following conditions:

- acute:
  - diagnostic: possible meningitis, encephalitis, or subarachnoid haemorrhage
  - therapeutic: to relieve sight- or life-threatening raised intracranial pressure
- chronic:
  - diagnostic: MS, other CNS inflammatory conditions, chronic meningitis, Guillain–Barré syndrome, CNS lymphoma, and dementia, especially Creutzfeldt–Jakob disease (neuronal and glial proteins; e.g. 14-3-3 and S100)
  - therapeutic: idiopathic intracranial hypertension, chronic cryptococcal meningitis, intrathecal chemotherapy delivery

Table 221.2 Cerebrospinal fluid results in common neurological conditions

Neurological condition	WCC	RBCs	Protein	Glucose*	Other tests
Bacterial meningitis	Neutrophilia	Absent	Raised	Reduced	Gram stain and culture
Viral meningitis/encephalitis	Lymphocytosis	Absent	Mildly raised/normal	Mildly reduced/normal	Viral PCR
Subarachnoid haemorrhage	Mildly raised/normal	Remains raised in sequential bottles†	Normal	Normal	Xanthochromia test
Multiple sclerosis	Mildly raised/normal	Absent	Normal	Normal	Oligoclonal banding*
Chronic infective meningitis	Lymphocytosis	Absent	Raised	Reduced	AAFB; tests for ACE, CMV, cryptococcus, and Whipple's disease
Guillain–Barré syndrome	Normal	Absent	Raised	Normal	
CNS lymphoma	Lymphocytosis	Absent	Normal	Normal	Cytology

Abbreviations: AAFB, acid- and alcohol-fast bacteria; ACE, angiotensin-converting enzyme; CMV, cytomegalovirus; CNS, central nervous system; CSF, cerebrospinal fluid; PCR, polymerase chain reaction; RBC, red blood cell; WCC, white-cell count.

*Always send a paired serum sample. Oligoclonal bands can be present in serum and CSF (matched), CSF only, or serum only. Bands which are present in CSF but not in serum (unmatched) are considered helpful in the diagnostic algorithm for CNS inflammatory conditions, particularly multiple sclerosis.

†Unlike the results from a traumatic tap.

Contraindications for lumbar puncture

Raised intracranial pressure is a relative contraindication for lumbar puncture, but is considered more absolute where non-communicating hydrocephalus is present. In addition, significant coagulopathy, depending on its importance/urgency, is a contraindication. Local cutaneous infection is another contraindication.

Procedure for lumbar puncture

The procedure for lumbar puncture is as follows:

1. Knowing that the iliac crests are at L4 means you can avoid the spinal cord, which ends at L1. Using this knowledge, you can plan to go in at an interspace from L2/3 to L4/5.
2. Make sure the spine of the patient is symmetrical about the midline in the left lateral position. This may require pillows between knees and under the neck.
3. Prepare the site using an aseptic technique and infiltrate 5 ml of 1%–2% lignocaine. Be generous and cover more than one interspace in the event of a failed first attempt.
4. Insert the spinal needle bevel up until you feel a 'give' as you leave the ligamentum flavum and enter the dura. We would estimate this sensation in around 50% of cases. Feel happy to remove the stylet to observe CSF flow if you have not felt a clear 'give'.
5. Measure the opening pressure with a manometer and collect CSF in four bottles for appropriate investigations (as under 'indications').

Complications/consent issues for lumbar puncture

Complications/consent issues for lumbar puncture are as follows:

- low-pressure headache (better when lying flat):
  - studies suggest rates between 20% and 40%
  - the incidence can be reduced by using atraumatic needles but there is limited evidence for bedrest or fluid intake
  - patients may require analgesia and caffeine
  - in severe cases, a blood patch may be necessary
- haemorrhage and infection are rare (<1%), but may lead to an epidural haematoma /abscess which can be surgically evacuated
- failure of procedure: not common in a thin, cognitively intact patient

Biochemistry

Serum electrolyte levels may be an important part of the diagnostic workup in a number of acute neurological settings. Specifically, serum sodium levels may be of importance in assessment of confusion and seizures, while potassium levels can be helpful in determining the cause of generalized muscle weakness or when diagnosing the periodic paralyses. The actual levels at which electrolyte disturbances cause neurological problems vary and, particularly in the case of sodium, the rate of change of serum concentration is an important factor.

Vitamin deficiencies/toxicity are associated with a variety of neurological disorders. Laboratory diagnosis may not rest on measurement of vitamin levels alone, but assays of active metabolites (e.g. pyridoxal phosphate for vitamin B_6) or specific enzymes (e.g. red cell transketolase for vitamin B_1).

Identification of porphyrins in urine or faeces in an acute attack can lead to a diagnosis of porphyria. Assays of the underlying defective enzyme are more helpful in defining the precise syndrome, particularly in the clinically quiescent state.

Serum ammonia levels may be helpful in investigating encephalopathy.

Immunology

Serum (and CSF) antibodies directed against certain neuronal proteins are of diagnostic importance in neurology. Most conditions associated with the following antibodies are immunotherapy responsive.

Skeletal muscle nicotinic acetylcholine receptor (AChR) antibodies are found in around 80% of cases of myasthenia gravis (MG). Lower rates of AChR-antibody positivity are seen in cases with pure ocular MG. These antibodies have been shown to be directly pathogenic, and titres correlate reasonably closely with clinical measures in an individual patient.

MuSK (for muscle-specific kinase) antibodies are found in 5%–10% of MG cases. This leaves around 10% of generalized MG cases without positive serology, but most of these antibodies are thought to be directed against the AChR and can be detected by using more sensitive assay techniques.

Ganglioside antibodies are associated with peripheral nerve inflammatory diseases within the Guillain–Barré syndrome spectrum. GM1 IgG antibodies are associated with *Campylobacter jejuni* infection and a motor syndrome. Also, GM1 IgM antibodies are found in around half of multifocal motor neuropathy patients. GQ1b antibodies strongly associate with the Miller–Fisher variant of Guillain–Barré syndrome (characterized by the triad of ataxia, ophthalmoplegia, and areflexia), being positive in 90%–95% of such cases.

Voltage-gated calcium channel (P/Q type) antibodies are seen in around 90% of cases of Lambert–Eaton myasthenic syndrome (LEMS). Like AChR antibodies, these are thought to be pathogenic. There is a low rate of positivity in patients with small cell lung cancer, which has a strong association with LEMS.

LGI1 (leucine-rich, glioma inactvated 1) and CASPR2 (contactin associated protein like-2) antibodies are tested for in patients with a variety of neurological syndromes. Testing for these directly offers improved sensitivity and specificity over testing for VGKC-complex antibodies, as VGKCs are – surprisingly – only rarely the direct target of these autoantibodies. LGI1 antibodies are known to associate with a predominantly non-paraneoplastic limbic encephliatis and a form of epilepsy known as 'faciobrachial dystonic seizures' CASPR2 anti-bodies are more commonly seen in neuromyotonia (peripheral nerve hyperexcitability), and in the rare Morvan's syndrome, which combines features of neuromyotonia and limbic encephalitis, also often with LGI1 antibodies. The latter two conditions are associated with a malignancy (commonly a thymoma) in around 25% of cases. CSF and serum should be sent to optimize assay sensitivity.

Table 221.3 Paraneoplastic antibodies and their associated clinical features and tumours

Antibody	Associated clinical syndrome (s)	Commonly associated tumours
Anti-Hu	Limbic encephalomyelitis Sensory neuronopathy Cerebellar degeneration Dysautonomia	SCLC Neuroblastoma Prostate
Anti-Ma2	Limbic brainstem encephalitis	Testicular (germ cell) Non-SCLC
Anti-CV2/CRMP5	Limbic encephalomyelitis Cerebellar degeneration Sensory neuronopathy Chorea Optic neuritis	SCLC Thymoma
Anti-Ma	Limbic brainstem encephalitis	SCLC Breast Others
Anti-amphiphysin	Encephalomyelitis Stiff person syndrome	Breast SCLC
Anti-Tr	Cerebellar degeneration	Hodgkin's disease
Anti-Ri	Ataxia +/− opsoclonus–myoclonus Brainstem encephalitis	Breast SCLC Bladder Gynaecological
Anti-Yo	Cerebellar degeneration	Breast Ovarian Uterine SCLC

Abbreviations: SCLC, small cell lung cancer.

Table 221.4 Common neurogenetic conditions, with their clinical features, diagnostic tests, chromosome affected, protein affected, and mode of inheritance

Condition	Clinical features	Diagnostic tests	Chromosome affected	Protein affected	Mode of inheritance
Muscle related					
Duchenne muscular dystrophy, or Becker's muscular dystrophy	Proximal weakness	Creatine kinase (raised) EMG (myopathic)	21 (X)	Dystrophin	X linked
Myotonic dystrophy type 1	Distal weakness and myotonia	EMG (myotonia ('dive bombing'))	19	Myotonic dystrophy protein kinase	Autosomal dominant (CTG repeat)
Mitochondrial	Ophthalmoplegia Retinopathy Diabetes Deafness	Many	Mitochondrial genome, or nuclear genes encoding mitochondrial proteins	Many	Autosomal dominant, or maternal
Peripheral nerve related					
Charcot–Marie–Tooth disease type 1A*	Peripheral motor and sensory loss	NCS (demyelination)	17	Peripheral myelin protein 22	Autosomal dominant (gene duplication)
Charcot–Marie–Tooth disease type 2A2	Peripheral motor and sensory loss +/− optic atrophy, tremor, and hearing loss	NCS (axonal pattern)	1	Mitofusin 2	Autosomal dominant or recessive
HNPP	Recurrent pressure palsies	NCS (generalized mild demyelination and focal slowing)	17	Peripheral myelin protein 22	Autosomal dominant (deletion)
Fabry's disease	Rash, renal dysfunction	Alpha-galactosidase activity	21 (X)	Alpha-galactosidase A	X linked
Ataxias					
Friedreich's ataxia	Ataxia Neuropathy Cardiomyopathy	NCS	9	Frataxin	Autosomal recessive (GAA repeat)
Spinocerebellar ataxia	Retinopathy Other neurology	Many	Many	Many	Autosomal dominant (triple repeats)
Fragile X-associated tremor/ataxia syndrome	Tremor Cognitive impairment Neuropathy	Many	21 (X)	Fragile X mental retardation protein 1	X linked (CGG repeat)
Episodic ataxia type 1	Brief attacks of ataxia +/− myokymia		12	Kv1.1 potassium channel	Autosomal dominant
Episodic ataxia type 12	Prolonged attacks of ataxia and nystagmus		19	P/Q-type calcium channel	Autosomal dominant
Dementia					
Huntington's disease	Choreiform and other involuntary movements Cognitive decline		4	Huntingtin	Autosomal dominant (CAG repeat)
CADASIL	Strokes Migraine with aura Cognitive decline	Skin biopsy (small vessel changes) MRI (subcortical infarcts)	19	Notch 3	Autosomal dominant
Prion disease	Ataxia Cognitive decline		20	Prion protein	Autosomal dominant
Motor nerve related					
Familial motor neuron disease	Global motor neuron dysfunction		21 (X)	Superoxide dismutase 1†	X linked
Kennedy's disease	Lower motor neuron dysfunction Gynaecomastia	Endocrine	21 (X)	Androgen receptor	X linked (CAG repeat)
Phakomatoses					
Neurofibromatosis type 1	Café au lait spots Lisch nodules Axillary freckling	MRI brain/ plexus/cord for neurofibromas	17	Neurofibromin	Autosomal dominant
Neurofibromatosis type 2	Bilateral acoustic neuromas		22	Merlin	Autosomal dominant

Abbreviations: CADASIL, cerebral autosomal dominant arteriopathy with subcortical infarcts and leucoencephalopathy; EMG, electromyography; HNPP, hereditary neuropathy with liability to pressure palsy; MRI, magnetic resonance imaging; NCS, nerve conduction study.

*The commonest form of Charcot–Marie–Tooth disease is the 1A subtype; other forms have alternative modes of inheritance. and mutations in different genes.

†The mutation affecting this protein is the commonest known mutation in familial motor neuron disease.

Glutamic acid decarboxylase antibody levels are mildly raised in diabetics, but are very high in cases with stiff person syndrome and in some cases of epilepsy and cerebellar ataxia.

Some of the aforementioned antibodies can be measured via a radioimmunoassay technique where a specific radioactively labelled ligand determines the antibody that can be detected (e.g. alpha-bungarotoxin, for AChR). ELISAs are used to detect ganglioside antibodies. In this assay, the gangliosides themselves are bound to the well of a polystyrene plate and probed with serum; binding is detected by way of an enzyme-linked secondary antibody and a colour change reaction. In contrast, LGI1, CASPR2 and the following antibodies are measured using a cell-based assay where the antigen of interest is expressed on the cell surface, and patient antibodies bind this exposed antigen.

NMDA-receptor antibodies target an excitatory receptor in the CNS and are increasingly recognized in an encephalopathy affecting young patients, often with a characteristic choreoathetoid movement disorder. A minority of cases have an underlying ovarian teratoma, and in some patients the syndrome arises after HSV encephalitis. Patients respond to (often prolonged) courses of immunotherapy. CSF and serum should be sent to optimize assay sensitivity.

Aquaporin-4 antibodies have been recently described in neuromyelitis optica (NMO; also known as Devic's disease), but not in MS. NMO produces severe optic neuritis and longitudinally extensive transverse myelitis. Hence, traditionally, there has been some confusion between this condition and MS. Differentiation between these conditions is of great importance, given the clear differential immunotherapy response seen in NMO. The importance of early immunotherapy in patients with faciobrachial dystonic seizures (Makuch et al. 2017).

The targets of the antibodies listed in Table 221.3 are all intracellular, so the antibodies are unlikely to be directly pathogenic. Furthermore, conditions associated with these antibodies are commonly associated with characteristic distant tumours (paraneoplastic) and often have a poor prognosis. The antibodies are typically detected by indirect immunohistochemistry (on rodent brain sections) followed by Western blotting for the specific antigen.

Genetics

Genetic testing and discussions with family members are often only performed with the help of a trained geneticist or genetic counsellor. A clear family history of neurological disease is often the most helpful pointer in assessment of an individual case, but awareness and recognition of the phenotype of neurological conditions with a strong genetic component is important when the family history is unhelpful. Genetic neurological diseases may affect any part of the nervous system. The majority of laboratory genetic testing is carried out on blood samples; however, supportive evidence from muscle and skin biopsies is important in certain diseases.

Modes of inheritance may be autosomal dominant, recessive, or X linked. Mitochondrial DNA is maternally inherited. Triplet repeat diseases are common causes of neurogenetic disorders and show anticipation: a lengthening of the triplet repeat through generations, and a more severe disease with earlier onset (see Table 221.4).

Polygenic inheritance

Many common CNS issues have a known genetic association which only accounts for a minority of cases of the disease. Such complex polygenic traits include Alzheimer's disease, where an association with the E4 allele of the APOE gene has been established; Parkinson's disease, where variants in the LRRK2 gene are present in a small proportion of sporadic cases; and MS, which has an established association with the HLA locus.

Further Reading

Bone I, Fuller G, et al. Neurology in practice: Neuroradiology. *J Neurol Neurosurg Psychiatry* 2005; 76: 1–63.

Bradly WG, Daroff RB, Marsden CD, et al. *Neurology: A Queen Square Text Book* (3rd edition), 1999. Butterworth–Heinemann.

Daroff RB, Fenichel GM, Jancovik J, et al. *Bradley's Neurology In Clinical Practice* (6th edition), 2012. Saunders.

Gozzard P and Maddison P. Which antibody and which cancer in which paraneoplastic syndromes? *Pract Neurol* 2010; 10: 260–70.

Irani SR, Gelfand JM, Al-Diwani A, et al. Cell-surface central nervous system autoantibodies: Clinical relevance and emerging paradigms. *Ann Neurol* 2014; 76: 168–84.

Makuch M, Bien CG, Chu K, Farooque P, Gelfand JM, Geschwind MD, Hirsch LJ, Somerville E, Lang B, Vincent A, Leite MI, Waters P, Irani SR; Faciobrachial Dystonic Seizures Study Group. *Brain*. 2017 Dec 18. doi: 10.1093/brain/awx323. [Epub ahead of print].

Misulis KE and Head TC. *Essentials of Clinical Neurophysiology*, 2003. Butterworth-Heinemann.

Rinaldi S and Willison HJ. Ganglioside antibodies and neuropathies. *Curr Opin Neurol* 2008; 21: 540–6.

Thompson J, Bi M, Murchison AG, et al. The importance of early immunotherapy in patients with faciobrachial dystonic seizures. *Brain* 2018; 141:348–6.

222 Demographics of neurological disease

Sarah Cader

Introduction

This chapter reviews the epidemiology of common neurological disorders. While neurological symptoms can potentially appear confusing, understanding which diseases affect particular groups can provide diagnostic guidance.

Epilepsy

Between 0.4% and 1% of the UK population have epilepsy, with an incidence of about 50 per 100 000 per year, affecting males slightly more than females. With treatment, most patients become seizure-free, but a poor prognosis is associated with epilepsy syndromes, early onset, or underlying cerebral disorder. Two-thirds of cases of epilepsy, which is defined as the occurrence more than one unprovoked seizure, have no identifiable cause.

There are different types of seizures that present at different ages, and this helps with classification of the epilepsy. The genetic epilepsy syndromes present in children, but secondary epilepsy will affect adults, especially in those suffering cerebrovascular disease.

Juvenile myoclonic epilepsy, characterized by myoclonus, tonic–clonic seizures, and absences, start around puberty. This has a strong genetic basis and is idiopathic.

Absence seizures tend to present before the age of 10, rather than in adults. Many of these children (about half) will go on to develop tonic–clonic seizures as adults.

Complex partial seizures usually arise from the mesial temporal lobe, and may indicate underlying sclerosis or other structural anomaly. They may present in early adult life, if not earlier.

Parkinson's disease and other movement disorders

Affecting approximately 70 000 patients in the UK, Parkinson's disease is a condition that leads to progressive disability due to a triad of bradykinesia, rigidity, and tremor. It is more common in men, and about 10% of patients have a relative with the condition. It has been reported to have a higher incidence in rural areas, and a reduced risk for smokers.

Parkinson's tends to affect individuals over the age of 55, with the prevalence increasing with age. However, in autosomal recessive juvenile parkinsonism, the onset is before the age of 40 years. This is caused by a mutation in the PRKN gene (Chromosome 6). While Parkinson's can lead to significant disability, average life expectancy is not significantly affected, and response to treatment with dopamine (L-DOPA) is usually good.

The other hypokinetic movement disorders, such as multisystem atrophy, progressive supranuclear palsy, and corticobasal degeneration, also usually begin in older adults. However, they are generally resistant to treatment, and prognosis is poor.

Huntington's disease is a genetic disorder causing writhing movements (chorea), ataxia, and dementia. It is a trinucleotide repeat disorder causing gene instability on Chromosome 4. Typically the onset is in the third decade, but 10% of those affected may not get symptoms until after 60 years old. The phenomenon of anticipation is seen, usually via paternal transmission, and can cause earlier onset and more fulminant course. These patients will have a particular large trinucleotide repeat. There is no currently available treatment.

Wilson's disease is an autosomal condition that presents in childhood, leading to copper deposition and causing a variety of movement disorders. It can present in adults with neurological or psychiatric features, but seldom beyond 40 years of age. Its importance, despite the rarity, is due to the potential for reversibility with chelating agents (penicillamine) if caught early.

Multiple sclerosis

Multiple sclerosis (MS) is a condition that is common in more northerly and southerly latitudes, but very rare in equatorial regions. Notable exceptions are the high prevalence in Italy, and the northwest to south-east gradient in the USA. This may reflect environmental factors that are still to be determined fully, but may be due to timing of exposure to viral insult.

Characterized by neurological disturbance anywhere in the CNS, it can present in discrete reversible episodes (relapsing–remitting) or progressive disability from onset (primary progressive) in 25% of patients. The peak incidence is at the age of 30, but MS does, rarely, affect children and those over 60 years. Women are twice as likely to be affected as men, and about 1 in 1000 people in the UK are affected.

One-third of patients will have a benign course, and about 20% of patients have marked disability within 20 years of onset. A poor prognosis is associated with older age of onset, in men, cerebellar symptoms at onset, and early progression.

There are some conditions that mimic MS. Devics's disease or neuromyelitis optica presents with optic neuritis or transverse myelitis. The age of onset is similar, but has less geographical variation. It most patients, antibodies to aquaporin-4 can be found, and the disease is characterized by frequent relapses that may respond to strong immunosuppression.

If the symptoms present in childhood or adolescence, then the demyelination may be due to a leukodystrophy, leading to a relentless progression in neurological disability with prominent dementia.

Motor neuron disease

Motor neuron disease is a degenerative condition causing progressive weakness and usually presents in the sixth decade. Men are slightly more affected than women. The incidence is around 1–2 per 100 000.

It is mostly a sporadic condition, but in a small proportion it is familial, although not all the mutations have been determined. In three-quarters of cases, the patients present with limb symptoms; the rest present with bulbar symptoms. Prognosis is usually poor, with median survival less than 5 years. Riluzole, the only licensed treatment, has a modest effect on life expectancy. However, in a small proportion with no bulbar involvement, the survival may be considerably longer.

Peripheral nerve disorders

Peripheral nerves disease can follow one of several patterns including mononeuropathies, radiculopathies, and polyneuropathies. Mononeuropathies are often caused by compression, and are most frequently seen in young adults. The most common is carpal tunnel syndrome, which predominates in women.

Guillain–Barré syndrome (GBS), an acute neuropathy, occurs at any age but is more common in the elderly and men. Two-thirds of patients will have onset within 6 weeks of an infection. It has a worse prognosis in older patients but, with good support and early treatment, there is usually a good recovery. The annual incidence is about 1–2 per 100 000.

There are number of conditions that are similar to GBS. Miller Fisher syndrome causes ataxia, ophthalmoplegia, and areflexia, and is also often preceded by a viral-like illness. Patients often have antibodies to GQ1b ganglioside. In acute axonal motor neuropathy, there can be antibodies to GM1 ganglioside, but the disease does not lead to the demyelinating neuropathy of GBS. The chronic relapsing variant of GBS, known as chronic inflammatory demyelinating polyneuropathy, may also have identifiable antibodies. Progression may occur, but usually responds to immunosuppressive treatment.

There are hereditary neuropathies that typically affect younger patients than the inflammatory and metabolic neuropathies do. Onset is usually before the age of 20, but the most severe types start in infancy, and some may present in later life. The progression is variable depending on the variant.

Myasthenia gravis, and related conditions

Myasthenia affects approximately 4 per 100 000. The distribution of myasthenia is bimodal, affecting young adults (20–25) and older individuals (over 40 years). It is a condition associated with antibodies to acetylcholine receptors, although it is more frequently seen in younger patients.

Myasthenia usually causes generalized weakness characterized by fatigability. However, in ocular myasthenia, there is isolated ptosis and ophthalmoplegia. This can occur at any age. Some patients with ocular myasthenia may progress to develop generalized symptoms. In those patients that are seronegative for receptor antibodies, a significant proportion are positive for the MuSK antibody. This can also present at any age, often with a different pattern of weakness that is predominantly ocular, facial, and bulbar.

In patients with late-onset myasthenia and ocular myasthenia, the ratio of men affected to women is 3:2. Otherwise, women tend to be affected more than men. There is an association with HLA A1, B8, and DR3, and other autoimmune conditions. There is a congenital form of myasthenia, which is autosomal recessive, and presents within the first 2 years of life.

Lambert–Eaton myasthenic syndrome is far less common than myasthenia gravis. Antibodies are found to presynaptic calcium channels that cause augmentation of motor contraction after sustained contraction or repetitive stimulation. In about half of patients, there is an underlying small cell lung cancer.

Dystrophies and other primary muscle diseases

Comprising a diverse range of acquired and genetic conditions, primary muscle disease affects about 50 000 people in the UK.

The age range can be wide but, broadly speaking, the genetic dystrophic conditions present early in childhood. The underlying defect in the muscle is present from birth, leading to muscle destruction, and so the less severe conditions may present in adolescence or early adult life. Other genetic muscle disorders with less deleterious effects may, therefore, also present in early adult life. Life expectancy depends on the phenotypic presentation, but is typically reduced due to problems with breathing or cardiac conduction defects.

Mitochondrial diseases can present at any age with most patients only suffering mild weakness, although they can suffer other problems such as deafness, visual loss, stroke-like episodes, and cardiac difficulties.

Inflammatory myopathies present later in life, although dermatomyositis does affect children also. Polymyositis and dermatomyositis affect women more than men. Immunosuppressive treatment is usually effective, but investigations should consider the possibility of associated underlying malignancies. Inclusion body myositis is more common in older men and tends to be progressively disabling, however.

Migraine and other headache disorders

Headache is a very common neurological presentation, representing at least 20% of neurology outpatient referrals. These are mostly due to migraine or tension headache.

The lifetime prevalence of migraine is about 15% ; over a 1-year period, it is approximately 10%. Migraine with aura is less common, affecting 4% in a 1-year period. Women are 2–3 times more likely to suffer with either form of migraine. There is a genetic predisposition, which has been demonstrated in twin studies, and there is a rarer familial form associated with hemiplegia. It commonly presents in the second or third decade, and is unusual over the age of 50. However, there is a variant of migraine accompaniment that occurs in late life without headache. Ophthalmolplegic migraine generally begins before the age of 10 years. It is more common in males and not usually familial.

Tension headache affects up to 3% of the population, and is also more common in women, most often presenting in the second decade. The prevalence declines with age.

Cluster headache is more often found in men (about 80%) but is far less common than migraine. In 2% there is a family history, and is sometimes associated with a structural brain lesion. It usually has onset in the late twenties.

Temporal arteritis presents with headache due to inflammation in arteries, almost invariably in Caucasians. Loss of vision may occur due to involvement of the posterior ciliary artery. It is usually seen in patients in their seventies, and is rare under the age of 50. It affects slightly more women than men.

Alzheimer's disease and other dementias

Alzheimer's is a neurodegenerative condition that causes progressive cognitive decline. Initially causing poor recollection of recent events, over time, it leads to wandering, irritability, worsening language skills, confusion, and, eventually, total dependence. There is an accumulation of characteristic amyloid plaques and neurofibrillary tangles, and gradual loss of neurons. It is not unsurprising that this is a disease that typically affects people over the age of 65. The incidence roughly doubles every 5 years after the age of 65, from about 1% to about 20% in those over the age of 85 years. Women are more likely to be affected than men. In a small number, there is onset before the age of 65 years; this is indicative of a genetic mutation.

Half of all dementias are due to Alzheimer's. Vascular dementia comprises the next largest proportion, affecting about 15% of all dementias. It is a rather heterogeneous group of patients, and the incidence does not increase with age, although doesn't usually present until after the age of 65.

Lewy body dementia presents at about the same age as Alzheimer's and Parkinson's. It shares features with both, and there is typically fluctuating cognition with vivid visual hallucinations.

Frontotemporal dementia may have an onset at an earlier age, but again tends to present at the age of 60 years. It is a rare form of dementia, and about a quarter of cases are familial.

Neurological infections

Meningitis can be caused by a variety of organisms and, as such, can affect a wide range of ages. However *Haemophilus influenzae* predominantly affects children under 5 years and *Neisseria menigitidis* is also common in children, but also affects adults. *Streptococcus pneumoniae* particularly affects the very young and very old, and the mortality can be as high as 20%. Other bacterial organisms, such as *Listeria monocytogenes*, are uncommon, and their presence raises the possibility of immunocompromise. Cryptococcus, tuberculosis, and fungal infections similarly tend to occur in those with predisposing conditions. However, tuberculous meningitis remains common in some developing countries, and may be present in immigrants from these regions.

Encephalitis is also caused by a large variety of organisms that vary according to geography, and there are some areas where rabies is a common cause of both encephalitis and paralysis. In the UK, herpes simplex is commonly seen. Following a measles infection, some individuals may develop subacute sclerosing panencephalitis. This affects about 1–3 per million, and does not occur after the age of 25 years.

Syphilis is still an important condition that is re-emerging in those not treated in the primary stage. It might present month to years later and so is more likely in older individuals. Similarly, Creutzfeldt–Jakob disease (CJD), a spongiform encephalopathy, also has a long latency, presenting in older adults, with dementia, involuntary movements, and seizures. There are about 50–100 cases a year of sporadic CJD. There are also familial forms that evolve slower, also presenting in older adults.

Many of the neurological infections tend to follow a pattern of exposure, and so may occur in travellers and those with bites. A detailed history is therefore important.

Further Reading

There is no one review that will cover all of the conditions discussed.

For further reading I would recommend reading *Practical Neurology* (BMJ journals), and *Continuum*, from the American Academy of Neurology (LWW publications).

GBD 2015 Neurological Disorders Collaborator Group. Global, regional, and national burden of neurological disorders during 1990–2015: A systematic analysis for the Global Burden of Disease Study 2015. *Lancet Neurol* 2017; 16: 877–97.

Hilton-Jones D and Turner MR (eds). *Oxford Textbook of Neuromuscular Disorders*, 2014. Oxford University Press.

'Neurological conditions', in Warrell DA, Cox TM, and Firth JD, eds, *Oxford Textbook of Medicine* (5th edition), 2010. Oxford University Press.

223 Neurogenetic disease

Tracey Graves

Introduction

There are many genetic diseases which affect the nervous system. Although some of these are extremely rare, several are quite common and, as a group, they comprise a significant proportion of neurological disease. Almost all clinical neurological syndromes can have a genetic cause. Not all of these have been genetically elucidated, but some have been extensively characterized in terms of clinical phenotype, molecular genetics, and cellular pathophysiology. Given the improvement in laboratory techniques and subsequent reduction in the cost of direct DNA sequencing, there is likely to be a rapid expansion over the next decade in the identification of causative genes and hence the availability of genetic tests. Thus, all clinicians should have a basic understanding about genetic disease; inheritance patterns; availability of genetic tests; genetic counselling; and ethics. Particular subspeciality areas where neurogenetic disease is common include neuromuscular disease and movement disorders.

The neurogenetic diseases have been categorized in Table 223.1. The four commonest conditions are discussed in detail in this chapter.

Huntington's disease

Definition of Huntington's disease

Huntington's disease (HD) is a neurodegenerative condition and is the archetypal polyglutamine expansion disorder.

Aetiology of HD

HD is due to a trinucleotide (CAG) expansion in the HTT gene and is inherited in an autosomal dominant manner.

Typical symptoms of HD, and less common symptoms

HD is characterized by a movement disorder, psychiatric features, and dementia. The movement disorder is usually choreiform; however, the juvenile onset form produces parkinsonism, and ataxia is also seen. The classical triad may not be present at presentation, but may develop during the course of the illness.

Demographics of HD

HD is globally distributed and there is no particular ethnic predilection.

Natural history of HD, and complications of the disease

HD is relentlessly progressive. The combination of dysphagia and catabolism lead to dramatic weight loss. Death is usually by progressive bulbar dysfunction and aspiration pneumonia or by suicide.

Approach to diagnosing HD

Those with the classical triad of HD symptoms should cause no diagnostic difficulty; however, monosymptomatic cases may be overlooked without a high index of clinical suspicion. A detailed family history including age and cause of death over two or three generations may show relatives with psychiatric disease, suicide, and institutionalization. Those with a known family history are now increasingly common, especially with the widespread availability of genetic testing.

Other diagnoses that should be considered aside from HD

There are HD mimics but, in practice, these are rare.

'Gold-standard' diagnostic test for HD

A clinical suspicion of HD can be readily confirmed by molecular genetic testing. The test is simple and inexpensive. However, the test should not be performed without adequate genetic counselling of the patient; this should include discussing the risk of diagnosing presymptomatic obligate carriers (i.e. the patient's parents) and the identification of at-risk individuals (siblings and offspring). Presymptomatic testing should only be carried out in a specialist genetics clinic with clinical expertise in counselling and after a cooling-off period, where the individual has had adequate time to contemplate the consequences of a positive test, with respect to life insurance, reproductive plans, and dealing with a positive test.

Acceptable diagnostic alternatives to the gold-standard test for HD

For HD, there are no acceptable diagnostic alternatives to genetic testing.

Other relevant investigations

There are no relevant investigations for HD, other than genetic testing.

Prognosis of HD, and how to estimate it

In general, the severity of HD and its age of onset are inversely proportional to CAG repeat length. However, this can be difficult to estimate in an individual. Lifespan is significantly reduced in younger onset cases.

Treatment of HD, and its effectiveness

For the treatment of HD, a multidisciplinary approach is required, with input from a physiotherapist, an occupational therapist, a dietician, a speech and language therapist, and, importantly, a clinical psychologist or psychiatrist. Chorea, although dramatic, often disturbs other family members more than it does the patient. It can be treated with tetrabenazine; however, this drug is contraindicated in those with psychiatric disease. Psychiatric complications should be treated in a standard manner.

Myotonic dystrophy type 1

Definition of myotonic dystrophy type 1

Myotonic dystrophy type 1 (DM1) is the commonest muscular dystrophy in adults. Although its clinical manifestations are largely in skeletal and cardiac muscle, it is a multisystem disease.

Aetiology of DM1

Like HD, DM1 is an autosomal dominant trinucleotide expansion disorder, but one where the CTG repeat is in the 3′ untranslated region of the DMPK gene, leading to aberrant RNA processing. This affects various gene products and is thought to underlie the multisystem nature of the condition. For example, abnormal RNA processing of the chloride channel protein CLC1 causes myotonia.

Typical symptoms of DM1, and less common symptoms

The classical phenotype of DM1 includes facial myopathic features (temporalis wasting, facial weakness), neck flexion, and finger extension weakness, with myotonia (delayed muscle relaxation after contraction). Cardiac involvement manifests as conduction abnormalities. Cataracts,

Table 223.1 Neurogenetic conditions

Disorder	Type	Examples	Genes
Nervous system disorders	Charcot–Marie–Tooth disease	Charcot–Marie–Tooth disease type 1 (autosomal dominant, demyelinating)	MPZ PNP22
		Charcot–Marie–Tooth disease type 2 (autosomal dominant, axonal)	MFN2
		Charcot–Marie–Tooth disease type 4 (autosomal recessive)	EGR2 PRX
		Charcot–Marie–Tooth disease type X (X linked)	GJB1
	Autonomic	Hereditary sensory and autonomic neuropathy	RAB7A SPTLC1
Muscle disorders	Dystrophies	Myotonic dystrophy type 1	DMPK
		Myotonic dystrophy type 2	ZFN9
		Duchenne muscular dystrophy	DMD
		Becker's muscular dystrophy	DMD
		Limb-girdle muscular dystrophy	Multiple genes
	Channelopathies	Non-dystrophic myotonias	CLCN1 SCN4A
		Periodic paralysis	CACNA1S KCNJ2 SCN4A
	Metabolic disorders	Pompe's disease	GAA
		McArdle's disease	PYGM
		Carnitine palmitoyltransferase II deficiency	CPT2
	Congenital myopathies	Nemaline myopathy	NEB
		Myotubular myopathy	MTM1
		Central core myopathy	RYR1
		Multicore myopathy	SEPN1
Neuromuscular junction and anterior horn disorders	Congenital myasthenic syndromes	Presynaptic	CHAT
		Synaptic	COLQ
		Postsynaptic	CHRNA1 CHRNE MUSK RAPSN
	Hereditary motor neuron disease		SOD1 ALS2 FUS SETX VAPB NEFH
	Spinal muscular atrophy	Spinal muscular atrophy	SMN1
		Kennedy's disease	AR
Ataxias	Dominant	Spinocerebellar ataxias 1–31	ATXN1 ATXN2 ATXN3 ANTX7 CACNA1A Others
		Episodic ataxias	CACNA1A KCNA1
		Dentatorubral–pallidoluysian atrophy	ATN1
		Fragile X-associated tremor/ataxia syndrome	FMR1
	Recessive	Friedreich's ataxia	FXN
		Ataxia with oculomotor apraxia	APTX SETX
		Ataxia–telangiectasia	ATM
		Abetalipoproteinaemia	MTTP
		Autosomal recessive cerebellar ataxia type 1	SYNE1
		Ataxia with vitamin E deficiency	TTPA

Table 223.1 (Continued)

Disorder	Type	Examples	Genes
Epilepsy	Structural	Neurocutaneous syndromes: • neurofibromatosis type 1 • tuberous sclerosis	NF1 TSC1 TSC2
		Migration defects: • lissencephaly • double cortex	RELN DCX
	Channelopathies	Autosomal dominant nocturnal frontal lobe epilepsy	CHRNA2 CHRNA4 CHRNB2
		Benign familial neonatal seizures	KCNQ2 KCNQ3 BFNC3
		Generalized epilepsy with febrile seizures plus	GABRG2 SCN1A SCN1B SCN2A
		Juvenile myoclonic epilepsy	CACNB4 CLCN2 EFHC1 GABRA1 GABRD
		Severe myoclonic epilepsy of infancy (Dravet syndrome)	SCN1A SCN1B
	Progressive myoclonic epilepsies	Dentatorubral–pallidoluysian atrophy	ATN1
		Lafora disease	EPM2A EPM2B
		Neuronal ceroid lipofuscinosis	CLN1
		MERRF syndrome	mtDNA 8344
		Sialidosis type 1	NEU1
		Unverricht—Lundborg disease	CSTB
Movement disorders	Dystonia	DYT1–DYT20	DYT1 GCH1 SGCE Other, unknown genes
	Parkinsonism	Genetic Parkinson's disease	LRRK2 PARK2 SNCA UCH-L1 PINK1 DJ-1 ATP13A2
	Chorea	Huntington's disease	HTT
		Dentatorubral–pallidoluysian atrophy	ATN1
		Chorea-acanthocytosis	CHAC
	Hereditary spastic paraparesis	SPG1–SPG42	SPAST ALT1 HSP60 KIF5A Other, unknown genes
	Multiple movement disorders	Wilson's disease	ATP7B
		Pantothenate kinase-associated neurodegeneration	PANK2
Dementia		Alzheimer's disease	PSEN1 PSEN2 APP
		Prion: familial Creutzfeldt–Jakob disease	PrP
		Frontotemporal dementia	PGRN MAPT
		Familial British dementia	ITM2B

(continued)

Table 223.1 (Continued)

Disorder	Type	Examples	Genes
Multisystem disease	Mitochondrial disorders	Multiple phenotypes	Mitochondrial DNA Nuclear genes: • POLG • TWNK • ANT1
	Lysosomal storage disorders	Tay–Sachs disease	HEXA
		Niemann–Pick type C	NPC1 NPC2
		Metachromatic leucodystrophy	ARSA
		Fabry's disease	GLA
	Peroxisomal disorders	Adrenoleukodystrophy	ABCD1
		Refsum disease	PAHX PEX7
	Leukodystrophies	Canavan disease	ASPA
		Alexander disease	GFAP

diabetes mellitus, premature balding, subfertility, and cognitive impairment may all occur. Congenital DM1 usually occurs when the repeat is inherited from the mother, with massive expansion occurring during meiosis. It is characterized by severe generalized weakness, hypotonia, and respiratory compromise, which may lead to death. Surviving infants have a gradual improvement in motor function and swallowing and can independently ventilate but develop learning difficulties.

Demographics of DM1

DM1 is globally distributed and there is no particular ethnic predilection.

Natural history of DM1, and complications of the disease

In DM1, the myopathy is slowly progressive and, as weakness ensues, myotonia becomes less prominent. Patients usually maintain ambulation, but have increasing problems with facial and hand weakness. A significant proportion of patients will develop cardiac conduction defects requiring placement of a permanent pacemaker. Cardiomyopathy is rare. Obstructive sleep apnoea or excessive daytime somnolence may also occur.

Approach to diagnosing DM1

The diagnosis of DM1 is clinical in those with a classic myopathic facies, frontal balding, and distal myotonia. The vast majority of adults who are found to have clinical or electrical myotonia will have DM1. Where this is not evident, the diagnosis may be delayed while other causes of myopathy are excluded.

Other diagnoses that should be considered aside from DM1

There are other causes of myotonia aside from DM1, but these do not lead to dystrophic features or multisystem involvement.

'Gold-standard' diagnostic test for DM1

A clinical suspicion of DM1 can be readily confirmed by molecular genetic testing. The test is simple and inexpensive. However, this should not be undertaken without adequate genetic counselling of the patient, including the risk of diagnosing presymptomatic obligate carriers (i.e. the patient's parents) and the identification of at-risk individuals (siblings and offspring).

Acceptable diagnostic alternatives to the gold-standard test for DM1

For DM1, there are no acceptable diagnostic alternatives to genetic testing.

Other relevant investigations for DM1

DM1 patients should have an annual ECG and referral to a cardiologist should conduction abnormalities appear. Blood or urine glucose should also be tested on an annual basis. Sleep studies can help elucidate the cause of excessive daytime somnolence.

Prognosis of DM1, and how to estimate it

In patients with DM1, lifespan is shortened by cardiac and respiratory involvement. A milder late-onset form with partial clinical manifestation is correlated with shorter CTG repeat length. However, in general, repeat length cannot be used to predict phenotype.

Treatment of DM1, and its effectiveness

There are no treatments to reverse muscle wasting and weakness in DM1. Myotonia is rarely disabling for patients. If prominent, it can be treated effectively with mexiletine (with regular ECG monitoring); phenytoin is less effective. Excessive daytime somnolence can be treated with modafinil or overnight continuous positive airway pressure, if there is a significant respiratory contribution. Conduction defects can be treated with permanent pacemaker implantation. Multidisciplinary involvement is useful in the later stages with input from a physiotherapist, an occupational therapist, a dietician, and a speech and language therapist.

Charcot–Marie–Tooth disease type 1a

Definition of Charcot–Marie–Tooth disease type 1a

Charcot–Marie–Tooth disease type 1a (CMT1a) is the commonest genetic neuropathy in adults.

Aetiology of CMT1a

CMT1a is an autosomal dominant demyelinating neuropathy due to a chromosomal duplication leading to duplication of PMP22.

Typical symptoms of CMT1a, and less common symptoms

The classical phenotype of CMT1a is of a slowly progressive sensory and motor neuropathy with onset in adulthood. This presents as foot weakness and deformity and leads to pes cavus, distal muscle wasting, and sensory loss.

Demographics of CMT1a

CMT1a is the commonest genetic neuropathy in Europe.

Natural history of CMT1a, and complications of the disease

The neuropathy in CMT1a is slowly progressive with weakness and sensory loss. Complications are usually of joint destruction (Charcot's joints) and subsequent loss of mobility. Pressure ulcers may also occur. There is no effect on lifespan.

Approach to diagnosing CMT1a

The diagnosis of Charcot–Marie–Tooth disease is clinical in those with the classic inverted-champagne-bottle legs, pes cavus, and stocking sensory loss. However, this does not elucidate what type of Charcot–Marie–Tooth disease a patient has. EMG and nerve conduction studies are required to determine whether the neuropathy is axonal or demyelinating. The genotype–phenotype correlation in this condition is poor.

Other diagnoses that should be considered aside from CMT1a

Other diagnoses that should be considered aside from CMT1a are other types of Charcot–Marie–Tooth disease.

'Gold-standard' diagnostic test for CMT1a

A clinical suspicion of CMT1a can be readily confirmed by molecular genetic testing. The test is simple and inexpensive. Over 98% of patients with CMT1a have a duplication of PMP22, and this can be detected using dosage techniques. However, around 2% have point mutations in PMP22, and this requires direct DNA sequencing to detect.

Acceptable diagnostic alternatives to the gold-standard test for CMT1a

For CMT1a, there are no acceptable diagnostic alternatives to genetic testing.

Other relevant investigations for CMT1a

For CMT1a, there are no relevant investigations other than genetic testing.

Prognosis of CMT1a, and how to estimate it

The lifespan of patients with CMT1a is not significantly reduced.

Treatment of CMT1a, and its effectiveness

There are no treatments to reverse muscle wasting and weakness in CMT1a. Multidisciplinary involvement is useful with input from physiotherapy, occupational therapy, and, in particular, the use of orthotics. Painful dysasthesiae are rare, but can be treated with amitriptyline, gabapentin, pregabalin, or duloxetine. Treatment trials are ongoing. Genetic counselling should be offered.

Friedreich's ataxia

Definition of Friedreich's ataxia

Friedreich's ataxia (FRDA) is the commonest autosomal recessive ataxia.

Aetiology of FRDA

FRDA is an autosomal recessive ataxia due to a trinucleotide repeat (GAA) expansion in the first intron of the FXN gene.

Typical symptoms of FRDA, and less common symptoms

FRDA begins in the first or second decade and is relentlessly progressive. It is characterized by ataxia, pyramidal signs, large fibre axonal neuropathy, skeletal abnormalities (pes cavus and scoliosis), cardiomyopathy, and, more rarely, optic atrophy, deafness, and diabetes mellitus. Patients are usually wheelchair bound by their twenties, and lifespan is considerably reduced, largely by the cardiomyopathy.

Demographics of FRDA

FRDA is the commonest hereditary ataxia amongst Caucasian populations and does not occur in non-Caucasians.

Natural history of FRDA, and complications of the disease

Most patients with FRDA will lose the ability to walk, stand, or sit unaided within 10–15 years of disease onset. The neuropathy is often subclinical. Hypertrophic cardiomyopathy occurs in around 10% of patients and may be asymptomatic. Diabetes mellitus occurs in about 10% of patients.

Approach to diagnosing FRDA

The diagnosis of FRDA is clinical in those with ataxia, scoliosis, pes cavus, absent reflexes, and pyramidal signs. Those who are less symptomatic may be harder to diagnose. With the advent of genetic testing, phenotypic variation has been noted, in particular, with later onset cases.

Other diagnoses that should be considered aside from FRDA

FRDA mimics include ataxia with oculomotor apraxia types 1 and 2, and ataxia–telangiectasia.

'Gold-standard' diagnostic test for FRDA

A clinical suspicion of FRDA can be readily confirmed by molecular genetic testing. The test is simple and inexpensive. Over 99% of patients with FRDA have two copies of the GAA expansion, and this can be detected using Southern blotting. However, around 1% have one GAA expansion and one point mutation in FXN, and this requires direct DNA sequencing to detect.

Acceptable diagnostic alternatives to the gold-standard test for FRDA

Other relevant investigations for FRDA

Patients with FRDA should have an annual ECG and echocardiography, and referral to a cardiologist should abnormalities occur. Blood or urine glucose should also be tested on an annual basis.

Prognosis of FRDA, and how to estimate it

The lifespan of patients with FRDA is significantly reduced. The GAA repeat size is inversely correlated with age of onset and age of confinement to wheelchair, and directly correlated with the incidence of cardiomyopathy.

Treatment of FRDA and its effectiveness

There are no treatments to reverse ataxia, muscle wasting, and weakness in FRDA. Multidisciplinary involvement is useful with input from physiotherapy, occupational therapy, and, in particular, the use of orthotics when patients are still mobile. When mobility is lost, wheelchair services are essential to prevent further complications from ill-fitting seats, arms, or foot rests. Dysarthria may be severe, and speech and language therapy can be extremely valuable. Orthopaedic intervention for scoliosis can reduce pain and disability. Treatment trials of idebenone (a coenzyme Q10 analogue) are ongoing.

Further Reading

Novak MJU and Tabrizi SJ. Huntington's disease. *BMJ* 2010; 340: 3109.

Pandolfo M. Friedreich ataxia: The clinical picture. *J Neurol* 2009; 256: 3–8.

Reilly MM and Shy ME. Diagnosis and new treatments in genetic neuropathies. *J Neurol Neurosurg Psychiatry* 2010; 80: 1304–14.

Shy ME and Patzkó Á. Axonal Charcot-Marie-Tooth disease. *Curr Opin Neurol* 2011; 24: 475–83.

Turner C and Hilton-Jones D. The myotonic dystrophies: Diagnosis and management. *J Neurol Neurosurg Psychiatry* 2010; 81: 358–67.

224 Neurocutaneous syndromes

Nerissa Jordan

Definition of the disease

The neurocutaneous syndromes are a diverse group of rare genetic disorders with both neurological and cutaneous manifestations. Each syndrome has a distinct phenotype. See Box 224.1 for a list of neurocutaneous syndromes.

Symptoms

Symptoms are variable and depend on the syndrome. See Table 224.1 for a summary of typical clinical and radiological features.

Demographics and aetiology

Neurocutaneous syndromes often present in childhood or adolescence; for example, tuberous sclerosis typically presents in early childhood. The age range of presentation is broad, depending on the specific condition and severity of expression. The majority are autosomally inherited conditions. De novo mutations can occur.

Natural history of the disease

Most are progressive conditions, such as tuberous sclerosis and neurofibromatosis. Others, such as Ehlers–Danlos, have milder phenotypes, with most symptoms due to intermittent complications, particularly haemorrhage.

Box 224.1 Neurocutaneous syndromes

- tuberous sclerosis
- neurofibromatosis type 1 and 2
- Ehlers–Danlos syndrome
- hereditary haemorrhagic telangiectasia
- Sturge–Weber syndrome
- ataxia–telangiectasia
- Fabry's disease
- von-Hippel–Lindau disease
- progressive facial hemiatrophy
- pseudoxanthoma elasticum
- kinky hair syndrome
- cerebrotendinous xanthomatosis
- epidermal naevus syndrome
- hypomelanosis of Ito
- neurocutaneous melanosis
- Wyburn–Mason syndrome
- xeroderma pigmentosum

Complications

There are two main groups of complications:

- complications of tumours, including local pressure effects and seizures
- vascular events, including stroke and haemorrhage

Approach to diagnosing the disease (including diagnostic pitfalls)

Most of these diseases may be diagnosed clinically, with characteristic skin lesions. Imaging may be helpful, for example, in identifying the typical cerebral lesions in tuberous sclerosis. The diagnosis may be clear at an early age. In other cases, the cutaneous lesions may be missed and diagnosed only when vascular lesions become symptomatic. For example, hereditary haemorrhagic telangiectasia may only be recognized following a cerebral haemorrhage in an individual with cutaneous telangiectasia. Genetic testing is available for confirmation for many of the disorders.

'Gold-standard' diagnostic test

Molecular genetic testing is the gold-standard test for diagnosing neurocutaneous syndromes (see Table 224.1 for known mutations).

Acceptable diagnostic alternatives to the gold standard

Clinical and radiological features can be highly suggestive.

Other relevant investigations

Other relevant investigations include MRI of the brain, with or without MRI of the spinal cord; angiography; EEG, for seizures; EMG, for peripheral neuropathy; an ophthalmology review, if relevant (e.g. cataracts); and audiometry, in neurofibromatosis type 2.

Prognosis, and how to estimate it

Severity of presentation and presence of complications will largely determine the prognosis.

Treatment and its effectiveness

Most neurocutaneous syndromes do not have a specific treatment, and management is predominantly supportive and aimed at symptom reduction and appropriate monitoring. This includes surgical excision of compressive tumours, radiation therapy, management of epilepsy, and surveillance for tumours. A multidisciplinary approach

Syndrome	Genetics	Cutaneous features	Neurological features	Systemic features	Imaging features
Tuberous sclerosis	TSC1/TSC2 gene Chromosome 9q34 Autosomal dominant Disorder of cellular differentiation/ proliferation	Hypomelanotic macules Shagreen patch* Ungual fibromas Facial angiofibromas	Seizures (80%–90%) Mental retardation Behavioural disorders (autism, aggressiveness, psychosis)	Retinal hamartomas Cardiac rhabdomyoma Renal angiomyolipomas Lymphangiomyomatosis	Calcified subependymal nodules Abnormal neural migration
Neurofibromatosis type 1	NF1 gene Chromosome 17q Autosomal dominant Cytoplasmic regulatory molecule	Café au lait spots Subcutaneous neurofibromas Axillary freckling	Peripheral neurofibromas Optic nerve gliomas Other CNS tumours	Pigmented iris hamartomas (Lisch nodules) Dysplasia of renal or carotid arteries Short stature Macrocephaly	Increased signal in basal ganglia, cerebellum, or brainstem
Neurofibromatosis type 2	NF2 gene Chromosome 22 Autosomal dominant Usually suppresses tumour function	Café au lait spots Peripheral neurofibromas	Bilateral vestibular schwannomas (deafness, brainstem compressive symptoms) Meningiomas, ependymomas		CNS tumours
Hereditary haemorrhagic telangiectasia	HHT1 gene/HHT2 Chromosome 9q34 Chromosome 12q13 Autosomal dominant TGF-beta receptor component	Telangiectasias of skin and mucous membranes	Arteriovenous malformations: CNS haemorrhage Pulmonary arteriovenous malformations: paradoxical embolism Cerebral abscess or meningitis from septic emboli	Organ telangiectasia: epistaxis Organ-related haemorrhage	Arteriovenous malformations Aneurysms
Ataxia–telangiectasia	ATM gene Chromosome 11q22–23 Autosomal recessive DNA repair	Telangiectasias of skin, especially of earlobes, sclera, and nasal bridge	Progressive ataxia followed by tremor, segmental myoclonus, and choreoathetosis	Sinopulmonary infections Increased risk of malignancy	Non-progressive cerebellar atrophy
Ehlers–Danlos syndrome	Multiple different defects of collagen subtypes	Hyperelastic or fragile skin Easy bruising	Intracranial aneurysms, particularly in the carotid artery Carotid–cavernous fistula	Hyperextensible joints	
Fabry's disease	Chromosome X q21.33–q22 X-linked recessive Alpha-galactosidase A deficiency	Punctate angiectatic lesions on trunk, buttocks, and legs	Peripheral neuropathy Severe limb pain Ischaemic or haemorrhagic strokes	Corneal opacification Cardiac and renal lesions	Left ventricular hypertrophy on echocardiography (may simulate hypertrophic cardiomyopathy)

*An area of yellowed, elevated, roughened skin with a texture of orange peel, often on the lower back.

is necessary. There are several new molecularly based treatments under investigation for conditions such as neurofibromatosis type 2; however, the role for these therapies is still being defined. Enzyme replacement is possible to treat Fabry's disease.

Further Reading

Asthagiri AR, Parry DM, Butman JA, et al. Neurofibromatosis type 2. *Lancet* 2009; 373: 1974–86.

Curatolo P, Bombardieri R, and Jozwiak S. Tuberous sclerosis. *Lancet* 2003; 372: 657–68.

Reynolds RM, Browning GGP, Nawroz I, et al. Von Recklinghausen's neurofibromatosis: Neurofibromatosis type 1. *Lancet* 2003; 361: 1552–4.

Stark Z, Campbell LJ, Mitchell C, et al. Spot diagnosis. *N Engl J Med* 2014; 370: 2229–36.

225 Congenital neurological disorders

Simon Rinaldi

Introduction

This chapter covers four congenital neurological disorders which may be encountered in adult medicine: cerebral palsy, Chiari malformations, spina bifida, and tethered cord syndromes.

Cerebral palsy

Cerebral palsy is a disturbance of motor function arising from damage to the developing fetal or infant brain. It usually refers to a disorder resulting from a non-progressive insult which occurred at less than 3 years of age. The term lacks specificity, and encompasses a wide range of clinical presentations and differing pathological processes.

In the developed world, cerebral palsy has a prevalence of around 2 per 1000 live births. It is substantially more common in premature births. The immature cerebral vasculature is at increased risk of failing to adequately perfuse certain areas of the brain, most notably the deep-lying periventricular white matter. This can result in periventricular leukomalacia and/or germinal matrix haemorrhage. In severe cases, the haemorrhage extends into the lateral ventricles or brain parenchyma. In contrast, vascular injuries in term infants more often affect the territory of the middle cerebral artery.

There is a widespread belief that cerebral palsy is solely a result of hypoxic–ischaemic birth injury. This is incorrect. In less than 10% of cases can 'birth asphyxia' be conclusively identified as the cause. In around 80%, the pathological process appears to have occurred prenatally. Congenital malformations, growth retardation, maternal hypotension, infection, thyroid disease, and exposure to toxins are part of a long list of prenatal, gestational risk factors. Even in these cases, the clinical deficit may not become apparent until much later in development.

Overall, around 30%–50% of cerebral palsy cases are associated with learning disability, and a similar proportion with epilepsy. The different clinical syndromes—spastic (80%), dyskinetic (10%–15%), or ataxic (<5%)—result from predominant damage to pyramidal, extrapyramidal, or cerebellar structures. Spastic cerebral palsy is further subdivided on the basis of the affected body regions into diplegic (affecting both legs, usually with lesser involvement of the arms), hemiplegic, and quadriplegic types. In premature infants, spastic diplegia is often a result of periventricular leukomalacia or haemorrhage. Pathological–clinical associations in term infants and for the other types of spastic cerebral palsy are less consistent.

Dyskinetic cerebral palsy is characterized by choreoathetoid movements, but combinations of dystonia, myoclonus, tremor, and hemiballismus can also be seen. Historically, kernicterus (neonatal hyperbilirubinaemia) was the most frequent cause. Current cases are usually attributed to hypoxic–ischaemic damage of the basal ganglia and/or thalamus.

The adult physician most usually encounters cerebral palsy in the context of an acute or subacute deterioration in functioning on the background of prior clinical stability. The challenge is then to identify and appropriately treat the cause of this deterioration. There are four broad possibilities.

First, intercurrent infections or metabolic disturbances can more profoundly affect patients with preexisting brain pathology than might otherwise be the case and, in this context, apparent new focal deficits can sometimes be seen. Second, like the wider population, cerebral palsy patients remain at risk of developing further neurological disease such as strokes, infective encephalitis, or even neurodegenerative pathology, and are at an increased risk of seizures.

Third, static pathological insults can cause clinical progression due to the additional effects of development (dyskinetic cerebral palsy especially can progress or even appear in adolescence) or normal ageing ('pseudodegeneration'). Finally, the label of cerebral palsy may be erroneous, and the patient instead suffers from a different, progressive pathology. Nevertheless, the priority of the acute medical team lies with assessing the first and second possibilities. Missed diagnoses of, for example, adrenoleucodystrophy, Wilson's disease, or metachromatic leucodystrophy, are uncommon but may need to be considered at a later time.

Chiari malformations

Chiari malformations are congenital abnormalities of the anatomy and structural relationships of the cerebellum, brainstem, and foramen magnum. They are numbered I to IV. Type III and IV malformations are rare, severe, well outside the domain of the adult physician, and are not further discussed.

In contrast, Chiari I malformations are by far the most common and least severe defects, and are often diagnosed in adult life. The key abnormality here is displacement of the cerebellar tonsils below the level of the foramen magnum. With the increasingly widespread availability of MRI, the diagnosis is made more frequently. Indeed, this often asymptomatic anomaly is found on up to 1 in every 200 MRI brain scans performed. Commonly, this is an incidental and unexpected finding but, on other occasions, symptomatic Chiari I malformations require surgical treatment. The adult physician therefore needs to be familiar with the neurological signs and symptoms which may result from a Chiari I malformation.

Herniation of the tonsils can compress the cerebellar structures themselves (resulting in dysmetria, ataxia, and other cerebellar signs and symptoms). In this context, the nystagmus is downbeating. The tonsils can additionally compress the cervicomedullary junction in the foramen magnum (giving lower cranial nerve dysfunction and/ or upper cervical myelopathy). The disruption of CSF flow through the foramen can result in hydrocephalus, but much more commonly induces a syrinx in the cervical cord. This leads to a suspended sensory level and motor weakness in the arms. CSF flow abnormalities are also the likely pathological mechanism for the cough-impulse headache which can be associated with Chiari I malformations. Here, a short-lived, severe, cervico-occipital headache occurs a fraction of a second or so after coughing or straining—the delay presumably reflecting the time taken for the CSF pressure wave to be transmitted to pain-sensitive structures.

When these symptoms can be correlated with the imaging abnormalities, surgical decompression is indicated, and can result in resolution of any associated syrinx. Surgical intervention is not warranted outwith this context or for the treatment of non-cough-impulse headaches or neck pain.

Type II malformations involve additional displacement of the lower brainstem structures through the foramen magnum, resulting in a more severe abnormality. As such, the diagnosis is usually made in infants who have signs and symptoms of brainstem dysfunction. Unlike type I malformations, type II malformations are frequently associated with hydrocephalus, and treatment of this with shunting is the surgical priority.

Dysraphism (spina bifida)

Dysraphism is a failure of opposition of anatomical structures which are normally fused. Spinal dysraphism is synonymous with spina bifida, a failure of embryological fusion of the neural tube. In all types, the vertebral arch fails to completely form. There is an association with maternal folate deficiency, pregestational diabetes, antiepileptic drug exposure (particularly sodium valproate), and certain chromosomal abnormalities.

Spina bifida occulta

Spina bifida occulta is usually an incidental and asymptomatic finding, and is likely to be very common. Although there is a defect in the vertebral arch, the meninges and neural tissue remain in the spinal canal. Progressive neurological symptoms can be seen, however, if there is an associated tethered cord (see 'Tethered cord syndromes') or other distortion of the cord and roots.

Spina bifida cystica

Spina bifida cystica involves protrusion of the meningeal sac through the vertebral defect. If the sac contains part of the spinal cord or roots it is termed a **myelomeningocele**. If these elements are absent, the term **meningocele** is used. Discounting spina bifida occulta, myelomeningocele is by far the most common type of spina bifida and, indeed, the most common major birth defect. Most often, lower lumbar segments are involved. With neurological involvement, the level of the defect generally relates to the resultant level of impairment. However, there may be additional contributions from coexistent syringomyelia, cerebral polymicrogyria, and/or hydrocephalus (sometimes with cerebellar herniation producing a Chiari II malformation).

Spina bifida cystica is treated with early neurosurgical closure to prevent infection and significantly improve survival. Existing myelopathic and radiculopathic symptoms are likely to persist, with varying degrees of lower limb paralysis and sensory loss. Incontinence is very common. If hydrocephalus is present, shunting allows the development of normal intelligence.

Complications arise from shunt obstruction, shunt infection, renal impairment, and urinary tract infections secondary to the neurogenic bladder, and from the long-term effects of reduced lower limb function, such as contractures and pressure sores.

Tethered cord syndromes

The tethered cord syndromes involve a restriction of the normal cephalad migration of the conus during life. This can occur both with and without spina bifida. On occasions, the cauda appears 'stuck' to an associated lipoma or dermoid. Combinations of upper and lower motor neuron signs, sensory disturbance in the legs, sphincter dysfunction, and scoliosis are found. Evolution of the symptoms in adulthood can be seen. Neurosurgical release of the cord is undertaken for progressive symptoms. A tethered cord is a contraindication to lumbar puncture, while spina bifida occulta itself is not, and may make the procedure easier.

Further Reading

Aisen ML, Kerkovich D, Mast J, et al. Cerebral palsy: Clinical care and neurological rehabilitation. *Lancet Neurol* 2011; 10: 844–52.

Badve CA, Khanna PC, Phillips GS, et al. MRI of closed spinal dysraphisms. *Pediatr Radiol* 2011; 41: 1308–20.

Chiapparini L, Saletti V, Solero CL, et al. Neuroradiological diagnosis of Chiari malformations. *Neurol Sci* 2011; 32: S283–6.

Murphy KP. The adult with cerebral palsy. *Orthop Clin North Am* 2010; 41: 595–605.

Sandler AD. Children with spina bifida: Key clinical issues. *Pediatr Clin North Am* 2010; 57: 879–92.

Sekula RF Jr, Arnone GD, Crocker C, et al. The pathogenesis of Chiari I malformation and syringomyelia. *Neurol Res* 2011; 33: 232–9.

CHAPTER 225 **Congenital neurological disorders**

226 Epilepsy

Yvonne Hart

Definition of the disease

Epilepsy is defined as the occurrence of at least two unprovoked or reflex seizures occurring more than 24 hours apart, an epilepsy syndrome, or a single unprovoked or reflex seizure where the chance of recurrence is at least 60%. A seizure can be defined as a transient excessive discharge of nerve cells within the brain, causing an event which is discernible to the person experiencing the seizure or to an observer. The term 'epilepsy' excludes provoked seizures, such as febrile seizures.

Symptoms

The symptoms of epilepsy vary according to the extent of the seizure activity, and the site of onset of the seizure. The 1981 classification of seizures developed by the International League Against Epilepsy (ILAE), shown in Box 226.1, is commonly used, but the ILAE has now published suggestions for a new 'organization' of seizures and epilepsies. Generalized seizures involve the rapid engagement of bilaterally distributed networks of seizure activity.

Generalized seizures

Generalized tonic–clonic seizures involve an initial tonic phase, usually lasting about 20 seconds, in which the patient becomes stiff, stops breathing and may cry out as air is forced out of the lungs, and tongue biting may occur. This is followed by a clonic phase often lasting 2–3 minutes, with jerking of the limbs and which is sometimes followed by incontinence of urine. A postictal phase follows, with headache, drowsiness, and confusion being common symptoms.

Absence ('petit mal') seizures usually develop in childhood or adolescence. The patient abruptly appears blank, as if in a trance, usually for around 10 seconds. Fluttering of the eyelids and swallowing may also occur.

Myoclonic jerks are brief muscle jerks involving part or all of the body, similar to the jerks sometimes seen as people are dropping off to sleep. They may occur in association with absence seizures and generalized tonic–clonic seizures in people with presumed genetic (idiopathic) generalized epilepsy.

Tonic seizures, in which patients develop a sudden generalized increase in muscle tone causing falling, and atonic seizures, in which the patient falls limply, are other forms of generalized seizures usually occurring in the context of severe childhood-onset epilepsy, such as Lennox–Gastaut syndrome. The seizures are usually brief but frequently cause injury due to the sudden falls. Clonic seizures are another form of generalized seizure.

Focal (partial) seizures

Focal (partial) seizures have their onset in a localized area of cerebral cortex, although they may spread to involve the rest of the cerebral cortex.

Focal seizures are described according to the symptoms experienced. Focal seizures without loss of awareness were previously termed simple partial seizures. They generally reflect the function of the area in which they arise; thus, occipital seizures commonly take the form of visual hallucinations (e.g. patients may complain of seeing coloured lights), frontal lobe seizures often take the form of motor seizures, and temporal lobe seizures may cause gustatory or auditory hallucinations, dysphasia, fear, and déjà vu or jamais vu.

Focal dyscognitive (complex partial) seizures occur when the seizure discharge spreads further such that loss of awareness occurs. They commonly (but not exclusively) arise in the temporal lobes, and may be characterized by a motionless stare, lip smacking or chewing, fiddling, rubbing, and undressing or wandering.

Focal seizures may progress further to become bilateral convulsive (secondarily generalized) seizures. These may appear identical to generalized tonic–clonic seizures, but symptoms occurring in the course of the preceding focal seizure may act as a warning or 'aura' to the attack.

Demographics and aetiology of epilepsy

Epilepsy occurs in all races and may develop at any time of life: it is most common in the elderly, probably due to the occurrence of cerebrovascular disease, with the second highest incidence being in childhood, where the most common causes are birth injury, developmental abnormalities, infection, and presumed genetic (idiopathic) epilepsy. Epilepsy is marginally more common in males than females. Overall, the incidence in the developed world is about 50–60 in 100 000 per annum; it is rather more common in the developing world, where it may exceed 100 in 100 000 per annum. The prevalence of active epilepsy is 0.5%–1.0%.

Other causes of epilepsy in adults include alcohol abuse, tumour, head trauma, infection, and, particularly in developing countries, parasitic infection.

Natural history of the disease

Approximately 50% of people experiencing a seizure do not have any recurrence, and it is therefore usual not to start treatment after a single seizure, unless there is an underlying condition (such as tumour) likely to significantly increase the risk of recurrence. Of those patients who do have a recurrence and are started on treatment, it will be possible to completely control the seizures in approximately 70%, while 20%–30% will be expected to have

---

Box 226.1 Classification of epileptic seizures (simplified)

1 *Focal seizures (partial seizures)*
   a. Without impairment of consciousness (e.g. focal motor) (simple partial seizures)
   b. Focal dyscognitive seizures (complex partial seizures)
   c. Bilateral convulsive seizures (secondarily generalised seizures)

2 *Generalised seizures*
   a. Absence seizures
   b. Myoclonic seizures
   c. Clonic seizures
   d. Tonic seizures
   e. Tonic clonic seizures
   f. Atonic seizures

3 *Unclassified epileptic seizures*

Reproduced with permission from Jean Bancaud et al. Proposal for Revised Clinical and Electroencephalographic Classification of Epileptic Seizures, *Epilepsia*, Volume 22, Issue 4, pp. 489–501, Copyright © 1981 John Wiley and Sons

seizures which are resistant to medication. Patients whose seizures fail to respond to the first two or three antiepileptic drugs often fail to respond to the addition of other antiepileptic drugs, although a small proportion (perhaps 4%) will find that a new antiepileptic drug will be effective. Approximately 50% of patients will eventually be able to discontinue medication without recurrence of seizures.

Epilepsy surgery may be feasible for patients with epilepsy which is refractory to medical treatment, where it is possible to identify the epileptic focus, and where the likely benefits of surgery outweigh the risks (e.g. of functional deficit as a result of surgery). In appropriately selected patients, the chance of becoming seizure-free may be of the order of 70%–80%.

Complications of epilepsy

Epileptic seizures, particularly where they cause falls without warning, are common causes of injury, with burns or scalds, dental injuries, head injuries, and fractures being particularly common. In one survey, a quarter of people having at least one seizure during the previous year had had such an injury. Dislocated shoulders and wedge fractures of the vertebrae may occur as a result of tonic–clonic seizures, as may aspiration pneumonia. Epilepsy is also associated with excess mortality, the standardized mortality ratio being of the order of 2–3, with the main causes of death being accidental death or drowning due to seizures, the underlying cause of the epilepsy, suicide, status epilepticus, and sudden unexpected death in epilepsy, the risk of which has been estimated at between 1 in 500 to 1 in 1000 (more for those with very severe epilepsy). Epilepsy is also responsible for considerable psychosocial morbidity.

Approach to diagnosing epilepsy

The diagnosis of epilepsy is essentially clinical, relying on the description of an eyewitness and of the patient himself.

Other diagnoses that should be considered

The most common conditions to be considered in the differential diagnosis of seizures are syncope (either vasovagal syncope or secondary to cardiac disorders), and psychogenic non-epileptic (dissociative or functional) seizures (formerly known as pseudoseizures). Hypoglycaemia, concussive seizures (seizures occurring within 2 seconds of a head injury and not causing long-term damage or predisposing to the development of epilepsy), and breath-holding attacks in children may also be confused with seizures causing loss of awareness. Focal seizures need to be distinguished from such conditions as migraine, transient global amnesia, panic attacks, and transient ischaemic attacks.

'Gold-standard' diagnostic test

The gold-standard diagnostic test is EEG videotelemetry, in which EEG and simultaneous video monitoring are carried out to record a seizure and confirm that the typical symptoms and signs of a seizure are accompanied by epileptic activity at the appropriate time on the EEG. In practice, this test is usually only helpful in people whose seizures are occurring so frequently that they can reliably recorded in a reasonable period of EEG videotelemetry recording (up to a week in most centres).

Acceptable diagnostic alternatives to the gold standard

As noted in 'Approach to diagnosing epilepsy', a clinical diagnosis of epilepsy frequently rests solely on the description of the event by the patient and an eyewitness, since it is often not possible to record a seizure, and investigations may be normal in between attacks.

Other relevant investigations

Diagnosis involves not only establishing that the patient is having epileptic seizures, but also diagnosis of the epilepsy syndrome, if possible, and of the underlying cause. Although the history is the most important factor in establishing the diagnosis of seizures, ECG is important in all patients to rule out cardiac causes of loss of consciousness, and a cardiology opinion may be appropriate. Interictal EEG only consistently shows epileptic abnormalities in 35% of patients with epilepsy while, in another 50% of patients, epileptic abnormalities will be present in some, but not all, interictal EEGs. On the other hand, only 0.5% of patients without epilepsy have interictal epileptic abnormalities on their EEG. Non-specific abnormalities (such as focal or diffuse slow waves) may be seen in 15%–25% of the normal population. The EEG may be helpful in classifying the type of epilepsy.

Blood tests are usually normal in people presenting with their first seizure, but may be helpful in ruling out infection or metabolic disorder. Liver function tests are useful in cases of suspected alcohol abuse, and should be checked as a baseline prior to starting antiepileptic drugs, many of which can have an effect on them. Neuroimaging should be carried out in all adults developing epilepsy, and in most children (except where the idiopathic nature of the epilepsy can be clearly established on EEG), to help establish the underlying aetiology.

Prognosis, and how to estimate it?

Approximately 50% of people having a single seizure will have a further seizure in the next 2 years, most commonly soon after the first. As noted in 'Natural history of the disease', epilepsy eventually becomes inactive in many patients, with up to 70% of all people developing epilepsy becoming seizure-free, and about half being able to successfully withdraw their medication. However, in about 30% of people developing epilepsy, the condition will become chronic and resistant to antiepileptic drugs. Most patients will have their seizures controlled by the first or second antiepileptic drug. However, if they fail to respond to the first thee antiepileptic drugs, the chance of becoming seizure-free with any new drug is of the order of 4%. Therefore, the possibility of using other methods of treatment such as epilepsy surgery should be considered in any person with epilepsy whose seizures persist despite medication.

In the UK, people having a single seizure are permitted to resume driving a car after 6 months in the absence of such factors as MRI or EEG abnormalities which might increase the risk of recurrence. People with epilepsy must be seizure-free for a year to be eligible to drive a car: special rules apply to those only having seizures which do not involve loss of consciousness or with seizures occurring in sleep.

Treatment and its effectiveness

In the UK, antiepileptic drugs are not usually prescribed after a single seizure in the absence of factors increasing the risk of recurrence (e.g. the presence of an underlying tumour). Prophylactic measures which may reduce the risk of recurrent seizures include avoiding sleep deprivation and excesses of alcohol. Those patients with epilepsy who are photosensitive (about 5% of the total) should avoid flashing lights.

The SANAD (Standard And New Antiepileptic Drugs) study compared valproate with topiramate and lamotrigine, and suggested that valproate was the most effective and best-tolerated drug in patients with genetic generalized epilepsy. However, it carries a relatively high risk of teratogenicity (of the order of 6%), and should preferably be avoided in women of childbearing age, in whom lamotrigine or levetiracetam may be a more appropriate choice. For patients with partial onset seizures, the SANAD study compared carbamazepine with lamotrigine, topiramate, gabapentin, and oxcarbazepine. While carbamazepine and lamotrigine appeared to be equally effective in controlling seizures, lamotrigine was better tolerated. However, response to antiepileptic drugs varies from person to person, and antiepileptic drug treatment should be tailored to the individual according to efficacy and adverse effects. At present, carbamazepine, lamotrigine, and levetiracetam appear to be the safest choices with respect to teratogenicity for women of childbearing age. Any woman taking antiepileptic drugs and planning a pregnancy should take folic acid 5 mg daily prior to conception and for the first trimester. Certain drugs, particularly enzyme-inducing drugs, can affect the efficacy of the oral contraceptive pill, and necessitate the use of an increased dose of the oral contraceptive or an alternative method such as a barrier method, intramuscular medroxyprogesterone, or the levonorgestrel-releasing intrauterine coil.

Further Reading

Berg AT, Berkovic SF, Brodie MJ, et al. Revised terminology and concepts for organization of seizures and epilepsies: Report of the ILAE Commission on Classification and Terminology, 2005–2009. *Epilepsia* 2010, 51: 676–85.

Hart YM. Epidemiology and classification of epilepsy. *Medicine* 2012, 40: 471–6.

Hart YM. Management of epilepsy. *Medicine* 2012, 40: 477–83.

227 Stroke

Victoria Haunton, Aung Sett, Amit Mistri, and Martin Fotherby

Definition of stroke

The World Health Organization defines stroke as 'a clinical syndrome consisting of rapidly developing clinical signs of focal (at times global) disturbance of cerebral function lasting greater than 24 hours (or leading to death) with no apparent cause other than that of vascular origin'.

Transient ischaemic attack (TIA) is defined as a rapid presentation of neurological deficit with complete recovery within 24 hours of the onset of symptoms. However, the 24-hour cut-off is arbitrary, has no biological basis, and is of limited use clinically. A shorter duration is now regarded as more appropriate, although it has yet to be universally accepted. In clinical practice, stroke and TIA are best thought of as comprising a continuum, as they have similar pathological mechanisms, etiologies, and management strategies.

While subarachnoid haemorrhage is a type of stroke, based on the above definition, it is not covered in this chapter, as its pathophysiology, clinical manifestations, and management are distinct from those of ischaemic stroke and haemorrhagic stroke.

Demographics of stroke

Stroke is a common medical emergency with an annual incidence of between 130 and 200 per 100 000. At least 46 000 people in the UK each year have a first TIA, and approximately 152 000 had a first or recurrent stroke in 2014. Stroke is the fourth-largest cause of death in the UK after cancer, heart disease, and respiratory disease, and is responsible for approximately 50 000 deaths per annum. At any one time, there are likely to be 25–35 patients with stroke as their primary diagnosis in an average UK general hospital and, at present, there are approximately 1.2 million stroke survivors in England, with around half being dependent on others for everyday activities. The costs of stroke are estimated to be between £3.7 billion and £8 billion, or 5% of the total NHS annual budget. If post-stroke-care community costs are taken into account, this figure rises to nearly 12%.

Although stroke was previously regarded as a disease of the developed world, its incidence in the developing world is rising because of the adoption there of unhealthier lifestyles. WHO data indicate that, globally, stroke is the second-commonest cause of death, being responsible for 6.7 million deaths worldwide every year. Of these, two-thirds are in the developing world.

While stroke can occur at any age, it is predominantly a disease of older people. Over two-thirds of cases occur in those over 65, and less than 15% occur in those under 45. The incidence of stroke increases progressively with each successive decade of life over the age of 55, with an overall rate of 0.2/1000 in those aged 45–54, and 10/1000 in those aged over 85. While stroke risk is higher in men, more women die from stroke, due to their overall greater life expectancy.

The incidence of stroke and the relative distribution of stroke subtypes vary amongst ethnic groups. African-Caribbean, Africans, and African descendants have a higher incidence of stroke, compared to Caucasians. Stroke incidence also appears to be higher in Chinese populations.

Ischaemic stroke

Aetiology of ischaemic stroke

Ischaemic stroke can be classified as being due to:

- large artery atherosclerosis
- cardioembolism
- small blood vessel occlusion (lacunar stroke)
- other determined etiologies, including arterial dissection, hereditary factors, vasculitis, haematological disorders, coagulopathies, moyamoya disease, and drugs
- undetermined aetiology

Atherosclerosis

Atherosclerosis is a well-recognized risk factor for ischaemic stroke and involves large and medium-sized arteries, most commonly, the aorta, the coronary arteries, the carotid artery at its bifurcation, and the basilar artery. Its prevalence increases with age, and hypertension, hyperlipidaemia, and diabetes mellitus are all predisposing risk factors for its development. Atherosclerotic plaques develop as a result of vessel wall injury and the deposition of lipids. Stroke occurs as these plaques rupture, promoting thrombus formation and subsequent occlusion of the cerebral arterial circulation.

Cardioembolism

Cardioembolism accounts for approximately 25% of all ischaemic strokes, and 36% of ischaemic stroke in young patients. Atrial fibrillation is the commonest cause of cardioembolic stroke and is usually associated with more severe stroke and higher mortality rates. Other causes of cardioembolic strokes are listed in Box 227.1.

Small blood vessel occlusion

Small vessel disease usually affects the arterioles and is associated with hypertension. It is caused by fibrosis and the sub-endothelial accumulation of a pathological protein, hyaline, which lead to narrowing and occlusion of these vessels.

Other determined etiologies

Arterial dissection

Arterial dissection is a common cause of stroke in younger patients, accounting for 20% of strokes in patients under the age of 45. It may be spontaneous or precipitated by neck trauma, which may be mild. A tear in the media or intima of the carotid or vertebral artery lumen leads to bleeding in the arterial wall. This may then track, creating

---

Box 227.1 Cardioembolic causes of stroke

High risk
- atrial fibrillation
- sick sinus syndrome
- mechanical prosthetic heart valve replacement
- mitral stenosis
- infective endocarditis
- myocardial infarction
- dilated cardiomyopathy
- atrial flutter
- left atrial thrombus
- left atrial appendage thrombus
- left ventricular myxoma

Low/uncertain risk
- subaortic hypertrophic cardiomyopathy
- aortic valve calcification
- patent foramen ovale
- mitral valve prolapse
- atrial septal aneurysm
- congestive cardiac failure

Box 227.2 Connective tissue disorders associated with carotid artery dissection

- Marfan syndrome
- collagen disorders
- Ehlers–Danlos syndrome type IV (vascular)
- osteogenesis imperfecta
- polycystic kidney disease
- fibromuscular dysplasia
- pseudoxanthoma elasticum

Box 227.3 Haematological disorders associated with stroke

- thrombotic thrombocytopenic purpura
- haemoglobinopathies
- paroxysmal nocturnal haemoglobinuria
- protein C deficiency
- protein S deficiency
- antithrombin III deficiency
- activated protein C resistance
- factor V Leiden mutation
- prothrombin gene mutation
- antiphospholipid antibody syndrome
- polycythaemia
- anaemia
- leukaemia
- essential thrombocytosis
- lymphoma
- disseminated intravascular coagulation

a false lumen, which may occlude the artery or predispose to the development of a thrombus which then embolizes.

Spontaneous arterial dissections are associated with a variety of connective tissue diseases, which are listed in Box 227.2.

Hereditary disorders

Several hereditary disorders have been implicated in stroke, including CADASIL (for **c**erebral **a**utosomal **d**ominant **a**rteriopathy with **s**ubcortical **i**nfarcts and **l**eukoencephalopathy) syndrome, Fabry's disease, homocystinuria, MELAS (for **m**itochondrial **e**ncephalopathy with **l**actic **a**cidosis and **s**troke) syndrome, and HERNS (for **h**ereditary **e**ndotheliopathy with **r**etinopathy and **s**troke) syndrome.

Vasculitis

Cerebral vasculitides may be primary or secondary, as outlined in Table 227.1.

Haematological disorders and coagulopathies

Various haematological disorders are associated with stroke, as outlined in Box 227.3

Moyamoya disease

Moyamoya disease is a progressive intracranial vasculopathy that usually becomes symptomatic in children or young adults. Angiographic studies reveal a tight stenosis or occlusion of the intracranial carotid arteries.

Drugs

Illicit drugs, including cocaine, amphetamines, ephedrine, and MDMA (ecstasy) have all been implicated in stroke. Of the prescribed drugs, antipsychotics (particularly atypical antipsychotics in elderly patients

with dementia) have been implicated, as has the oral combined or oestrogen contraceptive pill and oestrogen-containing hormonal replacement therapy.

Undetermined aetiology

The term 'undetermined aetiology' refers to strokes where the likely aetiology could not be determined despite an extensive evaluation, or where the treating physician felt that not all necessary investigations had been performed. As many as one-third of strokes may fall into this category.

Risk factors for ischaemic stroke

Multiple risk factors contribute to ischaemic stroke; these can be divided into modifiable and non-modifiable factors (see Box 227.4).

Signs and symptoms of ischaemic stroke

The typical presentations of anterior circulation and posterior circulation strokes are detailed in Box 227.5. However, the exact clinical presentation and stroke syndrome will depend upon which arterial territory is involved and the size and type of the lesion. These are explored in detail in this section. It should be noted that confusion and memory disturbance alone and syncope are rarely attributable to stroke, and their presence should prompt the clinician to consider alternative diagnoses.

Signs and symptoms of anterior circulation strokes

The anterior circulation refers to the area of the brain supplied by the carotid arteries. There are five main branches (see Figure 227.1): the ophthalmic artery, the posterior communicating artery, the anterior choroidal artery, the anterior cerebral artery, and the middle cerebral artery (MCA), which is further divided into the M1, M2, M3, and M4 segments.

Anterior choroidal strokes typically cause a lacunar-type syndrome with pure motor or sensorimotor hemiparesis. However, they may also give rise to the triad of contralateral hemiparesis, hyperaesthesia, and upper quadrantanopia.

Anterior cerebral artery infarcts usually lead to weakness and sensory loss of the contralateral lower limb but other presentations include urinary incontinence, mutism, anterograde amnesia, and behavioural disturbance secondary to frontal lobe dysfunction. Primitive reflexes may be elicited on clinical examination.

The MCA territory is the one most frequently affected by acute strokes. Complete MCA strokes give rise to contralateral hemiplegia, hemisensory loss, and homonymous hemianopia with a head and gaze preference away from the side of the hemiplegia (i.e. towards the lesion). Cognitive signs are usually present with dominant hemisphere infarcts, which result in a global aphasia and ideomotor apraxia, and non-dominant hemisphere infarcts, which result in a multimodal neglect and anosognosia (denial of illness). Segmental infarctions will give rise to some, but not all, of these features. A rare complication

Table 227.1 Cerebral vasculitides	
Primary vasculitis	Granulomatous, inflammatory, non-sarcoidotic, non-infectious vasculitis with giant cells
Secondary vasculitis in systemic disorders	Polyarteritis nodosa
	Churg–Strauss syndrome
	SLE
	Sjögren's syndrome
	Behçet's syndrome
	Sarcoidosis
	Inflammatory bowel disease
	Takayasu's arteritis
	Buerger's disease
	Eales disease
	Acute multifocal placoid pigment endotheliopathy
	Köhlmeier–Degos disease
Secondary vasculitis in infectious disorders	Tuberculosis
	HIV
	Syphilis
	Ophthalmic herpes zoster
	Lyme disease
	Malaria
	Cysticercosis
	Aspergillosis
	Cryptococcosis

Box 227.4 Ischaemic stroke risk factors

Box 227.4 Ischaemic stroke risk factors

Non-modifiable risk factors

Age
- most potent risk factor
- risk of stroke doubles with each decade of life after 55 years of age

Gender
- incidence higher in men
- prevalence higher in women, due to lower mortality

Ethnicity
- incidence higher in African-Caribbeans, Africans, African descendants, and Asian and Chinese populations

Hereditary disorders
- first-degree family history of premature atherosclerosis
- CADASIL syndrome
- HERNS syndrome
- MELAS syndrome
- Fabry's disease
- homocystinuria

Socio-economic status
- stroke risk is 60% higher for the lowest socio-economic class than for the highest social class

History of coronary heart disease or stroke
- prior history of coronary heart disease is a potent risk factor, indicating the need for better primary prevention

Modifiable risk factors

Hypertension
- most controllable risk factor
- risk doubles with each 5–7 mm Hg increase in systolic blood pressure

Diabetes
- diabetic patients have a 1.5- to 4-fold increased risk of stroke

High total cholesterol/LDL and low HDL
- high risk of atherosclerosis and ischaemic stroke
- greater risk in smokers and those with inactive lifestyles

Atrial fibrillation
- commonest cardioembolic cause

Smoking
- twofold increased risk of stroke
- risk diminishes 5 years after stopping

Alcohol consumption
- minimal alcohol consumption has some protective effect but heavy alcohol intake confers an increased risk of stroke

Obesity
- BMI ≥25 confers increased risk of stroke

Hyperhomocysteinaemia
- recognized risk factor
- no clear evidence of benefit from intervention

Box 227.5 Typical stroke presentations

anterior circulation
- unilateral hemiparesis and hemisensory impairment
- homonymous hemianopia
- dysphasia
- multimodal neglect/anosognosia

posterior circulation
- cranial nerve deficits
- ataxia
- diplopia
- cerebellar signs
- nystagmus
- bilateral or crossed signs

visual cortex. However, there is marked individual variability in the exact arterial anatomy of the posterior circulation, and persisting fetal circulations are not uncommon. Clinical features that suggest a posterior circulation stroke rather than an anterior circulation event include preceding TIAs in the days and hours prior to the event, and headache, which is typically ipsilateral to the side of the lesion. The most common symptoms are dizziness, diplopia, dysarthria, dysphagia, and ataxia, but the hallmark of a posterior circulation event is crossed signs with cranial nerve findings ipsilaterally and sensorimotor findings on the opposite side. However, patients may present with a wide variety of other

of large MCA infarction is the malignant MCA syndrome. This occurs in younger patients without brain atrophy and is caused by the development of life-threatening space-occupying oedema, which leads to raised intracranial pressure with subsequent subfalcine, uncal, and transtentorial herniation.

Signs and symptoms of posterior circulation strokes

The posterior circulation consists of the vertebral arteries, the basilar artery, and the posterior cerebral arteries with their branches. These arteries typically supply the brainstem (medulla, pons, and midbrain), the thalamus, the hippocampus, the cerebellum, and parts of the occipital and temporal lobes, including the

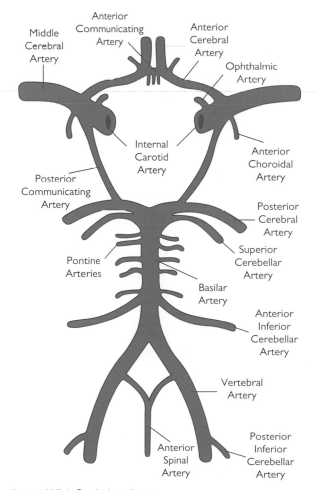

Figure 227.1 Cerebral circulation.
This article was published in *Gray's Anatomy*, Susan Standring, The Arteries of the Brain, p. 574, Copyright Elsevier (2008).

symptoms, including vertigo, fluctuating episodes of drowsiness, cranial nerve palsies, disorders of conjugate gaze, Horner's syndrome, and acute unilateral deafness.

Specifically, cerebellar strokes usually present with headache, vertigo, vomiting, nystagmus, and ataxia.

Lateral medullary syndrome, caused by sudden occlusion of the posterior inferior cerebellar artery, results in vertigo and vomiting with ipsilateral cranial nerve palsies, Horner's syndrome, and contralateral pain and temperature deficits.

Midbrain injury may produce coma, oculomotor nerve palsy, dilated pupils, and hemi- or quadriparesis.

Basilar artery occlusion is usually devastating, giving rise to massive brainstem dysfunction and death. However, if the medulla is spared, a significant number of syndromes can occur, including the 'locked-in' syndrome, in which patients are quadriplegic and communicate only by means of vertical eye movements.

Signs and symptoms of lacunar strokes

A lacunar infarct is a small, subcortical infarct of a perforating branch of a large cerebral artery. The most common clinical presentation of a lacunar stroke is a pure motor hemiparesis but they may also give rise to a pure sensory stroke, a sensorimotor stroke, dysarthria–clumsy hand syndrome, or an ataxic hemiparesis.

Haemorrhagic strokes

Aetiology of haemorrhage strokes

The causes of spontaneous intra-cerebral haemorrhage are listed in Box 227.6.

Signs and symptoms of haemorrhage strokes

Haemorrhagic strokes often have an apoplectic onset. Seizures, bilateral extensor plantars, and marked hypertension are common. However, these features are not specific and may also been seen with large infarcts. Furthermore, as with ischaemic strokes, the exact clinical presentation of a spontaneous intra-cerebral haemorrhage will depend on its site and size. The most common sites of haemorrhage, in order of frequency, are putaminal, thalamic, lobar, caudate, pontine, and cerebellar. The deep grey matter of the brain, including the basal ganglia and the thalamus, is the most common site for hypertensive haemorrhagic stroke, with cerebral amyloid intra-cerebral bleeds usually occurring in the white matter of brain parenchyma.

Putaminal haemorrhages typically give rise to contralateral limb weakness and hemisensory loss. Extension of the bleeding into the frontal lobe will cause conjugate eye deviation. Thalamic bleeding causes total hemisensory loss and dense hemiplegia. There may also be convergent downward gaze (the patient looks at the tip of their nose).

Progressive deterioration of the conscious level points to a growing haematoma, and sudden posturing and coma indicate bleeding into the lateral or third ventricle.

Classification of stroke

Several additional classification systems exist for stroke, including the Oxfordshire Community Stroke Project (OCSP) classification, which is often referred to as the Bamford classification, and the ICD-10 system.

Box 227.6 Causes of spontaneous intra-cerebral haemorrhage

- hypertension
- amyloid angiopathy
- arteriovenous malformation
- bleeding diatheses
- drugs (amphetamines, cocaine, anticoagulants, thrombolytics)
- tumours

Table 227.2 The Oxfordshire Community Stroke Project classification of stroke

FEATURES	CLASSIFICATION
All 3 present (see OCSP classification paragraph below)	TACS
2 out of 3 present	PACS
Drowsy + unilateral weakness (visual + higher cerebral involvement assumed)	TACS
Motor/Sensory/sensori-motor involvement affecting ≥2 of 3 body areas (arm/face/leg)	LACS
Cerebellar syndrome or brainstem involvement	POCS
Isolated speech or visual involvement	PACS
Restricted motor or sensory involvement—affecting only one body area (arm or face or leg)	PACS

Reprinted from *The Lancet*, Volume 337, J. Bamford, P. Sandercock, M. Dennis, C. Warlow, J. Burn, Classification and natural history of clinically identifiable subtypes of cerebral infarction, pp. 1521–1526, Copyright (1991), with permission from Elsevier.

OCSP classification

In the OCSP classification system (see Table 227.2), strokes are classified according to their constellation of symptoms and signs into four groups. These are:

- total anterior circulation stroke (TACS)
- partial anterior circulation stroke (PACS)
- lacunar stroke (LACS)
- posterior circulation stroke (POCS)

A stroke episode occurring in a patient with a current neurological deficit should never be labelled a 'TIA'. Classification depends on three main features:

- unilateral motor or sensory involvement (arm/face/leg)
- visual involvement (hemianopia, quadrantanopia, or visual neglect)
- higher cerebral dysfunction (dysphasia, dyscalculia, visuospatial disorder/inattention/neglect)

This is a clinical classification prior to any investigations. Once haemorrhage is excluded, the 'S' can be replaced by an 'I' (i.e. TACI, LACI, etc.), or 'H' indicating haemorrhage; however, the prognostic value of OCSP in PICH is uncertain.

Examples of OCSP classifications

The following are examples of OCSP classifications:

- weakness of left face, arm, and leg, expressive dysphasia, and left homonymous hemianopia: right TACS
- weakness of right face and arm, and right-sided sensory inattention: left PACS
- sensory loss in left arm and leg: right LACS
- sensory loss in left arm only: right PACS
- ataxic hemiparesis: LACS (contralateral to affected side)
- Horner's syndrome: POCS
- cerebellar syndrome: POCS

The four classical lacunar syndromes are: isolated hemimotor dysfunction, hemisensory dysfunction, hemi-sensori-motor dysfunction, and ataxic hemiparesis.

ICD-10 classification

The ICD-10 classification is outlined in Box 227.7.

Stroke prevention

Stroke prevention strategies can be classified as primary prevention, where there is no prior history of TIA or stroke, and secondary prevention, where there is such a history.

Primary prevention

All patients should have their cardiovascular risk assessed on a regular basis. In the UK, the National Institute for Health and Care Excellence

Box 227.7 ICD-10 classification of stroke

Acute stroke

I60 Non-traumatic subarachnoid haemorrhage
I61 Non-traumatic intracerebral haemorrhage
I63 Cerebral infarction
I64 Stroke, not specified as haemorrhage or infarction

Consistent with WHO definition of stroke, but considered distinct from a clinical viewpoint

I62 Other and unspecified non-traumatic intracranial haemorrhage (includes subdural, extradural and unspecified intracranial haemorrhages)

Other relevant codes

G45 Transient ischaemic attack, including transient global amnesia
I69 Sequelae of cerebrovascular disease
Z82.3 Family history of stroke

Reprinted from WHO, http://apps.who.int/classifications/icd10/browse/2015/en, Copyright (2015).

(NICE) recommends assessing a patient's 10-year cardiovascular risk with the Joint British Societies JBS3 Risk Calculator. Following this, lifestyle modifications and medical therapies should be instigated as appropriate.

Lifestyle modifications

All patients should be encouraged to stop smoking, maintain an appropriate weight (BMI between 20 and 25), and eat healthily. Dietary measures associated with stroke risk reduction include reduced total fat and cholesterol intake; increased consumption of fruits, vegetables, and fish oils; and reduced salt intake. Alcohol should be taken in moderation, with the weekly intake not exceeding 14 units per week. Exercise has a significant association with reduction in relative stroke risk, and the effect is even greater with strenuous activity. Patients should therefore be encouraged to take at least 30 minutes of exercise at least five times per week, or whatever they can achieve if they have limited mobility.

Hypertension

This is the most common risk factor for stroke, and is extremely treatable. Adults over 40, and those with other vascular risk factors, should therefore be screened regularly for raised blood pressure. Current British Hypertension Society and NICE guidelines classify hypertension as being Stage 1, Stage 2, or severe. Stage 1 hypertension refers to a clinic blood pressure of ≥140/90 mm Hg, and subsequent ambulatory blood-pressure monitoring (ABPM) daytime average or home blood-pressure monitoring (HBPM) average blood pressure of ≥135/85 mm Hg. Stage 2 hypertension is defined as a clinic blood pressure of ≥160/100 mm Hg, and subsequent ABPM daytime average or HBPM average blood pressure of ≥150/95 mm Hg. A clinic systolic blood pressure of >180 mm Hg or higher or clinic diastolic blood pressure of >110 mm Hg indicates severe hypertension. Antihypertensive drug treatment should be offered to all people aged under 80 who have Stage 1 hypertension and target organ damage, established cardiovascular disease, renal disease, diabetes, or a 10-year cardiovascular risk equivalent to 20% or greater and to people of any age with Stage 2 or severe hypertension. Current treatment targets are a clinic blood pressure <140/90 mm Hg in people aged under 80, and <150/90 mm Hg in people aged 80 and over.

Blood-pressure variability may be as important as average levels in predisposing to stroke risk, and further research is needed in this area.

Dyslipidaemia

Although hypercholesterolaemia is a weaker risk factor for stroke than for heart disease, trials have shown a clear positive effect of cholesterol-lowering therapy on the incidence of ischaemic stroke. The NICE guideline recommends pharmacological lipid modification in individuals with >20% 10-year risk of cardiovascular disease; lipid reduction is targeted at a total cholesterol level of <4 mmol/l, and

an LDL cholesterol level of <2 mmol/l. Dietary measures should be used for all patients, and pharmacological therapies added as needed. Niacin, fibrates, and statins can all be used, although statins have been shown to be most effective.

Diabetes

High-vascular-risk individuals should be screened for diabetes, and treatment instigated accordingly.

Atrial fibrillation

Atrial fibrillation is a strong independent risk factor for stroke; when atrial fibrillation is detected, serious consideration should be given to anticoagulant therapy. Various risk stratification tools are in use to guide such therapy, including the CHA_2DS_2-VASc score, which gives an estimate of embolic stroke risk, and the HASBLED score, which estimates bleeding risk. Antiplatelets are no longer considered adequate for prevention of cardioembolic stroke. There is strong evidence that dose-adjusted warfarin reduces the risk of stroke occurrence by approximately two-thirds, with only a slight increase in bleeding risk. The most common reasons for not prescribing warfarin are a high perceived risk of bleeding, and difficulties maintaining an international normalized ratio in the therapeutic range. Newer anticoagulants in the form of oral direct inhibitors have recently been evaluated by NICE and are available as alternatives to warfarin. These include Factor II inhibitors (dabigatran) and Factor X inhibitors (rivaroxaban, apixaban, edoxaban). Large clinical trials have demonstrated that these agents have effects that are broadly similar to those of warfarin, with a consistent reduction in intracranial haemorrhage risk. Their key advantage is their fixed dosing regimen with no requirement for anticoagulation monitoring. However, they are contraindicated in patients with a creatinine clearance less than 15 ml/min, and the current absence of an established antidote or rapid-reversal agent is considered a disadvantage.

Anticoagulant therapy

Outside the context of atrial fibrillation, anticoagulation is also recommended as primary prevention for various other patients who are at high risk of cardioembolic stroke. This includes patients who are at high risk of thromboembolism following acute myocardial infarction, particularly a large anterior myocardial infarction; patients with left ventricular aneurysm or thrombus; and patients with paroxysmal tachyarrhythmias, chronic heart failure, or a history of thromboembolic events. Anticoagulation is also indicated for patients with mechanical prosthetic heart valves or rheumatic mitral valve disease.

Antiplatelet agents

Antiplatelet agents provide no net benefit in the primary prevention of stroke, although they are widely accepted for secondary prevention.

Secondary prevention

While primary prevention of stroke is essential, it can be difficult to apply, as the population at risk is ill defined. Conversely, patients who have a history of stroke or TIA are a well-defined target population for secondary prevention, and come into contact with specialists as a result of the index event. Effective secondary prevention has the potential to reduce stroke risk by a half to two-thirds. The preventative strategies for long-term stroke prevention can be classified into three main categories: lifestyle modifications, medical therapies, and surgical intervention for carotid disease.

Lifestyle modifications

All patients should be educated regarding the same lifestyle modifications as recommended for primary prevention.

Medical therapies

Antithrombotic therapy

Overall, antiplatelet therapy reduces the risk of a recurrent vascular event by a fifth in people with a history of TIA or stroke. In the UK, aspirin, modified-release dipyridamole, and clopidogrel are the three drugs almost exclusively used in secondary prevention following TIA or ischaemic stroke. The recent Royal College of Physicians guideline recommends that clopidogrel 75 mg daily should be used first line and, if this is not tolerated, then aspirin 75 mg daily in combination with modified-release dipyridamole 200 mg twice daily should be offered.

Long-term dual antiplatelet therapy with aspirin and clopidogrel is not routinely used for stroke prevention. While prolonged use is associated with a reduction in ischaemic stroke, this is offset by an increased risk of major bleeding. There is some evidence for short-term use in those with significant symptomatic carotid atherosclerotic disease which is not amenable to surgery, and those at high risk of subsequent stroke (e.g. an $ABCD_2$ Score ≥4).

Anticoagulation should be initiated unless contraindicated in patients with cardioembolic stroke, after a suitable interval to avoid increasing the risk of early haemorrhagic transformation of cerebral infarcts.

Antihypertensives

The target blood pressure for stroke patients, as guided by the fifth edition of the *National Clinical Guideline for Stroke* (Royal College of Physicians London) and the American Stroke Association is <130/80 mm Hg, except for patients with severe bilateral carotid stenosis, for whom a systolic blood-pressure target of 130–150 mm Hg is appropriate. For patients aged 55 or over, and African or Caribbean patients of any age, antihypertensive treatment should typically be initiated with a long-acting dihydropyridine calcium channel blocker or a thiazide-like diuretic. If the target blood pressure is not achieved, an angiotensin-converting enzyme inhibitor or an angiotensin-II receptor blocker should be added.

For patients not of African or Caribbean origin, or younger than 55 years, the first choice for initial antihypertensive therapy should be an angiotensin-converting enzyme inhibitor or a low-cost angiotensin-II receptor blocker. Beta blockers are not routinely recommended as a first line antihypertensive therapy for stroke prevention unless there are associated comorbidities (e.g. ischaemic heart disease, heart failure, and atrial fibrillation). Blood-pressure-lowering treatment should be initiated after stroke or TIA. Thereafter, treatment should be monitored frequently and increased as necessary to achieve the target blood pressure as quickly as is tolerated and safe in primary care. Patients who do not achieve the target blood pressure should be referred for a specialist opinion.

Lipid-modifying agents Statin therapy should be initiated in almost everyone with a history of ischaemic stroke or TIA, unless the total cholesterol is <3.5 mmol/l. If statins are contraindicated or not tolerated, other agents such as fibrates (for elevated total cholesterol or high LDL) or niacin (for low HDL) should be used.

Glycaemic control

The general recommendation for the Hb A1c target level after a stroke is <7%, although a more stringent target of <6% may be considered in the early management of diabetes. More aggressive Hb A1c targets are not advised in the long-term management of glycaemic control, particularly in patients with high cardiovascular risk, as such targets are associated with increased mortality.

Surgical intervention for carotid artery disease

Early carotid ultrasound or angiogram is recommended for anterior circulation stroke and TIA patients with no significant dependency, either before or after the event. If an ipsilateral carotid artery stenosis of 50%–99% is detected, carotid artery revascularization (usually with endarterectomy) should be performed as soon as possible, but certainly within 2 weeks.

Approach to diagnosing stroke

Prompt diagnosis of stroke is crucial in order to commence appropriate treatment as quickly as possible. Several stroke screening tools are now in widespread use to help improve time to diagnosis, including FAST (for **F**ace **A**rm **S**peech **T**est; see Box 227.8), which is predominantly used outside hospitals, and the ROSIER (**R**ecognition of **S**troke **I**n the **E**mergency **R**oom) scale (see Table 227.3).

The diagnosis of stroke is predominantly clinical and, once stroke is suspected, the initial assessment should first to seek to establish

Box 227.8 FAST test

Facial weakness: Can the person smile? Has their mouth or eye drooped?
Arm weakness: Can the person raise both arms?
Speech problems: Can the person speak clearly and understand what you say?
Time to call '999'

Reproduced with permission from Harbison J, Hossain O, Jenkinson D, et al., Diagnostic accuracy of stroke referrals from primary care, emergency room physicians, and ambulance staff using the face arm speech test, *Stroke*, Volume 34, pp. 71–76, Copyright © 2003 Wolters Kluwer Health, Inc.

that there is indeed a clear history of **rapid** onset of **focal** neurological deficit. If these criteria are satisfied, the diagnosis of stroke will be correct in 95% of cases. Clinical assessment should then seek to establish what the mechanism of stroke is and where the lesion is, with a focused history and examination. As part of the clinical examination, a National Institutes of Health Stroke Scale (NIHSS) should be performed. This is a clinical evaluation instrument, with documented validity and reliability, and is used to assess the severity of a stroke and its likely prognosis. The NIHSS grades the following areas: conscious level, orientation, gaze, visual fields, facial weakness, limb weakness, ataxia, sensation, language, dysarthria, and inattention.

All patients should then undergo prompt brain imaging. The indications for immediate brain imaging are given in Box 227.9.

'Gold-standard' diagnostic test for stroke

CT perfusion scanning is the most sensitive for the detection of acute ischaemic stroke with a sensitivity of approximately 75% for ischaemic strokes and above 85% for non-lacunar supratentorial infarcts. In CT perfusion scanning, a baseline CT is followed by CT angiography of the head and neck and a contrast-enhanced CT of the brain using iodinated contrast. The perfusion CT images and their data are then used to create a map of the ischaemic area (infarct and penumbra).

Acceptable diagnostic alternatives to the gold-standard test for stroke

Despite the sensitivity of CT perfusion scanning in detecting early ischaemia, it is not yet widely enough available to be practicable. As prompt scanning is crucial for guiding emergency management in acute stroke, plain CT is currently the most practical and widely available modality available for imaging. A non-contrast CT brain scan can be performed in less than a minute with a helical CT scanner and is considered sufficient to select patients for IV thrombolysis. It is highly accurate for identifying acute intra-cerebral haemorrhage, which is present within minutes of onset and seen as hyperattenuation, but

Table 227.3 The ROSIER score	
Symptoms	**Points**
New onset of asymmetric facial weakness	1
New onset of asymmetric arm weakness	1
New onset of asymmetric leg weakness	1
Speech disturbance	1
Visual field defect	1
Loss of consciousness or syncope	−1
Any seizure activity	−1
Total	

If score totals >0, assume diagnosis of stroke. If score totals 0, −1, or −2, stroke diagnosis is unlikely but not excluded.

Reprinted from *The Lancet Neurology*, Volume 4, issue 11, Nor et al., The Recognition of Stroke in the Emergency Room (ROSIER) scale: development and validation of a stroke recognition instrument, pp. 727–734, Copyright (2005), with permission from Elsevier.

> **Box 227.9 Indications for immediate brain imaging**
>
> - indications for thrombolysis or early anticoagulation treatment
> - on anticoagulant treatment
> - a known bleeding tendency
> - a depressed level of consciousness (Glasgow Coma Score <13)
> - unexplained progressive or fluctuating symptoms
> - papilloedema, neck stiffness, or fever
> - severe headache at onset of stroke symptoms

only 5% of acute infarcts will be visible within the first 12 hours. Changes indicative of acute ischaemia include focal hypoattenuation, which is very specific and predictive for irreversible ischaemia, and oedema without hypoattenuation, in which case the tissue is potentially salvageable. The typical CT scan appearances of haemorrhage and ischaemia are shown in Figures 227.2 and 227.3, respectively.

MRI scanning is now being used in some centres as the sole modality for the emergency imaging of stroke, as it has been shown to be more effective than plain CT in the detection of acute ischaemia and can detect both acute and chronic haemorrhage. Typically, multiparametric sequences are obtained, including diffusion-weighted imaging, T1- and T2-weighted sequences, angiography, and fluid-attenuated inversion recovery. The advantage of this is that the extent of the lesion and the stroke mechanism can be clarified very early on.

It is likely that, with time, access to both immediate CT perfusion scanning and MRI will become more widely available.

Other investigations required following a stroke or a TIA

Other investigations required following a stroke or a TIA are outlined in Table 227.4.

Other diagnoses that should be considered aside from stroke

While the diagnosis of acute ischaemic stroke is often straightforward, there are several important stroke mimics (see Box 227.10). These should be considered in the differential diagnosis, and care taken to exclude them as appropriate.

Treatment for stroke

Stroke requires a multifaceted treatment approach, consisting of general measures including homeostatic control, drug therapies, prevention and

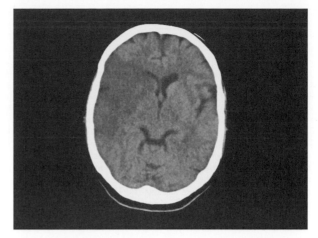

Figure 227.3 Acute right middle cerebral artery territory infarct; note the typical wedge shape.

Anonymised image obtained from University Hospitals of Leicester NHS Trust.

management of complications, and rehabilitation. Occasionally, neurosurgical intervention forms part of stroke treatment.

Stroke units

A stroke unit is defined as 'a geographically defined unit staffed by a coordinated multidisciplinary team with expertise in stroke'. All stroke patients should be treated in a stroke unit, as there is strong evidence that this significantly reduces death, dependency, and the need for institutional care. The gold standard is to admit patients with stroke directly to a stroke unit and continue care there until discharge.

Homeostasis

Oxygen

Patients should receive oxygen therapy if they are hypoxaemic (oxygen saturations <95%), as hypoxaemia can worsen cerebral ischaemia. However, the routine use of supplemental oxygen in patients who are not hypoxaemic is not currently recommended.

Blood pressure

Blood pressure is often elevated in acute stroke but usually returns to the patient's normal level within the first few days. Blood pressure

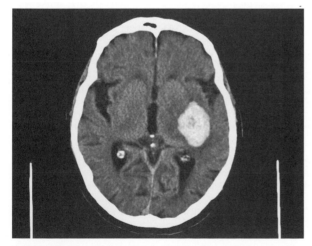

Figure 227.2 Acute left parenchymal haemorrhage with surrounding oedema.

Anonymised image obtained from University Hospitals of Leicester NHS Trust.

Table 227.4 Investigations required following a stroke or a transient ischaemic attack

Essential	To be considered	
Blood tests: • full blood count	Chest X-ray	If aspiration suspected
• renal profile • glucose	Arterial thrombophilia screen	In young patients or cryptogenic stroke
• cholesterol • lipid profile	Venous thrombophilia screen	
• clotting	HIV test	
• liver function test and creatine kinase test (prior to statin initiation)	Illicit drug screen	
	Autoimmune screen	
	Vasculitic screen	
Urine dip for proteinuria and haematuria	Cerebral angiography	
12-lead ECG	Holter ECG monitoring	If cardioembolic stroke suspected
Vascular imaging:	Echocardiography	
• carotid ultrasound • magnetic resonance angiography • CT angiography	Bubble echocardiogram or transcranial Doppler bubble scan	If paradoxical embolism suspected

Box 227.10 Stroke mimics

- complicated migraine
- hypoglycaemia
- hypertensive encephalopathy
- postictal paralysis
- cerebral neoplasm
- functional disorder
- subdural haematoma

Table 227.5 Inclusion and exclusion criteria for thrombolysis with alteplase*

Inclusion criteria	Exclusion criteria
CT scan appearances consistent with acute ischaemic stroke	Symptom onset greater than 4.5 hours before
	National Institutes of Health Stroke Scale ≤4 or ≥25
Onset of symptoms within 4.5 hours	Recent (less than 10 days) traumatic external cardiac massage, puncture of a non-compressible blood vessel, or lumbar puncture
Clinical diagnosis of ischaemic stroke causing a measurable neurological deficit	Fixed head or eye deviation
	Seizure at onset
	Pre-stroke Rankin score >3
	Blood pressure ≥185 mm Hg systolic or ≥110 mm Hg diastolic
Risks and benefits explained to patient or relative	Trauma with internal injuries, or visceral biopsy, within previous 4 weeks
	Serious head trauma or CNS surgery within 3 months
	Colitis, oesophageal varices, active peptic ulcer disease, aortic aneurysm, severe liver disease, or acute pancreatitis
	Proliferative diabetic retinopathy
	Blood glucose <3 or >22
	Hereditary or acquired bleeding disorder
	Recent severe or dangerous bleeding
	Platelet count <100 or haematocrit <25%
	Current anticoagulation therapy (unless patient's international normalized ratio <1.7 while on warfarin)

*Relative contraindications: pregnancy or childbirth within the last 4 weeks, or stroke within 3 months.

should not be lowered routinely in acute ischaemic stroke, as this may decrease cerebral perfusion and increase the infarct size. Current evidence suggests that it is probably safe to continue with antihypertensives that patients are already taking, but additional or new treatments should only be given if the blood pressure is persistently elevated above 200 mm Hg systolic or 120 mm Hg diastolic, or there are signs of cardiac failure, hypertensive encephalopathy, hypertensive nephropathy, aortic dissection, pre-eclampsia, or eclampsia.

In patients who are candidates for thrombolysis, the blood pressure should be lowered to ≤185/110 mm Hg.

In haemorrhagic stroke, however, intensively lowering systolic blood pressure to ≤140 mm Hg leads to reduced morbidity and increased quality of life at 90 days, although mortality rates are unchanged.

Temperature

Raised temperature is associated with a poorer outcome after stroke, as it may increase infarct volume. Pyrexial patients should be treated with paracetamol and cooling fans, and the cause of the pyrexia should be sought and appropriately treated.

Hyperglycaemia

Hyperglycaemia also appears to be associated with a poorer outcome, and blood glucose levels ≥11.1 should be treated with insulin. However, care should be taken to avoid overtreatment and hypoglycaemia.

Drug treatments

Thrombolysis

Thrombolysis with alteplase has been shown to improve outcomes in carefully selected patients. The main inclusion and exclusion criteria for its use are given in Table 227.5. It should only be used by trained, experienced physicians in centres which have immediate access to brain imaging and nursing staff who are trained in monitoring for complications. Although alteplase is currently only licensed for the thrombolysis of strokes in patients aged 80 or less, with a definite time of onset within 3 hours, there is growing evidence that it is safe both in older patients and in selected patients up to 4.5 hours after stroke onset. More recently, thrombectomy has been shown to dramatically improve outcomes in selected patients.

Antiplatelet therapy

Aspirin is safe, simple, and usually well tolerated and has been shown to improve long-term outcome. Indeed, treating 1000 patients for 2 weeks prevents 13 being dead or dependent at 6 months. All patients presenting with acute stroke who have had haemorrhage excluded with brain imaging should therefore be given aspirin 300 mg, either orally or rectally if they are unable to swallow.

Aspirin should be continued at this dose for 2 weeks and then patients should be switched to clopidogrel 75 mg daily, which they should remain on for the long term for secondary prevention.

Anticoagulants

There is no net benefit to be gained in the routine use of anticoagulants after acute stroke, except in the presence of venous thromboembolism and cardioembolic stroke (chiefly, atrial fibrillation). For patients with ischaemic stroke in atrial fibrillation, anticoagulation should be the standard treatment. However, it should not be commenced in patients with uncontrolled hypertension and, in patients with disabling ischaemic stroke, it should be deferred for at least 14 days, with aspirin 300 mg daily used in its place. In the case of

minor, non-disabling stroke, anticoagulation could be started sooner at the discretion of the treating clinician. In the case of TIA, once brain imaging has ruled out haemorrhage, an agent with a rapid onset, such as low-molecular-weight heparin or an oral direct thrombin or Factor Xa inhibitor, should be commenced.

In patients with proximal deep vein thrombosis or pulmonary embolus, anticoagulants should be given in preference to aspirin.

Patients who are taking anticoagulants for prosthetic heart valves and develop stroke require special consideration. In the case of ischaemic stroke, anticoagulation therapy can usually be continued unless there is a significant risk of haemorrhagic transformation. Patients who develop haemorrhagic stroke while taking anticoagulants for prosthetic heart valves may have their anticoagulation therapy temporarily withheld for a short period, with low risk of systemic embolism.

Stroke clinicians should weigh up the benefit and risk of initiating anticoagulation in patients who present with ischaemic stroke with haemorrhagic transformation, or those with mixed haemorrhagic and ischaemic strokes and atrial fibrillation, or those who have concurrent venous thromboembolism.

Statin therapy

As stated in 'Lipid-modifying agents', statin therapy should be initiated in almost everyone with a history of stroke or TIA, unless total cholesterol is < 3.5 mmol/l. Although there is evidence that statins are anti-inflammatory and may have beneficial effects on neuroprotection, endothelial function, and homeostasis, there is also a concern that they may increase the risk of haemorrhagic transformation. Statins should therefore only be considered 48 hours after the onset of an acute stroke if there is a high risk of haemorrhagic transformation (depending on the size of the infarct and the severity of stroke) and need not be given to patients with acute haemorrhagic stroke alone.

Prevention and management of complications

Prevention of venous thromboembolism

Despite traditionally held beliefs, there is no evidence to indicate any net benefit from the use of heparin or antiembolic stockings in preventing venous thromboembolism in acute ischaemic stroke. Indeed, these measures may be harmful. Evidence indicates that intermittent pneumatic compression significantly reduces major venous thromboembolism in patients with acute stroke, but robust health economics data have yet to be established. Simple measures including avoidance of dehydration and early mobilization should be encouraged for all stroke patients.

Pressure areas

Pressure areas should be checked regularly and care should be taken to reduce the risk of bedsores. This can be done by treating infections, maintaining nutrition, providing pressure-relieving mattresses, and turning immobile patients regularly.

Fluids and nutrition

Care must be taken to avoid dehydration as it can lead to electrolyte abnormalities, further vascular events, and urinary tract infection. If necessary, supplementary fluids should be given parenterally. Patients' swallowing should be screened at admission, by an appropriately trained professional person. If screening reveals a problem with swallowing, the patient should have a specialist assessment by a speech and language therapist. This should ideally be done within 24 hours. If swallowing is impaired, it may be possible for the patient to have food and fluids which have been modified in consistency (e.g. with thickener). However, if there is marked dysphagia, and the recovery of swallow is likely to be delayed, feeding should be commenced via a nasogastric tube. In the longer term, PEG tube insertion provides an easier route of feeding.

All patients with impaired swallow should be referred to the dietetics team, in addition to the speech and language team.

Continence

Urinary retention and constipation are relatively common in acute stroke and should be treated promptly. Care should, however, be given to ensuring that catheters are removed in a timely fashion, as they may lead to the development of urinary tract infection.

Early mobilization

Patients with acute stroke should be mobilized and helped to sit out of bed as soon as possible, as this helps to decrease the risk of complications, namely venous thromboembolism, orthostatic hypotension, infection, contractures, and subluxations.

Depression

The prevalence of post-stroke depression has been estimated to be as high as 61%. Stroke patients should therefore be screened carefully for depression via a validated method such as the Geriatric Depression Score, or the Aphasia Depression Rating Scale. Antidepressant therapy should then be initiated accordingly, as untreated depression may hinder rehabilitation and is associated with adverse outcomes.

Neurosurgery in acute stroke

Discussion with the neurosurgical team should be considered for most patients with intracerebral haemorrhage. However, patients with small, deep haemorrhages, lobar haemorrhages, multiple comorbidities, or a Glasgow Coma Score of ≤8 rarely benefit from surgical intervention and are usually managed medically.

Neurosurgical intervention should also be considered in patients with the malignant MCA syndrome in ischaemic stroke. It may be possible to treat such patients with decompressive hemicraniectomy, although there are strict selection criteria for the procedure (see Box 227.11).

Rehabilitation

Once the acute phase of their treatment is complete, and they are medically stable, stroke patients should receive ongoing neurorehabilitation. Such neurorehabilitation remains one of the key components

---

Box 227.11 Selection criteria for decompressive hemicraniectomy

- age ≤60
- National Institutes of Health Stroke Scale ≥15
- score of ≥1 or 1a on the National Institutes of Health Stroke Scale
- infarct size >50% of the middle cerebral artery territory on CT scan, or >145 cm³ on diffusion-weighted MRI

Data from National Institute for Health and Care Excellence 2007 Diagnosis and initial management of acute stroke and transient ischaemic attack (TIA). CG68. London: National Institute for Health and Care Excellence. Available at: http://www.nice.org.uk/nicemedia/live/12018/41363/41363.pdf

---

of stroke care today and is vital in decreasing the odds of death, institutionalization, and dependency. Specific neurorehabilitation allows patients to benefit from the skills and knowledge of a dedicated multidisciplinary team and, in much the same way that patients benefit from early specialized care on an acute stroke unit, they also benefit from specialized rehabilitation. Indeed, for every 100 patients treated by organized multidisciplinary neurorehabilitation, as compared to those treated on a general ward and in other non-specific rehabilitation facilities, an extra 5 will return home in an independent state.

The key aims of rehabilitation are to restore the individual to his or her fullest physical, mental, and social capability. This is achieved through:

- input from a multidisciplinary team consisting of medical, nursing, and therapy staff with expertise in stroke and rehabilitation, with the team's work coordinated through regular weekly meetings
- interdisciplinary goal setting
- involvement of patients and their families in the rehabilitation process

We shall now examine these key approaches in more detail.

A crucial aspect of successful rehabilitation is close multidisciplinary team working. For the team to be successful, the individuals must be motivated by a shared philosophy and goals and be prepared to coordinate their work. They must also recognize their complementary skills and have mutual respect for one another.

Typically, in stroke rehabilitation, the team comprises doctors, nurses, physiotherapists, occupational therapists, and speech and language therapists but it may also include neuropsychologists, social workers, and dieticians. Occasionally, lay people, such as previous stroke survivors or representatives from stroke charities and patient support groups, also form part of the team. The role of each team member is detailed in Box 227.12.

For this team to be effective, the team members must meet regularly. This helps to generate cohesion and allows careful coordination of patient care. Each team member may carry out different assessments and identify different problems. Multidisciplinary team meetings are therefore vital in ensuring that all members of staff have compatible goals and objectives and are providing a standard message to patients and carers. These meetings are also important to allow team members to get to know each other and discuss proposed practice changes. The meetings also provide a helpful forum for feedback and education.

Goal setting is crucial in rehabilitation. Goals are highly focused statements of intent that should be generated from the assessment processes. They may be physical, functional, psychological, or social but should be SMART (**S**pecific, **M**easurable, **A**chievable, **R**ealistic, and **T**imed). In ensuring that goals are measurable, a variety of assessment scales are used. These include the Rivermead Mobility Index, the Motor Assessment Scale, the Nine Hole Peg Test, and the Barthel index.

The Rivermead Mobility Index, a clinically relevant measure of disability, concentrates on body mobility. It consists of a series of 14 questions and one direct observation and covers a range of activities form turning over in bed to running. A modified version with a reduced number of test items has been developed specifically for use in stroke.

Box 227.12 Stroke multidisciplinary team members

Doctors
- provide medical care as appropriate for each patient
- need a good working knowledge of patients' diagnosis, prognosis, complications, and comorbidities
- it is often assumed that they are responsible for leading the multidisciplinary team but, in reality, this role should rotate

Nurses
- have a central role in stroke care, assisting with the daily care needs of patients
- help to prevent complications
- help to provide support for patients and their families

Physiotherapists
- largely responsible for the recovery of movement
- advise on positioning and handling issues
- provide mobility aids
- help prevent complications (particularly respiratory)

Occupational therapists
- dedicated to the recovery of functional tasks
- help patients gain independence with activities of daily living
- assess visuospatial function
- provide aids and appliances
- assess patients' abilities within the home

Speech and language therapists
- aid the recovery of function and speech
- provide detailed assessment of patients' swallow

Social workers
- help access and coordinate services and facilities within the community when patients are ready to leave hospital

Clinical psychologists
- help in the management of psychological and behavioural complications of stroke

Dieticians
- help to manage nutritional problems, dietary modification, and artificial feeding

Box 227.13 Indicators of a poor prognosis in stroke

- impaired consciousness
- gaze preference
- dense weakness
- cardiac comorbidity
- urinary incontinence
- pupillary abnormalities
- poor sitting balance at 2 weeks

stroke rehabilitation include poor postural control and sitting balance, advanced age, persistent bowel and bladder incontinence, prolonged hyporeflexia, prior stroke, visuospatial deficits, pre-stroke dependency, and initially decreased conscious level. Other barriers to rehabilitation include intercurrent medical illness, depression, and cultural reluctance to accept disability.

While the majority of stroke rehabilitation is provided in organized inpatient units, there is growing evidence that early supported discharge schemes are not only equally as effective but may actually improve physical function and decrease the economic burden of stroke care. In early supported discharge schemes, a qualified multidisciplinary team of healthcare professionals provides specialist stroke rehabilitation in the patients' home, with care initiated as soon as the patient is medically stable enough to leave hospital. This has several benefits. First, stroke patients undergoing rehabilitation at home have been shown to take the initiative more and express their desired goals more frequently than those undergoing hospital rehabilitation do. Second, therapists are able to observe the patient in a wider variety of roles and, consequently, identification of problem areas becomes more readily apparent both to the patient and the rehabilitation team. Third, in reducing hospital length of stay for stroke patients, early supported discharge schemes have been shown to lower hospital-related costs and overall care costs, with the saving in hospital-related costs being greater than the cost of the service. Such services, provided by a well-resourced, coordinated, specialist multidisciplinary team, therefore provide an acceptable alternative to hospital stroke unit care and are likely to become more widely available in the future.

Prognosis

After the first-ever stroke, death occurs in 12% at 1 week, 31% at 1 year, and 60% at 5 years. The risk of recurrent stroke amongst stroke survivors is 10%–16% at 1 year, thereafter falling to 4%–5% per year. The risk of not returning to independence varies with stroke type. Overall, 20%–30% of survivors are completely dependent at 1 year, and 40%–50% are independent. Indicators of a poor prognosis are given in Box 227.13.

Further Reading

Intercollegiate Stroke Working Party. National Clinical Guideline for Stroke (4th edition), 2012. Royal College of Physicians.

Lawton MT and Vates GE. Subarachnoid Hemorrhage. *N Engl J Med* 2017; 377: 257–66.

National Institute for Health and Care Excellence. *Stroke and Transient Ischaemic Attack in Over 16s: Diagnosis and Initial Management.* 2008. Available at http://www.nice.org.uk/CG068 (accessed 6 Jun 2017).

Saver JL. Cryptogenic Stroke. *N Engl J Med* 2016; 374: 2065–74.

The Motor Assessment Scale is a brief assessment of eight areas of motor function, and one area related to muscle tone. It is aimed at the functional capabilities of stroke patients.

The Nine Hole Peg Test is aimed at measuring manual dexterity and comprises a square board with nine pegs. The patient is instructed to take pegs from a container and place them into the holes on the board as quickly as possible.

The Barthel index is one of the numerous scales used to assess functional ability in activities of daily living. The activities assessed include feeding, bathing, grooming, toilet use, transfers, and mobility. While all these generic scales can be useful in helping to standardize rehabilitation, it is paramount that rehabilitation is ultimately tailored to each individual patient.

Rehabilitation is not passively 'done' to a patient, and there is no generic process that a patient goes through. Goals should be highly specific to each patient. Patients and their families should be fully informed about what the rehabilitation process entails and, while the multidisciplinary team should be optimistic and positive about rehabilitation, they should also be realistic, as false hope can be potentially devastating. The predictors for poor outcomes with

228 Dementia

Richard Armstrong

Definition of the disease

Dementia is a syndrome defined by a persistent, progressive decline in multiple cognitive functions to a degree sufficient to detrimentally impact activities of daily living and social function. The syndromic diagnosis of dementia remains useful, since the general management and economic burden of these patients remains similar, irrespective of aetiology. However, a more precise etiological diagnosis must be sought, since disease-specific treatment is increasingly likely to be appropriate.

The term 'mild cognitive impairment' (MCI) refers to objective impairment in a cognitive function (usually memory) which does not impair activities of daily living. The aim underlying the use of this term is to identify those with the early pathophysiological changes of neurodegenerative disease. Nonetheless, 'MCI' is not synonymous with 'early dementia', as a significant proportion of those with MCI will not worsen. The term should therefore be used cautiously.

Aetiology of the disease

Dementia results from progressive dysfunction of the cerebral cortex or its connections and may emerge from diverse disease processes. Most commonly implicated are the neurodegenerative diseases of ageing, but the relative importance of other causes is greater in the younger population (see Figure 228.1).

Molecular aetiology

Many neurodegenerative diseases share characteristic molecular pathological signatures. Insoluble, misfolded, aggregated proteins are found and they are of probable etiopathogenic importance. Multiple cellular processes may be affected but, ultimately, neuronal dysfunction and death ensues. Aggregates can be extracellular or intracellular, and the predominant protein component varies, although there is a considerable degree of overlap.

Genetic factors

Genotype is critical in determining the risk of developing a dementia. Classical genetic approaches in rare families with Mendelian inheritance of dementia have found that certain mutations confer very high risk, for example mutations in APP, PS-1, and PS-2 in Alzheimer's disease. These account for few (<5%) cases overall, but are instructive in disease neurobiology. Similar monogenic forms of other dementias exist.

Having two or more first-degree relatives with Alzheimer's disease confers around an 8× increased risk of developing the disease, attesting to the role of genetic factors in apparently sporadic cases. Modern genetic approaches, such as population-based genome-wide association studies, have identified frequently occurring low-risk polymorphisms that account for around 60% of the population-attributable risk of developing Alzheimer's disease. Similar studies are underway for other diseases. Soon, genetic tests will be available that give an individualized risk for developing a dementia.

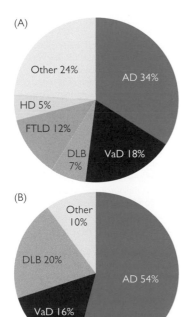

(A)

Other 24%
AD 34%
HD 5%
FTLD 12%
DLB 7%
VaD 18%

(B)

Other 10%
DLB 20%
AD 54%
VaD 16%

(C)

Neurodegenerative
Alzheimers Disease
Dementia with Lewy bodies
Parkinsons Disease dementia
Frontotemporal dementias
Creutzfeld-Jakob/Prion
Huntingtons Disease
Corticobasal syndrome

Vascular
Vascular dementia
Cerebral amyloid angiopathy
Vasculitis
CADASIL

Neoplastic
Strategic brain tumours
Intravascular lymphoma

Metabolic
Hypothyroidism
Hypercalcaemia
Thiamine-deficiency
B12 deficiency
Uraemia
Live failure

Other
Normal Pressure hydrocephalus
Obstructive sleep apneoa

Inflammatory/Infective
Multiple sclerosis
Antibody-mediated (eg VGKC, NMDA-R)
HIV, Neurosyphilis,
PML

Figure 228.1 The causes of dementia. Common cause of dementia in (A) those under 65 and (B) those over 65. Causes are listed in (C); this is not an exhaustive list of causes of global cognitive decline, but includes causes which are encountered on clinical practice; AD, Alzheimer's disease; DLB, dementia with Lewy bodies; FTLD, frontal temporal lobe dementia; HD, Huntington's disease; NMDA-R, NMDA receptor; PD, Parkinson's disease dementia; PML, progressive multifocal leukoencephalopathy; VaD, vascular dementia; VGKC, voltage-gated potassium channel.

Adapted with permission from Rossor et al., Dementia and cognitive impairment in *Neurology: A Queen Square Textbook*, pp. 245-289, Wiley-Blackwell, Oxford, UK, Copyright © 2009.

Environmental factors

Not all of the risk of dementia is currently explained by genetic factors. Other factors associated with an increased risk of developing dementia include diabetes, smoking, hypertension, hypercholesterolaemia, depression, and low social support. Conversely, high fruit and vegetable consumption, use of statins, low alcohol consumption, educational attainment, and physical activity have all been suggested to be protective. Overall, however, the quality of the scientific evidence is low for these factors, and interventional studies are lacking.

Typical symptoms of the disease, and less common symptoms

The end stage of most dementias is characterized by profound global impairment in all cognitive domains; behavioural disturbance; and functional dependence. The earliest symptoms and signs, however, reflect dysfunction in specific brain regions. These patterns are often characteristic and suggest the underlying cause of the dementia.

Memory

Memory is broadly represented in the brain, although deficits in the medial temporal lobes produce the well-recognized deficits in episodic memory in Alzheimer's disease. Episodic memory is the memory for autobiographical information (e.g. times, places, experiences, and contextual knowledge). Symptoms will include forgetting names, places, and facts about events that have occurred. Characteristically, there is a temporal gradient, with more recently experienced information being most vulnerable. Patients may therefore refer to such problems as 'poor short-term memory'. Such difficulties may lead to patients becoming repetitive. Difficulties in route finding reflect difficulties with topographical memory, a form of episodic memory. There is often difficulty in learning new tasks.

Semantic memory refers to concept-based knowledge ('general knowledge') unreliant on specific experiences, for example the knowledge that an elephant is an animal, not a plant. It is distinctively impaired in a form of frontotemporal dementia (FTD) termed semantic dementia. Patients will complain of 'word-finding difficulties', since they fail to link concepts of items to words.

Speech and language

Speech and language are subserved by distributed networks mainly located in the dominant frontal and temporal lobes. Language problems are a common symptom in many dementias. Difficulties in naming objects, comprehension of spoken or written language, misuse of grammar, word retrieval pauses, and circumlocutions are seen. Where speech dysfunction is early, isolated, or prominent, the syndrome is characterized as a primary progressive aphasia, in which case the underlying disease is usually FTD but occasionally is Alzheimer's disease.

Praxis and visuospatial function

Praxis and visuospatial function are prominently affected in conditions which have a posterior predominance and affect the parietal and occipital lobe. Posterior cortical atrophy refers to an early, isolated, or predominant posterior syndrome. Such posterior functions are commonly involved in Alzheimer's disease and Lewy body dementia (LBD) but spared in FTD and vascular dementia (VaD). Dyspraxia refers to the inability to execute complex motor programmes, for example being unable to work out how to dress or unlock a door. On examination, there are deficits in copying intersecting pentagons, mimicking meaningless hand gestures, and pantomiming actions. When visuospatial function is affected, patients may fail to recognize objects or even people, and there may be difficulty distinguishing objects such as coins, banknotes, or keys. On examination, there are difficulties in recognizing abstract representations such as fragmented letters/pictures. Calculation ability is susceptible to impairments in dominant parietal function, and these are often associated.

Executive function

Executive function refers to the ability to coordinate and sequence multiple cognitive functions and adapt them to the behavioural context. It is particularly susceptible to disease processes which affect the frontal lobe or its subcortical connections and thus deficits are prominently seen in behavioural variant FTD, Parkinson's disease, Huntington's disease, and VaD. There may be a slowing of thought and difficulty with tasks that require planning or flexibility. Examination tests which involve following simple rules or planning strategies are impaired.

Behavioural and psychiatric problems

Behavioural and psychiatric problems are common in advanced disease, irrespective of aetiology. Aggression, restlessness, and wandering can be troublesome. Psychotic features are seen.

In addition, symptoms often considered 'psychiatric' can be prominent early in certain circumstances. Hallucinations are a characteristic early feature of LBD and take a characteristic form of well-formed, silent, and usually non-threatening visual hallucinations. Visual misperceptions are also common.

When the pathological burden of disease falls mainly on frontal lobe circuits (e.g. in FTD, subcortical dementias, and VaD), behavioural disturbance may be an early problem: personality changes, emotional bunting, apathy, and a loss of empathy are characteristic. Patients may lose the ability to modulate their behaviour appropriately in the social context ('disinhibition'). Depression also frequently complicates dementia.

Demographics of the disease

Dementia becomes is more common with age. In the developed world, the prevalence below age 65 is around 1%, but increases exponentially to over 25% in those over 85, and data suggest little ethnic and geographical variation.

Natural history, and complications of the disease

There has been considerable emphasis on characterizing the natural history of MCI, giving hope that early disease-modifying therapy may soon be available. The risk of developing dementia in those with MCI is increased, but 20%–40% will never develop the full syndrome. Those with MCI have, on average, a 10%–15% annual risk of developing dementia, compared with a 1%–2% risk in the non-MCI population. Better objective markers of early disease and disease progression are therefore required. These 'biomarkers' will be of use in tracking the response to therapeutic interventions.

Practically, from clinical diagnosis, the decline in cognitive function is progressive and the tempo varies by aetiology. There is an average interval of 7 years between diagnosis and death in typical Alzheimer's disease, with the last couple of years characterized by dependency. LBD and VaD tend to progress faster, and FTD more slowly. A very rapidly progressive syndrome, over months, is not seen in the common neurodegenerative dementias and should lead one to consider non-degenerative (e.g. inflammatory) conditions or prion disease.

Late-stage disease is characterized by complications associated with frailty. Falls, fractures, malnutrition, and respiratory infections are common and usually contribute to death.

Approach to diagnosing the disease

The diagnosis of dementia and its cause currently remains largely clinical and criterion based and is made from the history obtained from the patient and an informant; this history should focus on symptoms from all domains specified in 'Natural history, and complications of the disease', together with an objective cognitive assessment. Further investigations (see 'Gold-standard' diagnostic test, alternatives, and other relevant investigations) provide support for underlying aetiology and serve to rule out reversible conditions that can produce a syndrome of global cognitive impairment.

Other diagnoses that should be considered

Cognitive impairment may result from non-neurodegenerative conditions which may be reversible. These conditions should be actively sought and excluded. Depression can result in complaints of subjective memory impairment and result in a 'pseudodementia'; cognitive testing may reveal inconsistencies but, occasionally, it can be very difficult to distinguish pseudodementia from early cognitive impairment and so longitudinal assessment will be required. Mass lesions rarely result in progressive global cognitive impairment in the absence of other neurological features, but tumours and subdural haematomas should be considered. Infective (e.g. HIV, syphilis), metabolic (e.g. hypothyroidism, B_{12} deficiency), and inflammatory (e.g. immune-mediated encephalitis, multiple sclerosis) conditions can all result in cognitive impairment but other symptoms usually suggest these diagnoses.

'Gold-standard' diagnostic test, alternatives, and other relevant investigations

As mentioned in 'Approach to diagnosing the disease', the diagnosis of dementia and its cause is criterion based, with most weight based on aspects of clinical history and objective cognitive assessment. Adjunctive investigations may allow more certainty, but currently established criteria allow a 'definite' (or gold-standard) disease-specific diagnosis only after pathological examination. Therefore, the choice of investigations must be tailored to the clinical scenario. All of the following investigations may be indicated in certain circumstances:

- objective cognitive assessment
- structural brain imaging
- nuclear/functional imaging
- CSF examination
- EEG
- blood work

Objective cognitive assessment

Objective cognitive assessment may take the form of 'bedside' cognitive tests or may involve detailed neuropsychological testing. Numerous validated cognitive tests are available for use in a clinic. The aim is to examine cognitive function across a number of domains. A given score can diagnose cognitive impairment with a given sensitivity and specificity. The Mini-Mental State Examination (MMSE) is widely used, with scores of ≤25/30 indicating impairment. Cognitive domains other than memory receive rather limited testing, however, and MMSE is less sensitive for the diagnosis of diseases other than Alzheimer's disease. The Montreal Cognitive Assessment is broader in scope and takes a similar amount of time to administer. It provides assessment of a number of domains, and is freely available for clinical use. The revised Addenbrooke's Cognitive Examination takes longer to administer but provides a fuller assessment. Multiple other assessments are available. Additional neuropsychological tests may be selected depending on dominant problems suggested in history taking.

Structural brain imaging

Structural brain imaging is mandatory in all cases. MRI is the most informative. While important to exclude alternative pathology, regional patterns of atrophy can suggest the underlying disease. The vascular burden can be estimated and diseases such as Creutzfeldt–Jakob disease have characteristic signal abnormalities. Serial volumetric imaging may be of use as a biomarker.

Nuclear/functional imaging

Nuclear/functional imaging may be used in specialist practice to reveal regional hypometabolism in the parietal and medial temporal lobes in Alzheimer's disease, and in the frontotemporal regions in FTD. Dopamine transporter imaging can reveal deficits in dopamine metabolism, suggesting LBD. It is likely that, in the near future, direct imaging of pathological proteins (e.g. amyloid beta 42) will become widely available.

CSF examination

CSF examination can be useful in restricted circumstances. Standard tests (e.g. cell count, protein, glucose) are normal in the common neurodegenerative dementias, and any abnormalities should suggest an alternative diagnosis. The 14-3-3 protein and S100 tests are sensitive for CJD but are non-specific, as these markers are raised in other circumstances where rapid cell death occurs, such as stroke. Specific assays are now available for amyloid beta 42 and tau in CSF. Amyloid beta 42 is reduced and tau is increased in Alzheimer's disease, and a significantly increased ratio of amyloid beta 42 to tau is specific for Alzheimer's disease pathology. Guidelines recommend these assays in young-onset cases.

EEG

EEG has restricted use but CJD gives a characteristic pattern of biphasic or triphasic spike discharges, although these can also be seen in metabolic encephalopathies. The common neurodegenerative dementias often show generalized slowing with a loss of alpha rhythm.

Blood work

Blood work has a role in excluding metabolic comorbidities which can, rarely, contribute to cognitive difficulty. A full blood count and renal, liver, calcium, and thyroid tests should be routinely performed. There may occasionally be cause to check HIV, syphilis serology, and vitamin B_{12} levels, but the yield from testing unselected patients is low.

Prognosis, and how to estimate it

A clearer understanding of the natural history of the individual diseases and the validation of biomarkers (see 'Natural history, and complications of the disease') will allow more accurate prognostication. Comorbidities such as diabetes mellitus and vascular disease worsen survival. In addition, for most acute medical conditions, the survival of those with advanced dementia is diminished with respect to unaffected individuals.

Treatment and its effectiveness

No proven treatments retard neurodegeneration or significantly alter the natural history of the neurodegenerative dementias, and all current treatments are considered symptomatic. Nonetheless, active management of symptoms can significantly improve quality of life and temporarily ameliorate cognitive function to some degree.

General and non-pharmacological measures

A multidisciplinary approach to care is requisite. The benefit of community specialist nurses, therapists, support groups, and social care workers to patients and their carers should not be underestimated. Caregiver stress must not be overlooked. There is some data to support a specific benefit of cognitive rehabilitation techniques and in improving cognitive function but standardized approaches need to be tested and validated.

Symptomatic treatment

Cognitive enhancers

A deficit in cholinergic neurotransmission is seen in Alzheimer's disease, and cholinesterase inhibitors (e.g. donepezil, rivastigmine, galantamine) are of clear (but temporary and modest) benefit on measures of cognitive function and activities of daily living. Adverse effects are relatively common and are largely gastrointestinal, but serious adverse events like heart block and seizures are well recognized. Meta-analyses suggest improvement on activities of daily living scales in mild–moderate dementia (an MMSE score of 10–26). This practically equates to preventing 2 months per year decline in typical Alzheimer's disease patients. It is doubtful whether there is any effect on long-term outcomes such as entry into institutionalized care. The benefit in advanced dementia (an MMSE score <10) is questionable, and standard practice is to withdraw treatment at this stage. A few patients will decline significantly when this is done. Practically, guidelines support consideration of individualized trials of these drugs in mild–moderate Alzheimer's disease, with objective regular assessment of benefit. In LBD and Parkinson's disease dementia, cholinesterase inhibitors are helpful in the treatment of hallucinations, and there is evidence for some benefit in VaD. They are of no proven benefit in any other condition. NMDA antagonists (e.g. memantine) may be of some modest benefit in moderate–advanced Alzheimer's disease, and some data suggest an additive benefit to cholinesterase inhibitors. Individualized trials may be considered in specialist practice.

Behavioural and psychiatric symptoms

If behavioural disturbance or psychotic features continue to present significant clinical risk despite sustained attempts at non-pharmacological solutions, then drug treatment should be carefully considered. There is evidence for a modest benefit of newer atypical antipsychotic drugs, but their use has recently been discouraged, since they are associated with a small increase in all-cause mortality when used in advanced dementia. Despite this, they retain some role after careful consideration and discussion of relative risks. Antipsychotic drugs can produce very significant worsening in patients with LBD and must be avoided. Benzodiazepines can provoke delirium or a worsening of cognitive function but are occasionally helpful to manage agitation. Comorbid depression should be treated with serotonin-specific reuptake inhibitors.

Disease-modifying treatment

A vast number of compounds proposed to modify pathways of neurodegeneration have been unsuccessfully trialled. Nonetheless, considerable optimism exists that more specific agents currently being developed and trialled will produce a more positive outcome.

Further Reading

Kester MI and Scheltens P. Dementia: The bare essentials. *Pract Neurol* 2009; 9: 241–51.

Mueller C, Ballard C, Corbett A et al. The prognosis of dementia with Lewy bodies. *Lancet Neurol* 2017; 16: 390–98.

Rosser M, Collinge J, Fox N, et al. 'Cognitive impairment and dementia' in Clarke C, Howard R, Rossor M, and Shorvon, SD, eds, *Neurology: A Queen Square Textbook*, 2009. Wiley-Blackwell.

Scheltens P, Blennow K, Breteler MMB et al. Alzheimer's disease. *Lancet* 2016; 388: 505–17.

229 Neurological infection

Tom Solomon and Benedict Michael

Definition of the disease

Neurological infections, affecting the central nervous system (CNS), can be broadly subdivided into chronic/subacute and acute. Chronic/subacute infection usually presents with global cognitive decline, with the prototypical disease being progressive multifocal leucoencephalopathy due to infection with the JC virus in immunocompromised patients. Acute neurological infections can be defined microbiologically, by the nature of the pathogen, clinically, by the presenting signs and symptoms and initial CSF findings, or anatomically. The anatomical definitions are those occurring intracranially ('meningitis', where infection involves the meninges overlying the brain; 'encephalitis', where the brain parenchyma is involved; or 'cerebral abscesses') and those affecting the spinal cord ('myelitis'). However, there is often both clinical and histological overlap between these syndromes; consequently, the terms 'meningoencephalitis' and 'encephalomyelitis' are often used.

Patients with acute intracranial CNS infections provide the greatest challenge to general physicians, because urgent investigation and appropriate treatment can save lives; they therefore form the focus of this chapter.

Aetiology of the disease

Acute CNS infections can be caused by a wide range of pathogens in the immunocompetent, and an even wider variety in the immunocompromised. There is significant global variation in the incidence of causal pathogens, reflecting endemic rates of HIV infection, TB infection, and malnutrition; viral vector prevalence; and vaccination programmes. Despite current diagnostic techniques, the causal pathogen is often not identified; for example, the causal pathogen in approximately 40% cases of encephalitis is not identified. A staged approach to the identification of the causal pathogen is outlined in Table 229.1.

Meningeal infection is subdivided into aseptic and purulent meningitis on the basis of the clinical presenting features and initial CSF findings (Table 229.2). Aseptic meningitis is typically caused by viruses, with enteroviruses, accounting for >90% of cases. Although accounting for fewer cases of aseptic meningitis, herpes simplex virus (HSV) 2 (HSV-2) is of particular importance as it can result in a recurrent meningitis (previously termed 'Mollaret's') and should direct investigation towards genital infection. Purulent meningitis is usually due to bacterial infection, with *Streptococcus pneumoniae* and *Neisseria meningitidis* making up >90% of cases in adults in the developed world. Since the introduction of the *Haemophilius influenza* and the measles, mumps, and rubella (MMR) vaccines, there has been a dramatic decline in the incidence of these pathogens, although they remain important in resource-poor countries. In addition, the recent decline in vaccination uptake in some developed countries has been accompanied by a rise in the incidence of these infections.

The most common infectious cause of encephalitis is viral, most commonly due to HSV-1 and varicella zoster virus (VZV) (approximately 19% and 5% of viral cases, respectively). A recent cohort study in the UK identified that HSV was the most common cause of acute CNS infections overall. However, in approximately 11% of cases, encephalitis follows infection or vaccination, causing an 'acute disseminated encephalomyelitis (ADEM)'. Additionally, antibody-mediated forms of encephalitis have been identified which often respond to immunomodulatory therapy; these are most commonly caused by the presence of anti-NMDA antibodies (accounting for 4% of cases) or antibodies against the voltage-gated potassium channel complex (accounting for 3% of cases).

The incidence of meningoencephalitis due to TB infection appears to be rising in the UK. It most often occurs in those exposed to the infection in Africa or India, or in the context of coexistent HIV infection. The clinical presentation is usually more subacute than for other CNS infections, and a longer prodrome of weight loss, malaise, and night sweats is typical. The CSF findings can be highly suggestive (Table 229.2), but the glucose is not *always* low, and the organism itself may be difficult to isolate.

Typical symptoms of the disease, and less common symptoms

Typical presenting symptoms include fever or an antecedent febrile illness, meningism (neck stiffness, nausea, and vomiting), headache, reduced or altered consciousness, seizures, and focal neurological signs. In encephalitis, there may be a reduced level of consciousness. However, the alteration in conscious is often a more subtle neuropsychiatric presentation of altered behaviour and cognition. Therefore, a collateral history is crucial. Evidence of focal neurological motor or sensory disturbance, including dysphasia or seizures, suggests brain parenchymal inflammation such as encephalitis, cerebral abscesses, or antibody-mediated encephalitides.

Effort should be undertaken to look for symptoms or signs which may suggest a particular pathogen. These include:

- a non-blanching purpuric rash in meningococcal septicaemia
- a dermatomal vesicular rash in varicella zoster infection
- stigmata of HIV infection (e.g. oral hairy leukoplakia and Kaposi's sarcoma)
- orchitis or pancreatitis in mumps virus infection
- lower cranial neuropathies and myoclonus suggesting a rhombencephalitis often due to listeria or some enteroviruses
- a longer prodrome including weight loss and night sweats; this suggests TB, and there may be multiple cranial nerve palsies and pyramidal signs in the meningitic phase
- movement disorders and extrapyramidal features, as seen in flavivirus infection such as West Nile or Japanese encephalitis virus infection

However, no clinical symptoms and signs, or combinations thereof, have been identified which can accurately diagnose or exclude CNS infection or accurately determine the aetiology. For example, the classical triad in meningitis of fever, meningism, and altered mental status is only present in 44% of cases. Even a rash which looks 'meningococcal' can be caused by other bacteria. Additionally, fever may be absent at presentation in up to 24% of patients with proven HSV encephalitis. Therefore, when the diagnosis of CNS infection is suggested by the presence of some, if not all, of the associated clinical features, further investigation is vital.

Demographics of the disease

The annual incidence is approximately 2.9–10.0 in 100 000 for viral encephalitis, 0.6–4.0 in 100 000 for purulent meningitis, and 5.2–7.6 in 100 000 for aseptic meningitis, although these are thought to be underestimates.

Acute CNS infections can occur at any age, but the young and the elderly are particularly at risk. While CNS infections often occur in the immunocompetent, individuals with immune compromise, such as patients with HIV infection or iatrogenic immune suppression, are at increased risk. Additionally, people with any chronic disease are

Table 229.1 A staged approach to pathogen identification in patients with suspected CNS infection

Diagnostic suspicion	Investigation	Indication	Items to test for
Suspected encephalitis	CSF PCR	All patients	HSV-1 HSV-2 VZV Enterovirus Parechovirus
		Immunocompromised patients	EBV CMV HHV6 HHV7 Adenovirus Influenza A Influenza B Parvovirus B19
		If clinically indicated	Measles Mumps Chlamydia
		If indicated by the travel history	Rabies West Nile virus and other flaviviruses Tick-borne encephalitis
	CSF and serum IgM and IgG antibody testing in acute and convalescent samples	If CSF PCR is negative	HSV-1 HSV-2 VZV CMV HHV6 HHV7 Enterovirus Parvovirus Adenovirus Influenza A and B
		If the patient is immune-suppressed	Cryptococcus Toxoplasma
	Serum antibody and antigen	Advised in all patients	HIV
	Serum antibody for autoimmunity	If psychiatric symptoms, seizures, movement disorder, subacute presentation, or known/suspected malignancy is present	Voltage-gated potassium channel complex antibodies Anti-NMDA receptor antibodies Further intra- or extra-cellular antibodies guided by clinical phenotype
		If associated with an atypical pneumonia	Mycoplasma serology Cold agglutinins Chlamydia serology
	Ancillary investigations: PCR and/or culture (these establish systemic infection, but not necessarily the cause of the CNS disease)	Respiratory tract symptoms: throat swab, nasopharyngeal aspirate Gastrointestinal symptoms: rectal swab Vesicular rash: vesicle swab	Enterovirus Mycoplasma Chlamydia Influenza Adenovirus HSV VZV
	Brain biopsy	Above investigations are negative and patient is deteriorating despite empirical treatment	Microscopy and immunohistochemistry Bacterial culture Extended fungal and mycobacterial culture Viral PCR (as above)
		Above investigations are negative and patient is deteriorating despite empirical treatment and is immune-suppressed	India ink stain for cryptococcus Ziehl–Neelsen stain for TB
Suspected meningitis	CSF culture	All patients	Microscopy, culture, and sensitivity for all pathogens
		Immune-suppressed patients	Extended culture for mycoplasma and fungi
	CSF PCR	If suspected viral meningitis	As for encephalitis
		If suspected bacterial meningitis and culture is negative	*Neisseria meningitidis* *Streptococcus pneumoniae* Listeria
	CSF cytological examination	Known or suspected systemic or CNS malignancy	Malignant cells Sample also for flow cytometry if haematological malignancy known/suspected

Abbreviations: CNS, central nervous system; CSF, cerebrospinal fluid; EBV, Epstein–Barr virus; HHV6, human herpes virus 6; HHV7, human herpes virus 7; HIV: human immunodeficiency virus; HSV, herpes simplex virus; PCR, polymerase chain reaction; TB, tuberculosis; VZV, varicella zoster virus.

Table 229.2 Cerebrospinal fluid analysis interpretation in patients with suspected CNS infection

Investigation	Normal	Purulent Meningitis	Aseptic Meningitis or Encephalitis	Tuberculous Meningitis	Fungal
Opening Pressure	10–20 cm*	High	Normal/High	High	High/Very High
Colour	Clear	Cloudy	'Gin' Clear	Cloudy/Yellow	Clear/Cloudy
Cells/mm³	<5**	High/Very High 100–50 000	Slightly Increased 5–1000	Slightly Increased 25–500	Normal–High 0–1000
Differential	Lymphocytes	Neutrophils	Lymphocytes	Lymphocytes	Lymphocytes
CSF/Plasma Glucose	66%***	Normal	Low	Low–Very Low (<30%)	Normal–Low
Protein (g/L)	<0.45	High >1	Normal–High 0.5–1	High–Very High 1.0–5.0	Normal–High 0.2–5.0

Abbreviations: CNS, central nervous system; CSF, cerebrospinal fluid; LP, lumbar puncture.

*Normal CSF opening pressure approximately <20 cm in adults and <10 cm in children under 8 years, but may be 'normal' at up to 25 cm.

**A bloody tap will falsely elevate both the CSF white-cell count and protein. To correct for a bloody tap; subtract 1 white cell/mm³ for every 700 red blood cells/mm³ and 0.1 g/dl of protein for every 1000 red blood cells/mm³.

***'Normal' CSF glucose ratio is typically quoted as 66%, although, in practice, only values below 50% are likely to be significant. Absolute CSF glucose levels can be misleading—a paired plasma glucose level is always required.

Some important exceptions
• In viral CNS infections, an early LP may show predominantly neutrophils, or there may be no cells in early or late LPs.
• If acute bacterial meningitis is partially treated with antibiotics (or patient <1 year old) the CSF cell count may not be very high and may be mostly lymphocytic.
• Tuberculous CSF may have predominant polymorphs early on.
• Listeria can give a similar CSF picture to tuberculous meningitis, although the history is shorter.
• CSF findings in cases of a bacterial abscess range from near normal to purulent depending on location and whether there is associated meningitis or rupture.
• A cryptococcal antigen test and India ink stain should be performed on all CSF samples of patients in whom cryptococcus is possible.

Reprinted from *Journal of Infection*, Volume 64, issue 5, R. Kneen, B. D. Michael, E. Menson, B. Mehta, A. Easton, C. Hemingway, P. E. Klapper, A. Vincent, M. Lim, E. Carrol, T. Solomon, Management of suspected viral encephalitis in children – Association of British Neurologists and British Paediatric Allergy, Immunology and Infection Group National Guidelines, pp. 449–477, Copyright (2012), with permission from Elsevier.

at increased risk, particularly if they have diabetes mellitus, chronic kidney disease, or a history of alcohol excess.

In the UK, bacterial infection is more common in the winter, respiratory viruses are more common in the winter and spring, and enteroviral infection is more common in the summer.

Natural history, and complications of the disease

Acute CNS infections have a mortality rate of 10%–28% in encephalitis and 3%–37% in bacterial meningitis, despite treatment. The national cost for patients hospitalized with encephalitis in the USA is estimated to be $630 million. Neurological and neuropsychiatric sequelae are common, particularly following encephalitis; they include seizures, focal neurological weakness, and cognitive and behavioural problems. Deafness is a common complication following bacterial meningitis.

If a patient with an acute CNS infection deteriorates despite treatment, look for complications, including:

• cerebral infarction
• cerebral oedema, brain shift, and herniation
• seizures, especially subtle motor status epilepticus
• venous sinus thrombosis
• subdural empyemas
• systemic shock
• aspiration pneumonia
• hyponatraemia or if delayed consider infection relapse or post-infectious autoimmunity

Hydrocephalus, vasculitis, tuberculomas, and radiculomyelopathy may additionally complicate TB infection.

Approach to diagnosing the disease

An approach to diagnosis is outlined in Figure 229.1.

All patients should undergo a lumbar puncture (LP), providing there are no clinical contraindications (Table 229.3). This can quickly confirm or refute the diagnosis and direct treatment towards a viral, bacterial, or mycobacterial pathogen. Additionally, the CSF culture can identify the pathogen and determine antibiotic sensitivities, which is of particular importance given the concerns of growing antibiotic resistance. Additionally, PCR allows for the rapid amplification of viral

nucleic acid and should also be requested in bacterial meningitis if the CSF culture is negative.

However, if clinical contraindications to an immediate LP are present urgent neuroimaging should be undertaken. While MRI is more sensitive for the identification of parenchymal lesions, CT is often more easily available urgently. As it is sufficient to identify significant brain shift precluding a LP, it is often the most pragmatic approach.

The initial CSF findings may be normal, for example in approximately 11% of patients who ultimately have proven HSV encephalitis. If clinical suspicion of CNS infection remains, the patient should be started on the appropriate antimicrobial regimen and the LP repeated 24–48 hours later.

The investigation and management of meningoencephalitis due to *Mycobacterium tuberculosis* infection is well described in the National Institute for Health and Clinical Excellence guideline and is beyond the scope of this chapter.

Other diagnoses that should be considered

Other causes of encephalopathy (altered consciousness) should be considered, including systemic sepsis, metabolic derangement, or toxaemia. However, be cautious of ascribing a previously healthy patient's altered mental state to an extra-CNS infection, such as a urinary infection, unless there is strong evidence for it. Additionally, hyponatraemia may often occur in CNS infection due to the syndrome of inappropriate antidiuretic hormone secretion and, when identified, may be a result of CNS infection rather than the cause of encephalopathy.

Two important diagnoses not to miss are venous sinus thrombosis and subtle convulsive status epilepticus. Venous sinus thrombosis should be considered, as it typically presents with headache, altered consciousness, and seizures, often in the context of a febrile illness such as sinusitis/otitis as the precipitant of the thrombosis. The diagnosis is confirmed by imaging of the venous system of the CNS. Subtle convulsive status epilepticus should be suspected in those with fluctuating levels of consciousness, particularly if there is evidence of subtle motor signs or a history suggestive of previous seizures. In this instance an EEG can be invaluable.

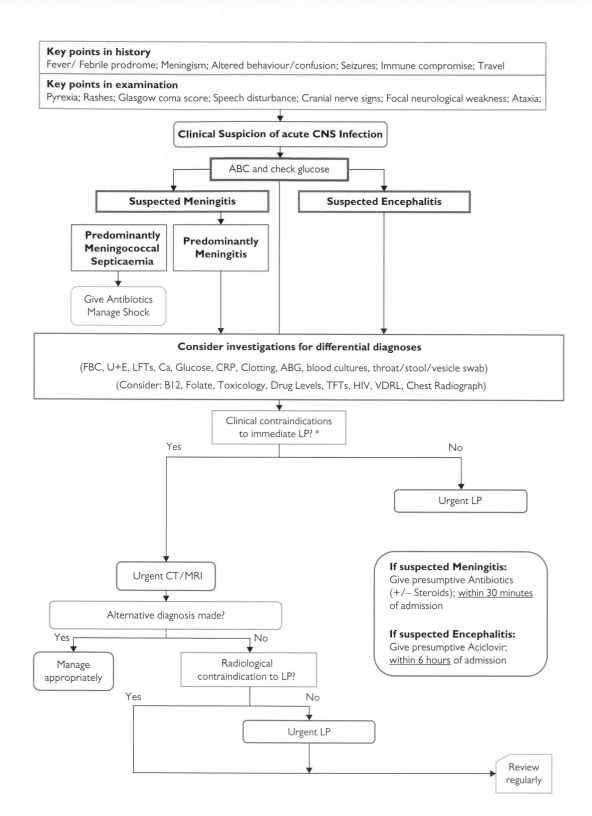

Key points in history
Fever/ Febrile prodrome; Meningism; Altered behaviour/confusion; Seizures; Immune compromise; Travel

Key points in examination
Pyrexia; Rashes; Glasgow coma score; Speech disturbance; Cranial nerve signs; Focal neurological weakness; Ataxia;

Clinical Suspicion of acute CNS Infection

ABC and check glucose

Suspected Meningitis

Suspected Encephalitis

Predominantly Meningococcal Septicaemia

Predominantly Meningitis

Give Antibiotics Manage Shock

Consider investigations for differential diagnoses

(FBC, U+E, LFTs, Ca, Glucose, CRP, Clotting, ABG, blood cultures, throat/stool/vesicle swab)

(Consider: B12, Folate, Toxicology, Drug Levels, TFTs, HIV, VDRL, Chest Radiograph)

Clinical contraindications to immediate LP? *

Yes — No

Urgent LP

Urgent CT/MRI

Alternative diagnosis made?

Yes — No

Manage appropriately

Radiological contraindication to LP?

Yes — No

If suspected Meningitis:
Give presumptive Antibiotics (+/– Steroids); within 30 minutes of admission

If suspected Encephalitis:
Give presumptive Aciclovir; within 6 hours of admission

Urgent LP

Review regularly

Abbreviations: FBC: Full blood count; U+E: Urea and electrolytes; Ca: Calcium; CRP: C-reactive protein; ABG: Arterial blood gases; LP: Lumbar puncture; CSF: cerebrospinal fluid; TFTs: Thyroid function tests; HIV: Human immunodeficiency virus; VRDL: Syphilis antibody testing; GCS: Glasgow coma score; CT: Computed tomography; MRI: Magnetic resonance imaging

Figure 229.1 An approach to the emergency management of acute CNS infections in adults; ABG, arterial blood gases; Ca, calcium; CRP, C-reactive protein; CSF, cerebrospinal fluid; CT, computed tomography; FBC, full blood count; GCS: Glasgow Coma Score; HIV: human immunodeficiency virus; LP, lumbar puncture; MRI, magnetic resonance imaging; TFTs, thyroid function tests; U+E, urea and electrolytes; VRDL, syphilis antibody testing.

Adapted from *Journal of Infection*, Volume 64, issue 5, R. Kneen, B. D. Michael, E. Menson, B. Mehta, A. Easton, C. Hemingway, P. E. Klapper, A. Vincent, M. Lim, E., Carrol, T. Solomon, Management of suspected viral encephalitis in children – Association of British Neurologists and British Paediatric Allergy, Immunology and Infection Group National Guidelines, pp. 449-477, Copyright (2012), with permission from Elsevier.

Table 229.3 Clinical contraindications to an immediate lumbar puncture in patients with suspected CNS infections*

Contraindication	Notes
Seizure(s)	New or persistent
Focal neurological signs	Hemiparesis
	Monoparesis
	Extensor plantar response
	Ocular palsies
Reduced level of consciousness	Glasgow Coma Scale score of <13 or a deterioration of >2
Signs of brain shift	Cushing's reflex
	Papilloedema
	Abnormal respiratory pattern
	Decorticate/decerebrate posturing
	Altered pupillary response
	Absent doll's eye reflex
Local superficial infection	At potential lumbar puncture site
Coagulation disorder	Including iatrogenic anticoagulation or platelets <40 × 10⁹/l
Known immune compromise	
Strong suspicion of meningococcal septicaemia	In a patient with sepsis, meningism, and a typical purpuric rash, a lumbar puncture is not needed, as the diagnosis may be made from blood cultures

* Clinical contraindications to lumbar puncture without neuroimaging.

'Gold-standard' diagnostic test

Traditionally, the gold-standard diagnostic investigation in encephalitis was histopathological examination of brain biopsy tissue demonstrating brain parenchymal inflammation with evidence of direct infection by a causal pathogen. However, due to the risks associated with brain biopsy and newer molecular diagnostic techniques, it is performed less often. Therefore, microbiological investigations identify the cause. In bacterial meningitis CSF culture and/or CSF PCR are used. As CSF viral culture has a lower sensitivity, PCR analysis of the CSF are used is the gold standard and has a high sensitivity (>95%) and specificity (>99%). Identification of viral nucleic acid in the CSF is diagnostic of active infection in the case of HSV-1, HSV-2, VZV, enterovirus, and parechovirus. However, ubiquitous lymphotrophic viruses such as EBV and human herpes viruses 6 and 7 may be identified due to latent infection or, in the case of human herpes virus 6, inherited viral DNA inclusions. Viral load determined by quantitative PCR may be useful.

Further investigation should be guided by the clinical, CSF, and neuroimaging features and by close collaboration between the attending clinicians, virologists, and infectious disease specialists.

Acceptable diagnostic alternatives to the gold standard

In the presence of the clinical features described in 'Approach to diagnosing the disease', identification of CNS inflammation on CSF findings and/or neuroimaging, if the features are classical, may be sufficient to establish the diagnosis of a CNS infection.

Other relevant investigations

All adults and teenage children with a CNS infection should have an HIV test. HIV seroconversion is a common cause of aseptic meningitis; alternatively, a CNS infection may be a clue that a patient is HIV positive.

Box 229.1 Risk factors for a poor prognosis

- age >60 years
- seizures
- immunocompromised patients
- abnormal brain imaging
- delays in treatment (e.g. due to inappropriate neuroimaging):
  - >6 hours from admission to starting treatment with antibiotics (in bacterial meningitis)
  - >1-2 day from admission to starting treatment with aciclovir (in viral encephalitis)

Young people and children should be tested for complement deficiency if they have any one of the following:

- more than one episode of meningococcal disease
- one episode of meningococcal disease caused by a serogroup other than B
- one episode of meningococcal disease, and a history of other recurrent bacterial infections

Patients with recurrent bacterial meningitis should undergo CT of the head, to look for dural defects, and an ear, nose, and throat specialist review. Patients with recurrent aseptic meningitis should be screened for systemic disease such as systemic lupus erythematosis.

Encephalitis, meningitis, and meningococcal septicaemia are notifiable conditions.

Prognosis and how to estimate it

There are no validated prognostic tools for clinical use for cases of CNS infection. However, cohort studies and case series have identified the risk factors for a poor prognosis (see Box 229.1).

Treatment and its effectiveness

In primary care, a single dose of IV or intramuscular third-generation cephalosporin should be given to patients in whom meningococcal infection is suspected and also in any patient with signs of severe sepsis or in whom there will be a dleay of >1 hr before ariving in hospital. Guidelines recommend that this therapy be started within 30 minutes of hospital admission and as guided by local microbiology policy for suspected meningitis. There is slightly less time pressure when treating encephalitis because patients with encephalitis do not appear to deteriorate as rapidly as those with bacterial meningitis. However, UK guidelines recommend aciclovir within 6 hours of admission and there is evidence of a worse prognosis in those in whom treatment is delayed beyond 1-2 days of admission. As it is often not possible to determine whether the infection is due to a virus or bacteria in the acute phase, it is reasonable to commence treatments for both. Nevertheless, due to the risks of opportunistic infection, antibiotic resistance, and nephrotoxicity, the prescription of antimicrobials should be regularly reviewed in light of test results.

Ideally, an LP should be undertaken prior to commencing treatment, to maximize the chance of establishing the diagnosis and identifying the pathogen. For example, in a recent study of 92 patients with suspected bacterial meningitis, a delay of 4 hours resulted in a significant decline in the detection rate; beyond 8 hours, no CSF culture was positive. Similar studies have identified CSF sterility between 2 and 10 hours following commencement of antibiotics. However, antibiotics should be commenced prior to the LP in two scenarios: first, if there is a strong clinical suspicion of meningococcal septicaemia, such as a septic patient with a widespread purpuric rash (blood cultures taken at the time of venous cannulation can often establish the diagnosis); second, in cases where there are clinical contraindications to an LP. In the latter case, antibiotics should not be delayed until neuroimaging and subsequent LP, as this is associated with increased morbidity and mortality. However, the time period during which it may be possible to detect infection following the commencement of antimicrobials is longer for PCR tests than for CSF culture, so the LP should still be performed urgently to maximize diagnostic sensitivity.

IV dexamethasone should be given immediately prior to the first antibiotic dose in patients with suspected streptococcal meningitis. Patients aged over 60yrs should also be given ampicillin or amoxicillin, to cover listeria infection.

Further Reading

Heyderman RS, Lambert HP, O'Sullivan I, et al. Early management of suspected bacterial meningitis and meningococcal septicaemia in adults. *J Infect* 2003; 46: 75–7.

McGill F, Heyderman R, Michael BD et al. Management of meningitis in immunocompetent adults: Association of British Neurologists and British Infection Association National Guideline. *J Infect* 2016; 72: 405–38.

Solomon T, Hart I, and Beeching NJ. Viral encephalitis: A clinician's guide. *Pract Neurol* 2007; 7: 288–305.

Solomon T, Michael BD, Smith PE, et al. Management of suspected viral encephalitis in adults: Association of British Neurologists and British Infection Association National Guideline. *J Infect* 2012; 64: 347–73.

230 Disorders of movement

Cris S. Constantinescu and Fahd Baig

Introduction

The neural pathways that control movement involve several structures, from the cerebral cortex through to the muscle. This allows for the maintenance of tone, posture, and volitional movement. Disruption of subcortical structures which modulate these pathways (such as the basal ganglia) can cause a variety of clinical presentations collectively termed movement disorders. They can be simply divided into hypokinetic disorders (e.g. parkinsonism) and hyperkinetic disorders.

Hypokinetic movement disorders

Parkinson's disease and parkinsonism

Definition of Parkinson's disease and parkinsonism

Parkinsonism is the collective term for a group of motor syndromes characterized by tremor, bradykinesia, rigidity, and postural instability. The most common cause is Parkinson's disease (PD), which is an idiopathic neurodegenerative disorder.

Aetiology of PD and parkinsonism

Dysfunction or loss of dopamine-containing cells in the substantia nigra causes the motor signs and symptoms of parkinsonism. Parkinsonian disorders can be divided into four subtypes, based on cause and clinical phenotype:

- PD (idiopathic)
- secondary parkinsonism (due to acquired causes, e.g. cerebrovascular disease, drugs, or toxins)
- familial parkinsonism (e.g. mutations in the genes LRRK2 and SNCA)
- Parkinson plus syndromes: these are idiopathic conditions in which parkinsonism is associated with the following additional clinical features:
  - progressive supranuclear palsy (restriction of voluntary eye movements and dementia)
  - multisystem atrophy (cerebellar or autonomic dysfunction)
  - corticobasal degeneration (dementia with features of frontal and parietal lobe dysfunction)

Typical symptoms of PD, and less common symptoms

Tremor at rest, bradykinesia (slowness in initiating and maintaining movements), rigidity, and postural instability are the cardinal features of PD. Patients with PD usually have asymmetric motor symptoms. They also commonly have anosmia, hypomimia, hypophonia, focal dystonia, constipation, hypersialorrhoea, and gait difficulty. In addition, cognitive impairment affects a significant proportion of PD sufferers and can lead to dementia.

Demographics of PD

In the UK, the prevalence of PD is estimated to be 100–180 per 100 000 population, with an incidence of 4–20 per 100 000. Both prevalence and incidence increase with age, and men are more likely to be affected than women.

Natural history of PD, and complications of the disease

PD is a chronic and progressive condition with symptoms, such as anosmia, sleep disturbance, depression, and constipation, starting up to 10 years prior to the diagnosis. Following diagnosis, patients develop worsening symptoms of bradykinesia, tremor, rigidity, and gait disturbance to varying degrees over several years. As the disease progresses, often 5–15 years post diagnosis, increasingly, motor complications (e.g. dyskinesias, gait freezing, axial deformities, dysarthria, and dysphagia) as well as non-motor complications (e.g. cognitive decline, depression, and autonomic dysfunction) become prominent.

Approach to diagnosing PD

Careful history taking and examination is the mainstay of diagnosis of PD, which is clinical. Particular focus should be paid to comorbidities (e.g. vascular risk factors), current and previous medications, drug use, family history, and non-motor features which patients may not think relevant to volunteer.

Other diagnoses that should be considered aside from PD

Wilson's disease, Huntington's disease, Hallervorden–Spatz disease, and neuroacanthocytosis can all present with parkinsonian features. In the context of cognitive impairment, Alzheimer's disease and Lewy body dementia should be considered.

'Gold-standard' diagnostic test for PD

As there is no reliable laboratory or imaging modality validated in isolation, clinical assessment remains the 'investigation' of choice.

Acceptable diagnostic alternatives to the gold-standard test for PD

DAT-SPECT (dopamine transporter single-photon emission CT) imaging, a SPECT that detects radioactively labelled dopamine transporters and shows initially asymmetrical decreased signal in PD, can be used to differentiate essential tremor, drug-induced parkinsonism, and vascular parkinsonism from PD. In the non-PD conditions, uptake is either unchanged or symmetrically reduced. Trials of treatment with medications such as levodopa are not useful.

Other relevant investigations for PD

MRI of the brain can identify structural causes of parkinsonism, such as cerebrovascular disease. This modality can also potentially identify features of Parkinson plus syndromes. SPECT imaging can differentiate dementia syndromes. Genetic screening for common mutations should be considered in young patients or when there is a family history. Laboratory tests for thyroid function, parathyroid function, heavy metals (e.g. Mn, Hg), acanthocytes (to look for neuroacanthocytosis), and copper can be useful in the appropriate clinical setting.

Prognosis of PD, and how to estimate it

Life expectancy in patients with PD is significantly reduced in patients with a younger age of onset, dementia, and dysphagia. Outside these groups, the life expectancy is near normal but the disability shows a predictable progressive pattern.

Treatment of PD, and its effectiveness

For effective management, a multidisciplinary approach to ameliorate the variety of disabling symptoms patients develop is required. The mainstay of drug therapy remains dopaminergic medications, which treat the motor features of PD. They have limited efficacy in treating the Parkinson plus syndromes and tend to be ineffective in secondary parkinsonism.

Levodopa preparations (in combination with a peripheral decarboxylase inhibitor to augment the half-life) are considered by many the most effective treatment. Side effects include confusion, hallucinations, gastrointestinal symptoms, orthostatic hypotension, and motor complications (such as dystonia and dyskinesia). Catechol-O-methyl transferase inhibitors are used to block the residual breakdown of levodopa in the gastrointestinal tract, thus extending the availability and half-life.

Dopamine agonists can be used synergistically in combination with levodopa or as monotherapy. The side effects are similar in nature to levodopa but can also cause additional neuropsychiatric symptoms, including obsessional behaviours, addiction (e.g. gambling, hypersexuality), hallucinations, and psychosis.

Other drug treatments include anticholinergics (particularly for tremor), amantadine, and monoamine oxidase inhibitors. Cholinesterase inhibitors have a role in patients with dementia.

Deep brain stimulation is effective in a select group of patients, mitigating motor symptoms and reducing medications (and therefore the side effects of medications).

Hyperkinetic disorders

Essential tremor

Definition of essential tremor

Tremor is the rhythmical oscillatory movement of any body part and may feature as a part of a number of disorders. The term 'essential tremor' is used to describe a progressive tremor syndrome which usually includes an upper limb tremor and for which no underlying cause or alternative diagnosis is identifiable.

Aetiology of essential tremor

About half of patients with essential tremor have a family member with tremor. Genetic studies have identified a number of candidate genes which need confirmation.

Typical symptoms of essential tremor, and less common symptoms

Nearly all patients with essential tremor have an upper limb tremor, but they can also have a tremor in the lower limbs, head, jaw, tongue, trunk, and voice. Typically, the tremor has a postural component (present on maintenance of a posture, such as when the arms are outstretched) and a kinetic component (present when moving a body part, such as a hand, towards a target).

Demographics of essential tremor

Essential tremor can start at any age but is more common in adults.

Natural history of essential tremor, and complications of the disease

In essential tremor, the tremor lasts for life, progressing slowly over time, and can cause some difficulty with embarrassment in social situations and possibly activities of daily living. Life expectancy is not affected.

Approach to diagnosing essential tremor

In essential tremor, careful assessment for features of alternative conditions is required, as this tremor can represent a number of other conditions.

Other diagnoses that should be considered aside from essential tremor

Enhanced physiological tremor (e.g. due to hyperthyroidism, anxiety, or medication) can mimic essential tremor. Additional neurological features such as pyramidal signs, extrapyramidal signs, cerebellar features, and dystonia can point to alternative diagnoses.

'Gold-standard' diagnostic test for essential tremor

There are no diagnostic investigations for essential tremor, aside from clinical assessment.

Acceptable diagnostic alternatives to the gold-standard test for essential tremor

In essential tremor, the response to alcohol or characterization of the tremor in terms of amplitude and frequency are not specific enough to be discriminatory.

Other relevant investigations for essential tremor

Thyroid function can exclude thyrotoxicosis. DAT-SPECT imaging can be used to discriminate PD from essential tremor in the case of indeterminate tremor.

Prognosis of essential tremor, and how to estimate it

Life expectancy is generally not affected by essential tremor, but some studies have linked essential tremor with alcoholism.

Treatment of essential tremor, and its effectiveness

Up to two-thirds of patients describe their tremor improves with alcohol, although this is not recommended as treatment. The first-line medications are propanolol and primidone, which both have trial data to support their use. Propranolol is less effective for head and voice tremor than for hand tremor. Topiramate, gabapentin, benzodiazepines, and other beta blockers have been studied and may also improve symptoms. Other anticonvulsants, botulinum toxin injection, and surgical therapies (such as deep brain stimulation) can be considered but remain controversial.

Tics

Definition of tics

Tics are sudden, often brief, involuntary movements (motor tics) or sounds (vocal tics) which occur intermittently and are often repetitive or stereotyped. Tourette's syndrome is the most common tic disorder. Lasting for at least 1 year after starting in childhood, it is characterized by a broad spectrum of motor and vocal tics as well as behavioural disorders.

Aetiology of tics

Most cases are idiopathic but a genetic basis is increasingly being recognized. The pathogenesis is uncertain but there is evidence for a neurological rather than psychogenic origin.

Typical symptoms of tics, and less common symptoms

Prior to expression, patients often describe a localized feeling of discomfort or a general urge, which settles after the tic. Simple motor tics can manifest as jerking, slow, forceful, or isometric muscle contractions. Simple vocal tics can be meaningless sounds such as coughing, sniffing, or throat clearing. Complex tics are coordinated sequenced movements or sounds, which can seem with or without purpose. Motor examples include facial grimacing, jumping, and pinching while vocal examples include parts of words or phrases repeated. They are usually voluntarily suppressible for at least a short time until the urge becomes overwhelming.

Demographics of tics

Onset of tics usually occurs in childhood, with a high male-to-female ratio. However, while the incidence is thought to be about 2%, accurate data is difficult to estimate, as perhaps up to a third of patients are unaware of their tic.

Natural history of tics, and complications of the disease

Tic disorders commonly occur transiently in childhood. Of these, up to a third will last for 2–3 years or longer. Symptoms starting in older children tend to persist longer and, in a minority, can last for life.

Other diagnoses that should be considered aside from tics

Secondary tic disorders are increasingly recognized. Drugs such as stimulants and dopaminergic or antiepileptic medication can cause or exacerbate tics. Infective, toxic, and neurodegenerative causes, amongst others, should be considered, with careful assessment for additional neurological features.

'Gold-standard' diagnostic test for tics

There are no diagnostic tests necessary for tics in the absence of additional neurological features.

Treatment of tics, and its effectiveness

Education of the condition for the patient, parents, and teachers or work colleagues is important to manage the symptoms. Counselling and behavioural therapies can achieve tolerable suppression of the tics. If daily life continues to be affected, dopamine-receptor-blocking drugs and monoamine-depleting drugs are the most effective medications, with a reduction in tic frequency of up to 80%.

Dystonia

Definition of dystonia

Dystonia is described as involuntary forceful or sustained contraction of muscles that can cause slow twisting movements, abnormal posturing, or rapid jerking movements, such as tremor.

Aetiology of dystonia

Dystonias can be primary or secondary. Primary dystonias are, by far, the most common and can be sporadic or inherited (usually in an autosomal dominant pattern).

Typical symptoms of dystonia, and less common symptoms

Dystonia can be focal, multifocal, segmental, or (rarely) generalized. Focal dystonias affect a single body part and are classified by location (e.g. cervical dystonia (spasmodic torticollis)). Task-specific dystonias are a subgroup of these, only occurring on a specific action, such as writer's cramp. Segmental dystonia affects two or more contiguous body parts. Generalized dystonia affects one or both legs, the trunk, and at least one other body part.

Stress and fatigue often worsen symptoms, while sensory tricks can relieve them (a 'geste antagoniste'). For example, touching the chin in cervical dystonia can correct the posture.

Demographics of dystonia

Symptoms of dystonia can start at any age, with no gender preference.

Approach to diagnosing dystonia

Family history and current and previous medications, as well as exposure to toxins, should all be carefully explored. Clinical assessment should focus on determining the presence of additional neurological features which could suggest a secondary cause.

Other diagnoses that should be considered aside from dystonia

Primary dystonia syndromes include dopa-responsive dystonia, myoclonic dystonia, and parkinsonian syndromes. Secondary causes include medications (including dopaminergic, antipsychotic, and anticonvulsant medications), toxins, and focal structural lesions (particularly in the basal ganglia). Inherited neurodegenerative and metabolic disorders can cause dystonia.

'Gold-standard' diagnostic test for dystonia

There are no confirmatory laboratory tests for sporadic dystonias, but genetic testing is available for certain forms of the inherited dystonias.

Other relevant investigations for dystonia

MRI of the brain and spinal cord is indicated to look for a structural lesion. Copper studies, including tests for caeruloplasmin and urinary copper, can exclude Wilson's disease. The presence of additional features would prompt investigation into specific secondary causes.

Prognosis of dystonia, and how to estimate it

Onset of limb dystonia in childhood is associated with an increased risk of developing generalized dystonia.

Treatment of dystonia, and its effectiveness

The first-line treatment for focal dystonia is botulinum toxin injected into the affected muscles. If this fails, then anticholinergics or muscle relaxants (such as baclofen or benzodiazepines) can be used as alternatives or adjuncts. For segmental and generalized dystonia, anticholinergics, tetrabenazines, and muscle relaxants can be tried. Intrathecal baclofen pump implantation, deep brain stimulation, and surgical denervation can be considered for refractory cases. For secondary dystonia, the underlying cause should be treated. Examples include removal of precipitating drugs or copper chelation in Wilson's disease.

Chorea and Huntington's disease

Definition of chorea and Huntington's disease

Chorea is defined as rapid, involuntary jerking movements which are irregular and purposeless. This is in contrast to athetosis, which is characterized by slow, writhing movements; a combination of the two is called 'choreoathetosis'. The most common cause for these movements is Huntington's disease (HD), which is a progressive, autosomal dominant genetic disorder.

Aetiology of chorea and HD

Insult to the corpus striatum (putamen, globus pallidus, and caudate) due to degeneration, structural abnormalities, or biochemical or metabolic disturbance can cause these symptoms.

Typical symptoms of HD, and less common symptoms

HD commonly causes chorea, dementia, and personality change. Imbalance, bradykinesia, dysarthria, dysphagia, dystonia, and depression may all occur as the disease progresses.

Demographics of HD

Precise figures are not known, but the figure in the UK is estimated to be 12.4 symptomatic patients per 100 000, based on figures from the Huntington Disease Association.

Natural history of HD, and complications of the disease

HD demonstrates anticipation, with each following generation which inherits the mutation likely to suffer symptoms earlier. Onset can vary but is often in the fourth or fifth decade of life.

Approach to diagnosing HD

To diagnose HD, clinical assessment with a detailed exploration of the family history is required.

Other diagnoses that should be considered aside from chorea and HD

Other causes of chorea include medications (such as dopaminergics or hormonal contraception), Sydenham's chorea (a manifestation of rheumatic fever), and chorea gravidarum (in association with pregnancy). Autoimmune conditions (such as SLE), neuroacanthocytosis, and polycythaemia vera can also be associated with chorea.

'Gold-standard' diagnostic test for HD

Genetic testing is available for the mutation which is diagnostic for HD: the expanded trinucleotide repeat in the IT15 gene, which is located on the short arm of Chromosome 4. Genetic testing should be done with appropriate counselling.

Other relevant investigations for chorea and HD

MRI of the brain can be done to look for structural damage to the basal ganglia. Other investigations, such as a blood film (to look for acanthocytes), thyroid function tests, and tests for glucose levels, copper levels (to exclude Wilson's disease), and antiphospholipid antibodies, should be guided by associated features.

Prognosis of HD, and how to estimate it

The neurological and psychiatric disability of HD is progressive, with life expectancy estimated to be limited to between 15–25 years following the onset of symptoms.

Treatment of chorea and HD and its effectiveness

A multidisciplinary approach is required for the treatment of chorea and HD, with input from neurologists, psychiatrists, and therapists. Treatment is supportive, with the focus on managing the symptoms individual to each patient. To date, there are no proven disease-modifying therapies. Tetrabenazine, haloperidol, and levetiracetam have all been used to treat chorea, with some success. Disruption of the sleep cycle can be disturbing, in which case lifestyle advice and medications (such as benzodiazepines) can be helpful.

Further Reading

Hobson P, Meara J, and Ishihara-Paul L. The estimated life expectancy in a community cohort of Parkinson's disease patients with and without dementia, compared with the UK population. *J Neurol Neurosurg Psychiatry* 2010; 81: 1093–8.

Hurwitz B. Parkinson's disease: what's in the name. *Lancet* 2017; 389: 2098–99.

Jankovic J. Treatment of hyperkinetic movement disorders. *Lancet Neurol* 2009; 8: 844–56.

National Institute for Health and Clinical Excellence. *Parkinson's Disease in Over 20s: Diagnosis and Management.* 2006. Available at https://www.nice.org.uk/Guidance/CG35 (14 Jun 2017).

Watts RL and Koller WC. *Movement Disorders: Neurologic Principles and Practice* (2nd edition), 2004. McGraw-Hill Companies.

231 Multiple sclerosis

Andrew Weir

Definition of the disease

Multiple sclerosis (MS) is an idiopathic inflammatory disorder of the CNS. The characteristic pathological feature is the occurrence of 'plaques': well-defined areas of myelin loss, with relative axonal preservation.

Aetiology of the disease

The cause of MS is not known.

Genetic factors play a role; the risk of MS is raised in relatives of patients, and varies with degree of genetic relatedness (25%–30% for monozygotic twins, 3% for siblings, and 2% for half-siblings). The most important specific genetic influences lie in the HLA region of Chromosome 6, and the Class II allele HLA-DRB1*1501 is the strongest genetic risk factor. The way the HLA region influences risk is complex and likely involves interactions between different parts of the region on both chromosomes. Genome-wide association studies have identified weaker modifiers of risk in other genes, including those for the IL2 and IL7 receptors.

Genetics, however, leaves much unaccounted for. Epidemiological patterns hint at various environmental factors. Current factors receiving research attention include vitamin D levels, and exposure to EBV.

Typical symptoms of the disease, and less common symptoms

The temporal pattern of symptoms in MS is important, and two major patterns are recognized. In a **relapse**, symptoms come on subacutely (typically over days or hours), stabilize, and then improve (rather more slowly than then they evolved), so that significant (sometimes complete) resolution occurs. In **progressive** disease, symptoms evolve over months and years (and do not recover); progression is therefore often only clear in retrospect.

MS that is causing relapses without progression is said to be 'relapsing–remitting'. MS that is progressive from onset is 'primary progressive'. When progression develops after a period of relapsing–remitting disease, MS has become 'secondary progressive'.

Typical sites for lesions causing relapse include the optic nerve, the spinal cord, and the brainstem (although many other areas may be involved and multifocal relapse also occurs). In optic neuritis, vision blurs and loses colour intensity in one eye, often with retro-orbital pain made worse by eye movement. In acute partial transverse myelitis (the 'partial' emphasizes that usually not all the cord structures at one level are affected), there may be weakness, but sensory symptoms often dominate, for example those ascending from leg to abdomen. A subjective sensory level ('like a belt hugging around my tummy'), and altered perineal sensation ('it feels odd when I wipe') are frequent complaints. Lhermitte's phenomenon (an electric shock sensation in the back or limbs on neck flexion) may occur. In brainstem relapse, typical symptoms are vertigo, diplopia, areas of facial numbness, and disequilibrium. Trigeminal neuralgia, especially in the young and if bilateral, may be the first presenting symptom.

Progressive-onset MS most often initially causes a subtle myelopathy, so patients complain of gait upset. Typical first symptoms are asymmetrical, with a leg that becomes stiff or drags after particularly long walks. Progressive cerebellar, sensory, or visual syndromes also occur.

Demographics of the disease

Across the UK, the prevalence of MS is 1–2 in 1000. Prevalence varies greatly around the world, likely due to a combination of genetic and environmental geographical effects. A latitudinal gradient has been described, with higher prevalence at greater separation from the equator. MS is commoner in women than men, and the sex ratio may be increasing towards 3F:1M. The peak age of onset lies in the late twenties/early thirties, although perhaps 5% of cases start under 16, and 5% over 50.

Natural history, and complications of the disease

MS usually runs its course over decades (early death or severe fixed disability can occur, but are rare). Eighty per cent of cases initially take a relapsing–remitting course. Secondary progression ensues in the majority but usually only after many years: after 20 years, half will be secondary progressive; 10%–20% of relapsing–remitting MS cases never become progressive.

MS can affect almost every aspect of neurological function. Typically, a patient becoming moderately disabled will have a spastic paraparesis, ataxic upper limbs, and sensory symptoms and signs. Pain may be neuropathic, although assuming this can lead one to miss other causes. Visual symptoms and signs are common. Bladder, bowel, and sexual function are frequently affected, but this may only be revealed on direct questioning. Cognitive problems are common on formal testing, and may contribute to the high rates of employment and relationship difficulties observed. Patients often rate fatigue as a major difficulty.

Approach to diagnosing the disease

The occurrence of episodes of neurological dysfunction affecting different parts of the CNS at different times ('dissemination in time and space'), with appropriate exclusion of other possibilities is the key. Paraclinical tests (MRI, and sometimes examination of CSF or evoked potential studies) provide support, but the diagnosis of MS remains clinical.

Other diagnoses that should be considered

The relevant differential varies greatly and depends on the mode of onset (relapsing or progressive) and the part of the CNS affected. For example, primary progressive MS causing a progressive myelopathy could be due to cervical spondylosis, primary lateral sclerosis, or a hereditary spastic paraparesis. Relapsing–remitting neurological syndromes can occur in the connective tissue diseases (especially SLE, Sjögren's syndrome, and the antiphospholipid syndrome), the vasculitides, and neurosarcoidosis. Neuromyelitis optica (Devic's disease) causes optic neuritis and transverse myelitis, and the brain MRI can also mimic MS.

'Gold-standard' diagnostic test

There is no gold-standard test for MS. Brain biopsy (done in rare circumstances to exclude other possibilities) can be hard to interpret, and the pathological features of MS are found in about 0.1% of routine post-mortems. Schemes to formalize the clinical diagnosis are used, especially for research purposes, but sometimes neurologists have to fall back on saying that 'multiple sclerosis is what a good clinician calls multiple sclerosis'.

Acceptable diagnostic alternatives to the gold standard

Several sets of diagnostic criteria have been proposed to help clinicians diagnose MS, for example the Schumacher criteria, the Poser criteria, and the Macdonald criteria. An innovation of the Macdonald criteria was to allow a changing MRI scan to satisfy 'dissemination in time', in some circumstances without a second clinical event. The current widely used criteria are a modification of these (Table 231.1). Future further modification seems likely.

Other relevant investigations

Other relevant investigations will be determined by the relevant differential. Imaging will rule out structural disease. Serological tests may indicate a connective tissue disorder or a metabolic cause for a myelopathy. Neuromyelitis optica is suggested by finding longitudinally extensive lesions on cord MRI (extending over more than three vertebral bodies); antibodies against aquaporin 4 are specific.

Prognosis and how to estimate it

Twenty years after onset the 'average patient' (i.e. someone with the median disability level) needs a stick to walk 100 m. The variation about this midpoint is, however, very considerable. A number of factors prognostic for the median course of groups of patients have been described (e.g. older patients tend to develop disability more quickly) but, even in combination, these do not allow accurate prediction of an individual's clinical state 5–10 years into the future.

Treatment and its effectiveness

Short courses of high-dose methylprednisolone (regimes recommended by the National Institute for Health and Care Excellence (NICE) include 500 mg orally for 5 days, or 1 g IV for 3 days) hasten recovery from relapse without changing final outcome. They are usually used therefore for relapses with significant impact on current function.

Interferon beta (as regular subcutaneous or intramuscular injections) and glatiramer acetate (as subcutaneous injections) are licensed in relapsing–remitting MS, and have been used for almost 20 years. They reduce the relapse rate by about a third. More recently, NICE have recommended three oral agents (fingolimod, dimethyl fumarate,

Table 231.1 The 2010 McDonald criteria for diagnosis of multiple sclerosis

Clinical Presentation	Additional Data Needed for MS Diagnosis
≥2 attacks[a]; objective clinical evidence of ≥2 lesions or objective clinical evidence of 1 lesion with reasonable historical evidence of a prior attack[b]	None[c]
≥2 attacks[a]; objective clinical evidence of 1 lesion	Dissemination in space, demonstrated by: ≥1 T2 lesion in at least 2 of 4 MS-typical regions of the CNS (periventricular, juxtacortical, infratentorial, or spinal cord)[d]; or Await a further clinical attack[a] implicating a different CNS site
1 attack[a]; objective clinical evidence of ≥2 lesions	Dissemination in time, demonstrated by: Simultaneous presence of asymptomatic gadolinium-enhancing and nonenhancing lesions at any time; or A new T2 and/or gadolinium-enhancing lesion(s) on follow-up MRI, irrespective of its timing with reference to a baseline scan; or Await a second clinical attack[a]
1 attack[a]; objective clinical evidence of 1 lesion (clinically isolated syndrome)	Dissemination in space and time, demonstrated by: For DIS: ≥1 T2 lesion in at least 2 of 4 MS-typical regions of the CNS (periventricular, juxtacortical, infratentorial, or spinal cord)[d]; or Await a second clinical attack[a] implicating a different CNS site; and For DIT: Simultaneous presence of asymptomatic gadolinium-enhancing and nonenhancing lesions at any time; or A new T2 and/or gadolinium-enhancing lesion(s) on follow-up MRI, irrespective of its timing with reference to a baseline scan; or Await a second clinical attack[a]
Insidious neurological progression suggestive of MS (PPMS)	1 year of disease progression (retrospectively or prospectively determined) plus 2 of 3 of the following criteria[d]: 1. Evidence for DIS in the brain based on ≥1 T2 lesions in the MS-characteristic (periventricular, juxtacortical, or infratentorial) regions 2. Evidence for DIS in the spinal cord based on ≥2 T2 lesions in the cord 3. Positive CSF (isoelectric focusing evidence of oligoclonal bands and/or elevated IgG index)

If the Criteria are fulfilled and there is no better explanation for the clinical presentation, the diagnosis is 'MS'; if suspicious, but the Criteria are not completely met, the diagnosis is 'possible MS'; if another diagnosis arises during the evaluation that better explains the clinical presentation, then the diagnosis is 'not MS'.

[a] An attack (relapse; exacerbation) is defined as patient-reported or objectively observed events typical of an acute inflammatory demyelinating event in the CNS, current or historical, with duration of at least 24 hours, in the absence of fever or infection. It should be documented by contemporaneous neurological examination, but some historical events with symptoms and evolution characteristic for MS, but for which no objective neurological findings are documented, can provide reasonable evidence of a prior demyelinating event. Reports of paroxysmal symptoms (historical or current) should, however, consist of multiple episodes occurring over not less than 24 hours. Before a definite diagnosis of MS can be made, at least 1 attack must be corroborated by findings on neurological examination, visual evoked potential response in patients reporting prior visual disturbance, or MRI consistent with demyelination in the area of the CNS implicated in the historical report of neurological symptoms.

[b] Clinical diagnosis based on objective clinical findings for 2 attacks is most secure. Reasonable historical evidence for 1 past attack, in the absence of documented objective neurological findings, can include historical events with symptoms and evolution characteristics for a prior inflammatory demyelinating event; at least 1 attack, however, must be supported by objective findings.

[c] No additional tests are required. However, it is desirable that any diagnosis of MS be made with access to imaging based on these Criteria. If imaging or other tests (for instance, CSF) are undertaken and are negative, extreme caution needs to be taken before making a diagnosis of MS, and alternative diagnoses must be considered. There must be no better explanation for the clinical presentation, and objective evidence must be present to support a diagnosis of MS.

[d] Gadolinium-enhancing lesions are not required; symptomatic lesions are excluded from consideration in subjects with brainstem or spinal cord syndromes.

MS—multiple sclerosis; CNS—central nervous system; MRI—magnetic resonance imaging; DIS—dissemination in space; DIT—dissemination in time; PPMS—primary progressive multiple sclerosis; CSF—cerebrospinal fluid; IgG—immunoglobulin G.

Reproduced with permission from Polman et al., Diagnostic criteria for multiple sclerosis: 2010 Revisions to the McDonald criteria, *Annals of Neurology*, Volume 69, Issue 2, pp. 292-302, Copyright © 2011 John Wiley and Sons.

CHAPTER 231 **Multiple sclerosis**

and teriflunomide) which reduce the relapse rate by about a half, and two monoclonal antibodies (natalizumab and alemtuzumab) which reduce it by about two-thirds, for subgroups of people with relapsing–remitting MS. Some of these agents are associated with a small risk of serious side effects, both infectious (including progressive multifocal leucoencephalopathy) and secondary autoimmune disorders. The effects of these agents on the risk of fixed disability in the long term (or the risk of transition to secondary progressive disease) are hard to confidently measure in trials lasting only a few years; the balance of risk and benefit, and cost-effectiveness, therefore, has been controversial. There are currently no agents that have been definitely shown to change the rate at which disability develops in primary or secondary MS.

Further Reading

Frohman EM, Racke MK, and Raine CS. Multiple sclerosis: The plaque and its pathogenesis. *N Engl J Med* 2006; 354: 942–55.
Ransohoff RM, Hafler DA, and Lucchinetti CF. Multiple sclerosis: A quiet revolution. *Nat Rev Neurol* 2015; 11: 134–42.

232 Motor neuron disease

Martin R. Turner

Definition of the disease

Motor neuron disease (MND) is characterized by progressive muscular weakness due to simultaneous degeneration of lower and upper motor neurons (L/UMNs). Involvement of LMNs, arising from the anterior horns of the spinal cord and brainstem, leads to secondary wasting as a result of muscle denervation. Involvement of the UMNs of the motor cortex and corticospinal tract results in hyperreflexia, sometimes with spasticity. In ~85% of cases, there is clinical involvement of both, and the condition is termed 'amyotrophic lateral sclerosis' (ALS; a term often used synonymously with MND). In ~13% of cases, there may be only LMN signs apparent, in which case the condition is termed 'progressive muscular atrophy', although such cases have a natural history similar to that for ALS. In a very small group of patients (~2%), there are only UMN signs for at least the first 4 years, in which case the condition is termed 'primary lateral sclerosis' (PLS); such cases have a uniformly slower progression. There is clinical, neuropathological, and genetic overlap between MND and some forms of frontotemporal dementia (FTD).

Aetiology of the disease

The causes of MND (which is a syndrome rather than one disease) are not clear, but in nearly all cases there are abnormal cytoplasmic inclusions of a protein TDP-43 in brain and spinal cord cells. Epidemiological studies have excluded a range of environmental insults as independent causes. It is possible that a complex genetic profile renders an individual at risk of MND, with as yet unidentified triggers. Approximately 5% of cases report a family history. Of these, up to 40% are associated with an intronic hexanucleotide expansion in C9ORF72, whose phenotype can be 'pure' FTD as well as ALS-predominant. A further 20% are found to have mutations of the gene SOD1 encoding superoxide dismutase-1, which is involved in the processing of free radicals. A smaller proportion (~5%) have mutations of the TARDBP and FUS genes, which encode proteins involved in RNA regulation.

Typical symptoms of the disease, and less common symptoms

The onset of MND is insidious, and the lack of a specific test results in a mean delay in diagnosis of 12 months. Those with an aggressive disease course tend to be diagnosed earlier.

The site of initial symptoms is approximately equally divided amongst the lower limb territory, the upper limb territory, and the 'bulbar' territory of the brainstem (cranial nerves IX, X, and XII). Limb onset is typically asymmetric prior to spread, which is usually to contiguous body regions. Tripping up, dragging the leg, weak shoulder abduction, and poor grip are all common early symptoms, and without prominent sensory involvement. Fasciculations, although characteristically florid in MND often go unnoticed by the patient.

Those with bulbar onset report dysarthria preceding dysphagia, and may be mis-referred to ENT or TIA clinic. Rarely, there may be a period of some months in which a patient who becomes rapidly anarthric remains ambulant with good limb function (historically referred to as 'progressive bulbar palsy').

In <3% cases, the presenting symptom may be respiratory, with orthopnoea due to diaphragm weakness. This may present as an emergency in the context of a secondary pneumonia.

Frank dementia affects up to 15% of MND cases (typically before the onset of motor symptoms). Milder cognitive deficits (particularly verbal fluency) may be detectable in up to 50%.

Demographics of the disease

MND has a global incidence of 1–2 in 100 000 per year, and a UK prevalence of ~5000. There is a slight male predominance, but more females amongst bulbar-onset patients.

The mean age of onset is the early sixties, and the majority of cases present in the sixth and seventh decades, but with rare cases seen as young as the teens. The perception of relative athleticism premorbidly in MND patients is unproven.

Natural history, and complications of the disease

Limb weakness leads to increasing dependency for activities of daily living. Loss of ambulation may be preceded by falls, and those with upper limb weakness are at high risk of head injury.

Bulbar involvement occurs in at least two-thirds of patients, with dysarthria limiting verbal communication, and dysphagia leading to poor nutritional intake and risk of aspiration. Choking is, however, exceptional as a mode of death. Sialorrhoea results from reduced swallowing frequency and can be treated with anti-cholinergic medication. While emotionality is common in MND (due to corticobulbar neuronal involvement), depression is rare. Progressive diaphragm weakness results in increasing dyspnoea with orthopnoea. Chronic nocturnal hypoventilation with hypercapnoea may cause sleep fragmentation, early morning headache, and daytime somnolence.

Death in MND typically occurs as a result of respiratory failure, often in the context of superimposed bronchopneumonia. Sudden death occurs in a small proportion of cases (<5%), some of whom may have occult pulmonary embolism.

Eye movements and bladder and bowel sphincters are generally spared in the course of MND, although oculomotor function may be impaired in the very late stages.

Approach to diagnosing the disease

The grave implication of a diagnosis of MND means it should not be suggested where there is significant doubt. Equally, however, fear of missing a treatable but implausible mimic leads to unnecessary delay in initiating community support, with loss of precious quality of life for those facing a life-shortening illness. A formal neurological opinion should therefore be sought as soon as possible in suspected cases.

MND should be considered in someone with a history of *progressive* muscle weakness over weeks or months without prominent sensory symptoms, particularly where there is wasting (which frequently involves the first dorsal interosseous) or dysarthria (especially with tongue wasting) and in the context of pathologically brisk reflexes in the same body territory. If signs are entirely confined to a single limb, then other causes are more likely.

Supportive examination features are the observation of florid fasciculations (commonly missed over the anterior shoulders and quadriceps if the patient is not undressed) and reduced vital capacity. Neck flexion weakness, emotionality, or primitive facial reflexes, are useful signs that limit the differential diagnosis considerably.

Other diagnoses that should be considered

There are few mimics of MND in its typical mixed UMN and LMN form, and particularly when there is clear bulbar involvement. Myasthenia gravis is usually possible to distinguish on clinical grounds, invariably due to ocular involvement in the context of bulbar symptoms.

Cervical spondylotic myeloradiculopathy may produce a syndrome of progressive limb weakness with relative sparing of sensory and sphincter functions, and mixed UMN and LMN signs. It should be considered in those with symptoms confined to the limbs, and excluded if necessary with MRI, bearing in mind that many patients in the age group for MND will have coincident cervical spine disease.

The rare autoimmune multifocal motor neuropathy may be considered in pure LMN presentations, especially involving finger extensors, and requires careful neurophysiological assessment to detect the characteristic (sometimes elusive) conduction block. Post-radiation lumbar radiculopathy may produce a syndrome similar to lower limb onset MND, with presentation occasionally delayed by decades. Inclusion body myositis is very rare and usually suggested by the predominant quadriceps or medial forearm involvement. HIV infection has been rarely associated with a motor neuropathy.

Progressive pure UMN syndromes need exclusion of a structural or inflammatory cause within the cord and brain, as well as exclusion of vitamin B_{12} and copper deficiencies. Primary progressive forms of multiple sclerosis occasionally mimic PLS.

The concept of 'paraneoplastic MND' is overstated and controversial as a distinct entity.

'Gold-standard' diagnostic test

The gold-standard diagnostic test for MND is post-mortem demonstration of characteristic motor neuronal cytoplasmic protein inclusions.

Acceptable diagnostic alternatives to the gold standard

An acceptable diagnostic alternative to the gold-standard test for MND is clinical examination by a neurologist, ideally one specializing in MND.

Other relevant investigations

Electromyography should not be considered a 'test for MND' but provides supportive evidence of LMN involvement in non-wasted muscles. It can be normal in isolated bulbar-onset MND.

Serum creatinine kinase level is neither sensitive nor specific but frequently mildly raised, reflecting muscle denervation. Values >2000 should prompt diagnostic re-evaluation.

Lumbar puncture and muscle biopsy are rarely indicated.

The lack of knowledge of the genes implicated in 30% of familial cases, the unreliability of a negative family history and the variable penetrance of those genes that are known, mean that genetic testing in established MND requires careful counselling.

Prognosis and how to estimate it

The median survival in MND is 3 years from the onset of symptoms. This tends to be shorter in patients with bulbar onset and those with associated FTD, and longer in those aged <40 at onset. In aggressive cases, survival can be as little as 6 months from diagnosis, but there is a marked variability in prognosis, with a small but consistent proportion of patients (10%) surviving more than 10 years from symptom onset. PLS patients characteristically survive for 10–20 years. The pace of deterioration in MND is generally fixed throughout the course of the disease, and no sustained 'plateau' should be expected.

Treatment and its effectiveness

The most useful intervention is early referral to a tertiary MND clinic, which can coordinate community-based palliative care (details via the Motor Neurone Disease Association UK; see http://www.mndassociation.org), which has been shown to improve survival as well as quality of life.

Riluzole is the only UK licensed disease-modifying drug for the treatment of MND (in its ALS form), at a dose of 50 mg twice daily. Thought to have broadly anti-glutamatergic properties, clinical trials suggests a <10% increase in overall survival, but this cannot be quantified for an individual, and neither will they experience improvement subjectively. The drug is usually well tolerated, but ~10% of patients may experience unacceptable lethargy or nausea. A full blood count and liver function tests are required at baseline and monthly for the first 3 months, 3-monthly for the first year, and annually thereafter. Significant rises in alanine transferase levels require initial dose reduction and withdrawal, if persistent.

Gastrostomy (typically percutaneous endoscopic gastrostomy) can improve the quality of life for patients with significant dysphagia. The device should ideally be inserted before the development of significant respiratory weakness (forced vital capacity >50%) in a centre with experience of this patient group.

Non-invasive ventilation is a valuable intervention for the effective relief of symptoms associated with hypercapnoea, and has an additional survival benefit. It requires close liaison with an experienced respiratory team, and those with prominent bulbar involvement may find it harder to use effectively. Invasive ventilation (tracheostomy) is rarely requested. Any perceived benefits are often unrealistic and do not take into account the inevitable total physical dependency, being 'locked in', or the possibility of dementia later in the course of the disease.

Further Reading

Burrell JR, Halliday GM, Kril JJ, et al. The frontotemporal dementia-motor neuron disease continuum. *Lancet* 2016; 388: 919–31.

Kiernan MC, Vucic S, Cheah BC, et al. Amyotrophic lateral sclerosis. *Lancet* 2011; 377: 942–55.

Talbot K, Turner M, Marsden R, and Botell RE. *Motor Neuron Disease: A Practical Manual*, 2009. Oxford University Press.

van Es MA, Hardiman O, Chio A et al. Amyotrophic lateral sclerosis. *Lancet* 2017; 390: 2084–98.

233 Spinal cord disease

Stephan Hinze and Paul Davies

Definition and aetiology of the disease

Injury to the spinal cord (myelopathy) can be due to many causes (see Table 233.1).

Typical symptoms of the disease, and less common symptoms

Symptoms will depend on the localization and extent of spinal cord damage and the nature of the pathology. Rapid damage, as in stroke or rapid inflammation, will cause spinal shock (flaccid paralysis and hypo/areflexia), which looks very different from the spasticity seen when there is slow onset of damage to the same area. Pathology progressing at intermediate rates (e.g. demyelination) often produces spreading numbness or weakness of appropriate anatomical distribution to the expanding lesion. Depending on the site of the lesion, the legs and arms can be affected to varying degrees, but strictly unilateral symptoms are uncommon. Weakness can affect both legs (paraparesis) or all four limbs (quadriparesis).

There are a number of classic patterns of symptoms due to the location of spinal cord damage (e.g. syringomyelia damages central crossing spinothalamic neurons and anterior horn cells in particular to produce a dissociated sensory loss and lower motor neuron signs; patients in this case might present with a history of burns and cuts to their hands and arms).

Table 233.1	Causes of myelopathy
Compression	Disc prolapse
	Cervical and lumbar spondylosis
	Rheumatoid disease
	Tumour
	Epidural abscess or haematoma
Inflammation	Inflammatory demyelinating diseases:
	• multiple sclerosis
	• neuromyelitis optica
	• idiopathic inflammatory demyelinating diseases
	Autoimmune conditions:
	• SLE
	• Sjögren's syndrome
	• systemic sclerosis
	Infections:
	• viral (e.g. HSV, VZV, CMV, Coxsackie virus (A and B))
	• bacterial (e.g. TB, mycoplasma)
	• parasitic (e.g. Lyme disease (borreliosis))
Metabolic causes	Vitamin B_{12} deficiency (subacute combined degeneration)
	Copper deficiency
	Vitamin E deficiency
Blood flow problems	Stroke (arterial and venous)
	Arteriovenous malformation
	Dural arteriovenous fistula
Degenerative causes	Motor neuron disease
Genetic causes	Familial/hereditary spastic paraparesis

Abbreviations: CMV, cytomegalovirus; HSV, herpes simplex virus; SLE, systemic lupus erythematosus; VZV, varicella zoster virus.

Patients with spinal cord problems often present with gait disturbance and imbalance. As a result of spasticity, they might report stiffness and jerking of their legs or loss of dexterity in their hands, although strength may be good or normal.

Autonomic symptoms can occur. Bladder symptoms are particularly important to recognize, as delayed treatment of cord compression may lead to permanent incontinence. Bowel symptoms and erectile dysfunction can be present as well. More infrequently, respiratory weakness can occur or paroxysms of hypertension and sweating.

Pain is often a prominent feature in degenerative and other compressive pathologies (e.g. spondylosis, disc prolapse, spinal metastasis, or epidural abscess) but can also occur with non-compressive etiologies like transverse myelitis, where it is especially located in the interscapular region.

The pathology may affect other parts of the nervous system (e.g. spinal cord) and there may be additional peripheral neuropathy, as in subacute combined degeneration of the cord, or an additional optic neuritis, as in neuromyelitis optica. There may also be systemic features, as in vasculitis.

Neurogenic claudication is often reported in lumbar spinal canal stenosis. It presents with cramping lumbar pain radiating to the legs; the pain occurs during walking and improves following flexion of the spine, for example when cycling. It does not improve, however, while standing (in contrast to vascular claudication). The patients often describe a feeling of heavy legs.

In the rare event of subarachnoid haemorrhage (SAH) of the spinal cord, patients can present with typical symptoms of cranial SAH (occipital headache, meningism, photophobia). Spinal cord tumours can occasionally produce papilloedema.

Although not in the scope of this chapter, there may be additional diseases below the level of L1 (the lower limit of the spinal cord), like cauda equina damage.

Demographics of the disease

Degenerative compressive causes are the most common spinal cord problems. They mainly occur in the older population (cervical spondylotic myelopathy, for example, especially in 40–60 year olds) with a predominance of men over woman (3:2). Symptomatic disc herniation affects 1500 per million in the US. Lumbar stenosis occurs in up to 50 per million. Degenerative changes on imaging of the cervical spine can be seen in over 50% of subjects older than 40, and in up to 89% of subjects over the age of 60. Asymptomatic cord compression can be seen in 7.5% of such patients. Cauda equine syndrome is fortunately relatively rare, occurring in only around 0.12% of all symptomatic disc herniations.

Also relatively common is spinal cord injury secondary to trauma; this mainly affects 20–40 year olds. The prevalence is estimated at 10–83 per million, and up to 1 in 40 of the patients admitted to trauma centres have spinal cord injury. The cervical cord is the most commonly affected region (in 55% of all cases).

Less common, but still relatively frequent, is acute transverse myelitis, with an incidence of 1–8 (or 24, if cases due to multiple sclerosis are included) new cases per million per year. It affects younger patients, with bimodal peaks at 10–19 and 30–39 years. There is no gender, family, or ethnic difference for the group as a whole.

The incidence of subacute combined degeneration (e.g. due to vitamin B_{12} deficiency (sometimes mimicked by copper deficiency)) has not been exactly established. Depending on the cut-off values, up to around 20% of people, especially white older woman, can be deficient in vitamin B_{12}. Not all develop neurological symptoms (74%

developed neurological symptoms, in one study which included all possible neurological symptoms).

Syringomyelia has an estimated prevalence of around 0.8 per million. It predominantly affects males in their third and fourth decade in life. It mainly occurs in conjunction with Chiari malformations, but also accompanies 25%–60% of all intramedullary tumours.

A similar prevalence has hereditary spastic paraparesis with up to around 1 per million. The mechanism is primarily autosomal dominant, but can also be X-linked recessive.

Natural history and complications of the disease

The main complications depend on the location and extend of the lesion. Motor and sensory function of the lower and/or upper limbs can be affected to varying degrees, the greatest concern being quadriplegia with higher cervical lesions. Care should be taken with regards to autonomic dysfunction involving loss of bowel function, urinary retention, and incontinence, as well as the potential, but fortunately rare, problems with lability of blood pressure and respiratory function. Severe damage causing paraplegia or quadriplegia, may lead to pressure sores, urinary infections, septicaemia, deep vein thrombosis, and pulmonary emboli.

Treatable diseases

Acute transverse myelitis reaches its maximum severity over 4 hours to 3 weeks, whereas vascular causes like stroke or acute compressive causes (e.g. disc prolapse) have a more rapid onset. Compressive degenerative myelopathy (cervical spondylotic myelopathy, lumbar spinal stenosis) tends to have a longer time course lasting over months to years.

Inflammatory/ infectious myelopathies are usually monophasic, with roughly one-third of cases recovering completely, one-third continuing to have residual symptoms, and the last third showing no great improvement at all. Neuromyelitis optica (NMO) in this group has to be highlighted in view of the often recurrent nature of myelitis or optic neuritis requiring early commencement of long-term immunosuppression.

Cervical spondylotic myelopathy tends to ultimately progress in an either gradual or stepwise progression in the majority of cases. But, initially, it can have a stable appearance for a few years, and a minority of patients might also improve.

Lumbar spinal stenosis, in contrast, has a more benign course, with an initially slow progression that reaches a plateau in the majority of cases with conservative management alone.

Subacute combined degeneration (vitamin B_{12} deficiency) often progresses over months to years to an ataxic paraplegia if untreated.

Palliative

Hereditary processes (e.g. familial spastic paraparesis) are often slowly progressive with an onset of symptoms frequently between the second and of forth decade of live. These patients often don't have a lower life expectancy.

In contrast, motor neuron disease frequently leads to death within a few years' time.

Approach to diagnosing the disease

Is it the spinal cord?

Localizing the pathology to the cord is an obvious but sometimes challenging clinical step in reaching a diagnosis. The presence of upper motor neuron signs (increased tone, sustained or asymmetric ankle clonus, hyperreflexia, and extensor plantar responses) and the presence of a sensory-level point towards a spinal cord problem. But, in the acute phase of a spinal shock, immediately after a stroke, for example, the reverse with presence of flaccid paralysis might be the case.

Ruling out other possible causes (e.g. a cauda equina syndrome (no upper motor neuron signs) or a brainstem cause (maybe only a brisk jaw jerk gives the game away)) might be one step. Just weakness of the legs (particularly proximal and symmetrical weakness)

with no sensory symptoms or signs might lead to a consideration of muscle disease (relatively rare) and, if there is variable weakness that becomes worse as the legs are used, consider myasthenia.

Where in the spinal cord?

If the legs are affected, but not the arms, a sensory level may locate the cord lesion. If all four limbs are affected and a cervical cord lesion is considered, the sensory level is often less helpful at precise localization, because the dermatomes C4 and T4 on the chest are close together. Sometimes an absent reflex locates the site (e.g. spastic legs and no biceps jerk suggests a disc at C5 (Table 233.2)). Consider diaphragmatic function in mid-cervical cord lesions.

Compression or not?

An early important question to answer is whether the underlying pathology is of acute compressive nature, since this will direct further management towards a possible urgent surgical referral. Imaging will often provide the answer. In order to determine which part of the spinal cord to image, the sensory level is an important tool. In cases of isolated leg involvement, it might not be sufficient to image the lumbar–sacral spine, since the underlying lesion could be in the thoracic region and thus one which a sensory-level examination might pick up.

Sudden onset of pain in the cervical or lumbar region, possibly with radiation along a specific nerve root and neurological deficits hint towards a compressive lesion (often prolapsed discs).

An asymmetric flaccid paresis of the lower limbs with reduced reflexes in the context of perianal/ saddle anaesthesia should raise the question of cauda equina syndrome, which often is caused by prolapsed discs but can also occur secondary to tumour, infection, stenosis, and hematoma. In suspected cases, the anal tone should be assessed.

Conus medullaris lesions, unlike cauda equina lesions, present with earlier sphincter dysfunction in context of sacral sensory loss with relatively milder motor disturbance. Here, the pathology is often inflammatory in nature.

What type of non-compressive pathology?

In non-compressive lesions, the clinical examination and history can guide towards the diagnosis.

Incomplete/partial lesions, like a hemicord syndrome (Brown–Séquard syndrome) make a final diagnosis of multiple sclerosis more likely. Brown–Séquard syndrome presents with ipsilateral pyramidal weakness and posterior column function loss (light touch, vibration, joint position) with contralateral loss of pain and temperature (crossed spinothalamic tract). In suspected multiple sclerosis, previous demyelinating events might be elicited in the history, and the MRI usually shows small (< 2 vertebral segments) and more peripheral (asymmetric) lesions. CSF examination in these cases shows unmatched oligoclonal bands (not present in a concurrent serum sample).

Table 233.2 Helpful pointers in determining the level of spinal cord involvement

Nerve root	Helpful clinical pointers in determining the level of spinal cord involvement
C5	Biceps jerk
C6	Brachioradialis jerk
C7	Triceps jerk
C8/T1	Finger jerk/Hoffmann's
T4/5	Nipple level
T10	Umbilical level
L1	Inguinal area
L2/3	Hip adductor jerk
L4	Knee jerk
L5	Hallux dorsiflexion
S1	Ankle jerk

With long lesions (>3 segments, central), neuromyelitis optica should be considered, and evidence of (past) optic neuritis should be sought, as well as further investigations with NMO antibodies thought of. In neuromyelitis optica, CSF does not show oligoclonal bands, but prominent pleocytosis instead.

Systemic markers of infection, confusion, meningism, or a rash should raise the suspicion of an infectious myelopathy. This should also be suspected in any immunocompromised patient. In infectious causes, the myelopathy is often complete, causing symmetric motor and sensory deficits with urinary dysfunction. It is important in these instances to think of CMV infections, even in immunocompetent patients.

What makes a vascular cause likely?

If clinical signs of **acute** bilateral flaccid weakness, loss of pain and temperature and sphincter function in the context of preserved dorsal column modalities (vibration, joint position) are found (anterior cord syndrome), a vascular cause should be considered, since the anterior spinal cord is supplied by a single anterior spinal artery (compared to two posterior arteries). An occlusion can occur in the context of aortic surgery or spinal angiography, but can also come from an embolic source. If an anterior cord syndrome occurs in the context of back pain and a history of physical exertion (often repeatedly), a diagnosis of fibrocartilaginous disc embolism might be present. Imaging evidence of reduced vertebral height in the area further aids this diagnosis. Sudden onset (recurrent) myelopathic symptoms during exercise or upright posture/walking are more commonly caused by an arteriovenous fistula, however. Formal angiography is often required for the diagnosis in these cases.

Other selective losses

A selective loss of posterior column function leading to unsteady gait (sensory ataxia) should raise the suspicion of vitamin B_{12} or copper deficiency (e.g. following bariatric surgery). If the level of vitamin B_{12} is in the lower range of normal, homocysteine and methylmalonic acid, both precursors for vitamin B_{12}-dependent chemical reactions, should be measured. Elevated levels would indicate vitamin B_{12} deficiency in this setting.

The presence of dissociated sensory loss and lower motor neuron signs should raise the suspicion of syringomyelia, a spinal cord cavity that can cause damage to the centrally crossing spinothalamic neurons and anterior horn cells of the affected levels.

Other diagnoses that should be considered

Brain causes

Paraplegia can sometimes be caused by a parasagittal meningioma, bilateral cerebral disease (commonly vascular or demyelinating), or brainstem lesions. If no cause can be found on investigation of the spine, brain imaging should be considered.

Muscle and neuromuscular junction causes

Just weakness of the legs (particularly proximal and symmetrical) with no sensory symptoms or signs might lead to a consideration of muscle disease (relatively rare) and, if there is variable weakness which is worse as the legs are used, consider myasthenia. If a myasthenic syndrome is considered, pay particular attention to the deep tendon reflexes, which are normal in myasthenia gravis but depressed yet augment on isometric contraction in Lambert–Eaton myasthenic syndrome.

Further hereditary conditions

Other genetic causes like the X-linked recessive condition of adrenoleukodystrophy (adrenomyeloneuropathy) can cause a progressive spastic paraparesis in association with adrenal insufficiency and possible peripheral neuropathy (decreased reflexes). Very long chain fatty acids will provide the diagnosis.

Musculoskeletal

If bilateral leg weakness in association with hip pain is present, the cause might also be found in the skeletal structures, like severe bilateral osteoarthritis of the hip.

'Gold-standard' diagnostic test

Ideally, an MRI with gadolinium of the clinically suspected area of the spinal cord should be undertaken. Sometimes imaging of the entire spinal cord is needed. A lumbar puncture can help further if no compressive cause can be elicited. Often, however, in practice, a plain MRI is undertaken in first instance. An MRI will not only show whether there is reduction in CSF space around a specific area of the spinal cord, suggesting a compressive problem, but it can also demonstrate myelopathic changes (high signal intensity on T2-weighted imaging). In non-compressive lesions, gadolinium enhancement would indicate an inflammatory cause, but can also be seen in neoplastic lesions. The absence of gadolinium enhancement together with an absence of pleocytosis or oligoclonal bands on CSF examination should lead to consideration of non-inflammatory causes like ischaemia or postradiation myelopathy, or rarer occurrences like fibrocartilaginous embolism.

Acceptable diagnostic alternatives to the gold standard

In situations where MRI imaging is not available or contraindicated or where the patient, due to pain or claustrophobia, is not able to lie still for the approximately 10 minutes required to perform the imaging, CT myelography provides an alternative. In contrast to plain CT imaging, which cannot visualize the spinal cord or nerve roots due to their similar densities compared to CSF, CT myelography allows evaluation of cord or nerve root compression by intrathecal administration of iodine. However, this benefit comes with risks of an allergic reaction to the contrast material, as well as potential complications of lumbar punctures like low pressure headache, aseptic meningitis, spinal hematoma, and arachnoiditis (inflammation of the arachnoid membrane that can lead to scarring and adhesions of spinal nerves with subsequent pain and focal neurological symptoms). CT myelography is useful in determining a compressive cause but, due to its inability to assess the spinal cord itself, it does not play a role in the differential diagnosis of non-compressive myelopathy. For surgical cases, however, it has an advantage over MRI in visualizing the bony anatomy more accurately.

Other relevant investigations

If initial investigations point towards an inflammatory origin, further MRI imaging of the brain might be indicated to determine whether the process is multifocal (e.g. multiple sclerosis, or acute disseminated encephalomyelopathy). Visual evoked potentials might also be useful in order to evaluate optic nerve involvement (neuromyelitis optica, multiple sclerosis).

If an infection is suspected, or generally in immunocompromised patients, HIV status, spinal fluid viral PCR, and VDRL (Venereal Disease Research Laboratory, syphilis), as well as bacterial and possibly fungal CSF cultures should be considered, in addition to TB screening and HTLV-1 serology.

If there are further clinical features of autoimmune problems, an autoimmune antibody screen (antinuclear antibodies, complement levels, double-stranded DNA, SS-A, SS-B, ACE, anticardiolipin, lupus anticoagulant) should be considered.

Vitamin B_{12}, methylmalonic acid, homocysteine, copper, and vitamin E levels might be indicated.

If the MRI shows a vascular anomaly (e.g. an arteriovenous dural fistula), then selective formal angiography can lead to diagnostic certainty and embolization treatment.

Prognosis, and how to estimate it

The prognosis for the individual patient is often difficult to determine.

Curable

Subacute combined degeneration of the cord (vitamin B_{12} deficiency) stops progressing, if treated. The prognosis is better in the absence of a sensory level and extensor plantar response, as well as with younger age and shorter duration. Cord atrophy and extended cord involvement (>7 segments) on imaging carry a poorer neurological prognosis.

Treatable: Medical

Acute transverse myelitis seems to have a better prognosis if the patient is younger, the onset of symptoms was slower (over days to weeks), recovery started earlier, and posterior column function (vibration, joint position sense), and deep tendon reflexes are spared. An acute onset of severe symptoms without recovery after 3 months, as well as the presence of incontinence and a cervical sensory level, seem to have a poorer prognosis. In addition, a positive CSF protein 14-3-3 (also found in CJD) has been associated with a poor prognosis.

The majority of idiopathic acute transverse myelitis and infectious or para-infectious myelitis run a monophasic course.

Neuromyelitis optica (NMO antibody positive with long spinal cord lesions, extending over three or more vertebral levels, and complete transverse myelitis, e.g. symmetrical motor and sensory deficits) tends to have a high risk (50%) of recurrence.

Further lesions on brain imaging and the presence of incomplete transverse myelitis (e.g. asymmetric incomplete loss of tracts) places patients at higher risk of being diagnosed with multiple sclerosis later on (88% within 20 years in the case of two or more typical multiple sclerosis brain lesions).

Treatable: Surgical

Cervical spondylotic myelopathy seems to ultimately progress in the majority of cases, whereas lumbar spinal stenosis seems to stabilize in the majority.

The prognosis of syringomyelia depends on the underlying cause (e.g. secondary to tumour vs secondary to trauma), as well as the degree of neurological deficit. The worse the deficit, the worse is the prognosis.

Palliative

Familial spastic paraparesis tends to slowly progress without affecting overall life expectancy. In contrast, motor neuron disease tends to lead to death within a few years.

Treatment and its effectiveness

Specific

Medical

No randomized controlled trials have been undertaken with regards to treatment in acute transverse myelitis (Table 233.3). High-dose IV steroids (methylprednisolone 1 g/day for 3–5 days) are usually given early in the disease course. Overall, 60%–70% of cases will improve completely or partially in the end.

In neuromyelitis optica, subsequent treatment with long-term immunosuppression, especially azathioprine, alone or with prednisolone, reduces the relapse frequency.

Subacute combined degeneration of the cord (vitamin B_{12} deficiency) tends to respond well to cobalamin injections, but neurological improvement can take up to 6–12 months.

Table 233.3 Symptomatic pharmacological treatment options

Spasticity	Diazepam: 2 mg twice daily to max 60 mg daily
	Baclofen: 5 mg twice daily to 40 mg three times per day
	Dantrolene: 25 mg twice daily to 100 mg four times per day
	Tizanidine: 2 mg daily to 8 mg three times per day
Neuropathic pain	Amitriptyline: 10–20 mg to 75 mg daily
	Nortriptyline: 10–20 mg to 75 mg daily
	Gabapentin: 300 mg daily to 1200 mg three times per day
	Pregabalin: 75 mg twice daily to 200 mg three times per day
To facilitate bladder emptying	Prazosin: 1 mg twice daily to 2 mg three times per day
	Tamsulosin: 0.4 mg daily
Urge incontinence/ frequency	Oxybutynin: 2.5 mg daily to 5 mg four times per day
	Tolterodine: 2 mg daily
	Imipramine: 25 mg to 75 mg daily

Surgical

A recent Cochrane review on the treatment of cervical spondylotic myelopathy did not provide reliable evidence with regards to long-term effects for surgical intervention over conservative management. But, especially in progressive markedly symptomatic cases, a neurosurgical referral is indicated.

Lumbar spinal stenosis due to its degenerative character is unlikely to be cured by surgery, and symptoms often tend to plateau. In cases of paresis or cauda equina syndrome, surgical intervention is indicated, however.

For cauda equina syndrome, early surgical intervention within 24 hours seems to provide a better outcome, at least for incomplete syndromes without urinary retention.

There are a number of surgical interventions available for syringomyelia, ranging from suboccipital/cervical decompression over cervical laminectomy to shunting procedures. Outcome depends on the underlying cause for the syrinx.

Non-specific

The most common non-specific problems will be that of spasticity, bladder problems, and neuropathic pain. General measures like physiotherapy are important with regards to spasticity, in addition to pharmacological treatment (Table 233.3). If spasticity is localized, then focal botulinum toxin injections might be of benefit. In case of ongoing bladder problems, intermittent self catheterization or a permanent urinary/suprapubic catheter might be needed. Neuropathic pain can be difficult to control.

Further Reading

Siebert E. et al. Lumbar spinal stenosis: Syndrome, diagnostics and treatment. *Nat Rev Neurol* 2009; 5: 392–403.

Jacob A and Weinshenker BG. An approach to the diagnosis of acute transverse myelitis. *Sem Neurology* 2008; 1:105–20.

Tracy JA and Bartleson JD. Cervical spondylotic myelopathy. *Neurologist* 2010; 10: 176–87.

234 Neuropathy

Liberty Jenkins

Definition of the disease

Neuropathy is disease of the peripheral nerve. The pathological process may affect the nerve at the root (radiculopathy), the dorsal root ganglion (ganglionopathy), the plexus (plexopathy), or anywhere along the terminal pathway, typically at sites of entrapment or in a length-dependent pattern. The cranial nerves may also be affected. The process may affect a single nerve (a mononeuropathy) or multiple discrete nerves (mononeuritis multiplex) or form a confluent, typically distal, and symmetrical pattern (polyneuropathy).

Aetiology of the disease

The causes of neuropathy are myriad. It is, therefore, pragmatic to approach the etiological diagnosis according to the clinical pattern, which is considered primarily in terms of the temporal course and its distribution. The predominance of symptoms, be they sensory, motor, or autonomic, may be also be helpful (Table 234.1). Any history of a general medical disorder or its treatment may be relevant.

Acute mononeuropathies are commonly due to pressure palsy or trauma, but a spontaneous lesion occurring at a site atypical for entrapment should raise the possibility of vasculitis. This is the commonest cause of acute mononeuritis multiplex. Acute symmetrical polyneuropathy, although rare, is a medical emergency, as death may occur from rapidly ensuing neuromuscular respiratory failure or dysautonomia. Table 234.2 summarizes the commoner causes of acute neuropathies.

Chronic peripheral neuropathies are common. Acquired causes (Table 234.3) may be easily identifiable from the history, particularly

Table 234.1 Causes of neuropathy by predominant symptomatology

Predominant symptomatology	Cause
Sensory	Diabetes mellitus
	Alcoholism
	Vitamin B_{12}, B_1, and B_6 deficiency
	Uraemia
	Leprosy
	Paraproteinaemic neuropathies
	Paraneoplasia
	Sjögren's syndrome
	Chronic idiopathic sensory neuropathy
Motor	Charcot–Marie–Tooth disease
	Guillain–Barré Syndrome
	Chronic inflammatory demyelinating polyradiculoneuropathy
	Multifocal motor neuropathy
	Lead toxicity
	Acute intermittent porphyria
	Diphtheria
	Hereditary distal motor neuropathy
Autonomic and small fibre (pain)	Diabetes mellitus
	Amyloidosis
	Fabry's disease
	Tangier's disease
	Hereditary sensory and autonomic neuropathy

Table 234.2 Causes of acute neuropathies

Clinical pattern	Cause
Mononeuropathy	Trauma
	Entrapment at common site, e.g. wrist or elbow
	Other extrinsic lesion, e.g. neoplasia, haematoma
	Infiltration, or primary nerve tumour
	Ischaemia secondary to vasculitis or diabetes mellitus
Mononeuritis multiplex	Vasculitis (primary systemic; systemic secondary to associated connective tissue disease, infection, or malignancy; or non-systemic, being confined to the peripheral nervous system)
	Diabetes mellitus
	Sarcoidosis
	Lyme disease
	Lymphomatous or carcinomatous infiltration
	Amyloidosis
	Leprosy
	Multiple pressure palsies, including hereditary neuropathy with liability to pressure palsies (although rarely acute)
Generalized polyneuropathy	Guillain–Barré syndrome
	Vasculitis
	Toxic or drug-induced acute neuropathy
	Critical illness neuropathy
	Thiamine deficiency
	Diabetes mellitus
	Acute intermittent porphyria
	Sarcoidosis
	Lymphomatous neuropathy
	Rabies
	Diptheria

in the context of diabetes, alcohol misuse, or certain drugs, as these account for the majority of cases in primary care. Nutritional deficiencies and metabolic, haematological, or endocrine derangements may be identified on simple investigation. Toxin exposure or infection may be relevant: leprosy is the commonest cause of peripheral neuropathy worldwide, while HIV is more frequently encountered in the UK. Paraneoplasia, malignancy, and inflammatory/immune-mediated causes may need particular consideration. Charcot–Marie–Tooth disease is the most frequent hereditary neuropathy. However, neuropathy may also be the sole manifestation of other genetic diseases or form part of a multisystem disorder. No cause is identified in 25% of cases.

Typical symptoms of the disease, and less common symptoms

Symptoms reflect the distribution of the nerve(s) involved and the predominant subpopulation of fibres affected.

Median nerve compression at the wrist (carpal tunnel syndrome) results in intermittent pain and tingling which is worse at night or on use or elevation of the hand and is relieved by shaking. The symptoms are not confined to the median innervated digits (although they are typically worse in these), with the pain often extending above the wrist. Ulnar nerve entrapment at the elbow results in tingling and numbness in the ring finger and the little finger. The degree of

Table 234.3 Causes of chronic neuropathies

Category	Cause
Hereditary	Charcot–Marie–Tooth disease
	Hereditary neuropathy with liability to pressure palsies
	Hereditary sensory and autonomic neuropathy
	Distal hereditary motor neuropathy
	Neuropathy associated with hereditary multisystem disease (e.g. metachromatic leukodystrophy, mitochondrial diseases, familial amyloid polyneuropathies, ataxia–telangiectasia)
Metabolic	Diabetes mellitus
	Uraemia
	Cirrhosis
Nutritional deficiencies	Deficiencies in:
	• thiamine
	• pyridoxine
	• vitamin E
	• vitamin B_{12}
	Possibly coeliac disease
Toxic	Alcohol
	Acrylamide
	Arsenic
	Lead
	Mercury
	Thallium
	Organophosphates
	Carbon disulphide
	Organic solvents
Drug induced	Amiodarone
	Amitriptyline
	Bortezomib
	Carboplatin
	Chloroquine
	Cisplatin
	Colchicine
	Dapsone
	Didanosine
	Disulfiram
	Docetaxel
	Doxorubicin
	Ethambutol
	Gold
	Hydralazine
	Isoniazid
	Metronidazole
	Misonidazole
	Nitrofurantoin
	Nitrous oxide
	Paclitaxel
	Phenytoin
	Podophyllin
	Pyridoxine
	Stavudine
	Suramin
	Thalidomide
	Vincristine
	Zalcitabine
Endocrine derangement	Hypothyroidism
	Acromegaly
Infection	Leprosy
	HIV

Category	Cause
Haematological	Paraprotein-associated neuropathy
	Amyloidosis due to plasma cell dyscrasia or myeloma
Malignancy related	Paraneoplasia
	Carcinomatous
	Lymphoma
Inflammatory/ immune	Chronic inflammatory demyelinating polyradiculopathy
	Multifocal motor neuropathy
	Sarcoidosis
	Sjögren's syndrome
	Rheumatoid arthritis
Idiopathic	

associated weakness is variable. Other less common mononeuropathies include radial nerve palsies (wrist and finger drop with impaired sensation over the anatomical snuffbox if occurring in the spiral groove of the humerus; finger drop without sensory disturbance if the lesion is more distal), compression of the lateral cutaneous nerve of the thigh (meralgia paresthetica: tingling and numbness over the lateral aspect of the thigh), and peroneal nerve palsies (foot drop with weak eversion and sensory disturbance affecting the lateral aspect of the lower leg and dorsum of the foot if the superficial branch is involved, or just the web between the first and second toe if the deep branch is solely affected).

Abrupt painful onset of a mononeuropathy or mononeuritis multiplex should raise the suspicion of vasculitis.

In the common chronic symmetrical polyneuropathies, distal paraesthesiae (tingling, prickling, or numbness) predominate. The feet are first affected, with gradual proximal extension prior to any upper limb symptoms, reflecting the length-dependent process. A sense of unsteadiness, particularly in the dark, is common. This 'sensory ataxia' is due to a loss of large-fibre sensory function. Impaired small-fibre function is associated with a prominent, painful, burning dysaesthesia, possibly with impaired autonomic function, resulting in symptoms of postural hypotension and impotence. Neuropathy predominantly or purely affecting the motor fibres is less common, but results in weakness, such that the patient may first complain of tripping when stepping up kerbs, before noticing a change in the sound when walking, with their feet slapping the ground. Later, upper limb involvement may result in difficulty opening jars or turning keys in a lock. Proximal weakness is unusual in neuropathy but can be seen in the rare demyelinating neuropathies. In the acquired form, these may also be distinguishable by a relapsing course. Hereditary neuropathies may be suggested by delayed motor milestones, difficulty fitting shoes, and failing to keep up with peers in school sports.

Acute symmetrical peripheral neuropathy is most commonly caused by Guillain–Barré syndrome (GBS). There is often an antecedent history of gastrointestinal or respiratory infection 1–2 weeks prior to the onset of distal paraesthesiae together with progressive weakness, evolving over hours. Pain, especially lower back pain reflecting radicular involvement, is common. Later onset of facial and bulbar weakness is typical, resulting in slurred speech and difficulty swallowing. The patient is unlikely to have symptoms of respiratory compromise even when neuromuscular respiratory failure is imminent. Autonomic dysfunction is common.

Demographics of the disease

The prevalence of a symptomatic chronic symmetrical peripheral neuropathy is 2400 in 100 000 (2.4%). This increases with age, being approximately 8% in those over 55. Reports of the prevalence in the diabetic population vary, but it is probably in the order of 35%. Charcot–Marie–Tooth disease has prevalence of 40 in 100 000. Carpal tunnel syndrome has a lifetime incidence of 10%. The annual incidence of GBS is 1–2 in 100 000.

Table 234.4 Investigation of neuropathy: A staged approach

Investigation	Test
Section A: Stage 1 investigations	
Blood tests	Full blood count
	Erythrocyte sedimentation rate
	Vitamin B$_{12}$
	Immunofixation/serum and urine protein electrophoresis
	HB A1C, fasting glucose +/− 2 hour glucose tolerance test instead of Glucose (fasting blood)
	Renal function
	Liver function
	Thyroid function
Urinalysis	Glucose
	Proteinuria
Basic autonomic function	Postural blood pressure measurement
	Pupillary responses
	ECG rhythm strip for presence of sinus arrhythmia
Section B: Stage 2 investigations	
Neurophysiology	
Blood tests	Protein electrophoresis
	Vasculitic screen:
	• antinuclear factor
	• rheumatoid factor
	• anti-extractable nuclear antigen antibodies
	• antineutrophil cytoplasmic antigen antibodies
	• eosinophil count
	Glucose (formal glucose tolerance test)
Radiology	Chest X-ray
Section C: Stage 3 investigations	
Immunological	Anti-neuronal antibodies
	Angiotensin-converting enzyme
	Anti-gliadin antibodies
	Antiganglioside antibodies
	Anti-myelin-associated-glycoprotein antibodies
	HIV testing
Search for neoplasia	Tumour markers
	Urine for Bence Jones protein
	Skeletal survey
	Bone marrow trephine
	Imaging:
	• ultrasound
	• mammography
	• CT
	• PET
Cerebrospinal fluid	Cells
	Protein
	Immunoglobulin oligoclonal bands
Testing for Sjögren's syndrome	Schirmer's test
	Rose Bengal test
	Anti-extractable antigen antibodies (anti-Ro and anti-La)
	Labial gland biopsy
Molecular genetics	For example:
	• peripheral nerve myelin protein 22 gene duplication (commonest cause of Charcot–Marie–Tooth disease type 1)
	• peripheral nerve myelin protein 22 deletion (hereditary neuropathy with liability to pressure palsies)
	• connexin 32 (X-linked Charcot–Marie–Tooth disease)
Detailed autonomic function	
Nerve biopsy	
Section D: Investigation in acute symmetrical neuropathy	
Neurophysiology	
Cerebrospinal fluid	Cells
	Protein
Blood	Acute and convalescent borrelia
	Mycoplasma
	Serology for EBV and CMV
	Antiganglioside antibodies
Stool	Campylobacter

Natural history, and complications of the disease

In patients with a chronic symmetrical axonal peripheral neuropathy, treatment of the underlying cause will usually halt progression, but the accumulated axonal damage may persist. In patients in whom investigation fails to identify a specific cause, an indolent course is to be anticipated. In demyelinating neuropathies, be they the acute symmetrical neuropathy of typical GBS or the focal entrapment mononeuropathies, treatment should result in remyelination of the affected segment, resolution of the conduction block, and, hence, a return to normal function. However, recovery of any axonal damage already sustained is protracted: peripheral nerve axons have the capacity to regenerate at a rate of 1 mm per day. Chronic axonal damage is often painful and results in secondary complications of ulceration and injury due to impaired sensory protective measures. The onset of neuropathy in childhood may result in deformity of the feet ('pes cavus').

Approach to diagnosing the disease

Having obtained a suggestive history, the clinical examination should be focused on detecting the classical lower motor neuron signs of a neuropathy. In the case of the common chronic symmetrical neuropathies, wasting of the small muscles of the feet, weakness of toe extension and (often subtly) of ankle dorsiflexion, loss of the ankle jerks, and impaired sensation in a stocking (and, later, glove) distribution should be anticipated with a positive Romberg's test. More widespread areflexia would be atypical and should alert the clinician to the possibility of a more unusual pathogenesis, such as demyelination. Areflexia is a classic finding in GBS but may not be present in the early stages. Wasting is not a feature of the acute neuropathies, typically taking weeks to months to develop. If the history is suggestive of a mononeuropathy or mononeuritis multiplex, then the function of the individual nerves should be mapped out. A general medical examination is imperative. Once a clinical diagnosis of a neuropathy has been established, investigations should be tailored appropriately.

Other diagnoses that should be considered

The cardinal history of distal numbness and paraesthesiae is strongly suggestive of peripheral neuropathy but, rarely, may reflect pathology of the CNS, particularly a myelopathy. Transient episodes of paraesthesia may also occur in hyperventilation. Distal weakness of the legs may infrequently be due to bilateral L5 radiculopathies. Distal myopathies are an even rarer cause. If proximal weakness is present, however, then myopathy or polyradiculopathy must be actively considered. Small-fibre neuropathies typically have a paucity of signs, and the pain needs to be distinguished from that arising from ischaemia or musculoskeletal disease.

'Gold-standard' diagnostic test

Nerve biopsy demonstrating typical pathological changes of the underlying process can be definitively diagnostic. However, demonstrating established non-specific axonal damage will not further the diagnostic process, and the procedure is not without associated morbidity. As such, biopsy is only performed in carefully selected cases, particularly where vasculitis is suspected and prompt but potentially toxic treatment is to be instigated.

Acceptable diagnostic alternatives to the gold standard

In the vast majority of cases, neurophysiological assessment is a satisfactory alternative, enabling the extent and type of neuropathy to be established (the principle aim being to distinguish the potentially specifically treatable demyelinating neuropathies from the axonal neuropathies). The motor and sensory function of accessible nerves can be studied using nerve conduction techniques to assess for points of entrapment, axonal loss, or demyelination. More proximal nerves can be studied indirectly by looking for secondary changes in the muscle as a result of denervation, using electromyography. The standard testing protocols are unable to assess small-fibre function and are normal in these cases. A typical history is usually sufficient.

Other relevant investigations

Given the multitudinous potential causes of a chronic symmetrical peripheral neuropathy, a staged approach to the investigations is recommended. A clinical diagnosis without investigation is appropriate in typical and proportional cases with a predictable cause, such as diabetes. All other patients should initially undergo the investigations in Table 234.4, Section A. If these fail to identify a cause or the case appears atypical, then specialist opinion should be sought. Of the second-tier investigations (Table 234.4, Section B), neurophysiological assessment is paramount. A third stage of investigations (Table 234.4, Section C) is performed selectively and reflects whether a demyelinating or axonal neuropathy has been identified electrophysiologically.

Acute symmetrical neuropathy requires urgent specialist investigation. Frequent vital capacity and cardiac monitoring are essential. In addition to routine medical investigations, specialist tests are likely to include those in Table 234.4, Section D.

Neurophysiological assessment provides the lynchpin of mononeuropathy investigation. Focused investigation for vasculitis should be rapidly instigated in cases of acute painful onset multiple mononeuropathies, together with a lower threshold for nerve biopsy.

Prognosis and how to estimate it

In general, recovery of axonal damage is protracted and often incomplete or with aberrant reinnervation. Clinically, this means that recovery is unlikely if marked muscle wasting is present or in proximal axonotmesis lesions. Neurophysiology can provide a more quantitative tool to guide prognosis, giving an indication of the pathophysiological process, degree of axonal damage, and secondary reinnervation that has occurred. In the established chronic axonal peripheral neuropathies, a guarded prognosis is recommended even on reversal of the cause, with the principle aim being to prevent progression. Conversely, should the neurophysiology show a purely demyelinating neuropathy, be it focal at a point of entrapment or generalized, one can be optimistic that treatment will be effective.

In GBS, poor prognostic factors include advanced age, onset following campylobacter infection, rapid onset and progression, severe muscular weakness, and the axonal variant.

Treatment and its effectiveness

The mainstay of treatment is reversal of the underlying cause.

Recognition of the demyelinating neuropathies is important, as specific treatment is effective. In chronic inflammatory demyelinating polyradiculoneuropathy, administration of corticosteroids, IV immunoglobulin, or plasma exchange is usually efficacious, with other immunosuppressive drugs used in refractory cases. In GBS, supportive medical care is paramount. IV immunoglobulin (or plasma exchange) hastens recovery and reduces long-term disability. Vasculitic neuropathy is commonly treated with a combination of corticosteroids and cyclophosphamide. Entrapment neuropathies may respond to conservative measures. In carpal tunnel syndrome, wrist splints and steroid injections may suffice, as may measures to prevent further insult to the nerve, for instance not leaning on the elbow in ulnar nerve entrapments. Persistent symptoms should prompt referral for consideration of surgical decompression.

Generic treatments to limit secondary complications include foot care, orthoses, and walking aids. Neuropathic pain is common and often responsive to a number of agents, including tricyclic antidepressants, duloxetine, and gabapentin. Autonomic features may be symptomatically ameliorated with compression stockings, raising the head of the bed, and sildenafil.

Further Reading

Smith C, Saint S, Price R, et al. Diagnosing one letter at a time. *N Engl J Med* 2015; 372: 67–73.

Willison HJ, Jacobs JBC, and van Doorn PA. Guillain-Barré syndrome. *Lancet* 2016; 388: 717–27.

Willison HJ and Winer JB. Clinical evaluation and investigation of neuropathy. *J Neurol Neurosurg Psychiatry* 2003; 74: 3–8.

Yuki N and Hartung H-P. Guillain–Barré Syndrome. *N Engl J Med* 2012; 366: 2294–304.

235 Myopathy

Liberty Jenkins

Definition of the disease

Myopathy refers to disease of skeletal muscle, which may be accompanied by cardiac or smooth muscle involvement.

Aetiology of the disease

The myopathies are a heterogeneous group of conditions of myriad and diverse aetiology. Box 235.1 provides a structure by which to classify these. An initial attempt to narrow the etiological diagnosis must be made, as no such list is exhaustive or of particular use to the clinician if approached blindly. Attention to the age of onset, family history, rate of progression or fluctuation, and any associated systemic disease or its treatment is, therefore, crucial.

In clinical practice, the commonest causes of significant secondary myopathy are alcohol misuse, corticosteroid administration (which results in a painless, slowly progressive myopathy with normal plasma creatine kinase (CK)), and, increasingly, statin-related myopathy. The latter may be associated with problems ranging from an asymptomatic raised CK, requiring no alteration in management, to significant myalgia and cramps, to acute necrosis with rhabdomyolysis. The inflammatory myopathies are treatable and, hence, an important diagnosis to consider. They may occur in isolation or in the context of systemic connective tissue diseases.

Typical symptoms of the disease, and less common symptoms

Muscle has a limited repertoire of response to damage, regardless of the causative insult. In the vast majority of cases, this is limited to **weakness** of the affected muscles. The **distribution** of this weakness may be suggestive of a specific diagnosis, particularly in the primary muscle diseases (be they inherited or acquired), but a non-specific pattern of symmetrical proximal limb–girdle weakness is much more common. The patient describes difficulty using the arms above shoulder height, such as when washing their hair or reaching up into cupboards, and of the legs, when rising from a chair or climbing stairs. The walk may be described as 'waddling'. In the secondary myopathies, the symptomatic weakness is typically restricted to this, but more widespread symptomatology may be present in the primary myopathies. Facial or bulbar weakness results in indistinct speech, weak eye closure, ptosis, difficulty using a straw, whistling, and swallowing. Distal weakness is uncommon but manifests as difficulty turning door handles or keys in a lock, and catching the toes when walking due to foot drop. Weakness of the ocular muscles may be seen on examination, but is infrequently symptomatic: complaints of double vision should raise the possibility of myasthenia gravis. Respiratory muscle weakness manifests as orthopnoea, excessive daytime sleepiness, and morning headache (due to hypercapnoea). Symptoms due to cardiac muscle involvement are those of heart failure and dysrhythmia, with dyspnoea, peripheral oedema, palpitations, and syncope.

The rate of **progression** of the weakness may be acute (as in some toxic myopathies and, infrequently, in the inflammatory myopathies), subacute (more typical of inflammatory cases and other secondary myopathies), or chronically progressive (as in the dystrophies). Alternatively, the weakness may be static over time (most congenital myopathies) or may be episodic, with or without insidious underlying progression (metabolic myopathies and channelopathies). The **age at onset** of the weakness may be indicated by reduced fetal movements, a 'floppy' baby at birth, poor feeding or respiratory

---

Box 235.1 Causes of myopathy

Primary muscle diseases

Inherited
- muscular dystrophies:
  - dystrophinopathies (Duchenne muscular dystrophy and Becker's muscular dystrophy)
  - myotonic dystrophy (types 1 and 2)
  - limb–girdle muscular dystrophy (types 1A–G and 2A–K)
  - Emery–Dreifuss muscular dystrophy
  - oculopharyngeal muscular dystrophy
  - facioscapulohumeral muscular dystrophy
  - scapulohumeral muscular dystrophy
  - congenital muscular dystrophies (including collagen VI disorders (e.g. Ullrich congenital muscular dystrophy, Bethlem myopathy), laminin-alpha-2 deficiency, Walker–Warburg syndrome, muscle–eye–brain disease, Fukuyama congenital muscular dystrophy, rigid spine syndrome)
  - distal myopathies/dystrophies (including Udd myopathy, Nonaka myopathy, Myoshi myopathy, Laing distal myopathy, and Welander distal myopathy)
- congenital myopathies:
  - central core disease
  - nemaline rod myopathy
  - myotubular myopathy
  - mini-core myopathy
  - type 1 fibre predominance
- metabolic myopathies:
  - mitochondrial disorders (including chronic progressive external ophthalmoplegia, Kearns–Sayre syndrome, MELAS, MERRF, Leber's hereditary optic neuropathy, and Leigh's syndrome)
  - disorders of beta oxidation (including carnitine pamitoyl-transferase deficiency and VCLAD)
  - disorders of carbohydrate metabolism (including acid maltase deficiency (Pompe's disease) and myophosphorylase deficiency (McArdle's disease))
- channelopathies:
  - periodic paralyses (hypo- or hyperkalaemic, and Andersen–Tawil syndrome)
  - myotonia congenita (Thomsen disease and Becker's muscular dystrophy)
  - paramyotonia congenita
  - potassium-aggravated myotonia
  - malignant hyperthermia
  - central core disease

Acquired
- inflammatory:
  - dermatomyositis
  - polymyositis
  - inclusion body myositis

Secondary muscle diseases
- toxic and drug induced:
  - alcohol
  - amiodarone
  - amphetamines
  - ciclosporin
  - cimetidine
  - cocaine
  - corticosteroids

Box 235.1 (Continued)

- fibrates
- gemfibrozil
- gold
- heroin
- hydralazine
- isoniazid
- labetalol
- lithium
- L-tryptophan
- nifedipine
- penicillamine
- procainamide
- propofol
- quetiapine
- salbutamol
- statins
- vincristine
- zidovudine
- endocrine derangement
  - thyroid disease (hypo- or hyperthyroidism)
  - adrenal disease (hypo- or hyperadrenalism)
  - vitamin D deficiency (osteomalacia)
  - hyperparathyroidism
  - hypopituitarism
  - acromegaly
- infective
  - viral (Coxsackie virus, influenza virus, parainfluenza virus, HIV, HTLV1, adenovirus, echovirus, CMV, herpes simplex, EBV)
  - bacterial (*Staphylococcus aureus, Streptococcus viridans, Streptococcus pyogenes, Streptococcus pneumoniae*), *Salmonella enteritidis, Klebsiella pneumoniae, Clostridium freundii*, bartonella, *Escherichia coli, Pseudomonas aeruginosa*, neisseria, yersinia, *Morganella morganii*, citrobacter, mycobacterium avium-intracellulare complex)
  - parasitic (cysticercosis, trypanosomiasis, Lyme disease, trichinosis, toxoplasmosis, toxocariasis, amoebiasis, echinococcosis)
  - fungal (cryptococcus, candida, histoplasma, coccidioides, aspergillus, pneumocystis, fusarium, actinomyces)
- electrolyte disturbance
  - hyper- or hypokalaemia
  - hypercalcaemia
  - hyper- or hypomagnesaemia
- inflammatory myopathy associated with connective tissue disease:
  - SLE
  - mixed connective tissue disease
  - scleroderma
  - Sjögren's syndrome
  - rheumatoid arthritis
- miscellaneous causes of inflammatory myopathy:
  - eosinophilic myositis
  - vasculitis associated with granulomatosis (sarcoidosis)
  - graft versus host disease
  - macrophage myofasciitis

Abbreviations: CMV, cytomegalovirus; MELAS, mitochondrial encephalomyopathy with lactic acidosis and stroke-like episodes; MERRF, myoclonic epilepsy with ragged red fibres; VCLAD, very long-chain acyl-coenzyme A dehydrogenase deficiency; HTLV1, human T-lymphotrophic virus 1.

effort, delayed motor milestones, failure to keep up with peers in school sports, or normal achievement until later in life.

Myalgia is common complaint in general practice, but muscular pain is, in fact, a relatively rare feature of the myopathies. It is reported by some patients with inflammatory myopathy and myotonic dystrophy, and, more frequently, in the toxic myopathies and those associated with hypothyroidism and vitamin D deficiency. Transient myalgia is common in the context of systemic infection.

Episodic pain with myoglobulinuria (dark 'coca-cola' coloured urine) is a particular feature of the metabolic myopathies but occurs with other causes of rhabdomyolysis.

Other symptoms of muscle disease are rare but may be more specific with regards to aetiology. Patients may report marked muscle **stiffness** (to be distinguished from common mild symptoms) due to myotonia. **Cramps** are more frequently a neurogenic symptom but occur in certain drug and metabolic myopathies. **Enlargement** of the muscles, most often of the calves, may result in difficulty fitting clothes. Pseudohypertrophy is marked in Duchenne muscular dystrophy and Becker's muscular dystrophy. True hypertrophy is rare but occurs in myotonia congenita and neuromyotonia. **Wasting** is common to many muscle diseases. A careful systemic enquiry is essential to identify **non-myopathic symptoms**. These may indicate a specific diagnosis and include, for example, those due to neuropathy, CNS disease, cataracts, retinopathy, endocrine dysfunction, or rash.

Demographics of the disease

There are approximately 50 000 people in the UK with a primary muscle disease. Many more have secondary muscle dysfunction but the prevalence is unknown. Duchenne muscular dystrophy is the commonest childhood-onset dystrophy, with an incidence of 1 in 3300 boys. Myotonic dystrophy occurs in 1 in 8000 people. The inflammatory myopathies have an incidence of approximately 5–10 in 100 000. Inclusion body myositis is the commonest primary myopathy in those over 50.

Natural history, and complications of the disease

The natural history depends on the etiological diagnosis. The spectrum ranges from transient, self-limiting symptoms to death in infancy. In the majority of patients with a secondary myopathy, reversal of the cause will ensure gradual restoration of normal muscle function. Inexorably progressive muscular weakness, regardless of aetiology, results in loss of mobility with the predictable **skeletal** complications of kyphoscoliosis (restricting respiratory function); contractures (although prominent, early contractures are a particular feature of some genetic myopathies); and skin damage. Pre-emptive management is required. **Respiratory** failure due to diaphragmatic weakness may be the presenting feature of the myopathy (as occurs in some inherited myopathies and occasional cases associated with hyperthyroidism or electrolyte dysfunction) or occur late in the disease. Interstitial lung disease complicates 10% of autoimmune inflammatory myopathies. **Cardiac** involvement, with heart failure and/or dysrhythmias, is common in specific genetic myopathies, and may be disproportionate to the limb weakness, but also occurs in secondary myopathies. Underlying **malignancy** is present in approximately 25% of patients with dermatomyositis (the association with polymyositis is weaker): screening is recommended in treatment-resistant cases in patients over the age of 40. **Rhabdomyolysis** may complicate acute severe muscle damage of any cause, with life-threatening renal complications, metabolic disturbance, and disseminated intravascular coagulation. **Malignant hyperthermia** is the commonest cause of death during general anaesthesia. Similar reactions may be seen in certain channelopathies, dystrophies, and metabolic muscle disease.

Approach to diagnosing the disease

Having established a suggestive history, the clinical examination should be focused on detecting the cardinal lower motor neuron signs of a myopathy. The classical clinical picture is of symmetrical proximal wasting (if chronic) and weakness. The pelvic girdle is more severely affected than the shoulder. The reflexes are preserved (except in advanced disease) and the sensory examination is normal. Functional assessment, for example the ability to stand from sitting, may be more useful than the documented Medical Research Council score in assessing this. Facial weakness is usually symmetrical and may be missed (look for failure to 'bury the eyelashes' on eye closure). Distal weakness is rare. However, weakness of the finger flexors and quadriceps is a hallmark of inclusion body myositis, and selective muscle weakness is a remarkable feature of the dystrophies. Muscle bulk, abnormal movements, contractures, and myotonia should be specifically examined for. A detailed general medical examination is imperative.

Given a clinical picture consistent with a myopathy, it is sensible to review parts of the history or examination that may narrow the differential diagnosis. If a satisfactorily explanatory secondary cause is apparent, then further investigation is unnecessary. In others cases, simple blood tests may suffice. In complex cases or where a primary muscle disease is suspected, early referral to a neurologist is warranted.

Other diagnoses that should be considered

The main differential diagnoses to be considered are other causes of lower motor neuron muscular weakness. Pure motor syndromes are likely to cause the greatest diagnostic challenge. Fatigable weakness is the hallmark of neuromuscular junction disorders, such as myasthenia gravis. Diplopia with complex external ophthalmoplegia is highly suggestive of this. Lambert–Eaton myasthenic syndrome is a rare disorder but typically presents with symmetrical leg weakness. The reflexes are absent on initial examination, being 'potentiated' by muscular contraction. Weakness with evidence of denervation (fasciculations and impaired deep tendon reflexes) and coexisting upper motor neuron signs is consistent with motor neuron disease, which is rarely as symmetrical as the classical myopathy picture. Spinal muscular atrophy may be difficult to distinguish clinically, especially in the neonatal population, but signs of denervation will again be present. Pure motor neuropathies are unusual, and the presence of any sensory symptoms is obviously inconsistent with a myopathy. In a neuropathy, the clinical picture is predominantly distal, and the reflexes are reduced or absent. Bilateral radiculopathies may result in proximal weakness but are associated with dermatomal sensory disturbance and loss of the innervated reflex arc. Upper motor neuron lesions are rarely troublesome but the asymmetry of some genetic myopathies, such as facioscapulohumeral dystrophy, may initially be misleading.

In general practice, symptoms of muscle pain, weariness, or fatigue are extremely common. The absence of demonstrable weakness (with a normal CK and no history of myoglobulinuria) makes an underlying myopathy unlikely. Fibromyalgia or chronic fatigue syndrome may need to be considered. Ill-defined global muscle dysfunction is common in the elderly, the immobile, and those with critical illness or cancer but rarely requires investigation in its own right.

'Gold-standard' diagnostic test

There is no single test that can be considered the 'gold standard'. In certain inherited myopathies, genetic testing or a specific enzyme assay is the only investigation required and can be considered 'first line' in the appropriate clinical setting. In other myopathies, muscle biopsy with immunohistochemical staining will prove definitively diagnostic. Selecting which muscle to biopsy is important: close collaboration with a muscle pathologist is essential. A histologically proven diagnosis should be considered a prerequisite in inflammatory myopathies, where potentially toxic immunotherapy is to be instigated.

Acceptable diagnostic alternatives to the gold standard

CK is useful as a non-specific marker of muscle damage. However, the degree of elevation is not a reliable indicator of the aetiology, or, in some cases, the severity (but changes in the level may be helpful in monitoring treatment response if used together with clinical

observation). Potentially misleading elevations are also 'normal' in Afro-Caribbeans, trauma, sepsis, exercise, hypothermia, myocardial injury, and severe denervating disorders.

Electromyography can also be useful but has similar caveats: the electrophysiological features of a myopathy are qualitative and non-specific. Neurophysiological assessment may, however, be valuable in excluding neuromuscular junction and neurogenic disorders and may identify myotonic discharges. Specific protocols are used in the assessment of the periodic paralyses.

Other relevant investigations

Given the multitudinous potential causes, directed, successive investigation is essential. Sensible 'screening' investigations include CK; full blood count; urea; electrolytes, including calcium, phosphate, and magnesium; liver function tests; and thyroid stimulating hormone. Other blood tests that may be pertinent include inflammatory markers, antinuclear factor, lactate, parathyroid hormone, vitamin D, cortisol, pituitary function tests, and serology, including HIV testing. Urinalysis for myoglobulinuria is useful in an acute attack. Additional specialist tests are probably best deferred to the neurologist or geneticist but may include specific assays for metabolic muscle disease, molecular genetics, MRI, and muscle biopsy. In myopathy patients at risk of cardiac or respiratory disease, regular electrocardiograms, echocardiograms, and vital-capacity monitoring are essential.

Prognosis and how to estimate it

Prognosis depends on the specific diagnosis. The inherited myopathies are incurable but life expectancy and disability vary widely, even, in some cases, within the same genotype. The majority are slowly progressive degenerative conditions. Boys with Duchenne muscular dystrophy are now surviving into adulthood but are rarely ambulant beyond the age of 12. Most patients with dermatomyositis and polymyositis are responsive to treatment, but a poorer prognosis is seen in older patients and those with underlying malignancy or associated respiratory or cardiac disease. Inclusion body myositis is chronically progressive and generally resistant to all therapy. Secondary myopathies are usually reversible on treatment of their underlying cause.

Treatment and its effectiveness

Specific treatments are available for a minority of myopathies. Corticosteroids form the mainstay of dermatomyositis and polymyositis treatment. An alternate day regime reduces side effects. Which steroid-sparing immunosuppressant is superior is unclear but methotrexate and azathioprine are most widely used. Steroids are now also frequently used in Duchenne muscular dystrophy. Respiratory and cardiac interventions prolong life expectancy. Exon skipping antisense oligonucleotide therapies are appropriate in some. Enzyme-replacement therapy is available for acid maltase deficiency. Several agents, particularly mexiletine, may be useful for myotonia. In a number of the metabolic myopathies and periodic paralyses, the frequency of attacks may be reduced with preventative measures. In most secondary myopathies, treatment of the underlying cause is effective. The management of rhabdomyolysis is largely supportive, with correction of the fluid and electrolyte abnormalities.

Generic treatment strategies to limit the complications of muscle disease are essential and require a well-integrated multidisciplinary team. Exercise, nutritional support, mobility aids, pain management, and skin care are all important. Surgical intervention for kyphoscoliosis and contractures may be required. Genetic counselling should be offered where appropriate.

Further Reading

Merrison AFA and Hanna MG. Muscle disease: The bare essentials. *Neurol Pract* 2009; 9: 54–65.

236 Vasculitis in neurology

Ben Wakerley

Definition

Vasculitis syndromes are characterized by inflammation of blood vessel walls, which may result in interruption of blood flow with resulting ischaemia or haemorrhage. Patients present with a variety of systemic and neurological symptoms which relate to the size and location of affected vessels.

Classification

Size (large, medium, small) and location (systemic, CNS, peripheral nervous system (PNS)) of affected vessels determine the symptoms associated with each specific vasculitis syndrome. Primary vasculitis occurs in isolation whereas secondary vasculitis is associated with underlying connective tissue disorders or infections (see Box 236.1).

Clinical manifestations

Clinical features vary considerably depending on which vessels are involved, and in each case specific differential diagnoses should be excluded. Localized visceral symptoms, relate to vessel size and location. Large and medium vessel vasculitis results in organ damage more often associated with ischaemia or haemorrhage and may mimic stroke or arterial occlusion. Small vessel vasculitis commonly affects the skin, kidneys, and peripheral nerves. Systemic manifestations of inflammation may include unexplained fever, generalized fatigue, and weight loss but are not always present.

Box 236.1 Classification of vasculitis

Primary

Large vessel vasculitis
- Takayasu arteritis
- giant cell arteritis

Medium vessel vasculitis
- polyarteritis nodosum
- Kawasaki disease
- primary angiitis of the CNS

Small vessel vasculitis
- microscopic polyangiitis
- Wegener's granulomatosis (granulomatosis with polyangiitis)
- Churg–Strauss syndrome
- Henoch–Schönlein purpura
- essential cryoglobulinaemic vasculitis
- non-systemic vasculitic neuropathy

Secondary

Connective tissue diseases
- SLE
- rheumatoid arthritis
- relapsing polychondritis
- Behçet's disease

Viral infections
- hepatitis B
- hepatitis C
- HIV
- CMV
- EBV
- parvovirus

Vasculitic strokes/encephalopathy

CNS vasculitis usually presents in one of two ways, depending on the distribution and size of vessels involved:

- stroke-like episodes indicate focal neurological deficit and occur with large vessel disease
- encephalopathy (reduced cognition, altered mental state, headaches and personality change) indicates more global neurological dysfunction and occurs with small vessel disease

Often, there is evidence of both processes and, in many cases, headache is the presenting feature with seizures occurring at any stage of disease.

Vasculitic neuropathy

Vasculitic neuropathy presents in three distinct patterns: mononeuritis multiplex, polyneuropathy, or radiculopathy/plexopathy. Onset can be abrupt or insidious and altered sensation and motor weakness is usually associated with pain.

Mononeuritis multiplex

Mononeuritis multiplex is the commonest presentation of vasculitic neuropathy and is defined as nerve damage in two or more peripheral nerves in separate parts of the body. The frequency of nerve involvement is length dependent, and involvement of the sciatic nerve, causing foot drop, is common. Other nerves commonly affected include the tibial, ulnar, and median nerves. With disease progression, other nerves may become involved and mimic symmetrical polyneuropathy.

Polyneuropathy

Vasculitic polyneuropathy is often difficult to distinguish from other distal symmetrical polyneuropathies.

Radiculopathy/plexopathy

When symptoms cannot be attributed to a single nerve then radiculopathy or plexopathy should be considered. This may be a feature of polyarteritis nodosa.

Diagnostic approach

Vasculitis is usually progressive but can be controlled with appropriate immunotherapy, which makes early diagnosis and treatment imperative. Vasculitis can be difficult to diagnose and may mimic other conditions; therefore, a detailed history and careful examination, including systems review, is essential. Serological tests and biopsy specimens are frequently negative, and imaging, including MRI and arteriography, can be non-specific. Important considerations to guide further investigations are:

- are symptoms limited to the nervous system or is there evidence of systemic disease (e.g. weight loss, fever, fatigue, hypertension, renal failure, skin rashes)?
- are there any features to suggest that vasculitis could be secondary to an atypical infection, connective tissue disease, or malignancy?

Investigations

All patients should have the following routine investigations:

- bloods (full blood count, clotting, urea and electrolytes, liver function tests, creatine kinase level, erythrocyte sedimentation rate (ESR), and C-reactive protein levels (CRP))
- urinalysis (protein, microscopy for blood cells/casts)
- ECG
- chest X-ray

A vasculitis blood screen is useful and should include antineutrophil cytoplasmic antibody (ANCA; myeloperoxidase (MPO)/proteinase 3 (PR3) if primary vasculitides are suspected or antinuclear antibodies, double-stranded DNA, complement, antiphospholipid/cardiolipin antibodies, anti-Ro, anti-La, anti-Sm, and rheumatoid factor for those associated with connective tissue disorders.

Blood/urine/tissue cultures to exclude *Treponema pallidum*, *Borrelia burgdorferi*, bartonella, and *Mycoplasma tuberculosis* can be useful.

Those presenting with features of CNS involvement should have CNS imaging (CT, MRI, angiography) and depending on the clinical picture, CSF analysis (microscopy/cell count, protein, glucose, viral PCR) and/or biopsy (temporal artery or brain) may be indicated. Arteriography is more sensitive than magnetic resonance angiography and may reveal beading, skip lesions, aneurysms, occlusions, or vessel wall irregularities in large and medium vessels.

Electroencephelography may demonstrate diffuse encephalopathy or epileptiform activity. Patients with mononeuritis multiplex should have nerve conduction studies and a nerve biopsy. A skin biopsy may determine the cause of a vasculitic rash, while a kidney biopsy is useful if there is renal involvement. A muscle biopsy can also be helpful. Additional blood tests including hepatitis serology, cryoglobulins, and HIV are often indicated.

Arteriography remains the most useful diagnostic test for large and medium vessel vasculitis, while the diagnosis of small vessel disease relies more on the presence of certain antibodies and immune complexes in the blood and characteristic histology on tissue biopsy (brain, nerve, skin, or kidney).

Differential diagnosis

The differential diagnosis of CNS vasculitis and mononeuritis multiplex is outlined in Box 236.2

Treatment: General principals

Vasculitis, by definition, has an inflammatory basis and therefore effective treatment only occurs if the immune system is adequately suppressed. In the case of large and medium vessel disease, this can usually be achieved with oral corticosteroids (prednisolone 1 mg/kg per day), which can be slowly reduced over several months once there is clinical and laboratory evidence of remission. Small vessel disease is usually treated with high-dose glucocorticoids (methylprednisolone 1 g for 3 days) followed by oral steroids. Frequently, especially if there is systemic involvement, remission can only be induced with more potent immunosuppressants such as cyclophosphamide or, in some cases, IV immunoglobulin or plasma exchange. Once the patient is in remission. steroid-sparing agents including azathioprine, methotrexate, or mycophenolate may need to be continued for several years. Patients should be carefully followed up to ensure adequate immunosuppression and identification of disease recurrence. Long-term immunosuppression increases the risk of infections and tumour formation, and treating physicians should be aware of drug-specific adverse reactions (Table 236.1). Bone protection is advocated in patients receiving prolonged courses of steroids, and prophylaxis against pneumocystis pneumonia should be considered in patients receiving more potent immunosuppressants.

Specific diseases

Large vessel vasculitis

Large vessel vasculitis affects the aorta and its main branches to the extremities, head, and neck and includes Takayasu arteritis and giant cell arteritis, which is sometimes called temporal arteritis.

Takayasu arteritis

Vessel wall inflammation results in stenotic lesions and aneurysms in the aorta and its major branches to the extremities, head, and neck. Takayasu arteritis is nine times more frequent in women, with peak

---

Box 236.2 Differential diagnosis of CNS vasculitis and mononeuritis multiplex

CNS vasculitis
Infections:
- bacterial (endocarditis, meningitis, syphilis, TB)
- viral (HIV, CMV, herpes zoster virus)
- fungal (histoplasmosis, aspergillus)

Drug use:
- cocaine
- amphetamines

Haematological causes:
- intravascular lymphoma*
- thrombotic thrombocytopenic purpura

Vasculopathy:
- malignant hypertension
- vasospasm with intracerebral haemorrhage
- radiation damage
- moyamoya disease
- atherosclerosis

Cardiac causes:
- atrial myxoma
- cardioembolic disease

Mononeuritis multiplex
Diabetes
Sarcoidosis
Infections:
- leprosy
- Lyme disease
- HIV
- hepatitis C

Nerve compression:
- multiple compression neuropathies
- hereditary neuropathy with a predisposition to pressure palsy

Multifocal motor neuropathy
Lymphoma

*Intravascular lymphoma is characterized by extra-nodal clonal expansion and proliferation of B-lymphocytes in small vessels, which may occlude, typically affecting the skin and CNS.

Table 236.1 Monitoring and adverse reaction in the treatment of vasculitis

Treatment	Monitoring	Adverse reactions
Steroids	Bone density Blood sugar Ocular pressures	Osteoporosis Diabetes Hypertension Cataract/glaucoma
Cyclophosphamide	Full blood count Liver function tests	Hepatic dysfunction Haemorrhagic cystitis Malignancy Infertility Cytopenia
Azathioprine	Full blood count Liver function tests	Hepatic dysfunction Cytopenia
Methotrexate	Full blood count Liver function tests	Hepatic dysfunction Cytopenia Teratogenic Interstitial pneumonia
IV immunoglobulin	Blood pressure	Hypertension Anaphylaxis Rashes
Plasma exchange	Blood pressure	Vascular instability Line infections

age of onset in the early twenties. Prevalence is highest in Japan and the Middle East.

Patients usually present with systemic features of inflammation and neck pain in conjunction with symptoms associated with ischaemia. Takayasu arteritis should always be considered in young Asian females presenting with stroke-like symptoms.

Symptoms of Takayasu arteritis

The major clinical features of Takayasu arteritis are as follows:

- carotid artery: neck pain, headache (25%), dizziness, visual impairment
- coronary/pulmonary arteries: shortness of breath, atypical chest pain
- subclavian artery: arm fatigue and sensory disturbance
- hypertension
- different blood pressures between arms
- absent/reduced peripheral pulses
- vascular bruits and heart murmurs

Diagnosis of Takayasu arteritis

There are no specific blood tests for Takayasu arteritis, although the presence of raised inflammatory markers correlates well with active disease. Demonstration of arterial damage in the great vessels by arteriography is highly suggestive, although three or more of the following six criteria are needed to establish diagnosis:

- age of onset <40 years
- claudication of extremities
- absent pulses
- difference in blood pressure of 10 mm Hg between arms
- subclavian/abdominal aorta bruits
- arteriographic narrowing of aorta/primary branches

Treatment/prognosis for Takayasu arteritis

In addition to immunosuppression, patients may require surgical intervention (aortic valve replacement, coronary artery bypass grafts, aortic root replacement, arterial grafts), which should be performed when in remission. Early diagnosis and treatment improve prognosis, although the outcome is poorer in patients with renal artery stenosis, aortic coarctation, aortic valve insufficiency, or aneurysms.

Giant cell arteritis

Giant cell arteritis characteristically affects large and medium vessels within the CNS. Histologically, inflamed arteries show evidence of mononuclear/multinucleated giant cell infiltrates. Women are more commonly affected and the age of onset is usually over 50.

The majority of patients feel constitutionally unwell with symptoms relating to ischaemia in large intracranial vessels, although extracranial involvement may also occur.

Symptoms of giant cell arteritis

The major clinical features of giant cell arteritis are:

- scalp tenderness over the temporal artery
- visual impairment (50%)
- jaw claudication
- pain and stiffness around the neck and shoulders, suggestive of polymyalgia rheumatica (30%)

Amaurosis fugax indicates involvement of the posterior ciliary, ophthalmic, or central retinal arteries. Arteritic anterior ischaemic optic neuropathy has a poor prognosis unless treated early and, in 10%–20%, visual loss is permanent. Less commonly, brainstem involvement may present as diplopia, and abdominal pain may occur if there is mesenteric ischaemia.

Diagnosis of giant cell arteritis

Early diagnosis and treatment are imperative if there are visual symptoms. Although giant cell arteritis is an uncommon cause of stroke, raised CRP and ESR confirm ongoing inflammation, and a temporal artery biopsy may confirm diagnosis. Temporal artery biopsies should be carried out before commencing glucocorticoids, if possible, and be >2 cm in length. False negatives are frequently >15% and, in such cases, MRI, ultrasonography, and PET are quite useful. The diagnosis is established if three or more of the following five criteria are present:

- age of onset > 50 years
- localized new-onset headache
- tenderness over scalp/temporal artery
- ESR > 50 mm
- arterial biopsy showing mononuclear cells/multinucleated giant cells

Treatment/prognosis for giant cell arteritis

Immunosuppression is usually with oral glucocorticoids, although cytotoxic drugs are advocated in resistant cases. It remains unclear whether low-dose aspirin helps reduce cerebral infarcts, which occur in 5% of patients. Prognosis is generally good and after steroid tapering, and treatment is usually complete within 2 years.

Medium vessel vasculitis

Polyarteritis nodosa

Polyarteritis nodosa is a systemic vasculitis characterized by necrotizing vasculitis in medium and small vessels but does not involve arterioles or capillaries and therefore does not cause glomerulonephritis. It is rarer than other forms of vasculitis and typically affects men. There is an association with hepatitis B in Europe and the US.

Symptoms of polyarteritis nodosa

Major clinical findings of polyarteritis nodosa include:

- prolonged fever (>38°C) and weight loss
- rapidly progressive renal failure, hypertension
- **cerebral haemorrhage/infarction (30%)**
- pleurisy
- gastrointestinal haemorrhage/infarction
- mononeuritis multiplex (>50%)
- subcutaneous nodules, purpura, livedo reticularis
- polyarthritis, myositis

Diagnosis of polyarteritis nodosa

There are no specific blood tests for polyarteritis nodosa, although there is an association with HBV and some patients (<20%) have ANCA. Characteristically, multiple aneurysms and strictures are seen in small/medium vessels with arteriography. Tissue biopsy (kidney, muscle, or nerve) demonstrates the presence of fibrinoid necrosis in small/medium vessels and helps to differentiate it from small vessel vasculitis (e.g. microscopic polyangiitis), in which inflammation is also present in capillaries.

Treatment/prognosis of polyarteritis nodosa

Immunosuppression with oral steroids or in some cases cytotoxic drugs is advocated. When in association with hepatitis B virus, then antivirals and plasma exchange may be beneficial. Early treatment improves outcome, although relapse is common (40%).

Kawasaki disease

Kawasaki disease is characterized by vasculitis of large, medium, and small blood vessels, especially those arising from the heart. Typically, it affects children, although cases have been reported in adulthood.

Symptoms of Kawasaki disease

Major clinical features of Kawasaki disease include:

- fever
- conjunctival injection, oral mucous membrane changes, palm erythema/oedema/desquamation, polymorphous rash
- cervical lymphadenopathy
- neurological involvement (stroke, seizures, or myositis; occurs in 1%)
- coronary vasculitis

Treatment of Kawasaki disease

Treatment of Kawasaki disease involves IV immunoglobulins and high-dose aspirin.

Primary angiitis of the CNS

Primary angiitis of the CNS (PACNS) is characterized by inflammation of small and medium vessels restricted to the brain and spinal cord. PACNS can occur at any age but is more common in middle-aged males.

Clinical manifestations vary considerably and the differential diagnosis is therefore wide. Diagnostic tests, including neuroimaging and brain biopsy, can be unrevealing; therefore, taking a detailed clinical history and excluding mimics is essential. PACNS should be suspected in patients presenting with features of chronic meningitis, unexplained focal neurological deficit, or unexplained diffuse brain dysfunction in the absence of systemic disease.

Symptoms of PACNS

Typically, symptoms progress over several weeks or months, with patients complaining of reduced cognition, altered mental state, headaches, and personality change. Focal neurological deficits may occur acutely secondary to ischaemic or haemorrhagic strokes, and seizures are common. Spinal cord disease may present as painful myelopathy.

Diagnosis of PACNS

Organs outside the CNS are not involved and therefore systemic features of vasculitis, including raised inflammatory markers (ESR, CRP) and active urinary sediment, are invariably absent. CSF is non-specifically abnormal (lymphocytosis, raised protein) in 80% of cases but is nevertheless useful to exclude infectious causes. MRI is not diagnostic and often demonstrates non-specific high-signal T2 lesions in grey and white matter areas but in the acute setting may show evidence of ischaemic or haemorrhagic stroke. Patients with normal CSF and imaging are unlikely to have vasculitis. Angiography is the gold standard but can be negative (specificity 60%, sensitivity 30%) and the presence of beading, aneurysms, or vascular irregularities may occur in other conditions. This includes reversible cerebral vasoconstriction syndrome, which is more common in women and characterized by headache, with or without focal neurological deficit but normal CSF and brain biopsy. Patients with suspected PACNS should have a brain biopsy, although vessel involvement is often patchy, and false negatives occur in up to 25% of cases. Higher yields are achieved in samples taken from radiologically abnormal areas.

Treatment/prognosis of PACNS

Untreated PACNS is usually fatal. Therapy should be individualized and tailored to disease severity. Acutely oral steroids (prednisolone 1 mg/kg per day) or pulsed steroids followed by oral steroids are indicated. These should be continued for 3–6 months before slowly tapering over 1 year. Invariably, patients require cyclophosphamide to halt disease progression.

Small vessel vasculitis

ANCA-positive small vessel vasculitis

Microscopic polyangiitis, Wegener's granulomatosis, and Churg–Strauss syndrome are systemic vasculitides which affect small vessels and cause ischaemic damage in various organs, including the brain and PNS. Males and females are equally affected, with onset typically in middle age in Wegener's granulomatosis and Churg–Strauss syndrome, and in those >50 years, in microscopic polyangiitis.

Symptoms of ANCA-positive small vessel vasculitis

Major clinical features of ANCA-positive small vessel vasculitis include:

- palpable purpura and skin ulceration
- hypertension, shortness of breath, haemoptysis, atypical chest pain
- mononeuritis multiplex
- headache, strokes, confusion, seizures

Patients with Wegener's granulomatosis frequently present with upper respiratory tract symptoms, including epistaxis, and cartilaginous necrosis may lead to saddle nose. Mononeuritis multiplex is more common in Churg–Strauss syndrome and, typically, these patients present with bronchial asthma or allergic rhinitis. Cerebral haemorrhage is less common but, together with gastrointestinal haemorrhage and myocardial infarction, frequently causes death.

Diagnosis of ANCA-positive small vessel vasculitis

Diagnosis of ANCA-positive small vessel vasculitis is based upon the clinical picture and the presence of ANCA in the blood (specifically, MPO in microscopic polyangiitis and Churg–Strauss syndrome, and PR3 in Wegener's granulomatosis). Additionally, patients with Churg–Strauss have eosinophilia (usually >10% white-blood-cell differential), although histological evidence of necrotizing vasculitis and eosinophilic infiltration is confirmatory. CNS vasculitis is common (10%–50%) in all three, but typically below the sensitivity of routine angiography.

Treatment/prognosis of ANCA-positive small vessel vasculitis

Early treatment with pulsed steroids, cyclophosphamide, or plasma exchange is indicated if major organs are involved, followed by oral glucocorticoids and milder immunosuppressants to maintain remission. Treatment should be continued for 1–2 years, and patients should be monitored for exacerbations, as active disease often recurs.

ANCA-negative small vessel vasculitis

Henoch–Schönlein purpura

Henoch–Schönlein purpura (HSP) is a systemic vasculitis characterized by small inflammation. Usually, it affects children between the ages of 4 and 7 years, although it may develop in adulthood. The disease process is thought to be mediated by IgA immune complex deposition and, in some cases, allergy towards microorganisms, food, and certain drugs can be demonstrated. Major clinical features of HSP include:

- fever
- non-thrombocytopenic palpable purpura
- abdominal pain, joint pain
- urinalysis demonstrating evidence of nephritis
- mononeuritis multiplex (less common)

Renal or nerve involvement advocates tissue biopsy to confirm diagnosis and treatment with immunosuppressants. Overall, prognosis for HSP is good, although a significant proportion of affected adults develop end-stage renal disease if nephritis has been a feature.

Essential cryoglobulinaemia

Essential cryoglobulinaemia is a systemic vasculitis characterized by small vessel inflammation that is secondary to deposition of immune complexes, and should be considered in patients with lymphoproliferative disorders, infections (e.g. hepatitis A, B, or C; Lyme disease; toxoplasmosis) or connective tissue disorders (e.g. rheumatoid arthritis, SLE) and who present with cerebral infarction or mononeuritis multiplex. Diagnosis is confirmed by the presence of cryoglobulins in serum. Treatment is often conservative but NSAIDs and glucocorticoids play a role. Prognosis is generally good, although a third of patients develop renal or hepatic failure.

Non-systemic vasculitic neuropathy

Non-systemic vasculitic neuropathy is characterized by inflammation of small vessels causing mononeuritis multiplex in the absence of other organ involvement. Patients present without features of systemic vasculitis, and early treatment with steroids or immunosuppressants is advocated to reduce permanent deficit.

Secondary CNS vasculitis

CNS vasculitis may also arise secondary to connective tissue disorders, infections, malignancy, and sarcoidosis.

Varicella zoster virus (VZV) angiitis sometimes occurs after trigeminal herpes zoster in the elderly or immunosuppressed, and diagnosis can be confirmed by the presence of VZV antibodies and positive VZV PCR in the CSF. Treatment with aciclovir and steroids is advocated. Other infectious agents, including HIV, syphilis, and hepatitis C virus (without underlying cryoglobulinaemia) can also cause vasculitis.

Vasculitis is not uncommon in SLE or antiphospholipid antibody syndrome, and neuropsychiatric symptoms may precede focal neurological deficit or global dysfunction by many months. Behçet's disease, Sjögren's syndrome, and sarcoidosis may present as relapsing–remitting or progressive diseases that are not dissimilar clinically and radiologically to multiple sclerosis. Rarely, it may complicate rheumatoid arthritis, mixed connective tissue disorders, relapsing polychondritis, or dermatomyositis.

Lymphoproliferative disorders, including lymphoma, may cause vasculitis and can be diagnosed on the basis of CSF cytology/flow cytometry and brain biopsy.

Further Reading

Birnbaum J and Hellmann DB. Primary angiitis of the central nervous system. *Arch Neurol* 2009; 66: 704–9.

Miller A, Chan M, Wiik A, et al. An approach to the diagnosis and management of systemic vasculitis. *Clin Exp Immunol* 2010; 160: 143–60.

CHAPTER 236 **Vasculitis in neurology**

237 Neurological tumours

Christine Elwell and Kufre Sampson

Definition of the disease

Neurological tumours are categorized as follows (Louis et al., 2016):

- neuroepithelial tumours (diffuse astrocytic and oligodendroglial tumours (gliomas), other astrocytic tumours (pilocytic astrocytoma), ependymomas, other gliomas, choroid plexus tumours, neuronal and mixed neuronal-glial tumours (ganglioglioma), pineal tumours, embryonal tumours (medulloblastoma))
- cranial and paraspinal nerve tumours (schwannoma, neurofibroma, melanocytic tumours)
- meningeal tumours (meningiomas and mesenchymal non-menigothelial tumours (solitary fibrous tumour, sarcomas)
- lymphomas
- histiocytic tumours
- germ cell tumours (germinoma, teratoma)
- sellar region tumours (craniopharingioma)
- metastases

CNS tumours were classified according to morphological features and grade. The WHO histological grading scheme used for astrocytomas is based on mitoses, nuclear pleomorphism, necrosis, and endothelial proliferation. WHO Grade I and II tumours (low grade) and WHO Grade III and IV (high grade). The 4th edition WHO classification of tumours of the central nervous system 2007 has since been updated (in 2016) to include both histopathological and molecular genetic information- 'integrated diagnosis'. This has made the greatest impact on the classification of diffuse gliomas (molecular markers are mandatory IDH, 1p19q, H3k27) and embryonal tumours as well as the recognition- of new brain tumour entities and deletion of others.

Aetiology of the disease

The aetiology of the disease is unknown. Increasing age, female gender, and high socio-economic status appear to be related to increased risk. The acquired immune deficiency syndrome (AIDS) is a recognized cause of cerebral lymphoma. Other known causative factors are ionizing radiation exposure and inherited cancer syndromes, including neurofibromatosis types 1 and 2, von Hippel Lindau disease, tuberous sclerosis, Li–Fraumeni disease, Cowden's disease, Gorlin syndrome (naevoid basal cell carcinoma), and Turcots's syndrome.

Typical symptoms of the disease, and less common symptoms

Typical symptoms of the disease include:

- symptoms of raised intracranial pressure:
  - headache (frontal/generalized); worse in mornings
  - nausea and vomiting
  - altered conscious level
- seizures
- cognitive or behavioural impairment
- progressive focal neurological deficit, including
  - weakness or sensory loss
  - speech abnormalities
  - cranial nerve palsies
  - unilateral visual field loss
- hormonal dysfunction (pituitary tumours)

Demographics of the disease

Primary CNS tumours are rare. In 2007, there were 4676 new cases (7 per 100 000 population) registered in the UK, accounting for 2% of new cases of all cancers (excluding non-melanoma skin cancer). Brain tumours can occur at any age and are the commonest site for solid tumours in childhood. There is a peak in incidence in childhood; this drops to a minimum in teenagers and rises to a larger second peak in people in their seventies. The age-standardized incidence rates for brain and CNS tumours increased between 1975 and 2007, mainly in the over-65 group.

Natural history, and complications of the disease

Gliomas

Gliomas account for 45% of all primary CNS tumours and rarely metastasize outside the CNS. Patients with low- grade gliomas tend to be young and relatively well and may have a long history of seizures. WHO Grade I tumours are usually discrete and have the potential for cure with surgery alone. WHO Grade II tumours can recur, with the potential to transform to higher grades. Patients with high-grade gliomas tend to be older and unwell, with a shorter history of symptoms. IDH mutations are implicated in the pathogenesis of malignant gliomas and are common in lower grade tumours.

Meningiomas

Meningiomas account for up to 39% of primary CNS tumours and most commonly arise in the skull vault. Most are low-grade tumours (WHO Grade I).

Primary CNS lymphoma

Primary CNS lymphoma tumours account for less than 2% of primary brain tumours; 90% are diffuse, large, B-cell lymphomas and tend to occur in the immunosuppressed. Lesions commonly occur in the brain parenchyma, although leptomeningeal, ependymal, or ocular disease may be noted. They rarely metastasize outside the CNS.

Medulloblastoma and embryonal tumours

Medulloblastomas and embryonal tumours are the commonest malignant brain tumours in childhood, accounting for 15%– 25% of all childhood primary CNS tumours. They usually occur in the posterior fossa and have a tendency to spread through CSF, with metastatic spread outside the CNS noted to bone, liver, and lungs.

Ependymoma

Ependymomas are the third most common childhood CNS tumour and usually occur in association with the ventricles. They can spread via CSF along the neuroaxis.

Pineal tumours and germ cell tumours

Pineal tumours and germ cell tumours are very rare in adults. There are three main histological types: germ cell tumours, astrocytomas, and pineal parenchymal tumours.

Pituitary tumours and pituitary-related tumours

Pituitary tumours may be functional and secrete hormones, or non-functional. The majority are pituitary adenomas (95%) with craniopharyngiomas, meningiomas, and Ranthke's cleft cysts accounting for the rest. Symptoms may include visual disturbance, as a result of pressure effects on the optic chiasm/nerves, or hormone imbalance, due to pressure effects on the pituitary gland and/or the hypothalamus.

Brain metastases

Brain metastases affect up to 20%–40% of patients with known cancer. The tumours that commonly metastasize to the brain include breast, lung cancer, melanoma, and renal cell cancers.

Spinal metastases

Common tumours causing spinal metastases include breast, lung, prostate, renal cancer, lymphoma, multiple myeloma, and sarcoma. Back pain, sensory loss, loss of sphincter function, and limb weakness are worrying signs requiring urgent oncological attention and, if left untreated, could result in paralysis and incontinence.

Approach to diagnosing the disease

The approach to diagnosing the disease should consist of the following:

- a good history, which may need to be corroborated
- physical examination
- subsequent investigation, which ideally should include imaging and, where possible, a biopsy for histological diagnosis

Other diagnoses that should be considered

Other diagnoses that should be considered include:

- metastases
- cerebrovascular event: haemorrhage or infarction
- infection: cerebral abscess
- demyelinating or inflammatory process: multiple sclerosis
- radiation necrosis

'Gold-standard' diagnostic test

The following are the gold-standard diagnostic tests for neurological tumours:

- radiology: MRI of the brain and the rest of the CNS if appropriate (the latter particularly in meduloblastomas and ependymomas)
- histology: whenever possible, a biopsy should be carried out for histopathological assessment

Acceptable diagnostic alternatives to the gold standard

CT is an acceptable diagnostic alternative for neurological tumours, if MRI is contraindicated or not tolerated.

Other relevant investigations

Other relevant investigations include:

- routine blood tests
- lumbar puncture: CSF examination (primary CNS lymphoma)
- pituitary function (pituitary tumours)
- viral serology: HIV, CMV, and HSV (primary CNS lymphoma)
- tests for alpha-fetoprotein and B-human chorionic gonadotrophin (germ cell tumours)
- visual field assessments (pituitary tumours)
- ophthalmology review (primary CNS lymphoma)
- whole-body CT (primary CNS lymphoma)

Prognosis, and how to estimate it

In general, low-grade tumours have a better prognosis than those of a higher grade, with 5-year survival rates varying from 5% (WHO Grade IV) to 65% (WHO Grade II).

Prognosis for low-grade glioma

Age (>40 years), astrocytoma histology, presence of neurological deficit before surgery, tumour diameter (>6 cm), and tumour crossing the midline are all unfavourable prognostic factors for survival, and the presence of more than two of these factors may prompt early intervention. Prognosis is often 10+ years.

Prognosis for high-grade glioma

Prognostic factors are tumour type, grade, age, fitness, presence or absence of seizures (patients presenting with fits have better prognosis than those that do not), and extent of resection. These tumours tend to have a poor prognosis (3–6 months) without intervention. Anaplastic oligodendrogliomas with chromosome deletions at 1p and 19q tend to have a better prognosis, as they are more chemosensitive; 5-year survival rates are between 5% and 25%.

Prognosis for meningioma

Most meningiomas are low-grade tumours and have a good prognosis.

Prognosis for primary CNS lymphoma

Primary CNS lymphoma is rapidly fatal if not treated. It has a 25% 5-year survival.

Prognosis for medulloblastoma and primitive neuroectodermal tumour

Prognostic factors for medulloblastomas and primitive neuroectodermal tumours include initial tumour size, brainstem infiltration, post-operative residual tumour, and metastatic disease.

Prognosis for ependymoma

The prognosis for ependymoma depends on the grade and type of the tumour. Local recurrence is a problem.

Prognosis for pineal tumour and germ cell tumour

The prognosis for pineal tumours and germ cell tumours is excellent with radical treatment.

Prognosis for brain metastasis

Brain metastasis is usually associated with a poor prognosis (months).

Prognosis for *spinal metastasis*

Patients who become paraplegic as a result of spinal metastasis have a poor prognosis and die within a few months.

Treatment and its effectiveness

The management of all patients with brain and other CNS tumours should be coordinated by the neuro-oncology multidisciplinary team with the aim of maximizing quality of life. Patients are likely to require physical, psychological, and social support. Treatment depends on patient fitness and the site, histological type, and grade of the tumour. The basis of treatment includes surgery, and radiotherapy with chemotherapy of proven benefit only in a select group of tumours. Surgery is often difficult due to the infiltrative nature of the tumours, which are likely to be close to vital structures.

Treatment for low-grade glioma

The treatment for low-grade glioma is 'watch and wait' and surgery, with radiotherapy if:

- there are persisting neurological symptoms and a significant residual tumour
- there is regrowth following surgery but re-excision is not an option
- there is evidence of tumour transformation to a high-grade tumour

Chemotherapy can be considered in patients with adverse prognostic factors (>40 years), residual disease).

Treatment for high-grade glioma

The treatment for high-grade glioma is as follows:

- corticosteroids
- surgery:
  - emergency decompression or ventriculoperitoneal shunts for hydrocephalus

- biopsy: partial or full debulking, depending on the site of the tumour; however, as these tumours are infiltrative, they tend to recur despite macroscopic resection
- radiotherapy: palliative or radical (the latter concurrent with chemotherapy (temozolamide) in younger, fitter patients)
- chemotherapy:
  - single agent: carmustine, lomustine, temozolamide (MGMT promoter methylation status is a good prognostic molecular marker of likely response to temozolamide in Glioblastomas).
  - carmustine implants in combination with surgical resection
  - combination therapy: PCV (procarbazine, lomustine, and vincristine)
- best supportive care (in some cases)

Treatment for meningioma

The treatment for meningioma is 'watch and wait' and surgery, with radiotherapy if:

- the tumour is WHO Grade II/III (even if the tumour is completely resected)
- there is local invasion of bone or vessels
- there is relapsed disease
- surgery is contraindicated

Treatment for primary CNS lymphoma

There is no clear consensus with regards to the management of primary CNS lymphoma:

- surgery has no role
- corticosteroids started after biopsy may relieve symptoms
- chemotherapy:
  - IV: high-dose methotrexate regimens (with leucovorin or vincristine and procarbazine)
  - intrathecal/intraventricular: for leptomeningeal disease
- radical radiotherapy:
  - can be given to the entire brain and meninges, with good responses
  - when given post chemotherapy, it may improve response rates
- palliative radiotherapy: for frail, immunosuppressed, or elderly patients

Treatment for medulloblastoma and primitive neuroectodermal tumour

The treatment for medulloblastoma and primitive neuroectodermal tumour is debulking surgery and then radiotherapy to the whole neuroaxis. Trials of chemotherapy continue.

Treatment for ependymoma

The treatment for ependymoma is debulking surgery followed by radiotherapy, sometimes to the whole neuroaxis. The role of chemotherapy has not yet been established.

Treatment for pineal tumour and germ cell tumour

The treatment for pineal tumour and germ cell tumour is as follows:

- surgery is the treatment of choice for parenchymal tumours
- radiotherapy may be required but a biopsy is needed to confirm this; note that:
  - germ cell tumours are very radiosensitive
  - craniospinal axis radiotherapy may be necessary in patients with pineoblastoma and metastatic germ cell tumours
- chemotherapy: bleomycin, cisplatin, and etoposide are used for germ cell tumours

Treatment for brain metastasis

Treatment for brain metastasis includes:

- symptom control:
  - corticosteroids
  - anticonvulsants (if the patient presents with seizures)
- palliative whole-brain radiotherapy: the main aims of this are symptom control and reducing dependence on steroid use
- stereotactic radiotherapy can be considered if there are fewer than three small metastases
- surgery: can be considered in patients with solitary metastases and a good performance status if systemic disease is controlled; is usually followed by whole-brain radiotherapy
- systemic treatment: usually ineffective for the brain

Treatment for pituitary tumour and pituitary-related tumour

Medical treatment for pituitary tumours and pituitary-related tumours includes:

- hormone replacement therapy (in the case of hyposecretion)
- somatostatin analogues (for acromegaly; in the case of hypersecretion)
- carbergoline (for prolactinomas)
- surgery (to control tumour mass effect and manage hypersecretion)

Radiotherapy can be used to treat:

- patients who are unfit for surgery
- patients with regrowth post surgery
- patients who are young and have residual disease post surgery
- patients with persistent hypersecretion

Small functional tumours can be treated via stereotactic radiotherapy. Side effects include hypopituitarism, which requires lifelong hormone replacement.

Treatment for metastatic spinal cord compression

Analgesia is very important in the treatment of metastatic spinal cord compression. In addition, corticosteroids reduce oedema and thus may help improve neurological function. Definitive treatment should be commenced within 24 hours of confirmed diagnosis. Radiotherapy is usually the preferred choice, as many of the patients with spinal cord compression are poor surgical candidates, due to advanced disease or multiple vertebral involvement. Surgery may be indicated in selected patients.

Further Reading

Kleihues P, Burger PC, Bernd W, et al. The New WHO classification of brain tumours 1. *Brain Path* 1993 3: 255–68.

Louis DN, Ohgaki H, Wiestler OD, et al. The 2007 WHO classification of tumours of the central nervous system. *Acta Neuropathol* 2007; 114: 97–109.

Louis DN, Perry A, Reifenberger G, et al. The 2016 World Health Organisation classification of tumors of the central nervous system: a summary. *Acta Neuropathol* 2016; 131: 803–20.

Stupp R, Hegi ME, Mason WP, et al. Effects of radiotherapy with concomitant and adjuvant temozolomide versus radiotherapy alone on survival in glioblastoma in a randomised phase III study: 5-year analysis of the EORTC-NCIC trial. *Lancet Oncol* 2009; 10: 459–66

Weller M, Stupp R, and Wick W. Epilepsy meets cancer: When, why, and what to do about it? *Lancet Oncol* 2012; 13: e375–e382.

238 Non-metastatic neurological manifestations of malignancy

Nerissa Jordan

Definition of the disease

Neurological complications of systemic malignancy are frequent. They may reflect direct local effects of the tumour; CNS infection; side effects of chemotherapy or radiotherapy; nutritional or metabolic derangements; or a paraneoplastic syndrome.

The 'paraneoplastic' neurological syndromes are a group of disorders associated with a malignancy outside the nervous system. The pathophysiology is immune mediated, with the tumour's expression of neuronal proteins invoking antibody formation, which in turn results in neurological symptoms. This chapter will mainly focus on these syndromes.

Symptoms

There are several well-defined paraneoplastic syndromes with classical symptoms and signs that can affect the central and peripheral nervous systems, the neuromuscular junction, and muscle (see Table 238.1 for the most common syndromes and their associated malignancies). Important syndromes to recognize are described in this section.

Lambert–Eaton myasthenic syndrome

Lambert–Eaton myasthenic syndrome (LEMS) is a disorder of the presynaptic neuromuscular junction, presenting with weakness which is usually maximal in the proximal lower limbs. Associated autonomic dysfunction (dry mouth, erectile dysfunction, constipation, urinary dysfunction, postural hypotension) is common. Examination findings of weakness with reduced reflexes that increase with muscle exercise are characteristic. EMG also has a characteristic low-amplitude compound muscle action potential which increases with high-frequency stimulation and muscle exercise.

Limbic encephalitis

Symptoms of limbic encephalitis are subacute onset of seizures, confusion, and psychiatric disturbance suggesting involvement of the limbic system. MRI of the brain may show high signal in the limbic system, and inflammatory changes in the CSF.

Cerebellar degeneration

Cerebellar degeneration is the development of a progressive cerebellar syndrome affecting all areas of cerebellar function (trunk and limb ataxia, nystagmus, eye movement abnormalities, and dysarthria). There is significant disability within 12 weeks of onset, and minimal cerebellar atrophy on early imaging.

Opsoclonus myoclonus

Opsoclonus myoclonus consists of rapid, arrhythmic conjugate eye movements in multiple directions, also known as 'dancing eyes'. Patients also have myoclonus of the limbs and trunk, and gait ataxia, and encephalopathy may be part of the syndrome.

Stiff person syndrome

Stiff person syndrome is characterized by generalized stiffness which is predominantly in axial muscles, with associated painful cramps.

Table 238.1 Neurological paraneoplastic syndromes and their most commonly associated malignancies and antibodies

Clinical syndrome	Associated malignancy	Antibodies	Frequency paraneoplastic (%)
Lambert–Eaton myasthenic syndrome	SCLC	Anti-VGCC	60
Limbic encephalitis	SCLC Testicular Breast	Anti-Hu Anti-amphiphysin	20
Subacute cerebellar ataxia	Ovarian Breast SCLC Hodgkin's lymphoma	Anti-Yo Anti Hu Anti-Tr	50
Opsoclonus myoclonus	Breast Ovarian SCLC Neuroblastoma	Anti-Ri Anti-Hu	20
Stiff person syndrome	Breast SCLC	Anti-amphiphysin Anti-GAD	20
Sensory ganglionopathy	SCLC	Anti-Hu Anti-CV2 Anti-amphiphysin	20
Dermatomyositis	Ovarian SCLC	–	30

Abbreviations: GAD, glutamic acid decarboxylase; SCLC, small cell lung cancer; VGCC, voltage-gated calcium channel.

Spasms in response to environmental stimuli are common. Psychiatric symptoms are often coexistent, including anxiety and depression. There is continuous motor unit activity on EMG in the affected muscles at rest.

Sensory ganglionopathy

Sensory ganglionopathy is characterized by asymmetrical numbness, which is often preceded by pain and paraesthesia. Examination findings are of areflexia and sensory loss, particularly loss of proprioception. There is electrophysiological evidence of a sensory neuropathy at the level of the sensory ganglion.

Dermatomyositis

Dermatomyositis is an inflammatory myopathy with progressive symptoms of muscle pain and weakness, especially proximally. Associated skin lesions assist with diagnosis. A violaceous rash over the eyes (heliotrope rash), Gottron's papules, periungual telangiectasia, and rashes over the shoulders and neck ('V sign' and 'shawl sign', respectively) are characteristic.

Demographics and aetiology

Paraneoplastic disorders are rare. LEMS is the most common, occurring in approximately 1% of patients with small cell lung cancer. Adults are more commonly affected, due to the higher incidence of malignancy. There are several syndromes more classically seen in children, such as opsoclonus myoclonus associated with neuroblastoma.

The formation of antineuronal antibodies by the immune system is the proposed underlying mechanism; however, the evidence for direct pathogenesis of the antibodies has not been found in many cases. Some antibodies, however, such as those directed at the voltage-gated calcium channels in LEMS, are directly pathogenic. Cytotoxic T-cells have been detected in the nervous system and are likely to play a role.

Natural history of the disease

Paraneoplastic syndromes may present acutely or subacutely, and typically are progressive. They may occur in patients with an existing diagnosis of cancer, or present prior to the detection of the malignancy.

Complications

Complications of the paraneoplastic syndromes are typically those of the underlying cancer.

Approach to diagnosing the disease (including diagnostic pitfalls)

Identification of symptoms suggestive of a paraneoplastic syndrome should prompt a search for an underlying malignancy. Certain malignancies are associated with particular syndromes and antibodies (see Table 238.1).

The diagnosis of a paraneoplastic neurological syndrome relies upon clinical symptoms and examination findings in association with an appropriate antibody. Paraneoplastic antineuronal antibodies may be detected at low levels in patients with a malignancy but without symptoms of a paraneoplastic neurological syndrome. Care must, therefore, be taken in the interpretation of these tests, and they should only be performed in the appropriate clinical context. Similarly, not all patients with a particular syndrome will have malignancy; for example, the majority of cases of stiff person syndrome with antibodies against glutamic acid decarboxylase are not paraneoplastic.

Diagnostic criteria have been proposed, considering the syndrome, antibody, and detection of malignancy. Patients can then be classified into categories of definite and probable paraneoplastic disorders (see 'Further Reading').

Other diagnoses that should be considered

As paraneoplastic disorders are rare, a direct effect of malignancy or treatment is much more common and must be included in the differential diagnosis. This includes metastases that may be difficult to detect, such as leptomeningeal disease or plexus infiltration. Other causes of neurological symptoms associated with cancer should be considered. This includes side effects of cytotoxic medications or radiotherapy, and nutritionally related neurological syndromes. The clinical syndromes are not always associated with cancer (see Table 238.1 for approximate frequency), and alternative causes of the condition should be sought, for example postinfectious opsoclonus myoclonus in a young adult.

'Gold-standard' diagnostic test

There is no gold-standard diagnostic test for paraneoplastic disorders. The diagnosis is made utilizing both clinical features and test results. Anti-neuronal antibodies are specific when positive in a patient with symptoms of a well-defined paraneoplastic syndrome. The tests can be performed on both the serum and CSF.

Other relevant investigations

Relevant investigations to define the syndrome should be performed, such as MRI, lumbar puncture, and EMG. Investigations to detect an underlying malignancy should be performed if the syndrome occurs in a patient prior to the diagnosis of a tumour. This can be tailored towards the most likely malignancy in the setting of the syndrome, and can include tumour markers, imaging including CT of the chest, abdomen, and pelvis; PET, for PET-avid malignancy; mammography; and endoscopy.

Prognosis and how to estimate it

The prognosis is largely dependent on the effectiveness of treatment for the underlying malignancy. Those not associated with malignancy often have a benign course.

Treatment and its effectiveness

For paraneoplastic disorders, treatment is focused on detection of and therapy for the underlying malignancy. Immune therapies have been trialled in many of the syndromes, including plasma exchange, IV immunoglobulin, steroids, and immune modulators, with some success. Certain conditions have specific therapies available, such as 3,4-diaminopyridine for LEMS, to increase the release of acetylcholine. For systemic disorders, correction of metabolic abnormalities, such as hypercalcaemia, or nutritional replacement for Wernicke's encephalopathy, may improve the relevant symptoms.

Further Reading

Falah M, Schiff D, and Burns TM. Neuromuscular complications of cancer diagnosis and treatment. J Support Oncol 2005; 3: 271–82.

Graus F, Delattre JY, Antoine JC, et al. Recommended diagnostic criteria for paraneoplastic neurological syndromes. J Neurol Neurosurg Psychiatry 2004; 75: 1135–40.

Honnorat J and Antoine JC. Paraneoplastic neurological syndromes. Orphanet J Rare Dis 2007; 2: 22.

239 Neurosurgery

Erlick A. C. Pereira, Jonathan A. Hyam, and Alexander L. Green

Introduction

Neurosurgery encompasses brain, spine, and peripheral nerve disorders that may benefit from operative management. These include congenital neurological diseases, epilepsy, stroke, neurological infection, movement disorders, spinal cord disease, neurological tumours, and pituitary disorders. This chapter focuses upon head injury and subarachnoid haemorrhage (SAH), two common neurosurgical disorders not detailed elsewhere in this book.

Head injury

Definition of head injury

Skull or brain damage due to direct or deceleration trauma can be classified as primary (immediate injury) or secondary (from complications like hypoxia, seizures, infection, and hydrocephalus). Patients with head injury are stratified by their level of consciousness (as determined by the Glasgow Coma Scale (GCS); see Table 239.1) as having mild (GCS >13), moderate (GCS 9–13), or severe (GCS <9) injury.

Aetiology of head injury

Blunt or penetrating head injuries are commonly caused by road traffic accidents, especially unhelmeted activities, combat, contact sports, and falls. Falls and accidents may be secondary to a primary event such as a seizure, aneurysmal SAH (see 'SAH') or cardiac arrhythmia, necessitating a careful collateral history.

Typical symptoms of head injury, and less common symptoms

Symptoms of head injury include headache, nausea, vomiting, visual disturbance, deterioration in GCS, and limb weakness. Hypertension,

Table 239.1 The Glasgow Coma Scale	
Event	**Score**
Best Motor response	
Commands are obeyed	6
Localises to pain	5
Flexion withdraws from pain	4
Abnormal flexion to pain	3
Extension to pain	2
No response	1
Verbal response	
Alert and orientated	5
Confused	4
Inappropriate	3
Incomprehensible	2
No response	1
Eye opening occurs	
Spontaneously	4
In response to voice	3
On painful stimulation	2
No response	1

Reprinted from *The Lancet*, Volume 304, issue 7872, Graham Teasdale, Bryan Jennett, ASSESSMENT OF COMA AND IMPAIRED CONSCIOUSNESS A Practical Scale, pp. 81–84, Copyright (1974), with permission from Elsevier.

bradycardia, and altered respiratory rate (Cushing's response) are late signs of brainstem compression.

Demographics of head injury

Every year, over a million patients with head injuries present to UK emergency departments; 5000 of them die from the injuries, some inevitably but many from preventable causes. Road traffic accidents cause just a quarter of the total number of head injury cases but account for two-thirds of those ending in death, with half of such patients dying before they reach the hospital.

Natural history, and complications of head injury

Complications include epilepsy; 5% of head injury cases have early seizures, which occur mostly in the first 24 hours after the injury, and 5% have late seizures, which occur within a year of injury and are more commonly seen with intracranial haematoma or compound depressed skull fracture. CSF leak with consequent meningitis is a particular risk in the first week of injury. Postconcussional problems of headache, dizziness, irritability, poor concentration, fatigue, depression, altered hearing, and a reduced sense of smell all occur. Dementia (dementia pugilistica) is a long-term consequence of repeated head injury.

Approach to diagnosing head injury

Taking a history and a collateral history regarding the mechanism of injury are vital. For traffic accidents, speed at impact, whether a seatbelt or helmet was used, details of the extrication, the state of the vehicle, and the fate of other victims are all relevant. After ensuring airways, breathing, and circulation, assess GCS, pupil size, equality and reactivity to light, and other signs of raised intracranial pressure, such as papilloedema. Assess limb movements and cranial nerves, in particular eye movements and, in the comatose, gag, cough, and corneal reflexes. For a penetrating injury, object/missile type and distance are important.

Inspect scalp lacerations for underlying skull fractures before considering closure.

Assess for evidence of basal skull fracture (e.g. raccoon's eyes (periorbital ecchymoses), Battle's sign (postauricular ecchymoses), CSF rhinorrhoea/otorrhea, haemotympanum). Examine for facial fractures, including an inspection for orbital rim step-off, and palpation for Le Fort fractures. Auscultate the carotids and eyes for bruits suggestive of dissection or carotid–cavernous fistula. Examine the cervical spine for tenderness or step deformity.

Clarify whether there is loss of consciousness, anterograde amnesia, persisting neurological deficit, vomiting, or visual disturbance. All justify CT head. Have a particularly low threshold for radiological investigation of a child or an elderly patient.

Other diagnoses that should be considered aside from head injury

Other diagnoses that should be considered aside from head injury include cervical spine injury, alcohol or recreational drug intoxication, and primary causes of secondary head injury (e.g. syncope, primary cardiac arrhythmias, primary seizure disorder).

'Gold-standard' diagnostic test for head injury

CT head scan is indicated if there is suspicion of a significant mechanism of injury or if there is a persisting deficit, amnesia, or vomiting, all of which are very established signs (see Table 239.2). CT cervical spine should similarly be performed. Fine-cut CT facial or skull-base/temporal bone views should be considered if such injuries are suspected.

Table 239.2 UK National Institute for Health and Care Excellence criteria for CT imaging in head injury; Comparison with observations of serious sequelae of head injury by Celsus, ancient Greek philosopher

NICE	Celsus
GCS <13 on initial hospital assessment	'Whether he has lain senseless as if asleep'
GCS <15 at 2 h after injury	'The mind wanders'
	'Stupor'
Any sign of basal skull fracture	'Bleeding from the nose or ears'
More than one episode of vomiting in adults; three or more episodes of vomiting in children	'Bilious vomiting'
Post-traumatic seizure	'Spasm'
Focal neurological deficit	'Obscurity of vision'
	'He has become speechless'
	'Paralysis'
Suspected open or depressed skull fracture	Not documented
Suspected or proven coagulopathy in context of loss of consciousness or amnesia	Not documented

Abbreviations: GCS, Glasgow Coma Scale.

Reprinted from *The Lancet*, Volume 373, issue 9675, Hyam JA, Green AL, Aziz TZ, NICE head injury guidelines pre-empted two millennia ago., pp. 1605–6, Copyright (2009), with permission from Elsevier.

Acceptable diagnostic alternatives to the gold-standard test for head injury

Skull radiographs are no longer considered adequate to exclude most intracranial injuries, and few hospitals lack a CT scanner. Cervical spine radiographs continue to be useful where the mechanism of injury is less worrisome but the patient presents with bony tenderness or step deformity.

Other relevant investigations for head injury

Other relevant investigations for head injury include the following:

- a full blood count
- clotting
- serum glucose
- electrolytes, including sodium, to assess for hyponatraemia
- anticonvulsant drug levels
- serum alcohol or drug level, if the patient is intoxicated
- CSF beta transferrin if there is suspicion of CSF otorrhoea/rhinorrhoea without imaging evidence

Prognosis for head injury, and how to estimate it

Head injuries are broadly classified radiologically as diffuse or focal, with the latter including contrecoup contusions, subdural haematomas, and extradural haematomas (see Figure 239.1A–C). In patients with a recent deterioration in conscious level and/or large subdural or extradural haematomas with mass effect and/or hydrocephalus or subfalcine herniation, urgent neurosurgery is indicated. Contraindications to surgery include fixed, dilated pupils unresponsive to medical measures; coagulopathies; and when a significant amount of time has passed since observation of a mass effect (more than several hours) in patients with comorbidities. Prognosis after craniotomy in the elderly (>75 years old) is poor, with high morbidity and mortality. In patients with focal deficits and/or reduced GCS, prognosis is improved by close neurological observation and expedient consideration of transfer to specialist neurosurgical care. A quarter of patients in coma with severe head injury die within 6 months. Most recovery occurs within 6 months of severe head injury, augmented by occupational and physical therapy; <2% enter a persistent vegetative state which, if it persists for more than 3 months, makes dependency inevitable. Table 239.3 correlates GCS with clinical outcome.

Treatment of head injury, and its effectiveness

Correct hypoxia, hypovolaemia, and suture skull lacerations once depressed skull fractures are excluded. Anticonvulsants should be administered if seizures occur. Intracranial pressure (ICP) should be monitored in the intubated and ventilated patient with severe head injury, and cerebral perfusion pressure maintained > 65 (cerebral perfusion pressure = mean arterial pressure − ICP). Raised ICP can be managed by diuretics such as mannitol and furosemide, hypertonic saline, barbiturate boluses, and controlled hypocapnia (partial pressure of CO_2 = 4.0–4.5). There is little convincing evidence for high-dose steroids for elevated ICP or for the use of prophylactic antibiotics in a CSF leak without meningitis in improving outcome in head injury. Space-occupying haematomas require urgent neurosurgical evacuation, with life-saving outcomes.

SAH

Definition of SAH

SAH is bleeding from intracranial vessels in the subdural space between the overlying arachnoid membrane and the underlying pia mater, usually involving vascular anastomoses of the circle of Willis and its branches (Figure 239.1D).

Aetiology of SAH

Rupture of one or more saccular aneurysms accounts for three-quarters of SAH cases. Arteriovenous malformations cause 5% of cases, and coagulopathies, vasculitis, and neoplasia cause <5% of cases, with the remaining 15% of cases being of unknown aetiology. Atherosclerosis, hypertension, smoking, pregnancy, oral contraceptive pill use, and polycystic kidney disease are identified associations.

Typical symptoms of SAH, and less common symptoms

Symptom severity is proportional to haemorrhage severity. The classic symptom is sudden-onset, severe headache, which is often bilateral and usually occipital, with the patient feeling as if they have been hit on the back of the head. Nausea and vomiting are common. Neck stiffness and photophobia are not unusual, with meningeal irritation, developing a few hours after the event. Seizures, focal neurological deficits, and a reduction in conscious level may be seen with more severe SAH. A mild headache may represent a warning/herald/sentinel bleed before a major bleed. Cranial nerve palsies may be seen, for example oculomotor nerve palsy due to irritation and compression after rupture of a posterior communicating artery aneurysm. Fundoscopy may reveal papilloedema and also vitreous haemorrhages in 10% of patients (Turson's syndrome), again correlated with bleed severity. Mild pyrexia and reactive hypertension may be observed.

Demographics of SAH

SAH has an annual UK incidence of 10–15 per 100 000. Saccular cerebral aneurysms are present in 2% of autopsies, with aneurysmal rupture occurring in 6–8 per 100 000 people per year. Male:female ratios are 2:3 overall, but SAH is more likely to occur in males >40 years of age. Aneurysmal SAH has some hereditary basis and is more common in Finland and Japan.

Natural history of SAH, and complications of the disease

Overall mortality from aneurysmal SAH is close to 50%; 10%–15% of people die before reaching hospital, and a further 10% within a few days of onset. Rebleeding is a major risk, at 15%–20% within 2 weeks of the first bleed. Other complications are vasospasm, which often presents with focal deficit and is of highest risk 4–10 days after first bleed, and hydrocephalus, which usually manifests as headaches that are worse on waking and lying flat, together with other signs of raised ICP (e.g. nausea, vomiting, Parinaud's phenomenon). One-third of SAHs occur during sleep, and some evidence suggests there is a higher risk of SAH in spring and autumn.

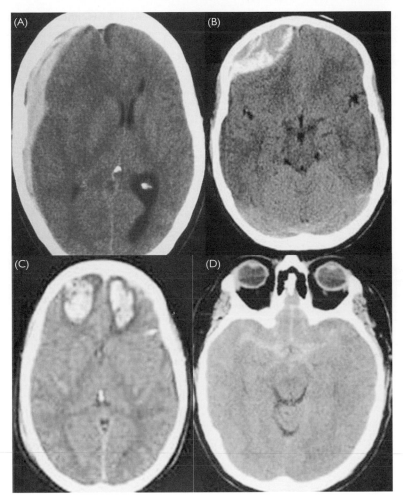

Figure 239.1 (A) 'Crescenteric' acute subdural haematoma. (B) 'Lenticular' acute extradural haematoma. (C) Contrecoup bifrontal contusions. (D) Subarachnoid haemorrhage.

Approach to diagnosing SAH

A history, together with symptoms and signs suggestive of SAI I, should encourage close neurological observations and urgent, unenhanced CT head. If no subarachnoid blood is seen on CT head imaging, confirming safety for lumbar puncture, a lumbar puncture should be performed between 12 hours and 2 weeks after the event and

assessed both for red blood cell count, in the first and third samples, and for xanthochromia, in the second sample. Oxyhaemoglobin and bilirubin content suggestive of or unable to exclude SAH determine its empirical treatment and transfer to a neurosurgical centre for cerebral angiography to find and treat any ruptured aneurysm or arteriovenous malformation.

Other diagnoses that should be considered aside from SAH

Other diagnoses that should be considered aside from SAH include migraine, cluster headache, benign coital and exertional headache syndromes, meningitis (bacterial and viral), stroke, alcohol intoxication, and head injury.

'Gold-standard' diagnostic test for SAH

Lumbar puncture 12 hours to 2 weeks after the event, for xanthochromia, is an extremely sensitive test for excluding SAH. Digital subtraction angiography is the gold standard for identifying intracerebral aneurysms. If intracranial blood extravasation obscures image clarity, repeat delayed angiography is indicated.

Acceptable diagnostic alternatives to the gold-standard test for SAH

Urgent CT head is the first line of investigation for suspected SAH. MRI is similarly sensitive. Should neither reveal blood, then lumbar puncture is indicated. Should lumbar puncture have been performed

Table 239.3 Glasgow Outcome Score, correlated with severity of head injury

During hospital admission	Poor outcome (dependent for care; GOS 1–3)	Favourable outcome (independent; GOS 4–6)
Coma >6 hours duration	61%	39%
Best GCS >11	18%	82%
Best GCS 8–10	32%	68%
Best GCS <8	73%	27%
Pupils reacting to light	50%	50%
Pupils unreactive to light	96%	4%
Age <20 years	41%	59%
Age >60 years	94%	6%

Abbreviations: GCS, Glasgow Coma Score; GOS, Glasgow Outcome Score.

Reproduced with permission from B. Jennett, Prognosis in Patients With Severe Head Injury, *Neurosurgery*, Volume 4, Issue 4, pp. 283–9, Copyright © 1979 Springer.

too early, late, more than once, or be equivocal in its results, then clinical suspicion should guide any decision to proceed to CT angiography or digital subtraction angiography.

Other relevant investigations for SAH

Other relevant investigations for SAH include:

- a full blood count
- a coagulation profile
- electrolytes, including sodium, for hyponatraemia
- ECG (T-wave changes sometimes seen)
- liver function tests
- chest X-ray (pulmonary oedema sometimes seen)
- close temperature and blood pressure monitoring
- ophthalmological investigations, if cranial nerve palsies are present

Prognosis for SAH, and how to estimate it

SAH can be graded by clinical severity (Table 239.4); clinical severity at presentation correlates with prognosis. Blood load on CT is also correlated with outcome.

Table 239.4 World Federation of Neurological Surgeons grading system for subarachnoid haemorrhage

Grade	GCS	Aphasia or hemiparesis
0	Unruptured aneurysm	No
1	15	No
2	13–14	No
3	13–14	Yes
4	7–12	Maybe
5	3–6	Maybe

Abbreviations: GCS, Glasgow Coma Score.
World Federation of Neurological Surgeons grading system for SAH.

Treatment of SAH, and its effectiveness

Best practice for SAH treatment is now considered to be early coiling or clipping of any ruptured aneurysm, to reduce the risk of rebleeding. Aneurysms amenable to coiling are managed accordingly. Clipping is usually reserved for complex aneurysms not readily amenable to coiling, or if there is an intra-cerebral haematoma which requires evacuation. Some still advocate late (after 10 days) over early clipping, as the brain is then less swollen, and the risk of vasospasm is reduced. Medical management includes analgesia; laxatives; anti-emetics; anticonvulsants, if required; aggressive hydration with 125 ml of normal saline per hour; close observation, including daily serum electrolytes to observe for hyponatraemia; administration of nimodipine 60 mg every 4 hours for 21 days post event; and ICP monitoring, if the patient is sedated. Early, aggressive treatment of suspected vasospasm is via IV fluid boluses, inotropes, and consideration of chemical angioplasty and emergent treatment of hydrocephalus by external ventricular drainage, lumbar drainage, or serial lumbar punctures. Limited evidence exists for use of statins to improve clinical outcomes. All patients with proven SAH should be investigated and managed in a neurosurgical centre; 85%–90% of people survive 5 years after coiling or clipping of a ruptured aneurysm, versus >50% mortality without initial treatment.

Further Reading

National Institute for Health and Care Excellence. *Head Injury: Assessment and Early Management.* 2014. Available at https://www.nice.org.uk/Guidance/CG176 (accessed 14 Jul 2017).

Serrone JC, Maekawa H, Tjahjadi M, et al. Aneurysmal subarachnoid haemorrhage: Pathobiology, current treatment. *Expert Rev Neurother* 2015; 15: 367–80.

Spetzler RF, McDougall CG, Zabramski JM, et al. The Barrow Ruptured Aneurysm Trial: 6-year results. *J Neurosurg* 2015; 123: 609–17.

240 Drug-induced neurological disease

Robin Ferner and Anthony Cox

Definition of the disease

The definition of an adverse drug reaction is 'an appreciably harmful or unpleasant reaction, resulting from an intervention related to the use of a medicinal product; adverse effects usually predict hazard from future administration and warrant prevention, or specific treatment, or alteration of the dosage regimen, or withdrawal of the product' (Aronson and Ferner, 2005, p. 851).

Scope of drug-induced neurological disorders

Adverse drug reactions can cause or contribute to central and peripheral nervous system disorders, including traumatic, infective, neoplastic, demyelinating, and vascular diseases.

Diagnosis of drug-induced disease

It can be difficult to differentiate adverse drug reactions from natural disease. The crucial diagnostic tools are a thorough drug history and a good database of potential adverse drug reactions (the *British National Formulary* is the obvious starting point). Features that are said to suggest a drug cause are:

- **challenge:** the condition started after treatment with the drug, or after a dose increase—but this ignores the possibility of disease aggravation
- **dechallenge:** the condition remitted after the drug was stopped—but this does not apply to irreversible adverse drug reactions (e.g. fatal adverse drug reactions)
- **rechallenge:** the condition recurs on re-exposure to the drug—but physicians would generally be foolish to re-expose patients to drugs that caused significant adverse drug reactions merely to make the diagnosis
- **drug specificity:** the observed condition is known to occur with the drug but is not a feature of the disease being treated—but this is only useful for well-recognized adverse effects, and well-characterized diseases.

It may be more useful to analyse reactions by '**DoTS**':

- **Do**se relation (did the adverse event occur at very low doses, very high doses, or standard therapeutic doses?)
- **T**iming of the reaction in relation to the start of treatment
- **S**usceptibility of the individual

A major challenge is to identify unknown adverse drug reactions in newly marketed drugs. Pre-marketing clinical trials cannot detect rare, yet important, adverse drug effects. This challenge is met in part by collecting data on suspicions of adverse drug reactions. In the UK, this is done via the Medicines and Healthcare Products Regulatory Agency (MHRA) Yellow Card Scheme (see http://yellowcard.mhra.gov.uk), which encourages reports from healthcare professionals and patients.

Drug-induced diseases of the CNS

Drug-induced unconsciousness

The differential diagnosis of patients admitted in an unconscious state should include drug-induced coma. In practice, common causes are opiates, GABA agonists of various sorts, and tricyclic antidepressants in deliberate overdose or as a result of error.

The clinical signs can help in differential diagnosis: pinpoint pupils and respiratory depression reversed by naloxone are the hallmarks of opiate intoxication; dilated pupils, tachycardia, and hyperreflexia are usual in tricyclic overdose. The GABA agonists include benzodiazepines, alcohol, and barbiturates, as well as the street drug gamma-hydroxybutyric acid. They tend to cause bradycardia and respiratory depression, and there may be nystagmus. Flumazenil is a specific antagonist of the effects of benzodiazepines. In addition to these, the street drug ketamine, an antagonist of the excitatory neurotransmitter glutamic acid, can cause rapid unconsciousness and seizures, with tachycardia and hypertension.

Important secondary causes include haemorrhage related to anticoagulants and hypoglycaemia, usually due to insulin or sulfonylureas.

Stroke

Young women who take the oral contraceptive pill are at increased risk of stroke, although the absolute risk is small. The threefold relative risk becomes much more significant in women with other risk factors, such as cigarette smoking, hypertension, and increasing age, and is more important with pills containing a high oestrogen dose. The risk is also significantly increased in postmenopausal women taking hormone-replacement therapy. Although the increase in relative risk is smaller, because the deleterious effects on thrombogenesis are partly balanced by favourable effects on lipids, the absolute increase in risk is still important. Tranexamic acid, used to treat menorrhagia, is an antifibrinolytic, and as a result, increases stroke risk. Stroke has also been associated with phenylpropanolamine, which is present in some cough and cold remedies in some countries.

Stroke is an important consequence of cocaine abuse, and may either be haemorrhagic, due to rupture of a preexisting intracranial aneurysm, or thrombotic, as a result of vasospasm. The effects are a consequence of the indirect sympathomimetic action of cocaine, which can cause sudden and extreme hypertension and vasospasm.

Drug-induced encephalitis and meningitis

Drugs derived from human tissue can introduce CNS infection. Human growth hormone derived from human pituitaries led to an outbreak of the fatal prion encephalopathy Creutzfeldt–Jakob disease in the 1980s.

Immune suppression, for example with high-dose corticosteroids, can increase the risks of tuberculous meningitis and virus encephalitis. In immune-suppressed patients, exposure to chickenpox can have a fatal outcome or cause irreversible brain damage. More recently, reactivation of the JC (for John Cunningham, the initial patient) polyomavirus has been recognized as a cause of the rare condition progressive multifocal leucoencephalopathy in patients treated with monoclonal antibodies, including natalizumab (for multiple sclerosis), infliximab, and rituximab. This demyelinating disease results from lytic infection of the oligodendrocytes, which produce myelin. It characteristically presents with the triad of progressive dementia, hemiparesis, and hemianopia.

Platinum compounds and other anticancer agents, as well as interferons and some other drugs, can cause a non-infective encephalopathy (see Table 240.1). Fluorouracil and its prodrug capecitabine can provoke patchy widespread demyelination. High-dose chemotherapy, for example with cisplatin, is a recognized cause of posterior reversible encephalopathy syndrome (PRES). The clinical features are headache, altered mental state, visual disturbance that can include cortical blindness, and tonic–clonic seizures. These are accompanied by symmetrical posterior cerebral and cerebellar white matter abnormalities on CT and MRI. PRES can be fatal, but less severe cases usually resolve after removal of the cause.

Aseptic meningitis presents with symptoms of headache and fever and signs of neck stiffness indistinguishable from infective meningitis. No organism can be cultured. The CSF can show an increase in

Table 240.1 Drug-induced encephalopathy

Common causes	Clinical features	Dose relation, time, susceptibilities
Antivirals: aciclovir	Aciclovir-induced encephalopathy in patients with renal failure resolves with haemodialysis	Usually within a few days High doses IV use Renal impairment Old age
Ciclosporin	Seizures and movement disorders occur	High doses Concurrent corticosteroids Hypomagnesaemia Systemic hypertension
Cisplatin Ifosfamide	Confusion Stupor Mutism Secondary to cerebral oedema	Renal impairment Hepatic impairment
Sodium valproate	Confusion Reduced consciousness Coma Associated with hyperammonaemia	Dose related

polymorphonuclear leucocytes or other cells, and in protein; glucose concentration is usually normal. Some drugs probably cause direct meningeal irritation. Type III delayed-type immunological hypersensitivity reaction can occur either by direct introduction into the CSF, or by crossing the blood–brain barrier. Some drug causes are listed (see Table 240.2). Even though they cause the reaction very rarely, NSAIDs are widely used and so constitute the commonest cause. The association is a potential source of confusion, as the analgesics are often taken for headache, which is an expected feature of meningitis. Patients with SLE seem to be especially susceptible, although this is hard to demonstrate, as aseptic meningitis can occur in SLE without a drug cause. Aseptic meningitis was also associated with the Urabe strain of mumps in a measles, mumps, rubella (MMR) vaccine withdrawn in 1992.

Drug-induced headache

Drug-induced headache is common, with up to 8% of headaches associated with drugs. Vasodilators, including calcium antagonists, nitrates, and hydralazine, cause the expected throbbing headache. Many patients develop the headache within an hour or two after taking standard-release calcium antagonists, when the peak plasma concentration occurs. Nitrate headache begins as soon as the nitrate is absorbed, and absorption is rapid with sublingual administration. It abates within several minutes after acute exposure, and after hours with continued exposure. However, asymmetric dosing regimens designed to reduce tachyphylaxis to the anti-anginal effect may also perpetuate the headache. Sildenafil, which inhibits nitric oxide

metabolism by phosphodiesterase type 5, can itself cause headache and can exacerbate nitrate-induced headache.

Intracranial hypertension ('pseudotumor cerebri') causes a characteristic headache that is worse with straining and on lying down, and so occurs typically after a night's sleep. The papilloedema that develops can lead to visual loss from pressure on the optic nerve. It is a recognized adverse effect of vitamin A and its derivatives, including isotretinoin and other retinoids, having been recognized in polar explorers who ate polar bear liver (which is rich in vitamin A). It may also occur with antibiotics (tetracyclines, penicillins, and nalidixic acid) and oestrogens.

'Medication-overuse headache' is a chronic headache occurring in patients with preexisting acute headache, usually migraine. In the condition, headaches occur on at least 15 days a month, in patients who have taken analgesics, ergot alkaloids, or triptans on more than 10 days each month for more than 3 months. Patients may develop a new type of headache, or their preexisting headache may be made markedly worse during overuse. Most sufferers are women. Treatment is to withdraw the medicines, but this is sometimes difficult, as the headache at first becomes worse and can persist for some months. The condition is common and under-diagnosed.

Seizures

Drugs can cause seizures by direct effects on the brain or neurotransmission (see Table 240.3) or secondarily to metabolic disturbances such as hyponatraemia (e.g. due to diuretics, antipsychotics, or selective serotonin-reuptake inhibitors), hypomagnesaemia (e.g. due to cisplatin or to proton-pump inhibitors), and hypoglycaemia (e.g. from anti-diabetic drugs).

Many drugs, even benzylpenicillin, can cause seizures at toxic doses. It is thought that the beta-lactam ring in penicillin binds to receptors for GABA, an inhibitory neurotransmitter. Tricyclic-antidepressant poisoning is commonly associated with seizures, at least in part as a result of central anti-cholinergic effects: other anti-cholinergic compounds (such as procyclidine) can also provoke seizures. The smoking cessation treatment bupropion causes seizures in 1 in 1000 patients, and the risk is increased in those with a prior history of seizures. Theophylline, another well-recognized cause of seizures in overdose, antagonizes the effects of adenosine, which is an inhibitory neurotransmitter. Local anaesthetic drugs, formerly used as anti-arrhythmics, cause seizures as a toxic effect related to blockade of sodium channels.

GABA agonists (e.g. alcohol, benzodiazepines, barbiturates) and antiepileptic drugs can provoke seizures on withdrawal.

CNS disturbance by drugs used to treat Parkinson's disease

'Punding'—from a Swedish slang term for the behaviour of amphetamine abusers—describes repetitive and often complex, purposeless, stereotyped behaviour: for example, arranging and rearranging coins in piles of different denominations. It is now recognized as part of a wider group of compulsive behaviours in patients treated with dopamine or dopamine agonists and who may also exhibit compulsive

Table 240.2 Drug-induced aseptic meningitis

Common causes	Clinical features	Dose relation, time, susceptibilities
Antibiotics; co-trimoxazole (sulfamethoxazole + trimethoprim) most common	Uncertain mechanism Excess mononuclear or polymorphonuclear cells in CSF	SLE HIV Sjögren's syndrome Crohn's disease
Cytarabine	Also associated with cerebellar dysfunction	
Immunoglobulins	Affects 1%–15% of those treated with high doses Inflammatory/immune mechanism	Usually within 2 days High dose History of migraine
Infliximab	Focal neurological deficit Loss of consciousness	Repeated administration
NSAIDs	Hypersensitivity Immune complexes and intrathecal IgG detected	Usually rapid onset SLE Prior history of aseptic meningitis

Table 240.3 Drug-induced seizures

Common causes	Clinical features	Dose relation, time, susceptibilities
Antipsychotic drugs	Reduced seizure threshold	SLE
Antidepressants (especially tricyclic antidepressants)	Direct seizure effect (especially tricyclic antidepressants)	Common in overdose Sudden doses changes or abrupt withdrawals
Antibiotics: penicillins and other beta-lactams; quinolones, isoniazid	Direct toxic effect	Large doses Intrathecal use
Carbamazepine	Can paradoxically increase seizure activity	High doses
Lidocaine	Partial and generalized tonic–clonic seizures Can occur with topical use of large amounts	Prior history of seizures High doses
Pethidine (meperidine)	Due to the norpethidine metabolite	High doses Renal failure
Theophylline	Generalized tonic–clonic seizures	High doses Co-prescription with cytochrome P450 isoenzyme inhibitors, especially macrolide antibiotics
Tramadol	Under 1% of users	Prolonged prescription Age 25–54 Alcohol abuse
Drugs of abuse: cocaine, ecstasy, amphetamines	May also cause haemorrhagic or thrombotic stroke	

gambling and compulsive sexual behaviour. Direct dopamine agonists, that is, ropinirole, pramipexole, and the ergot derivatives, can induce catalepsy and narcolepsy. These drugs induce 'sleep attacks' of sudden onset and are, therefore, potentially dangerous in drivers.

Spinal cord disease

Myodil® (Pantopaque™ in North America: ethyl-iodophenyl undecanoate), used as a radiocontrast medium for myelography from the 1940s to the 1970s, was an oily suspension that remained in the spinal canal and, in a minority of patients, caused a painful and sometimes disabling arachnoiditis with spinal cord damage. The contrast medium can still be seen on plain radiographs many years after injection. Its effects evolve slowly and are long-lasting.

Drug use in pregnancy carries the risk of neurological damage to the developing fetus. The rate of neural tube defects (spina bifida) is doubled in the offspring of women taking sodium valproate in pregnancy. Folate supplementation, particularly if commenced prior to conception, may reduce the risk.

Medication errors are an important cause of potentially preventable harm. Some are so egregious that they have been labelled 'never events'—events that should never be allowed to occur—by the UK National Health Service. One of these 'never events' is the intrathecal injection of the anticancer drug vincristine, usually in patients who were intended to receive intrathecal methotrexate and IV vincristine and in whom the routes of administration have been reversed. Vincristine causes a rapidly evolving, painful, and usually fatal arachnoiditis.

A more unexpected danger to the spinal cord is nitrous oxide, which is prone to abuse and which can lead to progressive ascending numbness in the legs and sometimes the arms, accompanied by loss of power and proprioception. These are the features of subacute combined degeneration of the spinal cord, a condition usually associated with vitamin B_{12} deficiency. While cord damage is commoner with prolonged or repeated inhalation, it has been reported after a single short exposure to nitrous oxide anaesthesia in the presence of vitamin B_{12} deficiency.

Peripheral neuropathy

Peripheral neuropathy can be due to damage to nerve cell bodies (neuronopathy), axons, or myelin. Symptoms can include pain, sensory loss, paraesthesia, and weakness, alone or in combination. Loss of proprioception can result in an abnormal gait.

Many drug-induced neuropathies are mixed, but pure types are sometimes found. Prolonged megadose therapy with vitamin B_6 (pyridoxine), at one time advocated for premenstrual tension, can cause a progressive neuropathy with sensory ataxia, loss of vibration sense, and paraesthesia. This is due to a direct and potentially reversible effect on cell bodies in the dorsal root ganglia.

Other causes include the antibiotics metronidazole and nitrofurantoin, the antituberculous drug isoniazid, and the antiarrhythmic amiodarone (see Table 240.4). Preexisting conditions such as diabetes mellitus, alcoholism, and vitamin deficiency, and impaired drug clearance, contribute to the risk. Nerve damage is a common adverse effect of cancer chemotherapy, occurring in over 20% of treated patients. Factors that increase the risk of chemotherapy-induced peripheral neuropathy include the cumulative chemotherapy dose, the administration of high single doses, rapid infusion times, and previous or concurrent use of neurotoxic drugs.

Vincristine is a common and important cause of peripheral neuropathy, which is often dose-limiting. Loss of deep tendon reflexes is an early sign and, while sensory changes precede motor changes,

Table 240.4 Drug-induced neuropathies

Common causes	Clinical features	Dose relation, time, susceptibilities
Amiodarone	Sensorimotor neuropathy Absent tendon reflexes Sensory ataxia	Reversible in some cases
Antiretrovirals	Needs to be distinguished from HIV-associated neuropathy	Low CD4 count
Cisplatin	Mainly sensory neuropathy, painful paraesthesia, and dysaesthesia	Cumulative dose
Ethambutol	Loss of visual acuity and visual field Colour blindness	Advanced age Renal insufficiency Diabetes
Isoniazid	Sensorimotor neuropathy	Slow acetylator status Pyridoxine deficiency
Metronidazole	Sensory axonal degeneration	Prolonged use High doses
Pyridoxine (vitamin B_6)	Paradoxical sensory neuropathy	High dose Long-term use
Statins	Rare Sensory axonal neuropathy	Prior history of neuropathy with a statin
Vincristine	Sensory neuropathy precedes motor neuropathy	High cumulative dose

sensory and motor neuropathies can coexist. Vincristine and other vinca alkaloids inhibit microtubular function, and this blocks axonal transport so that axons degenerate. Thalidomide, now used in the treatment of multiple myeloma, causes treatment-limiting peripheral neuropathy.

Demyelinating polyneuropathy and ascending paralysis with increased CSF protein concentration but without an increase in cells ('dissociation cyto-albuminique'), is the hallmark of Guillain–Barré syndrome, a delayed-type hypersensitivity disorder. It has been reported with gold, corticosteroids, penicillamine, and captopril. An outbreak of Guillain–Barré syndrome was attributed to swine influenza immunization in the United States. The attribution has been questioned. The cytotoxic T-lymphocyte antigen-4 checkpoint inhibitor ipilimumab, used to treat metastatic myeloma, can induce several autoimmune-related neurological adverse effects, including Guillain-Barré syndrome, a myaesthenia gravis-like condition, and an encephalitis.

Drug-induced movement disorders

Akathisia (motor restlessness) is a common adverse effect of phenothiazines and other rapidly acting dopamine antagonists given either for nausea or as antipsychotic medicines. In younger people, acute dopamine blockade can cause acute dystonic reactions, which are manifest as apparently bizarre hyperextension of the neck and trunk, with oculogyric crisis (upward rolling of the eyes). For this reason, the use of metoclopramide, prochlorperazine, and other dopamine antagonists should be avoided in children and young adults. The treatment for acute dystonic reactions, should they occur, is to administer a parenteral anti-cholinergic agent, such as procyclidine. In older adults, the same agents can cause parkinsonism. While this usually requires repeated administration, it can occur after a single dose. Anti-cholinergic agents were once prescribed as prophylaxis to patients treated with antipsychotic dopamine antagonists such as chlorpromazine and haloperidol, but are now reserved for treatment of overt parkinsonism.

If antidopaminergic treatment is continued over many years, patients can develop 'tardive dyskinesia', that is, abnormal involuntary movements, especially of the lips, face, and tongue. Unconscious chewing, sucking, and tongue protrusion are characteristic. The condition is commoner in older patients, perhaps because the duration of treatment has been longer; in women; and in those who have suffered from drug-induced parkinsonism. Tardive dyskinesia can persist after drug withdrawal.

Conclusion

Drug-induced disorders can affect the central, spinal, and peripheral nervous systems and their integration. They can be manifest as almost any neurological pathology, including infective, immunological, and thrombotic. The diagnosis rests on a careful and complete drug history supplemented by clinical examination and investigation, and by literature review. Treatment is primarily removal of the suspected drug. New, unusual, or serious reactions should be reported directly to MHRA via the Yellow Card Scheme.

Further Reading

Aronson JK. *Meyler's Side Effects of Drugs* (15th edition), 2006. Elsevier.

Aronson JK and Ferner RE. Clarification of Terminology in Drug Safety. *Drug Safety* 2005; 28(10): 851–70.

Butt T and Evans B. Drug-induced headache. *Adverse Drug React Bull* 2006; 240: 919–22.

Coleman JJ. Drug-induced seizures. *Adverse Drug React Bull* 2004; 227: 1–4.

Davies DM, Ferner RE, and de Glanville H. *Davies's Textbook of Adverse Drug Reactions* (5th edition), 1998. Hodder Arnold.

Jain KK. *Drug-Induced Neurological Disorders*, 1996. Hogrefe and Huber.

National Institute for Health and Clinical Excellence. *Headaches in over 12s: Diagnosis and Management*. 2012. Available at https://www.nice.org.uk/Guidance/CG150 (accessed 5 Sept 2017).

241 Functional and dissociative disorders in neurology

Jon Stone and Alan Carson

Definition of the disease

In this chapter, the focus is on patients who present with physical symptoms, such as weakness, or seizures, which can be positively identified as inconsistent with pathological diseases. These are called functional and dissociative neurological symptoms, although there are many other terms used, such as conversion disorder, psychogenic symptoms, somatization, hysterical symptoms, medically unexplained symptoms, non-organic symptoms, and pseudoseizures, to name a few.

Aetiology of the disease

The aetiology of functional and dissociative symptoms remains uncertain but is likely to be multifactorial. Studies consistently find emotional disorders in a proportion of patients, but not all of them. Likewise, the frequency of previous adverse life events (both childhood and recent) is higher in these patients than in matched disease controls, but many patients have no such history. Such features cannot be relied upon in making or excluding a functional diagnosis. Patients with weakness may develop their symptoms suddenly during an attack with features of panic or after a triggering event such as physical injury, or more gradually, in the context of fatigue. The prodromal symptomatology of dissociative seizures is often similar to that of panic attacks. Illness beliefs and iatrogenesis are important maintaining factors but the role of 'secondary gain' appears overestimated. Neurological disease itself is an important risk factor. Although these symptoms are traditionally conceived in purely psychological terms, there is a growing amount of literature on functional imaging and neural correlates.

Typical symptoms of the disease

Functional weakness typically presents with unilateral weakness or heaviness of limbs, although any pattern in the limbs may occur. Functional sensory symptoms are often hemisensory, and patients feel 'split in half'. Functional movement disorders include tremors, spasms, contractures, and jerks. Other functional symptoms include dysphonia, visual impairment, memory loss, and difficulty swallowing (globus).

Dissociation is a common accompaniment to many functional neurological symptoms, especially when acute, and is worth directly enquiring about if not volunteered. Depersonalization is a feeling of being disconnected from one's own body. Derealization is a feeling of disconnection from one's surroundings. Dissociative seizures involve an apparent alteration of consciousness, often preceded by dissociative or panic symptoms. Patients typically either display thrashing, large amplitude, sinusoidal movements (~70%) or lie motionless (~30%). Sudden, prolonged, motionless unresponsiveness does not occur in epilepsy and (apart from cardiac arrest) is almost pathognomonic of dissociative attacks.

Demographics of the disease

The female:male ratio for most functional neurological symptoms is 3:1, except for movement disorders, in which case it is 1:1. Functional weakness has a minimum incidence of 5 in 100 000 per year, like multiple sclerosis, with mean onset in the mid-thirties. Patients may present to a stroke unit and normally complain of fatigue and pain.

Dissociative seizures have a minimum incidence of 5 in 100 000 per year and account for up to 50% of patients admitted to hospital in apparent 'status'. Typically, the mean onset of dissociative seizures is in the twenties, with a history of other functional symptoms such as irritable bowel syndrome, but there is a subgroup with onset in middle age, equal sex distribution, and marked health anxiety (especially about heart disease).

Natural history, and complications of the disease

The spectrum of severity of functional and dissociative neurological symptoms is very wide. Some patients have only transient symptoms, while others become severely disabled and even bedbound. More severe cases may have a lifelong vulnerability to functional symptoms and multiple assessments, investigations, and repeated surgical interventions. In this case, the term 'somatization disorder' is used; this disorder has a poorer prognosis, often with onset before the age of 30. Patients with this disorder usually have a history of repeated presentation to medical services, with at least one neurological symptom, four pain symptoms, two gastrointestinal symptoms, and one sexual symptom.

Approach to diagnosing the disease

Functional and dissociative neurological symptoms should be diagnosed primarily on the basis of positive examination features of internal inconsistency, and incongruence with neurological disease. A history of multiple functional symptoms may be suggestive but is not diagnostic.

With functional weakness, some patients have a typical dragging gait with the hip inverted or everted. The key finding is internal inconsistency, for example being able to walk but having no leg power on the bed. Hoover's sign is positive when a weakness of hip extension (which in itself is unusual in neurological disease) returns to normal with contralateral hip flexion against resistance (see Figure 241.1); hip abduction can also be used. Hoover's sign may be falsely positive in cortical neglect, in mild weakness, or when there is a lot of pain. The weakness can have a 'give-way' quality. Tone and reflexes should be normal.

Functional movement disorders require particular experience to diagnose confidently, because of the sometimes unusual nature of 'organic' movement disorders. Functional tremor is typically variable in frequency, distractible (e.g. with complex motor tasks), or 'entrains' to the rhythm of copied voluntary movement in the opposite hand. Fixed dystonia usually presents with a clenched fist or a plantarflexed, inverted ankle after physical injury or immobilization, and its clinical presentation overlaps with complex regional pain syndrome type 1. Sudden jerky movements may also be functional.

Functional dysphonia is typically a whispering voice, often triggered by laryngitis. Functional word finding difficulties are common, but true dysphasia is not seen. Functional memory complaints present as attentional difficulties (e.g. failure to remember the reason for going up stairs) often accompanied by health anxiety, or as dense retrograde amnesia. Functional visual symptoms can be detected by a range of measures, including the use of tubular visual fields (e.g. the same restriction at 30 cm and 100 cm; visual fields are conical) or eliciting optokinetic nystagmus in functional blindness.

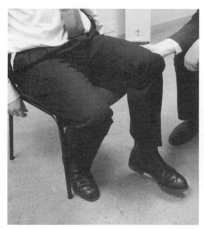
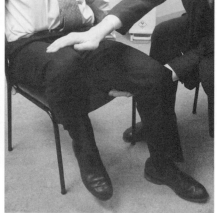

Test hip extension – it's weak

Test contralateral hip flexion against resistance – hip extension has become strong

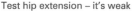

Figure 241.1 Hoover's sign for functional weakness.

Reproduced with permission from Jon Stone, Functional Symptoms in Neurology, *Practical Neurology*, Volume 9, pp 179–189, Copyright © 2009 The BMJ.

Diagnosing dissociative seizures needs a witness history; phone witnesses or ask carers to video an attack using a mobile phone. Table 241.1 describes clinical features, but any one feature in isolation may mislead.

Other diagnoses that should be considered

The differential for functional and dissociative neurological symptoms includes all neurological disorders. Comorbid neurological diseases are common (e.g. 5%–10% of patients with dissociative seizures also have epilepsy). Diagnosis is usually best confirmed by a neurologist.

Misdiagnosis occurs in less than 5% of patients in published series. It is more common in patients with frontal lobe epilepsy,

movement/gait disorder, and patients with severe psychiatric disturbance.

Factitious symptoms, symptoms deliberately simulated for medical care, and malingering symptoms simulated for material gain may present neurologically. Looking for major discrepancies in the history and using covert surveillance are the only methods for making these diagnoses.

Diagnostic tests

The diagnosis of functional and dissociative neurological symptoms is clinical and not one of exclusion. For dissociative seizures, a normal EEG during a customary attack is helpful, although this can be misleading in a patient with a deep epileptic focus. Many patients will require further investigation to exclude important alternative explanations (e.g. structural MRI in functional weakness). The patient should be forewarned that a negative result is expected.

Prognosis, and how to estimate it

The prognosis for functional and dissociative neurological symptoms is highly variable. Longer duration, personality disorder, and preoccupation with an exclusively physical aetiology appear to predict a worse outcome.

Treatment and its effectiveness

Explanation is the cornerstone of treatment. Patients are often bewildered, or frightened that they have multiple sclerosis or something similar. Make it clear that you believe the patient, that they have something common and potentially reversible, and that you do not think they are 'putting it on'. An explanation of how a positive diagnosis has been made, and, where appropriate, a demonstration of the patient's signs, for example the Hoover's sign, can help engagement with and acceptance of the diagnosis. Sensitivity about exploring psychological symptoms is required, because patients (and doctors) often connect these disorders with being 'imaginary' or 'malingering'. It is alienating, and probably scientifically inaccurate, to present a solely psychological explanation without reference to biological factors.

Symptomatic treatment of associated pain and mood symptoms, self-help (e.g. see http://www.neurosymptoms.org), and physiotherapy, especially for motor symptoms, is recommended. Hypnosis may be worth trying, especially for movement disorders. Studies of other functional symptoms support the use of antidepressants and cognitive behavioural therapy.

Before referral for assessment by psychiatry or psychology, ensure the clinician has specific expertise in the field.

Table 241.1 Dissociative versus epileptic seizures: Helpful and less helpful distinguishing features

	Dissociative seizures	Epileptic seizures
Helpful		
Duration over 5 minutes	Common	Rare
Gradual onset	Common	Rare
Fluctuating/relapsing course	Common	Rare
Eyes and mouth closed	Common	Rare
Resisting eye opening	Common	Very rare
Thrashing, violent movements	Common	Rare
Visible large bite mark on side of tongue	Very rare	Occasional
Respiration	Often fast	Ceases
Obeying commands during generalized shaking	Rare	Should not occur
Weeping/upset after a seizure	Occasional	Rare
Not so helpful		
Stereotyped attacks	Common	Common
Attack arising from sleep	Occasional	Common
Aura	Common	Common
Incontinence of urine or faeces	Occasional	Common
Injury	Common	Common
Report of tongue biting	Occasional	Common

Further Reading

Edwards MJ and Bhatia KP. Functional (psychogenic) movement disorders: Merging mind and brain. *Lancet Neurol* 2012; 11: 250–60.

Pula J. Functional vision loss. *Curr Opin Ophthalmol* 2012; 23: 460–5.

Reuber M. Psychogenic nonepileptic seizures: Answers and questions. *Epilepsy Behav* 2008; 12: 622–35.

Stone J, Carson A, and Sharpe M. Functional symptoms and signs in neurology: Assessment and diagnosis/management. *J Neurol Neurosurg Psychiatry* 2005; 76: i2–i12.

Definition of the disease

This chapter focuses on the management of patients with terminal neurological disease. The definition of the term 'terminal' varies but could be used to describe a patient who is in the last 6–12 months of their life. Some people prefer to reserve this term for patients in the last days to weeks of their life.

Aetiology of the disease

The definition of progressive neurological conditions is those conditions which are incurable and invariably result in ongoing deterioration without the prospect of improvement. The most commonly encountered conditions are parkinsonian syndromes, motor neuron disease, Huntington's disease, prion disease, cerebellar degeneration syndromes, and muscular dystrophies. Multiple sclerosis can follow a relapsing–remitting course but can also follow a progressive form where there are no remissions. Despite these conditions having many different pathologies, the symptoms relating to the end of life are very similar.

Typical symptoms of the disease, and less common symptoms

The symptoms experienced by this group of patients include weakness, immobility, constipation, nausea, pain, fatigue, hypersalivation (drooling or choking on excessive secretions), swallowing/speech difficulties, breathlessness, weight loss/anorexia, stiffness, anxiety, cognitive decline, agitation, and falls.

Demographics of the disease

In the UK, the incidence of neurological conditions is 625 per 100 000. The prevalence of neurological conditions within the population is approximately 1 million. Of these, approximately 20% are admitted to hospital, and 10% die each year (National Council of Palliative Care, 2010).

Natural history, and complications of the disease

The challenges faced when managing these patients include the multiple different pathologies which contribute to a variable level of physical, cognitive, and emotional decline. Some conditions (e.g. motor neuron disease, especially in the case of bulbar involvement) can be associated with a rapid deterioration from the onset of diagnosis. Other conditions can deteriorate slowly over many years, usually with a more rapid deterioration in the last weeks/months of life.
Complications include:

- swallowing problems
- recurrent infections
- weakness/falls
- hospital admissions

Approach to diagnosing the disease

Recognizing that a patient is dying can present quite a challenge, especially for patients that have deteriorated very slowly over many years. A multidisciplinary approach can often be helpful. Looking at

the literature, the following factors may be helpful symptoms or signs that may help to identify patients that are dying. These are:

- swallowing problems
- aspiration pneumonia
- recurrent infections
- marked decline in performance status
- cognitive difficulties
- weight loss

Other diagnoses that should be considered

When reviewing a patient who is thought to be dying, a thorough assessment including history, examination, and, if necessary, appropriate investigations may be required to identify/exclude reversible causes. The most likely reversible causes are:

- infection
- dehydration/with renal impairment
- other metabolic abnormalities (e.g. diabetes, hypothyroidism)
- depression

'Gold-standard' diagnostic test

It is difficult to accurately predict which patients are in the terminal phase of their illness. Often the most useful predictor of prognosis is the rate of deterioration and the associated comorbidity associated with this. The Gold Standards Framework identifies parameters that may allow the recognition of the terminal phase. The first of these is the so-called surprise question. This question asks the physician if they would be surprised if the patient died within the next 6–12 months. This in itself is an important recognition that the patient may be dying. In addition to this, there are disease-specific clinical indicators that may be suggestive that a patient is dying (see 'Prognosis, and how to estimate it').

Prognosis, and how to estimate it

As discussed earlier, neurological disease represents a wide range of pathological processes and clinical presentations. However, there are clinical indicators that can help to identify the patient who is thought to be dying. In motor neuron disease, a rapid onset and loss of neurological function is likely to represent that a patient will have a poor prognosis. Symptoms and signs suggestive of respiratory failure also are strongly suggestive of a poor prognosis. The prognostic indicator guidance as described in the Gold Standards Framework describes the following clinical indicators as markers for poor prognosis:

- disturbed sleep related to respiratory muscle weakness
- breathlessness at rest
- difficulty swallowing
- poor nutritional status
- poor performance status
- medical complications (e.g. infections)

Other specific issues

There are specific issues relating to patients with progressive neurological disease; these are associated with neurological decline and worsening neurological function. These tend to apply to patients in whom the condition causes predominantly muscle weakness and wasting (rather than stiffness or sensory changes). In these patients, there may be symptoms related to difficulty in swallowing and related to respiratory compromise.

In terms of nutrition, if a patient's deterioration is primarily related to an inability to eat due to weakness of the bulbar muscles (as in motor neuron disease), it may be important and appropriate to consider a feeding gastrostomy such as a percutaneous endoscopic gastrostomy (PEG) or radiologically inserted gastrostomy tube insertion if it is thought that the patient may still have many months left to live. The decision-making process is complex and must take into account the patient's premorbid condition prior to the problems with swallowing. It is also important to consider a PEG tube insertion as a palliative procedure to satisfy hunger and a route to enable administration of medications and water. The decision-making process needs to take into account the patient's wishes, as they may choose not to have a PEG tube inserted because not being able to eat by mouth may be impacting on their quality of life and, at this point in time, they may prefer symptom control measures rather than interventional procedures.

In terms of respiratory function, if a patient's deterioration is thought to be primarily related to respiratory muscle weakness and compromise, it may be important and appropriate to consider an assessment to see if non-invasive ventilation may be suitable for these patients (usually in the situation where a patient is expected to have many months left to live). Respiratory compromise can cause a lot of morbidity for a patient in terms of breathlessness, lethargy, fatigue, confusion, disturbed sleep, and headaches (due to the effects of hypoxia and hypercapnia).

Non-invasive ventilation in these patients may reduce their symptom burden and morbidity and improve the quality of life even in the last months of life. This needs to be weighed up against the morbidity caused travelling to a specialist respiratory centre for assessment and the burden of being attached to the ventilator. This process also involves the acknowledgement that the non-invasive ventilation may only provide temporary relief of symptoms and may need to be withdrawn if it is no longer effective, in which case pharmacological management of their symptoms will be more important (see 'Treatment and its effectiveness: Management of specific symptoms in the last weeks of life').

Treatment and its effectiveness: Management of specific symptoms in the last weeks of life

Symptom management will often involve the multidisciplinary team and include non-pharmacological and pharmacological measures. Weakness and immobility will require the input of occupational therapists and physiotherapists to improve the patient's function and symptoms using practical measures to provide comfort.

Pharmacological management may be challenging as the patient may be unable to swallow and therefore medications that cannot be swallowed in tablet form may need to be administered as syrups/suspensions. For other patients who have an existing gastrostomy tube in situ, medications may be administered via this route. For the patients who cannot use either of these routes, other routes of administration (e.g. subcutaneous, rectal, buccal, transdermal, or intra-nasal routes may need to be used).

Pain

Pain should be managed holistically, considering non-pharmacological management with input from the physiotherapists and occupational therapists. Pharmacological management should follow the WHO pain ladder, starting with simple analgesics and, if these are not effective, moving onto stronger analgesics.

Nausea

The management of nausea will need to take into account the pathophysiological process of the underlying condition. Haloperidol would be the drug of choice in most circumstances except for patients with parkinsonian conditions, where the dopamine-antagonist effect of this drug and other dopamine antagonists (e.g. metoclopramide/levomepromazine) may worsen the symptoms of the underlying condition and therefore contribute to worsening morbidity/symptoms (e.g. stiffness/tremor). Cyclizine, ondansetron or domperidone may be a better choice of drug for patients with parkinsonism. These drugs can be administered orally or subcutaneously (once daily or as an infusion over 24 hours via a syringe driver). The doses of these drugs are as follows:

- systemic cause: haloperidol 0.5–1.5 mg once daily and as needed (use above mentioned medications in parkinsonian patients)
- gastric stasis: metoclopramide 10 mg, as needed, or three times daily (use above mentioned medications in parkinsonian patients)
- levomepromazine: 6.25 mg once daily and as needed

Fatigue

Fatigue is a very common symptom in these patients and can be a very distressing symptom which impacts negatively on a patient's psychological well-being. Psychostimulants (e.g. methylphenidate) may have a role, even in the terminal phase, in improving the alertness and cognitive function of these patients, thereby allowing them to interact with family members. Psychostimulants are contraindicated in certain circumstances (e.g. in people with ischaemic heart disease) and therefore, if they are considered, specialist advice should be sought.

Secretions

Pharmacological management of secretions is as follows:

- glycopyrronium: 200–400 µg as needed (max 1200 µg in 24 hours)
- hyoscine hydrobromide: 200–400 µg as needed (max 1200 µg in 24 hours)

If these medications are ineffective and the patient is experiencing symptoms of choking (with severe distress), then use midazolam, 2.5–5.0 mg subcutaneously or bucally.

Breathlessness

Pharmacological management of breathlessness is as follows:

- low-dose opioids: morphine sulfate oral solution 2.5–5.0 mg four times daily and as needed (2 hourly)
- lorazepam: 0.5–1.0 mg sublingually (max 4 mg in 24 hours)
- morphine sulfate 1.25–2.50 mg as needed, subcutaneously
- midazolam 2.5–5.0 mg, subcutaneously

Anxiety

Pharmacological management of anxiety is as follows:

- lorazepam 0.5 mg–1.0 mg sublingually (4 mg in 24 hours)
- midazolam 2.5–5.0 mg as needed, subcutaneously/bucally

Further Reading

National Council of Palliative Care. *End of Life Care in Long Term Neurological Conditions*. 2010. Available at https://www.mssociety.org.uk/sites/default/files/Documents/Professionals/End%20life%20care%20long%20term%20neuro%20conditions.pdf (15 Jul 2017).

PART 11

Disorders of the skin

243 Normal skin function

Jenny Powell

Introduction

In simplest terms, our skin is a layer that separates and protects us from the external environment. This assumes the skin is a passive covering to keep the insides safe, and the outside out, and overlooks its enormous complexity. The skin is our largest organ and is constantly regenerating, but how efficiently it does so depends on a number of factors, some known, others unknown. It is an efficient mechanical barrier (designed for wear and repair), and a complex immunological membrane. It has a generous vascular, lymphatic, and nervous supply, all covering a considerable area. It has specialist structural and functional properties relating to specific areas, but also specialist cells within the layers of the skin. Most importantly, skin is the organ of display, an important part of social and sexual behaviour, immediately accessible to all, and often regarded as a barometer of the general state of health. Permanent scars inflicted on the skin may be a cause of great distress to the patient.

Skin structures

Skin consists of a superficial layer, 'the epidermis' (concerned with producing protective keratin and a pigment called melanin), which adheres closely to the deeper layer, 'the dermis' (which provides the strength of the skin, and houses the appendages), via the basement membrane. Loose connective tissue and fat underlie the dermis.

Structures found in the skin include:

- the epidermis
- the horny layer (stratum corneum)
- the granular layer
- the spinous cell layer
- the basal cell layer
- the basement membrane
- the dermis
- the papillary dermis
- the subpapillary network
- arterioles
- venules
- the deep vascular network
- lymphatics
- hair follicles
- subcutaneous fat
- sweat glands
- sebaceous glands
- melanocytes
- desmosomes
- hemidesmosomes

The structure and function of the different skin components are outlined in Table 243.1. Skin thickness varies according to function: for example, it is 0.1 mm thick over the eyelids but is 2 mm thick on the soles of the feet.

Epidermis

The epidermis is composed of stratified squamous epithelium, comprising layers of closely packed cells: the basal cell layer, the spinous layer, the granular layer, and the horny layer.

Table 243.1 Components of the skin	
Structure	**Functions**
Horny layer	Barrier protection against unregulated loss of salt and water and entry of particles (e.g. chemicals, microbes)
Keratinocytes	Cytokine production, keratin production, production of vitamin D, produce endogenous antibiotics.
Basal cell layer	Reduplication and repair
Langerhans cells	Immunological defence
Melanocytes	Protection against ultraviolet radiation including DNA damage
Basement membrane	Adhesion of epidermis to underlying zone supporting dermis
Dermis	Strength with suppleness, shock absorption, (toughness over back and soles of feet, elasticity over joints, delicacy of eyelids).
Sub-cutaneous fat	Cushioning trauma, insulation and calorie reserve. Also releases hormone leptin to regulate hunger and energy metabolism via the hypothalamus.
Blood vessels	Delivery of nutrients and removal of waste; temperature regulation
Peripheral nerves	Cutaneous sensation
Lymphatics	Drainage and removal of particulate waste
Eccrine sweat glands	Temperature regulation, over most of the body surface, more numerous on hands and feet.
Apocrine sweat glands	Production of pheromones, axillae, anogenital. Wax glands of ear. Milk glands of the breast.
Sebaceous glands	Waterproofing and moisturizing
Fibroblast cells	Synthesis of collagen, elastin, collagenase, fibronectin
Phagocytic cells	Engulf and destroy bacteria
Lymphocytes	Immunological defence
Mast cells	Mediator release under antigenic stimulation, chemotaxis
Nails	Protection and stabilization of terminal phalanx, important in pinching and prising objects
Hair	Display and attraction—social and psychological value; thermal properties

Surgery (Oxford), Volume 24, Issue 1, Pages 1-4 Copyright Elsevier Limited 2006. Author is the same as the original work.

Basal layer

Cells in the epidermis are produced by cell division in the basal cell layer (a single sheet of columnar cells at the lowest level of the epidermis). At any moment, 30% of these columnar cells are preparing for division. After division, one cell remains in position, continuing the task of reduplication, repair, and adherence to the underlying basement membrane. The other cell moves towards the surface suprabasally; it is unable to divide, but differentiates into a keratinocyte. As more cells are created from the basal layer, it is pushed upwards through the spinous and granular layers.

Spinous layer

The next level of the epidermis after the basal layer is the spinous layer, so-called because cells are joined by cohesive desmosomes that resemble 'spines' under the light microscope.

Granular layer

As a keratinocyte moves upwards, it becomes part of the granular layer, two to three layers of flatter cells containing many granules. These granules are lysosomes, containing hydrolytic enzymes that destroy the cell's nucleus and other organelles, resulting in cell death.

Horny layer

As the keratinocyte moves into the horny layer, which is the uppermost epidermal layer, it dies, loses its nucleus, and becomes flattened, with thick cell membranes that enable the cells in the horny layer to adhere to each other. Gradually, these cells flake off, and are replaced by underlying cells. The time from cell division to shedding is 28 days in normal skin. There is a close matching of rate of cell production with loss in healthy skin, and it is increased in response to injury and friction. This implies a local mechanism of repair within the skin.

The horny layer is an effective barrier to most organisms, chemicals, and fluids, although it is permeable to some substances (hence topical treatments). It also protects against uncontrolled loss of fluid from the body.

Keratins

Keratinocytes synthesize keratin, a triple-stranded helical molecule, which is the main structural protein of the epidermis. Keratin filaments form a 'basket' network around the nucleus, with spokes radiating through the cytoplasm to link the nucleus with the cell surface. This network of filaments forms the cytoskeleton. Keratinocytes are involved in the response to injury (see Figure 243.1).

Thirty different keratin molecules have been identified. Keratin molecules exist in pairs: one is acidic (type I), and one is basic (type II); they are transcribed from genes found on Chromosomes 17 and 12, respectively. The keratin pair 14 and 5 is found in basal cells. Production changes to keratins 10 and 1 as the basal cell divides, and the budded cell differentiates. Keratins 16 and 6 are expressed during wound healing, within 12 hours of injury. Mutation of keratin genes results in cell fragility and lysis. The resulting clinical phenotype depends on the keratin pair affected. For example, if mutation occurs in the genes transcribing for keratins 10 and 1, the epidermis is affected suprabasally, and this results clinically in congenital bullous icthyosiform erythroderma.

Keratinocytes are involved in the response to injury. They produce endogenous antibiotics (defensins and cathelicidins) providing an innate immune defence against bacteria, viruses, and fungi. Keratinocytes also synthesize cytokines.

Cytokines

Cytokines are chemical mediators, secreted by activated cells that affect other cells, usually by binding to cell surface receptors to modulate activity (including stimulation or inhibition of cell secretion, division, and migration, amongst other activities). Cytokines play a major role in inflammatory processes, immunoregulation, growth, and repair, allowing epidermal cells to communicate with and influence each other, and interact with dermal cells. Epidermal cells are also affected by cytokines secreted by other cells (e.g. white blood cells, mast cells, cells in vessel walls).

Cytokine production is stimulated by injury, including that caused by UV light or infection (endotoxins, antigen–T-cell reactions) and is reduced by the effect of corticosteroids. The earliest recognized cytokines include interleukin 1, interleukin 2, interleukin 3, interleukin 6, and interleukin 8; interferon alpha, interferon beta, and interferon gamma; tumour growth factor alpha and tumour growth factor beta; and platelet activators.

Tumour necrosis factor (TNF) has a central role in the immune response. It is released by cells of the immune system (e.g. macrophages, T-cells) when inflammation occurs, often after trauma or infection. Its action is mediated by two receptors, p55 and p75, which are found on the cell surface of various cells of the immune system and body tissues. Soluble p55 and p75 receptors are also found in serum and synovial fluid. Both receptors mediate the effects of fever, tissue damage, and shock. Tumour necrosis factor alpha (TNF-α) also stimulates cells in the surrounding tissue to produce chemokines, that cause the dilation of local blood vessels. TNF-α induces activation

Keratinocyte response to injury

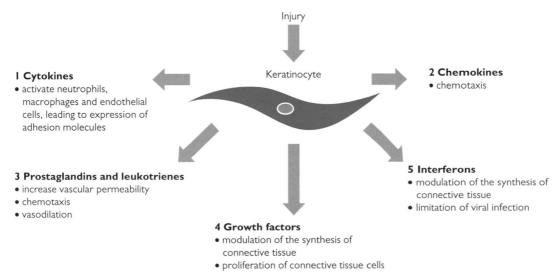

Figure 243.1 Keratinocyte response to injury.

Reprinted from Surgery (Oxford), Volume 24, issue 1, Jennifer Powell, Skin physiology, pp. 1-4, Copyright (2006), with permission from Elsevier.

of T- and B-cells and increases the production of cyclo-oxygenase 2. The latter is an enzyme that plays an important role in inflammation and is responsible for the production of inflammatory prostaglandins that stimulate the synthesis of other pro-inflammatory factors. TNF-α therefore acts physiologically to eradicate infection and repair damaged tissues by its direct and indirect actions. However, its central role in the propagation of the inflammatory process may become pathological if it occurs in excess, and tissue damage may result. Treatments have been developed that aim to reduce concentrations of TNF-α, and they may be effective in the treatment of rheumatoid arthritis, Crohn's disease, and psoriasis; for example, infliximab is a chimeric (human and mouse) monoclonal antibody against TNF-α, and it is an effective immunomodulator used singly or in combination. It can trigger complement-mediated lysis of cells expressing TNF in vitro.

Other epidermal cells

Melanocytes

Melanocytes are large dendritic cells that are interspersed amongst the basal cell layer. They originate from the neural crest in the embryo and migrate to the ectoderm, hair bulbs, retina, and pia arachnoid. Like neurons, they are terminally differentiated cells (i.e. they no longer divide under normal conditions). Melanocytes contain organelles called 'melanosomes' that synthesize the pigment melanin from the essential amino acid phenylalanine. Melanocytes are under the basal cell layer and send dendritic processes up between the basal cells. The tip of the dendrite is embedded in the cytoplasm of the basal cell and passes melanosomes directly into it. The size and number of melanosomes in the keratinocytes (and not the melanocytes) govern visible pigmentation. In dark-skinned people, there are no more melanocytes than in light-skinned people, but the melanosomes are larger and persist through the whole thickness of the epidermis. UV radiation increases melanocyte production and transfer of melanosomes, and the increased pigmentation or 'sun tan' helps to protect the skin from damage from UV light. Other influences on pigment formation include genetic factors, sex hormones, and melanocyte-stimulating hormone from the pituitary gland.

Langerhans cells

Langerhans cells are dendritic cells that are derived from bone marrow but migrate to the epidermis, and 2×10^9 of them persist in the epidermis, especially in the prickle cell layer. They are sentinel cells forming a network in the epidermis. They detect and collect exogenous antigen (i.e. anything coming through the skin), process it, and present it non-specifically to T-cells in the skin or lymph nodes. In this way, the T-cells specific for the antigen will receive some antigen, and be activated. Langerhans cells are part of the immunosurveillance system against viral and tumour antigens. They have lobulated nuclei and characteristic, racket-shaped organelles called 'Birbeck granules'. These granules arise from the cytoplasmic membrane by receptor specific endocytosis, thus internalizing human leukocyte antigen molecules from the cell membrane involved in antigen processing.

Langerhans cells possess surface receptors for the Fc portion of immunoglobulin-G and intracellular adhesion molecule 1, so they can adhere to other cells and thus permit communication. There are thousands of Langerhans cells per square centimetre of epidermis, and their interconnected dendritic arms form a network of communication through the skin. They can migrate from the epidermis to regional lymph nodes, and their mobilization is mediated through the interaction of their cell surface receptors with cytokines and chemokines. Langerhans cells can free themselves from the epidermis by the expression of and induced changes in adhesion molecules such as E-cadherin, CD44, and A6 integrins. Proteolysis must occur for the Langerhans cells to pass across the basement membrane.

Topical exposure of mice to contact allergens and skin irritants stimulates the expression of epidermal cytokines, including TNF, interleukin1 beta, granulocyte macrophage colony-stimulating factor, and interleukin 6. The first cytokine to be identified as a stimulus for migration of Langerhans cells was TNF-α, produced by keratinocytes acting via TNFr2 receptors on the Langerhans cell surface. Langerhans cells then produce interleukin 1 beta, which acts in an autocrine manner to stimulate migration. It also stimulates further production of TNF-α by keratinocytes.

Merkel cells

Merkel cells are not dendritic, and lie near hair follicles and unmyelinated nerve endings. It is thought that they may be transducers for fine touch, but their exact role is unclear.

Dermis

The dermis lies below the epidermis and supports it structurally and nutritionally. It primarily consists of fibroblasts and the collagen they produce. Collagen is a triple helix, comprising three polypeptide chains. Fibres are packed in bundles and give enormous tensile strength. The dermis also contains elastin fibres that provide stretch. The fibres sit within a matrix of amorphous mucopolysaccharide ground substance. This binds water to facilitate passage of nutrients and other chemicals, acts as a lubricant to allow skin movement, and provides bulk to aid shock absorption. The dermis contains blood vessels, lymphatics, and sensory nerves.

Blood vessels

Blood vessels form a deep plexus in the subcutaneous fat, to supply the sweat glands, the hair papillae, and a superficial plexus in the papillary dermis. Vasodilation can increase blood flow by a factor of 100, a reserve essential for thermoregulation, wound healing, and repair.

Lymphatics

Lymphatics collect tissue fluid and particulate matter by passive drainage and form part of the immune defence system. Lymphoedema results if they fail or are blocked or damaged, and can cause considerable disability.

Sensory nerves

Sensory nerves are abundant in the skin, and are used for touch, heat, pain, and itch. Mechanical, chemical, and cytokine stimuli affect fine, free nerve endings at the dermo-epidermal junction. Pruritus can be reduced by agents that interfere with the effect of cytokines on 'itch' fibres (e.g. topical corticosteroids, antihistamines).

Basement membrane zone

The basement membrane zone forms an adhesion complex between the dermis and epidermis, providing support for the basal cells to allow growth, multiplication, and migration, and allowing nutrients and cells to cross from the dermis (see Figure 243.2). Antibodies to specific components of the basement membrane zone may be found, via immunobiochemistry, in autoimmune blistering diseases and can be seen with fluorescein labelling. Antibody action leads to destruction or damage of the specific target component, which causes lack of cohesion and blistering (e.g. bullous pemphigoid). Blistering may also be genetic, and result from faulty production of one or more basement components (e.g. dystrophic epidermolysis bullosa).

Components of the basement membrane

Components of the basement membrane include:

- collagen types I and III (from the dermis)
- basal cells (from the epidermis)
- keratin intermediate filaments
- hemidesmosomes (on plasma membranes)
- the lamina lucida (electron-lucent zone), which contains laminin and fibronectin
- the lamina densa (electron-dense zone), which contains collagen type IV
- anchoring filaments:
  - anchoring fibrils, which are made up of collagen type VII
  - anchoring plaques, which are made up of collagen type IV

Keratinocyte response to injury

Keratinocytes respond to injury by secreting chemokines, cytokines, prostaglandins, leukotrienes, growth factors, and interferons. Chemokines mediate chemotaxis. Cytokines activate neutrophils,

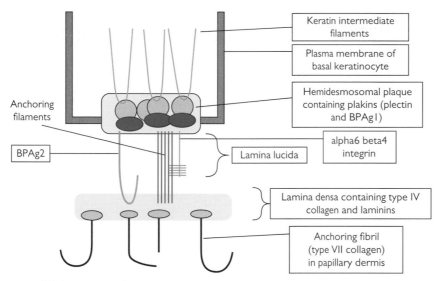

Figure 243.2 Components of the basement membrane.

Reproduced with permission from the Oxford Handbook of Medical Dermatology: Blisters, edited by Susan Burge, Dinny Wallis. Oxford University Press 2010.

macrophages, and endothelial cells, leading to the expression of adhesion molecules. Prostaglandins and leukotrienes increase vascular permeability, cause vasodilation, and mediate chemotaxis. Growth factors modulate the synthesis of connective tissue, and the proliferation of connective tissue cells. Interferons also modulate the synthesis of connective tissue, and act to limit viral infection.

The skin and psychological stress

Psychological stress may precipitate or aggravate chronic disorders of the skin (e.g. atopic eczema, psoriasis). Skin permeability is altered at times of stress; in animal studies, this coincides with corticosteroid secretion and can be reversed by giving anxiolytics or glucocorticosteroid receptor antagonists. In humans, there is a disruption of the epidermal barrier function during times of increased stress. This may explain why hypnosis is helpful in the treatment of psoriasis. It also explains the reduced resistance to the scratch reflex during times of stress.

Conclusion

Skin disease may be life-threatening. The incidence of fatal malignant melanoma is increasing, and erythroderma resulting from eczema, psoriasis, or lymphoma may cause death. Less well recognized is the disability caused by mild disease of the skin and minor blemishes, including scars. Skin is the organ of display, and abnormalities can disrupt patients' ability to physically and emotionally cope with themselves, their families, and their homes. Education, employment, and relationships may suffer if the patient perceives his or her skin as abnormal.

Further Reading

Burns T, Breathnach S, Cox N, et al. (eds). *Rook's Textbook of Dermatology* (8th edition), 2010. Wiley-Blackwell.

Gawkrodger D and Ardern-Jones MR. *Dermatology: An Illustrated Colour Text* (5th edition), 2012. Churchill Livingstone.

244 Approach to diagnosing skin disease

Jenny Powell

Introduction

Making a diagnosis in dermatology may seem daunting when there are 6 000 or more possibilities, and the terminology seems so complex. This chapter suggests a systematic approach to picking up clues from symptoms and signs, and understanding how to describe skin disease; this approach, together with experience (obtained through seeing patients, asking more experienced colleagues, and reading) will help with pattern recognition and, sometimes, lead to the answer.

The skin has such a wide range of structural and functional varieties that disorders of the skin are not only common but also very variable. However, it is important to be able to give a patient a diagnosis. This 'working label' means that the patient fits into a known group not only in their typical presentation but also as a guide for response to treatment, prognosis, and, sometimes, for explanation of aetiology and whether genetic or infective factors are important; that is, it is helpful in explaining the disease to the patient.

Despite the complexity of the skin, making a diagnosis in dermatology is no different from making a diagnosis in other areas; it is based on taking a history, examining the patient, and performing investigations, if indicated.

History

A complete history is made up of the following parts: the basic history, a past history, a family history, a social history, and treatments, as well as further enquiry, if necessary.

Basic history

The basic history gives an idea of the patients personality (and sometimes their theory of the diagnosis; this may or may not be helpful!) and establishes the onset and duration of the problem. It also establishes how the problem has evolved, changed, and spread; skin problems are often 'dynamic' and patients may bring photographs of previous stages of their evolving rash, as, for example, there may have been a 'herald patch' which has almost healed by the time the patient presents with the widespread smaller patches of pityriasis rosea. In addition, it allows the patient to admit how self-conscious they feel about the problem (this may be to the point of disgust and despair) and how it affects their quality of life at home or at school/work, their sleeping, and their personal relationships.

It is important to ask whether the problem is associated with itching, burning, or soreness. Pain is rare but can be diagnostic (e.g. pain on sun exposure with erythropoietic porphyria). Some lesions may be very tender or painful (e.g. lipoangiokeratoma, glioma). Itching (or 'pruritus') is a frequent complaint and can be further elucidated; when severe, it may be described as worse than pain, preventing sleep and interfering with work or school. The itch of Hodgkin's disease and that of dermatitis herpetiformis is very intense. The itch of scabies may be worse at night, whereas urticarial itch tends to be worst on waking. Many rashes cause no itching, but pruritus may occur with no rash, other than excoriations from scratching.

Past history

Past history enquiry may provide information about previous skin disease, allergies, and systemic illnesses, such as diabetes.

Family history

A family history may provide clues about genetic disorders (e.g. atopy, psoriasis, autoimmune diseases, skin type, skin cancer, etc.) and infectious diseases (e.g. warts, scabies, chicken pox).

Social history

A social history gives information on occupational risks, hobbies, and sun exposure.

Treatments

Treatments prescribed by medical practitioners, including complementary medicine, and those tried by the patients themselves may all affect the skin. These can include huge numbers of topical treatments and cosmetics, most of which patients may not mention or remember.

Further enquiry

Further enquiry is often made once the examination is underway. Detailed accounts of foreign travel, sexual history, and exposure to all possible allergens are only needed if unusual infection, sexually transmitted disease, or allergic contact dermatitis, respectively, are suspected

Examination

It is best to examine the whole of the patient's skin, inspecting and palpating, in daylight. The presenting problem may be a solitary warty lesion on the nose, but full inspection may reveal an unnoticed malignant melanoma on the back. It is important with rashes to know their extent and full distribution.

A dermatological assessment involves determining the answers to the following questions:

- How is the patient's general health?
- Where is the problem and how widespread is it?
- What type of lesion is involved?
- What are the characteristics of the lesion(s)?
- Are any other areas affected in similar or different ways ('secondary' sites)?
- Are special techniques for examination needed?
- Are further tests or investigations needed?

How is the patient's general health?

A general assessment of the patient's health often provides information that will help the diagnosis. The age, sex, race, shape, and mental state of the patient may be noted automatically but it still contributes to the arrival at a diagnosis of a skin complaint. Obese patients are more likely to have intertrigo (secondarily infected areas of skin in the sweaty skin flexures), whereas thin, cachectic patients are more likely to have a paraneoplastic skin problem related to an underlying malignancy. If anaemia is suspected, it may explain why the pruritus is so severe, since iron deficiency worsens the sensation of pruritus. Is there obvious sun damage to the skin, or a high tan? Many skin problems, including photosensitivity and skin malignancy, are sun related.

Ageing patients may develop multiple lesions that cause anxiety but are entirely benign. The most common of these are seborrhoeic keratoses, which are discrete lesions of benign epidermal hyperplasia, and Campbell de Morgan spots, which are benign haemangiomata. Darker skinned patients often show more variation in pattern of pigmentation than do Caucasians.

Where is the problem and how widespread is it?

Determining the site(s) and extent of the problem is very important; for example, atopic eczema occurs mostly in the flexures in children, whereas psoriasis affects the extensor surfaces of knees and elbows, as well as the scalp and sacrum. Acne appears mainly on the face and the upper back and chest, whereas basal cell carcinomas occur mostly on sun-exposed areas of the head and neck. Necrobiosis lipoidica causes circumscribed lesions on the shins of diabetic patients, whereas keratosis pilaris is most often found on the upper outer arms. A symmetrical rash suggests an endogenous underlying cause, whereas a unilateral rash may suggest an external aetiology, such as allergic contact dermatitis (e.g. jewellery and nickel dermatitis) or an infection (e.g. herpes simplex or tinea corporis). In addition, localization may occur with other external factors (e.g. the photosensitivity of porphyria cutanea tarda; blistering caused by footwear in epidermolysis bullosa; reactions to treatments seen in facial rosacea induced by topical steroids).

What type of lesion is involved?

Learning and using the correct terms to describe a skin lesion not only help to make a diagnosis but also help in recording the problems and communicating with colleagues. It is not really complicated, and the use of a systematic scheme of description soon becomes automatic.

The following terms can be used to identify the different types of lesions that can be seen:

- macule: a flat, impalpable, defined area of skin discolouration
- papule: a raised, palpable, defined area <0.5 cm in diameter
- nodule: a raised, palpable, and visible lump >0.5 cm in diameter
- vesicle: a small, visible, fluid-filled lesion (blister) <0.5 cm in diameter
- bulla: a large, visible fluid-filled lesion (blister) >0.5 cm in diameter
- pustule: a visible, pus-filled lesion
- plaque: a defined, raised, disc-shaped area of skin; considered large if >3 cm in diameter
- ulcer: a loss of epidermis and, in some cases, of dermis also
- weal: a well-defined area of raised cutaneous oedema (often called a 'hive')
- comedo: an open, raised lesion with a central white point (in which case the comedo is termed a 'whitehead') or a closed, dilated, blocked follicle (in which case the comedo is termed a 'blackhead'); both types of comedo are found in acne
- excoriation: a region of damage caused by scratching; may be linear
- horn: a raised projection of keratin
- telangiectasia: a visible small blood vessel in thinned skin, caused by sun damage or topical steroid use; also seen in benign spider naevi in children, or running over the pearly edge of a nodular basal cell carcinoma
- stria: a linear, atrophic (dermally thinned) lesion often secondary to increased growth at puberty; the expansion of the abdomen in pregnancy; or corticosteroid use

What are the characteristics of the lesion(s)?

The characteristics of a lesion include its size, shape, border, colour, and surface texture.

Size

Measure the size of the lesion in centimetres. Many clinicians also approximate the size to fruit, vegetables, or coins.

Shape

Record the shape of the lesion; it may be round, discoid, oval, annular (ringlike), linear, irregular, or regular. An annular shape often suggests that there has been central healing of the lesion, such as in the fungal infection tinea corporis (ringworm) or in granuloma annulare. Lichen planus that has moved or 'koebnerized' into a scratch or scar will have a linear shape. A dysplastic naevus with pigment spreading beyond the smooth border will have an irregular shape. A regular shape with straight edges suggests injury or an allergic response to an applied agent (e.g. allergic contact dermatitis to colophony, which is found in some sticking plasters).

Border

Look at the lesion's border; this may be well defined, as in psoriasis, or less so, as in eczema.

Colour

The colour of the lesion may be characteristic; for example:

- pink red: in common exanthems and inflammatory conditions such as eczema, psoriasis, and urticaria
- reddish-brown: in seborrhoeic dermatitis; pigmented purpuric dermatoses; and apple jelly nodules in cutaneous tuberculosis (lupus vulgaris)
- scarlet red: if there is a notable arterial component, as in pyogenic granuloma or spider naevus
- dark red: in vascular lesions such as haemangiomas and telangiectasias
- white: in post-inflammatory hypopigmentation, or depigmentation caused by vitiligo
- silvery: in psoriasis scale
- yellow: in xanthomatous disorders, jaundice
- orange: seen with haemosiderin in lichen aureus
- violet: seen in eyelids and dorsum of the fingers in dermatomyositis
- purple: in the pruritic, polygonal papules of lichen planus
- brown: in pigmented naevi, suntanned areas, or staining of the skin
- slate grey: in minocycline-induced pigmentation
- black: in malignant melanoma and dried, crusted blood
- blue-black: in rubber bleb and blue naevi

In addition, tattoos and bruising may introduce many other colours!

Surface texture

The surface texture of the lesion can help differentiate many diagnoses:

- smooth: if the lesion is superficial, it may be a macular lesion, such as a pigmented lentigo; if deep, it may be a dermal problem, such as granuloma annulare, or indicate swelling with no break in the epidermis, as occurs in urticaria
- scaly: a scaly texture results from the presence of flakes of accumulated epidermal cells, as occurs in psoriasis and fungal infections
- crusted: dried exudate forming a scab indicates a healing ulcerated lesion or wounds; alternatively, it may indicate impetigo, with serum crusting in bacterial infection
- macerated: softening and swelling of the skin occurs secondary to long-standing exposure to moisture
- lichenified: this is thickening and hardening of the skin and occurs in response to prolonged scratching
- blanching: this is loss of colour in response to pressure; it is seen with most inflammation but, importantly, is not seen in the palpable purpura of the vasculitis, as found in meningococcal septicaemia

Are any other areas affected in similar or different ways ('secondary' sites)?

Often it is possible to confirm a diagnosis by examining sites distant to that at which the patient has noticed a problem; for example:

- nails may be dystrophic with pits and onycholysis in psoriasis
- there may be telangiectasias in nail folds in dermatomyositis and lupus erythematosus
- the buccal mucosa may show a white lacy pattern and/or erosions in lichen planus
- the fingers may show burrows in scabies
- the genitalia may exhibit pallor, atrophy, and scarring in lichen sclerosus
- the toe web spaces may show 'athlete's foot' in fungal infections
- the iris may be flecked in atypical mole syndrome
- the appearance of a herpes simplex (a cold sore) on the lips may precipitate the widespread rash of erythema multiforme with target lesions
- lymph nodes may be enlarged from the secondary spread of malignant melanoma

Are special techniques for examination needed?

Special ways to examine the skin further are as follows:

- a hand lens and a dermatoscope can be used to magnify the changes seen on the skin and hair surface, to identify nits (head lice egg cases) and see fungal disease

- a Wood's lamp (UV light) can be used to show characteristic skin fluorescence in certain conditions, and urine fluorescence in some porphyrias
- skin scrapings may be looked at in clinic for fungi and yeasts, as well as being sent for culture
- smell can help in detecting anaerobic infection or the rare condition trimethylaminuria
- a wheal-and-flare reaction appearing after a scratch to the skin, or 'dermographism', is more commonly found in patients with urticaria
- a crust may be removed to ascertain the nature of the underlying lesion
- paring the skin may make it possible to differentiate between a wart and a corn
- a psoriatic plaque may be scratched to look for capillary bleeding
- if the lesions in a blistering disorder are superficial, as in pemphigus, the intact blister may be extended with gentle pressure (Nikolsky's sign)
- pinprick sensation may be lost in leprosy; the response to a light touch may be impaired in diabetic neuropathy
- glass slides may be used to look for blanching, as well as in diascopy, where pressure reveals the brown lesions of cutaneous tuberculosis when apple jelly nodules are flattened
- measuring the elasticity of the skin can be used to detect changes in growth of connective tissue; this skin will be more rigid in scleroderma but will exhibit extra mobility in Ehlers–Danlos syndrome
- sweating from the skin can be measured via the starch–iodine method; sweating will be increased in hyperhidrosis and reduced or absent in some ectodermal dysplasia syndromes
- the length, colour, and diameter of hair can be determined with a hand lens, and the surface of the hair can be examined via light and electron microscopy; growth can be assessed by looking at dye/bleach growth margins

Are further investigations needed?

Further investigations may be needed to make or confirm the diagnosis; these include:

- swabs, scrapes, and tissue samples, to look for infection
- blood tests, to look for underlying disease, or for genetic testing
- skin biopsy, for histopathology
- patch testing, to look for allergic contact dermatitis

Further Reading

Gawkrodger D and Ardern-Jones MR. *Dermatology: An Illustrated Colour Text* (6th edition), 2016. Elsevier.
Griffiths C, Barker J, Bleiker T, et al. (eds). *Rook's Textbook of Dermatology* (9th edition), 2016. Wiley-Blackwell.

245 Investigation in skin disease

Jenny Powell

Special investigation techniques in skin disease

When taking a history and examining the patient do not provide all the information required, further investigation is possible. This may be to provide a diagnosis, to add to prognostic information, to help with treatment required, or to find an associated systemic disorder or underlying genetic disorder.

Blood tests

Blood tests that may be used to investigate skin disease include:

- haematology and biochemistry:
  - for diagnosis and for monitoring the effect of systemic treatments
  - infections and inflammatory disorders may produce a neutrophilia and raised inflammatory markers (erythrocyte sedimentation rate and C-reactive protein)
  - eosinophilia (>0.44 x 10⁹/l) is seen in atopy, parasitic infestations, allergy to drugs, bullous disorders, eosinophilic fasciitis, and some cases of polyarteritis nodosa
- immunological studies:
  - to diagnose connective tissue disease
  - IgE and radioallergoabsorbent tests in allergy/atopic diseases
  - specific antibodies to diagnose autoimmune blistering disease
- genetic studies

Wood's lamp

A Wood's lamp is a UV lamp; in the light produced by it, visible rays are excluded via the use of a nickel oxide filter. Use of Wood's lamp aids in making a diagnosis in the following conditions:

- fungal infections: tinea capitis caused by *Microsporum* spp. appears fluorescent green, while pityriasis versicolor appears yellow; however, most fungi do **not** fluoresce
- bacterial infections: erythrasma caused by Gram-positive corynebacteria glows coral pink, while that caused by *Pseudomonas pyocyanea* appears yellow-green
- pigmentary change (e.g. vitiligo; ash leaf macules in tuberous sclerosis; café-au-lait patches in neurofibromatosis) is made more visible
- porphyrias: urine and faeces fluoresce in porphyria cutanea tarda; teeth fluoresce in erythropoietic porphyria; and blood fluoresces in protoporphyria

Identification of scabies mites

Scabies mites may be visualized with a dermatoscope (illuminated magnification), but it is possible to extract a mite from a burrow with a needle, see it using a microscope, and then show it to the patient to prove the diagnosis. Potassium hydroxide (10%) added to the scrapings under a coverslip helps dissolve the cell membranes. Gentle scraping of a burrow (e.g. in an affected interdigital space) may reveal the mite, its eggs, and its faecal pellets.

Swabs, scrapings, and clippings

Material from the skin, hair, or nails can be used for examination under the microscope or cultured to look for evidence of infection. This is especially useful in suspected fungal infections.

Skin biopsy

Microscopic examination of tissue in a skin biopsy is an important technique often used to confirm or establish a diagnosis and also to

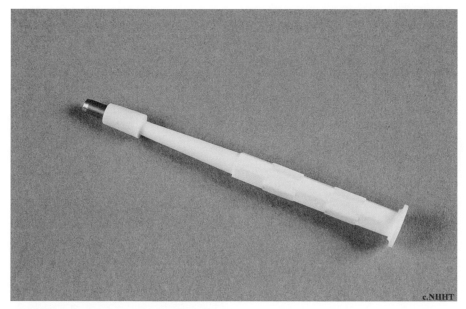

Figure 245.1 A punch biopsy.
Reproduced with permission from the Hampshire Hospitals NHS Foundation Trust.

remove malignant lesions. The procedure can be performed under local anaesthetic (1% or 2% lignocaine, with or without adrenaline to reduce bleeding, unless performed on the fingers or toes) in an outpatient setting with the patient's consent. It is important to check that the patient is not being treated with an anticoagulant and to warn that scars on the upper trunk may heal with keloid formation and that scars on the lower legs of elderly patients may suffer from slow healing.

A punch biopsy is a quick method used to obtain a small piece of skin. The biopsy is obtained by pushing a round, sharp-ended metal cylinder blade into an area of anaesthetized skin, with a downward twisting movement (Figure 245.1). The small plug of tissue is removed from the cylinder, and the base of the wound is treated with pressure, electrocautery, or a small suture to achieve haemostasis (Figure 245.2).

An elliptical biopsy provides larger samples for diagnosis or complete removal of even quite large lesions from an area of anaesthetized skin. An incisional diagnostic biopsy should be taken at right angles to the margin and include a margin of normal perilesional skin. Excisional biopsies require a wide-enough ellipse around the whole lesion, with a margin of normal skin. The edge must be cut vertically and not slant in towards the tumour. The long axis of the wound should follow the natural creases of the skin. The edges are brought neatly together with sutures, some subcuticular absorbable ones if necessary, and the finest possible sutures in the skin itself give a good cosmetic result with a fine linear scar.

Curettage is a useful device for removing hyperkeratotic lesions. A sharp-edged, spoonlike curette is used to remove the lesion from anaesthetized skin, and the wound is cauterized to achieve haemostasis. It may be difficult to assess the adequacy of removal.

A shave biopsy is used for the removal of protuberant superficial lesions; in this procedure, the lesion is removed with a sharp blade flat to the skin. A snip biopsy is used for the removal of skin tags.

Following the biopsy, the specimen is transported in a buffered formalin solution. It is processed, cut up, and stained, usually with haematoxylin and eosin, but there are numerous 'special' stains (e.g. Ziehl–Neelson stain for acid-fast bacilli; Congo Red stain for amyloid). In addition, there are many immunochemistry panels for specific cell markers (e.g. S-100 1, for melanocytes; tryptase 1, for mast cells; IgG and IgM for immunofluorescence labelling; and numerous markers for lymphoma and leukaemia). It is important to give the histopathologist good clinical information so the correct stains can be employed to confirm or refute the diagnosis.

Skin testing for suspected allergy

Substances introduced to the skin can give valuable information about immunological and pharmacological reactions. The significance of the results has to be interpreted according to each patient's individual clinical details.

Epicutaneous/patch tests are used to find out if a suspected allergic contact dermatitis exists; this is a test for delayed hypersensitivity. Possible allergens, diluted in suitable vehicles, are placed in small discs in contact with the skin, most often on the back (Figure 245.3). There are several 'batteries' of allergens, for specific conditions; some (e.g. standard, facial, and hairdressing batteries) may be applied together with one or two allergens prepared from suspected substances brought by the patient. The patch testing may be extended to include testing for photoallergy, and often for possible sunscreen allergy. The discs are removed at 48 hours, and the results are read at 48 and 96 hours. A positive reaction with erythema and palpable swelling at 48 and/or 96 hours confirms delayed hypersensitivity to the allergen in the disc at that site.

Intradermal injection or prick tests are used to see if there is an immediate hypersensitivity to a particular allergen. In this test, a drop of the test solution is placed on the skin, and a sharp needle is used to make a small prick through the drop. The size of any resulting weal-and-flare reaction is measured at 15 minutes and is compared to positive (histamine) and negative controls. When testing patients with severe allergic reactions (e.g. to peanuts), it is important to be prepared for the severe reactions that occasionally occur with prick

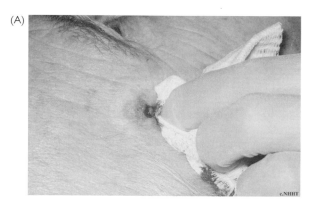

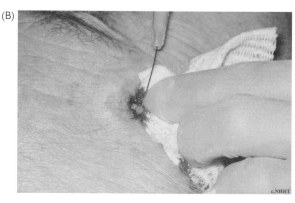

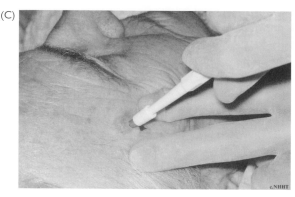

Figure 245.2 A punch biopsy procedure.
Reproduced with permission from the Hampshire Hospitals NHS Foundation Trust.

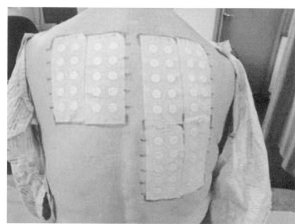

Figure 245.3 Patch tests, applied to the back.

testing. In addition, larger doses of allergen may be injected intradermally to test for delayed hypersensitivity to bacterial, fungal, and viral antigens indicating infection (e.g. the tuberculin test).

Moderate to large doses of corticosteroids may inhibit the positive response to patch tests but have no effect on prick-test reactions. Antihistamines, however, inhibit the weal-and-flare reaction of prick tests.

Radiology and imaging

In most patients with a skin problem, the skin can be seen and felt and further imaging is not necessary. However, imaging via X-rays, MRI, PET, and/or high-resolution ultrasound is useful for:

- detecting lymphadenopathy or metastatic skin cancer
- guiding biopsies
- determining the extent of an infection
- differentiating between cellulitis and necrotizing fasciitis
- detecting an internal disease that is linked to a skin condition (e.g. nervous system involvement in neurofibromatosis; muscle involvement in dermatomyositis; chest involvement in sarcoidosis)
- examining peripheral lower leg arteries (via Doppler assessment) before using high-compression bandaging in the treatment of venous leg ulcers

Photography and telemedicine

Photography may be used to document the size, extent, and nature of skin changes. This aids the detection of ongoing change in the skin (e.g. looking for worrying changes in atypical naevi, documenting improvement of a rash with treatment, showing healing or extension of a leg ulcer). Photography is also helpful when the patient suffers an intermittent rash, as a photograph is better than the patient's description in many cases.

Telemedicine can be effective if it is difficult for the patient to reach the dermatologist (because the patient is from abroad, live in a remote area, or has a disability) but is not as efficient or diagnostically reliable as the patient attending the dermatologist's clinic in person. Images may be sent electronically, and if the telemedicine consultation is set up well, with good photography and a primary care physician present (a 'real-time' teleconsultation), the accuracy of the diagnosis, as well as satisfaction with the consultation, is improved.

Further Reading

Ashton R, Leppard B, and Cooper H. *Differential Diagnosis in Dermatology* (4th edition), 2014. Radcliffe Publishing Ltd.

Griffiths C, Barker J, Bleiker T, et al. (eds). *Rook's Textbook of Dermatology* (9th edition), 2016. Wiley-Blackwell.

246 Skin infection and infestation

Christine Soon

Definition of the disease

An infection of the skin means a breach of the skin barrier has resulted in an organism gaining an opportunity to infect the area and causing inflammation, pain, erythema, and swelling. There can be associated systemic unwellness such as pyrexia, tachycardia, and hypotension.

An infestation occurs when creatures inhabit the skin, lay eggs, and multiply. These creatures are usually dependent on their host for food and transmission to others. They typically cause intense pruritus in the affected areas.

Aetiology of the disease

Organisms causing infection of the skin include bacteria, viruses, fungi, and yeast. Bacterial infection can lead to cellulitis, impetigo, cutaneous tuberculosis, leprosy, and others. Viral infections include herpes simplex, varicella, herpes zoster, HHV8, and HPV.

Fungi infections include trichophyton infections, microsporum infections, deep fungi infection, histoplasmosis, and so on. Yeast infections are caused by organisms such as candida, *Malassezia furfur*, and so on.

Infestations of the skin include scabies and those caused by lice and fleas.

Typical symptoms of the disease, and less common symptoms

Symptoms will depend on the aetiology. A bacterial infection such as cellulitis is typically caused by staphylococci or streptococci. The skin will become warm, erythematous, tender, and swollen. It may occur after a break in the skin barrier and can be associated with systemic symptoms such as malaise, pyrexia, nausea, tachycardia, and rigours. There may be associated lymphadenopathy. If the area affected becomes too swollen, blisters may occur.

Impetigo is a common skin infection in children. The causative agents are usually staphylococci or streptococci. The lesion is erythematous and often has a golden crust. It is contagious. In severe cases, blistering is seen.

Cutaneous tuberculosis has several different types of presentations: lupus vulgaris, scrofuloderma, tuberculid, military tuberculosis, and verrucosa cutis. It can be associated with lung tuberculosis or it can run a fairly indolent course.

Other mycobacterium infections include *Mycobacterium marinum* infection. It usually spreads in a sporotrichoid fashion up one limb such as the arm. It often lives in tropical fish tanks, and owners of tropical fish are more at risk.

Leprosy can present as hypopigmented patches of skin with loss of sensation and thickened nerves. It can also resemble a widespread erythematous rash with nodules, papules, and plaques.

Infestations with scabies mites, fleas, and lice are usually intensely pruritic. Patients may scratch themselves constantly and present with excoriations, bleeding on skin, scratch marks, and general distress. In scabies, burrows may be present. They sometimes have urticated lesions as well. Infants with scabies can have pustules on their palms and soles.

Flea bites often present as erythematous, itchy papules, especially on the lower limbs.

Head lice cause intense itching on the scalp. The eggs of the head lice, known as nits, may be seen on affected hair shafts. Nits and even the lice themselves may be extracted through the use of a very fine-toothed comb. Pubic lice cause itchy papules in the genital region. Bedbugs are experiencing resurgence. Their bites appear as itchy red papules, often grouped in a linear fashion and colloquially referred to as 'breakfast, lunch, and dinner'.

Viral infections of the skin may present as vesicles and erythema, as in varicella. Varicella affects the mucus membranes as well and may result in difficulty eating and drinking. It is also typically itchy. Shingles, or herpes zoster, is reactivation of the varicella virus. It tends to affect a single nerve root and, therefore, the appearance is of erythema, vesicles, and crusting affecting just one dermatome. It seems to be more common when a person's immunity is compromised or when there is increased stress. It affects the elderly more often and can result in post-herpetic neuralgia. This can persist despite the skin lesions settling.

Herpes simplex is commonly seen as a crusted nodule around the mouth or nose. It can also present in the genital area as a crop of intensely tender vesicles. Genital herpes is considered a sexually transmitted disease.

Fungus infection of the skin can appear as an itchy, erythematous, scaly, annular lesion with a well-defined ring. It can appear as numerous lesions or as a solitary lesion. It can also present as a scaly area on the scalp, often associated with some hair loss. When it affects the nails, the nails often become thickened, brittle, and yellow.

Less commonly, deep fungal infections of the skin occur, especially in the immunocompromised. This can present as erythematous nodules that may exude pus and ulcerate.

The most common yeast infection seen is thrush, caused by candida. It can affect the moist skin-fold areas and cause erythema and soreness. It is often associated with satellite lesions. Candida in the genital area is often accompanied by a white, cottage-cheese-like discharge. Oral candida appears as white patches on the tongue and oral mucosa. It can be very sore.

Malassezia can cause pityriasis versicolor. This presents as flaky, pigmented patches typically on the upper back and chest in a Christmas tree distribution. When it settles, it can leave hyperpigmentation or hypopigmentation of the skin.

Demographics of the disease

Cellulitis is more common in skin that has been damaged, creating an opportunity for the organism to invade the skin. It is also more common in patients with damaged lymphatic flow, such as patients with lymphoedema.

Scabies commonly occur in institutions where individuals are in close proximity with each other. This can be in residential and nursing homes, hospitals, or hostels.

Tinea capitis (fungal infection of the scalp), head lice, and impetigo are more common in children and are often passed on through close play and contact with others.

Pubic lice, genital herpes simplex, and HPV genital warts are sexually transmitted and seen more often in the sexually active.

Fleas tend to originate from animals, and flea bites are more common in pet owners, although fleas can survive in carpets and soft furnishing for many months after the pet has been removed.

Other animals such as cats, dogs, and horses can transmit fungal infection.

Leprosy and tuberculosis are more common in the developing world and are spread by droplet infection.

Bedbugs live in mattresses and soft furnishings such as carpets and cushions, and can be transmitted via suitcases and clothing to other areas.

Natural history, and complications of the disease

Most infections and infestations have a good prognosis. They are, however, contagious, and care should be taken to give adequate advice to patients and their close contacts. It is important to establish the diagnosis and treat appropriately. They can be more common in immunocompromised patients, the elderly, children, and patients with underlying conditions such as diabetes.

Most viral infections are self-limiting and will resolve on their own. Post-herpetic neuralgia is a complication of herpes zoster. Cervical and anal cancer can be a complication of HPV genital warts.

Bacterial infections can be more troublesome and often require a course of antimicrobials. It is helpful to establish the organism and treatments that it is sensitive to. Recurrent cellulitis can lead to damage of the lymphatic system and cause lymphoedema.

Leprosy can have long-term complicated sequelae, including mutilating disease such as deformation of digits. Both leprosy and tuberculosis may involve other systems of the body and, if inadequately treated, can result in significant morbidity.

Scabies requires a host to survive. It can spread amongst individuals. Norwegian scabies is a crusted form that is particularly virulent and spreads easily. Norwegian scabies is more common in the very old, the very young, and immunocompromised individuals.

Approach to diagnosing the disease

A careful history should be sought. This includes time of onset; duration of symptoms; area affected; distribution of the lesions; history of contact with other affected people and animals; social history; and systemic symptoms. Examination is important for making the diagnosis. In infestations, the mites, fleas, or lice may be seen. Close contacts may need to be examined, too.

Other diagnoses that should be considered

The differential diagnoses for cellulitis would include deep vein thrombosis. A history of recent long distance travel, major surgery, long periods of inactivity, oral contraceptives, or a family history of clotting disorders should help point towards this diagnosis.

Dermatitis can be difficult to differentiate from scabies, as scabies sufferers often have a widespread rash that is easy to mistake as dermatitis.

Granuloma annulare is often mistaken as ringworm. The clue is that granuloma annulare is usually asymptomatic and non-scaly.

Psoriasis can also cause discoloured, thickened nails. It is important here to examine other parts of the body, including the scalp, to look for signs of psoriasis plaques.

'Gold-standard' diagnostic test

The gold-standard diagnostic test for skin infection and infestation is the isolation and identification of the organism. In infestations, the offender can often be caught. It is important to look in the correct area; for example, look for scabies mites in burrows; fleas in the carpet, pets, and soft furnishings; bedbugs in the mattress, where blood stains can often be seen; and head lice in the hair, using a fine-toothed comb.

Skin scrapings can be taken of superficial fungal and yeast infections of the skin, nails, and scalp. Hair pluckings and nail clippings can also be taken. Often, hyphae and spores can be seen when examined under the microscope.

Skin swabs should be taken from bacterially infected skin and sent for microscopy, culture, and sensitivities. In deep fungal infections, tuberculosis, and leprosy, a skin biopsy could be sent for culture. PCR can also be carried out on the skin biopsies. In leprosy, split skin smears can be taken from the ear and sent for culture. Periodic acid–Schiff staining of skin biopsies may also help to identify fungal spores.

PCR can also be carried out on viral swabs for the identification of the virus.

Acceptable diagnostic alternatives to the gold standard

A good history and high clinical suspicion are very important. Blood tests are sometimes carried out to support the diagnosis. For example, a hot, red, swollen lower limb associated with a high white blood count and raised level of C-reactive protein would be a good pointer towards cellulitis as a diagnosis.

Other relevant investigations

In bacterial infections, blood tests with raised acute inflammatory markers and a white blood cell count will be helpful.

In tuberculosis, a chest X-ray, a T-spot test, or a Mantoux test should be carried out. Bronchoscopy, if there is chest involvement, may be helpful for obtaining further evidence of the infection.

Prognosis and how to estimate it

If treated appropriately, most infections and infestations will resolve. However, some such as tuberculosis and leprosy will require prolonged treatment for many months. Patient compliance can therefore be an issue. It is very easy to be reinfected in infestations, and education is important.

Treatment and its effectiveness

Head lice are becoming more resistant to topical insecticides. Treatment can be applied to wet hair and washed off after the recommended time. Retreatment is recommended after a week. It is important to check the hair of close contacts and treat them if they are affected as well. It is very easy to get reinfection with head lice. Avoiding close head-to-head contact with affected individuals is a good way of preventing reinfection. Using a hair conditioner and a fine-tooth comb to comb hair for a number of weeks may avoid the use of topical insecticides.

Body lice are spread through clothing. Pubic lice are spread through close contact and sexual contact. Washing clothes at 60°C should kill the lice and eggs. Affected individuals can be treated with topical insecticides.

Scabies causes intense itching. Symptoms appear 2–6 weeks after exposure in people affected for the first time, and 1–4 days after re-exposure. Treatment with topical insecticide such as malathion 0.5% liquid or permethrin 5% cream is commonly used in UK. All skin surfaces, including the genital areas, the soles of the feet, and under the nails, should be treated. In children, the scalp should be treated too. With malathion 0.5% liquid, treatment is left for 24 hours and then washed off. With permethrin 5%, treatment is left on for 8–12 hours. Retreatment a week later is recommended. All close contacts should be treated at the same time to prevent recurrence. Clothes should be washed at 60°C. It is common to have a post-scabies itch, which can persist for a few weeks despite successful eradication.

With fleas, pets in the family should be treated. The premises and soft furnishings should be treated as well. This is especially important for bedbugs. Suitcases have become a popular vector of transmission for bedbugs.

Bacterial infections should be treated with the appropriate antibiotics. As most skin bacterial infections are caused by streptococci or staphylococci, penicillin and flucloxacillin are usually the first choice to try. If cultures and sensitivities have been taken, it will be helpful to ensure that the antibiotic is sensitive to the particular strain of bacteria.

Impetigo can be treated with topical antiseptics and topical antibiotics such as fucidin.

Fungal infections can be treated with terbinafine cream. Nail fungal infections will require a course of oral antifungals such as oral terbinafine or pulsed itraconazole. Tinea capitis may require oral terbinafine or griseofulvin. Topical azoles can help in the treatment of yeast infections.

The treatment for tuberculosis and leprosy can involve a prolonged course with multiple agents. In the UK, these diseases are seen less commonly and it is important to seek the advice of experts who may be based in tertiary centres.

Antiviral such as aciclovir can be used in varicella, herpes zoster, and herpes simplex. However, treatment should be given promptly, ideally within 24 hours of the first symptoms occurring.

Further Reading

Britton WJ and Lockwood DNJ. Leprosy. *Lancet* 2004; 363; 1209–19.
Chambers HF, Moellering RC, and Kamitsuka P. Management of skin and soft-tissue infection. *N Engl J Med* 2008; 359: 1063–7.
Chosidow O. Scabies. *N Engl J Med* 2006; 354: 1718–27.
Heukelbach J and Feldmeier H. Scabies. *Lancet* 2006; 367: 1767–74.

247 Cutaneous vasculitis

Christine Soon

Definition of the disease

Vasculitis is inflammation of the blood vessels. It can affect large vessels, medium-sized vessels, or small vessels. Cutaneous vasculitis is inflammation of the blood vessels of the skin. This can include the capillaries, the venules, and the arterioles.

Aetiology of the disease

There are many possible causes of cutaneous vasculitis. These include infection, medication, and underlying disease such as connective tissue disease, solid-organ malignancies, haematological malignancies, inflammatory bowel disease, and other conditions. However, in many cases, an underlying cause is not found.

Typical symptoms of the disease, and less common symptoms

Purpura and petechiae are the common signs of cutaneous vasculitis. Symptoms usually present on the lower limbs first. Purpura is an area of extravasation of red blood cells under the skin. Petechiae are small areas of purpura. In severe cases, the overlying skin may become necrotic. The patient may complain of pain, bleeding, or itching. Livedo reticularis may be seen in association with connective tissue disease and is a lacelike, reddish-purple discoloration of the skin caused by capillary dilatation and the stagnation of blood within it. Occasionally, gangrene of the peripheries may be seen and necrotic ulcers may also be a feature. Oedema, nodules, vesicles, bullae, pustules, plaques, and urticated papules or plaques may also be noted.

Systemic symptoms such as fever, malaise, gastrointestinal symptoms, or arthralgia may also occur.

Demographics of the disease

Vasculitis can affect children or adults. A common childhood vasculitis is IgA vasculitis (Henoch–Schönlein Purpura). This is an IgA-mediated immune-complex vasculitis. It affects small blood vessels and may involve the gastrointestinal system, the skin, and the kidneys. It is usually self-limiting, and supportive treatment is usually enough. The lower limbs and buttocks tend to be affected.

Amongst adults, cutaneous small vessel vasculitis tends to be one of the most commonly seen forms of cutaneous vasculitis. It commonly affects women and tends to affect the lower limbs. It is a small vessel vasculitis. Urticarial vasculitis is a form of cutaneous vasculitis that presents as urticated papules and plaques which persist for more than 24 hours.

Erythema elevatum diutinum is a form of leucocytoclastic vasculitis that can be seen in adults. It appears as reddish-violaceous papules, plaques, or nodules that occur symmetrically over the dorsal surfaces of the knees, the hands, the Achilles tendons, and the buttocks.

Granuloma faciale is a rare cutaneous vasculitis characterized histologically by a prominent eosinophilic infiltrate that appears as nodules on the face. It typically affects white males.

Natural history, and complications of the disease

Cutaneous vasculitis without systemic involvement is usually a self-limiting condition.

Approach to diagnosing the disease

When diagnosing cutaneous vasculitis, a careful history is required. Systemic symptoms such as arthralgia, pyrexia, and general malaise are important. Dipstick of the urine should be carried out to detect any abnormalities. A comprehensive drug history must be taken. Family history and racial origins are important. Shortness of breath, chest pain, headaches, abdominal pain, and polyarthritis are all important to elucidate. A vasculitic screen is usually carried out to identify any underlying cause and to determine whether any internal organs are involved.

Other diagnoses that should be considered

Meningococcal septicaemia can present with a purpuric eruption. The speed of onset of the eruption and associated systemic symptoms such as headache, pyrexia, and photophobia are important clues to aid diagnosis.

Platelet and coagulation disorders can lead to purpura occurring in the skin. A full blood count, coagulation screen, and liver function tests should help in aiding the diagnosis.

Raised intravascular pressure can lead to petechiae or purpura appearing on lower legs, such as in gravitational or venous stasis, and on the face after prolonged coughing or vomiting.

Petechiae can be a sign of embolism from endocarditis, atrial myxoma, fat embolism after trauma, or cholesterol embolism.

In amyloidosis, pseudoxanthoma elasticum, and Ehlers–Danlos syndrome, the decreased vascular support can lead to purpura.

'Gold-standard' diagnostic test

Skin biopsies for histology and immunofluorescence would confirm the diagnosis.

Acceptable diagnostic alternatives to the gold standard

Acceptable diagnostic alternatives to the gold-standard diagnostic test are good history taking and examination, together with characteristic clinical appearances.

Other relevant investigations

Other relevant investigations include:

- chest X-ray
- ECG
- full blood count
- urea and electrolytes
- erythrocyte sedimentation rate
- C-reactive protein level
- antineutrophil cytoplasmic antibody assay
- antinuclear antibody assay
- extractable nuclear antigen antibody assay
- complement level
- immunoglobulin and serum electrophoresis
- urine dipstick test
- urine protein estimation
- T-spot test
- anti-streptococcal antibody test
- serology for hepatitis B and C
- cryoglobulins

Prognosis and how to estimate it

The prognosis will depend on the underlying cause. Leucocytoclastic vasculitis tends to be self-limiting, and patients generally do well. Cutaneous vasculitis occurring as part of a systemic vasculitis tends to run a more chronic course. Vasculitis can occasionally recur.

Treatment and its effectiveness

Supportive treatment to keep the patient symptom free is usually all that is required. This would include analgesia for pain, with rest and elevation of the lower limbs. In more severe cases, topical steroids or even systemic steroids might be required. Second-line agents such as dapsone and methotrexate have been used in refractory cases. If an underlying cause such as infection has been identified as the trigger, it is important to treat this, as treatment of the trigger usually helps the rash.

Further Reading

Burge S and Ogg GS. 'Cutaneous vasculitis, connective tissue diseases, and urticaria', in Warrell DA, Cox TM, and Firth JD, eds, *Oxford Textbook of Medicine* (5th edition), 2010. Oxford University Press.

248 Acne

Ben Esdaile

Definition of the disease

Acne vulgaris is a common, chronic inflammatory disorder of the pilosebaceous unit (the hair follicle and accompanying sebaceous gland). It can be classified as mild, moderate, or severe. Mild acne is characterized by comedones (non-inflammatory lesions: 'blackheads' and 'whiteheads') being the predominant lesions. Papules and pustules may also be present but are few in number. Moderate acne is defined by more inflammatory lesions such as papules and pustules, with comedones also usually present. Severe acne is defined as widespread inflammatory lesions, nodules, cysts, and scarring. Moderate acne that has not settled within 6 months of treatment, or acne that is causing serious psychological effects, is also categorized as severe.

Aetiology of the disease

The exact cause of acne vulgaris is not fully understood. The aetiology is complex with multifactorial influences on the pilosebaceous unit. There appears to be a genetic predisposition to acne, based on strong concordance in twin studies and family history. There appear to be four main contributors to the pathogenesis of the disease:

- blocking of the hair follicle with the formation of the comedone
- androgenic stimulation of the sebaceous gland, leading to increased sebum production
- colonization of the hair follicle with the gram-positive bacteria *Propionibacterium acnes*
- inflammation of the hair follicle and its surroundings

Typical symptoms of the disease, and the less common symptoms

The production of sebum form the sebaceous glands often results in 'greasy' skin. The skin lesions, namely comedones, papules, and pustules, are often asymptomatic but some of the large pustules, nodules, and cysts can become extremely tender. The prominent cosmetic distribution of acne can lead to a great psychological impact on the patient, and support groups can be extremely helpful.

A severe form of nodulocystic acne, acne fulminans, can produce severe systemic symptoms, including fever, arthralgia, and myalgia and requires urgent intervention.

Demographics and natural history of the disease

Acne vulgaris is the commonest skin condition to affect man. It is principally a disease of adolescence and it has been estimated to affect over 80% of those between 12 and 25. Although widely thought to be an adolescent disease, 3% of men and 12% of women will continue to have acne until their mid-forties.

Approach to diagnosing the disease

The diagnosis of acne vulgaris is a clinical one. Non-inflammatory acne is characterized by the presence of open (blackheads) and closed (whiteheads) comedones. Closed comedones are skin-coloured papules and are easily distinguished from the often black, discoloured, dilated follicular openings of the open comedone. When comedones become inflamed, they expand to develop pustules, inflammatory papules, nodules, and cysts. All of these lesions can result in scarring.

Acne fulminans is the most severe form of nodulocystic acne and is characterized by the abrupt onset of nodulocystic acne in association with systemic features, including fever, arthralgia, and myalgia. Severe eruptive nodulocystic acne without systemic features is known as acne conglobata.

Other diagnoses that should be considered

Although the diagnosis of acne vulgaris in adolescents is usually not difficult, in other age groups or when atypical features are present, other diagnoses may be considered. Rosacea is the most common differential diagnosis to acne vulgaris. Patients with rosacea often complain of both redness and spots. Important clues from the history are that sufferers often notice an exacerbation of their symptoms with alcohol, exercise, spicy foods, and emotion. They often also report easy flushing in their youth. Clinically, patients with rosacea have evidence of erythema, telangiectasia, and inflammatory papules and pustules. There may also be evidence of sebaceous hyperplasia, which can result in enlargement of the nose. A significant proportion of suffers have ocular involvement, with blepharitis and conjunctivitis.

Another cause of a red face is seborrhoeic dermatitis, which presents as a red, often scaly face, especially in the distribution of the nose and eyebrows, the so-called T-zone of the face. They usually also report scaling of the scalp; however, inflammatory pustules and papules are not usually present.

Table 248.1 summarizes possible differential diagnoses.

'Gold-standard' diagnostic test

There is no 'gold-standard' diagnostic test for acne vulgaris. It is a clinical diagnosis and it is therefore essential to perform a thorough history and examination of the patient. From the history, it is important to ascertain the use of all over-the counter preparations as well as comedogenic cosmetics, including pomades as well as topical steroids. In females, a menstrual and oral contraceptive history is important to evaluate the hormonal influence on the acne. It is important to establish the severity (using validated scoring system), the type of lesions (inflammatory or comedonal), and the presence of scarring.

Other relevant investigations

Usually no investigations are required; however, a skin swab from a pustule can provide sensitivities of *P. acnes* and hence can help tailor therapy. Skin and nasal swabs can also help to exclude a gram-negative folliculitis. In certain patients where a hormone abnormality is suspected (i.e. very irregular menstrual cycle, significant hirsutism), a sex hormone profile including testosterone, sex hormone-binding

Table 248.1 Differential diagnoses of acne vulgaris	
Comedonal acne	**Inflammatory acne**
Milia	Rosacea
Sebaceous hyperplasia	Perioral dermatitis
Miliaria rubra	Contact dermatitis
Syringomas	Folliculitis
Trichoepitheliomas	Keratosis pilaris
	SLE
	Steroid-induced acne

globulin, prolactin, follicular-stimulating hormone, and luteinizing hormone can be measured. In rare circumstances when a diagnosis of late-onset congenital adrenal hyperplasia is suspected, the 17-α-hydroxyprogesterone levels can be measured.

Treatment and its effectiveness

The treatment of acne is directed towards the four main areas in the pathogenesis of the disease. A summary of the treatments for acne vulgaris is shown in Table 248.2.

Topical treatments

Topical retinoids

Retinoids (e.g. adapalene, tazarotene, tretinoin) work by normalizing follicular keratinization and hence have anticomedonal properties. They also have significant anti-inflammatory affects and hence can be used as first-line treatments for both mild inflammatory and comedonal acne. Topical retinoids can be used as monotherapy or in combination with benzoyl peroxide or antibiotics. They can cause local drying, irritation of the skin, and thinning of the outer layer of the epidermis (stratum corneum). Some are also unstable in the sun; therefore, patients should be advised to apply them in the evening. Female patients should be advised not to become pregnant while using topical retinoids, as there is a theoretical risk of systemic absorption of this known teratogen.

Benzoyl peroxide

Benzoyl peroxide is a bactericidal agent and acts on the *P. acnes* within the hair follicle. It is available in multiple strengths, from 2.5% to 10%, as washes, soaps, gels, and lotions and in combinations with topical antibiotics. Patients should be warned that benzoyl peroxide can be an irritant as well as bleach clothes and bedding.

Topical antibiotics

Topical antibiotics (e.g. clindamycin, erythromycin, sodium sulfacetamide) should not be used in the long term due to the possibility of the development of bacterial resistance. They are available in combination with benzoyl peroxide or topical retinoids.

Salicylic acid

Salicylic acid has comedolytic and mild anti-inflammatory properties. It is available in strengths up to 2% in gels, creams, and lotions.

Azelaic acid

Azelaic acid is a naturally occurring dicarboxylic acid found in cereal grains. It has both anti-inflammatory effects and comedolytic activity. It also has the added benefit of helping post-inflammatory hyperpigmentation. It also has fewer side effects, compared to topical retinoids.

Oral treatments

Oral antibiotics

Oral antibiotics (e.g. oxytetracycline, tetracycline, doxycycline, lymecycline, minocycline, erythromycin, and trimethoprim) are prescribed for moderate-to-severe inflammatory acne. Their primary mechanism of action is the suppression of growth of *P. acnes* but they also possess intrinsic anti-inflammatory properties. There are increasing reports of resistance to erythromycin and some of the tetracyclines.

Hormonal manipulation

Hormone therapy is an established second-line therapy for female patients suffering from moderate-to-severe acne vulgaris. The oral contraceptive pill works by decreasing the production of both adrenal and ovarian androgens. A number of formulations that combine oestradiol with the anti-androgenic cyproterone acetate are widely used. Other formulations combine oestradiol with a low-androgenic progestin such as drospirenone.

Isotretinoin

Isotretinoin is a retinoid and an isomer of tretinoin. It is used for severe nodulocystic acne, significant acne that has not responded to adequate courses of antibiotic treatment or acne that is causing physical or psychological scarring. Its mechanism of action is not fully understood but it is known to inhibit maturation of the basal cells of the sebaceous gland, resulting in decreased sebum production. It also acts to normalize follicular keratinization as well as having anti-inflammatory and antimicrobial activity. It is the only treatment to target all four of the pathogenic contributors to acne.

Isotretinoin has a number of common side effects, including severe dryness of the skin and mucous membranes, causing nosebleeds, cracking of the lips, and intolerance of contact lenses. As it is teratogenic, it should not be prescribed in women of childbearing years unless they are registered with a pregnancy prevention programme. Therapy can also result in an elevation in serum triglyceride and cholesterol levels as well as abnormalities in liver enzymes.

A causal link between oral isotretinoin and psychological disturbance is not fully proven but it is prudent to get a specialist psychiatric opinion prior to initiating therapy if there are any mood concerns. Therapy should be stopped if there is any significant alteration in mood during therapy.

Surgical treatments

Comedones can be treated with a number of surgical techniques such as electrocautery, or the comedone can simply be expressed with a needle or scalpel blade. Deep, inflamed cystic lesions can be improved with steroid injections with triamcinolone acetonide. Low-concentration chemical peels have also been successful in the treatment of comedones.

Table 248.2	Acne vulgaris treatment algorithm				
Acne Treatment Algorithm					
	Mild		Moderate		Severe
	Comedonal (blackheads/ whiteheads)	Papular/ Pustular	Papular/ Pustular	Nodular	Nodular/ Conglobate
1st Choice	Topical Retinoid	Topical retinoid + topical antimicrobial	Oral antibiotic +/− topical retinoid +/− benzoyl peroxide	Oral antibiotic +/− topical retinoid +/− benzoyl peroxide	Oral Isotretinoin
Alternatives	Alternative topical retinoid or azelaic acid or salicylic acid.	Alternative topical antimicrobial + alternative topical retinoid or azelaic acid.	Alternative oral antibiotic + alternative topical retinoid +/− benzoyl peroxide	Oral Isotretinoin or alternative oral antibiotic + alternative topical retinoid +/− benzoyl peroxide/ azelaic acid.	High dose oral antibiotic + topical retinoid + benzoyl peroxide
Options for Females	Oral contraceptive/anti-androgen				
Maintenance	Topical retinoid		Topical retinoid +/− benzoyl peroxide		

Reprinted from *Journal of the American Academy of Dermatology*, Volume 49, issue 1, Harald Gollnick, William Cunliffe, Diane Berson, Brigitte Dreno, Andrew Finlay, James J. Leyden, Alan R. Shalita, Diane Thiboutot, Management of Acne A Report From a Global Alliance to Improve Outcomes in Acne, pp. S1-S37, Copyright (2003), with permission from Elsevier.

Acne scarring is difficult to treat satisfactorily. Chemical peels may be used to treat scars resulting from acne. Other techniques include dermabrasion and laser resurfacing, which aim to alter the contours of the scars.

Further Reading

Goodfield MJD, Cox NH, Bowser A., et al. Advice on the safe introduction and continued use of isotretinoin in acne in the UK 2010. *Brit J Dermatol* 2010; 162: 1172–9.

Nast A, Dreno B, Bettoli V, et al. European evidence-based guidelines for the treatment of acne. *J Eur Acad Dermatol* 2012; 26(S1): 1–29.

NHS Clinical Knowledge Summaries: *Acne Vulgaris* (http://cks.nice.org.uk/acne-vulgaris).

Zaenglein AL and Thiboutot DM. 'Acne vulgaris', in Bolognia JL, Jorizzo JL, and Rapini PR, eds, *Dermatology*, 2008. Mosby (Elsevier).

249 Psoriasis

Ben Esdaile

Definition of the disease

Psoriasis is a common, chronic inflammatory skin disease that is associated with joint disease in approximately 25% of patients. The most common variant of psoriasis is chronic plaque psoriasis (psoriasis vulgaris), which has the hallmark of well-demarcated erythematous plaques covered by silvery scale. There are a number of other variants of psoriasis, including guttate, inverse, palmoplantar, flexural, pustular, and erythrodermic.

Aetiology of the disease

Psoriasis is a polygenic disease. Twin studies have shown a 67% concordance for monozygotic twins versus 18% for dizygotic twins. Several susceptibility loci have so far been identified and the PSOR1 gene (C6p21.3), situated within the major histocompatibility complex (MHC) region of Chromosome 6, has been shown to be involved in around 50% of patients with psoriasis. The association of psoriasis with MHC alleles suggests an important role of T-lymphocytes in the pathogenesis. This has been confirmed as, once the disease is triggered, there appears to be a large recruitment of T-lymphocytes to the dermis and epidermis, resulting in the characteristic plaques. There is a resultant large production of pro-inflammatory mediators, including tumour necrosis factor alpha and interferon gamma, as well as numerous cytokines which have become targets for novel therapies.

Psoriasis can be triggered by external factors such as infection, physical trauma, or sunburn. The development of psoriasis in sites of trauma to the skin is known as the Koebner phenomenon. Other external factors include infections, especially streptococcal upper respiratory tract infections. Several drugs are known to trigger psoriasis, including beta blockers, lithium, and antimalarials.

Typical symptoms of the disease, and less common symptoms

Chronic plaque psoriasis is often asymptomatic but may itch or sting and can bleed easily when scratched (Auspitz sign). Psoriasis can have an enormous psychological impact and can limit normal social and leisure activities. This can be measured using the Dermatology Life Quality Index, which provides a score between 0 and 30. A score of greater than 10 is regarded as a severe impact on a patient's quality of life.

Demographics of the disease

In most reviews, the prevalence of psoriasis worldwide varies between 0.1% and 3%. In the UK, the prevalence is estimated at between 1% and 2%. There are certain parts of the world, such as Canada and the US, where the prevalence has been reported up to 4.7%. In contrast to this, there are some parts of Africa where the prevalence is estimated as low as 0.4%. Psoriasis affects both sexes equally.

Natural history, and complications of the disease

Psoriasis can first appear at any age but there appears to be two main peaks in a person's twenties and fifties; 75% of disease occurs before the age of 40. It tends to run a chronic relapsing and remitting course. Psoriasis can be complicated by its pustular and erythrodermic variants.

Psoriasis is associated with metabolic syndrome and its components, including diabetes, hypertension, and obesity. The increased risk of myocardial infarction in patient with psoriasis highlights the importance of addressing reversible risk factors.

Approach to diagnosing the disease

The diagnosis of psoriasis is usually made clinically and does not require histological confirmation. A full history is important and can reveal a family history of psoriasis, as well as details of all medications and recent illnesses which may be important triggers for the disease.

The most common variant of psoriasis is chronic plaque psoriasis (psoriasis vulgaris). Clinically, the patient presents with well-demarcated 'salmon-pink' symmetrical scaly plaques with an overlying silvery scale. The plaques classically present on extensor surfaces and can vary in size (from tiny papules to extremely large plaques). There are certain sites of predilection that can give clues to the diagnosis, such as the sacrum, the umbilicus, the nape of neck, the hairline of the scalp, and extensor surfaces. Approximately 50% will have nail changes such as pitting, onycholysis, and subungual hyperkeratosis. Plaques can occur in the flexures, in which case the condition is termed flexural psoriasis. When this is the only site of involvement, the term 'inverse' psoriasis is often used. The severity of chronic plaque psoriasis can be quantified using a scoring system known as the Psoriasis Area and Severity Index score.

Other variants of psoriasis include guttate psoriasis, which is common in children and young adults, with often an antecedent history of an upper respiratory tract infection. Clinically, patients present with a scattered 'rain-drop' appearance of small papules/plaques over the body.

Psoriasis can present with a pustular variant that is either localized (palmoplantar pustulosis/acrodermatitis of Hallopeau) or generalized. The generalized variant presents as multiple sterile pustules on an erythematous background. Importantly, this can be induced by the rapid cessation of oral steroids or the inappropriate use of topical steroids. Psoriasis is one of the causes of erythroderma, and patients can present with generalized erythema and desquamation from their psoriasis.

Other diagnoses that should be considered

The diagnosis of psoriasis is classical but differentials that may be considered are outlined in Table 249.1.

'Gold-standard' diagnostic test

The gold-standard diagnostic test for the diagnosis of psoriasis is a skin biopsy. In chronic plaque psoriasis, there is epidermal hyperplasia

Table 249.1 Differential diagnoses for chronic plaque psoriasis

Single plaque	Multiple plaques
Lichen simplex chronicus	Eczema
Bowen's disease (squamous cell carcinoma in situ)	Cutaneous T-cell lymphoma
	Lichen planus
Lichen planus	Tinea corporis
Tinea corporis/capitis	

(acanthosis), with flattening of the rete ridges and loss of the granular cell layer with cells in the stratum corneum still possessing flattened nuclei (parakeratosis). There are often neutrophils found in the epidermis in so-called Munro microabscesses.

Acceptable diagnostic alternatives to the gold standard

The diagnosis of psoriasis is usually made clinically without the need for histological confirmation or further investigations.

Other relevant investigations

Skins swabs can provide clues for potential triggers of flares of psoriasis. Patients who are commenced on systemic therapies need regular blood test monitoring that will be outlined in 'Systemic treatments'. The association of psoriasis and metabolic syndrome means that it is worth measuring lipids and other cardiovascular risk factors.

Prognosis, and how to estimate it

Chronic plaque psoriasis is a chronic disease that usually runs a relapsing and remitting course.

Treatment and its effectiveness

There are many factors that influence the choice of therapy in the management of psoriasis including patient choice, disease extent, lifestyle, and comorbidities. The different therapy choices available are detailed in this chapter.

Topical treatments

Vitamin D analogues

Vitamin D_3 analogues (e.g. calcipotriol, calcitriol, tacalcitol) act by inhibiting the proliferation of keratinocytes and inducing normal differentiation. They can have an effect on calcium homeostasis and so a maximum weekly dose of 100 g is recommended. They can also be combined with topical corticosteroids. They are used as monotherapy or in combination as a first-line agent for mild-to-moderate chronic plaque psoriasis.

Coal tar

The mechanism of action of coal tar is not understood but it has a range of anti-inflammatory properties. There are a number of preparations of tar used in creams, lotions, shampoos, gels, and ointments. It is also used in its crude form for special inpatient topical regimens. It is often combined with other products including salicylic acid, coconut oil, and corticosteroids. It is also occasionally used in combination with UV light.

Glucocorticoids

Topical corticosteroids have become one of the major first-line therapies for chronic plaque psoriasis. This is mainly due to their cosmetic acceptance and relative ease of use. Inappropriate use of topical steroids can not only lead to relapses and flares but can also induce pustular psoriasis. The topical corticosteroids are important in flexural disease due to their lack of irritancy.

Topical retinoids

Tazarotene is an acetylic retinoid which has an antiproliferative effect on the keratinocytes. Its use is limited by both efficacy and irritation.

Dithranol

Dithranol (anthralin) is derived from the bark of the araroba tree, which is indigenous to South America. It has a marked antiproliferative effect on the epidermis. It can cause burning and erythema to normal skin as well as stain clothes and bath enamel. It is rarely used on the flexures or face due to irritation. It is often used as part of an inpatient regimen but there are now some more 'short-contact' non-staining preparations that can be used in the day setting or even at home.

Phototherapy

It is well described that a number of patients note an improvement in their psoriasis after exposure to the sun. Phototherapy with UVA and UVB radiation is one of the mainstays of treatment of moderate-to-severe psoriasis. Phototherapy with broadband UVB has largely been replaced with narrow band UVB produced by TLO1 bulbs. UVA radiation is used in combination with photosensitizers 8-methoxypsoralen and 5-methoxypsoralen either orally or topically. Phototherapy does have side effects, with dose-dependent burning, photoageing, and the increased risk of skin carcinogenesis with cumulative doses.

Systemic treatments

When disease control fails with topical or light therapy, patients are often offered a systemic therapy. These drugs all have side effects and so the choice of agent is made after a balanced discussion between doctor and patient. Patients require careful monitoring.

Methotrexate

Methotrexate is the most commonly used systemic therapy for psoriasis in the UK. It is a derivative of folic acid and acts as an antimetabolite by inhibiting the enzyme dihydrofolate reductase and hence cell division. The drug also has anti-inflammatory properties on lymphocytes and neutrophils. Methotrexate is usually started at a dose of 5 mg weekly and a full blood count is recorded after 7 days to check for an idiosyncratic reaction of myelosuppression. The dose can then be increased, usually to a maximum of 15–25 mg weekly. Monitoring of liver tests, renal tests, and full blood counts takes place weekly for 2 weeks after any dose change and then 2–3 monthly once the dose is stable. Specific markers for liver fibrosis are the serum pro-collagen III N-terminal peptides levels, which are measured on a 3-monthly basis where available. This test has now superseded the previous invasive liver biopsies that were routinely performed before and after a cumulative 1.5 g dose. The co administration of 5 mg of folic acid is said to help reduce the main side effect of nausea.

Ciclosporin

Ciclosporin acts as a calcineurin inhibitor and prevents T-lymphocyte activation. It was originally used to prevent organ rejection in transplant patients. Ciclosporin is a highly effective drug in the treatment of psoriasis but its use is limited by its inevitable side effects. The major side effect is that of nephrotoxicity, which usually limits the therapy to short courses of 3–4 months. The usual starting dose is 2.5 mg/kg per day and can be increased up to a maximum of 4 mg/kg per day. Close monitoring of blood pressure and renal function is required during therapy.

Acitretin

Vitamin A (retinol) is an essential epithelial growth factor whose precise mode of action is not fully understood. A deficiency in vitamin A leads to reversible dry skin and squamous metaplasia. Acitretin is given in doses usually ranging from 10 mg to 50 mg daily. It is often combined with UVB therapy. Acitretin is useful in all forms of psoriasis but is especially in erythrodermic and pustular variants. The most important side effect is that of teratogenicity and it is therefore not usually used in women of childbearing age. It is important to monitor liver function and lipid metabolism during therapy.

Other systemic therapies

Other systemic therapies include the fumaric acid esters and hydroxyurea.

Biological therapy

Biologic therapies for psoriasis target specific molecules involved in the inflammatory cascade of psoriasis. There are now a number of licensed drugs which have transformed the lives of patients with psoriasis. Many of the biologics specifically target tumour necrosis factor and include infliximab, etanercept, and adalimumab. There are some newer monoclonal antibodies against other interleukins in the inflammatory cascade, such as ustekinumab, which targets interleukins 12 and 23. The long-term safety of these drugs is not proven, with potential long-term side effects including malignancy (e.g. lymphomas and skin cancers) and opportunistic infections (e.g. tuberculosis).

Further Reading

Cohen SN, Baron SE, and Archer CB. Guidance on the diagnosis and clinical management of psoriasis. *Clin Exp Dermatol* 2012; 37 (Suppl 1): 13–18.

Menter A and Griffiths CE. Current and future management of psoriasis. Lancet 2007; 370: 272–84.

National Institute for Health and Clinical Excellence. *Psoriasis: Assessment and Management.* 2012. Available at http://guidance.nice.org.uk/CG153 (accessed 15 Jul 2017).

Smith CG, Anstey AV, Barker JN, et al. British Association of Dermatologists' guidelines for biologic interventions for psoriasis 2009. Brit J Derm 2009; 161: 987–1019.

Van de Kerkhof PCM and Schalkwijk J. 'Psoriasis', in Bolognia JL, Jorizzo JL, and Rapini PR, eds, *Dermatology*, 2008. Mosby (Elsevier).

250 Eczema

Ben Esdaile

Definition of the disease

Eczema is a descriptive term for a set of symptoms and signs which usually involve itchy inflammation of the skin, and is subcategorized into many different forms. Atopic eczema (atopic dermatitis) is the most common chronic inflammatory disease amongst children. Other types of eczema include seborrhoeic eczema, discoid eczema, asteatotic eczema, contact allergic eczema, contact irritant eczema, pompholyx eczema, venous eczema, juvenile plantar dermatosis, and lichen simplex. In this chapter, we will cover atopic eczema, which is called 'atopic' due to its association with other atopic disorders such as asthma and allergic rhinitis.

Aetiology of the disease

The aetiology of atopic eczema has yet to be fully understood but it is known to have both genetic and environmental factors. A gene encoding a protein called filaggrin, which is involved in keratin aggregation, has been shown to be mutated in 20%–50% of children with the disease. The rising prevalence over the last few decades, with the simultaneous increasing levels of hygiene, led to the 'hygiene theory' that children who were exposed to more antigens were less likely to develop atopy. Factors that are known to exacerbate eczema include sweating, irritants such as detergents and solvents, infection, stress, and, in some cases, contact allergens, including aeroallergens.

Typical symptoms of the disease, and less common symptoms

The main symptom of atopic eczema is pruritus. Patients develop further symptoms from the sequelae of scratching (e.g. infection). Virtually all patients with atopic eczema have constitutional dry skin known as xerosis.

Demographics of the disease

Atopic eczema has an estimated prevalence of between 10% and 20% in Northern Europe and the US, with lower rates in Africa. It is slightly more common in girls. In the UK, it is associated with an estimated cost of over £500 million per year.

Natural history, and complications of the disease

The majority of patients with atopic eczema first develop their disease in early infancy, usually after 2 months. Many children with atopic eczema improve by the age of 3. Over 50% are disease-free by the age of 6, and up to 80% by the age of 14. Some may relapse in early adult life but most recover by their thirties. A small proportion will go on to suffer from lifelong disease.

Eczema can be complicated by infection, with bacteria being the most common offending agents. Secondary infection with herpes simplex virus can lead to eczema herpeticum with a characteristic (bullet-spray) appearance of punched-out erosions and vesicles. Patients can become systemically unwell, as well as have ophthalmic involvement. Eczema herpeticum can be life-threatening.

Patients with severe eczema can develop a generalized exfoliative erythroderma. This is a dermatological emergency, as patients can develop problems with temperature regulation, sepsis, and even cardiac failure.

Approach to diagnosing the disease

A diagnosis of atopic eczema is usually readily made from a history and clinical examination. The rash of atopic eczema is usually symmetrical, with ill-defined patches of erythema and scale and with serous exudate and vesiculation seen in acute states (the eczema usually starts on the face and then extends to involve the trunk and limbs). In infants, the face and extensor surfaces are mostly affected but, as children mature, it tends to involve the flexural areas, especially the antecubital fossae, the popliteal fossae, the wrists, and the neck. Chronic eczema leads to thickening of areas of scratching (lichenification) and post-inflammatory hyper- or hypopigmentation.

The decrease in epithelial/skin barrier function can result in secondary infection, with the classical yellow overlying crust of impetiginized eczema. Patients with eczema also appear to be more susceptible to viral infections, with higher incidences of molluscum contagiosum, warts, and herpes simplex viral infections (eczema herpeticum).

Other diagnoses that should be considered

In infancy, the main differential is seborrhoeic dermatitis. Seborrhoeic dermatitis is not usually pruritic and there is usually no associated family history of atopy. The main clue is the distribution, with seborrhoeic eczema being more prominent on the scalp (cradle cap), face, and nappy areas. In older children and adults, a diagnosis of scabies should always be considered in any itchy rash. When a patient presents with no family or personal history of eczema, one should always consider the possibility of an allergic contact dermatitis. Cutaneous T-cell lymphoma can mimic chronic eczema. It is sometimes difficult to differentiate eczema and psoriasis, especially when a patient presents with a hand/foot dermatitis.

'Gold-standard' diagnostic test

The diagnosis of atopic eczema is a clinical one and there is no 'gold-standard' diagnostic test. A skin biopsy is, therefore, rarely needed but the histological features of eczema will depend on the stage of the eczema. In acute eczema, there is oedema between the epidermal cells, known as spongiosis. In more chronic eczema, there is thickening of the epidermis with epidermal hyperplasia.

Acceptable diagnostic alternatives to the gold standard

As mentioned previously, the diagnosis of atopic eczema is a clinical one and rarely needs a skin biopsy. Patch testing is used to investigate any extrinsic allergens exacerbating the atopic eczema.

Other relevant investigations

Elevation of serum IgE levels and eosinophilia are often found in atopics, but approximately 25% will have normal levels. Total IgE levels are often elevated in atopic eczema patients but the usefulness of the detection of specific IgE-directed antibodies against certain allergens (radioallergosorbent testing (RAST)) in finding triggers of disease is controversial. RAST and skin prick testing can potentially provide some useful information about allergen avoidance but careful patient selection, based on their history, is advised (e.g. flares in exposed sites and associations with house dust mite allergy).

Prognosis, and how to estimate it

Prognosis is difficult to predict in atopic eczema but severe disease in infancy and disease on the extensor surfaces of the elbows and knees are poor prognostic markers.

Treatment and its effectiveness

Education plays a vital role in the management of eczema. A reduction of trigger factors such as harsh chemicals, the use of soaps, and avoidance of house dust mite are all beneficial. Cotton clothing appears to be less irritating to the skin than clothing made of other material. The importance of treating the xerosis of the skin and breaking the itch–scratch cycle is vital.

Topical treatments

Emollients

Emollients are an essential aspect of the treatment of atopic eczema. The xerosis and impaired barrier function are vital targets for therapy. There are numerous commercially available different emollients with varying ingredients, usually containing paraffin. The greasier the emollient, the more effective it will be but, usually, the less acceptable it will be to the patient. Emollients should be generously applied as many times a day as practical. They should also be applied after bathing, to damp skin.

Soap substitutes and bath additives

Soaps are irritating to the skin and so it is important to avoid them and use a soap substitute for washing. There are, again, a number of soap substitutes available, including *ones with emulsifying ointment and aqueous cream. In fact, many emollients can be used as a soap substitute. There are now a number of bath additives and shower gels designed for patients with eczema. Some are now combined with an antiseptic agent that can be useful in patients with recurrent infective exacerbations.

Topical corticosteroids

Topical glucocorticosteroids are the mainstay of treatment for atopic eczema. The choice of steroid is dependent on the age of the patient and the site and stage of the eczema. In general, low-potency steroids such as hydrocortisone and clobetasone butyrate are used on the face. Moderately potent steroids are used in the flexures. It is advised that a potent steroid is used at first to gain control, prior to reducing its strength. The vehicle of the active ingredient is important, as ointments lead to better absorption, compared to creams.

Inappropriate chronic daily use of topical corticosteroids can lead to complications of skin atrophy, telangiectasias, and striae. There is also a risk of cataract development if potent steroids are used near the eye for a prolonged duration.

A table summarizing the potency of some of the commonly used steroids is shown in Table 250.1.

Topical pimecrolimus and tacrolimus

Pimecrolimus and tacrolimus are licensed for mild-to-moderate and moderate-to-severe atopic eczema, respectively. They are steroid-sparing immunosuppressants that act via inhibition of the T-cell activator calcineurin. They have an important role in the long-term management of eczema (especially on the face) to reduce the use of topical steroids. They can cause stinging when first used but this effect fades after a number of applications.

Occlusive bandaging

Occlusive bandaging of the limbs can be extremely useful in the treatment of atopic eczema affecting the limbs. Steroids can be applied underneath the bandages, which can contain antipruritic substances such as zinc and ichthammol. The process of 'wet wrapping', a two-layer bandaging technique where the inner layer is soaked in warm water, is also useful in the paediatric setting.

Antihistamines

The sedating antihistamines do have a role in the treatment of atopic eczema. Their sedative properties can help break the itch–scratch cycle, especially at night. (It is the sedative properties that are useful.)

UV phototherapy

UVB TL01

There are a number of different phototherapy regimens that have been used with success in treating eczema but narrow-band UVB seems to be the safest and appears effective in some, but not, all patients.

Oral treatments

Systemic treatments are reserved for patients in whom optimal topical therapy does not result in disease control.

Oral corticosteroids

Systemic corticosteroids are used for acute severe flares of atopic eczema that fails to respond to topical therapy. Their use in protracted courses can result in systemic side effects.

Azathioprine

Azathioprine is an immunosuppressive corticosteroid-sparing agent that is an antimetabolite thought to inhibit the proliferation of lymphocytes. Note, however, that there is a genetic polymorphism for an enzyme called thiopurine methyltransferase (TPMT), which is important in the metabolism of azathioprine; although >1% of the population is homozygous for an allele of low activity of TPMT, they are at risk of profound myelosuppression at standard doses. For this reason, patients should have their TPMT levels checked prior to starting therapy.

Ciclosporin

Ciclosporin acts as a calcineurin inhibitor and prevents T-lymphocyte activation. It was originally used to prevent organ rejection in transplant patients. The major side effect is that of nephrotoxicity which usually limits the therapy to short courses. The usual starting dose is 2.5 mg/kg per day but can be increased up to a maximum of 4 mg/kg per day. Close monitoring of blood pressure and renal function is required during therapy.

Other systemics

There are many other agents that have been used with variable success in the long-term control of atopic eczema, including methotrexate and mycophenolate mofitil.

Further Reading

Kang K, Polster AM, Nedorost ST, et al. 'Atopic dermatitis', in Bolognia JL, Jorizzo JL, and Rapini PR, eds, *Dermatology*, 2008. Mosby (Elsevier).

Primary Care Dermatology Society and British Association of Dermatologists: *Guidelines for the Management of Atopic Eczema* (http://www.bad.org.uk)

Shams K, Grindlay DJC, and Williams HC. What's new in atopic eczema? An analysis of systematic reviews published in 2009–2010. *Clin Exp Dermatol* 201; 36: 573–7.

Williams, HC. Atopic dermatitis. *N Engl J Med* 2005; 352: 2314–24.

Table 250.1 The potency of some of the commonly used steroids

Generic name (brand names)	Potency
Hydrocortisone 0.5%–2.5%	Mild
Clobetasone butyrate 0.05%	Moderate
Betamethasone valerate 0.1%	Potent
Mometasone furoate 0.1%	Potent
Clobetasol propionate 0.05%	Very potent

251 Urticaria

Sarah Wakelin

Definition of the disease

Urticaria is an inflammatory complaint characterized by short-lived skin swellings termed 'weals' or 'hives'. It can be divided into acute urticaria, where the disease is short-lived and chronic urticaria, where weals occur on a regular basis for more than 6 weeks. Inducible or physical urticaria is a subgroup of chronic urticaria where an underlying external/physical trigger can be identified. Contact urticaria is a localized weal or swelling of the skin or mucosa following contact with a chemical substance.

Angioedema represents a similar process affecting the deeper dermal tissue and has a predilection for the skin around the eyes and mouth. It may occur in association with urticaria or as an isolated complaint.

Aetiology of the disease

The primary event is degranulation of activated dermal mast cells and release of pro-inflammatory mediators including histamine. These cause vasodilation and increased vascular permeability leading to leakage of plasma proteins and leukocytes into the perivascular tissue. Mast cell degranulation may occur in response to cross-linking of surface high-affinity IgE receptors by allergens or IgG autoantibodies or it can be directly triggered by non-immunological agents such as opiates, neuropeptides, and C5a anaphylaxotoxin.

An underlying cause may be identified in approximately 50% of patients with acute urticaria. In most cases, this is infective. Food allergy may need investigating if there is a temporal relationship. A detailed drug history is also mandatory. In chronic spontaneous urticaria, (CSU) some patients have evidence of underlaying autoimmunity especially autoimmune thyroid disease. It is seldom related to food allergy which can be excluded by taking a careful history. Parasite infection such as strongyloidiasis rarely causes urticaria in developed countries, but may be more significant in tropical regions.

Causes of inducible urticaria include friction (symptomatic dermographism), heat and sweating (cholinergic), stress (adrenergic), UV radiation (solar), pressure, and cold. Contact urticaria is usually mild and localized and may be caused by a range of environmental chemicals and proteins. Immunological contact urticaria (e.g. natural rubber latex allergy) is a manifestation of IgE-mediated, immediate-type hypersensitivity, and atopic individuals are predisposed to develop this complaint the aetiology of non-immunologic contact urticaria is not clear, but prostaglandins and other inflammatory mediators have been implicated.

Typical symptoms of the disease, and less common symptoms

Weals vary in size from a few millimetres to many centimetres (giant urticaria) and are raised, smooth red areas of skin, sometimes surrounded by pallor (see Figure 251.1). They are usually itchy and uncomfortable, and symptoms are aggravated by heat, sweating, and tight clothing. Weals of CSU are often round or annular, while those of symptomatic dermographism are typically linear and occur at sites of friction. Weal duration may be short-lived, as in contact urticaria and most forms of physical urticaria, where resolution usually occurs within an hour. However, in delayed pressure urticaria and delayed dermographism, the onset of weals is delayed for several hours and they can persist for over

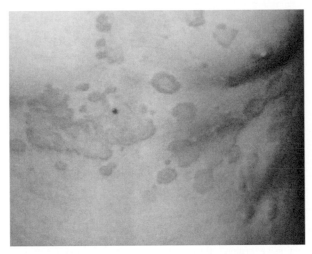

Figure 251.1 Widespread ordinary urticaria; the smooth erythematous papules and plaques may expand into annular shapes. Please see colour plate section.

Reproduced from Burge, S., Wallis, D, Oxford Handbook of Medical Dermatology (Copyright Oxford University Press 2010).

24 hours. Persistent, painful weals lasting for over 24 hours with residual bruising are a feature of urticarial vasculitis.

Exercise-induced (cholinergic) urticaria and immunological contact urticaria may, on rare occasions, progress to anaphylaxis with symptoms of hypotension and collapse.

Demographics of the disease

Statistics on the incidence of urticaria vary widely, depending on the age group studied and subtypes. The lifetime prevalence for all types of urticaria is around 10%, making this one of the commoner inflammatory dermatoses. Urticaria may affect all ages and races. Allergic urticaria is associated with atopy in childhood. CSU is commoner in women than men (2:1), while some forms of inducible urticaria such as delayed pressure urticaria are commoner in men.

Natural history, and complications of the disease

If acute urticaria and angioedema are caused by an underlying immediate-type hypersensitivity reaction, there may be associated systemic features, including bronchospasm and hypotension. CSU often coexists with a inducible urticaria, and both complaints are associated with a significant impairment in quality of life. NSAIDs and dietary pseudoallergens may exacerbate chronic urticaria.

Approach to diagnosing the disease

A careful history should be taken in patients with acute urticaria to identify any possible infective, dietary, or drug trigger. This may include over-the-counter medication. In chronic urticaria, enquiry about physical triggers and the duration of individual wheals is

Table 251.1 Typical duration of individual wheals in urticaria	
Type of urticaria	**Typical duration of individual wheals**
Physical urticaria	From minutes up to 2 hours
Delayed pressure urticaria (delay of 30 min to 12 hours)	From >24 hours to several days
Chronic spontaneous (idiopathic) urticaria	From 2 hours to 12 hours
Urticarial vasculitis	From 24 hours to several days

essential, as this will help distinguish the different types of urticaria (see Table 251.1).

Dermographism can be easily demonstrated as an exaggerated and pruritic wheal-and-flare response by firmly stroking the skin with a blunt, fine-tipped object such as an orange stick.

Other diagnoses that should be considered

Other intensely pruritic skin complaints include eczema, scabies, and insect bites. In these conditions, individual lesions persist for days to weeks and are usually excoriated. Bullous pemphigoid should be considered in elderly patients who present with fixed urticaria-like plaques and in pregnant women with an urticarial rash over the abdomen. Drug rashes may resemble urticaria, but lesions are typically polymorphic and persistent. A characteristic feature of acute eczema/dermatitis is that inflamed skin takes days to settle and resolves with surface changes of dryness and flaking.

Urticarial vasculitis is characterized by tender, long-lasting weals that leave bruising. Recurrent non-pruritic weals with arthralgia, fever, and a raised erythrocyte sedimentation rate are features of auto-inflammatory disease such as Schnitzler's syndrome, which is associated with an underlying IgM gammopathy.

Angioedema without urticaria may be a feature of hereditary or acquired C1-esterase inhibitor deficiency. It may also be induced by angiotensin-converting-enzyme inhibitors and can present many months after commencing the drug.

'Gold-standard' diagnostic test

Diagnostic tests are not usually required for urticaria, as the appearance is characteristic. In atypical cases, a skin biopsy can be helpful, especially to exclude urticarial vasculitis. Provocative testing can be carried out for inducible urticaria, for example the ice cube test for cold urticaria, and solar simulator exposure for solar urticaria.

Other relevant investigations

For inducible urticaria, no specific tests are required, with the exception of cold-urticaria, where underlying viral infections and coagulopathy should be excluded.

The routine investigations for CSU are full blood count, erythrocyte sedimentation rate, thyroid function tests, and thyroid autoantibodies.

In patients with a suspected underlying immediate-type allergy, further investigation with serological tests to measure antigen-specific IgE levels or with skin prick testing is indicated.

Prognosis, and how to estimate it

The prognosis depends on the underlying cause. Acute urticaria is usually an isolated and short-lived event, unless there is an unidentified allergen which is not avoided, in which case recurrent exposure can lead to further intermittent attacks.

The prognosis for CSU is variable. Studies have shown complete resolution in about a third of patients within 1–5 years, and partial improvement in another third. Patients who are under the age of 30 and have more severe symptoms and physical triggers fare less well. Associated angioedema is also a marker of chronicity.

Treatment and its effectiveness

Patients with acute urticaria and anaphylaxis require emergency management of this condition (see Chapter 75). Acute urticaria without systemic symptoms should be treated with oral antihistamines. Second-generation oral H1 antihistamines are the treatment of choice for CSU and inducible urticaria, as they are generally non-sedating at standard dosages, due to improved receptor selectivity and poor permeability across the blood–brain barrier. They are usually effective at reducing weal duration and pruritus. The aim is symptom control and they can be prescribed at increased doses in refractory cases. Simple advice includes wearing loose soft clothing, keeping cool, and avoiding alcohol because of its vasodilatory effects. Disease severity should be quantified for example with the UAS7 score and the dermatology life quality index. In patients with uncontrolled disease, addition of oral H2 antihistamines or leukotriene-receptor antagonists have been advocated but evidence for their effectiveness is limited. In a minority of patients, chronic urticaria runs a severe, recalcitrant course and may justify additional treatment with immunosuppressive drugs such as ciclosporin or methotrexate or the anti-IgE biological drug omalizumab which is licensed for severe CSU in patients aged 12 years and older. Corticosteroids, while effective for acute disease control, should be avoided for long-term treatment because of their adverse effects.

Low-salicylate or additive(pseudoallergen)-free diets have been advocated for chronic ordinary urticaria and may help a minority of individuals.

Further Reading

Powell RJ, Leech SC, Till S, et al. BSACI guideline for the management of chronic urticaria and angioedema. *Clin Exp Allergy* 2015; 45: 547–65.

Zuberbier T, Aberer W, Asero R, et al. The EAACI/GA(2) LEN/EDF/WAO Guideline for the definition, classification, diagnosis, and management of urticaria: the 2013 revision and update. *Allergy* 2014; 69: 868–87.

252 Bullous disorders

Emily Davies

Introduction

This chapter focuses on immunobullous diseases. Please refer to Chapter 69 for all other causes of bullous disorders.

Definition of the disease

The immunobullous disorders are a group of diseases in which pathogenic autoantibodies bind to target antigens either in intra-epidermal desmosomes (intercellular adhesion junctions) or in part of the basement membrane zone, resulting in loss of adhesion, and blister formation. The immunobullous disorders can be categorized by the level of blister formation (see Table 252.1).

This chapter will mainly focus on the following disorders: pemphigus vulgaris and pemphigus foliaceus; bullous pemphigoid; linear IgA disease and chronic bullous disease of childhood (CBCD); and dermatitis herpetiformis; it will also make mention of mucous membrane pemphigoid, pemphigoid gestationis, and epidermolysis bullosa acquisita.

Demographics of the disease

Pemphigus vulgaris and pemphigus foliaceus

Pemphigus is a chronic, blistering disorder affecting people of middle age (40–60 years). It has an equal sex distribution and affects all races, but pemphigus vulgaris is commonest in those of Jewish ancestry. Pemphigus folicaeus is very rare in the UK. Endemic pemphigus foliaceus (Fogo Selvagem) is common in parts of Brazil. It can be induced by some drugs.

Bullous pemphigoid

Bullous pemphigoid is a chronic, blistering disease affecting elderly people, usually with onset after the age of 60. Children can occasionally be affected. It is slightly commoner in men. Studies have found a higher frequency of neurological conditions such as multiple sclerosis in patients with bullous pemphigoid. It is the commonest immunobullous disease in Western Europe (2 per 100,000). Occasionally, it can be drug induced.

Linear IgA disease and CBCD

Linear IgA disease and CBCD are chronic, blistering diseases of adults and children, respectively. They are rare (1 per 2 million), with

a slight female predominance. They typically present in old age and in preschool children, respectively.

Dermatitis herpetiformis

Dermatitis herpetiformis is a rare, chronic, recurrent blistering disorder (1 per 15 000 in the UK). It affects all ages and has an equal sex distribution. Ireland has the highest incidence, with 600 per million people affected. It may be associated with coeliac disease.

Aetiology of the disease

The autoantibodies in patients with these disorders play a pathogenic role in inducing blister formation. The target antigens for many of these conditions have now been identified (see Table 252.2).

Typical symptoms of the disease, and less common symptoms

Pemphigus vulgaris and pemphigus foliaceus

Pemphigus vulgaris usually presents with painful erosions of the oral mucosa. Over 50% of patients also have cutaneous involvement with widespread flaccid blisters and erosions. The nasal and genital mucosae, the conjunctivae, and the oesophagus may also be involved.

Pemphigus foliaceus tends to be less severe than pemphigus vulgaris with a more insidious onset. Patients present with crusted, scaly lesions affecting the face, scalp, and upper trunk. Blisters are not usually seen as they are small and flaccid and easily rupture. There is no mucous membrane involvement, and the lesions heal without scarring.

Bullous pemphigoid

Bullous pemphigoid often presents with a prodrome of pruritus (may last for months), followed by development of urticated papules and plaques, and then tense bullae, on either erythematous or normal skin. Blisters most frequently appear on the central abdomen and limbs, often favouring the flexures. There may be mucosal involvement (usually the mouth), with blisters and erosions. The patient is systemically well.

Linear IgA disease and CBDC

In children, there is often an abrupt onset of CBDC. The rash affects the perineum, vulva, face, trunk, and limbs. The rash consists of annular polycyclic lesions with blistering around the edge, termed the 'string of pearls' sign.

The onset of linear IgA disease in adults may be insidious, but is usually abrupt. The trunk is always involved, but the limbs, face, and scalp are also commonly affected. The characteristic 'string of pearls' appearance is less common.

Pruritus in both age groups varies considerably. Blisters may arise from normal skin, and mucosal involvement is frequently seen.

Dermatitis herpetiformis

Dermatitis herpetiformis is an intensely pruritic, recurrent disease with a symmetrical distribution, and predilection for the extensor surfaces of knees, elbows, shoulders, and buttocks. Upon examination, only erosions may be seen. All patients have an underlying gluten-sensitive enteropathy, but this may be asymptomatic.

Table 252.1 Classification of immunobullous disorders by the level at which blisters form

Level of blister	Disease
Intra-epidermal	Pemphigus vulgaris (and foliaceus)
	IgA pemphigus
	Drug-induced pemphigus
Sub-epidermal	Bullous pemphigoid
	Linear IgA disease, and chronic bullous disease of childhood
	Dermatitis herpetiformis
	Mucous membrane pemphigoid
	Pemphigoid gestationis
	Epidermolysis bullosa acquisita
	Drug induced

Table 252.2 The target antigens in immunobullous disorders

Disease	Blister	Target antigen	Direct immunofluorescence	Indirect immunofluorescence
Pemphigus vulgaris	Intra-epidermal	Desmoglein 3 +/− 1	Intercellular deposition of IgG +/− C3	Positive
Pemphigus foliaceus	Subcorneal	Desmoglein 1	Intercellular deposition of IgG +/− C3	Positive
Bullous pemphigoid	Sub-epidermal	BP180 BP230	Linear deposition of IgG +/− C3	Positive
Linear IgA disease, and chronic bullous disease of childhood	Sub-epidermal	LAD285 BP180 BP230 Collagen VII	Linear deposition of IgA	Positive
Dermatitis herpetiformis	Sub-epidermal	Tissue transglutaminase	Granular deposition of IgA	Negative

Natural history, complications of the disease, and prognosis

The severity and disease duration of pemphigus vulgaris is variable. Disease activity usually decreases with time. The mortality is between 5% and 15%. This is related to disease severity, dose of prednisolone used for treatment, and comorbidities. The mortality rate was much higher before the use of corticosteroids. Pemphigus foliaceus is a much more benign, chronic disease. It responds well to treatment and may remit.

Bullous pemphigoid is a chronic, self-limiting disease with exacerbations and remissions. It is associated with significant morbidity and has a marked impact on a patient's quality of life. There is also an increased mortality rate in elderly patients, probably related to side effects from steroids and immunosuppressive agents.

Most cases of linear IgA disease and CBDC spontaneously remit after 3– 6 years. The vast majority of childhood cases resolve by puberty. In contrast, dermatitis herpetiformis is usually a lifelong condition and spontaneous remissions are rare (up to 10%).

In all these disorders, possible complications of cutaneous blistering may occur, such as secondary bacterial infections and scarring. Oral involvement can lead to severe pain and subsequent restriction of dietary intake and poor oral hygiene. The mouth and genital mucosa may become secondarily infected with candida.

Approach to diagnosing the disease

The clinician should take a history, including a detailed enquiry about the blisters, time course, any preceding itch or rash, previous episodes, and areas affected. A past medical history, a detailed drug history, a family history, and a systems enquiry including any gastrointestinal symptoms should be recorded (dermatitis herpetiformis). This should be followed by a thorough examination of the skin, hair, nails, and mucous membranes; look for blisters, excoriations, erosions, and evidence of scarring and/or secondary infection.

Other diagnoses that should be considered

The differential diagnosis for these conditions includes all causes of immunobullous disorders as well as other causes of blistering such as bullous impetigo and bullous erythema multiforme. Patients who have pemphigus but who only have oral involvement should have aphthous ulcers, herpes, mucous membrane pemphigoid, lichen planus, and erythema multiforme excluded. In the non-bullous phase of bullous pemphigoid, conditions such as eczema, scabies, and drug reactions should be considered. CBDC has sometimes been misdiagnosed as sexual abuse in cases with vulval involvement. Bullous drug reactions, as well as drug-induced pemphigus/bullous pemphigoid should be considered.

'Gold-standard' diagnostic test

All patients should have a skin biopsy performed. An incisional skin biopsy should be taken through an intact blister for histopathology. The level of the split (subcorneal, intra-epidermal or suprabasal) will help indicate possible diagnoses. The inflammatory infiltrate should also be recorded. A sample of perilesional, uninvolved skin should also be taken for direct immunofluorescence to look for deposition of immunoglobulins/complement.

Acceptable diagnostic alternatives to the gold standard

Indirect immunofluorescence is performed on serum or blister fluid and detects circulating immunoglobulins/complement. If a skin biopsy is not appropriate in a particular patient, this test will aid with diagnosis, depending on the pattern and type of immunoglobulin/complement deposition. This test is negative in dermatitis herpetiformis.

Other relevant investigations

All patients should have baseline blood tests performed, including a full blood count to assess for anaemia and evidence of any infection (elevated white-cell count). A swab should be taken if infection is suspected.

Treatment and its effectiveness

The general principle of treating immunobullous disease is to make the patient comfortable with the lowest dose of immunosuppression required. Most morbidity and mortality is from treatment rather than the disease and this has to be weighed up when making management decisions. In some patients, disease can be managed with superpotent topical steroids in combination with anti-inflammatory agents, such as a tetracycline, erythromycin, or nicotinamide. Many cases require oral steroids.

In most cases of bullous pemphigoid, oral prednisolone (0.5–1 mg/kg) will control the disease within a couple of weeks. When control is established, steroids should be tapered very slowly to avoid relapse. In those patients with more resistant disease and who are unable to come off steroids, an additional immunosuppressive agent, such as azathioprine or mycophenolate mofetil, is added.

Pemphigus is often more challenging to treat and therefore more frequently requires the addition of azathioprine or mycophenolate mofetil. Oral disease should be managed with good oral hygiene, topical antiseptics, and topical steroids (sprays/gels/mouthwashes). Any superimposed candida infection should be treated with oral fluconazole.

Treatment of dermatitis herpetiformis is usually with a combination of dapsone and a gluten-free diet. Pruritus is relieved within a couple of days of commencing dapsone, but the lesions will rapidly return if it is stopped. Dapsone has no effect on the enteropathy. Haemolysis and methaemoglobinaemia are present in virtually all patients on dapsone, although these are usually tolerable. Patients on a strict gluten-free diet may be able to reduce their dapsone dose or stop it completely. Sulfapyridine is used as an alternative in those patients who are unable to tolerate dapsone. All patients should be referred to gastroenterology.

Erythromycin is now used as the first-line treatment for CBDC. Those who do not respond require dapsone therapy. Dapsone or sulphapyridine are used to treat linear IgA disease.

Any patient with a suspected immunobullous disorder should be referred to dermatology for specialist investigation and treatment, although long-term management is often with a multidisciplinary team.

Other bullous disorders

Mucous membrane pemphigoid

Mucous membrane pemphigoid is a rare, chronic blistering disease which usually affects middle-aged or elderly people. It is predominantly a mucosal disease, most frequently affecting oral and conjunctival mucosa. Scarring can result in blindness. It runs a varied course and is often very treatment resistant. Patients should be managed by a multidisciplinary team, including ophthalmologists and oral surgeons. Oral and topical corticosteroids in combination with azathioprine or mycophenolate mofetil are used.

Pemphigoid gestationis

Pemphigoid gestationis is a rare blistering disorder, which occurs in association with pregnancy. The average onset is around 21 weeks gestation. The rash initially affects the periumbilicus and then spreads to involve the trunk, palms, and soles. The rash consists of urticated papules, plaques, and blisters. It usually remits after delivery, but can recur with subsequent pregnancies. Treatment is with topical or oral corticosteroids.

Epidermolysis bullosa acquisita

Epidermolysis bullosa acquisita is an extremely rare chronic blistering disorder with trauma-induced blistering. Scarring and deformities can result and treatment is difficult.

Further Reading

Roujeau JC, Lok C, Bastuji-Garin S, et al. High risk of death in elderly patients with extensive bullous pemphigoid. *Arch Dermatol* 1998; 134: 465–9.

Schmidt E and Zillikens D. The diagnosis and treatment of autoimmune blistering skin diseases. *Dtsch Arztebl Int* 2011; 108: 399–405.

Stanley JR and Amagai M. Pemphigus, bullous impetigo, and the staphylococcal scalded-skin syndrome. *N Engl J Med* 2006; 355: 1800–10.

Venning VA, Taghipour K, Mohd Mustapa MF, et al. British Association of Dermatologists' guidelines for the management of bullous pemphigoid 2012. *Br J Dermatol* 2012; 167: 1200–14.

Wojnarowska F, Kirtschig G, Highet AS, et al. Guidelines for management of bullous pemphigoid. *Br J Dermatol* 2002; 147: 214–21.

Inflammatory scalp diseases

Definition of inflammatory scalp diseases

Inflammatory diseases of the scalp can affect all epidermal surfaces or focus upon the follicle, with relative sparing of the interfollicular skin. Eczema and psoriasis are examples of the former; they affect the scalp in the manner of affecting skin elsewhere. The process is non-scarring in most instances, unless associated by bacterial infection. Other diseases, such as lichen planopilaris (LPP) or discoid lupus erythematosus (DLE) have a greater propensity to inflame the follicle than to cause inflammation in the surrounding skin. They can cause scarring. Some other follicular diseases, such as the family of diseases based on alopecia areata (alopecia areata (small areas of hair loss), alopecia totalis (whole scalp), and alopecia universalis (whole body)), cause barely visible follicular inflammation which results in hair loss but no scarring.

Aetiology of inflammatory scalp diseases

Eczema and psoriasis are lymphocyte-mediated diseases with significant inherited components. Atopic eczema is closely allied to mutations in the gene for filaggrin, an intermediate filament that contributes to the barrier structure of skin. In addition, there is a link with increased concentration and activity of IgE.

DLE and lichen planus are also lymphocyte mediated, characterized by a histological picture of lymphocytes interacting with the basal layer of the epidermis and causing keratinocyte death. Where this is associated with substantial damage to the basement membrane zone, there may be scarring. In some with DLE, sunlight plays an exacerbating factor.

Alopecia areata and related conditions are characterized by lymphocyte attack on the hair bulb—the deepest component of the hair follicle. Hair follicle function is halted by the attack, and the hair is lost. However, once the attack subsides, hair growth may recommence.

Typical symptoms of inflammatory scalp diseases, and less common symptoms

Eczema and psoriasis may present with itch, where scaling is particularly prominent in the latter. In some psoriatics, scale may build up to large, aggregated clumps of keratin matting the hair. In those with eczema, it is more likely to be exudative, especially if there is substantial itch which attracts scratching and secondary infection. In such instances, there may be regional lymphadenopathy. Scale and itch are less prominent with DLE and LPP, although new areas or disease activity may initially be indicated by slight itch. Symptoms are typically absent from those with alopecia areata, although, when there is rapid onset of severe disease, patients will often describe a preliminary tingling or slight discomfort of the scalp.

All of these diseases may present at other body sites with associated features characteristic of the diagnosis.

Demographics of inflammatory scalp diseases

Atopic eczema is most common in childhood, dropping to about 10% prevalence in adults, with a slight preponderance in women. Psoriasis is slightly more common in women than men, with a peak presentation age in the twenties. It is more common in Caucasians, with a prevalence in Western societies of about 2%. LPP is most common in women between the ages of 40 and 65. DLE is most common between the ages of 20 and 40 and seen twice as often in women as men. There is a slight excess in those of African origin over other races, with an overall prevalence of approximately 0.02%.

Alopecia areata can occur at any age or race and has no clear gender preference, with a prevalence of 0.1%–0.2%.

Natural history of inflammatory scalp diseases, and complications of these diseases

Eczema wanes with emerging adulthood, but then deteriorates again with senescence and the loss of skin barrier function. Psoriasis is less common with age, but may still present in the elderly. Neither cause scarring and so, with disease fluctuation, the scalp can return to normal during remission. With DLE and LPP, areas of more intense inflammation are associated with scarring, which means that remission leaves areas of permanent alopecia. Treatment aims to abbreviate and diminish the intensity of episodes of inflammation so that follicles are not lost. A single area of alopecia areata is said to have an 80% chance of remission. This is not the same as saying that the disease itself will fully remit, and patients often suffer intermittent periods of variable hair loss. The prognosis of recovery is inversely proportional to the amount of hair lost and the duration of its loss.

Approach to diagnosing inflammatory scalp diseases

Diagnosis is performed by assessing for local signs in the context of the history, and for signs elsewhere on the skin (see Table 253.1).

Other diagnoses that should be considered aside from inflammatory scalp diseases

Fungal scalp infection is the main differential for scalp disease where there is scaling and hair loss. This is most common in children, but can also present in adulthood. Folliculitis decalvans is an alternative scarring alopecia and usually presents with pustules mixed in with foci of hair loss and tufts of residual hair clumped into aggregated follicular opening.

'Gold-standard' diagnostic test for inflammatory scalp diseases

The gold-standard diagnostic test for inflammatory scalp disease is a scalp biopsy; ideally, this should be done using a 'double-punch' technique, where two 4 mm punch biopsies are taken and prepared for sections in the horizontal and vertical axes. Where DLE is suspected, half of a vertically bisected punch should be sent fresh for immunofluorescence.

Acceptable diagnostic alternatives to the gold-standard test for inflammatory scalp diseases

Often, the history and clinical examination provides a fully adequate basis for diagnosis with no histology. In any condition where there is scaling and uncertainty, scalp scale and hair should be sent for mycology. A biopsy of an affected body site may be a substitute in some instances.

Other relevant investigations for inflammatory scalp diseases

DLE can merge with SLE, either at presentation or with time. It is useful to test for autoantibodies (e.g. antinuclear antibodies, anti-double-stranded DNA antibodies, extractable nuclear antigen antibodies) to establish the antibody status at the outset. Where hair shedding accompanies any disease, it is advisable to check the full blood count, ferritin level, and thyroid function. The latter may be

Table 253.1 Diagnosis of inflammatory diseases

Disease	History	Local signs	Signs at other sites
Eczema	Family history common Atopy: asthma, hay fever, contact allergy	Redness Light scale Sometimes crust	Eczema at other sites, particularly the flexures if atopic Skin may be dry if the patient is elderly
Psoriasis	Family history common May have joint problems	Silvery scale that can build up and become matted Rash in patches and within and behind ears	Nail changes and rash on extensor surfaces
Discoid lupus erythematosus	50% have deterioration in bright sunlight Scalp irritation	Discoid red or purplish areas in scalp with prominent follicles as well as some rash between follicles Central zones may have scarring	Similar less follicular discoid patches may be seen at other sites and, in particular, on the head and neck
Lichen planopilaris	Scalp itch Progressive hair loss	Small cuff of redness and slight scale around the follicular openings in a zone of scalp which may be discoid or at a hair margin Pale scarred areas in zones of previous disease	Rarely have lichen planus at other sites, such as mucosae of mouth and genitals, or skin lichen planus on the wrists or other sites
Alopecia areata	History of previous episodes which have spontaneously remitted Family history in 20% of cases	Hair shed from circumscribed area with normal follicular openings May leave white hairs behind in early stages, or demonstrate regrowth of white hairs first with recovery Exclamation mark hairs seen at margins	Other patches of alopecia areata can be found at other body sites, such as the beard area, eyebrows, eyelashes, or limbs Nails can be involved, with pitting or a roughened surface and discoloration Alopecia totalis is the loss of all scalp hair Alopecia universalis is the loss of all body hair

particularly relevant to alopecia areata, as they are both thought to share an autoimmune basis.

Prognosis for inflammatory scalp diseases, and how to estimate it

Scalp eczema and psoriasis are chronic relapsing and partially remitting conditions. They are unlikely to go away completely unless there is systemic treatment. However, they can become well controlled. DLE and LPP both demonstrate the tendency to 'burn out' after an unpredictable period of activity, causing irreversible hair loss. It is rare to see either disease progress to the extent that it creates substantial baldness, and wigs are rarely needed. Alopecia areata is thought to be worse if there is an onset in childhood and possibly worse if there is associated atopy. Overall prognosis is dependant on how much hair is lost—such severe disease means a poor prognosis.

Treatment of inflammatory scalp diseases, and its effectiveness

Scalp eczema and psoriasis can be treated with the same products used on the skin elsewhere—typically, a range of steroids and, with psoriasis, calcipotriol. Tar and emollient can be used with both diseases, especially psoriasis, where the emollient can help lift scale. Treatments applied in the evening and retained overnight with a shower cap can be very effective. For cosmetic ease, people may choose a vehicle such as a gel, alcohol liquid, or thin emollient base. These do not mess up the hair as much as the heavier cream or ointment bases. Systemic therapy with immunosuppression can be indicated for very severe disease.

DLE and LPP both respond to some extent to potent topical steroid, usually applied as a cream or gel as, focally, there is no hair to make greasy. Injected triamcinolone acetonide can be useful, and systemic treatment with hydroxychloroquine can help DLE. Systemic prednisolone or ciclosporin are short-term options for LPP.

Topical and injected steroids are the mainstay of treatment for alopecia areata. Systemic steroid is rarely used due to the high relapse rate and the risks of the treatment if used long term.

Hair shedding: Telogen effluvium and pattern hair loss

Definition of hair shedding

Some patients present with hair shedding or change of hair pattern as their primary complaint, with no scalp disease. Patterned loss, when manifest, is characteristic of ageing.

Aetiology of hair shedding

Shedding is continuous and normal in humans and, in most instances, occurs at a rate of 150 hairs a day. When a significant event increases the proportion of hair follicles entering the resting phase (telogen), then more hairs will be shed. This event can be physiological, for example occurring 1–3 months after a fever or haemorrhage, and is termed telogen effluvium. Alternatively, it can be toxicological, as with the ingestion of a poison such as a chemotherapy agent. In some instances, it is where a normal medication may have an adverse effect of impairing follicular function, as occurs with some forms of synthetic vitamin A (retinoids).

Other patients, without conspicuous shedding, present with an altered pattern of scalp hair. This is usually following a period during which the normal rate of shedding has exceeded the rate of regrowth such that there is an overall decline in scalp coverage. This is the basis for patterned hair loss, which is seen in both men and women. Women are more likely than men to seek medical advice to determine whether there is a cause or treatment for the hair loss.

Typical symptoms of hair shedding, and less common symptoms

Hair shedding is noted in the shower and sink and also commented on by social partners. There are rarely any physical associations unless there is a clear recollection of a preceding event or causal medication. Change of hair pattern is usually based on gradual realization.

Demographics of hair shedding

All people and ages appear susceptible to telogen effluvium. Men and women suffer patterned hair loss with age, starting as early as mid-adolescence. There is a strong but ill-defined genetic basis. Those of Chinese origin are thought to have less marked patterned balding than those of other origins.

Natural history of hair shedding, and complications of the disease

Telogen effluvium evolves 1–3 months after the event and may take a further 2–3 months to peak. Return towards normal takes a further 3 months, such that it is common for people to be affected to some extent for a year. Patterned hair loss in men and women may be highlighted by a period of shedding that does not fully reverse. By the age of 70, 70% of men will have significant balding. By menopause, 30% of women will have a degree of male pattern balding with frontal recession. Most of the rest of the women will have some thinning on the crown, but will retain their frontal margin.

CHAPTER 253 **Hair disorders**

Approach to diagnosing hair shedding

A history of shedding is normally clear and substantiated by gently pulling strands of hair on the scalp as part of the examination. If these easily pluck, then it confirms the account. If it does not, it does contradict the account, but may mean that the period of active shedding is passed and regrowth can be anticipated.

Diagnosing patterned hair loss is one of recognizing the pattern and ensuring that there are no other features in the history or examination.

Other diagnoses that should be considered aside from hair shedding

Fungal scalp infection can be considered if there is hair breakage or scalp scaling, but is not common in the age group presenting with these problems. Endocrine problems with masculinization can be relevant with androgen-secreting tumours and will usually present with features such as amenorrhoea, evolution of hirsutism, and altered body habitus. A milder version of this pathology is represented by polycystic ovary syndrome.

'Gold-standard' diagnostic test for hair shedding

In the presence of normal periods and no change in body habitus, the main test for telogen effluvium is the hair pull test. Where multiple hairs come out with the lightest pull, the diagnosis is confirmed.

Patterned hair loss is characterized by miniaturization of the hair follicles and their hairs and can be confirmed by scalp biopsy. This needs to be done with horizontal sections of 4 mm punch biopsies in order that the number, hair cycle status, and bore of the hairs can be determined.

Acceptable diagnostic alternatives to the gold-standard test for hair shedding

Biopsy is rarely needed, and clinical assessment usually provides all that is needed.

Other relevant investigations for hair shedding

Iron deficiency and thyroid disease can be contributory and would normally be checked. Any other investigation would be done on the basis of some relevant part of the history or examination such as a testosterone if there were a degree of hirsutism or altered periods.

Prognosis for hair shedding, and how to estimate it

Telogen effluvium has a good prognosis over a 12-month period. As people age, they may find that the reversal is not complete and there has been a stepped reduction in the bulk and extent of their hair. Prognosis for those with either male or female pattern hair loss is that it will gradually progress with time. Women do not go bald, although, with advanced age, there can be considerable loss of coverage.

Treatment of hair shedding, and its effectiveness

Any medical abnormalities detected should be addressed. Telogen effluvium is self-limiting. If medication is thought to play a part (e.g. atenolol, oral retinoids, some anticonvulsants, progesterone-containing medication), then alternatives might be sought.

Many argue that ferritin should be maintained significantly above the lower range of normal described by most laboratories, such that it is 70 ng/ml. This may require iron supplementation.

Anti-androgens, such as the oral contraceptive pill with a synthetic progestogen (not norethisterone), cyproterone acetate, or spironolactone, are advocated by some. The potential for iatrogenic disease related to treatment for a normal variant should be considered with these options. Also, the end point of treatment and hence its duration is difficult to determine.

In men, finasteride is licensed for use in male pattern balding and can result in some regrowth for 60% of men within 2 years. Over the subsequent 5 years, this improvement tails off, but probably the person will have some additional retained hair for as long as they take the medication. Data on improvement for women with other anti-androgens (finasteride is not licensed in women) is not so definite.

Topical minoxidil 2% and 5% is available over the counter as a liquid applied twice daily to affected areas for a minimum of 6 months, to be continued as long as any benefit accrued is desired to be maintained. There is technical evidence of increased hair growth in men and women, although the change in front of the mirror is seldom marked.

Further Reading

Harries MJ, Sinclair RD, Macdonald-Hull S, et al. Management of primary cicatricial alopecias: Options for treatment. *Br J Dermatol* 2008; 159: 1–22.

Macbeth A and Harries M. Hair loss in hospital medicine: A practical guide. *Br J Hosp Med (Lond)* 2012; 73: 372–9.

Miteva M and Tosti A. Treatment options for alopecia: An update, looking to the future. *Expert Opin Pharmacother* 2012; 13: 1271–81.

Sinclair R, Patel M, Dawson TL Jr, et al. Hair loss in women: Medical and cosmetic approaches to increase scalp hair fullness. *Br J Dermatol* 2011; 165 (Suppl 3): 12–8.

254 Nail disorders

David de Berker

Definition of the disease

Nail diseases present as alteration of the nail plate, alteration of the periungual tissues, or as a combination of the two. Most commonly, external agents, such as fungus or trauma, affect the nail alone, whereas all inflammatory and neoplastic processes affect the surrounding tissues as a primary process giving rise to secondary nail plate alteration.

Aetiology of the disease

The most common inflammatory diseases of nail are psoriasis, eczema, and lichen planus, which, in turn, are amongst the most common inflammatory disease of the rest of the skin.

The most common infections arise through fungal invasion of the nail plate and the nail bed, which is the skin underlying the nail. Fungi are of two main families, dermatophytes and non-dermatophytes. For dermatophytes, skin is a natural medium for existence, whereas non-dermatophytes are more typically found in the soil, but may rarely become pathological to skin, nail, and hair.

Trauma represents the third most common cause of nail abnormalities, with an increasing prevalence of traumatic disease affecting toenails as people age. Some trauma is directly upon the nail, made vulnerable through its location on the dorsal distal tip of the toe. Other trauma may be related to foot mechanics, which alter with time. Trauma to fingernails is less commonly a cause of significant dystrophy, outside the specific area of self-inflicted damage arising from nail biting or a form of self-mutilation known as onychophagia.

Both benign and malignant neoplasia can present with nail changes. The former cause a space-occupying effect, distorting the position of the nail. If the mass is proximal and pressing on the nail matrix, then it will alter the nail during its creation. More distal or lateral tumours will impinge on the nail following generation and will usually just alter its position. Glomus tumours, subungual exostoses, or periungual fibromas of the type seen in tuberous sclerosis can be found in either location.

Malignancy of the nail unit presents as squamous cell carcinoma or malignant melanoma. The former is typically in situ in the first instance and has a very long prodrome before invasion. HPV 16 and 18, seen in genital squamous cell carcinoma, can be present. Malignant melanoma of the nail unit is rare and represents about 2% of all melanoma, with an incidence in the UK of 1 per million population per year. It is diagnosed later than melanoma on other skin sites and, consequently, is usually deeper and has a worse prognosis.

Typical symptoms of the disease, and less common symptoms

All nail disease evolves from minor changes in appearance to more major alterations of nail integrity. Depending on the focus and inflammatory basis of the disease, there may be associated pain and loss of function. Onychomycosis is mainly associated with asymptomatic thickening and white-to-yellow nail discoloration extending from the distal edge.

Less common diseases present with features such as sterile pustulation in psoriasis or chronic ooze from beneath the nail for a squamous cell carcinoma of the nail bed. Malignant melanoma most commonly presents initially as a dark longitudinal streak in the nail in a pale-skinned person. When someone has a single such streak, it warrants close and expert assessment.

An important factor in any presentation of nail disease identifying a pattern. Disease that affects multiple digits is more likely to yield significant clues at other body sites. For psoriasis, the presence of pits in the nail, lifting of the nail (onycholysis), and nail thickening may be corroborated by scaling on the elbow, on the scalp, and in the ears. For eczema, the presence of itching and a typical rash at other body sites may illustrate the disposition. Conversely, if the pathology is limited to a single digit, then neoplasia or infection is more likely and, given that some neoplasias can be malignant, it is important to obtain a clear diagnosis.

Demographics of the disease

Different nail diseases have their own demographic. Eighty percent of patients with psoriasis of the skin will develop nail psoriasis at some point in their lives, but only 30%–40% will have it at any one time. It is not common in childhood and becomes particularly prevalent amongst those patients who have psoriatic arthritis of the distal interphalangeal joints. The demographic for eczema of the nail is only partly related to the peak of atopic manifestation. Whereas the latter occurs mainly in childhood, it is common for irritant and occupational factors to become major factors once people enter the workforce and are subject to repetitive activities, like wet work or building, that disturb periungual skin.

Fungal nail infection (onychomycosis) is mainly a disease of middle age and beyond. It is more common in subgroups where there is a predisposing factor, such as psoriatics, the immunosuppressed, or those with damage to the nail. The accumulation of damage to the nail is a feature of time, so onychomycosis increases in prevalence in the elderly.

Malignancy of the nail primarily is seen in those 40 and older. However, immunosuppression predisposes to squamous cell carcinoma, in which case people may present with malignancy of the nail at an earlier age.

Natural history, and complications of the disease

All the inflammatory diseases are fluctuating, except for those with scarring potential, such as lichen planus, where the nail matrix and, consequently, the nail plate may be permanently lost. Onychomycosis is gradually progressive such that it will usually destroy a nail plate over 20 or more years, or immunity may hold it in check. Malignancy of the nail is slow to progress in most instances, save for where nodular variants present at the outset or evolve on the background of indolent disease. In such instances, the outcome can be fatal, especially for melanoma, where 5-year survival rates are reported at around 50%–70%.

Approach to diagnosing the disease

Diagnosis is by assessment for characteristic signs within the digit, all other digits, and the rest of the skin. Some diseases may give clues through other systems, such as the joints for psoriasis, or asthma for atopic eczema. Where onychomycosis is a potential diagnosis, generous clippings of nail and subungual debris should be obtained for mycological examination and culture. It is only with the results of this that the clinician is equipped to prescribe oral antifungal medication. The presence of fungus does not rule out coexisting disease. Where pathology presents with a single digit, the author would advocate close attention to detail in order to not miss malignancy or some treatable structural abnormality. This objective may entail imaging with all soft tissue and bone modalities and taking an incisional diagnostic biopsy under local anaesthetic.

Other diagnoses that should be considered

Some nail changes are manifestations of systemic disease. Examples include clubbing, splinter haemorrhages, and paraneoplastic changes within the nail unit. The latter may mimic psoriasis, but come about through internal malignancy. Hence, anyone presenting with a marked inflammatory change in their nails, usually in later life, in the absence of an obvious cause, should be assessed for internal malignancy.

'Gold-standard' diagnostic test

If there were one test that the clinician could do, and no other, then it would be the incisional biopsy. However, usually there is enough information from the clinical examination and history, supplemented by a generous mycology sample, to conclude the diagnosis. In widespread nail disease, when a diagnosis cannot be made, it may be warranted to take a diagnostic biopsy in order to ensure that any proposed systemic therapy is appropriate. Such therapies are usually immunosuppressant and may be intermittently long term with side effects. To give such treatment without a clear diagnosis would be questionable. For diagnosis of the single digit, it is possibly more understandable to resort to biopsy, given the risk of malignancy.

Who does the biopsy, what pattern of biopsy is done, and who interprets the histology make a difference. It is best that such tests are undertaken by those who do them frequently.

Acceptable diagnostic alternatives to the gold standard

Clinical acumen with only marginal confidence may be adequate when balanced against complete confidence. This holds as long as the sequelae of the proposed treatment are not problematic, or as long as the significance of the diagnosis being missed because of a failure to obtain histological certainty is not a grave one. Mycology should be undertaken several times to ensure that fungus is not missed, as laboratory standards acknowledge a false-negative rate for mycology of the nail at around 40%.

Other relevant investigations

Skin biopsy or mycology of abnormal non-nail tissue can sometimes provide enough information to give confidence to the interpretation of the nail problems.

Prognosis and how to estimate it

The prognosis of non-scarring nail disease is that it will progress at approximately the same rate as that of the skin disease at other sites. It will fluctuate and respond well but variably to treatment. Compliance with treatment plans will make a difference and, typically, people tire of prolonged regimens of hand care and topical therapies. The prognosis of scarring nail disease will depend upon the natural aggressiveness of the disease and the intensity of immunosuppression. At times, the consequences of treatment will not be acceptable. Dermatophyte onychomycosis is cured in about 60% of people after systemic treatment but in more like 20% of those who have milder disease eligible for topical therapy. However, topical therapy may hold the disease back and render it manageable. Relapse after systemic therapy is about 20% over 5 years.

Treatment and its effectiveness

Hand and foot care is important in all nail diseases, save possibly malignancy. It entails keeping nails short, using copious amounts of emollient, and wearing gloves during wet work. Where toenails are involved, this may be achieved for the elderly with the help of a podiatrist and carefully fitted footwear.

Topical treatments for psoriasis are calcipotriol ointment with or without betamethasone valerate or dipropionate. This is applied to the affected periungual area; at times, in order to do this, the nail plate may have to be clipped back to expose the nail bed. For eczema, the steroid alone may be sufficient. In resistant cases, it is possible to inject steroid into the nail matrix. Systemic therapy is as for the disease in general, and the most successful for psoriasis has been ciclosporin or biologics such as infliximab and etanercept.

Onychomycosis is usually treated with oral terbinafine, although there is a significant side-effect profile that includes liver failure. Death has been reported. Malignancy is treated with surgery and, in more advanced cases, this may require distal or ray amputation to ensure adequate clearance.

Further Reading

Braun RP, Baran R, Le Gal FA, et al. Diagnosis and management of nail pigmentations. *J Am Acad Dermatol* 2007; 56: 835–47.

de Berker D. Clinical practice. Fungal nail disease. *N Engl J Med* 2009; 360: 2108–16.

de Berker D. Management of psoriatic nail disease. *Semin Cutan Med Surg* 2009; 28: 39–43.

255 Mucosal disease

Kathy Taghipour

Pemphigus vulgaris

Definition of pemphigus vulgaris

Pemphigus vulgaris is an autoimmune disease that affects the skin and the mucosal membranes with blisters and erosions.

Aetiology of pemphigus vulgaris

In pemphigus vulgaris, autoantibodies target components of desmosomes, the structures that provide cell-to-cell adhesion in the skin. An intra-epidermal cleavage results from this immune reaction, leading to blister formation.

Typical symptoms of pemphigus vulgaris, and less common symptoms

In pemphigus vulgaris, flaccid and thin-walled blisters and/or erosions are present on the skin and mucosal membranes, including in the oropharynx and the genital area. The oral lesions often present on buccal and palatal mucosa and are painful.

Demographics of pemphigus vulgaris

Pemphigus vulgaris commonly affects individuals in their middle age. The incidence in the UK is 7 per million per year and both sexes are equally affected. It is more common in Eastern Europe, Middle East, India, and amongst Ashkenazi Jews, and certain HLA associations have been described.

Natural history of pemphigus vulgaris, and complications of the disease

The clinical course of pemphigus vulgaris varies between individuals but, in most cases, immunosuppressive treatment is required for years to control the disease. Painful mouth lesions may lead to malnutrition. Most complications are, however, related to long-term treatment with systemic steroids.

Approach to diagnosing pemphigus vulgaris

A diagnosis of pemphigus should be considered when patients present with painful, non-healing oral or genital erosions. A full skin examination is important in confirming the clinical diagnosis. Pemphigus has a predilection for scalp, face, and flexures, although mucosal erosion may be the only presenting sign. A full history of drug intake should be taken to exclude drug-induced pemphigus.

Other diagnoses that should be considered aside from pemphigus vulgaris

Other diagnoses that should be considered aside from pemphigus vulgaris include erosive lichen planus and mucous membrane pemphigoid. Erosive lichen planus presents with erosions of the oral and/or genital mucosa. It may be associated with a skin rash and white, lacy streaks on buccal mucosa, namely Wickham striae. Mucous membrane pemphigoid is a rare sub-epidermal bullous disease that leads to erosions and gingivitis in the mouth and may affect the genital mucosa, skin, conjunctivae, and gastrointestinal tract, leaving scars on the affected areas. Drug-induced reactions such as Stevens–Johnson syndrome (see 'Stevens–Johnson syndrome') should also be considered when the history is suggestive of a recent relevant drug intake, in particular if conjunctivae are involved. Other differential diagnoses include infections and systemic disease (Box 255.1).

Box 255.1 Common disorders that affect mucosal membranes

Infections

Viral
- herpes simplex
- herpes zoster virus
- Coxsackie virus (e.g. hand, foot, and mouth disease)
- HIV

Bacterial
- gram-negative bacteria
- anaerobes

Fungal
- candida

Treponemal
- syphilis

Skin diseases
- erosive/oral lichen planus
- autoimmune bullous diseases (e.g. pemphigus vulgaris, linear IgA disease, mucous membrane pemphigoid)
- erythema multiforme
- Stevens–Johnson syndrome
- Sweet's syndrome
- lichen sclerosus et atrophicus of vulva

Systemic diseases

Gastrointestinal tract
- inflammatory bowel disease
- coeliac disease

Rheumatology
- SLE
- Behçet's syndrome
- Reiter's syndrome

Drug induced
- chemotherapy
- other drugs (e.g. nicorandil, NSAIDs, angiotensin-converting-enzyme inhibitors)

Malignancy
- leukaemia
- squamous cell carcinoma
- other malignancies

Iatrogenic
- radiotherapy

'Gold-standard' diagnostic test for pemphigus vulgaris

The gold-standard diagnostic tests for pemphigus vulgaris are immunofluorescence studies on a perilesional skin biopsy (direct immunofluorescence) and on serum (indirect immunofluorescence), to confirm the presence of IgG antibodies in the intercellular space.

Acceptable diagnostic alternatives to the gold-standard test for pemphigus vulgaris

An acceptable diagnostic alternative to the gold-standard test for pemphigus vulgaris is light microscopy of the lesional biopsy, showing rounding and separation of the keratinocytes (acantholysis) and intra-epidermal cleavage. In addition, circulating antibodies to desmogleins 1 and 3 can be detected with ELISA.

Other relevant investigations for pemphigus vulgaris

In pemphigus vulgaris, it is important to have a haematology and biochemistry workup and a relevant infection and malignancy screen before patients are commenced on immunosuppressive treatment. A baseline bone densitometry scan is useful when long-term oral steroids are considered.

Prognosis for pemphigus vulgaris, and how to estimate it

Prognosis varies amongst individuals but, in general, older patients, patients with extensive disease, and those who require high doses of systemic steroids have poorer prognosis. Relapse and mortality is more common within the first 2–5 years of diagnosis than at other times.

Treatment of pemphigus vulgaris, and its effectiveness

In pemphigus vulgaris, topical treatment with steroids and good oral care is important in providing comfort for patients. Systemic steroids provide the mainstay of treatment and are often required to reach disease control. Adjuvant immunosuppressants are usually used while steroids are tapered, and the most common agents include azathioprine, mycophenolate mofetile, and cyclophosphamide. More recently, an anti-B-cell monoclonal antibody (rituximab) has been used successfully in refractory disease.

Lichen planus

Definition of lichen planus

Lichen planus is a cell-mediated immunological mucocutaneous disease. Oral lichen planus may present with erosions, white streaks, or plaques in the oral cavity.

Aetiology of lichen planus

The exact aetiology of lichen planus is unknown. An association with hepatitis C virus has been documented in patients from Italy and is likely to be related to immunogenetics. Mercury in dental amalgam fillings has been suggested as an immunogenic or irritant factor that may trigger oral lichen planus.

Typical symptoms of lichen planus, and less common symptoms

Oral lichen planus may be asymptomatic, and the onset may be insidious. It may present with rough plaques, sensitivity to acidic or hot food, soreness of the oral cavity and gums, and erosions and ulceration. A pruritic skin rash consisting of violaceous, flat-topped papules may be present, and genitals may be affected. Associated frontal alopecia and nail involvement is less common.

Demographics of lichen planus

There is no significant racial or geographical preponderance of lichen planus. Oral lichen planus is rare in childhood.

Natural history of lichen planus, and complications of the disease

The disease course of lichen planus is chronic, with waxing and waning over years. Stress and anxiety may trigger exacerbation. Squamous cell carcinoma may rarely complicate oral lichen planus.

Approach to diagnosing lichen planus

Asymptomatic oral lichen planus is usually detected by dental practitioners. A detailed drug history is important in differentiating lichen planus from lichenoid drug reactions. Examination of skin, scalp, genital mucosa, and nails should be performed to look for other manifestations of lichen planus.

Other diagnoses that should be considered aside from lichen planus

When considering a diagnosis of lichen planus, important differential diagnoses include oral manifestations of autoimmune bullous diseases, contact dermatitis, oral candidiasis, viral infection, and drug reaction.

'Gold-standard' diagnostic test for lichen planus

The diagnosis of lichen planus is clinical and can be confirmed with a biopsy from the affected area. The hallmark of the histology is a lichenoid (band-like) lymphocytic infiltrate at the dermoepidermal junction, and basal cell layer degeneration. Immunofluorescence studies may help differentiate lichen planus from lupus or autoimmune bullous disease.

Acceptable diagnostic alternatives to the gold-standard test for lichen planus

There are no acceptable diagnostic alternatives to the gold-standard test for lichen planus.

Other relevant investigations for lichen planus

There are no other relevant investigations for lichen planus, aside from the gold-standard test.

Prognosis of lichen planus, and how to estimate it

Oral lesions in lichen planus are slow to heal, and complete remission is rare.

Treatment of lichen planus, and its effectiveness

The treatment of lichen planus aims at symptomatic relief. Good oral hygiene and well-fitting dentures to reduce trauma are important aspects of the treatment. Potent topical steroids and steroid oral rinses accelerate the healing, and anaesthetic mouthwash provides pain relief. Extensive ulceration requires systemic treatment with steroids or other agents such as retinoids and ciclosporin.

Stevens–Johnson syndrome

Definition of Stevens–Johnson syndrome

Stevens–Johnson syndrome is an emergency dermatological condition in which an immunological hypersensitivity causes erosions and inflammation of mucosal membranes and the skin.

Aetiology of Stevens–Johnson syndrome

The main trigger factor for Stevens–Johnson syndrome is drug intake. Antibiotics (e.g. sulpha-group antibiotics and penicillin), NSAIDs, allopurinol, antiepileptics, and some antiretrovirals may cause Stevens–Johnson syndrome. Certain HLA classes are associated with increased risk of developing drug-induced Stevens–Johnson syndrome. Idiopathic and infection-related forms of Stevens–Johnson syndrome are less common.

Typical symptoms of Stevens–Johnson syndrome, and less common symptoms

In Stevens–Johnson syndrome, non-specific symptoms such as flu-like symptoms, fever, and soreness of eyes and throat may precede erosions and blistering of the skin and mucosa. Trunk and face as well as acral skin are most commonly affected, and oral, genital, and conjunctival mucosa are involved. In severe cases, the mucosal lining of the respiratory and gastrointestinal tract are also affected. Detachment of epidermis may be present in <10% of body surface area.

Demographics of Stevens–Johnson syndrome

The incidence of Stevens–Johnson syndrome is estimated at 1–2 per million per year; the disease affects both sexes and all age groups.

Natural history of Stevens–Johnson syndrome, and complications of the disease

In Stevens–Johnson syndrome, the erosions on the skin and mucosa are painful and may be complicated by infection. Pneumonitis, urinary retention, and renal failure are other complications; however, the most common sequelae is damage to the eyes, including symblepharon, corneal ulcerations, and opacities.

Approach to diagnosing Stevens–Johnson syndrome

The diagnosis of Stevens–Johnson syndrome is based on the clinical picture and a detailed history of any drug intake, including over-the-counter drugs, in the period of 1–3 weeks preceding the symptoms.

Other diagnoses that should be considered aside from Stevens–Johnson syndrome

Toxic epidermal necrolysis should be considered if >30% of the skin is denuded in addition to oral, genital, or respiratory mucosal involvement. It is important to note that Stevens–Johnson syndrome may evolve into toxic epidermal necrolysis. Staphylococcal scalded skin syndrome and some autoimmune bullous diseases such as paraneoplastic pemphigus and linear IgA disease may mimic Stevens–Johnson syndrome.

'Gold-standard' diagnostic test for Stevens–Johnson syndrome

In Stevens–Johnson syndrome, a skin biopsy complements the clinical diagnosis.

Acceptable diagnostic alternatives to the gold-standard test for Stevens–Johnson syndrome

There are no acceptable diagnostic alternatives to the gold-standard test for Stevens–Johnson syndrome.

Other relevant investigations for Stevens–Johnson syndrome

In Stevens–Johnson syndrome, in addition to routine haematology and biochemistry tests, skin swabs and blood cultures are useful in cases of secondary infection and sepsis. Renal function should be monitored for haematuria and renal failure.

Prognosis of Stevens–Johnson syndrome, and how to estimate it

Mortality in Stevens–Johnson syndrome is estimated at 1%–5% and is mainly due to sepsis. Prognosis worsens when erosions and denuded skin involve larger body surface area, and with transition of Stevens–Johnson syndrome to toxic epidermal necrolysis. When epidermal detachment occurs over more than 10% of skin surface area, the prognosis and severity of the condition should be estimated with a validated scoring system (SCORTEN) that evaluates age, malignancy, tachycardia, body surface area involved, serum urea, bicarbonate, and glucose. A patient with a SCORTEN score of 3 or above should be managed in intensive care. The outcome improves with early withdrawal of the culprit drug, although drugs with long half-life are associated with a higher risk of death. The commonest sequelae in survivors of Stevens–Johnson syndrome are ophthalmological complications.

Treatment of Stevens–Johnson syndrome, and its effectiveness

Following discontinuation of the causative drug, patients with Stevens–Johnson syndrome often require admission and symptomatic treatment. There is no specific treatment for Stevens–Johnson syndrome, and supportive treatment should address haemodynamic, respiratory, and infectious complications. Topical care of skin, conjunctivae, and oral mucosa provides further symptom relief.

Further Reading

Thong BY. Stevens-Johnson syndrome/toxic epidermal necrolysis: An Asia-Pacific perspective. *Asia Pac Allergy* 2013; 3: 215–23.

Wolff K and Johnson R. *Fitzpatrick's Color Atlas and Synopsis of Clinical Dermatology* (6th edition), 2009. McGraw-Hill Professional.

CHAPTER 255 **Mucosal disease**

256 Genital disease

Susan Cooper and Tess McPherson

Definition of the disease

The term 'genital disease' refers to a spectrum of diseases. Certain systemic diseases preferentially affect mucous membranes. Local factors including warmth, occlusion, irritants, and friction are important and contribute to skin disease in this region and increase risk of certain infections. Skin conditions may be difficult to diagnose as they may have atypical appearances. Therefore, the diagnosis of disease in the anogenital region may be complex.

This chapter will focus on the most common genital diseases seen in the dermatology clinic: lichen sclerosus, lichen planus, eczema, genital pain syndromes, and pre-malignant and malignant disease. Other less common dermatological conditions seen in this area will be briefly covered.

Definition and aetiology of the most common diseases

Lichen sclerosus is a chronic inflammatory disease of unknown aetiology, preferentially affecting the anogenital region. There appears to be a genetic component, with a positive family history in some patients and a relationship with certain HLA types. Lichen sclerosus appears to be related to other autoimmune conditions such as vitiligo and thyroid disease.

Lichen planus is a chronic inflammatory disease which affects skin, nails, and mucous membranes. The aetiology is unknown but probably represents T-cell-mediated damage to epidermal cells.

In patients with genital eczema, a mixed picture of both endogenous (e.g. atopic) and exogenous eczema is frequently seen. Atopic eczema may be associated with history of eczema in other sites or other atopic disease (asthma and hay fever). Contact dermatitis can be due to irritants or allergens and is an important contributor to genital eczema. Allergens seen on patch testing include rubber and fragrance. Haemorrhoid creams and medicated toilet paper are also frequent culprits. Lichen simplex chronicus is chronic dermatitis with skin changes caused by itching/rubbing.

Vulvodynia and scrotodynia may be localized (vestibulodynia) or generalized. These both probably represent a regional pain syndrome.

Typical symptoms of the disease, and less common symptoms

There are only a limited number of symptoms in the anogenital area. Therefore, pruritus or itch and pain may be the presenting feature of a wide variety of diseases.

Itch and soreness are presenting features of lichen planus, lichen sclerosus, and vulval eczema. The patient may report an abnormal clinical appearance, and this can be primary or secondary to scratching.

A normal clinical appearance with localized pain or persistent burning is a presenting feature of vulvodynia and scrotodynia. Depression may be a feature of any chronic pain syndrome.

Demographics of the diseases

Lichen sclerosus is more common in females; the female:male ratio is reported to be 6–10:1. It may occur at any age, but two peaks of onset are during childhood and after menopause. In men, it most frequently occurs in the fourth or fifth decades, with an estimated prevalence of 1 in 660.

Like lichen sclerosus, lichen planus is more common in females. It can present any time but is more common in the sixth decade. In the UK, lichen planus accounts for around 1% of referrals to dermatologists.

Dermatitis is an extremely common condition, with a lifetime risk of over 30%.

Natural history, and complications of the disease

Lichen sclerosus, lichen planus, and vulval eczema can be chronic or resolve after a period of time with or without treatment. An important complication of lichen sclerosus and lichen planus is an increased risk of malignancy.

Approach to diagnosing the disease

In diagnosing genital disease, a full history of symptoms and their time course is required. Examination of all skin, as well as the mouth and nails, can lead to a clinical diagnosis and help differentiate between conditions that may present similarly in the genital area. Full examination of the mouth is essential and can show typical features of lichen planus (white lacy streaks on buccal mucosa) or evidence of other conditions, such as autoimmune bullous disorders. The nails and the scalp should be examined for evidence of lichen planus or psoriasis. Additionally, the presence of other autoimmune conditions, such as vitiligo, may be associated with lichen sclerosus. Other areas affected by dermatitis would be relevant.

Lichen sclerosus preferentially affects the genitals and only rarely affects other cutaneous sites. On examination of the anogenital area, clinical findings for lichen sclerosus include pallor, atrophy, fissures, and foci of hyperkeratosis. Scarring may cause loss of architecture.

Genital lichen planus can be seen with or without cutaneous disease; 50% of women with cutaneous lichen planus, and 25% of men with cutaneous lichen planus, have genital involvement. The most frequent finding is the classical violaceous papules and plaques on the labia minora and majora in woman, and on the glans or the shaft of the penis in men. Erosive lichen planus is a distinct subtype characterized by severe, scarring, erosive disease of the vestibule, the introitus, the vagina, and the oral cavity. Lacy white streaks, as seen orally, may be seen in these areas as well. Hypertrophic and lichen planopilaris are the least frequent forms of this disease.

Genital eczema appearances range from mild erythema to extreme thickening and lichenification. Typical sites affected are the labia majora and the mons pubis in women, and the crura and the scrotum in men.

Pain on examination may be feature of vulvodynia. This typically has normal clinical findings but there is overlap of some syndromes, and patients with lichen sclerosus may have vulvodynia.

A skin biopsy of lesional (abnormal) tissue can be very useful in clarifying the clinical diagnosis. In particular, it is useful for distinguishing between an interface dermatosis, such as lichen planus and lichen sclerosus, and a spongiotic dermatitis, such as dermatitis. Histological analysis is also vital to distinguish malignant from inflammatory conditions.

Perilesional skin can be biopsied for immunofluorescence if an autoimmune blistering disorder is suspected.

Swabs may be important for diagnosing candida infection, which can complicate all anogenital pathology.

Other diagnoses that should be considered

If there is any clinical doubt when diagnosing genital disease, a biopsy will help differentiate between diagnoses.

Other causes of pale patches/plaques

Other causes of pale patches/plaques in genital disease include morphoea and vitiligo. Morphoea presents with hypopigmented atrophic plaques. Vitiligo presents with asymptomatic hypopigmented patches. There may be cutaneous lesions elsewhere.

Other causes of erythematous patches/plaques

Pre-malignant and malignant causes

Vulval intra-epithelial neoplasia and penile intra-epithelial neoplasia

The majority of intra-epithelial neoplasias in genital disease are HPV related or occur in association with lichen sclerosus or lichen planus. The natural history of these conditions is unclear but an increased risk of malignancy would be expected.

Squamous cell carcinoma

Squamous cell carcinoma is the most common vulval tumour and is most frequently seen in elderly patients. It is very rare in circumcised men.

Extra-mammary Paget's disease

Extra-mammary Paget's disease is a rare intra-epithelial adenocarcinoma of apocrine gland-bearing sites. It may be primary or secondary to underlying malignancy. It is seen most commonly in the vulva (in women) or in the perianal region (in men). There may be pruritus/burning, or it may be asymptomatic. A slowly expanding erythematous plaque is typical. Erosions and scale cause a 'strawberries and cream' appearance. Because of the association of this disease with malignancy, if Paget's disease is diagnosed, a systemic evaluation is required.

Inflammatory causes

Psoriasis

Psoriasis presents with erythematous, well-defined plaques with slight scale. It may look different from psoriatic areas on the rest of the body, with the typical silver scale being not present (as in other flexural sites). It is usually confined to hair-bearing areas, so the labia minora are unaffected. Painful fissuring of the perianal and intergluteal clefts is a problem in both sexes. The presence of typical lesions elsewhere can help in the diagnosis of this disease.

Reiter's disease

Reiter's disease may present on the penis with psoriasiform lesions.

Zoon's (plasma cell) balanitis/vulvitis

Zoon's (plasma cell) disorders predominantly affect males. Clinically, the disorders present with erythematous, moist, speckled, discrete plaques. Involvement of adjacent surfaces produces 'kissing lesions' in men. Circumcision is curative.

Causes of blistering

Acquired autoimmune blistering disorders

Bullous pemphigoid

Bullous pemphigoid has a propensity for flexural sites. It presents with tense blisters on urticated plaques. There is mucosal involvement in 50% of patients.

Mucous membrane pemphigoid

Mucous membrane pemphigoid is a scarring, blistering disorder.

Erythema multiforme and Stevens–Johnson syndrome

Both erythema multiforme and Stevens–Johnson syndrome may present as a bullous eruption, particularly in the genital region. An association with herpes simplex virus is important in recurrent disease.

Fixed drug eruption

A fixed drug eruption presents as recurrent, erythematous, blistered or eroded plaques that, upon exposure to the drug, recur at exactly same site.

'Gold-standard' diagnostic test

The gold-standard diagnostic tests for genital disease include clinical findings and skin biopsy.

Acceptable diagnostic alternatives to the gold standard

An acceptable diagnostic alternative to the gold-standard tests for genital disease is a response to an appropriate treatment (e.g. strong topical steroids in lichen planus and lichen sclerosus).

Other relevant investigations

In genital disease, if pruritus is a predominant symptom, a screen for any other underlying causes of pruritus (e.g. systemic disease, such as liver or renal disease) would be relevant. If a diagnosis of lichen sclerosus or lichen planus is suspected, investigations should screen for other autoimmune diseases.

Prognosis, and how to estimate it

The risk of vulval squamous cell carcinoma is increased in both lichen sclerosus and lichen planus. It is estimated at approximately 2%–5% in lichen sclerosus, although the risk has not been quantified in men. There is also thought to be an increased risk of squamous cell carcinoma in lichen planus. The natural history of intra-epithelial neoplasia is not fully understood but an increased risk of squamous cell carcinoma is expected. Therefore, longitudinal evaluation is recommended for lichen sclerosus, lichen planus, and vulval intra-epithelial neoplasia. Self-examination should be taught. Any non-healing ulcers, fissures, or nodules should be biopsied for histological evaluation.

Treatment and its effectiveness

In genital disease amongst women, general care of the vulva can help all conditions. This includes avoidance of irritants and appropriate emollients. Lichen sclerosus responds well to strong topical steroids. Lichen planus tends to be a self-limiting condition and responds to strong topical steroids, although genital disease can be more resistant to treatment than cutaneous disease is. Hypertrophic lichen planus may benefit from interlesional corticosteroids. Erosive lichen planus is more challenging to treat and may need longer maintenance with topical steroids.

Eczema improves with soap/irritant avoidance, and use of emollients and topical steroids for flares. It can be a chronic condition and challenging to manage. Allergic contact dermatitis is investigated by patch testing and managed by avoidance of proven allergens.

Vulval pain improvement can be seen with the use of bland emollients and the avoidance of irritants and fragrance. Topical local anaesthetic agents and tricyclic antidepressants are the mainstays of treatment.

Pre-malignant and malignant conditions require an appropriate biopsy for diagnosis, together with education of the patient, and longitudinal observation for any risk of malignancy.

Further Reading

Wojnarowska F and Cooper SM. 'Anogenital (non-venereal) diseases', in Bolognia JL, Jorizzo JL, and Rapini RP, eds, *Dermatology*, 2012. Elsevier

Wolff K and Johnson R. *Fitzpatrick's Color Atlas and Synopsis of Clinical Dermatology* (6th edition), 2009. McGraw-Hill Professional.

CHAPTER 256 **Genital disease**

257 Polymorphic light eruption and actinic prurigo

Jane McGregor

Definition of polymorphic light eruption and actinic prurigo

Polymorphic light eruption (PLE) is an acute photodermatosis affecting approximately 10% of the population, predominantly women. It is almost always itchy and comprises erythema (redness) and papules which appear within a few hours of sufficient sun exposure to trigger the eruption. It usually lasts a few days to a few weeks, when it resolves spontaneously without scarring, unless re-exposure occurs. It is a seasonal eruption in temperate climates between the months of March and September.

Actinic prurigo is a much less common photodermatosis, but is probably related to PLE. It is a more long-lasting, excoriated eruption that can leave scarring.

Aetiology of PLE and actinic prurigo

The aetiology of PLE and actinic prurigo are unknown, but there appears to be a genetic element. A high proportion of patients with systemic and cutaneous lupus present with symptoms of PLE, but transformation of PLE into lupus is uncommon. About 10% of patients with PLE will have mildly elevated antinuclear antibodies, nonetheless.

Typical symptoms of PLE and actinic prurigo, and less common symptoms

PLE typically presents as an acute itchy papular eruption confined to sun-exposed sites, some hours after sufficient exposure. It resolves within a few days, to weeks without sequelae.

Rarely, PLE can present as facial swelling and erythema (redness) or with blistering on sun-exposed sites. Such cases should be investigated thoroughly for systemic lupus.

Actinic prurigo may at first resemble PLE, but then patients develop more widespread itching and excoriation. The eruption may resemble eczema in its more chronic form. It resolves to leave small scars on exposed sites. It more frequently involves the face than PLE does.

Demographics of PLE and actinic prurigo

PLE is the most common of the photodermatoses and accounts for approximately 90% of all cases of photosensitivity (excluding sunburn). It is most common in temperate climates, but can affect all races, irrespective of skin type.

Actinic prurigo is very rare and usually requires a specialist to confirm the diagnosis as it can be difficult to distinguish from PLE in some cases. It can affect all races.

Natural history of PLE and actinic prurigo, and complications of the diseases

PLE and actinic prurigo typically present in young adulthood, but can be seen as early as at a few months of age or present for the first time in elderly patients. Both conditions appear to last several years and then remit, although more persistent forms do occur.

A very small percentage of patients presenting with PLE will go on to develop systemic or cutaneous forms of lupus, and lupus serology should be undertaken at first and then periodically thereafter, particularly if symptoms worsen or change.

Approach to diagnosing of PLE and actinic prurigo

The diagnosis of PLE is clinical, but lupus serology should be undertaken to exclude cutaneous forms of lupus, especially before phototherapy desensitization.

The diagnosis of actinic prurigo is more challenging and must be distinguished from PLE. HLA typing can be helpful in supporting a diagnosis of actinic prurigo, since HLA-DRB1 0407 is prevalent in this population, but rare in those with PLE and in the general population.

Other diagnoses that should be considered aside from PLE and actinic prurigo

Subacute lupus erythematosus, discoid lupus erythematosus, and SLE can all mimic PLE.

Occasionally, it is difficult to distinguish PLE from actinic prurigo.

'Gold-standard' diagnostic test for PLE and actinic prurigo

The gold standard for the diagnosis of PLE and actinic prurigo is clinical; it therefore relies on an experienced clinician.

Prognosis of PLE and actinic prurigo, and how to estimate it

Both PLE and actinic prurigo have a good prognosis if managed well. A tiny percentage (<1%) of patients with PLE will develop cutaneous or systemic lupus.

Actinic prurigo leaves scarring, but this is usually mild and will improve once the disease has remitted, which it usually does within a few years.

Treatment of PLE and actinic prurigo, and its effectiveness

Sun avoidance and sunblock remain mainstays of treatment for PLE and actinic prurigo. Desensitization with low-dose phototherapy in specialist units is advised when simple measures are insufficient. Occasionally, patients with PLE require immunosuppression with agents such as azathioprine or cyclosporin, to control symptoms.

Actinic prurigo is more challenging to treat. Simple measures are usually ineffective and desensitization rarely works sufficiently well as a monotherapy. Thalidomide is the treatment of choice, and is highly effective at doses of between 50 and 100 mg daily. Treatment holidays can occasionally be taken over the winter months. Monitoring for neuropathy by EMG is mandatory.

Sunburn, and sunburn-related disorders

Definition of sunburn

Sunburn is usually a consequence of overexposure of the skin to solar UV light. The sunburn spectrum is within the UVB wavelengths (290–320 nm) of terrestrial solar radiation. Sunburn presents as reddening of the skin at exposed sites.

Aetiology of sunburn and sunburn-related disorders

Sunburn is usually caused by overexposure of the skin to sunlight. The paler the skin type, the more readily sunburn occurs. Darkly pigmented races require much higher doses of sunlight in order to produce erythema (redness) or sunburn.

Easy sunburn, defined as erythema or redness out of proportion to the perceived exposure, is a cause for investigation. The most common cause of disproportionate sunburn is drug phototoxicity. Many drugs, including antibiotics, diuretics, painkillers, and antipsychotics, are phototoxic.

If easy sunburn occurs in a young child, although the most likely cause is straightforward overexposure of unprotected fair skin, a DNA-repair-deficient dermatosis should be considered, namely xeroderma pigmentosum (XP).

Typical symptoms of XP, and less common symptoms

Typical symptoms of XP in a very young, previously unexposed child are of disproportionate sunburn. Later signs include freckling, dryness of the skin, poikiloderma (pigmentation and atrophy), and, in subsequent years, the development of premalignant and malignant skin cancers, including melanoma.

Demographics of XP

XP is very rare but occurs in all races and all skin types.

Natural history of XP, and complications of the disease

XP is a repair-deficient genodermatosis which ultimately leads to the development of multiple skin cancers caused by a failure to repair UV-induced DNA damage. Some patients also develop neurological complications independent of sun exposure.

Approach to diagnosing XP

The most important approach is to consider the diagnosis of XP, since the signs at an early age, where intervention can quite literally be life-saving, are very subtle. In cases of easy sunburn or freckling in a young child, if in doubt, refer for a specialist opinion.

Other diagnoses that should be considered aside from XP

Easy sunburn occurs in children because their skin has not had the opportunity to harden—this involves keratinization as well as constitutive tanning following sun exposure. Nonetheless, if a child appears to burn easily, XP is an important diagnosis to consider. Distinguishing easy sunburn in a fair-skinned child from potential XP is **very** difficult and requires specialist referral.

Drug phototoxicity should be considered in all cases of easy sunburn. Take a standard and over-the-counter history of drugs. Occasionally, foodstuffs can also cause phototoxicity—celery, for example, contains psoralen and has been documented as causing phototoxicity after a patient ate homemade celery soup!

'Gold-standard' diagnostic test for XP

The gold-standard test for XP is excision-repair testing in ex vivo fibroblasts and so requires a skin biopsy to be performed. This is an expensive and detailed test available in only a handful of centres in the UK.

Prognosis of XP, and how to estimate it

The prognosis for children with XP depends on the complement type that they have inherited (certain XP complements are more severe than others), and the vigilance of their carers and themselves in enforcing sun avoidance.

Most patients with XP, despite best care, will develop skin cancers early in life. Although survival rates have improved, the commonest cause of death is from metastatic skin cancer, sometimes in young adulthood.

Treatment of XP, and its effectiveness

Treatment for XP is complete sun avoidance. UV face shields and UV screening of windows is standard treatment. A recent product, a T4 endonuclease, applied to the skin daily, showed some promise in reducing skin cancer frequency in trials, but its use is not widespread.

Further Reading

Kraemer KH and DiGioyanna JJ. Forty years of research on xeroderma pigmentosum at the US National Institutes of Health. *Photochem Photobiol* 2015; 91: 452–9.

Warwick L and Morison WL. Photosensitivity. *N Engl J Med* 2004; 350: 1111–17.

Disorders of pigmentation

David J. Gawkrodger

Introduction

Skin colour is due to a mixture of the pigments melanin, oxyhaemoglobin (in blood), and carotene (in the stratum corneum and subcutaneous fat). Pigmentary diseases are common and particularly distressing to those with darker skin. Disorders of pigmentation often involve melanocytes. Vitiligo is the commonest disease of reduced pigmentation, and melasma is the commonest of hyperpigmentation.

Vitiligo

Definition of vitiligo

Vitiligo is an acquired idiopathic disorder showing white non-scaly macules.

Aetiology of vitiligo

In vitiligo, melanocytes are absent from affected skin on histology. An autoimmune aetiology is suggested by the association with thyroid disease and Addison's disease in some cases, and the presence of antibodies to melanocytes in the blood.

Typical symptoms of vitiligo, and less common symptoms

In vitiligo, sharply defined, white, often symmetrical macules are seen, often involving the hands, wrists, knees, neck, and areas around the mouth or eyes (see Figure 258.1). Occasionally, vitiligo is segmental (e.g. down an arm), generalized, or universal. In light-skinned individuals, vitiligo may only be discernible in summer, when the non-vitiliginous areas become tanned.

Demographics of vitiligo

Vitiligo affects 1% of the population. It is seen in all races but is most troublesome in those with a dark skin. The sex incidence is equal. The onset is usually between 10 and 30 years of age. About 20% of patients have a family history of vitiligo.

Natural history of vitiligo, and complications of the disease

Vitiligo may be precipitated by injury or sunburn. Areas may remain static, spread, or (infrequently) repigment. The condition is usually relentlessly progressive over several years.

Approach to diagnosing vitiligo

In the diagnosis of vitiligo, when taking the history, enquire about any precipitants, any personal history of other autoimmune disease, and any family history of vitiligo or autoimmune disease. Examine the entire skin surface, including with a Wood's light.

Other diagnoses that should be considered aside from vitiligo

Other diagnoses that should be considered aside from vitiligo include inflammatory skin disease, chemical leucoderma, leprosy, albinism, and phenylketonuria (see Table 258.1). Post-inflammatory hypopigmentation may occur with inflammatory skin disease. In chemical leucoderma, a history of exposure to phenolic chemicals should be sought. The hypopigmented macules of leprosy normally are anaesthetic. Albinism is a group of autosomal recessive conditions in which the melanocytes fail to synthesize pigment in the epidermis, hair bulb, and eye due to defects in the enzyme tyrosinase. It is uncommon (1 in 20 000) and usually presents in infancy with white or pink skin, white hair, and eyes that lack pigmentation. Phenylketonuria is an autosomal recessive defect of phenylalanine hydroxylase and is usually detected after birth by a routine screening test (incidence 1 in 10 000). Patients have fair hair and skin, due to impaired melanin synthesis. If phenylketonuria is left untreated, mental retardation and choreoathetosis develop.

'Gold-standard' diagnostic test for vitiligo

The gold-standard diagnostic test for vitiligo is Wood's light, a hand-held UVB light source, which can show up areas of vitiligo not visible to the naked eye.

Table 258.1 Other causes of hypopigmentation	
Cause	**Disease or example**
Chemical	Substituted phenols
	Hydroquinone
Genetic	Albinism
	Phenylketonuria
	Tuberous sclerosis
	Piebaldism
Infection	Leprosy
	Yaws
	Pityriasis versicolor
Post inflammatory	Cryotherapy
	Eczema
	Psoriasis
	Morphoea
	Pityriasis alba
Other	Lichen sclerosus
	Halo naevus
	Scarring

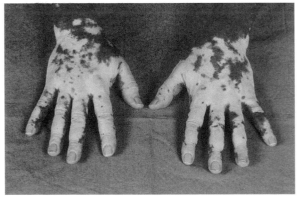

Figure 258.1 Extensive vitiligo of the hands. Please see colour plate section.

Acceptable diagnostic alternatives to the gold-standard test for vitiligo

There are no acceptable diagnostic alternatives to the gold-standard test for vitiligo. The diagnosis is usually clinical.

Other relevant investigations for vitiligo

In vitiligo, it is recommended to perform thyroid function tests.

Prognosis of vitiligo, and how to estimate it

The course of vitiligo is usually relentlessly progressive, with episodes of exacerbation alternating with times of inactivity.

Treatment and its effectiveness

The currently available treatment for vitiligo is unsatisfactory. Camouflage cosmetics are of limited use. Sunscreens help reduce tanning of non-vitiligo skin. Potent topical steroids (e.g. betamethasone valerate) or calcineurin inhibitors (e.g. tacrolimus or pimecrolimus) can induce repigmentation. UVB or photochemotherapy (psoralen and UVA) may induce repigmentation but it may take months. Rarely, depigmentation using hydroquinone derivatives is considered when vitiligo is very extensive.

Melasma

Definition of melasma

Melasma is a common patterned macular facial pigmentation especially occurring with pregnancy and in women on oral contraceptives.

Aetiology of melasma

In melasma, there is an increase in the amount of melanin in the skin from an increased melanin synthesis by melanocytes, often stimulated by hormonal factors.

Typical symptoms of melasma, and less common symptoms

In melasma, the pigmentation is symmetrical and often involves the forehead.

Demographics of melasma

Women are mostly but not exclusively affected by melasma.

Natural history of melasma, and complications of the disease

Melasma usually progresses during the twenties and thirties but may improve spontaneously.

Approach to diagnosing melasma

When diagnosing melasma, determine whether there are any underlying hormonal factors that might be treatable.

Other diagnoses that should be considered aside from melasma

Other diagnoses that should be considered aside from melasma are listed in Table 258.2; they include:

- freckles: small, light-brown macules, typically facial, which darken on sun exposure
- lentigines: brown macules that are scattered and do not darken in the sun; in Peutz–Jeghers syndrome, lentigines are found around the lips, buccal mucosa, and fingers and are associated with small bowel polyps
- Addison's disease: excess adrenocorticotropic hormone stimulates melanogenesis; addisonian-like pigmentation is also seen in Cushing's syndrome, hyperthyroidism, and acromegaly

Table 258.2 Other causes of hyperpigmentation

Cause	Disease or example
Drugs	Psoralens
	Oestrogens
	Phenothiazines
	Minocycline
	Amiodarone
Endocrine	Addison's disease
	Cushing's syndrome
	Graves' disease
Genetic	Racial
	Freckles
	Neurofibromatosis
	Peutz–Jeghers syndrome
Metabolic	Biliary cirrhosis
	Haemochromatosis
	Porphyria
Nutritional	Carotenaemia
	Malabsorption
	Malnutrition
	Pellagra
Post inflammatory	Eczema
	Lichen planus
	Systemic sclerosis
	Lichen amyloidosis
Other	Malignant melanoma
	Chronic renal failure
	Argyria

- drug-induced pigmentation: may be due to stimulation of melanogenesis or deposition of the drug in the skin, but often the mechanism is not well understood.

In addition, sometimes other pigments can colour the skin in a generalized manner, such as iron (with melanin), in haemochromatosis, and carotene (causing an orange discoloration), in carotenaemia (usually due to eating too many carrots).

'Gold-standard' diagnostic test for melasma

There is no gold-standard diagnostic test for melasma.

Other relevant investigations for melasma

Usually, there are no other relevant investigations for melasma, but consider a skin biopsy in atypical cases.

Prognosis of melasma, and how to estimate it

Melasma is usually a persistent condition. It darkens with sun exposure.

Treatment of melasma, and its effectiveness

In melasma, topical tretinoin, azelaic acid, or hydroquinone can reduce pigmentation. Sunscreens and camouflage cosmetics can also help.

Further Reading

Grimes P, Nordlund JJ, Pandyra AG, et al. Increasing our understanding of pigmentary disorders. *J Am Acad Dermatol* 2006; 54: S255–S261.

Nordlund J, Boissy R, Hearing V, et al. (eds). *The Pigmentary System* (2nd edition), 2006. Oxford University Press.

Taieb A and Picardo M. The definition and assessment of vitiligo. *Pigment Cell Res* 2007; 20: 27–35.

Definition of the disease

Skin cancer is very common in the UK, and its incidence is rising rapidly. There are two broad classes of primary skin cancer: non-melanoma and melanoma. Non-melanoma skin cancer is the commonest form (100 000 cases diagnosed annually in the UK), accounting for nine out of ten skin cancers and includes basal cell carcinoma (BCC) and squamous cell carcinoma (SCC). Cutaneous melanoma is less common (10 000 cases diagnosed in the UK annually) but confers a significantly worse prognosis and accounts for 75% of skin cancer related deaths. There are also a number of other, rarer, non-melanoma skin cancers (e.g. appendageal carcinomas, Merkel cell carcinoma, sarcomas, vascular malignancies, and cutaneous lymphomas); however, these account for less than 1% of all skin cancers in the UK and so will not be specifically discussed here.

Cutaneous metastases can occur secondary to any internal cancer or, indeed, to skin cancer (e.g. melanoma). In most cases, cutaneous metastasis occurs after the diagnosis of a primary cancer and usually in late stages of the disease but, in some cases, it may be the first presentation, in which case it should prompt a thorough investigation for the primary malignancy.

Aetiology of the disease

Aetiology of non-melanoma skin cancer

Aetiology of BCC

BCCs are tumours of basal epidermal keratinocytes and occasionally arise from the outer root sheath of a hair follicle, specifically, from hair follicle stem cells residing just below the sebaceous gland duct in an area called the bulge. The most significant etiological factors are exposure to UV radiation, and genetic predisposition. Intense, intermittent sun exposure in childhood is particularly important, and the most commonly involved sites are the head and neck. Increasing age, male sex, fair skin type, a positive family history, immunosuppression, and arsenic exposure are other recognized risk factors. Multiple BCCs are a feature of a rare genodermatosis, basal cell naevus (Gorlin) syndrome. Following development of a BCC, patients are at significantly increased risk (approximately 40%–50%) of developing subsequent BCCs at other sites and are also at increased risk of SCC and melanoma.

Genetic studies have shown somatic mutations in the PTCH gene in 40%–70% sporadic BCCs. These are predominantly UV-signature mutations, supporting the role of UV radiation in the pathogenesis of these skin cancers.

Aetiology of SCC

SCC is a malignant tumour arising from epidermal keratinocytes. Its occurrence is usually related to chronic UV-radiation exposure and is therefore especially common in people with fair, sun-damaged skin, and in UV-sensitive genodermatoses such as oculocutaneous albinism and xeroderma pigmentosum. It may also develop as a result of previous exposure to ionizing radiation or to arsenic, or at sites of chronic inflammation (chronic wounds, scars, burns, ulcers, or sinus tracts). It may arise de novo or against a background of clinically apparent intra-epidermal keratinocyte dysplasia (full thickness intra-epidermal SCC or Bowen's disease; partial thickness intra-epidermal dysplasia or actinic keratosis).

Individuals with impaired immune function, for example those receiving immunosuppressive drugs following allogeneic organ transplantation or for autoimmune or inflammatory diseases, are at significantly increased risk of SCC. In organ transplant recipients, the risk of SCC increases 65–250-fold and the risk of BCC 10 to 16-fold, compared to that in the non-transplanted population, with consequent reversal of the usual BCC:SCC ratio of 3–4:1. Age, duration of immunosuppression, skin phototype, and a history of high UV exposure are key risk factors in the pathogenesis of post-transplant non-melanoma skin cancer. However, complex genetic factors can determine individual risk. The risk of SCC with the new wave of 'biological' therapies (for inflammatory and haematological disease) has yet to be quantified. Patients with HIV/AIDS or non-Hodgkin lymphoma, specifically chronic lymphocytic leukaemia, may also develop aggressive SCC. Increased cutaneous HPV infection in these immunosuppressed groups, together with the occurrence of SCC in up to 60% patients with the rare genodermatosis epidermodysplasia verruciformis (which is associated with widespread cutaneous HPV infection) indicates a possible association between HPV and SCC.

Aetiology of Kaposi's sarcoma

Kaposi's sarcoma (KS) is a vascular malignancy of spindle-cell origin, thought to be derived from the endothelial cell lineage, which is characterized by mucocutaneous violaceous lesions and oedema. Any organ can be affected. It is caused by human herpesvirus-8. Immunosuppression appears to be a significant cofactor (e.g. in HIV/AIDS (see Chapter 296) and post-organ transplantation). The four main types of KS are detailed in Table 259.1.

Aetiology of cutaneous melanoma

Melanoma arises in genetically susceptible individuals exposed to environmental agents, principally UV radiation. Risk factors for melanoma are detailed in Table 259.2. Major risk factors for melanoma are a past history of melanoma (especially if under the age of 40), a history of eight moles >6 mm diameter, atypical mole syndrome (particularly with a family history of melanoma), large congenital melanocytic naevi (>15 cm in diameter), and the nucleotide excision repair genodermatosis, xeroderma pigmentosum. Mutations in several high-penetrance genes have been identified as influencing melanoma risk: in particular, CDKN2A (chromosomal location: 9p21), which encodes a p16 tumour suppressor protein, and CDK4 (chromosomal location: 12q13). Polymorphisms in low-penetrance genes have also been identified, including the melanoma susceptibility gene, MC1R (chromosome location: 16q24.7).

Typical symptoms of the disease, and less common symptoms

Symptoms of non-melanoma skin cancer

Symptoms of BCC

BCCs usually arise on chronically and intermittently sun-exposed skin of individuals over age 40, but can occur in younger people. Clinicopathological subtypes include nodular, superficial, infiltrating, and morphoeic. Nodular BCC accounts for 60%–70% of cases. It is most common on the head and neck and presents as a pearly or translucent papule or plaque with rolled edges and overlying telangiectasia. It may ulcerate centrally and there may be a history of recurrent bleeding or crusting. Some lesions have cystic centres. In darker skin types, BCCs may be pigmented and simulate melanoma.

Superficial BCC accounts for 15% of all BCCs and commonly affect the trunk of younger patients. They present as scaly papules or plaques with a pink to red-brown colour and often have a characteristic thread-like, pearly border. They are often misdiagnosed as patches of eczema, psoriasis, or tinea.

Table 259.1 Typical appearance of common primary skin cancers

BCC	SCC	KS	MM
Nodular: skin-coloured nodule with prominent overlying telangiectasia Soft in consistency Easily damaged by trauma Superficial BCC are scaly erythematous patches/papules with a thin pearly border; they can be mistaken for patches of eczema, psoriasis, or tinea Infiltrative/morphoeic subtypes may present with a scar-like appearance	Indurated, crusted, nodular, or ulcerated lesion arising on sun-damaged skin On lip or genitalia, presents as fissure or non-healing ulcer	Classic KS: affects those of Jewish Ashkenazi/ Mediterranean descent African endemic KS: adult male predominance, 1.3%–10% of black Africans affected; lymphadenopathic variant seen KS in immunosuppression: observed in all iatrogenically immunosuppressed individuals, including post-transplantation individuals AIDS-related epidemic KS: high incidence in certain regions of Africa and the Caribbean	Changing or new mole (defined by ABCDE criteria*)

Abbreviations: BCC, basal cell carcinoma; KS, Kaposi's sarcoma; MM, malignant melanoma; SCC, squamous cell carcinoma.

*ABCDE criteria are used to identify early melanomas: **A**symmetry, **B**order irregularity, **C**olour variation, **D**iameter > 6 mm, **E**levation.

Infiltrative/morphoeic subtypes are perhaps the most difficult to diagnose clinically as they may present with a scar-like appearance. Because of their histological characteristics, with cords of tumour cells infiltrating beyond the apparent clinical margins of the BCC, they are the type most likely to recur after surgery.

Symptoms of SCC

SCC commonly arises on chronically sun-exposed skin of elderly Caucasians over the age of 60. The usual sites for SCC are the dorsa of the hands; the forearms; the upper face; the lower lip; and the ears. SCCs most commonly present as indurated, keratotic nodules or plaques, which may ulcerate and are often tender on palpation. They may also present as a fissure or a non-healing indurated ulcer on the lip or genitalia. Regional lymph nodes may be enlarged due to infection/inflammation of the tumour (dermatopathic lymphadenopathy) or as a result of metastases (with harder, irregular, matted nodes).

Symptoms of KS

KS usually begins as macules, which evolve into papules, plaques, nodules, and tumours which may range in colour from violaceous, pink, red, or tan and become purplish-brown. Lesions are usually palpable and firm to hard in consistency. Lesions may originate at a site of trauma and ulcerate or form an overlying crust. Skin lesions may be associated with deeper involvement of the lymphatic system or lymph nodes, resulting in lymphoedema, which common affects the lower limbs. Skin changes secondary to lymphoedema, including papillomatosis and hyperkeratosis, may then complicate the clinical picture. Mucocutaneous lesions are usually asymptomatic.

Symptoms of cutaneous melanoma

All lesions suspected of being a melanoma should be urgently referred to a clinician trained in their diagnosis and management, usually a dermatologist. There are a number of presenting signs and symptoms for which urgent referral to the local skin cancer multidisciplinary team is indicated:

- a new mole which appears after the onset of puberty and which is changing in shape, colour, or size
- a long-standing mole which is changing in shape, colour, or size
- any mole which has three or more colours or has lost its symmetry
- a mole which is itching or bleeding
- any new persistent skin lesion, especially if growing, pigmented, or vascular in appearance, and if the diagnosis is not clear
- a new pigmented line in a nail, especially where there is associated damage to the nail
- a suspicious lesion growing under a nail

Symptoms of cutaneous metastases

Most skin metastasis occurs in a body region near the primary tumour. The first sign of skin metastasis can be a firm, round or oval, mobile, non-painful nodule. The nodules are rubbery, firm, or hard in texture and can vary in size. These may be skin-coloured,

Table 259.2 Risk factors for the common skin cancers

Risk factor	RR for developing BCC*	RR for developing SCC*	RR for developing melanoma*
UV exposure: history of blistering sunburn	+	1.9	2.5
Fitzpatrick skin type I (burns without tanning)†	+	2	1.7
Keratotic lesions >50	4	12.1	
Multiple benign naevi	NA	NA	11
Multiple atypical naevi	NA	NA	11
Strong family history of melanoma§	NA	NA	35–70
Previous history of melanoma	NA	NA	8.5
Previous history of non-melanoma skin cancer (BCC and/or SCC)	10	10	2.9
Immunosuppression: • HIV • Transplant recipients	10-fold	+ 50–100-fold	1.5 2–17
Ionizing radiation	3.6	2.94	?+
Tanning beds	1.5	2.5	2.86–4.44
Arsenic exposure	+	+	
Tobacco smoking		+	
Photosensitizing drugs, e.g. fluoroquinolones, voriconazole	+	+	

Abbreviations: BCC, basal cell carcinoma; RR, relative risk; SCC, squamous cell carcinoma.

*Where quantifiable relative risk is not available, + confirms evidence of increased relative risk.

†Fitzpatrick skin types: I: always burns/never tans; II: usually burns/sometimes tans; III: usually tans/sometimes burns; IV: always tans/rarely burns; V: Asian; VI: Black African and Afro-Caribbean.

§Defined as ≥3 family members affected.

Table 259.3 Commonest primary tumours giving rise to skin metastases

Primary tumour	Demographics	Common sites affected	Features
Breast	Commonest primary cancer in females of all ages	Trunk/scalp	Firm, scar-like area May appear as inflammatory plaques with well-demarcated elevated margin
Colon/stomach	Males > females	Abdomen/pelvis	Nodule at umbilicus (Sister Mary Joseph nodule) is a sign of extensive colorectal carcinoma
Melanoma	Males (<40 years) > Females (>40 years)	Trunk and extremities (males) Lower limbs (females)	Pigmented papules and dermal nodules
Lung	Commonest primary cancer in males (>40 years)	Trunk	Firm, erythematous nodules which tend to follow intercostal vessels when on the chest
Squamous cell carcinoma oral cavity/larynx	Males > 40 years	Head and neck	

red, or, in the case of melanoma, blue or black. Sometimes, multiple nodules appear rapidly. The skin metastases may break down and ulcerate through the skin. Depending on the location of the primary tumour, skin metastasis display certain characteristic features (see Table 259.3). More unusual patterns of cutaneous involvement by metastases include:

- carcinoma erysipeloides: sharply demarcated red patches that occur when the local spread of a primary cancer blocks lymphatic blood vessels in the adjacent skin
- en cuirasse or sclerodermoid carcinoma: indurated, fibrous, scar-like plaques due to cancer cells infiltrating collagen in the skin
- carcinoma telangiectoides: red patches with telangiectasia or lymphatic vessels (lymphangioma-like)

Demographics of the disease

Demographics of non-melanoma skin cancer

In 2007 more than 84 000 cases of non-melanoma skin cancer were registered, but it is estimated that the actual number of new cases each year is at least 100 000, a figure which is steadily increasing. By 2030, the number of cases presenting to dermatologists could increase by an estimated 50%. The incidence of non-melanoma skin cancer increases with age, and 80% of cases occur in people over the age of 60 years. In addition, the incidence is higher in men than in women.

Demographics of BCC

BCC is the most common cancer in Europe, Australia, and the US and is showing a worldwide increase in incidence. Poor BCC data collection by many tumour registries means that accurate figures for the incidence of BCC in the UK are difficult to obtain.

Demographics of SCC

SCC is the second most common skin cancer and, in many countries, its incidence is rising. It accounts for the majority of non-melanoma skin cancer-related deaths. The BCC:SCC ratio is approximately 3-4:1 in most countries, but is often reversed in immunosuppressed populations.

Demographics of KS

Classic KS was first described as a slow-growing endothelial cell tumour in elderly men of Mediterranean or Eastern European descent; subsequently, a slightly more aggressive form of the disease (so-called endemic KS) was recognized at higher rates in African populations. With the onset of the AIDS epidemic, the worldwide incidence of this cancer has increased dramatically in the past 25 years, and a much more aggressive form of KS is now the commonest tumour amongst HIV-infected people in Africa (>10/100 000 males). KS became common amongst a subset of HIV patients in the West, but the incidence is now falling with the introduction of effective anti-HIV drug therapy. An increased incidence of KS is also observed in organ transplant recipients and other iatrogenically immuonosuppressed individuals.

Demographics of cutaneous melanoma

The incidence of cutaneous melanoma is rising faster than for any other major cancer, and rates are set to treble over the next 30 years.

More than 10 400 cases of melanoma are diagnosed annually in the UK, with over 2000 deaths attributable to melanoma. In 2006, melanoma was more common in females than males, with a male:female ratio of 4:5. Although the incidence of melanoma rises with age, a disproportionately high incidence of melanoma is observed amongst young people; almost a third of cases (31%) occur in people aged <50 years and it is the commonest cancer amongst 15–34 year olds. For females, it is the sixth most common cancer and, for males, it is the eighth. The current lifetime risk for males in the UK is about 1:91; for females, it is 1:77.

Demographics of cutaneous metastases

The incidence of skin metastases is 3%–10% for all primary cancers. Although most cancers can metastasize to the skin, some cancers are more likely to than others and this is also dependent on gender and age of the individual (see Table 259.3).

Natural history and complications of the disease

Natural history of non-melanoma skin cancer, and complications of the disease

Although non-melanoma skin cancer is very common, in the vast majority of cases it is not life-threatening.

Natural history of BCC, and complications of the disease

BCC is a slow-growing, locally invasive, malignant epidermal skin tumour predominantly affecting Caucasians. Metastasis is extremely rare, and morbidity results from local tissue invasion and destruction particularly to the face, head, and neck (giving rise to the lay term of 'rodent ulcer').

Natural history of SCC, and complications of the disease

SCCs are also locally invasive but, unlike BCCs, have the potential to metastasize to lymph nodes and other organs. Patients with impaired immune function are at higher risk of metastasis. Spread by bloodstream is uncommon. The risk of metastasis is also associated with the size of the tumour (>2 cm), the depth of invasion (>6 mm confers a 16% risk of metastasis), differentiation state (poor differentiated tumours fare worse), the rate of growth, and the anatomical location: tumours on the ear and lip have a worse prognosis than tumours elsewhere. Mucosal SCCs have a greater tendency to recur and metastasize than SCCs located on the glabrous sun-exposed skin. Tumours arising in actinic keratoses on the dorsa of hands are indolent and late in metastasizing. Lesions in sun-exposed areas have a better prognosis than those arising from non-sun-exposed areas. There is an increased risk of a second primary SCC within 5 years after therapy for the first malignancy; this risk is approximately 30% for the general population, but up to 75% in immunosuppressed individuals.

Natural history of KS, and complications of the disease

Although the skin is the most frequent organ of involvement, internal lesions of KS are commonly seen (e.g. affecting the lungs, abdominal viscera, or lymph nodes). Overall mean survival is 10–15 years.

Classic or European KS is typically slowly progressive. African endemic KS has been described in two age groups: young adults (mean age 35) with generally benign cutaneous nodular disease, and young children (mean age 3) with fulminant lymphadenopathic disease, which is fatal within 3 years.

Natural history of cutaneous melanoma, and complications of the disease

Cutaneous melanoma arises from epidermal melanocytes. It is one of the most aggressive skin cancers, occurring in all ages but predominantly affecting adults. Prognosis is closely related to the depth of the tumour (Breslow thickness), as well as tumour ulceration, mitotic rate, and nodal status (see Table 259.4). It accounts for 75% of all skin cancer-related deaths. It is assumed that most melanomas increase in size with time and that early recognition and excision provides the greatest opportunity for cure. Moreover, melanoma is notoriously chemoresistant and often proves to be radiotherapy resistant. Over the last 30 years, there have been no new therapeutic approaches that have improved overall survival rates in metastatic disease but there are recent indications that new targeted and immunotherapy-based therapeutic interventions (e.g. BRAF-targeted therapy and PDL-1 inhibition) may improve this dismal situation.

Approach to diagnosing the disease

Take a thorough history

The following features must be established and can help with diagnosis:

* duration of the lesion: BCCs are usually slow-growing; SCCs often have a more rapid growth pattern
* change in size: a pigmented lesion which is growing or changing in shape or colour is likely to be evolving and could be an early sign of malignant change
* change in colour
* change in shape
* symptoms: itchiness or bleeding in long-standing melanocytic naevi may be suggestive of malignant change, particularly if associated with changes in size, colour, or shape

Assess risk factors

Skin phototype and a UV-exposure history should be established. Individuals deemed to have had high UV exposure would be those with an outdoor occupation for >5 years, those who have lived in a sunny climate for >6 months, or 'sun worshippers' who have actively sought a suntan for >2 weeks per year for >10 years and/or have ever used sunbeds. Conversely, a low-UV-exposure category would include individuals with indoor occupations, those who have

not lived in sunny climates, and those who avoid the sun or do not actively sunbathe. Intermediate UV exposure falls between these two categories.

Patients with a history of long-standing ulcers or wounds (e.g. burns), previous radiotherapy, UV therapy (e.g. psoralen and UVA therapy, for psoriasis), chronic immunosuppressive therapy, or arsenic ingestion are also more likely to develop skin cancers.

Physical examination

Examination of the individual lesion should be undertaken, detailing the following:

* site: this can influence treatment options and prognosis
* size (maximum diameter): this is important to determine further treatment based on surgical margins
* colour (flesh-coloured, erythematous, pigmented); variability of colour should also be noted
* elevation (palpable, nodular)
* margins/border (regular, irregular)
* surface (smooth, scaling, roughened, crusted, ulcerated, bleeding)

When skin cancer is suspected, regional lymph nodes should also be examined to determine any nodal spread. A complete examination of the entire skin should also be undertaken to identify any other pre-malignant or malignant lesions.

Other diagnoses that should be considered

Common differential diagnoses for skin cancers according to type are detailed in Table 259.5.

'Gold-standard' diagnostic test

'Gold-standard' diagnostic test for BCC and SCC

The gold-standard diagnostic test for all skin cancers is histological assessment. There are now well-defined criteria for reporting of histological features to confirm the diagnosis and to determine the prognosis. For smaller tumours, primary excision may be both diagnostic and therapeutic. For larger lesions and for those in cosmetically sensitive sites, an initial diagnostic biopsy (incision or punch biopsy) may be required to confirm the diagnosis and histological subtype (e.g. superficial vs infiltrative BCC; well-differentiated vs poorly differentiated SCC) before planning definitive treatment.

'Gold-standard' diagnostic test for KS

The diagnosis of KS is usually confirmed on skin biopsy.

Table 259.4 Prognosis of melanoma		
Stage	**Characteristics**	**5 year survival**
1a	Melanoma cells confined to the epidermis	95% +
1b	<1 mm thick Not ulcerated No spread elsewhere	
2a	1–2 mm and ulcerated, or 2–4 mm and not ulcerated No spread elsewhere	Men 80% Women 90%
2b	2–4 mm + ulcerated or >4 mm and no ulceration	Prognosis worsens with higher-grade tumour (i.e. worse for 2c than for 2a)
2c	> 4 mm and ulcerated, confined to skin, and no spread	
3a	Spread into up to three lymph nodes near the primary, only detectable microscopically Melanoma not ulcerated	Men 50% Women more than 50%
3b	Ulcerated melanoma + 1–3 microscopic lymph node spread **or** non-ulcerated melanoma + 1–3 lymph nodes, which are enlarged, **or** non-ulcerated melanoma + local skin spread but no lymph node involvement	Prognosis worsens with higher-grade tumour (i.e. worse for 3c than for 3a)
3c	Melanoma in lymph nodes + local skin **or** spread to 1–3 lymph nodes which are enlarged or spread to 4+ nearby lymph nodes or spread to lymph nodes which have joined together	
4	Spread away from origin and local lymph nodes	Men 10% Women 25%

Data from http://www.cancerresearchuk.org/about-cancer/type/melanoma/treatment/melanoma-statistics-and-outlook.

Table 259.5 Common differential diagnoses for skin cancers according to type

Non-melanoma skin cancer	Cutaneous melanoma
Actinic keratoses: • rough, scaly erythematous papules on chronically sun-exposed skin • if hyperkeratotic, may simulate an early SCC Bowen's disease (intra-epidermal squamous cell carcinoma): • fixed, erythematous, scaly plaque which gradually expands • usually on sun-exposed skin but characteristically on the lower legs • may be difficult to differentiate from a superficial BCC, although BCCs often has a thread-like rolled edge Benign intradermal naevus: • usually very long history of a stable lesion • may simulate nodular BCC Keratoacanthoma: • usually very rapidly growing nodule on sun-exposed skin with symmetrical configuration, 'shouldered' erythematous/translucent margins, and a central keratotic plug • SCCs tend to be more irregular in shape and slower growing and do not regress spontaneously	Melanocytic naevi: • benign or dysplastic • any naevus in which there is a history of change or which is clinically suspicious should be excised for histological examination Seborrhoeic keratosis (basal cell papillomas): • can mimic many of the features suggestive of melanoma but have a 'stuck-on appearance', and patients often have multiple similar lesions on the body • dermoscopy can be a useful adjunct to diagnosis Dermatofibroma: • usually a firm nodule which may be pigmented • often on limbs • a history of insect bite may be given Vascular lesions: • may simulate melanoma, e.g. angiokeratomas (dark red/black scaly papules), pyogenic granuloma (rapidly growing, bright red/purple ulcerated, rounded nodule, surrounding skin is normal)

Abbreviations: BCC, basal cell carcinoma; SCC, squamous cell carcinoma.

'Gold-standard' diagnostic test for cutaneous melanoma

A lesion suspected to be a melanoma should be photographed and then excised completely by a trained specialist. The axis of excision should be orientated to facilitate possible subsequent wide local excision. The excision biopsy should include the whole tumour, with a clinical margin of 2 mm around normal skin, and a cuff of fat. This allows for examination of the entire lesion, such that subsequent definitive treatment can be based on Breslow thickness. With few exceptions, diagnostic shave biopsies or partial removal of lesions must be avoided, as these can lead to incorrect diagnosis due to sampling error.

Acceptable diagnostic alternatives to the gold-standard tests

Although complete excision is the gold standard for diagnosis of melanoma, in a few circumstances, incisional biopsies may be acceptable (e.g. for large lesions on cosmetically sensitive sites). It should be emphasized that, while this approach may assist in confirming whether a lesion is indeed a melanoma, it cannot provide an accurate Breslow thickness, which is required for planning definitive surgical excision, and, occasionally, false negatives may arise from sampling error.

Other relevant investigations

Dermoscopy

Experienced specialists can make a clinical diagnosis of BCC in many cases. Diagnostic accuracy is enhanced by good lighting and magnification, and the dermatoscope can be helpful in some cases. The dermatoscope allows a closer examination of the surface of pigmented lesions with 10× magnification, and a glass plate/oil interface or polarized light to minimize reflection from the surface. A dermatoscopic score takes into account features such as asymmetry, number of colours, pigment structure, and irregular border; this scoring can be correlated with risk of malignancy. Dermoscopy is a specialized tool, usually most successfully used by trained and experienced dermatologists.

Radiological imaging

Imaging is not routinely indicated to aid diagnosis of non-melanoma skin cancers or cutaneous melanoma. However, it may be required to establish involvement of underlying structures (e.g. bony involvement), prior to planning definitive treatment. For melanoma, no routine imaging is recommended unless the disease is Stage IIC/III or above; in these circumstances, staging should be determined using whole-body CT or CT–PET scans. Ultrasound or CT scanning is indicated for patients with a diagnosis of KS, to exclude visceral or lymphatic involvement.

Investigation of suspicious lymph nodes

Sentinel lymph node biopsy

Sentinel lymph node biopsy (SLNB) was developed as a means to identify the first lymph node draining the skin in which a melanoma arises. This investigation is usually performed at the same time as definitive wider excision of a primary melanoma. It is usually considered as a staging procedure for melanomas for which the Breslow thickness is between 1 mm and 4 mm, as sentinel node positivity is associated with a worse prognosis in such melanomas. As yet, there is no therapeutic value associated with the procedure. Patients with a positive SLNB usually proceed to complete lymphadenectomy. The procedure is associated with 5% morbidity and, in 5% of cases, it is not possible to identify the sentinel lymph node.

As an alternative to SLNB, ultrasound surveillance of lymph node basins can be used but it is only available in specialist centres. Nodes clinically suspicious for metastatic disease should be sampled using fine-needle aspiration cytology or ultrasound-guided biopsy. Prior to lymph node dissection, staging CT scan should be performed.

Prognosis, and how to estimate it

Prognosis of non-melanoma skin cancer

There are a number of well-defined prognostic factors, which affect the outcome of non-melanoma skin cancers (see Table 259.6).

Prognosis of BCC

The histological subtype of BCC may influence the prognosis: morphoeic/infiltrative, micronodular, and basosquamous variants are associated with aggressive tissue invasion and destruction. Perivascular or perineural invasion are features associated with increased aggression and recurrence. Metastasis is extremely rare (1:50 000), but may occur in the setting of tumours exceeding 5 cm in diameter.

Prognosis of SCC

Most patients with primary cutaneous SCC have a very good prognosis. Conversely, metastatic disease has a poor long-term prognosis; patients with regional lymphadenopathy have a <20% 10-year survival rate, and patients with distant metastases have <10% 10-year survival rate. Factors predicting metastatic potential include anatomical site, size, tumour thickness, level of invasion, rate of growth, aetiology, degree of histological differentiation, and host immunosuppression.

Table 259.6 Factors influencing prognosis of non-melanoma skin cancer

Feature	Effect on prognosis of BCC	Effect on prognosis of SCC
Tumour site	Lesions on central face, especially around eyes, nose, lips, and ears are at higher risk of recurrence	SCC arising in areas of radiation or thermal injury, chronic ulcers or pre-malignant lesions > in non-sun-exposed sites > ear > lip (increasing metastatic potential)
Tumour size	Increasing size confers higher risk of recurrence	Tumours >2 cm are twice more likely to recur locally and 3× more likely to metastasize
Tumour depth	–	Tumours <2 mm virtually never metastasize
		Tumours >6 mm in depth or extending into or beyond the subcutis are more likely to recur and metastasize (risk 16%)
Defined clinical margins	Poorly defined lesions are at higher risk of recurrence	
Histological subtype	Morphoeic, micronodular, infiltrative, and basosquamous histological subtypes confer higher risk of recurrence	Poorly differentiated tumours have a worse prognosis, with >2× local recurrence rates and 3× metastatic rate compared with well-differentiated tumours
		Certain subtypes (e.g. desmoplastic SCC) have a 24% risk of local recurrence vs 1% for non-desmoplastic SCC
Perivascular or perineural invasion	Confers higher risk of recurrence	More likely to recur and to metastasize (rates up to 50%)
Failure of previous treatments	Recurrent lesions have increased risk of further recurrence	Locally recurrent disease is a risk factor for metastatic disease
	Local recurrence is lower with Mohs micrographic surgery	
Host immunosuppression	Tenfold increased incidence risk	Worse prognosis, increased risk approximately 100-fold, increased risk of metastasis 5%–7%

Abbreviations: BCC, basal cell carcinoma; SCC, squamous cell carcinoma.

Adapted: a) with permission from Telfer, N.R., G.B. Colver, and C.A. Morton, Guidelines for the management of basal cell carcinoma, The British journal of dermatology, Volume 159, Issue 1, pp. 35–48, Copyright © 2008.

b) Reproduced with permission from R. Motley, P. Kersey, C. Lawrence, Multiprofessional guidelines for the management of the patient with primary cutaneous squamous cell carcinoma, The British journal of dermatology, Volume 146, Issue 1, pp. 18/25, Copyright © 2002 John Wiley and Sons.

Prognosis of cutaneous melanoma

The prognosis of melanoma is dependent on several factors:

(a) Breslow thickness (the deepest contiguous point of the tumour in millimetres)
(b) mitotic count (the number of mitoses per square millimetre)
(c) ulceration status (ulcerated tumours have a worse prognosis)
(d) nodal involvement (the prognosis of tumours is dependent on the presence and number of involved nodes)
(e) LDH level
(f) host immunosuppression
(g) site of melanoma (limb melanomas have a better prognosis than truncal melanomas do)
(h) age (younger patients have a better prognosis than older patients)
(i) gender (males fare worse than females)

Factors (a)–(e) have a significant effect when determining prognosis and are included in the seventh edition of the American Joint Committee on Cancer (AJCC) classification for prognostic staging of melanoma (summarized in Table 259.4). More recently, a website has been set up that provides a tool for predicting the clinical outcome of an individual patient with localized or regional cutaneous melanoma (http://www.melanomaprognosis.net). The prediction tools can be used to predict the 1-, 2-, 5-, and 10-year survival rates from initial diagnosis (with a 95% confidence interval) for an individual patient, based on his/her relevant clinical and pathological information. The predictive models were developed and validated using a combined database (n = 28 047) from 11 major institutions and study groups participating in the development of the AJCC Melanoma Staging System.

Treatment and its effectiveness

Treatment of non-melanoma skin cancer

Although surgical excision remains the gold standard for the treatment of non-melanoma skin cancer, there are a range of other surgical and non-surgical management options for selected non-melanoma skin cancers (see Table 259.7). The choice offered to the patient will depend on the anatomical location of the cancer, its size, its clinical appearance, the histological diagnosis, and the availability of the options.

Treatment of BCC

The range of possible treatments for BCC is listed in Table 259.7.

Treatment of SCC

Prevention of SCC

Individuals at risk of SCC should be given advice regarding photoprotection (e.g. use of protective clothing and effective sunscreens), as this may reduce the incidence of both actinic keratoses and SCC. Although there is good evidence linking SCCs with chronic actinic damage, there is no definite evidence that the treatment of actinic keratosis prevents the development of SCC.

These measures are particularly important for immunosuppressed individuals and those individuals who have rare genodermatoses and so are at increased risk of developing SCC. Education on self-skin surveillance for early detection and treatment should be part of routine care. Topical agents such as imiquimod may have a useful role in preventing the development of skin dysplasia in high-risk renal transplant recipients but substantive evidence is awaited.

Management of SCC

Management of SCC entails surgical excision with a margin of normal skin removed from around the tumour. For clinically well-defined, low-risk tumours (<2 cm in diameter), surgical excision with a minimum 4 mm margin around the tumour border is advised. Narrower margins of excision are more likely to leave residual tumour. In order to maintain the same degree of confidence of adequate excision, high-risk tumours (e.g. tumours >2 cm in diameter; tumours classified as moderately differentiated, poorly differentiated, or undifferentiated; tumours extending into the subcutaneous tissue; tumours on the ear, lip, scalp, eyelids, or nose) should be removed with a wider margin (≥6 mm), and the tissue margins examined histologically or with Mohs micrographic surgery. In cases where the margins of the tumour are ill-defined (e.g. in poorly differentiated SCCs), tumour extent may not be accurately predicted. After excision of high-risk SCCs, patients should be kept under regular review for at least 2 years, with particular attention to the possibility of recurrence at

Table 259.7 Summary of treatments of skin cancers

Treatment	BCC	SCC	KS	Melanoma	Cutaneous metastases
Surgical excision	Nodular ++ Morphoeic ++ Superficial +	Well++ Moderate ++ Poor ++	+	Primary cutaneous, recurrent, and metastatic disease	+
Curettage/shave excision	Superficial subtype ++	Well differentiated +	–	–	–
Cryotherapy /cryosurgery	Superficial+	In situ (Bowen's disease)+	+	–	+
Mohs micrographic surgery*	Morphoeic, cosmetically sensitive sites, recurrent BCC ++	High-risk SCCs (SCC of lip/ ear, recurrent SCC, SCC arising in non-sun-exposed sites or in chronic ulcers/inflammation)	–	Lentigo maligna	–
Radiotherapy	Primary treatment for BCCs not amenable to surgery or as an adjunctive therapy, e.g. after incomplete surgical excision	Adjunctive for tumours with perineural invasion or where surgical excision is inadequate/impossible	+	Metastatic disease	+
Topical 5-fluorouracil	Superficial	Actinic keratosis, Bowen's disease	–	–	–
Topical imiquimod	Superficial	Actinic keratosis	–	Small lentigo maligna (in the context of a clinical trial)	+
Photodynamic therapy	Superficial BCCs and some nodular subtypes	Actinic keratosis and Bowen's disease	–	–	+

Abbreviations: BCC, basal cell carcinoma; KS, Kaposi's sarcoma; SCC, squamous cell carcinoma.

*Mohs micrographic surgery is a surgical technique used to treat skin cancers which allows precise microscopic margin control by using horizontal frozen sections. The advantages are superior cure rates, maximal tissue conservation, ability to trace perineural or infiltrating tumours histologically, and negligible risk of anaesthetic complications because of the almost exclusive use of local anaesthesia.

the original site and in the draining lymph nodes. Lower-risk tumours may not require such prolonged follow-up, but all patients should be educated about the risk of further SCCs and the importance of self-skin surveillance and photoprotection.

In immunologically or genetically predisposed individuals (e.g. organ transplant recipients and patients with xeroderma pigmentosa) who have multiple SCCs, making surgical management difficult, systemic retinoids (acitretin) or nicotinamide may reduce the rate of development of new lesions. Where appropriate, reduction of immunosuppression or switching to mTOR inhibitor-based immunosuppression may also reduce SCC risk.

Treatment of KS

The aim of treatment of KS is to control the symptoms of the disease, as it is not 'curable'. Various modalities have been used and are detailed in Table 259.7. In addition, intra-lesional and systemic chemotherapies are also used (e.g. bleomycin, vinblastine, doxorubicin, etoposide). In the setting of iatrogenic KS, reduction of immunosuppression and switching from calcineurin inhibitors to mTOR-based immunosuppression (e.g. rapamycin) are additional therapeutic strategies.

Treatment of cutaneous melanoma

Prevention of cutaneous melanoma

The role of photoprotection in melanoma prevention was recently confirmed in a randomized controlled trial in Australia. This demonstrated that, amongst adults aged 25–75, regular application of SPF15+ sunscreen in a 5-year period appeared to reduce the incidence of a new primary melanoma (as well as of SCC) for up to 10 years.

Management of cutaneous melanoma

Management of primary cutaneous melanoma

Surgery is the only curative treatment for primary melanoma. Following excision for diagnosis and for measurement of microscopic Breslow thickness, a wider and deeper margin is taken to ensure complete removal of the primary lesion, and to remove any micro-metastases. Lateral surgical excision margins for invasive melanoma depend on Breslow thickness and are based on five randomized clinical trials including about 3300 patients, and a National Institutes of Health Consensus Panel (see Table 259.8).

Table 259.8 Recommended lateral surgical excision margins for cutaneous melanoma

Tumour thickness	Surgical excision margins (cm)
In situ	0.5
<1.00 mm	1.0
1.01–2.00 mm	1.0–2.0
2.01–4.00 mm	2.0–3.0
>4.00 mm	2.0–3.0

Management of lymph node basins in melanoma patients should be carried out by specialist skin cancer multidisciplinary teams so that surgical treatment planning and investigations can be run in parallel. Clinically node-negative patients can be investigated using ultrasound or SLNB in specialist centres in the UK. Patients should have access to a skin cancer nurse specialist. There is no evidence of a survival benefit for adjuvant chemotherapy in patients with melanoma.

Management of secondary cutaneous melanoma

Surgery is the treatment of choice for single local or regional metastases. Excision should be clinically and histologically clear but a wide margin is not required. The treatment of locoregional recurrence in a limb is palliative. Multiple small dermal lesions may be treated surgically; CO_2 laser and electrochemotherapy with bleomycin may also be useful palliative strategies. Regional chemotherapy with isolated limb infusion (melphalan and dactinomycin D) should be considered for dermal disease which is progressing despite surgery or laser, and for subcutaneous/deeper limb metastases. Isolated limb perfusion may be suitable for larger volume disease. Surgery should be considered for oligometastatic disease at sites such as the skin, the brain, or the bowel or to prevent ulceration. Radiotherapy may have a palliative role in the treatment of metastases.

Patients with Stage IV melanoma should be considered for entry into clinical trials. Due to a better understanding of melanoma cell signalling and immunological response first line agents include immunotherapies either as monotherapy (PD1 inhibitors) or in combination with anti-CTLA4 antibodies. Targeted therapies are second line agents also as monotherapy (BRAF inhibitors) or in combination with MEK inhibitors. Over the next decade, it is likely that further developments will change the face of managing locoregional and metastatic disease.

Treatment of cutaneous metastases

In the case of cutaneous metastases, the underlying primary tumour should be treated but, in most cases when skin metastases have developed, the cancer is usually widespread and only palliative care is appropriate. Treatment options include debridement or palliation by debulking or removing symptomatic/ulcerative lesions and radiotherapy (see Table 259.7).

Further Reading

Bichakjian CK, Halpern AC, Johnson TM, et al. Guidelines of care for the management of primary cutaneous melanoma. *J Am Acad Dermatol* 2011; 65: 1032–47.

Green AC and Olsen CM. Cutaneous squamous cell carcinoma: an epidmiological review. *Br J Dermatol* 2017; 177: 373–81.

Madan V, Lear JT, and Szeimies RM. Non-melanoma skin cancer. *Lancet* 2010; 375: 673–85.

Marsden JR, Newton-Bishop JA, Burrows L, et al. Revised UK guidelines for the management of cutaneous melanoma 2010. *Br J Dermatol* 2010; 163: 238–56.

Miller AJ and Mihm MC Jr. Melanoma. *N Engl J Med* 2006; 355: 51–65.

Charles M. G. Archer and Clive B. Archer

Introduction

Some of the most interesting aspects of dermatology are seen when internal medicine and dermatology overlap. Skin lesions may be part of a systemic disease, as occurs in sarcoidosis or SLE, or may be a manifestation or 'marker' of an underlying disease or process, as seen in acanthosis nigricans. Here, we will focus on the diagnosis and treatment of selected skin markers of internal medicine.

Erythema nodosum

Erythema nodosum (Figure 260.1) is a form of septal panniculitis in which the inflammatory changes also involve the overlying dermis. There are usually painful bruise-like lesions on the shins. Erythema nodosum may be provoked by a number of stimuli, including streptococcal infection, drugs (including oral contraceptives and sulphonamides), sarcoidosis, and tuberculosis, although often a cause is not found. The patient may be unwell with fever and arthralgia, and the lesions usually resolve in a few weeks.

Granuloma annulare and necrobiosis lipoidica

The non-infectious granulomatous disorders include granuloma annulare and necrobiosis lipoidica, as well as sarcoidosis.

Granuloma annulare

Granuloma annulare (see Figure 260.2) is a reaction pattern in the skin, with a well-established morphology and natural history, although the aetiology and pathogenesis are unclear. A number of potential antigenic trigger factors have been suggested. There is an association between granuloma annulare and diabetes mellitus but this is seen uncommonly. Granuloma annulare can occur at any age but most patients are under 30 years old, and women are affected more frequently than men.

Localized granuloma annulare is the commonest form of granuloma annulare and presents as reddish collections of papules which form annular lesions with palpable edges, often over the knuckles and on the elbows. Other areas of the skin may be involved, and a diffuse or generalized pattern occurs uncommonly. In the generalized pattern, there are numerous skin-coloured or erythematous, slightly palpable, coalescing papules, arranged symmetrically on the trunk and limbs. Annular lesions may be violaceous in colour, and itching is often a feature of the generalized form. Perforating (referring to extrusion of material through the epidermis) and subcutaneous granuloma annulare are uncommon patterns, with the latter sometimes being difficult to distinguish from rheumatoid nodules.

It is reasonable to exclude diabetes mellitus in patients with granuloma annulare but this probably occurs in only about 5% cases of localized granuloma annulare, rising to up to 20% in the generalized form. The association of granuloma annulare with diabetes mellitus is debatable, however, and some relatively small studies have not shown a definite association. The distinction from necrobiosis lipoidica, which is more strongly associated with diabetes mellitus, is usually made histologically but granuloma annulare and necrobiosis lipoidica can occur in the same patient.

The sporadic occurrence of granuloma annulare and its tendency to remit spontaneously makes it difficult to assess the efficacy

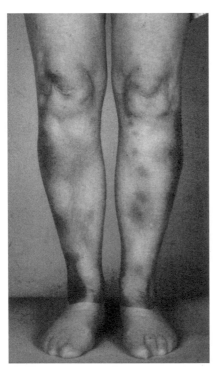

Figure 260.1 Erythema nodosum, with painful bruise-like lesions on the shins. Please see colour plate section.

From: *Ethnic Dermatology: Clinical Problems and Skin Pigmentation*, Archer CB, Copyright 2008, Informa Healthcare, reproduced by permission of Taylor & Francis Books UK.

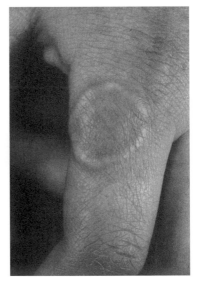

Figure 260.2 Granuloma annulare, showing an annular dermal lesion on the dorsum of the hand. Please see colour plate section.

From: *Ethnic Dermatology: Clinical Problems and Skin Pigmentation*, Archer CB, Copyright 2008, Informa Healthcare, reproduced by permission of Taylor & Francis Books UK.

of treatment; in addition, in many cases, no treatment is needed. Spontaneous remission occurs in about 50% of patients within 2 years but recurrence, usually at the same sites, occurs in 40%.

Treatment of granuloma annulare, and its effectiveness

Potent topical corticosteroids may hasten resolution of localized granuloma annulare, and intra-lesional triamcinolone can be effective if treatment is required. Cryotherapy has also been used. Psoralen plus UVA (PUVA) therapy seems to be effective for generalized granuloma annulare. Other treatments reported to be of benefit include retinoids, ciclosporin, local injections of low-dose recombinant interferon gamma, and topical imiquimod or tacrolimus. However, better clinical studies are required in what is a sporadic disorder. In one clinical trial of generalized granuloma annulare treated with oral potassium iodide, the active drug had no advantage over placebo.

Necrobiosis lipoidica

The precise pathogenesis of necrobiosis lipoidica (see Figure 260.3) is unknown but impaired vascularity of the microcirculation is considered to play a role. The occurrence of diabetes mellitus in up 60% patients who have necrobiosis lipoidica was probably overestimated previously in tertiary referral populations. Necrobiosis lipoidica may precede the development of diabetes in about one in ten individuals. However, it does not occur exclusively in diabetes, and the term necrobiosis lipoidica diabeticorum is no longer used. It can occur at any age but usually develops in young adults and in early middle age. There is a female to male ratio of 3:1. Only about 0.3% patients with diabetes mellitus will have necrobiosis lipoidica.

Necrobiosis lipoidica occurs as reddish-yellow shiny plaques on the shins, with atrophy and telangiectasia, but early lesions are less obvious. Lesions may ulcerate and a chronic course is usual. In most cases, lesions are bilateral, and they are similar in appearance whether occurring in diabetic or non-diabetic patients.

The differential diagnosis includes granuloma annulare, in which there is less necrobiosis on histology. The yellowish appearance may resemble xanthomatous lesions but this will be distinguished on histology.

Treatment of necrobiosis lipoidica, and its effectiveness

Treatment with a super-potent topical corticosteroid under polythene occlusion is effective in settling the active inflammatory process of necrobiosis lipoidica but the chronic atrophic changes are not reversible and the lesions persist. Early treatment is therefore recommended. Intra-lesional triamcinolone has been used with good effect, and some dermatologists use perilesional triamcinolone to prevent extension of the process centrifugally. Short courses of prednisolone have been reported to arrest the process but are usually not required.

PUVA using a topical psoralen has been beneficial, as has excision and grafting in severe cases. Other treatments which have been tried in the past with limited success include nicotinamide, clofazamine, pentoxifylline, ciclosporin, mycophenolate mofetil, and, more recently, infliximab.

Other skin disorders in diabetes mellitus

Skin disorders in diabetes mellitus include diabetic dermopathy, which is the commonest skin disorder associated with diabetes; cutaneous infections which occur as a consequences of diabetic neuropathy; acanthosis nigricans (related to insulin resistance); and, as discussed in 'Granuloma annulare and necrobiosis lipoidica', necrobiosis lipoidica and probably generalized granuloma annulare. Anogenital pruritus in diabetes mellitus may be caused by candidiasis or streptococcal infection but diabetes is not a proven cause of generalized pruritus.

Diabetic dermopathy (diabetic shin spots)

Diabetic dermopathy occurs in about half of the patients with diabetes, with men being more commonly affected than women. Diabetic dermopathy is thought to be due to microangiopathy and possible neuropathy. Reddish oval macules and slightly scaly plaques are seen on the shins, forearms, and thighs and over bony prominences, later evolving into brownish atrophic scars, where the brown pigment is due to haemosiderin deposition. The presence of these lesions has been suggested to correlate with other internal complications of diabetes, including retinopathy, nephropathy, and neuropathy.

Acanthosis nigricans and insulin resistance

Acanthosis nigricans (Figure 260.4), in which there is hyperpigmentation and hyperkeratosis of the flexures (e.g. a velvety appearance in the axillae), exists in two forms. In the absence of obesity, acanthosis nigricans may be an important clinical sign of an underlying

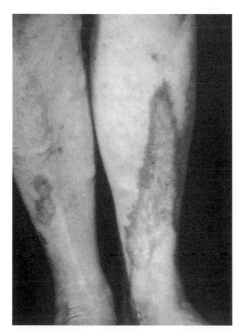

Figure 260.3 Necrobiosis lipoidica, showing atrophic plaques on the shins. Please see colour plate section.

From: *Ethnic Dermatology: Clinical Problems and Skin Pigmentation*, Archer CB, Copyright 2008, Informa Healthcare, reproduced by permission of Taylor & Francis Books UK.

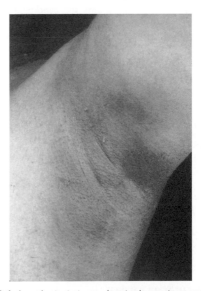

Figure 260.4 Acanthosis nigricans, showing hyperpigmentation and hyperkeratosis of the axillary skin. Please see colour plate section.

From: *Ethnic Dermatology: Clinical Problems and Skin Pigmentation*, Archer CB, Copyright 2008, Informa Healthcare, reproduced by permission of Taylor & Francis Books UK.

adenocarcinoma (e.g. carcinoma of the stomach). The changes of acanthosis nigricans in younger obese patients, in whom the nape of neck and the antecubital fossae are often involved, are associated with insulin resistance (hyperinsulinaemia) and sometimes overt diabetes mellitus. There are considered to be two syndromes of insulin resistance: type A, which occurs in hyperandrogenic women due to a genetic defect affecting insulin receptor function, and type B, which occurs in older women with signs of immunological dysfunction.

Xanthomata

There are different forms of xanthoma. Eruptive xanthomata of the skin, often on the buttocks and limbs, may develop in patients with hyperlipoproteinaemia in association with diabetes mellitus. Control of the hyperlipoproteinaemia and diabetes usually leads to resolution of the yellowish papules.

Skin markers of liver diseases

Pruritus in liver disease

Generalized pruritus is the most common symptom associated with liver disease. It may precede the onset of jaundice and may be a feature of hepatitis. Itching is most prominent in primary biliary cholangitis, sclerosing cholangitis, and other forms of biliary tract obstruction, being less of a problem in alcoholic cirrhosis, autoimmune chronic active hepatitis, and haemochromatosis. Improvement in hepatic itching by drugs which block the action of opiates suggests that endogenous opiates may be important in the mechanism of itching.

Treatment of pruritus, and its effectiveness

Treatment of pruritus is directed at the underlying cause (e.g. drug withdrawal, in drug-induced cholestasis; surgery, for mechanical biliary obstruction). Antihistamines are usually ineffective. Other approaches have included colestyramine, rifampicin, and various forms of phototherapy.

Pigmentary changes in liver disease

Jaundice is first seen in the sclerae before it becomes generalized. Carotenaemia and drugs, including mepacrine, can also cause yellowing of the skin.

A grey hyperpigmentation may occur in chronic liver disease of any cause. There may be a yellowish tinge due to associated jaundice. The pigmentation is usually more prominent on sun-exposed sites, including the face, with perioral and periorbital accentuation. Pigmentation sometimes localizes to the palmar creases, and men sometimes have increased pigmentation of the areola in association with gynaecomastia.

Vascular changes in liver disease

Some of the recognized vascular changes in liver disease are non-specific, including spider naevi (spider telangiectasias/spider angiomas) and palmar erythema. Finger clubbing, thought to be due to increased digital pulp blood flow and dilation of arteriovenous anastomoses, occurs in about 15% of patients with cirrhosis.

Hair, nail, and collagen changes in liver disease

The body hair is often thinned and men tend to develop a female pubic-hair pattern, due to increased production and decreased metabolism of oestrogens and associated with decreased production and increased metabolism of testosterone. Extensive loss of scalp hair may be due to zinc deficiency.

Nail colour changes include diffuse white colour; proximal white colour and distal reddish-pink colour; and white bands. Nail plate changes include clubbing, flattened nails, or koilonychia, associated with poor nutrition or altered iron metabolism.

Porphyria cutanea tarda

Porphyria cutanea tarda is associated with chronic liver disease. In this form of porphyria, there is photosensitivity with blisters, scarring, milia (small epidermal cysts), and hyperpigmentation on sun-exposed areas (e.g. backs of hands and forearms) and hypertrichosis of the face (e.g. the temples).

Skin markers of chronic renal failure

Uraemic pruritus

Generalized severe pruritus occurs in about one-third of patients with renal failure (chronic kidney disease), particularly in patients on haemodialysis, with many more patients experiencing less troublesome pruritus. There seems to be a correlation between pruritus and pre-dialysis plasma urea levels, but a less obvious relationship between itching and dry skin (xerosis) and secondary hyperparathyroidism. The mechanism of pruritus is complicated, since a reduction in uraemia often does not improve the itching, and pruritus is unusual in acute renal failure. Uraemic neuropathy affects about 60% of patients with renal failure or on long-term haemodialysis and may play a role in uraemic pruritus.

The incidence of uraemic pruritus has been reported to be decreasing, which in part may be due to the use of more sophisticated techniques and equipment for dialysis.

Treatment of uraemic pruritus, and its effectiveness

In dialysis, lowering the magnesium concentration of the dialysate has been reported to be helpful. In intractable itching, emollients and UVB radiation are reported to be the most effective therapy. Other treatments have included UVA (without psoralen), colestyramine, activated charcoal, and erythropoietin therapy.

Pigmentary changes in chronic renal failure

Anaemia presenting as pallor is an early and common sign of chronic renal failure, resulting from reduced haemopoiesis and increased haemolysis. A greyish-brown discolouration develops in many cases, due to deposition of melanin. Increased nail pigmentation usually confined to the distal nail occurs in a proportion of patients. This distal brown or reddish colour, combined with a proximal white appearance, gives rise to the term 'half-and-half nails', a distinctive pattern seen in about 10% of patients with renal failure.

Purpura due to mild thrombocytopenia or more marked platelet dysfunction is common and may be partly corrected by dialysis.

Calcific arteriolopathy (calciphylaxis)

Calcific arteriolopathy (sometimes called 'calciphylaxis' or 'calcific uraemic arteriolopathy') is a disorder in which patients, usually with renal failure, develop large painful areas of ulceration.

Recent studies have shown that the calcification seen in this condition is not the same as that seen in patients with skin necrosis, so the term 'calciphylaxis' is now considered inaccurate. The term 'calcific uraemic arteriolopathy' indicates the site of the calcification and the usual clinical state of the patients. However, a similar type of arteriolopathy has been reported in patients with minimal or no renal failure, hence our preferred use of the term 'calcific arteriolopathy'.

In addition to renal failure, the other major risk factors include female gender, white race, diabetes mellitus, obesity, warfarin use, and clotting disorders such as protein C and protein S deficiency. It has also been shown that the use of calcium salts and vitamin D in chronic renal failure is a risk factor. There does not seem to be a direct role of hyperparathyroidism in the development of calcific arteriolopathy, the disease having been described in the presence of normal parathormone levels.

The usual presentation of calcific arteriolopathy is of areas of ulceration on the legs, buttocks, abdomen, or breasts; these areas are painful and may be extensive. Livedo reticularis around the ulcers may be present. Acral ulceration can also occur, causing autoamputation. The differential diagnosis is any cause of ulceration, and especially vasculitis, in which livedo reticularis may also be present. Increasing awareness of the condition is allowing the diagnosis of calcific arteriolopathy at an earlier, non-ulcerative stage, before the subcutaneous indurated plaques develop into ulcers.

The diagnosis of calcific arteriolopathy is usually by biopsy, with the histology showing calcification of the media of small arterioles in the skin. The outcome is poor, with a mortality of about 60% for proximal disease and about 20% for distal disease, usually from overwhelming sepsis.

Treatment of calcific arteriolopathy, and its effectiveness

Since there is such a high mortality in calcific arteriolopathy, the approach should be to aim for prevention. The control of the hyperphosphataemia is thought to be fundamental to this. Phosphate binders are used, with some evidence showing that the non-calcium-containing binders are better. Parathyroidectomy has been found to be useful in the control of calcific arteriolopathy in some series but not in others.

Nephrogenic fibrosing dermopathy

Nephrogenic fibrosing dermopathy (NFD) is a fibrotic disease occurring in patients with renal disease. NFD was initially reported in patients with established renal failure, either on dialysis or having had a transplant, but it has since been reported in patients with chronic renal insufficiency not requiring renal replacement therapy. An association with the IV injection of gadolinium-based radiocontrast media (particularly containing gadodiamide) has been suggested.

The clinical presentation of this rare disorder is of plaques of indurated skin on the extensor surfaces of the limbs, and scleral involvement has been described. The limbs are affected in a symmetrical manner with skin-coloured papules coalescing to form brawny plaques with a 'peau d'orange' appearance, occasionally with swelling of the hands and feet. Patients may complain of pain, pruritus, and causalgia. Most patients do not have systemic involvement but, when this is present, the disease may be rapidly fatal.

Treatment of NFD, and its effectiveness

The mainstay of treatment of NFD is improvement of the renal function but transplantation is not guaranteed to cure the disease.

Addison's disease

The autoimmune diseases include Addison's disease (adrenal insufficiency), in which one sees melanin pigmentation of the buccal mucosa and skin, particularly the palmar creases. This may be associated with vitiligo, alopecia areata, and other autoimmune diseases, including pernicious anaemia and thyroiditis.

Thyroid disease and the skin

There are a number of cutaneous manifestations of both hypothyroidism and hyperthyroidism. Skin features associated with hypothyroidism include pale and cold extremities; absence of sweating; puffy oedema of the hands and the face; eczema craquelé and pruritus; xanthomatosis (secondary to hyperlipoproteinaemia); coarse sparse hair; brittle/striated nails; purpura/ecchymoses; punctuate telangiectasia on arms and fingertips; and delayed wound healing. Features associated with hyperthyroidism include soft and dry skin, palmar erythema, flushing, increased sweating, fast nail growth, pruritus, urticaria, pretibial myxoedema (see Figure 260.5), acropachy, and diffuse Addisonian hyperpigmentation.

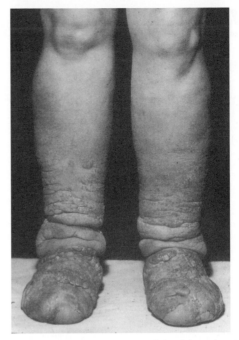

Figure 260.5 Pretibial myxoedema associated with hyperthyroidism. Please see colour plate section.

From: *Ethnic Dermatology: Clinical Problems and Skin Pigmentation*, Archer CB, Copyright 2008, Informa Healthcare, reproduced by permission of Taylor & Francis Books UK.

Pruritus without a rash

Individuals presenting with itch in the absence of skin disease should be carefully assessed. It can sometimes be difficult to distinguish secondary changes associated with excoriation from primary skin disease. However, a detailed history (including drug history) and a thorough systemic examination are crucial. Routine initial investigations might include renal function tests, a full blood count with differential and haematinics, thyroid function tests, and liver function tests, with consideration of other investigations, such as a chest X-ray, HIV testing, and screening for malignancy, dependent on the clinical findings.

Further Reading

Caccavale S and Ruocco E. Acral manifestations of systemic diseases: Drug-induced and infectious diseases. *Clin Dermatol* 2017; 35: 55–63.

Finucane KA and Archer CB. Dermatological aspects of medicine: Recent advances in nephrology. *Clin Exp Dermatol* 2005; 30: 98–102.

Gawkrodger D and Ardern-Jones MR, *Dermatology: An Illustrated Colour Text*, (5th edition), 2012. Churchill Livingstone.

Wolff K and Johnson RA. *Fitzpatrick's Color Atlas and Synopsis of Clinical Dermatology* (6th edition), 2009. McGraw-Hill Medical.

261 Drug-induced skin disease

Muthu Sivaramakrishnan

Introduction

Drug-induced skin disease is one of the commonest dermatological presentations in both hospitalized and ambulatory patients. It affects 2%–3% of hospitalized patients and it is estimated that 1 in 1000 hospitalized patients has a serious cutaneous drug reaction. The clinical presentation can mimic any skin disease and should be considered in the differential diagnosis of any acute-onset symmetrical skin eruption. It is important to make a correct diagnosis, as removal of the offending drug results in clinical resolution in most instances.

Etiopathogenesis

Cutaneous drug reactions can be caused by both immunological and non-immunological mechanisms. The immunological mechanism can be due to the various types of hypersensitivity reactions classified by Gell and Coombs. Non-immunological mechanisms include irritant reactions caused by topical agents, dose-dependent toxic reactions, phototoxic reactions, and idiosyncratic reactions.

Clinical features

Cutaneous drug reactions can mimic any form of skin disease. Most of the reactions are mild and often settle after removing the offending drug. The commonest clinical presentations are exanthematous reactions; urticaria and angioedema; erythema multiforme; lichenoid eruptions; bullous eruptions; and drug hypersensitivity syndrome. Bullous eruptions present in various forms, including fixed drug eruptions, drug-induced vasculitis, Stevens–Johnson syndrome, toxic epidermal necrolysis, drug-induced porphyrias, pseudoporphyria, pemphigus, and pemphigoid. Severe drug reactions can be recognized from their cutaneous and systemic features.

Features of severe cutaneous drug reactions include skin and systemic manifestations. For the skin, extensive reddening, facial swelling, pain, palpable purpura, blisters (especially if extensive), involvement of mucous membranes, and a swollen tongue may be seen. Systemic features include a high temperature; swollen lymph nodes (indicating extensive skin inflammation); joint pains or swelling; respiratory symptoms (particularly breathlessness); and, ominously, low blood pressure.

Individual types of drug-induced skin disease

Common drugs causing cutaneous drug reactions are listed in Table 261.1.

Fixed drug eruption

A fixed drug eruption is characterized by the occurrence of one or more erythematous patches, plaques, bullae, or erosions that are present at the same site and were caused by the ingestion of a drug.

Causes of a fixed drug eruption

The following agents can cause a fixed drug eruption:

- antibacterial agents (e.g. sulfonamides, tetracyclines, penicillin, quinine)
- barbiturates
- NSAIDs
- oral contraceptives
- food substitutes

Table 261.1 Common drugs causing cutaneous drug reactions

Drug reaction	Drugs
Fixed drug eruption	Sulfonamides
	Tetracyclines
	Penicillin
	Quinine
	Barbiturates
	NSAIDs
Erythema multiforme	Cephalosporin
	Sulfonamides
	Penicillin
	Rifampicin
	Barbiturates
	Carbamazepine
	Phenothiazines
	Thiazide diuretics
Stevens–Johnson syndrome and toxic epidermal necrolysis	Sulfonamides
	Penicillin
	Ethambutol
	Rifampicin
	Tetracyclines
	NSAIDs
	Barbiturates
	Carbamazepine
	Lamotrigine
	Phenytoin
	Terbinafine
	Griseofulvin
Exanthematous drug eruption	Penicillin
	Ampicillin
	Co-amoxiclav
	Sulfonamides
	Phenytoin
	Carbamazepine
Drug hypersensitivity syndrome	Anticonvulsants
	Co-trimoxazole
	Minocycline
	Allopurinol
	Terbinafine
	Dapsone
Urticaria and angioedema	Antibiotics
	Antifungal agents
	Angiotensin-converting enzyme inhibitors
	NSAIDs
	Muscle relaxants
	Food additives
Lichenoid drug eruption	Gold salts
	Antimalarials
	Penicillamine
	Frusemide
	Thiazides
	Sulfasalazine

Clinical features of a fixed drug eruption

Lesions are usually single on the limbs but can be multiple and can occur at any site, including mucous membranes. The initial lesion is an erythematous macule developing then into a patch, plaque, or bulla with erosion. The lesions heal with post-inflammatory pigmentation.

Diagnosis of a fixed drug eruption

Diagnosis is usually done by clinical signs but, occasionally, a skin biopsy may be necessary.

Management of a fixed drug eruption

With a fixed drug eruption, stopping the offending drug will help the lesions heal in few weeks. Potent topical steroids will be helpful for localized lesions, but systemic steroids may be essential for generalized and painful mucosal lesions.

Erythema multiforme

Erythema multiforme is characterized by multiple macules, papules, or urticarial lesions, along with target lesions mainly affecting the distal extremities. It is more often by caused by viral infections (e.g. by herpes simplex virus) but can occasionally be caused by the ingestion of a drug.

Causes of erythema multiforme

The following agents can cause erythema multiforme:

- antimicrobials (e.g. cephalosporin, sulfonamides, penicillin, rifampin)
- barbiturates
- carbamazepine
- phenothiazines
- thiazide diuretics

Clinical features of erythema multiforme

In erythema multiforme, the characteristic lesion is a target lesion which is less than 3 cm in diameter, is round in shape, and has three zones: a central area of erythema or purpura, which is surrounded by a pale zone of oedema, which in turn is surrounded by well-defined erythema. Other lesions may be in the form of macules, papules, or urticarial lesions. The commonest site of involvement is the distal extremities, with rare involvement of mucous membranes (erythema multiforme minor). However, some patients may have a prodromal illness with severe generalized disease and mucous membrane involvement (erythema multiforme major).

Diagnosis of erythema multiforme

The diagnosis of erythema multiforme is usually made with clinical signs but a skin biopsy may be necessary on occasion. The cutaneous biopsy may show vacuolar degeneration of lower epidermis, individual necrotic epidermal cells, and dermal, perivascular lymphohistiocytic infiltrate.

Treatment of erythema multiforme

When treating erythema multiforme, it is important to stop the offending drug. Ocular involvement requires urgent help from an ophthalmologist. Good skin nursing care is essential in severe cases. Potent topical steroids may be helpful in localized lesions. The use of systemic steroids is debated, although they can help in the relief of systemic symptoms and in severe cases. Thalidomide, dapsone, azathioprine, and ciclosporin may be helpful in recurrent cases.

Stevens–Johnson syndrome and toxic epidermal necrolysis

Stevens–Johnson syndrome is a severe, acute-onset disease characterized by a prodromal illness, erythema multiforme of the trunk, and skin blisters involving less than 10% of the body's surface area. Toxic epidermal necrolysis is also a severe, acute-onset illness but is characterized by a prodromal illness, sheets of erythema, and skin peeling involving more than 30% of the body's surface area.

Causes of Stevens–Johnson syndrome and toxic epidermal necrolysis

The following agents can cause Stevens–Johnson syndrome and/or toxic epidermal necrolysis:

- antibiotics (e.g. sulfonamides, penicillin, ethambutol, rifampicin, tetracyclines, thioacetazone)
- NSAIDs
- anticonvulsants (e.g. barbiturates, carbamazepine, lamotrigine, phenytoin)
- antiretroviral agents
- antifungal agents (e.g. terbinafine and griseofulvin)
- others (e.g. allopurinol, thiazide diuretics, gold, vaccines)

Clinical features of Stevens–Johnson syndrome and toxic epidermal necrolysis

In Stevens–Johnson syndrome, patients usually have a severe prodromal illness with fever, myalgia, and arthralgia, following which they develop extensive erythema multiforme lesions on the trunk. They also develop blisters and erosions both on the skin and on mucosal areas. The oral mucosa is commonly involved, followed by the mucosae in the eyes and the genitalia, but any mucosal membrane can be affected. Involvement of lungs and kidneys has been reported. The mortality rate is 5%–15% in untreated patients, due to renal damage, infection, and toxaemia. In treated patients, the eruption usually heals well but permanent damage can be caused to mucous membranes, particularly in the eyes.

In toxic epidermal necrolysis, patients have a severe prodromal flu-like illness followed by sheets of erythema leading to painful erosions involving the skin and mucous membrane. Mucous membranes are involved in all patients; the oral mucosa is particularly involved, but any mucosal areas can be affected. Acute complications include sepsis, renal failure, induction of a hypercatabolic state, and pneumonitis. Chronic complications are mainly due to permanent damage to mucous membranes. The mortality rate is around 30%–40% in untreated cases.

Diagnosis of Stevens–Johnson syndrome and toxic epidermal necrolysis

Skin biopsy and histopathology of toxic epidermal necrolysis will reveal full thickness necrosis of skin in established lesions with perivascular mononuclear cells in the dermis. The histology of Stevens–Johnson syndrome more often resembles erythema multiforme.

Management of Stevens–Johnson syndrome and toxic epidermal necrolysis

In Stevens–Johnson syndrome and toxic epidermal necrolysis, early diagnosis and stopping the offending drug are the most important steps in management. Patients are best managed in specialized dermatology unit or burns unit (particularly patients with toxic epidermal necrolysis).

Fluid and electrolyte replacement and maintaining body temperature is important, as often these patients can develop renal failure and hypothermia. Specialist involvement should be sought early if mucosal areas are involved to prevent complications.

Good skin care with emollients and topical antibacterial agents is necessary. Systemic steroids in high doses and early in the disease might be helpful but their use is controversial. IV immunoglobulins early in the disease might help further progression. Appropriate early treatment of complications (like sepsis) is essential.

Exanthematous drug eruptions

Exanthematous drug eruptions are the most common of all cutaneous drug reactions (about 75% of all drug rashes) and can occur between 3 days to 2 weeks of ingesting a drug. An exanthematous drug eruption is characterized by an erythematous maculopapular eruption and scaly patches commonly affecting the trunk and extremities. Purpuric lesions of the legs and erosive stomatis can occur in some patients. Some patients may have fever, itching, and peripheral eosinophilia.

The commonly implicated drugs are penicillin, ampicillin, co-amoxiclav, sulfonamides phenytoin, and carbamazepine. Removal of the offending agent, together with the use of moderately potent to potent topical steroids and antihistamines, will usually help to resolve the situation.

Drug hypersensitivity syndrome

Drug hypersensitivity syndrome, also known as DRESS syndrome (drug rash with eosinophilia and systemic symptoms), consists of fever, lymphadenopathy, organ involvement (e.g. hepatitis, nephritis, pneumonitis, and encephalitis), haematological abnormalities, and a cutaneous rash. The skin eruption is usually in the form of papules or a papulopustular or exanthematous rash leading to erythroderma. Haematological abnormalities include eosinophilia and atypical lymphocytes.

This condition is usually caused by anticonvulsants but can also be caused by co-trimoxazole, minocycline, allopurinol, terbinafine, and dapsone. Treatment includes stopping the offending drug and administering systemic corticosteroids.

Urticaria and angioedema

Urticaria is characterized by itchy, transient, oedematous papules, and plaques. These lesions are called 'wheals' and are caused by superficial oedema in the papillary dermis. Angioedema involves oedema of the deeper tissues, including the dermis and subcutaneous tissue.

The common causative drugs in urticaria and angioedema are antibiotics, antifungal agents, angiotensin-converting enzyme inhibitors, NSAIDs, muscle relaxants, and food additives. Management involves stopping the offending drug and administering antihistamines and systemic corticosteroids (in severe cases).

Lichenoid drug eruption

A lichenoid drug eruption is characterized by scaly violaceous papules and plaques on the trunk and extremities, sometimes leading to erythroderma. Mucosal involvement is uncommon in a lichenoid drug eruption, unlike the case with lichen planus. The common causative drugs include gold salts, antimalarials, penicillamine, furosemide, thiazides, and sulfasalazine. Quinine and tetracyclines can cause such eruptions on the photo-exposed areas of the skin. Management involves stopping the offending drug and administering potent topical steroids and systemic corticosteroids (in severe cases).

Further Reading

Burns T, Breathnach S, Cox N, et al. (eds). *Rook's Textbook of Dermatology* (8th edition), 2010. Wiley-Blackwell.

Duong TA, Valeyrie-Allanore L, Wolkenstein P et al. Severe cutaneous adverse reactions to drugs *Lancet* 2017; 390: 1996–2011.

Stern RS. Exanthematous drug eruptions. *N Engl J Med* 2012; 366: 2492–501.

Wolff K and Johnson RA. *Fitzpatrick's Color Atlas and Synopsis of Clinical Dermatology* (6th edition), 2009. McGraw-Hill Medical.

262 Psychocutaneous medicine

Anthony Bewley

Introduction

The links between the mind and the skin have long been recognized. The skin has been described as the mirror of the mind, and so it is not surprising that the interface between dermatology and psychiatry ('psychocutaneous medicine' or 'psychodermatology') is emerging as a specific subspeciality of dermatology. Psychodermatological conditions can be classified as either primarily psychiatric disorders which manifest via skin disease, for example delusional infestation, or primarily dermatological disorders, for example psoriasis, which may be caused by, or associated with profound psychiatric morbidity (e.g. anxiety, depression; see Table 262.1).

Delusional infestation

Delusional infestation is a well-recognized uncommon condition in which patients hold a fixed belief that they are infested with organisms (parasites, bacteria, viruses) or fibres. When referred to a purely psychiatric clinic, patients with delusional infestation often default their appointments, but they are also difficult to manage in a standard dermatology clinics. Older terms such as 'delusional parasitosis' and 'acaraphobie' have been replaced by the term 'delusional infestation'. Delusional infestation can be classified into primary and secondary disorders. Primary delusional infestation is classified by DSM-IV as 'delusional disorder of somatic type', and in ICD-10 as 'persistent delusional disorder'. It is uncommon (about 20 new cases per million population); the female-to-male ratio under the age of 50 years is similar, but that for those over 50 is 2:1. There is a bimodal distribution with respect to age, with one peak occurring between 20 and 30 years of age, and then another at over 50, and there are frequent reports of the delusions being shared with a relative or close friend (folie-a-deux; 8%–12% of cases), and occasionally more than one person (folie-a-trois).

Secondary delusional infestation may follow a real infestation, be associated with recreational drug use (alcohol, cannabis, etc.), be a precursor to dementia, and be associated with other organic disease. But also delusional infestation may be secondary to 'functional' psychiatric diseases (such as schizophrenia). It is therefore essential that a full medical history (including a dermatological history, a history of substance abuse, and a psychiatric history) and a physical examination are undertaken to identify potential organic disease and make an accurate diagnosis.

Many patients bring containers with samples of 'infested material' (the 'matchbox sign') to the doctor. Patients may take extreme measures to eradicate the organisms from their bodies, and frequently cause severe damage to their skin through applying noxious substances or even burning the skin.

Patients with delusional infestation are notoriously difficult to manage due to their lack of insight and resistance to psychiatric referral. Joint working between psychiatrists and dermatologists is therefore vital. Exclusion of organic cause is mandatory. This may include a pruritus screen (thyroid, renal, and liver function tests, blood count, vitamin B_{12}, folate, and syphilis serology). But clinical assessment will inform whether these or other investigations may be relevant.

It is important **not** to confront the patient with the falsity of their delusional belief, as this leads to loss of any therapeutic alliance, and the patient will simply move to find someone who will take their concern 'seriously'. All samples should be sent for analysis, first, to support the patient, second, to provide a template for discussions about why treatment with antimicrobials is inappropriate, and, last, to exclude genuine infestation. Empathizing with patients is crucial. Patients with delusional infestation have usually seen a large number of doctors, are often frustrated with the perceived lack of help they have received, and are frequently hostile. But it is important not to collude with patients, too. Instead, letting patients know that you understand the seriousness of their condition, and that there are effective therapeutic options for their symptoms, is often enough to engage the patient in a clinical dialogue.

Conventional antipsychotics are probably effective. Pimozide was considered the treatment of choice; however, in view of its cardiotoxic side effects, atypical antipsychotics are now considered a better choice. There are no random controlled trials but case reports, case series, and clinical experience suggest that atypical agents such as risperidone, olanzapine, quetiapine, and amilsulpride are effective. Typically, patients respond to smaller doses (e.g. 0.5 mg risperidone twice daily, increasing if necessary to 1 mg twice daily). The prognosis of delusional infestation is highly dependent on the clinical environment. In joint dermatology–psychiatry clinics, successful treatment of delusional infestation can be expected in over 75% of patients.

Body dysmorphic disorder

Body dysmorphic disorder (BDD; also, inaccurately, called dysmorphophobia) is characterized by a preoccupation with a perceived or real visible difference in which the patient's concern is out of proportion to the 'defect'. There is a spectrum from patients with overvalued ideas to those whose beliefs are held with delusional conviction (in DSM IV, 'delusional disorder-somatic type'; in ICD 10, 'other persistent delusional disorders').

BDD is common, affecting 1%–2% of the population (although many of us have a lesser degree of dissatisfaction with our bodies), especially in adolescence, and is known to be associated with mood disorders, obsessive compulsive disease, and social phobia. The condition is extremely disabling for patients and their relatives, as the 'defect' may seem, objectively, to be minor and the reaction to the 'defect', extreme. Many patients spend long periods in front of mirrors, while others have extensive rituals simply to build enough confidence to look in a mirror. Many become socially isolated, and many seek repeated aesthetic surgery, only to be dissatisfied with the results, or to find another perceived 'defect'.

Table 262.1 Psychocutaneous medicine	
Primary psychiatric disorders which present with skin disease	**Primary dermatological disorders caused by or associated with psychiatric comorbidity**
Delusional infestation	Psoriasis
Body dysmorphic disorder	Eczema
Dermatitis artefacta	Alopecia (e.g. areata)
OCD (e.g. repeated handwashing)	Acne
Trichotillomania	Rosacea
Neurotic excoriation	Urticaria
Others	Vitiligo
	Visible differences (disfigurements)
	Inherited skin conditions (e.g. ichthyosis)
	May be caused, exacerbated by, or associated with:
	• depression
	• anxiety
	• body image disorder
	• social anxiety

Treatment may be tricky, as most patients lack insight and will not accept psychiatric treatment or referral. Affected individuals are therefore best seen in a joint psychodermatology clinic, where they can be supported, and gradually encouraged to accept psychological interventions. Their surgery-seeking behaviour can also be contained. The limited evidence base indicates that serotonergic antidepressants (fluoxetine, citalopram, fluvoxamine) may be effective, particularly in higher doses and for longer periods. Importantly, CBT can be effective in BDD patients, and may be pivotal in allowing the patient to regain a healthier perspective of their 'defect'. Untreated, the condition tends to be chronic, and there is a high suicide risk.

Dermatitis artefacta

Dermatitis artefacta (DA) describes the condition whereby a patient creates skin lesions but denies knowledge of self-infliction (as opposed to deliberate self-harm, where the patient will be able to acknowledge the self-infliction, and will usually indicate that 'cutting' gives the individual a sense of control over their body, and/or relieves some emotional tension). In DA, patients produce their artefacts secretly, deny complicity, and may be unaware of their psychological motivations. They and their relatives are often puzzled about the aetiology of their skin lesions, and may be angry with doctors' inability to diagnose and treat the mysterious problem. The skin lesions, themselves, may be very varied in character (e.g. linear tears, bruises, cuts, non-healing ulcers) and in severity (minor erosions to widespread, severe, deep ulceration).

DA is probably common and under-reported. It is more common in women (at least 3:1), and the incidence is greatest in the late teens or early twenties. Often, there is a connection between the patient or their family and some aspect of healthcare (such as a recent illness). In addition, studies suggest an association with physical or sexual abuse in some patients.

The first rule of managing patients with DA is to be absolutely certain that the diagnosis of DA is accurate and that non-self-induced disease has been comprehensively excluded. A non-confrontational approach is essential. Focusing on how the skin lesions are generated is of less importance than finding out why they are there. Although DA is primarily a dermatological diagnosis, management should involve close cooperation with specialists in mental health. Management is of the skin as well as the underlying psychological issues. General measures such as emollients and topical antibacterials can all be used, depending on the presenting lesions. Occlusion has been used as a diagnostic and therapeutic tool with variable success. Psychological and psychopharmacological approaches are started at the same time as the dermatological treatments. CBT and psychotherapy are probably pivotal, but there is a wide range of efficacy. Patients are often unwilling to accept the psychiatric nature of the disorder and lack the awareness of their circumstances that trigger the drive to produce the lesions. In such circumstances, dermatology/liaison psychiatry clinics may be beneficial. Often, it is important to simply wait until the patient has enough confidence to relate the underlying psychological issues (there is almost always an underlying issue; this may be relatively minor, such as pressure from examinations, or may be

> **Box 262.1 Management of the psychosocial aspects of chronic skin disease**
>
> 1. **Listen to the patient.** This is by far the easiest and most important aspect of psychosocial care. It is easily overlooked.
> 2. **Engage patients with support groups:**
>   - http://vitiligosociety.org.uk
>   - http://www.psoriasis-association.org.uk
>   - http://www.changingfaces.org.uk
> 3. **Assess any suicidal ideation.**
> 4. **Consider a referral to a 'psychodermatology clinic'.** Unfortunately, these are few and far between, but local dermatology units may have either someone with psychodermatological experience, or will be able to refer to a local (usually liaison) psychiatrist.
> 5. **Discuss the possibility of CBT.** This may be invaluable for some patients. Person-centred psychotherapy is probably the most appropriate, as it may focus on thought and behaviour patterns which are unhelpful.
> 6. **Consider psychotropic medication.** Sometimes medication for affective disorders may be a useful part of the patient's holistic care. SSRIs (e.g. citalopram) are usually the medication of choice.

devastating, such as sexual abuse). SSRIs can be used where there is an underlying or associated affective disorder. The prognosis of this condition is probably much, much better when patients are engaged with their healthcare professional team.

Psychological comorbidities of chronic skin disease

Psychological comorbidities of chronic skin disease are often underestimated by healthcare professionals. The anxiety, disempowerment, and frustration felt by patients with, for example, psoriasis and vitiligo is only beginning to be recognized. The commonest psychological implication of cutaneous disease is impaired self-esteem, to the extent that some patients will even consider suicide.

Inclusive management of the dermatology patient's psychosocial comorbidities (Box 262.1) is a newer, under-recognized and emerging area of holistic care.

Further Reading

Brown GE, Malakouti M, Sorenson E, et al. Psychodermatology. *Adv Psychosom Med* 2015; 34: 123–34.

Mohandas P, Bewley A, and Taylor R. Dermatitis artefacta and artefactual skin disease: The need for a multi-disciplinary psycho-cutaneous medicine team to treat a difficult condition. *Br J Dermatol* 2013; 169: 600–6.

Raff AB and Kroshinsky D. Cellulitis: a review. *JAMA* 2016; 316: 325–37.

PART 12

Disorders of the musculoskeletal system

263 Normal function of the musculoskeletal system

Shireen Shaffu and James Taylor

Introduction

The musculoskeletal system consists of specialized connective tissue whose primary function is to allow locomotion. The tissues of the musculoskeletal system are bones, muscles, tendons, and ligaments. In particular, the bony skeleton also has the task of protecting vital internal organs, contains the bone marrow, and is an intrinsic part of the metabolic pathways involved in calcium homeostasis. Motion is allowed by specialized articulating structures, the joints. This chapter contains a brief description of all the components.

Bone

Bone is a collagen-rich connective tissue matrix (mainly collagen type I) that is calcified to provide rigidity. Some bones are laid down as a matrix that then calcifies, in a process called **membranous ossification** (e.g. skull, collarbone), but the majority are laid down as a cartilage model which then gets remodelled and replaced by bone in a process called **endochondral ossification** (e.g. long tubular bones of the limbs). Initially, the shaft diaphysis calcifies, but the ends of the bones maintain a cartilage architecture which allows further elongation of the bone, resulting in linear growth. These cartilaginous growth plates (epiphyses) eventually calcify as the skeleton matures, so further longitudinal growth ceases.

Bone is not an inert tissue; it is in a constant cycle of resorption and formation to allow microarchitectural repair of bone. Bone contains most of the body stores of calcium and therefore is an integral part of calcium homeostasis, which is principally under the control of parathyroid hormone and vitamin D. These hormones control intestinal absorption of calcium, calcium exchange with the principal body stores in bone, and renal excretion of calcium. Abnormalities of these hormone systems can therefore have substantial impacts on the calcified bone matrix and, therefore, the overall bone strength.

There are many genetic disorders which affect bone growth and structure and which result in short stature, disproportionate growth, or deformity (e.g. achondroplasia). Genetic alteration of the collagen 1 production results in very low bone mass prone to fracture, a condition known as osteogenesis imperfecta. The common acquired diseases affecting bone metabolism are:

- **osteoporosis**, which is an idiopathic reduction in bone mass which becomes increasingly prevalent with age; risk factors for premature osteoporosis include early menopause, chronic steroid use, rheumatoid arthritis, thyroid/parathyroid and adrenal disorders, and malabsorption syndromes of any cause
- **osteomalacia**, which is defined as a failure to calcify the connective tissue matrix of bone due to reduced availability of calcium or phosphorus, most usually as a result of vitamin D deficiency

Cartilage

Cartilage is a specialized and largely avascular connective tissue, rich in collagen type II, which in the adult skeleton covers the articulating surfaces of bone of synovial joints. Cartilage is rich in highly charged hydrophilic molecules (glycosaminoglycans) attached to a large hyaluronic acid molecule, which allows cartilage to maintain a high water content. In the growing skeleton, cartilage also forms a matrix scaffold of future long bones, which are further remodelled by endochondral

ossification into mature bone. Some structures in the body remain as cartilage (e.g. the pinna of the ear and the nasal septum). Idiopathic inflammation of cartilage structures is the hallmark of the rare disease **relapsing polychondritis.** More commonly in degenerative arthritis (**osteoarthritis**), there is degeneration of cartilage within the joint; this progresses from fibrillation of the surface to fissuring of cartilage and eventual thinning of the cartilage layer, resulting in exposed bone.

Muscle

Muscle is a specialized connective tissue that is able to contract. This is a metabolically active process directed by a neurological signal. Acetylcholine released at the nerve ending crosses the neuromuscular junction and engages a receptor to trigger calcium-dependent actin/myosin interactions which allow the muscle fibres to shorten. Further requirements are a supply of oxygen, a source of fuel, such as glycogen, and a well-maintained balance of potassium and calcium, all of which are essential for normal muscle function. **Voluntary muscle** (sometimes referred to as **striated muscle** due to its appearance under the microscope) requires an intact neurological supply and neuromuscular junction to initiate movement. This type of muscle is made up of two principal types of muscle fibre cell: type 1, fast-twitch muscle fibres, and type 2, slow-twitch muscle fibres. Some muscles are not under voluntary control. These **involuntary muscles** (sometimes referred to as **smooth muscle** due to their appearance under the microscope) are largely controlled by the autonomic nervous system and are generally found in the muscular walls of some arterial, bronchiolar, and intestinal tissues, as well as tissues of the urogenital tract. Some specialized muscles (e.g. **cardiac muscle**) are able to contract autonomously but still require some neuronal control for appropriate function.

Alterations in muscle function are caused by depravation of oxygen or by metabolic abnormalities that alter the metabolism or availability of the muscle's fuel sources. Biochemical imbalances and neurological disease also result in impaired muscle function. Genetic abnormalities can result in muscular dystrophies or myotonic syndromes. However, the principal manifestation of muscle disorders in rheumatology are due to direct tissue injury by an inflammatory process, **myositis.**

Tendons

Tendons are non-calcified collagen-rich connective tissues that attach muscle to bone. Tendons transmit the force generated by muscles to the moving parts of the skeleton through a specialized attachment called an enthesis. Inflammation of these attachment points, **enthesitis**, is a common feature of the inflammatory spondyloarthritides. The tendon itself can become inflamed, resulting in a condition known as **tendonitis**, as part of a more general inflammatory disorder, or as a specific localized event. Tendons sometimes have a sheath which can also become inflamed; this condition is referred to as **tenosynovitis**. However, the principal cause of localized tendon damage is usually secondary to mechanical loading which exceeds the capabilities of the tendon and commonly results in a degenerative process referred to as **tendinosis** but occasionally progresses to catastrophic failure: tendon rupture.

Ligaments

Ligaments are non-calcified connective tissues attaching adjoining bones together across a joint. By providing constraints, ligaments can define congruency of adjoining joint surfaces and the number of possible planes of movement. Ligament strains are frequent causes of pain following injury. Ligament rupture often results in instability, and the abnormal motion can accelerate cartilage degradation in the joint due to the alteration in joint biomechanics.

Disorders which affect the connective tissue components of tendons and ligament frequently result in **hypermobility** and, in extreme cases, recurrent dislocation of joints is sometimes associated with arterial fragility and rupture (e.g. **Ehlos-Danlos syndrome**—of which there are many types).

Joints

Synovial joints allow significant movement between two adjacent bones. The joint is enclosed by a capsule lined by **synovium** on its inner surface. Ligaments reinforce the capsule and hold the bones which make up the joint together. The ligaments and the articulating surfaces define the planes of movement possible at that joint. Movement is facilitated by a reduction in friction of the joint surfaces due to the formation of a cartilage cap at the end of each bone, thus allowing cartilage–cartilage articulation. The **synovium** is a layer of specialized connective which secretes joint fluid, which in small quantities is present in all joint spaces. Joint fluid provides a boundary fluid layer which further helps to reduce the coefficient of friction between cartilage surfaces. As well as secreting joint fluid, the cells of the synovium also take part in the immune response by taking on tissue macrophage roles and allowing the generation of germinal centres if required. In inflammatory arthritides, the synovium is the target for the inflammatory process which results in **synovitis**.

In synovitis, the synovium thickens due to the accumulation of chronic inflammatory cells involved in the immune response and the generation of inflammation. The synovitic tissue can have locally invasive effects eroding into the cartilage of the joint; this mass of synovial tissue in contact with cartilage and bone within the joint is often referred to as a **pannus**. Synovial lining cells also secrete large quantities of joint fluid which can result in a **joint effusion**.

Arthritis is said to exist if the joint is swollen and tender on palpation and if there is limitation of movement on examination. In inflammatory synovitis, the joint will, in addition, often be warm to the touch and, in acute onset, may have overlying skin colour changes (particularly if the joint is close to the skin surface).

Ageing and the musculoskeletal system

Any discussion of normal musculoskeletal function should include an understanding of how the normal ageing process affects both normal homeostatic mechanisms for normal musculoskeletal function, and the types of diseases one is likely to encounter at different ages. Our genes programme development in utero and affect the growth and development of the skeleton into the mid-twenties. Some tissues retain the capability to repair (e.g. soft tissue, bone) and some do not or only retain a limited capacity to repair (e.g. cartilage). In general, genes determine our maximum capacity to develop traits (e.g. bone mineralization, muscle strength/endurance). Whether or not an individual achieves this maximum capacity predetermined by our genes depends on subsequent nurture and avoidance of disease (e.g. a child affected by inflammatory arthritis through pre-teen and teenage life will struggle to achieve maximum bone mineralization and will therefore be at higher risk of osteoporosis in later life).

Further Reading

Hochberg MC, Silman AJ, Smolen JS, et al. *Rheumatology* (6th edition), 2014. Mosby.

264 Diagnosis in suspected rheumatological disease

Rachel Jeffery

Introduction

Musculoskeletal symptoms may be the sole presenting complaint of a rheumatological disease or may be a minor part of a presenting symptom complex. Determining whether or not these symptoms reflect serious pathology requiring specialist management relies on careful history taking and a thorough examination. The majority of rheumatic conditions are chronic, and a holistic approach to patient management is required to establish how the illness affects the physical and psychological functioning of the patient, and to explore how symptoms may be managed.

In assessing the patient with musculoskeletal symptoms, you must consider the following questions:

- are the symptoms due to an inflammatory process or a non-inflammatory process?
- do the symptoms reflect a primary rheumatological disease or are they secondary to another pathology (e.g. infection or malignancy)?
- are the symptoms a complication of the disease or a complication of treatment?
- is there evidence of non-articular disease, which may be relevant to diagnosis or management?

This chapter focuses on how elements of the history and examination can help answer these questions. Investigation, dealt with in Chapter 265, provides additional information on diagnosis and prognosis.

History taking

When the history is being taken, the age, gender, and ethnicity of the patient should be noted, as well as whether the patient is pregnant, whether the patient smokes, and the presence of any psychosocial factors that may have an impact. Symptoms should be recorded and a history of preceding symptoms, a travel history, a sexual history, and a family history should be taken.

Age

When diagnosing rheumatological disease, the following age-related factors should be taken into consideration:

- most autoimmune rheumatic disease can present at any age, although peak incidence varies with condition
- osteoarthritis is uncommon below the age of 45, unless there has been specific trauma or congenital deformity at one site
- calcium pyrophosphate crystal arthropathy (pseudogout) is rare in patients under the age of 60, unless there is a familial association
- malignancy as cause of musculoskeletal or systemic symptoms is more common in those over the age of 65
- polymyalgia rheumatica and giant cell arteritis rarely occur in those <50
- the onset of ankylosing spondylitis typically occurs before the age of 40
- the juvenile onset of rheumatic disease (occurring before the age of 16) has separate classification criteria
- Kawasaki disease is an acute vasculitis predominantly affecting infants and young children
- the incidence of primary systemic vasculitis in adults increases with age (peak onset at ages 65–74)

- the risk of complications varies less with age than with duration of disease (e.g. in diffuse systemic sclerosis, the highest risk of pulmonary hypertension and renal crisis is in the first 5 years; with rheumatoid arthritis, early diagnosis and treatment is associated with better functional outcome)
- in lupus, the pattern of disease may differ with age; there is some evidence that, when onset occurs over the age of 55, the disease is more insidious, with less renal and neurological disease but more interstitial lung disease, serositis, and overlap syndromes
- polypharmacy is more common in older age and can be associated with a higher risk of drug interactions and side effects, with implications for the treatment and cause of symptoms (e.g. statins and toxic myopathy)
- osteoporosis risk factors, for patients on long-term corticosteroids or with falls risk, should be considered in all age groups; the risk is highest for postmenopausal women

Gender

When diagnosing rheumatological disease, the following gender-related factors should be taken into consideration:

- there is a female predominance in SLE, rheumatoid arthritis (which occurs less frequently in older age groups), polymyalgia rheumatica, giant cell arteritis (which occurs mainly in older Caucasians), Takayasu's arteritis (which occurs mainly in young Asians), systemic sclerosis (although there is less sex difference with the diffuse subtype), Sjögren's syndrome, and fibromyalgia
- gout may be the most common inflammatory arthritis in men and is associated with obesity, family history, alcohol, renal insufficiency, and hypertension; its onset in men occurs at a younger age than it does in females, where it is rare prior to menopause
- men tend to develop rheumatoid arthritis at a later age than females do; in addition, while more men are seropositive (a feature associated with extra-articular disease), with more rheumatoid nodules, more lung, large joint and proximal joint involvement, and more secondary vasculitis, women tend to have more sicca symptoms and worse joint disease activity and functional scores
- male survival with diffuse systemic sclerosis is worse than female survival, and pulmonary fibrosis is more common in men than in women
- ankylosing spondylitis is more prevalent in men than in women, and occurs with more spinal fusion; however, peripheral joint involvement is more common in women
- primary systemic vasculitis of medium vessels is more common in men than in women
- Behçet's syndrome has an equal sex distribution but tends to run a more severe course in men than in women
- osteoarthritis has female predilection in the hands and knees

Ethnicity

When diagnosing rheumatological disease, the following ethnicity-related factors should be taken into consideration:

- rheumatoid arthritis has higher prevalence in Northern Europe than in Southern Europe; in the UK, it seems less common in those of Afro-Caribbean descent than in other ethnic groups
- while SLE is more prevalent in those of Asian descent than it is in those of Caucasian descent, it is most prevalent in those of Afro-Caribbean descent; in addition, renal disease is associated with a worse outcome in those of Afro-Caribbean descent, and this

group responds less well to certain drug therapies (e.g. IV cyclo-phosphamide, angiotensin-converting-enzyme inhibitors)
- cultural factors may influence use of health resources

Pregnancy

When diagnosing rheumatological disease, the following pregnancy-related factors should be taken into consideration:

- musculoskeletal pain (back pain, symphysis pubis pain, sacro-iliac pain) is common in pregnancy, particularly during the third trimester
- vitamin D sufficiency is important, as insufficiency fractures can occur
- pregnancy influences the drugs that can be used
- autoimmune disease can present in pregnancy (especially lupus)
- lupus can deteriorate during pregnancy, with renal complications being particularly serious
- early and diffuse systemic sclerosis is associated with an increased risk of renal crisis
- renal involvement from connective tissue disease can be hard to distinguish from pre-eclampsia
- anti-Ro and anti-La antibodies can cause fetal heart block or neo-natal lupus and can be the first presentation of rheumatological disease; if these antibodies are known to be present, fetal cardiac monitoring should be arranged
- pregnancy loss, intrauterine growth retardation, thrombosis, pre-eclampsia, and premature delivery occur in higher incidence with SLE and antiphospholipid syndrome (anticardiolipin antibody or lupus anticoagulant positive); specialist obstetrics advice should be sought
- rheumatoid arthritis often improves symptomatically during preg-nancy but can relapse in the post-partum period

Cigarette smoking

When diagnosing rheumatological disease, if the patient smokes, the following should be taken into consideration:

- smokers have an increased risk of developing autoimmune disease (e.g. the risk of developing rheumatoid arthritis is doubled)
- smokers have a poorer prognosis for rheumatoid arthritis:
  - they have an increased risk of being seropositive (which is asso-ciated with erosive and extra-articular disease)
  - they have a reduced response to some drugs (e.g. methotrexate, hydroxychloroquine, anti-tumour necrosis factor therapy)
- they have an increased risk of cardiovascular disease, which occurs at a higher incidence in autoimmune rheumatic disease

Psychosocial factors

Psychosocial factors, such as employment, depression, relationships, and coping strategies, impact on outcome and disability; in addition, there is a two-way interaction, as disease impacts on psychosocial factors. Obtaining information in the history is important in anticipat-ing these issues.

Employment

Manual workers are less likely to retain employment than those in professional or managerial roles. Length of time off work (>6 weeks) reduces the likelihood of returning to work. Financial problems pre-dict depression, disability, and relationship problems.

Depression

Depression is common in chronic rheumatologic conditions and is often missed. It is predicted by level of disability rather than severity of disease. Deformity, negative self-image, loss of independence, and control also contribute.

Relationships

Social support from family, friends, healthcare workers, and patient groups is associated with lower levels of depression. Problems arise when there are reduced opportunity for social contacts; increased isolation and dependence; sexual problems; mood changes; and loss of income.

Table 264.1 Features suggesting inflammatory versus non-inflammatory causes

Inflammatory	Non-inflammatory
Pain improves with activity	Pain worse on activity
Pain worse with rest	Pain better with rest
Early morning stiffness >30 min	Early morning stiffness <30 mins
Stiffness improves with exercise, worse with rest	Stiffness less responsive to exercise and rest

Coping strategies

The belief of self-control over pain is associated with higher well-being and lower disability scores. In contrast, catastrophizing, fear-avoidance behaviour, and reduced levels of activity are associated with lower psychological well-being and higher disability scores.

Symptoms

Determining the presence of specific symptom complexes helps to narrow the differential diagnosis and classification and will guide decisions on further investigations and management. Classification criteria for rheumatic disease should not be confused with diag-nostic criteria. Once information about pain and stiffness has been obtained, it should be possible to decide whether the condition is more likely to be inflammatory or non-inflammatory (mechanical; see Table 264.1).

This distinction is important, as it will influence the rest of the his-tory taking. For inflammatory conditions, systemic and extra-articular features, as well as clues as to classification of the condition, will be looked for in both the history and the examination. For non-inflam-matory conditions, aggravating factors and ways of managing the symptoms within the patient's lifestyle will be considered. In addition, 'red flags', which would indicate the need for urgent further investiga-tion to exclude infection and malignancy, need to be excluded (see Box 264.1).

Pain

Pain is the most common rheumatological symptom. Several patterns of pain are recognizable:

- pain which is worse with or following movement and which is often worse later in the day is suggestive of a mechanical process, such as degenerative arthritis
- pain which is worse in the early morning, is often associated with prolonged early morning stiffness, is worse after rest, and is relieved by exercise is suggestive of an inflammatory process
- pain associated with neurological symptoms suggests a neuro-pathic element; radicular pain that is sharp, electric-shock-like, and often aggravated by cough (due to raised intrathecal pressure) suggests nerve root entrapment; pain associated with significant neurological dysfunction suggests neural injury and is often worse at night-time
- well-localized bone pain suggests an injury and, if severe at rest or at night, may be indicative of a malignancy
- poorly defined pain localized to a single area but not affected by movement of that area suggests referred pain (e.g. right shoulder pain in cholecystitis; left arm pain in acute coronary syndrome)
- musculoskeletal pain associated with systemic/constitutional symptoms should prompt a search for infection, malignancy, or features of connective tissue disease or vasculitis

Box 264.1 'Red flags'

- pain worse at night
- associated systemic features (fever, sweats)
- unexplained weight loss
- new neurological symptoms
- previous history of malignancy
- immunocompromise
- extremes of age (<16 years, >70 years)

- increasing muscle pain during the use of a limb suggests vascular claudication and, when in unusual locations (upper limb or jaw), could suggest a vasculitis
- hyperalgesia (more pain than expected from a noxious stimulus) and allodynia (pain from a non-noxious stimulus) suggests a more complex central pain-processing problem; this can be generalized pain in fibromyalgia, or localized pain in complex regional pain syndrome

Stiffness

Stiffness is another common symptom of rheumatological disease, but it can be difficult to characterize precisely, as patients will often equate it with pain. Significant stiffness, particularly early morning stiffness of more than 30 minutes duration, is more in keeping with inflammatory disease and will usually improve with activity through the day.

Mechanical disorders can cause stiffness but this is often short-lived, start-up pain/stiffness.

Some neurological conditions cause stiffness following upper motor neuron lesions (e.g. cervical cord compression) or extrapyramidal disease (e.g. parkinsonism).

Swelling

Swelling is often reported but must be corroborated by examination (e.g. patients with areas of numbness often report a feeling of swelling). When swelling of a joint is fixed and bony, this suggests osteoarthritis. When swelling of a joint is soft and boggy, it may be inflammatory. When swelling of a limb occurs with pitting on pressure, this suggests oedema.

Colour changes

Redness (erythema) associated with a joint or bursa should be considered a sign of infection until proven otherwise. Non-specific skin redness of a limb should be considered a possible sign of cellulitis. Once infection has been excluded, other possible causes include crystal arthropathy, seronegative spondyloarthropathy, erythema nodosum, ruptured Baker's cyst, and DVT. Palmar erythema can be seen in rheumatoid arthritis and vasculitis, although other non-rheumatological causes need to be considered.

Vascular changes in Raynaud's disease typically follow a triphasic colour change of white (the initial vasoconstrictive phase), blue (deoxygenated blood flow), and red (erythralgia, usually painful, as compensatory vasodilatation occurs). Raynaud's disease is more likely to be primary if it is of young onset (age <20), occurs in female patients with low BMI, and is triggered in cold environment and recovers quickly on warming, without associated skin changes. It will be aggravated by smoking and some drugs (e.g. beta blockers). Chilblains can occur. Secondary Raynaud's disease is more likely with older onset (age >40), digital ulceration, persistence even in a warm environment, and systemic symptoms. Unilateral Raynaud's disease or vascular changes should prompt a search for occlusive causes (extravascular, mural, or intravascular).

Livedo reticularis, producing a characteristic purple criss-cross pattern over the skin, is more commonly pathological if the upper limbs are involved and if it persists in warm environment. This can be associated with vasculitis or antiphospholipid syndrome.

Joint range of movement

Joint range of movement is not a particularly helpful feature of the history, as movement may be restricted by pain from any area of the limb. This feature is more useful and specific on examination.

Fatigue

Fatigue is a very common symptom in association with chronic rheumatologic conditions, both inflammatory and non-inflammatory (reported in up to 90% of patients). The aetiology is multifactorial and often there is a history of sleep disturbance either in the duration or the quality of sleep. This is not always associated with pain and often does not respond to treatment of the underlying condition. Fatigue can affect pain experience, mood, and coping ability and impact on functional outcome.

Systemic symptoms

Systemic symptoms of fever, sweats, or unexplained weight loss can occur with severe inflammatory arthritides and systemic autoimmune rheumatic disease, but infection and malignancy must be excluded.

Generalized myalgia (pain in the muscles) and arthralgia (pain in the joints) can occur with systemic illness and fever, due to systemic cytokine release, without the musculoskeletal system being the primary location of inflammation, as in response to a viral' flu-like' illness. A history of associated and preceding symptoms as well as the duration of the symptoms will provide pointers to possible infectious aetiology.

Preceding symptoms, travel, and sexual history

A history of upper or lower respiratory tract infection, acute gastroenteritis, genitourinary symptoms, or risk of exposure to sexually transmitted disease may help identify a reactive arthritis (likely if multiple joints involved) or secondary septic arthritis (essential to consider, particularly if only one joint is involved). In addition, note that an individual who already has one autoimmune disease has a 1 in 5 risk of developing a second one.

The spectrum of infectious agents considered will be influenced by the travel history, for example travel to areas endemic for Lyme disease (e.g. New Forest and Norfolk in the UK; Germany; northern parts of North America). HIV infection can be associated with autoimmune disease presentation at seroconversion, as part of the AIDS complex of symptoms and during immune reconstitution on antiretroviral treatment. Diffuse infiltrative lymphocytosis syndrome (DILS), presenting with Sjögren's type glandular swelling, should not be missed. Psoriasis and spondyloarthropathies can present in HIV infection, and there is a higher risk of septic arthritis.

Family history

The following factors should be taken into consideration when taking the family history:

- there is a 20% increased risk of autoimmune disease if the patient has a first-degree relative with an autoimmune disease; the impact of this will depend on the incidence of the disease
- in spondyloarthropathies, there is a strong dominant association with HLA-B27:
  - of Caucasian patients with ankylosing spondylitis, >90% are positive for HLA-B27 (the percentage is less for non-Caucasians)
  - of patients with reactive arthritis with sacroiliitis, 80% are positive for HLA-B27
  - of patients with peripheral arthritis without sacroiliitis, 25%–40% are positive for HLA-B27
- there is a familial association for early onset gout without traditional associated risk factors
- periodic syndromes (acute remitting attacks of fever and serositis) have strong family associations
- benign joint hypermobility and pathological hypermobility associated with specific syndromes (e.g. Marfan syndrome and Ehlers–Danlos syndrome) usually present in familial clusters
- in osteogenesis imperfecta, the most common types (Types I and IV) are usually inherited in an autosomal dominant fashion, whereas the more severe forms (including Types II and III) usually occur as the result of sporadic mutations, with no family history
- polyarticular generalized nodal osteoarthritis is increasingly recognized as having familial associations

The penetrance of phenotype may vary between individuals.

Examination

The history will establish whether the symptoms are likely to have an inflammatory or non-inflammatory cause. The musculoskeletal system is then examined with this in mind, looking for features to confirm or refute the suspected diagnosis. These findings then inform the general examination.

Examination of the musculoskeletal system

Inspect the joints and limbs, looking for:

- swelling, its localization to the joint or surrounding tissue/bursa and whether it arises from one compartment or arises more diffusely in the limb
- the pattern of joint swelling: whether it occurs in one joint or multiple joints, and the symmetry and size of joint involvement (see Figure 264.1)

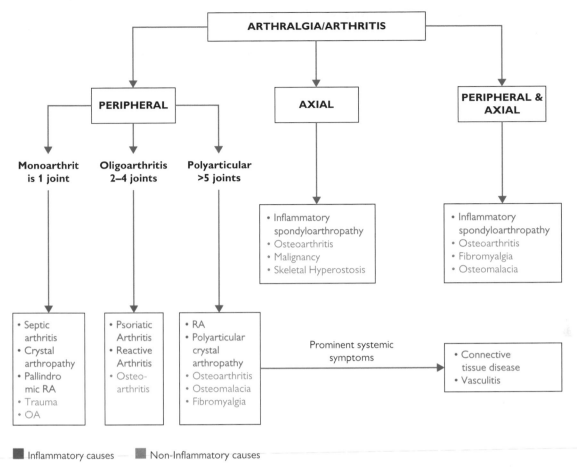

Figure 264.1 Approach to the diagnosis of joint pain; OA, osteoarthritis; RA, rheumatoid arthritis.

- deformity: bone distortion (post fracture, osteophytes, remodelling in Paget's or osteomalacia), subluxation (joint failure due to soft tissue damage), and/or Boutonniere (fixed flexion of the proximal interphalangeal joint, with hyperextension of the distal interphalangeal joint) or swan neck (fixed flexion of the distal interphalangeal joint, with hyperextension of the proximal interphalangeal joint) deformities of fingers (characteristic of chronic rheumatoid arthritis)
- local skin changes or trauma
- muscle changes (e.g. wasting, indicating disuse)

Palpate the joints and muscles, looking for:

- tenderness and the site of tenderness:
  - tenderness at the joint line is more specific for joint disease
  - tenderness over entheses occurs in spondyloarthropathies but also with generalized chronic pain syndrome (fibromyalgia)
  - tenderness over muscles; identify the pattern and localization (see Chapter 63)
- specific bony tenderness at one site (suggests a local bone problem)
- the nature of the swelling:
  - is it bony?
  - is it boggy (suggesting inflammation)?
  - is there fluid within the joint (fluctuance; e.g. test with a patella tap) and/or in the surrounding soft tissue (pitting oedema)?
- the temperature of the overlying skin: (e.g. is it raised, due to inflammation, or cold, due to reduced circulation?)

Examine the movement of the joints and muscles:

- compare the range of movement on both sides and in similarly sized joints, as the exact flexibility will vary between individuals and between joints and will usually reduce with age
- mild hyperextension is normal for most joints in children and young adults but is classified as hypermobility when this is more marked

- inability to achieve a normal range of movement is considered restricted movement

In addition, confirm the nature of deformity and identify any restrictions. Observing both passive and active ranges of movement makes it possible to distinguish between fixed deformities and restrictions (arising from bone and cartilage changes within the joint, from restrictions from soft tissue surrounding the joint, or from skin restrictions), and reversible deformities (arising from altered muscle balance—primary to the muscle or secondary to neurological disease—or from tendon rupture or subluxation)

General examination

Specific further local and systemic examination will be determined by the findings from the examination of the musculoskeletal system and by features from the history. If systemic/inflammatory causes are a possibility, then a full systems examination is mandatory. Looking for localizing signs of infection or malignancy is essential.

Neurological system

When examining the neurological system, look for the following features:

- muscle weakness, which can present as inability to move a joint; this necessitates neurological examination of the limb
- numbness or neuropathic pain; if present, a full neurological assessment is indicated
- new-onset headache (unusual for the patient), which is unilateral, involving temple, jaw claudication, visual symptoms (partial or complete loss of vision), with associated systemic symptoms; this suggests giant cell arteritis and requires immediate corticosteroids and further investigation

- headaches with features of meningitis or encephalitis occurring in a patient with known or suspected autoimmune disease; need to exclude these or treat infective causes

Cardiovascular system

When examining the cardiovascular system, look for the following:

- infective endocarditis, which can present with joint pains, swelling, heart murmur, and haematuria; note that heart murmur can also be a feature of vasculitis and lupus (Libman–Sacks endocarditis) or secondary aortic valve incompetence with aortitis from arteritis or ankylosing spondylitis; rheumatic fever is less common with antibiotic treatment of throat infections
- signs of right-sided cardiac failure in association with pulmonary hypertension or constrictive pericarditis, as these are possible complications of connective tissue disease
- absence of peripheral pulses (can occur in arteritis)
- peripheral oedema in cardiac failure, nephrotic syndrome, or liver disease

Respiratory system

When examining the respiratory system, look for the following:

- pneumonia; note that, particularly in the elderly and immunocompromised, this may present with systemic features without localizing symptoms
- pulmonary fibrosis in association with inflammatory arthritides, connective tissue disease, or vasculitis, or as complication of treatment (methotrexate, leflunomide)
- pulmonary embolism; usually associated with antiphospholipid syndrome, but also there is increased risk of this in connective tissue disease and from immobility due to musculoskeletal symptoms
- pleural effusion associated with serositis
- late-onset asthma in Churg–Strauss syndrome

Gastrointestinal system

When examining the gastrointestinal system, look for the following features:

- hepatosplenomegaly; mild enlargement can occur with autoimmune rheumatic disease, usually in association with reactive lymphadenopathy, although this finding should prompt exclusion of malignancy (lymphoma can occur at increased incidence in association with autoimmune disease, especially Sjögren's syndrome)
- liver disease, as a feature of autoimmune disease or drug therapy
- blood or mucous in the stool, or malabsorptive stool, in association with infective or inflammatory colitis, coeliac disease, or upper gastrointestinal dysmotility or bacterial overgrowth (e.g. in systemic sclerosis)

Urogenital system

When examining the urogenital system, look for the following features:

- peripheral oedema with nephrotic syndrome (suggests lupus, vasculitis, amyloidosis)
- the following urine dipstick results:
  - proteinuria and haematuria, suggesting glomerular inflammation
  - leucocytes and nitrites, suggesting infection
  - glucose suggesting diabetes mellitus
- genital ulcers (see 'Oral and genital ulceration')

Skin, nails, and mucosa

Typical diagnostic skin features

Typical diagnostic skin features include:

- butterfly malar rash (SLE)
- discoid rash (discoid lupus)
- rheumatoid nodules (seropositive rheumatoid arthritis)
- psoriasis and nail dystrophy (psoriatic arthritis)
- plantar palmar pustulosis (reactive arthritis)
- tophi (gout)
- heliotrope rash and Gottron's papules (dermatomyositis)

- sclerodactyly and scleroderma changes (systemic sclerosis; changes can be subtle)
- lupus pernio (sarcoidosis)

Features suggestive of autoimmune disease but not specific to one condition

Features suggestive of autoimmune disease but not specific to one condition include:

- pyoderma gangrenosum
- livedo reticularis
- photosensitivity
- purpura (including palpable); look for the more specific Henoch–Schönlein purpura distribution on lower limb, extensor aspects
- erythema nodosum

Other diagnostic clues

Other diagnostic clues include:

- erythema marginatum (streptococcal infection)
- erythema migrans (Lyme disease)

Oral and genital ulceration

If there is oral and/or genital ulceration, note the following:

- duration, frequency, severity, and size can help distinguish pathological ulcers
- it is important to exclude infectious causes, especially with genital-only ulcers (e.g. from herpes simplex, lymphogranuloma venereum)
- autoimmune causes include SLE, Behçet's syndrome, inflammatory bowel disease, reactive arthritis, and Stevens–Johnston syndrome (including reaction to drugs)
- lichen planus can be oral or genital; it is associated with Sjögren's syndrome

Eyes

When examining the eyes, look for the following:

- conjunctivitis or episcleritis (red eyes with itching, mild photophobia, and normal visual acuity)
- uveitis (red eyes with pain and loss of visual acuity); requires urgent ophthalmology review (NB: in children, uveitis is commonly asymptomatic, and all children with known or suspected inflammatory arthritis or connective tissue disease should be screened and monitored by an experienced ophthalmologist)
- dry, gritty eyes with or without dry mouth can occur with primary or secondary Sjögren's syndrome; Schirmer's test (the rate of tear chromatography down filter paper) and a wafer test (time to dissolve a thin wafer orally) can give a more quantitative assessment

ENT

When examining the ears, nose, and throat, be aware of the following:

- rhinosinusitis can occur with vasculitides but it is also a common allergic symptom, so it is non-specific
- nasal crusting, nosebleeds, nasal stuffiness, and conductive hearing loss can occur in Wegener's granulomatosis
- destructive cartilage changes can occur in the nasal septum or upper airways (in Wegener's granulomatosis and relapsing polychondritis) or pinna (in relapsing polychondritis); other causes such as trauma, surgery, cocaine abuse, or risk of leprosy need to be excluded
- parotid and salivary gland enlargement in Sjögren's syndrome, sarcoidosis, and DILS
- lymphadenopathy (with or without hepatosplenomegaly (see 'Gastrointestinal system')); exclude malignancy and infection

Prognosis

The prognosis of rheumatological disease is predominantly influenced by disease type and natural history, with the outcome modified by the extent of organ involvement and the degree of reversible versus permanent tissue damage. Extent of involvement forms part of the assessment of a patient with rheumatic disease and informs decisions on management. The extent of disability from symptoms is influenced not only by the severity of organ involvement but also by a wider range of functional factors.

Further Reading

Cawston TE. 'Structure and function: 'Joints and connective tissue', in Warrell, DA, Cox TM, and Firth JD, eds, *Oxford Textbook of Medicine* (5th edition), 2010. Oxford University Press.

Doherty M and Lanyon PC, 'Clinical investigation', in Warrell, DA, Cox TM, and Firth JD, eds, *Oxford Textbook of Medicine* (5th edition), 2010. Oxford University Press.

Hochberg MC, Silman AJ, Smolen JS, et al. *Rheumatology* (6th edition), 2014.

Russell AS and Ferrari R. 'Clinical presentation and diagnosis of rheumatic disease', in Warrell, DA, Cox TM, and Firth JD, eds, *Oxford Textbook of Medicine* (5th edition), 2010. Oxford University Press.

Introduction

In suspected rheumatological disease, the findings on careful clinical assessment, as detailed in Chapter 264, are crucial to the interpretation of test results. Investigation should not be used as a screening tool, but rather to clarify the differential diagnosis. In established disease, investigation should also be used to assess the extent and severity of organ involvement, establish prognosis, and guide treatment choices.

Full blood count

The full blood count is often affected by rheumatological diseases and their treatments. The haemoglobin concentration may be low because of anaemia of chronic disease, iron deficiency, or macrocytic anaemia. For example, in uncontrolled rheumatoid arthritis (RA), anaemia of chronic disease may be seen. If there is coexisting celiac disease, the patient may have an iron-deficiency anaemia. A macrocytic anaemia may be seen if there is folate deficiency related to methotrexate toxicity.

White blood cell count

The white blood cell count is useful in monitoring for neutrophilia from infection and neutropenia related to active disease or disease-modifying anti-rheumatic drugs (DMARDs). The platelet count may be raised in active RA. Felty's syndrome, a complication of untreated or poorly controlled RA, is associated with neutropenia, splenomegaly, and thrombocytopenia. SLE may result in leucopenia, lymphopenia, and thrombocytopenia

Liver function tests

Liver function tests are used to monitor for liver injury due to DMARDs such as methotrexate and leflunomide.

Acute phase reactants

Acute phase reactants are described as 'positive' or 'negative' depending on whether they rise or fall in the presence of an inflammatory state. They are usually driven by cytokines such as interleukin-6, tumour necrosis factor alpha, interferon gamma, and transforming growth factor beta. Positive acute phase reactants include the erythrocyte sedimentation rate (ESR), C-reactive protein (CRP), and ferritin. Negative acute phase reactants include albumin and transferrin.

The two most widely used acute phase reactants are ESR and CRP. Both are elevated in most inflammatory diseases, and are helpful in assessing disease activity. In polymyalgia rheumatica, giant cell arteritis, and RA, ESR and CRP are indicators of severity, prognosis, and response to treatment. However, in early psoriatic arthritis and ankylosing spondylitis, these acute phase reactants can be normal. In SLE, a raised ESR with a normal CRP is typical; a raised CRP in SLE may reflect infection, lupus serositis, or vasculitis.

Procalcitonin is an emerging positive acute phase reactant which may have utility in differentiating bacterial infection from disease progression.

Uric acid

The plasma level of uric acid is useful in the diagnosis of gout. In a patient with risk factors for gout, and an acutely swollen joint or joints, the presence of a raised uric acid confirms the diagnosis of gout. However, it is important to note that plasma uric acid may be normal during an acute attack of gout, and so this does not exclude the diagnosis. In this setting, an aspirate of the swollen joint is needed for crystal analysis.

Rheumatoid factor, and anti-cyclic citrullinated peptide antibodies

Rheumatoid factor (RF) is an antibody against the Fc portion of IgG in the patient's serum. The most commonly measured and clinically useful class of RF is IgM RF. Five per cent of a healthy population can be RF positive, and the prevalence increases with age. Testing for RF is useful in the diagnosis and management of RA, but RF positivity is not a necessary diagnostic criterion. RF positivity is associated with more severe joint disease, systemic disease (extra-articular features), and responsiveness to biological DMARDs such as rituximab. RF can also be seen in a number of other rheumatic diseases, as well as in non-rheumatic diseases.

Anti-cyclic citrullinated peptide (anti-CCP) antibodies are directed against citrulline residues formed in post-translational modification of arginine.

In patients with RA, anti-CCP antibodies have a sensitivity comparable to that of RF but with a much higher specificity of 95%–98%. The presence of anti-CCP antibodies can predate the onset of RA and may be positive in patients who are RF negative. Thus, these antibodies, if present, can help in making the diagnosis of RA, given their high specificity. Their presence is also associated with a more severe disease course and more extra-articular features. Unlike RF, anti-CCP antibodies are rarely found in patients with non-rheumatic disease.

Antinuclear antibodies

Antinuclear antibodies (ANAs) are autoantibodies that bind to components of the cell nucleus and (despite their name) cytoplasm. The most commonly used technique to detect ANAs is indirect immunofluorescence, in which HEp-2 cells (obtained from a human epithelial tumour line) are made permeable and incubated first with the patient's serum, and then with anti-human antibodies conjugated to a fluorescent molecule. The cells are then examined by microscopy, and the staining pattern noted. The results are reported as positive or negative and include a titre.

The presence or absence of ANAs is not sufficient to confirm or exclude any rheumatic disease. For example, nearly all patients with untreated SLE have a positive ANA test but not all people with a positive ANA have SLE. Given the low prevalence of SLE, the positive predictive value of a positive ANA for SLE is also low, at around 11%.

ANA titres of 1:160 or more are usually regarded as significant. However, amongst healthy people, 25%–30% have a positive ANA test with a titre of 1:40, 10%–15% have a titre of 1:80, and 5% have a titre of 1:160 or more. The positivity of the test also increases with age, particularly in women. An ANA titre of 1:40 is seen in 25%–30% of relatives of patients with rheumatic disease. In Raynaud's phenomenon, a positive ANA test increases the risk of developing an associated rheumatic disease from 19% to 30%, and a negative test decreases this risk to 7%. Table 265.1 summarizes the prevalence of ANAs in rheumatic diseases.

Table 265.1 Utility of autoantibodies in the diagnosis of rheumatological disease

Disease	Sensitivity (True positive rate)	Specificity (True negative rate)
SLE	93%	57%
Systemic sclerosis	85%	54%
Polymyositis/dermatomyositis	61%	63%
Rheumatoid arthritis	41%	56%
Sjögren's syndrome	48%	52%
Secondary Raynaud's phenomenon	64%	41%

Adapted with permission from Daniel H. Solomon, Arthur J. Kavanaugh, Peter H. Schur, Evidence-based guidelines for the use of immunologic tests: Antinuclear antibody testing, Arthritis & Rheumatology, Volume 47, Issue 4, pp. 434–444, Copyright © 2002 John Wiley and Sons.

Extractable nuclear antigens

In a patient with a positive ANA test, it is important to determine the target antigen of the ANA. These target antigens, also called extractable nuclear antigens, are soluble nuclear and cytoplasmic components that leach from the cell when extracted with saline. Table 265.2 summarizes the prevalence of extractable nuclear antigen antibodies in rheumatic diseases.

SLE-associated autoantibodies

SLE-associated autoantibodies include:

- anti-double-stranded DNA antibodies:
  - most strongly associated with SLE
  - important in the diagnosis and assessment of the disease, as their levels correlate with disease activity
  - also associated with the development of lupus nephritis
- the anti-Smith antibody:
- high specificity but low sensitivity for SLE
- associated with renal involvement and poor prognosis
- antiribonucleoprotein antibody:
  - high specificity for mixed connective tissue disorder and is an essential criterion in making this diagnosis
  - often present before the onset of disease

Table 265.2 Autoantibodies and their associated rheumatological disease

Antibody	Associated condition	Sensitivity (True positive rate)	Specificity (True negative rate)
Anti-dsDNA Ab	SLE	57%	97%
Anti-Smith Ab	SLE	25%—0%	High*
Anti-Ro/SS-A Ab	Sjögren, SCLE, neonatal lupus syndrome	8%–70%	87%
Anti-La/SS-B Ab	Sjögren, SCLE, neonatal lupus syndrome	16%–40%	94%
Anti-Scl-70 Ab	Systemic sclerosis	20%	100%
Anticentromere Ab	Limited cutaneous systemic sclerosis	65%	99.9%
Anti-U3-RNP Ab	Scleroderma	12%	96%

Abbreviations: Ab, antibody; anti-dsDNA, anti-double-stranded DNA antibody; RNP, ribonucleoprotein; SCLE, subacute cutaneous lupus erythematosus.

*Precise data not available.

Adapted from Sheldon J., Laboratory testing in autoimmune rheumatic diseases, Best Practice & Research Clinical Rheumatology, volume 18, issue 33, pp. 249–269, copyright © 2004 with permission from Elsevier.

- anti-SS-A/Ro and anti SS-B/La antibodies:
  - female patients with SLE who become pregnant must have blood testing for these antibodies because of the associated risk of congenital heart block in the fetus or neonate, or neonatal lupus

Sjögren's syndrome antibodies

Antibodies associated with Sjögren's syndrome include the anti-SS-A/Ro and anti-SS-B/La antibodies. They are of importance in making a diagnosis of Sjögren's syndrome, as they are rarely seen in healthy people, although they may be present in other rheumatic diseases such as RA, SLE, and polymyositis.

Scleroderma-associated antibodies

Scleroderma-associated antibodies include anticentromere antibodies, the anti-Scl-70 antibody, and anti-U3-ribonucleoprotein antibodies.

Anticentromere antibodies

Anticentromere antibodies are associated with limited cutaneous systemic sclerosis, which was previously called CREST (**c**alcinosis, **R**aynaud's phenomenon, **o**esophageal dysmotility, **s**clerodactyly, **t**elangectasia) syndrome, and have high specificity but limited sensitivity for the diagnosis. They are rarely found in patients with other connective tissue diseases or in healthy people, Their presence distinguishes patients with limited systemic sclerosis from those with diffuse systemic sclerosis or primary Raynaud's phenomenon.

Anti-Scl-70

The anti-Scl-70 antibody is also very useful in diagnosing diffuse systemic sclerosis. This antibody is highly specific for diffuse disease, although not very sensitive. Anti-Scl-70 and anticentromere antibodies rarely coexist in the same person. The presence of anti-Scl-70 antibodies is useful in predicting a greater likelihood for the development of diffuse cutaneous involvement and pulmonary fibrosis.

Anti-U3-ribonucleoprotein antibodies

Anti-U3-ribonucleoprotein antibodies are antinucleolar antibodies which have high specificity but low sensitivity for scleroderma.

Myositis-associated antibodies

Tests for myositis-associated antibodies are helpful in the diagnosis of polymyositis and dermatomyositis (Table 265.3). They have high specificity but low sensitivity for these diseases.

Antineutrophil cytoplasmic antibodies

Neutrophils contain enzymes including proteinase 3 (PR3), myeloperoxidase (MPO), and elastase, which are components of the immune response. Antibodies directed against these enzymes are associated with certain small vessel vasculitides. Antineutrophil cytoplasmic antibodies (ANCAs) are detected by indirect immunofluorescence and have two main patterns of immunofluorescent staining in patients who are ANCA positive: cytoplasmic (cANCA) and perinuclear (pANCA).

Following the finding of cANCA or pANCA positivity, an enzyme immunoassay (i.e. ELISA) is done to determine the presence or absence of antibodies directed against either PR3 or MPO. A cANCA staining pattern in combination with a positive PR3 ANCA result from an ELISA is highly specific (99%) for small vessel vasculitis. A pANCA staining pattern in combination with a positive MPO ANCA is also highly specific for small vessel vasculitis. However, a pANCA staining pattern on indirect immunofluorescence can be seen in a number of non-rheumatic diseases. Table 265.4 summarizes the sensitivities of ANCA in selected rheumatic and non-rheumatic diseases.

Table 265.3 Myositis-associated antibodies

Antibodies	Significance
Anti-Jo1 antibody	Associated with rarer antisynthetase syndrome: interstitial lung disease, non-erosive symmetrical arthritis, Raynaud's phenomenon, and mechanic's hand
Anti-signal recognition particle antibody	Associated with acute onset severe illness with minimal evidence of inflammation on muscle biopsy, requiring aggressive immunosuppression
Anti-Mi2 antibody	Associated with classical dermatomyositis (erythroderma/shawl sign)

Human leukocyte antigen B27

Human leukocyte antigen B27 (HLA-B27) is a Class I surface antigen encoded by the B locus in the major histocompatibility complex on Chromosome 6. HLA-B27 is strongly associated with the seronegative spondyloarthritides, including psoriatic arthritis, ankylosing spondylitis, reactive arthritis, and inflammatory-bowel-disease-related arthritis.

HLA-B27's association with this group of diseases is strongest in ankylosing spondylitis. It is important to note, however, that the presence of HLA-B27 alone cannot be taken as indicating rheumatic disease: 8% of the healthy white population is HLA-B27 positive, while 4% of the healthy African-American population is HLA-B27 positive. HLA-B27 should only be tested in an individual with a strong clinical suspicion of seronegative spondyloarthritis.

Blood tests for monitoring DMARDs

Patients with rheumatic disease require monitoring via blood tests, to prevent medication-related complications. Table 265.5 highlights important DMARDs, with some comment on their adverse effects.

Urinalysis

Urinalysis is an effective method of detecting renal involvement in rheumatological disease (e.g. SLE, scleroderma) or a renal complication of therapy (e.g. gold and d-penicillamine in RA (see Table 265.6).

Urinary Bence Jones protein (monoclonal free kappa or lambda light chains) should be measured if the differential diagnosis includes myeloma (because of bone pain, increased plasma alkaline phosphatase, renal impairment, or a monoclonal band on serum protein electrophoresis).

Table 265.4 Prevalence of antineutrophil cytoplasmic antibodies findings in vasculitic disease

Disease	cANCA/PR3	pANCA/MPO
Granulomatosis with polyangiitis (formerly Wegener's granulomatosis)	85%	10%
Microscopic polyangiitis	45%	45%
Allergic granulomatosis and angiitis (formerly Churg–Strauss syndrome)	10%	60%
Idiopathic crescentic glomerulonephritis	25%	65%
Polyarteritis nodosa	5%	15%
Anti-GBM disease (Goodpasture's disease)		20%–30%

Abbreviations: cANCA, cytoplasmic antineutrophil cytoplasmic antibody; GBM, glomerular basement membrane; MPO, myeloperoxidase; pANCA, perinuclear antineutrophil cytoplasmic antibody; PR3, proteinase-3.

Adapted from Sheldon J., Laboratory testing in autoimmune rheumatic diseases, Best Practice & Research Clinical Rheumatology, volume 18, issue 33, pp. 249–269, copyright © 2004 with permission from Elsevier.

Table 265.5 Adverse effects of disease-modifying agents in rheumatological disease

DMARD	Major adverse effects
Methotrexate	• oral ulcers (patient may need to increase dose of folic acid) • marrow suppression (patient may need folinic-acid rescue therapy) • hepatotoxicity (presents as deranged LFTs) • pulmonary toxicity (ask patient about symptoms of dyspnoea) • rashes • alopecia
Sulphasalazine	• GI discomfort (nausea and vomiting) • rashes • headaches, also mood alterations • oligospermia (reversible once medication is stopped) • marrow suppression (rare) • major allergic reaction with Stevens–Johnson syndrome (rare) • hepatotoxicity (rare)
Hydroxychloroquine	• ophthalmology: abnormal colour vision, macular pigmentary changes, loss of visual acuity • rash and photosensitivity (ask about sun-exposed areas) • diarrhoea (not common) • nausea
Azathioprine TPMT levels (pretreatment)	• marrow suppression • hypersensitivity hepatitis with cholestasis • GI intolerance • increased risk of infections
Ciclosporin Creatinine clearance (pretreatment)	• hypertension (patient will need regular BP checks) • hyperkalaemia and renal toxicity • hypercholesterolemia (patient will need 3-monthly fasting lipids) • increased hair growth (female patients may find this cosmetically unacceptable) • gum hypertrophy
Leflunomide BP check (preferably <140/90 pretreatment)	• marrow suppression (patient may need colestyramine rescue therapy) • hepatotoxicity • hypertension
Mycophenolate mofetil	• marrow suppression • increased infection risk
Biological therapies (anti-TNFα, rituximab (CD19 levels, Ig levels pretreatment for rituximab), tocilizumab}	• marrow suppression • hepatitis (usually with rituximab) • increased infection risk

Abbreviations: BP, blood pressure; DMARD, disease-modifying anti-rheumatic drug; GI, gastrointestinal; LFTs, liver function tests; TPMT, thiopurine methyltransferase; TNFα, tumour necrosis factor alpha.

Data from BSR/BHPR DMARD guidelines.

Joint aspiration

Joint aspiration is done to diagnose the cause of acute mono- or oligoarthritis, in particular to confirm or exclude septic or crystal arthritis (see Table 265.7).

Imaging

Plain radiography

Plain radiography of peripheral joints is useful in well-established disease but may fail to detect abnormalities early in its course (see

Table 265.6 Urinary dipstick findings in rheumatological disease

Abnormality	Significance in rheumatological disease	Action	Comment
RBC	Important clue for glomerulonephritis, SLE, and vasculitis but other causes (e.g. renal, urological) need to be excluded	Address the cause	In **glomerular disease** (usually RBC casts, proteinuria, and dysmorphic RBCs) Microscopic haematuria in suspected vasculitis or glomerulonephritis with or without renal impairment (urea and electrolytes can be normal) Fresh urine sample for microscopy and cytology should be sent to see RBC casts in glomerulonephritis In females, think of period
WBC	Found in inflammation or infection	If infection is present, treat	
Nitrite positive	Organism : urinary infection	To treat	In patients on DMARDs or biologics, the infection must be treated aggressively May need to withhold biologics temporarily
Protein	Urine dipstick will primarily detect albumin and may not detect low concentrations of gamma globulins or Bence Jones proteins	Increase in urinary **protein** is an indication of kidney involvement Further evaluation of urinary proteinuria can done via either 24-hour urinary protein excretion or spot-urine protein:creatinine ratio, which allows quantification	Persistent proteinuria may be due to primary glomerular disease (glomerulonephritis), secondary glomerular disease (e.g. SLE, drugs (e.g. NSAIDs, penicillamine, gold, ACE-I)), or some other, general cause
Glucose	Urine dipstick is positive for DM	If diabetic, then treat	Can be positive in tubular renal acidosis in patient with Sjögren's syndrome

Abbreviations: ACE-I, angiotensin-converting enzyme inhibitor; DM, diabetes mellitus; DMARDs, disease-modifying anti-rheumatic drugs; NSAIDs, non-steroidal anti-inflammatory drugs; SLE, systemic lupus erythematosus, RBC, red blood cell; WBC, white blood cell.

Table 265.8). Findings on spinal radiography are summarized in Table 265.9, and those on chest radiography in Table 265.10. The diagnostic yield of high-resolution CT (HRCT) of the chest is substantially greater than that of chest radiography; HRCT should be considered if interstitial lung disease is suspected but the chest X-ray is normal.

Musculoskeletal ultrasonography

Ultrasonography can detect early inflammatory arthritis and can also detect erosions before they are evident on plain radiographs. Ultrasonography is also used to detect joint effusion and tendon rupture, and can guide joint aspiration or injection.

Table 265.7 Findings on joint aspiration in acute arthritis

Synovial fluid	Colour	Cell	Comments
Normal	Transparent, straw colour	Contains <200 cells/mm³	
Inflammatory	Slight turbid	Count can go up >2000 leucocytes/mm³	Inflammatory arthritis, SLE, etc.
Septic	Turbid	>100 000 leucocytes/mm³	In suspected septic joint, urgent aspiration and immediate Gram staining is essential Even few drops of fluid are adequate for WCC (count, differential), Gram staining, culture, and sensitivity and, if an adequate amount of fluid is available, then crystals Negative joint aspiration does not rule out septic arthritis; the entire clinical picture needs to be taken into consideration In suspected septic arthritis, consider routine FBC, renal function tests, liver function tests, CRP level, blood culture, synovial fluid culture, and urine culture Immunosuppression, steroid therapy, and diabetes are risk factors for septic arthritis
Crystal arthropathy	Can be slightly turbid	20 000–50 000 leucocytes/mm³	**Monosodium urate crystals** cause gout (monosodium urate crystals are negatively birefringent, needle-shaped crystals seen in polarized microscopy) **Calcium pyrophosphate dihydrate crystals** are associated with pseudogout, and the deposition of these crystals may be superimposed on osteoarthritis X-ray may show chondrocalcinosis in pseudogout Other causes are **calcium oxalate crystals** (if the patient is on dialysis) and **calcium phosphate crystals** (Milwaukee shoulder/knee) Important reminder: crystals and infection can coexist
Haemorrhagic synovial fluid	Bloody, fluid Haematocrit >10% will appear grossly bloody	Predominantly RBC	Can be due to trauma, bleeding disorder, or pigmented villonodular synovitis

Abbreviations: FBC, full blood count, RBC, red blood cell; WCC, white-cell count.

Table 265.8 Findings on peripheral-joint radiography

Disease	Value of peripheral-joint radiography	Finding	Comment
Early inflammatory arthritis	May be uninformative in early disease	May show soft-tissue swelling and/or periarticular osteoporosis	High-frequency ultrasound or MRI may be more useful
Established rheumatoid arthritis or other inflammatory arthritis	Evidence of joint damage and structural deformity	In established rheumatoid arthritis, may show loss of cartilage, and bone erosion In a rheumatoid arthritis hand, MCP joints and PIP joints are more affected than DIP joints Erosion suggests late-stage disease, but erosion can be seen in other conditions (e.g. psoriatic arthritis, gout) In connective tissue disease, a peripheral-joint X-ray will show a non-erosive arthropathy	High-frequency ultrasound may be still of value for active disease
Osteoarthritis	Usually the first-line investigation	A plain X-ray may reveal loss of joint space, subchondral sclerosis, and cyst and osteophyte formation	In osteoarthritis of the hand, DIP joints are more affected than PIP joints; in the thumb, the carpometacarpal joint is commonly affected Other joints (e.g. hip, knee (medial compartment common), spine) may also be affected
Crystal arthropathy	Some value	In gout, soft-tissue swelling or punched-out erosion may be seen Nodular deposits of calcium urate can occur in the synovium In calcium pyrophosphate dihydrate crystal deposition (pseudogout), cartilage or meniscal calcification can be seen, especially in the knee	Joint aspiration for the presence of crystals is the gold-standard investigation
Osteoporosis	Limited value	A plain X-ray may show diffuse osteopenia with cortical thinning	FRAX score and DEXA scan
Osteomalacia	Value in advanced stages	A plain X-ray may show Looser zones (pseudofractures)	Looser zones most commonly seen in the medial femoral neck, the axillary border of scapula, the ribs, and the pubic rami Rare in the Western world
Paget's disease	Diagnostic value	A plain X-ray may show enlarged, sclerotic bones with a trabecular pattern	Stress fracture Bone softening Sarcomatous changes (1%) may occur

Abbreviations: DIP, distal interphalangeal; MCP, metacarpophalangeal; PIP, proximal interphalangeal.

CT

CT is superior to plain radiography in assessing disorders of the bone cortex (e.g. cortical fractures or metastases). It can detect fractures of the cervical spine, the hip, the wrist, and the foot when these are not evident on plain radiographs.

MRI

MRI shows non-calcified tissues that cannot be assessed by plain radiography or CT. Thus, it can demonstrate abnormalities present in synovium, tendons, and muscles and which may precede joint involvement. For example, in early RA, pre-erosive changes like bone marrow oedema, synovitis, and tendinosis can be seen on MRI.

In suspected myopathy or myositis, MRI can be used to identify muscle inflammation and the best site for biopsy.

Dual X-ray absorptiometry

Dual X-ray absorptiometry (also called 'DEXA scan') measures bone mineral density (BMD) and is used to confirm or refute a diagnosis of osteoporosis and predict the fracture risk in patients with radiographic osteopenia or vertebral deformity.

Table 265.9 Findings on spinal radiography

Disease	Value of spinal X-ray	Findings	Comment
Spondyloarthropathy-like ankylosing spondylitis	Useful	An X-ray of sacroiliac joint may pick up early or advanced sacroiliitis In ankylosing spondylitis, an X-ray might show 'squaring of endplates', Romanus lesions, osteopenia, calcification, and, in late stages, bamboo spine	MRI may be useful early in diagnosis (other causes of sacroiliitis are inflammatory bowel disease, psoriatic spondyloarthropathy, and Reiter's syndrome)
Degenerative spinal disease	Limited value	Presence of osteophytes Lower cervical/lumbar findings	MRI is useful for radiculopathy
Osteoporosis	Limited value	X-ray of spine in an osteoporotic individual may show a wedge fracture Fracture to site previously may result in kyphosis of the spine	FRAX score and DEXA scan

Table 265.10 Findings on chest radiography

Disease	Possible findings	Comment
Rheumatoid arthritis	Rheumatoid nodules (typically peripheral location in lower zones) Interstitial lung disease Pleural effusion (usually unilateral) Pneumonitis as complication of methotrexate therapy	Chest X-ray should be done as a baseline before methotrexate started
SLE	Pleural effusion (often bilateral) Acute pneumonitis Interstitial lung disease Pericardial effusion (enlarged cardiac silhouette)	SLE may present with pulmonary disease
Ankylosing spondylitis	Apical fibrosis	Apical fibrosis also seen in tuberculosis, in sarcoidosis, and after radiotherapy
Systemic sclerosis	Interstitial lung disease Oesophageal dilatation	Pulmonary involvement occurs in >80% of patients Echocardiography is needed to screen for pulmonary hypertension
GPA (formerly Wegener's granulomatosis)	Nodules that may be cavitary Lobar or segmental atelectasis Pleural opacities	Upper respiratory tract involvement (nasal, sinus, or ear) occurs in 90% of patients with GPA

Abbreviations: GPA, granulomatosis with polyangiitis; SLE, systemic lupus erythematosus.

The T-score compares individual results to those in a young population (aged 20–30) of the same gender and ethnic background, while the Z-score compares individual results to those in an age-matched population. BMD is classified by the WHO as being normal (T-score within one standard deviation (SD) of the BMD of an average 25-year-old) or indicating the presence of osteopenia (T-score between −1 and −2.5 SD), osteoporosis (T-score below −2.5 SD), or established osteoporosis (T-score below −2.5 SD, with one or more fragility fractures). The risk of bone fracture is slightly increased in patients with osteopenia and considerably increased in those with osteoporosis.

Bone scan

A bone scan using technetium-99m-labelled methyl diphosphonate can be useful in the diagnosis of bone metastases, infection, occult fracture, and other bone disorders (e.g. fibrous dysplasia). In Paget's disease, a bone scan may show intense activity but, in sarcomatous change, there may be lower uptake.

PET–CT

PET–CT can be used to diagnose large vessel vasculitis (e.g. Takayasu arteritis). It can also be used to screen for cancer in patients with dermatomyositis and polymyositis.

Echocardiography

Echocardiography can be used to assess for cardiac and aortic involvement in diseases such as SLE, ankylosing spondylitis, and vascular Ehlers–Danlos syndrome. It is also used to screen for pulmonary hypertension complicating diseases such as systemic sclerosis.

Further Reading

Cawston TE. 'Structure and function: Joints and connective tissue', in Warrell DA, Cox TM, and Firth JD, eds, *Oxford Textbook of Medicine* (5th edition), 2010. Oxford University Press.

Doherty M. 'Clinical investigation' in Warrell DA, Cox TM, and Firth JD, eds, *Oxford Textbook of Medicine* (5th edition), 2010. Oxford University Press.

Hochberg MC, Silman AJ, Smolen JS, et al. *Rheumatology* (6th edition), 2014. Mosby.

Russell AS and Ferrarri R. 'Clinical presentation and diagnosis of rheumatic disease', in Warrell DA, Cox TM, and Firth JD, eds, *Oxford Textbook of Medicine* (5th edition), 2010. Oxford University Press.

Michael Doherty

Definition of osteoarthritis

Osteoarthritis (OA) is a disorder of synovial joints and is characterized by the combination of (1) **focal hyaline cartilage loss**, and (2) accompanying subchondral **bone remodelling** and **marginal new bone formation** (osteophyte). It has genetic, constitutional, and environmental risk factors and presents a spectrum of clinical phenotypes and outcomes.

OA commonly affects just one region (e.g. knee OA, hip OA). However, multiple hand interphalangeal joint (IPJ) OA, usually accompanied by posterolateral firm swellings (nodes), is a marker for a tendency towards polyarticular **generalized nodal OA**.

Etiology of OA

OA is a dynamic, metabolically active condition involving all joint tissues. It is regarded as the inherent repair process of synovial joints. A variety of insults may trigger the need to repair, and often this slow but efficient process compensates for the insults, resulting in an anatomically remodelled but functioning asymptomatic joint. However, in some cases, due to overwhelming insult or inefficient repair, the OA process cannot compensate, resulting in pain, disability, and presentation as a patient with clinically relevant OA.

Risk factors vary according to joint site, and differ according to development and progression. For example, high bone mineral density (BMD) is a risk factor for development of hand, knee, and hip OA, but low BMD is a risk factor for more rapid progression of hip and knee OA. There are three main categories of risk factors:

- genetic factors: OA shows strong heritability (40%–60% for hand, knee, and hip OA), although the specific associations are currently poorly defined (specific associations, such as COL2A1 mutations, are identified for some rare monogenic disorders causing premature polyarticular OA (e.g. Stickler's syndrome))
- generalized, constitutional factors, such as age, obesity, female gender, bone density, and low muscle strength
- localized mechanical factors that cause abnormal joint loading, such as abnormalities of joint shape (dysplasia) or alignment; trauma; meniscectomy; instability; and occupational/recreational overloading

Some factors (e.g. obesity, muscle function, and occupation) may be modified and thus offer scope for primary, secondary, and tertiary prevention.

Typical and less common symptoms of OA

The two main symptoms of OA are pain and restricted activity and function. The pain is characteristically worse on usage/movement and is relieved by rest, typically being worst at the end of the day and best in the morning. The joint may feel stiff in the morning or after rest ('gelling') but, unlike inflammatory joint pain, it quickly 'loosens up' on moving. Pain is usually restricted to just one or a few joints. It is often variable, with 'good days' and 'bad days', and any progression is slow over many months or years.
Restricted activity and function often reflects pain severity but may be the presenting symptom, even in the absence of marked pain. The severity of pain and functional impairment are greatly influenced by psychosocial factors (anxiety, depression), daily activity requirements, and the presence of comorbidity.

Cartilage changes in OA facilitate crystal deposition, so superimposed symptoms of **acute crystal synovitis** are not uncommon (especially at the knee, for calcium pyrophosphate dihydrate crystal deposition disease, and at peripheral lower and upper limb joints in gout).

Less common symptoms are **mechanical locking** and **rapid progression** of hip (less commonly, knee) symptoms.

Demographics of OA

OA has a higher prevalence than that of all other arthropathies considered together. Structural OA is frequently asymptomatic, so radiographic OA is always more prevalent than symptomatic OA. In general:

- OA increases markedly with age (especially after 40) and is more common in women than men at all sites other than the hip (equal prevalence)
- the prevalence is highest for hand OA, then knee OA, and then hip OA, with other joints (e.g. feet, shoulders, elbows) affected less commonly
- although hand OA is most prevalent, it only occasionally causes significant disability, and symptomatic knee and hip OA present the major burden
- knee OA alone is the single most common cause of disability in those aged over 65, and knee and hip OA together affect >20% of the older population

With the increasing proportion of older people, large-joint OA will become an even more important healthcare problem.

Natural history of OA, and complications

The natural history of OA, as well as its complications, varies according to joint site.

Natural history of hip OA

Symptomatic hip OA commonly progresses, eventually requiring surgery. **Superior pole** OA (i.e. maximal cartilage narrowing superiorly) is the usual pattern in men and usually progresses more rapidly, with superolateral femoral head migration, than other patterns. **Medial** and **axial** hip OA, mainly restricted to women, often associate with nodal OA and have a better prognosis.

Natural history of knee OA

Symptoms are often intermittent and sometimes improve and the correlation between clinical outcome and radiographic change is less strong than at the hip. In those that worsen, clinical progression is variable but is usually only slowly progressive and the transition from mild to severe typically takes many years.

Natural history of hand OA

The overall prognosis is good. Nodal hand OA typically improves symptomatically once nodes are fully developed, often after several years. The exception is thumb-base involvement (first carpometacarpal joint and trapezioscaphoid joint), which sometimes progresses to require surgery.

Complications of OA

Complications of OA include poorly controlled pain, joint restriction, and deformity.

Approach to diagnosing OA

The diagnosis of OA is essentially clinical and depends on a full history and examination. Patients are usually over age 40 and have predominantly usage-related or 'mechanical' (non-inflammatory) symptoms (see 'Etiology of OA') in one or a few joints. More widespread signs of asymptomatic OA are commonly present in older patients. The main findings are those of joint damage, which may include:

- restricted movement, with or without pain
- bony joint enlargement
- coarse, palpable crepitus, sometimes also audible, on movement (mainly large joints)
- weakness and wasting of muscles acting over the joint
- deformity (instability is uncommon, due to capsular thickening)
- varying degrees of inflammation (effusion, increased warmth)

There may be joint-line tenderness, but periarticular tenderness is also common with knee and hip OA.

Diagnosing hip OA

Pain from hip OA is typically felt maximally deep in the anterior groin but may be referred over a wide area including the lateral thigh and buttock, anterior thigh, knee, and as far down as the ankle. Pain is mainly a problem when walking but can occur at rest and disturb sleep. The gait is typically an antalgic limp, with less time spent weight bearing on the arthritic side. The usual first sign is painful restriction of internal rotation with the hip flexed, although, with advanced OA, there may be more widespread restriction, a fixed flexion and external rotation deformity, and leg length narrowing due to marked cartilage and bone attrition.

Diagnosing knee OA

Knee OA is usually bilateral and symmetrical, mainly targeting the medial tibiofemoral and patellofemoral compartments. Pain is usually well localized to the affected compartment, and quadriceps weakness, with frequent 'giving way', is common. Patellofemoral OA causes localized anterior knee pain which is worse on inclines or stairs, particularly when going down. Examination may reveal restricted flexion/extension, coarse crepitus, joint-line tenderness (with or without periarticular tenderness, especially over the upper medial tibia region), and small-to-moderate knee effusions. With advanced OA, there may be bony swelling (femoral condyles, tibial plateaux), flexion and varus (bow-legged deformity), or, less commonly, valgus (knock-knee deformity).

Diagnosing nodal hand OA

Nodal hand OA is a polyarticular arthropathy of hand IPJs and is characterized by multiple Heberden's nodes (see Figure 266.1) and Bouchard's nodes (proximal IPJs), mainly affecting women and often with a family history. It causes intermittent pain and stiffness and is well localized to the involved joints; it commonly starts around menopause but becomes less symptomatic once nodes are fully developed. Typical end-stage deformity is lateral (ulnar/radial) deviation without instability. Thumb-base OA may cause more persistent, aching pain which is maximal at the thumb base but often radiates distally up the thumb and proximally to the wrist. Advanced cases may show

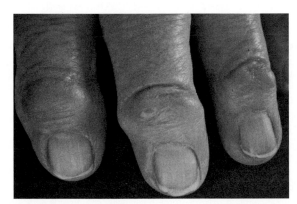

Figure 266.1 Heberden's nodes: posterolateral hard swellings of distal interphalangeal joints.

Reproduced with permission from Watts et al. *Oxford Textbook of Rheumatology*, fourth edition, Oxford University Press, Oxford, UK, Copyright © 2013.

thumb-base 'squaring' caused by subluxation, osteophyte, and bone remodelling.

Other diagnoses that should be considered

OA and **gout** co-associate, so gout should be considered in patients with OA if they develop typical acute attacks of crystal synovitis, if they have more pronounced symptoms and signs of joint inflammation, or if their established finger nodes become more swollen and symptomatic in older age. Other types of **inflammatory arthritis** (e.g. rheumatoid arthritis, seronegative spondyloarthritis) can be distinguished usually by pronounced early morning and inactivity stiffness, involvement of several or multiple joints, and frequent systemic upset. However, some cases of OA may have a lesser inflammatory component, and combined synchronous symptoms in hands and other sites. The presence of predominantly soft tissue rather than bony swelling and high inflammatory markers in the blood are more suggestive of inflammatory arthritis.

In patients with apparently **young-onset OA** (occurring at age <45) affecting just one or a few joints, the usual explanation is overt prior trauma (e.g. meniscectomy, subchondral fracture). However, in younger people with oligo- or polyarticular 'OA', especially with an atypical distribution, the following may need consideration:

- epiphyseal or spondylo-epiphyseal dysplasia
- haemochromatosis (predilection for hips, knees, carpus, metacarpophalangeal joints, sometimes with chondrocalcinosis)
- acromegaly (OA signs, often with normal or increased range of movement)
- osteonecrosis (hips, shoulders, knees, elbows)

Calcium crystals, notably calcium pyrophosphate and basic calcium phosphates such as apatite, commonly occur in cartilage and synovial fluid of OA joints. **OA with calcium pyrophosphate deposition** predominates in older people and may show an atypical distribution and more inflammatory features, as well as superimposed acute calcium pyrophosphate crystal arthritis.

Apatite-associated destructive arthritis

Apatite-associated destructive arthritis occurs in elderly women, is almost totally confined to the hips, shoulders (Milwaukee shoulder), and knees, and has a poor outcome. It typically presents as painful, rapidly progressive OA with large cool effusions, progressive instability, and atrophic radiographic changes with marked cartilage and bone attrition. Although modest amounts of apatite are present in most OA joints, large amounts occur in this condition.

'Gold-standard' diagnostic test

For OA, the gold-standard diagnostic test is a good clinical assessment. Asymptomatic radiographic OA is very common, and only careful enquiry and examination can determine the cause of pain. Generally, imaging and special investigations are not required, as they do not confirm the clinical diagnosis or alter decision-making.

Acceptable diagnostic alternatives to the gold standard

With good clinical assessment, the diagnosis of OA should be clear. If there is diagnostic uncertainty in a patient with significant or progressive symptoms in a large joint, then imaging (e.g. radiographs, MRI) and/or arthroscopy may be helpful in confirming focal cartilage fibrillation/loss and in excluding other causes of joint pain (e.g. internal derangement, inflammatory arthritis).

Other relevant investigations

Other relevant investigations for OA include:

- a full clinical assessment, including BMI and blood pressure, with screening for common comorbidities
- a plain radiograph; OA changes include focal loss of joint space; marginal osteophytes; subchondral sclerosis; subchondral 'cysts'; and small osteochondral 'loose' bodies (Figure 266.2)

CHAPTER 266 **Osteoarthritis**

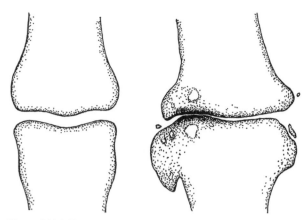

Figure 266.2 Diagram of a normal (left) and an osteoarthritic (right) joint, showing focal joint-space narrowing, adjacent subchondral sclerosis, marginal osteophyte, cysts, and osteochondral bodies typical of osteoarthritis.
With permission from MD.

- synovial fluid analysis, for patients with more inflammatory-component or progressive OA; OA synovial fluid is usually clear, viscous, and low in volume; calcium pyrophosphate crystals may be identified by polarized light microscopy
- OA causes no abnormality in routine blood tests (e.g. full blood count, erythrocyte sedimentation rate, C-reactive protein, autoimmune profile) but blood tests may be helpful to screen for comorbidities, such as chronic renal impairment, prior to selection of treatment

Prognosis, and how to estimate it

Risk factors for OA progression vary according to joint site:

- for hip OA: superior pole involvement on radiographs, high BMI, low BMD, and chondrocalcinosis
- for knee OA: synovial fluid calcium pyrophosphate crystals, varus, instability, and high BMI
- for hand OA: radiographic subchondral erosions (so-called erosive OA), IPJ instability, thumb-base involvement

Not all OA patients worsen and many improve symptomatically (especially those with hand and knee OA). Rapidly progressive joint damage is uncommon in OA. However, if OA is not treated adequately, the quality of a patient's life can significantly deteriorate from pain and loss of mobility, with negative effects on activities and physical and mental health.

Treatment and its effectiveness

Objectives of management

The accepted objectives of management in OA are:

- to educate the patient and provide access to information about OA and its treatment
- to control pain
- to optimize function and reduce participation restriction
- to beneficially modify the OA process

Management principles

Guidelines for OA concur in recommending the following principles:

- non-pharmacological measures should be central to the management plan of any patient with OA
- pharmacological agents are mainly adjunctive, optional treatments
- management of a patient with OA needs to be **individualized and patient centred**; there is no algorithm that is applicable to all patients, and **a holistic approach is essential**
- although research evidence often examines monotherapy, **a package of combined therapies** is used successfully in clinical practice; although the individual effect of each component may

be small, the combined effects of the whole programme may be clinically significant

The National Institute for Health and Clinical Excellence (NICE) examined all three major forms of evidence relating to OA management (research evidence, expert opinion and experience, and patient opinion and acceptability) and, additionally, considered cost-effectiveness estimations. They found that the data reinforced the concept that key factors to be taken into account when treating individual patients include:

- the patient's perceptions and knowledge of OA and its treatment
- balancing the efficacy and side effects of appropriate evidence-based interventions
- the costs, availability, and logistics of treatment delivery
- the presence of comorbid disease, and its treatment
- the treatments and coping strategies already tried by the patient
- the patient's daily activity requirements and work and recreational aspirations

Core treatment for OA

NICE concluded that the following core non-pharmacological measures should be considered for all patients with OA (Figure 266.3):

- access to information about OA and its treatment: this can be provided to the patient in a variety of ways, is completely safe, and can reduce pain and disability in the long term
- weight loss, if the patient is overweight or obese: this reduces the risk of progression and further incident OA, improves functioning, and may reduce pain and low affect in the long term
- local muscle-strengthening exercise and aerobic fitness training: these act in different ways to reduce pain and disability in large-joint OA; initial instruction and subsequent reinforcement by a physiotherapist is beneficial

There is good research evidence to support these lifestyle changes, all of which are safe, increase self-efficacy, and may avoid, or reduce, the requirement for drug therapy. Unfortunately, undue emphasis on short-term symptomatic treatments such as NSAIDs and coxibs may deflect attention from these more important long-term measures.

Initial analgesics to consider

The following two agents are can provide simple and safe analgesia and are recommended to be considered first for pain relief of peripheral joint OA (e.g. OA in the hands and/or knees):

- paracetamol: in view of its efficacy, safety, and cost effectiveness, paracetamol is the preferred oral analgesic for symptomatic OA
- topical NSAIDs (usually applied three times daily over the area of pain); these are safe, very popular with patients, and, when directly compared to the equivalent oral NSAID, may give equal analgesic benefit, with many fewer adverse events; since topical NSAIDs vary considerably with respect to formulation, additives, and carrier/delivery systems, the evidence for each type needs to be assessed separately

Additional non-surgical treatments to consider

The addition of other systemic or local pharmacological agents and physical treatments for OA should be considered, depending on individual patient factors. The following are recommended for consideration, in no specific hierarchical order:

- topical capsaicin
- oral NSAIDs/coxibs
- mild- to moderate-strength opioids
- intra-articular long-acting corticosteroids
- reduction of adverse biomechanical measures

Topical capsaicin

Topical capsaicin (0.025%, three times daily) can provide very safe analgesia and is especially suited to hand and knee OA. Effectiveness should be judged after 2 weeks of daily application. Any initial burning sensations usually wear off after the first few days.

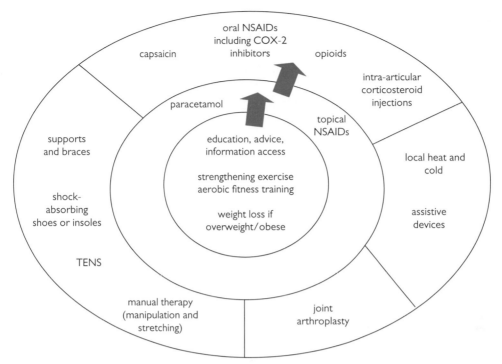

Figure 266.3 Summary of NICE treatment recommendations.

National Guideline Centre (2014) Osteoarthritis: Care and management in adults, Clinical guideline 177.

Published by the National Guideline Centre at The Royal College of Physicians, 11 St Andrews Place, Regent's Park, London, NW11 4LE.

Copyright © NGC. Reproduced by permission.

Oral NSAIDs/coxibs

The magnitude of benefit from oral NSAIDs in OA is usually modest and at a similar or slightly higher level to paracetamol or topical NSAIDs. However, they have potential for serious toxicity from gut bleeding/perforation, renal impairment, cardiovascular safety, and drug interactions. NICE guidance recommends these be considered only after topical NSAIDs and paracetamol have been unsuccessful and after careful consideration of potential risk factors for toxicity. If used, they should be co-prescribed with a proton-pump inhibitor. These drugs are contraindicated in many older patients with OA.

Mild- to moderate-strength opioids

Mild- to moderate-strength opioids may be used alone but may also achieve additive symptomatic benefit for OA patients when combined with paracetamol. Unfortunately, constipation and CNS side effects are common in the older OA population and often limit the use of these drugs.

Intra-articular long-acting corticosteroids

The use of intra-articular long-acting corticosteroids is an excellent and safe treatment for patients with OA of the knee, thumb base, and other joints (ultrasound guidance is recommended for hip OA). Controlled studies confirm an often marked and rapid reduction in pain (within 24–48 hours), although it is usually short-lived (less than 6 weeks). Steroid injection is therefore best reserved to obtain temporary control of moderate-to-severe pain, for example to enable a patient to participate in a special event such as a holiday or wedding.

Reduction of adverse biomechanical measures

Reduction of adverse biomechanical measures, such as via pacing of activities, use of appropriate footwear (e.g. footwear with a thick, soft sole, no raised heel, and a broad forefoot), can help prevent excessive loading of the OA joint. Local assistive devices (e.g. a walking stick, other walking aids, hinged knee braces, wedged insoles) are also safe options to consider.

Joint surgery

At present, no drug has a licence for disease modification in OA. Suitable patients who fail to respond to conservative measures should be referred for a surgical opinion. For patients with severe, disabling hip or knee OA, total hip arthroplasty and total knee arthroplasty are acknowledged as appropriate and reliable interventions to control pain, restore function, and improve quality of life. Evidence for their efficacy is based on uncontrolled, observational studies and several large cohort studies, but also on a wealth of expert and patient experience. Over 95% of joint replacements continue to function well into the second decade after surgery, and most provide lifelong, pain-free function. However, around one in five patients are not satisfied with their replacement, and a minority obtains little or no pain relief following this procedure. Importantly, referral should be made before there is prolonged and established functional limitation and severe pain, since these often compromise a good outcome from surgery. Age and comorbidity (e.g. obesity, smoking status) are not reasons to defer referral for a surgical opinion. Surgery may also be useful for refractory thumb-base OA (simple trapeziectomy) and when OA in other joints is resistant to medical treatments.

Further Reading

Felson DT. Osteoarthritis of the knee. *N Engl J Med* 2006; 354: 841–8.
Glyn-Jones S, Palmer AJR, Agricola R, et al. Osteoarthritis. *Lancet* 2015; 386: 376–87.
National Institute for Health and Care Excellence. *Osteoarthritis: The Care and Management of Osteoarthritis in Adults*. 2008. Available at http://www.nice.org.uk/CG059 (accessed 19 Jul 2017).

267 Rheumatoid arthritis

Karim Raza, Caroline Cardy, and Elizabeth Justice

Definition of rheumatoid arthritis

Rheumatoid arthritis (RA) is a chronic systemic inflammatory disorder. It is characterized by inflammation of the synovium with consequent cartilage and bone destruction. Extra-articular manifestations are not uncommon.

Symptoms of RA

Joint inflammation is the characteristic feature. Patients typically present with symmetrical joint pain and swelling of the small joints of the hands (metacarpophalangeal (MCP), proximal interphalangeal (PIP), and wrist; see Figure 267.1) and feet (metatarsophalangeal). However, larger joints (e.g. ankle, knee, and elbow) are frequently involved and, in very early disease, asymmetric joint involvement is not unusual. Early morning stiffness of at least an hour is usual. Joint symptoms may improve with gentle activity. Constitutional systems such as fatigue are common. Extra-articular manifestations are summarized in Table 267.1. They are generally associated with long-standing disease, being relatively rare at presentation.

Demographics of RA

The worldwide prevalence of RA is 0.5%–1.0%. It is two to three times more common in females than males. It affects all ethnic groups, although an increased prevalence has been found in certain Native American populations. Patients can present at any age, with a peak incidence at 35–50 years.

Etiology of RA

In established RA, the inflamed synovium consists of a network of leukocytes (T-cells, B-cells, and macrophages) and stromal cells (fibroblasts). Cytokine and cell-contact-dependent interactions drive the persistence of inflammation, with fibroblasts playing a central role in leukocyte retention and survival. Synovial fibroblasts and macrophages drive joint destruction. Although mechanisms underlying disease persistence are reasonably well defined, those causing the disease remain elusive.

Susceptibility to RA is strongly associated with certain HLA-DRB1 alleles, which encode DR beta 1 molecules with a conserved amino acid sequence (the shared epitope) in the third hypervariable region. An additional important and non-HLA linked risk factor is a single nucleotide polymorphism in the gene encoding the protein tyrosine phosphatase non-receptor 22 (PTPN22). These genetic risk factors define a subgroup of RA which is characterized by the presence of anti-citrullinated protein/peptide antibodies (ACPAs). Smoking, the best defined environmental risk factor for RA, also associates with ACPA-positive disease, supporting the concept that ACPA-positive and ACPA-negative RA are discrete subsets with etiological differences.

Natural history of RA, and complications

RA is a chronic progressive condition. It typically follows a relapsing and remitting course, with patients experiencing less symptomatic periods followed by disease flares. It is a heterogeneous condition and can range from mild to severe disease. Untreated, the presence of persistent joint synovial inflammation damages the underlying cartilage and bone resulting in joint deformity. Inflammation of the synovial lining of tendon sheaths can result in tendon damage and rupture. Classic deformities in the hands and feet may develop, such as ulnar deviation of the MCP joints, swan neck and Boutonniere deformities of the fingers, and hammer toes (see Figure 267.1). Muscle atrophy, often due to disuse, is common. Functional impairment with limitation of activities of daily living is frequent. Depression is a common sequel.

Abnormal joint structure predisposes RA patients to both secondary osteoarthritis and joint infection. Septic arthritis is a serious complication with a high mortality, and diagnosis requires a high degree of clinical suspicion. RA patients are also at increased risk of osteoporosis due to a combination of chronic systemic inflammation, immobility, and corticosteroid use.

Cervical spine involvement can be seen but is uncommon. Joint and ligament destruction of the upper cervical spine can result in

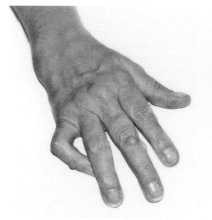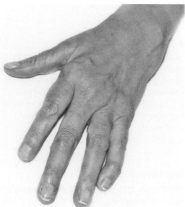

Figure 267.1 Hands of a patient with rheumatoid arthritis. Synovitis of the wrists and metacarpophalangeal joints is apparent. Rheumatoid nodules (present here over the right middle finger proximal interphalangeal joint) and fixed deformity (present here at the right little finger proximal interphalangeal joint) are unusual in early disease. Please see colour plate section.

Table 267.1 Extra-articular manifestations of rheumatoid arthritis

Site	Manifestation
Cutaneous	Subcutaneous nodules
	Vasculitis (palpable purpura, ulcers)
Ocular	Episcleritis
	Scleritis
	Keratoconjunctivitis sicca
Pulmonary	Interstitial lung disease
	Pleural effusion
	Pulmonary nodules
	Bronchiolitis obliterans
Cardiac	Ischaemic heart disease
	Pericarditis
	Myocarditis
	Coronary vasculitis
Neurological	Entrapment neuropathies (e.g. carpal tunnel syndrome)
	Peripheral neuropathy
	Mononeuritis multiplex
	Cervical myelopathy
Haematological	Felty's syndrome (rheumatoid arthritis, splenomegaly, leukopenia)

atlantoaxial instability and subluxation. This in turn may result in impingement of the spinal cord (cervical myelopathy), presenting a neurosurgical emergency.

Pulmonary involvement is one of the most frequent extra-articular manifestations of RA. Clinically significant interstitial lung disease occurs in around 5%–10% of patients, although radiographic evidence of disease is more common. Systemic vasculitis is probably the most serious extra-articular complication of RA. It appears to be on the decline, with the current incidence estimated at two to three patients per million per year. Typical features include fever, weight loss, cutaneous ulceration, and mononeuritis multiplex. Clinically significant involvement of the endocardium, myocardium, and pericardium are rare but there is a significantly increased risk of cardiovascular disease, explaining, in large part, the reduced life expectancy associated with RA.

Approach to diagnosing the disease

Classification criteria exist to identify cases of RA for inclusion in clinical studies. The 1987 American College of Rheumatology criteria (Table 267.2) were developed using hospital-based populations with long-standing disease (mean disease duration, 7.7 years) and they are of limited use in the early phase of RA. Reliance on these classification criteria to diagnose RA in clinical practice will lead to under-recognition of early disease as erosive change and subcutaneous nodules

Table 267.2 Summary of the 1987 American College of Rheumatology classification criteria for rheumatoid arthritis

1	Morning Stiffness (lasting at least one hour)
2	Swelling (soft tissue/fluid) in at least three joint areas
3	Swelling (soft tissue/fluid) in hand joints (wrist, MCP or PIP joints)
4	Symmetric joint swelling
5	Rheumatoid nodules
6	Positive rheumatoid factor
7	Typical changes of RA (erosions and/or periarticular osteopenia) on plain radiographs of the hand and wrists

Patients must have at least 4 of these 7 criteria. Criteria 1–4 must have been present for at least 6 weeks.

Reproduced with permission from Arnett FC, Edworthy SM, Bloch DA, McShane DJ, Fries JF, Cooper NS, et al., The American Rheumatism Association 1987 revised criteria for the classification of rheumatoid arthritis, *Arthritis & Rheumatology*, Volume 31, Issue 3, pp. 315-324, Copyright © 1988 John Wiley and Sons and American College of Rheumatology.

usually reflect advanced disease, and up to 40% of RA patients are rheumatoid factor (RF) negative at presentation.

Early diagnosis of RA is important, allowing rapid initiation of disease-modifying anti-rheumatic drugs (DMARDs), to reduce progression of radiological damage and loss of function. In 2010, new criteria were developed in a collaboration between the American College of Rheumatology and the European League Against Rheumatism, to facilitate the early identification of RA patients. These criteria consist of four domains (pattern and extent of joint involvement, serology (for both RF and ACPAs), duration of synovitis, and acute phase reactants). These criteria identify patients with RA at an earlier stage of disease than the 1987 criteria although a greater proportion of patients whose disease may resolve without therapy (e.g. patients with post viral arthritis) will fulfil the 2010 criteria as compared with the 1987 criteria. It is however important to appreciate that the 1987 criteria and the 2010 criteria are classification criteria, primarily for research purposes, and formal diagnostic criteria have not been developed for RA.

A major challenge is to predict which patients with early undifferentiated arthritis (UA) will develop RA and which will experience spontaneous remission (~50% of all cases of UA). Predictive models exist which utilize clinical variables related to joint assessment (mostly variants of criteria from the 1987 set) and other variables such as age, sex, C-reactive protein (CRP) levels, and presence of ACPAs to determine the probability of a patient with UA developing RA.

A pragmatic approach to diagnosing RA requires taking a careful history from the patient, eliciting symptoms of an inflammatory arthritis, looking at the pattern of joint involvement and examining the patient for articular and extra-articular features. The duration of the symptoms is important; their presence for at least 6 weeks is predictive of the development of persistent inflammation.

Other diagnoses that should be considered

Non-inflammatory conditions such as osteoarthritis can present with polyarthralgia (pain in five or more joints), but significant synovitis and protracted early morning stiffness are uncommon. There are, however, many conditions which can associate with an inflammatory arthritis and should be considered in the differential diagnosis of RA.

Reactive arthritis

An infective antecedent can point to a reactive etiology.

Reactive arthritis is usually oligoarticular and asymmetric and often affects the large joints of the lower limbs. Pain and stiffness of the lower back and sacroiliac regions is common. Other symptoms may include urethritis and conjunctivitis. Infections are often of the gastrointestinal (*Salmonella* spp., *Shigella* spp., and *Yersinia* spp.) or genitourinary (*Chlamydia trachomatis* and *Neisseria gonorrhoea*) tracts. The articular symptoms usually resolve within 6 months and may require NSAIDs and intra-articular steroids in the short term. Rarely (<10% of cases), symptoms persist and DMARDs may be warranted.

Several viral infections (e.g. parvovirus B19) can be associated with an inflammatory arthritis. In these cases, the pattern of synovitis is more consistent with RA (with a symmetric inflammatory polyarthritis), although the disease usually resolves within a few months.

Crystal arthritides

Gout results from the intra-articular deposition of monosodium urate crystals. Episodes of arthritis are usually monoarticular (the great toe is most commonly affected) and begin suddenly, often overnight. The joint is very painful, warm, and swollen with overlying erythema. Occasionally, gout can present in an oligo- or polyarticular manner and this can cause particular diagnostic confusion. Pseudogout is caused by the deposition of calcium pyrophosphate dihydrate crystals into joints. The presentation of pseudogout is similar to that of gout, although the knees and wrists are most commonly affected.

Psoriatic arthritis

Psoriatic arthritis (PsA) can present in five distinct ways: asymmetric oligoarthritis, distal interphalangeal arthritis, axial arthritis, arthritis mutilans, and 'rheumatoid-like' disease. No widely accepted diagnostic criteria exist for PsA. **Clas**sification criteria for **p**soriatic **ar**thritis (CASPAR), developed in 2006, require patients to have inflammatory disease of peripheral joints, the spine, or the entheses, together with at least three of the following:

- a personal or family history of psoriasis
- psoriatic nail dystrophy
- RF negativity
- dactylitis (sausage digits)
- juxta-articular new bone formation (excluding osteophytes)

The skin changes can be quite subtle (e.g. the appearance of minor plaques around the scalp and umbilicus).

Ankylosing spondylitis

Approximately 30% of patients with ankylosing spondylitis (AS) will have a peripheral arthritis. The most commonly affected joints are the hips and the shoulders, although more distal joints such as the knees and ankles can be involved. A history of inflammatory back pain, early morning stiffness of the back, and reduced spinal movement, when in a young patient, should alert the clinician to the diagnosis of AS, which is confirmed if sacroiliitis is evident on radiographs.

Connective tissues diseases

Connective tissues diseases (CTDs) such as SLE can present with arthritis alongside other systemic features. The arthritis found in association with SLE usually affects the small peripheral joints and is rarely erosive; in addition, when joint deformity does occur, it is usually due to ligament laxity (termed Jaccoud's arthropathy). CTDs are typically associated with elevated serum levels of antinuclear antibodies.

Polymyalgia rheumatica

In the elderly, RA can be preceded by a polymyalgia rheumatica (PMR)-like onset. The presence of synovitis of the wrist, MCP, and PIP joints and the presence of ACPAs (which should be checked in the presence of synovitis) is predictive of PMR-like onset RA.

'Gold-standard' diagnostic test

There is no gold-standard diagnostic test for RA. Clinically detectable synovitis affecting the small joints of the hands and wrists in a symmetrical pattern in the absence of any other features associated with an alternative diagnosis is the most reliable way to diagnose RA. Identification of serological markers for RA aids the diagnosis. RF (an immunoglobulin molecule that binds to the Fc portion of immunoglobulin G) is routinely measured by ELISA or latex agglutination techniques and has a sensitivity of ~75% and specificity of ~85%. Its specificity is limited because of its detection in other autoimmune conditions such as Sjögren's syndrome, following infections (e.g. hepatitis B and EBV), and in the healthy ageing population. The development of cyclic citrullinated peptides for use in ELISAs has allowed the development of commercially available assays (e.g. the anti-CCP2 test) for the identification of patients with circulating ACPAs. The presence of anti-CCP2 has an extremely high specificity for RA (~95%), with a sensitivity approaching that of RF. Anti-CCP2 antibody testing combined with RF has a particularly high specificity (~98%) for RA.

Other relevant investigations

Blood tests

Measurements of the full blood count, renal function, and liver function are essential. Anaemia may be the consequence of chronic disease, and renal impairment can be seen as a consequence of therapy (e.g. with NSAIDs). Furthermore, many DMARDs affect these parameters, and renal impairment is associated with an increased risk of toxicity associated with several DMARDs (e.g. methotrexate). Consequently, measurement before and during therapy is required. Inflammatory markers (e.g. erythrocyte sedimentation rate (ESR) and CRP levels) are helpful in assessing the extent of disease activity and form a component of the widely used Disease Activity Score (DAS; see 'Treatment and its effectiveness'). Antinuclear antibodies should be checked if a connective tissue disease is suspected.

Urinalysis

Urinalysis can be useful to detect proteinuria, casts, and red cells, all of which may point to a nephritis associated with a CTD.

Synovial fluid analysis

Synovial fluid analysis should be carried out if the diagnosis is uncertain and fluid is available, particularly if a septic arthritis is suspected. A cell count on the fluid can identify if the process is inflammatory (>1000 white blood cells/mm³), and polarized microscopy allows the identification of crystals.

Imaging

Plain radiographs

Plain radiographs of the hands and feet should usually be performed in patients with a symmetrical inflammatory arthritis. Radiographic features of RA include periarticular osteopenia, joint space narrowing, and erosive change. The latter usually occurs after several years of the disease; however erosions are occasionally evident within the first year of symptoms, and the initial radiographs serve as a baseline for comparison with future films.

Ultrasound

There is increasing interest in the ability of ultrasound to detect and quantify synovitis and to detect early erosive change not evident on plain radiographs. Ultrasound detection of synovitis in clinically uninvolved joints may be useful in identifying patients who present with joint pain and features suggestive of inflammation (e.g. prolonged early morning stiffness) but without clinically apparent synovitis.

MRI

As with ultrasound, MRI can be used to detect and quantify synovitis. Bone marrow oedema (which may precede erosive change) and early erosions can also be visualized. MRI is not used routinely in a clinical setting and is less practical than ultrasound for imaging large numbers of joints.

Prognosis and how to estimate it

RA causes joint destruction and functional impairment. About a third of patients stop working within 5 years of diagnosis. In addition, life expectancy is reduced (by ~10 years); accelerated cardiovascular disease is an important cause of this. Seropositivity (for RF and, in particular, ACPAs) and high disease activity at presentation are markers of worse articular outcomes. The early control of disease activity is associated with improved outcomes, and delays in diagnosis or the commencement of DMARDs are associated with worse prognosis.

Treatment and its effectiveness

DMARD therapy should be initiated as soon as a diagnosis of RA is made. Methotrexate is the DMARD of choice for initial management and should be used unless there are specific contraindications (e.g. pregnancy is planned in the near future, pulmonary fibrosis is present). Alternative DMARDs include sulfasalazine, hydroxychloroquine, and leflunomide. There is evidence that a combination of DMARDs may be more effective than DMARD monotherapy in the initial management of RA, and some national guidelines advocate this approach. The time from the initiation of DMARDs to an effect being apparent is typically 8 weeks. Approaches to control synovitis in the interim include steroids (which can be administered orally, intramuscularly or intra-articularly); NSAIDs can also be helpful. The aim of therapy is to induce disease remission, and DMARD treatment should be escalated to achieve this. Disease activity should be monitored using the DAS28 score (which incorporates measures of clinically apparent joint swelling and tenderness in 28 predefined joints; the patient's perspective on the extent and impact of their inflammatory arthritis; and the ESR or CRP).

If disease cannot be adequately controlled with oral conventional synthetic DMARDs, biologic drugs or targeted synthetic DMARDs (e.g. Janus kinase (JAK) inhibitors) should be used. Potential biologic agents include those that target tumour necrosis factor alpha (e.g. etanercept, adalimumab, infliximab, golimumab and certolizumab pegol), interleukin 6 (tocilizumab), B-cells (e.g. rituximab), and T-cell co-stimulation (abatacept). The high cost of these drugs means that regulatory authorities typically restrict their availability to subgroups of patients with difficult-to-control, severe RA.

Attention must be paid to management of the comorbidities that accompany RA, particularly cardiovascular disease. There is evidence that the effective control of synovitis reduces the risk of accelerated cardiovascular disease. However, modifiable cardiovascular risk factors such as smoking, hypertension, and hypercholesterolaemia should be appropriately managed.

Input from clinical nurse specialists, physiotherapists, occupational therapists, and podiatrists is essential and should be sought at an early stage.

Further Reading

McInnes IB and Schett G. The pathogenesis of rheumatoid arthritis. *N Engl J Med* 2011; 365: 2205–19.

National Institute for Health and Clinical Excellence. *Rheumatoid Arthritis: The Management of Rheumatoid Arthritis in Adults*. Available at http://www.nice.org.uk/nicemedia/pdf/cg79niceguideline.pdf (accessed 6 May 2015).

Scott DL, Wolfe F, and Huizinga TW. Rheumatoid arthritis. *Lancet* 2010; 376: 1094–108.

Smolen JS, Aletaha D, and McInnes IB. Rheumatoid arthritis. *Lancet* 2016; 388: 2023–38.

Definition of the disease

Spondyloarthropathies consist of several rheumatic conditions, initially grouped together on the basis of shared clinical features, later reinforced by their strong association with HLA-B27. The distinctive features are axial involvement, including sacroiliac joints, and enthesitis—inflammation at ligament and tendon insertions—together with certain extra-articular manifestations.

The presentation of a patient with combinations of inflammatory spinal pain, peripheral synovitis and/or enthesitis, and typical extra-articular manifestations, often with a family history, is characteristic (Box 268.1).

The principal spondyloarthropathies are:

- ankylosing spondylitis
- reactive arthritis
- psoriatic arthritis
- arthropathy of inflammatory bowel disease (enteropathic arthritis)
- undifferentiated spondyloarthropathy
- juvenile spondyloarthropathy (enthesitis-related arthritis)

Classification criteria have been developed which cover the entire spectrum of spondyloarthropathy. The Amor criteria and the European Spondyloarthropathy Study Group criteria for spondyloarthropathies provide helpful algorithms which can be used to aid diagnosis (Sieper et al., 2009; see Table 268.1 and Box 268.2).

Etiology of the disease

The etiology of spondyloarthropathies is not yet fully understood. A complex interaction between genetic (e.g. HLA-B27) and environmental factors (e.g. infective triggers) is clearly implicated. The role of HLA-B27 has not been resolved. Initial theories postulated that HLA-B27 presented an 'arthritogenic' peptide to (CD8$^+$) T-cells, possibly a bacterial peptide resembling a component of the joint or enthesis, thereby initiating autoimmunity through molecular mimicry. Evidence of involvement of CD8$^+$ T-cells and for autoimmunity has been sparse, and more recent theories take note of atypical features of HLA-B27 such as the ability of HLA-B27 heavy chains to be expressed in unusual forms on the cell surface, and how their inefficient folding and assembly in the endoplasmic reticulum affects cytokine production in antigen-presenting cells.

Table 268.1 Amor criteria for spondyloarthropathy*

Criterion	Points
Clinical symptoms or past history	
Lumbar or dorsal pain during the night, or morning stiffness of lumbar or dorsal spine	1
Asymmetric oligoarthritis	2
Buttock pain • if affecting buttocks alternately	1 2
Sausage-like digit	2
Heel pain, or any other well-defined enthesopathy	2
Iritis	2
Non-gonococcal urethritis or cervicitis accompanying, or within 1 month of, the onset of arthritis	1
Acute diarrhoea accompanying, or within 1 month of, the onset of arthritis	1
Presence or history of psoriasis, balanitis, or inflammatory bowel disease (ulcerative colitis or Crohn's disease)	2
Radiological findings	
Sacroiliitis (Grade >2 if bilateral; Grade >3 if unilateral)	3
Genetic background	
Presence of HLA-B27, or familial history of ankylosing spondylitis, reactive arthritis uveitis, psoriasis, or inflammatory bowel disease	2
Response to treatment	
Good response to NSAIDs within 48 hours, or relapse of pain within 48 hours if NSAIDs discontinued	2

*A patient is considered to have spondyloarthritis if the sum of the points is 6 or more. A total point score of 5 or more is classified as probable spondyloarthritis.

Adapted by permission from BMJ Publishing Group LTD [The assessment of Spondyloarthritis international society (ASAS) handbook: a guide to assess spondyloarthritis, J Sieper M Rudwaleit, X Baraliakos, J Brandt, J Braun, R Burgos-Vargas, M Dougados, K-G Hermann, R Landewe, W Maksymowych and D van der Heijde, Annals of the Rheumatic diseases, 2009;68;ii1-ii44].

Box 268.1 Common characteristics of spondyloarthropathies

- inflammatory spinal pain
- sacroiliitis
- peripheral arthritis (asymmetrical, predominantly lower limb)
- enthesopathy
- dactylitis
- skin lesions (psoriasis, balanitis, keratoderma)
- inflammatory bowel disease
- family history
- HLA-B27 positivity
- eye inflammation: uveitis or conjunctivitis
- urethritis and/or cervicitis; acute diarrhoea and vomiting

Adapted from Watts R, Clunie G, Hall F, Marshall T (2009). Oxford Desk Reference Rheumatology. Oxford University Press, Oxford UK

Box 268.2 European Spondyloarthropathy Study Group criteria

Inflammatory spinal pain **or** synovitis (asymmetrical or predominately lower limbs), **and** one or more of the following:

- positive family history
- psoriasis
- inflammatory bowel disease
- urethritis, cervicitis, or acute diarrhoea within 1 month of the onset of arthritis
- buttock pain alternating between right and left gluteal areas
- enthesopathy
- sacroiliitis

Adapted by permission from BMJ Publishing Group LTD [The assessment of Spondyloarthritis international Society (ASAS) handbook: a guide to assess spondyloarthritis, J Sieper, M Rudwaleit, X Baraliakos, J Brandt, J Braun, R Burgos-Vargas, M Dougados, K-G Hermann, R Landewe, W Maksymowych and D van der Heijde, Annals of the Rheumatic disease, 2009;68;ii1-ii44]

Typical symptoms of the disease

While spondyloarthropathies share common clinical features, each condition has a distinct set of symptoms. However, inflammatory back pain is a central feature, common to all the spondyloarthropathies and the most typical symptom. The term is applied to back or neck pain present most days for more than 3 months (except in reactive arthritis, where it may be acute). The pain, which is insidious in nature, improves with exercise, and worsens or does not improve with rest. Pain occurring at night is consistent, and the age of onset is typically before 40 years.

Ankylosing spondylitis presents with typical symptoms of inflammatory back pain in a young person (often male) and is typically insidious, often leading to diagnosis being delayed for many years. Associated symptoms, requiring careful questioning, include:

- alternating buttock pain
- enthesitis (e.g. heel pain), with plantar fasciitis or Achilles tendonitis
- decreased spinal movements
- fatigue or systemic features
- history of uveitis (painful red eye), inflammatory bowel disease, or psoriasis.

Reactive arthritis is characterized by inflammatory spinal pain and/or peripheral arthritis **within** 4–6 weeks of specific infections, principally bacterial gastroenteritis and genitourinary infection (usually chlamydia). Gastrointestinal symptoms vary in severity according to the triggering infection—severe with shigella, often mild with yersinia—while chlamydia infection is often asymptomatic, although symptoms of urethritis/cervicitis should be sought. Enthesitis is common, and dactylitis (diffuse swelling of a digit) may occur. Extra-articular features include mucocutaneous lesions, such as oral or penile ulcers, and keratoderma blennorrhagica (hyperkeratotic psoriatic lesions on hands and feet), as well as conjunctivitis or, occasionally, uveitis.

Psoriatic arthritis symptoms include peripheral inflammatory arthritis, which is often asymmetric and can occur with or without inflammatory back pain. Peripheral arthritis is subdivided into oligo- and polyarthritis, with the latter being commonest, and some patients have only distal interphalangeal joint disease. The presence of psoriasis at presentation or at any time in the past, or a family history of psoriasis, is key. Other spondyloarthropathy features, including dactylitis and enthesitis, occur frequently.

Arthropathy of inflammatory bowel disease (enteropathic arthritis) may present with typical axial and peripheral features of spondyloarthropathy, in addition to intestinal symptoms or a known diagnosis of inflammatory bowel disease. Other extra-intestinal manifestations include mouth ulcers, fatigue, systemic features, erythema nodosum, and pyoderma gangrenosum.

Undifferentiated spondyloarthropathy can include any of the symptoms of other forms of spondyloarthropathy, but the condition fails to satisfy classification criteria for any of them.

Juvenile spondyloarthropathy symptoms can include the spectrum of clinical characteristics of adult spondyloarthropathy. They tend to occur in children over 10 years of age, mostly boys, often with a family history of spondyloarthropathy.

Demographics of the disease

Spondyloarthropathy may present at any age but young adults are primarily affected. The prevalence of spondyloarthropathy as a whole is 1%–2% in the Caucasian population.

Natural history, and complications of the disease

Spondyloarthropathies are often progressive chronic conditions with long-term complications, both musculoskeletal and extra-articular. However, they may also be self-limiting, as in reactive arthritis, with 75% cases in remission at 2 years. Spondyloarthropathies often follow a relapsing–remitting course with short or extended symptom-free periods.

In ankylosing spondylitis, chronic spinal inflammation leads to bony ankylosis, resulting in progressive restriction of spinal movement.

Significant morbidity and mortality results from spinal disease, and complications arising include spinal fractures with or without neurological complications. The fractures occur due to spinal osteoporosis, which is often marked and related to chronic inflammation. Iritis may result in visual loss, while less common manifestations, including conduction defects, aortic valve incompetence, upper lobe lung fibrosis, renal complications, and amyloidosis, may result in poor outcomes.

Reactive arthritis is self-limiting in the majority of cases but may relapse or persist. Persistent arthropathy, axial involvement, and extra-articular manifestations may represent evolution into other forms of spondyloarthropathy in predisposed patients.

Psoriatic arthritis complications depend on the pattern of joint involvement and its severity, with a wide spectrum of outcomes ranging from mild, non-destructive polyarthritis to severe joint destruction with bone loss (arthritis mutilans; rarely seen now). Progressive joint destruction, or axial disease combined with significant skin disease, can produce significant disability and considerable psychosocial morbidity.

Approach to diagnosing the disease

The diagnosis of spondyloarthropathies can be difficult, due to the evolution of symptoms over time, as well as the overlap between different forms. In approaching the diagnosis of the disease you should:

- take a thorough history to identify **key or classical features** (e.g. a classical description of inflammatory back pain, with dactylitis or monoarticular joint swelling, and a preceding history of recent diarrhoea, is highly suggestive of reactive arthritis)
- consider the appropriate demographic group (e.g. ankylosing spondylitis primarily affects males under 40)
- perform relevant clinical examination looking for characteristic joint and entheseal inflammation, together with extra-articular manifestations (see Figure 268.1)
- obtain appropriate investigations, including radiology and blood tests, as well as others

Radiology includes plain X-rays and/or MRI of the following:

- sacroiliac joints: note that
  - plain X-rays demonstrate chronic changes and are not suitable for early diagnosis but are useful in established disease; sclerosis, erosions, bony bridges, and ankylosis are common findings
  - MRI is helpful in early diagnosis, with demonstration of bone marrow oedema, capsulitis, synovitis, and enthesitis, as well as of later progression to the more chronic changes
- spine: look for ankylosis, syndesmophytes, and spinal fractures in more advanced disease
- affected peripheral joints: look for evidence of periarticular osteopenia, erosions, and chronic joint deformity, as well as periosteal reaction or enthesitis (Sieper et al., 2009)

Blood tests can be used as follows:

- to find evidence of the acute phase response (e.g. elevated erythrocyte sedimentation rate (ESR) or C-reactive protein levels (CRP) and decreased haemoglobin levels)
- HLA-B27 typing
- to find serological evidence of infection by organisms associated with reactive arthritis (e.g. yersinia, campylobacter, and salmonella)

Other tests include:

- culture of stool, and culture/PCR of urine or genital tract, with or without rectal swabs for organisms associated with reactive arthritis
- skin biopsy, where clinical diagnosis is uncertain
- colonoscopy, to investigate possible inflammatory bowel disease

Other diagnoses that should be considered

Given the wide and varied presentation of spondyloarthropathies, other inflammatory arthritides (e.g. rheumatoid arthritis) should be considered when inflammatory peripheral arthritis predominates. A monoarthritis should always raise the suspicion of septic arthritis

Ankylosing Spondylitis: Extra-articular Manifestations

Authors:
Payam Pournazari
Reviewers:
Yan Yu
Scott Rapske
Liam Martin*
*MD at time of publication

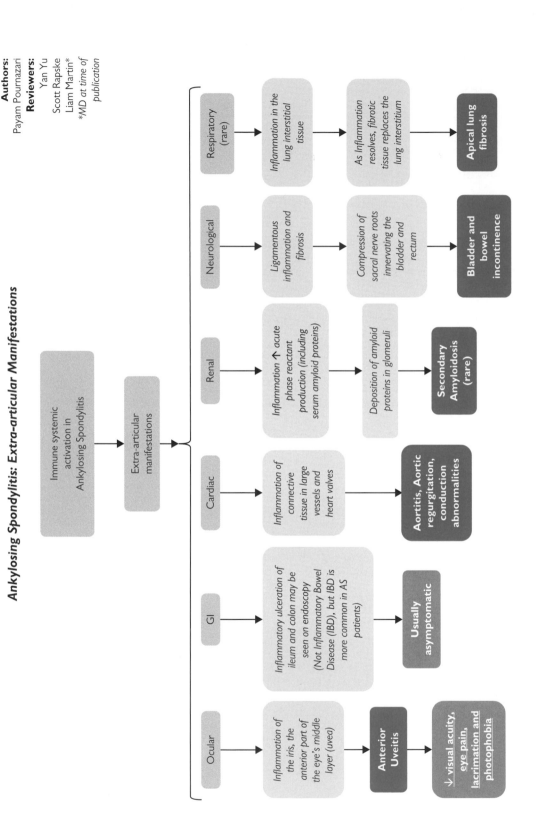

Legend: Pathophysiology | Mechanism | Sign/Symptom/Lab Finding | Complications

Figure 268.1 Ankylosing spondylitis: extra-articular manifestations; AS, ankylosing spondylitis; GI, gastrointestinal.

Reproduced with permission from The Calgary Guide to Understanding Disease, a collaborative student/faculty project of the University of Calgary. For this, and other materials which illuminate the connection between pathophysiology and clinical manifestation of disease, visit www.thecalgaryguide.com.

Copyright (c) 2012 The Calgary Guide to Understanding Disease.

or a crystal arthropathy. Sarcoidosis can also present with dactylitis and/or enthesitis. In addition, mechanical back pain and diffuse idiopathic skeletal hyperostosis are diagnoses to be considered as alternatives to inflammatory spinal pain.

'Gold-standard' diagnostic test

There is no 'gold-standard' diagnostic test for seronegative spondyloarthropathy; diagnosis is made using the framework detailed in 'Approach to diagnosing the disease'.

Acceptable diagnostic alternatives to the gold standard

As there is no 'gold-standard' diagnostic test for seronegative spondyloarthropathy, there are also no acceptable diagnostic alternatives to the gold-standard test; instead, diagnosis is made using the framework detailed in 'Approach to diagnosing the disease'.

Other relevant investigations

For seronegative spondyloarthropathy, only investigations used to clarify the diagnosis and exclude the differentials are relevant.

Prognosis and how to estimate it

The prognosis of seronegative spondyloarthropathy depends principally on its form; for any given disease, severity varies considerably, and it is not currently possible to give an accurate prognosis.

In the early phase of ankylosing spondylitis, elevated acute phase reactants, hip involvement, and osteoporosis are markers of poor prognosis. As the disease progresses, extra-articular manifestations, spinal fracture, continued elevation of ESR/CRP, and anaemia are associated with a worse outcome.

Patients who have reactive arthritis and are HLA-B27 positive tend to have more severe and more persistent disease, with a higher likelihood of axial disease and extra-articular manifestations.

Indicators of poor outcome in psoriatic arthritis include polyarticular involvement, early decline in functional abilities, and HIV positivity (Watts et al., 2009).

Treatment and its effectiveness

Management of spondyloarthropathy is according to disease subset, its activity, and the possibility of progression.

Initial conservative management includes NSAIDs and non-pharmacological measures such as education and physiotherapy. An escalation in treatment is often required and tailored according to the presence of peripheral or axial disease, as well as severity of symptoms and initial response to treatment.

Recently, international criteria for the management of ankylosing spondylitis have been established (Sieper et al., 2009). Both pharmacological and non-pharmacological management should run in parallel. In recent times, the use of anti-tumour necrosis factor (anti-TNF) agents has dramatically improved the quality of life of patients with ankylosing spondylitis, as these agents treat both peripheral and axial symptoms as well as extra-articular manifestations.

Psoriatic arthritis treatment aims for peripheral joint remission, symptom control, and prevention of disease progression. Initial management with NSAIDs, escalating to both oral and intra-articular steroids, is appropriate. Disease-modifying anti-rheumatic drugs (DMARDs), including methotrexate, sulfasalazine, and leflunomide, have been shown to be beneficial for peripheral disease but **not** for axial disease. For polyarthritis, very active oligoarthritis, or enthesopathy, DMARDs are introduced early in disease, as for the treatment of rheumatoid arthritis, although the rationale for doing this is less well established than in rheumatoid arthritis. Anti-TNF agents, used when DMARDs fail to control peripheral disease, treat both peripheral and axial symptoms. Additional biologic drugs, especially those targeting IL-17 and IL-23 are proving useful in psoriatic arthritis and ankylosing spondylitis.

The management of reactive arthritis involves treatment of the triggering infection, although there is no definitive evidence that this approach affects the outcome of the condition. Arthritis is controlled initially with full-dose NSAIDs, aspiration of affected joints, and intra-articular steroids. Short courses of oral steroids may be required. If synovitis fails to resolve by 4–6 months, particularly in HLA-B27-positive patients, or if there are flares, treatment with DMARDs (e.g. sulfasalazine, methotrexate, or leflunomide) may be used. In a proportion of these cases, the DMARD can be discontinued after ~2 years if the patient is asymptomatic, but 5%–10% of reactive arthritis patients have persistent disease which continues to require DMARD treatment; in severe cases, the use of anti-TNF agents can be effective without unmasking latent infection.

Spondyloarthropathy associated with inflammatory bowel disease requires optimal management of the colitis/enteritis. NSAIDs may aggravate inflammatory bowel disease and worsen anaemia and so must be used with caution. Intra-articular steroids are useful for individual active joints. DMARDs such as sulfasalazine and methotrexate must be tailored to treat both joint and bowel symptoms (note that drugs that are used in inflammatory bowel disease but do not contain a sulfonamide component (e.g. mesalazine) are ineffective for arthritis). When DMARDs are inadequate, anti-TNF drugs can be used and are also effective for Crohn's disease.

Undifferentiated spondyloarthropathy can also be managed via these strategies, according to whether peripheral or axial disease predominates.

Juvenile spondyloarthropathy requires a multidisciplinary approach to treatment, which generally uses the same agents as for adult disease. As for all patients with juvenile arthritis, monitoring for eye disease is recommended, although anterior uveitis, which is the commonest complication, is usually symptomatic.

Further Reading

Braun J and Sieper J. Ankylosing spondylitis. *Lancet* 2007; 369: 1379–90.

Sieper J, Rudwaleit M, Baraliakos X, et al. The Assessment of SpondyloArthritis International Society (ASAS) handbook: A guide to assess spondyloarthritis. *Ann Rheum Dis* 2009; 68 (Suppl. 2): 1–44.

Taurog JD, Chhabra A, and Colbert RA. Ankylosing Spondylitis and Axial Spondyloarthritis. *N Engl J Med* 2016; 374: 2563–74.

Watts R, Clunie G, Hall F, et al. *Oxford Desk Reference Rheumatology*, 2009. Oxford University Press.

269 Systemic lupus erythematosus

Robert Stevens and Chee-Seng Yee

Definition and etiology of the disease

Systemic lupus erythematosus (SLE) is a chronic multisystem autoimmune inflammatory disorder of unknown etiology. Numerous abnormalities within the innate and adaptive immune system have been described. The hallmark of this disease is B-cell hyperactivity resulting in autoantibody production, abnormal T-cell function, impaired clearance of immune complexes (resulting in their deposition in tissues), complement activation, and defective cellular apoptosis. However, these abnormalities of the immune system are not uniform across patients and within the same patient at different stages of the disease, resulting in heterogeneity in its presentation and progress. The pathogenesis is complex, involving genetic, environmental, and hormonal factors.

Genetic factors

SLE is considered a complex genetic trait, with a lack of correlation between phenotype and genotype. The genetic basis is supported by the fact that there are ethnic differences in disease incidence/prevalence, the disease has a tendency for familial clustering, a higher concordance rate in monozygotic twins than in dizygotic twins, and several genetic associations. Genetic factors are a major determinant of susceptibility to the disease and possibly of disease severity as well.

Environmental factors

Environmental factors are thought to be involved in triggering the autoimmune process in a genetically susceptible individual. The three main environmental factors are UV light, infections (especially with Epstein–Barr virus), and drugs. Many drugs have been implicated in drug-induced lupus but the most recognized are procainamide and hydrallazine.

Hormonal factors

The role of oestrogen is suggested by the strong female preponderance of this disease, the timing of disease onset (occurring mainly after puberty), and the increased risk of flare of disease during pregnancy.

Demographics and epidemiology

SLE has been reported worldwide, with differences in the incidence, prevalence, pattern of organ involvement, and severity of disease across different ethnic groups. Any age can be affected but it predominantly affects women of childbearing age, with a female to male ratio of 11:1. This is an uncommon disease, with a prevalence of about 1 in 2000 and an incidence of 7 per 100 000 per year amongst adult women in the UK. It is more common in those of Afro-Caribbean and South Asian descent than in those of Caucasian descent. There appears to be a trend towards increasing prevalence and incidence of the disease over time.

Clinical manifestations

SLE is a chronic disease that is characterized by periods of exacerbations with variable course. Recognized triggers of flare of disease activity are UV light, infection, oestrogen, and stress.

SLE is a multisystem disease that can affect any parts of the body, with protean manifestations. As any organ system can be involved, the disease may present in variable combinations of organ system manifestations that can vary both between patients and within the same patient over time.

Fatigue

Fatigue is the most common symptom of SLE and can be disabling. Another contributory factor is fibromyalgia, which is common in SLE patients and tends to be persistent, even when the disease is under controlled.

Non-specific mucocutaneous manifestations

Non-specific mucocutaneous manifestations of SLE include:

- mucosal ulcers (nasal or oral)
- photosensitivity
- cutaneous vasculitis (e.g. purpuric rash, urticaria, subcutaneous nodules, and ulcers)

Lupus-specific mucocutaneous lesions

Lupus-specific mucocutaneous lesions are characterized by deposition of IgG along the dermal–epidermal junction (known as positive lupus band test); this occurs both in obvious lesions and in normal-appearing skin. Lesions can be classified into three types:

- acute cutaneous lupus, which can be erythematous (including malar rash), exanthematous (resembling erythema multiforme), or bullous
- subacute cutaneous lupus, which can be psoriasiform or annular/polycyclic
- chronic cutaneous lupus, which can lead to scarring; this commonly manifests as discoid lesions with follicular plugging or, in the case of lupus profundus, as tender subcutaneous nodules

Musculoskeletal disorders

Musculoskeletal manifestations of SLE include:

- arthralgia/myalgia, which is very common but non-specific
- inflammatory arthritis, which is usually non-erosive
- Jaccoud's arthropathy, which is a deforming arthropathy that can be rheumatoid-like but is correctable

Serositis

Both pleurisy and pericarditis can occur in SLE.

Renal manifestations

Renal involvement in SLE is commonly asymptomatic or non-specific, especially in the early stages. It is most commonly picked up with urine dipstick testing (e.g. as proteinuria, haematuria, and/or pyuria). Hence, it is crucial that urine dipstick testing is performed as part of the routine assessment of SLE patients.

Haematological disorders

The following haematological disorders are common in SLE but are usually asymptomatic:

- anaemia (this is usually the anaemia of chronic disease)
- leucopenia with neutropenia and/or lymphopenia
- thrombocytopenia

Approach to diagnosis

There is no specific diagnostic test for SLE. Although classification criteria have been devised by the American College of Rheumatology, the criteria were developed for research studies and are not intended for diagnostic purposes.

The two key features of SLE are systemic involvement and the presence of autoantibodies.

Evidence of systemic involvement

As there is no diagnostic test, a good clinical assessment is essential to determine the pattern of systemic involvement. A high index of suspicion is required, particularly when there is multisystem involvement and the following common manifestations of SLE are present:

- mucocutaneous features (especially mouth ulcers, alopecia, rash, and photosensitivity)
- inflammatory arthritis
- renal involvement (as indicated by proteinuria and active urinary sediment)
- pleurisy or pericarditis
- haematological manifestations (especially haemolytic anaemia, leucopenia, neutropenia, lymphopenia, and thrombocytopenia)

As renal and haematological involvement may be asymptomatic, it is important to perform the following tests during the diagnostic workup:

- a urine test for proteinuria and active urinary sediment (a urine dipstick test on its own is not sufficient, as it is not accurate and is associated with a high level of false-positive results)
- a full blood count

Other investigations will be dictated by patient's presentation and are performed mainly to exclude other causes for the manifestation(s). These include:

- biopsy (e.g. renal biopsy, skin biopsy)
- imaging (e.g. MRI of the head/spine; high-resolution CT of the chest)
- electrophysiological tests (e.g. nerve conduction studies, electromyography)
- blood tests (e.g. Coomb's test, hepatitis serology, muscle enzymes)

Presence of autoantibodies

As B cell hyperactivity is the hallmark of SLE, the absence of autoantibodies in an untreated patient makes the diagnosis unlikely (good negative predictive value). Autoantibodies that are specific to SLE are anti-double-stranded DNA antibodies (present in 60%–70% of cases) and anti-Sm antibodies (present in 10%–30% of cases).

Autoantibodies to be tested for include:

- antinuclear antibody (ANA), which is the most common type of autoantibody found in SLE (>95% of cases)
- extractable nuclear antigens, including anti-Ro, anti-La, and anti-Sm
- anti-double-stranded DNA antibodies
- antiphospholipid antibodies (anticardiolipin antibodies and lupus anticoagulant)

Two further important points to note regarding autoantibodies are that:

- ANA is not specific to SLE, as many different conditions can cause a positive result for the ANA test, and up to 5% of the normal population is positive for ANA; hence, a positive ANA test does not equate to a diagnosis of SLE
- a patient being treated for SLE can become negative for autoantibodies

Other diagnosis to be considered

As SLE is a multisystem disease with protean manifestations, of which most are not specific to the disease itself, the clinical presentation can mimic other conditions.

The main differential diagnoses are other multisystem conditions, in particular:

- sepsis (it is important to note that SLE patients have an increased risk of infection (in part due to immunosuppressive treatment) and that infection itself could trigger a flare of disease activity)
- primary systemic vasculitis (e.g. antineutrophil cytoplasmic antibody-associated vasculitis, and Behçet's syndrome)
- other connective tissue diseases (note that it is not uncommon for there to be overlapping features of other connective tissue

diseases (e.g. Sjögren's syndrome, dermatomyositis, polymyositis, and systemic sclerosis), termed overlap syndrome and mixed connective tissue disease)
- antiphospholipid syndrome (note that this can occur as part of SLE (secondary antiphospholipid syndrome))
- sarcoidosis
- other inflammatory arthritis (such as rheumatoid arthritis and seronegative spondyloarthropathy)

Assessment of disease

In assessing SLE patients, there are three outcome domains to be considered: disease activity, damage, and the health status of patient. Disease activity is the immune-mediated process that is potentially reversible or 'inflammation', while damage is an irreversible process or 'scarring'. Damage can be a result of uncontrolled disease activity but, more commonly, it is multifactorial, due to a combination of disease activity, treatment, and comorbidities. Examples of damage are myocardial infarctions, joint erosions, and scarring alopecia. The health status of the patient is the person's sense of physical, emotional, and social well-being associated with the disease or its treatment; it is perhaps better known as the 'health-related quality of life'. These three outcome domains are managed differently; hence, it is crucial to differentiate these domains with regards to attribution of manifestations. In particular, immunomodulators are used to treat manifestations of disease activity but not manifestations of damage or health-related quality of life.

Assessing SLE can be challenging, particularly when trying to attribute clinical manifestations to disease activity. This is due to the lack of a good biomarker and the complexity of this multisystem disease, with its myriad of presentations that can vary between patients and within the same patient over time.

Complications

Organ damage

Organ damage caused by SLE includes skin scarring (including scarring alopecia), avascular necrosis of bone (especially hip), chronic kidney disease, and pulmonary fibrosis.

Premature atherosclerosis

SLE patients are at much higher risk of developing cardiovascular disease, compared to the general population. Furthermore, in women, the premenopausal protective effect for cardiovascular disease appears to be abrogated by the disease. It should be noted that the traditional Framingham risk calculator underestimates the risk of cardiovascular disease in SLE patients. It has been suggested that SLE patients should be considered to have the same level of risk for cardiovascular disease as those with diabetes mellitus.

Malignancy

SLE patients have an increased risk of cancer, compared to general population. This is even more so for:

- non-Hodgkin's lymphoma
- lung cancer
- cervical cancer

Pregnancy comorbidities

Comorbidities seen during pregnancy in SLE patients include:

- neonatal lupus syndrome
- pregnancy loss
- flare of disease activity

Prognosis

Before the advent of corticosteroids, the 5-year survival for SLE was less than 55%. Over the last few decades, survival has improved considerably; currently, the 10-year survival rate is ~90%. However, SLE patients still have much lower life expectancy, compared to the general population, and this is most pronounced in those under the age of 45. The most common causes of deaths are cardiovascular disease, infection, and malignancy. The more damage a patient has accumulated, the higher is the risk of death.

Treatment

The treatment of SLE is aimed at controlling disease activity (through immunomodulation), prevention of development of damage, and management of complications.

The treatment options for disease activity are:

- symptomatic treatment (e.g. NSAIDs)
- antimalarials (e.g. hydroxychloroquine, chloroquine, and mepacrine)
- corticosteroids (e.g. topical, oral, intra-lesional, or parenteral)
- immunosuppressives (in particular, azathioprine, methotrexate, mycophenolate, and cyclophosphamide)
- biologicals (e.g. rituximab and belimumab)
- plasmapheresis
- IV immunoglobulins
- others (e.g. thalidomide, prasterone, dapsone, and retinoids)

The management of disease activity is tailored to the patient, and the major determinant of treatment option is the level of disease activity. Severe disease activity is defined as manifestations that are life-threatening or result in significant organ dysfunction, such as seizure, nephrotic syndrome, and inability of the patient to perform the activities of daily living. On the other end of the spectrum, mild disease activity refers to minor manifestations that cause some discomfort but leave the patient able to continue with their daily routines.

Severe disease activity requires treatment with high-dose corticosteroids and usually with immunosuppressives and/or biologicals. IV immunoglobulins and plasmapheresis are mainly reserved for life-threatening manifestations.

Moderate disease activity is commonly treated with lower doses of corticosteroids, and immunosuppressives may be added in. Antimalarials are also commonly used and have been shown to be effective in controlling mucocutaneous manifestations and inflammatory arthritis. For certain manifestations, local treatment with corticosteroids (and occasionally immunosuppressives) could be used, such as intra-articular injection of methylprednisolone for inflammatory arthritis, and corticosteroid cream for discoid rash. Thalidomide, retinoids, and dapsone are used for the treatment of refractory skin lesions. Prasterone (an androgen) has been shown to have steroid-sparing properties and reduce the number of SLE flares.

Mild disease activity usually only requires symptomatic treatment. Due to their low toxicity, antimalarials are also used to treat recurrent or persistent milder mucocutaneous and musculoskeletal manifestations. There is also evidence supporting the ubiquitous use of hydroxychloroquine, as long-term usage is associated with lower cardiovascular events and improved survival.

Apart from managing disease activity, other measures that deserve special mention are:

- photoprotection (in the form of protective clothing and high-factor (at least SPF 30) sun cream); many SLE patients are photosensitive, and UV light is a well-recognized trigger of disease activity flare
- smoking cessation; this is important, as SLE patients have an increased risk of cardiovascular disease and lung cancer
- aggressive management of cardiovascular risk factors, given the increased risk of cardiovascular disease in SLE
- physiotherapy and occupational therapy; these non-pharmacological measures may help with inflammatory arthritis, fatigue, and fibromyalgia (commonly associated with SLE)

Further Reading

Lisnevskaia L, Murphy G, and Isenberg D. Systemic lupus erythematosus. *Lancet* 2014; 384: 1878–88.

Rahman A and Isenberg DA. Systemic lupus erythematosus. *N Engl J Med* 2008; 358: 929–39.

270 Crystal arthropathy

Michael Doherty

Definition of crystal arthropathy

Three main crystals associate with arthritis:

- monosodium urate (MSU)
- calcium pyrophosphate, the usual cause of cartilage calcification (*chondrocalcinosis* **(CC)**)
- basic calcium phosphates (BCP), including hydroxyapatite

Gout is a true crystal deposition disease caused by MSU. **Calcium pyrophosphate crystal deposition (CPPD)** is the umbrella term for calcium pyrophosphate deposition. Calcium pyrophosphate crystals cause inflammation in **acute calcium pyrophosphate crystal arthritis** and **chronic calcium pyrophosphate crystal inflammatory arthritis.** However, osteoarthritis (OA) commonly associates with calcium pyrophosphate **(OA with CPPD)** and BCP crystals and, in this context, it is unclear if the crystals are pathogenic.

Aetiology of crystal arthropathy

Crystals only form when the saturation point for crystallization is exceeded. A serum uric acid (SUA) of 360 μmol/L (6.0 mg/dl) approximates to the saturation point for MSU. Extracellular pyrophosphate (ePPi) in cartilage is the key determinant of CPPD but cannot be measured clinically.

Uric acid (UA), produced from xanthine by xanthine oxidase (XO), is the end product of purine breakdown. About two-thirds of UA is produced endogenously, with the rest coming from dietary purines. UA is excreted mainly via the kidney. Risk factors for SUA elevation and gout are shown in Table 270.1. MSU preferentially deposits in and around joints, mainly feet, knees, hands, and elbows.

Most ePPi comes from the breakdown of nucleoside triphosphates, although some comes from intracellular pyrophosphate transported outside by the progressive ankylosis protein homolog protein, which is encoded by the ANKH gene. ePPi is converted to orthophosphate by alkaline phosphatase (with magnesium as a cofactor). Moderate increases in ePPi stimulate, but high levels inhibit, BCP crystal formation, making ePPi a key regulator of normal mineralization (bones, teeth) and an inhibitor of unwanted BCP (cartilage, urine, saliva). High ePPi levels in hyaline and fibrocartilage predispose to CPPD, particularly in knees. Risk factors for CPPD are shown in Table 270.2.

Typical symptoms of crystal arthropathy, and less common symptoms

Acute gout and acute calcium pyrophosphate crystal arthritis

Acute gout and acute calcium pyrophosphate crystal arthritis present as acute mono-arthritis characterized by:

- rapid-onset severe pain ('worst ever'), reaching a maximum in 6–24 hours
- marked tenderness—even to clothing over the joint
- swelling, effusion, increased warmth (± erythema)

The 'attack' resolves within a few days or weeks. Occasionally, several joints are affected simultaneously. Milder, short-lived episodes

Table 270.1 Risk factors for gout

Risk factor	Mechanism
Hereditary, genetic risk	Inefficient renal excretion (>95%) due to polymorphisms related to URAT1 and other renal ion transporter systems
	Overproduction due to purine enzyme mutation (very rare)
Metabolic syndrome:	
• obesity	Increased endogenous production
• hypertension	Reduction in renal efficiency of urate clearance
• hyperlipidaemia	Reduction in renal efficiency of urate clearance
• insulin resistance	Reduction in renal efficiency of urate clearance
Dietary risk factors:	
• excessive beer, spirits	Increased exogenous uric acid production (from guanosine in beer)
• diet high in red meat, shellfish, offal, etc.	Increased exogenous uric acid production
Renal impairment:	
• chronic renal impairment	Reduction in renal efficiency of urate clearance
• drugs (e.g. diuretics, ciclosporin)	Reduction in renal efficiency of urate clearance
Ageing, osteoarthritis	Altered balance between tissue inhibitors/ promotors for crystal nucleation and growth (particularly in osteoarthritis)
	Age-related reduction in renal efficiency of urate clearance

Table 270.2 Risk factors for calcium pyrophosphate dihydrate deposition disease

Risk factor	Mechanism
Ageing	Unclear; possible increase in pyrophosphate, alteration of tissue factors
Prior joint insult	Increased production of ePPi by hypertrophic chondrocytes
Osteoarthritis	Increased production of ePPi by hypertrophic chondrocytes
	Reduction in normal crystal inhibitors (e.g. proteoglycans)
	Increase in promotors of crystallization (e.g. osteopontin, collagen X)
Metabolic disease:	All of the following lead to increased ePPi levels:
• haemochromatosis	Iron inhibits alkaline phosphatase; iron is also a nucleating factor
• hyperparathyroidism	Ca^{++} inhibits alkaline phosphatase and increases the ionic product
• hypophosphatasia	Reduced breakdown of ePPi to orthophosphate
• hypomagnesaemia	Reduced breakdown of ePPi by alkaline phosphatase
Diuretics	Possibly due to diuretic-induced hypomagnesaemia
Familial CPPD	Rare; families with polyarticular CC and variable arthropathy
	Some cases due to a mutation in the ANKH (CCAL2) gene

Abbreviations: CPPD, calcium pyrophosphate dihydrate deposition; ePPi, extracellular pyrophosphate.

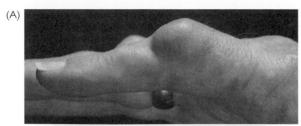

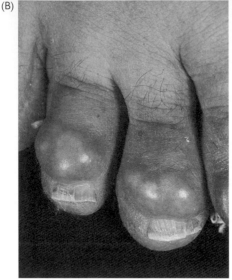

Figure 270.1 Tophi on a finger (A) and toes (B) of a patient with chronic tophaceous gout; in some cases, the white colour of monosodium urate crystals can be seen, allowing distinction from rheumatoid nodules.

('petite attacks') are common. Gout also causes acute self-limiting bursitis, tenosynovitis, or cellulitis.

Acute gout targets the first metatarsophalangeal joint (1MTPJ), the mid-foot, the ankle, the knee, the wrist, the metacarpophalangeal (MCP) joints, the finger joints, and the elbows. First attacks often affect feet (1MTPJ especially). Acute calcium pyrophosphate crystal arthritis targets knees and, less commonly, wrists, MCP joints, elbows, and shoulders (rarely, it occurs in other joints).

Both conditions can be triggered by intercurrent illness, surgery, or joint trauma. Initiation of urate-lowering drugs can trigger gout.

Recurrent and chronic tophaceous gout

Acute attacks usually recur, become more frequent, and involve new sites. With continuing deposition, enlarging crystal concretions (tophi) damage cartilage and bone, causing chronic pain, stiffness, and disability. Tophi may be clinically evident (Figure 270.1) mainly over extensor surfaces of feet, knees, hands, and elbows, sometimes discharging pus-like fluid containing white MSU. Occasionally, tophi occur without preceding attacks.

OA with CPPD and chronic calcium pyrophosphate crystal inflammatory arthritis

OA with CPPD is identical to OA (see Chapter 266). It may be asymptomatic or associate with usage-related pain and functional limitation, with or without superimposed attacks. Chronic calcium pyrophosphate crystal inflammatory arthritis resembles OA but with more inflammation (stiffness, effusion) and involvement of joints (e.g. wrists, MCP joints) atypically affected by OA.

Demographics

Gout is the most common inflammatory arthritis in men, and in women aged >65. Overall prevalence is 1.4% but it is more common

in men (~5:1) and increases with age, rising to 7% prevalence in older men. Usually, it presents after age 30 and is rare before the menopause (oestrogen is uricosuric).

Knee CC is rare under the age of 50, but increases from 4% in those aged 50–60 to 20% in those over the age of 80, affecting both sexes equally.

Natural history, and complications of crystal arthropathy

Untreated gout typically progresses through an asymptomatic phase to presentation with acute gout, to recurrent attacks separated by asymptomatic inter-critical periods and, finally, to chronic tophaceous gout. Evolution is slow, usually taking several decades to reach tophaceous gout.

Renal complications include nephrolithiasis (UA, but also common calcium stones) and chronic interstitial nephritis (due to MSU deposition). There is growing evidence that high SUA is an independent risk factor for cardiovascular disease and renal impairment, unrelated to MSU deposition.

The natural history of CPPD is variable. Acute attacks usually occur only a few times in a patient's lifetime.

Approach to diagnosing crystal arthropathy

For typical attacks, clinical features alone permit a diagnosis. Factors such as age, the joint involved, comorbidity, drug history and presence of joint damage/OA usually allow distinction between MSU and calcium pyrophosphate. However, for atypical presentations and chronic disease, crystal identification becomes increasingly important.

Other diagnoses that should be considered

For atypical attacks, the following require consideration:

- septic arthritis (see Chapter 271): this is subacute and progressive; crystals and sepsis can coexist so, if sepsis is suspected, microbiological investigation should still be undertaken, despite identification of synovial fluid (SF) crystals
- psoriatic and reactive arthritis (see Chapter 264)
- palindromic rheumatism: this produces progressive synovitis with adjacent inflammation and erythema over 1–3 days and which resolves in a similar amount of time
- acute haemarthrosis: this presents a tense effusion with no periarticular inflammation or erythema

Both chronic gout and chronic calcium pyrophosphate crystal inflammatory arthritis may superficially resemble rheumatoid arthritis. A routine search for SF crystals should be undertaken in any undiagnosed inflammatory arthritis.

'Gold-standard' diagnostic test

The gold-standard test for crystal arthropathy is crystal identification in SF or a tophus aspirate, using compensated polarized microscopy. MSU crystals are needle shaped and brightly birefringent (negative sign). Calcium pyrophosphate crystals are smaller rhomboid crystals with weak (positive) or no birefringence.

Acceptable diagnostic alternatives to the gold standard

In the absence of crystal confirmation, diagnosis may be supported by imaging, via radiographs or ultrasound.

Radiographs

Radiographs may show CC (Figure 270.2) and, occasionally, synovial/capsular calcification, with or without OA. Radiographic changes in gout occur late and are mainly those of OA. More specific are para-articular 'punched-out' cortical erosions and well-defined cysts (intra-osseous tophi; see Figure 270.3).

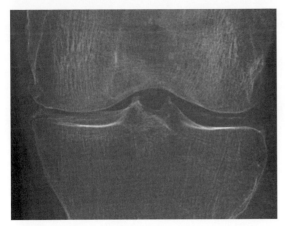

Figure 270.2 Radiographic knee chondrocalcinosis, with predominant involvement of the fibrocartilaginous menisci.

Ultrasound

Crystals can produce hyperechogenicity in cartilage of peripheral joints (e.g. 1MTPJs, knees). MSU occurs at the cartilage surface, whereas CPPD targets the midzone, allowing differentiation. Elevated SUA is a strong risk factor for gout but is unhelpful in diagnosis.

Other relevant investigations

Renal function and SUA are relevant to gout, and X-rays of clinically abnormal joints help assess damage. Metabolic screening (of e.g. calcium, ferritin, alkaline phosphatase, magnesium) is recommended for polyarticular CC and for patients presenting with CC but are under the age of 60.

Prognosis, and how to estimate it

A therapeutic aim for troublesome gout is elimination of the crystals. Therefore, the main prognostic factor, as for CPPD, is the degree of irreversible damage (OA), which is assessed clinically and by radiographs.

Treatment and its effectiveness

Acute gout and acute calcium pyrophosphate crystal arthritis

The following treatments are recommended for acute gout and acute calcium pyrophosphate crystal arthritis:

- **rest the joint** and apply **ice packs**
- if possible, **aspirate** the affected joint and **inject a long-acting steroid** (e.g. methylprednisolone) into it; this gives rapid relief and

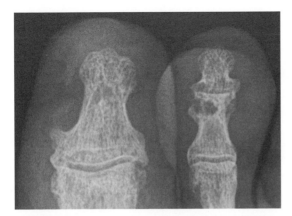

Figure 270.3 Foot radiograph of a patient with chronic tophaceous gout, showing cyst-like bone lesions, cortical erosion, cartilage loss, and the soft-tissue swelling of the clinically evident tophi.

is the preferred treatment in hospital; also, the SF can be examined to confirm the diagnosis and, if required, exclude sepsis
- **an oral NSAID** (naproxen, diclofenac, etoricoxib) plus a proton-pump inhibitor; although widely used, NSAIDs often are contraindicated in older patients due to comorbidity (e.g. renal impairment) or concomitant drugs (e.g. warfarin, diuretics)
- **oral colchicine:** this alkaloid effectively reduces the neutrophil-driven inflammation of crystal synovitis; its main side effect of severe diarrhoea is dose dependent, so use only low doses (0.5 mg twice daily for elderly or those with renal impairment; up to three to four times daily for more robust patients)
- **systemic steroids**: A short course of prednisolone (e.g. 15 mg daily for 5 days) or single intramuscular injection of methylprednisolone (80–120 mg) may be considered for oligo-articular attacks and for patients with contraindications or intolerance to NSAIDs and colchicine, if aspiration/injection is impractical

Long-term management of gout

The following are recommended for long-term management of gout:

- provide **information** concerning gout and its management
- **modify risk factors** (e.g. advise the patient to lose weight, if the patient is obese, and to reduce excessive intake of high purine foods, beer, and spirits; stop diuretics, if possible)
- initiate **urate-lowering therapy** (ULT): this is indicated for frequent attacks, tophi, joint damage, or urolithiasis, with the aim being to reduce SUA well below the saturation point (360 μmol/l), to prevent further crystal formation and dissolve existing crystals; with the increasing realization that microtophi (seen on ultrasound or MRI) are widespread at first presentation, the trend is towards earlier definitive treatment (see 'Drugs used for ULT')
- **treat comorbidity**: treatment of hypertension, hyperlipidaemia, and insulin resistance helps lower SUA; the antihypertensive losartan and the lipid-lowering agent fenofibrate have an additional beneficial, mild, uricosuric effect

Drugs used for ULT

Allopurinol, the first-line ULT, is a purine, non-specific, XO inhibitor that reduces UA production. Its active metabolite oxypurinol is excreted via the kidney. The recommended starting dose is 100 mg daily (50 mg in older patients or those with impaired renal function). SUA is measured every 3–4 weeks, and the dose increased in 100 mg increments (50 mg if elderly or with renal impairment) until this is achieved (maximum 900 mg; algorithms allow calculation of the lower maximum in renal impairment). The reduction in UA following the initiation of ULT can partially dissolve MSU crystals, encouraging crystal shedding and triggering of attacks. The patient should be warned of this and told to continue ULT if an attack occurs. This triggering is minimized by slow upward titration, or by prophylaxis for several months using daily colchicine (0.5 mg 12 hourly) or NSAIDs (plus a proton-pump inhibitor). Allopurinol is usually well tolerated but 10% of patients experience gastrointestinal upset, a headache, or mild rashes. Vasculitic rashes and allopurinol hypersensitivity syndrome are serious but rare (mainly in renal impaired patients). Annual SUA monitoring is advised to ensure continuing effective treatment. ULT usually is required indefinitely.

Febuxostat is a new, non-purine, specific XO inhibitor that undergoes hepatic metabolism, requiring no dose adjustment in renal impairment. It is recommended for patients intolerant of allopurinol or in whom allopurinol is contraindicated (e.g. those with severe renal disease). It usually provokes attacks at the starting dose (80 mg), so prophylaxis with colchicine/NSAID is advised. It has just two dose options (120 mg daily being the maximum).

Uricosuric drugs such as **sulfinpyrazone** or **prebenecid** have restricted availability, are less efficient than allopurinol, require high fluid intake to avoid UA crystallization in renal tubules, and are contraindicated in patients with renal impairment or urolithiasis. Benzbromarone (50–200 mg daily) is a very efficient uricosuric that is effective and safe in mild-to-moderate renal impairment. Because of rare hepatotoxicity, it has limited availability and is used on a named-patient basis.

Long-term management of CPPD

No drugs are available to modify CPPD. Principles of management of OA with CPPD are identical to those for OA (see Chapter 266). For frequent flares or chronic calcium pyrophosphate crystal inflammatory arthritis, oral colchicine (0.5 mg twice daily) or NSAIDs (plus a proton-pump inhibitor) may be helpful, and hydroxychloroquine or low-dose methotrexate is sometimes used empirically.

Further Reading

Mulay SR and Anders HJ Crystallopathies. *N Engl J Med* 2016; 374: 2465–76.

Neogi T. Gout. *N Engl J Med* 2011; 364: 443–52.

Qaseem A, Harris RP, and Forciea MA. Management of Acute and Recurrent Gout: A Clinical Practice Guideline From the American College of Physicians. *Ann Intern Med* 2017; 166: 58–68.

Richette P and Bardin T. Gout. *Lancet* 2009; 375: 318–28.

Zhang W, Doherty M, Bardin T, et al. EULAR evidence-based recommendations for calcium pyrophosphate crystal associated arthritis. Part I: Diagnosis. *Ann Rheum Dis* 2011; 70: 563–70.

Zhang W, Doherty M, Pascual E, et al. EULAR evidence-based recommendations for calcium pyrophosphate crystal associated arthritis. Part II: Management. *Ann Rheum Dis* 70: 571–5.

271 Infection of joints and bones

Benjamin Bloch

Definition and classification of infection

Infection can arise at any time within the bone or soft tissues, and sepsis should always be a consideration in the assessment of an acutely swollen, painful joint. A variety of organisms can be responsible (Table 271.1). An acute infection is an orthopaedic emergency, and prompt assessment should always be sought.

Infection can affect either joints (septic arthritis) or bones (osteomyelitis).

Septic arthritis can affect either a native joint or a prosthetic one, and the presentation can be acute or chronic. Similarly, osteomyelitis can present acutely or chronically, and can be due to haematogenous spread (particularly affecting the long-bone metaphyses in children, and the vertebral bodies in adults), direct inoculation via trauma or surgery, or communication from a contiguous infection site.

Presentation

Acute septic arthritis is usually as a result of haematogenous infection, and presents typically with pain, swelling, restriction of movement, and fever. Care should be taken when assessing patients who are immunocompromised or taking immunosuppressive drugs, as their inflammatory response may be depressed and they may not show the same pyrexia, leucocytosis, or elevation of serum C-reactive protein (CRP) levels as healthy patients would.

Chronic septic arthritis is rare, but generally presents with a more prolonged course, and may not have as dramatic a rise in blood parameters as acute septic arthritis. In these cases, other organisms such as mycobacteria or atypical bacteria should be considered.

Septic arthritis following a prosthetic joint replacement may present acutely or some time after the joint is replaced. Acute presentations tend to be due to local contamination and will present with a hot, red, swollen joint that is usually discharging, as the wound will not have healed fully. A joint replacement that becomes infected many years down the line will have done so either due to an indolent infection that has been present long term or, more commonly, due to haematogenous spread from another source.

Acute osteomyelitis is more commonly seen in children, and is typically rapid in onset and severe in presentation. In adults, acute osteomyelitis is usually associated with the presence of lowered resistance to infection due to conditions such as diabetes or immunosuppression secondary to chemotherapy, HIV/AIDS, or post-transplant suppression. Finally, those patients with sickle cell disease are at risk of developing salmonella osteomyelitis.

The cardinal signs of osteomyelitis are pain, fever, acute tenderness, and inflammation. Radiographs will look normal in the acute stage, and MRI is more useful for diagnosing osteomyelitis.

Chronic osteomyelitis is a more indolent process, often as a result of open fractures, surgery, or (in the foot) the sequelae of diabetes. Patients often have sinuses or scars of previous surgery, and will present with recurrent flares of pyrexia, redness, and swelling. The sinus may recommence drainage. The overlying tissues are usually of poor quality and are tethered and adherent to the underlying bone. Plain radiographs may show the typical features of sequestrum (sclerotic, avascular bone) and involucrum (new bone formation as a result of lifting of the periosteum. Further imaging can include the use of radioisotope bone scans, which will show increased uptake in osteomyelitis, and CT and MRI scans are both useful for preoperative planning, particularly in showing the surgeon how much of the bone is involved.

Diagnosis and treatment

In all cases, a history and examination is the starting point. The duration of symptoms is important, as it may guide further treatment.

Haematological investigations include a full blood count, particularly looking at the white-cell count, the erythrocyte sedimentation rate, and the CRP level.

Radiological investigations generally start with plain X-rays of the affected bone or joint. However, acute infections rarely show any changes on plain radiographs and, if there is any doubt about the diagnosis, an MRI scan can be beneficial. For those joints that are deep, such as the hip, an ultrasound scan can help to detect an effusion and these can also be aspirated under ultrasound guidance.

Septic native joints should be aspirated, and the fluid sent for microscopy, culture, and sensitivities. It is possible to aspirate the shoulder, elbow, wrist, knee, and ankle without radiological guidance. The aspirate should also be examined for the presence of crystals, but infection can, of course, coexist with crystal arthropathy. Whenever possible, aspiration should be done before the administration of antibiotics, to maximize the possibility of identifying the responsible organism.

Table 271.1 Causative organisms

Infection	Acute	Chronic
Native septic arthritis	*Staphylococcus aureus* *Streptococcus pyogenes* *Neisseria gonorrhoeae* Gram-negative organisms such as *Escherichia coli* and *Pseudomonas* sp. (in elderly and immunocompromised patients) Anaerobes (rare; associated with penetrating trauma)	In addition to those causing acute infection: • *Mycobacterium tuberculosis* • low-virulence organisms (e.g. coagulase-negative staphylococci)
Prosthetic septic arthritis	*Staphylococcus aureus* (including MRSA) *Streptococcus pyogenes* *Enterococcus* sp. Gram-negative organisms (*Escherichia coli*, *Pseudomonas* sp.)	Coagulase-negative staphylococci *Staphylococcus aureus* (including methicillin-sensitive *Staphylococcus aureus* and MRSA) *Streptococcus pyogenes* *Enterococcus* sp. Corynebacteria Gram-negative bacilli Anaerobes Mycobacteria (rare) Fungi (even rarer) **Up to 50% of infections are polymicrobial**
Osteomyelitis	*Staphylococcus aureus* *Streptococcus pyogenes* *Streptococcus pneumoniae* *Haemophilus influenzae* type b (more common in children) Salmonella (sickle cell) *Pseudomonas aeruginosa*	*Staphylococcus aureus* *Streptococcus pyogenes* *Escherichia coli* *Pseudomonas aeruginosa* *Enterobacter* sp. **>30% of infections are polymicrobial**

A prosthetic joint should never be aspirated without prior orthopaedic discussion, and it should be done in the operating theatre in a clean environment.

The treatment of an acutely septic joint is urgent washout and debridement. In the case of an acutely infected prosthetic joint, it may be possible to salvage the joint by aggressive debridement and exchange of easily accessible parts such as polyethylene bearings. A chronically infected prosthetic joint is likely to need a planned revision, and this may be done either as a single-stage revision or as a two-stage revision in which the first stage is removal of the infected replacement and implantation of a temporary spacer, usually with antibiotics given both locally and systemically.

In the case of osteomyelitis, a biopsy of the infection may be required for diagnostic purposes, and this drainage can also be therapeutic. Acute osteomyelitis, if appropriately treated, can be arrested before it becomes chronic and the bone becomes necrotic. Chronic osteomyelitis exhibits the radiographic changes of sequestrum (dead bone) and involucrum (an encasing sheath of live bone walling off the sequestrum). Both acute and chronic osteomyelitis require prolonged antibiotic treatment, usually of 6 weeks' duration, and microbiological advice should be sought for the most appropriate regime.

The treatment of chronic osteomyelitis is more complex and requires aggressive surgical debridement of dead bone, removal of infected metalware, and reconstruction of any bony defects. This may involve the use of bone grafts or Ilizarov frames and bone transport techniques, and amputation may be required.

Chronic osteomyelitis is commonly seen in diabetic patients with ulcers, particularly affecting the metatarsal heads and the calcaneus. In these patients, following initial debridement, the most appropriate treatment may be amputation. Depending on the level of involvement, it may be possible to preserve part of the foot through the use of ray or partial foot amputations but, if not, then a below-knee amputation would be required. Management of these patients is best done in a multidisciplinary setting, with input from diabetologists, vascular surgeons, orthopaedic surgeons, prosthetists, and podiatrists.

Further Reading

Mathews CJ, Kingsley G, Field M, et al. Management of septic arthritis: A systematic review. *Postgrad Med J* 2008; 84: 265–70.

Mathews CJ, Weston VC, Jones A, et al. Bacterial septic arthritis in adults. *Lancet* 2010; 375: 846–55.

Matthews PC, Berendt AC, McNally MA, et al. Prosthetic joint infection. *BMJ* 2009; 338: b1773.

Solomon L, Warwick D, and Nayagam S. *Apley's System of Orthopaedics and Fractures* (9th edition), 2010. Hodder Arnold.

272 Vasculitis

Raashid Luqmani, Joanna Robson, and Ravi Suppiah

Definition of the disease

The vasculitides are a heterogeneous group of disorders that can range from mild inflammation of blood vessels in the skin, to organ- and life-threatening diseases. The term 'vasculitis' is a pathological description of blood vessel wall inflammation which leads to ischaemia and infarction of the target organs. Definitions and classifications of the primary vasculitides are mainly based on the predominant calibre of the blood vessels involved but incorporate clinical, pathological, and laboratory features. The secondary vasculitides usually occur in the context of other connective tissue diseases and are not discussed further in this section. Anti-glomerular basement membrane disease (previously known as Goodpasture's disease) is not usually included in the primary vasculitides, but has compatible clinical features of pulmonary capillaritis and glomerulonephritis. The definitions of the most common types of primary vasculitis proposed at the Chapel Hill Consensus Conference are given in Table 272.1. The 2013 conference advised changing the name of 'Wegener's granulomatosis' to 'granulomatosis with polyangiitis' and 'Churg–Strauss syndrome' to 'eosinophilic granulomatosis with polyangiitis'.

Aetiology

Hepatitis B virus infection and resulting immune complex deposition cause hepatitis B-related polyarteritis nodosa. Hepatitis C virus is the cause of over 90% of mixed cryoglobulinaemia. For all other forms of primary vasculitis, the aetiology is unknown. Antineutrophil cytoplasm antibodies (ANCAs) may play a role in the pathogenesis of granulomatosis with polyangiitis and microscopic polyangiitis; furthermore, *Staphylococcus aureus* infection is implicated in granulomatosis with polyangiitis.

Symptoms

The specific symptoms listed in Table 272.2, some alone but especially in combination, may occur in patients with systemic vasculitis. Non-specific symptoms such as fever, weight loss, myalgia, and arthralgia are common but not very discriminatory between vasculitis and other conditions.

Demographics of the disease

The demographics depend on the type of systemic vasculitis and are shown in Table 272.3. We have not discussed isolated cutaneous vasculitis any further.

Natural history and complications of the disease

The natural history of untreated multisystem vasculitis is likely to be death within the first year. Giant cell arteritis can result in blindness from ischaemic optic neuropathy (in up to 60% of untreated patients) and, rarely, strokes (especially brainstem infarcts). Takayasu arteritis can result in limb ischaemia, gangrene, aortic aneurysms, aortic dissections, aortic ruptures, and potentially death. The ANCA-associated vasculitides, especially granulomatosis with polyangiitis and microscopic polyangiitis, are associated with acute renal failure from rapidly progressive glomerulonephritis and/or fulminant pulmonary haemorrhage due to pulmonary capillaritis, both of which can cause long-term morbidity such as end-stage renal failure or death.

Anti-glomerular basement membrane disease has a poor untreated outcome (most cases will die from pulmonary haemorrhage and renal failure). Henoch–Schönlein purpura in childhood is usually a self-limiting disease but in adulthood only has 75% survival at 5 years (mainly due to renal disease). Kawasaki disease is associated with coronary aneurysms in 15%–25% of untreated cases; in the short term, these can be fatal in approximately 1% of children and, in the remainder, can cause complications such as premature atherosclerotic disease and myocardial infarction later in life.

Approach to diagnosing the disease

A high index of suspicion and a detailed history and examination are the key to making an accurate diagnosis. In some cases, the clinical history will be highly suggestive. For example, in a patient over the age of 50, the presence of a new-onset headache with temporal tenderness, jaw claudication, and raised inflammatory markers implies giant cell arteritis. The temporal artery biopsy is the gold standard but may be negative in around 40% of cases. Other patients can present in a more subtle way, and a systematic approach is required to evaluate these patients. It is very important to consider the differential diagnoses and avoid either missing the diagnosis of vasculitis or, conversely, over-diagnosing it. Ideally, patients should be identified before potentially organ- and life-threatening features develop, but this can be difficult in the early, non-specific stages. A systematic approach to the patient with multisystem disease is shown in Table 272.4. Where there is a high clinical suspicion, a biopsy from an affected organ is then obtained to try and confirm the diagnosis and exclude other conditions.

Other diagnoses that should be considered

The differential diagnosis of primary systemic vasculitis is wide and can be broadly divided into the following categories: infection (e.g. HIV, subacute bacterial endocarditis), malignancy (e.g. lymphoma, atrial myxoma), drugs (e.g. cocaine, ciprofloxacin, allopurinol), secondary forms of vasculitis (e.g. connective tissue diseases), and other miscellaneous causes (e.g. thromboembolic disease, calciphylaxis, amyloid).

'Gold-standard' diagnostic test

Although there is no gold standard for the diagnosis of systemic vasculitis, a confirmatory biopsy from an involved organ such as a kidney, a lung, or a nerve demonstrating active vasculitis should always be sought. In practice, histological findings can be inconclusive, possibly because of early disease, patchy involvement in a particular organ, or the effect of previous treatment with corticosteroids or other immunosuppressants (which may have to be started promptly in severe life- or organ-threatening disease). Histology and microbiology are important to exclude as far as is possible the presence of infection or malignancy but clinical judgement is still essential, especially when the pathological findings are non-diagnostic. ANCA testing can be very helpful in patients with clinical features suggestive of systemic small vessel vasculitis, but its indiscriminate use is not encouraged. Furthermore, not all cases of granulomatosis with polyangiitis, eosinophilic granulomatosis with polyangiitis, or microscopic polyangiitis are ANCA positive. There is a strong association between the presence of anti-glomerular-basement-membrane antibodies and Goodpasture's disease.

Table 272.1 Definitions for vasculitides adopted by the 2012 International Chapel Hill Consensus Conference on the Nomenclature of Vasculitides

CHCC2012 name	CHCC2012 definition
Large vessel vasculitis (LVV)	Vasculitis affecting large arteries more often than other vasculitides. Large arteries are the aorta and its major branches. Any size artery may be affected.
Takayasu arteritis (TAK)	Arteritis, often granulomatous, predominantly affecting the aorta and/or its major branches. Onset usually in patients younger than 50 years.
Giant cell arteritis (GCA)	Arteritis, often granulomatous, usually affecting the aorta and/or its major branches, with a predilection for the branches of the carotid and vertebral arteries. Often involves the temporal artery. Onset usually in patients older than 50 years and often associated with polymyalgia rheumatica.
Medium vessel vasculitis (MVV)	Vasculitis predominantly affecting medium arteries defined as the main visceral arteries and their branches. Any size artery may be affected. Inflammatory aneurysms and stenoses are common.
Polyarteritis nodosa (PAN)	Necrotizing arteritis of medium or small arteries without glomerulonephritis or vasculitis in arterioles, capillaries, or venules, and not associated with antineutrophil cytoplasmic antibodies (ANCAs).
Kawasaki disease (KD)	Arteritis associated with the mucocutaneous lymph node syndrome and predominantly affecting medium and small arteries. Coronary arteries are often involved. Aorta and large arteries may be involved. Usually occurs in infants and young children.
Small vessel vasculitis (SVV)	Vasculitis predominantly affecting small vessels, defined as small intraparenchymal arteries, arterioles, capillaries, and venules. Medium arteries and veins may be affected.
ANCA-associated vasculitis (AAV)	Necrotizing vasculitis, with few or no immune deposits, predominantly affecting small vessels (i.e., capillaries, venules, arterioles, and small arteries), associated with myeloperoxidase (MPO) ANCA or proteinase 3 (PR3) ANCA. Not all patients have ANCA. Add a prefix indicating ANCA reactivity, e.g., MPO-ANCA, PR3-ANCA, ANCA-negative.
Microscopic polyangiitis (MPA)	Necrotizing vasculitis, with few or no immune deposits, predominantly affecting small vessels (i.e., capillaries, venules, or arterioles). Necrotizing arteritis involving small and medium arteries may be present. Necrotizing glomerulonephritis is very common. Pulmonary capillaritis often occurs. Granulomatous inflammation is absent.
Granulomatosis with polyangiitis (Wegener's) (GPA)	Necrotizing granulomatous inflammation usually involving the upper and lower respiratory tract, and necrotizing vasculitis affecting predominantly small to medium vessels (e.g., capillaries, venules, arterioles, arteries, and veins). Necrotizing glomerulonephritis is common.
Single-organ vasculitis (SOV)	Vasculitis in arteries or veins of any size in a single organ that has no features that indicate that it is a limited expression of a systemic vasculitis. The involved organ and vessel type should be included in the name (e.g., cutaneous small vessel vasculitis, testicular arteritis, central nervous system vasculitis). Vasculitis distribution may be unifocal or multifocal (diffuse) within an organ. Some patients originally diagnosed as having SOV will develop additional disease manifestations that warrant redefining the case as one of the systemic vasculitides (e.g., cutaneous arteritis later becoming systemic polyarteritis nodosa, etc.).
Eosinophilic granulomatosis with polyangiitis (Churg-Strauss) (EGPA)	Eosinophil-rich and necrotizing granulomatous inflammation often involving the respiratory tract, and necrotizing vasculitis predominantly affecting small to medium vessels, and associated with asthma and eosinophilia. ANCA is more frequent when glomerulonephritis is present.
Immune complex vasculitis	Vasculitis with moderate to marked vessel wall deposits of immunoglobulin and/or complement components predominantly affecting small vessels (i.e., capillaries, venules, arterioles, and small arteries). Glomerulonephritis is frequent.
Anti-glomerular basement membrane (anti-GBM) disease	Vasculitis affecting glomerular capillaries, pulmonary capillaries, or both, with GBM deposition of anti-GBM autoantibodies. Lung involvement causes pulmonary hemorrhage, and renal involvement causes glomerulonephritis with necrosis and crescents.
Cryoglobulinemic vasculitis (CV)	Vasculitis with cryoglobulin immune deposits affecting small vessels (predominantly capillaries, venules, or arterioles) and associated with serum cryoglobulins. Skin, glomeruli, and peripheral nerves are often involved.
IgA vasculitis (Henoch–Schönlein) (IgAV)	Vasculitis, with IgA1-dominant immune deposits, affecting small vessels (predominantly capillaries, venules, or arterioles). Often involves skin and gastrointestinal tract, and frequently causes arthritis. Glomerulonephritis indistinguishable from IgA nephropathy may occur.
Hypocomplementemic urticarial vasculitis (HUV) (anti-C1q vasculitis)	Vasculitis accompanied by urticaria and hypocomplementemia affecting small vessels (i.e., capillaries, venules, or arterioles), and associated with anti-C1q antibodies. Glomerulonephritis, arthritis, obstructive pulmonary disease, and ocular inflammation are common.
Variable vessel vasculitis (VVV)	Vasculitis with no predominant type of vessel involved that can affect vessels of any size (small, medium, and large) and type (arteries, veins, and capillaries).
Behçet's disease (BD)	Vasculitis occurring in patients with Behçet's disease that can affect arteries or veins. Behçet's disease is characterized by recurrent oral and/or genital aphthous ulcers accompanied by cutaneous, ocular, articular, gastrointestinal, and/or central nervous system inflammatory lesions. Small vessel vasculitis, thromboangiitis, thrombosis, arteritis, and arterial aneurysms may occur.
Cogan's syndrome (CS)	Vasculitis occurring in patients with Cogan's syndrome. Cogan's syndrome characterized by ocular inflammatory lesions, including interstitial keratitis, uveitis, and episcleritis, and inner ear disease, including sensorineural hearing loss and vestibular dysfunction. Vasculitic manifestations may include arteritis (affecting small, medium, or large arteries), aortitis, aortic aneurysms, and aortic and mitral valvulitis.
Vasculitis associated with systemic disease	Vasculitis that is associated with and may be secondary to (caused by) a systemic disease. The name (diagnosis) should have a prefix term specifying the systemic disease (e.g., rheumatoid vasculitis, lupus vasculitis, etc.).
Vasculitis associated with probable aetiology	Vasculitis that is associated with a probable specific aetiology. The name (diagnosis) should have a prefix term specifying the association (e.g., hydralazine-associated microscopic polyangiitis, hepatitis B virus–associated vasculitis, hepatitis C virus–associated cryoglobulinemic vasculitis, etc.).

Reproduced with permission from J. C. Jennette et al., 2012 Revised International Chapel Hill Consensus Conference Nomenclature of Vasculitides, Arthritis & Rheumatology, Volume 65, Issue 1, pp. 1-11, Copyright © 2012 John Wiley and Sons.

Table 272.2 Symptoms that may suggest a diagnosis of vasculitis

Vessel size	Symptoms	Comments
Large vessel	New-onset/unaccustomed headache Jaw claudication Tongue pain Limb claudication Sudden onset of blindness	Any of these symptoms alone should raise the suspicion of vasculitis
Medium vessel	New-onset hypertension Abdominal ischaemic symptoms Ischaemic chest pain Polyneuropathy	Hypertension in itself is not very discriminatory, but in combination with abdominal ischaemia and polyneuropathy is very suggestive
Small vessel	Pulmonary haemorrhage or haemoptysis New-onset asthma or treatment-resistant asthma Chronic upper respiratory symptoms (e.g. nasal crusting, discharge) Sensory or motor peripheral neuropathy (mononeuritis multiplex) Haematuria, proteinuria, and/or oliguria Inflammatory arthritis Purpura	A combination of these symptoms is suggestive of vasculitis but other causes such as infection should be excluded first

Table 272.3 Incidence of vasculitis in Europe

Disease	Incidence per million population	Age distribution	Notes
Giant cell arteritis	37–350 (for patients older than 50 years of age)	Almost always over the age of 50	Incidence is in the higher range in northern Europe, and in the lower range in central and southern Europe Female-to-male ratio is 3:1
Takayasu arteritis	0.4–2.6	Usually below the age of 10, but cases reported as old as 60	Prevalence is thought to be higher in Turkey and Asia but there is no epidemiological data to support this
Kawasaki disease	55–146 (for children less than 5 years of age and living in the UK)	Usually children under 5	Incidence is lowest in children of Caucasian ancestry and highest in children of Asian origin A significantly higher incidence is reported in China and Japan
Polyarteritis nodosa	0.0–0.9	Any age, but peak in 40–60-year-old age group	Incidence has been dramatically reduced in the past two decades due to widespread vaccination and better screening of blood products for hepatitis B virus
Granulomatosis with polyangiitis	4.9–10.5	Any age	Prevalence is higher in northern Europe
Microscopic polyangiitis	2.7–11.6	Any age	Prevalence is higher in southern Europe
Eosinophilic granulomatosis with polyangiitis	0.5–4.2	Any age	
Henoch–Schönlein purpura	62–240 (for children under the age of 17 and living in the UK)	Usually children under 15, but can occur in adults	Lowest incidence observed in children of black Caribbean descent, and highest in children with Asian ancestry

Table 272.4 A systematic approach to the assessment of the patient with systemic vasculitis

General: Myalgia, arthralgia/arthritis, fever >38°C, weight loss			
Skin	Infarcts, purpura, ulcers, gangrene	**Respiratory**	Wheeze, nodules or cavities, effusions, infiltrates, haemoptysis, haemorrhage, respiratory failure
Mucous membranes/eyes	Mouth or genital ulcers, uveitis, scleritis, episcleritis, retinal changes	**Cardiovascular**	Valvular disease, loss of pulses, pericarditis, IHD, cardiomyopathy, CCF
Ear nose and throat	Bloody nasal discharge, crusts, granulomata, deafness, subglottic stenosis, sinusitis	**Gastrointestinal**	Peritonitis, bloody diarrhoea, ischaemic abdominal pain
Neurological	Headache, meningitis, confusion, seizures, cranial nerve and peripheral nerves, spinal cord lesions, CVA	**Renal**	Hypertension, proteinuria, haematuria, rise in creatinine

Abbreviations: CCF, congestive cardiac failure; CVA, cerebral vascular accident; IHD, ischaemic heart disease.

Reproduced from *Annals of the Rheumatic Diseases*, Mukhtyar C, et al, Modification and validation of the Birmingham Vasculitis Activity Score (version 3), volume 68, issue 12, pp. 1827–1832, copyright © 2008 BMJ Publishing Group Ltd.

Table 272.5 Mortality in systemic vasculitis: Five-year survival compared with age-matched population

Diagnosis	5-year survival (%)
Granulomatosis with polyangiitis	75
Microscopic polyangiitis	45–75
Eosinophilic granulomatosis with polyangiitis	68–100
Adult-onset Henoch–Schönlein purpura	75
Polyarteritis nodosa	75–80
Kawasaki disease	>99
Giant cell arteritis	100
Takayasu arteritis	70–93

Data from Phillip R and Luqmani R. Mortality in systemic vasculitis: a systematic review. *Clin Exp Rheumatol*, 2008. 26(5 Suppl 51): p. S94–104.

Acceptable diagnostic alternatives to the gold standard

Temporal artery ultrasound is more sensitive but less specific than temporal artery biopsy for the diagnosis of giant cell arteritis. In Takayasu arteritis and in polyarteritis, the use of MRI and magnetic resonance angiography for diagnosis and monitoring of the disease is now replacing invasive conventional angiography. PET scans may prove valuable in suspected large vessel disease but have a considerable radiation load, especially when used in conjunction with CT.

Table 272.6 Recommendations for the treatment of vasculitis

Vasculitis type	Recommendations for treatment
Large vessel vasculitis (giant cell arteritis and Takayasu arteritis)	For suspected giant cell arteritis, treatment should be initiated even before the biopsy or scan has been obtained and may be continued despite a negative biopsy or scan if the clinical suspicion is high
	Early use of high-dose corticosteroids (approximately 1 mg/kg of prednisolone (maximum 60 mg) per day or equivalent) to achieve remission; continue with this high dose for 1 month
	Taper steroids to achieve a target daily dose of 10–15 mg per day by 3 months
	Do not use alternative-day steroids, as this is more likely to lead to relapse of disease
	Immunosuppressive therapy (e.g. methotrexate or azathioprine) can be considered as an adjunct to treatment with corticosteroids
	There is growing evidence of benefit from anti-cytokine therapy, targeting interleukin-6, and in some cases from targeting interleukin -12
	Adequate bone protection (e.g. bisphosphonates) should be considered because patients are likely to require several years of glucocorticoid therapy
Small or medium vessel vasculitis (including granulomatosis with polyangiitis; microscopic polyangiitis; eosinophilic granulomatosis with polyangiitis; polyarteritis nodosa (not hepatitis B related); and non-infectious essential mixed-cryoglobulinaemia vasculitis)	Induction therapy in generalized disease (to induce remission):
	• cyclophosphamide and rituximab are equivalent in efficacy for treatment of GPA and MPA
	• IV pulse cyclophosphamide 15mg/kg (maximum 1.2g) fortnightly for first three doses, then 3 weekly for the next 3–7 doses; less commonly, continuous oral cyclophosphamide 2mg/kg/day (maximum 200mg/day) for 3–6 months may be given
	• daily prednisolone 1 mg/kg per day (maximum 60 mg/day) for the first months, and then taper to a target of 15 mg/day by the end of the third month
	• consider an initial pulse of IV methylprednisolone (0.5–1.0 g) as a single dose at the start of therapy, in addition to oral steroids
	• plasma exchange should be used as an adjunct to cyclophosphamide and steroid therapy in patients with severe renal disease (creatinine >500 μmol/l)
	• trimethoprim/sulfamethoxazole (800/160 mg on alternate days) should be used to prevent *Pneumocystis jiroveci* infection, which can result from severe immunosuppression
	• oral or IV mesna should be given to patients receiving pulse cyclophosphamide, to reduce the risk of bladder toxicity
	• consider rituximab, mycophenolate mofetil, 15-deoxyspergualin, anti-thymocyte globulin, infliximab, or IV immunoglobulin in patients who are refractory to induction therapy with cyclophosphamide
	Induction therapy in limited disease (to induce remission):
	• methotrexate (20–25 mg/day) can be used as an alternative to cyclophosphamide to induce remission in patients with mild disease and normal renal function
	Maintenance therapy (to maintain remission once this is achieved with induction therapy) in limited and generalized disease:
	• azathioprine (2 mg/kg per day), methotrexate (20–25 mg/week), mycophenolate mofetil (2–3g per day), or leflunomide (20–30 mg/day) should be used to maintain remission; continue for a minimum of 18 months
	• taper glucocorticoids to 10 mg/day by 6 months and then slowly taper further by 18 months
	• the addition of trimethoprim/sulfamethoxazole (800/160 mg twice daily) may reduce the risk of relapse in granulomatosis with polyangiitis
Hepatitis B-associated polyarteritis nodosa	Combination therapy utilizing high-dose glucocorticoids, antiviral therapy, and plasma exchange
	Hepatitis B can usually be cured with antiviral therapy
Hepatitis C-associated mixed-cryoglobulinaemia vasculitis	Antiviral therapy; usually, long-term dual therapy with ribavirin and interferon alfa, due to chronic persistence of infection despite antiviral therapy
Henoch–Schönlein purpura	In children, supportive therapy only
	Adults may be managed using immunosuppressive therapy +/− plasma exchange as for small vessel vasculitis, although there is no evidence base for effectiveness
Kawasaki disease	IV immunoglobulin 2 g/kg as a single infusion as soon as diagnosis is made
	High-dose aspirin 80–100 mg/kg per day in four divided doses for a minimum of 14 days and patient afebrile for >72 hours, then reduce dose to 3–5 mg/kg per day for 6–8 weeks; if there is evidence of coronary aneurysm, continue low-dose aspirin indefinitely

Data from:

Lapraik C, Watts R, Bacon P, et al. BSR and BHPR guidelines for the management of adults with ANCA associated vasculitis. Rheumatology (Oxford), 2007. 46(10): p. 1615–6.

Mukhtyar C, Guillevin L, Cid MC, et al. EULAR recommendations for the management of large vessel vasculitis. Ann Rheum Dis, 2009. 68(3): p. 318–23.

Mukhtyar C, Guillevin L, Cid MC, et al. EULAR recommendations for the management of primary small and medium vessel vasculitis. Ann Rheum Dis, 2009. 68(3): p. 310–7.

Newburger JW, Takahashi M, Gerber MA, et al. Diagnosis, treatment, and long-term management of Kawasaki disease: a statement for health professionals from the Committee on Rheumatic Fever, Endocarditis and Kawasaki Disease, Council on Cardiovascular Disease in the Young, American Heart Association. Circulation, 2004. 110(17): p. 2747–71.

Other relevant investigations

Baseline investigations in all patients with suspected vasculitis should include a full blood count, tests for urea and electrolytes, liver function tests, inflammatory markers, urinalysis, a chest radiograph, and an ECG. Further investigations, such as CT scans, can then be arranged as indicated from the pattern of organ involvement.

Prognosis and how to estimate it

Historically, patients with untreated systemic vasculitis had an 80% mortality rate. Improved recognition of these diseases and immunosuppressive therapy has reversed this to a 5-year survival of approximately 80%. Table 272.5 summarizes the outcome from a variety of studies of vasculitis over the last 50 years. Early deaths are usually secondary to uncontrolled vasculitis and highlight the need for aggressive early therapy in life- or organ-threatening disease. The other major cause of early death is infection. Due to more patients surviving the initial presentation, the effects of immunosuppressive therapy and comorbidities such as cardiovascular disease become important causes of death in the long term. A five-factor score (FFS) which comprises renal impairment, proteinuria, cardiomyopathy, CNS involvement, and gastrointestinal involvement predicts prognosis in polyarteritis nodosa and eosinophilic granulomatosis with polyangiitis. Patients with a FFS of 0 have a 5-year mortality of 12%, whereas, in patients with three or more factors, the mortality is 46%.

Treatment and its effectiveness

The treatment recommendations differ between the types of vasculitis but, in general, large vessel vasculitis is treated with moderate-to-high doses of corticosteroids alone, whereas most small and medium-sized vessel vasculitides require stronger immunosuppression in conjunction with steroids. The choice and intensity of immunosuppressive treatment for small vessel vasculitis is dependent on the severity of disease and the distribution of the organs involved. The exceptions are childhood-onset Henoch–Schönlein purpura, which is normally self-limiting, and Kawasaki disease (which requires aspirin and IV Ig). Antiviral strategies are necessary for the vasculitides associated with an infectious cause such as hepatitis B-associated polyarteritis and hepatitis C-related mixed-cryoglobulinaemia vasculitis.

Modern treatment strategies are usually very effective at treating acute disease, but patients are still prone to recurrent flares and long-term sequelae from low-grade, grumbling disease, from relapse, or from the therapy itself. Table 272.6 is based on the current recommendations from the European League Against Rheumatism and the American Heart Association.

Further Reading

Guillevin L, Lhote F, Gayraud M, et al. Prognostic factors in polyarteritis nodosa and Churg-Strauss syndrome. A prospective study in 342 patients. *Medicine (Baltimore)*, 1996; 75: 17–28.

Lane SE, Watts R, and Scott DG. Epidemiology of systemic vasculitis. *Curr Rheumatol Rep* 2005; 7: 270–5.

Lapraik C, Watts R, Bacon P, et al. BSR and BHPR guidelines for the management of adults with ANCA associated vasculitis. *Rheumatology (Oxford)* 2007; 46: 1615–16.

Mukhtyar C, Guillevin L, Cid MC, et al. EULAR recommendations for the management of large vessel vasculitis. *Ann Rheum Dis* 2009; 68: 318–23.

Mukhtyar C, Guillevin L, Cid MC, et al. EULAR recommendations for the management of primary small and medium vessel vasculitis. *Ann Rheum Dis* 2009; 68: 310–17.

Phillip R and Luqmani R. Mortality in systemic vasculitis: A systematic review. *Clin Exp Rheumatol* 2008; 26: S94–S104.

273 Osteomalacia

Kassim Javaid

Definition of the disease

Osteomalacia is a disorder of bone mineralization and is due to a lack of vitamin D.

Aetiology of the disease

Vitamin D is a prohormone formed by the action of UV radiation on the vitamin's precursor (7-dehydrocholesterol) in the skin. It then undergoes two hydroxylation steps to become an active hormone: the step to become 25-hydroxyvitamin D (25-OH vitamin D) occurs in the liver, and the second conversion takes place in the kidney to produce 1,25-dihydroxyvitamin D (1,25-OH vitamin D; also known as calcitriol), which is the active form. Conversion to calcitriol also occurs in most tissues for auto-/paracrine functions.

The commonest cause of osteomalacia is vitamin D deficiency due to a lack of UVB skin exposure. This is likely in those with darker skin, a reduced cutaneous exposure to the sun due to cultural clothing or lifestyle restrictions, or an ageing-associated reduced cutaneous capacity to metabolize vitamin D. Other causes include malabsorption (due to coeliac disease or pancreatic insufficiency), obesity, and chronic kidney disease. Rarer causes include Fanconi syndrome, distal renal tubular acidosis, drugs (e.g. phenytoin, carbamazepine, aluminium), cancer, and monogenic diseases that present in early life (e.g. X-linked hypophosphataemic rickets, autosomal dominant hypophosphataemic rickets).

Typical symptoms of the disease, and less common symptoms

The typical symptoms of osteomalacia are non-specific bone pain, proximal myopathy (which can be severe), fatigue, and polyarthralgia. The presence of unexplained groin pain may reflect an underlying insufficiency fracture of the proximal femur. Hypocalcaemia is uncommon but may lead to fits if severe. In patients with vitamin D deficiency, serum calcium is usually maintained by a secondary rise in parathyroid hormone (PTH), which resorbs bone to release calcium. If however, there is then a sudden substantial pharmacological block to resorption with drugs, such as with IV bisphosphonates or RANKL inhibitors, subclinical vitamin D deficiency can lead to clinically severe hypocalcaemia.

Oncogenic osteomalacia is due to ectopic production of fibroblast growth factor (FGF23) by benign, small, mesenchymal tumours. Patients present with profound proximal weakness with skeletal complications of vitamin D deficiency. Treatment is aimed to remove the tumour(s) with supportive with use of phosphate supplements and calcitriol. However, tumour localization can be challenging and may involve whole-body MRI, 18F-labelled FDG-PET, and octreotide scintography.

Demographics of the disease

Clinical osteomalacia is uncommon and usually seen in specific ethnic groups. In contrast, biochemical vitamin D deficiency (<50 nmol/l 25-OH vitamin D) has a much higher prevalence of 10%–65% in the UK population throughout the life course.

Natural history, and complications of the disease

The natural history of the osteomalacia, if untreated, is progressive bone pain and weakness leading to falls or pathological fracture. If severe, the secondary hyperparathyroidism can transform to tertiary hyperparathyroidism.

Approach to diagnosing the disease

The key is to establish abnormalities blood bone chemistry such as hypocalcaemia, hypophosphataemia, raised alkaline phosphatase levels, and raised PTH in conjunction with a low level of 25-OH vitamin D. Levels of 1,25-OH vitamin D are only helpful in cases of oncogenic osteomalacia, in which case FGF23 should also be measured. The 1,25-OH vitamin D level in patients with osteomalacia is elevated in early cases and then declines to within and then below the normal range with time and therefore is of no use, except in oncogenic osteomalacia. Radiology is indicated if there is a suspicion of insufficiency fracture, such as a Looser zone on the medial femoral neck.

Other diagnoses that should be considered

As the symptoms of osteomalacia are non-specific, the differential is wide and includes osteoporotic fracture, fibromyalgia, and polymyalgia rheumatica.

'Gold-standard' diagnostic test

The gold-standard diagnostic test for osteomalacia is a transiliac trephine bone biopsy to demonstrate excess osteoid.

Other relevant investigations

In osteomalacia, the creatine kinase level is normal. If there is concomitant iron deficiency or a history of malabsorption, then a coeliac screen should be requested.

Prognosis and how to estimate it

With effective treatment of osteomalacia, symptoms usually remit.

Treatment and its effectiveness

There is little agreement on the optimal strategy for treating vitamin D deficiency. Current evidence favours an oral rather than an intramuscular route, cholecalciferol rather than ergocalciferol, and only using concomitant calcium if required. Proposed dosing strategies include 50 000 IU weekly for 8 weeks, or 4000 IU daily for 12 weeks. Response to treatment is variable and can take 6–9 months. Following loading, maintenance therapy with 800–2000 IU per day is needed. If the vitamin D level is to be rechecked, this should be done at the end of the winter or in early spring, when it is at its nadir.

Further Reading

Bikle D. 'Vitamin D: Production, metabolism, and mechanisms of action', in De Groot LJ, Chrousos G, Dungan K, et al., eds, *Endotext*, 2000. MDText.com, Inc.

Rosen CJ. Vitamin D insufficiency. *N Engl J Med* 2011; 364: 248–54.

274 Paget's disease of bone

Kassim Javaid

Definition of the disease

Paget's disease of bone is an uncommon bone disorder with increased bone resorption and disorganized bone formation of woven bone.

Aetiology of the disease

The aetiology of Paget's disease of bone is unclear. There is a clear genetic component, with an eightfold increase in risk with an affected sibling. Additional environmental factors are important, given the reduction in severity and prevalence in the UK. Half of familial adult cases and 10% of non-familial cases are due to mutations in seques-tosome 1, which is part of the intracellular RANK signalling pathway. The genetic causes are better characterized for the less common subtypes of Paget's. Mutations in RANK are important for the early onset type of Paget's, which is characterized by severe polyostotic disease and osteoarthritis of the hands. Juvenile Paget's is due to abnormalities in osteoprotogerin, the antagonist of the RANK ligand, and is characterized by childhood onset with accelerated cardiovascular disease. Paget's associated with inclusion body myopathy and frontotemporal dementia is due to mutations in valosin-containing protein.

Typical symptoms of the disease, and less common symptoms

Paget's disease is usually asymptomatic and detected by an unexplained raised level of alkaline phosphatase (ALP) on routine biochemistry. Symptoms include focal bone pain, including headache, which can be severe, nocturnal, and associated with bony tenderness. The most commonly affected bones are the pelvis, then the lumbar spine, the femur, the thoracic spine, the sacrum, the skull, the tibia, and then, finally, the humerus.

Other symptoms include bone deformity and complications such as fracture and nerve conduction. Paget's disease can rarely present with immobilization-associated hypercalcaemia or high-output cardiac failure. Rarely, Paget's disease can transform into an osteosarcoma in the sixth and seventh decades, most commonly at the humerus.

Demographics of the disease

Paget's disease of bone affects up to 5% of the population aged over 55 years, with an equal gender risk. It is commonest in the UK and rare in Japan.

Natural history and complications of the disease

The natural history of the disease, if the disease is left untreated, is progressive bone pain and local deformity with resulting local symptoms and complications. Common local complications include:

- nerve compression (auditory nerve, optic nerve, spinal cord)
- secondary osteoarthritis (due to loss of joint congruity)
- pathological fracture

Approach to diagnosing the disease

Paget's has characteristic radiographic features of cortical expansion with disorganized trabeculation. The main stay of diagnosis is radiographic imaging of the affected area and a technetium-99 isotope bone scan. In the early lytic phase, Paget's may be difficult to distinguish from other lytic bone disease. For those identified by a raised ALP level, the key issue is to first ascertain whether the increase in ALP is due to bone isoenzymes and not hepatobiliary in origin. The next stage is to ascertain the sites affected, which do not change with the natural history of disease, using plain radiography and an isotope bone scan. Skull involvement highlights the potential for auditory or, less commonly, optic nerve compression and the potential for headaches which can become severe; the involvement of bones forming an articular surface raises the risk of secondary osteoarthritis, and the involvement of load-bearing bones raises the possibility of insufficiency fractures. For this reason, it is important to X-ray affected loading-bearing bones.

Other diagnoses that should be considered

When diagnosing Paget's disease of bone, important diagnoses to exclude include primary and secondary bone malignancy as well as local osteomyelitis. However, the radiological findings and lack of systemic features usually make the diagnosis.

'Gold-standard' diagnostic test

While bone biopsy is the gold-standard test for Paget's disease of bone, the presence of both radiographic and/or nuclear medicine findings is usually definitive. In cases of possible transformation to osteosarcoma, the biopsy may not be definitive and may require serial imaging with correlation with clinical features (increasing bone pain, local heat, and markedly raised ALP).

Other relevant investigations

Other investigations relevant for Paget's disease include the measurement of serum calcium (usually normal), ALP (raised; if possible, test for the bone isoenzyme), and 25-hydroxyvitamin D (to exclude concomitant osteomalacia raising ALP), and a renal profile (to guide treatment).

Prognosis and how to estimate it

The prognosis of Paget's disease has been revolutionized by the advent of bisphosphonates. However, late presentation or diagnosis may lead to bone complications.

Treatment and its effectiveness

The first line of treatment is patient education, as this is an uncommon disease, and, in the UK, linking the patient to the Paget's Association. Current first-line treatment is with a single infusion of 5 mg zoledronic acid. This requires an estimated glomerular filtration rate of >35 ml/min per 1.73 m², normocalcaemia, and a 25-hydroxyvitamin D level of more than 50 nmol/l. Zoledronic acid is highly effective in this disorder, and a single infusion appears to result in a sustained improvement in symptoms for many years. It is unusual for the markers of bone turnover (ALP or other bone turnover markers) to not suppress after treatment; if this is the case, one would want to exclude vitamin D deficiency and then repeat the infusion. For those with ongoing joint symptoms, where it is unclear if symptoms are due to Paget's disease or secondary osteoarthritis, if pain persists following zoledronic acid infusion, it is likely that secondary osteoarthritis is established. The patient's treatment pathway should then focus on analgesics, physiotherapy, and referral for consideration of arthroplasty. For those unable to take zoledronic acid, 30 mg daily of oral risedronate for 2 months is recommended. Other treatments such as calcitonin are no longer used except in exceptional circumstances. Treatment of asymptomatic Paget's disease of bone is controversial, and some wait for symptoms to occur before initiating treatment.

Further Reading

Ralston SH. Paget's disease of bone. *N Engl J Med* 2013; 368: 644–50.

Singer FR. 'Paget's disease of bone', in De Groot LJ, Chrousos G, Dungan K, et al., eds, *Endotext*, 2000. MDText.com, Inc.

Osteoporosis and fragility fracture

Kassim Javaid

Definition of the disease

Osteoporosis is defined as a systemic bone disease with reduction in both bone density and microarchitectural integrity, resulting in an increase in fragility fracture risk.

Aetiology of the disease

Osteoporosis is a multifactorial disease, through effects on bone formation and resorption on both the peak bone mass achieved during early adulthood and on rates of bone loss in later adulthood. Regulation of bone mass is currently thought to involve mechano-sensing by osteocytes, which regulate osteoblast activity through sclerostin and DKK1 inhibition of the WNT pathway. Osteoblasts then regulate osteoclast proliferation and activity through a balance of pro-osteoclastic RANKL and anti-osteoclastic osteoprotegerin. There is a significant genetic component for osteoporosis, with studies identifying pathways including WNT, RANKL, osteoprotegerin, and the oestrogen receptor. Environmental factors are thought to influence fracture risk across the life course, including vitamin D deficiency during in utero life, inadequate physical exercise, and vitamin D and calcium deficiency during childhood. In later adulthood, the commonest cause is sex hormone deficiency, including deficiency due to menopause, premature menopause (menopause occurring before the age of 45), testosterone deficiency, drug-induced gonadal deficiency (via the use of progesterone-only contraception, aromatase inhibitors, or androgen deprivation therapy), glucocorticoid excess (iatrogenic or due to Cushing's disease), current smoking, excess alcohol intake (greater than 3 units per day), and secondary diseases (malabsorption (e.g. coeliac disease), inflammatory diseases (e.g. inflammatory arthritides, inflammatory bowel disease, asthma), endocrine disorders (e.g. hyperparathyroidism, hyperthyroidism, diabetes)). Falls are an important risk factor for fracture and it is important to differentiate contributors such as syncope, poor balance, poor gait, postural hypotension, medication, and neurological diseases. Finally, there are rare genetic causes of osteoporosis, such as osteogenesis imperfecta and Turner's syndrome.

Typical symptoms of the disease, and less common symptoms

Osteoporosis is clinically silent until a fragility fracture occurs, as defined as due to a fall from standing height or less. The commonest sites are the distal forearm, the proximal femur, the thoracic/lumbar vertebra, the ribs, and the proximal humerus. However, recent evidence such as a fracture in an older person from any level of trauma should raise the suspicion of osteoporosis. Fractures of the digits, the face, the skull, the scaphoid, and the ankle, by some, are not usually considered osteoporotic. While fractures in the young typically heal with limited ongoing morbidity and excess mortality, osteoporotic fractures are associated with poorer healing and excess mortality (hip, spine, and pelvis). The morbidity after fracture depends on the site and includes chronic back pain for vertebral fracture, and wrist pain and weakness after distal forearm fracture. Progressive kyphosis from vertebral fracture reduces respiratory reserve.

Demographics of the disease

There are 3 million patients with osteoporosis in the UK, with over 200 000 fractures per year and 80 000 hip fractures. Fractures are commoner in those over 65 years and in women. A 50-year woman has a 1:2 lifetime risk of future fracture, with the risk being 1:5 for men. While, with an ageing population, the absolute number of fractures is set to rise, for reasons not completely understood, the age-specific rate of fracture is reducing in the USA and Northern Europe while still increasing in other parts of the world.

Natural history, and complications of the disease

Initially, patients present with peripheral fractures and then vertebral fractures before proximal femoral fractures. Half of patients with a proximal femoral fracture have a history of previous first fracture. Without therapy, bone mineral density (BMD) progressively declines with age. The outcomes after hip fracture are 50% fail to return home, with a significant reduction capacity to independently mobilize, and a 30% 1-year mortality. Further, only half of patients with a distal forearm fracture report a satisfactory recovery. Vertebral fractures lead to chronic back pain but only rarely lead to neurological compromise.

Approach to diagnosing the disease

The key issue is the ascertainment of primary versus secondary fracture prevention. The next stage is to determine BMD at the hip and spine using DEXA and then to exclude secondary causes and establish the most appropriate therapy according to patient-specific factors. The identification of a fragility fracture after the age of 40 years substantially increases the risk of future fracture and guides therapy. However, identification of occult vertebral fragility fractures can be challenging and requires radiological confirmation. The presence of one of the risk factors listed in 'Aetiology of the disease' warrants DEXA measurement. Those over 75 years with a fracture or with two or more risk factors can start treatment without a BMD test if DEXA imaging is clinically not appropriate. It is also important to rule out secondary causes of osteoporosis as well as ensure that patients are calcium and vitamin D replete.

Other diagnoses that should be considered

Osteoporosis is effectively a disease of exclusion. Important diagnoses to exclude include those diseases listed in 'Aetiology of the disease' as well as myeloma, malabsorption, osteomalacia, hyperthyroidism, chronic-kidney-disease-associated metabolic bone disease, and Cushing's syndrome.

'Gold-standard' diagnostic test

The gold-standard diagnostic test for osteoporosis is a BMD T-score for the lumbar spine, total hip, or femoral neck area of −2.5 or lower, as measured by DEXA. Some DEXA scanners can also measure the lateral and anterior posterior thoracolumbar X-ray as part of instant vertebral assessment, which often detects occult vertebral fractures. Care must be taken to exclude fractured vertebra(e) from the BMD assessment and to ensure optimal positioning.

Acceptable diagnostic alternatives to the gold standard

Patients over 75 years old with a fragility fracture or two or more risk factors for osteoporosis can start treatment. Peripheral DEXA and ultrasound may also be used as screening tools in experienced departments or as part of research.

Other relevant investigations

Other investigations that are relevant to osteoporosis include measurements of:

- serum calcium
- serum phosphate
- serum alkaline phosphatase
- serum 25-hydroxyvitamin D
- serum parathyroid hormone
- thyroid-stimulating hormone

Other tests include:

- a renal profile
- a liver profile
- full blood count
- erythrocyte sedimentation rate

Optional investigations include:

- a coeliac screen
- a myeloma screen
- the urinary calcium/creatinine ratio

- 24-hour urinary calcium excretion
- 24-hour urinary cortisol

Prognosis and how to estimate it

The prognosis of osteoporosis can now be assessed using the online FRAX tool. This uses readily ascertained risk factors with or without BMD measurement to provide an estimate of the 10-year risk of major fracture and hip fracture. Caveats for its use are that it does not include measurements of the lumbar spine BMD, dose of glucocorticoids, or measures of fracture number or site. There is some evidence that FRAX predicts fracture risk both off and on therapy.

Treatment and its effectiveness

Treatment for osteoporosis is aimed at reducing future fracture risk. As there is no symptomatic benefit from therapy, and oral treatment requires complex administration regimens, it is important to ensure adequate patient information using the National Osteoporosis Society literature. The first line of treatment is to ensure patients are calcium (>800 mg/day) and vitamin D (25-hydroxyvitamin

Table 275.1 NICE guidance for primary and secondary prevention of osteoporotic fragility fractures in postmenopausal women

Age	50/54	55/65	65/69	70/74	75+
Primary prevention					
Alendronic acid	T-score ≤ −2.5, 1 CRF*, and 1 BRF†	T-score ≤ −2.5, 1 CRF, and 1 BRF	T-score ≤ −2.5, and 1 CRF	T-score ≤ −2.5, and 1 CRF/BRF	2 CRFs/BRFs
Risedronate	Not recommended	Not recommended	T-score ≤ −3.5, and 1 CRF T-score ≤ −3, and 2 CRFs	T-score ≤ −3.5 T-score ≤−3.0, and 1 CRF T-score ≤−2.5, and 2 CRFs	T-score ≤ −3.0 T-score ≤ −2.5, and 2 CRFs
Denosumab	Not recommended	Not recommended	T-score ≤ −4.5, and 1 CRF T-score ≤ −4.0, and 2 CRFs	T-score ≤ −4.5 T-score ≤ −4.0, and 1 CRF T-score ≤ −3.5, and 2 CRFs	T-score ≤−4.0 T-score ≤−3.0, and 2 CRFs
Strontium	Not recommended	Not recommended	T-score ≤ −4.5, and 1 CRF T-score ≤ −4.0, and 2 CRFs	T-score ≤ −4.5 T-score ≤ −4.0, and 1 CRF T-score ≤−3.5, and 2 CRF	T-score ≤ −4.0 T-score ≤ −3.0, and 2 CRFs
Secondary prevention					
Alendronic acid	T-score ≤ −2.5	T-score ≤ −2.5	T-score ≤ −2.5	T-score ≤ −2.5	No DEXA threshold
Risedronate	T-score ≤ −3.0, and 1 CRF T-score ≤ −2.5, and 2 CRFs	T-score ≤ −3.0 T-score ≤ −2.5, and 2 CRFs	T-score ≤ −3.0 T-score ≤ −2.5, and 1 CRF	T-score ≤ −2.5	No DEXA threshold
Denosumab	Intolerant to alendronate or risedronate	Intolerant to alendronate or risedronate	Intolerant to alendronate or risedronate	Intolerant to alendronate or risedronate	Intolerant to alendronate or risedronate
Strontium or raloxifene	T-score ≤ −3.5, and 1 CRF	T-score ≤ −4.0 T-score ≤ −3.5, and 1 CRF	T-score ≤ −4.0 T-score ≤ −3.5, and 1 CRF T-score ≤ −3.0, and 2 CRFs	T-score ≤ −3.0 T-score ≤ −2.5, and 2 CRFs	T-score ≤ −3.0 T-score ≤ −2.5, and 1 CRF
Teriparatide		T-score ≤ −4.0, and ≥ 3 fractures	T-score ≤ −4.0 T-score ≤−3.5, and ≥ 3 fractures	T-score ≤ −4.0 T-score ≤−3.5, and ≥ 3 fractures	T-score ≤ −4.0 T-score ≤−3.5, and ≥ 3 fractures

Abbreviations: BRF, bone risk factor; CRF, clinical risk factor for parental hip fracture.

*Clinical risk factors for parental hip fracture: alcohol ≥4 units/ day; rheumatoid arthritis.

†Bone risk factors: BMI < 22 kg/m²; diseases like Crohn's disease or ankylosing spondylitis; prolonged immobility; untreated premature menopause.

Data from

NICE: Alendronate, etidronate, risedronate, raloxifene and strontium ranelate for the primary prevention of osteoporotic fragility fractures in postmenopausal women (2008)

http://www.nice.org.uk/guidance/ta160.

NICE: Alendronate, etidronate, risedronate, raloxifene, strontium ranelate and teriparatide for the secondary prevention of osteoporotic fragility fractures in postmenopausal women (2008) http://www.nice.org.uk/guidance/ta161.

NICE: Denosumab for the prevention of osteoporotic fractures in postmenopausal women (2010).

http://www.nice.org.uk/guidance/ta204.

D >50 nmol/l) replete. Diet is a good source of calcium, with 600 mg in a pint of milk, and 200 mg in a small pot of yoghurt or a small matchbox of cheese. The ideal intake is 800–1200 mg/day. Vitamin D is difficult to find in the diet and often requires use of supplements.

Next requires selection of the optimal bone therapy and the National Institute for Health and Clinical Excellence (NICE) have produced intervention thresholds based on primary versus secondary prevention, BMD, clinical risk factors, and patient tolerability (see Table 275.1). Most of the agents show fracture reductions in the range of 30% for non-vertebral fracture, and 50%–70% for vertebral fracture.

The first-line agent is 70 mg oral alendronate weekly. This is an amino bisphosphonate that inhibits farnesyl transferase and osteoclast function. As it has a very poor bioavailability (0.7%), there are four keys aspects for administration: (1) to take it first thing in the morning after an overnight fast with a large glass of tap water; (2) not to take any other drink, food, or medication for the next 30 minutes; (3) to remain upright (standing, sitting, and/or walking) for the next 30 minutes; and (4) to take any calcium supplements in the afternoon on the day that the oral bisphosphonate is taken. Alendronic acid is contraindicated in those with significant upper gastrointestinal pathology, hypocalcaemia, an estimated glomerular filtration rate (eGFR) of less than 30 ml/min, and pregnancy. Dyspepsia is common and should be managed by switching to another agent rather than adding an proton-pump inhibitor (PPI), as there is evidence that PPI use blunts the fracture reduction benefit.

Alternative oral therapies include risedronate (35 mg weekly with similar administration and contraindications) and strontium ranelate. Strontium ranelate 2 g is taken in the middle of a 4-hour calcium- and magnesium-free dietary fast. Typically, it is given at bedtime after a 2-hour fast. It is an insoluble powder that patients suspend in water and then take. Common unwanted effects are loose stool to diarrhoea. Rarely, a DRESS syndrome (**d**rug **r**ash with **e**osinophilia and **s**ystemic **s**ymptoms) can occur, and patients should be advised to stop and consult their doctor if they develop a rash on treatment.

Given the poor adherence to oral therapies, three groups of parenteral therapy are available. Denosumab is a monoclonal antibody that binds RANKL and inhibits osteoclast proliferation and function. It is given every 6 months as a subcutaneous injection and has efficacy with an eGFR of greater than 15 ml/min. Unwanted effects are uncommon and we await Phase 4 analyses for more information. Zoledronic acid is an IV bisphosphonate given as a short infusion every year for 3–6 years. It is slightly renally toxic and so is contraindicated in patients with an eGFR of less than 35 ml/min. It commonly causes flu-like symptoms for up to 7 days but, in some cases, it leads to an acute inflammatory response in specific organs, causing iritis or colitis. Both denosumab and zoledronic acid as well as oral bisphosphonates have been associated with osteonecrosis of the jaw (ONJ). This is an exposure of the mandible for more than 6 weeks, despite antibiotic therapy, usually after an invasive dental procedure. However, cases are usually cancer patients receiving 3–12-times-higher doses of bone agents than are used in osteoporosis therapy. Currently, the risk of ONJ is considered rare in osteoporosis therapy.

Teriparatide is a humanized 1-34 parathyroid hormone analogue. It is the only pure anabolic agent available and is given as a daily subcutaneous injection, for 18 months. It is usually reserved for those with severe osteoporosis, as evidenced by a T-score less than −3.5, the presence of more than two fractures, and intolerance/fracture on treatment with oral agents. The higher cost of teriparatide is offset by its observed greater fracture reduction, especially at the spine. The duration of therapy with bone-specific therapies is only clear for teriparatide, for which 24 months is the licensed duration. In the absence of evidence, currently, the recommendation is 5 years' treatment and then a drug holiday for 2 years before considering another cycle of therapy. In those with a vertebral fracture, 10-year cycles are appropriate. For those who refracture while on treatment, a switch in therapy, usually to a parenteral therapy, should be considered.

Atypical subtrochanteric fractures are a growing concern in the field of osteoporosis. They are typically preceded by atypical thigh pain and lead to a spontaneous or minimal-trauma horizontal femoral fracture with a characteristic breaking on one side and relatively thickened femoral shaft cortices. They appear to be associated with prolonged use of bisphosphonates. Key principles in their management are effective orthopaedic intervention, given that the bone is likely to be brittle; early imaging of the contralateral side with radiographs; MRI of the whole femur, to exclude a contralateral fracture; and cessation of bisphosphonate therapy. If the patient remains at risk of fracture at other sites, strontium ranelate or teriparatide therapy should be considered. The role of denosumab in this patient group is not known. The estimated rate of subtrochanteric fracture is 5 per 10 000 patient years of treatment, and the risk rapidly diminishes with cessation of bisphosphonate therapy.

Vertebroplasty and kyphoplasty are used to manage painful vertebral fractures but currently undergoing NICE reappraisal, as two sham-controlled trials have not replicated the benefits of usual care-controlled trials.

Further Reading

Lewiecki EM. 'Osteoporosis: Clinical evaluation', in De Groot LJ, Chrousos G, Dungan K, et al., eds, *Endotext*, 2000. MDText.com, Inc.

National Institute for Health and Clinical Excellence. Osteoporosis: Assessing the risk of fragility fracture. 2012. Available at http://www.nice.org.uk/guidance/cg146 (accessed 8 Sep 2017).

Seibel MJ, Cooper MS, and Zhou H. Glucocorticoid-induced osteoporosis: Mechanisms, management, and future perspectives. *Lancet Diabetes Endocrinol* 2013; 1: 59–70.

Introduction

Genetic conditions affecting the skeleton and supporting structures are individually rare and heterogeneous. This chapter suggests approaches to assessing patients for suspected skeletal dysplasia, osteogenesis imperfecta, Marfan syndrome, and Ehlers–Danlos syndrome.

Skeletal dysplasia

Aetiology of skeletal dysplasia

Skeletal dysplasias are caused by abnormalities of bone growth and modelling. Many are linked to mutations in genes for particular collagens or for growth factors and their receptors.

Typical symptoms of skeletal dysplasia, and less common symptoms

Skeletal dysplasias predominantly cause short stature and deformity. However, the affected sites are linked to different complications.
   Conditions affecting the epiphyses (the area of secondary ossification at the ends of long bones) affect articulation and predispose to early arthritis, requiring joint replacement.
   The metaphysis is adjacent to the epiphysis and is the main growth region. **Conditions affecting metaphyses** (including achondroplasia) shorten long bones, compromising eventual height.
   The diaphysis is the central shaft and is affected by conditions, like osteogenesis imperfecta, that alter the early collagen bone model.
   The term 'spondylo' is used where the spine is affected. The spine may be short, with kyphosis or scoliosis.
   The skeletal dysplasias can be classified clinically, radiologically, or by the causative genetic mutation. One such classification, which is regularly revised, is from the International Skeletal Dysplasia Society and is referred to as the International Nomenclature and Classification of the Osteochondrodysplasias.

Demographics of skeletal dysplasia

Each specific type of skeletal dysplasia is individually rare. The commonest non-lethal type is achondroplasia, with an incidence of 1/10 000 to 1/30 000.

Natural history of skeletal dysplasia, and complications of the disease

In achondroplasia, disordered endochondral bone formation can result in compression of the cervical cord and medulla at the foramen magnum, spinal stenosis, atlantoaxial subluxation, and macrocrania, with or without hydrocephalus.

Approach to diagnosing skeletal dysplasia

When diagnosing skeletal dysplasia, take a three-generation history with details of adult height, joint replacement, and specific questions about consanguinity. Document whether growth was normal in pregnancy and try to obtain early growth records. Ask about fractures and developmental delay.
   Assess whether the growth problem is proportionate or disproportionate. Measure span, height, and lower segment length. If the growth problem is disproportionate, is the shortening proximal (rhizomelic) or distal (mesomelic)? Is there any bowing of the bones or contractures? There are many other features that can be linked to specific dysplasias, particularly polydactyly or abnormal thumbs; cleft palate; abnormal teeth and hair; cataract or myopia; and congenital heart disease. Many patients with skeletal dysplasia will have lax joints.

Other diagnoses that should be considered aside from skeletal dysplasia

When considering a diagnosis of skeletal dysplasia, exclude other causes of short stature (e.g. chromosomal or syndromic causes). These will often have proportionate short stature. Storage disorders and a wide range of other metabolic and hormonal conditions can affect growth.

'Gold-standard' diagnostic test for skeletal dysplasia

A definitive diagnosis of skeletal dysplasia is generally made after specialist review of a skeletal survey; this is often most helpful in childhood. Mutation analysis may then be possible. A skeletal survey should include the following X-rays:

- skull AP and lateral
- chest PA
- spine AP and lateral
- pelvis with hips
- unilateral humerus, radius, ulna, femur, tibia, and fibula
- hand carpal bones and phalanges

Acceptable diagnostic alternatives to the gold-standard test for skeletal dysplasia

When skeletal dysplasia is suspected, an acceptable diagnostic alternative to a skeletal survey is a descriptive diagnosis based on family history and examination findings, with patients classified according to the following clinical diagnostic groups:

- those with short limbs but in whom the trunk less affected: hypochondroplasia, achondroplasia, and pseudoachondroplasia
- those with short limbs and trunk: diastrophic dysplasia
- those with epiphyseal dysplasias: multiple epiphyseal dysplasia
- those with a short trunk but in whom the limbs are less affected; spondyloepiphyseal and spondylometaphyseal disorders
- metaphyseal disorders: metabolic disease
- abnormal bone density: osteogenesis imperfecta

Other relevant investigations for skeletal dysplasia

Other relevant investigations for skeletal dysplasia include:

- a metabolic screen, if a metaphyseal disorder is suspected
- MRI of the brain with the cervical and lower spine, if there are neurological signs or there is evolving hydrocephalus
- molecular analysis (e.g. FGFR3 in achondroplasia and hypochondroplasia)
- cytogenetic screen for X-chromosome deletions

Prognosis of skeletal dysplasia, and how to estimate it

In skeletal dysplasia, severe conditions can present in utero, and many are lethal because of reduced lung capacity or evolving hydrops. Prognosis in terms of eventual height and complications is condition specific.

Treatment of skeletal dysplasia, and its effectiveness

As treatment for skeletal dysplasia, surgical management of deformities to improve function and, occasionally, operations to lengthen limbs may be suggested. Growth hormone treatment is of no benefit to the majority of children. Exercise can be helpful, to maintain range of movement and build strength. A referral for mobility aid assessment can be considered.

Osteogenesis imperfecta

Aetiology of osteogenesis imperfecta

Most patients with osteogenesis imperfecta have mutations in COL1A1 or COL1A2. Abnormal collagen production gives a more open meshwork to the early bone model, and this eventually leads to reduced mineralization. There are four main types of osteogenesis imperfecta (see 'Natural history of osteogenesis imperfecta, and complications of the disease'); osteogenesis imperfecta types I and IV are dominantly inherited, type II is generally caused by a de novo dominant mutation, and type III is mostly dominant, although some recessive families have been described.

Typical symptoms of osteogenesis imperfecta, and less common symptoms

The typical presentation of osteogenesis imperfecta is with multiple fractures, sometimes prenatally. There may be associated short stature, bone deformity, dentogenesis imperfecta, blue sclera, and hearing loss. This is a collagen disease, and patients can have the soft skin, lax joints, scoliosis, and mitral valve prolapse seen in other conditions affecting collagen. Spinal deformity can cause neurological and respiratory compromise.

Demographics of osteogenesis imperfecta

The most common form of osteogenesis imperfecta, osteogenesis imperfecta type 1, has a frequency of 2–5/100 000.

Natural history of osteogenesis imperfecta, and complications of the disease

The natural history of osteogenesis imperfecta is linked to the severity of the condition, but also the degree of osteoporosis in later life. The clinical classification of osteogenesis imperfecta (called the Sillence classification) is useful in predicting severity and outcome. The main types are:

- type I:
  - mild
  - non-deforming
  - mild short stature
  - blue sclera
  - normal teeth
- type II:
  - perinatally lethal due to respiratory compromise
  - multiple rib and long-bone fractures present at birth, with deformity and dark sclera
  - low bone density
  - separated into types IIA, IIB, and IIC, depending on the radiographic appearance
- type III:
  - severe
  - deforming
  - very short stature
  - scoliosis
  - multiple fractures
  - patient must often use a wheelchair
  - grey sclera
  - dentogenesis imperfecta
  - triangular facies
- type IV:
  - moderately deforming
  - moderate short stature
  - patient may have scoliosis
  - grey/white sclera
  - dentogenesis imperfecta

Hearing loss is common, being found in ~50% of cases by 30 years of age, and 95% of cases in later life, but is not usually seen in those under 10 years old. About 10% of cases will have asymptomatic mitral valve prolapse, and 24% of affected males (but only 4% of affected females) have non-progressive aortic dilatation.

Approach to diagnosing osteogenesis imperfecta

When diagnosing osteogenesis imperfecta, take a three-generation family history of fracturing, deformity, and the associated features. It is generally possible to diagnose the type on history and examination findings alone.

Other diagnoses that should be considered aside from osteogenesis imperfecta

Recurrent childhood fractures require sensitive questioning, given the possible confusion with non-accidental injury. Juvenile and premature osteoporosis can lead to fractures, as can hypophosphatasia. Bruck syndrome is a recessive condition linking blue sclera, Wormian bones, and congenital contractures of large joints.

'Gold-standard' diagnostic test for osteogenesis imperfecta

The following are gold-standard diagnostic tests for osteogenesis imperfecta:

- skin biopsy for examination of fibroblast collagens via electron microscopy
- COL1A1, COL1A2 and rarer gene mutation testing

Acceptable diagnostic alternatives to the gold-standard for osteogenesis imperfecta

Wormian bones on a skull X-ray are often seen in osteogenesis imperfecta type I but bone density generally can be variable and often normal. For more severe forms of osteogenesis imperfecta, a full skeletal survey will be helpful. Offer hearing tests throughout life, and an initial biochemistry screen to exclude metabolic bone disease.

Other relevant investigations for osteogenesis imperfecta

Another investigation that is relevant in osteogenesis imperfecta is echocardiography, to assess for valve involvement.

Prognosis of osteogenesis imperfecta, and how to estimate it

The prognosis of osteogenesis imperfecta will be related to the severity of the bone disease, but also the site of fractures (e.g. if they affect the joints). Often, children with osteogenesis imperfecta fracture recurrently until puberty, when the condition improves. Multiple fractures in childhood may predict later osteoporosis, and bone density scanning in adult life is indicated.

Treatment of osteogenesis imperfecta, and its effectiveness

Treatment of osteogenesis imperfecta requires prompt, specialist, orthopaedic management of fractures, with full physiotherapy and rehabilitation support. The use of bisphosphonates is under assessment; these drugs can reduce osteoclast bone reabsorption. However, they are used in specialist centres only, and for severer types of the disease.

Marfan syndrome

Aetiology of Marfan syndrome

Between 66% and 91% of individuals with Marfan syndrome have a mutation in fibrillin 1 (FBN1; locus: 15q21). Some families have mutations in TGFBR1 or TGFBR2. Marfan syndrome is a dominantly inherited condition, but up to a third of cases are caused by a spontaneous mutation.

Typical symptoms of Marfan syndrome, and less common symptoms

Marfan syndrome is a connective tissue disease with a pattern of symptoms related to the presence of fibrillin in tissues. Typically affected individuals are of tall, thin stature, with long fingers and toes (arachnodactyly), a pectus deformity, and scoliosis. They may have a high palate with dental crowding; lax joints; excessive striae; and a history of recurrent herniae or pneumothoraces.

Demographics of Marfan syndrome

The estimated prevalence of Marfan syndrome is 1/3000 to 1/5000.

Natural history of Marfan syndrome, and complications of the disease

In Marfan syndrome, joint hypermobility can give chronic pain and early arthritis. There may be bilateral ectopia lentis (in ~50% of cases), myopia (in 30% of cases), and, rarely, retinal detachment. However, the most serious complication is aortic dilatation, and an annual echocardiogram is requested for affected individuals. Particular care is needed in pregnancy.

Approach to diagnosing Marfan syndrome

When diagnosing Marfan syndrome, take a three-generation family history detailing symptoms of Marfan syndrome. Measure height, weight, arm span, and lower segment length. A standard examination scoring system for assessing individuals with suspected Marfan syndrome is used. This is referred to as the Ghent criteria and has been shown to detect about 86% of individuals carrying a fibrillin 1 mutation (see Table 276.1); however, this system is less reliable in children. The system scores common features in the skeleton, eyes, heart, lungs, and skin, and notes the presence or absence of dural ectasia or a family history. There are major and minor criteria; in the absence of a family history, two of the major criteria and one of the minor criteria must be present to confirm a clinical diagnosis. An echocardiogram (to measure the aortic root diameter at the level of the sinuses of Valsalva and screen for mitral prolapse) and eye examination (to look for refractive error and lens instability) will be requested. Mutation detection can be undertaken where resources allow, and can be useful for defining screening in large families.

Other diagnoses that should be considered aside from Marfan syndrome

Other diagnoses that should be considered aside from Marfan syndrome are summarized in Table 276.1. If there is learning difficulty, homocystinuria should be excluded. Mild Ehlers–Danlos syndrome can give similar joint hypermobility.

'Gold-standard' diagnostic test for Marfan syndrome

The gold-standard diagnostic test for Marfan syndrome is fibrillin 1 mutation testing.

Acceptable diagnostic alternatives to the gold-standard test for Marfan syndrome

An acceptable diagnostic alternative to fibrillin 1 mutation testing is an assessment of family history and the application of Ghent criteria.

Other relevant investigations for Marfan syndrome

Relevant investigations for Marfan syndrome include monitoring the ratio of the aortic diameter to the body surface area, as this can be used to assess the progression of aortic dilatation over time. In addition, an X-ray of the hip or spinal MRI may be relevant if these features would alter assessment using the Ghent criteria.

Prognosis of Marfan syndrome, and how to estimate it

Untreated, unscreened people with Marfan syndrome have a 40% reduced life expectance from aortic complications, predominantly dissection. Plotting the aortic root diameter over time helps to plan if aortic replacement is indicated.

Treatment of Marfan syndrome, and its effectiveness

The major complication of Marfan syndrome is aortic root dilatation, which predisposes to aortic dissection. Regular surveillance of the aortic root by echocardiography, the use of beta blockers and angiotensin-receptor blockers to retard dilatation, and aortic root repair when the diameter reaches 5.0 cm improve the prognosis. Contact sports and sports causing high cardiovascular stress should be avoided. Regular ophthalmic review is suggested until adolescence.

Ehlers–Danlos syndrome

Aetiology of the disease

Classical Ehlers–Danlos syndrome (types I and II) is caused by dominant mutations in COL5A1 and COL5A2. Hypermobility (Ehlers–Danlos syndrome type III) is dominantly inherited and molecularly undefined. Vascular Ehlers–Danlos syndrome (type IV) can be dominantly or recessively inherited with mutations in COL3A1. Kyphoscoliosis (Ehlers–Danlos syndrome type VI) is a recessive condition caused by mutations in PLOD1. Arthrochalasia (Ehlers–Danlos syndrome types VIIA and B) is linked to dominant exonic deletions in COL1A1 and COL1A2. Dermatosporaxis (Ehlers–Danlos syndrome type VIIC) is caused by recessive mutations in a collagen N-peptidase (ADAMTS2).

Table 276.1 Differential diagnosis of Marfan syndrome

Differential diagnosis	Gene	Discriminating features
Loeys–Dietz syndrome (LDS)	TGFBR1/2	Bifid uvula/cleft palate, arterial tortuosity, hypertelorism, diffuse aortic and arterial aneurysms, craniosynostosis, clubfoot, cervical spine instability, thin and velvety skin, easy bruising
Shprintzen–Goldberg syndrome (SGS)	FBN1 and other	Craniosynostosis, mental retardation
Congenital contractural arachnodactyly (CCA)	FBN2	Crumpled ears, contractures
Weill–Marchesani syndrome (WMS)	FBN1 and ADAMTS10	Microspherophakia, brachydactyly, joint stiffness
Ectopia lentis syndrome (ELS)	FBN1 LTBP2 ADAMTSL4	Lack of aortic root dilatation
Homocystinuria	CBS	Thrombosis, mental retardation
Familial thoracic aortic aneurysm syndrome (FTAA)	TGFBR1/2, ACTA2	Lack of Marfanoid skeletal features, levido reticularis, iris flocculi
FTAA with bicuspid aortic valve (BAV)		
FTAA with patent ductus arteriosus (PDA)	MYH11	
Arterial tortuosity syndrome (ATS)	SLC2A10	Generalised arterial tortuosity, arterial stenosis, facial dysmorphism
Ehlers–Danlos syndromes (vascular, valvular, kyphoscoliotic type)	COL3A1, COL1A2, PLOD1	Middle sized artery aneurysm, severe valvular insufficiency, translucent skin, dystrophic scars, facial characteristics

Reproduced from *Journal of Medical Genetics*, Loeys et al., The revised Ghent nosology for the Marfan syndrome, volume 47, issue 7, pp. 476–485, copyright © 2010 with permission from BMJ Publishing Group Ltd.

Typical symptoms of Ehlers–Danlos syndrome, and less common symptoms

All forms of Ehlers–Danlos syndrome present with variable thinning and fragility of skin, leading to easy bruising and poor scar formation. There is skin and joint laxity. In severe forms, blood vessels and internal organs are affected.

Demographics of Ehlers–Danlos syndrome

The incidence of Ehlers–Danlos syndrome (as a group) is about 1 in 5000.

Natural history of Ehlers–Danlos syndrome, and complications of the disease

In Ehlers–Danlos syndrome, the degree of hypermobility can decrease with age and move to more stiffness related to arthritis. Vascular Ehlers–Danlos syndrome causes increasing complications with age.

Approach to diagnosing Ehlers–Danlos syndrome

When diagnosing Ehlers–Danlos syndrome, take a three-generation family history of joint dislocation/early arthritis and abnormal scarring. Examine all joints for range of mobility to give a Beighton score, which is calculated as follows:

- passive extension of little finger beyond 90°: score 1 for each hand
- passive opposition of thumb to the flexor surface of forearm: score 1 for each hand
- hyperextension of elbow beyond 10°: score 1 for each elbow
- hyperextension of knee beyond 10°: score 1 for each knee
- flex the spine; if the patient's hands are flat on the floor, score 1

Therefore, the total Beighton score could be at most 9.

Assess the skin for softness, elasticity, and atrophy. The Villefranche classification is used to describe the various patterns of Ehlers–Danlos syndrome. A shortened summary of main types is as follows:

- classical Ehlers–Danlos syndrome (types I and II):
  - soft hyperextensible skin
  - lax joints
  - easy bruising
  - thin scars
  - varicose veins
  - risk of prematurity in affected fetuses
- hypermobility (Ehlers–Danlos syndrome type III):
  - merges into the general population
  - use if Beighton score >5/9
- vascular (Ehlers–Danlos syndrome type IV):
  - more serious condition
  - patients tend to look aged, with deep-set eyes and thin skin
  - little joint laxity, but high risk for rupture of blood vessels, bladder, bowel, or uterus
- kyphoscoliosis (Ehlers–Danlos syndrome type VI):
  - soft skin
  - joint hypermobility
  - muscle hypotonia
  - scoliosis
  - rupture of the optic globe
- arthrochalasia (Ehlers–Danlos syndrome types VIIA and B):
  - normal scars
  - severe joint problems, including hip dislocation
- dermatosporaxis (Ehlers–Danlos syndrome type VIIC):
  - affects the skin which is sagging, redundant, and fragile

Other diagnoses that should be considered aside from Ehlers–Danlos syndrome

Other diagnoses that should be considered aside from Ehlers–Danlos syndrome include cutis laxa and Marfan syndrome, which share some features, and benign hypermobility, which is common.

'Gold-standard' diagnostic test for Ehlers–Danlos syndrome

The gold-standard diagnostic tests for Ehlers–Danlos syndrome are a skin biopsy, to provide a fibroblast culture for electron microscope analysis of collagen fibres, and targeted collagen mutation testing, particularly when Ehlers–Danlos syndrome vascular type is being considered.

Acceptable diagnostic alternatives to the gold-standard tests for Ehlers–Danlos syndrome

An acceptable diagnostic alternative to the gold-standard tests for Ehlers–Danlos syndrome is clinical classification.

Other relevant investigations for Ehlers–Danlos syndrome

Other relevant investigations for Ehlers–Danlos syndrome are an echocardiogram, to look for aortic diameter and mitral valve prolapse in classical, hypermobile, and kyphoscoliotic Ehlers–Danlos syndrome, and MRI of major vessels in vascular Ehlers–Danlos syndrome, although it is still unclear if aneurysm repair is indicated, given the extreme tissue fragility.

Prognosis of Ehlers–Danlos syndrome, and how to estimate it

The majority of individuals with Ehlers–Danlos syndrome are primarily affected by morbidity from skin and joint problems. Only the vascular type is associated with high mortality. About 25% of affected individuals will have serious complications by 20 years of age, and 50% by 40 years of age. The median life expectancy is around 48 years, with most dying of arterial rupture. Pregnancies are very high risk.

Treatment of Ehlers–Danlos syndrome, and its effectiveness

The management of Ehlers–Danlos syndrome is largely supportive, with surgical treatment of dislocation and careful management of wounds. Celiprolol has been shown (in one randomized controlled trial) to reduce the risk of complications in vascular Ehlers–Danlos syndrome.

Further Reading

Loeys BL, Dietz HC, Braverman AC, et al. The revised Ghent nosology for the Marfan syndrome. *J Med Genet* 2010; 47: 476–85.

Malfait F. The 2017 International Classification of Ehlers danlos Syndromes. *Am J Med Genet C Semin Genet.* 2017; Mar: 175(1) 8–26.

Murphy-Ryan M, Psychogios A, and Lindor NM. Hereditary disorders of connective tissue: A guide to the emerging differential diagnosis. *Genet Med* 2010; 12: 344–54.

Radke RM and Baumgartner H. Diagnosis and treatment of Marfan syndrome: An update. *Heart* 2014; 100: 1382–91.

The Brittle Bone Society (http://www.brittlebone.org)

The Restricted Growth Association (www.restrictedgrowth.co.uk)

PART 13

Haematological disorders

Chris Bunch

Introduction

Haematology concerns blood, its formation, function, and disorders. It holds a special position in clinical medicine, as many diseases affect the blood at some stage of their course, and disorders of the blood itself often have effects on one or more of the other organ systems. The accessibility of blood and its cells has allowed the pathophysiology of many haematological disorders to be unravelled in detail, before that of many other diseases, at both the cellular and the molecular level. Indeed, many of the analytical techniques now widely used in molecular biology and genetics were developed for, and first applied to, the study of the blood.

The composition and function of blood

Blood consists of cells of three main types, suspended in a nutrient fluid called plasma. The cellular component comprises about 40%–50 % of the total volume, and consists of red cells (erythrocytes), white cells (leucocytes), and platelets (see Table 277.1).

Red cells and haemoglobin

The red cell is a biconcave disc about 7 μM in diameter. It lacks a nucleus and contains a concentrated solution of **haemoglobin** — an iron-containing protein responsible for oxygen transport from the lungs to the tissues—together with a few enzymes necessary to maintain the function and integrity of the haemoglobin and the cell membrane. The biconcave shape maximizes the cell's surface area in relation to volume—important for gas exchange—and contributes to the cell's flexibility and deformability, allowing it to pass easily through narrow capillaries.

In a normal stained blood film, the red cells appear reasonably similar in size, shape, and colour. Abnormal appearances are seen in a variety of conditions (see Table 277.2).

Table 277.1 Indicative reference ranges for haematological values in normal adults

Parameter (unit)	
Haemoglobin (g/dl)	Men: 14–18
	Women: 12–16
Haematocrit (packed cell volume)	Men: 0.40–0.52
	Women: 10.35–0.47
Red-cell count (× 10^{12}/l)	Men: 4.5–6.0
	Women: 13.8–5.2
Mean red-cell volume (fl)	80–100
Mean red-cell haemoglobin (pg)	27–33
Mean cell haemoglobin concentration (g/dl)	31.5–36.5
White cells (leucocytes) (× 10^9/l)	4.00–10.00
• neutrophils	2.00–7.00 (40%–80%)
• lymphocytes	1.00–3.00 (20%–40%)
• monocytes	0.20–1.00 (2%–10%)
• eosinophils	0.04–0.40 (1%–6%)
• basophils	0.00–0.10 (0%–2%)
Platelets (× 10^9/l)	150–450

Note: These values are typical, but may vary between laboratories; results marginally outside these ranges are not necessarily abnormal, and should be evaluated in the clinical context.

Table 277.2 Common abnormalities of red-cell morphology

Abnormality	Meaning	Associations
Anisocytosis	Variation in cell size (usually red cells)	Iron deficiency
		Thalassaemia
Poikilocytosis	Variation in cell shape (usually red cells)	Often associated with Anisocytosis
		Myelosclerosis
Hypochromia	Pale red cells	Reduced haemoglobin content
		Iron deficiency
		Thalassaemia
Microcytosis	Small red cells	Reduced haemoglobin content
		Iron deficiency
		Thalassaemia
Macrocytosis	Large red cells	Various
Spherocytes	Spherical rather than biconcave red cells	Membrane defect leading to loss of surface area
Schistocytes	Fragmented red cells	Microangiopathy
		Disseminated intravascular coagulation

Reticulocytes are young red cells (less than 2–3 or less days old) recently released from the marrow. They contain residual traces of globin mRNA, which gives the cells a bluish tinge **(polychromasia)** that contrasts with the normal red colour in a stained blood film. The reticular RNA strands can be demonstrated directly with suitable stains, facilitating estimation of the reticulocyte percentage.

Structure of haemoglobin

The haemoglobins are a family of molecules with a basically similar structure consisting of two pairs of globin chains, each associated with a haem moiety. Normal adult haemoglobin (Hb A) is formed from two alpha (α) and two beta (β) globin chains ($α_2β_2$). Interaction between the amino acid side chains leads to complex folding of the globin molecule to give a quaternary structure, with the haem molecules tucked inside the folds of the chains (see Figure 277.1).

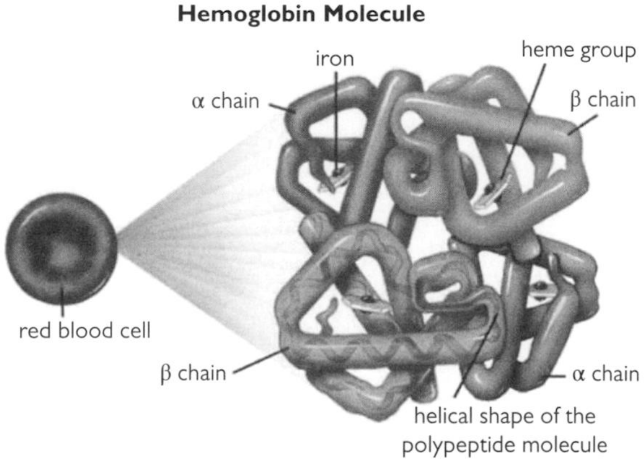

Hemoglobin Molecule

Figure 277.1 A haemoglobin molecule, showing the position of one of the haem molecules in a cleft formed by the globin chain.
http://www.mhhe.com/biosci/genbio/maderinquiry/234329.html.

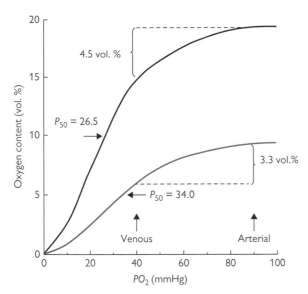

Figure 277.2 Oxygen dissociation curves for a normal patient (black line) and an anaemic patient (blue line), showing enhancement of oxygen loading by decreased red-cell oxygen affinity in the latter: the anaemic patient, with a 50% reduction in haemoglobin concentration, has only a 27% reduction in oxygen unloading, compared to a normal patient; P_{50}, partial pressure of oxygen in the blood at which the haemoglobin is 50% saturated; PO_2, partial pressure of oxygen in the blood.

Reproduced with permission from Weatherall &Hatton, Anaemia: pathophysiology, classification, and clinical features, in Oxford Textbook of Medicine, Fifth Edition Oxford University Press, Oxford, UK, Copyright © 2010.

Reprinted from Chest, volume 62, issue 5, Robert A. Klocke, Oxygen Transport and 2, 3-Diphosphoglycerate (DPG), pp. 79S-85S, Copyright (1972), with permission from Elsevier.

Haem consists of a porphyrin ring, with an iron atom at its centre. It has a certain affinity for oxygen, which is sensitive to the surrounding pH and CO_2 concentration: as blood passes through the lungs, the pH is relatively high and the CO_2 concentration is relatively low, so oxygen readily binds to haem. In the tissues, the reverse is true: oxygen dissociates from haem and becomes available to the surrounding milieu. This can be illustrated by an oxygen-dissociation curve, which has a characteristic sigmoid shape (see Figure 277.2). The affinity of haem for oxygen, and the position of the dissociation curve, are also profoundly affected by intracellular levels of 2,3-bisphosphoglycerate (2,3-BPG, previously known as 2,3-diphosphoglycerate or 2,3-DPG).

Adaptation to anaemia

The amount of oxygen extracted from the blood by the tissues depends primarily on:

- the circulating haemoglobin level
- blood flow
- the difference in oxygen tension between the red cell and the tissues
- the affinity of the haemoglobin for oxygen

Under resting conditions, the tissues require about 250 ml of oxygen per minute. Normal blood carries 20 ml of oxygen per 100 ml (1.34 ml of oxygen per gram of haemoglobin). Thus, at a resting cardiac output of 5 l per minute, about 1 l of oxygen per minute would be available to the tissues. As blood flows through the capillaries, the lower oxygen tension in the tissues promotes the release of oxygen from haemoglobin. Extraction of 250 ml of oxygen is associated with a reduction in the red-cell oxygen tension from 100 mm Hg (13.5 kPa) at the arterial end of the capillary to 40 mm Hg (5.5 kPa) at the venous end.

In anaemia, the extraction of the same amount of oxygen from a reduced amount of haemoglobin would involve a greater degree of oxygen desaturation and would eventually lead to tissue hypoxia if a number of compensatory mechanisms did not come into play. These include:

- increased cardiac output: this becomes evident once the haemoglobin level has fallen to around 7–8 g/dl. The output then rises progressively as the level falls further, and may reach four to five times the normal output
- increased blood flow: this is partly due to a rise in cardiac output, but is facilitated by the reduced blood viscosity and a decrease in peripheral vascular resistance; there is a redistribution of blood flow in favour of tissues such as the brain and the myocardium, for which oxygen delivery is especially critical
- reduced red-cell oxygen affinity: this is reflected in a right shift in the haemoglobin oxygen dissociation curve and is mainly due to an increase in the levels of red-cell 2,3-BPG, which interacts with the haemoglobin molecule to reduce its affinity for oxygen, allowing greater oxygen release at similar oxygen tensions

Developmental changes in haemoglobin production

Other normal human haemoglobins consist of α or the α-like ζ chain, combined with one of the β-like chains, ε or γ. The first haemoglobins to appear in the embryo are haemoglobin Gower 1 ($\zeta_2\varepsilon_2$), haemoglobin Portland ($\zeta_2\gamma_2$), and haemoglobin Gower 2 ($\alpha_2\varepsilon_2$). These are replaced in the fetus by fetal haemoglobin (Hb F; $\alpha_2\gamma_2$). Shortly before birth. production switches to HbA, which largely replaces Hb F by the end of the first year of life. In postnatal life, a minor adult haemoglobin, HbA_2 ($\alpha_2\delta_2$), accounts for less than 2.5 % of total haemoglobin. The switch from fetal to adult haemoglobin is affected by some of the molecular lesions responsible for the thalassaemias, and may lead to continued or increased production of HbF, with some amelioration of the expression of the disease.

Genetic control of haemoglobin synthesis

The genes for the α chains are found on chromosome 16, together with the embryonic ζ chain gene. The α gene is duplicated on each haploid chromosome, making four in all. The non-α genes are clustered on Chromosome 11, closely linked and in order of developmental expression: $3'$-ε-γ^G-γ^A-δ-β-$5'$. These genes are sequentially activated and then repressed during fetal development to ensure the appropriate developmental changes in haemoglobin production. In addition, α-chain synthesis and non-α-chain synthesis are synchronized, with haem being incorporated into each chain by a separate pathway before they are combined to form the complete haemoglobin molecule.

The genetic control of haemoglobin production has several important consequences. First, abnormalities affecting individual globin genes may be inherited from one or both parents (heterozygosity and homozygosity, respectively). Second, different abnormalities can be inherited from each parent (double heterozygosity). Third, abnormalities affecting the β chain will not become apparent until after the first 3–6 months of life, when β-chain synthesis supersedes γ-chain production. On the other hand, disorders affecting α-chain production may become apparent during fetal life, although duplication of the α-chain gene affords protection from limited abnormalities.

White cells (leucocytes)

The white cells are a group of cells whose principal collective function is defence against infection. This role is principally played out in the tissues, and the white cells' presence in the blood is largely transitory. There are three main groups of white cells:

- **polymorphonuclear cells (polymorphs) or granulocytes**, which have multilobed, condensed nuclei and contain prominent cytoplasmic granules; they are classified according to the staining characteristics of the main granule type as **neutrophils, eosinophils, or basophils**
- **lymphocytes**, which are the cells of the immune system
- **monocytes**, which are the precursors of tissue macrophages.

Neutrophils are the predominant granulocytes and are phagocytic cells primarily concerned with defence against bacterial invasion. They spend just a few hours in the bloodstream before migrating into the tissues, where they become attracted to sites of infection and inflammation, by a process of **chemotaxis** along a gradient of soluble mediators released by other inflammatory cells at the affected site. A reduction in the concentration of neutrophils in the blood is termed **neutropenia**; an increase is a **neutrophil leucocytosis**,

Box 277.1 Quantitative alterations in circulating neutrophil and eosinophils

Increased neutrophils: Neutrophilia
- infection
- inflammation
- stress/exercise
- corticosteroids
- malignancy
- tissue damage/infarction

Decreased neutrophils: Neutropenia
- marrow failure
- severe infection
- endotoxin
- hypersplenism
- immune destruction

Increased eosinophils: Eosinophilia
- parasitic infestations
- allergies: asthma, drugs, hay fever, polyarteritis nodosa
- skin disorders: eczema, urticaria, pemphigus, dermatitis herpetiformis
- sarcoidosis
- malignancy: carcinoma, lymphoma
- hypereosinophilic syndrome

Reduced eosinophils: Eosinopenia
- hypercortisolaemia: Cushing's disease, steroids, stress
- adrenaline
- congenital (very rare)

or **neutrophilia**. Causes of neutropenia and neutrophilia are shown in Box 277.1.

Eosinophils have granules that stain deep red with eosin and represent 2% or less of total leucocytes. They are phagocytic but less so than neutrophils. They are important in the defence against certain parasitic infestations, and in modulating hypersensitivity reactions. Common causes of an increase in circulating eosinophils (eosinophilia) are given in Box 277.1.

Basophils are the least numerous of the leucocytes. They have deeply basophilic granules containing a variety of substances including histamine, heparin, a factor chemotactic for eosinophils, and one that promotes platelet aggregation and degranulation. They are probably related to tissue mast cells. They have membrane receptors for the Fc portion of IgE, and participate in immediate hypersensitivity reactions.

Platelets

The platelets are small discoid bodies that are primarily concerned with haemostasis. Their morphology, function, and disorders are described in Chapter 281.

Plasma

Plasma is the liquid phase of blood and normally makes up around 55% of blood volume. It consists of a variety of proteins and salts suspended in water. The predominant proteins are albumin (35–45 g/dl), immunoglobulins (IgG, IgA, IgM), coagulation factors, and a number of transport proteins such as caeruloplasmin and transferrin. Serum is that part of plasma that remains after blood (or plasma) has clotted: the principal difference is the absence of fibrinogen in serum.

The formation of blood cells: Haemopoiesis

Blood cells are formed from progenitor cells in the bone marrow by haemopoiesis, which is a process of proliferation and differentiation. This process is carefully regulated throughout life to ensure both the steady replacement of ageing blood cells, and to provide a brisk increase in production when required. Given the central role

that erythrocytes, leucocytes, and platelets have in sustaining life and maintaining the body's integrity, it is not surprising that failure of marrow function can have serious consequences.

Normal haemopoiesis

All peripheral blood cells arise from progenitor cells known as stem cells (see Figure 277.3). Stem cells have the responsibility for providing all the blood cells required in a lifetime: to do this, they must maintain their own numbers by proliferation, as well as regularly 'committing' some to differentiate down the pathways that lead to mature cells. The number of stem cells is very small: differentiation and proliferation go hand in hand at first, so that each stem cell eventually gives rise to a large number of mature, non-dividing cells.

Regulation of haemopoiesis

Growth and differentiation of haemopoietic progenitors is to a large extent governed by a series of glycoprotein hormones, or **growth factors**. These react with specific cell-surface receptors to stimulate proliferation and differentiation, and some also enhance granulocyte function. Growth factors are produced by cells that are in a good position to 'sense' the need for increased haemopoietic activity. For example, specialized cells in the juxtaglomerular region of the kidney (an organ with very high oxygen demand) sense reduced oxygen delivery and release erythropoietin, a hormone which stimulates erythropoiesis. Analogous granulocytic growth factors are produced by a wide range of connective tissue cells, macrophages, and activated T-cells, which are all cells that are affected by tissue injury or infection.

Most of the haemopoietic growth factors have been isolated and their genes molecularly cloned. This has enabled several factors to be synthesized and made available for clinical use, via recombinant DNA techniques.

Erythropoietin

Erythropoietin is secreted by the kidney in response to reduced oxygen delivery. It acts both to expand the committed erythroid progenitor pool and to stimulate differentiation, increasing the output of red cells. Reduced erythropoietin production leads to reduced red-cell production. This is largely responsible for the anaemia of renal failure and contributes to the anaemia of infection and chronic inflammatory disorders. On the other hand, increased erythropoietin production leads to erythrocytosis or polycythaemia.

Recombinant human erythropoietin is now widely used to treat the anaemia of chronic renal failure, and clinical studies are currently under way in the anaemia of chronic disorders and in myelodysplasia.

Granulocyte colony-stimulating factor

Granulocyte colony-stimulating factor (G-CSF) is produced by macrophages and stimulates granulocyte production and release from the marrow. Recombinant human G-CSF accelerates granulocyte recovery after chemotherapy for malignant disease and bone marrow transplantation, and reduces the risks of infection after these treatments.

Granulocyte–macrophage colony-stimulating factor

Granulocyte–macrophage colony-stimulating factor (GM-CSF) is also produced by macrophages, but has a wider spectrum of action than G-CSF does, stimulating the production of monocytes as well as granulocytes. Recombinant GM-CSF has also been used to stimulate granulocyte recovery after chemotherapy for malignancy, but has more pronounced side effects of fever, fluid retention, bone pain, pruritus, and possibly thrombosis.

Interleukin-3

Interleukin-3 has an even broader spectrum of action than G-CSF and GM-CSF do. It acts on a more primitive cell, and is able to stimulate erythroid and megakaryocytic as well as granulocytic activity. It is currently undergoing clinical trials in a range of marrow failure states.

Other factors affecting haemopoiesis

Proliferating cells require both vitamin B_{12} and folate for DNA synthesis. Lack of either results in megaloblastic haemopoiesis (see Chapter 279).

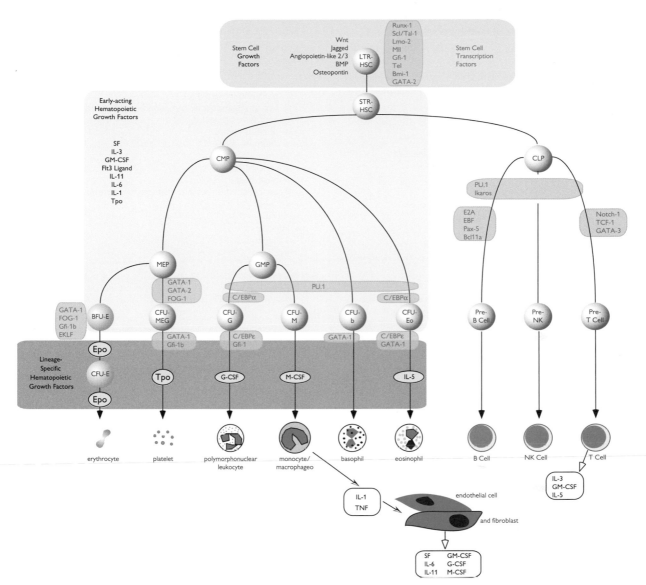

Figure 277.3 Major cytokine sources and actions and transcription factor requirements for haemopoietic cells. Cells of the bone-marrow micro-environment, such as macrophages, endothelial cells, and reticular fibroblastoid cells, produce macrophage-colony-stimulating factor (M-CSF), granulocyte–macrophage-colony-stimulating factor (GM-CSF), granulocyte-colony-stimulating factor (G-CSF), interleukin 6 (IL-6), and probably stem cell factor after induction with endotoxins (macrophages) or interleukin 1 (IL-1)/tumour necrosis factor (TNF; endothelial cells and fibroblasts). T-cells produce interleukin 3 (IL-3), GM-CSF, and interleukin 5 (IL-5) in response to antigenic and IL-1 stimulation. These cytokines have overlapping actions during haematopoietic differentiation, as indicated and, for all lineages, optimal development requires a combination of early acting and late-acting factors. Transcription factors important for survival or self-renewal of stem cells are shown at the top, and stages of haemopoiesis blocked after the depletion of indicated transcription factors are shown for multipotent and committed progenitors; CLP, common lymphoid progenitor; CMP, common myeloid progenitor; EPO, erythropoietin; GMP, granulocyte–macrophage progenitor; LTR-HSC, long-term repopulating haematopoietic stem cell; MEP, megakaryocyte–erythrocyte progenitor; NK, natural killer; SF, scatter factor; STR-HSC, short-term repopulating haematopoietic stem cells; TNF, tumour necrosis factor; Tpo, thrombopoietin.

Reproduced with permission from Sieff, Stem cells and haemopoiesis, in *Oxford Textbook of Medicine*, Fifth Edition Oxford University Press, Oxford, UK, Copyright © 2010.

A further important regulatory factor for erythropoiesis is the **iron supply**. Developing erythroblasts acquire iron for haemoglobin synthesis directly from adjacent marrow macrophages. Iron availability is reduced not only in iron deficiency (see Chapter 279), but also in inflammation and infection, when macrophages retain iron and the serum iron falls. Why this happens is a matter of some controversy, but sequestration of body iron may disadvantage bacteria, which depend on iron for their growth.

Disorders of haemopoiesis

Disorders of haemopoiesis may involve over- or underproduction of one or more cell types by the marrow (see Box 277.2). Intrinsic or primary disorders affecting haemopoietic progenitors themselves are discussed here. Megaloblastic haemopoiesis and anaemia is covered in Chapter 279, and disorders of red-cell production due to abnormal haemoglobin synthesis in Chapter 280.

The majority of primary haemopoietic disorders are acquired and arise from a single defective progenitor. Congenital disorders are rare and often associated with other congenital abnormalities (see Box 277.2).

The concept of clonality

One of the central concepts in cell biology is that every individual differentiated cell originates from a single progenitor, or stem cell and,

Box 277.2 Disorders of haemopoiesis

Clonal disorders originating in pluripotent stem cells and so affecting all three cell lines
- myeloproliferative disorders: chronic granulocytic leukaemia, polycythaemia rubra vera, thrombocythaemia, myelofibrosis
- paroxysmal nocturnal haemoglobinuria
- acute myeloid leukaemia (some)
- myelodysplastic syndromes
- congenital cyclical neutropenia (rare)

Clonal disorders affecting committed progenitors
- acute myeloid leukaemia (some)
- myelodysplasia (some)
- acute lymphoblastic leukaemia
- chronic lymphocytic leukaemia
- myeloma
- lymphomas

Non-clonal disorders affecting all cell lines
- aplastic anaemia (some cases may have underlying clonal abnormality)
- megaloblastic haemopoiesis

Non-clonal disorders affecting primarily a single cell line
- selective cytopenias (autoimmune or drug induced)
- thalassaemias
- iron-deficiency anaemia
- congenital dyserythropoietic anaemia
- pure red-cell aplasia
- parvovirus infection (erythroid progenitors)

conversely, that each stem cell gives rise to a family (or 'clone') of differentiated daughter cells. Once a pluripotent haemopoietic stem cell becomes committed to differentiation, it ultimately produces a number of red cells, granulocytes, platelets, and lymphoid cells, which thus belong to the same clone. Similarly, each committed granulocyte progenitor (for example) gives rise to a single clone of granulocytes, which is therefore a subclone of the parent pluripotent stem cell.

Box 277.3 Some drugs and other toxic agents causing bone marrow failure

Predictable (dose related)
- radiation
- cytotoxic drugs
- chloramphenicol

Idiosyncratic (not dose related)

Agents causing granulocytosis
- antithyroid drugs
- dapsone
- amidopyrine
- NSAIDs
- co-trimoxazole
- chlorpromazine

Agents causing thrombocytopenia
- heparin
- quinine
- quinidine
- gold
- NSAIDs
- co-trimoxazole

Agents causing aplastic anaemia
- chloramphenicol
- phenylbutazone and other NSAIDs
- benzene and derivatives
- gold
- penicillamine
- pesticides

Box 277.4 Causes of aplastic anaemia

- drugs:
  - antibiotics (chloramphenicol, penicillin, cephalosporins, sulfonamides)
  - anti-inflammatory agents (phenylbutazone, indomethacin, penicillamine, gold)
  - hypoglycaemics (chlorpropamide, tolbutamide)
  - antithyroid drugs
  - phenothiazines
  - antimalarials
  - antiepileptics
- chemicals and toxins:
  - pesticides
  - benzine derivatives and related solvent compounds
  - dyes
- radiation
- infections:
  - hepatitis
  - EBV
  - CMV
  - rubella
- pregnancy

From time to time, an individual progenitor sustains genetic damage which alters its potential for growth and differentiation. This may give the cell and its progeny a growth advantage over normal cells, allowing **clonal expansion** of the affected line. The consequences of this will depend upon the nature of the mutant cell, the nature of the damage, and its effect on growth and differentiation. Uncontrolled clonal expansion of this sort is the basis of virtually every malignant neoplastic disorder.

Clonal disorders of haemopoiesis include frank haematological malignancies such as leukaemia and lymphoma, as well as less obviously malignant myelo- and lymphoproliferative disorders (see Box 277.2).

Bone marrow failure

Failure of haemopoiesis usually results from damage to proliferating marrow cells by cytotoxic drugs or radiation, haemopoietic malignancy, or a combination of the two. Much less commonly, damage to one or more cell lines can occur in patients taking other medication, due to immune mechanisms, certain viral infections, or for unknown reasons (see Box 277.3). Marrow replacement by metastatic malignancy may also result in marrow failure.

The result is a varying degree of anaemia, neutropenia, and thrombocytopenia; reduction in all three cell types is known as **pancytopenia**. The term **aplastic anaemia** is reserved for primary marrow failure with pancytopenia that is **not** obviously due to cytotoxic drugs or radiation.

Anaemia

Cessation of erythropoiesis leads to anaemia (see Chapter 279). The normal erythrocyte life span is 120 days, so interruption of production will lead to a fall in haemoglobin of about 1% per day (1 g/dl per week). Infection and bleeding, secondary to neutropenia and thrombocytopenia, are therefore often earlier and more serious manifestations of marrow failure.

Anaemia can be corrected by red-cell transfusions. In general, the aim is to maintain a haemoglobin level compatible with good health, normally above 9 g/dl. Below this level, there is a significant risk of optic fundal haemorrhage, which may occur in any form of anaemia but which can be particularly troublesome if infection and thrombocytopenia are also present.

Transfusion should be with packed red cells or red-cell concentrates, given slowly, and with diuretics if necessary, to avoid circulatory overload.

Neutropenia

Unlike red cells and platelets, neutrophil granulocytes have a predominantly extravascular role, and circulate in the blood for only a few hours, before passing into the tissues. The generation of mature neutrophils from pluripotent stem cells takes 10–14 days, although the last few days in the marrow are spent in a non-mitotic **maturation compartment** which can be mobilized into the circulation rapidly in response to infection. Neutrophil lifespan in the tissues is only 2–3 days, so neutropenia is usually the earliest and most pronounced feature of marrow failure, reaching a nadir 7–10 days after haemopoiesis has been arrested.

The principal function of the neutrophil is bacterial phagocytosis and, in the steady state, most neutrophils scavenge for normal commensal gut organisms and other organisms which gain access to the body through breaks in the skin or gut mucosa. Bacterial infection is thus the major consequence of neutropenia, and will occur in around one-half of patients with peripheral blood neutrophil counts less than $0.5 \times 10^9/l$, and virtually all those with less than $0.2 \times 10^9/l$, lasting more than 10–14 days.

Gram-negative organisms of bowel origin are most commonly involved but, in hospitalized patients, the normal gut flora is often supplemented by resistant pathogens, such as *Klebsiella* spp. and *Pseudomonas* spp. Gram-positive organisms, such as *Staphylococcus epidermidis*, are commonly associated with the use of implanted central venous catheters for vascular access.

The earliest and often only manifestation of serious infection is fever. Local inflammatory signs are impaired, and focal signs may be minimal. Pulmonary, soft tissue, and urinary infections may occur. Septicaemia is common, although positive blood cultures are obtained in less than one-third of patients with a temperature higher than 38°C.

Suspected infection must be treated promptly, as delay may prove rapidly fatal. If a temperature >38°C develops, blood and urine cultures should be taken, and a chest radiograph performed. IV broad-spectrum antibiotics should be started immediately, following local protocols which should reflect the local pattern of organisms. Antibiotic therapy may be subsequently modified by the results of cultures.

Modern antimicrobials are capable of curing the majority of bacterial infections in neutropenic patients. Problems occur when neutropenia is particularly prolonged, especially in association with aggressive cytotoxic therapy, which may damage mucosal barriers and impair macrophage, as well as neutrophil production. Deep-seated fungal infections may develop in this situation and are often difficult to diagnose in vivo. Empirical IV antifungal therapy (e.g. with amphotericin) is advisable when fever or signs of infection persist, despite broad-spectrum antibiotic cover.

Infection may be prevented in severely neutropenic patients by strict isolation in a sterile environment, together with rigorous decontamination of skin and gut with disinfectants and antibiotics. In general, however, such measures do not improve the overall outcome, and their expense and poor patient acceptability has led most centres to abandon such regimes. Certain oral antibiotics, such as co-trimoxazole, ciprofloxacin, and norfloxacin may reduce the incidence of systemic infection and are often recommended in prolonged neutropenia, although there is potential risk of antibiotic resistance.

Recombinant growth factors (e.g. G-CSF) can reduce the period and severity of neutropenia after cytotoxic therapy, and thereby the morbidity and mortality from infection. Alternatively, by reducing myelotoxicity, they may permit the safe use of higher, and thus perhaps more effective, doses of cytotoxic therapy for malignant disease.

Thrombocytopenia

Platelets survive in the circulation for an average of 9–10 days, but are consumed more rapidly in the presence of bleeding, infection, or fever. The likelihood of abnormal bleeding depends upon the platelet count and the nature of the injury: spontaneous haemorrhage is uncommon unless the count falls below $20 \times 10^9/l$. At levels below this, petechial haemorrhages occur in the skin and mucous membranes, and in the internal organs.

Bleeding is aggravated by minor trauma and is most noticeable in dependent areas (because of hydrostatic pressure) and in pressure areas. The most serious risk from thrombocytopenia is cerebral haemorrhage.

Bleeding can be treated and prevented by transfusion of platelet concentrates. In an average adult, a transfusion of 5–6 units of platelet concentrate will raise the platelet count by $10–30 \times 10^9/l$. Transfused platelets have a slightly shorter life span than normal, and 2–3 transfusions weekly may be required—increasing to daily in the presence of active bleeding or infection, both of which increase platelet consumption.

The major problem with repeated platelet transfusions is sensitization to foreign human leucocyte antigens (HLA) and platelet-specific antigens, which may lead to rapid platelet destruction, and ineffectiveness of transfusions from random donors. In this situation, good responses may be obtained by using platelets from HLA-matched donors, often as single-donor transfusions (collected on a cell separator), from the outset of thrombocytopenia to reduce the subsequent risk of sensitization. Since the responsible HLAs are most strongly expressed on leucocytes, an alternative approach is to use high-efficiency in-line filters at the time of transfusion to remove any leucocytes. Despite such measures, however, sensitization to platelet-specific antigens may still occur.

Drug-induced cytopenias

A variety of drugs may damage the marrow (see Box 277.3). Myelotoxicity is a well-recognized (and often intended) dose-dependent effect of the cytotoxic drugs used to treat malignant disease or as immunosuppressants. Other drugs may, on rare occasions, produce a severe reduction in the production of one or more cell types, in a non-dose-dependent or idiosyncratic fashion.

Prompt recovery usually follows withdrawal of the offending drug, provided this is rapidly identified. Prognosis is good except in patients who present with severe infection, and in whom mortality is high. Full supportive measures should be given as outlined in 'Neutropenia'.

Aplastic anaemia

Aplastic anaemia is a rare form of marrow failure leading to pancytopenia with a hypocellular or acellular bone marrow. In the majority of cases, no specific cause can be found, although various factors may be implicated in a minority (see Box 277.4).

Most cytotoxic drugs can produce severe pancytopenia, but this is usually recoverable, as the pluripotent stem cell population is relatively resistant to permanent damage. However, the alkylating agent busulphan, when used carelessly, can lead to prolonged or permanent aplasia, as can high doses of whole-body irradiation. Several drugs and chemicals have been associated with severe aplastic anaemia, presumably through an idiosyncratic and possibly immune-mediated mechanism.

The diagnosis of aplastic anaemia requires demonstration of the severely hypocellular marrow, preferably on two separate trephine examinations. Aplastic anaemia is said to be **severe** when, over a period of at least 3–4 weeks, the following findings are observed:

- the neutrophil count remains less than $0.5 \times 10^9/l$
- platelets are less than $20 \times 10^9/l$
- the **absolute** reticulocyte count (red blood cell count × per cent reticulocytes) is less than $20 \times 10^{12}/l$

Untreated, severe aplastic anaemia is almost always ultimately fatal, although spontaneous recovery may occur occasionally.

Management involves supportive care, but with particular attention to the risk of sensitization to HLAs by transfusion, as this may impair platelet support and increase the risk of graft rejection if bone marrow transplantation (BMT) is undertaken. BMT is the treatment of choice in patients who are under the age of 50 and who have an HLA-compatible sibling donor. Two-thirds of transplanted patients will be cured permanently; the major problem is graft-vs-host disease, which tends to be less severe in younger patients.

An alternative to BMT is antithymocyte globulin (ATG). This was initially used as an immunosuppressant in the early days of BMT, but apparent early success of BMT in some patients was shown to be due to autologous recovery of the patient's own marrow, following failure of engraftment. Infusion of ATG over 5 days produces a response in about one-half of patients; the response is complete in about one-quarter and is sustained in over two-thirds. Age is not a factor influencing response, and ATG therapy is the treatment of choice over the age of 50, and in younger patients without a marrow donor.

The success of ATG therapy suggests a possible immune basis for aplasia in those who respond, although other non-myelotoxic immunosuppressive agents, such as corticosteroids and cyclosporin A, have only occasionally produced a response.

Pure red-cell aplasia

Rare causes of severe anaemia occur in which the marrow shows complete absence of erythroid activity, but normal white-cell and platelet production. A congenital form, Diamond–Blackfan anaemia, is apparent at or shortly after birth and is associated with a variety of other, mainly skeletal, deformities in about one-third. There is a reduction in erythroid progenitors, which are also relatively insensitive to erythropoietin.

Acquired red-cell aplasia is thought to be autoimmune, with cytotoxic immune reactions directed against developing erythroblasts or, rarely, autoantibodies to erythropoietin. There is an association with thymoma, and it is worth doing a CT scan of the chest in affected patients, as removal of a thymoma may reverse the red-cell aplasia. Treatment is otherwise with corticosteroids. It is also occasionally seen in patients with chronic lymphocytic leukaemia (see Chapter 287).

Transient erythroblastopenia of childhood is an uncommon condition in which sudden onset of anaemia is associated with the erythropoiesis being temporarily suppressed.

Leukaemia

Leukaemias are clonal malignant proliferations of leukocytes and/or their precursors. **Acute** leukaemias (see Chapter 286) are characterized by uncontrolled growth of immature haemopoietic progenitor cells, at the expense of normal marrow function, and most of the clinical features are therefore those of marrow failure. They are of either myeloid (more common in adults) or lymphoblastic (more common in childhood) origin, and are rapidly fatal if untreated, but potentially curable with appropriate treatment.

Chronic leukaemias are clonal proliferations of haemopoietic cells that have not completely lost the ability to differentiate. Chronic myeloid (granulocytic) leukaemia has features in common with myeloproliferative disorders, while chronic lymphocytic leukaemia is best considered as a form of low-grade non-Hodgkin lymphoma.

Myeloproliferative disorders

The myeloproliferative disorders are a group of clonal disorders arising in haemopoietic or pluripotent stem cells characterized by uncontrolled growth but relatively normal differentiation—predominantly (but not always exclusively) down one of the three main haemopoietic pathways. The result is a significant expansion of red cells, granulocytes, or platelets and their precursors, alone or in combination.

Clinically, the myeloproliferative disorders may be classified according to the predominant cell type:

- **polycythaemia rubra vera**: red cells
- **essential thrombocythaemia**: platelets
- **myelofibrosis**: fibroblasts proliferating in response to growth factors, produced by an immature haemopoietic clone
- **chronic granulocytic leukaemia**: granulocytes

Further Reading

Boxer LA. How to approach neutropenia. *Hematology* 2012; 2012: 174–82.

Carson JL Triulzi DJ, and Ness PM. Indications for and Adverse Effects of Red-Cell Transfusion. *N Engl J Med* 2017; 399: 1261–72.

Koury MJ and Rhodes M. How to approach chronic anemia. *Hematology* 2012; 2012: 183–90.

Stasi R. How to approach thrombocytopenia. *Hematology* 2012; 2012: 191–7.

278 Diagnosis and investigation in haematology

Chris Bunch

The full blood count

A routine full blood count performed by the haematology laboratory will include the following parameters (some of these are measured directly, while others are derived by calculation; typical reference ranges are given in Table 278.1):

- **haemoglobin (Hb)**: the concentration of haemoglobin in whole blood (expressed as grams per decilitre)
- **red-cell count (RCC)**:
  - the concentration of red cells ($\times 10^{12}$/l)
  - changes in the RCC tend to parallel changes in the haemoglobin and haematocrit
  - a decrease in the RCC is called **anaemia**
  - an increase in the RCC is called **erythrocytosis** or **polycythaemia**
- **mean corpuscular volume (MCV)**:
  - the average volume of individual red cells (expressed in femtoliters)
  - a low MCV indicates **microcytosis**
  - a high MCV indicates **macrocytosis**
- **haematocrit**, or **packed cell volume**:
  - the proportion of red cells in a unit volume of blood, usually expressed as a ratio (e.g. 0.45) or a percentage
  - derived from MCV × RCC
- **mean cell haemoglobin (MCH)**:
  - the average amount of haemoglobin per cell (expressed in picograms)
  - derived from Hb/RCC
- **mean cell haemoglobin concentration (MCHC)**:
  - the mean concentration of haemoglobin per cell (expressed as grams per decilitre of red cells)
  - derived from Hb/(MCV × RCC)

Table 278.1 Normal values for full blood count

Variable	Normal range
Hemoglobin	Male: 13.5–17.5 g/dl
	Female: 12.0–16.0 g/dl
Hematocrit	Male: 41–53%
	Female: 36–46%
Mean corpuscular volume (MCV)	80–100 fl
Red cell distribution width (RDW)	11.5–14.5%
Reticulocyte count	0.5–2.5% red cells
White blood cell count	4.5–11.0 · 10^9/L
Neutrophils	40–70%
Lymphocytes	22–44%
Monocytes	4–11%
Eosinophils	0–8%
Basophils	0–3%
Platelet count	150–350 · 10^9/L

Reproduced from David C. Sprigings, John B. Chambers, *Acute Medicine: A Practical Guide to the Management of Medical Emergencies*, 4th Edition, Chambers, Wiley-Blackwell, UK, Copyright © 2007.

Data from Kratz et al., Laboratory reference values, New England Journal of Medicine, volume 351, pp. 1548–63. Copyright 2004.

- the MCHC tends to remain fairly constant but may be reduced in severe iron deficiency or thalassaemia
- pale (hypochromic) red cells on a blood smear may indicate small red cells (low MCV and MCH) but is more striking when MCHC is also reduced
- **white-cell (leucocyte) count**:
  - the total concentration of leucocytes ($\times 10^9$/l)
  - an increase is called a **leucocytosis**
  - a decrease is **leucopenia**
- **differential leucocyte count**:
  - either the absolute concentration ($\times 10^9$/l) or the percentage of each type of white cell
  - this may be derived manually by examination of a stained blood smear or by automated counters which differentiate cells by size, staining, or other characteristics
  - automated counters are potentially more accurate numerically (especially with low counts), but may misclassify some abnormal leucocytes
- **platelet count**: the concentration of platelets ($\times 10^9$/l)

The blood film or smear

Examination of a stained blood film is one of the key investigations in haematology, as alterations in the appearances of red cells, white cells, and platelets may give clues to the cause of any blood count abnormality, while the presence of abnormal cells, for example immature leucocytes in leukaemia, may be diagnostic (see Tables 278.2–6 and Box 278.1).

Unfortunately, the automation of blood counts has led to blood film examination becoming less routine in many laboratories, but a film should always be requested if a blood count abnormality cannot readily be explained by the clinical context.

The reticulocyte count

The reticulocyte count can give valuable information about the dynamics of erythropoiesis. In the normal, steady state, 1%–2% of red cells are reticulocytes. A normal marrow will respond to anaemia by increasing red-cell production and, thereby, the proportion of reticulocytes. This effect is most marked when red-cell lifespan is also reduced, as in haemolysis.

Because anaemia implies a reduction in the absolute RCC, a small increase in reticulocyte percentage does not necessarily indicate a healthy marrow response to anaemia, and calculation of the absolute reticulocyte count (% reticulocytes × RCC: normally 25×10^9/l to 85×10^9/l) is a more accurate guide.

The erythrocyte sedimentation rate, and plasma viscosity

When anticoagulated whole blood is left to stand, the red cells, white cells, and platelets sediment over time. The rate of red-cell sedimentation is directly proportional to the concentration of macromolecules such as fibrinogen and immunoglobulins in the plasma; so, any condition that increases these will increase the **erythrocyte sedimentation rate (ESR)**. In practice, the ESR is measured by timing the extent of red-cell sedimentation

Table 278.2 Clues from the blood film

Finding	Interpretation/causes
Red cells	
Microcytes	Iron deficiency
	Anaemia of chronic disease
	Thalassemia
	Sideroblastic anaemia
Macrocytes	Drug induced
	Vitamin B_{12}/folate deficiency
	Haemolysis
	Primary bone disorder
	Alcohol
	Hypothyroidism
	Chronic liver disease
Red cell aggregation	Rouleaux, seen in:
	• high polyclonal immunoglobulin
	• monoclonal immunoglobulin (paraprotein, e.g. myeloma)
	• high fibrinogen
	Agglutination, reflecting the presence of cold agglutinin, seen in:
	• mycoplasma infection
	• infectious mononucleosis
	• lymphoproliferative disorder
	• idiopathic
Fragmented red cells (schistocytes)	Microangiopathic haemolytic anaemia, seen in:
	• disseminated intravascular coagulation
	• thrombotic thrombocytopenic purpura/haemolytic uremic syndrome
	• disseminated cancer
	• pre-eclampsia/eclampsia with HELPP syndrome
	• malignant phase hypertension
	Prosthetic heart valve
	Severe burn
'Bite cells' (keratocytes)	Acute haemolysis induced by oxidant damage (e.g. in glucose-6-phosphate dehydrogenase deficiency)
Target cells	Iron deficiency
	Thalassemia
	Liver disease
	Postsplenectomy
Nucleated red cells	Marrow replacement, due to:
	• carcinoma (most commonly of breast or prostate origin)
	• myelofibrosis
	• myeloma
	• tuberculosis
White cells	
Blast cells	Leukemias
	Lymphomas
	Marrow replacement
Platelets	
Platelet clumps	EDTA-induced platelet clumping may cause spurious thrombocytopenia
Other findings	
Abnormal cells	Lymphoma cells
	Myeloma cells

Data from Bain, B.J. Diagnosis from the blood smear. *N Engl J Med* 2005; 353: 498–507; and Tefferi, A. et al. How to interpret and pursue an abnormal complete blood cell count in adults. Mayo Clinic Proc 2005;80: 923–36.

after 1 hour in a standardized calibrated tube, and the result is expressed in millimetres per hour. The upper limit of normal is age- and sex-dependent, ranging from 17 mm/h in men aged 17–50, and 30 mm/h in men over 70, with acceptable values being 5–10 mm/h higher in women.

The ESR is most commonly raised in infections and inflammation, reflecting predominantly increased levels of fibrinogen, an 'acute phase reactant'. In this respect, it gives information similar to that provided by C-reactive protein (CRP) levels. However, it is a very non-specific test and may be raised in a range of underlying disorders, including malignancy. It will usually be higher than normal with significant anaemia (reflecting the reduced haematocrit).

The ESR can be significantly elevated when immunoglobulin levels are high, as in polyclonal hypergammaglobulinaemia (suggestive of chronic infection or inflammation), or monoclonal paraproteinaemia due to myeloma. Very high ESR levels (>100 mm/h) are highly suggestive of myeloma, Waldenstrom's macroglobulinaemia, tuberculosis, or vasculitic conditions, such as polymyalgia rheumatica or giant cell arteritis. The CRP level can sometimes help differentiation, as it is elevated in 'acute phase' conditions (inflammation or infection) but is usually unaffected by monoclonal paraproteinaemia.

The ESR is simply an indirect measure of plasma viscosity, which is increased by the same macromolecules, and some laboratories offer plasma viscosity measurements by preference. The information obtained is the same, and just as non-specific.

Iron, vitamin B_{12}, and folate studies

Iron-deficient erythropoiesis occurs when the iron supply to developing erythroblasts is reduced, typically due to iron deficiency or the anaemia of chronic disorders (ACD) and results in anaemia with a reduced MCV (microcytosis). Serum iron estimation alone is insufficient, as it is reduced in both cases, and proper evaluation requires serum ferritin and transferrin levels and/or transferrin saturation as well. In iron deficiency, ferritin is low and transferrin high; in ACD, transferrin is normal or low, and ferritin normal or raised (ferritin is also an 'acute phase reactant').

Serum vitamin B_{12} and folate levels are required to determine the cause of megaloblastic anaemia and to elucidate macrocytic anaemia generally. Low folate levels in dietary folate deficiency can be rapidly reversed by refeeding, and the diagnosis missed. If this is suspected, then red-cell folate estimation may be helpful, as low levels recover much more slowly.

Vitamin B_{12} levels are often requested in the investigation of dementia, but the interpretation of low levels in the absence of anaemia or typical neurology is a matter of some debate. Low levels may be associated with increased risk of falls in the elderly. High vitamin B_{12} levels are seen in patients receiving intramuscular vitamin B_{12} replacement, and in some myeloproliferative disorders, but are not diagnostic.

Radioisotopic studies

Radiation protection regulations have severely limited the availability of radioisotopes for haematological investigation. Traditional uses include blood volume estimations (red cells labelled with ^{51}Cr; plasma with ^{125}I), red-cell survival (^{51}Cr-labelled red cells), and the Schilling test for pernicious anaemia (absorption of ^{57}Co- or ^{58}Co-labelled cobalamins, with and without bound intrinsic factor).

Bone marrow examination

Although the nature of many haematological disorders can be determined from the blood count and film, examination of the bone marrow is essential to the proper evaluation and diagnosis of many disorders (see Box 278.2). The simplest form of marrow examination involves needle aspiration of marrow cells from the posterior iliac crest, after infiltrating the skin and periosteum with local anaesthetic. Smears are made and stained in the same way as a blood film and allow quantitative and qualitative assessment of the developing blood cells. Marrow can also be biopsied for histological examination, by using a special trephine biopsy needle. This can be performed at the same time as marrow aspiration from the iliac crest.

A marrow aspirate is usually sufficient to diagnose qualitative and quantitative defects in blood cell precursors, although it must be recognized that it only provides a 'snapshot' of a dynamic process. On occasions, marrow cells cannot be aspirated, and the attempt yields just a 'dry' or 'blood' tap. This may occur in myelofibrosis with a

Table 278.3 Microcytic anaemia (mean corpuscular volume <78 fl)

Cause	Clues from full blood count and film	Other blood results	Causes/comment
Iron deficiency	Increased red-cell distribution width Anisocytosis Increased platelet count	Low iron Increased transferrin Low ferritin	Commonest cause of microcytic anemia, caused by inadequate dietary intake, malabsorption (e.g. celiac disease) or blood loss
Anemia of chronic disease (ACD)	Film usually unremarkable	Low iron Low/normal transferrin Normal/increased ferritin	~20% ACDs are microcytic: causes include Hodgkin disease and renal cell carcinoma
Thalassemia	Polychromasia Target cells	Normal ferritin Hemoglobin electrophoresis normal in alpha-thalassemia trait, and abnormal in beta-thalassemia trait and other thalassemia syndromes	Hematocrit usually >30% and MCV <75 fl in beta-thalassemia trait
Sideroblastic anemia	Siderocytes may be seen: hypochromic red cells with basophilic stippling that stain positive for iron (Pappenheimer bodies)	Increased ferritin	Rare Hereditary and acquired forms

Abbreviations: MCV, mean corpuscular volume.

Reproduced with permission from David C. Sprigings, John B. Chambers, *Acute Medicine: A Practical Guide to the Management of Medical Emergencies*, 4th Edition, Chambers, Wiley-Blackwell, UK, Copyright © 2007.

Table 278.4 Normocytic anaemia (mean corpuscular volume 78–100 fl)

Cause	Clues from full blood count and film	Other blood results	Causes/comment
Bleeding	Polychromasia Anisocytosis	Falling hemoglobin without evidence of hemolysis	Occult bleeding may occur from gut or into retroperitoneal space
Hemolysis	Polychromasia (reflecting increased reticulocyte count) Spherocytes Keratocytes ('bite' cells, due to acute hemolysis induced by oxidant damage, as may occur in G6PD deficiency) Fragmented red cells seen in microangiopathic hemolytic anemia	Increased unconjugated bilirubin, increased LDH and reduced serum haptoglobin seen in hemolysis of all causes	Hemolysis is due either to abnormalities of red cells (e.g. G6PD deficiency, sickle cell anemia), or to extrinsic factors (immune and non-immune causes)
Anemia of chronic disease	Film usually unremarkable	Normal/increased ferritin Abnormalities related to underlying cause	Seen in acute and chronic infection, cancer, renal failure, inflammatory disorders (e.g. rheumatoid arthritis, systemic lupus erythematosus), endocrine disorders, and chronic rejection after solid organ transplantation
Bone marrow disorder	Other cytopenias Leukocytosis Monocytosis Thrombocytosis Blast cells	Paraproteinemia in myeloma	Myelodysplasia, myeloma, leukemia

Abbreviations: G6PD, glucose-6-phosphate dehydrogenase; LDH, lactate dehydrogenase; MCV, mean corpuscular volume.

Reproduced with permission from David C. Sprigings, John B. Chambers, *Acute Medicine: A Practical Guide to the Management of Medical Emergencies*, 4th Edition, Chambers, Wiley-Blackwell, UK, Copyright © 2007.

Table 278.5 Macrocytosis (mean corpuscular volume >100 fl)

Cause	Clues from full blood count and film	Other blood results	Causes/comment
Drug-induced	Usually unremarkable	No specific abnormality	Many drugs, e.g. azathioprine, zidovudine
Vitamin B₁₂/folate deficiency	Oval macrocytic red cells, hypersegmented neutrophils, pancytopenia	Low serum B₁₂/red-cell folate Positive intrinsic factor antibodies in pernicious anaemia	B₁₂ deficiency: pernicious anemia/malabsorption Folate deficiency: inadequate dietary intake/malabsorption
Hemolysis	Hemolytic anemia is usually normocytic, but can be macrocytic if there is marked reticulocytosis		
Primary bone marrow disorder	MCV usually >110 fl Other cytopenias Leukocytosis Monocytosis Thrombocytosis Blast cells	No specific abnormality	Myelodysplasia, leukemia
Alcohol	Alcohol excess may also cause lymphopenia and thrombocytopenia	Abnormal liver function tests, with raised AST (>ALT) and γGT	
Hypothyroidism	Usually unremarkable	Raised TSH, low free T4/free T3	Hypothyroidism may also cause normocytic anemia
Chronic liver disease	Associated thrombocytopenia may be seen in cirrhosis with portal hypertension and splenomegaly	Abnormal liver function tests/prothrombin time	

Abbreviations: ALT, alanine aminotransferase; AST, aspartate aminotransferase; γGT, gamma-glutamyl transferase; MCV, mean corpuscular volume; T3, triiodothyronine; T4, thyroxine; TSH, thyroid-stimulating hormone.

Reproduced with permission from David C. Sprigings, John B. Chambers, *Acute Medicine: A Practical Guide to the Management of Medical Emergencies*, 4th Edition, Chambers, Wiley-Blackwell, UK, Copyright © 2007.

Table 278.6 White blood cell abnormalities

Finding	Possible causes
Neutrophilia	Sepsis
	Metastatic cancer
	Acidosis
	Corticosteroid therapy
	Trauma, surgery, burn
	Myeloproliferative disorders
Neutropenia	Drugs (e.g. carbimazole)
	Infections (e.g. viral, severe bacterial, HIV)
	Vitamin B_{12} and folate deficiency
	Systemic lupus erythematosus
	Felty syndrome
	Hematological disorders (e.g. leukemia)
Lymphocytosis	Infections (e.g. infectious mononucleosis)
	Chronic lymphocytic leukemia
Lymphopenia	Infections (e.g. viral, HIV, severe bacterial)
	Immunosuppressive therapy
	Systemic lupus erythematosus
	Alcohol excess
	Chronic renal failure
Monocytosis	Infections
	Myeloproliferative disorders (e.g. chronic myelomonocytic leukemia)
	Metastatic cancer
Eosinophilia	Drug allergy
	Parasitic infestation
	Hematological disorders (e.g. lymphoma, leukemia)
	Churg–Strauss vasculitis
	Disorders with eosinophilic involvement of specific organs
	Adrenal insufficiency
	Atheroembolism

Reproduced with permission from David C. Sprigings, John B. Chambers, *Acute Medicine: A Practical Guide to the Management of Medical Emergencies*, 4th Edition, Chambers, Wiley-Blackwell, UK, Copyright © 2007.

Box 278.1 Causes of pancytopenia

Aplastic anemia
• Idiopathic
• Cytotoxic drugs and radiation
• Idiosyncratic drug reaction
• Viral infections

Acute leukemia
Marrow replacement
• Cancer
• Myelofibrosis
• Military tuberculosis

Vitamin B_{12}/folate deficiency
Paroxysmal nocturnal hemoglobinuria
Myelodysplasia
HIV

Reproduced with permission from David C. Sprigings, John B. Chambers, *Acute Medicine: A Practical Guide to the Management of Medical Emergencies*, 4th Edition, Chambers, Wiley-Blackwell, UK, Copyright © 2007

Box 278.2 Indications for examination of bone marrow

• haematological malignancy, including leukaemia, lymphoma, myeloma, chronic granulocytic leukaemia, and myelodysplasia
• pancytopenia, or selective thrombocytopenia or neutropenia, where cause otherwise is not evident
• refractory anaemias (those not due to or responding to iron, vitamin B_{12}, folate replacement, or to obvious red-cell production disorders, such as thalassaemia
• unexplained protracted fever; may rarely demonstrate tuberculosis, kala azar, or underlying malignancy
• leucoerythroblastic anaemia; to detect metastatic carcinoma, or myelofibrosis
• to confirm megaloblastic anaemia (rarely necessary)

hypercellular or 'packed' marrow—as in some cases of leukaemia or other haematological malignancies—or if the marrow is severely hypocellular. Trephine biopsy is necessary in these circumstances and is also helpful if marrow infiltration with metastatic malignancy is suspected. Where haematological malignancy is suspected or being investigated, a sample for cytogenetics may be taken for karyotyping and/or molecular studies.

Marrow aspirate and biopsy are invasive and unpleasant procedures and should not be undertaken lightly. It is important to consider carefully what information is being sought and to plan the samples and sample handling accordingly. Formal consent should be obtained: although the risks are low, occasional fatalities have occurred; extensive bleeding may occur in patients with recognized or unrecognized coagulation, or platelet function abnormalities, and inadvertent puncture of internal organs or blood vessels may occur if an unduly long biopsy needle is used. Particular care should be taken in the elderly, who may have a degree of osteopenia.

Further Reading

Bain BJ. Diagnosis from the blood smear. *N Engl J Med* 2005; 353: 498–507.
Boxer LA. How to approach neutropenia. *Hematology* 2012; 2012: 174–82.
Chabot-Richards DS and Foucar K. Does morphology matter in 2017? An approach to morphologic clues in non-neoplastic blood and bone marrow disorders. *Int J Lab Hematol* 2017; 39 Suppl 1: 23–30.
Koury MJ and Rhodes M. How to approach chronic anemia. *Hematology* 2012; 2012: 183–90.
Stasi R. How to approach thrombocytopenia. *Hematology* 2012; 2012: 191–7.

279 Deficiency anaemias

Chris Bunch

Definition

Erythropoiesis requires an adequate supply of iron for haem formation, as well as vitamin B_{12} and folic acid (folate) to support high levels of DNA synthesis, and a lack of any of these will result in anaemia. Iron-deficient anaemias are typically microcytic, while a deficiency in vitamin B_{12} or folate results in megaloblastic haemopoiesis and a macrocytic anaemia.

Aetiology

Iron deficiency

When iron loss exceeds iron intake, the body stores of iron are mobilized for haemoglobin production. As the stores become depleted, the ability to absorb iron from the diet is increased, and serum ferritin falls. As stores are further depleted, the serum iron level falls, and the total iron binding capacity (transferrin) rises. If a negative iron balance continues, the stores become exhausted, and tissue iron deficiency and anaemia will develop.

Iron deficiency will result from poor dietary iron intake, poor absorption, increased demands, blood loss, or combinations of these.

Diet

The bioavailability of iron in the diet is low for many people worldwide, although poor diet is rarely the sole cause of iron deficiency in Western societies, except in the very poor and the elderly. Even in populations whose diet is largely vegetarian and is poor in available iron, deficiency may only develop at times of increased losses or physiological demands.

Increased physiological demands

Increased physiological demands will commonly lead to a degree of iron deficiency in infants (6–24 months), adolescents (especially at the time of the growth spurt and puberty), and in menstruating women who are also childbearing. The additional requirements during pregnancy, amounting to about 500 mg, include iron supply to the fetus, the expanded maternal red-cell volume, and blood losses at delivery.

Blood loss

Menstruating women form the largest group of people who suffer sufficient blood loss to cause iron deficiency. Losses of up to 80 ml a month may be tolerated by increased absorption, provided the diet is adequate. However, worldwide, this is often not the case and, with the additional stresses of pregnancy, menstruating women are frequently iron deficient. Even in Western societies, where only 5% of women are overtly iron deficient as assessed by haemoglobin measurements, some 30% may respond to iron supplementation with a rise in haemoglobin.

Gastrointestinal bleeding accounts for the majority of other cases involving blood loss. The normal insensible loss in the gastrointestinal tract amounts to 1 ml/day. Since tests for occult bleeding are insensitive below about 20 ml/day, and bleeding is often intermittent, even moderate intestinal bleeding cannot always be documented. The most important benign causes of gastrointestinal bleeding are:

- haemorrhoids
- hiatus hernia
- NSAID use
- diverticulosis
- peptic ulceration
- angiodysplasia (especially in the elderly)

The possibility of occult bowel malignancy is always a major concern in postmenopausal women and adult males. Such patients should have upper gastrointestinal endoscopy and colonoscopy, or barium studies if these are not available. Hookworm infestation is a major cause of blood loss in developing countries, and should always be considered in recent immigrants.

Malabsorption

Malabsorption of iron occurs in coeliac disease, and may be its only manifestation, although there is usually also folate deficiency. Iron deficiency secondary to gastric atrophy is common in association with pernicious anaemia, but simple atrophic gastritis may respond to iron therapy, and thus be a result, rather than a cause, of iron deficiency.

Megaloblastic anaemias

Megaloblastic haemopoiesis produces a macrocytic anaemia with a slow and pernicious onset. This allows time for compensatory mechanisms to develop, and symptoms may not be apparent until the haemoglobin is very low, often below 6 g/dl. The principal complaint is therefore of progressive lassitude, with shortness of breath. Angina pectoris may occur in patients with coexistent impairment of myocardial function or coronary blood flow. Increased bilirubin production, associated with ineffective erythropoiesis and a shortened red-cell survival, may give rise to mild jaundice which, combined with extreme pallor, gives rise to a 'lemon-yellow' appearance.

Anaemia due to vitamin B_{12} deficiency

Vitamin B_{12} is synthesized only by microorganisms, and is obtained in man by ingestion of other animal products, or from bacterially contaminated vegetable matter. Pure dietary deficiency is therefore rare, and seen only in strict vegans.

Dietary vitamin B_{12} binds to R factor in saliva and gastric juices. In the duodenum, it dissociates from R factor, and binds to intrinsic factor (IF) in the presence of pancreatic enzymes. The IF–B_{12} complex is taken up by receptors (cubilin) in the terminal ileum and then released into plasma, bound to transcobalamins TC I, II, or III. Vitamin B_{12} enters cells by receptor-mediated endocytosis and is metabolized into two coenzymes: adenosylcobalamin and methylcobalamin.

The usual cause of severe vitamin B_{12} deficiency in Western countries is an autoimmune atrophic gastritis, in which there is a loss of gastric parietal cell numbers and an absence of intrinsic factor production, which effectively prevents vitamin B_{12} absorption. This is the classical **pernicious anaemia**, and it is often seen in association with other autoimmune disorders, such as myxoedema (hypothyroidism), Addison's disease (hypoadrenalism), and vitiligo.

Vitamin B_{12} deficiency may result from infestation with the fish tapeworm *Diphyllobothrium latum*. More rarely, it may result from total gastrectomy; surgery or disease (e.g. Crohn's) affecting the terminal ileum, or congenital deficiencies of intrinsic factor, cubilin (the IF–B_{12} receptor), or transcobalamins.

Anaemia due to folate deficiency

Folate deficiency may result from a poor diet, from malabsorption, or when demand for folate is increased, for example during pregnancy or with increased haemopoiesis in haemolytic anaemias or myeloproliferative disorders.

Dietary sources of folate are varied, with high amounts in liver, kidney, green vegetables, yeast, nuts, and fruit. Cooking at high temperatures and in large volumes of water largely destroys it. Alcoholics whose caloric intake is in large part derived from ethanol are particularly prone to folate deficiency.

Folate malabsorption occurs in gluten-sensitive enteropathy (coeliac disease), and most untreated patients will have low serum and red-cell folate levels. Clinical anaemia is more often due to combined iron and folate depletion, but folate deficiency may be sufficiently severe to lead to pure megaloblastic anaemia. Dermatitis herpetiformis may also be associated with folate malabsorption. Less common causes are jejunal resection; partial gastrectomy; extensive Crohn's disease involving the small bowel; lymphoma; and severe systemic infection. Tropical sprue is an important cause on a worldwide basis.

Typical symptoms of the disease, and less common symptoms

The symptoms and signs of anaemia due to deficiency in iron, vitamin B_{12}, or folate are principally those of any associated anaemia—tiredness, fatigue, pallor—and may occasionally presage the development of anaemia. Deficiency of iron or folate is associated with slowed growth and impaired cognitive development in infants and young children, and with premature birth and low birthweight in pregnancy. In addition, folate deficiency is linked to neural tube defects.

Severe iron deficiency may also be associated with pica (an abnormal appetite for non-nutritional substances such as clay, or for food ingredients such as raw meat or vegetables), mucous membrane inflammation affecting the tongue (glossitis) and sometimes the pharynx and oesophagus (Plummer–Vinson/Paterson–Brown–Kelly syndrome), brittle, ridged nails (koilonychia), or hair loss.

Severe vitamin B_{12} deficiency may be complicated by a symmetrical peripheral neuropathy, with predominant signs in the lower limbs. A classical and often irreversible complication of vitamin B_{12} deficiency is **subacute combined degeneration of the spinal cord**. Psychiatric disturbance and optic atrophy may also occur. Recently, low blood levels of vitamin B_{12} have been linked to postural hypotension and falls in the elderly in the absence of anaemia. The biochemical basis of these neurological complications is unclear. Low vitamin B_{12} and folate levels have also been linked to depression.

Folate in the 5-methyltetrahydrofolic acid form is a cosubstrate for methionine synthase in the conversion of homocysteine to methionine; consequently, homocysteine accumulates in folate deficiency and is strongly associated with atherosclerotic vascular disease such as coronary artery disease and stroke.

Demographics of the disease

Demographics of iron deficiency

Iron deficiency is a worldwide problem, reflecting the heavy physiological demands for iron and its limited bioavailability in many diets. Overall, more than 500 million people are thought to be affected. Even in 'advanced' Western societies, around 10% of infants, adolescents, and menstruating women are iron deficient, with anaemia evident in around a quarter of these. Both chronic blood loss and poor diet play a part.

Demographics of folate deficiency

Like iron deficiency, folate deficiency is a worldwide problem associated with inadequate nutrition. Dietary lack may be aggravated by previous gastric or abdominal surgery, gastrointestinal disorders such as chronic tropical sprue, and chronic inflammatory conditions, such as rheumatoid arthritis and chronic infections, which appear to inhibit absorption. Pure dietary deficiency may also occur in infants fed goats' milk (which is very low in folate) as a substitute for mother's or cows' milk.

Since 1998, food fortification with folic acid has been compulsory in the US, and this has been accompanied by a reduction in the prevalence of low serum folate levels from 16% to 0.5%

Demographics of vitamin B_{12} deficiency

Nutritional vitamin B_{12} deficiency is much less common than iron or folate deficiency, reflecting the widespread availability of vitamin B_{12} in all but the strictest vegan diets. However, the risk of developing vitamin B_{12} deficiency increases with age for a number of reasons, including cognitive dysfunction, social isolation, mobility limitations, and poverty.

Pernicious anaemia, which is vitamin B_{12} malabsorption due to a lack of gastric intrinsic factor, is the commonest form of vitamin B_{12} deficiency. It is most common in Caucasians of Northern European descent, affecting up to 3% of individuals over 60.

Natural history and complications of the disease

Deficiency anaemias are progressive until the deficiency is corrected. As the onset is usually slow, adaptive mechanisms can mitigate the symptoms of anaemia, which in extreme cases may only become symptomatic at very low haemoglobin levels (2–4 g/dl). However, anaemia is likely to aggravate coexisting coronary or cerebrovascular disease.

Approach to diagnosing the disease

Iron deficiency should be considered in any anaemia that is microcytic, and vitamin B_{12} or folate deficiency in any anaemia that is macrocytic. The aim of investigation is to establish whether or not a deficiency exists, as well as the underlying cause. The former can usually be achieved by laboratory tests. The latter depends on the clinical picture, so a full clinical history, covering diet as well as bleeding history, together with a full clinical examination (including neurology) is important and will dictate subsequent investigation.

Other diagnoses that should be considered

Causes of red-cell microcytosis and macrocytosis are given in Table 279.1.

'Gold-standard' diagnostic test

The diagnosis of deficiency anaemias is made on the basis of the clinical and haematological picture, together with measurement of serum levels of iron, ferritin, and transferrin (iron deficiency); serum and red-cell folate levels (folate deficiency); and serum vitamin B_{12} levels (vitamin B_{12} deficiency). A bone marrow aspirate stained for iron has long been considered the gold-standard test for iron deficiency, but it is invasive, painful, and rarely justified for this purpose alone. On the other hand, while the blood film may reveal features of megaloblastic anaemia (e.g. macrocytosis, circulating megaloblasts, hypersegmented neutrophils), a bone marrow aspirate may occasionally be necessary to confirm the presence of megaloblastic haemopoiesis in vitamin B_{12} or folate deficiency, if these features are not unequivocally present.

Acceptable diagnostic alternatives to the gold standard

Acceptable diagnostic alternatives to the gold-standard test for iron deficiency

A low serum iron and ferritin, with a raised serum transferrin, is virtually diagnostic of iron deficiency. In practice, the ferritin level is more useful than iron or transferrin levels, although it is an acute phase

Table 279.1 Causes of red-cell microcytosis and macrocytosis	
Microcytic	**Macrocytic**
Iron deficiency	Alcohol
Anaemia of chronic disease	Pregnancy
Thalassaemias (alpha and beta)	Reticulocytosis
Abnormal haemoglobins (haemoglobin C, S/C, or E)	Liver disease
	Hypothyroidism
	Liver disease
	Myeloma
	Myelodysplasia
	Cytotoxic drugs
	Vitamin B_{12} deficiency
	Folate deficiency

reactant and is raised in the presence of infection or inflammation. In the presence of microcytic anaemia, a ferritin of <15 μg/l confirms iron deficiency, while a level of >100 μg/l virtually excludes it.

Acute or chronic inflammation, infection, or malignancy can confuse the picture, as these may cause a mild-to-moderate anaemia that is normocytic to microcytic with a reduced serum iron but, typically, a raised ferritin and normal or low transferrin—the **anaemia of chronic disease**. For this reason, a trial of oral iron therapy should be considered in anaemic patients with a serum ferritin of <40 μg/l, or <70 μg/l in the presence of infection, inflammation, or malignancy.

Acceptable diagnostic alternatives to the gold-standard test for folate deficiency

Folate status is normally assessed by measurement of serum and red-cell folate concentrations. A normal serum folate more or less excludes significant folate deficiency, but a reduced level does not in itself make a diagnosis of deficiency. This is because serum folate levels reflect recent folate intake and may be depressed after a short period of inadequate intake, while red-cell folate reflects folate status over the previous 2–3 months, and a low level is a more reliable indicator of tissue folate depletion. As a single meal can improve a low serum folate level within a few hours, red-cell folate should be measured in patients who have been admitted to (and fed in) hospital.

Low folate levels reflect poor dietary intake or absorption, while high levels may be associated with blind loop syndrome (bacterial production), active liver disease (release of stored folate), or folate supplementation.

Acceptable diagnostic alternatives to the gold-standard test for vitamin B₁₂ deficiency

Serum vitamin B_{12} levels in megaloblastic anaemia due to vitamin B_{12} deficiency are usually significantly reduced, and the diagnosis is then straightforward. More difficult to interpret are marginally reduced vitamin B_{12} levels in the absence of significant anaemia or macrocytosis. This is a fairly common situation in the elderly, who are also prone to falls, a condition which is thought by many to be a consequence of mild, subclinical deficiency.

A diagnosis of pernicious anaemia (vitamin B_{12} malabsorption due to gastric atrophy and intrinsic factor deficiency) as the cause of anaemia due to vitamin B_{12} deficiency normally rests on the demonstration of a reduced absorption of radioactive vitamin B_{12} administered orally, and increased absorption when the dose is combined with intrinsic factor—the **Schilling test**. However, tougher regulation of medical radioisotope use has all but completely eliminated the availability of this test, and the diagnosis rests on probabilities. The presence of other autoimmune conditions such as thyroid disease and adrenal insufficiency (Addison's disease), as well as the presence of gastric parietal cell antibodies or intrinsic factor antibodies, are strong pointers to pernicious anaemia being the cause.

Other relevant investigations

Less commonly available investigations that may be helpful in diagnosing the presence of deficiency anaemias include:

- circulating transferrin receptor levels, which parallel tissue receptor levels and are increased in iron deficiency
- serum or urinary hepcidin levels, which are low in iron deficiency but raised in anaemia of chronic disease
- methylmalonic acid and homocysteine levels, which may be useful in the evaluation of slightly reduced or low-normal vitamin B_{12} or folate levels; a raised methylmalonic acid and/or homocysteine level gives some support to the diagnosis of vitamin B_{12} and folate deficiency

Prognosis

Deficiency anaemias are usually easily correctable by replacement of the missing substance, so the main determinant of prognosis is the underlying cause.

Treatment and its effectiveness

Treatment for iron deficiency

In most cases, iron deficiency responds well to oral replacement: ferrous sulfate 200 mg or ferrous fumarate 300 mg daily, raising to twice, and then three times daily if tolerated. In uncomplicated iron deficiency, a rise in haemoglobin of 1 g/dl per week may be expected. Treatment should continue for 6 months after the anaemia is corrected, in order to replenish iron stores. If this is not done, the risk of recurrence is high.

Response to iron therapy may be suboptimal in the presence of infection, inflammation, renal impairment, cancer, or continuing blood loss. Oral iron commonly causes gastrointestinal symptoms such as nausea, epigastric pain, and diarrhoea; in addition, iron supplementation turns the stools black, so that they are commonly mistaken for melaena. Ideally, for maximal absorption, iron should be taken between meals, although side effects are likely to be worse. Concomitant administration of vitamin C improves absorption of a given dose. Alternative oral preparations (liquid, slow release) may cause fewer side effects but are less effective because they contain less iron and/or release most of it beyond the duodenum and upper jejunum, where iron is absorbed.

In rare cases of complete intolerance or refusal to take oral iron, it may be given intravenously. Earlier IV iron preparations were high-molecular-weight carbohydrate complexes (e.g. iron dextran) and were associated with serious (and sometimes fatal) side effects. Newer preparations such as iron sucrose appear to be more effective and safer.

Treatment of folate deficiency

Folate is easily replaced orally in a dose of 5–15 mg of folic acid daily, with no side effects. IV replacement is necessary, only in patients receiving total parenteral nutrition.

Treatment of vitamin B₁₂ deficiency

Vitamin B_{12} is usually replaced by regular intramuscular injection of hydroxocobalamin, which is available in 1 mg ampoules. This is about 1000 times the normal daily requirement, but this is not a problem as the vitamin is inexpensive and safe, and most of it is excreted in the urine. For this reason, initial treatment should be 1 mg on alternate days for a fortnight and then monthly thereafter.

Indications for blood transfusion

There is sometimes a temptation to perform a blood transfusion on a patient with severe or even moderate anaemia that is clearly due to a deficiency in iron, vitamin B_{12}, or folate. This temptation should be resisted in most instances, and is usually only justified if there is ongoing bleeding, when iron replacement may be insufficient to correct the anaemia. Indeed, transfusion may be dangerous: deficiency anaemias usually develop gradually over weeks or months, giving plenty of time for adaptive mechanisms to develop. Such red cells, that are circulating, are actually highly attuned to optimal oxygen delivery. Transfused red cells are the opposite: they have been refrigerated, are metabolically inert, and have lost much of their 2,3-diphosphoglycerate, shifting the oxygen-dissociation curve in favour of retaining rather than delivering oxygen.

Further Reading

Camaschella C. Iron-deficiency anemia. *N Engl J Med* 2015; 372: 1832–43.

Devalia V, Hamilton M, and Molloy AM. Guidelines for the diagnosis and treatment of cobalamin and folate disorders. *Brit J Haematol* 2014; 166: 496–513.

Stabler SP. Vitamin B12 deficiency. *N Engl J Med* 2013; 368: 149–60.

280 Haemolytic anaemia

Chris Bunch

Introduction

Haemolytic anaemias occur when the rate of red-cell breakdown is increased and exceeds the marrow's capacity to generate new cells. The normal red-cell lifespan averages 120 days: by this time, the cells' metabolic activity is no longer able to maintain membrane integrity, resulting in removal by macrophages, predominantly in the spleen. Increased red-cell destruction, or **haemolysis**, may occur for a variety of reasons (Box 280.1). Some involve intrinsic defects in the red cell itself; in others, the red cells are normal but subjected to external factors which lead to premature destruction. Many of the intrinsic defects are due to inherited disorders affecting the red-cell membrane, its enzymes, or haemoglobin. Some of these represent major worldwide health problems.

The marrow can normally compensate for moderate haemolysis by increasing red-cell production up to tenfold. Only when haemolysis is severe and the red-cell lifespan is reduced to less

than about 15 days, or the marrow is unable to compensate, will anaemia occur.

General features of haemolysis

The clinical effects of haemolysis can be divided into those of increased red-cell breakdown, and those related to compensatory marrow activity. The breakdown of haemoglobin generates bilirubin, which is transported to the liver, where it is conjugated with glucuronic acid and excreted in the bile. The conjugation pathway is easily saturated, leading to mild jaundice due to increased levels of circulating unconjugated bilirubin. This is sometimes called **acholuric jaundice** (literally, 'no bile in the urine' jaundice).

In most cases, haemolysis is **extravascular**: the red cells are destroyed after phagocytosis by fixed macrophages lining the sinusoids of the spleen, liver, and bone marrow. Less commonly, red-cell destruction is **intravascular**, with release of haemoglobin into the circulation. Free haemoglobin binds to circulating haptoglobins, and the complex is removed by the liver. Haptoglobins can normally bind 100–140 mg of haemoglobin per 100 ml of plasma: a fall in haptoglobin level is thus a sensitive indicator of intravascular haemolysis, although some reduction usually also occurs in severe extravascular haemolysis. Large amounts of haemoglobin may exceed the binding capacity of haptoglobin, so that free haemoglobin appears in the circulation, is filtered by the glomerulus, and appears in the urine. Small amounts are reabsorbed and metabolized by the tubular cells to haemosiderin, which may be detected in a urine deposit due to shedding of tubular cells. This is a particularly sensitive measure of chronic intravascular haemolysis.

Anaemia occurs in severe haemolysis or when the marrow is unable to compensate normally. The appearance of the red cells may give some clue to the nature of the haemolysis. For example, there may be spherocytes, sickle cells, deposits of precipitated haemoglobin (**Heinz bodies**), and so on.

Increased red-cell production is reflected by a **reticulocytosis** greater than the normal level of 2%. This produces polychromasia (the reticulocytes stain with a bluish tinge on routine blood smears) and a mild macrocytosis, as reticulocytes are larger than mature red cells. The marrow shows erythroid hyperplasia. In long-standing or severe haemolysis, increased folate utilization may lead to deficiency, with superadded megaloblastic change.

Patients with haemolytic anaemia may suffer sudden and profound falls in haemoglobin in association with human parvovirus infection; such events are termed '**aplastic crises**'. The virus infects erythrocyte progenitors in the marrow, and red-cell production ceases completely for 48–72 hours. The effect is insignificant in normal individuals but, with haemolysis, when red-cell survival is very short, sudden failure of compensation produces catastrophic anaemia with reticulotopenia. The leucocyte and platelet counts may be affected to a lesser degree. The infection is self-limiting, but transfusion may be needed.

Red-cell membrane disorders

The red-cell membrane has important functions in maintaining the cell shape and deformability, in controlling the osmotic equilibrium of the cell by energy-dependent cation transport systems, and in governing the permeability and other properties of the cell via the structural organization of its proteins, lipids, and terminal sugar residues. Interference with any of these functions increases red-cell fragility and can lead to haemolysis. This is usually the result of an inherited structural or metabolic defect.

Box 280.1 Causes of haemolysis

Intrinsic red-cell defects

Red cell membrane disorders
- hereditary spherocytosis
- other rare inherited membrane disorders (e.g. hereditary elliptocytosis, stomatocytosis, hereditary pyropoikilocytosis, acanthocytosis)
- paroxysmal nocturnal haemoglobinuria
- other acquired membrane disorders (e.g. myelodysplasia, lipid defects)

Red cell metabolic disorders
- abnormalities of the pentose phosphate pathway (e.g. glucose-6-phosphate-dehydrogenase deficiency)
- abnormalities of the glycolytic pathway (e.g. pyruvate kinase deficiency)
- abnormalities in glutathione metabolism
- acquired abnormalities (e.g. in myelodysplasia)

Haemoglobin disorders
- disorders of globin chain synthesis: the thalassaemias
- structural globin chain variants: sickle cell disease, haemoglobin E, etc.

Extrinsic factors causing haemolysis

Immune haemolysis
- alloimmune haemolysis
- autoimmune haemolysis
- drug-induced haemolysis

Haemolysis secondary to red-cell damage
- damage from infections (e.g. malaria, toxoplasmosis, *Clostridium welchii*)
- damage from drugs or chemicals (e.g. phenylhydrazine, dapsone, sulfasalazine, arsine, chlorate)
- damage from mechanical trauma (e.g. artificial heart valves, march haemoglobinuria, microangiopathic haemolytic anaemia)
- damage from other causes (e.g. fibrinoid necrosis, vasculitis, tumour cell invasion (especially from mucin-secreting carcinomas), burns (from direct heat damage and, secondarily, disseminated intravascular coagulation))

Hereditary spherocytosis

Hereditary spherocytosis (HS) is characterized by red cells that are spherical rather than biconcave and have increased osmotic fragility and a shortened life span. The condition is heterogeneous both in clinical severity and in terms of the underlying defect. In the majority of cases, the defect is inherited in an autosomal dominant fashion, although recessive forms are also recognized. It is the commonest form of haemolytic anaemia due to a red-cell membrane abnormality, and the commonest inherited haemolytic anaemia in Northern Europeans, affecting 1:5000 of this population.

Aetiology of HS

HS results from a molecular defect in one or other of the membrane cytoskeleton proteins (e.g. spectrin, actin, band 3 protein, protein 4.2). The cell is unable to maintain its normal biconcave shape and becomes spherical and prone to early destruction, predominantly in the spleen.

Clinical features of HS

The severity of HS is variable but is often similar in the affected members of a given family. It usually presents in childhood, sometimes as neonatal jaundice but, in mild cases, may only be recognized in an adult after identification of an affected offspring or grandchild, or when pigment gallstones are found at cholecystectomy.

In HS, anaemia is mild (haemoglobin levels of 8–12 g/dl) or absent. The reticulocyte count is elevated and the blood film shows spherocytes and polychromasia. Mild jaundice is common, with bilirubin levels of 16–20 mmol/l, which may be accentuated at times, such as during infection, when haemolysis increases. A high bilirubin turnover can lead to the formation of pigment gallstones. The spleen is usually just palpable.

Diagnosis of HS

The diagnosis of HS is confirmed by an **osmotic fragility test**, in which cell lysis is assessed in solutions of differing osmotic strength. In spherocytosis, the fragility curve characteristically shows two cell populations, with a 'tail' of fragile cells.

Management of HS

Splenectomy markedly reduces the rate of haemolysis in HS and produces almost complete reversal of the anaemia. It is recommended in symptomatic patients, especially if recurrent transfusion has been required. However, its role is more debatable in asymptomatic patients with a well-compensated low-grade haemolysis, and the risks of post-splenectomy infection must be borne in mind. The risk of infection is much greater in children, and splenectomy should therefore be delayed as long as possible. The spleen should be removed at the time of cholecystectomy in patients with gallstones.

Other inherited membrane disorders

Haemolytic anaemia is associated with a variety of other rare red-cell membrane disorders. These include:

- **hereditary elliptocytosis**:
  - this is a fairly common but mild defect with autosomal dominant inheritance
  - it is rarely a clinical problem
  - some forms are linked to the rhesus D group loci
  - occasional homozygotes may have severe disease
- **stomatocytosis**: in this disorder, the membrane defect gives the cell a characteristic 'stoma', or mouth-like appearance
- **hereditary pyropoikilocytosis**: in this disorder, the red-cell membrane is unusually temperature sensitive, which leads to red-cell fragmentation
- **acanthocytosis**: in this disorder, a membrane lipid defect produces cells with characteristic 'spiky' projections, which can be seen on a fresh blood film

Paroxysmal nocturnal haemoglobinuria

Definition of paroxysmal nocturnal haemoglobinuria

Paroxysmal nocturnal haemoglobinuria (PNH) is a rare acquired haemolytic disorder characterized by exquisite sensitivity of the red cells to intravascular lysis by complement, resulting in haemoglobinuria. Sufferers also have an increased tendency to thrombosis.

Aetiology of PNH

The abnormality in PNH arises from a mutation in a haemopoietic stem cell: it is thus a clonal disorder which affects red cells, white cells, and platelets, although the most obvious clinical manifestations arise from red-cell lysis. The abnormal clone coexists with normal cells, with the proportion of abnormal cells determining the severity of the disease.

The defect is caused by the absence of glycosyl-phosphatidylinositol (GPI)-anchored proteins which normally protect against complement-mediated lysis. The absence of two of these proteins, CD55 and CD59, is fundamental to the pathophysiology of PNH. The enzyme phosphatidylinositol glycan A (PIG-A), which is needed for GPI synthesis, is deficient in PNH. The gene for PIG-A resides on the X chromosome: in males, cells contain only one X chromosome while, in females, there is random inactivation of one of each pair at an early stage of development. Thus, just a single PIG-A mutation is required to disrupt the GPI anchor.

The thrombotic tendency is thought to be due to a similar membrane defect in platelets.

Clinical features of PNH

PNH classically presents with early morning haemoglobinuria, as haemolysis is more active during sleep. There may also be exacerbations during infection or following surgery. In many patients, however, the brief paroxysms of haemoglobinuria go unnoticed, and the condition presents as unexplained anaemia or jaundice. For this reason, several years may ensue from the first onset of symptoms to eventual diagnosis. In some patients, the disease comes to light because of thrombotic complications: these often involve unusual sites, such as the mesenteric and hepatic veins (Budd–Chiari syndrome), or the intracranial venous sinuses.

A PNH clone, and other features of the disease, may appear in some patients with aplastic anaemia. Most patients with PNH have a degree of pancytopenia at some stage in their illness, and recurrent infections may occur. Recurrent haemoglobinuria commonly leads to iron deficiency.

Diagnosis of PNH

The major barrier to the diagnosis of PNH is not thinking of the disorder in the first place. It should be considered in patients with unexplained pancytopenia, bizarre thromboses, or jaundice. The diagnosis is confirmed by the demonstration of reduced membrane CD55 and CD59 in red or white cells by flow cytometry, or by the fluorescein-labelled proaerolysin test (proaerolysin binds to GPI.) Screening the urine for haemosiderin is a useful indicator of low-grade chronic intravascular haemolysis.

Treatment of PNH

Many PNH patients require no treatment. Transfusion may occasionally be necessary but can precipitate haemolysis unless the red cells are washed free of plasma before transfusion. Patients who have experienced thrombosis should take oral anticoagulants for life. Steroids may be of benefit in acute exacerbations but are not indicated in the long term. Oral iron supplements should be given if iron deficiency occurs. Marrow transplantation should be considered in severe cases, especially in those with predominant pancytopenia.

Recently, use of the monoclonal antibody eculizumab has been advocated for the management of PNH. Eculizumab is directed against the complement protein C5, which inhibits terminal activation, and it is effective in preventing intravascular haemolysis in PNH. However, its precise role has not yet been determined.

Prognosis of PNH

Most patients with PNH survive for many years. The major hazards are thrombotic events, and pancytopenia, which tends to progress with time. Acute myeloid leukaemia may occasionally occur, reflecting clonal evolution of the abnormal clone. Many years of chronic haemoglobinuria may eventually lead to renal failure.

Other acquired membrane disorders

Alterations in the red-cell environment can lead to the development of abnormal membrane characteristics, which then result in mechanical destruction of the cell and a shortened lifespan. **Lipid disorders** and **liver disease** may alter the red-cell lipid content by passive exchange. **Zieve's syndrome** is a severe haemolytic anaemia with abdominal pain, cirrhosis, hyperlipidaemia, and jaundice, seen in chronic alcoholics. **Vitamin E deficiency** in the newborn allows auto-oxidation of the membrane lipids and haemolysis.

Haemolysis is a feature of a number of acquired haematological dysplasias. It may arise because of ineffective erythropoiesis with defective cell formation, or because of clonally acquired red-cell membrane defects due to inherited disorders such as PNH. Both **megaloblastic anaemia** and **iron-deficiency anaemia** are associated with ineffective erythropoiesis and a slightly shortened red-cell lifespan. In the **myelodysplasias**, acquired abnormalities of red-cell shape, metabolism, or surface components may reduce the red-cell lifespan.

Red cell metabolic disorders

The red cell is anucleate and lacks most intracellular structures such as ribosomes and mitochondria. It cannot replace lost or damaged proteins or use oxidative phosphorylation as an energy source. It therefore relies on anaerobic glycolysis and the hexose monophosphate shunts to provide its energy and reducing power. Consequently, abnormalities in these pathways are associated with haemolysis.

The enzymes most commonly implicated in haemolytic anaemia are glucose 6-phosphate dehydrogenase (G6PD) and pyruvate kinase (PK).

G6PD deficiency

G6PD deficiency is by far the most important red-cell enzyme deficiency worldwide; as many as 100 million people carry a mutation leading to this deficiency. The deficiency is inherited as an X-linked characteristic which is only fully expressed in males, with females having varied expression depending upon the random X-chromosome inactivation in the red-cell precursor population. The condition is particularly prevalent in the populations of Africa, the Mediterranean, the Middle East, and South East Asia, probably because carriers of mutant G6PD alleles are afforded some protection from falciparum malaria.

Pathophysiology of G6PD deficiency

G6PD deficiency results from the inheritance of one of the 400 or so known variant forms of the enzyme. Only two of these occur with any frequency: the unstable A⁻ variant in the African population, and the structural Mediterranean variant. The precise mechanism by which G6PD deficiency causes haemolysis is not completely understood. In outline, there is failure to reduce glutathione which allows oxidative damage to haemoglobin, leading to its precipitation as Heinz bodies. Haemolysis is most apparent in the presence of oxidant drugs and chemicals, which would normally be adequately dealt with by the cells' reducing capacity.

Clinical features of G6PD deficiency

G6PD deficiency has the following clinical features:

- drug-induced haemolysis
- favism
- neonatal jaundice
- chronic haemolysis

Drug-induced haemolysis

In G6PD-deficient individuals, intravascular haemolysis can occur within a few days of ingestion of an oxidant drug. The pattern and severity of the haemolysis depend upon the drug, its dose, and the G6PD variant in question. Anaemia and jaundice develop rapidly and, in severe cases, are associated with shivering, backache, and the passage of dark urine. In the A⁻ variant, G6PD levels are lowest in older red cells, and the episode may be self-limiting, as the reticulocytes produced in response to the haemolysis have relatively normal amounts of the enzyme. On the other hand, G6PD activity is virtually absent in the Mediterranean type, and haemolysis may be progressive and fatal.

Favism

Favism refers to a severe haemolytic reaction that occurs in individuals with the Mediterranean G6PD deficiency when they are exposed to the fava bean (*Vicia faba*) or its pollen. It is not known how the haemolysis is precipitated or why some individuals are spared while others have recurrent attacks or only have an attack after multiple exposures.

Neonatal jaundice

Neonatal jaundice, occasionally leading to kernicterus, is seen in some individuals with G6PD deficiency. However, other factors seem to be involved, as the haemolysis observed does not fully account for the clinical picture.

Chronic haemolysis

Chronic haemolysis with jaundice and splenomegaly is seen in some G6PD-deficient individuals. In addition, haemolysis can occur or become apparent during an intercurrent illness or infection.

Laboratory diagnosis of G6PD deficiency

Heinz bodies will be detectable in the red cells during period of haemolysis but, in their absence, diagnosis depends on the demonstration of reduced levels of G6PD in red cells. The diagnosis is difficult in a patient with the A⁻ variant during the recovery phase from a haemolytic episode because of the high proportion of reticulocytes containing normal levels of the enzyme. Tests may need repeating in the stable state. More sophisticated analysis is required to identify the G6PD subtype.

Treatment of G6PD deficiency

Avoidance of drugs precipitating acute episodes is most important. Supplementary folic acid should be given in chronic haemolysis, and transfusion may be required during acute haemolysis, with exchange in the neonatal period.

PK deficiency

Although deficiencies of each of the enzymes in the Embden–Meyerhof pathway have been described, the only clinically important deficiency is PK deficiency. PK deficiency is a relatively rare disorder, with autosomal recessive inheritance, and shows considerable molecular heterogeneity. PK catalyses the final reaction in the glycolytic pathway: deficiency slows the overall glycolytic rate, reduces levels of ATP, and leads to accumulation of all metabolic intermediates including 2,3-bisphosphoglyceric acid. Haemoglobin oxygen affinity is thereby reduced, ameliorating to some extent the clinical effects of the anaemia.

Clinical features of PK

Most patients present in the neonatal period or in infancy with a moderate-to-severe anaemia (haemoglobin levels of 4–10 g/dl) that is relatively well tolerated. The spleen may be enlarged and there is jaundice. Haemolysis may increase during intercurrent infection; aplastic crises and gallstones may also occur.

Management of PK

In patients with PK, transfusion should be reserved for times of stress, such as infection or pregnancy. Splenectomy is indicated occasionally and can lead to an overall clinical improvement associated with a marked rise in the reticulocyte count. Folic acid should be given to prevent secondary deficiency.

Deficiencies of enzymes in the glutathione cycle

The glutathione cycle is important in the oxidoreductive balance of the red cells, and there is a link between its reactions, the reduced NADPH of the hexose monophosphate pathway, and the oxidation reactions affecting haemoglobin and the red-cell membrane. Deficiencies of glutathione synthetase and glutathione reductase are both rare causes of haemolytic anaemia.

The only other important red-cell defect—although not associated with haemolysis—is **NADH:methaemoglobin reductase deficiency**. In homozygotes, this causes congenital methaemoglobinaemia, with cyanosis from birth. It is important to differentiate the condition from other causes of cyanosis which may need intervention. Heterozygotes may be unusually susceptible to the action of drugs known to cause methaemoglobinaemia.

Acquired red-cell metabolic disorders

As mentioned in 'Other acquired membrane disorders', in the myelodysplasias, an acquired abnormality of red-cell metabolism may reduce red-cell lifespan.

Haemoglobin disorders

The haemoglobins are a family of molecules with a basically similar structure consisting of two pairs of globin chains, each associated with a haem moiety. Normal adult haemoglobin (Hb A) is formed from two alpha globin chains and two beta globin chains. Interactions between the amino acid side chains lead to complex folding of the globin molecule to give a quaternary structure, with the haem molecules tucked inside the folds of the chains.

Other normal human haemoglobins consist of an alpha chain or the alpha-like zeta chain, combined with one of the beta-like chains: epsilon or gamma (there are two gamma chains: gamma G (which is predominant at birth) and gamma A). The first haemoglobins to appear in the embryo are haemoglobin Gower 1, which is made up of two zeta chains and two epsilon chains; haemoglobin Portland, which is made up of two zeta chains and two gamma chains; and haemoglobin Gower 2, which is made up of two alpha chains and two epsilon chains. These are replaced in the fetus by fetal haemoglobin (Hb F), which is made up of two alpha chains and two gamma chains. Shortly before birth, production switches to Hb A, which largely replaces Hb F by the end of the first year of life. In postnatal life, a minor adult haemoglobin, haemoglobin A_2 (Hb A_2), which is made up of two alpha chains and two delta chains, accounts for less than 2.5% of total haemoglobin. The switch from fetal to adult haemoglobin is affected by some of the molecular lesions responsible for the thalassaemias and may lead to continued or increased production of Hb F, with some amelioration of the expression of the disease.

The genes for the alpha chains are found on Chromosome 16, together with the embryonic zeta chain gene. The alpha gene is duplicated on each haploid chromosome so, in each individual, there are four copies of the alpha gene. The non-alpha genes are clustered on Chromosome 11, closely linked and in order of developmental expression: their order is, from 3′ 5′, epsilon, gamma G, gamma A, delta, and beta. These genes are sequentially activated and then repressed during fetal development, to ensure the appropriate developmental changes in haemoglobin production. Alpha and non-alpha chain synthesis is synchronized, with haem being incorporated into each chain by a separate pathway before the chains are combined to form the complete haemoglobin molecule.

The genetic control of haemoglobin production has several important consequences. First, abnormalities affecting individual globin genes may be inherited from one or both parents (heterozygosity and homozygosity, respectively). Second, different abnormalities can be inherited from each parent (double heterozygosity). Third, abnormalities affecting the beta chain will not become apparent until after the first 3–6 months of life, when beta chain synthesis supersedes gamma chain production. On the other hand, disorders affecting alpha chain production may become apparent during fetal life, although duplication of the alpha chain gene affords protection from limited abnormalities.

The thalassaemias

The term 'thalassaemia' comes from the Greek θαλασσα, meaning 'the sea', and refers to a group of genetic anaemias that was first recognized in patients of Mediterranean origin. It has subsequently become clear that the thalassaemias are heterogeneous disorders with a worldwide distribution and which result from a reduced rate of production of one or other of the two globin chains of the haemoglobin molecule. Study of these conditions has made a major contribution to our understanding of cellular and molecular biology and genetics, both of haemoglobin and more generally.

Molecular genetics of thalassaemia

The thalassaemias are classified according to which globin chain genes are affected and by how much globin production is reduced (Table 280.1). A wide variety of molecular lesions have been uncovered and complex interactions can occur. In beta thalassaemia, most of the molecular lesions are small—often single base-pair changes—which may interfere with RNA transcription, post-translational modification of RNA, or its translation into protein. In alpha thalassaemia, deletion mutations are more common. The clinical effects depend upon whether synthesis of the particular globin chain is completely or partially suppressed, and whether or not the switch from fetal to adult haemoglobin production is affected.

Pathophysiology of the thalassaemias

Beta thalassaemia is the more important disorder clinically, and results from reduction (beta[+] thalassaemia) or failure (beta[0] thalassaemia) of beta chain synthesis. This only comes to light a few months after birth, when Hb A production takes over from Hb F production.

Failure of beta chain production leads to an excess of alpha chains, which cannot be incorporated into Hb A and so precipitate in the cell, producing large inclusion bodies. These interfere with cell maturation of the cell and may lead to cell death in the marrow (ineffective erythropoiesis) or to premature destruction of the cells which have been released into the circulation (shortened red-cell lifespan). Both factors contribute to the anaemia, which stimulates erythropoietin production, leading to expansion of the erythropoietic marrow to an extent that may produce gross skeletal deformities. Peripheral red-cell destruction leads to splenomegaly, and this may further exaggerate the anaemia and also cause thrombocytopenia.

Those cells which continue to produce some gamma chains are able to 'mop up' some of the excess alpha chains to make Hb F. These cells have fewer inclusion bodies and thus a survival advantage, leading to a relative increase in Hb F levels. A similar effect leads to increased levels of Hb A_2, unless the molecular lesion extends to the delta gene (delta beta thalassaemia).

Table 280.1 Classification of thalassaemias

Type of thalassaemia	Findings in homozygote	Findings in heterozygote
α[0]	Hb Bart's hydrops	Thalassaemia minor
α[+](deletion)	Thalassaemia minor	Normal blood picture[2]
α[+](nondeletion)	Hb H disease[1]	Normal blood picture[2]
β[0]	Thalassaemia major[3,4] Hbs F and A_2	Thalassaemia minor Raised Hb A_2
β[+]	Thalassaemia major[3,4] Hbs F, A, and A_2	Thalassaemia minor Raised Hb A_2
δβ	Thalassaemia intermedia Hb F only	Thalassaemia minor Hb F 5–15%; Hb A_2 normal
(δβ)[+]	Thalassaemia major or intermedia	Thalassaemia minor
(Lepore)	Hbs F and Lepore	Hb Lepore 5–15%; Hb A_2 normal
εγδβ	Not viable	Neonatal haemolysis Thalassaemia minor in adults, with normal Hbs F and A_2

Abbreviations: Hb, haemoglobin.

[1] Haemoglobin H disease more commonly results from the compound heterozygous inheritance of α[0] and either variety of α[+] thalassaemia.

[2] There may be very mild red-cell hypochromia.

[3] Occasionally have thalassaemia intermedia phenotype.

[4] Many patients with thalassaemia are compound heterozygotes for different molecular forms of β[0] or β[+] thalassaemia.

Reproduced with permission from Weatherall, Disorders of the synthesis or function of haemoglobin, in *Oxford Textbook of Medicine*, Fifth Edition Oxford University Press, Oxford, UK, Copyright © 2010.

In alpha thalassaemia, alpha chain production is reduced or absent, and there is relatively excess production of gamma chains during fetal life, and of beta chains after birth. Above a certain level of chain imbalance, gamma and beta chains can form tetramers, producing haemoglobin Barts (Hb Barts), which consists of four gamma chains, and haemoglobin H (Hb H), which consists of four beta chains, respectively. If all four copies of the alpha chain gene are affected, the fetus is unable to make any alpha chains and only Hb Barts is formed: this is physiologically useless, and severe anaemia leading to hydrops fetalis and fetal loss results. In milder forms of alpha thalassaemia—involving one, two, or three of the four copies of the alpha chain gene—alpha chain synthesis is reduced rather than absent. Excess non-alpha chains form Hb Barts in infancy, and Hb H in adult life. There is, therefore, less globin chain precipitation in the marrow cells than in beta thalassaemia, and less ineffective erythropoiesis and marrow expansion. However, there is some precipitation of excess globin, leading to a degree of haemolysis in all the alpha thalassaemia variants.

Geographical distribution of the thalassaemias

Some beta thalassaemia occurs sporadically in all populations, but the high incidence zones lie in a band from the Mediterranean and North and West Africa through the Middle East and Indian subcontinent to South East Asia. The highest incidences (up to 30% gene frequency) are seen in South East Asia.

Severe forms of alpha thalassaemia only occur with any frequency in South East Asia, in some parts of the Middle East, and in isolated Mediterranean populations. Mild alpha thalassaemia has a high incidence in West Africa, and in some immigrant populations originating from this area.

The high frequencies of thalassaemic alleles in these populations seems to have resulted from a relative protection of heterozygote carriers from falciparum malaria, and population genetic studies clearly show that the allelic frequency reflects changing malaria endemicity. How this protection may be afforded by thalassaemia alleles is not clearly understood.

Beta thalassaemia

The beta thalassaemias fall into two groups: those with no beta chain production (beta^0), and those with some beta chain production (beta$^+$). The beta$^+$ thalassaemias are extremely heterogeneous, with beta chain production ranging from being virtually absent to being near normal levels. The clinical phenotype usually depends on the amount of beta chain synthesized, although this may be modified in patients who have also inherited other forms of thalassaemia or one of the haemoglobinopathies. In practice, three broad clinical phenotypes are recognized:

- beta thalassaemia major: this is a homozygous or compound heterozygous state, with severe, transfusion-dependent anaemia
- beta thalassaemia intermedia: this is also a homozygous or heterozygous state, but with mild-to-moderate moderate anaemia requiring only occasional transfusion
- beta thalassaemia minor or trait: this is the heterozygous state; it is usually asymptomatic, but affected individual may have a severely affected child

Beta thalassaemia major

Beta thalassaemia major is clinically the most important form of thalassaemia. It presents in the first year of life, with failure to thrive, poor feeding, and intermittent fever. The infant is usually pale and has splenomegaly. There is severe anaemia with small misshapen red cells. The bilirubin is raised and haptoglobins are reduced, because of haemolysis. Haemoglobin electrophoresis shows only Hb F and Hb A$_2$ in beta^0 thalassaemia, with variable amounts of Hb A in beta$^+$ thalassaemia.

Untreated or inadequately treated children progressively fail to thrive and have reduced growth rate and slow development. The spleen enlarges massively and hypersplenism leads to exaggeration of the anaemia and additional thrombocytopenia. The expansion of the bone marrow leads to disfiguring deformities, and bossing of the skull and expansion of the zygomata lead to a typical facial appearance. Radiologically, there is a fine, lacy trabecular pattern to the long bones, and the classical 'hair-on-end' appearance of the skull. The long bones are fragile, and fractures are common, while the skull deformities can be complicated by malocclusion and poor sinus drainage, with infection and deafness.

Reduced resistance to infection leads to further chronic malaise and intermittent additional falls in the haemoglobin. The massive expansion of the marrow with the ineffective erythropoiesis puts the children into a hypermetabolic state leading to folic acid depletion, hyperuricaemia, and gout. A bleeding tendency from liver abnormalities adds to the thrombocytopenia secondary to hypersplenism.

Without transfusion, death occurs in the first year of life. Those who receive inadequate transfusions will often succumb to overwhelming infection in early childhood.

With early diagnosis and adequate transfusion, early growth and development is normal. However, transfusional iron overload is inevitable by the end of the first decade unless long-term iron chelation is undertaken. Iron overload produces endocrine, hepatic, and cardiac complications, with growth spurt failure, diabetes, hypothyroidism, adrenal insufficiency, progressive liver failure, and cardiac failure. The commonest mode of death is either sudden arrhythmia or intractable cardiac failure, which occurs in the teens or the early twenties.

Intensive chelation therapy may avoid these complications and should be introduced as early as is practicable. A subcutaneous infusion of desferrioxamine for five or six nights a week, started early and maintained indefinitely, may prevent iron overload altogether. However, compliance may be poor, especially in teenage children.

Beta thalassaemia minor

In heterozygous beta thalassaemia, excess alpha chains are readily degraded, and damage to the developing red cells is minimal. Affected persons are usually asymptomatic, although symptomatic anaemia may develop during pregnancy or at other times of stress. Anaemia is mild or absent (haemoglobin levels of 9–12 g/dl), but the blood film shows hypochromia and microcytosis with moderate anisocytosis and some target cell change. The amount of Hb that is Hb A$_2$ is elevated to 4%–6%, and the amount that is Hb F to 1%–3%. Diagnosis can be difficult if there is concomitant iron deficiency, in which case iron supplementation, monitoring of the serum ferritin, and repeat haemoglobin electrophoresis and quantitation may be necessary.

It is important to recognize beta thalassaemia trait so that the patient can be counselled about the risk of having a severely affected child if their partner is also a carrier. Once the diagnosis is established, further investigation and unnecessary iron therapy can be avoided.

Beta thalassaemia intermedia

There are various ways in which the severity of homozygous beta thalassaemia is ameliorated in some way, giving rise to a less severe or intermediate clinical phenotype with reduced or absent transfusion requirement. These include the production of large amounts of Hb F, the co-inheritance of an alpha thalassaemia allele which reduces the degree of chain imbalance, or a variety of other situations. These patients usually maintain haemoglobin levels of 6–10 g/dl, although anaemia may become more severe during intercurrent illness or during pregnancy. Iron absorption is increased, and loading can occur. Chelation may be required.

Beta thalassaemia interactions with haemoglobin variants

The beta thalassaemia allele and the alleles for structural haemoglobin variants (e.g. beta^S, which encodes the beta chain in sickle haemoglobin (Hb S); beta^C, which encodes the mutant beta chain leading to the formation of haemoglobin C (Hb C); beta^D, which encodes the mutant beta chain leading to the formation of haemoglobin D (Hb D); and beta^E, which encodes the mutant beta chain leading to the formation of haemoglobin E (Hb E); see 'The haemoglobinopathies') occur at high frequencies in similar populations, so co-inheritance of a different abnormality from each parent is not infrequent. Three interactions are clinically important:

- sickle cell beta thalassaemia
- Hb C thalassaemia
- Hb E thalassaemia

Sickle cell beta thalassaemia produces a variable picture depending upon whether the beta thalassaemia allele is beta$^+$ (as it is in many of African descent) or beta⁰. The clinical picture in the former may be almost normal or be that of a mild sickling trait. The red-cell indices will be hypochromic and microcytic, and the film will show anisopoikilocytosis with target cells and occasional sickle cells. Hb S will account for about 70% of the haemoglobin, and Hb A for about 25%. The level of Hb A_2 will be raised. Sickle cell beta thalassaemia is clinically indistinguishable from sickle cell anaemia (see 'Sickle cell disease'). Haemoglobin electrophoresis shows a complete absence of Hb A, with Hb S and raised levels of Hb A_2 and Hb F.

Hb C thalassaemia is a mild disorder that is similar to Hb C disease (see 'The haemoglobinopathies'). There is mild anaemia and splenomegaly, and the blood film shows thalassaemic changes with large numbers of target cells. Haemoglobin electrophoresis shows predominantly Hb C, with some Hb F and Hb A_2 and variable amounts of Hb A. Hb C thalassaemia is largely restricted to West Africans, with occasional North African and Mediterranean cases.

Hb E thalassaemia is the commonest severe thalassaemic syndrome in South East Asia and India. The inefficiency of production of the Hb E structural haemoglobin variant leads to a severe beta thalassaemia major syndrome when the allele for this variant is co-inherited with the beta⁰ thalassaemia allele. The overall spectrum of disease varies greatly. Haemoglobin electrophoresis shows only Hb E and Hb F.

Delta beta thalassaemias

The delta beta thalassaemias comprise a group of disorders involving reduction or absence of synthesis of both delta and beta chains. The molecular defects at the genetic level may be very varied. Clinically, homozygotes present with thalassaemia intermedia, although in homozygotes for one variant, haemoglobin Lepore, the disease behaves more like thalassaemia major. Hb F is the only haemoglobin detectable. Heterozygotes are asymptomatic but have raised level of Hb F (5%–15%) with a normal Hb A_2 level.

Another African variant is characterized by a failure to switch off gamma chain synthesis, producing homozygotes that have a normal haemoglobin level consisting only of Hb F, and heterozygotes with 20%–30% Hb F and a normal Hb A_2 level. This disorder is known as **hereditary persistence of fetal haemoglobin**.

Alpha thalassaemia

Four different alpha thalassaemia phenotypes are recognized, depending on how many of the four copies of the alpha gene are affected:

- **single gene deletion**:
  - a single copy of the alpha gene is affected
    - this produces a 'silent' carrier state
    - affected persons are clinically and haematologically normal
- **alpha thalassaemia trait**:
  - two copies of the alpha gene are affected
  - there is a mild microcytic hypochromic anaemia
- **Hb H disease**:
  - three copies of the gene are affected
  - excess beta chains produce Hb H, which can be demonstrated after precipitation by brilliant cresyl blue
  - there is a variable degree of anaemia, with splenomegaly and a typical thalassaemic blood picture
  - haemoglobin electrophoresis shows Hb A with variable amounts of Hb H and some Hb Barts
- **Hb Barts hydrops syndrome**
  - this occurs when all four alpha chain genes are affected
  - it is a common cause of stillbirth in South East Asia
  - the absence of alpha chain production leads to severe anaemia, with haemoglobin consisting mainly of the beta chain tetramer Hb Barts
  - hydrops fetalis, with gross oedema, splenomegaly, and extra-medullary haemopoiesis occurs, and affected babies are still-born at 36–40 weeks gestation
- **haemoglobin Constant Spring thalassaemia**:
  - this form of thalassaemia occurs when a single base mutation in the termination codon for haemoglobin leads to the (rather inefficient) formation of elongated alpha chains and, consequently, an abnormal haemoglobin, haemoglobin Constant Spring (Hb CS)

- co-inheritance of this abnormality with the alpha thalassaemia trait can lead to a disorder that is similar to Hb H disease
- the heterozygous state is clinically and haematologically silent, apart from the presence of trace amounts of Hb CS

The haemoglobinopathies

Whereas thalassaemias result from a reduced rate of production of the globin chains that make up the haemoglobin molecule, the haemoglobinopathies are disorders resulting from a structural abnormality of the haemoglobin molecule. A large number of structural haemoglobin variants have been described. Some are without obvious effect, while others may impair the integrity of the red cell and lead to haemolysis.

The most common abnormal haemoglobin is Hb S, which causes haemolytic anaemia in homozygotes or when co-inherited with another abnormal haemoglobin or a thalassaemic trait. The only other relatively common abnormal haemoglobins are Hb C, Hb D, and Hb E, although several rare unstable haemoglobins are known. Inheritance of a single abnormal haemoglobin gene is not usually associated with significant problems.

Sickle cell disease

The generic term 'sickle cell disease' refers to the disease that occurs when the sickle beta chain (betaˢ) allele is inherited from one parent, and an allele for another abnormal beta chain (e.g. a second betaˢ or a betaᶜ, betaᴰ, or betaᶠ allele) or one of the forms of beta thalassaemia is inherited from the other parent. Heterozygote carriers of betaˢ do not, in the main, suffer the recognized consequences of the disease, but are important as potential parents of affected children.

Pathophysiology of sickle cell disease

Hb S results from a single base substitution leading to the replacement of glutamic acid by valine at Position 6 in the beta globin chain. Hb S has unusual solubility properties, forming liquid crystals—'tactoids'—when it becomes deoxygenated. These further aggregate into parallel rod-like structures. The end result is that the cells become rigid and distort into a sickle shape (sickling). Initially, this is reversible on reoxygenation, but repeated cycles of sickling and unsickling lead to a loss of membrane and membrane permeability and, eventually, to irreversible sickling.

Sickled erythrocytes have a shortened lifespan resulting from increased mechanical fragility. They also tend to form aggregates, especially in the microcirculation; these increase blood viscosity and reduce flow, causing hypoxia (which aggravates sickling) and, eventually, tissue infarction.

The presence of other haemoglobins may affect the behaviour of Hb S. For example, Hb C, Hb D, and Hb E will all form tactoids with Hb S, while Hb A, Hb A_2, and Hb F inhibit tactoid formation. These differences explain the involvement of the haemoglobins in the first group in the sickling syndromes, and the protective effect of those in the second group, especially Hb F.

Clinical features of sickle cell disease

Sickle cell disease is a chronic haemolytic anaemia with a course that is punctuated by painful crises and other less common manifestations. It may run a variable clinical course in any individual and is occasionally undiagnosed into adulthood. This variability is related in some degree to factors such as climate, socio-economic status, and the level of Hb F present, but still remains largely unexplained. Hb S has a low oxygen affinity, so anaemia is well tolerated, with most patients asymptomatic at their steady state level (6–10 g/dl).

Children with sickle cell disease are well at birth because of the protective effect of the high levels of Hb F, but will present in infancy with anaemia, jaundice, susceptibility to infection, and recurrent painful crises. The **hand–foot syndrome** of painful dactylitis resulting from multiple microinfarcts in the digital bones is a classic feature of sickle cell disease in childhood (and may lead to permanent shortening if the epiphyses are affected).

Sickle cell trait (which occurs when the patient is heterozygous for betaˢ) rarely causes any clinical problems. Extremes of anoxia, such as those encountered when flying in unpressurized aircraft, when scuba diving or, occasionally, during anaesthesia, can, rarely, precipitate a crisis. Some individuals may also experience renal papillary necrosis, reflecting the relative hypoxia deep in the renal medulla.

Complications of sickle cell disease

Most patients with sickle disease will experience complications at some point, although the nature of the complication will vary with factors such as the specific defect and the age of the patient. Complications include those seen in any chronic haemolytic state, such as jaundice, gallstones, and aplastic crises. Those specifically related to the sickling process include:

- painful veno-occlusive episodes
- sequestration syndromes
- stroke
- priapism
- infection

Painful veno-occlusive episodes result from tissue infarction caused by the sickling of cells in the microvasculature. Painful crises may be precipitated by cold, dehydration, and infection. In the younger child, they tend to affect the long bones but, later, they appear more often in the axial skeleton. The episodes are characterized by severe pain, fever, and tachycardia. Treatment involves adequate pain control (often requiring opiates) and maintenance of hydration, intravenously if necessary. Antibiotics may be required, as the fever of crisis is not easily distinguished from that of infection.

Sequestration syndromes are the most serious and immediately life-threatening of the sickling complications. All are associated with massive 'sequestration' of sickle cells into some part of the circulation, leading to a rapid fall in haemoglobin. The cause is not known but, if they are unrecognized, the patient may deteriorate rapidly and succumb in a surprisingly short time. Sequestration of sickled red cells in the spleen usually occurs in young children in association with severe infection. There is rapid enlargement of the spleen and a life-threatening fall in the haemoglobin. The mortality is high. In older children and young adults with splenic atrophy, sequestration into the liver may occur, with rapid enlargement and progressive anaemia. Lung sequestration produces the 'sickle chest syndrome', in which there is acute breathlessness with back or chest pain; initial patchy lung consolidation may progress extremely rapidly and is accompanied by a rapidly falling haemoglobin and platelet count, increasing hypoxia, and possibly infection. Sequestration may also involve the circulation of the gastrointestinal tract, sometimes with involvement of the lungs and the liver—the 'girdle syndrome'. The abdomen is painful, distended, and often silent. Differentiation from other causes of abdominal catastrophe is difficult. All the sequestration crises are medical emergencies and require intervention with intensive supportive therapy, hydration, oxygen, antibiotics, and exchange transfusion.

Cerebral thrombosis and the signs of acute stroke may be seen in up to 7% of affected children. The treatment is with exchange transfusion, and subsequent regular transfusion to maintain Hb S at a low level for 3 years to cover the highest risk period for recurrence.

Priapism presents in adult males as a painful erection, occurring either as multiple brief episodes or as a major attack. Initial treatment of the stuttering phase with cyproterone may prevent a major attack, which will require exchange transfusion and sometimes surgical intervention. Subsequent impotence is common.

Infection is commonly seen in patients with sickle cell disease, as they have an increased susceptibility for it. This may relate to splenic malfunction in some manner, but the reasons are not fully understood. Overwhelming pneumococcal infection is particularly common in young children, and penicillin prophylaxis is recommended at least until early adulthood. Septicaemias with salmonella, *E. coli*, and/or *Staphylococcus aureus* are common and may be accompanied by osteomyelitis.

Other complications specifically related to sickle cell disease include:

- **aplastic crisis**: infection with parvovirus may lead to transient erythropoietic arrest and a dramatic fall in haemoglobin levels
- **splenomegaly**: this is present in most children with sickle cell disease but, usually, progressive infarction leads to splenic atrophy by the age of 10; in a minority of patients who are homozygous for beta^s, and a larger number of patients who carry one copy of beta^s

and one copy of beta^c (termed 'Hb SC patients'), splenomegaly will persist into adult life

- **proliferative retinopathy**: this is common in the sickling syndromes, particularly in Hb SC patients; regular review by an ophthalmologist, together with laser treatment, may prevent many severe complications
- **renal problems**: sickle cell disease patients frequently lack renal concentrating ability and so can be susceptible to enuresis in childhood and have a predisposition for rapid dehydration, which may aggravate sickling crises; in addition, urinary tract infections, papillary necrosis, nephrotic syndrome, and chronic renal failure are all common in these patients
- **growth problems and delayed puberty**: most children with sickle cell disease will be thin and grow relatively poorly in comparison to normal siblings; in addition, puberty in patients with sickle cell disease is usually delayed, although complete failure of puberty rarely occurs

Fertility is usually normal in patients with sickle cell disease. However, pregnancy may lead to an increase in the frequency of crises and there is an excess of miscarriage and stillbirth. Many babies are also small for gestational dates. Regular transfusion during pregnancy will often reduce the maternal complications, but the evidence for any significant alteration in the outcome for the fetus is scanty.

Diagnosis of sickle cell disease

The diagnosis of sickle cell disease is made in adults and older children based on the results from a full blood count, the blood film, the solubility test (which demonstrates the presence of Hb S in a sample but does not differentiate between heterozygosity and homozygosity), and haemoglobin electrophoresis.

In disease resulting from two copies of beta^s, there will be a partially compensated haemolytic anaemia, with a haemoglobin level of 6–10 g/dl, reticulocytosis of 10%–20%, sickled red blood cells on the blood film, a positive sickle test, and an electrophoresis showing only Hb S.

The other sickling syndromes are variable in the degree of anaemia, the appearance of the blood film, the haemoglobin electrophoresis, and clinical features.

Management of sickle cell disease

It is important that sickle cell disease patients and their relatives understand the nature of the disease and its complications. The manoeuvres that can be used to avoid crises or curtail minor ones should be explained. The signs that a major event is occurring should alert those concerned that hospital admission is needed.

Minor surgery may be safely performed if there is careful attention to hydration and the maintenance of oxygenation. However, major procedures should only be performed after transfusion, to reduce the proportion of Hb S cells to less than 30%. Some operations, particularly orthopaedic operations, may require maintenance transfusion post-operatively to allow adequate healing.

Simple blood transfusion will be required to correct the profound anaemia of an aplastic crisis or a sequestration syndrome but should probably be avoided at other times. Exchange transfusion can be used preoperatively and may be necessary in some crises in order to reduce the percentage of sickle haemoglobin rapidly. Hypertransfusion may be used for limited periods to avoid crises or allow healing but should not be continued indefinitely because of the dangers of iron overload, and sensitization to red-cell antigens.

Immune haemolysis

Immune haemolysis occurs when antibodies or complement are bound onto the red-cell membrane. The Fc portion of the IgG antibody and the C3d component of the complement system induce phagocytosis of the red cells by fixed macrophages in the spleen, liver, and bone marrow. IgM antibodies may lead to complement binding and activation, which produces direct intravascular red-cell lysis in addition to stimulating removal of the red cells by phagocytosis.

Antibodies bind to red cells by a variety of mechanisms; there may be specificity for red-cell membrane antigens themselves, or the antibody may bind to complexes formed between certain drugs and the red-cell membrane. Damage may also occur following passive binding of certain immune complexes.

Immune haemolysis may occur with allo- or autoantibodies to red cells.

Alloimmune haemolysis

Alloantibodies are responsible when haemolysis follows transfusion of plasma or red cells, for example when Group O blood containing anti-A antibodies is transfused into a Group A individual or when Kell-positive red cells are transfused into a previously sensitized patient, who will have anti-Kell antibodies. Alloantibodies are also involved in haemolytic disease of the newborn when maternal immune IgG antibodies cross the placenta and cause haemolysis in the fetus.

Autoimmune haemolysis

Haemolytic anaemias due to autoantibodies directed against normal red-cell constituents may be idiopathic or associated with lymphoproliferative malignancy or other immune disorders such as SLE and rheumatoid arthritis. Such haemolytic anaemias may be further classified according to antibody type, the complement-fixing ability of the antibody, and whether the antibody is more active at body temperature (a 'warm antibody') or reduced temperatures (a 'cold antibody'), as follows:

* Ig-mediated autoimmune haemolytic anaemia
* paroxysmal cold haemoglobinuria
* chronic cold haemagglutinin disease
* acute cold haemagglutinin disease

IgG-mediated autoimmune haemolytic anaemia

IgG-mediated autoimmune haemolytic anaemia usually involves a 'warm' IgG autoantibody that is most active at 37°C. It is associated with low-grade lymphoproliferative malignancies such as non-Hodgkin lymphoma and chronic lymphocytic leukaemia, and also with other autoimmune disorders. Initially idiopathic cases may in fact precede the development of an associated condition, sometimes by many years. The incidence increases with age, probably reflecting the increase in the incidence of the associated lymphoid malignancies.

The onset is usually insidious, with progressive anaemia and mild jaundice, but it may occasionally be fulminant. The spleen is usually moderately enlarged. There is anaemia and reticulocytosis, with spherocytosis and, in extreme cases, nucleated red cells in the blood film. The direct antiglobulin test shows IgG and sometimes C3d bound to the membrane.

Treatment is aimed at reducing haemolysis and correcting anaemia. Haemolysis may cease when any underlying condition is treated, and idiopathic cases may 'burn out' after a time. Symptomatic cases are treated with prednisolone, 1 mg per kilogram of body weight initially, tailing after 2–3 weeks to a maintenance dose. Transfusion may be necessary in severe cases provided compatible blood can be found. Refractory cases may be managed with rituximab with or without azathioprine or cyclophosphamide. Splenectomy may also be considered, but is successful in only half of cases. Folic acid supplementation should also be given.

Paroxysmal cold haemoglobinuria

Paroxysmal cold haemoglobinuria, which is a rare condition, is caused by an IgG antibody with peculiar thermal characteristics: the Donath–Landsteiner antibody. It was once typically associated with congenital syphilis but is now more commonly seen after certain viral infections, usually in childhood. There is acute intravascular haemolysis, with haemoglobinuria, on exposure to cold. The condition is usually self-limiting and the patient should be kept in a warm environment until remission occurs. Blood transfusion, when required, should be given through a warmer.

Chronic cold haemagglutinin disease

Chronic cold haemagglutinin disease is usually a primary disorder affecting older patients, although it is occasionally associated with lymphoma. There may be chronic intravascular haemolysis which is aggravated by a cold environment, but the main problem is often a painful peripheral acrocyanosis due to stasis and agglutination in the cold extremities. There is striking red-cell agglutination in the specimen tube and blood film; this may produce an artificially high mean corpuscular volume unless the blood is tested at 37°C. The direct antiglobulin test is positive with complement only. The antibody is always an IgM monoclonal kappa paraprotein with anti-I activity. Treatment is directed at avoiding haemolysis by keeping the patient (and especially their hands and feet) warm and, if necessary, lowering the level of antibody with chlorambucil. Steroids and splenectomy are not useful in this condition. Transfusions should be given using a blood warmer.

Acute cold haemagglutinin disease

Acute cold haemagglutinins are seen as transient phenomena after certain infections in patients of any age, most commonly mycoplasma pneumonia or infectious mononucleosis.

Drug-induced immune haemolysis

A number of drugs have been associated with immune haemolysis (true autoimmune mechanisms are uncommon, and the red cells are usually damaged in some indirect way.)

Immune complex formation

Drug-induced haemolysis associated with immune complexes was originally described with stibophen but has been seen on occasion with a large number of drugs. The antibody is directed against the drug, or a complex of the drug and a plasma component, and the antibody–drug complex then binds to the red cells. The antibody is IgG or IgM and fixes complement, leading to brisk intravascular haemolysis on second and subsequent exposures to the drug. This mechanism has been described as an 'innocent bystander' effect. The direct antiglobulin test is positive with complement alone, and the antibody is only lytic in the presence of the drug.

Hapten-membrane-induced antibodies

Hapten-membrane-induced antibodies are responsible for the haemolysis occasionally seen with penicillin administration. The drug is bound covalently to the cell membrane, and an IgG antibody against the complex is responsible for the haemolysis. The antibody will only bind to red cells in the presence of the drug. The direct antiglobulin test is positive with IgG, and the haemolysis ceases on withdrawal of the drug.

'Autoimmune' drug-induced haemolysis

Therapy with methyldopa, and sometimes levodopa and mefenamic acid, leads to the development of a positive direct antiglobulin test in up to 20% of users. The antibody involved is an IgG which is directed against red-cell membrane constituents, most often in the rhesus system, and is thus a true autoantibody. In a minority of cases, haemolysis will occur, which ceases on withdrawal of the drug, although the direct antiglobulin test may remain positive for some time.

Diagnosis of immune haemolysis

Antibody or complement bound to the red-cell surface may be detected by the direct (Coombs) antiglobulin test, while free antibody in the serum may be detected by an indirect antiglobulin test. Antibody bound to the red cell may be eluted for further investigation of its nature and specificity. For a complete diagnosis, the class of the antibody, its thermal amplitude, and its activity in the presence of any suspect drug must also be assessed.

Haemolysis secondary to red-cell damage

Haemolysis may result from red-cell damage secondary to infections, the oxidative effects of drugs or chemicals, or by physical or mechanical means.

Damage from infections

Malaria causes haemolysis as the parasites burst out of the red cells. Falciparum malaria occasionally causes acute massive intravascular haemolysis (blackwater fever) or disseminated intravascular coagulation. **Toxoplasmosis** may cause a severe haemolytic anaemia in congenitally infected newborns. **Bacterial infection** with Gram-negative organisms which produce endotoxin may lead to disseminated intravascular coagulation with intravascular haemolysis. *Clostridium welchii* septicaemia is associated with the production of a lecithinase which can directly damage red cells. This results in an intense haemolysis with microspherocytes and red-cell fragments in the blood film.

Damage from drugs or chemicals

Drugs or chemicals which are powerful oxidizing agents may overcome the red cell's normal reducing capacity. These effects are exaggerated in persons with deficiencies of these enzymes systems. The clinical effects produced will reflect the nature of the oxidant substance and the dose administered. Acute intravascular haemolysis and renal failure will result from exposure to strongly oxidizing substances such as arsine or chlorate, but there will be less intense responses with drugs such as phenylhydrazine (which was once used to treat polycythaemia). Chronic intravascular haemolysis is seen in association with the use of dapsone and sulfasalazine used in the treatment of inflammatory bowel disease.

Damage from mechanical trauma

Certain conditions lead to the physical breakup of the red cell by mechanical trauma. For example, **artificial heart valves** cause fragmentation of the red cells when there is turbulent flow in relation to prosthetic inserts. This rarely occurs with homografts and is more common with aortic than mitral prostheses. The basis is usually a small leak around the attachment of the valve, allowing a high-pressure jet to flow from the ventricle to the atrium. When it arises, it may be aggravated by conditions increasing cardiac output and turbulent flow. Anaemia of varying degree results and the blood film shows fragmented and distorted red cells and spherocytes. Haemolysis is intravascular, and haemosiderin may be detected in the urine, and iron deficiency may develop. Surgical correction may be required in severe cases. Haemolysis in association with endocarditis on a valve needs to be distinguished from simple fragmentation haemolysis.

March haemoglobinuria is a benign condition seen usually in young men after vigorous exercise. It is usually asymptomatic but may be associated with loin discomfort through an unknown mechanism. The condition appears to be due to fragmentation of the red cells on a hard surface and can be avoided by the use of shoes with a springy sole, which cushions the impact of the ground on the feet and actually reduces red-cell breakup.

Microangiopathic haemolytic anaemia is a term used to describe the red-cell fragmentation seen in a variety of conditions in which the underlying defect is probably damage to the microvasculature. This may be due to microthrombi, fibrinoid necrosis, necrotizing arteritis, or invasion by malignant cells. The precise means by which any of these conditions lead to red-cell fragmentation are poorly understood. The clinical features will reflect the underlying cause, and the presence of haemolysis (anaemia, jaundice, low serum haptoglobins). The blood film shows fragmented red cells and microspherocytes, and the direct antiglobulin test is negative. There may also be thrombocytopenia, especially when microangiopathy is associated with disseminated intravascular coagulation, haemolytic–uraemic syndrome, or thrombotic thrombocytopenic purpura). The treatment of microangiopathic haemolysis is directed primarily at the underlying cause, with red-cell transfusion to correct the anaemia if required.

Damage from other causes

Other situations which may produce red-cell fragmentation and haemolysis include

- **fibrinoid necrosis** from malignant hypertension and pre-eclampsia
- **vasculitis** in SLE, Wegener's granulomatosis, and polyarteritis nodosa
- **invasion** of small blood vessels by tumour cells; this occurs especially with mucin-secreting carcinomas
- **burns**, following direct heat damage to the red blood cells and, secondarily, from disseminated intravascular coagulation

Further Reading

Brodsky RA. Paroxysmal nocturnal hemoglobinuria. *Blood* 2014; 124: 2804–11.

GBD 2015 Neurological Disorders Collaborator Group. Global, regional, and national burden of neurological disorders during 1990–2015: a systematic analysis for the Global Burden of Disease Study 2015. *Lancet Neurol* 2017; 16: 877–97.

Go RS, Winters JL, and Kay NE. How I treat autoimmune hemolytic anemia. *Blood* 2017; 129: 2971–79.

George JN and Nester CM. Syndromes of thrombotic microangiopathy. *N Engl J Med* 2014; 371: 654–66.

Piel FB and Weatherall DJ. The α-thalassemias. *N Engl J Med* 2014; 371: 1908–16.

Ware RE, De Montalembert M, Tshilolo L, et al. Sickle cell disease. *Lancet* 2017; 390: 311–23.

281 Normal platelet function

Nicola Curry and Raza Alikhan

Introduction

The platelet is a small (2–4 μm in diameter), discoid, anucleate cell that circulates in the blood. In health, it plays a vital role in haemostasis, and in disease it contributes to problems with bleeding as well as thrombosis.

Platelets are produced from the surfaces of megakaryocytes in the bone marrow. Each megakaryocyte has the ability to produce 2000–3000 platelets over its lifetime. The number of platelets produced in the body is under tight homeostatic control, and is regulated by the cytokine thrombopoietin. Thrombopoietin binds to its receptor, c-Mpl, which is found on the megakaryocyte, and platelet surfaces and is then internalized by these cells. It acts to stimulate megakaryopoiesis, and platelets are released into the blood stream. A normal platelet count lies between 150×10^9 platelets/l and 450×10^9 platelets/l.

Platelets have a lifespan of approximately 7–10 days, and they usually circulate in the bloodstream in a quiescent state. Intact, undamaged vessel walls help to maintain the platelets in this inactive state by releasing nitric oxide, which acts both to dilate the vessel wall and to inhibit adhesion, activation, and aggregation of the platelet.

However, after a traumatic insult to the blood vessel wall, the platelet becomes activated (see 'Platelet physiology'). The activated platelet then acts in concert with coagulation factors and the endothelium to form a stable clot. The single aim is to minimize blood loss (see Figure 281.1).

Structure of the platelet

The platelet can be thought of as a bag stuffed full with goodies which enable it to rapidly transform from a resting to fully activated state. There are several components that help this process:

- specialized membrane receptors
- a phospholipid-rich outer membrane

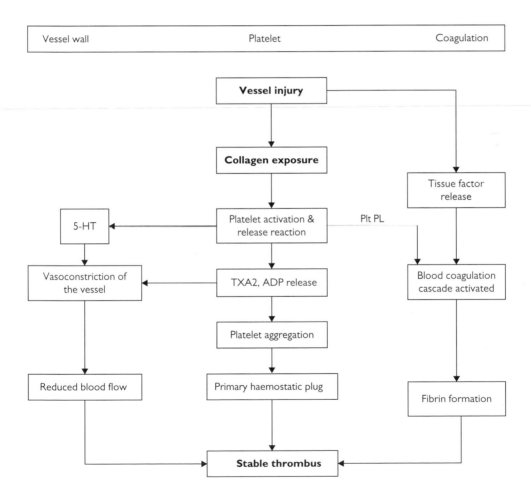

Plt PL: platelet phospholipid surface supports coagulation

Figure 281.1 The central role of the platelet in the blood-clotting process. The platelet phospholipid surface supports coagulation; ADP, adenosine diphosphate; 5-HT, serotonin; Plt PL: platelet phospholipid; TXA2, thromboxane A2.

- the platelet's canalicular system
- specialized storage granules
- adaptations in the platelet's cytoskeleton

Platelet membrane receptors

Platelet integrins are membrane receptors made up of glycoproteins (GPs) that enable the platelet to adhere to the endothelium, as well as to other platelets. They include:

- the GPIa/IIa complex (receptor for collagen)
- GPIb (receptor for von Willebrand factor (vWF); deficiency in this causes Bernard–Soulier syndrome)
- the GPIIb/IIIa complex (receptor for fibrinogen; deficiency in this causes Glanzmann thrombasthenia)
- GPVI (another receptor for collagen)

Phospholipid-rich outer membrane

The platelet membrane is rich in phospholipids, and this helps to support the assembly of several important procoagulant complexes—namely factor tenase (which contains factors VIIIa and IXa, which convert factor X to factor Xa) and prothrombinase (made up of factors Va and Xa, which convert factor II to factor IIa (thrombin)). The end result is the generation of thrombin right at the site of injury. Thrombin has two roles: first, to convert fibrinogen to fibrin and, second, to provide positive feedback to the platelets by encouraging further activation.

The importance of the phospholipid membrane in assisting coagulation can be seen in the autosomal recessive bleeding disease known as Scott syndrome. In this syndrome, the ability of platelets to promote tenase and prothrombinase activity is significantly reduced, and patients present with a moderately severe bleeding disorder.

Canalicular system

The platelet surface has extensive invaginations, collectively known as the canalicular system, which connect the inside of the platelet to the external environment. This interconnecting network of small tubes enables rapid secretion of platelet granule contents to the outside, as well as easy access for plasma proteins to the inside of the platelet.

Platelet granules

There are three main storage granules found in the platelet:

- alpha granules
- dense granules
- lysosomes

Alpha granules

Alpha granules are the most numerous (approximately 80 per platelet), and are important both in haemostasis and host defence. They contain fibrinogen, factors V and VIII, fibronectin, vWF, and platelet factor 4, as well as many other important factors. Deficiency leads to grey platelet syndrome, Quebec platelet disorder, and Paris–Trousseau syndrome.

Dense granules

Dense granules, of which there are usually less than ten per platelet, contain the nucleotides ADP and ATP, as well as calcium and serotonin. Their role is to support platelet activation and to contribute to vasoconstriction of the surrounding vessel, thereby aiding reduction of blood loss. Deficiency leads to delta storage pool disease, Hermansky–Pudlak syndrome, and Chediak–Higashi syndrome. Deficiency of both alpha and dense granules leads to alpha delta storage pool disease.

Lysosomes

Lysosomes are the third type of granule in platelets. They act as part of the host defence mechanisms against invading microorganisms

Platelet cytoskeleton

The cytoskeleton is made up of a circumferential band of microtubules (containing spectrin and actin fibrils), which respond to changes in the intracellular calcium concentration in the platelet. The cytoskeleton enables the platelet to change shape during the process of activation.

Platelet physiology

Vessel injury initiates a set of highly regulated and specialized responses from the platelet. These include adhesion, activation, granule release reactions, and platelet aggregation. The process is complex, but a simplified schematic of it is shown in Figure 281.1.

When a vessel is damaged, the resultant exposure of subendothelial matrix proteins, such as collagen, starts the process of platelet activation. First, vWF, which normally circulates in the blood and which is also released from damaged endothelial cells, quickly binds to the exposed collagen. Platelets then can bind to vWF using the GPIb receptor.

Platelets are able to make initial contact with vWF because of their small size and discoid shape, both of which enable them to circulate in the bloodstream in a position that is close to the periphery of the blood vessel. Platelets will bind under conditions of high shear stress to vWF, using the platelet glycoprotein receptor GPIb. This forms a weak bond, but one that enables the platelet to slow down in the blood vessel. In conditions of low shear, such as in the venous system, platelets can bind directly to collagen and fibrinogen.

Once the platelet has slowed down, it can bind to collagen using another glycoprotein; the GPVI receptor. This is of importance, because it results in conformational changes to two of the important glycoproteins, namely GPIIb/IIIa and GPIa/IIa. Once these protein receptors have changed shape, they are able to bind avidly to the subendothelial matrix, binding to vWF and collagen, respectively. This is vital, since these bonds are very strong and anchor the platelet more firmly.

The next step in platelet activation is the granule release reaction. This happens after agonists such as ADP, thrombin, and thromboxane A2 (which are in the surrounding plasma milieu) bind to their respective platelet surface membrane receptors. Many of these platelet receptors are coupled to G proteins, and activation results in changes in intracellular platelet calcium concentrations. The contents of the granules are released when calcium levels rise within the platelet. (Conversely, granule release is inhibited by substances that lead to increased cAMP platelet activity, such as prostacyclin.)

The contents of the alpha and dense granules are released into the canalicular system to enable rapid delivery of the contents. The granules contain many important factors (see 'Structure of the platelet'), the majority of which support ongoing haemostasis, and provide positive feedback to the platelet.

At the same time that the granule release reaction occurs, the platelet undergoes a shape change. This is again facilitated by alterations in calcium levels within the platelet and the resulting activation of enzymes that regulate myosin activity. The cytoskeleton affects the shape changes.

The changes in shape enable platelets to adhere more easily to the endothelial surfaces and also to each other. In addition, agonists in the plasma, in particular ADP and thromboxane A2, encourage more platelets to adhere to the site of injury, resulting in platelet aggregation. Platelets are said to aggregate when they bind to each other, using fibrinogen as the glue. (The platelets bind to fibrinogen with the GPIIb/IIIa receptors.)

The end product is the formation of a thrombus which is rich in platelets and fibrinogen. During these latter stages, fibrinogen is converted to fibrin under the action of thrombin, and this increases the stability of the platelet plug. Finally, the clot undergoes retraction, which helps the clot to withstand high shear forces within the blood vessels.

The platelet therefore contributes heavily to the formation of a stable clot at the site of vessel injury, a process often called primary haemostasis. Under normal circumstances, this whole process takes approximately 3–5 minutes.

Wider roles of the platelet

The platelet not only is important in the formation of the thrombus but also plays several other important roles which highlight the close relationship seen between coagulation and inflammation. These include:

- promotion of vessel constriction, brought about by release of serotonin from dense granules (this helps reduce blood loss)
- vessel wall repair
- leucocyte recruitment
- promotion of inflammatory processes, in particular atherosclerosis

Further Reading

Gardiner EE and Andrews RK. Structure and function of platelet receptors initiating blood clotting. *Adv Exp Med Biol* 2014; 844: 263–75.

Golebiewska EM and Poole AW. Platelet secretion: From haemostasis to wound healing and beyond. *Blood Rev* 2014; 29: 153–62.

282 Platelet disorders

Nicola Curry and Raza Alikhan

Definition of the disease

The term 'platelet disorder' covers a very large and heterogeneous group of diseases that have a multitude of causes. Platelet disorders are either inherited or acquired, and are due to:

- an abnormality of platelet number (quantitative disorder; see Box 282.1 and Box 282.2; e.g. thrombocytopenia (platelet count <150 × 10^9/l) and thrombocytosis (platelet count >450 × 10^9/l))
- an abnormality of platelet function (qualitative disorder; see Table 282.1 and Box 282.3)
- a combination of quantitative and qualitative abnormalities

Aetiology of the disease

For the aetiology of the disease, see Boxes 282.1–282.3 and Table 282.1.

Typical symptoms of the disease, and less common symptoms

The symptoms of a platelet disorder include:

- mucosal surface bleeding, i.e.:
  - bleeding into the skin: easy or spontaneous bruising, ecchymoses, purpura
  - petechial haemorrhages
  - gum bleeding
  - epistaxis
  - menorrhagia
  - gastrointestinal bleeding
- immediate and continued bleeding after injury (in contrast to bleeding due to coagulation factors, which is often delayed)

There may be no symptoms at all until a patient bleeds excessively after a haemostatic challenge such as surgery, dental extraction, or childbirth. Less commonly, a patient may present with symptoms of anaemia, due to continued occult blood loss and the development of iron deficiency.

Approach to diagnosing the disease

The most important part of the assessment is to take a detailed history, particularly focusing on:

- family history (to look for evidence of an inherited disease)
- bleeding history

Box 282.1 Inherited disorders of platelet number

Thrombocytopenia
- small platelets (mean platelet volume <7 fl)
  - Wiskott–Aldrich syndrome
  - X-linked thrombocytopenia
- normal-sized platelets (mean platelet volume 7–11 fl)
  - thrombocytopenia with absent radii
  - congenital amegakaryocytic thrombocytopenia
- large platelets (mean platelet volume >11 fl)
  - MYH9 disorders: May–Hegglin anomaly, Fechtner syndrome, Epstein syndrome, Sebastian syndrome
  - velocardiofacial/DiGeorge syndrome
  - grey platelet syndrome
  - Bernard–Soulier syndrome

Thrombocytosis
- familial essential thrombocytosis

Box 282.2 Acquired disorders of platelet number

Thrombocytopenia
- autoimmune
  - immune thrombocytopenia purpura
  - connective tissue disease
  - lymphoproliferative disease
- drugs
  - heparin (heparin-induced thrombocytopenia)
  - quinine
  - co-trimoxazole
  - gold
  - cytotoxic drugs
- infection
  - viral: HIV, hepatitis C, CMV, parvovirus
  - severe sepsis
- microangiopathic diseases
  - thrombotic thrombocytopenia purpura
  - haemolytic–uraemic syndrome
  - disseminated intravascular coagulopathy
- alloimmune thrombocytopenia
  - neonatal alloimmune thrombocytopenia
  - post-transfusion purpura
- bone marrow infiltration
  - many haematological diseases such as leukaemia
- malignancy
- pregnancy related
  - pre-eclampsia
  - HELLP syndrome
- liver disease
- aplastic anaemia
- radiation
- vitamin B$_{12}$ deficiency
- folate deficiency
- massive transfusion

Thrombocytosis
- bleeding
- infection
- inflammation
- splenectomy
- malignancy
- iron deficiency
- myeloproliferative diseases:
  - essential thrombocythaemia
  - polycythaemia rubra vera
  - chronic myeloid leukaemia
  - myelofibrosis

It must be remembered that a bleeding history is a very subjective method of assessment, and mild platelet disorders can be difficult to distinguish from normality.

There are some standardized guides, or 'bleeding questionnaires', that can improve the accuracy of taking a bleeding history: such as the ISTH bleeding assessment tool (BAT). In women with menorrhagia, pictorial menstrual blood loss charts are a useful method of quantifying bleeding.

Inherited or acquired disease

A patient is more likely to have an inherited disease if they give a positive family history of bleeding or they present at a young age.

Box 282.3 Acquired disorders of platelet function

Drugs

NSAIDs
- aspirin
- ibuprofen
- indometacin
- naproxen

Anticoagulants
- heparin

Cardiovascular drugs
- propranolol
- furosemide
- calcium-channel antagonists
- angiotensin-converting enzyme inhibitors

Antimicrobials
- beta-lactam antibiotics

Pyschotropics
- haloperidol
- amitriptyline
- chlorpromazine

Chemotherapy
- daunorubicin
- mitomycin

Conditions
- uraemia
- liver disease
- myeloma
- leukaemia
- myelodysplasia
- myeloproliferative disorders: polycythaemia vera, essential thrombocythaemia
- cardiopulmonary bypass

Previous platelet counts can prove invaluable as they may provide evidence of a long-standing thrombocytopenia, suggesting an inherited disease, or may show a rapid recent fall in a platelet count more in keeping with an acquired problem.

Remember, some of the inherited platelet disorders are autosomal recessive, and you should ask if the patient's parents are in a consanguineous relationship.

Disease severity

Questions that relate to the severity of disease are important. The following points are suggestive of more severe disease:

- mucosal bleeding taking a significant length of time to stop, i.e. >30 minutes, and/or requiring intervention such as packing, pressure dressings, etc.

- bleeding following routine surgery or childbirth, sufficient to require a blood transfusion
- a single or repeated episode of iron deficiency, due to recurrent bleeding
- significant bleeding at one site on three separate occasions

Mild bleeding disorders are more likely to present at a later stage in life, and often only become apparent after invasive procedures.

In patients with thrombocytopenia, spontaneous bleeding is rare with counts that are greater than $50 \times 10^9/l$, and bleeding only tends to become a problem when counts fall below $20 \times 10^9/l$. However, platelet dysfunction in combination with a reduced number of platelets may mean that a patient will bleed with a much higher platelet count.

Drug history

It is important to take a full drug history and, specifically, to ask about over-the-counter medicines, that may contain aspirin or other anti-platelet agents, such as NSAIDs, the use of which is one of the most common reasons for an acquired platelet abnormality.

Other diagnoses that should be considered

von Willebrand's disease presents with symptoms that are indistinguishable from platelet disorders and should therefore be excluded during your investigation. It is important to remember that von Willebrand's disease is much more common than many of the inherited platelet disorders.

Connective tissue disorders such as Ehlers–Danlos syndrome can present with problematic bruising and should at least be considered in the differential.

Purpura is a presenting feature of vasculitis, but the purpura is palpable. Purpura in platelet disorders is not palpable.

'Gold-standard' diagnostic test

Although platelet aggregometry is said to be the gold-standard test to assess platelet function, there is no single diagnostic test that informs a clinician which platelet abnormality is affecting their patient. This is partly due to the diversity of the underlying causes, but is also because the tests are unable to look at all of the functions of the platelet in one go.

Therefore, a group of tests will often need to be requested for patients under investigation. Many of the tests are specialized, and can only be performed at certain laboratories. One should consider whether the patient would benefit from referral to a haemostasis specialist centre.

Acceptable diagnostic alternatives to the gold standard

Routine laboratory tests

Full blood count and blood film

A full blood count should be performed and a blood film examined, to determine the platelet count, the mean platelet volume, and the haemoglobin concentration (see Table 282.2). It is best to look at the

Table 282.1 Inherited disorders of platelet function

Platelet abnormality	Defect	Disorder
Platelet receptors	Glycoprotein IIb/IIIa	Glanzmann thrombasthenia
	Glycoprotein Ib/IX/V	Bernard–Soulier syndrome
Platelet granules	Dense granules	Hermansky–Pudlak syndrome
	Alpha granules	Chediak–Higashi syndrome
	Combined defects	Delta storage pool disease
		Grey platelet syndrome
		Quebec platelet disorder
		Paris–Trousseau syndrome
		Alpha delta storage pool disease
Platelet membrane phospholipids	Inability to support coagulation proteases	Scott syndrome

Table 282.2 Full blood count and blood film

Test	Uses	Limitations
Platelet count	Usually accurate, unless count very low	Unusually large platelets may be counted as red blood cells Red-cell fragments may be counted as platelets Platelet clumps
Mean platelet volume	Platelet size (high in immune thrombocytopenic purpura)	
Haemoglobin concentration	Associated anaemia	

Box 282.4 Bleeding time

Test

- bleeding time

Use

- screen for severe platelet disorders

Limitations

- painful
- operator dependent
- affected by low haematocrit, skin laxity, subject age
- leaves a scar
- will not pick up mild disease; therefore, it cannot be used as a standalone screening test

results of as many full blood count tests as possible for a patient, as trends often provide clues to the underlying problem.

Coagulation screen

The activated partial thromboplastin time, prothrombin time, thrombin time, and Clauss fibrinogen assays should be performed. These will provide information about the coagulation factors, and whether the bleeding abnormality is more complex than an isolated platelet problem. For example, disseminated intravascular coagulation (DIC) may cause bleeding, and tests will demonstrate a thrombocytopenia, as well as prolonged clotting results.

von Willebrand testing

von Willebrand's disease must be excluded. To do so the following tests should be taken:

- factor VIII:Ag assay
- von Willebrand factor:Ag assay
- von Willbrand factor ristocetin cofactor assay
- ristocetin induced platelet aggregation (RIPA)

Bleeding time

Methods such as the 'Ivy' or the 'template' bleeding time can be used to assess primary haemostasis (the interaction between the platelet and the vessel wall; see Box 282.4). This test is rarely used nowadays – a blood pressure cuff is wrapped around the upper arm, and inflated to 40 mm Hg. Using a special blade to cut the skin, often on the forearm, incisions are made to a specified depth and length. The puncture sites are blotted with absorbent gauze every 30 seconds, until bleeding stops. The bleeding time depends slightly on the method used, but averages between 1 and 9 minutes. Greater than 15 minutes is recognized as abnormal.

Platelet function analyser-100

The platelet function analyser-100 test goes someway to replacing the bleeding time and providing an automated means of assessing primary haemostasis, but again it cannot be used to exclude a platelet disorder when used as a standalone test (see Box 282.5). Two cartridges are used for each test; an ADP/collagen cartridge, and an epinephrine/collagen cartridge. Both of these cartridges have a small hole or aperture in the centre of them, and the patient's blood flows through these holes

Box 282.5 Platelet function analyser-100 test

Test

- PFA-100

Use

- severe platelet disorders

Limitations

- will not pick up mild disease
- affected by haematocrit, thrombocytopenia, diet, aspirin
- cannot therefore be used as a single screening test

under shear stress. The cartridges activate the platelets in the blood sample, and the time taken for the holes in the cartridges to be closed by a platelet plug is measured. This time is called the 'closure time'.

More specialized tests

The following tests are usually performed in specialist coagulation laboratories. Tests that look at platelet function should be performed within 2 hours from the time of venepuncture. This is because the platelets can undergo in vitro activation or desensitization if left in blood bottles.

Platelet aggregation

This test involves analysing the response of a patient's platelets to the addition of a variety of known platelet agonists. The aggregometer monitors changes in light transmission through a sample of platelet rich plasma over time. Light transmission increases as platelet aggregation increases.

The following are commonly used as platelet agonists:

- ADP
- collagen
- ristocetin
- arachidonic acid
- epinephrine

Typical patterns of aggregation are found with various platelet disorders.

Platelet nucleotide testing

The nucleotides ADP and ATP are found in the dense granules of the platelet. Assessment of platelet ADP and ATP levels may be useful in helping in the diagnosis of storage pool disorders.

Platelet flow cytometry

Flow cytometry can be used to assess several areas of the platelet, but it is most commonly used to measure numbers of glycoproteins found on the surface of the platelet. For example, Glanzmann's thrombasthenia is caused by a deficiency in glycoprotein IIb/IIIa receptors in the platelet membrane. Flow cytometry is able to detect this deficiency.

Electron microscopy

Electron microscopy can be used to assess platelet granule defects and other changes in the structure of the platelet. For example, the platelet in a patient with Hermansky–Pudlak syndrome contains no dense granules.

Molecular analysis

Families with inherited disorders of platelets may benefit from molecular analysis to determine their underlying genetic defect. This information may then be used for antenatal diagnosis. There is an increasing interest in the genetics of platelet disorders, helped by the introduction of Next Generation Sequencing and GWAS, which has led recently to the elucidation of many new causative mutations being discovered.

Treatment and its effectiveness

Acquired platelet disorders

Once a cause for the platelet dysfunction is found, any bleeding symptoms are likely to improve when treatment of the underlying condition commences. For example, dialysis improves the bleeding from platelet dysfunction associated with uraemia. On the other hand, if bleeding is caused by drugs such as NSAIDs, they should be discontinued where possible and alternative medication prescribed.

Bleeding in patients with acquired platelet dysfunction can be treated in a variety of ways (see Table 282.3). When making decisions as to which therapy to use, you must take into consideration the risks of the bleeding and weigh this against the benefits and risks of the treatment. Many of the more common acquired disorders of platelets will not require any treatment at all. For example, there would be no reason to treat a patient with mild thrombocytopenia but who has no bleeding symptoms. If you are in any doubt, a haematologist will be able to provide advice.

Table 282.3 Management options for bleeding due to platelet disorders

Therapy	Dose	Precautions
Tranexamic acid	Orally: 15–25 mg/kg three times per day IV: 10–15 mg/kg three times per day Mouthwash: 10 ml of a 5% solution four times per day	Care in patients with increased thromboembolic risk Reduce dose with renal failure Contraindicated with haematuria (risk of clot retention)
Desmopressin	Subcutaneous: 0.3 µg/kg IV: 0.3 µg/kg Intranasal: 300 µg for adults, 150 µg for children Note: tachyphylaxis occurs with repeated doses Doses can be repeated after 12 hours	Can cause fluid retention/hyponatraemia Should not be given to the elderly, or patients with atherosclerosis (increased risk of myocardial infarction) Do not use in children <2 years old, due to risk of hyponatraemia and fits Ask adults to restrict fluids for 24 hours after dose
Platelets	Adult dose: 1 unit of platelets usually, but may depend on indication	Low risk of transfusion-transmitted infection Allergic reaction risk HLA-sensitization; HLA-matched platelets may be given to some patients with hereditary diseases

Inherited platelet disorders

These disorders should be managed within a haemophilia and haemostasis comprehensive care centre, where specialist care can be provided. This is particularly important for management of surgery and pregnancy.

General advice for all patients with platelet disorders

Patients with platelet disorders should:

- avoid aspirin, other antiplatelet agents, and NSAIDs (note: aspirin may be given to patients for whom the benefit outweighs the risk)
- avoid intramuscular injections
- avoid contact sports if they have severe disease

Platelet dysfunction

Mild platelet dysfunction disorders

Most patients with mild platelet disorders are unlikely to bleed spontaneously. They will require treatment for interventional procedures. For minor surgery or dental extraction:

- care should be taken at the site of surgery; e.g. stitches should be placed for dental extractions, packing for nasal bleeding, etc.
- desmopressin should be given as a single dose prior to surgery; if rebleeding occurs, a patient may be given a second dose 12 hours later
- tranexamic acid may also be used in combination with desmopressin
- mouthwashes are often very effective for oral bleeding

For major surgery:

- desmopressin may not provide adequate cover for major surgery
- platelet transfusion is likely to be required; in the case of inherited disease, these may be HLA-matched platelets
- tranexamic acid should also be considered
- measures local to the operated area should be taken, such as careful suturing, pressure dressings, the use of fibrin sealants if appropriate, etc.

Severe platelet dysfunction disorders

For dental extraction:

- local measures, such as suturing, should be employed
- oral tranexamic acid should be commenced 24 hours prior to a procedure and continued for 5–7 days afterwards
- if bleeding persists, consider the use of platelets or, in the case of Glanzmann's thrombasthenia, NovoSeven® may be used; these cases should be discussed with a haematologist

For minor surgery:

- NovoSeven® may be used for patients with hereditary platelet disorders, in particular Glanzmann's thrombasthenia, but this must be discussed with a haematologist
- if bleeding persists, platelets should be given
- platelets may be considered for patients with acquired disease
- tranexamic acid should be given in addition

For major surgery:

- platelets are the mainstay of treatment
- tranexamic acid should be given in addition

Thrombocytopenic disorders

For those patients **without** platelet dysfunction, management of invasive procedures is dependent upon the platelet count. Follow the guidance in Table 282.4

Notable exceptions

Several specific acquired platelet conditions require different management to that outlined; these include immune thrombocytopenia (ITP), thrombotic thrombocytopenic purpura (TTP), DIC, and heparin-induced thrombocytopenia (HIT). If you think that your patient may have one of these diseases, contact your haematologist for further advice.

ITP

ITP is one of the commoner acquired platelet disorders, and may have an acute or chronic onset. The important thing to remember with ITP is that platelet transfusion should be avoided, unless the patient is bleeding, and treatment is most often with oral corticosteroids.

TTP

TTP is an uncommon microangiopathic disorder, with a high mortality rate. The mainstay of treatment for these patients is plasma exchange. Again, platelet transfusion should be avoided.

HIT

HIT is due to an immune response to a neoantigen formed by heparin and PF4. The result is platelet destruction and thrombocytopenia. It typically occurs 5–10 days after starting heparin, and platelet counts usually fall by greater than 50% from the baseline. HIT often leads to thrombosis, and treatment involves discontinuation of the heparin and anticoagulating the patient with an alternative agent, such as lepirudin or danaparoid.

Table 282.4 Recommended minimum platelet counts for invasive procedures

Procedure	Recommended platelet count (× 10⁹/l)
Dental extraction	>30
Minor operations, i.e. • liver biopsy • laparotomy • central venous catheter insertion	>50
Major surgery	Variable recommendations >50 to >80
Surgery on the eye or brain	>100

DIC

DIC is a clinicopathological diagnosis that requires evidence of a disease process that is known to predispose to DIC, and laboratory tests to support this diagnosis. Treatment for patients who are bleeding involves treating the underlying disease, and transfusing fresh frozen plasma, platelets, and cryoprecipitate as necessary.

Further Reading

Harrison P, Mackie I, Mumford A, et al. Guidelines for the laboratory investigation of heritable disorders of platelet function. *Brit J Haematol* 2011; 155: 30–44.

Hunt BJ. Bleeding and coagulopathies in critical care. *N Engl J Med* 2014; 370: 847–59.

283 Normal haemostatic function

Raza Alikhan

Introduction

Humans have evolved an intricate system that maintains blood in a fluid state. This relies on an intact vascular endothelium modulating vascular tone and forming a barrier between blood components and reactive subendothelial components. It also involves the production of inhibitors of both blood coagulation and platelet aggregation. In addition, haemostatic systems are primed to convert blood from its fluid state to a solid state, to allow the formation of a haemostatic plug, following vessel injury, to stem the flow of blood from or within a blood vessel.

It is convenient to divide these haemostatic processes into:

- primary haemostasis:
  - vasoconstriction
  - platelet activation and aggregation at the site of vessel injury
- secondary haemostasis:
  - stimulation of protein serine enzyme coagulation pathways, resulting in thrombin generation, and formation of a fibrin clot at the site of vessel injury
- fibrinolysis:
  - a process whereby the size of the fibrin clot is initially limited to the site of injury, by plasmin, and is then broken down once vessel wall healing has occurred

It is important to remember that these processes often occur simultaneously, rather than in a stepwise manner.

These haemostatic systems exist in a dynamic state of equilibrium in the majority of people, but disturbances in this balance may result in bleeding disorders (see Chapter 284) or thrombotic disorders (see Chapter 285).

Endothelium

The normal vascular endothelium maintains blood fluidity by producing inhibitors to platelet aggregation and blood coagulation, by promoting fibrinolysis, and by regulating vascular tone.

The endothelium inhibits platelet aggregation by releasing:

- prostaglandin I2 (PGI2, or prostacyclin)
- nitric oxide (NO)

The endothelium inhibits blood coagulation by synthesizing and secreting:

- thrombomodulin
- heparin sulphate

The endothelium promotes fibrinolysis by synthesizing and secreting:

- tissue plasminogen activator
- urokinase plasminogen activator
- plasminogen activator inhibitor

In addition to their effects on platelet aggregation, both PGI2 and NO (also known as endothelium-derived relaxing factor) exert vasodilatory effects on smooth muscle cells in the vessel wall, to modulate vascular tone and help to maintain blood flow.

Platelets

Following injury to the blood vessel wall, platelets become activated and begin to aggregate, forming a haemostatic plug to stem the flow of blood. In addition, the platelet phospholipid membrane provides a surface for the assembly of the procoagulant complexes tenase and prothrombinase, which are central to the production of thrombin

and the fibrin clot. Chapter 281 describes normal platelet synthesis and function, including their roles in haemostasis (see Figure 283.1).

Coagulation

Historically, the coagulation system has been divided into an extrinsic pathway (tissue factor–factor VIIa complex) and an intrinsic pathway (contact factors). However, such a division does not occur in vivo. There are essentially two linked phases of coagulation: an initiation phase and a propagation phase (see Figure 283.2).

Initiation of clotting arises when tissue factor, expressed on damaged endothelium or activated monocytes, comes into contact with the active form of the vitamin K-dependent factor VII, factor VIIa. Approximately 1%–2% of factor VII circulates in the active form. The tissue factor–factor VIIa complex converts two other vitamin K-dependent factors, factor IX and factor X, to factor IXa and factor Xa, respectively. Factor Xa cleaves prothrombin and generates a small amount of thrombin, which activates factors V, VIII, and XI. These activated factors are crucial to the development of the tenase and prothrombinase complexes and the propagation phase of coagulation.

Tenase complex

Once factor VIIIa is formed, factor IXa, generated by the tissue factor–factor VIIa complex, combines with factor VIIIa on the platelet phospholipid membrane, in the presence of calcium, to form 'factor Xase'. This 'tenase' complex is the major activator of factor X.

Prothrombinase complex

Factor Xa binds to factor Va (which is generated by the small amount of thrombin during the initiation phase). In the presence of calcium and membrane-bound phospholipids, the 'prothrombinase' complex is formed. This prothrombinase complex is 300 000-fold more active than factor Xa alone in catalysing the conversion of prothrombin and results in a 'thrombin burst' that is responsible for more than 95% of the thrombin activity generated.

Thrombin has a number of roles in haemostasis. The primary role of thrombin is to cleave fibrinogen to form a fibrin clot. This clot is further stabilized by cross linkage in the presence of factor XIII, which is activated by thrombin. Thrombin activation of factors V, VIII, and XI allow formation of the tenase and prothrombinase complexes.

Inhibition of coagulation

The presence of natural anticoagulants regulates and localizes the formation of the haemostatic plug to the site of endothelial damage.

Antithrombin (AT), also known as heparin cofactor I, is a serine protease inhibitor (or serpin) that inactivates the serine proteases thrombin (factor IIa) and factors IXa, Xa, and XIa. AT binds irreversibly, via an arginine residue in its active site, to the active serine site of the serine proteases. In the presence of heparin or vessel wall heparan sulphate, a conformational change of AT results in potentiation of its inhibition of thrombin. Congenital deficiency of AT results in a significantly increased risk of venous thromboembolism (VTE; see Chapter 285).

Heparin cofactor II, another serpin, can also be activated by heparin or dermatan sulphate and selectively inhibits thrombin (but not factor Xa).

Protein Z, a vitamin K-dependent protein, is a cofactor for the inhibition of factor Xa by Z protease inhibitor.

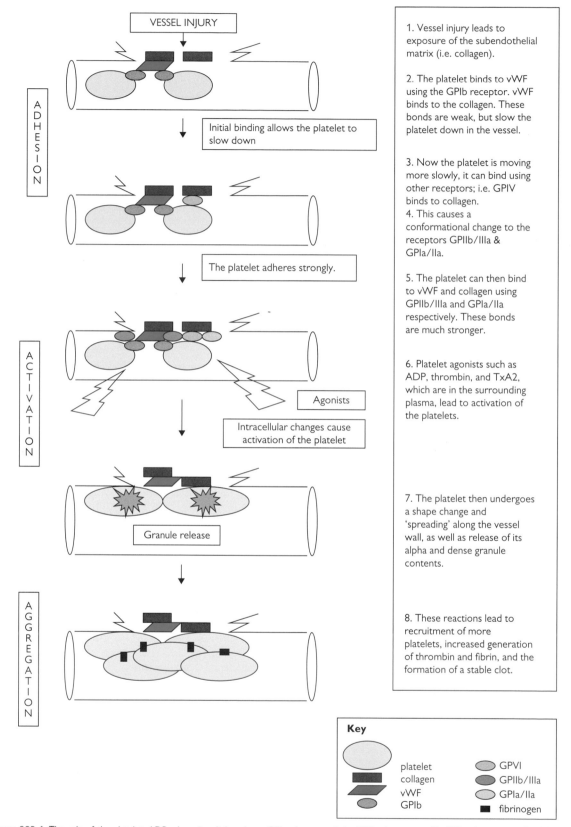

Figure 283.1 The role of the platelet; ADP, adenosine diphosphate; GPIa, glycoprotein Ia; GPIb, glycoprotein Ib; GPIIa, glycoprotein IIa; GPIIb, glycoprotein IIb; GPIIIa, glycoprotein IIIa; GPIV, glycoprotein IV; TXA2, thromboxane A2; vWF, von Willebrand factor.

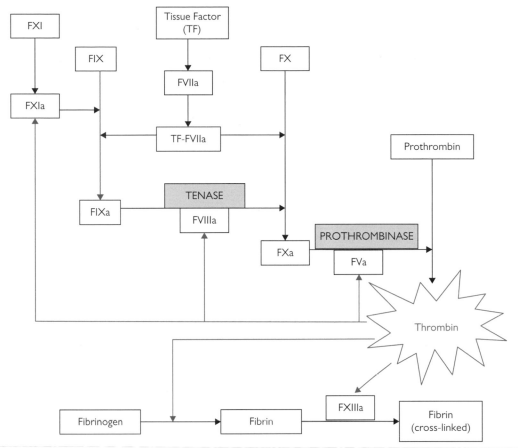

Figure 283.2 Haemostasis pathway; FVa, factor Va; FVIIa, factor VIIa; FVIIIa, factor VIIIa; FIX, factor IX; FIXa, factor IXa; FX, factor X; FXa, factor Xa; FXI, factor XI; FXIa, factor XIa; FXIIIa, factor XIIIa; TF-FVIIa, tissue factor–factor VIIa complex.

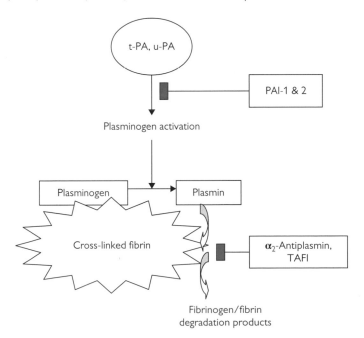

t-PA –tissue plasminogen activator, u-PA –urokinase plasminogen activator,
PAI –plasminogen activator inhibitor, TAFI –thrombin activatable fibrinolysis inhibitor

Figure 283.3 The fibrinolysis pathway; PAI, plasminogen activator inhibitor; TAFI, thrombin-activatable brinolysis inhibitor; t-PA, tissue plasminogen activator; u-PA, urokinase plasminogen activator.

Thrombomodulin forms a complex with thrombin and enhances thrombin's activation of protein C.

Protein C, a vitamin K-dependent protein, is activated by thrombomodulin to activated protein C (APC) and inhibits factors Va and VIIIa. Hereditary resistance to APC (factor V Leiden) arises due to a mutation in factor V, which prevents APC from inactivating factor Va. This results in a procoagulant state and is associated with an increased risk of VTE (see Chapter 285).

Protein S, a vitamin K-dependent protein, is a cofactor for activated protein C. Protein S deficiency is also associated with an increased risk of VTE (see Chapter 285).

Tissue factor pathway inhibitor (TFPI) inhibits both the tissue factor–factor VIIa complex and the conversion of factor X to factor Xa. TFPI may serve a potentially crucial role in maintaining the endothelium in a thromboresistant state. However, unlike the case with the other natural anticoagulants, an inherited deficiency of TFPI with an increased risk of VTE has not yet been described.

Alpha-2 antiplasmin is the primary inhibitor of plasmin. It limits the fibrinolytic response and allows the haemostatic plug to remain intact until healing has occurred. Deficiency of alpha-2-antiplasmin results in dissolution of the haemostatic plug before healing is complete and results in a haemorrhagic disorder.

Alpha-2-macroglobulin is a secondary or backup inhibitor for plasmin and thrombin. No clinical disorder of alpha-2-macroglobulin deficiency has yet been described.

The fibrinolytic system

The fibrinolytic system contributes to the localization of the haemostatic plug to the site of vessel injury and ensures that the clot is removed once healing has occurred.

During the initial period of haemostatic plug formation, platelets and endothelial cells release plasminogen activator inhibitors 1 and 2, alpha-2 antiplasmin, alpha-2 macroglobulin, and thrombin activatable fibrinolysis inhibitor, which facilitate fibrin formation by inhibiting both the conversion of plasminogen and the action of plasmin (see Figure 283.3).

By a poorly understood but timely orchestrated process, tissue plasminogen activator and, to a much lesser extent, urokinase plasminogen activator convert plasminogen to the serine protease active form, plasmin, by cleavage of a single peptide bond.

Both fibrinogen and fibrin are substrates for plasmin, leading to the production of specific fragments collectively known as fibrinogen/fibrin degradation products. Cleavage of fibrinogen produces transient X fragments, which degrade into D and E fragments. Cleavage of fibrin leads to a different pattern of fragments, because of the cross linkage of fibrin by factor XIIIa. These fragments, DY, YY, and DD (D-dimer), are characteristic of fibrin breakdown.

The measurement of D-dimer levels has been incorporated into clinical decision models for the diagnosis of VTE. Normal D-dimer levels in a patient with a low clinical probability of VTE can be used to exclude the presence of deep vein thrombosis or pulmonary embolism, without the need for further investigation.

Further Reading

Mackie I, Cooper P, Lawrie A, et al. Guidelines on the laboratory aspects of assays used in haemostasis and thrombosis. *Int J Lab Hem* 2013; 35: 1–13

Versteeg HH, Heemskerk JWM, Levi M, et al. New fundamentals in hemostasis. *Physiol Rev* 2013; 93: 327–58.

Wahad A. *Coagulation: the bare essentials*. http://hemepathreview.com/Heme-Review/Chap26-Coagulation.pdf

284 Bleeding disorders

Raza Alikhan

Introduction

From the rabbinical writings in the second century AD, to the spread of haemophilia within the royal families of Europe, there have been reports of bleeding disorders throughout history. The most common inherited bleeding disorders are haemophilia and von Willebrand's disease. There are also a number of rarer inherited bleeding disorders, which are summarized in Table 284.1.

Haemophilia

Definition of haemophilia

Haemophilia, from the Greek *haima* ('blood'), and *philia* ('friend'), is the most common of the severe bleeding disorders. Haemophilia A and B arise as a result of deficiencies of factors VIII and IX, respectively, and are inherited in an X-linked recessive fashion.

Aetiology of haemophilia

The factor VIII gene, F8, is located on the long arm of the X chromosome (Xq28). It is a large gene, spanning 186 000 base pairs of DNA, and is comprised of 26 exons. This accounts for its greater risk of mutation, compared with the gene for factor IX, F9, which is also located on the long arm of the X chromosome (Xq27), but is only 34 000 base pairs long. A number of mutations have been described in *F8*. The most common is the Intron 22 inversion mutation, which occurs in 20% of haemophilia A patients, and always produces severe disease, accounting for up to 50% of cases of severe haemophilia A.

Typical symptoms of haemophilia, and less common symptoms

Affected haemophiliac males suffer from joint and muscle bleeds, as well as easy bruising, the severity of which is closely related to the concentration or level of activity of the affected coagulation factor (see Table 284.2). Haemophilia A and B have an identical presentation, and can only be distinguished by measuring the specific factor levels.

Although factor VIII or IX deficiency is present at birth, spontaneous bleeding during the neonatal period is uncommon. Children with severe haemophilia tend to present this within the first year of life. In contrast, those suffering with mild or moderate haemophilia may not present with symptoms until adolescence or adulthood. The most common presenting symptoms are oral bleeding, either when teeth begin to erupt at age 6–9 months, or associated with a bitten tongue or lip. Bleeding from the frenulum of the upper or lower lip is

Table 284.1 Rare coagulation disorders

Deficiency	Diagnosis	Treatment	Prevalence	Genetics
Factor I (fibrinogen)	↑ PT ↑ APTT ↑ TT ↓ Fibrinogen	Fibrinogen concentrate Cryoprecipitate	1 in 1 000 000	Autosomal recessive Chromosome 4
Factor II (prothrombin)	↑ PT ↑ APTT ↓ Factor II	Prothrombin complex	1 in 2 000 000	Autosomal recessive Chromosome 11
Factor V	↑ PT ↑ APTT Normal TT ↓ Factor V	Fresh frozen plasma	1 in 1 000 000	Autosomal recessive Chromosome 1
Combined Factor V + Factor VIII	↑ PT ↑ APTT ↓ Factor V ↓ Factor VIII	Fresh frozen plasma + Factor VIII concentrate	1 in 1 000 000	Autosomal recessive Chromosome 18
Factor VII	↑ PT Normal APTT ↓ Factor VII	Recombinant Factor VIIa (Novoseven)	1 in 500 000	Autosomal recessive Chromosome 13
Factor X	↑ PT ↑ APTT Normal TT ↓ Factor X	Prothrombin complex	1 in 1 000 000	Autosomal recessive Chromosome 13
Factor XI	Normal PT ↑ APTT Normal TT ↓ Factor XI	Factor XI concentrate	1 in 1 000 000	Autosomal recessive Chromosome 4
Factor XIII	Normal PT Normal APTT ↓ Factor XIII	Factor XIII concentrate	1 in 1 000 000	Autosomal recessive Chromosome 6

Abbreviations: APTT, activated partial thromboplastin time; PT, prothrombin time; TT, thrombin time.

Table 284.2 Presentations of haemophilia		
Severity of haemophilia	Activity of coagulation factor	Presentation
Severe	<1 IU/dl	Spontaneous bleeds
Moderate	1–5 IU/dl	Bleeds after mild trauma
Mild	>5 to <40 IU/dl	Bleeds after surgery or trauma

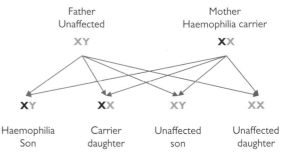

Figure 284.2 Inheritance of haemophilia when father is unaffected and mother carries the haemophilia gene.

also common, often caused by the child chewing or exploring objects with his mouth.

Once the child becomes mobile and begins crawling or walking, they are prone to hitting their heads against various objects, such as tables or chairs, causing large bruises of the forehead, often out of keeping with the severity of the injury. While learning to walk, children tend to fall into a sitting position, possibly onto hard objects such as toys, resulting in haematomas of the buttocks. These haematomas may be painful and extend into the scrotum or perineum.

Spontaneous joint bleeds (haemarthroses) are a classic feature of severe haemophilia. This usually starts at age 18 months and continues intermittently, sometimes as often as once or twice a week if untreated, throughout the patient's life. The common sites for bleeding are ankles, knees, and elbows and, less frequently, hips and shoulders.

Muscle bleeds are also characteristic of severe haemophilia, commonly affecting the flexor muscles of the limbs, as well as the calf, gluteal, and iliopsoas muscles. In addition to causing pain, swelling, and loss of function, muscle bleeds may press on important blood vessels and/or nerves and result in compartment syndrome.

Demographics of haemophilia

Haemophilia A affects approximately 1 in 5000 live male births, and haemophilia B affects approximately 1 in 30 000. Haemophilia is inherited in an X-linked recessive fashion. However, approximately one-third of cases has no family history and arises due to de novo mutations in F8 or F9.

All daughters of a man with haemophilia will be obligatory carriers of haemophilia, whereas all sons will be unaffected (see Figure 284.1).

The children of a haemophilia-carrier woman have a 50:50 chance of being either unaffected or affected by haemophilia if male, and a 50:50 chance of being unaffected or a carrier if female (see Figure 284.2). When an affected male has children with a carrier female, all children born will have a 50% chance of having haemophilia. This, therefore, is one of the rare situations where a female may present with haemophilia.

Natural history of haemophilia, and complications of the disease

Intracranial haemorrhage (ICH), although uncommon, is a serious complication of haemophilia and may be precipitated by mild trauma, but can also occur spontaneously. ICH is the most common cause of death in children with severe haemophilia.

Recurrent haemarthroses result in the deposition of haemosiderin into synovial tissue, and results in the formation of new vessels in the subsynovial layer and proliferation of the synovium. This results in inflammation of the synovium (synovitis). The friable and highly vascular synovium is more susceptible to further bleeding, and becomes progressively hypertrophic. In addition to synovial proliferation, iron deposition from blood results in destruction of the articular cartilage. The thickened synovium and damaged cartilage lead to bony erosions, which eventually lead to arthropathy. Haemophiliac arthropathy is characterized by joint stiffness, chronic pain, and a reduced range of movement in the affected joint.

Calf muscle bleeds may result in shortening of the Achilles tendon and subsequent equinus deformity of the ankle. Iliopsoas muscle bleeds clinically present with pain in the groin, hip flexion, and loss of sensation across the anterior thigh, and may result in femoral nerve palsy, and weakness and wasting of the quadriceps muscle.

Approach to diagnosing haemophilia

If a patient presents with unusual bruising or bleeding, particularly into the joints or muscles, a diagnosis of haemophilia should be considered. Equally, when faced with an unusual pattern of bleeding that is out of context with the precipitating injury, or, more importantly, when faced with a serious condition such as ICH in a neonate, a bleeding disorder should be considered as part of the differential diagnosis.

It is important to document the patient's bleeding history, and any family history of bleeding that may suggest the presence of an inherited bleeding disorder. A family history of haemophilia is an indicator for referral and further investigation.

First-line tests include a full blood count, prothrombin time, activated partial thromboplastin time (APTT), and liver function tests. If the APTT is prolonged, a mixing test with pooled normal plasma should be performed. Correction of the APTT with normal plasma implies a deficiency of a clotting factor or fibrinogen. Further tests should include a fibrinogen concentration and factor assay(s).

Factor assays and mutation testing is generally performed in affected males, and then confirmed or excluded in female relatives. Prior to genetic testing it is advisable that counselling is provided by a healthcare professional experienced in the management of haemophilia.

Other diagnoses that should be considered aside from haemophilia

If there is no family history and only a mild reduction in the factor level, it is important to test the ABO blood group and measure von Willebrand factor (vWF) levels and activity. Patients with Group O blood have lower levels of factor VIII and vWF than those with non-Group O blood.

It is also important to exclude von Willebrand's disease, in particular, type 2N von Willebrand's disease. These patients have low levels of factor VIII, and may be misdiagnosed as having mild haemophilia A (see 'Approach to diagnosing von Willebrand's disease').

In a patient with a bleeding history, a prolonged APTT which corrects on mixing, and normal levels of factor VIII and IX, it is important to measure factor XI levels. The bleeding manifestations in factor

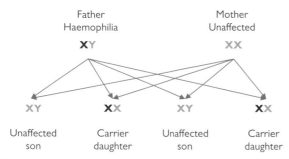

Figure 284.1 Inheritance of haemophilia when father has haemophilia and mother is unaffected.

XI deficiency, which is sometimes referred to as haemophilia C, are much less predictable than those in haemophilia A or B.

'Gold-standard' diagnostic test for haemophilia

DNA sequencing is the gold-standard test for mutation detection. A candidate mutation is first identified in a male haemophiliac, and then DNA sequencing can be used to determine the presence or absence of an abnormality in at-risk family members.

Acceptable diagnostic alternatives to the gold-standard test for haemophilia

The F8 Intron 22 inversion can be detected by Southern blotting or by a long-PCR-based protocol. The long-PCR method allows results to be obtained within 24 hours and only uses small amounts of DNA. This is an important consideration when performing prenatal diagnosis on a limited quantity of chorionic villus biopsy material.

Prognosis of haemophilia, and how to estimate it

In the 1920s, the median life span for a boy with haemophilia was approximately 10 years; however, by the 1980s, this had been extended to 55 years. However, this has not been without cost, as highlighted by the tragic infection of haemophiliac patients with hepatitis and HIV, and the chronic morbidity and mortality that has resulted. In the new millennium, the expected lifespan of a newly born haemophiliac is close to that of the general population.

Treatment of haemophilia, and its effectiveness

The goals of modern haemophilia management are to minimize joint disease, and maximize quality of life. The common standard of care falls into one of two categories:

- 'on demand' treatment: this involves treating bleeding episodes once they arise
- prophylaxis: many patients with severe haemophilia receive regular prophylactic infusions of factor VIII or factor IX to prevent bleeding episodes; this is based on the observation that patients with moderate haemophilia (factor level >1%) suffer from significantly less spontaneous bleeds; the aim of prophylactic treatment is to maintain trough factor levels above 1 IU/dl

Once bleeding has started, it is important to raise factor VIII or factor IX to a haemostatic level, with the appropriate factor replacement concentrate, to arrest bleeding and prevent complications. Factors VIII and IX are currently available as both plasma-derived and recombinant factor concentrates. For patients presenting with a joint bleed, the aim of treatment is to raise the level of factor VIII or factor IX to above 50 IU/dl; for a major bleed, such as ICH, the aim is to raise factor levels above 100 IU/dl.

In addition to factor replacement, the 'PRICE regime' is recommended following an acute bleed:

- P (protection): reduced weight bearing on the affected joint or muscle for the first 24–48 hours
- R (rest): the affected area should initially be rested completely; this allows swelling to settle and prevents further bleeding
- I (ice): helps to reduce swelling, prevents further bleeding, and eases pain
- C (compression): due to increased volumes of fluid, the more swollen an affected area, the more painful it becomes; compression reduces swelling and eases pain
- E (elevation): this also helps to reduce swelling and reduces blood flow to the affected area

von Willebrand's disease

Definition of von Willebrand's disease

von Willebrand's disease is a bleeding disorder caused by inherited defects in the concentration, structure, or function of vWF. vWF has two essential functions:

- primary haemostasis: vWF enables platelets to adhere to injured vascular endothelium, and then to form platelet aggregates

- secondary haemostasis: vWF binds to and stabilizes factor VIII; in the presence of vWF, the half-life of factor VIII is 8–12 hours; in its absence, it is <1 hour

Aetiology of von Willebrand's disease

The vWF gene is located on the short arm of Chromosome 12 (12p13.2). Mutations in this gene result in quantitative or qualitative defects of vWF. The current international classification of von Willebrand's disease is as follows:

- quantitative classification:
  - type 1 von Willebrand's disease: partial loss of vWF
  - type 3 von Willebrand's disease: total loss of vWF
- qualitative classification:
- type 2 von Willebrand's disease defects:
  - type 2A: absence of high-molecular-weight (HMW) multimers of vWF
  - type 2B: increased affinity of vWF for platelet glycoprotein Ib (GpIb) causing removal of HMW multimers from plasma, and associated with thrombocytopenia
  - type 2M: defective interaction between vWF and platelets, and no loss of HMW multimers
  - type 2N: defect in the N terminal region of vWF where the binding domain for factor VIII is located, resulting in reduced binding of vWF to this factor; no loss of HMW multimers

Typical symptoms of von Willebrand's disease, and less common symptoms

Bleeding manifestations are those suggestive of a defect in primary haemostasis:

- easy bruising
- epistaxis
- oral mucosa bleeding
- menorrhagia

Demographics of von Willebrand's disease

von Willebrand's disease is the commonest of the inherited bleeding disorders, with up to 1% of the population having reduced vWF levels commensurate with a diagnosis of von Willebrand's disease. However, only 125 per million of the population has a clinically significant bleeding disorder.

The plasma level of vWF in normal individuals varies between 40 and 240 IU/dl, and is affected by various genetic and environmental factors:

- ABO blood group: people with Group O blood have a lower vWF level than people with non-Group O blood
- ethnicity: Africans appear to have higher vWF levels than Caucasians and Asians do
- age: neonates have a raised vWF level at birth, which falls to baseline by 6 months
- pregnancy: the level of vWF increases during pregnancy in women without von Willebrand's disease, and in most women with type 1 von Willebrand's disease; there is no increase in vWF in women with type 3 von Willebrand's disease, and variable increased levels in women with type 2 von Willebrand's disease
- thyroid disease: vWF levels are raised in hyperthyroidism, decreased in hypothyroidism (acquired von Willebrand's disease), and resolve when the patient is treated and becomes euthyroid

Natural history of von Willebrand's disease, and complications of the disease

The clinical expression of von Willebrand's disease is usually mild in type 1 von Willebrand's disease, with increasing severity in type 2 and type 3.

Approach to diagnosing von Willebrand's disease

A personal and/or family history of bleeding and the pattern of bleeding are central to a diagnosis of von Willebrand's disease. Bleeding events that may suggest von Willebrand's disease include:

- prolonged epistaxis, without a history of trauma and which is not stopped within 20 minutes by compression, leads to anaemia, or requires a blood transfusion

- cutaneous haemorrhage and bruising, with minimal or no apparent trauma
- prolonged bleeding from trivial wounds, lasting >15 minutes
- oral cavity bleeding, such as gingival bleeding, bleeding with tooth eruption, or bites to lips and tongue, that requires medical attention
- heavy, prolonged, or recurrent bleeding after dental extraction, tonsillectomy, or adenoidectomy
- menorrhagia not associated with structural lesions of the uterus

Preliminary investigations include:

- full blood count: the platelet count should always be performed when investigating a suspected bleeding disorder; patients with type 2B von Willebrand's disease may have a moderate thrombocytopenia
- APTT: this is often prolonged in von Willebrand's disease; however, a normal APTT does not exclude a diagnosis of von Willebrand's disease
- prothrombin time, thrombin time, and fibrinogen are all normal in von Willebrand's disease
- PFA-100: this allows a rapid and simple determination of platelet-vWF function; it simulates primary haemostasis in the high sheer stress environment that occurs after small vessel injury

Other diagnoses that should be considered aside from von Willebrand's disease

Platelet-type (pseudo-) von Willebrand's disease is a rare disorder resulting from mutations that affect the platelet glycoprotein Ib/glycoprotein IX receptor complex and causes increased binding between vWF and platelets (i.e. the defect is in the platelets rather than in vWF). Laboratory findings are similar to those found for type 2B von Willebrand's disease (thrombocytopenia, increased ristocetin-induced platelet aggregation (RIPA), and decreased HMW multimers). Therefore, to differentiate type 2B von Willebrand's disease from pseudo-von Willebrand's disease, cryoprecipitate (containing normal vWF) is added to the patient's plasma; it will result in aggregation of platelets in pseudo-von Willebrand's disease, but not in type 2B von Willebrand's disease.

'Gold-standard' diagnostic test for von Willebrand's disease

There is no single diagnostic test for von Willebrand's disease; it requires a series of tests to be performed and interpreted in a step-wise manner, as described in Figure 284.3.

- Factor VIII functional assay: factor VIII is frequently reduced in von Willebrand's disease, as the half-life of this factor is regulated by vWF

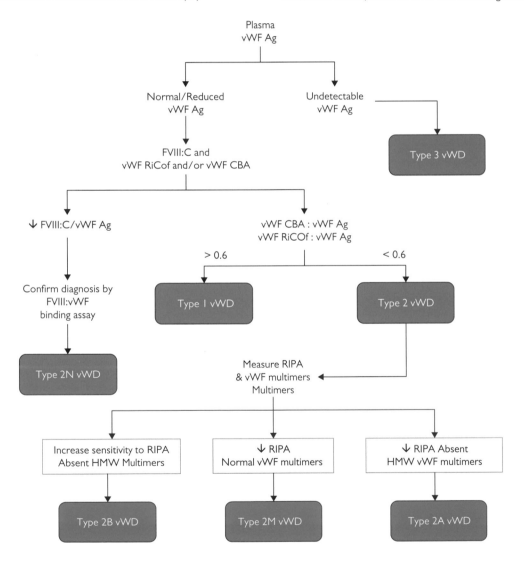

vWF: von Willebrand factor, FVIII: factor VIII, RiCof: risctoceitin cofactor; CBA: collagen binding activity; RIPA: ristocetin induced platelet aggregation

Figure 284.3 Sequence of tests in the diagnosis of von Willebrand's disease subtypes; Ag, antigen; CBA, collagen-binding activity; FVIII, factor VIII; FVIII:C, factor VIII antigen; HMW, high molecular weight; RiCof, risctoceitin cofactor; RIPA, ristocetin-induced platelet aggregation; vWD, von Willebrand's disease; vWF, von Willebrand factor.

- vWF antigen (vWF:Ag): vWF antigen levels are measured by immunological methods, such as ELISA assays
- vWF ristocetin cofactor activity (vWF:RiCof): addition of the antibiotic ristocetin promotes the binding of vWF to platelet glycoprotein Ib; this is a functional assay, rather than an antigen assay (like vWF:Ag), which only measures the level of vWF present
vWF collagen-binding activity: this is another functional assay
RIPA: in this assay, ristocetin is added at several concentrations (ranging from 0.2 to 1.5 mg/ml) to platelet-rich plasma from the patient, to assess the affinity of vWF for platelets by determining the lowest ristocetin concentration that induces agglutination; aggregation at concentrations <0.5 mg/ml indicates vWF/platelet hyper-reactivity, and is an essential diagnostic criterion for type 2B von Willebrand's disease
- multimeric analysis of vWF: this has a role in the subclassification of von Willebrand's disease
- vWF–factor VIII binding assay: reduced binding of factor VIII to vWF is diagnostic of type 2N von Willebrand's disease
- molecular analyses: in some circumstances, the identification of a molecular defect in the vWF gene can help with diagnosis and classification

Treatment of von Willebrand's disease, and its effectiveness

Desmopressin (1-deamino-8-D-arginine vasopressin; Desmopressin) is a synthetic analogue of vasopressin. It causes vWF to be released from endothelial stores, and increases factor VIII and vWF levels to 3–5 times their baseline level, 30–60 minutes after IV or subcutaneous administration. Side effects include headache, facial flushing, hypotension, and hyponatraemia. It should be avoided in patients with cardiovascular disease, as it has been associated with myocardial infarction and stroke.

Desmopressin (0.3 μg/kg) is most effective in patients with type 1 von Willebrand's disease, where increasing levels by three- to fivefold is sufficient for haemostasis. It is of no use in type 3 von Willebrand's disease. Patients with type 2 von Willebrand's disease have a variable response, and a trial of Desmopressin should be considered in type 2A and 2M von Willebrand's disease. Desmopressin is usually avoided in patients with type 2B von Willebrand's disease, because it appears to exacerbate thrombocytopenia.

Tranexamic acid is an antifibrinolytic agent that binds to the lysine-binding sites of plasminogen and therefore inhibits the binding of plasminogen to fibrin. Like desmopressin, it is useful for the management of epistaxis and menorrhagia and following dental extraction. It can be given orally (15–25 mg/kg three times per day), intravenously (10 mg/kg three times per day), or as a mouthwash (10 ml of a 5% solution four times per day).

Patients unresponsive to desmopressin require transfusion with vWF/factor VIII concentrates derived from plasma, as there is no recombinant vWF currently available. There are a number of vWF/factor VIII concentrates available: Haemate P, Alphanate, and Fanhdi. The aim of treatment is to raise the vWF:RiCof and factor VIII levels to above 100 IU/dl for a major surgical procedure, or to treat a significant bleed. The vWF:RiCof and factor VIII levels are then maintained above 50 IU/dl until wound healing has occurred.

Rare inherited bleeding disorders

Rare coagulation disorders are outlined in Table 284.1.

Further Reading

Berntorp E and Shapiro AD. Modern haemophilia care. *Lancet* 2012; 379: 1447–56.
GUIDELINES FOR THE MANAGEMENT OF HEMOPHILIA 2nd edition Prepared by the Treatment Guidelines Working Group, on behalf of the World Federation of Hemophilia (WFH) http://www1.wfh.org/publications/files/pdf-1472.pdf
Laffan MA, Lester W, O'Donnell JS, et al. The diagnosis and management of von Willebrand disease: A United Kingdom Haemophilia Centre Doctors Organization guideline approved by the British Committee for Standards in Haematology. *Brit J Haematol* 2014; 167: 453–65.
Leebeek FW and Eikenboom JC. Von Willebrand's Disease. *N Engl J Med* 2016; 375: 2067–80.
Mumford AD, Ackroyd S, Alikhan R, et al. Guideline for the diagnosis and management of the rare coagulation disorders: A United Kingdom Haemophilia Centre Doctors' Organization guideline on behalf of the British Committee for Standards in Haematology. *Brit J Haematol* 2014; 167: 304–26.
Peyvandi F, Garagiola I, Young G. et al. The past and future of haemophilia: diagnosis, treatments, and its complications. *Lancet* 2016; 388: 187–97.

Definition of the disease

The term thrombophilia is used to describe an individual who has a tendency to develop thrombosis. Arterial thrombosis is usually linked with classical risk factors such as age, smoking, hypertension, hyperlipidaemia, or diabetes; a thrombophilia assessment and workup is not usually considered in cases of arterial thrombosis. A clinically useful approach to the diagnosis and management of a patient with a venous thrombotic process is to categorize the disorder as either a primary (inherited) or a secondary (acquired) hypercoagulable state (see Table 285.1).

Aetiology of the disease

Inherited hypercoagulable states

Antithrombin deficiency

Antithrombin (AT) is synthesized by the liver. In addition to inhibiting thrombin, it inhibits the activated clotting factors IXa, Xa, XIa, XIIa, and tissue factor bound VIIa. Two important functional regions have been identified: a heparin-binding domain and a thrombin-binding domain. There are two types of AT deficiency, and both cause a reduction of AT activity:

- type I: due to a quantitative reduction in the AT protein
- type II: due to a qualitatively (functionally) abnormal AT protein; subclassified according to the site of the molecular defect:
  - reactive site (RS): abnormality in the reactive (thrombin-binding) site
  - heparin-binding site (HBS)
  - pleiotropic: abnormality in both the RS and the HBS

Type I and II deficiencies can be differentiated by comparing the results of an immunological assay (quantitative level) with those of a heparin cofactor assay (functional level). The distinction between

subtypes is of clinical relevance, as the incidence of thrombosis is higher with type I and type II RS deficiencies.

Protein C deficiency

Protein C is a vitamin K-dependent protein synthesized in the liver. Activated by a complex of thrombin and thrombomodulin, it inhibits activated clotting factors Va and VIIIa. Activated protein C (APC) requires the presence of a cofactor, protein S, to exert its inhibitory effects. Protein C deficiency is classified into two subtypes on the basis of functional and immunological assays. However, subtyping serves no clinical purpose, as there is no difference in thrombotic risk. Acquired deficiencies of protein C activity occur in patients with disseminated intravascular coagulopathy (DIC), patients with liver disease, and patients on warfarin therapy.

Protein S deficiency

Protein S, another vitamin K-dependent protein synthesized in the liver, is a cofactor for APC. Two-thirds of the plasma protein S is bound to C4b-binding protein; the remaining third, free protein S, is unbound and has functional activity. Three types of protein S deficiency have been described:

- type I, which is due to a quantitative defect (reduced levels of total and free protein S)
- type II, which is due to a qualitative (functional) defect
- type III, which there are normal levels of total protein S but reduced levels of free protein S

Protein S levels are lower in women than in men and fall both during pregnancy and with the use of oestrogen-containing contraceptive pills or hormone replacement therapy. Acquired deficiency of protein S also occurs in patients with DIC, liver disease, antiphospholipid antibodies, or SLE, as well as with warfarin therapy.

APC resistance/factor V Leiden mutation

The majority of patients with inherited APC resistance have the same point mutation (G1691A) in the gene that codes for clotting factor V: the 'factor V Leiden' (FVL) mutation. Acquired APC resistance occurs with advancing age, in the presence of antiphospholipid antibodies, during pregnancy, and in women using oestrogen-containing contraceptive pills or hormone replacement therapy.

APC resistance is measured using an activated partial thromboplastin time (APTT), with samples tested with and without added APC; the resulting clotting time is expressed as a ratio, the APC sensitivity ratio. The FVL mutation can be detected by amplifying the DNA around the mutation site using a polymerase chain reaction (PCR) and then performing a restriction digest with an enzyme. This recognizes the sequence GAGG, which is present in normal factor V but is lost in the FVL form of the protein. The resulting cleaved fragment is then electrophoresed on an agarose gel to separate the fragments and visualized directly after staining. DNA testing clearly identifies those who have the normal form of the gene, those who are heterozygotes for the FVL mutation, and those who are homozygotes for the FVL mutation.

The FVL mutation is the most common inherited cause of thrombophilia, with a prevalence of 5% in Caucasian populations. The FVL mutation is identified in 20% of patients presenting with a first venous thromboembolism (VTE) and in more than 50% with recurrent VTE. Heterozygous carriers have a three- to eightfold increased risk of VTE, and homozygous have an 80-fold increased risk.

Prothrombin G20210A mutation

The prothrombin G20210A mutation is a guanine (G) to adenine (A) base substitution at nucleotide position 20210 in the

Table 285.1 Hypercoagulable states	
Inherited (primary) hypercoagulable state	**Acquired (secondary) hypercoagulable state**
Antithrombin deficiency	Surgery
Protein C deficiency	Immobility
Protein S deficiency	Malignancy
Activated protein C resistance/factor V Leiden mutation	Advancing age
	Pregnancy
Prothrombin gene mutation	Oestrogen
Hyperhomocysteinaemia	• oral contraceptive
Dysfibrinogenaemia	• hormone replacement therapy
	Obesity
	Acute medical illness
	• acute heart failure
	• acute respiratory failure
	• sepsis
	Antiphospholipid syndrome
	Nephrotic syndrome
	Myeloproliferative disorders
	• polycythaemia vera
	• essential thrombocythaemia
	Paroxysmal nocturnal haemoglobinuria

Table 285.2 Prevalence of inherited thrombophilia in the general population, and the risk of venous thrombosis

Thrombophilia	Prevalence in population (%)	Relative risk of VTE
Antithrombin deficiency	0.0002	25–50
Protein C deficiency	0.2000	10
Protein S deficiency	0.0800	2–10
FVL heterozygous mutation	5.000	5
FVL homozygous mutation	0.0002	50–80
Prothrombin G20210A mutation	2.000	2–3
Hyperhomocysteinaemia	5.000–10.000	2

Abbreviations: FVL, factor V Leiden; VTE, venous thromboembolism.

Table 285.3 Level of thromboembolic risk in surgical patients without thromboprophylaxis

Procedure	DVT %	Clinical PE %	Fatal PE %
Low risk			
Minor surgery in patients <40 years old with no additional VTE risk factors	<10	<1	<0.01
Moderate risk			
Most general, open gynaecological or urological procedures	10–40	1–4	0.1–1.0
High risk			
Major trauma, surgery in patients with multiple VTE risk factors	40–80	1–10	0.1–5.0
Hip arthroplasty	40–60	1–10	0.1–2.0
Knee arthroplasty	40–80	1–10	0.1–2.0
Hip fracture surgery	50–60	3–10	2.0–5.0

Abbreviations: DVT, deep vein thrombosis; PE, pulmonary embolism; VTE, venous thromboembolism.

3′ untranslated region of the prothrombin gene. Following PCR of the target region, the presence of the mutation can be determined by cleaving the fragment with a restriction enzyme. In normal individuals, the PCR product will not be cleaved, while the product from those possessing the mutation will be cleaved. The cleaved material is then electrophoresed on an agarose gel to separate the fragments and visualized directly after staining.

The prothrombin G20210A mutation causes elevated levels of prothrombin, resulting in enhanced thrombin generation and an increased risk of VTE (see Table 285.2). The gain of function mutation is almost exclusively found in Caucasians. As FVL and the prothrombin gene mutation are common, compound heterozygotes are often encountered and they have a 20-fold increased risk of thrombosis when compared to individuals with neither mutation.

Hyperhomocysteinaemia

Elevated homocysteine levels in the blood, hyperhomocysteinaemia, are associated with both arterial disease and VTE. Homocysteine is an amino acid derived from methionine during its metabolism. There are two types of hyperhomocysteinaemia:

- primary hyperhomocysteinaemia: an inherited deficiency affecting one of the following two enzymes:
  - cystathionine beta synthase: a deficiency in this enzyme occurs in 1 in 100 000 live births and leads to the inherited metabolic disorder homocysteinuria
  - methylene tetrahydrofolate reductase: this enzyme is involved in the remethylation pathway by which homocysteine is converted to methionine; approximately 10% of the population have a mutation in this enzyme, with resultant elevated homocysteine levels
- secondary hyperhomocysteinaemia: this is acquired and is caused by a deficiency in one of the following three vitamins:
  - folic acid
  - pyridoxine (vitamin B_6)
  - cobalamin (vitamin B_{12})

Homocysteine increases the activation of procoagulant factors such as tissue factor and factor V and decreases levels of anticoagulant factors such as protein C and thrombomodulin. It also promotes platelet activation and inhibits fibrinolysis. The presence of elevated homocysteine levels in the blood result in a doubling of the risk of VTE and a two- to fourfold increase in the risk of premature arterial disease. However, there is currently no convincing evidence that reducing homocysteine levels reduces either arterial or venous thrombosis.

Acquired hypercoagulable states

Surgery

All patients admitted to hospital should be assessed for risk factors for VTE (see Table 285.2). The type and duration of surgery, in association with additional risk factors for VTE, contribute to the overall thrombotic risk (see Table 285.3).

Age

VTE affects 1 in 1000 individuals annually. The risk of VTE increases steadily with age, affecting approximately 1 in 100 of the population over the age of 75 years. Although the exact mechanism for this increase in risk is uncertain, there are a number of plausible explanations. The levels of procoagulants increase without a concomitant increase in natural anticoagulant levels; activity decreases, with increased periods of immobility due to illness, and the frequency of acute infections increase as do serious cardiovascular and respiratory conditions. There also appears to be the development of a hypercoagulable state with age, suggested by the rise in levels of D-dimers and prothrombin fragments.

Malignancy

Armand Trousseau first described the association between thrombosis and cancer, stating that 'there appears in the cachexia … a particular condition of the blood which predisposes it to spontaneous coagulation' (Trousseau, 1865). Cancer and its associated treatments (central venous lines, chemotherapy) increase the risk of VTE by six- to tenfold. Venous thromboembolic events are one of the leading causes of death in patients with cancer.

Tumours shed membrane particles that contain procoagulant activity, including tissue factor, and membrane lipids that propagate the coagulation response. The risk of VTE appears to be highest for tumours affecting the brain, the ovaries, the pancreas, and the lungs. Approximately 10% of patients presenting with idiopathic VTE are diagnosed with malignancy within a year of their thrombotic event.

Pregnancy

Physiological changes in the haemostatic and fibrinolytic systems increase the risk of VTE during pregnancy. There are increased levels of coagulation factors (von Willebrand factor, factor VIII, and fibrinogen). There is also a reduction in protein S levels, and a third of pregnant women acquire resistance to APC. In addition, venous stasis during pregnancy, and endothelial damage of the pelvic vessels during vaginal or operative delivery, contribute to the thromboembolic risk.

Overall, approximately 1 in 1000 pregnancies is complicated by VTE. Pulmonary embolism is one of the most common causes of maternal death. The incidence of antenatal deep vein thrombosis (DVT) is 0.6 per 1000 maternities in women aged less than 35 years of age, and 1.2 per 1000 maternities in women over 35 years of age (see Table 285.3). For post-partum DVT, the incidence is 0.3 per 1000 maternities in women under 35 years of age, and 0.7 per 1000 maternities in women over 35 years of age. The DVT event rate is highest during the 6-week puerperal period. As well as age, obesity appears to be a significant risk factor for VTE during pregnancy.

Table 285.4 Risk of venous thromboembolism

Demographics	Relative risk	VTE cases per 100 000 women per year
Non-pregnant Not on combined OCP	–	5
Second-generation OCP	3-fold increase	15
Third-generation OCP	5-fold increase	25
Pregnant (age < 35)	12-fold increase	60
Pregnant (age > 35)	24-fold increase	120

Abbreviations: OCP, oral contraceptive pill; VTE, venous thromboembolism.

Table 285.5 Criteria for antiphospholipid syndrome

Clinical criteria	Laboratory criteria
1. Vascular thrombosis • arterial • venous • small vessel thrombosis 2. Pregnancy morbidity • one or more unexplained death of a morphologically normal fetus at/or beyond the 10th week of gestation, or • one or more premature birth of a morphologically normal fetus before the 34th week of gestation, or • three or more unexplained consecutive spontaneous abortions before the 10th week of gestation	1. Lupus anticoagulant • present in plasma, on two or more occasions at least 12 weeks apart 2. Anticardiolipin antibody • IgG and/or IgM in serum/plasma • present in medium or high titre (>40 G phospholipids or M phospholipids), on two or more occasions at least 12 weeks apart 3. Anti-beta-2 glycoprotein 1 antibody • IgG and/or IgM in serum/plasma • present on two or more occasions at least 12 weeks apart

Hormones

Combined oral contraceptive pill

All combined oral contraceptive pills (OCPs) contain two hormones: oestrogen and progestogen. The different types of OCP are known as second- or third-generation contraceptives, depending on the type of progestogen they contain. Third-generation OCPs contain progestogen in the form of either deogestrel or gestodene. Second-generation OCPs contain progestogen as levonorgestrel or norethisterone. All women taking combined OCPs have a small increased risk of VTE; this risk is greater with third-generation OCPs than with second-generation OCPs (see Table 285.4). There does not appear to be an increased risk of VTE with progestogen-only contraceptive pills.

The presence of an inherited thrombophilia increases the risk of VTE in women who use OCPs. Heterozygous FVL carriers have a 20–30-fold increased risk of VTE and, in homozygous carriers, oral contraceptives confer an even higher risk. Prothrombin G20210A carriers who use OCPs have a 16-fold increased risk, compared with non-users. In addition to the risk of VTE from OCP use, the presence of obesity (BMI >30 kg/m²) or smoking increases the risk of venous thrombosis by a further twofold in those using OCPs.

Progestogen-only contraception

Progestogen-only pills, injectables, levonorgesterol implants, or levonorgesterol-releasing intrauterine devices have not been shown to increase the risk of VTE. In addition, the WHO and UK medical eligibility criteria for contraceptive use state that progestogen-only contraception may be used in patients with a personal or family history of VTE and in patients with an identified inherited thrombophilia.

Hormone replacement therapy

Women with hypo-oestrogenic symptoms may suffer with marked impairment in their quality of life that may be improved with hormone replacement therapy. However, hormone replacement therapy is associated with severe side effects such as stroke, myocardial infarction, and breast cancer. In addition, the risk of VTE in women receiving oral oestrogen appears to be double that of those not receiving oestrogen. The risk is highest in the first year of treatment. However, recent evidence suggests that women receiving transdermal hormone replacement therapy do not appear to be at an increased risk of VTE.

Antiphospholipid syndrome

Antiphospholipid syndrome (APS) is present if at least one of the clinical criteria for it **and** one of the laboratory criteria for it are present (see Table 285.5).

Antiphospholipid antibodies are present in 1%–5% of apparently healthy subjects and in up to 30% of patients with SLE. For healthy subjects, it is uncertain how many will go onto develop a thrombotic or pregnancy-related complication. In contrast, 50% of patients with SLE and antiphospholipid antibodies develop APS.

The pathogenesis of thrombosis, associated with the presence of antiphospholipid antibodies, appears to be multifactorial and includes interference with the natural anticoagulant proteins C and S, inhibition of fibrinolysis, induction of tissue factor, promotion of platelet aggregation, and activation of complement. Thrombosis may affect the arterial system, the venous system, or both. The most common presentation is with lower limb DVT, but other sites such as cerebral veins and abdominal veins (portal, hepatic, mesenteric) may be affected. Arterial thrombosis usually presents as stroke or transient ischaemic attacks and rarely as myocardial infarction.

APS should be considered in all patients who present with unprovoked VTE, in young patients with arterial thrombosis, and following pregnancy complications that fulfil the criteria in Table 285.5.

Nephrotic syndrome

Nephrotic syndrome is characterized by proteinuria (>3.5 g/day), hypoalbuminaemia, hyperlipidaemia, and peripheral oedema. The leaking of protein from the kidney may be associated with the loss of AT, resulting in an acquired AT deficiency. The incidence of VTE in nephrotic syndrome appears to be approximately 20 events per 1000 patient years.

Paroxysmal nocturnal haemoglobinuria

Paroxysmal nocturnal haemoglobinuria (PNH) is an acquired clonal stem cell disorder, characterized by the triad of chronic intravascular haemolytic anaemia, hypercoagulability, and deficient haematopoiesis. It arises due to the loss of the cell membrane protein anchors CD55 and CD59. As a result, there is excessive activation of factor X, increased complement activation of platelets, and impaired fibrinolysis. In addition to lower limb DVT, patients with PNH often present with thrombosis of the inferior vena cava, the portal vein, the sagittal sinus, or the hepatic vein (Budd–Chiari syndrome).

Typical symptoms of the disease, and less common symptoms

The symptoms and signs of VTE depend on the site of thrombosis. The most common site of thrombosis is the lower limb. Less common sites include the upper limbs, the abdominal (splanchnic) veins, and the cerebral vessels. It is important to appreciate that the clinical features suggestive of venous thrombosis may be non-specific and fit a long list of differential diagnoses. Objective testing confirms the presence of DVT in less than a third of patients with suspected thrombosis. However, it is equally important to realize that the diagnosis is often missed or not considered in clinical practice, as indicated by the significant incidence of VTE at post mortem.

What is clear from Table 285.6, which lists the symptoms and signs of VTE, are the non-specific features of venous thromboembolic disease. The clinician needs to have a high index of suspicion and should consider thrombotic events as part of the differential diagnosis of a wide spectrum of disorders.

Approach to diagnosing the disease

The initial investigation of a patient with thrombosis should include the following:

- a full blood count, looking for:
  - elevation of the haematocrit/packed cell volume; if present, consider polycythaemia

Table 285.6 Site-related clinical features of venous thromboembolism

Symptoms	Signs
Limbs (lower > upper)	
Pain; no specific characteristics; the location of the pain is not necessarily related to the site of thrombosis; it varies from: • aching to cramping • dull to sharp • mild to severe Swelling Tender Red skin	Homans' sign: • pain in the calf on forced dorsiflexion • Lowenberg's sign • pain in the calf on inflation of cuff to 180 mm Hg at the thigh Moses' sign: • pain from compression of calf in a forward/backward motion is greater than that from lateral compression Unilateral pitting oedema Tender to palpation Erythema, if associated inflammation
Splanchnic vessels (hepatic, portal, mesenteric veins)	
Upper abdominal pain: • all patients present with a varying degree of this very non-specific symptom • sudden onset of pain/post-prandial abdominal pain is suggestive of mesenteric artery thrombosis • gradual onset of pain is more suggestive of venous thrombosis Nausea + vomiting Bloody stools	Abdominal pain + hepatomegaly + ascites: • need to consider obstruction of the hepatic vein: Budd–Chiari syndrome Splenomegaly • portal vein thrombosis • portal hypertension
Cerebral vein thrombosis	
Headache Lethargy Fits Stroke Coma	Focal neurological signs
Pulmonary embolism	
Chest pain: • often pleuritic in nature, worse on deep inspiration Dyspnoea: • subjective experience of hampered breathing Haemoptysis Cough	Circulatory collapse: • right ventricular dysfunction Tachypnoea: • objective observation of increased respiratory rate Hypoxia Tachycardia

• elevation of the platelet count; if present, consider essential thrombocythaemia, or a cause of reactive thrombocytosis, such as sepsis or malignancy
• reduction of the platelet count: this may be a feature of drug-induced thrombocytopenia (due to heparin), thrombotic thrombocytopenia purpura (TTP), SLE, or PNH
• a blood film; look for red cell fragments, as these may indicate DIC or TTP
• the following coagulation tests:
  • prothrombin time
  • APTT, using a lupus sensitive reagent; this will provide an initial screen for the presence of a lupus anticoagulant
  • fibrinogen: to screen for dysfibrinogenaemia

The following tests may also be requested, depending on the suspected clinical disorder:

• special coagulation tests, such as:
  • protein C activity (followed by protein C antigen level if the activity is low)
  • protein S activity (followed by free protein S antigen level if the activity is low; the total protein S antigen level may be helpful if the level of free protein S antigen is low)
  • AT activity
  • the APC resistance ratio; if the ratio is abnormal (low), test for the FVL mutation
  • a test for the prothrombin G20210A mutation
• selective special tests, such as:
  • tests for anticardiolipin and anti-beta-2-glycoprotein 1 antibodies (IgG and IgM), to exclude APS
  • tests for platelet anti-PF4/glycosaminoglycan antibodies, to exclude heparin-induced thrombocytopenia

• a test for the JAK2 mutation, to exclude myeloproliferative disorder (portal or splanchnic vein thrombosis)
• a test for plasma ADAMTS13 activity, to exclude acquired or familial TTP
• flow cytometry, to detect PNH

In addition, the following selective general tests may be requested:

• renal function tests
• liver function tests:
  • abnormal results occur in the Budd–Chiari syndrome, which is characterized by ascites, hepatomegaly, and obstruction of the hepatic venous circulation
  • hypoalbuminaemia occurs in nephrotic syndrome
• urinalysis:
  • protein, to exclude nephrotic syndrome
  • bilirubin, to exclude PNH

In addition, if associated symptoms are suggestive of malignancy, the following tests may be requested:

• tests for tumour markers (e.g. prostate-specific antigen, carcinoembryonic antigen, cancer antigen 125)
• imaging:
  • chest X-ray
  • ultrasound of abdomen/pelvis
  • CT abdomen/pelvis

'Gold-standard' diagnostic test

The gold-standard diagnostic test for DVT (upper or lower limb) is venography. The gold-standard diagnostic test for cerebral and splanchnic vein thrombosis is magnetic resonance angiography. The gold-standard diagnostic test for pulmonary embolism (PE) is pulmonary angiography.

Thrombophilia testing should not be performed during an acute thrombotic episode because interpretation during such an event is difficult, as levels of e.g. protein C or S are affected by the present of thrombosis and anticoagulants. In addition, note that thrombophilia results do not alter the initial treatment.

Acceptable diagnostic alternatives to the gold standard

Acceptable diagnostic alternatives to the gold-standard test for DVT are Doppler ultrasound and compression ultrasound. MRI is an acceptable diagnostic alternative to the gold-standard test for cerebral vein thrombosis. Acceptable diagnostic alternatives to the gold-standard test for splanchnic vein thrombosis are Doppler ultrasound and CT.

Acceptable diagnostic alternatives to the gold-standard test for PE are CT pulmonary angiography and ventilation/perfusion scintigraphy (also known as a V/Q scan).

Treatment and its effectiveness

The initial treatment of VTE should be with a rapidly acting anticoagulant such as:

- unfractionated heparin (UFH)
- low-molecular-weight heparin (LMWH)
- fondaparinux

Selected patients with extensive acute proximal DVT but who have a low risk of bleeding, and patients with PE and haemodynamic compromise, should be considered for catheter-directed or systemic thrombolysis. Vena caval filters should not be used routinely and are only indicated for patients in whom anticoagulation is contraindicated.

In addition to UFH, LMWH, or fondaparinux, a vitamin K antagonist (e.g. warfarin) or direct-acting oral anticoagulant should be started, with duration of treatment as given in Table 285.7.

Table 285.7 Duration of anticoagulation for specific clinical conditions

Condition	Duration	Target INR (range) for warfarin
First idiopathic VTE: proximal DVT or PE	>3 months*	2.5 (2.0–3.0)
First proximal DVT or PE, with precipitating factors (e.g. surgery, trauma, pregnancy)	3 months	2.5 (2.0–3.0)
First idiopathic calf DVT	3 months	2.5 (2.0–3.0)
First calf vein DVT, with precipitating factors (e.g. surgery, trauma)	6 weeks to 3 months	2.5 (2.0–3.0)
Recurrent VTE	Long term	2.5 (2.0–3.0)
VTE while on warfarin	Long term	3.5 (3.0–4.0)

Abbreviations: DVT, deep vein thrombosis; INR, international normalized ratio; PE, pulmonary embolism; VTE, venous thromboembolism.

*Patients with unprovoked DVT or PE should be treated for a minimum of 3 months. After 3 months, all patients should be evaluated for the risk–benefit ratio of long-term treatment. Patients with unprovoked VTE and in whom risk factors for bleeding are absent and good anticoagulant monitoring is achievable should receive long-term treatment.

Further Reading

Connors JM. Thrombophilia testing and venous thrombosis. *N Engl J Med* 2017; 377: 2298.

Martinelli I, De Stefano V, and Mannucci PM. Inherited risk factors for venous thromboembolism. *Nat Rev Cardiol* 2014; 11: 140–56.

Piazza G. Thrombophilia testing, recurrent thrombosis, and women's health. *Circulation* 2014; 130: 283–7.

Trousseau A. 'Phlegmasia alba dolens', in *Clinique Medicale de l'Hotel-Dieu de Paris*, 1865. JB Balliere et Fils.

Watson HG, Keeling DM, Laffan R, et al. Guideline on aspects of cancer-related venous thrombosis. *Br J Haematol* 2015; 170: 640–8.

Sciascia S, Baldovino S, Schreiber K et al. Thrombotic risk assessment in antiphospholipid syndrome: the role of new antibody specificities and thrombin generation assay. *Clin Mol Allergy* 2016; 14: 6.

286 Acute leukaemia

Graham Collins and Chris Bunch

Definition of the disease

Acute leukaemia is a rapidly progressive, clonal haematopoietic stem cell disorder resulting in the accumulation of immature blood cell precursors (known as blasts) in the bone marrow. There are two main types of acute leukaemia:

- acute myeloid leukaemia (AML), which is defined by the presence of myeloid lineage markers on the blast cells
- acute lymphoblastic leukaemia (ALL), which is defined by the presence of lymphoid markers on the blast cells

Occasionally, the blast cells express markers from both lineages. Such cases are referred to as 'biphenotypic'.

Aetiology of the disease

AML is associated with a number of predisposing factors:

- other haematological conditions such as myelodysplasia or myeloproliferative conditions can transform into AML
- previous chemotherapy agents predispose to AML (e.g. topoisomerase II inhibitors, alkylating agents)
- toxins (e.g. benzene)
- ionizing radiation
- inherited predisposition: Down's syndrome is associated with a significantly increased risk of developing a rare subtype of AML called acute megakaryoblastic leukaemia

Frequently, however, no etiological factors can be identified.

ALL can also arise from chronic myeloid leukaemia and is also associated with Down's syndrome. In the vast majority of cases, no cause can be identified.

Typical symptoms of the disease, and less common symptoms

Acute leukaemia frequently presents with symptoms and signs of bone marrow failure:

- anaemia: fatigue, shortness of breath, headache, palpitations
- leucopenia: bacterial or fungal infections
- thrombocytopenia: purpuric rash, mucosal haemorrhage

In children, a very important symptom of ALL is bone pain, which can often be rather vague and simply present as a limp.

Less commonly, a very high white-cell count can cause symptoms of leucostasis: shortness of breath, retinal haemorrhages, confusion, and priapism. In certain forms of leukaemia, disseminated intravascular coagulation can result in catastrophic haemorrhage and, in other forms, tissue infiltration by blast cells can produce gum hypertrophy, skin lesions (called chloromas), organomegaly, and lymphadenopathy.

Demographics of the disease

Demographics of ALL

ALL is the commonest childhood cancer, although, overall, it is an uncommon disease. ALL accounts for only 20% of adult acute leukaemia. In childhood, there is a clear peak in incidence between 1 and 6 years of age with the highest incidence between ages 2 and 3. In adults, the incidence increases with age. Childhood ALL is 30% more frequent in boys than in girls.

Demographics of AML

The incidence of AML peaks between 60 and 70 years of age; 80% of cases are diagnosed in the over-50 group. It also can occur in children, although it is uncommon in that age group.

Natural history, and complications of the disease

Acute leukaemia is a rapidly progressive condition which rapidly causes deterioration and death if left untreated. Progressive bone marrow failure causes worsening anaemia with subsequent organ failure, increased risk of severe haemorrhage, and a high risk of life-threatening bacterial and fungal infections.

Numerous complications are associated with the treatment of the disease. Potentially curative chemotherapy is intensive and associated with hair loss, fatigue, gastrointestinal disturbances, reduced fertility, and specific organ damage. The most frequent complication encountered is infection. Prolonged episodes of neutropenia result in a high risk of invasive bacterial infections (especially with *Pseudomonas* and other Gram-negative bacteria, although the incidence of Gram-positive sepsis is increasing) and fungal infections (especially with *Aspergillus*). In ALL, high-dose steroids form an integral part of treatment but frequently result in infections, mood swings, and bony avascular necrosis.

In acute leukaemia patients with very high white counts, tumour lysis syndrome (TLS) is a potential complication in which biochemical disturbances caused by rapid cell death, such as hypocalcaemia, hyperkalaemia, hyperuricaemia, and hyperphosphataemia, are seen. Renal failure may ensue unless prompt action is taken. Treatment is focused on prevention by identifying at-risk patients, initiating IV fluids, and using allopurinol or rasburicase (recombinant urate oxidase). Treatment of established TLS is by correcting clinically important biochemical disturbances and possibly initiating renal dialysis.

In some patients, an allogeneic stem cell transplant is offered as part of the treatment strategy. In addition to infection, graft-vs-host disease (GvHD) is an important complication of this procedure. Acute GvHD (within 100 days of the transplant) typically causes a rash, diarrhoea, and jaundice. GvHD is also immunosuppressive and is frequently complicated by bacterial, fungal, and/or viral infections, including reactivation of CMV. Chronic GvHD (after 100 days from the transplant) can result in numerous manifestations such as mouth ulcers, sclerodermatous skin changes, pulmonary involvement, and neuropathies.

Approach to diagnosing the disease

Acute leukaemia should be considered in the following clinical situations:

- rapidly falling blood counts (more than one lineage involvement should raise suspicion further)
- a rapidly rising white-cell count with blasts seen on the blood film
- deterioration of a previously stable haematological condition (e.g. a rapidly enlarging spleen in a patient with chronic myeloid leukaemia or myelofibrosis)
- a child who is non-specifically unwell and has vague bony symptoms or signs (such as a mild limp)

Other diagnoses that should be considered

A serious underlying infection or solid tumour can cause a reactive blood picture associated with circulating immature blood cell precursors, including blast cells. This is called a 'leukaemoid reaction', and care should be taken not to diagnose acute leukaemia in these cases.

Acute viral infections such as infectious mononucleosis frequently result in atypical lymphocytes being seen on a blood film. Occasionally, these can be hard to distinguish from blast cells. A bone marrow aspirate in these cases can also be hard to distinguish from acute leukaemia. Clinicians should have a low threshold for performing a monospot test.

'Gold-standard' diagnostic test

Acute leukaemia is a disorder of the bone marrow, and accurate diagnosis requires a bone marrow biopsy; an aspirate will often suffice, although a trephine may be helpful in some situations. Morphological examination will give a diagnosis of acute leukaemia but immunophenotyping (by flow cytometry or immunohistochemistry) will allow accurate subtyping.

Acceptable diagnostic alternatives to the gold standard

In some cases (particularly when curative treatment is not appropriate), sufficient diagnostic material may be obtained from the peripheral blood. Although superseded by immunophenotyping, cytochemistry is an acceptable alternative to enable accurate subtyping.

Other relevant investigations

Other relevant investigations for acute leukaemia include:

- a full blood count: to determine the extent of bone marrow failure or leucocytosis; a blood film may or may not show circulating blast cells
- a coagulation screen: some acute leukaemias (especially acute promyelocytic leukaemia) may present with disseminated intravascular coagulation
- a blood group and antibody screen: blood transfusion is highly likely due to the disease or its treatment
- biochemistry: patients may be acutely unwell at diagnosis, with renal and/or liver impairment; renal impairment increases the risk of TLS
- serum calcium: may be elevated in a subset of patients
- inflammatory markers: may indicate an underlying infection
- viral serology including monospot: to exclude acute viral infection in the differential
- serum urate: raised levels increase the risk of TLS
- cytogenetics (preferably from a bone marrow aspirate): can provide important prognostic information from molecular testing which looks for certain genetic mutations and is also important in prognostication and in guiding subsequent disease monitoring and treatment
- septic screen, including blood cultures, chest X-ray, urinalysis
- ECG: in preparation for receiving cytotoxic chemotherapy

Prognosis and how to estimate it

When acute leukaemia is diagnosed in a patient who is unfit for potentially curative treatment, life expectancy is in the order of a few months to a few years. In younger adults with acute leukaemia, intensive chemotherapy with or without allogeneic stem cell transplantation results in 5-year survival rates of approximately 40%. In children, intensive treatment of ALL results in long-term remission rates of 80%.

In childhood ALL, a number of parameters indicate prognosis. Factors associated with a worse prognosis include:

- male sex

- age <1 or >9 years of age
- white-cell count at diagnosis of >50 × 10⁹/l
- CNS involvement
- certain cytogenetic findings (e.g. Philadelphia chromosome, complex karyotype, low hypodiploidy, t(4:11), t(8:14))
- poor response to initial treatment, as assessed by clearance of blasts from the bone marrow, or failure to eliminate the presence of minimal residual disease, as assessed by molecular techniques

For AML, poor prognostic factors include:

- increasing age and comorbidities
- cytogenetic features (e.g. complex karyotype, monosomy 5 or 7, abnormal 3q)
- antecedent myelodysplastic syndrome or myeloproliferative disease
- specific genetic mutations, such as internal tandem duplications involving the FLT3 gene
- poor response to initial chemotherapy

Treatment and its effectiveness

Wherever possible, patients with any malignancy should be treated within the context of a clinical trial. This is especially true in acute leukaemia, for which national clinical trials are designed to incorporate the broadest possible spectrum of patients, including childhood ALL, adult ALL, adult AML, and elderly AML.

Treatment of ALL

Treatment of ALL typically consists of three main phases:

- remission induction: this uses agents such as corticosteroids (prednisolone or dexamethasone), vincristine, asparaginase, and daunorubicin
- intensification: this involves multidrug chemotherapy regimens, including treatment directed to the CNS; agents used include cyclophosphamide, cytarabine, etoposide, and methotrexate
- maintenance: this phase of treatment lasts for 2 years in girls, and 3 years in boys; typical regimens include daily oral mercaptopurine, weekly oral methotrexate, and occasional IV vincristine

Approximately 80% of children achieve long-term remission, although the figure is much less in adults. Current clinical trials are aimed at using the technique of minimal residual disease (a genetic test which can pick up very small amounts of residual leukaemia) to identify those patients who are responding well to treatment and those that are responding poorly. Poor responders may benefit from intensification of treatment, and good responders may benefit from de-escalation.

Treatment of AML

Potentially curative treatment of AML involves one or two courses of remission induction chemotherapy followed by one or two courses of consolidation chemotherapy. In fit patients with a poor prognosis and with a suitable donor, allogeneic bone marrow transplant may form part of the consolidation. Standard induction chemotherapy generally consists of cytarabine and daunorubicin. Alternative agents include fludarabine and idarubicin.

Induction and consolidation chemotherapy is intense and associated with profound myelosuppression. Most patients have a central venous cannula (such as a Hickman line) to avoid repeated venepuncture and peripheral cannula insertion. Most patients achieve an initial remission with standard chemotherapy, although relapse remains a major problem.

Allogeneic bone marrow transplantation is the most effective strategy for prevention of relapse, as demonstrated by a number of studies. However, the treatment-related mortality of these procedures is high and limits their use to relatively young and fit patients and to those with a suitable donor. Conventional allogeneic transplants involve high-dose chemotherapy, often with total body irradiation. The intensity of the regimen limits its use to those aged under

45. More recent developments include the use of reduced-intensity conditioning transplants which utilize conditioning protocols which are better tolerated. The efficacy of these procedures relies on a graft-vs-leukaemia effect.

In patients unfit for standard chemotherapy, supportive care or low-dose cytarabine are options. The focus of clinical trials is shifting towards targeting specific types of AML, using small molecule inhibitors of deregulating cellular pathways. Alternatively, monoclonal antibodies are being used to deliver chemotherapy in a more targeted way.

Further Reading

Döhner H, Estey E, Grimwade D et al. Diagnosis and management of AML in adults: 2017 ELN recommendations from an international expert panel. *Blood* 2017; 129: 424–47.

Guidelines and management recommendations of the European Leukaemia Net (http://www.leukemia-net.org/content/physicians/recommendations/index_eng.html)

Guidelines and management recommendations of the American Society of Hematology (http://www.hematology.org)

Terwilliger T and Abdul-Hay M. Acute lymphoblastic leukemia: a comprehensive review and 2017 update. *Blood Cancer* J 2017; 7: e577.

Definition of the disease

Leukaemia is, in broad terms, a 'cancer of the blood'. However, this is inaccurate, as the malignant process primarily occurs outside of the bloodstream. In acute leukaemias, it occurs in the bone marrow within immature blood-forming cells. In the two forms of chronic leukaemia, leukaemogenesis occurs in two completely different cell types (and possibly even two different anatomical sites), leading to two very different forms of the disease: chronic myeloid leukaemia (CML) and chronic lymphocytic leukaemia (CLL).

CML is best thought of as a myeloproliferative disorder. It is a clonal disorder of the haematopoietic stem cell, leading to overproduction of the myeloid cells: neutrophils and their precursors, basophils and eosinophils.

CLL is best thought of as a low-grade lymphoma. It is a clonal disorder of mature B-lymphocytes (possibly memory B-cells). The site of initiation of this disorder is unclear; it could be within lymph nodes or within the bone marrow.

Aetiology of the disease

Aetiology of CML

A higher incidence of CML is associated with heavy radiation exposure but this applies to the minority of patients. CLL is the only leukaemia that is not associated with radiation exposure and it also shows the strongest degree of familial clustering, although, again, this applies to the minority.

Much is understood of the pathobiology of CML. CML was the first malignant disease in which a recurrent chromosomal translocation was described, between Chromosomes 9 and 22. This forms an abnormal derivative chromosome termed the Philadelphia chromosome. At the molecular level, this leads to the juxtaposition of the 3′ end of the c-ABL proto-oncogene on Chromosome 9 with the 5′ end of the BCR gene from Chromosome 22. This fusion gene is transcribed and produces a constitutively active tyrosine kinase. This protein then phosphorylates a number of substrates, leading to changes in cell proliferation, differentiation, adhesion, and survival. Interestingly, mouse models indicate that the Philadelphia chromosome is both necessary and sufficient for the development of CML. The result is an inappropriate expansion of the myeloid component of the bone marrow. This leads to an increasing white-cell count and, often, pronounced splenomegaly.

Aetiology of CLL

The pathobiology of CLL is much less well understood than that for CML. No single chromosomal aberration is found in CLL cells. However, recurrent cytogenetic changes of various types are found in up to 80% of cases, suggesting that the familiar morphology of CLL cells may represent the final state of a number of different acquired genetic anomalies. Some cytogenetic changes define specific clinical groups. For example, deletion of the short arm of 17p (which results in loss of the tumour suppressor gene p53) is associated with a clinically aggressive course and resistance to standard chemotherapy agents. Although CLL is a clonal disorder of B-cells, the type of B-cell giving rise to CLL remains a matter of some debate. Genetic analysis of the immunoglobulin genes shows that some cases of CLL have very few mutations affecting these genes, suggesting it has not experienced antigen and traversed the germinal centre. However, other cases show a higher burden of mutations, suggesting a post-germinal centre origin. These do not represent two clear groups, however, as there is a spectrum of mutational events affecting this gene. Also, gene expression profiling experiments suggest that the closest normal cell is actually a memory B-cell, leading some to think that this may be the cell of origin.

Typical symptoms of the disease, and less common symptoms

Symptoms of CML

CML typically presents with one or more of the following:

- systemic symptoms: anorexia, weight loss, sweats
- symptoms of splenomegaly: abdominal bloating, early satiety, haemorrhoids
- symptoms of leucostasis: breathlessness, blurred vision, priapism, confusion, seizures

Patients are usually symptomatic, although a routine blood test may also pick up the condition. It is most common to present in the chronic phase of the disease, although, occasionally, patients may present in blast crisis. Blast crisis is really a form of acute leukaemia and most commonly presents with symptoms and signs of bone marrow failure (anaemia, infections due to leucopenia, and bleeding/bruising due to thrombocytopenia).

Symptoms of CLL

CLL is much more commonly picked up incidentally from a blood test taken for an unrelated reason (40%–50% of cases). In such situations, there is usually a lymphocytosis with a normal haemoglobin and platelet count. Symptomatic patients usually complain of one or more of:

- systemic symptoms: fevers, weight loss, anorexia, night sweats
- lymphadenopathy (e.g. a lump in the neck, axilla, and/or inguinal regions)
- symptoms of bone marrow failure, especially anaemia; it should be borne in mind that CLL is associated with autoimmune haemolytic anaemia and so anaemia should not be immediately ascribed to bone marrow involvement
- symptoms of organomegaly (e.g. abdominal bloating); however, the spleen is rarely as large as that typically seen in CML

CLL is also associated with a number of autoimmune conditions and may present with one of these. Most commonly, this would be autoimmune haemolytic anaemia, although idiopathic thrombocytopenic purpura and pure red cell aplasia are also sometimes seen.

Demographics of the disease

Demographics of CML

For CML, the median age at presentation is 50–60 years of age, and the disease affects men slightly more often than it does women. The incidence is 1–2 per 100 000 per year.

Demographics of CLL

For CLL, incidence increases with age, with the median age at presentation being 60–70 years of age. Like CML, CLL affects men more than women. The annual incidence of CLL is approximately 10–20 per 100 000 per year.

Natural history and complications of the disease

Natural history and complications of CML

CML has defined phases of disease, although the natural history has been significantly altered by improvements in treatment. Most patients present with chronic phase disease, which is characterized clinically by slowly evolving symptoms and in the laboratory by a neutrophilia and circulating immature granulocytes called myelocytes (but a relatively small number of circulating primitive cells, or blasts). Without treatment using modern tyrosine kinase inhibitors (TKIs), the risk of progressing to the accelerated or blast phase is 10% per year for the first 2 years but this rises to 30% per year thereafter. This means that a typical duration for the chronic phase before the advent of TKIs was 3–4 years.

The onset of the accelerated phase of CML is characterized by the progression of symptoms and haematological abnormalities, despite escalation of treatment. At the molecular level, there is an accumulation of additional genetic alterations and genomic instability. The accelerated phase proceeds to blast crisis, which is the accumulation of primitive cells in the bone marrow, leading to bone marrow failure. The prognosis for blast crisis remains poor.

Natural history and complications of CLL

CLL has a much less predictable clinical course than CML. Patients who are diagnosed incidentally, at a very early stage, may never progress to the point where they need treatment. However, a proportion will and, despite advances in prognostication, it is not easy to identify those with an indolent course from those with an aggressive course. In those who do progress, treatment is not curative but frequently results in a remission. CLL then becomes a relapsing and remitting illness, although the benefit obtained from treatment tends to become less the higher the number of previous treatment courses used. It is not unusual for patients with CLL to develop extremely high white-cell counts (>300 × 10⁹/l). However, leucostasis due to such a high count is extremely uncommon, and treatment is rarely initiated purely due to a high white-cell count.

Other well-known complications of CLL include haematological autoimmune disorders. Autoimmune haemolytic anaemia is a relatively common occurrence during the course of the disease and its incidence is increased by treatment with fludarabine monotherapy. Immune thrombocytopenic purpura is the second most common autoimmune manifestation, followed by pure red cell aplasia, whereby there is immune attack against red cell precursors, resulting in profound anaemia with low reticulocytes. It is also becoming appreciated that the incidence of solid cancers is increased in CLL, although the mechanism is unclear. Finally, infections are common in CLL, mainly due to hypogammaglobulinaemia (although bone marrow failure and drug-related immunosuppression also contribute). The most common organism involved is *Pneumococcus*.

Approach to diagnosing the disease

Diagnosing CML

In diagnosing CML, a clinical history should be taken and the examination and investigations should be performed to exclude other causes of splenomegaly with or without hepatomegaly and to search for solid malignancies, as, in a blood film test, these can sometimes produce a so-called leukaemoid picture which can be similar to that seen in CML. Specific investigations for CML should then be undertaken.

Diagnosing CLL

In diagnosing CLL, a clinical history should be taken and the examination and investigations should be performed to exclude other causes of lymphadenopathy. Specific diagnostic tests should then be performed.

Other diagnoses that should be considered

Other diagnoses that should be considered aside from CML

Other diagnoses that should be considered aside from CML include:

- myelofibrosis (another cause of massive splenomegaly in developed countries)
- a solid tumour (which can produce a 'leukaemoid' blood film appearance)
- essential thrombocythaemia (CML and essential thrombocythaemia can present with isolated thrombocythaemia)

Other diagnoses that should be considered aside from CLL

Other diagnoses that should be considered aside from CLL include:

- a solid tumour with regional lymphadenopathy (e.g. head and neck cancer causing cervical nodes)
- infections (endocarditis, TB, viral infections):
  - note that, in children, a raised lymphocyte count is never indicative of CLL, as children have a higher lymphoctye:neutrophil ratio than adults
  - pertussis is also well known to cause a very elevated lymphocyte count
- other lymphoproliferative disorders can present with a lymphocytosis (e.g. follicular lymphoma, mantle cell lymphoma)

'Gold-standard' diagnostic test

Gold-standard diagnostic test for CML

The gold-standard diagnostic tests for CML are:

- PCR for the BCR–ABL fusion gene on peripheral blood and/or bone marrow aspirate
- fluorescent in situ hybridization (FISH) for t(9;22) on peripheral blood or bone marrow aspirate

Gold-standard diagnostic test for CLL

The gold-standard diagnostic tests for CLL are:

- immunophenotyping of peripheral blood lymphocytes
- bone marrow aspirate with immunophenotyping of lymphocytes

Acceptable diagnostic alternatives to the gold standard

Acceptable diagnostic alternatives to the gold-standard test for CML

An acceptable diagnostic alternative to the gold-standard test for CML is conventional karyotyping to identify the Philadelphia chromosome.

Acceptable diagnostic alternatives to the gold-standard test for CLL

An acceptable diagnostic alternative to the gold-standard test for CML is lymph node excision or core biopsy with immunohistochemistry. This is usually not needed, as blood or bone marrow will usually give the diagnosis. Rarely, only lymph nodes are involved (a condition often called small lymphocytic lymphoma rather than CLL). In these cases, a lymph node biopsy is required.

Other relevant investigations

Other relevant investigations for CML

Other relevant investigations for CML include:

- a full blood count and a blood film:
  - patients will often be anaemic at presentation
  - blast count, basophil count, and platelet count also give an idea as to the prognosis of the disorder
- bone marrow aspirate and cytogenetic evaluation: in addition to establishing the diagnosis, cytogenetic changes in addition to t(9;22) may give prognostic information
- CT chest, abdomen, and/or pelvis **if** there is diagnostic doubt, looking for a solid tumour giving rise to a 'leukaemoid' reaction
- PCR for BCR–ABL: if not already performed to establish the diagnosis, a baseline is needed in order to monitor response to treatment
- biochemistry, including liver function tests: note that the TKIs can cause liver toxicity, so baseline readings are important

Other relevant investigations for CLL

Other relevant investigations for CML include the following:

- a full blood count and a blood film:
  - the classic blood film picture shows numerous mature lymphocytes with smear cells; while this is characteristic, it is not pathognomonic and should not be considered diagnostic

- the film may also show evidence of haemolysis (polychromasia and spherocytes)
- a direct Coombe's test, a bilirubin test, a lactate dehydrogenase test, and a reticulocyte count, to look for the presence of coexisting autoimmune haemolysis
- biochemistry, including renal and liver function tests: these measurements are needed to calculate the correct doses of chemotherapy drugs to use and to monitor for side effects
- FISH (or, preferably, mutation analysis) for p53: although not required at diagnosis, it is required before treatment, as p53 deletion or mutation is strongly predictive of resistance to standard chemotherapy agents
- immunophenotyping for CD38 and Zap70: expression of these markers has been associated with a worse prognosis
- analysis of the mutational status of immunoglobulin heavy chain genes: mutated cases have a better prognosis than unmutated ones
- serum beta 2 microglobulin is raised in more aggressive disease
- CT chest, abdomen, and/or pelvis: may be helpful in cases characterized more by lymph node involvement than blood or marrow involvement (e.g. cases of small lymphocytic lymphoma)

Prognosis, and how to estimate it

Prognosis for CML

For CML, various factors at diagnosis indicate a worse prognosis, although these are less important in the era of TKI therapy. The two most commonly used prognostic scores are the Sokal score and the Hasford score. Poor prognostic factors include advancing age, increasing spleen size, raised platelet count, raised basophil count, and raised blast count. However, the most important factor is the response to treatment. Patients who respond to TKIs have an excellent prognosis. Overall, current estimates are of a 90% 5-year survival rate for a newly diagnosed patient with CML treated with TKIs. In those who respond well (defined as achieved a stable cytogenetic remission in which the t(9;22) translocation cannot be detected by FISH on bone marrow samples), the 8-year survival rate is in excess of 95%.

Prognosis for CLL

In CLL, the following factors at diagnosis confer a worse prognosis:

- deletion or mutation of the p53 gene
- an 11p deletion
- a rapid lymphocyte doubling time (less than 12 months)
- CD38 expression
- Zap70 expression
- a raised level of beta-2 microglobulin
- an unmutated immunoglobulin heavy chain gene
- advanced clinical stage (by the Rai or the Binet staging system)

Overall, the average life expectancy of a patient with CLL is in the region of 10–12 years. However, this is highly variable. A Binet stage A patient with mutated immunoglobulin heavy chains has a life expectancy of 25 years, whereas this falls to 8 years when the heavy chains are unmutated. In cases of p53 mutation or deletion, the average life expectancy is only on the order of 3 years.

Treatment and its effectiveness

Treatment for CML

The standard treatment for patients with CML is with TKIs (e.g. imatinib). This is highly effective at inducing haematological remission (normal blood count) and cytogenetic remission (no evidence of t(9;22) by FISH). In some patients, it also produces a molecular remission (no evidence of BCR–ABL on PCR testing). Drug resistance can be present at diagnosis or can evolve. Depending on the mechanism of resistance, a number of novel TKIs (e.g. dasatinib, nilotinib) remain effective in many of these cases. These drugs have transformed the outlook of CML and are generally well tolerated. Before TKIs, the life expectancy of a patient with CML was 3–5 years, unless the patient had an allogeneic bone marrow transplant. With TKIs, the 5-year survival rate is approximately 90%. However, they are not considered curative, as most patients who stop them do relapse, even when they achieved a molecular remission. TKIs also should not be taken in pregnancy; interferon is the drug of choice in this situation. The treatment of blast crisis, however, is poor and consists of high-dose chemotherapy followed by an allogeneic stem cell transplant if the patient is young and fit enough to tolerate this approach.

Treatment for CLL

Asymptomatic CLL is usually not actively treated. However, the development of symptoms or evidence suggesting critical organ involvement does warrant treatment. Treatment is in the form of chemo-immunotherapy. In younger patients with a good performance status, fludarabine and cyclophosphamide combined with rituximab is considered to be the gold-standard treatment, due to clinical trial evidence showing superior survival outcomes. In older patients, drugs such as bendamustine or chlorambucil (again, usually in combination with rituximab) may be more appropriate, due to a more favourable toxicity profile. Treatment of relapsed disease is more difficult, relying mainly on similar chemo-immunotherapy agents. In younger patients with more aggressive disease, an allogeneic stem cell transplant offers a potential cure but at relatively high risk of morbidity and mortality. In p53 mutated or deleted cases, treatment with the anti-CD52 antibody alemtuzumab followed by a stem cell transplant is considered optimal therapy. Novel agents which are being trialled include novel monoclonal antibodies (e.g. ofatumumab) and immunomodulatory drugs such as lenalidomide. Chemo-immunotherapy is not considered curative.

Further Reading

Apperley JF. Chronic myeloid leukaemia. *Lancet* 2014; 385: 1447–59.
Guidelines and management recommendations of the American Society of Hematology (http://www.hematology.org)
Guidelines and management recommendations of the European Leukaemia Net (http://www.leukaemia-net.org/content/physicians/recommendations/index_eng.html)
Hallek M. Chronic lymphocytic leukemia: 2017 update on diagnosis, risk stratification, and treatment. *Am J Hematol* 2017; 92: 946–65.

288 Myelodysplasia

Chris Bunch

Introduction

The myelodysplastic syndromes (or myelodysplasias) comprise a spectrum of disorders characterized by dysplastic or ineffective haemopoiesis that leads to variable anaemia, neutropenia, and thrombocytopenia. There is often a degree of red-cell macrocytosis. The majority are clonal stem cell disorders in which the abnormal clone predominates and expands only slowly over a number of years. Myelodysplasias have a tendency to develop ultimately into acute leukaemia in some patients; for this reason, they are sometimes referred to as 'preleukaemias', even though two-thirds of patients will never develop this complication.

Classifications of myelodysplasia have traditionally focused on clinical and pathological features but now take into account other prognostic features, notably cytogenetics (see Box 288.1). Additional risk classifications, including multiple scoring systems, have been used to define prognosis in myelodysplasia and to evaluate its potential for transformation to acute myeloid leukaemia. The International Prognostic Scoring System takes into account specific cytopenias, age, and cytogenetics, in addition to bone marrow morphology. It defines four risk categories, Low, Intermediate-1, Intermediate-2, and High, which indicate both survival and evolution to acute myeloid leukaemia.

General features

Myelodysplasia is mainly a disease of the elderly, and is becoming more common as the population ages. The median age at diagnosis is 70–75, and comorbidities are common and have a significant effect on prognosis. Most cases arise de novo, but myelodysplasia develops occasionally in patients who have been treated with radiation and/or cytotoxic chemotherapy for some other condition. These secondary cases occur mostly 5–10 years after the original therapy and, again, are more frequent in older patients.

The condition usually presents as a mild symptomatic, refractory anaemia or comes to light following a routine blood count. This may be normocytic but typically shows a mild macrocytosis (mean corpuscular volume, 95–110 fl) with frequent red-cell abnormalities on the blood film. There may also be mild-to-moderate thrombocytopenia and/or neutropenia. Platelets and neutrophils may also be morphologically abnormal with giant platelets and neutrophil hypogranularity with reduced nuclear lobulation. Bleeding and infection may occur in severe cases.

The marrow is usually hypercellular and shows abnormal cellular and nuclear maturation with evidence of ineffective haemopoiesis and intra-medullary cell death (i.e. dysplasia). Thus, despite apparent increased cellular activity, output of blood cells is reduced. In around 10% of cases, the marrow is hypocellular; here, there is overlap with aplastic anaemia.

An abnormal karyotype is found in at least one-half of primary cases and 85%–90% of secondary cases and generally has an adverse effect on prognosis. Over 600 different cytogenetic abnormalities have been described, although only a few occur commonly.

Box 288.1 The World Health Organization classification of myelodysplasia (2008)

Refractory cytopenia with unilineage dysplasia (RCUD)
Refractory anemia with ring sideroblasts (RARS)
Refractory cytopenia with multilineage dysplasia (RCMD)
Refractory anemia with excess blasts-1 (RAEB-1) (<5% marrow blasts)
Refractory anemia with excess blasts-2 (RAEB-2) (5–19% marrow blasts)
Myelodysplastic syndrome—unclassified (MDS-U)
MDS associated with isolated del(5q)

Reprinted from Blood, Volume 114, issue 5, Vardiman et al., The 2008 revision of the World Health Organization (WHO) classification of myeloid neoplasms and acute leukemia: rationale and important changes, pp. 937-951. Copyright (2009) World Health Organization

Translocations are rare: the commonest affect Chromosome 8 (gain), Chromosome 5 (deletion or loss), and Chromosome 7 (deletion or loss). There is a tendency for abnormalities to accumulate as the disease progresses, and complex (multiple) abnormalities carry a worse prognosis. Isolated deletion of the long arm of Chromosome 5—del(5q)—is associated with a specific form of refractory anaemia characterized by a high prevalence in elderly females and a relatively good prognosis. It is characterized by a macrocytic anaemia, a normal or high platelet count, a modest leucopenia without excess blasts in the marrow, and a particular megakaryocyte appearance.

The risk of leukaemic transformation is about 30% overall in primary myelodysplasia but much higher in secondary cases. Leukaemia occurs less often and at a later stage in the 'refractory anaemia' subgroup. Acute myeloid leukaemia arising from myelodysplasia responds very poorly to chemotherapy, and cure is realistically only feasible following allogeneic bone marrow transplantation.

Treatment is supportive in the early stages, with blood and platelet transfusion and prompt treatment of infection as required. Erythropoietin may help the anaemia in some patients. The thalidomide analogue lenalidomide has shown a beneficial effect on anaemia in ~80% of patients with del(5q) and in ~50% of other low-risk patients. Cytotoxic therapy is inappropriate (and usually harmful) in most cases unless acute leukaemia develops, and is usually unsuccessful when it does. An exception may be younger patients (less than 65 years) who have a suitable donor, in which case they should be considered for bone marrow transplantation.

Further Reading

Adès L, Itzykson R, and Fenaux P. Myelodysplastic syndromes. *Lancet* 2014; 383: 2239–52.
Bulycheva E, Rauner M, Medyouf H, et al. Myelodysplasia is in the niche: Novel concepts and emerging therapies. *Leukemia* 2015; 29: 259–68.

289 Lymphoma

Graham Collins and Chris Bunch

Definition of the disease

Lymphoma is a cancerous disorder characterized by a clonal proliferation of lymphocytes. There are two broad categories: Hodgkin lymphoma and non-Hodgkin lymphoma (NHL), with Hodgkin lymphoma defined by the presence of Reed–Sternberg cells on histological examination of affected tissue. Within the NHLs, there are the much more common B-cell lymphomas and the uncommon T-cell lymphomas. Within the B-cell non-Hodgkin lymphomas, there are clinically aggressive (high-grade) forms and much more indolent (low-grade) forms.

Aetiology of the disease

In most cases of lymphoma, no cause can be identified. Less often, one or more of the following factors may be involved:

- infectious agents
- immunosuppression
- inflammatory conditions

Infectious agents

Infectious agents associated with lymphoma include:

- HIV
- EBV
- *Helicobacter pylori*
- other agents

HIV

HIV infection is associated with a much higher incidence of high-grade B-cell lymphomas such as diffuse large B-cell lymphoma, Burkitt's lymphoma, and primary CNS lymphoma. There is also a more moderate association with Hodgkin lymphoma. In some cases, HIV infection predisposes to co-infection with other viruses such as EBV, which are thought to be directly involved in lymphomagenesis.

EBV

EBV infection is associated with 100% of cases of endemic Burkitt lymphoma (a condition predominantly affecting African children) and around 50% of cases of Hodgkin lymphoma in developed countries. It is also linked with other types of lymphoma such as diffuse large B-cell lymphoma in the elderly, and lymphomas arising in the setting of immunosuppression such as HIV infection or following organ transplantation.

Helicobacter pylori

Infection with *Helicobacter pylori* is associated with a low-grade B-cell lymphoma called gastric MALT (**m**ucosa-**a**ssociated **l**ymphoid **t**issue) lymphoma. In some cases, eradication of the infection is sufficient to cure the lymphoma.

Other agents

Human T-lymphotropic virus 1 is associated with adult T-cell leukaemia/lymphoma. Hepatitis C has been associated with some cases of splenic marginal zone lymphoma (a low-grade B-cell NHL). *Campylobacter jejuni* has been implicated in immunoproliferative small intestinal disease (otherwise known as alpha-heavy chain disease), and *Chlamydia psittaci* has been linked with ocular adnexal MALT lymphoma (although this is controversial).

Immunosuppression

Lymphoma is associated with the following immunosuppressive conditions:

- HIV infection
- immunosuppression following organ transplantation; this may lead in some cases to clonal outgrowth of EBV-infected B-cells which are no longer inhibited by the host's T-cell response, leading to post-transplant lymphoproliferative disease
- other, rare, immunosuppressive conditions (e.g. common variable immunodeficiency, X-linked lymphoproliferative syndrome, and Wiskott–Aldrich syndrome)

Inflammatory conditions

Other MALT lymphomas are associated with organ-specific autoimmune conditions such as Hashimoto's thyroiditis (which may give rise to thyroid MALT lymphoma) and Sjögren's syndrome (which may give rise to a salivary or lacrimal gland MALT lymphoma).

Typical symptoms of the disease, and less common symptoms

Lymphoma usually presents in one of two main ways:

- lymph node enlargement
- systemic symptoms

Lymph node enlargement

Lymph node enlargement may present either as a lump (if the node is superficial) or with symptoms due to compression of surrounding structures. In these cases, mediastinal nodal enlargement may present with cough, breathlessness, or superior vena cava obstruction; porta hepatis nodal enlargement may present with obstructive jaundice; and pelvic nodal enlargement may present with a deep vein thrombosis or bilateral lower limb oedema.

Systemic symptoms

Common symptoms include fatigue, anorexia, weight loss, fever, and night sweats. Pruritus is also not uncommon, and alcohol-induced pain is a rare but characteristic feature of lymphoid malignancy.

Lymphoma may, however, present in any number of ways, depending mainly on the sites of involvement. For example, involvement of the gastrointestinal tract may lead to gastrointestinal bleeding, CNS involvement may lead to headaches and focal neurological symptoms, and bone involvement may cause a pathological fracture. Less common systemic effects of lymphomas are also well documented, including a paraprotein-induced peripheral neuropathy and a nephrotic syndrome caused by unknown mechanisms.

Demographics of the disease

The incidence of lymphoma is roughly 19 per 100 000 of the population per year, representing the fifth most common form of cancer. Overall, the incidence of lymphoma increases with age. However, Hodgkin lymphoma peaks in the 20–35 age group. Lymphoma in children is uncommon but, when it occurs, it is usually either Hodgkin's lymphoma (especially in adolescents) or high-grade B-cell lymphomas. Overall, lymphoma is 50% more common in men and affects white Americans 50% more than black Americans.

Table 289.1 Natural history and response to treatment of the various broad categories of lymphoma

	Hodgkin lymphoma	Low-grade B-cell non-Hodgkin lymphoma	High-grade B-cell non-Hodgkin lymphoma	Systemic T-cell non-Hodgkin lymphoma
Disease tempo	Usually fairly rapid	Indolent	Rapid	Rapid
Life expectancy with no treatment	Months to years	Often several years	Months	Months
Cure rate with chemotherapy	>75%	<20%	50%–60%	<20%

Certain lymphoma subtypes have a strong geographical association. For example, endemic Burkitt lymphoma is found almost exclusively in equatorial Africa, whereas adult T-cell leukaemia/lymphoma is most common in Japan and the Caribbean basin. These locations are thought to provide exposure to specific etiological factors.

Natural history, and complications of the disease

Table 289.1 illustrates the fact that, although indolent, low-grade B-cell lymphomas are relatively resistant to chemotherapy, the majority of high-grade B-cell NHLs can be cured. A proportion of indolent lymphomas will, however, undergo a large-cell transformation and then behave as aggressive, high-grade lymphomas. Systemic T-cell lymphomas are usually rapidly progressive and generally respond poorly to treatment. Cutaneous T-cell lymphomas (which will not be dealt with further) often have excellent outcomes, however.

Approach to diagnosing the disease

Lymphoma should be suspected in any patient with lymphadenopathy persisting for more than 6 weeks; or with persisting systemic symptoms with no other identifiable cause (including pruritus).

In a patient suspected of having a lymphoma, the following principles of diagnosis should be adhered to:

- CT and/or PET scanning of the chest, abdomen, and pelvis may show up areas of disease that are not detected on clinical examination and may facilitate biopsy; it is also required to stage the disease
- biopsy material should, where possible, be obtained from an affected lymph node or extra-nodal mass; bone marrow biopsy is a much less sensitive technique for both diagnosing and subtyping the disease
- a biopsy should be either an excision of an affected lymph node (most preferable) or a core biopsy; fine-needle aspiration does not provide sufficient material to diagnose, or exclude, lymphoma
- blood tests are helpful in assessing prognostic factors but are rarely helpful in diagnosing lymphoma; in particular, a raised lactate dehydrogenase (LDH) is very non-specific and is in no way diagnostic of an underlying lymphoma

Other diagnoses that should be considered

Lymphoma can mimic many other diseases. In particular, when a patient presents with generalized lymphadenopathy, the following conditions should be considered:

- viral infections (e.g. EBV, CMV, HIV)
- other infections (e.g. toxoplasmosis, tuberculosis, cat scratch disease)
- generalized skin diseases (e.g. eczema, which causes dermatopathic lymphadenopathy)
- autoimmune conditions (e.g. SLE, rheumatoid arthritis, sarcoidosis)
- other malignancy (usually cause is local lymphadenopathy)
- Kikuchi's disease (necrotizing lymphadenitis)

'Gold-standard' diagnostic test

The gold-standard diagnostic test for lymphoma is an excision nodal biopsy or a core biopsy of affected tissue.

Acceptable diagnostic alternatives to the gold standard

There is really no alternative to obtaining good quality biopsy material. Occasionally, the diagnosis can be made on bone marrow trephine only but biopsy of a lymph node or extra-nodal mass is usually preferable first.

Other relevant investigations

Other relevant investigations for lymphoma include:

- a full blood count: to detect bone marrow infiltration; occasionally, lymphoma cells circulate in the blood and can be identified using flow cytometry
- biochemistry: depending on the site of involvement, lymphoma can affect many biochemical parameters
- serum LDH: a raised LDH is a poor prognostic factor
- serum protein electrophoresis: some lymphomas are associated with a paraprotein
- beta-2 microglobulin: raised levels are associated with a worse prognosis
- HIV test: some lymphomas are associated with underlying HIV infection
- CMV, EBV, and toxoplasma serology: to exclude these common infections from the differential
- antinuclear antibodies: to exclude SLE from the differential
- ECG: in preparation for receiving anthracycline-containing chemotherapy regimens
- echocardiography: if the ECG is abnormal or there is a cardiac history (to assess suitability for anthracyclines)
- chest X-ray: to detect mediastinal masses, which are not uncommon in lymphoma
- CT and/or PET of chest/abdomen/pelvis: to stage the disease
- bone marrow trephine: to stage the disease

Prognosis and how to estimate it

In NHL, prognosis is estimated by the International Prognostic Index (IPI). An individual patient scores a point for each of the following:

- age > 60
- Stage III or IV
- LDH above the upper limit of normal
- two or more extra-nodal sites
- ECOG performance status ≥2

Table 289.2 outlines how the final score relates to the prognosis of the commonest type of high grade B-cell NHL: diffuse large B-cell lymphoma treated with R-CHOP chemotherapy which is the gold standard chemotherapy regimen for this disease. This is called the Revised-IPI score (R-IPI) since it has been modified from the original IPI score which was published prior to the routine use of rituximab.

Table 289.2 Association of international prognostic scoring system with 5-year survival in patients with diffuse large B-cell lymphoma treated with CHOP chemotherapy

Score	Prognostic group	4 year overall survival when treated with RCHOP (%)
0	very good risk	94% 4y overall survival
1, 2	good risk	79% 4y overall survival
3, 4, 5	poor risk	55% 4y overall survival

Note: The addition of rituximab has significantly improved the 5-year survival rates in each prognostic category.

Modifications of the IPI have been used to stratify prognosis in low-grade B-cell NHLs such as follicular lymphoma and mantle cell lymphoma. In the low-grade conditions, average life expectancy is typically on the order of 12–15 years.

Treatment and its effectiveness

Treatment of Hodgkin lymphoma

Treatment is generally with combination chemotherapy regimens such as ABVD (**a**driamycin® [doxorubicin], **b**leomycin, **v**inblastine, and **d**acarbazine). Important side effects include neuropathy (from the vinblastine) and lung toxicity (from the bleomycin). Fertility is usually preserved. Adjunctive involved field radiotherapy may be used at sites of bulk disease or at extra-nodal sites. Overall long-term survival rates are in excess of 80%. Due to the high survival rates, concern has shifted to the late toxic effects of treatment. In particular, rates of heart disease and second malignancies are raised in survivors of Hodgkin's lymphoma. Efforts are being made to reduce toxicity of treatment while maintaining the excellent disease control.

Relapsed Hodgkin lymphoma is treated where possible with salvage chemotherapy (consisting of different agents from those initially used to minimize the effects of drug resistance). If the disease remains chemo-responsive, the patient usually receives high-dose chemotherapy with autologous stem cell support. This procedure enables high-dose chemotherapy to be given while minimizing the resulting period of myelosuppression. Cure rates in the relapsed setting are on the order of 40%–60%.

Treatment of high-grade B-cell NHL

The standard treatment for the commonest form of high-grade B-cell NHL is R-CHOP chemotherapy (rituximab combined with cyclophosphamide, doxorubicin, vincristine, and prednisolone). CHOP has been in use since the 1980s, and efforts to improve its efficacy have not been successful until the introduction of the anti-CD20 monoclonal antibody rituximab. The addition of rituximab to CHOP is associated with increased overall survival rates of high-grade B-cell NHL in nearly all patient groups tested. As for Hodgkin lymphoma, involved field radiotherapy is used in some centres to sites of bulky or extra-nodal disease.

Relapsed high-grade B-cell NHL is still considered potentially curable with non-cross-reactive chemotherapy, which is often based on a platinum drug such as cisplatin. In patients who are fit enough, second remissions are then consolidated with high-dose chemotherapy combined with autologous stem cell support. If patients are not deemed fit enough to undergo this procedure, a palliative approach is frequently adopted.

Treatment of low-grade B-cell NHL

Low-grade B-cell NHL is generally considered incurable apart from in a minority of patients who can undergo an allogeneic stem cell transplant. Therefore, the aim of treatment is to keep the patient as healthy as possible for as long as possible. Initiation of treatment is only indicated for symptoms or critical organ impairment such as bone marrow failure. This means that early stage disease is often managed with a 'watch and wait' policy whereby no active treatment is given. This can be psychologically difficult for a patient who has recently been diagnosed with 'cancer'. When treatment is indicated, chemotherapy combined with rituximab is given. The chemotherapy is often in the form of CHOP or related regimens such as CVP (**c**yclophosphamide, **v**incristine, and **p**rednisolone). As for high-grade disease, the addition of rituximab has been demonstrated to improve responses and survival.

Subsequent relapses are treated with further rounds of chemotherapy, although subsequent remissions tend to be of reducing duration. Certain interventions may prolong subsequent remissions, such as the use of high-dose chemotherapy with autologous stem cell support, the use of maintenance rituximab infusions, or the use of radioimmunotherapy (which utilizes a monoclonal antibody conjugated to a radioisotope).

T-cell NHL

Systemic T-cell lymphomas are aggressive and are associated with poor treatment outcomes (except anaplastic large-cell lymphoma associated with the expression of anaplastic lymphoma kinase). Treatment is generally with CHOP chemotherapy. Although initial responses are often seen, relapses are frequent and difficult to treat. Experimental approaches are being investigated.

Further Reading

Armitage JO, Gascoyne RD, Lunning MA et al. Non-Hodgkin lymphoma. *Lancet* 2017; 390: 298–310.

Guidelines of the British Committee for Standards in Haematology (http://www.bcshguidelines.com)

Shankland KR, Armitage JO, and Hancock BW. Non-Hodgkin lymphoma. *Lancet* 2012; 380: 848–57.

Townsend W and Linch D. Hodgkin's lymphoma in adults. *Lancet* 2012; 380: 836–47.

290 Multiple myeloma and related conditions

Graham Collins and Chris Bunch

Definition of the disease

Multiple myeloma is a cancerous disorder of the bone marrow and arises from a clonal proliferation of plasma cells, resulting in end-organ damage (e.g. renal failure, hypercalcaemia, bone disease, and bone marrow failure). When a plasma cell clone is only detected in one site (either bony or soft tissue), it is termed a plasmacytoma. Monoclonal gammopathy of uncertain significance (MGUS) is also a clonal proliferation of plasma cells but, by definition, does not result in end-organ damage. Primary amyloidosis is dealt with in Chapter 181.

Aetiology of the disease

Cumulative exposure to ionizing radiation increases the risk of myeloma. Exposure to certain chemicals, such as dioxin and other pesticides, also increases the risk. However, in most cases, no etiological agent can be identified.

Typical symptoms of the disease, and less common symptoms

Associated symptoms are either due to the local effect of malignant plasma cells or due to the effect of the monoclonal immunoglobulin produced (see Table 290.1)

Demographics of the disease

Incidence

MGUS is relatively common, with a monoclonal paraprotein being present in 3% of those over 70. Myeloma is the second most common haematological malignancy (after non-Hodgkin's lymphoma), with an incidence in the UK of 4–5 cases per 100 000 per year.

Age

Myeloma is a disease of the elderly, with the peak incidence occurring at 65–70 years of age.

Gender difference

Myeloma is nearly twice as common in men as it is in women.

Racial variations

Myeloma is more common in African Americans than in Caucasians.

Natural history and complications of the disease

Although chemo-responsive in the majority of patients, myeloma is generally considered to be incurable. Until recently, the average life expectancy for those with myeloma was 3–4 years. The introduction of new agents which have proven activity in this condition is thought to extend life expectancy, although the follow-up has not been long enough to determine their precise impact. Complications are related to the disease process itself and the effect of treatment. Renal failure is common at presentation but less common in subsequent phases of the disease. Bone disease with or without fractures or hypercalcaemia frequently occurs with disease progression. Other particularly common complications include:

- infections:
  - myeloma is associated with immunoparesis (i.e. panhypogammaglobulinaemia) due to replacement of normal plasma cells by malignant, clonal plasma cells; this results in increased infection risk, especially with pneumonia
  - treatment is also immunosuppressive and can substantially increase risk of infection; for example, long-term, high-dose steroid treatment is associated with *Pneumocystis jiroveci*

Table 290.1 Myeloma symptoms due to the local presence of malignant plasma cells or due to monoclonal immunoglobulins produced by the malignant plasma cells

Symptoms due to the local presence of malignant plasma cells	Symptoms due to monoclonal immunoglobulins produced by malignant plasma cells
Bone disease, causing: • generalized osteopenia (which is in itself asymptomatic) • lytic lesions (may be asymptomatic or painful) • pathological fractures; most commonly vertebral (causing back pain)	Renal failure (most common cause being cast nephropathy due to precipitation of light chains; can also be caused by light chain deposition disease, amyloid deposition, NSAID ingestion due to pain, or sepsis)
Bone marrow failure, causing: • anaemia (fatigue, shortness of breath, headaches, palpitations) • leucopenia (infections) • thrombocytopenia (bleeding)	Amyloid deposition, causing: • nephrotic syndrome • heart failure • neuropathy • organomegaly
Hypercalcaemua, causing: • polyuria and polydipsia • constipation and abdominal pain • confusion • renal failure	Less commonly, the monoclonal immunoglobulin may cause an autoimmune condition such as acquired von Willebrand's disease, paraprotin-associated neuropathy, or acquired C1 esterase inhibitor deficiency; these syndromes may be associated with underlying myeloma or monoclonal gammopathy of unknown significance
Immunoparesis increases susceptibility to infections, especially by encapsulated organisms such as penumococcus	

infection, and alkylating agents frequently used in this disorder cause myelosuppression and possibly neutropenia, increasing the risk of bacterial and fungal infections

- neuropathy:
  - many of the treatments for myeloma can cause neuropathy, especially thalidomide and bortezomib
  - amyloid deposition frequently affects the nerves, causing a peripheral neuropathy, often with autonomic involvement
  - occasionally, the monoclonal immunoglobulin can possess auto-immune activity against nerve components, causing a peripheral neuropathy
- spinal cord compression:
  - due to bone disease and resulting in vertebral fracture
  - symptoms usually include back pain; weakness and paraesthesiae in the legs; and bowel and bladder dysfunction
  - urgent radiotherapy or surgical decompression is indicated
- venous thromboembolism (VTE):
  - any malignancy is associated with an increased risk of VTE; however, an additional increase in risk is observed when myeloma is treated with thalidomide or lenalidomide
  - prophylactic anticoagulation is indicated, with aspirin, heparin, or warfarin
- anaemia:
  - this is often multifactorial
  - the presence of malignant plasma cells in the bone marrow can cause a degree of myelosuppression
  - renal impairment leads to a reduced erythropoietin level, and underlying chronic infection can lead to anaemia of chronic disease

Approach to diagnosing the disease

Myeloma should be considered in the presence of the following:

- pathological fractures (especially vertebral)
- acute renal failure (especially in the context of a high or normal calcium)
- hypercalcaemia
- recurrent infections
- unexplained anaemia, with or without other cytopenias
- the finding of a serum or urine paraprotein

Other diagnoses that should be considered

The differential diagnosis for myeloma is broad and relates to the presenting features:

- bony pains: consider other malignant conditions or musculoskeletal pathologies
- hypercalcaemia: consider other malignant conditions or hyperparathyroidism
- bone marrow failure: consider other infiltrative conditions of the bone marrow, or primary bone marrow disorders
- recurrent infections: consider other causes of acquired immunodeficiency

An important differential of a paraprotein is an alternative lymphoproliferative condition such as a low-grade lymphoma. Although IgG paraproteins can be associated with myeloma or lymphomas, an IgM paraprotein is almost never associated with myeloma.

'Gold-standard' diagnostic test

Bone marrow aspirate and trephine will usually diagnose myeloma, with more than 10% plasma cells considered diagnostic in the appropriate clinical context. However, myeloma can be a patchy disease, so false negatives are not uncommon.

An isolated plasmacytoma can only be accurately diagnosed by biopsy of the affected region.

MGUS can be accurately diagnosed in patients with a small paraprotein in the absence of end-organ damage.

Acceptable diagnostic alternatives to the gold standard

A diagnosis of myeloma is highly suggestive in the presence of a significant paraprotein detected on serum protein or urine electrophoresis; note that 15%–20% of cases are associated with a urine paraprotein in the absence of a serum paraprotein.

Rarely, myeloma is not associated with a paraprotein (so-called non-secretory myeloma). In most of these cases, a monoclonal free light chain can be detected in the serum by using the Freelite assay.

Lytic lesions demonstrated on plain imaging (usually a skeletal survey) or on MRI are suggestive but other malignancies can produce similar findings.

Note that a bone scan is not an appropriate investigation, as lytic lesions usually appear as 'cold' due to the suppression of osteoblast activity by the malignant plasma cells. For similar reasons, levels of alkaline phosphatase in the bone are normal in the presence of lytic lesions, unless a fracture has occurred.

Other relevant investigations

Other relevant investigations for myeloma include:

- a full blood count: to detect bone marrow failure
- urea and electrolytes: to assess for renal impairment
- calcium: to assess for hypercalcaemia
- beta-2 microglobulin: a raised level suggests poor prognosis disease
- serum albumin: a low level suggests poor prognosis disease
- 24-hour urine collection for quantification of Bence Jones proteinuria: a baseline is required to properly assess response to treatment
- free light chain assay can detect light chain only myeloma which is otherwise missed on a serum electrophoresis
- subcutaneous fat biopsy: if amyloid is suspected
- ECG/echocardiogram: to assess for cardiac amyloid if clinically suspected
- bone marrow cytogenetics: may have prognostic significance

Prognosis, and how to estimate it

The International Staging System (ISS) for myeloma was published in 2005 and replaces the complex Durie–Salmon staging system previously in place. The ISS divides patients into three stages at presentation, based on serum albumin and beta-2 microglobulin levels. Patients with a serum albumin level ≥35 g/l and a beta-2 microglobulin level <3.5 mg/l are in the most favourable prognostic group, with a median survival of 62 months, while those with a serum beta 2-microglobulin ≥5.5 mg/l are in the least favourable, with a median survival of 29 months.

Cytogenetics is increasingly being used to determine prognostic groups. Monosomy 13 and translocations involving Chromosome 14 are associated with a poor prognosis.

Treatment and its effectiveness

In the presence of established end-organ damage, treatment is indicated. This is usually in the form of combination chemotherapy, which frequently includes:

- a corticosteroid, such as dexamethasone or prednisolone
- an alkylating agent, such as cyclophosphamide or melphalan
- thalidomide
- bortezomib containing regimes (see below)

Thalidomide-containing regimens are associated with an increased risk of VTE, and suitable prophylaxis should be considered (usually in the form of prophylactic- or treatment-dose heparin or adjusted-dose warfarin).

In fit patients, remissions are frequently consolidated with high-dose chemotherapy with autologous stem cell support, which, in the majority of trials, is associated with an increase in life expectancy by about 1 year. Subsequent treatments include bortezomib (a proteasome inhibitor) and lenalidomide (an immunomodulatory agent). Bortezomib containing regimens are also being used more commonly in the front line setting especially for patients with renal impairment or high risk cytogenetics. Recently, the anti-CD38 antibody daratumumab has found to have significant activity in myeloma and is likely to play a role in future treatment regimens.

Radiotherapy is indicated for localized painful disease or for spinal cord compression. Surgical decompression is also appropriate for some cases of spinal cord compression.

In young patients with a suitable donor, allogeneic stem cell transplant may be considered as a potentially curative strategy.

This procedure is, however, associated with significant morbidity and mortality.

Further Reading

Bird JM, Owen RG, D'Sa SD, et al. *Guidelines for the Diagnosis and Management of Multiple Myeloma 2014* (http://www.bcshguidelines.com).

Rollig C, Knop S, and Bornhauser M. Multiple myeloma. *Lancet* 2015; 385: 2197–208.

291 Myeloproliferative disorders

Graham Collins and Chris Bunch

Definition of the disease

Myeloproliferative disorders (also called myeloproliferative neoplasms) can be defined as clonal haematopoietic disorders resulting in excess production of one or more blood cell lineage. The four main conditions are:

- primary polycythaemia, which is characterized by excess red-cell production
- essential thrombocythaemia, which is characterized by excess platelet production
- chronic myeloid leukaemia, which is characterized by excess granulocyte production
- myelofibrosis, which is characterized by excess megakaryocyte proliferation which results in a reactive fibroblast proliferation, causing marrow fibrosis and failure

Chronic myeloid leukaemia will not be discussed further in this chapter—see Chapter 287.

Aetiology of the disease

Apart from exposure to radiation, no causative factors for the myeloproliferative disorders being discussed here have been identified. However, much progress into their pathogenesis has been made in recent years. In 2005, several groups reported the finding of a mutation in the gene encoding the signalling protein JAK2 in the majority of cases of primary polycythaemia. Since then, it has also become clear that the same mutation is found in approximately 50% of cases of essential thrombocythaemia and myelofibrosis. JAK2 is normally involved in mediating a proliferative response of red-cell precursors to the binding of erythropoietin to its surface membrane receptor. The single base pair mutation (V617F) produces a constitutively active tyrosine kinase which delivers a proliferative signal to the cell irrespective of erythropoietin binding. Further work on primary polycythaemia has shown that, in almost all of the rare V617F-negative cases, a different activating JAK2 mutation is present within Exon 12 of the gene. Subsequent analysis of other candidate genes in essential thrombocythaemia has identified an activating mutation in the gene encoding the thrombopoietin receptor (MPL) to be present in about 3%–4% of mostly JAK2-negative cases. Most recently, groups have identified mutation in the last exon of the gene encoding Calreticulin as the most common mutation in Jak2 wild type and MPL negative essential thrombocythaemia and myelofirbosis. This makes it the second commonest mutation in these disorders.

Despite the progress made, many unanswered questions remain. It is unclear why an identically mutated JAK2 gene produces primary polycythaemia in some patients but essential thrombocythaemia or myelofibrosis in others. It may be to do with the cell in which the mutation first occurred, the genetic background of the patient, or the extent to which the JAK2 protein becomes activated. There is also convincing data that, in some patients, there is a pre-JAK2 event resulting in a pool of cells which would only go on to produce a myeloproliferative disorder if JAK2 becomes mutated.

Typical symptoms of the disease, and less common symptoms

In recent years, many patients are presenting with no symptoms. Rather, abnormal blood counts have been detected from blood tests taken for an unrelated reason. When symptoms do occur, they can be thought of as:

- symptoms due to a hypercatabolic state (e.g. weight loss, anorexia, night sweats, gout due to hyperuricaemia)

- symptoms due to raised red cells or platelets (e.g. pruritus (typically after a hot bath), erythromelalgia (painful discolouration of the extremities), headaches, visual disturbances, dizziness, venous or arterial thrombosis); in essential thrombocythaemia, bleeding may also occur which is thought to be due to a low level of circulating von Willebrand factor, secondary to adsorption of this factor onto the increased platelet surface area

It is important to be aware that the red cells and/or platelets being produced are not functionally normal. They are often more thrombogenic than their normal counterparts; this explains why a raised platelet count due to a reactive phenomenon almost never predisposes to thrombosis, whereas a raised platelet count due to essential thrombocythaemia certainly does.

Myelofibrosis often presents rather differently from essential thrombocythaemia or primary polycythaemia. Due to marrow fibrosis, patients offer suffer symptoms from bone marrow failure, especially anaemia. Breathlessness and fatigue are common. Extra-medullary haematopoiesis causes a very large spleen which can cause symptoms such as early satiety, abdominal distension, and haemorrhoids.

Demographics of the disease

Collectively, myeloproliferative disorders are uncommon. The total incidence is approximately 3–5 in 100 000 per year. Generally, they are regarded as conditions which increase with age, although childhood cases are well recognized.

Primary polycythaemia and myelofibrosis are more common in men; essential thrombocythaemia is more common in women. The most common myeloproliferative disorder is essential thrombocythaemia, with primary polycythaemia being the next commonest, and myelofibrosis being very rare.

Natural history and complications of the disease

Primary polycythaemia, essential thrombocythaemia, and myelofibrosis are biologically related conditions. As such, they can evolve into one another. Approximately 5% of patients with an original diagnosis of essential thrombocythaemia will develop a raised red-cell count that puts them into the diagnostic category of primary polycythaemia. Although, by definition, primary polycythaemia does not formally evolve into essential thrombocythaemia, a substantial proportion of patients with primary polycythaemia will present with or subsequently develop a raised platelet count which needs treating. Myelofibrosis is thought by some as the inevitable outcome of primary polycythaemia or essential thrombocythaemia, given enough time. However, the time to myelofibrosis can be very long, meaning that only approximately 5%–10% of cases will develop clinically significant marrow fibrosis.

The most feared complication of the myeloproliferative disorders, however, is acute myeloid leukaemia. Happily, the incidence of acute myeloid leukaemia in patients with primary polycythaemia and essential thrombocythaemia is low (approximately 1%–3% lifetime risk). However, for myelofibrosis, this rises to around 20%–30%.

Approach to diagnosing the disease

For primary polycythaemia and essential thrombocythaemia, the approach to diagnosis should involve a thorough history and examination to exclude secondary causes of a high haematocrit or platelet count respectively. Specific investigations should then be performed to come up with a definitive diagnosis.

Other diagnoses that should be considered

Secondary causes for a raised haematocrit or a raised platelet count should always be considered.

Secondary causes of a raised haematocrit

Secondary causes of a raised haematocrit include:

- relative erythrocytosis due to plasma volume contraction seen with high alcohol intake, diuretic use, and stressful lifestyle factors
- absolute erythrocytosis due to appropriately raised serum erythropoietin:
  - severe lung disease with associated hypoxia
  - cyanotic congenital heart disease (e.g. tetralogy of Fallot)
  - living at a high altitude
  - sleep apnoea
- absolute erythrocytosis due to inappropriately raised serum erythropoietin:
  - renal disease: renal cell carcinoma, renal cysts, diffuse parenchymal disease, renal artery stenosis, post renal transplant
  - other tumours: Wilms' tumour, lymphoma, cerebellar haemangioblastoma, hepatoma
- absolute erythrocytosis due to other drugs:
  - androgens
- absolute erythrocytosis due to genetic conditions:
  - high-affinity haemoglobins
  - activating erythropoietin receptor mutations
  - Chuvash polycythaemia

Secondary causes of a raised platelet count

Secondary causes of a raised platelet count include:

- infections: especially occult abscess, TB
- inflammatory conditions (e.g. lupus, rheumatoid arthritis)
- underlying malignancy
- iron deficiency

Other primary haematological disorders can also present with a raised platelet count. These include the other myeloproliferative conditions, such as primary polycythaemia, chronic myeloid leukaemia, and myelofibrosis , and certain forms of myelodysplastic conditions.

'Gold-standard' diagnostic test

The finding of an activating JAK2 mutation (V617F or an Exon 12 mutation) in the context of a raised haematocrit (>0.52 in men; >0.48 in women) or raised platelet count (≥450 × 10^9/l) is the current gold standard for diagnosis of primary polycythaemia and essential thrombocythaemia respectively. It ET and MF which are negative for Jak2, mutations in the MPL gene and Calreticulin gene can also confirm the diagnosis. For myelofibrosis, the result of a bone marrow biopsy is more crucial in the diagnosis. Findings of megakaryocytic proliferation and/or atypia plus increased marrow fibrosis in conjunction with an activating JAK2 mutation or other clonal marker is diagnostic of myelofibrosis.

Acceptable diagnostic alternatives to the gold standard

Diagnostic criteria for primary polycythaemia and essential thrombocythaemia where the JAK2 mutations is either negative or unavailable are published.

For primary polycythaemia, the first step is to prove that the raised haematocrit is due to an absolute erythrocytosis (as opposed to a relative erythrocytosis). A haematocrit of ≥0.60 in a man and ≥0.56 in a woman cannot be due to plasma volume depletion and is diagnostic of an absolute erythrocytosis. In patients with raised values less than these levels, a red-cell mass analysis has to be performed which must show a mass of >25% above predicted. Secondary causes must then be excluded and, if these patients also have a palpable spleen or a cytogenetic abnormality on bone marrow aspirate, then the diagnosis is secure. If neither of these last two conditions is met, other supportive criteria are needed, such as a raised platelet count, a raised neutrophil count, or radiological evidence of splenomegaly.

For JAK2-negative essential thrombocythaemia, which are also negative for MPL and calreticulin mutations, the first step in diagnosis is to exclude as far as possible secondary causes. These include inflammatory, infectious, or malignant conditions, iron deficiency, other myeloproliferative conditions such as primary polycythaemia, chronic myeloid leukaemia, and myelofibrosis and some cases of myelodysplastic conditions.

For myelofibrosis in the absence of a clonal marker such as an activating JAK2 mutation, the diagnosis is supported by the finding of a leucoerythroblastic blood film (in which circulating red- and white-cell precursors are observed), an increased serum lactate dehydrogenase, anaemia, and palpable splenomegaly.

Other relevant investigations

A blood film can be helpful in determining whether a high red-cell count or platelet count is primary or secondary. Features suggest of a myeloproliferative condition include marked variation in platelet size and a basophilia.

In some situations, a bone marrow trephine can provide useful evidence for a primary myeloproliferative condition.

Cytogenetic evaluation can provide evidence for myeloproliferative disorders and is also helpful in excluding other diagnoses such as the myelodysplastic syndrome known as 5q− syndrome.

The serum erythropoietin level can also sometimes be helpful in distinguishing between a primary and a secondary raised haematocrit. Primary polycythaemia is associated with a low erythropoietin level, whereas a high or inappropriately normal level can be associated with secondary causes.

An ultrasound scan of the abdomen can be helpful in detecting radiological enlargement of the spleen (a criterion for JAK2-negative primary polycythaemia diagnosis) and also to exclude renal cell carcinoma as a cause of secondary polycythaemia.

An oxygen saturation estimation and a chest X-ray may aid the diagnosis of a primary lung pathology leading to hypoxia and a raised haematocrit. Echocardiography may identify cyanotic congenital heart disease. A sleep study may be needed to diagnose sleep apnoea.

Exclusion of a secondary cause of thrombocytosis may require abdominal CT scanning in order to detect occult infection or abscess.

Prognosis and how to estimate it

For cases of primary polycythaemia and essential thrombocythaemia at diagnosis, the prognosis is excellent, although thrombotic risk is significantly raised. Life expectancy is roughly equivalent to the normal population. In the rare cases which transform to myelofibrosis or acute myeloid leukaemia, however, the prognosis is much worse. Transformation risk is increased by certain agents such as busulphan and ^{32}P. Hydroxycarbamide may be associated with a small increased risk of acute myeloid leukaemia, although this remains controversial. The platelet-lowering agent anagrelide is associated with a slightly increased risk of myelofibrosis.

In myelofibrosis, the prognosis is highly variable. Lower-risk patients have a median survival of around 12 years, whereas high-risk patients have a median survival of 2–3 years. A worse prognosis is associated with:

- age > 60
- abnormal karyotype of cytogenetic analysis
- presence of constitutional symptoms
- elevated white-cell count
- increased circulating immature precursors
- circulating blast cells

Treatment and its effectiveness

Treatment of primary polycythaemia

Reduction of the haematocrit is achieved by repeated venesections. In cases of primary polycythaemia, the target haematocrit is <0.45. Although there is little evidence to directly support this target, it reflects the fact that patients with primary polycythaemia are prothrombotic even when their haematocrit is in the upper end of the normal range. Recurrent venesections can lead to iron deficiency with increasing microcytosis. This, however, stabilizes the haematocrit and results in a reduction in the need for venesections. Iron supplementation should **not** be given, as this would lead to a rapid haematocrit rise, which would possibly be associated with thrombosis.

Aspirin should be given to all primary polycythaemia patients unless there is a contraindication. This practice is supported by randomized clinical trial evidence showing low-dose aspirin was associated with a reduction in thrombosis.

The platelet count should be controlled. Primary polycythaemia is often associated with thrombocytosis, which may need controlling in order to reduce thrombotic risk. This can be achieved using a gentle cytoreductive agent such as hydroxycarbamide.

In the elderly, control of the haematocrit and the platelet count can be achieved by administration of busulphan or ^{32}P. These both increase the long-term risk of acute leukaemia, which is less of a concern in the elderly.

Treatment of essential thrombocythaemia

Not all cases of essential thrombocythaemia require platelet-lowering therapy. In young patients (less than 60 years of age) with a platelet count of <1000 × 10^9/l and no history of major thrombosis or bleeding, such therapy is generally not indicated. In patients <60 years of age and with a predisposition to thrombosis or significant cardiovascular risk factors, platelet-lowering therapy may be indicated, as it may also be for patients with severe vasomotor symptoms despite antiplatelet therapy. However, there is little consensus on when to use platelet-lowering therapy in the more borderline cases. A target platelet count of <400 × 10^9/l should be used except when toxicity is a major issue. When platelet-lowering therapy is recommended, the following agents can be used:

- hydroxycarbamide
- anagrelide
- interferon alfa
- alkylating agents

Hydroxycarbamide

Hydroxycarbamide is cytoreductive and is generally well tolerated, although it may rarely cause ulceration. A raised mean corpuscular volume almost invariably occurs on this drug and is simply a reflection of its mechanism of action. Concerns have been raised over a slight increased risk of transformation to acute myeloid leukaemia. For this reason, interferon is often used initially in young patients.

Anagrelide

Anagrelide works specifically as an inhibitor of megakaryocyte proliferation and is effective at lowering platelet counts. In a randomized trial of hydroxycarbamide versus anagrelide in essential thrombocythaemia, anagrelide use was associated with a slightly increased risk of major bleeding and marrow fibrosis. However, both drugs were used with aspirin, and anagrelide is known to have an intrinsic antiplatelet effect which may account for the bleeding risk. Based on these results, anagrelide is generally used as a second- or subsequent-line agent. Palpitations are a frequent side effect, so anagrelide should be used cautiously in patients with a cardiac history.

Interferon alfa

Subcutaneous injection of interferon alfa at 3 × 10^6 to 6 × 10^6 units three times per week effectively controls platelet counts, splenomegaly, and constitutional symptoms associated with essential thrombocythaemia. However, it is expensive, inconvenient, and associated with sometimes severe side effects such as fatigue and depression. For this reason, use is usually limited to women who wish to have children, as this is considered the only safe agent to be on during pregnancy.

Alkylating agents

Alkylating agents (e.g. busulfhan) may be used in the elderly. The use of these agents is associated with an increased risk of transformation to acute leukaemia and they should not be used in younger patients.

Use of antiplatelet agents in patients with essential thrombocythaemia

Antiplatelet agents should be considered in all patients with essential thrombocythaemia who have no contraindications, although no randomized controlled trials exist for the use of this therapy. Results in primary polycythaemia are generally considered to also apply to essential thrombocythaemia. Antiplatelet agents should be used with caution in those with platelet counts >1500 × 10^9/l, as coexisting acquired von Willebrand's disease may greatly increase the bleeding risk.

Further Reading

Stein BL, Gotlib J, Arcasoy M, et al. Historical views, conventional approaches, and evolving management strategies for myeloproliferative neoplasms. *J Natl Compr Canc Netw* 2015; 13: 424–34.

Tefferi A and Pardanani A. Myeloproliferative neoplasms: A contemporary review. *JAMA Oncol* 2015; 1: 97–105.

Chandramouli Nagarajan

Introduction

Care of terminally ill haematology patients presents a unique challenge, due to the complexity of treatment decisions in an era of newly developing therapeutic options, and the speed of change in patients' condition from a potentially curable to a terminal phase. Terminal illness is defined as progressive disease for which curative treatment is neither possible nor appropriate and from which death is inevitable, although this may not be impending and the prognosis can vary from a few days to many months. The focus of this chapter is to try and bring together various palliative treatment options that should be made available to this cohort of patients with terminal disease.

Many forms of haematological cancers are treatable and, indeed, advances in treatment over the last two decades, such as the use of monoclonal antibodies, transfusion support, and stem cell transplantation, have made it possible to achieve cure in many types of leukaemias and lymphomas. The general principle in the treatment of most haematological malignancies is to get the disease into remission (remission induction) and then consolidate this with further treatment (chemotherapy, radiotherapy, or a stem cell transplant), either up front or when the disease relapses. Most cancers indeed go into a period of 'remission' for months to years but may relapse at any time. At this time, the disease will be reassessed (radiologically, repeat biopsies, cytogenetically as appropriate) and a decision on further treatment taken. Many young or fit elderly patients will go through further intensive or even escalated treatments with the aim of achieving a second remission but in others this may not be possible and the management has to be palliative. Some patients may go through such treatments and relapse again to reach a terminal phase either due to disease itself or due to treatment-related complications. It can be difficult to judge when to stop using intensive forms of treatment; clinicians, patients, and their families often find it difficult to acknowledge when remission induction is no longer possible. This is a complex decision that needs a careful reassessment of the patient's age, history, performance status, comorbid states, and tolerability of further available treatment options in the light of any organ dysfunction, balancing the risks of treatment against the benefits of and potential survival from the regime. The decision to change to a palliative approach may be taken too late or not at all, and persistence with aggressive treatment can cause great distress. This change in approach has to be sensitively, openly, and honestly discussed with the patient and family so that their aims and expectations are correctly set.

Management of patients during the last phase of their illness includes control of physical symptoms such as pain, nausea, and so on, as well as holistic attention to the psychosocial, cultural, spiritual, and social needs of the patient, with the aim of easing suffering and enabling dying patients to live and die with dignity, as well as offering support to their families and carers. Although much of the care is provided by palliative-care professionals, it is best delivered in an integrated multidisciplinary manner with close cooperation amongst haematologists, palliative-care doctors, nurses, psycho-oncologists, GPs, pain control teams, occupational therapists, alternative and complementary therapy practitioners, dieticians, and other clinical/primary-care support staff.

Uncontrolled symptoms in a terminally ill patient not only significantly impair the patient's quality of life but are also believed to impact on the family's subsequent resolution of grief. Hence, it is paramount to achieve symptom control by appropriate intervention (pharmacological, psychological, spiritual, etc.) and referral to specialists where symptoms prove difficult to control.

Common symptoms encountered in the terminal phase

Symptom control in terminal illness is dealt with in more detail elsewhere in this book, and the principles in terminal haematological illnesses are the same as in management of terminal care due any other malignancy.

Pain

Pain is a multidimensional symptom frequently feared by terminally ill patients, occurring in up to 75% of patients with advanced cancer. Uncontrollable pain can affect all aspects of a patient's life, impacting upon mood, family relations, social life, sleep, appetite, and so on. It is important to note that pain may not be directly related to tissue pathology, and its perception can be modified by various elements, including psychological factors.

Practically, it is useful to differentiate opioid responsive pain from opioid insensitive pain, such as neuropathic and bone pain. Management should start with simple non-opioid analgesics (e.g. NSAIDs, paracetamol), proceeding to weak opiates (e.g. codeine) and then to strong opiates (e.g. morphine, oxycodone) in accordance with the WHO analgesic ladder (see Chapter 329).

In some, management of pain in terminal illness can be complex and requires specialized assessment (e.g. pain control teams) and this ensures that most up-to-date evidence based treatments are offered. Where the oral route is not possible or dependable, syringe drivers can be used to deliver medications.

Nausea and vomiting

Nausea and vomiting are other common symptoms at the end of life, experienced by up to two-thirds of people dying of cancer. Diagnostic assessment and management are considered in detail elsewhere in this book. In addition to pharmacological measures, practical steps (e.g. well-presented, small portions of favourite foods eaten 'little and often'; cold, carbonated drinks; the avoidance of strong odours) also can help. Careful consideration of the route of anti-emetic (subcutaneous drivers) should be made when oral delivery is unreliable—such as in bowel obstruction or repeated vomiting.

Dyspnoea

The term 'dyspnoea' is defined by the American Thoracic Society as 'a subjective experience of breathing discomfort' (Rose, 1999, p. 3259). It can be a distressing symptom for dying patients. Although management depends on the cause, since further investigations to find a cause may not be appropriate, management sometimes has to be empiric. Patients with progressive haematological diseases may have bone marrow failure and resulting anaemia leading to dyspnoea and tiredness. Reversible causes of anaemia such as haematinic deficiencies must be looked for and treated. The decision to transfuse should be made on an individual basis after discussions with the patient and family, and these discussions should be regularly reviewed. The focus should be to improve symptoms and quality of life, with minimum adverse effects. It must be remembered, however, that, as the disease progresses, the degree of symptomatic improvement is likely to abate, and the increasing frequency of required transfusions may significantly impair any quality of life that the patient may have. Furthermore, transfusion is not without risks, such as circulatory overload and various transfusion reactions, to name but a few. Hence, regular discussions with patient and family must be undertaken not only to assess the response to transfusion but also to identify adverse effects on patient's quality of life.

The decision to discontinue transfusion support for a patient already on a transfusion programme is a difficult one but must be considered as a part of the management of these patients. The parameters that may guide one's decision to do so include:

- lack of symptomatic benefit from the intervention
- inability to keep up replacement with ongoing blood loss
- difficulty obtaining IV access
- difficulty in obtaining appropriate blood products due to antibodies

At each stage in the decision-making, the involvement of the patient and their family is important.

Opiates at much lower doses than are usually needed for analgesia can relieve the distress associated with dyspnoea. Oxygen is not indicated for every breathless patient and needs assessing on an individual basis. Avoidance/minimizing fluids may decrease and serve as treatment of pulmonary congestion and provide comfort. Treatment of other contributory factors like anxiety and pain can also decrease the feeling of dyspnoea. Patients with large pleural effusions should be considered for chest drains with pleurodesis.

Bleeding

Patients with bone marrow failure may have significant thrombocytopenia and, while some patients may be asymptomatic, some may have significant haemorrhagic symptoms. Prophylactic platelet transfusions in those with no bleeding symptoms are not recommended. Those with petechial rashes or minor nose or mouth bleeds can be managed with oral tranexamic acid or topical application using soaked gauze. Where patients have ongoing bleeding, platelet transfusions may be considered, to improve patient comfort and reduce distress. Patients with major haemorrhagic symptoms must be managed sensitively with appropriate sedation and analgesia as required, using dark-coloured blankets to reduce the distressing visual impact this may have on family and carers. Reassurance and explanation to patients and their families are paramount here.

Other symptoms in terminally ill patients

Fever sometimes associated with chills and sweating can occur due to cytokine release. Simple interventions like tepid sponging and using fans for cooling, as well as administering paracetamol, help relieve the distress associated with fever. NSAIDs may be used but are contraindicated in patients with renal impairment or thrombocytopenia.

Declining social and physical function due to debility and cachexia can be a source of significant discomfort to some of these patients. Reversible causes should be identified and treated (e.g. oro-mucosal candidiasis). Nutritional interventions may be indicated if appropriate, but artificial feeding is controversial and there is no evidence that it provides any comfort or clinical benefit. Families of dying patients may request this in the belief that it will provide comfort or may be due to cultural beliefs. On the other hand, cessation of eating and drinking is a normal part of dying and, by educating the families to understand this, their time and attention can be focused into providing other comforts.

Patients can become delirious due to medications, metabolic changes, infections, and so on. If an obvious reversible cause cannot be found, haloperidol at doses of 1.0–2.5 mg IV or subcutaneously can be used. Benzodiazepines are often ineffective and can potentially worsen delirium.

Psychological/emotional symptoms and their management

The recognition and discussions regarding the terminal phase of a patient's illness pose a considerable professional challenge but are central to enable the healthcare team to provide appropriate psychological support to the patient and family. This aspect of the terminal care is complex in that it is unique to each individual, and time must be allowed for the patient and family to express their feelings, expectations, and fears so that these can be dealt with sensitively. Haematology clinical nurse specialists are often well placed to support patients and their families, having supported them through the active phase of treatment, and often already have a good relationship with patients. Regular, clear communication between the medical team and patient as well as their family is crucial.

Alternative therapies

Complementary therapies such as acupuncture, spiritual healing, herbal medicine, massage, aromatherapy, reflexology, hypnosis, and meditation have all been applied in the palliative-care setting in managing difficult symptoms. The success rate of these therapies is variable but the side-effect profile tends to be low. The last decade has seen an increase in use and provision of complementary therapies, both within the hospital settings and within hospices. Careful consideration of patient's symptoms and referral to appropriate complementary health practitioners must form a part of the terminal care of patients willing to try these therapies.

Where to manage patients in the terminal phase

There are various settings in which patients can be managed in the terminal phase of their disease and it is important to try and establish the patient's preference and work towards this if possible. Although up to 50%–70% of patients with cancer would prefer to be cared for or die at home, a lot fewer are able to achieve this for various reasons. The establishment of domiciliary palliative-care teams which are usually composed of Macmillan nurses has improved the feasibility of this goal.

Finally, hospices with inpatient facilities may be an appropriate place for some patients. Usually, these units are run by medical and nursing staff specializing in palliative care and symptom control, with high nurse-to-patient ratios. They may admit patients for symptom control, respite, or terminal care if the patient and family cannot manage at home.

Working closely with the patient and family, it is possible to explore the various options and achieve the most suitable place for patient care at the end of life.

To summarize, provision of terminal care in the haematological setting is a complex, challenging process encompassing identification of the onset of the terminal phase of the disease, communicating this to the patient and family effectively, making difficult treatment decisions about what treatments to continue and which ones to abandon, managing complex symptoms, and maintaining good communication within the multidisciplinary team to provide the best possible care to each individual. The importance of patient and family involvement in each stage of this process cannot be highlighted enough.

Further Reading

Rose VL. American Thoracic Society issues consensus statement on dyspnea. *Am Fam Physician* 1999; 59: 3259–60.

Scottish Palliative Care Guidelines (http://www.palliativecareguidelines.scot.nhs.uk/)

PART 14

Disorders of the immune system

Introduction

The environment contains a whole range of pathogenic organisms and toxic substances which constantly challenge the health and well-being of human beings though a variety of pathological mechanisms. The immune system in humans has evolved to provide a defence mechanism against these microbial challenges.

The immune system is divided into two main branches, namely innate and adaptive. In addition, there are physical and chemical barriers, including skin, mucous membrane, mucous secretions, saliva, and various enzymes, and these contribute to the first line of defence against pathogens. The innate immune system provides the initial quick response for rapid recognition and elimination of pathogens, as opposed to the adaptive immune system, which has evolved to provide a more definitive and finely tuned response. The common central feature of both of these systems is the ability to distinguish between self and non-self. The recognition of non-self or 'foreign' pathogens and the subsequent immune response is orchestrated by a whole range of cells and soluble (humoral) factors in both innate and adaptive immune systems.

Components of the immune system

Innate immune system

Cells

Cells in the innate immune system include:

- neutrophils/phagocytes
- monocytes/macrophages
- dendritic cells
- mast cells
- eosinophils
- natural killer (NK) cells

Soluble factors

Soluble factors in the innate immune system include:

- complement
- cytokines
- chemokines
- toll-like receptors (TLRs)

Adaptive immune system

Cells

Cells in the adaptive immune system include:

- T-cells
- B-cells
- NK cells

Soluble factors

Soluble factors in the adaptive immune system include:

- receptors
- other surface molecules
- cytokines

Lymphoid organs

The individual components of the immune system function coherently within the structure of distinct anatomical lymphoid organs. Lymphoid organs play an important role in the development of lymphocytes and their subsequent survival. They form the site of initial lymphocyte education, as well as site of initiation of the adaptive immune responses and interaction between the cells of the innate and adaptive immune system. Lymphoid organs are divided into two groups:

- central or primary lymphoid organs, where lymphocytes are generated; these include:
  - bone marrow
  - thymus
- peripheral or secondary lymphoid organs, where adaptive responses are initiated and lymphocytes are maintained; these include:
  - lymph nodes
  - spleen
  - mucosal lymphoid tissues

Once T- and B-lymphocytes mature in the thymus and the bone marrow, respectively, they circulate through the secondary lymphoid organs in a coordinated fashion (see Figure 293.1). This movement is guided by adhesion molecules (e.g. L-selectin) and chemokine receptors which are present on the lymphocyte surface and which act as homing receptors.

White pulp
Central arteriole
Periarteriolar lymphoid sheath (T)
Follicle (B)

Red pulp

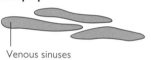

Venous sinuses
(plasma cells, macrophages)

Figure 293.1 The recirculation pathways of lymphocytes in a secondary lymphoid organ (in this case, the spleen). The majority of native T-cells entering the spleen from blood will leave the node immediately via efferent lymphatics (in this case, the periarteriolar lymphoid sheaths in the white pulp of the spleen). Naive T-cells that recognize a specific antigen while in the periarteriolar lymphoid sheath differentiate into effector T-cells and re-enter the circulation. B-cell recirculation follows a similar route; when B-cells, which accumulate in the follicles of the white pulp, encounter a specific antigen, they proliferate to form germinal centres; memory B-cells form a surrounding marginal zone. The red pulp of the spleen contains venous sinuses, which contain plasma cells and macrophages.

Reproduced with permission from Chapel, Helen, Haeney, Mansel, Misbah, Siraj, Snowden, Neil, *Essentials of Clinical Immunology*. 6th ed, Wiley-Blackwell, Oxford, UK, Copyright © 2014.

Function of the immune system: Recognition of 'non-self'

Closely integrated functioning of both innate and adaptive immune systems is required for adequate and timely host defence. Although each system plays a distinct role in host defence, there is a considerable degree of interplay and crosstalk between different components of the innate and adaptive immune system to provide efficient immune responses.

Innate immune system

The innate immune response characteristically lacks immunological memory and, as a consequence, remains unchanged even after repeated encounters with the same pathogen or antigen. Cells of the innate immune system, particularly phagocytic cells, recognize highly conserved, invariant structures that are shared across entire classes of microorganisms. These structures are called pathogen-associated molecular patterns (PAMPs) and are usually essential for the survival or pathogenicity of these organisms. Examples of PAMPs are given in Box 293.1.

PAMPs are small, conserved molecular motifs that are present in microbes. They include structures of cell walls and cell membranes or intracellular components, including nucleic acids (DNA, RNA, CpG).

The receptors that recognize PAMPs are known as pattern recognition receptors (PRRs; Figure 293.2). PRRs are expressed in

---

Box 293.1 Pathogen-associated molecular patterns

- bacterial lipopolysaccharides
- peptidoglycans
- lipotechoic acid
- mannans
- heat-shock proteins
- bacterial flagellin
- bacterial DNA
- single-/double-stranded RNA
- CpG repeats

---

many cells, important amongst them being macrophages, dendritic cells, and B-cells. Structurally, PRRs contain several different protein domains, such as leucine-rich repeat domains, calcium-dependent lectin domains, and scavenger-receptor protein domains. Functionally, they are divided into three main classes:

- secreted PRRs:
  - these function mainly as opsonins
  - examples are complement receptors and mannan-binding lectin
- endocytic PRRs:
  - these receptors are present on the surface of macrophages
  - they mediate uptake and delivery of pathogens into lysosomes
  - examples include the macrophage mannose receptor and the macrophage scavenger receptor
- signalling PRRs:
  - these activate signal transduction pathways that induce expression of immune response genes, including pro-inflammatory cytokines
  - examples include toll-like receptors and NOD-like receptors.

In addition, NK cells, which constitute an important component of the innate immune system, recognize their targets via different sets of receptors: Fcγ receptors and killer receptors.

Fcγ receptors

Fcγ receptors are surface receptors that bind the IgG molecule. NK cells recognize target cells that have been opsonized by IgG molecules and destroy them by a process known as antibody-dependent cellular cytotoxicity.

Killer receptors

The second system of receptors that is characteristic to NK cells is composed of the killer-activating receptors and the killer-inhibitory receptors. These receptors recognize a number of different molecules, including major histocompatibility complex (MHC) Class I molecules, which are normally expressed by all nucleated cells. Expression of these surface molecules may be absent or disrupted in virally infected cells or certain malignant cells. These receptors thus play a very important role in immune surveillance and in recognition between 'self' and 'non-self'. Downstream signalling from these receptors instructs NK cells to either 'kill' or 'not kill' the target cells.

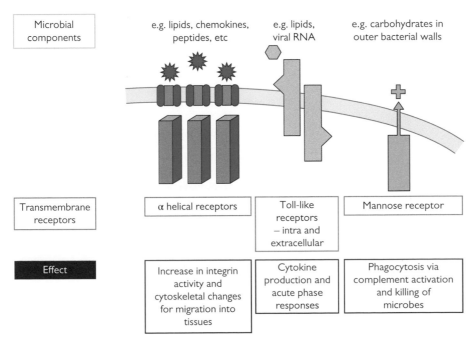

Figure 293.2 Pattern recognition receptors and their functions in mononuclear phagocytic cells.

Reproduced with permission from Chapel, Helen, Haeney, Mansel, Misbah, Siraj, Snowden, Neil, *Essentials of Clinical Immunology*. 6th ed, Wiley-Blackwell, Oxford, UK, Copyright © 2014.

Adaptive immune system

In contrast to the innate immune system, the adaptive immune response has evolved to provide a refined and specific immune response. The main distinguishing feature is the development of immunological memory, which enhances the subsequent response to the same antigen. The cells of the adaptive immune system, namely T-cells and B-cells, recognize specific antigenic epitopes via cell surface receptors, referred to as the T-cell receptor (TCR) and the B-cell receptor (BCR), respectively.

TCRs are membrane-bound receptors that are present on the surface of T-cells. Most TCR are heterodimers consisting of an alpha chain and a beta chain and recognize protein epitopes from pathogens that are processed and presented in relation to the MHC Class I and II by professional antigen-presenting cells (macrophages, dendritic cells, and B-cells). A small proportion of TCRs are made up of gamma and delta chains and recognize antigens either directly or in relation to MHC-like CD1 molecules; these are not discussed further in this chapter.

MHC molecules are specialized host-cell glycoproteins that bind foreign peptides and transport them to the cell surface for presentation to the host T-cells. They are encoded in a large cluster of genes. There are two classes of MHC molecules, which differ in structure, cellular expression, and function, as detailed in Table 293.1.

BCRs, on the other hand, exist in membrane-bound states on the surface of B-cells, as well as in a soluble state in the peripheral circulation. The soluble BCRs are known as immunoglobulins (Igs) or antibodies and mainly function as opsonins and/or complement activators. They exist as different isotypes with slightly variable individual properties and function, as discussed in 'Functions of the immune system: The role of individual components'.

Both TCRs and BCRs are formed by random recombination of different gene segments, each encoding for different portions of the receptor protein, and this results in the generation of a hugely variable and diverse repertoire of receptors capable of mounting a specific immune response against the large number of pathogenic epitopes that are present in the environment. It is beyond the scope of this chapter to discuss the details of receptor development.

Functions of the immune system: The role of individual components

Neutrophils

Neutrophils are derived from myeloid precursors and are the most numerous in peripheral circulation, forming an important cellular component of the innate immune system. Neutrophils are rapidly recruited to sites of infection and provide the first line for defence. Pathogens are phagocytosed and killed intracellularly via the generation of lysosomal NADPH oxidases and other enzymes in a process known as the respiratory burst. Neutrophils are short-lived cells and die after one round of phagocytosis and form a major component of pus at the site of infection.

Macrophages

Macrophages and newly recruited monocytes, which differentiate into macrophages, also function like neutrophils and destroy microorganisms by phagocytosis and intracellular killing. Once activated, macrophages produce inflammatory mediators, including tumour necrosis factor alpha, prostaglandins, and leukotrienes. Unlike neutrophils, macrophages are long-lived and continue to generate new lysosomes and enzymes. In addition, macrophages also act as antigen-presenting cells, presenting processed pathogenic protein epitopes to T-lymphocytes in the context of the MHC Class I and Class II molecules and appropriate cytokines, which are required for the induction of adaptive immune responses.

Dendritic cells

Along with neutrophils and macrophages, dendritic cells are a type of phagocytic cell found in the innate immune system. They are distributed all over the body and are strategically located in the skin, mucous membranes, and surfaces that are exposed to the environment. On activation, dendritic cells express increased levels of MHC Class I and Class II molecules, as well as co-stimulatory molecules, and migrate to the local lymph nodes, where they function as antigen-presenting cells.

Eosinophils

The main physiological role of eosinophils is thought to be in the host defence against parasitic infections, predominantly via the release of cationic proteins, reactive oxygen metabolites, inflammatory mediators, and cytokines into the extracellular space. Their role in the delayed phase of the allergic response is being increasingly recognized.

Mast cells and basophils

Mast cells and basophils play a critical role in mounting allergic responses to innocuous environmental agents, and have a lesser role in host defence against pathogens. However, recent reviews suggest that both these cells may have a wider role in shaping the adaptive immune response, particularly with regards to autoimmune disorders. Mast cells and basophils express high affinity receptors for IgE and are coated with specific IgE following initial sensitization with allergens. The subsequent response, on repeat exposure to the allergen, is mediated by cross-linking of the cell-bound IgE molecules, leading to mast cell degranulation, which is a hallmark of allergic reactions.

NK cells

Although derived from a lymphoid lineage, NK cells lack antigen-specific receptors and are considered to be a part of the innate immune system. They circulate in peripheral blood as large lymphocytes with distinctive cytotoxic granules and play an important role in immune surveillance and destruction of virus-infected cells and tumour cells.

Complement system

The complement system is made up of a large number of distinct plasma proteins, which function as proteases and activate each other in a cascade resulting in an inflammatory immune response. Complement proteins act as a bridge between the innate and adaptive immune systems. There are three different activating pathways that initiate the complement cascades (see Figure 293.3); these are known as:

- the classical pathway
- the alternative pathway
- the mannan-binding lectin pathway

All three initiating pathways converge with the formation of C3 convertase, which in turn cleaves C3 to generate large amounts of C3b, the main effector molecule of the complement system. Subsequent effector functions and activation of the terminal

Table 293.1 MHC molecules

Characteristics	MHC Class I	MHC Class II
Structure	Two polypeptide chains; a larger alpha chain and a smaller beta-2 microglobulin chain, which is not encoded in the MHC locus	Non-covalent complex of two equal sized chains; alpha and beta chains, both encoded within the MHC locus
Cellular expression	All nucleated cells	Mainly on dendritic cells, macrophages, and B-cells
Peptide binding	Peptides from cytosolic pathogens, commonly viruses	Peptides from intra-vesicular pathogens, extracellular bacteria, and toxins
Antigen presentation	To CD8+ T-cells	To CD4+ T-cells

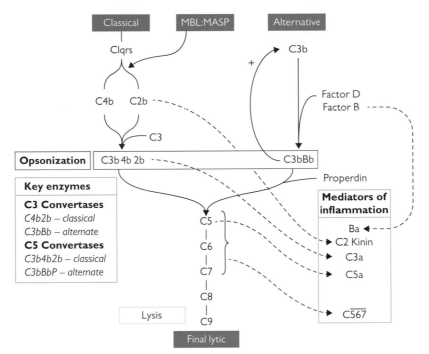

Figure 293.3 Functions of complement pathways; MASP, mannan-binding-lectin-associated serine protease; MBL, mannan-binding lectin.
Reproduced with permission from Chapel, Helen, Haeney, Mansel, Misbah, Siraj, Snowden, Neil, *Essentials of Clinical Immunology.* 6th ed, Wiley-Blackwell, Oxford, UK, Copyright © 2014.

components are common to all the pathways. The three main effector functions of the complement system are:

- opsonization of pathogens and subsequent clearance of the immune complexes
- recruitment of inflammatory cells and other mediators via chemoattraction
- direct lysis and killing of pathogens via the formation of a membrane-attack complex

The clinical consequences of complement deficiency are discussed in Chapter 299.

T-cells

T-cells are mainly divided into CD4+ T-cells (T helper cells) or CD8+ T-cells (cytotoxic T-cells), based on the surface expression of CD4 or CD8 molecules, respectively. CD4+ T-cells recognize peptides presented by MHC Class II molecules expressed by antigen-presenting cells. In contrast, cytotoxic T-cells recognize peptides presented by MHC Class I molecules, which are expressed by all nucleated cells. T-cells are responsible for cell-mediated adaptive immune responses, and their main effector functions are:

- direct killing of virally infected cells
- destruction of intracellular pathogens by activation of macrophages
- destruction of extracellular pathogens by activation of B-cells
- epithelial and mucosal immunity

Direct killing of virally infected cells

Direct killing of virally infected cells is mediated by CD8+ cytotoxic T-cells, which kill infected cells either via the death receptor-dependent pathway or the perforin/granzyme-dependent pathway.

Destruction of intracellular pathogens by activations of macrophages

Destruction of intracellular pathogens by activation of macrophages is mediated by a subset of CD4+ T-cells known as Th1 cells (see Table 293.2). Th1 cells produce large amounts of interferon gamma (IFNγ) and activate macrophages via the IFNγ–interleukin 12 pathway, with resultant destruction of intracellular pathogens.

Destruction of extracellular pathogens via activation of B-cells

Destruction of extracellular pathogens is mediated by T-cell dependent B-cell activation leading to opsonization and subsequent destruction of extracellular pathogens.

Epithelial and mucosal immunity

Epithelial and mucosal immunity is mediated by a recently described subset of CD4+ T-cells, the Th17 cells. These cells can rapidly initiate an inflammatory response which is dominated by neutrophils, and they are thought to play a significant role in maintaining immunity at epithelial and mucosal surfaces.

Table 293.2 Subsets of CD4+ T-cells based on cell surface receptors and cytokine profile

Subset	Surface marker*	Cytokine profile	Cellular target and function
Th1 cells	IL-12 receptor	IFN gamma	Activation of macrophages via IFN gamma–IL12 pathway and B-cells to produce opsonizing antibodies (IgG1/IgG3)
Th2 cells	IL-4 receptor	IL-4 IL-13 IL-5	Activation of B-cells to produce immunoglobulins of other classes (IgM, IgA, IgE) Activation of eosinophils and basophils
Th17 cells	IL-23 receptor	IL-17 IL-21 IL-22	Predominantly neutrophils Actively initiate inflammatory response Important role in immunity at epithelial and mucosal surfaces

Abbreviations: IL, interleukin; IFN, interferon; Th, T helper.
*These surface markers are not specific for each subset, but are characteristically co-expressed along with other cell surface markers that define the cell.

B-cells

B-cells produce different classes of antibodies or immunoglobulins (IgG, IgA, IgM, IgD, IgE) and are responsible for the humoral immune response against extracellular pathogens (see Chapter 297). The main effector mechanisms constituting humoral defence against pathogens are:

- neutralization
- opsonization
- complement fixation

Neutralization

In neutralization, antibodies neutralize extracellular pathogens and toxins by binding to them and forming immune complexes, which are subsequently cleared. Neutralization prevents bacterial adherence to target cells and cell entry.

Opsonization

In opsonization, extracellular pathogens are coated by antibody molecules facilitating ingestion by phagocytic cells (with receptors for the Fc portion of immunoglobulin molecules) and subsequent destruction.

Complement fixation

Following opsonization, antibody molecules can also activate the complement system with resultant complement-mediated destruction of the pathogen.

Antigen presentation

In addition to providing humoral defence against extracellular pathogens, B-cells also act as professional antigen-presenting cells and can present protein epitopes to CD4+ T-cells in relation to MHC Class II molecules. This interaction between T-cells and B-cells results in isotype switching and affinity maturation of the B-cell response via processes known as class-switch recombination and somatic hypermutation, respectively.

Conclusion

This chapter provided a brief overview of the function of the immune system. It is clear from this that human host defence is a complex, dynamic process involving a variety of interactions between key cells of the immune system and soluble mediators acting in concert to combat infection.

It is therefore understandable that even minor defects in any arm of the immune system may have far-reaching clinical consequences. It is beyond the scope of this chapter to discuss defects in the immune system and associated diseases. This is covered to a greater extent in Chapters 294–300.

Further Reading

Chapel H, Haeney M, Misbah S, et al. *Essentials of Clinical Immunology*, (6th edition), 2014. Wiley-Blackwell.

Crotty S. A brief history of T cell help to B cells. *Nat Rev Immunol* 2015; 15: 85–189.

Iwasaki A and Medzhitov R. Control of adaptive immunity by the innate immune system. *Nat Immunol* 2015; 16: 343–53.

Kurosaki T, Komtani K, and Ise W. Memory B cells. *Nat Rev Immunol* 2015; 15: 149–59.

294 Clinical features and diagnosis of immunological disease

Siraj Misbah

Definition of the disease

Immunological disease can be broadly defined as a spectrum of problems ranging from failure of the immune system (primary or secondary immunodeficiency) to the clinical consequences of an overzealous immune system, manifesting clinically as autoimmunity, allergy, or, rarely, as an autoinflammatory syndrome.

Aetiology of the disease

Immunological disease is frequently a reflection of the complex interactions between genetics and environmental factors. Over 150 primary immune deficiency disorders now have clearly defined molecular bases, where environmental influences in the form of infection are responsible for disease manifestations.

For common autoimmune diseases such as SLE and rheumatoid arthritis (RA), observations on increased concordance rates in monozygotic twins have been complemented by genome-wide association studies highlighting significant contributions from a number of genes. Approximately 50% of the risk of developing RA is attributable to genetic factors, with over 30 single nucleotide polymorphisms being associated with disease susceptibility. Some susceptibility loci such as PTPN22 and STAT4 are associated with multiple autoimmune diseases, including SLE and RA. The significant female preponderance of autoimmune diseases underscores the importance of oestrogen on disease susceptibility, although its causal role remains a matter of debate.

For allergy, genome-wide association studies have identified multiple markers located at chromosomal position 17q21 and which are strong and reproducible loci associated with childhood asthma. Allied to genetic predisposition, the role of the environment in skewing immune responses has been the focus of the 'hygiene hypothesis', which states that the lack of immunological priming in childhood by way of infections may divert the immune system away from protective Th1 responses to allergy-prone Th2 responses.

Typical symptoms of the disease

Although there may be overlap in some presenting symptoms, clinical presentation of disease is best considered under the broad headings of immunodeficiency, systemic autoimmune disease, and allergy. In all of these disease categories, disease may be asymptomatic or subclinical until unmasked by a triggering event such as infection.

Immunodeficiency

Patients with immunodeficiency are particularly prone to infections whose characteristics are summarized by the mnemonic SPUR, which stands for severe, persistent, unusual, or recurrent. The pathogens causing these infections range from common ones such as *Streptococcus pneumoniae*, which is responsible for a significant proportion of the infective burden faced by patients with primary and secondary B-cell deficiency, to opportunistic pathogens such as *Pneumocystis jiroveci* in patients with T-cell defects.

In order to deal with the array of pathogens that challenge the immune system, there is a degree of immunological subspecialization that helps deal with various pathogens. This is clinically reflected in the correlation between different types of infections and underlying immunological defects (Figure 294.1).

Just as infections unmask immunodeficiency, iatrogenic disease caused by live vaccines is a strong pointer to immune system failure. Examples of vaccine-induced disease in this context include the development of BCG vaccine-induced disease in babies with severe combined immune deficiency (SCID), and paralytic poliomyelitis in agammaglobulinaemia.

Paradoxically, some patients with B-cell immune defects are capable of mounting immune responses to self-antigens, leading to autoimmune disease manifesting as immune thrombocytopenia or autoimmune haemolytic anaemia. It is not uncommon to encounter patients who have primary antibody deficiency and present with a combination of recurrent infections and autoimmune disease.

Autoimmune disease

The presenting symptoms of autoimmune disease will depend on the extent of organ involvement. Fatigue is frequently a prominent feature of both organ-specific and systemic autoimmune disease. While in the former, fatigue may be the only symptom, as in Addison's disease and gluten-sensitive enteropathy, in the latter, fatigue may be accompanied by arthralgia, skin rashes, Raynaud's phenomenon, and pleuritic pain, as exemplified by SLE. In patients affected by lupus-overlap disorders such as mixed connective tissue disease, additional symptoms suggestive of inflammatory myositis (proximal muscle weakness), and scleroderma (skin tightening, dysphagia) may be present.

Patients afflicted with small vessel vasculitides of the Wegener's–microscopic polyangiitis spectrum frequently present with sinusitis, epistaxis, haemoptysis, and renal impairment.

Allergy

The symptoms of IgE-mediated allergic disease are influenced by the route of entry of the allergen and driven by the products of mast cell degranulation, in particular the release of histamine, leukotrienes, and platelet-activating factor. Consequently, systemic allergic reactions are characterized by urticaria, bronchospasm, hypotension, and angioedema. The rapid onset of symptoms within 30 minutes of exposure to the offending allergen is a characteristic feature of IgE-mediated allergy.

Demographics

While immunological disease affects all ages, inherited immune deficiencies predominantly present in early infancy or childhood. SCID occurs in approximately 1 in 60 000 births, and is considered an immunological emergency because of the urgency of stem cell transplantation or gene therapy. X-linked agammaglobulinaemia occurs with an incidence of 1 in 200 000, and characteristically presents after 3–6 months of age, once protective maternal IgG (acquired transplacentally) has dissipated. Common variable immunodeficiency (CVID) is estimated to occur with a frequency of 1 in 10 000 to 100 000, and is considered to be the commonest treatable immunodeficiency. A history of parental consanguinity is a common feature of many autosomal recessive immunodeficiency disorders.

For autoimmune disease, a significant female preponderance attests to the importance of female sex hormones on disease pathogenesis. Autoimmune disease affects approximately 5% of the population, with the prevalence of SLE estimated at 40 cases per 100 000 in Northern Europe.

Natural history, and complications of the disease

The natural history of immunological disease is strongly influenced by the time taken to reach a diagnosis and instigate appropriate treatment.

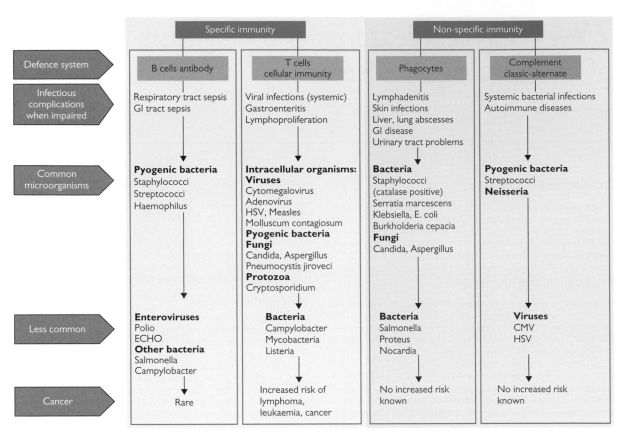

Figure 294.1 Defects in immunity suggested by infections with certain organisms; GI, gastrointestinal; HSV, herpes simplex virus.
Essentials of Clinical Immunology, Sixth edition, Helen Chapel, Maneel Haeney, Siraj Misbah and Neil Snowden. 2014. John Wiley & Sons Ltd.

Immunodeficiency

Failure to treat a baby with SCID or gene therapy results in a high mortality rate (>80%) during infancy. Conversely, successful transplantation from a HLA-matched sibling donor offers an 80% chance of cure, whiles fully matched unrelated transplant offers a 70% chance.

For adults with CVID, early diagnosis and instigation of adequate immunoglobulin replacement has resulted in substantial improvements in morbidity and mortality, with life expectancy only a decade below that of the normal population.

Autoimmune disease

Early diagnosis and optimal hormone replacement therapy enables most patients with organ-specific autoimmune disease such as Hashimoto's thyroiditis and Addison's disease to enjoy a virtually normal quality of life, with only a minimal reduction in life expectancy. For systemic autoimmune diseases such as SLE, prognosis is determined by the extent of renal involvement, the risk of infection associated with immunosuppressive therapy, and the increased cardiovascular mortality associated with accelerated atherosclerosis. Advances in disease management have led to significant improvements in life expectancy, with a 15-year survival rate of 80% today, in contrast to a 4-year survival rate of 50% in the 1950s.

Allergy

Identification and avoidance, wherever possible, of the offending allergen, prevents a recurrence of acute allergic reactions without any impairment in quality of life. However, occasional fatalities occur in patients with nut allergy and poorly controlled asthma, due to inadvertent ingestion of nuts leading to irreversible bronchospasm.

When to refer patients for an immunological opinion

The need for an immunological opinion or investigations will be self-evident in patients presenting with recurrent infections, symptoms

suggestive of multisystem autoimmune disease, and anaphylaxis, respectively. While immunologists will be the lead physicians in assessing patients with suspected immunodeficiency or allergic disease, patients with systemic autoimmune disease are best served by the relevant organ-based specialist working in conjunction with an immunologist.

The symptoms which merit immunological referral are detailed in 'Typical symptoms of immunological disease' and 'Differential diagnosis'. In addition, it would be worthwhile considering an immunological opinion in cases of immunodeficiency or allergy.

Immunodeficiency and autoimmunity

Failure to mount an appropriate acute phase response, despite invasive bacterial infection, is a pointer to defective innate immunity, as evidenced by patients with mutations in the IRAK4 component of the toll-like receptor pathway. Such patients fail to mount a rise in C-reactive protein levels or the erythrocyte sedimentation rate, despite having pneumococcal septicaemia.

Patients who develop recurrent infections in the setting of autoimmune disease may be thought to have impaired immunity, as a consequence of immunosuppressive therapy. While this is a frequent occurrence, it is equally possible for autoimmune disorders such as immune thrombocytopenia and autoimmune haemolytic anaemia to be the presenting manifestation of primary immunodeficiency disoders (see Chapter 297). The detection of hypogammaglobulinaemia in these patients should prompt immunological referral in such cases.

Allergy

While conventional antihistamines targeting H1 and H2 receptors will be sufficient to control symptoms in the majority of patients with chronic urticaria, a minority will have severe disease requiring high doses of multiple antihistamines coupled with steroids. These patients merit immunological assessment to explore the possibility of autoimmune urticaria or urticarial vasculitis (see 'Differential diagnosis'). Although it is recognized that the majority of patients with uncomplicated allergic problems can be adequately managed in primary care, patients with severe food, drug, or insect-venom allergy merit specialist investigation and, where appropriate, assessment for immunotherapy.

Approach to diagnosing immunological disease

As in the rest of clinical medicine, the history is crucial in guiding the selection of investigations for the diagnosis of immunological disease. In most patients, the history alone will suffice to suggest whether a patient should be investigated for allergy, autoimmune disease, or immunodeficiency (see 'Typical symptoms of immunological disease').

Table 294.1 summarizes the key investigations that would be useful in investigating patients with suspected immunological disease.

Table 294.1 Summary of key investigations in suspected immunological disease

Disease	Key investigations	Comments
Allergy		
IgE-mediated allergy	Skin tests: prick and intradermal tests or specific IgE antibodies to suspected allergens	Selection of skin tests and allergen-specific IgE should be guided entirely by the clinical history
		Blanket screens for allergy are wasteful, and frequently lead to inappropriate management
	Total IgE	Marker of allergic diathesis, but a normal total IgE does not exclude type I allergy
	Tryptase	Sensitive marker of mast cell degranulation
		Useful in the assessment of suspected anaphylaxis and mastocytosis
		Normal tryptase does not exclude anaphylaxis
Immunodeficiency		
B-cell defects	Total serum immunoglobulins	Hypogammaglobulinaemia associated with absent circulating B-cells is suggestive of arrested B-cell development
	IgG subclasses (in selected cases)	
	Specific antibodies to routine immunizations and common pathogens	
	Circulating lymphocyte subsets	
T-cell defects	Circulating lymphocyte surface markers	
	Lymphocyte transformation (selected cases)	
Combined T- and B-cell defects	As for T- and B-cell defects individually	
Complement	Haemolytic complement activity of classical and alternative pathways (CH50, AP50)	Assesses integrity of entire complement pathway
	Quantification of individual complement components (C3, C4) and others of interest	
Neutrophil defects	Dihydrorhodamine reduction	Reliable screening test for suspected chronic granulomatous disease
	CD11/CD18	For suspected leucocyte adhesion deficiency
Defects in the TLR pathway	Assessment of pro-inflammatory cytokine release	Failure to mount an appropriate acute phase response is an important clue to TLR defects
Systemic autoimmune disease		
SLE	ANA followed by anti-ENA and anti-DNA	Negative ANA at presentation effectively excludes SLE
	Complement C3, C4	
	Anti-cardiolipin	
	Lupus anticoagulant	
	Skin biopsy (selected cases)	
Scleroderma	ANA	Anti-Scl 70 and anticentromere antibodies tend to be mutually exclusive
	Anti-Scl 70 antibody	
	Anticentromere antibody	
Vasculitides		
WG–MPA spectrum of small vessel vasculitides	ANCA	cANCA is associated with antibodies to proteinase-3
	Tissue biopsy	pANCA is associated with antibodies to myeloperoxidase
		The positive predictive value of ANCA for a diagnosis of small vessel vasculitis varies from 50% to 80%, depending on the patient population
		ANCA is frequently found in non-vasculitic disorders
Mixed cryoglobulinaemia	Cryoglobulins	Over 80% of patients with type II cryoglobulinaemia have a low C4 and are positive for rheumatoid factor
	Rheumatoid factor	
	Complement C3, C4	
Inflammatory myositis	Muscle biopsy	Active myositis may be present with a normal creatinine kinase level
	Creatinine kinase	Anti-Jo-1 (Jo-1 is a transfer RNA synthetase) is a marker of interstitial lung disease associated with dermatomyositis
	ANA	
	Anti-Jo-1	
Autoinflammatory syndromes	Genetic analysis to detect mutations in genes for mevalonate kinase, familial Mediterranean fever, and the tumour necrosis factor receptor	

Abbreviations: ANCA, antineutrophil cytoplasmic antibody; ANA, antinuclear antibody; cANCA, cytoplasmic antineutrophil cytoplasmic antibody; ENA, extractable nuclear antigen antibody; pANCA, perinuclear antineutrophil cytoplasmic antibody; SLE, systemic lupus erythematosus; TLR, Toll-like receptor; WG–MPA, Wegener's granulomatosis–microscopic polyangiitis.

Differential diagnosis

Given the fundamental involvement of immunological mechanisms in disease across the whole of clinical medicine, the possibility of immune-mediated disease needs to be considered in many different clinical scenarios.

Immunodeficiency

The clinical situations in which a diagnosis of various immunodeficiencies should be considered are discussed in the chapters dealing with antibody deficiency (Chapter 297), acquired T-cell deficiency (Chapter 296), combined B- and T-cell deficiencies (Chapter 298), complement deficiency (Chapter 299), and neutrophil defects (Chapter 295).

Autoimmune disease

Systemic autoimmune diseases, such as SLE and small vessel vasculitides, often feature as possible differential diagnoses in the workup of patients presenting with multisystem disease. For example, while joint pains and photosensitivity would be suggestive of SLE, other possible causes should also be considered (see Box 294.1).

If the presenting constellation of problems is widened to arthralgia, joint pains, and renal impairment, the list of differential diagnoses includes SLE, Wegener's granulomatosis, microscopic polyangiitis, mixed cryoglobulinaemia, rheumatoid vasculitis, and Henoch–Schönlein purpura.

Allergy

In the workup of patients presenting with urticaria and angioedema, occurring either singly or in combination, the possibility of allergic drivers (food, drugs, venom) should be considered. A significant proportion of patients (up to one-third) will be labelled as having idiopathic disease in the absence of a clear underlying diagnosis, with a small minority (<5%) having autoimmune disease due to IgG antibodies directed against IgE or the IgE receptor. In patients presenting with recurrent isolated angioedema, the possibility of C1 inhibitor deficiency, albeit rare, should be considered.

The differential diagnoses that should be considered in the workup of patients with anaphylaxis has been considered in Chapter 75.

> **Box 294.1 Causes of joint pains and rash**
> - SLE
> - infections (e.g. parvovirus, rheumatic fever, Lyme disease)
> - dermatomyositis
> - psoriatic arthritis
> - small vessel vasculitides

Further Reading

Chapel H, Haeney M, Misbah S, et al. *Essentials of Clinical Immunology* (6th edition), 2014. Wiley-Blackwell.

Kurts C, Panzer U, Anders H-J, et al. The immune system and kidney disease: Basic concepts and clinical implications. *Nat Rev Immunol* 2013; 13: 738–53.

CHAPTER 294 Clinical features and diagnosis of immunological disease

Malini Bhole

Definition of the disease

Neutrophils are an important component of the innate immune system, forming the first line of defence against bacterial invasion. Abnormalities in either neutrophil numbers or function lead to immunodeficiency disorders affecting the innate immune system (see Table 295.1) with a predisposition towards developing serious and often life-threatening infections. Alterations in neutrophil numbers and function may also be noted secondary to systemic diseases, where they may act as markers for ongoing disease processes.

Most of the primary neutrophil disorders discussed in this chapter will present in childhood. In adults, acquired neutropenia is the commonest neutrophil abnormality encountered in clinical practice, although rarely, some primary neutrophil defects may present.

Aetiology of the disease

Primary immunodeficiency disorders, due to neutrophil abnormalities, result from genetic mutations affecting the development, maturation, or function of the neutrophils. The inheritance may be X linked, autosomal recessive, or autosomal dominant, as detailed in Table 295.1. Sporadic mutations, although rare, may be seen in certain conditions.

Inherited neutropenias

Neutropaenia is defined as an absolute reduction in the number of circulating neutrophils (absolute neutrophil count (ANC)) to less than 1.5×10^9/l. In primary phagocytic disorders, this results from a decrease in bone marrow storage pools, either due to decreased total marrow cellularity, arrested maturation at the promyelocyte stage, the myelocyte stage, or both.

Abnormalities of neutrophil function

Abnormalities of neutrophil function may result from genetic disorders that affect the migration of neutrophils, phagocytosis, and intracellular killing.

Acquired neutropenia

The normal ANC in an adult ranges from 1.5 to 8.0 (1500–8000/mm³). Neutropenia, defined as an abnormally low neutrophil count, is divided into mild, moderate, or severe, based on the ANC:

- mild neutropenia (ANC: 1.0–1.5): minimal risk of infection
- moderate neutropenia (ANC: 0.5–1.0) : moderate risk of infection
- severe neutropenia (ANC: <0.5): severe risk of infection

The main causes of acquired neutropenia in an adult are:

- autoimmune neutropenia
- immunosuppressive drugs and chemotherapeutic agents, used in the treatment of autoimmune disease and cancer

Typical symptoms of the disease, and less common symptoms

Patients with neutrophil defects typically manifest in infancy or early childhood, with an increased susceptibility to infections, particularly catalase-positive microorganisms and fungi. In general, these children may present with:

- malaise and lethargy
- skin infections, including cellulitis and skin abscesses
- mucosal infections, such as gingivitis, stomatitis, aphthous ulcers, and periodontitis
- respiratory tract infections, including otitis media and pneumonias
- serious infections, including septicaemia, meningitis, and deep-seated abscesses

Although rare, inherited neutrophil defects such as chronic granulomatous disease (CGD) may manifest as overwhelming aspergillus infection, associated with inhalation of aerosolized mulch or organic material, in mulch pneumonitis.

Table 295.1 Immunodeficiency disorders caused by neutrophil abnormalities

Disease	Mutation/genetic defect	Inheritance
Abnormalities in neutrophil numbers		
Cyclical neutropenia	ELA2	Autosomal dominant, or sporadic
Severe congenital neutropenia/Kostmann syndrome	HAX1 ELA2	Autosomal recessive or autosomal dominant
Schwachman–Diamond syndrome	SBDS	Autosomal recessive, or sporadic
Defects in neutrophil migration		
Leucocyte adhesion defect types 1–3	Type 1 due to mutations in INTG2	Autosomal recessive
Hyper-IgE syndrome	STAT3/TYK2	Autosomal dominant or autosomal recessive
X-linked neutropenia	WAS	X linked
Defects in respiratory burst/ killing		
Chronic granulomatous disease	CYBB NCF NCF2 CYBA	X linked or autosomal recessive
Myeloperoxidase deficiency	MPO	Autosomal recessive
Neutrophil glucose-6-phosphate dehydrogenase deficiency	G6PD	X linked
Defects in neutrophil granules		
Chédiak–Higashi syndrome	LYST	Autosomal recessive

Table 295.2 Clinical features of neutrophil disorders

Disease	Specific clinical manifestation
Cyclical neutropaenia	Periodic/cyclical fever episodes, occurring every 21 days
Schwachman–Diamond syndrome	Pancreatic insufficiency
	Skeletal abnormalities
Leukocyte adhesion defects	Delayed separation of cord
Hyper-IgE syndromes	Skeletal involvement
	Distinctive facies
Chronic granulomatous disease	Granuloma formation in both cutaneous and hollow viscera
Myeloperoxidase deficiency	Disseminated candidiasis in patients with diabetes mellitus
Neutrophil glucose-6-phosphate dehydrogenase deficiency	Haemolytic anaemia
Chédiak–Higashi syndrome	Partial ocular and cutaneous albinism
	Mental retardation
	Peripheral neuropathy
Specific granule deficiency	Bleeding diathesis

Common organisms include:

- *Staphylococcus aureus*
- *Pseudomonas/Burkholderia aeruginosa*
- *Burkholderia cepacia*
- Gram-negative enteric bacteria
- *Aspergillus* species

In addition to the common clinical features associated with neutrophil abnormalities, there are some clinical features that are typically seen in certain disorders, as detailed in Table 295.2.

Febrile neutropenia as a complication of chemotherapy

Febrile neutropenia is the development of fever, usually associated with other signs of infection, in patients with neutropenia. Febrile neutropenia and neutropenic sepsis is most commonly recognized as a complication of chemotherapy. This is a medical emergency, as the infection may progress within hours and result in shock and death. Rapid and timely recognition with prompt use of appropriate antibiotics are the mainstay of treatment. Appropriate bacterial, viral, and fungal cultures must be requested prior to antibiotic treatment.

Demographics of the disease

Inherited disorders of neutrophil numbers or function are rare, with a variable frequency ranging from 1 to 2 cases per million people for cyclic neutropaenia, to 8.5 per million live births for CGD (UK registry). Most of the inherited neutrophil disorders present in infancy and early childhood.

Natural history, and complications of the disease

The natural history and complications associated with primary neutrophil disorders depends on the underlying genetic mutation.

Cyclical neutropaenia

Patients with cyclical neutropenia develop oropharyngeal and skin infections associated with fever episodes which occur in a regular 21-day cycle.

Severe congenital neutropenia

It is estimated that about 2% of patients with severe congenital neutropenia undergo malignant transformation every year. Patients progress to develop myelodysplasia (MDS) or acute myelogenous leukaemia (AML), and this has been linked to partial or complete loss of Chromosome 7 and abnormalities in Chromosome 21.

Shwachman–Diamond syndrome

Shwachman–Diamond syndrome is associated with exocrine pancreatic insufficiency and metaphyseal dysplasia (25% of cases). Survival to adulthood has been reported in approximately 50% of patients, and up to one-third of these survivors progress to develop AML or MDS. Progression to MDS or AML has been associated with abnormalities in Chromosome 7.

CGD

Patients with the X-linked variety of CGD present in early infancy and tend to have a more severe clinical course. Autosomal recessive forms of CGD may present later in childhood and often have a milder clinical phenotype. Prior to the development of antibiotics, survival beyond childhood was unusual. The introduction of antibiotic and antifungal prophylaxis has increased the survival of patients with CGD to the fourth decade. The overall survival is still low without definitive treatment, and patients succumb to serious fungal infections or obstructive complications due to granuloma formation.

Leukocyte adhesion molecule deficiency

Leukocyte adhesion molecule deficiency may present in the neonatal period, with delayed umbilical cord separation beyond 21 days. The condition is characterized by absence of pus at infected sites, despite a pronounced peripheral blood neutrophilia. Survival beyond 5 years of age is unusual without a bone marrow transplant.

Approach to diagnosing the disease

An important approach to diagnosing neutrophil abnormalities is an accurate clinical history, and a high degree of clinical suspicion. Repeated full blood counts with differential white-cell count may detect a persistent or chronic abnormality in neutrophil numbers. Abnormally high neutrophil counts, especially in the presence of poor wound healing and lack of pus formation, must raise the suspicion of leucocyte adhesion defects. Patients with recurrent superficial or deep abscess must be investigated further for defects in innate immunity, particularly neutrophil functional defects including CGD.

Differential diagnosis

Alterations in neutrophil numbers due to secondary causes such as ongoing infections, inflammation, medications, or malignancy are more common than primary defects and form an important differential diagnosis. Bone marrow examination may be required in selected cases to rule out other causes such as aplastic anaemia, leukaemia, or malignant infiltration. Serum immunoglobulin levels must be checked to exclude other causes for recurrent infections.

The cause of acquired neutropenia in adults is usually relatively easy to diagnose since it predominantly occurs in the setting of autoimmune disease such as systemic lupus erythematosus or in conjunction with immunosuppressive drug therapy or chemotherapy.

'Gold-standard' diagnostic test

Detection of a known genetic mutation, associated with the particular neutrophil defect would be the gold-standard test for diagnosis. However, a strong clinical history supported by the appropriate flow cytometric tests is acceptable for a working diagnosis.

Acceptable diagnostic alternatives to the gold standard

Acceptable alternatives to support the diagnosis of a neutrophil defect would depend up on the condition that is clinically suspected; these include:

- cyclical neutropenia: demonstration of a cyclical fall in neutrophil counts every 21 days by maintaining a record of twice weekly neutrophil counts for a period of at least 6 weeks

- severe congenital neutropenia and Shwachman–Diamond syndrome: bone marrow biopsy
- CGD: abnormal dihydrorhodamine assay on flow cytometry, or abnormal nitro-blue tetrazolium test
- leucocyte adhesion defects: deficient CD11/CD18 expression on flow cytometry
- hyper-IgE syndrome: total IgE levels >5000 with clinical features suggestive of the syndrome
- X-linked neutropenia: abnormal expression of WASP protein

Other relevant investigations

Other relevant investigations would depend on the suspected condition. Screening for periodic fever syndromes would be appropriate while investigating cyclical neutropenia and, similarly, assessing pancreatic function would be appropriate for Shwachman–Diamond syndrome. Patients with suspected CGD may need relevant imaging for deep-seated abscesses or fungal infections, or endoscopy to rule out inflammatory bowel disease. Family screening is appropriate in X-linked or autosomal recessive conditions.

Prognosis and how to estimate it

The overall prognosis for neutrophil defects is poor and, for many conditions, survival beyond childhood is rare without definitive treatment. Although the use of recombinant granulocyte-colony stimulating factor (G-CSF) has significantly increased the life expectancy in severe congenital neutropaenia, many of these children progress to develop AML or MDS. Similarly, improved antibiotic and antifungal prophylaxis for CGD patients has improved life expectancy to the fourth decade, but patients still succumb to invasive aspergillus infection or complications due to granuloma formation.

Treatment and its effectiveness

The definitive treatment for many inherited neutrophil defects is bone marrow transplantation. Prophylactic antibiotic and antifungal treatments have been effective therapeutic interventions for both chronic neutropaenias and functional neutrophil defects. Prompt identification and treatment of infections is essential for the management of these patients. Regular recombinant G-CSF has been used successfully in the treatment of patients with severe congenital neutropenia and Shwachman–Diamond syndrome.

Neutropenic sepsis post chemotherapy requires aggressive treatment with broad-spectrum antipseudomonal antibiotics, combined with an aminoglycoside. Appropriate bacterial, viral, and fungal cultures must be requested prior to antibiotic treatment.

Further Reading

American Society of Hematology: Hematology, The Education Program. Evidence-Based Approaches to Cytopenias (http://asheducation-book.hematologylibrary.org/search?tocsectionid=Evidence-Based+Approaches+to+Cytopenias&sortspec=date&submit=Submit)

Bouma G, Ancliff PJ, Thrasher AJ, et al. Recent advances in the understanding of genetic defects of neutrophil number and function. *Br J Haematol* 2010; 151: 312–26.

Boxer LA. How to approach neutropenia. *Hematology* 2012; 2012: 174–82.

Malini Bhole, Mas Chaponda, and Nick Beeching

Introduction

Since its discovery in the 1980s, infection with the human immunodeficiency virus (HIV) has rapidly spread across the world, especially to large parts of the African continent. By the end of 2013, an estimated 35 million people were living with HIV worldwide. In the UK, this figure was close to 108 000 (a prevalence of 2.8 per 1000 population aged 15–59 years (1.9 per 1000 women and 3.7 per 1000 men)).

Significant progress has been made in diagnosis, and current treatments are life-saving. However, there is still no cure and no vaccine. This chapter will predominantly concentrate on the clinical features and management of HIV infection.

Aetiology of the disease

HIV is an RNA virus with reverse transcriptase activity. There are two distinct types: HIV-1 and HIV-2. Both viruses cause similar immune defects and are associated with similar clinical disease. They originated in the chimpanzee and sooty mangabey, respectively, which carry the simian immunodeficiency virus (SIV). It is likely that HIV-1 and HIV-2 infected humans as a result of these primates being hunted for food. Theories linking the introduction of HIV into humans via polio vaccination campaigns in Africa in the 1950s have been disproved. The replicative cycle of HIV is summarized in Figure 296.1.

The virus gains entry into cells as a result of high-affinity binding of the viral envelope protein gp120 with the CD4 molecule on T-cells. In addition to the CD4 molecule, the virus uses chemokine receptors as cofactors for cellular entry; these are CXCR4, which is expressed on T-cells (T-tropic HIV), and CCR5, which is expressed on macrophages (M-tropic HIV). Binding of gp120 to CD4 molecule and CXCR4/CCR5 allows HIV to adhere to the cell and to effect conformational change in the gp120/gp41 complex to allow membrane fusion and cell entry. Following entry, the reverse transcriptase enzyme allows transcription of double-stranded DNA from viral RNA, which integrates into the host genome. Viral protein elements are transcribed, translated, and assembled within the affected cell. The virus uses the host's lipid cell wall to form the envelope, and progeny virus is formed.

HIV disease classification and progression

Initial infection with HIV via the mucosal or parenteral route results in a high viral load (viraemia) and may be associated with a brief, acute, flu-like illness. This phase of high viral replication soon resolves to a lower 'set point' of viraemia (see Figure 296.2), which varies between patients. This is followed by a variable period of asymptomatic chronic infection, during which there is an uncontrolled proliferation of HIV within the cells of the immune system, particularly CD4+ T-cells. HIV infection is characterized by a profound decrease in the number of CD4+ T-cells, resulting in immune failure and a predisposition to infections with a wide range of pathogens and malignancies, including Kaposi's sarcoma and non-Hodgkin's lymphoma (see Table 296.1). Most untreated patients with HIV infection eventually progress to develop advanced/symptomatic HIV. The term

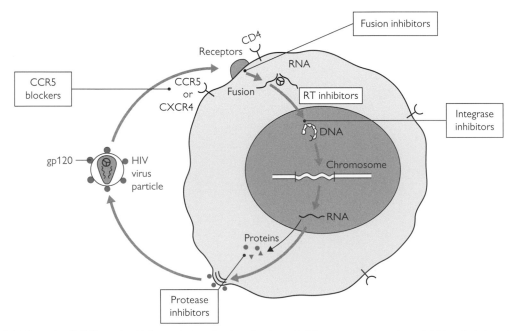

Figure 296.1 Schematic of HIV life cycle with five main sites of action of antiretroviral drugs; reverse transcriptase inhibitors include nucleot(s)ide reverse transcriptase inhibitors and non-nucleot(s)ide reverse transcriptase inhibitors; RT, reverse transcriptase.

Adapted with permission from Luzzi, HIV/AIDS, in *Oxford Textbook of Medicine*, Fifth Edition Oxford University Press, Oxford, UK, Copyright © 2010.

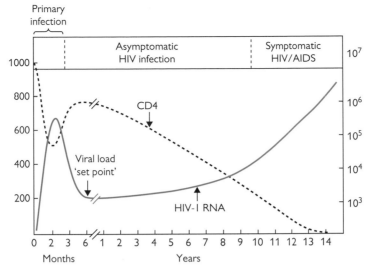

Figure 296.2 HIV disease classification and progression: typical changes in CD4 count (left axis, x 10^6 cells/l) and plasma HIV-1 RNA (right axis, copies per millilitre) with time, during the natural history of HIV infection.

Reproduced with permission from Luzzi, HIV/AIDS, in *Oxford Textbook of Medicine*, Fifth Edition Oxford University Press, Oxford, UK, Copyright © 2010.

'acquired immune deficiency syndrome' (AIDS) was previously used to classify the medical progression or the presence of specific clinical complications. There are now much better measures of diseases progression, and it is more common to refer to advanced/symptomatic HIV disease.

A small minority of HIV-infected patients (<0.5%) remain clinically well without needing antiretroviral therapy after 20 years or more of infection. These patients are known as 'long-term non-progressors'

(LTNPs) or 'elite controllers' and are defined on the basis of remaining healthy with CD4 counts exceeding 500 × 10^6 cells/l for 10 or more years and having a very low viral load without antiretroviral treatment. The low level of viral replication in the LTNP group has been attributed to a combination of host genetic factors that prevent HIV from gaining entry to host CD4+ T-cells, changes in the host immune response, and, very rarely, infection with attenuated or defective virus.

Table 296.1 Principal complications of untreated HIV infection

Infections	Neoplasms	Direct HIV effects
Early/intermediate HIV infection (CD4 >200x10⁶ cells/l)		
Varicella zoster (shingles)	Non-Hodgkin's lymphoma[a]	Persistent generalized lymphadenopathy
Oral hairy leucoplakia	Cervical intraepithelial neoplasia	Atopy; eczema
Oral candidiasis; candidal vaginitis	Anal intraepithelial neoplasia	Recurrent aphthous ulcers (oral and gastrointestinal tract)
Pulmonary tuberculosis[a]		Immune thrombocytopenia
Bacterial pneumonia, especially pneumococcal		Neutropenia
Bacteraemia, especially pneumococcal and salmonella		Neuropathy (mononeuritis multiplex; Guillian–Barré syndrome)
Bacillary angiomatosis		HIV-associated nephropathy (HIVAN)
		Lymphocytic interstitial pneumonitis (LIP)
Late HIV infection (CD4 <200x10⁶ cells/l)		
Pneumocystis pneumonia[a]	Kaposi's sarcoma[a]	HIV enteropathy
Candidal oesophagitis[a]	Primary cerebral lymphoma[a]	Peripheral neuropathy (distal, axonal)
Cerebral toxoplasmosis[a]	Hodgkin's lymphoma	Autonomic neuropathy
Cryptococcal meningitis[a]	Conjunctival carcinoma	Myelopathy
Chronic cryptosporidial diarrhoea[a]	Cervical carcinoma[a]	HIV dementia[a]
Chronic cystoisosporiasis[a], microsporidiosis	Anal carcinoma	Wasting syndrome[a]
Chronic HSV[a] ulceration		Cardiomyopathy
Extrapulmonary tuberculosis[a]		
Disseminated *M. avium* complex (MAC)[a]		
CMV (retinitis and disseminated)[a]		
Progressive multifocal leucoencephalopathy[a]		
Recurrent bacterial pneumonia[a]		
Recurrent bacteraemia, especially salmonella[a]		
Disseminated histoplasmosis[a], and *Talaromyces (Penicillium) marneffei*		

[a] AIDS-defining conditions; incomplete list.

Many of the early/intermediate manifestations also occur in late-stage HIV disease; non-Hodgkin's lymphoma is more common during the later stages.

Reproduced with permission from Luzzi, HIV/AIDS, in *Oxford Textbook of Medicine*, Fifth Edition Oxford University Press, Oxford, UK, Copyright © 2010.

Immunopathogenesis

The primary immunological effect of HIV infection is the dramatic depletion of CD4+ T-cells. Emerging concepts regarding the immune pathogenesis of HIV infection and the development of AIDS suggest that chronic systemic immune activation is an important feature of progressive HIV infection and differentiates it from non-pathogenic SIV infection in primates. Immune activation is seen in both CD4+/CD8+ T-cells and B-cells, which are polyclonally activated. T-cell proliferation is beneficial in the early stages of the disease, with partial restoration of CD4+ T-cell numbers, but sustained rapid turnover of immune cells imposes a strain on the homeostatic mechanism, resulting in a shorter cell half-life and clonal exhaustion. In addition, activated T-cells are targets for the virus itself, and this allows further replication of the virus, and the infection of more immune cells. Cytotoxic CD8+ T-cells only partially limit (but do not stop) viral replication, and neutralizing antibodies have little effect on viral replication. Thus, the clinical manifestations of the disease depend on the balance and interplay between host immune activation and viral replication. Clonal exhaustion leads to the progressive depletion of immune cells, as well as their loss of function, resulting in an immunodeficiency syndrome (AIDS).

Risk factors and transmission

HIV can affect both sexes equally and affects people of all ages. The virus is transmitted via blood and body fluids amongst adults. It is also transmitted vertically via maternofetal transfer and through breast milk. Although widespread across the world, endemicity is variable, with the highest rates in parts of Africa and increasing rapidly in Asia. Screening of blood donors for HIV has greatly reduced the chance of HIV transmission through transfusion. There is a small risk to healthcare workers exposed to HIV-infected blood through needle stick injury (about 0.3% for a high-risk deep needle stick injury); this figure is probably much lower if the health worker takes post-exposure prophylaxis very soon after the injury.

Staging of disease

As immunodeficiency progresses, there is an increased susceptibility to a variety of fungal, viral, bacterial, and protozoal infections. The absolute CD4 count is a useful way of staging HIV infection. The disease manifestations and susceptibility are inversely proportional to the absolute CD4+ T-cell levels, as shown in Figure 296.2. A count of <200 ×10^6 cells/l indicates advanced immunosuppression (previously referred to as AIDS) and renders a patient susceptible to a wide range of opportunistic infections The most common invasive pathogens occurring at any stage of infection are *Mycobacterium tuberculosis*, *Streptococcus pneumoniae*, and non-typhi *Salmonellae*. There is early increase in frequency and severity of mucosal and skin infections with pathogens such as herpes simplex, varicella zoster, candida, and dermatophytes, and bacteria such as staphylococci.

Clinical suspicion and triggers for testing

The availability of effective antiretroviral agents has increased the importance of early diagnosis. This requires a high index of clinical suspicion, to recognize early disease during seroconversion, and awareness of high-risk groups and high-risk behaviour patterns predisposing to HIV infections. Early recognition allows for prompt therapeutic interventions, including disease monitoring and treatment, which dramatically improve patient survival and quality of life and reduce infectivity to others. This is not only beneficial for the individual patient, but also has implications for wider public health.

Historically, HIV testing has been the subject of much political debate, with excessive emphasis on the need for protracted 'counselling' of individuals perceived to be at risk due to lifestyle or other factors. However, HIV infection is now recognized to be a treatable infection that all may contract, and all healthcare workers should be capable of offering the test routinely in any healthcare setting. HIV testing in the UK is now recommended for specific groups with identifiable behavioural risks, and for all patients with medical conditions that are more common or more severe in HIV-positive individuals (see Box 296.1). The presence of any of these should prompt the clinician to suggest that an HIV test be performed. Universal HIV testing is recommended in all antenatal services; genitourinary medicine or sexual health services; abortion services; and drug dependency

---

Box 296.1 Clinical indicator diseases for adult HIV infection; patients with the following specific indicator conditions should be routinely offered an HIV test

Respiratory
- aspergillosis
- bacterial pneumonia
- pneumocystis pneumonia
- tuberculosis

Gastroenterology
- chronic diarrhoea of unknown cause
- cryptosporidiosis
- hepatitis B infection
- hepatitis C infection
- oesophageal candidiasis
- oral hairy leucoplakia
- persistent oral candidiasis
- proven salmonella, shigella, or campylobacter infection
- weight loss of unknown cause

Neurology
- cerebral toxoplasmosis
- cryptococcal meningitis
- dementia
- Guillain–Barré syndrome
- leucoencephalopathy
- primary CNS lymphoma
- transverse myelitis

Dermatology
- Kaposi's sarcoma
- severe acne
- severe psoriasis
- severe seborrhoeic dermatitis
- varicella zoster especially recurrent or multidermatomal presentations

ENT
- chronic parotitis
- lymphadenopathy of unknown cause
- parotid cysts

Haematology
- unexplained lymphopenia
- unexplained neutropenia
- unexplained thrombocytopenia

Oncology
- anal intraepithelial neoplasia
- Castleman's disease
- Hodgkin's disease
- lung cancer
- non-Hodgkin's lymphoma
- seminoma

Gynaecology
- cervical cancer
- vaginal intraepithelial neoplasia

Ophthalmology
- cytomegalovirus retinitis
- infective retinal diseases, including herpes virus infection
- toxoplasmosis

Other
- any sexually transmitted infection
- mononucleosis-type syndrome
- pyrexia of unknown origin

programmes. In some parts of the UK with a higher prevalence of HIV in the adult population (>2/1000), all patients presenting for hospital admission should be offered testing.

Evidence suggests that requesting HIV testing on a routine or opt-out basis is easier for healthcare workers and acceptable to patients, as it is perceived as non-judgemental. Although risk should be discussed without prejudgement, it is appropriate to offer the test to anyone who might be at risk. Those considered at risk include men who have had sex with men; female sexual contacts of men who have sex with men; persons from an area with high prevalence of HIV; those who have had multiple sexual partners, a history of sexually transmitted infection, or of injecting drug use; those having been raped; those having had blood transfusions, transplants, or other risk-prone procedures in countries without rigorous procedures for HIV screening; and those who may have had an occupational exposure.

Verbal consent for testing should be recorded in the case notes, and specific arrangements should be agreed on how the result will be given to the patient and who may know about the result. For the small number of people who feel challenged by being asked to have an HIV test, local infectious disease or genitourinary medicine specialists (usually nurses/counsellors/health advisers) can assist. Before giving a patient a positive or equivocal result (always in person, never over the telephone), make arrangements for immediate review by a specialist healthcare worker experienced in HIV.

The most widely used tests identify specific anti-HIV antibodies in blood or saliva. This is done by laboratory ELISA testing. The WHO no longer recommends Western blotting for confirmation, suggesting instead that, if it is necessary, the combination of ELISA with a simple or rapid assay is as reliable. Antibodies to HIV typically appear 4–6 weeks after infection, but this may occasionally take as long as 12 weeks. During acute HIV infection, also known as the seroconversion or 'window' period, antibody tests may be negative, weakly positive, or discordant. The CD4 cell count should not be used as a surrogate marker for the diagnosis of HIV infection.

Clinical staging depends on the presence or absence of complications of immunosuppression, and simple laboratory parameters, particularly the full blood count and CD4 cell count. Response to treatment is evaluated primarily by the response of the plasma HIV viral load to therapy and secondarily by the rise in CD4 count following treatment.

Principles of treatment

There is currently no cure or successful vaccine for HIV infection. Current treatment for HIV infection consists of highly active antiretroviral therapy (HAART). The only effective prevention is to take appropriate measures to avoid primary infection. Interventions supporting safer sex and improving knowledge of HIV and transmission risk have had some success.

Over 20 antiretroviral drugs are licensed for clinical use as antiretroviral therapy (ART). The WHO now recommends that most patients should receive ART when HIV is diagnosed, irrespective of the presence or absence of symptoms or the CD4 cell count, as this prevents the immune system from deteriorating to a point where the individual becomes very susceptible to infections. It also greatly reduces the risk of onward transmission of HIV to others. Since its introduction in 1996, HAART has dramatically reduced patient mortality. The preferred options are combinations containing at least two or three different classes of antiretroviral agents, namely nucleoside analogue reverse transcriptase inhibitors, protease inhibitors, and non-nucleoside analogue reverse transcriptase inhibitors. Newer classes of drugs include CCR5 inhibitors, integrase inhibitors, and fusion inhibitors (see Table 296.2).

Treatment with HAART reduces HIV-associated morbidity, mortality, and infectivity to others. Many antiretroviral drugs are safe to use during pregnancy, to prevent mother-to-child transmission. However, the HIV viral load rises on discontinuation of treatment, and resistance to medication develops, so the clinical effectiveness in suppressing HIV viraemia falls dramatically if patient adherence is less than 90%. Much of the clinic follow-up of patients with HIV is aimed at supporting adherence to ART. Adherence is maximized by altering the daily lifestyle around medication times, minimizing the pill burden by using once-daily combinations of as few pills as possible, and tailoring therapy to minimize side effects. This is one of the areas in which the specialist multidisciplinary team have much to offer in the care of people with HIV.

Some antiretroviral drugs have profound effects on metabolism and have many side effects. These include hypersensitivity, hyperlipidaemia, lipodystrophy, renal impairment, renal stones, insulin resistance, peripheral neuropathy, bone marrow suppression, lactic acidosis, and hepatotoxicity.

Post-exposure prophylaxis following accidental occupational or sexual HIV exposure should be universally available and is about 80% effective in reducing transmission. When prescribing post-exposure prophylaxis after occupational exposure, local protocols should be followed. Following an injury, the wound should be washed and encouraged to bleed. The source patient and the healthcare worker should be tested for HIV but, if the test is not immediately available, there should be no delay in giving prophylaxis, which is only effective if initiated within 72 hours, and preferably within 4 hours of the exposure.

Pre-exposure prophylaxis (PrEP) is available in some countries, including the UK, for HIV negative individuals who identify themselves as having a high risk for acquiring HIV infection.

Table 296.2 Principal antiretroviral agents			
Nucleoside reverse transcriptase inhibitors	**Non-nucleoside reverse transcriptase inhibitors**	**Protease inhibitors**	**Entry inhibitors**
Zidovudine	Nevirapine	Lopinavir[a]	*Fusion inhibitor*
Lamivudine	Efavirenz	Ritonavir	Enfuvirtide (T20)
Emtricitabine	Etravirine	Atazanavir[a]	
	Rilpivirine		
Abacavir		Saquinavir[a]	*CCR5 antagonist*
Didanosine		Fosamprenavir[a]	Maraviroc
Stavudine		Indinavir[a]	
Nucleotide reverse transcriptase inhibitor		Tipranavir[a]	*Integrase inhibitors*
Tenofovir		Darunavir[a]	Raltegravir
			Elvitegravir[a]
			Dolutegravir[a]
			Carbotegravir

Other compounds (not shown) are at earlier phases of development and evaluation.

[a]Given with low-dose ritonavir or cobicistat for pharmacokinetic enhancement.

Adapted with permission from Luzzi, HIV/AIDS, in *Oxford Textbook of Medicine*, Fifth Edition Oxford University Press, Oxford, UK, Copyright © 2010.

Immune reconstitution inflammatory syndrome

Immune reconstitution inflammatory syndrome (IRIS) occurs in a proportion of HIV patients (10%–30%) after introduction of ART. This is thought to be due to the restoration of the host immune system to mount an inflammatory response following treatment and may result from a dysregulated balance between the number and function of T-cells, pro-inflammatory cytokines, and T-regulatory cells.

The factors associated with an increased risk of developing IRIS are:

- low CD4 cell count at the start of ART
- good virological response to ART (>2 log drop in plasma HIV viral load within 90 days)
- preexisting antigenic burden of opportunistic infection prior to starting ART
- early initiation of ART after opportunistic infection

The clinical manifestations are varied and are predominantly driven by the type of underlying opportunistic infection prior to starting ART. There is no diagnostic test for IRIS. Early initiation of ART prior to the development of significant immunosuppression and opportunistic infection may reduce the risk of development of IRIS. The suggested approaches for the treatment of IRIS, either as monotherapy or in combination, include:

- use of corticosteroids or NSAIDs
- pathogen-specific treatment (e.g. antituberculous treatment)

Prognosis and how to estimate it

In the absence of HAART, the median time from infection with HIV to progression to advanced symptoms is about 10 years, and median survival after diagnosis of AIDS is less than 1 year. The range is wide: poor prognostic indicators include low CD4 count at diagnosis, male gender, age >40, and concurrent morbidities. The use of HAART has increased the life expectancy of a newly diagnosed individual by at least two decades, as evidenced by the survival of patients diagnosed in the late 1980s and early 1990s. However, together with increasing survival, there is an increased incidence of complications such as lymphoma, other cancers (e.g. lung, cervix), and non-infectious comorbidities (e.g. renal disease, myocardial disease, and metabolic syndromes). People with diagnosed HIV infection should follow safer sex and safer drug use practices. Delays in diagnosis can increase transmission of HIV and lead to decreased life expectancy, death, and increased morbidity.

Further Reading

Aidsmap: extensive information on treatments and general management and lifestyle issues, including updates on the latest research; database of HIV organizations worldwide; useful for patients and healthcare workers (http://www.aidsmap.com)

British HIV Association Guidelines (http://www.bhiva.org/Guidelines.aspx)

Cihlar T and Fordyce M. Current status and prospects of HIV treatment. *Curr Opin Virol* 2016; 18: 50–6.

Drug Interactions, University of Liverpool: up-to-date interactions of most drugs with antiretroviral therapy, with relevant advice for dose modification; includes free apps for mobile devices (http://www.HIV-druginteractions.org)

Medical Foundation for HIV and Sexual Health: website with various free resources, including illustrated handbooks for recognition and testing of HIV in primary and secondary care, and other practical resources around testing (http://www.medfash.org.uk)

Definition of the disease

Antibody deficiencies comprise a heterogeneous group of disorders characterized by a failure of antibody production and recurrent infections. Antibody deficiency may be primary or secondary to other medical conditions such as B-cell lymphoid malignancies, drugs, and urinary or gastrointestinal loss of IgG.

Aetiology of the disease

Antibody deficiencies result from inherited or acquired disorders that lead to abnormalities in the development, maturation, and/or function of B-lymphocytes. Impaired functioning of B-cells leads to decreased immunoglobulin production, which manifests clinically as an increased susceptibility to infections. Some of these diseases occur due to single-gene mutations which affect the development or function of B-lymphocytes. Key steps in B-cell development, and known genetic defects responsible for arrested B-cell development, are summarized in Figure 297.1. B-cells are derived from the common lymphoid progenitor and develop within the bone marrow. Mature, naive B-cells leave the bone marrow and circulate within the bloodstream. The final stages of maturation occur within the germinal centre of secondary lymphoid organs (lymph nodes, spleen) on encounter with the specific antigen. This process requires interaction with CD4+ T-cells, resulting in class switch recombination and somatic hypermutation, which leads to formation of antigen-specific high-affinity antibodies (immunoglobulins).

The most common group of symptomatic antibody deficiencies, common variable immunodeficiency (CVID) disorders, are, however, likely to be polygenic disorders resulting from yet unidentified environmental triggers in genetically predisposed individuals.

From the point of view of clinical investigation, it is useful to classify antibody deficiency in terms of circulating B-cell numbers and the pattern of reduction of serum immunoglobulins (see Table 297.1). While the absence of B-cells is highly suggestive of an inherited defect interfering with B-cell development, an elevated serum IgM in association with reduced IgG and or IgA points to a defect in immunoglobulin

class switching, as exemplified by the spectrum of hyperimmunoglobulin M (HIGM) syndromes.

Typical symptoms of the disease, and less common symptoms

Typically, patients with inherited antibody deficiencies are protected for the first 6 months of life because of transplacental transmission of maternal IgG. Many of the single-gene defects and primary defects that result in pan-hypogammaglobulinaemia (severe reduction in all three major immunoglobulin isotypes) present later in infancy or early childhood. However, CVID may not clinically manifest until adolescence or early adulthood.

Recurrent bacterial infections of the respiratory tract are a common feature of all types of antibody deficiency. In addition, up to 40% of patients with CVID develop inflammatory gastrointestinal disease, concomitant lymphoproliferative disorders, autoimmune phenomena, or granulomatous inflammation.

Demographics of the disease

The overall prevalence of clinically significant primary antibody deficiency is estimated to vary from 1: 25 000 to 1: 110 000. The commonest immunodeficiency is selective IgA deficiency with a prevalence of 1:500 to 1:700, but a majority of these patients remain asymptomatic. CVID occurs with an estimated incidence of 1: 25 000 to 1:50 000. HIGM syndromes are estimated to occur in 1:1 000 000 to 1:2 000 000 live births. Other single-gene defects are even rarer, with only few reported cases for some conditions.

Natural history, and complications of the disease

Bronchiectasis is a frequent consequence of recurrent sino-pulmonary infections with encapsulated organisms, commonly, *Streptococcus pneumonia, Haemophilus influenza,* and *Staphylococcus*

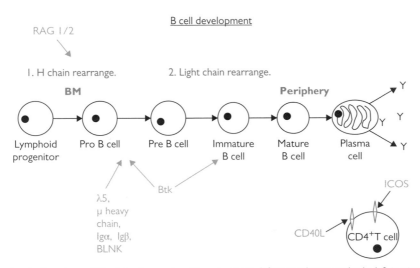

Figure 297.1 Diagram showing key stages of B-cell development, and known genetic defects resulting in antibody deficiencies; BLNK, B-cell linker; Btk, Bruton's tyrosine kinase; RAG, recombination activating gene.

Table 297.1 Inherited disorders resulting in antibody deficiency

Disease	Genetic disorder	Inheritance
I. Severe reduction in all Immunoglobulin isotypes with absent B-cells		
1. X-linked agammaglobulinaemia (XLA)	Mutations in *BTK*	X-linked recessive (XL)
2. Autosomal recessive agammaglobulinaemia	Mutations in μ heavy chain or λ5	Autosomal recessive (AR)
3. Ig heavy chain defect	Mutations in Igα or Igβ	AR
4. BLNK deficiency	Mutations in *BLNK*	AR
II. Reduction in at least 2 isotypes with normal or decreased B-cells		
1. Common Variable Immunodeficiency disorders (CVIDs)	Possible polygenic disease. Associated polymorphisms in TACI, BAFFR and Msh5 reported	AD/AR, 10% positive family history
2. ICOS deficiency	Mutation in ICOS	AR
3. CD19 deficiency	Mutation in CD19	AR
III. Single isotype deficiencies with normal B cell numbers		
1. Selective IgA deficiency	Unknown	Variable
2. Isolated IgG subclass deficiency	Unknown	Variable
3. IgA with IgG subclass deficiency	Unknown	Variable
IV. Hyperimmunoglobulin M (HIGM) syndromes		
1. CD40L deficiency	Mutations in *CD40L* (CD154)	XL recessive
2. CD40 deficiency	Mutations in CD40	AR
3. AID deficiency	Mutations in *AICDA* gene	AR
4. UNG deficiency	Mutations in *UNG* gene	AR

Abbreviations: AD, autosomal dominant; AR, autosomal recessive.

Reprinted from *Journal of Allergy and Clinical Immunology*, volume 124, issue 6, Notarangelo et al, Primary immunodeficiencies: 2009 update, pp. 1161–78, Copyright (2009), with permission from Elsevier.

aureus. Other sites of infection include the skin, the joints, the gastrointestinal tract, and the urinary tract. Chronic fungal or viral infections are rare. However, enteroviral meningoencephalitis has been reported in patients with X-linked agammaglobulinaemia. The current practice of maintaining a higher-trough IgG level has significantly reduced the incidence of this complication. *Pneumocystis jiroveci* (*carinii*), which is an unusual pathogen in pure antibody deficiency, has been reported in patients with HIGM syndromes, in keeping with the combined B- and T-cell defects seen in these patients.

Despite the inability to mount antibody responses against exogenous antigens, some patients with CVID mount paradoxical immune responses to self-antigens, resulting in autoimmune disease.

Other non-infectious complications include polyclonal lymphocytic infiltration, frank lymphoma, enteropathy, and liver abnormalities.

Recent data from CVID patients collected from seven European centres showed that the highest mortality in this cohort was seen in patients with enteropathy or polyclonal lymphoid infiltration.

Approach to diagnosing the disease

A good clinical history, a high degree of suspicion, and awareness of the possibility of a new diagnosis of primary antibody deficiency in any age group are important for the diagnosis of this condition. Antibody deficiencies must be considered in patients with SPUR (**s**evere, **p**ersistent, **u**nusual, or **r**ecurrent) infections.

First-line investigations are:

- full blood count, including lymphocyte count
- serum immunoglobulin levels
- specific antibodies and vaccine responses to protein and polysaccharide antigens
- serum and urine electrophoresis
- renal and liver function tests, including albumin levels
- quantification of circulating T-cells, B-cells, and natural killer cells
- B-lymphocyte memory panels for naive and switched memory B-cells

Second-line or specialized tests for known single-gene defects include:

- BTK protein expression and mutation analysis for the BTK gene
- CD40L/CD40 expression by flow cytometry, a technique by which the surface and intracellular characteristics of single cells

are analysed via a combination of lasers and fluorochrome-tagged antibodies
- mutation analysis for known genetic defects
- genetic tests for other known single-gene defects and polymorphisms

Screening for complications includes:

- radiology: baseline CT scan, ultrasound scan of abdomen (if clinically indicated)
- pulmonary function tests and gas transfer
- investigation for autoimmune diseases as appropriate

Differential diagnosis

Primary antibody deficiency must be differentiated from antibody deficiency, due to secondary causes such as loss of protein from the gut or urinary tract, chronic infections (HIV, persistent EBV), and disorders where the function of B-lymphocytes may be affected due to a malignant process (myeloma or lymphoma) or as a side effect of medications (including immunosuppressive agents and anticonvulsants). In children with recurrent bacterial infections, it is important to consider other causes of impaired immune function, such as:

- transient hypogammaglobulinaemia of infancy
- leaky severe combined immunodeficiency
- undefined combined immunodeficiency
- cystic fibrosis

'Gold-standard' diagnostic test

The gold standard for diagnosis of primary antibody deficiencies due to single-gene defects is demonstration of the genetic defect. The diagnosis of CVID still remains a diagnosis of exclusion, after ruling out other known causes of antibody deficiencies (see Box 297.1).

Acceptable diagnostic alternatives

The initial working diagnosis of primary antibody deficiency can be established with a good clinical history and supporting evidence from initial blood tests, including serum immunoglobulin levels, specific antibody responses, and lymphocyte surface markers

Flow cytometric analysis for expression of proteins (BTK and CD40L) may be required in selected cases. These results are usually

Box 297.1 Diagnostic criteria to define common variable immunodeficiency disorders

- less than 4 years of age
- serum IgG level less than 4.5 g/l for adults or the 2.5th percentile for age; serum IgA level less than the lower limit of normal for age and/or serum IgM level less than the lower limit of normal for age
- lack of antibody responses to protein antigens from exposure or immunization
- exclusion of all other known causes of failure of antibody production

Chapel H, Cunningham-Rundles C. Update in understanding common variable immunodeficiency disorders (CVIDs) and the management of patients with these conditions. Br J Haematol 2009; 145: 709–727

sufficient to institute appropriate management while further investigations are carried out to establish a definitive diagnosis.

Prognosis and how to estimate it

Treatment of patients with antibody deficiency syndromes with replacement immunoglobulin therapy and aggressive antibiotic treatment significantly improves the prognosis, with a reduction in the number of infection episodes and infection-related complications, such as the development or progression of bronchiectasis. This, however, does not alter the natural course of the condition or the development of non-infectious complications.

Although it is impossible to make accurate prognostic judgements for individual patients with primary antibody deficiency, there is sufficient evidence to support the contention that maintenance of adequate trough IgG levels, rapid treatment of infections, and close monitoring for complications such as lymphoproliferative disease have resulted in long-term survival that is only a few years below that of the actuarial curves of the normal population.

Treatment and its effectiveness

The mainstay of treatment for primary antibody deficiency is replacement immunoglobulin therapy, along with judicious use of antibiotics for the treatment of acute infections as well as for prophylaxis in individual patients. Currently, immunoglobulin replacement can be achieved effectively either intravenously or subcutaneously. Both methods have been shown to be safe and efficacious in decreasing the incidence and severity of infections in patients with antibody deficiencies. The recommended starting dose is 0.4–0.6 g/kg per month, titrated in each individual patient to achieve optimal protection against infections.

Further Reading

Durandy A, Kracker S, and Fischer A. Primary antibody deficiencies. *Nat Rev Immunol* 2013; 13: 519–33.

Lucas M, Lee M, Lortan J, et al. Infection outcomes in patients with common variable immunodeficiency disorders: Relationship to immunoglobulin therapy over 22 years. *J Allergy Clin Immunol* 2010; 125: 1354–60.

298 Combined T- and B-cell immunodeficiencies

Siraj Misbah

Definition of the disease

Combined defects in the functioning of T- lymphocytes and B-lymphocytes are predominantly disorders of childhood, and are encompassed by the term severe combined immunodeficiency (SCID). SCID comprises a heterogeneous group of inherited disorders characterized by fundamental defects in T-cell development, accompanied by severe impairment of B-cell function. Although SCID is largely a paediatric problem, prompt diagnosis followed by early haemopoietic stem cell transplantation (HSCT) has resulted in many adult survivors, who are followed up by clinical immunologists.

Aetiology of the disease

Several different molecular defects which lead to SCID have been identified (see Table 298.1). These comprise mutations in genes encoding for purine pathway enzymes, and a range of molecules involved in signal transduction, including tyrosine kinases, cytokine receptors, and key cell surface receptors. Of the different molecular defects responsible for SCID, X-linked SCID (due to mutations in the gene encoding the common gamma chain of cytokine receptors (γc) shared by five interleukins (interleukins 2, 4, 7, 9, and 15)) accounts for 40% of all cases of SCID in the US. Deficiency of adenosine deaminase (ADA), a key enzyme in the purine salvage pathway, accounts for approximately 15% of cases. While lymphopenia is characteristic of all forms of SCID, analysis of the exact numbers of circulating T-cells, B-cells, and natural killer (NK) cells provides useful clues as to the underlying genetic defect. For example, ADA deficiency causes severe global lymphopenia (T-cell negative, B-cell negative, NK-cell negative), while γc deficiency causes T-cell and NK-cell lymphopenia (T-cell negative, B-cell positive, NK-cell negative).

Apart from SCID, a rare group of patients with the hyperimmunoglobulin M (HIGM) syndrome have combined T-cell and B-cell defects, which are characterized by defective immunoglobulin class switching. Typically, patients have elevated serum IgM levels, accompanied by reduced IgG and IgA, due to a failure to switch from IgM to other classes of immunoglobulin when mounting a secondary immune response against pathogens. The commonest form of the HIGM syndrome affects males, due to transmission in an X-linked recessive manner, and is due to mutations in the gene encoding for the CD40 ligand on T-cells. Defective expression of the CD40 ligand interferes with crosstalk between T-cells and B-cells, leading to impaired antibody production (Figure 298.1).

CD40 deficiency results in a clinical picture identical to CD40 ligand deficiency but is inherited in an autosomal recessive fashion.

Typical symptoms of the disease

Children with SCID typically present in the first few months of life, with recurrent viral and fungal infections on a background of lymphopenia. The latter is an important diagnostic clue which is present in most cases. Awareness of the importance of persistent lymphopenia in the context of a baby with recurrent infections is enabling earlier diagnosis and, consequently, has improved the chances of curative treatment with HSCT or gene therapy.

In keeping with the profound T-cell and B-cell defects associated with SCID, infection with a range of intracellular pathogens (CMV, varicella, adenovirus, respiratory syncytial virus, EBV), fungi (*Pneumocystis jiroveci, Candida* sp.), and bacteria (*Pseudomonas* sp., *Streptococcus pneumoniae*) are a prominent part of the clinical picture. Contrary to popular belief, some babies with SCID may show no evidence of growth retardation.

In keeping with the lack of functioning T-cells and B-cells, babies with SCID are unable to reject foreign tissue and are at serious risk of transfusion-associated graft-vs-host disease (TA-GvHD). All babies with suspected or confirmed SCID should, therefore, only receive irradiated blood which has been screened to be CMV negative. Equally, immunization with live vaccines is contraindicated, to avoid the risk of vaccine-induced disease, as evidenced by the development of BCG-induced mycobacterial disease in SCID.

Boys and adults with the X-linked HIGM syndrome present with recurrent bacterial infections, neutropenia, and pneumocystis infection. Defective T-cell function is associated with chronic intestinal and biliary colonization with *Cryptosporidium* spp., leading to enteritis and ascending cholangitis. The lack of lymph node germinal centres due to defective interaction between T-cells and B-cells is a characteristic histological feature.

Demographics of the disease

SCID is rare, with an estimated incidence of 1 in 50 000 to 1 in 100 000 live births. This figure is likely to be higher in those populations with a high degree of consanguineous marriages. Although the disease predominantly presents in infancy, less severe forms of combined T-cell and B-cell deficiency (leaky SCID) may present in adulthood, as seen in ADA deficiency. The preponderance of genes encoding important immunological functions on the X-chromosome leads to a predominance of affected boys.

Table 298.1 Common causes of severe combined immunodeficiency

Site of deficiency	Inheritance	Phenotype	Percentage of cases
Common gamma chain (γc) of T cell receptor	X-linked recessive	T−, B+, NK−	~40%
Adenosine deaminase (ADA)	Autosomal recessive	T−, B−, NK−	~15%
Alpha chain of IL-7 receptor	Autosomal recessive	T−, B+, NK+	~10%
Janus kinase3 (Jak3)	Autosomal recessive	T−, B+, NK−	<10%

Abbreviations: B, B-cell; NK, natural killer cell; T, T-cell.

Reproduced with permission from Warrell, Cox and Firth, *Oxford Textbook of Medicine*, Fifth Edition, Oxford University Press, Oxford, UK, Copyright © 2010.

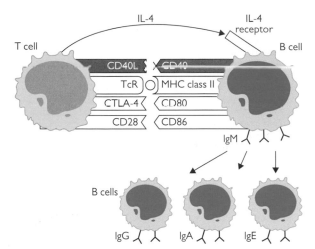

Figure 298.1 Interaction between the CD40 ligand on T-cells, and CD40 on B-cells, under the influence of interleukin 4, leading to isotype switching; CD40L, CD40 ligand; IL-4, interleukin 4; TcR, T-cell receptor. *Essentials of Clinical Immunology*, Sixth edition, Helen Chapel, Mansel Haeney, Siraj Misbah and Neil Snowden. 2014. John Wiley & Sons Ltd.

Natural history, and complications of the disease

Until the advent of HSCT, SCID was invariably fatal during infancy. The only exceptions to this dictum were rare cases of spontaneous reversion of gene mutations, as described with SCID associated with γc deficiency. Lack of awareness of the possibility of SCID in an ill baby may lead to unirradiated blood transfusions with the attendant risk of TA-GvHD. Iatrogenic disease may also result from the use of live vaccines in babies before the diagnosis of SCID has been made; for example, a newborn baby with SCID may receive a BCG vaccine due to a failure to grasp the significance of a family history of previous siblings affected with SCID.

Approach to diagnosis

The combination of recurrent infections and lymphopenia in a baby should prompt serious consideration of SCID as a possible diagnosis. In pursuing this diagnosis, it is essential to obtain evidence of combined T-cell and B-cell dysfunction, as evidenced by the presence of T-cell lymphopenia, impaired lymphocyte proliferation, and hypogammaglobulinaemia. The key investigations required to demonstrate these features are circulating lymphocyte surface marker analysis to quantify numbers of T-cells, B-cells, and NK cells. Simultaneous analysis of key cell surface markers, such as human leukocyte antigen (HLA) Class II proteins, may provide additional clues regarding the precise form of SCID. Measurement of serum immunoglobulins and specific antibodies serve as markers of B-cell function. While the circulating lymphocyte surface marker profile provides useful clues as to the underlying molecular defect, definitive diagnosis requires sequencing of the relevant gene to identify disease-causing mutations.

The diagnosis of HIGM syndrome should be considered in any patient with the characteristic immunoglobulin profile of elevated or normal serum IgM, low serum IgG, and low serum IgA on a background of recurrent bacterial infections or chronic cryptosporidial enteritis. Suspicion of the X-linked HIGM syndrome should be investigated by the demonstration of the absence of CD40 ligand expression on activated T-cells.

Other diagnoses that should be considered

The main alternative diagnosis that should be considered in the setting of recurrent infections and lymphopenia is HIV infection, because of similarities in the clinical presentations of vertically transmitted HIV infection and SCID. Indeed, it is good practice to exclude the possibility of HIV infection in the workup of any baby with suspected SCID. Very rarely, intestinal lymphangiectasia may be associated with T-cell lymphopenia and a low serum IgG as a direct consequence of loss of IgG and efflux of lymphocytes via aberrant lymphatic channels. These cases are distinguishable from SCID by the characteristic clinical picture and low albumin accompanying an isolated low-IgG and low-T-cell lymphopenia.

Clinically significant drug-induced combined T-cell and B-cell defects may occur in some patients who have received chemotherapy for cancer or immunosuppressive therapy for autoimmune disease. Drugs responsible for such iatrogenic immune defects include corticosteroids, cyclophosphamide, fludarabine, methotrexate, azathioprine, mycophenolate mofetil, and ciclosporin. Interestingly, while ciclosporin interferes with CD40 ligand expression on human T-cells, this is not associated with clinical features suggestive of the HIGM syndrome. Where significant drug-induced immune deficiency associated with T-cell and B-cell defects does develop, they do not usually pose a diagnostic challenge because of the clinical context in which immunodeficiency develops.

'Gold-standard' diagnostic test

The demonstration of arrested T-cell development, by way of T-cell lymphopenia, accompanied by evidence of severe B-cell deficiency in the form of hypogammaglobulinaemia in the context of a baby with recurrent infections, is sufficient to establish a diagnosis of SCID. However, precise molecular diagnosis is essential for purposes of genetic counselling, prenatal diagnosis, assessing prognosis, and, in the future, using gene therapy. The selection of which genes to focus on is heavily influenced by the circulating lymphocyte profile in terms of T-cells, B-cells, and NK cells (see Table 298.1).

Confirmation of suspected X-linked HIGM syndrome requires sequencing of the CD40 ligand gene.

Acceptable diagnostic alternatives to the gold standard

In view of the ease with which serum immunoglobulins and circulating lymphocytes can be measured, there is little need for alternative surrogate tests of T-cell and B-cell function. In a resource-limited setting where access to flow cytometry may be limited, the finding of an absolute lymphopenia would be highly indicative of T-cell lymphopenia, since T-cells constitute approximately 70% of the circulating lymphocyte count. Similarly, the absence of a thymic shadow on a chest X-ray would point to a T-cell defect, but its utility as a diagnostic marker is limited by the occurrence of thymic atrophy in acutely ill babies.

Other relevant investigations

In the assessment of a child with suspected SCID or HIGM syndrome, a thorough microbiological investigation is essential to make a precise diagnosis of infective pathogens and institute appropriate treatment. Imaging of the chest followed by bronchoalveolar lavage, where possible, is important to explore the possibility of pneumocystis infection. A chest X-ray may also yield additional diagnostic clues regarding thymic size and the presence of chondro-osseous dysplasia, which is a feature of ADA deficiency. Measurement of ADA activity should be performed in any baby with profound lymphopenia affecting all classes of lymphocytes (T-cells, B-cells, and NK cells). Once the diagnosis of SCID is confirmed, HLA typing of the patient and family members will be required in a search for a suitable bone marrow donor.

Prognosis and how to estimate it

Speed is of the essence in making a diagnosis of SCID in order to enable prompt and potentially curative HSCT or gene therapy to be performed. The donor source and extent of HLA matching is a strong influence on the outcome of HSCT, with the best results being obtained with a HLA-matched, genotypically identical transplant, where survival rates of 80% at 20 years have been achieved. While HSCT is curative in the majority of patients, a significant minority will experience long-term problems with persistent chronic TA-GvHD and autoimmune and inflammatory complications.

In CD40 ligand deficiency, 40%–50% of patients treated with immunoglobulin replacement therapy and antibiotics will not survive beyond the fourth decade.

Treatment and its effectiveness

Currently, HSCT from an HLA-matched sibling donor offers an 80% chance of cure, while a fully HLA-matched unrelated donor transplant offers a 70% chance of cure. A minority of patients will fail to achieve adequate B-cell reconstitution, thus requiring long-term immunoglobulin replacement even after HSCT.

For babies with SCID due to a clearly defined single-gene defect, where a suitable HLA-matched donor is unavailable, gene therapy offers great promise, as shown in some children with ADA deficiency or common γc-chain deficiency, with clear evidence of T-cell, B-cell, and NK-cell reconstitution in the former, and T-cell and NK-cell reconstitution in the latter. Gene therapy does, however, carry with it the risk of insertional mutagenesis, as exemplified by the development of T-cell lymphoproliferative disease in some babies with common γc-chain SCID, due to integration of the retroviral vector close to a known T-cell proto-oncogene, LMO2. While this serious adverse event proved to be a temporary setback to gene therapy, the development of new strategies to minimize the risk of insertional mutagenesis and allow better regulation of gene expression has allowed gene therapy trials for SCID to continue.

In CD40 ligand deficiency, while the B-cell defect is managed by regular immunoglobulin infusions, correction of the fundamental defect requires HSCT. Currently, HSCT is curative in approximately 60% of cases. The mortality in the remainder of cases has been due to severe infection, with reactivated cryptosporidial disease being a particular problem.

Further Reading

Chapel H, Haeney M, Misbah S, et al. *Essentials of Clinical Immunology* (6th edition), 2014. Wiley-Blackwell.

Immune Deficiency Foundation *Patient & Family Handbook for Primary Immunodeficiency Diseases* (http://primaryimmune.org/)

Pai S-Y, Logan BR, Griffith LM, et al. Transplantation outcomes for severe combined immunodeficiency, 2000–2009. *N Engl J Med* 2014; 371: 434–46.

Definition of the disease

The complement system comprises a group of heat-labile proteins which form part of the innate immune system. There are three early complement pathways: namely, the classical pathway, the alternative pathway, and the mannan-binding-lectin (MBL) pathway, all of which converge with the cleavage of C3 (see Figure 299.1). The main physiological functions of the complement system include defence against pyogenic bacterial infections, clearance of immune complexes and products of inflammatory damage, and acting as a bridge between the innate and adaptive immune system (see Table 299.1).

The complement system is regulated by various complement inhibitors (regulatory proteins) that are present in both the classical pathway and the alternate pathway and which regulate and prevent spontaneous activation of the complement system, thereby preventing complement-mediated damage to tissues under normal circumstances. Inherited deficiency of complement proteins or inhibitors may result in disease.

Acquired complement deficiency may occur as a consequence of autoantibody-mediated inhibition of complement proteins, as evidenced by anti-C1-inhibitor and acquired angioedema and anti-C3 nephritic factor and mesangiocapillary glomerulonephritis.

Aetiology of the disease

Genetic defects are described for nearly all the components of the complement system. Most of the defects in the classical complement pathway are inherited as autosomal recessive traits. Defects in the alternative pathway are rare. Properdin deficiency (affecting the alternative pathway) is an X-linked recessive condition, and the mode of inheritance of factor D deficiency is not known. Inherited defects affecting the inhibitors or regulatory proteins of the complement system, namely C1-inhibitor and factors H and I, have also been described. C1-inhibitor deficiency is the most well characterized; it is inherited in an autosomal dominant manner and is associated with hereditary angioedema. Mutations in the gene coding for C1-inhibitor result in either an absent or a non-functional protein. C1-inhibitor deficiency may be acquired secondary to a range of lymphoproliferative conditions, including chronic lymphocytic leukaemia and multiple myeloma.

In addition to disease-causing mutations, genetic polymorphisms have been described for many complement components.

Typical symptoms of the disease, and less common ones

Recurrent infections

Patients with inherited complement defects have an increased susceptibility to pyogenic infections. Properdin deficiency and defects in the components of the terminal lytic pathway are particularly associated with an increased susceptibility to neisserial infections, indicating the importance of the cytolytic property of the terminal membrane attack complex in host defence against *Neisseria*.

SLE-like syndrome

Deficiency of the early components of the classical pathway (C1q, C1r, C1s, C2, and C4) is associated with SLE, in keeping with the role

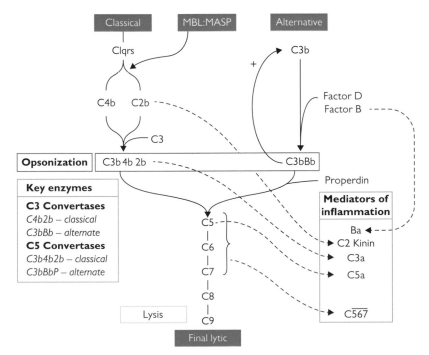

Figure 299.1 Schematic representation of complement pathways.

Essentials of Clinical Immunology, Sixth edition, Helen Chapel, Maneel Haeney, Siraj Misbah and Neil Snowden. 2014. John Wiley & Sons Ltd.

Table 299.1 Physiological role of complement

Function	Complement component
Host defence	
Opsonization	C3b covalently bound fragments of C3
Chemotaxis and chemoattraction	C3a C5a C4a
Bacterial lysis	Terminal lytic complex (C5b–C9)
Bridge between innate and adaptive	
Complement antibody responses	C3b and C4b C3 receptors on B-cells
Enhance immunological memory	C3 receptors on antigen-presenting cells
Waste disposal	
Clearance of immune complexes and apoptotic cells	C1q Covalently bound fragments of C3

of these components in clearing immune complexes and apoptotic debris.

Angioedema

Congenital and acquired C1-inhibitor deficiency results in spontaneous, episodic angioedema but this is not primarily due to dysregulation of the early classical complement pathway. C1-inhibitor is also a major regulator of kallikrein (contact system), plasmin (fibrinolytic pathway), and factor XII. Deficiency of C1-inhibitor leads to inappropriate generation of bradykinin, with resultant increased vascular permeability.

Dysregulation of the alternative pathway

Factors H and I are the main regulators of the alternative pathway, and deficiency of either of them result in an uncontrolled activation of this pathway with consumption of C3. Deficiencies in these factors are associated with an increased susceptibility to develop atypical haemolytic–uraemic syndrome (HUS) in children and adults. The clinical features of atypical HUS are renal failure due to glomerular thrombotic microangiopathy; thrombocytopenia; and microangiopathic haemolytic anaemia. Factor H deficiency is also associated with membranoproliferative glomerulonephritis or dense deposition disease, predominantly in children.

Demographics of the disease

Defects and deficiencies of complement components are rare, but are being increasingly recognized and reported. Inherited complement deficiencies form only a very small proportion of patients with SLE, but over 75% of patients with defects in the C1 complex and C4 have lupus or lupus-like syndromes.

Homozygous C3 deficiency is a rare autosomal recessive disease which is associated with recurrent bacterial infections and defects in adaptive immune responses. Approximately 1 in 10 000 individuals are reported to be deficient in one of the terminal complement components, but geographical and ethnic differences in prevalence and incidence have been noted.

MBL deficiency is considered to be the most common congenital immunodeficiency, with an estimated frequency of between 5% and 10% of the general Caucasian population. Individuals with MBL deficiency, however, remain healthy and are only susceptible to recurrent infections when the deficiency is associated with other immunodeficiencies or occurs prior to the maturation of the adaptive immune system.

Properdin deficiency is the most common defect associated with the alternative pathway and is transmitted as an X-linked recessive condition.

Hereditary angioedema due to C1-inhibitor deficiency is the best-studied inherited defect of complement regulators. The prevalence is

estimated to be 1:10 000 to 1:50 000, and the disease occurs in both sexes. Spontaneous de novo mutations occur in up to 25% of cases.

Defects in the components of the alternative pathway, including in factor H, factor I, factor B, membrane cofactor protein, and CD59 are very rare, with only individual cases or a few families currently reported.

Natural history and complications of the disease

Natural history of infections in complement disorders, and their complications

The most common presentation of patients with complement deficiencies is an increased susceptibility to recurrent infections by encapsulated bacteria, particularly *Neisseria meningitides* (Table 299.2). Homozygous C3 deficiency is also associated with increased susceptibility to *Streptococcus pneumoniae* and *Haemophilus influenza* sino-pulmonary infections and meningitis. While the majority of the infections occur in childhood, there is a reduction in frequency and severity of infections as the adaptive immune response matures.

Patients with MBL deficiency are generally asymptomatic. MBL concentrations correlate with gestational age, as reflected by a high prevalence of MBL deficiency in preterm neonates. MBL deficiency is clinically relevant in certain cohorts, including preterm neonates and other immunocompromised patients, including patients on chemotherapy.

Natural history of SLE-like syndrome in complement deficiencies, and its complications

There appears to be a hierarchy for deficiencies of the early components of the classical complement pathway, with respect to the risk of development of SLE or SLE-like disease, with the highest risk being in patients with C1q deficiency and the lowest risk associated with C2 deficiency: 90% of individuals with C1q and C1r/C1s deficiency develop a SLE-like disorder, while the estimated incidence in individuals with C2 deficiency is 10%–20%. Patients with C1-complex or C4 deficiency present early in life, and both sexes may be equally affected. In contrast, the disease in C2-deficient patients is similar to classical SLE but starts later and occurs more frequently in females

Table 299.2 Presentations of complement deficiencies

Deficiency	Clinical phenotype
Complement components	
C1q C1r C1s C2 C4	SLE-like syndrome Infections
C3 C2 C4 Mannose-binding lectin MASP	Recurrent pyogenic infections
C5–C9 Properdin Factor D Factor B	Neisserial infections
Regulatory proteins	
C1 Inhibitor	Hereditary angioedema
Factor H	Atypical haemolytic–uraemic syndrome Membranoproliferative glomerulonephritis
Factor I	Atypical haemolytic–uraemic syndrome Membranoproliferative glomerulonephritis
CD59 Decay accelerating factor	Paroxysmal nocturnal haemoglobinuria

Note: All of the above disorders may present either in children or in adults.

than in males (7:1). Renal involvement may be seen in about 30% of patients. Individuals with early complement defects, however, do not have an increased risk of development of any other systemic or organ-specific autoimmune disease.

Natural history of angioedema in complement deficiencies, and its complications

There is wide phenotypic variation amongst patients with inherited or acquired C1-inhibitor deficiency even within the same family, ranging from almost asymptomatic disease to frequent episodes of subcutaneous and/or mucosal angioedema and severe abdominal attacks. Patients may develop symptoms at any age, but the disease commonly manifests during adolescence or during periods of stress or trauma. It is potentially life-threatening when associated with laryngeal involvement. Patients with severe, unexplained abdominal episodes may be subject to unwanted exploratory laparotomies prior to diagnosis of the condition, especially in the absence of a family history. Certain medications, including oestrogen-based contraceptive pills and angiotensin-converting-enzyme inhibitors, are associated with an increased frequency of symptoms.

Approach to diagnosing the disease

Assessment of the integrity of the entire pathway should be made by testing for haemolytic complement activity (using the CH50 assay for the classical pathway, and the AP50 assay for the alternative pathway), coupled with quantitative measurement of serum C3 and C4. These initial results will help determine which part of the complement pathway might be defective, and help direct further, more detailed testing. Normal CH50 and AP50 values effectively exclude significant complement deficiency in most patients. In rare cases where the clinical history is compelling, further testing will be required, even with normal CH50 and AP50 values.

In most patients with recurrent angioedema a normal C4 test effectively excludes the diagnosis of C1-inhibitor deficiency. Additional tests of the complement pathway include:

- quantification of individual complement components
- C1-inhibitor quantitative and functional assays
- functional assays of classical and alternative pathway
- molecular analysis for underlying gene mutations

Differential diagnosis

The differential diagnosis includes:

- recurrent infections: primary antibody deficiency
- defects in innate immune system
- other causes for recurrent meningitis
- SLE
- idiopathic angioedema
- allergy
- medications

'Gold-standard' diagnostic test

The gold standard for complement defects is to establish a molecular diagnosis and identify the disease-causing genetic mutation for the condition. Complement deficiencies are rare conditions, and a registry of complement deficiencies has been established recently in Europe with the support of the European Complement Network. The aim of the registry is to collect information regarding complement defects from participating countries in order to define the prevalence, distribution, and disease associations in different populations and ethnic groups.

Acceptable diagnostic alternatives

A working diagnosis of complement defects may be established using the clinical history supported by appropriate functional assays, but definitive testing requires referral to a specialist complement laboratory.

Other relevant investigations

The following additional investigations may be of value in the appropriate clinical context:

- C3 nephritic factor (in cases of marked C3 hypocomplementaemia)
- anti-C1q antibodies (in hypocomplementaemic urticarial vasculitis)
- demonstration of complement and immunoglobulin deposition on renal biopsy (in immune-complex-mediated glomerulonephritis)

Prognosis and how to estimate it

The long-term prognosis with regard to infections is good, with a reduction in severity and frequency of bacterial infections with age, reflecting the maturity of the adaptive immune system. Thirty per cent of patients with early complement defects and SLE-like symptoms develop renal involvement, and the long-term prognosis depends on the extent of renal disease.

The natural history and prognosis of hereditary angioedema due to C1-inhibitor deficiency is unpredictable and varies from patient to patient, even in those with the same genetic mutation.

Treatment

Treatment of recurrent bacterial/neisserial infections

The treatment for recurrent bacterial/neisserial infections is:

- antibiotic treatment/supportive care
- penicillin prophylaxis/immunization

Treatment of SLE-like syndrome

The treatment for SLE-like syndrome is:

- use of corticosteroids and immunosuppressive treatment
- replacement of C1q using fresh frozen plasma in selected cases

Treatment of angioedema

The treatment for angioedema is:

- use of C1-inhibitor concentrate (for acute attacks/short-term prophylaxis)
- use of synthetic androgens/antifibrinolytic agents (for long-term prophylaxis)
- use of a bradykinin receptor antagonist (a new alternative to C1-inhibitor for the treatment of acute attacks)
- use of a kallikrein inhibitor/recombinant human C1-inhibitor (under development)

Further Reading

Brodsky RA. Paroxysmal nocturnal hemoglobinuria. *Blood* 2014; 124: 2804–11.

Caccia S, Suffritti C, and Cicardi M. Pathophysiology of hereditary angioedema. *Pediatr Allergy Immunol Pulmonol* 2014; 27: 159–63.

Chapel H, Haeney M, Misbah S, et al. *Essentials of Clinical Immunology* (6th edition), 2014. Wiley-Blackwell.

300 Hypersensitivity diseases

Malini Bhole

Definition of the disease

Hypersensitivity reactions are aberrant immune responses that are provoked by innocuous extrinsic or self-antigens, are mediated by B-cells or T-cells, and may result in tissue or organ damage.

Aetiology of the disease

Coombs and Gell classified hypersensitivity reactions into four types, based on the different immune responses, as shown in Table 300.1.

Pathophysiology of hypersensitivity reactions

Pathophysiology of type I hypersensitivity reactions

Type I hypersensitivity reactions result from IgE-mediated mast cell degranulation, with resultant release of early (preformed) mediators, newly formed mediators, and cytokines, predominantly interleukins 4, 5, 6, and 13. The important mediators include histamine, tryptase, leukotrienes, prostaglandin D2, and platelet-activating factor. Release of these mediators leads to vasodilatation, bronchial constriction, increased vascular permeability, smooth muscle contraction, increased mucus production, and pruritus.

Pathophysiology of type II hypersensitivity reactions

Type II hypersensitivity reactions are caused by autoantibodies that are directed against cell membrane-bound antigens. The cells may then be destroyed by different mechanisms, including:

- complement-mediated cytolysis
- antibody-dependent cell-mediated cytotoxicity
- phagocytosis

Pathophysiology of type III hypersensitivity reactions

In type III hypersensitivity reactions, antibodies react with soluble antigens and form immune complexes, which are deposited on the vascular endothelium or the glomerular membrane. The ensuing complement activation via the classical pathway leads to tissue damage and destruction.

Pathophysiology of type IV hypersensitivity reactions

Type IV hypersensitivity reactions are T-cell-mediated delayed hypersensitivity reactions directed against persistent antigens or foreign bodies. The main effector cells include cytotoxic T-cells and macrophages, which drive chronic inflammation and granuloma formation.

Typical symptoms of the disease, and less common ones

Typical symptoms and clinical manifestations of a hypersensitivity reaction depends on the type of reaction it is, as well as the route of entry of the allergen and/or the site of the antigen–antibody reaction.

Symptoms of type I hypersensitivity reactions

The symptoms of type I hypersensitivity reactions may vary in severity and manifest clinically as anaphylaxis, urticaria (generalized or local), angioedema, allergic rhinitis, or asthma. These reactions can occur in response to:

- inhaled aeroallergens (e.g. pollen, dust, mould, animal dander):
  - allergic rhinitis
  - allergic asthma
- ingestion of medications or food:
  - food allergies
  - drug allergies
- injection (e.g. venom stings):
  - local urticaria and angioedema
  - generalized reactions
  - anaphylaxis
- skin contact (e.g. poison ivy, animal scratches, pollen, latex):
  - urticarial rash
  - dermatitis

Symptoms of type II hypersensitivity reactions

The symptoms of type II hypersensitivity reactions manifest clinically as:

- autoimmune cytopenias
  - autoimmune haemolytic anaemia
  - immune thrombocytopenia

Table 300.1 Types of hypersensitivity reactions

Hypersensitivity reactions	Immune mechanism	Cells/mediators involved	Typical clinical features
Type I, or immediate hypersensitivity	Antigen cross-linking IgE molecules bond to mast cell membrane	Mast cell degranulation and release of mediators like histamine, tryptase, and leukotrienes	Urticarial rash Bronchoconstriction Hypotension
Type II, or antibody-mediated (humoral) cytotoxicity	Antibodies directed against cell or membrane-bound antigens	Complements Neutrophils Macrophages Natural killer cells	Haemolysis Cytopenias
Type III, or immune-complex disease	Antibody binds to soluble antigens with resultant formation of immune complexes	Immune complexes activate complement cascade leading to recruitment of neutrophils and macrophages, and local inflammation at site of deposition	Cutaneous and systemic vasculitis
Type IV, or delayed hypersensitivity	Autoreactive T-cells recognize antigens in relation to self-MHC molecules	Cytotoxic CD8+ T-cells, macrophages, and cytokines	Contact dermatitis Granuloma formation

Data from Gell PGH, Coombs RRA, *Clinical Aspects of Immunology*. 1st ed. Oxford, England: Blackwell; 1963.

- bullous pemphigoid
- Goodpasture's disease (anti-basement membrane antibody)
- some drug reactions

Symptoms of type III hypersensitivity reactions

The symptoms of type III hypersensitivity reactions manifest clinically as:

- systemic disease, such as:
  - serum sickness (following certain drugs or injection of foreign serum)
  - arthus reaction (a localized immune-complex reaction; e.g. extrinsic allergic alveolitis)
- organ-specific manifestations, such as:
  - glomerulonephritis
  - vasculitis
  - arthritis

Symptoms of type IV hypersensitivity reactions

The symptoms of type IV hypersensitivity reactions manifest clinically as:

- contact dermatitis (in response to an epidermal antigen, e.g. metals, poison ivy, organic chemicals, etc.)
- a tuberculin reaction (in response to an intradermal antigen, e.g. tuberculin administered during a Mantoux test)
- granuloma formation (in response to a persistent antigen)

Demographics of the disease

Hypersensitivity reactions, in general, result from a complex interplay between genetic predisposition and environmental factors. The overall prevalence of allergies, or IgE-mediated type I hypersensitivity reactions, appear to be increasing, especially in relation to food and aeroallergens (see Chapter 75). Atopy is defined as the genetic predisposition to make IgE antibodies in response to allergen exposure, and patients prone to IgE-mediated allergic reactions are said to be atopic.

Natural history and complications of the disease

The natural history and complications vary with the type of hypersensitivity reaction.

Natural history of type I hypersensitivity reactions, and their complications

A type I hypersensitivity reaction typically occurs within 15–30 minutes from the time of exposure to the antigen. A delayed phase may occur 2–6 hours after exposure. The severity of the reaction is unpredictable and may vary from minor localized reactions to severe, generalized manifestations, including anaphylaxis and death. The factors affecting the natural history and complications of type I hypersensitivity reactions include the nature and amount of the allergen, the site of allergen entry, the duration of the exposure, and the degree of sensitization of the individual patient.

Natural history of type II hypersensitivity reactions, and their complications

The reaction time for a type II hypersensitivity reaction is usually minutes to hours and primarily involves autoantibody- and complement-mediated injury directed against endogenous or exogenous (commonly, drug haptens) membrane-bound antigens. The natural history and complications depend on the site(s) involved in the reaction (e.g. haematopoietic cells; the skin; renal or lung basement membrane).

Natural history of type III hypersensitivity reactions, and their complications

A type III hypersensitivity reaction may manifest several hours after exposure (3–10 hours) and is mediated by soluble immune complexes. The natural history of this type of reaction, and the complications associated with it, depend upon the size of the immune complexes and their site of deposition (joints, blood vessels, kidneys, etc.).

Natural history of type IV hypersensitivity reactions, and their complications

A type IV hypersensitivity reaction is a delayed hypersensitivity reaction, which typically manifests 48–72 hours after exposure. The natural history and course of reaction depends upon the antigen and the site of contact. Granuloma formation is a more chronic manifestation of a type IV reaction to a persistent antigen or foreign body and may present 3–4 weeks after initial exposure. Complications of this reaction are directly related to the site of granuloma formation.

Approach to diagnosing the disease

The initial approach to the diagnosis of hypersensitivity diseases is based on a detailed clinical history and examination for typical clinical manifestations (see Figure 300.1). The important points in the clinical history would include details of the reaction, the nature of the exposure, the route of entry, the time period between exposures, and the clinical manifestations. Obtaining these allows an early differentiation between the four main types of hypersensitivity

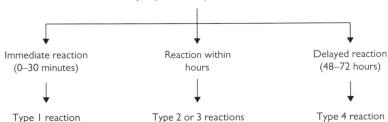

Approach to Hypersensitivity diseases

History
- Timing of reaction in relation to exposure to suspect agent
- Type of manifestations
- Duration of reaction
- History of background atopy
- History of previous exposure/reaction

Immediate reaction (0–30 minutes)	Reaction within hours	Delayed reaction (48–72 hours)
Type I reaction	Type 2 or 3 reactions	Type 4 reaction

Appropriate immediate management and further investigations and long term treatment according to manifestations

Figure 300.1 Initial approach to hypersensitivity diseases.

Table 300.2 Gold-standard diagnostic tests for hypersensitivity diseases

Type of reaction	Gold-standard test	Risks/difficulties
Type I hypersensitivity	Double-blind, placebo-controlled allergen challenge	Potentially life-threatening, with inherent risk of severe reaction Time consuming
Type II hypersensitivity	Biopsy and direct immunofluorescence of involved tissue The staining pattern is typically **smooth and linear**, and contains antibodies, complement, and neutrophils	Accessibility of tissue Expertise to interpret findings
Type III hypersensitivity	Biopsy and direct immunofluorescence of involved tissue The staining is granular, and contains primarily deposits of immune complexes and complement	Accessibility of tissue Expertise to interpret findings
Type IV hypersensitivity	Biopsy of involved tissue Typical granulomatous infiltrates containing lymphocytes and macrophages	

reactions; this is then confirmed with further specific investigations (see Table 300.2 and 'Acceptable diagnostic alternatives to the gold standard').

Differential diagnosis

Differential diagnosis for type I hypersensitivity

The differential diagnosis for type I hypersensitivity includes:

- non-IgE-mediated direct mast cell degranulation
- vasovagal symptoms and panic attacks
- systemic mastocytosis
- chronic idiopathic urticaria/angioedema

Differential diagnosis for type II hypersensitivity

The differential diagnosis for type II hypersensitivity includes:

- non-antibody-mediated causes of haemolytic anaemia
- other causes of pulmonary–renal syndrome (e.g. Goodpasture's disease, Wegener's granulomatosis, microscopic polyangiitis)

Differential diagnosis for type III hypersensitivity

The differential diagnosis for type III hypersensitivity includes other causes of glomerulonephritis and vasculitis

'Gold-standard' diagnostic test

'Gold-standard' diagnostic tests for hypersensitivity diseases vary according to the immunological process involved in the pathogenesis. These tests, as detailed in Table 300.2, are not always practical or feasible. Acceptable alternative investigations and tests are therefore used in the diagnosis of these conditions (see 'Acceptable diagnostic alternatives to the gold standard').

Acceptable diagnostic alternatives to the gold standard

Acceptable diagnostic alternatives to the gold-standard test for type I hypersensitivity

Acceptable diagnostic alternatives to the gold-standard test for type I hypersensitivity are:

- serial measurement of serum mast cell tryptase at 1, 6, and 24 hours, to demonstrate immediate mast cell degranulation
- measurement of specific IgE antibodies against the suspected allergen(s)
- newer in vitro tests, including basophil activation tests and component-resolved diagnostics, which are still under investigation
- skin prick tests and intradermal tests with the suspected allergen(s)

Acceptable diagnostic alternatives to the gold-standard test for type II hypersensitivity

Acceptable diagnostic alternatives to the gold-standard test for type II hypersensitivity are:

- detection of circulating antibody against tissues involved (via indirect immunofluorescence, ELISA)
- direct Coomb's test, for autoimmune cytopenias

Acceptable diagnostic alternatives to the gold-standard test for type III hypersensitivity

Acceptable diagnostic alternatives to the gold-standard test for type III hypersensitivity are serum complement levels, to demonstrate hypocomplementaemia.

Acceptable diagnostic alternatives to the gold-standard test for type IV hypersensitivity

Acceptable diagnostic alternatives to the gold-standard test for type IV hypersensitivity are:

- intradermal tests
- patch tests

Other relevant investigations

Other relevant investigations for hypersensitivity diseases are tests to rule out other immunological conditions that form the differential diagnosis of hypersensitivity disease. Depending on the clinical context, the following investigations should be considered:

- screening for C1-inhibitor deficiency (e.g. C3, C4, and C1-inhibitor concentrations)
- tests to exclude systemic mastocytosis (e.g. baseline serum tryptase, bone marrow examination)
- tests to exclude chronic urticaria (e.g. thyroid function tests, autoimmune screening)
- tests to exclude other causes of cytopenia (e.g. bone marrow examination)
- tests to exclude vasculitic syndromes (e.g. tests for antineutrophil cytoplasmic antibodies; renal biopsy)
- tests to exclude granulomatous conditions such as tuberculosis and sarcoidosis

Treatment

Treatment for type I hypersensitivity reactions

Treatment for type I hypersensitivity reactions includes:

- allergen avoidance
- use of antihistamines
- administration of adrenalin for acute severe reactions (see Chapter 75)
- allergen immunotherapy
- desensitization

Treatment for type II/III hypersensitivity reactions

Treatment for type II/III hypersensitivity reactions includes:

- use of anti-inflammatory agents
- use of immunosuppressive agents

Treatment for type IV hypersensitivity reactions

Treatment for type IV hypersensitivity reactions includes:

- avoidance of the trigger, if the trigger can be identified
- treatment of underlying condition
- use of steroids and immunosuppressive agents

Further Reading

Igea JM. The history of the idea of allergy. *Allergy* 2013; 68: 966–73.
Rive CM, Bourke J, and Phillips EJ. Testing for drug hypersensitivity syndromes. *Clin Biochem Rev* 2013; 34: 15–38.

Introduction

Therapeutic immunoglobulin is produced from plasma pooled from approximately 10 000 to 15 000 blood donors. As a direct consequence, a single unit of immunoglobulin has a vast array of antibody specificities (of the order of 10^{15}) which enable it to fulfil its function of antibody replacement in patients with B-lymphocyte immunodeficiency (primary or secondary hypogammaglobulinaemia). Following on from the use of immunoglobulin in immunodeficiency over the past two decades, high-dose immunoglobulin has emerged as an important form of immunomodulatory therapy for patients with various autoimmune diseases.

Although pooled immunoglobulin is largely composed of IgG, there is a range of other immunologically active molecules, including cytokines (interferon gamma, transforming growth factor beta), anti-cytokine antibodies (anti-interleukin 1 alpha), and soluble cell surface glycoproteins (CD4, CD8), which are also likely to influence the therapeutic efficacy of immunoglobulin as an immunomodulator.

Preparation of therapeutic immunoglobulin

Therapeutic immunoglobulin is produced by fractionating plasma from donors who have undergone a rigorous screen for blood-borne viruses, including HIV1, HIV2, hepatitis B, and hepatitis C. The plasma fractionation process using cold ethanol has been shown to inactivate both HIV and hepatitis B, thus providing an added level of safety preventing transmission of these viruses. Because hepatitis C, an enveloped RNA virus, has proved resistant to ethanol fractionation, additional antiviral steps based on solvent–detergent or low pH treatment were introduced in the mid-1990s, following the last outbreak of hepatitis C transmission by IV immunoglobulin (IVIg). Using PCR to perform random testing of plasma minipools for hepatitis C antigen is an additional safety measure that has helped prevent any further outbreaks of hepatitis C in immunoglobulin recipients.

Concerns regarding the remote possibility of prion transmission by blood products have led the UK's department of health to institute leucodepletion of red-cell transfusions and to ban the use of British plasma for the production of therapeutic immunoglobulin.

Mechanisms of action

The efficacy of immunoglobulin therapy in patients who have a B-cell deficiency and so are unable to produce protective antibodies is easily explained by the replacement of missing antibodies. In contrast, multiple mechanisms of action, often variable by disease, are likely to be operational when high-dose IVIg is used for immunomodulation. These include Fc receptor blockade, induction of inhibitory Fcγ receptors, neutralization of cytokines, and accelerated removal of autoantibodies via the FcRn (Fc receptor of the neonate) receptor, expressed on endothelium and monocytes. Although initially identified as a placental receptor, responsible for transplacental passage of IgG in the third trimester of pregnancy, FcRn plays an important role in regulating IgG half-life by acting as a protective receptor preventing lysosomal degradation of IgG (see Figure 301.1).

Indications for therapeutic immunoglobulin

Until the 1980s, the use of immunoglobulin as a therapeutic agent was confined to replacement therapy in patients with primary or secondary antibody deficiency. Its role as an effective immunomodulator was discovered serendipitously, when IVIg was shown to consistently increase the platelet count in a child with antibody

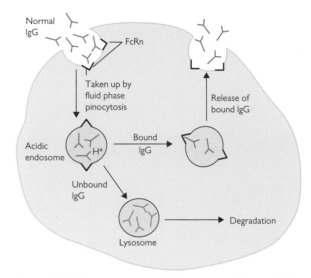

Figure 301.1 Schematic representation of the role of the endothelial FcRn receptor in IgG homeostasis.

Essentials of Clinical Immunology, Sixth edition, Helen Chapel, Maneel Haeney, Siraj Misbah and Neil Snowden. 2014. John Wiley & Sons Ltd.

deficiency and immune thrombocytopenic purpura. Since then, the use of high-dose IVIg as an immunomodulator has become established as an important therapeutic option in many immune-mediated diseases (see Table 301.1). The key difference in the

Table 301.1 Evidence-based indications for therapeutic immunoglobulin

Condition	Evidence
Immunology	
Primary antibody deficiency	Not subjected to placebo-controlled trials when first used as IMIg in the 1950s
	IVIg subsequently shown to be as efficacious or superior to IMIg as infection prophylaxis
Neurology	
Guillain–Barré syndrome	Demonstrated in RCTs to be as efficacious as plasmapheresis in patients with paralytic disease
Chronic inflammatory demyelinating polyneuropathy	Demonstrated in RCTs to be as efficacious as plasmapheresis
Multifocal motor neuropathy	Immunoglobulin has been shown to be the treatment of choice (evidence from RCTs)
Myasthenia gravis	Of proven benefit in myasthenic crises (evidence from RCTs)
Paediatrics	
Kawasaki disease	High-dose aspirin combined with IVIg is the treatment of choice (evidence from RCTs)
Haematology	
ITP	IVIg equally efficacious as steroids, in both adult and childhood ITP

Abbreviations: ITP, immune thrombocytopenia; IMIg, intramuscular immunoglobulin; IVIg, intravenous immunoglobulin; RCT, randomized control trial.

use of immunoglobulin for antibody replacement versus its use for immunomodulation relates to the dose. Although the dose of immunoglobulin required for immunomodulation (2 g/kg) is five times higher than that required for antibody replacement (0.4 g/kg), it is important to be aware that these doses have been derived empirically. In practice, many patients receiving maintenance high-dose IVIg for autoimmune diseases derive benefit from 1 g/kg administered at variable infusion intervals (3–6 weeks). The lower doses of immunoglobulin used for antibody replacement can also be administered effectively weekly via the subcutaneous route, which eliminates the peaks and troughs associated with IV bolus doses.

Adverse effects

Based on pathogenesis, immunoglobulin-induced adverse effects are classified into the following categories:

- immediate infusion-related adverse effects
- complications attributable to a sudden increase in serum IgG
- transmission of infective agents

Immediate infusion-related adverse effects

Immediate infusion-related adverse effects can occur with any immunoglobulin preparation, irrespective of the dose. These comprise self-limiting backache, chills, headaches, and flu-like symptoms, and, rarely, anaphylaxis. The latter is associated in some patients with the presence of anti-IgA antibodies complexing with the small amounts of IgA contained in some immunoglobulin preparations.

Complications attributable to a sudden increase in serum IgG

Complications attributable to a sudden increase in serum IgG are largely confined to patients receiving high-dose IVIg for immunomodulatory therapy. Haematological adverse effects include arterial or venous thrombosis in patients with preexisting cardiovascular disease or with disorders associated with increased viscosity and acute haemolysis due to passive transfer of anti-blood group antibodies contained in IVIg. Reversible renal impairment due to osmotic renal tubular vacuolopathy caused by the carbohydrate stabilizer (sucrose) found in some immunoglobulin preparations was a particular problem in some patients with preexisting renal disease. The development of sucrose-free preparations has led to a dramatic decrease in nephrotoxicity. Patients with type II mixed cryoglobulinaemia are at particular risk of immune-complex-mediated renal failure arising from the deposition of complexes composed of the IgM component of cryoglobulin (containing rheumatoid factor activity) when combined with infused IgG. High-dose IVIg may also cause a self-limiting acute aseptic meningitis which has been attributed to the sudden increase in the IgG gradient at the blood–brain barrier, and the consequent perturbation of meningeal endothelium.

Box 301.1 Checklist for safe use of intravenous immunoglobulin

- for elective use, exclude IgA deficiency; if the patient is totally deficient in IgA and has high titres of anti-IgA antibodies, consider IgA-depleted preparation of IVIg
- check liver and renal function prior to infusion
- check hepatitis C PCR/antibody status pre-Rx
- proceed with caution in the elderly and in patients with preexisting cardiovascular disease, hyperviscosity, and thrombophilia
- avoid use of IVIg in mixed cryoglobulinaemia and rapidly progressive renal disease
- beware potential risk of haemolysis
- adhere to manufacturer's recommendations regarding reconstitution and rate of infusion
- record batch number of IVIg preparation

Abbreviations: IVIg, intravenous immunoglobulin; PCR, polymerase chain reaction.

Transmission of infective agents

Given its origins as a plasma product, transmission of blood-borne viruses has always been a concern with IVIg. As previously discussed, the main concern is regarding the risk of transmission of hepatitis C. Although no precise estimates of risk of transmission are available for IVIg, the stringency and rigour of current plasma screening methods renders the risk of hepatitis C transmission with a single unit of blood at approximately 1 in 1 million. The risk with pooled IVIg is therefore likely to be even lower.

Minimizing immunoglobulin-associated adverse effects

Used correctly, pooled immunoglobulin has proven to be an effective therapeutic agent in a wide range of immune-mediated disorders. With its increasing use as an immunomodulator, adverse effects associated with high-dose immunoglobulin are gaining prominence. Close attention to the checklist provided in Box 301.1 will minimize the risk of adverse effects.

Further Reading

Lunemann JD, Nimmerjahn F, and Dalakas MC. Intravenous immunoglobulin in neurology: Mode of action and clinical efficacy. *Nat Rev Neurol* 2015; 11: 80–9.

Schwab I and Nimmerjahn F. Intravenous immunoglobulin therapy: How does IgG modulate the immune system? *Nat Rev Immunol* 2013; 13: 176–89.

Definition

The term immunosuppressive therapy encompasses all forms of treatment that dampens function of the recipient's immune system, with a view to controlling severe autoimmune, inflammatory, or allergic disease.

All immunosuppressive agents carry an inherent risk of increasing a patient's susceptibility to infection. Hence, given the trade-off between expected therapeutic benefit and possibility of adverse effects, a careful risk assessment and informed discussion with the patient should precede initiation of treatment.

Classification and mechanisms of action

Despite the structural heterogeneity of current immunosuppressive agents, the predominant targets of these drugs are T-lymphocytes, with multiple downstream effects including containment of T-cell activation, inhibition of cytokine production, restriction of clonal expansion, and varying degrees of suppression of B-cell function. Despite inhibition of B-cell function, many patients are still able to mount clinically useful, albeit somewhat blunted, antibody responses. More pronounced effects on B-cell function, leading to frank hypogammaglobulinaemia, may be seen in up to 5% of patients receiving cyclophosphamide, mycophenolate mofetil, or therapeutic monoclonal antibodies targeted at B-cell surface antigens, as exemplified by rituximab (see 'Therapeutic monoclonal antibodies').

The mechanism of action of commonly used immunosuppressive drugs is summarized in Figure 302.1.

Therapeutic monoclonal antibodies

Conventional immunosuppressive agents are unselective in their effects, with the potential for harm. This has driven the search for safer agents directed at an antigenic target pivotal to the relevant disease process. Therapeutic biologics (monoclonal antibodies or receptor-fusion proteins), which are based on Kohler and Milstein's Nobel Prize-winning hybridoma technology, are a superb example of true translational science which has revolutionized the treatment of many autoimmune and inflammatory diseases. Presciently, Kohler and Milstein envisaged that hybridoma technology, in which specific antibody-producing B-cells from immunized animals (or humans) are fused with a myeloma cell line conferring immortality, thus producing cell lines capable of secreting monoclonal antibodies, would have medical and industrial use. However, the technology was never patented, leading to the loss of millions of pounds to the British economy.

The recent explosion of therapeutic monoclonal antibodies has been led by rituximab, a chimaeric antibody licensed for the treatment of B-cell lymphoma by virtue of its selective targeting of the CD20 surface glycoprotein on B-lymphocytes. Rituximab exemplifies three important criteria for the development of therapeutic monoclonal antibodies:

- the target antigen should be largely restricted to cells or mediator(s) that are pivotal to disease causation (e.g. malignant cells or cells involved in immunopathogenesis)
- the target antigen should not be internalized by cells
- the target antigen should not be soluble (for cancer therapy)

The use of rituximab in a patient with B-cell lymphoma and concomitant rheumatoid arthritis (RA) led to the serendipitous observation of regression of RA, which in turn has spurred the use of rituximab in a variety of autoimmune diseases associated with B-cell overactivity. Rituximab is currently licensed for the treatment of severe RA that has proven to be unresponsive to monoclonal antibodies or receptor-fusion proteins targeted against tumour necrosis factor (TNF). Table 302.1 lists some therapeutic monoclonal

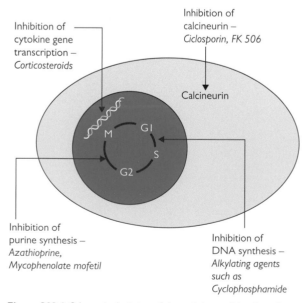

Figure 302.1 Schematic depiction of the main intracellular sites of action of the major groups of immunosuppressive drugs.

Essentials of Clinical Immunology, Sixth edition, Helen Chapel, Maneel Haeney, Siraj Misbah and Neil Snowden. 2014. John Wiley & Sons Ltd.

Table 302.1 Some therapeutic monoclonal antibodies used in the treatment of autoimmune, inflammatory, and neoplastic disorders

Monoclonal antibody	Indications	Molecular target
Adalimumab Infliximab Golimumab	Inflammatory bowel disease Ankylosing spondylitis Psoriatic arthritis Psoriasis Rheumatoid arthritis Juvenile idiopathic arthritis	Tumour necrosis factor alpha
Alemtuzumab	Relapsing-remitting multiple sclerosis	CD52 receptor
Rituximab	Rheumatoid arthritis Non-Hodgkin's lymphoma	CD20 receptor
Trastuzumab	HER2-positive breast cancer HER2-positive gastric cancer	HER2

Abbreviations: HER2, human epidermal growth factor receptor 2.

antibodies licensed for use in the UK in the treatment of autoimmune, inflammatory, and neoplastic disorders.

Although rituximab depletes a wide range of B-cells expressing CD20, it spares fully differentiated plasma cells, thus accounting for the lack of significant hypogammaglobulinaemia in the majority of recipients. However, a minority of patients may develop hypogammaglobulinaemia and recurrent bacterial infections following repeated courses of treatment, thus highlighting the importance of monitoring serum immunoglobulin levels in patients receiving rituximab. Other serious infective challenges posed by rituximab include reactivation of hepatitis B in patients previously infected with hepatitis B, despite their being negative for the hepatitis B surface antigen, and the development of progressive multifocal leucoencephalopathy (PML) due to the JC virus. While pretreatment hepatitis viral screens are able to identify and ensure pre-emptive antiviral treatment for hepatitis B, the onset of PML can be neither predicted nor prevented at present.

While the precise mechanism of rituximab awaits elucidation, it is likely that B-cell depletion by a number of routes (see Figure 302.2), coupled possibly with the potentiation of regulatory T-cells, accounts for the therapeutic success of the antibody in autoimmune diseases.

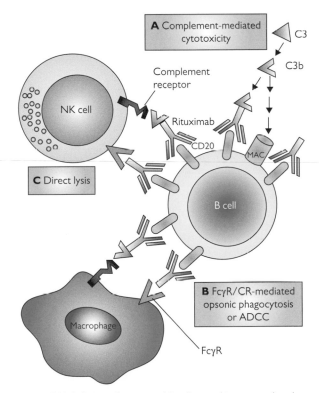

Figure 302.2 Rituximab-opsonized B-cells are subject to attack and killing via at least three pathways. (A) Binding of rituximab causes activation of the complement cascade, which generates the membrane attack complex that can directly lyse B-cells by complement-mediated cytotoxicity. (B) Complement activation also deposits C3b/iC3b fragments on the B-cell. The Fc portion of rituximab and the deposited C3b/iC3b fragments allow for recognition by both Fc gamma receptors and complement receptors 1 and 3 on macrophages, leading to phagocytosis and antibody-dependent cell-mediated cytotoxicity. (C) Binding of rituximab allows interaction with natural killer cells via Fc gamma RIII and complement receptor 3, leading to antibody-dependent cell-mediated cytotoxicity; ADCC, antibody-dependent cell-mediated cytotoxicity; CR, complement receptor; FcγR, Fc gamma receptor; MAC, membrane attack complex; NK, natural killer.

Reprinted by permission from Macmillan Publishers Ltd: Nature Reviews *Rheumatology*, Ronald P Taylor and Margaret A Lindorfer, Drug Insight: the mechanism of action of rituximab in autoimmune disease-the immune complex decoy hypothesis, volume 3, issue 2, pp. 86–95, copyright (1969).

An example of monoclonal antibodies targeting cytokines to induce disease remission is the use of anti-TNF based therapy, which has dramatically improved the management of RA. In view of the pivotal position of TNF in the pathogenesis of RA, interruption of TNF production induces further downstream suppression of other pro-inflammatory cytokines, such as interleukin 1 and interleukin 6. However, the neutralization of TNF in RA carries with it the risk of reactivating TB, reflecting the key role of TNF in the protective immune response to *Mycobacterium tuberculosis*. In order to minimize this risk, patients are screened for latent TB by interferon-gamma-based assays prior to commencing treatment with anti-TNF blockers. Based on the success of TNF blockade in RA, a range of other autoimmune diseases, including ankylosing spondylitis, psoriatic arthritis, juvenile chronic arthritis, and Crohn's disease, have been shown to benefit from the same therapeutic concept.

Selection of immunosuppressive agents

The selection of immunosuppressive drugs in the initial treatment of autoimmune or inflammatory diseases is predominantly guided by disease severity and the need to induce rapid remission, in addition to being informed by knowledge of disease pathogenesis. In practice, this entails the use of corticosteroids, either in combination with other drugs or, occasionally, singly.

High-dose corticosteroids are frequently used to induce disease remission, followed by maintenance immunosuppressive treatment to prevent disease relapse. An example of the use of steroids alone to control disease would be in a patient with giant cell arteritis and presenting with headache and nasal symptoms, as, in this case, urgent treatment would be critical for preventing loss of vision. In contrast, a patient with Wegener's granulomatosis and presenting with a pulmonary–renal syndrome would require steroids and cyclophosphamide to induce disease remission. Where cyclophosphamide is used for induction therapy in small vessel vasculitis, evidence from randomized controlled trials shows that remission can be maintained by switching to azathioprine at 3 months, thus limiting cyclophosphamide-induced toxicity. This model of treatment is increasingly being adopted when planning immunosuppressive regimens for other autoimmune diseases. Alternatives to the use of azathioprine in maintaining disease remission are mycophenolate mofetil, and methotrexate.

Although a knowledge of the immunopathogenesis of the disease being treated is essential, its influence on the choice of immunosuppressive agent is largely nullified by the broad-ranging immunological actions of conventional agents. In contrast, the choice of therapeutic monoclonal antibody is predominantly guided by the immunopathogenesis of the disease being treated, as clearly exemplified by the use of anti-TNF agents in RA, and rituximab in B-cell-driven autoimmune disease.

Adverse effects, and strategies to minimize them

The brief discussion of adverse effects in the ensuing paragraphs is designed to complement the adverse effects listed in Table 302.2. Anticipating and preventing adverse effects is of paramount importance when using immunosuppressive therapy. All immunosuppressive agents increase susceptibility to infection. Where adverse effects are predictable by virtue of the mechanism of action or metabolism of the drug, steps should be taken to prevent or detect them at the earliest opportunity. For example, assessing a patient's thiopurine methyltransferase (TPMT) status would make it possible to avoid using azathioprine in those patients with a homozygous TPMT deficiency, as bone marrow suppression in these patients would be a virtual certainty. The lack of specificity of most immunosuppressive agents means that regular full blood counts are required to monitor therapy.

Cyclophosphamide therapy carries with it particular risks of inducing haematological (acute myeloid leukaemia) and bladder malignancy (with oral therapy). It is important to monitor the cumulative doses

Table 302.2 Adverse effects of immunosuppressive therapy

Class	Examples	Major adverse effects
Glucocorticoids	Prednisolone	Adrenal suppression
		Glucose intolerance/diabetes
		Osteoporosis
Alkylating agents	Cyclophosphamide	Marrow suppression
		Bladder toxicity
		Gonadal toxicity
Antimetabolites	Methotrexate	Marrow suppression
		Liver toxicity
		Pneumonitis
	Azathioprine	Gastrointestinal intolerance
		Marrow suppression
		Liver toxicity
Drugs acting on immunophilins	Ciclosporin	Nephrotoxicity
		Hyperkalaemia
		Hypomagnesaemia
	Tacrolimus	Neurotoxicity
		Cardiotoxicity
Interferons	–	Influenza-like symptoms
		Cardiovascular effects
Mycophenolate	–	Marrow suppression
		Increased susceptibility to infection
Fingolimod	–	Bradycardia
		Atrioventricular block
		QT prolongation

of cyclophosphamide received, to identify those patients at greatest risk of these adverse effects. Susceptibility to infections during cyclophosphamide therapy is minimized by the use of prophylactic co-trimoxazole.

Further Reading

Faurschoul M and Jayne DRW. Anti–B cell antibody therapies for inflammatory rheumatic diseases. *Ann Rev Med* 2014; 65: 263–78.

Glassman PM and Balthasar JP. Mechanistic considerations for the use of monoclonal antibodies for cancer therapy. *Cancer Biol Med* 2014; 11: 20–33.

PART 15

Infectious diseases

Innate, cellular, humoral, and combined defences

The immune system is classified into a series of component parts, each specialized to defend the host against infection (see Box 303.1); consideration of the acquired and rare congenital immune deficiencies provides insight into this defence (see Table 303.1). Cells of the innate immune system are distributed throughout the body, in the tissues, and in the circulation, to defend against the first signs of danger, combining the acute inflammatory response with the ability to kill and remove invading pathogens. Monocytes, macrophages, and neutrophils phagocytose and kill exogenous and endogenous targets, using both oxygen-dependent and oxygen-independent mechanisms. Some species such as *Mycobacterium tuberculosis* avoid these mechanisms and can grow intracellularly. The fundamental role of neutrophils is illustrated in chronic granulomatous disease, where a lack of oxidative killing leads to bacterial and fungal infection and excessive inflammation. Neutrophil deficiency increases risk of bacterial sepsis and may be acquired from some medications, or occur in autoimmunity or in haematological malignancies. Inherited complement deficiencies are rare, but infection with *Neisseria meningitidis* occurs in patients unable to form the membrane attack complex, the final step in the complement pathway.

The adaptive immune system creates a structurally specific and prolonged response mediated by lymphocytes to clear infection and generate immunological memory. It is instigated by antigen presentation, often by dendritic cells. T-thymocytes (thymic lymphocytes, or T-cells) are responsible for cellular immunity and comprise an array of subsets which are broadly described as T-helper cells (Th cells), T-cytotoxic cells (T_C cells), and T-regulatory cells. Aplasia of the thymus and failure of T-cell development (DiGeorge syndrome) results in a predisposition to chronic viral and fungal infections. B-lymphocytes (bone marrow cells, or B-cells) are present but, without Th-cell help, antibody production is abnormal. Natural killer (NK) cells kill virally infected and tumour cells; in Chédiak–Higashi syndrome, which is associated with severely depressed NK cell function, patients respond abnormally to EBV infection and have abnormal lymphoproliferation but normal immunoglobulin responses. B-cells create the humoral immune response. They express membrane-bound antibody specific for an antigen, which triggers the generation of antibody-secreting plasma cells. Some antigen–B-cell interactions require help from Th cells for this process to occur. Congenital plasma cell deficiency and hypogammaglobulinaemia (common variable immune deficiency) lead to recurrent infections. Hypogammaglobulinaemia may also be acquired in later life.

Routine testing for immunodeficiency is often not undertaken in the acute phase of an infection, as it is difficult to interpret the results and may be non-contributory. If immunodeficiency is felt to be a strong possibility, then the clinician should liaise closely with the local immunology service, as immunodeficiency is a specialized area. Table 303.2 provides a broad overview of the different types of tests that should be considered for the different forms of immunodeficiency.

Causes of acquired immunodeficiency

HIV infection

The most common acquired immune deficiency is infection with HIV. In 2013, there were 35 million people living with HIV. Since the start of the epidemic, around 78 million people have become infected with HIV, and 39 million people have died of AIDS-related illnesses. The reason for the extreme virulence of HIV is manifest in its evasive multifaceted interaction with the human immune system. Untreated, HIV infection results in severe immune deficiency and infection with pathogens that would be controlled by an immunocompetent host. Cells bearing the CD4 receptor, including Th cells, dendritic cells, and monocytes–macrophages, are susceptible to infection. The destruction of CD4$^+$ T-cells is profound during primary infection, after which there is a slow decline over 5–10 years, towards clinical immunodeficiency. Innate and cellular immune processes are affected early in infection; later, there is evidence of a combined immunodeficiency. Infection with HIV-1 conveys early susceptibility to progression of latent TB infection to active disease. Fungal infections (e.g. oral candidiasis) and viral recrudescences (e.g. varicella zoster virus), along with early malignancies such as cervical dysplasia, herald advancing immunosuppression. Late-stage disease is characterized by opportunistic infection that may be fungal (e.g. cryptococcosis), viral (e.g. CMV infection), bacterial (e.g. salmonella septicaemia), and protozoan (e.g. cryptosporidium infection). Treatment with highly active antiretroviral therapy

---

Box 303.1 Basic immunology

Innate responses

Phagocytosis

- monocytes–macrophages: circulate as monocytes; upon contact with antigen, mature into phagocytic macrophages; includes tissue-specific forms (e.g. Kupffer cells in the liver)
- neutrophils: granulocyte; phagocytosis and killing of bacteria
- eosinophils: granulocyte; phagocytosis and parasitic defences

Immune modulation

- basophils: granulocyte; release preformed immune mediators
- mast cells: differentiate in tissues where they can release preformed immune mediators (e.g. histamine)

Complement

- a cascade of serum proteins which have intrinsic antipathogenic function, and interact with cellular and humoral responses

Antigen presentation

- dendritic cells: professional antigen presentation to instigate the adaptive response, includes a minority circulating population, and a majority tissue-resident population (e.g. Langerhans cells)

Adaptive responses

Cellular

- cytotoxicity:
  - natural killer cells: capable of antibody dependent and independent cell-mediated cytotoxicity
  - cytotoxic CD8$^+$ T-cells: recognize antigen bound to MHC Class I molecules, and destroy infected cells
- T-cell help:
  - helper CD4$^+$ T-cells: recognize MHC Class II molecules, secrete cytokines and chemokines, and provide help to macrophages, cytotoxic T-cells, and B-cells; several subtypes described

Humoral

- B-cells: mature B-cells produce membrane-bound antibody and, upon activation, divide to form memory cells and antibody-secreting plasma cells

---

Table 303.1 Acquired and inherited immune deficiencies

Immunity	Acquired	Examples of resulting infection	Inherited	Examples of resulting infection
Innate	HIV-1	TB	Chronic granulomatous disease	Susceptibility to bacterial and fungal infection due to lack of oxidative killing, except organisms that generate hydrogen peroxide (e.g. pneumococcus)
	Neutropenia secondary to autoimmune diseases (e.g. SLE) or iatrogenic causes (e.g. chemotherapeutic drugs)	Serious bacterial infections due to extracellular organisms (e.g. *Staphylococcus aureus*, *Escherichia coli*), and systemic fungal infection (e.g. *Candida* spp.)	Chédiak–Higashi syndrome	Recurrent bacterial infections due to failure of phagocytes to kill bacteria
	Steroids	Neutrophil adhesion deficiency Increased infection with *Staphylococcus* spp. and Gram-negative bacteria		
Cellular	HIV-1	Viral (e.g. CMV, herpes simplex virus 1 and 2, EBV) Bacterial (e.g. non-typhi *Salmonella* spp., TB) Fungal (e.g. *Cryptococcus neoformans*, *Candida* spp.)	DiGeorge syndrome	Defective or absent T-cell responses result in viral and fungal infections and chronic diarrhoea
	Iatrogenic causes Anti-tumour necrosis factor alpha therapy Steroids Other immunosuppressive agents (e.g. ciclosporin, tacrolimus)	Failure of cellular control of latent tuberculosis infection Viral, fungal, or opportunistic infection		
	Protein–calorie malnutrition	Infection with helminths, viruses (e.g. influenza), or protozoa (e.g. malaria)		
	Chronic infections (e.g. TB)			
Humoral	Acquired humoral immune deficiency	Recurrent bacterial infection (e.g. *Campylobacter* spp., *Mycoplasma* spp.)	Common variable immunodeficiency	Failure of B-cells to mature into plasma cells causes recurrent bacterial infections
	Hyposplenism	Encapsulated bacteria (e.g. *Neisseria meningitidis*) Protozoans (e.g. *Babesia* spp.)		
Combined cellular and humoral	HIV-1	Broad range of infections depending on the severity and underlying disorder, including bacterial, fungal, viral, and protozoan	Severe combined immunodeficiency	Severe recurrent infections, usually as a result of defective T-cell immunity (e.g. fungi and viruses), although defective B-cell immunity is also present
	Chronic morbidities Chronic renal failure Diabetes mellitus	Broad range of infections depending on the severity and underlying disorder, including bacterial, fungal, viral, and protozoan		
	Disorders of consumption Alcohol dependency Micronutrient malnutrition (e.g. zinc deficiency)	Broad range of infections depending on the severity and underlying disorder, including bacterial, fungal, viral, and protozoan		

Table 303.2 Initial investigation of immunodeficiency

Type of suspected immunodeficiency	Specific investigations
All	Full blood count with differential white-cell count
Antibody deficiency	Immunoglobulin levels, especially IgG, IgA, IgM IgG subclass analysis
B/T-cell deficiency: • number • B-cell function • T-cell function	Quantification of B- and T-cell numbers Antibodies to routine immunizations (e.g. *haemophilus influenzae* type b, pneumococcus) Skin tests for delayed-type hypersensitivity, cell response to mitogens
Neutrophil/phagocyte deficiency	Absolute numbers of full blood count (may be neutropenic) Reduction of nitro blue tetrazolium chloride
Complement deficiency	Total serum classic haemolytic complement test/alternative haemolytic complement test

suppresses viral replication, to prevent and partially reverse the immune destruction.

Other acquired immunodeficiencies

Other acquired immunodeficiencies include the cellular immune deficiency of chronic renal failure, which is due to chronic immune activation, reduced immune function, vitamin D deficiency, and lymphopaenia. The latter may be mediated by uraemia, predisposing T-cells and B-cells to apoptosis. Progression of latent TB to active disease is increased in these patients and is exacerbated by advancing age, low body mass index (BMI), and the presence of diabetes mellitus. Uraemia affects the innate immune responses; macrophage cytotoxicity is impaired in vitro and neutrophils are less able to kill organisms intracellularly, increasing bacterial sepsis. Patients may also have an underlying hypogammaglobulinaemia, and vaccine responses are impaired.

Diabetes mellitus

Diabetes mellitus predisposes to infection through uncontrolled blood sugar, minor trauma, and immune suppression. The immune dysfunction in diabetes is wide-ranging, including deficiencies in complement, and impaired monocyte phagocytosis and chemotaxis. Glycosaemia leads to increased immune activation and basal cytokine levels, but neutrophil, monocytes–macrophage, and T-cell functions are all depressed. Patients commonly experience fungal infections, such as candidiasis, and bacterial infections of the extremities, as well as frequent urinary tract and respiratory infections.

Steroids and other immunosuppressive drugs

Steroids and other immunosuppressive drugs are agents that have broad-reaching immunological effects. Long-term use of steroids such as prednisolone causes neutrophil and cellular immune dysfunction, and hypogammaglobulinaemia may occur, although the functional significance of this is unclear. Bacterial and yeast infections, such as candidiasis, are more common and more severe. Azathioprine causes dose-related bone marrow suppression with neutropenia and a high risk of bacterial sepsis. Mycophenolate, used post organ transplantation, increases susceptibility to opportunistic infections, especially CMV. The calcineurin inhibitors ciclosporin and tacrolimus affect T-cell immunity and may reduce antiviral immunity. Finally, therapy with drugs blocking tumour necrosis factor-alpha (TNF-alpha) or its receptor, to reduce the inflammatory process in rheumatoid arthritis, has inadvertently revealed the importance of TNF-alpha in the control of *Mycobacterium tuberculosis* infection. Where therapy is considered, screening for and treatment of latent TB infection will reduce the risk of progressive disease.

Malnutrition

Malnutrition is a common cause of immunodeficiency worldwide; protein–calorie malnutrition causes thymic damage and a reduction in T-cell memory responses; skin test reactivity is reduced, and there is an increased risk of viral, bacterial, parasitic, and opportunistic infection. Micronutrient deficiencies cause patterns of immune dysfunction: zinc deficiency alters thymic and T-cell functions; copper deficiency is associated with lymphopaenia and a reduced interleukin-2 response; and selenium and vitamin E deficiencies damage antioxidant defences. Vitamin C is necessary for phagocyte function, and its deficiency increases the risk of infections. Nutritional insufficiency, chronic immune activation, and liver dysfunction contribute to the immune deficiency seen in chronic heavy alcohol intake. Long-term alcohol dependents are at much greater risk of post-operative infection; this may be related to downregulation of the pro-inflammatory Th type 1 response. Progression from latent to active disease and death from TB are both associated with alcohol dependence.

Organs and tissues involved in defence against infection

The spleen

Disorders of splenic function greatly affect the immune response. The spleen removes senescent red blood cells and traps antigen for presentation. It is important for phagocytosis and antibody production,

as T-cells are found in the white pulp surrounding the splenic arterioles, and B-cells are found in the marginal zones. Infectious causes of splenic enlargement include malaria, EBV infection, leishmaniasis, TB, and bacterial infections such as *Salmonella typhi*, resulting in hypersplenism, pancytopenia, and, in some cases, a functional immune deficiency. Hyposplenism from surgical removal, trauma, or splenic atrophy in coeliac disease increases the susceptibility to infection with encapsulated bacteria (e.g. *Neisseria meningitidis*). Patients with hyposplenism should be given vaccination for pneumococcus, *Haemophilus influenza* type b, meningococcus, and influenza. Oral prophylaxis with phenoxymethylpenicillin or erythromycin is recommended.

The skin

Human skin forms a barrier defence that contains a network of immune cells. The outer epidermal layer consists of a tightly knit keratinized layer, which prevents the entry of microorganisms; breakdown secondary to conditions such as eczema or burns greatly increases the risk of localized infection. The keratinocytes express major MHC Class II molecules and can produce cytokines such as interleukin-23 which enhances Th type 1 responses. The second dermal layer includes sebaceous glands that form acidic sebum (pH 3–5) to inhibit microbial growth. Skin-associated dendritic cells (Langerhans cells) are migratory and can move to draining lymph nodes to present antigen. Immune reactions manifesting in skin can form useful diagnostic tools; for example, the delayed-type hypersensitivity (type IV hypersensitivity) reaction has been used for a century in the diagnosis of tuberculosis, and the wheal and flare of atopic urticaria (type I hypersensitivity) is used in the assessment of response to common allergens; these reactions are depressed in conditions associated with cellular immune suppression (e.g. HIV-1 infection, and uraemia). Breaches of the integumental defences, either through instrumentation or via indwelling devices such as IV lines (e.g. Venflons, central lines), are common sources of nosocomial infection. Localized pyogenic collections may occur, or more serious disseminated bacteraemia or fungal infection. To reduce this risk, such devices should only be used where absolutely necessary, should be placed using an aseptic technique, and should be changed regularly as a matter of course or at the first sign of infection.

The gastrointestinal system

Gut-associated lymphoid tissue forms a network throughout the gastrointestinal tract. A large population of CD8+ T-cells are found in the small intestine. The lamina propria contains many subtypes of immune cells. Below the lamina propria are Peyer's patches, which are loose aggregation of dendritic cells, T-cells, and germinal follicles. Specialized M cells, which are similar to enterocytes, transport antigens across the Peyer's patches. Primary HIV infection causes preferential and, to some extent, irreversible loss of CD4+ cells in the gut mucosa.

Mucous membranes

The mucous membranes lining the conjunctivae, respiratory, genitourinary, and gastrointestinal tracts use secretions to prevent pathogen binding to the epithelium. The secretions contain defensive proteins, including large amounts of IgA antibody, and lysozyme, which cleaves components of bacterial cell walls. Secretory IgA from plasma cells is able to form complexes with large viral and bacterial antigens, which are then removed with the rest of the secretions. Secretions are reduced in volume in cystic fibrosis; in the respiratory tract, this encourages colonization, infection with pathogenic bacteria such as *Pseudomonas aeruginosa*, and inflammation.

Conclusion

Where there are deficiencies in the immune system, either present from birth or acquired through other disease processes or treatment, there is vulnerability to infection which can be often fatal. A basic understanding of the cellular, humoral, integumental, and secretory defences against infection is fundamental both to the recognition of pathological immune deficiency and to the recognition of infectious processes. Congenital defects are rare but their specificity has provided insight into the immune system's components. Acquired immune deficiencies are common but often overlooked, to the detriment of patient care. Understanding how the immune system defends the body and recognizing when it is likely to be deficient can promote prescient action for the treatment and support of affected patients.

Further Reading

Iwasaki A and Pillai PS. Innate immunity to influenza virus infection. *Nat Rev Immunol* 2014; 14: 315–28.

Weiss G and Schaible UE. Macrophage defense mechanisms against intracellular bacteria. *Immunol Rev* 2015; 264: 182–203.

304 Nature and demographics: Epidemiology of infective organisms

Andrew Lever and Sian Coggle

Definition of disease

An infection is an interaction between a host and a parasitic microorganism, with the interaction being deleterious to the host. Its occurrence and outcome are a combination of the nature of the organism, the site at which it is found, and the competence of the host defensive (immune) system. There are around 1500 documented agents that are infectious for man. The majority of the microorganisms in the world do not cause disease in humans. An organism which in one bodily compartment may be a beneficial commensal (such as some gut bacteria) may become a pathogen if it escapes into the blood. Similarly, a benign organism, such as the BCG mycobacterium used as a vaccine, may become a life-threatening infection in a patient with a serious immunodeficiency. Many microorganisms cause disease by accident. *Neisseria meningitidis*, despite its name, is designed to be a throat commensal. Invasion of the blood and subsequently the cerebrospinal fluid is a mistake, and a dead-end niche for the bacterium, as well as being highly lethal to the host.

Infectious agents are incredibly diverse, in their physical nature, in their complexity (from a prion to a helminth), and in the diseases they cause (from the 'common cold' to the haemorrhagic fever caused by Ebola virus).

Demographics of infectious disease

In resource-poor settings, infectious diseases are associated with poverty and overcrowding, and lead to a greater proportion of the morbidity and mortality than in the developed world. As antimicrobial use has increased in the latter, the burden of disease has decreased, but it has also resulted in new problems emerging, such as antibiotic-resistant organisms (e.g. methicillin-resistant *Staphylococcus aureus* (commonly referred to as MRSA), or the depletion of commensals and thus allowing the overgrowth of disease-producing organisms such as *Clostridium difficile*.

The global epidemiology of infectious diseases has changed rapidly over the last few decades. Increased air travel has meant that new epidemics can spread much more rapidly around the world (e.g. SARS) and also that diseases such as malaria, which were traditionally thought of as 'tropical' diseases, now must be included in some differential diagnoses in more temperate countries. New infectious diseases are constantly appearing —approximately one per year for the last 25 years—such as HIV or H1N1 'swine flu', and some old problems are re-emerging (e.g. drug-resistant forms of TB). In addition, climate change is likely to influence epidemiology in the future, as vector habitats and breeding patterns are altered.

Pathogenic organisms

There are four categories of causative organisms recognized for infectious diseases: prions, viruses, bacteria, and eukaryotes.

Prions

Prions consist of only a single protein. They contain no nucleic acid, and disease arises as a consequence of their inducing the homologous host protein to physically mutate into a prion protein. Diseases caused by prions have been recognized for many years, but their biological nature was established only recently, and their properties are still being fully elucidated.

Viruses

Viruses contain either RNA or DNA as their genetic material, and have to utilize host cell machinery to replicate; they are obligate intracellular parasites. They range in size from 20 nm to 300 nm. They cause disease either by direct cytopathicity or as a consequence of the damage caused by the immune system in trying to clear them. Viral infections can be diagnosed in a variety of ways, including through the use of PCR or serological tests.

Bacteria

Bacteria have a genome encoded by DNA. They have a cell membrane, and most are able to replicate independently of their host. They are generally larger than viruses. Bacteria can cause disease by direct damage to tissue, through the secretion of exotoxins, or by endotoxin-mediated hyperactivation of the immune system. They can generally be diagnosed by culture, although some require special media or may be extremely difficult to grow. In some cases, serology is an alternative and, when appropriate, the toxins can be used in diagnosis. Generic PCR methods, such as 16S ribosomal PCR, are becoming more widely used.

Eukaryotes

Eukaryotes infecting man are the most complex of the causative organisms and are extremely diverse, from unicellular amoebae, to fungi, or multicellular helminths. They all have function-specific organelles. Diagnostics for this category are equivalently diverse, ranging from microscopic examination of a 'hot' stool specimen for amoebae to macroscopic identification of a tapeworm, as well as including serology.

Modes of transmission

There are many possible modes of transmission of infectious agents. Commensal organisms can, under certain circumstances, cause infection in their hosts (e.g. coliform bacteria from the gut leading to a urinary tract infection). Other organisms only cause an infection when they are transmitted to a new and susceptible host, by one of the methods detailed in this section.

Environmental reservoir

Organisms may have a reservoir in the soil (e.g. *Clostridium tetani*), where they are able to exist independently of a human host. Some parasites, such as *Strongyloides stercoralis*, have a stage of their life cycle which involves soil-living larvae, although the adult worms require a vertebrate host. Organisms with an environmental reservoir are rarely capable of direct person-to-person spread.

Animal reservoir

Zoonotic infections are transmitted from another vertebrate host to a human, in a number of different ways (e.g. via eating an infected foodstuff (*Salmonella enteritidis*) or through inoculation of saliva into a bite (rabies)). Examples of zoonoses can be found from all forms of causative organisms, and they can often be transmitted onwards from person to person.

Vector-mediated transmission

Arthropod vectors can transmit disease from animal to person, or person to person. Usually part of the life cycle of the pathogen occurs inside the vector, and a specific arthropod is required for each organism (e.g. *Plasmodium falciparum* inside the gut lining of the female *Anopheles* mosquito). Vector-borne diseases are generally a problem in tropical climates, but this has the potential to change if the correct vector is present (e.g. the Chikungunya outbreak in Italy in 2007, transmitted by the *Aedes albopictus* mosquito).

Direct person-to-person transmission

Direct person-to-person transmission encompasses several modes of transmission. Airborne spread of droplets or droplet nuclei is a common method of transmission of respiratory tract infections (e.g. influenza). Direct contact with skin infections or infestations may lead to transmission (e.g. scabies). All sexually transmitted infections rely on direct contact during sexual intercourse. Blood-to-blood contact can occur (e.g. during delivery, or as a result of sharing needles) and transmit agents such as HIV and the hepatitis B and C viruses.

Indirect person-to-person transmission

Sometimes organisms can survive for a period of time outside their host, and this means they can be transmitted via an intermediate surface (e.g. via a fomite or a stethoscope). Examples include typhoid or cholera.

Epidemiology

Epidemiology is the study of the aetiology, distribution, and control of a disease in a defined population. By knowing the epidemiology of infectious organisms, it is possible to refine a differential diagnosis, and limit the number of investigations needed. Certain specific definitions pertain:

- **incidence:** the number of new cases of a specific disease in a designated population over a defined time period, usually expressed as a proportion of the total study population
- **prevalence:** the total number of cases in a designated population at a specific point in time, expressed as a proportion of the total study population
- **endemic infection:** one which remains at a relatively constant rate, with respect to both incidence and prevalence, in a population over a prolonged period of time
- **epidemic infection:** occurs when there is a significant increase from the expected incidence of a disease over a defined time period
- **pandemic:** a worldwide epidemic
- **incubation period:** the time from a patient becoming infected with a specific disease, to the development of clinical symptoms
- **latent or pre-infectious period:** the time from a patient becoming infected with a specific disease, to them becoming infectious to others; this is often slightly shorter than the incubation period, and can have important implications for contact tracing
- **secondary attack rate:** a measure of the transmissibility or infectiousness of a disease; it is the risk of developing a secondary case amongst all those exposed to a primary case; thus, if four people were exposed to an infection, and two of them developed the disease, the secondary attack rate would be 2/4, or 50%
- **case reproductive number:** the average number of secondary cases that are caused by a single case of the infection; for example, a single patient with measles will infect, on average, 12 other susceptible people (note: in an endemic infectious disease, the net reproductive number needs to be greater than 1 for the rates to be maintained, so the aim of many disease control programmes is to decrease the reproductive number to less than 1)
- **herd immunity:** this occurs if there are sufficient people immune to a specific disease in a population so that the infection rates are very low and thus those who are susceptible are indirectly protected from infection; this phenomenon is part of the rationale behind mass vaccination programmes

Diagnostic approach to a patient with a possible infection

Infections can affect any system of the body and may be multisystemic. They can therefore present in a huge variety of ways. Not all infections lead to a fever, and not all fever is a result of infection. It is important to remember other causes, such as neoplasia or autoimmune disease, in the differential diagnosis. If infection is suspected, it is essential to consider where the patient may have acquired the disease, and also the patient themselves. Community-acquired infections from outside the hospital environment may be due to a diverse group of organisms. Nosocomial (hospital-acquired) infections result from a patient's admission. Between 5% and 10% of all hospital patients will acquire a nosocomial infection. Factors which increase this probability include a prolonged admission, intensive care treatment, and the use of prosthetic devices (e.g. intravascular catheters). The main types of nosocomial infection are lower respiratory tract infections, urinary tract infections, wound infections, and intravascular catheter-site infections. The heavy use of antimicrobial therapy in hospitals imposes a selection pressure towards resistant organisms, which must be considered in the treatment of nosocomial infections.

A patient with a compromised immune system will be susceptible to a wider range of infections, including unusual pathogens such as fungi or mycobacteria. A patient may have a weakened immune system as a result of a concurrent illness (e.g. HIV infection or leukaemia), due to treatment they are receiving (e.g. chemotherapy), or because of their age or nutritional status. It is important to recognize this, as the differential diagnosis will be different from that of an immunocompetent patient, and they may have more than one infectious disease simultaneously. Specific immune defects predispose to specific infections (e.g. hypogammaglobulinaemia and mycoplasma/ureaplasma infection).

The keys to the diagnosis of an infection, as in all of medicine, are a detailed history and a thorough clinical examination. Specific investigations for certain infectious diseases will be detailed elsewhere. Some key points to note are detailed in this section.

History

Within the detailed history, knowledge of likely epidemiological risk factors should trigger specific lines of inquiry:

- a full travel history: this is vital, as exposure to some pathogens (e.g. *Plasmodium falciparum*) will only occur if a patient has visited the appropriate geographical area
  - details about dates of travel, the conditions in which the patient stayed, as well as their activities and dietary habits while away
  - a vaccination history and appropriate prophylaxis use
- any exposure to animals, both domestic and wild, for zoonotic infections
- occupational history: this may reveal important exposures
- hobbies (e.g. canoeing may lead to exposure to water-borne pathogens)
- a full sexual history: this is important not only in the case of suspected sexually transmitted infections but also to help assess the patient's risk for HIV and any associated immune suppression
- previous or current IV drug use: this is associated not only with the acquisition of blood-borne viruses, but also with an increase in some bacterial or fungal diseases, due to the skin penetration; tattoos, piercings, and blood transfusions should also be noted if there is a possibility of blood-borne virus infection
- recent food history and source water: this may be relevant in certain cases
- close contact with children under 5 years old: this can increase the risk of certain viral infections

Clinical examination

A thorough general examination is required, particularly including assessment for lymphadenopathy, and ear, nose, and throat examination. Many infections cause a rash, so careful observation of the skin is necessary. If a sexually transmitted disease is being considered, a full genital examination should be performed.

A full set of observations should be obtained to help assess the severity of any possible infection; in addition, check for signs of septic shock.

Basic investigations

Basic investigations will vary, depending on the clinical picture, but the vast majority of patients with a suspected infection should have the following investigations:

- blood tests (see Table 304.1):
  - a full blood count, including a differential white-cell count
  - a coagulation screen
  - renal and liver function tests
  - C-reactive protein level, and erythrocyte sedimentation rate
- microscopy and culture:
  - all febrile patients should have a blood culture, and urine dipstick and culture where appropriate

- where clinically indicated, sputum samples should be cultured and, if TB is on the differential, the sputum should be examined and stained for acid-fast bacilli
- in patients with diarrhoea, faecal samples should also be taken for routine culture and examination for ova, cysts, and parasites if there is an appropriate history
- any other clinically indicated specimens, such as CSF or wound swabs, should be sent for microbiological examination
- radiology: depending on the clinical presentation, X-ray, ultra-sonography, CT, MRI, PET CT, or radionuclide scanning should be used to help localize infection
- echocardiography, if bacterial endocarditis is suspected
- culture of samples from aspiration/biopsy of infected sites is often the critical diagnostic procedure

Treatment and prognosis

Most infections never come to medical attention, and are cleared by the immune system. If, however, treatment is needed, there are therapeutics for most bacterial and fungal infections. Fewer treatments are available for eukaryotic and viral pathogens (in some cases, none), with a few exceptions. The outcome of infection with HIV, for example, has been revolutionized from certain death 30 years ago to there now being over 25 therapeutics, in 6 drug classes, available, and a normal life expectancy if drug adherence is good. For other infections, particularly rare ones in the developing world, the picture is very different, and economic circumstances define access to many drugs. The competence of the host immune system is critical. Pathogens with the capacity to persist in human hosts often can mutate to become resistant to drugs and can evade the immune system. There has been far too slow acceptance of the fact that, for most, if not all, of these diseases, combination therapy is the only way to ensure successful treatment.

Further Reading

Cohen J, Vincent J-L, Adhikari NKJ, et al. Sepsis: A roadmap for future research. *Lancet Infect Dis* 2015; 15: 581–614.

GBD 2013 Mortality and Causes of Death Collaborators. Global, regional, and national age–sex-specific, all-cause, and cause-specific mortality for 240 causes of death, 1990–2013: A systematic analysis for the Global Burden of Disease Study 2013. *Lancet* 2015; 385: 117–71.

World Health Organization overview of infectious disease (http://www.who.int/topics/infectious_diseases/en/)

Table 304.1 Interpretations of common blood test results in the context of infection

Result of investigation	Causes to consider
Anaemia	Malaria
	Helminth infection
	Overwhelming sepsis
Neutrophilia	Bacterial infection
Neutropaenia	Overwhelming sepsis
	Viral infection
Lymphocytosis	Viral infection
Lymphopaenia	Viral infection, particular consideration to HIV
Atypical lymphocytes	Infectious mononucleosis
Eosinophilia	Helminths
Thrombocytosis	Abscess
Thrombocytopaenia	Overwhelming sepsis
	Malaria
	HIV
Deranged coagulation	Overwhelming sepsis
	Hepatitis
Markedly elevated transaminases	Viral hepatitis
Raised C-reactive protein level and erythrocyte sedimentation rate	Non-specific sign of infection or inflammation.

305 Diagnosis in suspected infective disease: The history and examination

Ajit Lalvani, Katrina Pollock, and Manish Pareek

Introduction

Physicians assessing a patient with a suspected infective disease should bear in mind that the clinical presentation primarily results from the interaction between organism(s) and host, although this can be modulated by the environment. Therefore, while the critical elements of the diagnostic process for an infective disease follow the same basic tenets as for any clinical assessment—in other words, history, examination, and supportive investigations—this should be tailored when assessing patients who are presenting with an infectious disease, so that appropriate antimicrobial and supportive therapy can be commenced.

History

Obtaining a coherent history from the patient with a suspected infective disease requires a holistic outlook whereby the clinician should aim to collate information about the following aspects:

- the patient's background
- potential exposures to infectious organisms
- details about the illness

Patient's background

A full understanding of the patient's background can help to quickly narrow down the list of potential diagnoses.

Age

One of the most important questions to ask is the patient's age. Risk of infection, the likely causative organism, and the clinical pattern of disease change according to the subject's age.

Age modulates immunity against infection, with individuals at the extremes of life more prone to infection. Neonates (particularly when maternal antibodies have waned) and young children have immature immune systems, while the elderly are immunocompromised, either due to immunity waning over time or, more usually, due to coexisting medical conditions (such as diabetes mellitus) or medications (such as steroid therapy).

The types of organisms causing clinical disease also changes with age. Broadly speaking, children and young adults present with viral infections (such as infection with respiratory syncytial virus, CMV, and EBV), whereas more elderly patients are prone to bacterial infections—especially urinary tract and lower respiratory tract infections. However, this does not mean that children and young adults do not develop bacterial sepsis; the difference simply is that the spectrum of causative bacteria changes. This is highlighted if one considers the case of which organisms cause bacterial meningitis (see Table 305.1).

Clinical presentation of disease may also differ according to age. While children and young adults with established infection would usually be expected to present with a high-grade fever (>38°C), elderly patients can often present non-specifically without fever or, in some cases, with hypothermia. This is likely to be due, at least in part, to the host immune response—where a vigorous response results in marked symptomatology.

Preexisting medical conditions

Preexisting conditions can increase the chance of a patient developing an infection, and it is important to enquire about this in the history. It is useful to consider these conditions under two main headings:

- conditions which affect host immunity
- conditions which allow infection to become established

Underlying immunocompromise can be caused by a medical condition (such as diabetes mellitus or HIV infection) or due to the medication an individual is receiving (such as chemotherapy for neoplasia, or azathioprine for inflammatory bowel disease). The immunocompromised host can be difficult to manage clinically, but making the correct diagnosis is critical as they are more prone to acquiring infections, developing disseminated disease/complications, and becoming infected with a wider range of pathogens.

HIV deserves special mention. As HIV infection becomes more advanced and cellular immunity is affected, individuals become more prone to atypical infections, which are unlikely in those with an intact immune system. Therefore, it is important to enquire about an individual's HIV status (if known) or to test for it, as it will affect the clinical decision-making process. For example, if an individual has fever and headache, a potential diagnosis is bacterial or viral meningitis if the individual is not HIV-positive whereas, for HIV-infected individuals, the differential diagnosis would also include tuberculous meningitis, cryptococcal meningitis, and CNS toxoplasmosis. This clearly will affect the investigations that are undertaken, as well as the empiric therapy that will need to be commenced.

Aside from the host's immune function, it is also important to enquire about other risk factors that render increased host susceptibility to infection. This encompasses individuals with prosthetic devices (such as heart valves, joint replacements, and semi-permanent central venous catheters), which can become foci of infection; those with chronic suppurative lung infection (such as cystic fibrosis, where thick sputum becomes infected); and individuals with anatomical abnormalities, such as strictures within the renal tract (where the slow flow of urine results in the tract becoming infected).

Sociodemographic factors

Certain infections are also more common in those who were born in developing-world nations but have since migrated to the developed

Table 305.1 Common organisms causing bacterial meningitis in different age groups

Age group	Common organisms
Neonates	Group B streptococci
	Escherichia coli (carrying K1 antigen)
	Listeria monocytogenes
Young children	*Neisseria meningitidis*
	Streptococcus pneumoniae
	Haemophilus influenzae
Adults	*Streptococcus pneumoniae*
	Neisseria meningitidis
	Haemophilus influenzae
Older adults	*Streptococcus pneumoniae*
	Neisseria meningitidis
	Listeria monocytogenes (if >50 years of age)
	Aerobic Gram-negative bacilli

world. It is useful to ask the patient where they were born, where they grew up, when they migrated, and how long they have been living in the receiving country. The pattern of disease seen in immigrants is likely to be very different from that seen in the locally born population. Much of this can be attributed to the different type and quantity of exposure to pathogens during childhood and young adulthood (as most migrants will leave their country of origin as young adults). As a consequence, it is clear that a number of infections are more common in immigrants, including latent TB infection, active TB, hepatitis B/C, and gastrointestinal helminths. An additional point to note is that immigrants are also more likely to continue returning to developing countries to visit friends and relations, which puts them at risk of travel-associated infections such as malaria, dengue, and typhoid fever (see 'Travel history').

Exposure to infectious agents

The clinician should make a point of asking about all aspects of the patient's life, even if some of the questions may be considered intimate, to understand the nature and risk of potential exposure to infectious pathogens. Specific areas to enquire about include travel history; recent operations or antibiotic therapy; lifestyle choices (including occupation); and a family history of infectious diseases.

Travel history

International air travel to all parts of the world has increased hugely and become much more affordable to the general public. As a consequence, enquiring about recent travel is undoubtedly important in an individual presenting with a suspected infective disease. Physicians should ask very detailed questions about the dates of travel, the specific countries (and areas) visited, the type of stay (e.g. a business visit to a 5-star hotel is very different from backpacking), and personal behaviour (such as avoiding local street foods, drinking bottled water, and avoiding mosquitoes). It is also important to establish whether the patient took pre-travel medical advice with respect to travel vaccinations and malaria prophylaxis (as well as whether they were compliant during and after the trip with the medication).

Recent medical procedures/antibiotics

Conventional history taking often overlooks previous contact the patient has had with medical professionals. However, this should be specifically asked if infection is present. For example, if the patient has had recent dental work or a colonoscopy of the bowel and presents with fever and a murmur, infective endocarditis should be included in the differential diagnosis. Similarly, in a patient presenting with diarrhoea, it is important to specifically ask about any recent courses of antibiotics (enquire about the name and duration) as *Clostridium difficile* is a possibility.

Lifestyle factors

Understanding the personal behaviour of the patient is also important. This includes a number of areas, but specific enquires should include blood-borne virus risk (through recreational drug use as an IV drug user, as this increases the risk of hepatitis B/C and HIV infection) and sexual history (if appropriate from the clinical presentation).

Occupation is also important. Certain occupations have an increased risk of exposure to specific pathogens, and clinicians should make sure this is established during the history. For example, healthcare workers will be at a higher risk of occupational exposure to blood-borne viruses (such as hepatitis B/C and HIV) and respiratory infections (such as influenza and tuberculosis), while individuals who work in drains/sewers are at an increased risk of acquiring leptospirosis.

Family history/contact with pathogens

Infectious diseases are, by definition, communicable, and can occur from a single infectious source. In this respect, family structure is relevant, as infections can spread rapidly from member to member, but also because they may all be linked, epidemiologically, to a source of infection (e.g. food poisoning from a restaurant meal). It is important to directly enquire about other family members who are unwell or have already been diagnosed with an infection (e.g. pulmonary TB or a diarrhoeal illness). In this way, the admitting physician can narrow down the differential diagnosis, and instigate therapy more rapidly while also limiting the spread of the infection.

Features of the presenting illness

With a fuller understanding of the patient's background and potential source(s) of exposure, the clinician must go on to establish the symptoms and signs of the presenting illness, so that appropriate investigations can be ordered.

Chronology of illness

On encountering the patient, the clinician should first attempt to delineate illness onset, including its date and nature (abrupt vs indolent). A further important point to establish is when the exposure/infection has occurred in relation to the onset of the symptoms, as this provides an indication of the incubation period (see Table 305.2).

The next step is to try and understand the course of the illness over time. One of the fascinating things about the clinical features of infectious diseases is how they evolve. While some illnesses usually result in rapid deterioration after initial presentation (e.g. meningococcal meningitis), others, such as TB, usually progress more slowly and symptoms may wax and wane. This must be established early in the history, as it will give important clues as to the etiological infectious agent.

A complicating factor is that the course of the illness can be modulated by previous antimicrobial/antipyretic therapy, and it is important to directly enquire about this from the patient.

Symptoms

Detailed questions about the symptoms are critical to the history-taking process. Physicians should ensure that they take time to get a clear understanding of the main symptoms, and the order in which they have appeared. Clinical features of infectious disease can be categorized as systemic or localized/organ specific.

An ongoing difficulty with diagnosing infectious diseases is that systemic symptoms, which are non-specific and non-contributory, often

Table 305.2 Common infectious diseases, their causative organisms, and the lengths of their incubation periods

Type of organism	Disease	Causative organism	Incubation period
Virus	HIV	HIV	2–4 weeks for acute seroconversion illness; many years until advanced HIV/AIDS
	Influenza	Influenza virus	1–5 days
	Dengue fever / Dengue haemorrhagic fever	Dengue flavivirus	3–14 days
	Measles	Measles virus (paramyxovirus)	6–19 days
	Mumps	Mumps virus (paramyxovirus)	15–24 days
	Rubella	Rubella virus (togavirus)	14–21 days
	Chicken pox	Varicella zoster virus	10–21 days
Bacteria	Diphtheria	*Corynebacterium diphtheriae*	2–5 days
	Tetanus	*Clostridium tetani*	3–21 days
	Typhoid	*Salmonella typhi*	7–14 days
Protozoa	Malaria (falciparum)	*Plasmodium falciparum*	1–4 weeks

predominate. As a consequence, they are not that useful at distinguishing different types of infection or, indeed, alternative differential diagnoses. Common systemic symptoms include fever, malaise, lethargy, anorexia/weight loss, and myalgia.

Fever is almost always present in patients who have an underlying infection. Although the definition of fever varies, a temperature above 38°C is generally considered to be abnormal. If the patient does complain of fever, it is useful to try and establish if it is constant or whether the temperature spikes at a certain time of the day. It is also important to determine if there are any associated symptoms with the fever—such as rigors. Rigors are episodes of severe, uncontrollable shivering, and characteristically occur in biliary sepsis, pyelonephritis, malaria, and visceral abscesses. They are less common in viral infections.

Other systemic symptoms, such as anorexia/weight loss, malaise, and lethargy, are fairly common in most infections and are indication of the underlying inflammatory response. Myalgia is also seen in a number of infections, although its severity will vary. While it may be relatively mild in influenza, it may be very severe in dengue, malaria, or leptospirosis.

Localized, site-specific symptoms (such as dysuria and cough) are important to elucidate, as they usually help to identify the specific organ system involved (see Table 305.3 for common localizing syndromes). Armed with this information, the clinician can focus the clinical examination and ensure that site-specific samples are obtained which will increase the chance of identifying the infecting organism. However, it must be understood that some symptoms which appear to be localizing may, in fact, not be. For example, in the returning traveller with fever and diarrhoea, it is tempting to consider this to be simply due to gastroenteritis, even though malaria presents in this way and will be rapidly fatal if not diagnosed and treated appropriately.

After completion of the history, the next step for the physician is to use the information that has been gathered, to underpin a thorough examination of the patient.

Examination

A thorough physical examination is essential in the assessment of suspected infective disease; the physiological state of the patient is gauged, and clinical signs are elicited that, with the constellation of symptoms, build the initial differential diagnosis. This is the major opportunity to comprehensively characterize the patient's condition and enables the clinician to tailor the subsequent investigation plan to be relevant, directive, and brief.

Examination of the patient with suspected active disease should focus on the following areas:

- general appearance
- the lymph system
- the skin
- cardiovascular status
- the respiratory system
- the abdomen
- the eyes, and neurological assessment
- the ears, the nose, and the throat

Findings of particular significance in the examination of the immunocompromised patient are summarized in Box 305.1.

General appearance

The severely unwell patient should be quickly recognized by assessment of pallor or erythema, sweating, ambulatory ability, cognitive functional status, and conscious level (see Box 305.2). Body temperature should be recorded.

The lymph system

The pattern and nature of lymphadenopathy is a useful tool in the diagnosis of infectious disease (see Table 305.4), and examination can identify nodes suitable for biopsy. Examination of the tonsils and the submandibular, preauricular, cervical, clavicular, axillary, epitrochlear, and inguinal lymph nodes for palpable lymphadenopathy should be coupled with inspection of the skin for visible causes such as a

Table 305.3 Localizing symptoms, and the differential diagnoses associated with each one

Organ system	Clinical symptoms	Differential diagnosis
Cardiac	Chest pain	Infective endocarditis
		TB
Respiratory	Dyspnoea	Pneumonia
	Cough	Pleural effusion
	Haemoptysis	TB
		Malaria
		Influenza
		Respiratory syncytial virus
		Parainfluenza
Gastrointestinal	Diarrhoea	Viral gastroenteritis
	Abdominal	Malaria
	pain	Clostridium difficile
	Jaundice	Bacterial diarrhoea (Escherichia coli, Salmonella sp., Shigella sp.)
		Typhoid
		Giardia
		Amoebic dysentery
		TB
		Hepatitis (A/B/C/E)
		Infectious mononucleosis (EBV)
		CMV
		Leptospirosis
		Pyogenic liver abscess
Neurological	Headache	Meningitis (bacterial, viral, tuberculous, fungal)
	Meningism	Encephalitis (viral)
	Confusion	Malaria
		Leptospirosis
		Dengue
		Any infection can cause confusion, as part of the sepsis syndrome
Genitourinary	Dysuria	Urinary tract infection (bacterial)
	Haematuria	TB
	Discharge	Malaria
	Ulceration	Schistosomiasis
		Sexually transmitted infection
Dermatological	Rash	Wide range of conditions
		Specific type of rash will allude to underlying cause

cellulitis or an infective lesion (e.g. for *Bartonella henselae*). If lymphadenopathy is found, the major differential diagnosis for infection is neoplasia. Generalized lymphadenopathy due to infection is less common than localized eruptions and should immediately alert the physician to the possibility of the persistent generalized lymphadenopathy of HIV infection. Other common causes of generalized lymphadenopathy include infectious mononucleosis; disseminated bacterial infection, such as brucellosis; and rare fungal infections, such as histoplasmosis.

The skin

Infection often manifests in the skin, and descriptive classification detailing the distribution, colour, form, and location (including in the mouth, the nails, and the genitalia) of the infection can aid in the identification of the infectious disease (see Table 305.5).

Pyogenic collections are relatively common, ranging from folliculitis of hair follicles to larger abscesses; lesions are pustular, painful, and erythematous. Spreading forms of bacterial infection of the skin due to *Streptococcal* spp. and *Staphylococcal* spp. include cellulitis, which is common in diabetic patients; erysipelas; and necrotizing fasciitis. The latter is a surgical emergency, recognizable by extreme tenderness, failure to respond to IV antibiotics, tissue

Box 305.1 Examination of the immunocompromised patient

HIV infection causes the most common acquired immunodeficiency worldwide. Elucidating the signs of immunocompromise can aid this often subtle diagnosis. As part of a full examination, the following areas should be focused on:

- the general appearance
- the mouth
- the lymph system
- the respiratory system
- the genitalia
- the nervous system

General appearance

There is evidence of wasting and cachexia in advanced disease. Infections are present in unusual distributions (e.g. facial *Molluscum contagiosum*).

The skin

Exacerbation of underlying skin conditions (e.g. psoriasis) is common. Other associated conditions include eosinophilic pustular folliculitis; skin manifestations of opportunistic fungal and mycobacterial infection; seborrheic dermatitis; and Kaposi's sarcoma. Seroconversion gives rise to a maculopapular rash.

The mouth

A thorough examination of the mouth is essential; signs of candidiasis, oral hairy leukoplakia, gingivitis, aphthous ulcers, and Kaposi's sarcoma should be sought.

The lymph system

Lymphadenopathy may occur at any stage of infection due to HIV (persistent generalized lymphadenopathy: enlarged lymph nodes in two or more extra-inguinal sites, for more than 3 months). Kaposi's sarcoma, TB, and lymphoma are also common causes. With more advanced disease, opportunistic and unusual infections, including atypical mycobacterial disease, bacillary angiomatosis, systemic fungal infection, and toxoplasmosis, are possible causes.

The respiratory system

Acute bronchitis and chronic sinusitis are common at all stages of disease. Pulmonary infection is one of the most common complications of HIV infection, either bacterial or due to *Pneumocystis jiroveci* (pneumocystis pneumonia; often referred to as PCP). Mycobacteria and fungi (e.g. *Cryptococcus* sp.) can cause florid pulmonary signs.

The genitalia

Manifestations of dermatological conditions may be found in the genitalia. Genital and rectal lesions due to HSV-1 and HSV-2 are common, as well as lesions of Kaposi's sarcoma, intra-epithelial neoplasia, and condylomata acuminata.

The nervous system

Central and peripheral neurological manifestations of HIV warrant careful examination and investigation, even if signs are subtle. The altered inflammatory response can reduce the signs of florid infection, and mild signs of headache or meningism may belie life-threatening pathology. Fundoscopy may reveal signs of CMV retinitis in late disease.

Box 305.2 Recognition of the patient in septic shock

Sepsis is the physiological response to a major insult that is usually infective in origin. Septic shock is severe sepsis plus hypotension not reversed with fluid resuscitation. Recognition of the early stages of sepsis, before irretrievable organ damage has occurred, is crucial to patient survival. The examination should focus on:

- temperature
- general appearance and the skin
- the CNS
- the cardiovascular system
- the respiratory system
- the abdomen

Temperature

Look for fever (temperature >38.3°C) or hypothermia (temperature <36.0°C)

General appearance and the skin

Look for tissue perfusion, which is assessed from the capillary refill time, and the presence of mottling and cool peripheries. Rashes may represent a response to infection (e.g. the purpura of disseminated intravascular coagulation), haematogenous seeding of organisms (e.g. meningococcal or staphylococcal sepsis), or the source of infection (e.g. cellulitis).

The CNS

Altered mental status is common; evidence of alcohol or illicit drug use frequently confuses this picture and should not be assumed as the primary cause. Signs of meningitis should be carefully sought.

The cardiovascular system

Tachycardia (heart rate >90/min or more than two standard deviations above the normal value for age) is common, and the pulse may be hyperdynamic. Assess for the presence of arterial hypotension (systolic blood pressure <90 mm Hg, mean arterial pressure <70 mm Hg, or systolic blood pressure decreased by >40 mm Hg in adults or more than two standard deviations below the normal value for age), and a postural drop in blood pressure.

The respiratory system

Tachypnoea is common; signs of respiratory compromise may be the respiratory response of normal lungs to lactic acidosis or incipient acute respiratory distress syndrome, secondary to sepsis as well as indicating a pulmonary focus of infection.

The abdomen

Ileus with absent bowel sounds may occur and there may be signs of underlying infection (e.g. diverticular abscess, subphrenic abscess, *Clostridium difficile*). Hyperglycaemia in the absence of diabetes is indicative of sepsis. Acute oliguria with urine output <0.5 ml/kg per hour for at least 2 hours despite adequate fluid replacement indicates renal dysfunction.

---

maculopapular rash or wart-like condylomata lata, and tertiary syphilis as skin gummata.

Cardiovascular status

Assessment of the circulatory status can indicate shock, abnormal fluid balance, or a hyperdynamic state as evidenced by skin temperature, capillary refill time, pulse rate, pulse character, jugular venous pressure, and blood pressure. Examination of the mouth and the conjunctivae for signs of anaemia should be undertaken, as anaemia of chronic disease (e.g. in TB), iron-deficiency anaemia (e.g. from intestinal parasites), or anaemia due to haemolysis (e.g. in *Treponema pallidum* infection, malaria, or haemophagocytosis secondary to certain viral infections) or bone marrow failure (e.g. in parvovirus B19 infection or following marrow replacement (e.g. due to disseminated fungal infection)) may be present.

Cardiac auscultation may indicate a murmur, due to infective endocarditis or viral myocarditis. Endocarditis is an important cause of

---

fluctuance, and warmth. Some rashes, such as shingles, which is a dermatomal vesicular rash caused by recrudescent varicella zoster virus (VZV) infection, are diagnostic; other skin manifestations (e.g. erythema multiforme) have many etiologies. Rashes that appear generalized at first may have a pattern of involvement that can hint at the underlying cause, such as scabies or dermatophyte infection. Lastly, infections such as syphilis mimic other conditions and change throughout the natural history of the disease; primary syphilis may appear as a painless, highly infectious ulcer at the site of inoculation, while secondary syphilis manifests as a generalized

Table 305.4 Major causes of lymphadenopathy

Distribution	Classification	Examples of aetiology
Localized	Viral	Acute self-limiting viral infection (e.g. adenovirus; cervical/axillary)
	Bacterial	Staphylococci and streptococci
		Acute bacterial lymphadenitis
		TB (e.g. cold abscess)
		Bartonella henselae (cervical/axillary)
		Lymphogranuloma venereum (inguinal)
		Tularaemia
	Protozoan	*Toxoplasma gondii* (occipital/cervical)
	Inflammatory	Reactive hyperplasia (e.g. rheumatoid arthritis)
	Neoplastic	Metastatic tumour (e.g. melanoma) Virchow's node
		Early stages of Hodgkin's and non-Hodgkin's lymphomas
Generalized	Viral	Persistent generalized lymphadenopathy of HIV infection
		EBV
		CMV
		HHV8 (Kaposi's sarcoma)
	Bacterial	Brucellosis
		TB
	Fungi	Histoplasmosis
		Coccidiodomycosis
	Inflammatory	Dermatopathic (e.g. eczema)
		Sarcoidosis
		Medications
	Neoplastic	Late stages of Hodgkin's and non-Hodgkin's lymphomas

cardiovascular infection and should not be missed. Features include fever, evidence of valvular surgery, evidence of injecting drug use, splenomegaly, and vascular, embolic, or immunological signs, such as Osler's nodes in the extremities, and Roth spots on fundoscopy.

Lastly, assessment of pitting peripheral oedema may indicate poor physiological status, due to infection. Non-pitting oedema may be related to infectious lymphatic obstruction, which is sometimes florid in lymphatic filariasis (due to *Wuchereria bancrofti* infection).

The respiratory system

The respiratory examination may reveal a source of infection, or the physiological response to infection in the normal lung. The presence of chronic lung pathology such as bronchiectasis will alter the pattern and extent of disease. Measurements of pulse oximetry and respiratory rate are essential assessments of respiratory function. However, the respiratory rate is often raised in the presence of infection or pain and is not a specific sign of lung pathology (see Box 305.2). Unequal chest expansion can indicate unilateral compromise of one lung due to infection. The apices should be examined, as infection with mycobacteria or fungi can occur in this region. Pulmonary infections are common in the developed world, and classic signs of fever, hypoxia, and consolidation (bronchial breathing, reduced air entry) may be coupled with gastrointestinal symptoms and changes in mental status. Pleuritic chest pain may indicate an effusion, and the overlying area should be percussed for dullness and carefully auscultated. Common causes of pneumonia in the UK include *Streptococcus pneumoniae*, *Mycoplasma pneumoniae*, and *Haemophilus influenzae*, although causative viruses (e.g. influenza virus, VZV) and organisms associated with immunocompromise (e.g. *Pneumocystis jiroveci*), should not be overlooked. The simple CURB-65 prediction rule (**c**onfusion; **u**rea >7 mmol/l; **r**espiratory rate ≥30/minute; low systolic (<90 mm Hg) or diastolic (≤60 mm Hg) **b**lood pressure; **age** ≥**65** years) is a useful tool for assessing the severity of pneumonia within the context of the full clinical picture.

The abdomen

General inspection may have revealed signs of abdominal involvement in the infectious process; frank jaundice is obvious, but mild discolouration requires closer inspection of the mouth and conjunctivae. Infectious intra-hepatic causes to consider are viral hepatitides, infectious mononucleosis, and leptospirosis. Post-hepatic obstruction may be infective in origin or complicate non-infectious causes such as gallstones.

Examination of the mouth should look for anaemia, candida, and gingivitis, tonsillar infection, and palatial purpura. The source of infection may be found on general palpation and per rectal examination, including intestinal infections (e.g. with *Salmonella typhi*) or complications of diverticular disease, such as diverticulosis. Fever and lower abdominal tenderness are generally present in pyelonephritis, and one or both renal angles may be tender. Acute pelvic inflammation due to a sexually transmitted infection may be distinguished by cervical excitation tenderness (pain on movement of the cervix) with or without adnexal tenderness. Percussion and palpation of abdominal organs for enlargement or tenderness may reveal organomegaly, which has a large differential diagnosis (see Table 305.6). Finally, a genital exam may be required for assessment of inguinal lymphadenopathy, local tissue involvement, and signs of sexually transmitted infection. Serious soft tissue infections of the inguinal, genital, or perianal region (e.g. Fournier's gangrene) should not be missed for want of proper examination.

The eyes, and neurological assessment

Examination of the eyes, including of the visual fields, the pupils, and eye movements, aids the localization of CNS or cavernous sinus infection. Infection of the conjunctiva is common and may have a viral (erythematous, non-pyogenic) or bacterial (erythematous, pyogenic) origin. Clues for infectious diseases can be found by careful fundoscopy and should be performed on all patients; retinal haemorrhages with a white centre (Roth spots), initially described in infective endocarditis, are found in association with other conditions, including diabetes and haematological malignancies. TB can infect the eyes or give rise to several forms of inflammation, including anterior uveitis, which is a valuable indication in those without typical tuberculous symptoms.

A thorough neurological examination should identify level of consciousness, cognitive function, and foci of infection, centrally and peripherally. Any patient with a headache should be examined for signs of meningism, including neck stiffness, photophobia, and Kernig's sign. Encephalitis can be difficult to distinguish clinically, and examination of cognitive function can be key. Florid meningitis may be bacterial in origin, with *Haemophilus influenzae* type b, *Streptococcus pneumoniae*, and *Neisseria meningitidis* being the principal causes worldwide. Clinical suspicion following history and examination is sufficient to initiate antibiotic treatment, which should not be delayed for the results of investigations. Viral meningitides are generally more indolent, but can be indistinguishable, especially where bacterial meningitis has been partially treated. Tuberculous meningitis, while rare in low-incidence countries such as the UK, has an extremely high mortality, and early intervention is essential.

The ears, the nose, and the throat

Examination of the ears, the nose, and the throat completes the examination of the patient with suspected infectious disease. Visualization of a bulging erythematous tympanic membrane can localize a previously elusive febrile infection. Vesicles of varicella zoster infecting the geniculate ganglion may be seen in association with facial paralysis (indicating Ramsay–Hunt syndrome). Viral and bacterial tonsillitis are common and usually easily visualized. Occasionally, a bacterial abscess known as a quinsy may form.

Conclusions

Diagnosing a patient with suspected infective disease can be challenging—particularly as it is not a protocol-driven specialty. As a consequence, the encounter with the patient must be undertaken in a systematic manner so that crucial elements of the history and examination can be gleaned. This directs immediate management and informs the requesting of appropriate investigations.

Table 305.5 A descriptive approach to identifying causes of common skin manifestations of infectious disease

Distribution	Colour	Location	Description	Possible infectious causes
Generalized	Erythematous	NA	Confluent Desquamation	Bacterial: • Group A Streptococcus (scarlet fever) • toxic shock syndrome • staphylococcal scalded-skin syndrome
		NA	Maculopapular or macular	Viral: • primary HIV • EBV • HHV6 (spares face) • measles • rubella (begins facially) • dengue (initially diffuse flushing) Bacterial: • secondary syphilis • rickettsial disease • leptospirosis • typhoid fever (rose spots on trunk)
		NA	Vesicular	Viral: • primary varicella zoster virus
	Purpuric	NA	Papular or maculopapular	Bacterial: • meningococcal sepsis • septic emboli (e.g. *Staphylococcus aureus*) • disseminated gonococcal infection
	Hyper- or hypopigmented	Trunk and proximal extremities	Scaly macules	Tinea versicolor
Localized	Erythematous	Facial	Confluent	Viral: • parvovirus B19 (slapped cheek) Bacterial: • erysipelas (*Streptococcus* spp.)
		Dermatomal	Vesicular	Recrudescent varicella zoster virus
		Oral /mucocutaneous	Vesicular ulcerative	Herpes simplex virus 1 and 2 (genital lesions common) Coxsackie virus (herpangina)
		Trunk in Christmas tree distribution Groin Axillae Scalp Toes	Scaly patches Scaly patches (annular)	Pityriasis rosea (causative organism unclear) Dermatophytes
		Groin Fingers Feet	Papules Excoriation	Scabies (evidence of burrows)
	Erythematous; purple then greenish yellow	Lower limbs, often bilateral	Nodules or papules	Erythema nodosum, many etiologies: • bacterial: *Mycobacterium* spp. (including TB), *Streptococcal* spp. *Brucella* spp., *Campylobacter* spp., *Corynebacterium diphtheriae*, *Klebsiella pneumoniae*, etc. • viral: CMV, hepatitis B and C viruses, EBV, HIV, measles virus • fungal: *Coccidioides immitis*, dermatophytes • protozoal: *Entamoeba* spp., *Giardia lamblia*
	White–erythematous	Hair-bearing skin	Pustular	Folliculitis (*Staphylococcal* spp.)
	Erythema with central clearing	Site of tick bite	Erythema chonicum migrans	Lyme disease (*Borrelia burgdorferi*)

Table 305.6 Examples of infectious causes of organomegaly

Organomegaly	Infectious aetiology
Hepatomegaly	Acute infections: • viral: viral hepatitides, EBV, CMV • bacterial: pneumococcal pneumonia, pyomyositis, bacterial abscess, *Leptospira* spp. • protozoan: malaria Chronic infections: • viral: hepatocellular carcinoma secondary to hepatitis B • bacterial: TB, *Coxiella burnetii* (chronic Q fever), brucellosis, *Bartonella henselae* • protozoan: leishmaniasis, amoebic abscess • fungal: histoplasmosis • helminthic: schistosomiasis, liver flukes, toxocariasis, *Echinococcus granulosus* (hydatid disease)
Splenomegaly: mild to moderate (<5 cm or 5–10 cm below costal margin)	Acute infections: • viral: viral hepatitides • bacterial: bacterial sepsis, *Rickettsia* spp. (e.g. epidemic typhus) • protozoan: malaria, toxoplasmosis Chronic infections: • bacterial: TB, infective endocarditis, brucellosis, syphilis • fungal: histoplasmosis
Splenomegaly: massive (>10 cm below costal margin)	Protozoan: • hyper-reactive malarial splenomegaly • leishmaniasis Helminths: • schistosomiasis
Genitourinary organomegaly (renal and bladder enlargement)	Bacterial: • renal pyogenic abscess • obstruction secondary to pyelonephritis Helminths: • chronic urinary schistosomiasis, with bladder and genital involvement

Further Reading

British Infection Association Guidelines (http://www.britishinfection.org/guidelines-resources/published-guidelines/)

Infectious Diseases Society of America Practice Guidelines (http://www.idsociety.org/idsa_practice_guidelines/)

Long B and Koyfman A. Clinical Mimics: An Emergency Medicine-Focused Review of Cellulitis Mimics *The J Emerg Med* 2017; 52(1): 34–42.

NICE guideline 51 Methods, evidence and recommendations. Sepsis: recognition, assessment and early management, 2016.

306 Investigation in infection

Ajit Lalvani and Manish Pareek

Introduction

Making a diagnosis in a patient with a suspected infection is dependent on obtaining a comprehensive history complemented by a thorough examination; these crucial elements narrow down the potential causative agent(s) and the organ systems affected, thereby guiding the clinician in undertaking appropriate investigations.

Investigating a patient with a suspected infectious disease necessitates understanding the multitude of tests that are available to clinicians and being able to interpret and integrate the results.

Investigations in infection can be subclassified into three distinct areas:

* baseline investigations: these are undertaken in all patients and provide an indication of the impact of infection on the host
* specific investigations: these are undertaken to identify the causative organism(s)
* additional investigations: these add weight to the diagnosis of infection and can provide further information about the host/causative organism

Baseline investigations

Admitting clinicians suspecting infection in a patient should undertake simple baseline investigations which provide an initial assessment of the host response to infection—in terms of organ systems affected, disease severity, and its chronicity. These usually consist of urine tests, blood tests, and simple radiology.

Urine and blood tests

Routine urine dipstick and blood investigations, including haematology and biochemistry, are often undertaken in the acute phase.

Table 306.1 outlines the blood tests which should be undertaken as a baseline, as well the commonly seen abnormalities where a patient has an underlying infection.

Radiology

In the acute stage, chest radiographs are useful in patients presenting with respiratory symptoms or as part of a workup in those cases where the source of a fever cannot be localized. The specific abnormalities that are seen include bronchopneumonia, lobar pneumonia, cavitation, or a pleural effusion.

Tests aimed at identifying the infectious agent or categories of infectious agents

Simple baseline investigations only provide an indication of the underlying pathological process. Making the correct diagnosis depends on identifying the causative organism(s) either within the host or tissues/fluids (e.g. sputum). These site-specific specimens can be tested for protein, white cells, red blood cells, and pH (e.g. in pleural fluid, a low pH suggests an empyema). These results can tell us two things:

* whether an infection is present
* if so, what type of infection is present (e.g. if lymphocytes predominate, then TB is more likely, whereas a predominance of neutrophils would suggest a bacterial aetiology)

Determining these allows the clinician to commence antimicrobial therapy while awaiting more specific diagnostic tests which identify the organism directly or indirectly.

Methods of direct identification

Direct identification of the causative organism stems from obtaining samples from sites of disease, as indicated by the history and

Table 306.1 Commonly seen abnormalities on baseline blood investigations in patients with underlying infection

Type of test	Specific investigations	Commonly seen abnormalities in infection
Urine	Urine dipstick	Usually, presence of blood, protein, nitrites, and leucocytes
		If urinary tract infection suggested, the sample should be sent for culture
Full blood count	Haemoglobin	Anaemia; may be seen both in acute infection and chronic disease
	White-cell count	Raised white-cell count common
		Neutrophilia present in bacterial infections
		Lymphocyotis or lymphopaenia present in viral infections
		In certain infections, neutropenia (e.g. malaria and tuberculosis) or lymphopenia (tuberculosis, HIV infection) may be present
		Eosinophilia present in parasitic infections
	Platelets	Thrombocytosis
		Thrombocytopenia (may be seen in infection with or without the presence of disseminated intravascular coagulation)
	Blood film	Leucoerythroblastic blood film in severe sepsis
Biochemistry	Urea and electrolytes	May be non-specifically increased, especially if renal tract infection present
	Liver function tests	May indicate hepatitis if the liver is directly affected
		May be non-specifically raised when sepsis is at a site other than the liver
		Albumin level decreases as part of the acute phase response*
	C-reactive protein	Usually raised in bacterial infection
		Can be used to monitor the response to antimicrobials

*The acute phase response is often seen in infection and results in the following specific abnormalities: an **increase** in the erythrocyte sedimentation rate and in the levels of C-reactive protein, globulins, and ferritin, with a **decrease** in albumin and transferrin.

examination. When obtaining samples, clinicians should closely liaise with the laboratory to ensure that specimens are correctly taken in the appropriate media, handled appropriately, and delivered in a timely manner so that they can be appropriately processed by the microbiologists.

Amongst direct methods of identification, common modalities include microscopy, culture, antigen detection tests, and nucleic acid amplification-based modalities.

Microscopy

Microscopy on sterile, site-specific host samples is a common method of identifying bacteria and protozoa (but not viruses). These specimens can be examined directly as wet mounts or after they have been stained.

Wet mounts are used in stool examination for gastrointestinal parasites or their ova (e.g. in giardia), or in microscopy of blood (e.g. peripheral smears for malaria parasites and whole blood to look for microfilaria which cause lymphatic filariasis).

The performance of microscopy can be enhanced with the use of specific stains. One commonly used stain is Gram's stain, which identifies, and differentiates, bacteria according to their cell walls: Gram-positive bacteria have a peptidoglycan cell wall and stain purple; Gram-negative bacteria have a thin cell wall and stain pink. Table 306.2 highlights other important stains in microscopy.

Microscopy is useful as it rapidly indicates the causative pathogen before definitive culture results can be obtained, thus allowing targeted antimicrobial therapy to be prescribed.

Culture

Culture complements microscopy. Specimens are plated on growth media and allowed to multiply, with results generally available in 24–48 hours. When interpreting culture results, clinicians should consider the following key questions:

- Where was the sample taken from? Was the site sterile (e.g. in the case of CSF) or non-sterile (e.g. skin/sputum)?
- Does the result reflect contamination? (This is important for specimens such as skin swabs (where coagulase-negative staphylococci reside as commensals)).
- Has the patient received antibiotics prior to the specimen being sent for culture? (This can result in false-negative culture results.)

Culture is the gold-standard test for infection, as it has superior sensitivity to microscopy alone. Specific advantages include the ability to identify the organism, and the ability to perform drug susceptibility testing. However, drawbacks of culture include the fact that some organisms are slow-growing and difficult to culture (e.g. *Mycobacterium tuberculosis*) and, thus, alternative diagnostic modalities are required. Culture is rarely used for viruses, as it has been superseded by antibody-based and nucleic acid amplification tests.

Table 306.2 Different stains used in microscopy when investigating a patient with an infection

Name of stain	Specimen	Common organisms identified by stain
Gram	Blood CSF	Most bacteria, classified as Gram positive (purple) or Gram negative (pink)
Ziehl–Nielsen	Sputum Pleural fluid Lymph node aspirates Pus	Mycobacteria species
Giemsa	Blood Marrow aspirates	Malaria Trypanosomes
Wright's stain	Blood	Malaria
India ink	CSF	*Cryptococcus neoformans*
Silver stain	Sputum	*Pneumocystis jiroveci*

Table 306.3 Different antigen detection tests currently in use

Name of organism	Specimen
Cryptococcus neoformans	Blood CSF
Streptococcus pneumoniae	Urine CSF
Legionella pneumophila	Urine
Clostridium difficile	Stool (for toxin)
Influenza A/B	Nasopharyngeal swab/aspirate
Plasmodium falciparum (malaria)	Blood

Antigen detection tests

Antigen detection tests detect the antigen/pathogen itself or the toxin it is producing (e.g. *Clostridium difficile* toxin) and can be undertaken on various specimens, including blood, CSF, urine, and stool, to identify a range of different organisms (Table 306.3).

Several types of antigen detection tests are available, of which latex agglutination and enzyme immunoassays are commonly used. Latex agglutination tests use antibodies to test for the presence of antigen in the clinical specimen (e.g. a cryptococcal antigen test). With enzyme immunoassays, the specimen containing the antigen is mixed with a specific antibody which is linked to an enzyme which produces a detectable signal, such as colour. These tests are relatively cheap and fast with moderate/high sensitivity.

Nucleic acid amplification tests

Recently, traditional methods of identifying organisms are being supplemented by molecular techniques. Nucleic acid amplification tests, of which PCR is the commonest method, are increasingly being used to detect the presence of pathogen DNA/RNA in clinical specimens.

PCR is based on the amplification of pathogen DNA/RNA and is particularly useful for those organisms which are difficult or, in some cases, impossible to culture, such as viruses (e.g. hepatitis C, HIV) and certain bacteria (e.g. chlamydia). PCR can be qualitative or quantitative (e.g. used for determining the HIV viral load or the hepatitis C viral load) and so can be used for staging disease and monitoring response to treatment. While PCR has a very high sensitivity and specificity, it is unable to differentiate between live and dead organisms and is sensitive to contamination.

Methods of indirect identification

While direct identification of the causative organism is preferable, this is often difficult or may take a long time. Consequently, indirect methods that identify pathogen-specific immune responses are used.

Serological diagnosis

Serological tests derive from the normal antibody response to infection in an immunocompetent individual. Following infection with an organism, there is often some delay before antibody production commences. When it does, IgM antibody is initially produced; however, IgM production will eventually wane over time and be replaced by IgG production. It is the antibodies, directed against specific organisms, which are measured by serologically based methods.

The presence of IgM suggests a recent/current infection, while IgG positivity represents a past/already established infection. Having an understanding of this is critical for the physician, although complications in interpretation can arise, as the biology and natural history of infection vary for different pathogens. Antibody results should be interpreted carefully, and, in difficult situations, discussion with a virologist/microbiologist in difficult situations.

An additional method for determining whether the infection is recent is to collect two samples—one at the beginning of the illness (an acute sample) and another 10–14 days later (a convalescent sample)—which can be tested together. A greater than fourfold rise in the antibody titre indicates that disease is present (e.g. mumps and legionella).

Common serological techniques include ELISAs, complement fixation, and agglutination. These are widely used in virological diagnosis (e.g. for infection with HIV or with hepatitis A/B/C) and also to determine whether an individual is immune to certain pathogens (e.g. rubella virus, in pregnant women).

T-cell-based diagnosis: Interferon gamma release assays

Significant advances made over the last decade have resulted in the development of interferon gamma release assays to diagnose latent TB infection. These blood tests, which measure in vitro interferon gamma levels, have been shown to be more specific and sensitive than the tuberculin skin test. In addition, recent longitudinal studies have demonstrated, as with the tuberculin skin test, that a positive result from an interferon gamma release assay predicts the future development of active TB.

Additional investigations to undertake in the patient suspected to have an infection

Aside from the generic initial tests, the investigations described in 'Baseline investigations' aim to identify the infectious organism. However, diagnosing an infectious disease often requires additional tests which, in combination with the clinical findings and other tests, add weight to the diagnosis, provide further information about the host/causative organism, and rule out alternative differential diagnoses.

Blood tests

One of the difficulties with infectious diseases is that the symptoms are often non-specific (e.g. fever) and, hence, the differential diagnosis is wide. Therefore, it is important to rule out alternative diagnoses. Clearly, which blood tests to undertake will depend on the clinical syndrome, but important tests to consider include an autoimmune screen; tests for immunoglobulins; a liver autoantibody screen (if the patient presents with hepatitis); and an ESR.

However, further blood tests may also be the logical sequelae of a diagnosis previously made. For example, once HIV infection is diagnosed, the clinician should ascertain how advanced the HIV infection is by undertaking a CD4 cell count and determining the HIV viral load. Similarly, blood tests may be necessary to monitor the patient's response to treatment; for example, in patients who are diagnosed with *Plasmodium falciparum* malaria, the percentage parasitaemia should be monitored to ensure that the antimalarial treatment is having the desired effect.

Radiology

Detailed radiological examinations have revolutionized the diagnosis of infectious disease and are often undertaken soon after the patient presents to medical care. Usually, the history and examination findings will guide the clinician to the specific area which should be imaged, although more extensive scanning may sometimes be required (such as when investigating a fever of unknown origin).

Cross-sectional imaging is very important, as it can delineate the pathological process, such as with ring-enhancing lesions in a CT/MRI scan. Moreover, imaging can identify the specific focus of infection (if sampling is required), as well as the response to treatment (e.g. it can

be used to look at the change in size of mediastinal lymph nodes in a patient being treated for tuberculosis).

Histology

In some cases, if the initial microscopy results are negative, clinicians will have to wait for several weeks before the culture results are known. In this case, it is recommended that the same sites of disease samples (pus, pleural/peritoneal fluid, CSF, bone marrow) which were sent for culture are also sent, in large volumes, for cytological/histological analysis. The advantage of this is that certain organisms result in such characteristic histological findings that, if these are seen, even while formal culture results are awaited, they may provide enough evidence to commence therapy. TB exemplifies this most clearly; if histology shows caseating granulomas with epithelioid macrophages and multinucleate giants cells, the clinician should strongly consider commencing antituberculous treatment, as any delays may result in clinical deterioration of the patient.

Tests of immune function

In some situations, it is useful to consider if an underlying disorder of immune function has affected the subject's ability to fight infection and resulted in their presentation with the infectious disease.

Immunodeficiency can be primary (usually inherited) or secondary (usually due to external disease/medications). Primary immunodeficiency mainly affects children and is suggested by the history and examination findings. The actual spectrum of disease depends on which element of the immunological system is not functioning appropriately and can include, amongst others, antibody deficiency, T-cell deficiencies, B-cell deficiencies, and complement deficiency (see Chapter 303).

Conclusion

Undertaking investigations in a patient with a suspected infectious disease should complement the history and examination findings. There are several aims of investigation in infection, including identifying the causative organism, elucidating the host response to infection, identifying any underlying susceptibility to infection, and, finally, ruling out non-infectious causes which may present with similarly non-specific features.

As a huge range of tests are available to the physician, it is advisable to liaise closely with the microbiology/virology laboratory so that the correct test is used in the correct situation. However, it must be borne in mind that clinical suspicion remains critical—particularly as all diagnostic tests can suffer from false-negative results. Therefore, even negative test results should not dissuade the clinician, as the diagnostic process is an ongoing one; tests may often need to be repeated over the course of the patient's illness to confirm the diagnosis or, indeed, observe a response to treatment.

Further Reading

British Infection Association Guidelines (http://www.britishinfection.org/guidelines-resources/published-guidelines/)
Infectious Diseases Society of America Practice Guidelines (http://www.idsociety.org/idsa_practice_guidelines/)

307 Treatment of infection

Ian Bowler and Matthew Scarborough

Treatment and its effectiveness

Background

The healthy human body is colonized by a complex mix of microorganisms which numerically outnumber human cells by a factor of 10. These resident flora, located primarily in the gut, respiratory tract, and skin, rarely invade to cause disease unless host surfaces are damaged, for example by viral infection, trauma, or surgery. They play an important role in protecting the host from infection by preventing the establishment of more virulent organisms which might initiate disease. This is called colonization resistance. The distinction between colonization and infection is vital to the interpretation of microbiological investigations.

Infection

Infection can be regarded as a struggle between the host and the infecting organism, which may be a bacterium, virus, protozoan, or fungus. The likelihood that an infection will occur will depend on the number of organisms, their virulence, and the quality of the host defences. Organisms causing the greatest burden of disease in the UK are respiratory viruses, such as rhinovirus, respiratory syncytial virus (RSV), and influenza. Their virulence enables them to initiate disease in healthy hosts. Once mucosae have been damaged by these agents, commensal bacteria may invade. There are strong temporal links between peak influenza activity and the incidence of pneumococcal pneumonia and meningococcal meningitis in the winter in temperate climates. 'Treatment' involves shifting the balance in favour of the host. This might involve:

- supporting the host (e.g. providing oral rehydration solution to patients with gastroenteritis)
- removing the pathogen (e.g. drainage of abscess, excision of osteomyelitic bone, starting antimicrobial therapy)
- modulation of the host immune response (e.g. administration of steroids in TB and pneumococcal meningitis)

The approach to the potentially infected patient

The history and the physical examination are used to formulate a differential diagnosis that is tested using laboratory and radiological investigations. This process includes:

- an assessment of host competence; for instance, the degree of organ dysfunction, which helps to predict:
  - the level of support required (i.e. whether the patient can be managed as an outpatient or requires inpatient care or admission to an ICU)
  - how quickly and comprehensively interventions should be carried out
  - the likely course and outcome of the illness
- an assessment of the presenting features, the pattern of the illness, and which systems are affected; this helps predict the nature of the pathogen and therefore guides initial therapy
- an understanding of the epidemiological context: local travel, sexual history, animal contact, and local epidemiology of infection, including antibiotic resistance patterns (i.e. US vs UK for community-acquired MRSA)
- an awareness of local treatment guidelines based on local epidemiological data; this will ensure that patients are managed according to best practice

- an assessment of infectivity of the patient so that care can be given in a way which minimizes the risk of transmission to other patients and to staff:
  - negative-pressure ventilation rooms can be used to manage patients with open pulmonary TB and chicken pox
- patients with infection caused by varicella zoster virus should be nursed by staff who are immune to the virus, in order to help prevent transmission

Discussion of interventions

Patients with infection may require a variety of interventions to improve their chance of a good outcome in their struggle with the infecting organism; these include:

- supporting the host
- removing or reducing the dose of the pathogen
- immunomodulation

Supporting the host

Patients with a sepsis syndrome characterized by fever and hypotension will benefit from fluid repletion and temperature control by fanning or the use of antipyretics such as paracetamol. Oral rehydration is usually used in the outpatient setting. For more severely affected patients, IV fluids may be required. In those with persisting hypotension, the use of a pressor agent such as noradrenaline may be appropriate. Additional support such as ventilation and haemofiltration may also be necessary.

Removing or reducing the dose of the pathogen

Source control

There are a wide variety of interventions aimed at physically removing the invading pathogen. Examples of 'source control' include:

- laparotomy, for the repair of a perforated viscus, drainage of collections, or diversion of the faecal stream (Hartman's procedure)
- relieving obstruction (e.g. placement of urinary bladder catheter in the setting of acute obstruction due to prostatic enlargement; insertion of a nephrostomy into the renal pelvis when there is obstruction due to a renal stone; sphincterotomy of the duodenal ampulla to release a biliary stone)
- removing non-viable tissue (e.g. in the setting of necrotizing fasciitis or osteomyelitis)
- removing intravascular lines and other foreign bodies that may harbour biofilms on their surface, as biofilms render bacteria insusceptible to antibiotic therapy

These therapeutic interventions have the benefit of providing clinical material for confirmation of diagnosis by histology, culture, or molecular probes via PCR.

Appropriate antimicrobials

Treatment strategy and choice of antimicrobials

The choice of antimicrobial agent depends on the organism, the host, and the pharmacokinetics of the drug.

The identity and the antimicrobial sensitivities of the organism are usually determined by culture or molecular techniques. These diagnostic tests are not rapid; so, in most settings, antimicrobial therapy will be given on an empirical basis before the nature of the infecting agent is known. The spectrum of cover required will depend in part on the severity of illness, with a broader spectrum being appropriate for the sickest patients. It is important that the initiation of treatment is not delayed while awaiting results of laboratory tests, as there is evidence that early intervention improves outcome in life-threatening infections such as meningitis and pneumonia, and in neutropenic sepsis.

Once the infecting agent has been characterized, the spectrum of antibacterial therapy can be narrowed, thus avoiding side effects, reducing cost, and limiting disturbance to the normal flora. In this way, the risk of *Clostridium difficile* infection, which occurs when the gut flora is disturbed, can be minimized.

Diseases mediated by bacterial toxins are best treated with antimicrobials that are able to inhibit toxin formation. Clindamycin is chosen for this reason in cases of necrotizing fasciitis caused by organisms such as *Streptococcus pyogenes* or *Clostridium* spp.

Most antimicrobials are either excreted via the kidneys or metabolized in the liver. The dose will therefore depend on the glomerular filtration rate or liver function of the host. Further determinants of dosage include tissue distribution of the drug (e.g. vancomycin does not cross the blood brain barrier well) and the concentration of drug required to inhibit the target pathogen(s); the latter is known as the minimum inhibitory concentration (MIC).

The dosing interval will depend on the pharmacokinetics and mode of action of the drug. Some antimicrobials, such as aminoglycosides, display concentration-dependent killing and so are best used in large, once-daily doses. Others, like the penicillins and cephalosporins, display time-dependent killing, where the aim of dosing is to keep the drug concentration above the MIC for as long as possible. The ratio of the MIC to the area under the curve of drug serum concentration plotted against time has been found to be predictive of outcome in animal models of infection and in observational studies in humans.

Antimicrobial choice may be affected by a history of allergy. The most common allergic response is a skin reaction to penicillin; in patients who have this reaction, a cephalosporin can usually be given safely. In a patient giving a history of type 1 allergy to penicillin with collapse or bronchospasm, nearly all beta-lactam antibiotics should be avoided.

Route of antimicrobials

Antimicrobials are usually given by the IV route in severely ill patients or if oral absorption is unreliable. As soon as the patient is well enough, IV therapy can be switched to oral therapy. The oral route is preferred, as it is more convenient and cheaper and it does not expose the patient to the risks associated with IV cannulation, such as phlebitis and infection.

Duration of antimicrobial therapy

There are many determinants for duration of therapy but there is increasing evidence that many infections respond to shorter courses of antibiotics than originally thought. This has been most extensively studied in urinary tract infections. In female patients with cystitis (urinary frequency, and dysuria without fever or loin pain), 3 days of oral therapy is effective. In female patients with pyelonephritis, 7 days of therapy with a quinolone is as effective as 2 weeks of therapy with co-trimoxazole. In children, males, and pregnant females. treatment courses shorter that 14 days have not been shown to be effective but, in practice, treatment may be shortened to 10 days. Asymptomatic bacteriuria in pregnancy is usually treated for 7 days, although there is little evidence base for this.

Patients who have mild-to-moderate community-acquired pneumonia and require admission to hospital can be treated for 3 days. Hospital-acquired pneumonia, including in the ITU, is usually treated for 5– 7 days, although the evidence base for this is poor.

The optimal duration of therapy for endocarditis depends on the infecting pathogen and the presence of a prosthetic valve. For native valve disease caused by 'viridans' streptococci with an MIC <0.01 mg/l to penicillin, 2 weeks of therapy with penicillin and a synergistic aminoglycoside (e.g. gentamicin) is effective. For prosthetic valve endocarditis caused by the same organism, 6 weeks of therapy is usually required. In bacterial meningitis, studies show that 7 days of therapy is effective for the treatment of uncomplicated meningococcal meningitis, but 10 days of therapy is recommended for pneumococcal meningitis.

In most other settings, the duration of antibiotics is decided empirically depending on the patient's response. For instance, treatment of skin and soft tissue infection may vary from 5 to 21 days, depending on the structures involved and the response to therapy.

Where organisms have a persisting phenotype and are not easily killed by antimicrobials, therapy may need to be prolonged. The treatment for pulmonary TB is usually extended to 6 months. In settings where the organism cannot be eliminated, the aim of therapy is suppression; examples of scenarios where this approach is used include the treatment of HIV infection, and the suppression of metalware-related infection in orthopaedic practice, when the metalwork cannot be removed.

Immunomodulation

In some infection scenarios, the host's immune response to the pathogen is overactive and causes tissue damage. The aim of therapy in this instance is to modify the immune response in order to avoid this damage while allowing sufficient response to eliminate the pathogen. Steroids are potent immunomodulators. In patients with acute bacterial meningitis and in chronic meningitis due to *Mycobacterium tuberculosis*, steroid therapy reduces mortality and reduces the risk of complications amongst survivors. Some patients who present with advanced HIV 1 become unwell when their immune system begins to recover with antiretroviral therapy. This immune reconstitution inflammatory syndrome is often directed against *Mycobacterium tuberculosis* and usually responds well to steroid therapy.

In other settings, the immune response is poor but can be boosted to help overcome the pathogen. Patients receiving cadaveric renal transplant require potent immunosuppressive therapy to prevent rejection of the graft. This may allow latent viruses to escape immune control and cause end-organ damage. CMV may cause colitis, hepatitis, and pneumonitis in this way. Treatment is with antivirals to limit viral replication, as well as a reduction in immunosuppressive therapy to allow the immune response to re-establish control.

Some diseases are caused by toxins produced by the infecting pathogen. These toxins are antigenic, and treatment can be given with antibodies raised in animals or human volunteers. Both tetanus and botulism are treated in this way. The role of normal human immunoglobulin for the treatment of necrotizing fasciitis due to *Streptococcus pyogenes* is controversial, as only one small randomized study has been done. Recently, monoclonal antibodies to the *Clostridium difficile* toxin have been shown to be effective in reducing the risk of relapse in patients with recurrent *Clostridium difficile* disease.

Monitoring effectiveness of interventions

Monitoring of patients' progress is important to assess whether therapy is effective. This is done by monitoring vital signs such as blood pressure, pulse rate, fluid balance, and degree of hydration. Pulse oximetry and blood pH monitoring can be used to assess tissue oxygenation and perfusion. The function of the kidneys and the liver is monitored, in case these require support. Regular monitoring of the white blood cell count and serum C reactive protein can be used to assess response to therapy. In chronic viral infections such as HIV and hepatitis B or C, measurement of viral load in the blood can be helpful in assessing response to therapy.

Approach to the patient not responding to treatment

In patients who are responding poorly to therapy, the initial diagnosis should be reviewed. There should be a renewed search for uncontrolled foci of infection, such as drainable collections or infected prosthetic material such as intravascular lines which could be removed. It is more common for patients to fail therapy for these reasons than because of inappropriate empirical antimicrobials or because of the emergence of antimicrobial resistance during therapy. However, a prior history of colonization or infection with an antibiotic-resistant organism such as MRSA or *Pseudomonas aeruginosa* should be sought in order to ensure that empiric antibiotic cover is appropriate. Persisting fever despite several days of appropriate therapy should prompt consideration of either thromboembolic disease or an allergic response to the antimicrobial therapy.

Wider impact of antimicrobial therapy

All diseases and their therapies carry with them risks of complications and side effects. Infection and antimicrobials hold two additional threats: transmission of infection, and the development of drug resistances. The disciplines of infection control and antibiotic stewardship are directed at countering these concerns, and both have increasing public and political sensitivity.

Minimizing the spread of antibiotic resistance in hospitals and community

Antimicrobials save millions of lives and have contributed significantly to the gains in life expectancy seen since their introduction in the 1940s. However, these advances are now seriously threatened by the emergence of drug resistance.

Antimicrobial resistance emerges as a result of the selective pressure of exposure through the use and abuse of antimicrobials in hospitals and the community, and also in the animal industry as growth promoters.

There are many examples of evolution of antimicrobial resistance. For *Staphylococcus aureus*, penicillin resistance emerged 4 years after its introduction in the 1940s. As a result, meticillin (closely related to flucloxacillin) was developed but, in the 1960s, meticillin resistance was detected. Currently, MRSA accounts for approximately 50% of the bloodstream isolates in the UK. Vancomycin is now the mainstay of therapy for MRSA but, in the 1990s, vancomycin resistance emerged. In 2002, a strain of MRSA with complete resistance (MIC >16 mg/l) to vancomycin was isolated form a patient in the US. There is now increasing concern over the emergence of *Staphylococcus aureus* strains resistant to all glycopeptides antibiotics.

Gram-negative organisms similarly have evolved resistance mechanisms as a result of exposure to antimicrobials. In 2010 there were reports of imported cases of organisms expressing an enzyme, the New Delhi metallo-beta-lactamase NDM1, to the UK and USA. These organisms are resistant to treatment with carbapenem antibiotics. There is a worrying void in the development of new drug classes to combat resistant Gram-negative infections, and current trends suggest that, over the next decade or so, organisms will emerge which will have no effective therapy.

Similar stories of emergent resistance are seen in many other microorganisms including TB—so-called XDR TB—malaria and HIV. All are thought to be driven by exposure to antimicrobial therapies. Prudent and appropriate use of antimicrobials is a key component in managing such resistance.

Antimicrobial stewardship

A critical factor in the evolution of resistance is the total consumption of antimicrobials. Currently, it is thought that up to 30% of prescriptions for antibiotics are inappropriate or unnecessary. Where it is required, antibiotic therapy should be optimized to provide the best chance of cure while minimizing cost, risks of toxicity, and the selection of resistance. In most infections, this is best achieved by using the narrowest spectrum of antibiotic at the lowest dose and for the shortest duration necessary to effect a cure. Antimicrobial stewardship programmes incorporate several strategies to improve prescribing patterns, including:

- public and prescriber education (e.g. campaigns explaining that most sore throats are viral in origin and will therefore not respond to antibiotics)
- the formulation and promotion of appropriate antibiotic guidelines, governed by local epidemiology and resistance patterns
- formulary restriction or prior approval by an infection specialist: mechanisms whereby access to certain antimicrobial classes is carefully controlled in order to prevent inappropriate prescribing and preserve efficacy

- computer-assisted prescribing: software programmes that ensure that the prescription is appropriate for the indication

Antimicrobial stewardship should be supported by a robust surveillance system to identify trends and emerging threats.

Infection prevention and control procedures

Infection prevention and control programmes can minimize the spread of antibiotic-resistant bacteria from patient to patient. It is estimated that, at any one time, 10% of all hospital inpatients suffer from a nosocomial or healthcare-associated infection. Infection control is the discipline concerned with reducing nosocomial infection rates through prevention (education, cleaning, hand hygiene, vaccination, isolation), surveillance (MRSA screening, root cause analyses, contact tracing), and management. Common nosocomial infections include intravascular-device-related bacteraemia, urinary and respiratory tract infections, and surgical-site infections. Nosocomial infection rates have recently become the target of considerable scrutiny by the public and the media and are now used as an important metric against which quality of care is measured.

Many interventions known to be effective in reducing the risk of nosocomial infection are well recognized but poorly deployed. The importance of hand hygiene was established in the mid-19th century by Semmelweiss and Holmes but has been notoriously difficult to implement. Similarly, it has been difficult to convince the medical profession of the considerable risks associated with intravascular devices and urinary catheters.

Central and peripheral IV cannulae cause almost 50% of all hospital-acquired bloodstream infections, half of which are due to *Staphylococcus aureus*. The attributable mortality is thought to be between 12% and 25%, and the cost of a single episode has been estimated to be over £6000. The risks associated with cannulae are best managed by ensuring that staff are appropriately trained in their insertion and aftercare.

Urinary tract infections account for a fifth of all hospital-acquired infections, and 60% are related to catheter insertions. Urinary catheters become colonized by bacteria at a rate of 4% per day, and the odds of a septic death in a catheterized patient as compared to a matched non-catheterized patient is about 30:1. Appropriate use and improved care of urinary catheters is likely to limit the associated risks.

In addition to providing appropriate training for clinical staff, infection control teams play an important role in limiting transmission of infections within the hospital. They frequently advise, for example, on the isolation and management of patients with *Clostridium difficile* diarrhoea; MRSA colonization or infection: shingles: TB; hepatitis viruses; and RSV. Through a series of audit programmes, they advance good clinical practice in relation to hand hygiene, hospital cleaning, and surgical-site infections. Infection control teams also serve to protect staff through the promotion of universal precautions and the safe disposal of sharps.

In recognition of the importance of infection prevention and control, the UK government has mandated the implementation of a new code of practice in all healthcare institutions (The Health and Social Care Act 2008 Code of Practice on the prevention and control of infections and related guidance). The code states that 'effective control and prevention of healthcare related infection must be embedded into everyday practice and applied consistently by everyone'. All staff are therefore bound by law to engage with local infection prevention and control policies.

Further Reading

British Infection Association Guidelines (http://www.britishinfection.org/guidelines-resources/published-guidelines/)
Infectious Diseases Society of America Practice Guidelines (http://www.idsociety.org/idsa_practice_guidelines/)
National Institute for Health and Care Excellence. Infection Prevention and Control. 2014. Available at https://www.nice.org.uk/guidance/qs61 (accessed 13 Sep 2017).

308 Viral infection

Graham Cooke and Richard Lessells

Definition of the disease

Viral infection includes any clinical illness caused by a pathogenic virus. This chapter deals primarily with acute viral infections in immunocompetent individuals.

Aetiology of the disease

Acute viral infections are amongst the most common illnesses of humans, and numerous viruses can cause disease in humans. Specific syndromes can be identified that have certain viruses as potential causative agents (Table 308.1).

Table 308.1 Common syndromes associated with viral infection and the causative agents

Syndrome	Symptoms	Virus
Respiratory viral infection	Sore throat Rhinorrhoea Cough Wheeze Otalgia Headache	Influenza Parainfluenza Respiratory syncytial virus Adenovirus Rhinovirus Coronavirus
Gastroenteritis	Diarrhoea Vomiting	Norovirus Rotavirus Adenovirus
Infectious mononucleosis	Sore throat Fatigue/malaise Lymph node enlargement	Epstein-Barr virus Cytomegalovirus HIV: acute infection
Oral–genital ulceration	Oral ulceration Anogenital ulceration	Herpes simplex virus 1 and 2
Exanthema	Skin rash	Varicella zoster virus Human herpesvirus 6 Measles virus Rubella virus Enterovirus Poxviruses Parvovirus B19 Dengue virus
Encephalitis	Headache Confusion Seizures	Herpes simplex virus 1 Varicella zoster virus Enterovirus
Acute hepatitis	Jaundice Abdominal pain Anorexia Nausea/vomiting	Hepatitis A virus Hepatitis B virus Hepatitis C virus Hepatitis E virus Cytomegalovirus Epstein-Barr virus
Viral haemorrhagic fever	Headache Dizziness Myalgia Petechial rash Oedema Shock	Dengue virus Arenavirus (e.g. Lassa virus) Bunyavirus (e.g. Ebola virus, Marburg virus) Filovirus (e.g. Crimean–Congo haemorrhagic fever virus)

Typical symptoms of the disease

Symptoms of viral infections will usually include fever, with more specific symptoms dependent on the site of infection and causative agent (symptoms listed in Table 308.1).

Demographics of the disease

Viral infections can affect individuals of any age, gender, and ethnicity. The host–pathogen response determines different outcomes for specific viral infections. After infection with some viruses (e.g. measles virus, rubella virus) protective immunity develops, there is no latency or chronic carriage, and reinfection is prevented. Other viruses (e.g. herpes simplex virus (HSV), varicella zoster virus (VZV)) enter latency (when viral replication ceases but the virus lies dormant within cells), and reactivation of the virus can cause symptoms at a later stage—a good example of this is VZV, which, after initial infection (chickenpox), enters latency in the trigeminal and dorsal root ganglia and can reactivate many years later to cause herpes zoster disease (shingles). Another group of viruses, in the presence of inadequate immune response, can cause chronic infection (e.g. hepatitis B and C viruses).

Natural history and complications of the disease

Respiratory viral infections

Respiratory viral infections in immunocompetent adults are usually mild, self-limiting, and without complication. In the elderly and other high-risk groups (e.g. those with chronic heart disease or chronic lung disease), respiratory viral infections can cause more significant morbidity, either through the development of pneumonia or through secondary bacterial infection. In recent years, there have been notable outbreaks of respiratory viral infections associated with more severe morbidity and mortality (e.g. infections with SARS coronavirus or influenza H1N1)

Infectious mononucleosis

Mild forms of infectious mononucleosis can resolve within a few days but most cases resolve over 2–3 weeks. Serious complications are rare but include splenic rupture, haemolytic anaemia, thrombocytopenia, and Guillain–Barré syndrome.

Oral–genital ulceration

Primary infection with HSV is asymptomatic in approximately 50% of cases. Primary HSV-1 infection can manifest with orolabial vesicles and ulceration, often accompanied by fever, pharyngitis, and cervical lymphadenopathy. Primary HSV-2 infection can manifest with vesicles and ulceration of genitalia or perineum, often accompanied by fever and inguinal lymphadenopathy.

Both HSV-1 and HSV-2 enter latency in sensory nerves, and reactivation causes recurrent orolabial lesions ('cold sores') or anogenital lesions. Severe complications of HSV infection are rare but include neurological infections (see 'Encephalitis').

Exanthema

Primary infection with VZV causes varicella (chickenpox), which, in children, is usually a self-limiting illness. In adults (particularly, pregnant females), there is a higher risk of severe disease and complications such as pneumonia and encephalitis. VZV reactivation causes herpes zoster (shingles), which manifests as a vesicular rash in a single dermatome. Complications of herpes zoster include herpes zoster ophthalmicus (zoster affecting the ophthalmic branch of the trigeminal nerve, causing conjunctivitis, keratitis, or uveitis) and post-herpetic neuralgia.

Encephalitis

Acute encephalitis is a serious and potentially fatal consequence of viral infection and can be caused by primary infection or reactivation of HSV-1, HSV-2, or VZV. It needs to be distinguished from meningitis, which can be commonly caused by the same viruses and many others (e.g. enteroviruses), but which generally has a benign course.

Mortality from untreated herpes encephalitis is approximately 70% and, even with appropriate treatment, fewer than 50% recover with no neurological sequelae. Varicella zoster encephalitis is less well understood but is thought to have a more benign course.

Acute hepatitis

The natural history of acute viral hepatitis varies quite considerably between individuals. The hepatitis viruses differ in their propensity to cause liver failure or chronic infection. The majority of hepatitis A virus infections are self-limiting: the case fatality rate is <0.1%, and chronic infection does not occur. Hepatitis B virus infection causes fulminant liver failure in approximately 1% of cases. The rate of chronic carriage of hepatitis B depends on the age at infection: if infected in adulthood, the rate of chronic infection is 5%–10%. Acute hepatitis C virus infection is often asymptomatic. Acute infection rarely causes liver failure, but 70%–80% of those infected develop chronic infection. Hepatitis E can cause fulminant liver failure, particularly in pregnant women, with consequent high mortality rates, but does not cause chronic infection (except in rare cases of immunosuppression).

Viral haemorrhagic fever

Tropical viral infections can be imported into the UK by persons travelling in areas endemic for certain viruses. Viral haemorrhagic fever is a syndrome with a number of causative viral agents. These imported infections are extremely rare in the UK, but retain importance due to the high mortality and the potential for onward spread of the virus. Since 1971, there have been 12 confirmed cases of Lassa fever in the UK (all from West Africa) and one case of Crimean–Congo haemorrhagic fever. During the West African outbreak of Ebola virus (2013–2016), there were three cases of imported Ebola virus disease in the UK, all in health care workers directly involved in the response to the epidemic. Dengue virus infection is more common and can be acquired in sub-Saharan Africa, South America, and Asia. Classical dengue has an incubation period of 3–14 days, is characterized by fever, headache, myalgia, and rash, and is usually self-limiting. Dengue haemorrhagic fever is characterized by more severe haemorrhagic manifestations and circulatory failure (due to vascular leak).

Approach to diagnosing the disease

The principles in diagnosing acute viral infections are, first, recognize the syndrome, then identify key features that might suggest a specific diagnosis, and, finally, consider laboratory investigations to elucidate the specific causative agent. Many of the syndromes are not clearly identifiable as viral infections at initial presentation so the differential diagnosis will often include bacterial infections, other infections (fungal, parasitic), and other conditions (e.g. malignant disease or autoimmune disease). As with any infection, a detailed history is paramount. A travel history in particular might identify a risk for rare but potentially serious infections. Febrile illness in a patient with history of recent overseas travel should always prompt specialist advice, to guide investigation and management.

For many self-limiting viral infections (e.g. respiratory viral infections), there will be no need for specific laboratory diagnosis, as treatment will be largely supportive. Similarly, viral infections with unique features (e.g. herpes zoster) rarely require laboratory confirmation, and treatment can be given based on clinical features alone.

Table 308.2 Important differential diagnoses for common viral syndromes

Syndrome	Differential diagnosis
Respiratory viral infection	Bacterial upper/lower respiratory tract infection
Gastroenteritis	Bacterial gastroenteritis
	Inflammatory bowel disease
Infectious mononucleosis	Bacterial/viral upper respiratory tract infection
	Acute toxoplasmosis
	Haematological malignancy (e.g. lymphoma)
Oral–genital ulceration	Aphthous ulcers
	Behçet's disease
	Inflammatory bowel disease
	Syphilis
	Chancroid
Exanthema	Meningococcal sepsis
	Staphylococcal or streptococcal sepsis
	Scarlet fever (Group A Streptococcus)
	Rickettsial infection
	Drug hypersensitivity
	Kawasaki disease
Encephalitis	Bacterial meningitis
	TB meningoencephalitis
	Brain abscess
	HIV-related opportunistic infections
	Cerebral vasculitis
Acute hepatitis	Cholecystitis/cholangitis
	Liver abscess
	Drug-induced hepatitis
	Leptospirosis
	Autoimmune hepatitis
Viral haemorrhagic fever	Malaria
	Leptospirosis
	Enteric fever (typhoid, paratyphoid)
	Rickettsial infection

Other diagnoses that should be considered

Certain viral infections have such a classical presentation (e.g. herpes zoster) that there are usually no other potential diagnoses. The majority of presentations of viral infection, however, are not specific to viral diseases, and the differential diagnosis may be broad. Table 308.2 summarizes some key diagnoses to consider for each of the syndromes previously described.

The differentiation between viral and bacterial causes of upper and lower respiratory tract infection is extremely difficult based on history and physical examination alone. Even the use of inflammatory markers in peripheral blood (white blood cell count, C-reactive protein) does not reliably discriminate between a viral and bacterial aetiology.

'Gold-standard' diagnostic test

Laboratory diagnosis of viral infections encompasses two main forms of diagnosis:

- direct detection of virus in blood or tissue (via PCR)
- detection of virus-specific antibodies in blood (serology); usually requires paired acute and convalescent samples (the latter taken 10–14 days later)

Other diagnostic methods that might be used include virus detection by immunofluorescence or electron microscopy, and viral culture. PCR has surpassed serology as the gold-standard tests for many infections, as it can confirm diagnosis earlier in the illness and it eliminates confusion in interpreting serology results. Testing for resistance to antiviral therapy is not commonplace in the treatment of acute viral infection but is likely to play a greater role in the future as the

Table 308.3 'Gold-standard' diagnostic tests for common viral infections

Syndrome	Recommended samples	Diagnostic tests
Respiratory viral infection	Nasopharyngeal aspirate Nose/throat swabs Bronchoalveolar lavage Tracheal aspirate	Influenza (PCR) Parainfluenza (PCR) Respiratory syncytial virus (PCR) Adenovirus (PCR) Rhinovirus (PCR) Coronavirus (PCR)
Gastroenteritis	Stool (only in outbreaks and in young children or immunocompromised)	Norovirus (PCR) Rotavirus (PCR) Adenovirus (PCR)
Infectious mononucleosis	Serum	Epstein-Barr virus (serology)* Cytomegalovirus (serology) HIV (fourth-generation ELISA)
Oral–genital ulceration	Aspirate/swab from lesion	Herpes simplex virus 1 (PCR) Herpes simplex virus 2 (PCR)
Exanthema	Aspirate/swab from lesion Serum Throat swab	Varicella zoster virus (PCR or immunofluorescence) Human herpesvirus 6 (serology) Measles virus (PCR on throat swab) Rubella virus (serology) Enterovirus (serology) Poxviruses (clinical diagnosis or biopsy) Parvovirus B19 (serology and PCR)
Encephalitis	CSF	Herpes simplex virus 1 and 2 (PCR) Varicella zoster virus (PCR) Enterovirus (PCR)
Acute hepatitis	Serum	Hepatitis A virus (serology) Hepatitis B virus (serology and PCR) Hepatitis C virus (serology and PCR) Hepatitis E virus (serology) Cytomegalovirus (serology and PCR) Epstein-Barr virus (serology and PCR)
Viral haemorrhagic fever	Serum	Specialist investigations (reference laboratory)†

*Monospot (or heterophile antibody test) commonly used but should not be considered gold standard for specific diagnosis.

†In the UK, Public Health England should be contacted in any suspected case of viral haemorrhagic fever prior to any laboratory tests, as there are special requirements for specimen handling, transport, and so on.

impact of viral mutations on treatment response is better understood (e.g. in the management of influenza)

The gold-standard diagnostic tests for common viral infections are given in Table 308.3.

Acceptable diagnostic alternatives to the gold standard

In most cases, it is also possible to use serology for diagnosis of viral infection. The main drawback of serology is that it often requires a comparison of acute and convalescent sera and, hence, diagnosis is delayed. It can, however, be useful to confirm diagnoses retrospectively and is especially useful in epidemiological investigations.

Other relevant investigations

Other forms of investigation will be warranted for certain syndromes, to assist with the diagnosis or to search for other causes of the presentation. Investigations may include other microbiological tests (e.g. bacterial culture), imaging procedures (e.g. X-ray, CT, MRI), and histopathology. Some examples of other investigations that might be considered for the presentations described are as follows:

- for respiratory infections: sputum culture (bacterial), chest X-ray
- for gastroenteritis: stool culture, stool microscopy, *Clostridium difficile* toxin testing, sigmoidoscopy
- for infectious mononucleosis: throat swab (bacterial), full blood count

- for oral–genital ulceration: syphilis serology, biopsy
- for exanthema: blood cultures, anti-streptolysin titre, rickettsial serology, skin biopsy
- for encephalitis: MRI brain, EEG, CSF bacterial culture, TB culture, cryptococcal antigen test
- for acute hepatitis: abdominal ultrasound, blood cultures, *Leptospira* serology, autoantibodies (antinuclear antibody, anti-smooth muscle antibody, anti-liver–kidney microsomal antibody, anti-mitochondrial antibody)

Prognosis and how to estimate it

The prognosis for the majority of viral infections in immunocompetent individuals is extremely good, even in the absence of specific therapy. However, certain viral infections and their complications (e.g. herpes simplex encephalitis) are associated with high mortality and thus require rapid identification and rapid initiation of specific treatment.

Treatment and its effectiveness

There are few specific antiviral therapies (aside from antiretroviral therapy for HIV infection) available to treat viral infections. The available therapies and their licensed indications are illustrated in Table 308.4. Certain agents may be used outside of their licensed indications (e.g. IV ribavirin for viral respiratory infections and for viral haemorrhagic fever).

Otherwise, for most viral infections, treatment is supportive and symptomatic. Adjunctive treatment might include analgesics and antipyretics.

Table 308.4 Commonly used antiviral therapies and their main indications

Medication	Indication	Dose	Duration
Aciclovir	Herpes simplex (treatment)	200 mg five times per day	10 days (primary)
			5 days (recurrence)
	Varicella or herpes zoster	800 mg five times per day	7 days
	Herpes simplex encephalitis	10 mg/kg three times per day, IV	14–21 days
Valaciclovir	Herpes simplex (treatment)	500 mg twice daily	10 days (primary)
			5 days (recurrence)
	Herpes zoster	1 g three times per day	7 days
Ganciclovir	CMV disease in immunocompromised patients	5 mg/kg twice daily, IV	14–21 days
Valganciclovir	CMV retinitis	900 mg twice daily	21 days
Oseltamivir	Influenza	75 mg twice daily	5 days
Zanamivir	Influenza	10 mg twice daily, inhaled	5 days
Amantadine	Influenza	100 mg once daily	5 days

Further Reading

British Infection Association Guidelines (http://www.britishinfection.org/guidelines-resources/published-guidelines/)

Department of Health and Public Health England. Viral haemorrhagic fever: ACDP algorithm and guidance on management of patients. https://www.gov.uk/government/publications/viral-haemorrhagic-fever-algorithm-and-guidance-on-management-of-patients (accessed 13 Sep 2017).

Paules C and Subbarao K. Influenza. *Lancet* 2017; 390: 697–708.

Infectious Diseases Society of America Practice Guidelines (http://www.idsociety.org/idsa_practice_guidelines/)

309 Sepsis

Graham Cooke and Jaime Vera

Definition of the disease

Sepsis is a clinical syndrome resulting from infection that is characterized by activation of the the immune and coagulation systems. The pathogenesis of sepsis is complex and may differ according to the host's immunological and physiological statues prior to infection.

Symptoms of the disease

Sepsis syndrome can be associated with a range of signs and symptoms that differ from patient to patient (see Box 309.1). There are general symptoms indicative of systemic inflammation (e.g. sweating, confusion, lethargy, fatigue, myalgia) that should alert the clinician to the development of sepsis syndrome. In addition, there can be localizing symptoms, such as pain, vomiting, diarrhoea, ileus, erythema, and headache, which can all provide important clues to the infectious source.

Aetiology of the disease

Sepsis occurs in 2% of hospitalized patients and up to 75% of intensive care (ICU) patients. The presence of underlying diseases, and the physiological health status of the patient, are important determinants of the outcome of severe sepsis. Important risk factors for sepsis include the presence of bacteraemia, advanced age (>65), impaired immune system function (due to AIDS, neutropenia, splenectomy, neoplasm, renal or hepatic failure, diabetes, alcohol dependence, or malnutrition), IV drug use, and prolonged use of intravascular and indwelling urinary catheters. A comprehensive list of pathogens causing sepsis is beyond the scope of this chapter; however, some of the most common infections and microbes responsible for causing sepsis in the community and hospitalized patients are shown in Table 309.1.

Natural history, and complications of the disease

The clinical spectrum usually begins with infection (bacteraemia) that leads to sepsis, organ dysfunction, and septic shock. Complications develop as a result of organ damage, and their clinical presentation usually is superimposed on the signs and symptoms of the systemic response. Findings indicative of organ dysfunction may be the first symptoms noticed by clinicians when assessing the patient. Common complications of sepsis include toxic metabolic encephalopathy; acute respiratory distress syndrome; myocardial dysfunction and decreased ejection fraction; renal failure; impaired gut mobility; elevation in the levels of transaminases; hyperbillirubinaemia; disseminated intravascular coagulation; pancytopenia; a rise creatinine kinase levels, together with critical illness myopathy; and adrenal haemorrhage resulting in Addison's disease.

Approach to diagnosis

The cornerstone of the management of sepsis is early recognition and prompt initiation of supportive therapy combined with antimicrobial therapy. Emergency management should be focused on simultaneous evaluation and resuscitation. The evaluation of the patient should begin with a carefully taken history focused on the assessment of any underlying or predisposing disorder such as an impaired immune system, recent surgery, chemotherapy, transplantation, trauma, or any treatment given. Special attention should be devoted to any history of previous infections and antimicrobial treatment, along with any microbiological data that may be available from previous studies. In addition, an accurate travel history, a recreational drugs history, and history of exposure to infectious agents, whether from contacts or in the environment, can be valuable to the clinician in the identification of an infectious process.

A comprehensive physical examination should be undertaken looking for clues to the source of infection. For instance, cutaneous manifestations of Gram-positive or Gram-negative infections, such as cellulitis, erythroderma, bullae, ecthyma, petechia, or splinter haemorrhages, can provide an opportunity for early diagnosis and initiation of specific antimicrobial therapy.

Other diagnosis that should be considered

Non-infectious etiologies of SIRS to be considered include pancreatitis; trauma; burns; pulmonary embolism; anaphylaxis; drug overdose; dissecting or rupture aortic aneurysm; occult haemorrhage; myocardial infarction; and adrenal insufficiency.

Box 309.1 Diagnostic criteria for sepsis syndrome

Infection
Presence of documented or suspected infection

General response
Fever (>38°C)
Hypothermia (<36°C)
Heart rate: >90 beats/min
Tachypnea: >30 breaths/min
Altered mental status
Decrease capillary filling or mottling, chills

Inflammatory parameters
Leukocytosis
Leukopenia
White blood cell count with >10% immature forms
Plasma C-reactive protein >2 S.D. normal parameters
Hyperlactatemia (>3 mmol/l) and acidosis

Organ dysfunction parameters
Arterial hypotension (systolic blood pressure of >90mmHg, mean arterial pressure <70)
Arterial hypoxaemia (PaO2)
Acute oliguria (urine output <0.5 ml per kg per h)
Creatinine increase
Ileus (absent bowel sounds)
Hyperbilirubinaemia (plasma total bilirubin of more than 70mmol/l)
Coagulation abnormalities (INR>1.5 APTT> 60 s)
Thrombocytopenia (platelet count <100,000/ul)

Abbreviations: APTT, activated partial thromboplastin time; INR, international normalized ratio; PaO2, partial pressure of oxygen in arterial blood.

Reproduced with permission from Mitchell M. Levy et al., 2001 SCCM/ESICM/ACCP/ATS/SIS International Sepsis Definitions Conference, *Intensive Care Medicine*, Volume 29, Issue 4, pp. 1250-6, Copyright © 2003 Springer

Table 309.1 Common organisms

Suspected focus of infection	Most likely organism	Possible empiric therapy*
Unknown	Gram-negative bacteria Gram-positive bacteria Anaerobe species	Community acquired: third-generation cephalosporin + metronidazole; consider aminoglycoside Hospital acquired: piperacillin–tazobactam + aminoglycoside; add vancomycin if MRSA colonized or suspected
Community-acquired pneumonia	*Streptococcus pneumoniae* *Haemophilus influenzae* *Chlamydophila pneumoniae* *Mycoplasma pneumoniae*	Third-generation cephalosporin + clarithromycin or doxycycline
Hospital-acquired pneumonia	*Klebsiella* spp. *Staphylococcus aureus* *Pseudomonas aeruginosa* Enterobacteriaceae Anaerobes	Piperacillin–tazobactam; add vancomycin if MRSA colonized or suspected; add metronidazole or clindamycin if aspiration pneumonia
Urinary tract infection	*Escherichia coli* Enterobacteriaceae Enterococci	Co-amoxiclav + aminoglycoside or third-generation cephalosporin
Intra-abdominal sepsis	*Escherichia coli* *Bacteroides fragilis* *Peptostreptococcus* ssp. *Clostridium* spp.	Piperacillin–tazobactam + metronidazole + consider aminoglycoside
Septic arthritis	*Staphylococcus aureus* Streptococci Aerobic Gram-negative bacilli	Third-generation cephalosporin; add vancomycin if MRSA suspected
Biliary sepsis (cholangitis)	*Escherichia coli* *Klebsiella pneumoniae* *Pseudomonas* spp. *Enterococcus faecalis*	Piperacillin–tazobactam + aminoglycoside; add metronidazole if severe pancreatitis is present
Skin and soft tissue	*Staphylococcus aureus* *Streptococcus pyogenes* Coagulase-negative staphylococci *Clostridium* spp. in necrotizing infections	Flucloxacillin; add vancomycin if MRSA suspected If necrotizing fasciitis is present, third-generation cephalosporin + clindamycin + aminoglycoside
Meningitis and encephalitis	*Neisseria meningitides* *Streptococcus pneumoniae* *Haemophilus influenzae*	Third-generation cephalosporin + vancomycin in areas with resistant pneumococci
AIDS	*Pneumocystis jiroveci* *Streptococcus pneumoniae* *Salmonella* spp. *Pseudomonas* spp.	Co-trimoxazole for pneumocystis pneumonia Third-generation cephalosporin + metronidazole or clindamycin
Neutropenic sepsis	Gram-positive bacteria (*Staphylococcus aureus*, coagulase-negative staphylococci, enterococci) Gram-negative bacteria (*Escherichia coli*, *Klebsiella pneumoniae*, *Pseudomonas aeruginosa*)	Piperacillin–tazobactam + aminoglycoside

*Local guidelines will differ according to local organisms and variations in practice.

'Gold-standard' diagnostic test

There is no specific test that confirms the diagnosis of sepsis syndrome or severe sepsis. However, the combination of physical, clinical, and laboratory parameters should prompt the clinician to conclude that a patient is 'septic'.

The selection of laboratory studies should be based on the physical findings and the overall clinical presentation. Definitive etiologic diagnosis requires isolation of the microorganism from blood or a local site of infection. An attempt should be made to obtain infected secretions or body fluids or to aspirate an area that is suspicious for infection. Blood cultures are essential, and a minimum of two sets of blood cultures (10 ml each) taken at different venous sites are strongly recommended.

Other relevant investigations

In order to aid the diagnosis and assess the severity of the disease, all patients with suspected sepsis syndrome should be considered for the following investigations:

- a full blood count
- urinalysis
- coagulation profile
- liver function tests
- electrolytes
- blood glucose
- urea
- creatinine
- arterial blood gas
- plasma C-reactive protein
- ECG
- chest X ray
- HIV test

Base excess and blood lactate can be useful as prognostic markers of severity in sepsis and should be included in the initial laboratory screening. Based on the clinical presentation, other investigations may be appropriate; for instance, CSF testing for glucose, protein, cell count, and culture, if meningitis is suspected.

Prognosis

Twenty to thirty-five per cent of patients with severe sepsis, and 50%–75% of patients with septic shock, die within 30 days. Poor prognostic factors are advanced age, impaired host immune status, infection with a resistant organism, poor prior functional status, and an APACHE II score ≥25. Although 50% of patients with severe sepsis have bacteraemia at the time of infection, the presence or absence of positive blood cultures does not appear to influence the outcome. Similarly, case fatality rates are similar for culture-positive and culture-negative severe sepsis.

Treatment

Initial resuscitation

Establishing vascular access and initiating resuscitation are the first priorities when managing patients with severe sepsis or septic shock. Early resuscitation should be initiated as soon as tissue hypoperfusion is recognized and should not be delayed pending ICU admission. There is evidence from randomized control trials that early, goal-directed resuscitation improves survival for patients presenting to emergency with Septic shock. Early resuscitation comprises:

* fluid therapy
* support of respiratory function

Fluid therapy

Large volumes of IV fluids are indicated to correct the relative vascular hypovolaemia typical of sepsis. IV fluids should be administered in rapid infused boluses. Clinical trials have found no consistent difference between colloids and crystalloid in the treatment of septic shock. IV fluid challenges can be repeated until tissue perfusion is acceptable but, in patients at risk of pulmonary oedema, must be done with caution. Target a central venous pressure of ≥8 mm Hg, a mean arterial pressure of ≥65 mm Hg, and a urine output of ≥0.5 ml/kg per hour. The rate of fluid administration should be reduced if cardiac filling pressures increase without concomitant hemodynamic improvement.

Support of respiratory function

Assessment of airway intubation for high-risk patients, as well as oxygen supplementation to all patients with sepsis, is indicated. Oxygenation should be monitored continuously with pulse oximetry.

Antimicrobial treatment

Antimicrobial treatment should be initiated as soon as possible, ideally after cultures have been obtained. The choice of antibiotics would depend on the patient's history, the most likely source of infection, the clinical context (hospital or community acquired) and local resistance patterns (see Table 309.1). Reassessment of antibiotic regime is important to optimize efficacy and minimize toxicity.

Other therapies

Corticosteroids

Corticosteroids do not prevent the development of shock, reverse shock, or improve mortality at 14 days. Therefore, high doses of corticosteroids should not be used in patients with severe sepsis unless the patient's endocrine or corticosteroid history warrants it. In the presence of severe refractory sepsis shock (unresponsive to fluid resuscitation and vasopressors), corticosteroid therapy may be beneficial.

Recombinant human activated protein C

Recombinant human activated protein C (rhAPC) was a drug therapy proposed for the treatment of sepsis. The first evidence concerning the use of a form of rhAPC, drotrecogin alfa, in adults was based on two randomized control trials that suggested early administration was associated with better outcomes. In those studies, drotrecogin alfa was of greater benefit in the most acutely ill patients (APACHE II score >25). However, a later Cochrane review found that using drotrecogin alfa did not improve survival rates and, instead, increased the risk of bleeding (Martí-Carvajal et al., 2012). The drug was withdrawn from the market in 2011 (Kylat and Ohlsson, 2012).

Control of the sepsis focus

Identification of the site of infection should be achieved as soon as possible. Prompt drainage of abscesses, debridement of infected necrotic tissue, and removal of potentially infected devices are usually in the best interest of the patient but clinical judgement is required to balance risks of source control with those of procedures.

Further Reading

Angus DC and van der Poll T. Severe sepsis and septic shock. *N Engl J Med* 2013; 369: 840–51.

Dellinger RP, Levy MM, Carlet JM, et al. Surviving sepsis campaign: International guidelines for management of severe sepsis and septic shock: 2008. *Critical Care Med* 2008; 36: 296–327.

Kaukonen K-M, Bailey M, Pilcher D, et al. Systemic inflammatory response syndrome criteria in defining severe sepsis. *N Engl J Med* 2015; 372: 1629–38.

Kylat RI and Ohlsson A. Recombinant human activated protein C for severe sepsis in neonates. *Cochrane Database Syst Rev* 2012; 12: CD005385.

Long B and Koyfman A. An emergency medicine-focused review of sepsis mimics. *J Emerg Med* 2017; 52: 34–42.

Martí-Carvajal AJ, Solà I, Gluud C, et al. Human recombinant protein C for severe sepsis and septic shock in adult and paediatric patients. *Cochrane Database Syst Rev* 2012; 12: CD004388.

National Institute for Health and Clinical Excellence, *NICE Guidelines: Sepsis: recognition, assessment and early management.* 2016. Available at https://www.nice.org.uk/guidance/ng51/evidence/full-guideline-2551523297.

Vincent JL, Mira JP, and Antonelli M, Sepsis: older and newer concepts. *Lancet Respir Med* 2016; 4: 237–40.

310 Bacterial infection

Tony Bentley

Staphylococci

Staphylococci are Gram-positive cocci which grow in clusters. *Staphylococcus aureus*, which can be distinguished from *Staphylococcus epidermidis* and other less pathogenic species by a positive coagulase test, is capable of producing numerous toxins that act as virulence factors.

Toxins and other pathogenic molecules produced by *Staphylococcus aureus* include:

- teichoic acid: an adhesin responsible for binding the organisms to fibronectin present on epithelial cell membranes
- fibronectin-, fibrinogen-, and collagen-binding proteins: thought to explain *Staphylococcus aureus*'s predilection for diseased tissue
- protein A: binds to the Fc component of immunoglobulin, resulting in resistance to phagocytosis
- catalase: a peroxidase enzyme that helps the organism survive the host's oxygen-dependent bactericidal system
- coagulase: causes a fibrinous capsule to form around the localized infection
- hyaluronidase: causes local tissue destruction
- DNAse: causes nucleic acid damage
- haemolysins: cause red-cell damage
- Panton–Valentine leucocidin (PVL): a pore-forming toxin that results in leakage of leucocyte contents
- enterotoxins A–E: cytotoxins that stimulate receptors in the gastrointestinal tract, interfering with peristalsis and leading to emesis and diarrhoea
- pyrogenic exotoxin: causes fever, intense inflammation, and rash
- exfoliative toxin: causes superficial splitting of the granular layer (scalded skin syndrome in children)
- toxic shock syndrome toxins: act as superantigens

Staphylococcus aureus is well adapted to the human body and colonizes the nasopharynx of approximately 30% of the normal population. It may also colonize the skin, the perineum, the vagina, and the gastrointestinal tract. It is capable of person-to-person spread and causes pyogenic, septicaemic, and superficial cutaneous disease. It is able to survive intracellularly.

Some staphylococcal infections are toxin mediated (e.g. food poisoning (vomiting induced by ingestion of preformed toxin), scalded skin syndrome (extensive skin disease following localized staphylococcal infection), and toxic shock syndrome (systemic symptoms following localiaed infection)). In other situations, the severity of the infection may be increased due to toxin production by organisms growing in a pyogenic focus (e.g. extensive necrotic skin infection, or pneumonia associated with PVL-positive strains).

Staphylococcus aureus is a major cause of healthcare-associated and true community-acquired bacteraemia. True community-acquired bacteraemia affects younger people, is less frequently associated with a primary focus of infection, is more commonly associated with a secondary focus of infection (such as endocarditis and osteomyelitis), and has a higher mortality. The majority of *Staphylococcus aureus* bacteraemias are healthcare associated. In modern healthcare, however, the majority of these develop in patients living outside hospital. The most common healthcare-associated sources of *Staphylococcus aureus* bacteraemia are vascular catheters and wound, skin, and soft tissue infections.

Staphylococcus epidermidis and other coagulase-negative staphylococci are organisms of much lower virulence but are common causes of infection of intravascular devices and prosthetic joints. They are associated with the production of biofilm, which makes their eradication by antibiotic either difficult or impossible. *Staphylococcus saprophyticus* is a recognized cause of urinary tract infection in young women.

Staphylococcus aureus infection is most commonly treated with flucloxacillin or co-amoxiclav. Culture and sensitivity testing should be undertaken to confirm any empirical choice. Success relies on the strain being reported by the laboratory as meticillin sensitive. Alternative agents for meticillin-sensitive strains include erythromycin and tetracyclines. MRSA is detected in less than 1% of the overall population but in about 7% of those recognized as being at higher risk (e.g. individuals having multiple comorbidities, individuals having had multiple hospital admissions, and those from residential and nursing homes). Many meticillin-resistant strains are also erythromycin resistant; for these strains, alternative agents include tetracyclines, the glycopeptides vancomycin and teicoplanin, and linezolid. Combination therapy with oral rifampicin and fusidic acid is also commonly used.

Streptococci

Streptococci are Gram-positive cocci that grow in chains. They are catalase negative. When grown on blood agar, streptococci may produce a green-coloured zone (alpha haemolysis) or a clear zone (beta haemolysis), or be non-haemolytic. Streptococci may also be classified according to their Lancefield group antigen. In addition, each strain may be given a species name. This complexity of nomenclature can lead to some confusion.

Most alpha-haemolytic or 'viridans' streptococci are normal inhabitants of the mouth. Common species include *Streptococcus mutans*, *Streptococcus mitis*, *Streptococcus sanguis*, and *Streptococcus salivarius*. *Streptococcus mutans* is the bacterial cause of dental caries. All are potential causes of infective endocarditis, which, when caused by these organisms, is usually subacute in onset.

Streptococcus pneumoniae is a particular alpha-haemolytic streptococcus recognized in the laboratory by its capsulate appearance, bile solubility, and sensitivity to optochin. The pneumococcus causes many types of infection in addition to pneumonia. These include primary bacteraemia, meningitis, brain abscess, acute sinusitis, otitis media, septic arthritis, septic osteomyelitis, peritonitis, and pericarditis. The capsule, of which over 90 different serotypes have been characterized, is the most important virulence factor. Eight to ten capsular types cause about 60% of the serious infections in adults, and 80% of the invasive infections in children. The pneumococcal polysaccharide vaccine contains purified capsular polysaccharide from 23 capsular types and is thought to be 50%–70% effective in preventing pneumococcal bacteraemia but ineffective against non-bacteraemic disease. It is ineffective in children under 2 years of age. It is recommended for adults over 65 years of age in at-risk groups (e.g., those with splenic absence or dysfunction; chronic respiratory, heart, liver, or renal disease; diabetes; or immunosuppression). The pneumococcal conjugate vaccine, however, is immunogenic in children over 2 months of age. It was first introduced into the childhood immunization programme in the UK in 2006 and originally contained polysaccharide from seven capsular types conjugated to a protein molecule. This has recently been replaced by a new conjugate vaccine covering a further six pneumococcal serotypes and which is indicated for active immunization for the prevention of invasive pneumococcal disease in adults aged 50 years and over and for the prevention of invasive disease, pneumonia, and acute otitis media caused by *Streptococcus pneumoniae* in infants and children from 6 weeks to 5 years of age.

Streptococcus milleri is the name commonly applied to a group of three closely related alpha-haemolytic streptococci (*Streptococcus anginosus*, *Streptococcus constellatus*, and *Streptococcus intermedius*).

These organisms are seen as causes of abscess formation in the brain, liver, and other sites.

The most important beta-haemolytic streptococcus is Lancefield Group A or *Streptococcus pyogenes*. This organism is responsible for a wide range of infections, including localized skin infections (impetigo, cellulitis, and erysipelas), more extensive skin infections (e.g. necrotizing fasciitis), tonsillitis, and associated abscess formation (quinsy), puerperal sepsis, wound infection, and, more rarely, overwhelming sepsis. *Streptococcus pyogenes* can be further classified by the serological characteristics of the surface M proteins (which may prevent opsonization) and T antigens (pili used for bacterial attachment). Streptococcal pyrogenic exotoxins A and C are superantigens secreted by many strains of *Streptococcus pyogenes* that are responsible for the rash of scarlet fever and many of the symptoms of streptococcal toxic shock syndrome. Serological evidence of *Streptococcus pyogenes* infection can be sought by detection of anti-streptolysin O and anti-DNAse antibodies. The combination of tests is more sensitive than either alone, and interpretation of single test results, particularly in children, should be undertaken with care due to high background levels in some populations. *Streptococcus pyogenes* can also cause postinfectious, autoimmune-mediated complications such as rheumatic fever and glomerulonephritis.

Group B beta-haemolytic streptococcus or *Streptococcus agalactiae*, originally recognized as a vetinary pathogen causing bovine mastitis, has been reported with increasing frequency as a cause of sepsis in adult patients. In particular, it has been found in those with diabetes and liver disease, as a cause of bone and joint infections and spontaneous bacterial peritonitis. It is a commensal organism of the gastrointestinal tract and vagina and a cause of neonatal sepsis, causing both bacteraemias and meningitis.

The commonest non-haemolytic streptococci are the enterococci (i.e. *Enterococcus faecalis* and *Enterococcus faecium*). Associated diseases include urinary tract infection and, less commonly, endocarditis. Unlike other streptococci, enterococci are resistant to cephalosporins.

Neisseria species

Neisseria are Gram-negative cocci that have a characteristic paired arrangement that resembles coffee beans. Numerous species exist of which two are important human pathogens: *Neisseria meningitidis* and *Neisseria gonorrhoeae*. Antibiotic culture media for the recovery of *Neisseria meningitidis* and *Neisseria gonorrhoeae* are made selective by the use of an antibiotic cocktail to aid recovery from mixed throat and genital tract flora. The organisms are then identified by Gram stain, a positive oxidase test, and by at least two of the following modes of identification: utilization of sugars, detection of specific preformed enzymes, or immunological tests.

Gonorrhoea is a sexually transmitted infection primarily of the mucous membranes of the urethra, the endocervix, the rectum, the pharynx, and the conjunctiva. Common symptoms include urethral and/or cervical discharge and dysuria, but infection may be asymptomatic in up to 50% of cases. Complications include epididymitis, pelvic inflammatory disease, and haematogenous spread. In addition to routine microscopy and culture methods, molecular amplification techniques are increasingly being used for the detection of *Neisseria gonorrhoeae*. However, only culture enables sensitivity tests to be performed. As resistance profiles continue to change over time, these are a key part of the management of both the individual patient and his or her contacts, and the maintenance of up-to-date local and national treatment guidelines.

Meningococcal infection most commonly presents as either meningitis or septicaemia or a combination of both. Haematogenous spread can result in arthritis, pneumonia, and cardiac infection. Localized infection of mucous membranes can occur. Disease usually occurs from 2 to 7 days after acquisition of the organism in the nasopharynx. However, approximately 10% of adults, and a higher proportion of adolescents, carry meningococci without developing disease. When disease occurs, there may be a prodrome, but the disease is often acute with symptoms that include pyrexia, malaise, headache, neck stiffness, photophobia, and vomiting. A petechial or purpuric non-blanching rash may accompany meningococcal

septicaemia. In developed countries, overall mortality remains at around 10% with a further 10%–20% developing permanent sequelae.

Meningococci remain fully sensitive to penicillin. Treatment should be initiated promptly upon suspicion with either IV benzyl penicillin given in high and frequent doses such as 2.4 g 4 hourly or with one of the long-acting cephalosporins such as ceftriaxone 2 g 12 hourly or cefotaxime 2 g 6 hourly. Secondary cases of meningococcal disease are known to occur. The local consultant in communicable disease control should be informed immediately on clinical suspicion of meningococcal disease. The consultant in communicable disease control will make arrangements for all recent close family and other contacts to receive antibiotic prophylaxis aimed at eradicating *Neisseria meningitidis* from the nasopharynx. The most common agents used in adults are rifampicin 600 mg orally 12 hourly for 2 days, single-dose ciprofloxacin 500 mg orally, or cefotaxime 500 mg intramuscularly.

Of the 13 distinct serogroups of meningococci, the most common in the UK are B and C, while A, Y, and W135 occur less frequently. The decline in the number of cases of serogroup C disease seen since the introduction of the MenC conjugate vaccine in 2000–2 should be regarded as a major achievement of the UK immunization programme. Group B strains now account for 80% of laboratory confirmed isolates in the UK. Group A strains are seen predominantly in sub-Saharan African. In the countries of this 'meningitis belt', the disease is seasonal occurring in sudden, severe epidemics at the end of the dry season.

Haemophilus influenzae

Haemophilus influenzae is a pleomorphic, Gram-negative bacillus that is fastidious in its cultural requirements, needing the cofactors haemin and NAD for growth. These are provided in routine culture media by the heating of horse blood to 56°C—a process that changes the pigmentation from red to brown, producing so-called chocolate agar. Capsulate strains (typed as a–f) are more virulent than non-capsulate ones, the capsular polysaccharide of serotype b *Haemophilus influenzae* being recognized as a major virulence factor in relation to invasive disease such as bacteraemia, meningitis, pneumonia, and epiglottitis. Non-capsulate strains of *Haemophilus influenzae* are a commonly recognized cause of both pneumonia and acute exacerbations of chronic obstructive pulmonary disease.

The *Haemophilus influenzae* type b vaccine (Hib vaccine) was introduced to the UK in late 1992. The Hib vaccine was the first where the capsular polysaccharide, extracted from Hib cultures, was conjugated to a carrier protein molecule to increase the immunogenicity particularly in young children. In the previous 3 years, there had been approximately 900 cases reported of invasive Hib disease in England and Wales. By 1995, this had been reduced to fewer than 100.

Due to the production of beta-lactamase by many strains of *Haemophilus influenzae*, antibiotic therapy is usually with co-amoxiclav or a cephalosporin.

Bacterial enteric pathogens

Acute infectious diarrhoea may be caused by any one of a number of bacterial pathogens. Each one requires a somewhat different culture technique to recover it from a faecal sample, making the routine microbiological investigation of this common syndrome both complex and expensive. Nevertheless, the importance of understanding the cause of acute infectious diarrhoea both for the patient and for epidemiological purposes justifies routine investigation.

The commonly sought bacterial causes are *Campylobacter* spp., *Salmonella* spp., *Shigella* spp., and enterohaemorrhagic (verocytotoxin-producing) *E. coli* O157. Additionally, laboratories will attempt culture of *Vibrio* spp., provided appropriate clinical details are made available, and will test for *Clostridium difficile* toxins in hospital patients and those with a history of recent antibiotic use. In order for laboratories to comprehensively yet cost-effectively search for relevant bacterial, viral, and protozoal pathogens, faecal samples must be accompanied by appropriate clinical detail, including the patient's age and location, the duration of the patient's symptoms, and a travel and antibiotic history.

Campylobacter spp. are the most frequently identified cause of acute gastroenteritis. They are curved or spiral Gram-negative rods that require a culture medium made selective by antibiotics, an atmosphere of 5%–10% oxygen (microaerophilic), and incubation at 42°C for 48 hours. The common species that cause human gastrointestinal infection are *Campylobacter jejuni* and *Campylobacter coli*. These pathogens cause acute diarrhoea which is often associated with severe abdominal pain and malaise. *Campylobacter* species do not multiply in food. However, the infective dose is small, and transmission to humans usually occurs from undercooked poultry or unpasteurized milk. There is an unexplained seasonality associated with *Campylobacter* infection, with a peak incidence in late spring.

Salmonella species (other than *Salmonella typhi* and *Salmonella paratyphi*) cause gastrointestinal infection via the consumption of contaminated food. As *Salmonella* bacteria colonize the gastrointestinal tracts of many farm animals, food contamination can occur in uncooked or undercooked meat, poultry, eggs, and unpasteurized milk. In addition, contamination of green vegetables and fruit can occur on the farm, and contamination of shellfish can occur from the contamination of seawater with sewage. *Salmonella* are sought by examination of faecal samples for non-lactose fermenting coliforms on selective agar plates. Faecal samples are also enriched by using a specialized broth and then subculture, to ensure any small numbers of *Salmonella* bacteria present are recovered. *Salmonella* species are identified using serological tests to confirm the antigenic structure of the capsule and flagellae. The most commonly isolated serospecies are *Salmonella enteritidis* and *Salmonella typhimurium*. Many other serospecies are known, often bearing the name of the place where that strain was first identified. Some less common species can be acquired from the gastrointestinal tracts of reptiles kept as pets. *Salmonella* species are capable of infecting patients of all ages. Infants, the elderly, and the immunosuppressed are at greater risk of more serious infection.

The four species of *Shigella* responsible for bacillary dysentery are *Shigella dysenteriae*, *Shigella flexneri*, *Shigella boydii*, and *Shigella sonnei*. All are non-lactose fermenting and are sought from faecal samples in much the same way as *Salmonella* spp. The common clinical feature of infection is bloody diarrhoea. *Shigella sonnei* accounts for most cases of bacillary dysentery seen in the UK. It produces a more mild disease and is often caught by faecal–oral spread from household or institutional cases, particularly children. Since the peak of an epidemic seen in the early 1990s, the incidence in the UK has fallen significantly to under 1000 reported cases per annum. The other strains are most commonly seen in the UK as imported cases. Infection with *Shigella dysenteriae* may be severe and be complicated by haemolytic–uraemic syndrome, due to the production of Shiga toxin.

A toxin closely related to Shiga toxin is produced by some strains of *E. coli* serotype O157. Infection with these verocytotoxin-producing organisms is the commonest cause of haemolytic–uraemic syndrome in the UK. Infection can occur in any age group but is more severe in young children. The inoculum required for infection with these organisms is small compared to that for other enteric pathogens. Infection is associated with contaminated milk, contaminated water, undercooked minced beef, and undercooked beef burgers. Children have acquired *E. coli* O157 infection by petting small animals at open farms. *E. coli* O157 are sought using a selective agar and can be recognized by their inability to ferment sorbitol.

Uropathogens

Urinary tract infection accounts for 1%–3% of GP consultations in the UK and affects half of all women at some time during their life. Sexually active women aged 20–50, pregnant women, the elderly, diabetics, and young girls are particularly susceptible to urinary tract infections. Prostatic enlargement in older men may cause obstruction of the urinary tract, thereby increasing the risk of infection. Urinary tract infections are most commonly caused by coliforms, including *E. coli* and *Proteus* spp. (which, together, cause about 83% of urinary tract infections); *Enterococcus* spp. and Group B beta-haemolytic streptococci (which cause about 10% of urinary tract infections); *Staphylococcus epidermidis* and *Staphylococcus saprophyticus* (which cause about 4% of urinary tract infections); and *Pseudomonas aeruginosa*.

Urinary tract infection is confirmed by a combination of microscopy and semi-quantitative culture. Laboratory microscopy is now frequently undertaken by an automated system, either one based on flow cytometry or one based on high-speed microphotography with image recognition. The key elements reported are white blood cells, red blood cells, epithelial cells, and casts. Some automated systems perform a 'small particle' count that may act as a surrogate for an estimate of the number of bacteria present. This will not be reported but, together with the cell counts, may aid the laboratory in determining the chance of bacterial growth being found on culture and, therefore, the utility of performing a full culture.

Semi-quantitative culture usually relies on the use of a calibrated bacteriological loop. If a loop delivers 1 µl on to a CLED or chromogenic agar plate, and more than 100 colonies of the same organism are grown after 18 hours incubation, then the original specimen can be said to have $>10^5$ colony-forming units/ml. This number is said to represent significant bacteriuria (i.e. lesser numbers than this may be regarded as not significant and dismissed as contaminants). It must be remembered, however, that, with suprapubic aspirates or other surgically obtained urine samples, a pure growth of 10^4 colony-forming units/ml may be clinically significant.

It is not necessary to send a urine specimen to the laboratory from every patient. Non-pregnant women who are between teenage years and menopause and who have urinary tract infection symptoms (e.g. dysuria, frequency, urgency, or nocturia) may instead have an early morning midstream urine specimen tested using a multitest dipstick. The four principal analytes are nitrite (bacteria reduce dietary nitrates to nitrites), leucocyte esterase (an enzyme present in white blood cells), protein, and blood. While these tests have very low sensitivity and specificity individually, the negative predictive value of an overall negative test (i.e. when all four indicators are negative) is very high. In patients with a negative urine dipstick, other causes of the patient's symptoms should be considered (e.g. candidal vulvovaginitis or chlamydial urethritis).

The ability of the multitest dipstick to predict a positive culture result is lower. However, in premenopausal non-pregnant women with clear symptoms of urinary tract infection, the positive dipstick test can be seen as confirmation of infection and empirical antibiotic therapy can be started. A 3-day course of either trimethoprim 200 mg twice daily, nitrofurantoin 50–100 mg four times per day, co-amoxiclav 625 mg three times per day, or cephalexin 500 mg twice daily can be prescribed. These agents are active in vitro against approximately 70%–90% of urinary tract infection isolates.

Urinary tract infection occurring in pregnant women, children, men, or the elderly, or one that either recurs or ascends to the upper tract, should be considered complicated. Infection of the upper tract produces symptoms such as fever, nausea, malaise, or loin pain. All patients with complicated urinary tract infection should have a midstream urine sample sent for microscopy, culture, and sensitivity, and treatment should be based on the results. In general, treatment of complicated urinary tract infection should be for 7 days. This should be extended to 14 days for acute pyelonephritis, for which nitrofurantoin should not be used but ciprofloxacin 500 mg twice daily may be considered.

A midstream urine sample should be sent if symptoms of urinary tract infection occur in a pregnant woman and 7 days of treatment begun with either cephalexin or nitrofurantoin. If cultures remain positive after treatment, or symptoms recur, then prophylaxis may be indicated for the remainder of the pregnancy. Pregnant women who develop a urinary tract infection due to Group B beta-haemolytic streptococcus (*Streptococcus agalactiae*) should, in addition to treatment being given at the time of infection, be offered intrapartum antibiotic prophylaxis against neonatal Group B beta-haemolytic streptococcal infection.

In older women, clinical symptoms may be less specific (e.g. fever, anorexia, or confusion). Furthermore, up to 20% of elderly women may have asymptomatic bacteriuria that does not justify treatment. Consequently, the diagnosis requires both bacteriological evidence and careful clinical judgement prior to treatment. Similar care is needed when prescribing for catheterized patients, who will almost certainly have bacteriuria; antibiotic therapy will not eradicate this and will select resistant organisms.

Further Reading

Barnett R. Typhoid fever. *Lancet* 2016; 388: 2467.

Gotts Jeffrey E and Matthay Michael A. Sepsis: Pathophysiology and clinical management. *BMJ* 2016; 353 :i1585

McGill F, Heyderman RS, Michael BD et al. The UK joint specialist societies guideline on the diagnosis and management of acute meningitis and meningococcal sepsis in immunocompetent adults. *J Infect* 2016; 72: 405–38.

Polat G, Ugan RA, Cadirci E, and Halici Z. Sepsis and Septic Shock: Current Treatment Strategies and New Approaches. *Eurasian J Med* 2017; 49:53–8.

Public Health England. *Immunisation Against Infectious Disease.* Accessible at https://www.gov.uk/government/collections/immunisation-against-infectious-disease-the-green-book (accessed 14 Sep 2017).

Torok E, Moran E, and Cook F. *The Oxford Handbook of Infectious Diseases and Microbiology*, 2009. Oxford University Press.

311 Mycobacterial infection other than tuberculosis

Stephen Aston, Geraint Davies, and Nick Beeching

Introduction

Mycobacteria are aerobic bacilli with a lipid-rich cell wall and are widespread both in the environment and in animals. Many species within the genus cause disease in humans, most notably those of the *Mycobacterium tuberculosis* complex, which cause tuberculosis, and *Mycobacterium leprae*, the causative agent of leprosy. Several other species, termed non-tuberculous mycobacteria, can cause chronic cutaneous, pulmonary, and disseminated infections. This chapter will briefly review infection with non-tuberculous mycobacteria and *Mycobacterium leprae*; tuberculosis is the focus of Chapter 130.

Non-tuberculous mycobacterial infection

Definition and aetiology of non-tuberculous mycobacteria infections

Non-tuberculous mycobacteria (NTM) are resilient microorganisms widely distributed in both soil and water. The number of recognized species is steadily rising, with more than 125 catalogued to date, although most human disease is due to a relatively limited number of species (Table 311.1). NTM infection is rare, with an estimated incidence in industrialized countries of 4.0–6.1 cases per 100 000. Significant under-reporting is probable, since the condition is not notifiable.

Natural history of NTM infections

Infection is acquired from environmental sources via respiratory, gastrointestinal, or cutaneous routes. Human-to-human transmission of NTM has traditionally been considered unlikely, although recent studies suggest this may be an important mechanism for acquisition of *M. abscessus* by individuals with cystic fibrosis. As for *Mycobacterium tuberculosis* infection, macrophages are key to an effective host immune response. Resident macrophages phagocytose the invading mycobacteria, but then require stimulation with interferon gamma and other cytokines to activate intracellular killing mechanisms and eradicate the infection. Most infections are asymptomatic and, unlike the case with tuberculosis, latent infection with NTM has not been shown to occur. Many NTM species are of low pathogenic potential and, if identified to be the cause of symptomatic illness, would indicate significantly impaired host immunity.

Typical disease syndromes of NTM infections, and their management

NTM lung disease

Aetiology and natural history of NTM lung disease

Lung disease is the most common clinical manifestation of NTM infection. There is some geographic variation in the predominant causal species, but *Mycobacterium avium* complex (MAC), *Mycobacterium kansasii*, *Mycobacterium abscessus*, and *Mycobacterium xenopi* are frequently implicated (Table 311.1). Classically, NTM lung disease has been recognized as complicating chronic lung conditions such as COPD and bronchiectasis. More recently, it has been described in individuals without structural lung disease and, in this setting, post-menopausal Caucasian women are predominantly affected.

Typical symptoms of NTM lung disease

The clinical features of NTM lung disease are highly variable, influenced by the presence of concurrent lung disease, the immunological status of the individual, and the virulence of the relevant NTM species. Virtually all patients have chronic cough. Sputum production, dyspnoea, haemoptysis, chest pain, and weight loss are variably reported; systemic feature become more prominent as the disease progresses.

Approach to diagnosing NTM lung disease

Diagnosis of NTM lung disease requires the demonstration of persistently positive sputum culture results in the presence of compatible clinical and radiological features. Investigation of a patient suspected of having NTM lung disease should include a chest X-ray, high-resolution CT of the chest, and examination of three or more sputum specimens. However, the diagnosis of NTM lung disease is frequently challenging. The clinical features may resemble those of concurrent chronic lung disease, and radiological changes may be equally non-specific. Environmental contamination of clinical specimens yielding false positive results is common, and even repeatedly positive sputum culture may occur in the absence of progressive clinical or radiological features. The following techniques may be used in the diagnosis:

- Radiology:
  - Two main patterns of pulmonary disease are recognized: nodular/bronchiectatic disease, characterized by nodules and bronchiectasis predominantly affecting the mid- and lower lung fields; and fibrocavitary disease that resembles the typical upper zone changes of post-primary TB.

Table 311.1 Main non-tuberculous mycobacterial species causing human disease

Lung disease	Skin, soft tissue, and bone disease	Disseminated disease	Lymphadenitis
Mycobacterium avium complex	Mycobacterium marinum	Mycobacterium avium complex	Mycobacterium avium complex
Mycobacterium kansasii	Mycobacterium ulcerans	Mycobacterium kansasii	Mycobacterium malmoense
Mycobacterium xenopi	Mycobacterium abscessus	Mycobacterium chelonae	Mycobacterium scrofulaceum
Mycobacterium abscessus	Mycobacterium chelonae	Mycobacterium abscessus	Mycobacterium genavense
Mycobacterium malmoense	Mycobacterium avium complex	Mycobacterium haemophilum	
Mycobacterium fortuitum	Mycobacterium kansasii	Mycobacterium genavense	
	Mycobacterium terrae		

- The features of any underlying chronic lung disease will also be evident.
- It is not possible reliably to distinguish NTM lung disease from pulmonary TB on the basis of radiological features alone.
- Microscopy:
  - Sputum microscopy may reveal acid-fast bacilli (AFB); nucleic acid amplification tests can then be employed to rapidly differentiate NTM species from those of the *Mycobacterium tuberculosis* complex.
  - In areas of low TB endemicity, AFB seen in sputum are more likely to be NTM.
- Culture:
  - NTM commonly contaminate microbiological samples; therefore, a single positive sputum culture sample in isolation is insufficient to prove a diagnosis of NTM lung disease.
  - At least three sputum samples should be collected on separate days.
  - Consistently culture-positive specimens are predictive of NTM disease, but need to be correlated with clinical and radiological features.
- Histology:
  - Granulomatous inflammation evident on biopsy provides further supportive evidence of NTM disease in individuals with NTM culture-positive sputum specimens.

Treatment of NTM lung disease

The management of NTM lung disease varies according to the species involved and the clinical presentation of the disease. Generally, medical therapy with combinations of antimicrobial agents is used and continued for at least 12 months after achieving negative sputum cultures. Preferred regimens for disease due to MAC and *Mycobacterium kansasii* are defined. For MAC pulmonary disease, these are combination regimens which include a macrolide, ethambutol, a rifamycin, and, for patients with cavitary or previously treated disease, an aminoglycoside is added. For other NTM species, treatment regimens are generally extrapolated from those used for MAC. It should be remembered that, for many NTM species, the results of in vitro drug susceptibility tests do not correlate with the clinical response to therapeutic agents.

For symptomatic individuals with AFB-positive sputum and presenting with progressive pulmonary disease, commencement of empirical TB treatment while awaiting the results of sputum culture or nucleic acid amplification testing is often appropriate (see Chapter 130). Conversely, treatment may be deferred for individuals whose sputum cultures are persistently positive for NTM but who have no relevant symptoms or radiological evidence of disease progression. These patients should be observed closely with repeated sputum cultures and appropriate interval lung imaging. For patients with disease predominantly localized to one lung, there is a role for resectional surgery in the circumstances of inadequate response to drug therapy, infection with resistant organisms, or the development of significant local complications (e.g. haemoptysis).

Skin and soft tissue NTM disease

Skin and soft tissue NTM disease develops after direct inoculation of mycobacteria into the skin as a result of local trauma. It is most commonly due to *Mycobacterium fortuitum*, *Mycobacterium abscessus*, *Mycobacterium chelonae*, *Mycobacterium marinum*, and *Mycobacterium ulcerans* (Table 311.1). It typically manifests as a chronic, nodular, ulcerating eruption. Deeper inoculation of mycobacteria may occur through accidental trauma or surgery and may result in tenosynovitis, arthritis, or osteomyelitis. The diagnosis of NTM disease is confirmed by biopsy of the skin or affected tissue, in which AFB and granulomata are usually evident. Recommended antimicrobial treatment regimens vary with the NTM species involved and the extent of disease. Surgical debridement may be indicated for extensive disease, abscess formation, or circumstances where adequate drug therapy is difficult. For small isolated lesions, surgical excision alone may be curative.

Disseminated NTM disease

Disseminated NTM disease is only seen in severely immunocompromised individuals, most commonly those with advanced HIV infection. Prior to the introduction of highly active antiretroviral therapy (HAART), it was noted in 40% of patients with advanced HIV. The widespread use of HAART has led to significant falls in incidence. In non-HIV patients, disseminated NTM disease has been described in the context of malignancy, chemotherapy, long-term corticosteroids, and genetic defects of the interferon gamma pathway. More than 90% of cases of disseminated NTM cases are caused by MAC (Table 311.1).

Disseminated NTM disease typically presents with fever, night sweats, weight loss, and malaise. Hepatosplenomegaly and lymphadenopathy are often evident on imaging, if not detectable on clinical examination. Laboratory tests reveal non-specific abnormalities, including anaemia, leucopaenia, and elevated alkaline phosphatase levels. In more than 90% of cases, blood cultures are positive. For the remaining cases, disseminated NTM disease may be established by culture of a bone marrow or liver biopsy specimen. The possibility of multiple concurrent infectious pathologies should always be remembered, as the affected patients are usually highly immunocompromised.

Disseminated MAC disease is treated with either azithromycin or clarithromycin in combination with ethambutol. Rifabutin may be added for highly immunocompromised or symptomatic patients. For HIV-infected patients, HAART should be initiated promptly after diagnosis. Following the completion of treatment, secondary prophylaxis with either azithromycin or clarithromycin should be continued until adequate immune reconstitution has occurred. The mortality rate due to disseminated NTM infection is around 30% in both HIV-infected and uninfected patients.

Lymphadenitis due to NTM

Lymphadenitis due to NTM is most commonly seen in young children and usually involves the submandibular, cervical, and preauricular lymph nodes. In the absence of HIV infection, it rarely occurs in adults. MAC currently accounts for approximately 80% of culture-proven cases of NTM lymphadenitis (Table 311.1).

The typical clinical presentation of non-tender, unilateral lymphadenopathy with minimal systemic symptoms is largely indistinguishable from that of tuberculous lymphadenitis which is the main differential diagnosis. In a low TB endemicity setting such as the UK, tuberculous lymphadenitis accounts for only 10% of mycobacterial lymphadenitis in children, but more than 90% in adults. For both tuberculous and NTM disease, histological examination of lymph node material typically shows caesating granulomata with or without visible AFB. A definitive diagnosis may be made on mycobacterial culture, but results are delayed by several weeks and, frequently, no organism is cultured. Lack of reactivity to a tuberculin skin test is supportive of disease due to NTM.

Complete surgical excision of the affected lymph nodes is the recommended treatment for most localized NTM lymphadenitis. Antimycobacterial chemotherapy is usually reserved for recurrent disease or cases where surgical excision is impossible or incomplete.

Leprosy

Definition and aetiology of leprosy

Leprosy is a chronic granulomatous infection of the skin and peripheral nerves caused by the intracellular bacillus *Mycobacterium leprae*. It is characterized by anaesthetic skin lesions and peripheral neuropathy with nerve thickening. Left untreated, affected individuals may develop disfiguring and disabling deformities as a result of repeated trauma and secondary infection of anaesthetic areas.

Demographics of leprosy

The WHO reports the global prevalence of leprosy as the number of individuals currently on registered treatment programmes. Following the introduction of multidrug treatment, the global prevalence of leprosy has fallen dramatically from an estimated 12 million registered cases in 1985 to fewer than 200 000 at the start of 2011. However, disease transmission continues to occur at substantial levels in some countries. In recent years over 200 000 new cases of leprosy have been detected each year, with over 80% occurring in four countries—India, Brazil, Indonesia, and the Democratic Republic

Box 311.1 WHO diagnostic criteria for leprosy

The presence of one or more of these features is considered diagnostic of leprosy:

One or more hypopigmented or reddish patches with definite loss of sensation

Thickened peripheral nerves

Acid-fast bacilli identified in slit-skin smears or biopsy

Reproduced with permission of Public Health England

of Congo. Persistent disability resulting from nerve damage adds to the global burden of disease and means that leprosy remains a leading cause of neurological disability in developing countries. About ten new cases are currently diagnosed each year in the UK, all imported. The last documented case of transmission within the UK occurred over 50 years ago.

Natural history of leprosy

The means of transmission and natural history of *Mycobacterium leprae* infection are not completely understood. Individuals with lepromatous disease produce minute particles laden with bacilli that are presumed to be the vehicle of airborne person-to-person transmission. Only a small minority of exposed individuals develop clinical disease. Bacilli are taken up via the upper respiratory tract mucosa and then demonstrate a specific tropism for Schwann cells and macrophages, to establish a slowly replicating intracellular infection. The emergence of mycobacterial antigens from infected cells induces a specific host immune response, which may result in a chronic inflammatory process affecting the skin and peripheral nerves.

Typical symptoms of leprosy, and less common symptoms

The cardinal diagnostic features of leprosy are summarized in Box 311.1.

The nature of the host cell-mediated immune response determines the clinical manifestations of leprosy. The Ridley–Jopling classification categorizes leprosy into five types on the basis of clinical and histological features and the bacillary load. This is shown in Table 311.2, together with the simplified WHO case definition, which divides the clinical spectrum into paucibacillary disease (≤5 lesions) and multibacillary disease (≥6 lesions in the skin and/or the nerves).

Cutaneous features of leprosy

Tuberculoid leprosy

A robust cell-mediated immune response results in tuberculoid leprosy (the 'TT' form in the Ridley–Jopling classification), which is characterized by localization of infection within one or few nerves, and/or a small number of well-demarcated, hypopigmented, anaesthetic patches; this is also termed paucibacillary disease by the WHO. Histological examination demonstrates well-formed granulomas with an abundance of CD4+ T-lymphocytes surrounding dermal nerves, and an absence of visible bacilli.

Lepromatous leprosy

Unlike tuberculoid leprosy, lepromatous leprosy (the 'LL' form in the Ridley–Jopling classification) occurs when the cell-mediated immune response is poor. Lesions are generally macular, poorly defined, and widely and symmetrically distributed. Diffuse dermal infiltration and skin thickening may result in a classical 'leonine facies' appearance. Histological examination demonstrates diffuse infiltration of the deeper dermis with foamy macrophages laden with bacilli but few granulomata.

Borderline forms of leprosy

Between these polar extremes, several forms of disease are recognized which have intermediate clinical and histological features (the 'BT', 'BB', and 'BL' forms in the Ridley–Jopling classification). Moving from tuberculoid towards lepromatous disease, there is a reduction in the cellular immune response and a corresponding increase in the bacillary load and the number of skin lesions present. Histological examination reveals small granulomata that become more diffuse on progression towards lepromatous disease. The skin lesions of intermediate forms are highly variable and may be macular, papulonodular, plaque-like, or geographic. The term 'multibacillary disease' includes lepromatous disease and borderline disease states near the lepromatous end of the disease spectrum (see Table 311.2).

Nerve involvement in leprosy

Peripheral nerve involvement in leprosy is extremely common. Sensory nerve dysfunction usually predominates, characterized by anaesthetic skin lesions. Motor and autonomic nerves may also be affected, resulting in weakness and reduced sweating, respectively. Affected nerves are usually thickened and palpable but, occasionally, significant nerve dysfunction occurs in the absence of obvious inflammation. Some patients have purely neural leprosy, without visible skin lesions.

Eye involvement in leprosy

Blindness is a relatively common complication of leprosy. Motor and sensory damage lead to impaired eye closure and reduced corneal sensation, predisposing to corneal ulceration, repeated trauma, and secondary cataract formation.

Reactional states in leprosy

The immune response in leprosy is dynamic, and spontaneous fluctuations can result in rapid alterations in clinical status. Type 1 (reversal) reactions follow spontaneous increases in T-cell reactivity and are characterized by inflammation of skin lesions and acute neuritis, often associated with rapid deterioration in nerve function. Inflammation must be rapidly controlled in order to prevent permanent nerve damage. Type 1 reactions occur in one-third of individuals with borderline disease and may be evident at presentation.

Erythema nodosum leprosum (Type 2) reaction is an acute onset systemic disorder with multiple organ involvement that typically occurs in individuals with multibacillary disease. It arises as a result of extravascular deposition of immune complexes and consequent complement and neutrophil activation. Typical features include fever, painful skin nodules, uveitis, arthritis, and dactylitis.

Table 311.2 Classifications and features of leprosy

WHO Classification	Paucibacillary (PB) ———→		←——— Multibacillary (MB) ———————→		
Bacteriological Index	0	0–1+	1–3+	3–5+	5–6+
Type of leprosy	Polar tuberculoid	Borderline			Polar lepromatous
Ridley–Jopling Classification	TT	BT	BB	BL	LL
Skin lesions	Increasing number of skin lesions ———————————————————→				
Nerve lesions	Increasing number of enlarged nerves & nerve involvement ———————→				
Stability	Stable	Unstable—may develop reactions and new nerve damage			Stable

Reproduced with permission of Public Health England.

Table 311.3 WHO-recommended multidrug therapy regimens

Type of leprosy	Drug treatment		Minimum duration of treatment (months)
	Monthly supervised	Daily, self-administered	
Paucibacillary	Rifampicin 600 mg	Dapsone 100 mg	6
Multibacillary	Rifampicin 600 mg	Clofazimine 50 mg	12
	Clofazimine 300 mg	Dapsone 100 mg	12

Reproduced with permission of Public Health England.

Approach to diagnosing leprosy

In an endemic area, leprosy should be considered in any patient presenting with peripheral neuropathy or persistent skin lesions. In the UK, leprosy is frequently missed and should be considered in any patient who has ever lived abroad and who presents with peripheral anaesthesia and nerve thickening (which should always be sought in immigrants with supposed diabetic neuropathy), unusual skin lesions, or unexplained acute rheumatological presentations. All suspected patients should be referred to a national specialist in leprosy (see https://www.gov.uk/government/uploads/system/uploads/attachment_data/file/334363/Memorandum_on_leprosy_2012.pdf for a list of UK consultant advisers in leprosy).

Histological diagnosis is the gold-standard test, with the presence of neural inflammation distinguishing leprosy from other granulomatous disorders. Microscopy of slit-skin smears for bacilli is useful for identifying infectious patients and to monitor the response to treatment, but is of little value in diagnosis since it is negative in many patients with leprosy. The bacillary load is measured by counting the average number of bacilli seen in 6–8 slit-skin smear preparations, yielding a 'bacterial index' (BI). In this semi-quantitative logarithmic scale, a BI of 1+ indicates at least 1 bacillus per 100 microscopic fields, and the maximum possible BI of 6+ found in polar lepromatous leprosy indicates 1000 or more bacilli per field (Table 311.2).

Other diagnoses that should be considered aside from leprosy

The varied manifestations of leprosy lead to a broad differential diagnosis including sarcoidosis, cutaneous leishmaniasis, post-kala-azar dermal leishmaniasis, cutaneous TB, syphilis, granuloma annulare, vitiligo, post-inflammatory hypopigmentation, pityriasis versicolor, dermatophyte infection, and hereditary neuropathies associated with nerve thickening.

Treatment of leprosy, and its effectiveness

Antimicrobial therapy for leprosy

All patients diagnosed with leprosy should receive multidrug combination treatment. WHO recommends two first-line regimens corresponding to its simplified classification system (Table 311.3).

Prior to the adoption of current treatment guidelines, 24 months of antimicrobial therapy was recommended for multibacillary disease but this has been reduced to 12 months for field use in endemic settings. Reported relapse rates following directly observed multidrug therapy are very low. All treatment should be managed in conjunction with a leprosy specialist. Contact details for designated consultant advisers in leprosy in the UK are available at https://www.gov.uk/government/uploads/system/uploads/attachment_data/file/334363/Memorandum_on_leprosy_2012.pdf.

Management of reactional states in leprosy

Reactional states require urgent assessment and treatment in order to prevent permanent nerve dysfunction. Type 1 reactions are treated with oral corticosteroids, which are gradually tapered over 3–5 months. Decompressive surgery is occasionally used to relieve mechanical obstruction caused by nerve oedema if nerve dysfunction persists despite medical treatment. Similarly, high-dose corticosteroids are initially used to treat erythema nodosum leprosum reactions but alternative agents such as thalidomide may be required to achieve sustained control. Reactions may continue to occur for years after successful antimicrobial therapy, and patients must be educated about the possibility and nature of reactions and the need to contact their physician immediately if symptoms arise.

Prevention of disability in leprosy

Rapidly identifying nerve dysfunction and early institution of steroid therapy are essential in preventing disability. Hence, a detailed neurological assessment should be performed at each clinical encounter. If neuropathy occurs, prevention of secondary tissue damage is the primary objective. Patients should be educated to avoid activities that put neuropathic areas at risk, provided with appropriate orthotics, and advised to undertake regular self-examination. Secondarily infected tissues require prompt antibiotic treatment and possibly surgical debridement to minimize tissue damage.

Further Reading

Alvarez-Uria G. Lung disease caused by nontuberculous mycobacteria. *Curr Opin Pulm Med* 2010; 16: 251–6.

Griffith DE, Aksamit T, Brown-Elliott BA, et al. An official ATS/IDSA statement: Diagnosis, treatment, and prevention of nontuberculous mycobacterial diseases. *Am J Respir Crit Care Med* 2007; 175: 367–416.

Haworth CS, Banks J, Capstick T et al. British Thoracic Society guidelines for the the management of non-tuberculous mycobacterial pulmonary disease. *Thorax* 2017; 72: ii1–ii64.

Johnson MM and Odell JA. Nontuberculous mycobacterial pulmonary infections. *J Thorac Dis* 2014; 6: 210–20.

Public Health England. *Memorandum on Leprosy.* Departments of Health, 2012. https://www.gov.uk/government/uploads/system/uploads/attachment_data/file/334363/Memorandum_on_leprosy_2012.pdf.

Lastória JC and Abreu MA. Leprosy: Review of the epidemiological, clinical, and etiopathogenic aspects—Part 1. *An Bras Dermatol* 2014; 89: 205–18.

Rodrigues LC and Lockwood DNJ. Leprosy now: Epidemiology, progress, challenges, and research gaps. *Lancet Infect Dis* 2011; 11: 464–70.

Introduction

Spirochaetes are slender, helical, Gram-negative rods. The group includes *Treponema*, *Leptospira*, and *Borrelia*, which are further classified as summarized in Table 312.1. This chapter focuses on leptospirosis and Lyme disease; syphilis is covered in Chapter 313. Discussion of the non-venereal treponematoses and relapsing fevers is beyond the scope of this text; they are rarely encountered in the UK.

Leptospirosis

Definition of leptospirosis

Leptospirosis is a zoonotic infection caused by *Leptospira interrogans*. There are over 250 serovars associated with infection in different animals, for example *Leptospira interrogans icterohaemorrhagiae* (rats) and *Leptospira interrogans hardjo* (cattle).

Aetiology of leptospirosis

Animals excrete leptospires in their urine. Humans are incidental hosts and acquire infection through contact with animal urine or contaminated fresh water. Transmission occurs across mucous membranes or damaged skin and possibly via ingestion or inhalation of contaminated water.

Typical symptoms of leptospirosis, and less common symptoms

Most infections are asymptomatic or only mildly symptomatic and self-limiting. The incubation period is usually 7–12 days (range 2–30 days). Illness typically follows a biphasic course, with an acute bacteraemic phase, which lasts for approximately 1 week, and then an immune phase. During the bacteraemic phase, patients may present with a flu-like illness with headache, fever, and vomiting. Conjunctival suffusion and myalgia, often affecting the calves, are characteristic. Less frequent findings include hepatosplenomegaly, meningism, and a rash.

Patients may show signs of recovery before progressing to the immune phase, when fever and rigors recur with clinical deterioration. Aseptic meningitis is common, while Weil's disease (jaundice, acute renal failure, and haemorrhage) develops in only a minority.

Demographics of leptospirosis

Leptospirosis occurs worldwide, with the highest incidence in tropical and subtropical regions. In the UK, infection is associated with occupational or recreational activities carrying a risk of exposure, such as farming, fishing, sewer work, canoeing, windsurfing, and freshwater swimming. Imported cases in adventure travellers are increasingly recognized.

Natural history of leptospirosis, and complications of the disease

The bacteraemic phase may resolve without treatment, and only a minority develop biphasic disease. The immune phase can last up to 30 days, and recovery may take up to 3 months after severe disease; however, most patients recover within 2–6 weeks with appropriate treatment. Complications include renal failure, haemorrhage, hepatic dysfunction, myocarditis, rhabdomyolysis, pulmonary haemorrhage, and acute respiratory distress syndrome.

Approach to diagnosing leptospirosis

Diagnosis requires a high index of suspicion in a febrile patient with headache, myalgia, conjunctival suffusion, or jaundice, and possible exposure to leptospires.

Other diagnoses that should be considered aside from leptospirosis

Depending on the travel history, the differential diagnosis may include influenza, dengue, yellow fever, hantavirus, malaria, typhoid fever, rickettsial disease, viral hepatitis, meningococcal disease, and relapsing fever.

'Gold-standard' diagnostic test for leptospirosis

Most cases of leptospirosis are identified through serology. Antibodies to leptospires may be detected 5–10 days after symptom onset. An IgM ELISA is used to screen all sera, with positive results confirmed by a microscopic agglutination test. At least two serum specimens are required, taken at least 7 days apart.

Acceptable diagnostic alternatives to the gold-standard test for leptospirosis

PCR is used on clinical samples (e.g. blood, urine, CSF, bronchoalveolar lavage, and tissue) taken within 7 days of symptom onset. Leptospira culture can be performed from blood culture and samples of blood, CSF, and tissue. Culture is performed on clinical samples that have tested PCR positive.

Other relevant investigations for leptospirosis

Patients may have a leucocytosis or leucopenia, and about half have mild-to-moderate elevations in hepatic transaminases and creatine kinase. In Weil's disease, the bilirubin may be very high, and there is often thrombocytopenia and renal impairment. CSF may show raised white cells and protein, and normal glucose.

Prognosis of leptospirosis, and how to estimate it

For leptospirosis, mortality is <1% in anicteric disease, 5%–15% in Weil's disease, and even higher in severe pulmonary haemorrhage. Acute renal failure, respiratory insufficiency, hypotension, arrhythmias, and altered mental status are poor prognostic factors. Males suffer more severe illness.

Treatment of leptospirosis, and its effectiveness

The value of antimicrobial therapy is debated due to a lack of evidence. We strongly recommend early initiation of antibiotics, whenever there is clinical suspicion of leptospirosis. Mild disease can be

Table 312.1 Principal spirochaetes associated with human disease

Genus	Species	Clinical disease
Treponema	Treponema pallidum subspecies pallidum	Syphilis
	Treponema pallidum subspecies pertenue	Yaws
	Treponema pallidum subspecies endemicum	Bejel
	Treponema careteum	Pinta
Leptospira	Leptospira interrogans	Leptospirosis
Borrelia	Borrelia burgdorferi	Lyme disease
	Borrelia recurrentis	Epidemic relapsing fever
	Various Borrelia spp.	Endemic relapsing fever

treated with oral doxycycline (100 mg twice daily) or amoxycillin (500 mg four times daily) for 7–10 days. IV benzylpenicillin (600 mg (=1 million IU) every 4 hours) or ceftriaxone (1 g once daily) should be used in severe cases. Adequate supportive care is essential, including renal replacement therapy and ventilation if required. A Jarisch–Herxheimer reaction, which is a reaction to bacterial antigens released from disrupted organisms, may complicate the early phase of treatment. It usually manifests as abrupt worsening of the patient, with hypotension and sometimes features of immune-complex disease, typically within the first 24–48 hours after starting antimicrobial therapy.

Lyme disease

Definition of Lyme disease

First described in Lyme, Connecticut, Lyme disease is the most common tick-borne infection in Europe and North America. It is caused by *Borrelia burgdorferi*, a spirochaete transmitted by *Ixodes* ticks. Ticks are only just visible at the time of attachment and are easily missed by the patient, so a definitive history of tick bite is often absent.

Aetiology of Lyme disease

Several pathogenic species of *Borrelia* have been identified in Europe, principally *Borrelia garinii, Borrelia afzelii*, and *Borrelia burgdorferi* sensu stricto. In North America, the disease is caused exclusively by *Borrelia burgdorferi* sensu stricto.

Typical symptoms of Lyme disease, and less common symptoms

Infection may be asymptomatic. The most common manifestation is erythema migrans, an expanding rash which spreads from the site of a tick bite after 3–30 days. Central clearing develops producing an annular pattern. Fever, myalgia, arthralgia, and headache may accompany the rash.

Without treatment, infection may disseminate to the nervous system, joints, and heart. In the UK the most common complications involve the nervous system (neuroborreliosis). Unilateral or bilateral facial nerve palsy, lymphocytic meningitis, and radiculoneuritis are seen in adults, usually within 3–12 weeks of infection. Radiculoneuritis may not be apparent until several months after infection and produces severe shingles-like pain with altered sensation or paresis. Less commonly, neuroborreliosis may present as an encephalitis or myelitis.

Lyme carditis mainly presents with conduction defects within a few weeks of infection. Lyme arthritis usually affects the knee, producing synovitis, effusion, and pain. It is more frequently associated with *Borrelia burgdorferi* sensu stricto infection acquired in North America or central Europe.

Demographics of Lyme disease

Lyme disease occurs predominantly in temperate regions of Europe, North America, and Asia. Woodland areas are the usual habitat for ticks, as well as animal species which act as reservoir hosts for *Borrelia burgdorferi*. Occupational and recreational activities associated with exposure to tick bites include forestry, farming, deer handling, hiking, and mountain biking, particularly in highly endemic areas such as central and eastern Europe.

Natural history of Lyme disease, and complications of the disease

Clinical Lyme disease can be considered to consist of three stages: early localized disease, early disseminated disease, and late disease. Only a minority of untreated patients develop late-stage disease, which arises months to years later and affects the skin, the musculoskeletal system, and/or the nervous system. Neuroborreliosis complicates 5%–10% of infections. It is classified as early (i.e. neurological symptoms lasting for <6 months) or late (i.e. lasting for >6 months).

Approach to diagnosing Lyme disease

Erythema migrans can be diagnosed reliably by clinical examination alone, if a typical rash occurs following potential exposure to ticks. Patients may not recall having been bitten. Antibody tests are positive in only 30%–70% of patients at this early stage, and are not recommended unless the rash is atypical. All other manifestations of Lyme require laboratory confirmation.

Other diagnoses that should be considered aside from Lyme disease

Anaplasmosis, babesiosis, Q fever, and tick-borne encephalitis are also transmitted by tick bites in areas where these infections are endemic. The differential diagnosis for rashes resembling erythema migrans includes cellulitis, insect/tick-bite reactions, ringworm, granuloma annulare, and erythema multiforme.

'Gold-standard' diagnostic test for Lyme disease

Lyme disease is usually diagnosed by serology. Samples should be sent to the national reference laboratory at Public Health England at Porton Down, where a validated, two-tier testing methodology is used. The screening test is a C6-antigen-based ELISA (combined IgG and IgM), followed by a confirmatory Western blot (separate IgG and IgM). Antibodies develop slowly; thus, negative serology in early disease does not exclude infection. A second sample taken 2–4 weeks later may confirm seroconversion.

Acceptable diagnostic alternatives to the gold-standard test for Lyme disease

Detection of borrelial DNA in synovial fluid by PCR is useful in suspected Lyme arthritis. PCR examination of CSF has a low yield, and detection of intrathecal antibodies specific to *Borrelia burgdorferi* is more useful in suspected neuroborreliosis.

Other relevant investigations for Lyme disease

In neuroborreliosis, the CSF leucocyte count is typically 10–1000 cells/mm³ and the protein count often elevated.

Prognosis of Lyme disease, and how to estimate it

More than 90% of patients with early disease respond to treatment. Patients with late manifestations usually respond to antibiotics but improvement may take weeks to months.

Table 312.2 Management of Lyme disease		
Clinical manifestation	**Preferred antibiotic regimens**	**Comments**
Erythema migrans or isolated facial palsy	Doxycycline* 100 mg twice daily orally for 14 to 21 days, or amoxicillin 500 mg three times per day orally for 14 to 21 days	
Neuroborreliosis†	Ceftriaxone 2 g once per day IV for 14 days	Treat for 21 days if late neuroborreliosis
Lyme arthritis	Doxycycline* 100 mg twice per day orally for 28 days, or amoxicillin 500 mg three times per day orally for 28 days	Ceftriaxone 2 g once per day IV 14–28 days if arthritis progresses despite oral therapy
Lyme carditis	If the patient is hospitalized: ceftriaxone 2 g once per day IV for 14 to 21 days If the patient does not require admission: treat as for erythema migrans	Admit for cardiac monitoring if the patient is symptomatic, there is second-/third-degree heart block, or the PR interval is ≥300 milliseconds Temporary pacing may be required

*Avoid in pregnancy and breastfeeding.

†In light of recent evidence, European guidelines recommend that oral doxycycline (200 mg daily) can be used as an alternative to IV ceftriaxone for patients with neurological involvement confined to the meninges, cranial nerves, nerve roots, or peripheral nerves. Patients with myelitis, encephalitis, or cerebral vasculitis should receive IV ceftriaxone.

Neurological sequelae following neuroborreliosis are more common if symptoms are prolonged prior to treatment and in those with CNS involvement.

Treatment of Lyme disease, and its effectiveness

Table 312.2 summarizes antibiotic recommendations for Lyme disease in adults. Treatment success should be judged on clinical response, as antibodies can persist for years. Antibiotics may not hasten the resolution of facial palsy or carditis but should be given to prevent further sequelae. Complete heart block usually resolves within 1 week, and lesser conduction disturbances within 6 weeks.

Further Reading

British Infection Association. The epidemiology, prevention, investigation and treatment of *Lyme borreliosis* in United Kingdom patients: A position statement by the British Infection Association. *J Infect* 2011; 62: 329–38.

Forbes AE, Zochowski WJ, Dubrey SW, et al. Leptospirosis and Weil's disease in the UK. *QJM* 2012; 105: 1151–62.

NICE guidance on Lyme disease. Expected 2018. www.nice.org.uk

313 Syphilis

Martyn Wood and Marilyn Bradley

Definition of the disease

The term 'syphilis' describes the wide-ranging clinical manifestations of infection with the slowly dividing spirochete bacterium *Treponema pallidum* subsp. *pallidum*.

Aetiology and demographics of the disease

T. pallidum infection is mainly sexually acquired; it is thought the bacterium enters through microabrasions in the skin or mucosa. Congenital infection via mother-to-child transmission is also recognized. The driving force of the clinical manifestations of all stages of syphilis is an underlying and often multisystem vasculitis.

The incidence of syphilis in the general British population rapidly declined following the widespread introduction of penicillin in the 1940s. Increasing levels of syphilis were seen again in the 1960s and 1970s, mainly in men who have sex with men (MSM). With the emergence of the HIV epidemic in the 1980s, syphilis infections declined, along with other sexually transmitted infection rates, as people adopted safer sexual practices.

The end of the twentieth century again saw large rises in syphilis incidence, reaching epidemic proportions, which continue today. The majority of cases are seen in MSM. However, infection levels continue to rise in heterosexual men and women, the majority acquiring their infection in the United Kingdom.

Natural history of the disease

Acquired syphilis can be divided into early and late presentations. In early stage infection, the *T. pallidum* infection has been acquired within 2 years of the diagnosis. This early stage includes the symptomatic primary and secondary stages of infection, and the asymptomatic early latent stage. Late infection of over 2 years' standing includes all the manifestations of tertiary syphilis, and asymptomatic late latent infection.

T. pallidum has an incubation period of approximately 9–90 days. The primary stage of infection often goes unnoticed or is truly asymptomatic. Classically, primary syphilis presents with a painless indurated ulcer (chancre) at the site of *T. pallidum* inoculation in genital areas such as the penis, the vulva, the cervix, and the rectum. Regional lymphadenopathy soon follows, with systemic spread of infection then occurring. Atypical presentations such as painful lesions, balanitis, vulvitis, oral lesions, or multiple lesions are frequently described and often go undiagnosed.

Secondary syphilis occurs approximately 4–10 weeks after the primary infection. In the majority of cases, it presents as a rash which is commonly maculopapular but can have many appearances, including psoriaform or pustular. The rash preferentially affects the trunk in most cases and occurs on the palms and soles in around half of infections. The primary lesion may not have healed by the time secondary syphilis symptoms develop, and the two may be present simultaneously. There are multiple other potential, less common, but clinically significant presentations of secondary syphilis; these are summarized in Table 313.1.

Complications of the disease

Tertiary stage syphilis is the result of untreated, long-standing infection. Pre-antibiotic-era studies suggest that 40% of untreated individuals will advance to tertiary stage infection. If the tertiary stage occurs, it can present anywhere from 2 to 15 years after the initial infection. This stage includes gummatous, cardiovascular, and neurological syphilis. Gummatous syphilis is often erroneously referred to as benign tertiary syphilis, but lesions can be destructive or infiltrative and can cause significant organ or tissue damage, depending on which system is involved. Neurosyphilis (encompassing tabes dorsalis and general paralysis of the insane) presents as small vessel vasculitis, with meningeal or cortical involvement. Syphilitic retinitis is classified as neurosyphilis due to optic nerve involvement but can present early as part of the secondary syphilis stage. Cardiovascular syphilis involves the aortic arch and root, leading to aortic aneurysm and valve dysfunction. Coronary ostial involvement can also precipitate myocardial ischaemia.

Approach to diagnosing the disease

If syphilis is suspected or a patient's presentation is unexplained, a sexual history should be taken, specifically assessing timing and type of sexual risk. This will guide the clinician as to which diagnostic tests to perform and will allow correct interpretation of results. In those individuals who are at higher risk for syphilis acquisition, regular serological screening should be undertaken. To interpret serological tests appropriately, a history of previous syphilis testing and treatment and the current timing of symptoms should be ascertained. Other treponemal infections can give rise to false-positive serological screening tests and should be enquired about.

Other diseases that should be considered

Syphilis can present very non-specifically and can resemble multiple other pathologies. In general, any systemic vasculitic process should be considered in the differential diagnosis. The risks for HIV and syphilis infection are very similar, and the two often coexist. HIV infection is known to rapidly accelerate and exacerbate syphilis complications. If syphilis testing is undertaken, HIV testing should also be routinely performed.

'Gold-standard' diagnostic test

If a lesion consistent with primary infection is present, appropriately taken samples can be examined for treponemes via dark-field contrast microscopy. Certain manifestations of secondary syphilis can be sampled for microscopy, such as condylomata lata (wart-like genital lesions) and mucous patches. As dark-field microscopy requires an experienced clinician and microscopist, its general application is limited.

The majority of syphilis diagnoses are made via interpretation of a combination of serological investigations, which include specific treponemal antibody/antigen tests (e.g. IgM and IgG EIA, and TPHA/TPPA) and non-specific cardiolipin tests (VDRL/RPR), which can be used to diagnose and assess response to treatment. Common test results corresponding to stages of infection are summarized in Table 313.1.

Acceptable diagnostic alternatives to the gold standard

For syphilis, there is no substitute for diagnosis made by serology, but PCR techniques are starting to be used in place of dark-field microscopy. Specimens analysed by PCR are less susceptible to sampling error and transport conditions; in addition, PCR analysis allows testing of lesions at non-genital sites. Multiplex PCR is available, allowing combination testing for several infective genital ulcerative conditions to be carried out on a single sample.

Table 313.1 Summary of common clinical and serological manifestations of syphilis infection, by stage

Clinical stage	Symptoms/signs	IgM EIA	IgG EIA	TPHA/TPPA	VDRL/RPR
Primary	Balanitis or vulvitis Oral lesions Painless indurated ulcer (chancre; single or multiple) Regional lymphadenopathy	Positive	Positive in majority	Negative in majority or positive at low titre	Positive at low titre
Secondary or early latent (i.e. asymptomatic and infected <2 years)	Alopecia Anterior uveitis Arthralgia/periosteitis Cranial nerve palsies Fever Glomerulonephritis Hepatitis Lymphadenopathy Meningitis Mucous lesions Rash Retinitis Snail-track ulcers	Positive Can be negative in latent infection	Positive	Positive at high titre	Positive at high titre
Tertiary (40% of untreated) or late latent (asymptomatic and infected >2 years (60% of untreated cases))	Gummatous (15% of untreated): skin and joint involvement common Cardiovascular (15% of untreated): aortic root, aortic arch, and coronary ostial involvement Neurological (10% of untreated): meningovascular (stroke syndromes), parenchymal (general paresis and tabes dorsalis)	Negative	Positive	Positive at low titre	Positive at low titre, or negative
Treated or incompletely treated (from previous antibiotic exposure)		Negative	Positive	Positive at low titre	Negative or positive at low titre

Other relevant investigations

When late latent syphilis is suspected, an assessment for end-organ damage should be made, specifically cardiovascular involvement with ECG and chest X-ray, proceeding to echocardiography as necessary. If neurological syphilis is suspected (and the patient has positive serum serological tests), neurological imaging and CSF sampling should be undertaken. The majority of patients with symptomatic neurosyphilis have a raised CSF white-cell count (>5 cells/mm³). A negative direct treponemal test (TPPA or TPHA) on CSF (without blood contamination) excludes neurosyphilis in the majority of cases; however, it can be negative in cortical disease. A positive test has a high sensitivity for CNS infection. It must be noted that CSF TPPA/TPHA tests are prone to false-positive results (poor specificity) due to immunoglobulins crossing the blood–brain barrier.

Prognosis and how to estimate it

If treated in the early stages of infection, syphilis has an excellent prognosis and is curable. If treatment is delayed for several years, disabling and life-threatening complications can result; therefore, individuals at high risk should undergo regular screening.

Treatment and its effectiveness

The mainstay of treatment is parenteral penicillin, given for a sufficiently long period to cover the slow replication time of *T. pallidum*. Other agents such as cephalosporins and tetracyclines have also been shown to be effective. Treatment duration is based on the stage of clinical infection. National guidelines for the treatment of syphilis exist, and an expert opinion should also be sought prior to initiating treatment.

Further Reading

Kingston M, French P, Higgins S, et al. UK national guidelines on the management of syphilis 2015. *Int J STD & AIDS* 2016; 27: 421–46.

Mattei PL, Beachkofsky TM, Gilson RT, et al. Syphilis: A reemerging infection. *Am Fam Physician* 2012; 86: 433–40.

Singh AE and Romanowski B. Syphilis: Review with emphasis on clinical, epidemiologic, and some biologic features. *Clin Microbiol Rev* 1999; 12: 187–209.

Timmermans M and Carr J. Neurosyphilis in the modern era. *J Neurol Neurosurg Psychiatry* 2004; 75: 1727–30.

Unemo M, Bradshaw CS, Hocking JS et al. Sexually transmitted infections: challenges ahead 2017. *Lancet Infect Dis* 2017; 17: e235–79

314 Rickettsial infection

Tom Fletcher and Nick Beeching

Introduction

Rickettsial infections are caused by a variety of obligate intracellular, Gram-negative bacteria from the genera *Rickettsia, Orientia, Ehrlichia,* and *Anaplasma*. *Rickettsia* is further subdivided into the spotted fever group and the typhus group. *Bartonella* and *Coxiella burnetii* bacteria are similar to rickettsiae and cause similar diseases. The range of recognized spotted fever group infections is rapidly expanding, complementing long-recognized examples such as Rocky Mountain spotted fever (*Rickettsia rickettsii*) in the US, and Australian tick typhus (*Rickettsia australis*), as well as those in southern Europe and Africa.

Animals are the predominant reservoir of infection, and transmission to people is usually through ticks, mites, fleas, or lice, during blood-feeding or from scarification of faeces deposited on the skin. In this chapter, we will focus on the two of the most relevant infections encountered in UK practice: African tick typhus, and Q fever.

African tick typhus

Definition of African tick typhus

African tick typhus is a collective name used for two distinct spotted fever group rickettsial infections that occur in Africa: African tick-bite fever and Mediterranean spotted fever (MSF; also known as 'fièvre boutonneuse'). There has been considerable overlap historically between the two, but it is now well recognized that they are distinct diseases, with different epidemiology, bacteriology, and disease presentations.

Aetiology of African tick typhus

African tick-bite fever is caused by *Rickettsia africae* and is transmitted by hard ticks (*Amblyomma* spp.) that feed on a wide range of domestic and wild animals. MSF is caused by *Rickettsia conorii* and is transmitted by the brown dog tick (*Rhipicephalus sanguineus*). The ticks act as both vectors and reservoirs of the disease, and humans are accidental hosts.

Typical symptoms of African tick typhus, and less common symptoms

The majority of patients with African tick typhus present with features common to most rickettsial infections, including fever, severe headache, and malaise. Inoculation eschars (ulcerated lesions with a central dark scab or 'tâche noire' at the site of the tick bite) are present in the majority of patients but can be easily overlooked, especially within the hairline. In addition, in African tick-bite fever there is often prominent neck muscle myalgia, regional lymphadenitis (43%), and multiple eschars (49%). A generalized cutaneous rash is much more common in MSF (97% vs 49%), and generally occurs on day 3 of the illness.

Demographics of African tick typhus

Epidemiological data suggest that *Rickettsia africae* exists widely throughout sub-Saharan Africa and the eastern Caribbean. It is the most widespread and commonest of the pathogenic spotted fever group of rickettsiae. It is thought that most rural indigenous populations are infected in childhood with mild clinical disease. However, it is increasingly reported amongst travellers to endemic areas, and seroprevalence studies in travellers have shown incidence rates of up to 5%.

In Africa, *Rickettsia conorii* occurs mainly in Algeria, Morocco, Egypt, and Libya, but has also been isolated in countries such as Kenya, Zimbabwe, and South Africa. Infection in humans in sub-Saharan Africa is much less common, however, as the ticks are more host specific.

Natural history of African tick typhus, and complications, of the disease

The mean incubation period is usually 6 days for both infections and, in African tick-bite fever, complications, such as reactive arthritis, are rare. However, in MSF, severe forms of the infection occur in up to 6% of cases; in addition, neurological, renal, and cardiovascular complications are common, with a mortality rate as high as 2.5%.

Approach to diagnosing African tick typhus

African tick typhus should be considered in any febrile traveller returning from sub-Saharan Africa, particularly when an eschar, lymphadenitis, or rash is present.

Other diagnoses that should be considered aside from African tick typhus

Common infections in febrile returning travellers must be considered, particularly malaria (which does not cause a rash or lymphadenopathy), typhoid, other rickettsioses, and meningococcal disease. A risk assessment should also be undertaken for the possibility of a viral haemorrhagic fever.

'Gold-standard' diagnostic test for African tick typhus

Serology with immunofluorescence is the most commonly utilized technique for diagnosing African tick typhus and is available in specialist centres. Diagnostic antibody titres are often only seen in convalescent samples and may not appear in those treated early with appropriate antibiotics.

Other diagnostic methods for African tick typhus

PCR of serum and in tissue, such as from a biopsy or swab of an eschar site, is increasingly utilized in diagnosing African tick typhus. Cell culture can also be performed from clinical specimens but has several limitations and is not routinely undertaken.

Other relevant investigations for African tick typhus

In African tick typhus, elevated levels of C-reactive protein and liver enzymes are often seen in combination with mild thrombocytopenia and lymphopenia.

Treatment of African tick typhus, and its effectiveness

The treatment of African tick typhus should be based on clinical suspicion and should not be delayed for confirmatory serology. The tetracycline class of antibiotics is most commonly utilized, with a high degree of efficacy and minimal toxicity. A standard regimen is doxycycline 200 mg daily for up to 14 days. Alternatives include chloramphenicol and macrolides.

Q fever

Definition of Q fever

Q (for 'query') fever is so called because, for many years, its cause was unknown. It is a zoonosis caused by the Gram-negative intracellular coccobacillus *Coxiella burnetii*. Its diagnosis can be difficult, due to the variety of clinical presentations, and the delay involved in serological confirmation.

Aetiology of Q fever

Coxiella burnetii is widespread globally, except in New Zealand, and has a resistant spore-like form which survives for prolonged periods in the environment. A wide variety of ticks, birds, rodents, and wild mammals can be infected, but domestic ruminants (sheep, cattle, and goats) are the most frequent sources of human infection.

Aerosols are the major route of transmission to humans, either from direct exposure to infected tissues or from indirect exposure through contaminated dust. However, direct contact with animals is not required.

Typical symptoms of Q fever, and less common symptoms

The most typical manifestation of Q fever is an undifferentiated febrile illness similar to influenza, but other common presentations include atypical pneumonia and hepatitis. The hepatitis is usually asymptomatic; however, patients with only mild biochemical abnormalities may have significant histological changes, and hepatic coma and death has been reported.

Neurological symptoms are recognized in 4%-22% of all Q fever cases, with meningoencephalitis, meningitis, and myelitis being the most common neurological presentations. Chronic malaise and fatigue may persist for months after the acute illness.

Demographics of Q fever

In the UK, 5% of the population have serological evidence of past exposure to Q fever, rising to ~15% in farmers. However only 50–100 cases of Q fever are reported each year, due to many cases being asymptomatic, or mild and under-investigated. Outbreaks have occurred in a variety of settings.

Q fever is associated with certain risk occupations, including farming, working in an abattoir, and meat packing, but, frequently, there is no history of obvious exposure. Pregnancy, valvular heart disease, and immunosuppression are factors associated with more severe disease and progression to chronic infection.

Natural history of Q fever, and complications of the disease

The incubation period of Q fever is between 7 and 30 days; most patients make a complete recovery, and death is rare. The main complication is chronic infection that presents months to several years after the initial infection. This occurs in 1%–5% of patients, and in 60%–70% results in endocarditis, which develops more slowly than other forms of infective endocarditis and which frequently relapses, despite prolonged antibiotic treatment.

Approach to diagnosing Q fever

Q fever should be considered in any acute febrile illness, atypical pneumonia, or aseptic meningitis. Laboratory clues include raised transaminases and thrombocytopenia. Chronic infection should also be considered in all those with a 'culture-negative' endocarditis.

'Gold-standard' diagnostic test for Q fever

Serology using indirect immunofluorescence is the most accurate and readily available diagnostic test for Q fever. Antibodies may be detected 2–3 weeks after the onset of the disease, and tests should be performed on both acute and convalescent samples. Phase I IgG of ≥1:800 at 6 months is considered diagnostic of chronic infection and is one of the major modified Duke criteria for endocarditis.

Other diagnostic methods for Q fever

Culture for Q fever is not routine, and requires Biosafety Level 3 laboratories, but is available from specialist laboratories. PCR can also identify *Coxiella burnetii* in blood, urine, and tissue samples. Complement fixation tests are available but are less specific and sensitive.

Other relevant investigations for Q fever

All patients with confirmed Q fever should have a transthoracic echocardiogram, but it is recognized that cardiac vegetations are evident in only 12% of patients with chronic infection. Repeat serological testing looking for evidence of progression to chronic infection should be undertaken.

Prognosis for Q fever

Death is rare in acute infection and, with effective antibiotic therapy for endocarditis, mortality is less than 10%. However, relapse rates of over 50% after cessation of antibiotic therapy can occur, and delay in diagnosis has an important effect on the prognosis of chronic Q fever.

Treatment of Q fever, and its effectiveness

Tetracycline or doxycycline is the treatment of choice in acute Q fever, but fluoroquinolones should be used for patients with neurological symptoms because of their better penetration of the CNS. Co-trimoxazole is used in women who are pregnant or breast feeding, and in children under 12.

Rarely, severe cases of hepatitis may require additional treatment with corticosteroids. The first line treatment of Q fever endocarditis is a combination of doxycycline and hydroxychloroquine, for a minimum of 18 months depending on serological response.

Further Reading

Jensenius M, Fournier PE, Kelly P, et al. African tick bite fever. *Lancet Infect Dis* 2003; 3: 557–64.

Kersh GJ. Antimicrobial therapies for Q fever. Expert Rev *Anti Infect Ther* 2013; 11: 1207–14.

Paris DH and Dumler JS. State of the art of diagnosis of rickettsial diseases: the use of blood specimens for diagnosis of scrub typhus, spotted fever group rickettsiosis, and murine typhus. *Curr Opin Infect Dis* 2016; 29: 433–9.

Schneeberger PM, Wintenberger C, van der Hoek W, et al. Q fever in the Netherlands - 2007-2010: what we learned from the largest outbreak ever. *Med Mal Infect* 2014; 44: 339–53.

315 Fungal infection

Stacy Todd and Nick Beeching

Introduction

Fungi, comprising yeasts, moulds, and higher fungi have a worldwide distribution and are uncommon causes of disease in healthy individuals. However, over the last 20 years invasive fungal disease (IFD) has become an increasing cause of morbidity and mortality. This is probably due to the increasing numbers of patients with underlying host conditions, which predispose to opportunistic IFD (e.g. transplant and anti-tumour necrosis factor immunosuppression, HIV, or chronic lung disease), and to increased recognition of endemic IFD (e.g. histoplasmosis), which cause disease in both immunocompetent and immunocompromised hosts in selected geographic locations.

Diagnosis of IFD remains a challenge. Symptoms are often non-specific, and a definite diagnosis requires invasive sampling with appropriate laboratory testing of these samples. Non-invasive tests are being developed, but their positive and negative predictive values still need validation. Diagnostic criteria ('proven, probable and possible' (see Table 315.1) established primarily for use in research, and clinical trials can also prove useful in clinical environments. However, the most important step in identifying patients with IFD is to consider the diagnosis in those at risk.

This chapter will focus on the commonest causes of IFD: *Candida* spp., *Aspergillus* spp., *Cryptococcus* spp., and histoplasmosis.

Aspergillus infection

Definition of aspergillosis

Aspergillosis is classically divided into invasive, saprophytic, and allergic disease. Invasive aspergillosis typically enters via the respiratory tract, sinuses, or skin, and can reach other tissues via direct extension or haematogenous spread. Saprophytic disease includes otomycotic disease and aspergilloma. Allergic disease includes aspergillus sinusitis and allergic bronchopulmonary aspergillosis (ABPA).

Aetiology of aspergillosis

Aspergillus spp. comprise a globally recognized family of moulds which grow in oxygen-rich environments such as air-conditioning units, hospital environments, and decaying vegetation. *Aspergillus fumigatus* is the most common pathogenic species, but an increasing number of non-fumigatus species are known to cause disease.

Typical symptoms of aspergillosis, and less common symptoms

Invasive aspergillosis typically presents with non-specific features of pneumonia, such as fever, cough, and dyspnoea. Pleuritic chest pain and haemoptysis are reported, particularly when there has been vascular invasion. Tracheobronchitis can cause lobar collapse if pseudomembranes develop. In neutropenic patients, persistent fever may be the only symptom of invasive aspergillosis.

Extra-pulmonary aspergillosis can cause sinusitis or skin lesions, progressing to local invasion to cause meningitis, renal, and hepatic dysfunction. Chronic saprophytic disease presents with haemoptysis, or may be found incidentally when imaging is performed for other reasons. Osteomyelitis, prosthetic device infections, and endophthalmitis have been reported.

ABPA presents with wheeze, chronic productive cough, fever, and anorexia, or may be suspected due to inappropriately high eosinophilia in asthmatics.

Demographics of aspergillosis

Host factors which predispose to invasive aspergillosis include:

- decreased quantity or function of neutrophils due to myeloablative chemotherapy and corticosteroids
- immunological biological agents such as anti-tumour necrosis factor agents
- haemopoetic stem cell transplant patients, particularly those who have acquired cytomegalovirus or have severe graft versus host disease
- solid organ transplant patients.

Invasive aspergillosis has also been reported in critically ill patients without preexisting immunocompromise.

Conditions which increase the risk of other forms of aspergillus disease include preexisting structural lung disease (bronchiectasis/previous tuberculosis) leading to a chronic necrotizing aspergillosis, and/or aspergilloma. Patients with asthma and cystic fibrosis are at increased risk of ABPA, although there is likely to be a genetic component involved in whether a patient will go on to develop ABPA after colonization.

Natural history of aspergillosis, and complications of the disease

Invasive aspergillosis is almost universally fatal if it is not identified and if appropriate treatment is not commenced early. The initial presentation is normally with pulmonary disease, which can progress to haemorrhagic infarction and necrotizing pneumonia. Inadequate therapy can lead to CNS involvement or direct extension into intrathoracic structures. Recent improvements in survival have been due to alterations in the levels of immunosuppression used for transplantation, increased awareness of the disease, use of prophylaxis, and early empirical treatment.

Approach to diagnosing aspergillosis

There is a high index of suspicion of aspergillosis in patients who are potentially at risk of the disease.

Other diagnoses that should be considered aside from aspergillosis

Other diagnoses that should be considered aside from aspergillosis are other causes of pneumonia, including bacterial community and

---

Table 315.1 Diagnostic classification of non-endemic invasive fungal disease

Diagnostic Classification of IFD	Diagnostic Criteria
PROVEN (a OR b)	a. Histopathological documentation of infection
	b. Culture of fungal species from a normally sterile site
PROBABLE (c, d AND e) **POSSIBLE** (2 from c, d OR e)	c. Host factors including immunosuppression (neutropenia, corticosteroid use, anti-TNF agents)
	d. Clinical manifestations
	e. Microbiological evidence (direct/indirect tests, not meeting proven diagnostic criteria)

Abbreviations: IFD, invasive fungal disease; TNF, tumour necrosis factor.

Reproduced with permission from Ben De Pauw et al., Revised Definitions of Invasive Fungal Disease from the European Organization for Research and Treatment of Cancer/Invasive Fungal Infections Cooperative Group and the National Institute of Allergy and Infectious Diseases Mycoses Study Group (EORTC/MSG) Consensus Group:, Clinical Infectious Diseases, Volume 46, Issue 12, pp. 1813–21, Copyright © 2008 Oxford University Press.

nosocomial organisms (e.g. *Nocardia* spp.), mycobacterial, and viral causes. Pulmonary emboli and adult respiratory distress syndrome can also present with similar symptoms in critically ill patients.

'Gold-standard' diagnostic test for aspergillosis

The gold-standard diagnostic test for aspergillosis is a fungal culture and/or histopathology from tissue samples, typically taken at bronchoscopy or rhinoscopy, or samples taken from a normally sterile environment (e.g. pleural fluid).

Acceptable diagnostic alternatives to the gold-standard test for aspergillosis

Chest X-rays are often normal, so it is important to perform to chest CT early. Characteristic (but not pathognomonic) changes of invasive aspergillosis include early pulmonary nodules, macro-nodules with surrounding ground-glass changes ('halo sign'), and air crescent signs. Other non-specific pulmonary signs include consolidation, infarcts, and cavitation. In patients with tracheobronchitis, collapse and pseudomembranes are seen, along with 'tree and bud' appearances. Fungal balls and cavities can also be seen on CT, when investigating aspergillomas.

Increasing availability of galactomannan antigen testing provides a useful adjunct to diagnosis of invasive aspergillosis. It can be measured in bronchoalveolar lavage fluid, CSF, plasma, and fluid, with a sensitivity of 71% and specificity of 89% in serum for patients with haemopoetic stem cell transplants. False positives occur with concomitant use of piperacillin/tazobactam, and there is cross-reactivity with other fungal species. Serial testing is preferred.

Identification of fungal elements in sputum, bronchoalveolar lavage fluid, and sinus aspirate can also indicate invasive aspergillus disease.

Other relevant investigations for aspergillosis

CT of the head and sinuses may also be helpful. Bronchoscopy is useful, not only to obtain samples for culture and histology, but also to look for typical macroscopic appearances of tracheobronchitis.

Elevated IgE aspergillus-precipitins are useful for the diagnosis of ABPA, but not for the diagnosis of invasive aspergillosis. Blood cultures are seldom positive, even in cases of endocarditis.

Prognosis of aspergillosis, and how to estimate it

Invasive aspergillosis can rapidly be fatal. Improved outcomes at 6 weeks are reported in those not having myeloablative treatments, and those not requiring invasive ventilation or renal support.

Treatment of aspergillosis and its effectiveness

First-line treatment for invasive aspergillosis is normally with voriconazole, which is superior to liposomal amphotericin B. Newer agents such as caspofungin and other echinocandins can be used as salvage therapy. Oral itraconazole has been used particularly in chronic cavitatory pulmonary aspergillosis. Fluconazole is not effective against *Aspergillus* spp., but there may be a role for newer agents such as posaconazole or isavuconazole in some patients.

Aspergillomas do not respond to antifungal medication and may require surgical resection. ABPA is usually treated with corticosteroids alone; occasionally, systemic antifungal drugs such as itraconazole are used, but only in the context of severe disease and after consultation with experts.

Candida infection

Definition of candidiasis

Candidiasis can be divided into mucocutaneous disease, focal infection in specific organs, or fungaemia/invasive disease.

Aetiology of candidiasis

Candida spp. are the commonest cause of IFD worldwide. Although the dominant pathogen has been *C. albicans*, other species including *C. glabrata*, *C. tropicalis*, and *C. krusei* have emerged over the last 15 years. *Candida* spp. are commensal organisms of the gastrointestinal tract and, occasionally, of the skin. Infection is normally due to invasion by these commensal organisms, rather than new infection.

Typical symptoms of candidiasis, and less common symptoms

Typical symptoms depend on the site of infection. In mucocutaneous disease, classical white plaques are seen on the hard palate; dysphagia and odynophagia are the hallmarks of oesophageal candidiasis. Genitourinary candidiasis presents with dysuria, vaginal discharge, and itch. Visual loss is a presenting feature of endophthalmitis.

Invasive candidiasis normally presents as fever and/or sepsis syndrome with no obvious source. Some patients, particularly those who are neutropenic, can present with a disseminated papulonodular rash, which is a sign of disseminated disease.

Demographics of candidiasis

As the pathogen is normally a commensal, the precipitating factor is a change in the patient's own host defences, especially the development of neutropenia. Others at a higher risk include those who have had broad-spectrum antibiotics, or who have total parenteral nutrition, recent gastrointestinal surgery, haemodialysis, or indwelling vascular catheters. Although mucocutaneous candidiasis is relatively common in HIV, invasive candidiasis only tends to occur when a patient is extremely immunosuppressed.

Natural history and complications of candidiasis

Untreated candidaemia has a high mortality. Even with treatment, mortality can be as high as 50% in neutropenic patients. Candidaemia which is not detected early can result in dissemination to other tissues, leading to endophthalmitis, endocarditis, bone and joint involvement, and meningitis.

Chronic mucocutaneous candidiasis can be a sign of underlying immunosuppression, and should prompt further investigation. Depending on the cause, it does not normally affect mortality, but can cause considerable morbidity and distress to patients.

Approach to diagnosing candidiasis

There is a high index of suspicion of candidiasis in patients who are potentially at risk of this disease. Ophthalmoscopy should be performed in all patients with suspected or proven candidaemia.

Other diagnoses that should be considered aside from candidiasis

Other diagnoses that should be considered aside from candidiasis are other causes of fever in neutropenic patients, including bacteria (community and nosocomial organisms (e.g. *Nocardia* spp.)), mycobacteria, and viruses. Non-resolving mucocutaneous lesions should also prompt investigations for underlying malignancy, HIV, and diabetes mellitus.

'Gold-standard' diagnostic test for candidiasis

Candida spp. grow readily in standard culture media and on blood agar plates, as well as special media such as Sabouraud's agar. Identification of these organisms in normally sterile fluids such as blood or CSF should prompt early treatment. Production of germ tubes in culture is a simple test to distinguish *C. albicans* from other species, which are more likely to have antifungal resistance.

Acceptable diagnostic alternatives to the gold-standard test for candidiasis

Identification of *Candida* spp. in environments such as sputum, bronchoalveolar lavage fluid, urine, and skin swabs should be interpreted with caution, as most isolates will be commensals rather than pathogens. When *Candida* spp. have been isolated, clinicians should consider whether the patient is in a high-risk group, whether the organism has been isolated on more than one occasion, and whether there are any other causes for the symptoms.

Other relevant investigations for candidiasis

Histological findings consistent with candidiasis, such as hyphae and pseudohyphae in tissue samples, can help with diagnosis. However, there is no role at present for serological assays in the diagnosis of candidiasis, although tests are in development.

Prognosis of candidiasis, and how to estimate it

Invasive candidiasis has a poor outcome. Patients with a *Candida* spp. isolated from blood cultures have a twofold higher mortality rate than those with non-candidal blood stream infection. Worse outcomes are associated with delayed commencement of therapy and inadequate antifungal regimens.

Treatment of candidiasis and its effectiveness

Empirical treatment for candidaemia/invasive candidiasis is with an echinocandin agent such as caspofungin. Fluconazole can be considered for non-neutropenic patients who are not critically ill and who are not considered to be at high risk for fluconazole resistance. Liposomal amphotericin B is an alternative in the case of intolerance or lack of availability of other treatments. Best practice is to remove all invasive venous catheters and to treat for a minimum of 14 days after blood culture clearance. Oral step down to fluconazole can be considered once the patient is clinically stable but should be managed in consultation with an infection specialist.

For oesophageal candidiasis, oral fluconazole or amphotericin are the first choice, although echinocandins may be used. A single dose of fluconazole is normally sufficient for uncomplicated vaginal candidiasis.

Cryptococcal infection

Definition of cryptococcosis

Cryptococcosis, also known as cryptococcus disease, is caused by dissemination of *Cryptococcus* spp.

Aetiology of cryptococcosis

Cryptococcus neoformans and *C. gatti* are the major causes of disseminated cryptococcosis. They are encapsulated yeasts, which are inhaled from the environment. *C. neoformans* is found worldwide and, although *C. gatti* was thought to be tropical and subtropical in origin, it has recently been implicated in outbreaks in the north-west United States and Canada. The clinical disease pattern caused by these organisms is similar, and laboratories do not normally speciate further than *Cryptococcus* spp.

Typical symptoms of cryptococcosis, and less common symptoms

The primary route of infection is via inhalation and subsequent haematogenous dissemination. CNS infection is the most dangerous presentation, and often has a prolonged, indolent course with headache, mild confusion, or behavioural change. Focal neurological signs are a sign of late disease and should prompt rapid investigation and treatment. Pulmonary disease can vary from asymptomatic infection, to typical pneumonic symptoms, to disease patterns which can mimic pneumocystis pneumonia. Cutaneous manifestations of disseminated disease are relatively common, with pustular, nodular, umbilicated, or ulcerated lesions.

Cryptococcal infection can also disseminate to other organs, including the long bones, the liver, the kidneys, and the spleen. However, it is unusual for such dissemination to present symptomatically in the absence of other signs. There is a relative lack of inflammation associated with invasive cryptococcosis, so high fever and very high inflammatory markers are not common.

Demographics of cryptococcosis

The majority of patients presenting with cryptococcosis are immunosuppressed in some way, but some patients with invasive disease (particularly *C. gatti*) have a normal immune system. Cryptococcal disease is an AIDS-defining illness, and its increase in prevalence over the last 35 years has mainly followed the HIV pandemic.

Natural history and complications of cryptococcosis

Untreated cryptococcal meningitis is universally fatal. Since the introduction of antiretroviral therapy and combination antifungal treatment, this has improved dramatically, but there is still an acute mortality of 6%–15% related to complications, such as raised intracranial pressure and immune reconstitution inflammatory syndrome (IRIS). In non-HIV immunosuppressed states, acute mortality is 15%–21%. Up to 40% of patients who survive the initial illness have significant neurological complications such as hydrocephalus, blindness, and cognitive impairment. Relapses can occur in 20%–25% of patients, particularly if they remain immunosuppressed.

Approach to diagnosing cryptococcosis

There is a high index of suspicion in patients who are potentially at risk of invasive cryptococcosis.

Other diagnoses that should be considered aside from cryptococcosis

In CNS disease, other causes of meningoencephalitis with a long prodrome, such as syphilis, toxoplasmosis, and tuberculosis, should be considered, in addition to cryptococcosis. Pulmonary cryptococcosis can easily be confused with pneumocystis pneumonia or other causes of pneumonia in the immunocompromised host. Skin manifestations of cryptococcosis can easily be mistaken for malignancy, molluscum contagiosum, or invasive yeast infections other than cryptococcosis, such as histoplasmosis or talaromycosis (penicilliosis). HIV testing should always be performed.

'Gold-standard' diagnostic test for cryptococcosis

The gold-standard diagnostic test for cryptococcosis is fungal culture from CSF, blood, urine, or skin.

Acceptable diagnostic alternatives to the gold-standard test for cryptococcosis

An acceptable diagnostic alternative to fungal culture is the cryptococcal antigen (CrAG) assay, which is available for testing both serum and CSF. Serum tests are positive in >99% of patients with disseminated invasive cryptococcosis. Although this assay is highly sensitive when used to test the CSF, it may be negative when there is non-meningeal disseminated cryptococcosis.

India ink stains of the CSF are less sensitive than the CrAG assay but may be more readily available in low-income settings.

Other relevant investigations for cryptococcosis

CT or MRI brain scans are useful to rule out cryptococcomas and should be considered prior to lumbar puncture, due to risks associated with raised intracranial pressure. When a lumbar puncture is performed, there is generally a marked increase in opening pressure with mild increase in protein, lymphocytosis (although the white-cell count can be normal), and low glucose ratio.

For pulmonary disease, chest CT should be considered.

Prognosis for cryptococcosis, and how to estimate it

CNS cryptococcosis can be rapidly fatal if not identified. Better outcomes can be expected if immunosuppression can be reversed. Patients with positive CrAG and evidence of disease elsewhere should have a lumbar puncture, even in the absence of CNS symptoms, to assess for evidence of meningitis.

Treatment of cryptococcosis, and its effectiveness

For patients with CNS disease and/or severe respiratory disease, the standard first-line treatment is IV amphotericin (liposomal if high risk of renal disease), with IV/oral flucytosine for a minimum of 2 weeks. This should be followed by up to 8 weeks' oral fluconazole 400 mg daily, to give a total 10-week induction course. This is then followed by long-term prophylaxis oral fluconazole 200 mg daily for at least 12 months, and until the CD4 cell count is >100 x 10⁶/l. For mild/moderate pulmonary disease, treatment is with fluconazole 400 mg daily for 6–12 months, and then prophylaxis until the CD4 cell count is >100 x 10⁶/l.

In HIV-negative immunosuppression, treat CNS disease with a 10-week induction period. Fluconazole prophylaxis should continue for 6–12 months after this induction phase.

Most immunocompetent people who have only pulmonary disease will settle with no treatment, but some require short courses of fluconazole to prevent haematogenous spread.

Management of complications such as raised intracranial pressure (via therapeutic lumbar puncture, often repeatedly) and IRIS (via corticosteroids) should always be considered.

Histoplasmosis infection

Definition of histoplasmosis

Histoplasmosis is caused by infection with variants of the fungus *Histoplasma capsulatum*.

Aetiology of histoplasmosis

Histoplasma capsulatum is an endemic dimorphic fungus that is found worldwide. The disease is most commonly reported in North and Central America (var. *capsulatum*), and Africa (var. *duboisii*).

Typical symptoms of histoplasmosis, and less common symptoms

Acute pulmonary histoplasmosis most commonly occurs when an individual is exposed to histoplasma organisms for the first time. Symptoms typically include dry cough, chest tightness, fevers, headaches, and malaise. Joint and skin involvement is seen in 5% of patients, and erythema nodosum or erythema multiforme can occur. In more severe cases, it can progress to acute respiratory distress syndrome.

Chronic cavitatory histoplasmosis presents with symptoms and signs similar to pulmonary TB with apical cavitatory changes. Disseminated histoplasmosis involves an indolent course with progressive hepatosplenomegaly, bone marrow involvement, and non-specific symptoms of fever, malaise, and weight loss.

Less commonly, histoplasmosis can cause pericarditis, meningitis, and granulomatous mediastinitis. Compared with other disseminated fungal diseases, histoplasmosis is more likely to cause peri-oral or mucous membrane involvement. It can present with addisonism, due to adrenal necrosis. Disseminated skin lesions may be papular or umbilicated.

Demographics of histoplasmosis

Within endemic areas, up to 80% of the population have serological evidence of exposure. The fungus is found in nitrogen-rich soil, in association with bird or bat faeces. Disease tends to occur when a person from an endemic area becomes immunosuppressed, or in non-immune visitors to endemic settings. Outbreaks have been reported when soil has been disturbed on a large scale, causing aerosolization. Exploration of bat-infested caves is a risk factor.

Natural history and complications of histoplasmosis

Histoplasmosis is usually a self-limiting condition which does not require treatment, but is occasionally fatal in severe disease. Chronic cavitatory disease is often fatal, because of pulmonary damage, rather that unopposed infection. Progressive disseminated disease is fatal in >90% of patients if untreated.

Approach to diagnosing histoplasmosis

There is a high index of suspicion of histoplasmosis in patients who are potentially at risk of the disease.

Other diagnoses that should be considered aside from histoplasmosis

In acute pulmonary disease, other causes of atypical pneumonia, aside from *Histoplasma capsulatum*, should be considered, including other fungi and *Mycoplasma pneumoniae*. In chronic cavitatory disease, major differential diagnoses include TB, non-TB mycobacteria, sarcoidosis, malignancy, and other chronic fungal lung conditions. Disseminated histoplasmosis can mimic a variety of conditions (e.g. miliary TB), particularly in the immunocompromised. Skin lesions due to histoplasmosis can mimic umbilicated lesions from other infections, such as cryptococcosis. HIV testing should be done.

'Gold-standard' diagnostic test for histoplasmosis

The gold-standard diagnostic test for histoplasmosis is fungal culture from blood or body tissue. The CSF usually remains sterile in histoplasma meningitis.

Acceptable diagnostic alternatives to the gold-standard test for histoplasmosis

An acceptable diagnostic alternative to fungal culture is histology of body tissue, as this will often show the characteristic appearances of histoplasmosis (small, oval budding yeasts), especially when silver-based or other special stains are used. Paired antigen testing of urine and serum has proved helpful in diagnoses, but there is cross-reactivity with other fungal diseases; in addition, these tests are not readily available.

Other relevant investigations for histoplasmosis

Other relevant investigations in histoplasmosis include plain chest X-rays or CT scans, as these can show a diffuse reticulonodular picture in acute disease with some perihilar lymphadenopathy. However, these changes are often fleeting, and may be absent by the time the patient presents. Chronic disease typically causes calcified cavities in the apices. In disseminated disease, other infected tissues beyond the lungs can also be abnormal. In meningitis, multiple enhancing lesions are often located around the basal meninges.

Prognosis for histoplasmosis, and how to estimate it

Histoplasmosis is usually a self-limiting condition, but patients on immunosuppressive treatments and those with HIV have a more rapid disease onset and worse prognosis. Even with treatment, up to 50% of HIV-positive patients die from disseminated disease. Other predictors of a worse outcome include fungaemia, renal impairment, and extremes of age.

Treatment of histoplasmosis and its effectiveness

Acute pulmonary histoplasmosis

For mild-to-moderate acute pulmonary histoplasmosis, no treatment is required, unless symptoms persist for >1 month; in this case, use itraconazole 200 mg three times daily for 3 days, and then 200 mg daily for 6–12 weeks. For moderately severe to severe disease, use liposomal amphotericin B (3–5 mg/kg) daily for 1–2 weeks, and then itraconazole 200 mg, initially three times daily for 3 days and then daily for a total of 12 weeks; methylprednisolone should also be used during the first 1–2 weeks if severe respiratory compromise is a problem.

Chronic cavitatory pulmonary histoplasmosis

For chronic cavitatory pulmonary histoplasmosis, use itraconazole 200 mg three times daily for 3 days, and then once or twice daily for 12 months (some recommend for 18–24 months).

Disseminated histoplasmosis

For mild-to-moderate disseminated histoplasmosis in adults, use itraconazole 200 mg three times daily for 3 days, and then twice daily for 12 months. For moderately severe to severe disease, use liposomal amphotericin B (3 mg/kg) daily for 1–2 weeks, then itraconazole 200 mg three times daily for 3 days, and then daily for total of at least 12 months. Patients may need to stay on long-term suppressive therapy if it is not possible to correct/stop immunosuppression.

Complications, such as joint involvement and skin manifestations, should be treated with NSAIDs or prednisolone if uncontrolled.

Further Reading

Adams P. Cryptococcal meningitis: a blind spot in curbing AIDS. *Lancet* 2016; 387: 1605–6.

Denning DW and Chakrabarti A. Pulmonary and sinus fungal diseases in non-immunocompromised patients. *Lancet Infect Dis* 2017; 17: e357–e366.

De Pauw B, Walsh TJ, Donnelly JP, et al. Revised definitions of invasive fungal disease from the European Organization for Research and Treatment of Cancer/Invasive Fungal Infections Cooperative Group and the National Institute of Allergy and Infectious Diseases Mycoses Study Group (EORTC/MSG) Consensus Group. *Clin Infect Dis* 2008; 46: 1813–21.

Pappas PG, Kauffman CA, Andes DR, et al. Clinical practice guideline for the management of candidiasis: 2016 update by the Infectious Diseases Society of America. *Clin Infect Dis* 2016; 62: e1–e50.

Perfect JR, Dismukes WE, Dromer F, et al. Clinical practice guidelines for the management of cryptococcal disease: 2010 update by the Infectious Disease Society of America. *Clin Infect Dis* 2010; 50: 291–322.

Patterson KC and Strek ME. Diagnosis and treatment of pulmonary aspergillosis syndromes. *Chest* 2014; 146: 1358–68.

Patterson TF, Thompson GR, Denning DW, et al. Practice guidelines for the diagnosis and management of aspergillosis: 2016 update by the Infectious Diseases Society of America. *Clin Infect Dis* 2016; 63: e1–e60.

Segal BH. Aspergillosis. *N Engl J Med* 2009; 360: 1870–84.

Wheat LG, Freifeld AG, Kleiman MB, et al. Clinical practice guidelines for the management of patients with histoplasmosis: 2007 update by the Infectious Diseases Society of America. *Clin Infect Dis* 2007; 45: 807–25.

316 Protozoal infection: Gut organisms

Pavithra Natarajan and Nick Beeching

Definition of the diseases

Protozoa are single-celled (unicellular) eukaryotic organisms. There are many protozoa causing parasitic infection in humans. This chapter will concentrate on the three that most commonly cause gastrointestinal disease worldwide and have the biggest impact in the UK: *Giardia lamblia*, *Cryptosporidium* spp., and *Entamoeba histolytica*.

These three infections are of great significance worldwide, but are less common in Western settings. In the UK, they tend to be seen in more commonly in travellers returning from endemic countries, migrant populations, men who have sex with men, and the immunocompromised. The clinical features of all three infections vary from asymptomatic small- or large-bowel carriage with passage of cysts to infect others, to more serious manifestations.

Giardiasis

Aetiology of giardiasis

Giardia lamblia (also known as *Giardia intestinalis* and *Giardia duodenalis*) is a flagellated, binucleated protozoan that attaches to the small bowel mucosa and can cause subtotal villous atrophy. Infection is complicated by transient lactase intolerance. Transmission is by ingestion of cysts that are relatively resistant to chlorination and remain viable for several weeks in water, and is most commonly from contaminated water. Person-to-person spread can occur in settings of poor faeco-oral hygiene; less commonly, food-borne spread can occur. Chronic recurrent infections complicate inherited disorders of immunoglobulin production (e.g. Bruton's disease.) but not HIV infection.

Typical symptoms of giardiasis, and less common symptoms

The incubation period for giardiasis is 1–2 weeks. The spectrum of disease ranges from asymptomatic infection to chronic diarrhoea or steatorrhoea, with cramping upper abdominal pain and flatulence. This may result in malabsorption and weight loss, especially in children with a poor underlying level of nutrition, or those with preexisting lactase small bowel deficiency. Prolonged illness can cause folate and vitamin B_{12} deficiency.

Demographics of giardiasis

Giardiasis has a worldwide distribution, with an estimated 2–3 million infections per year. It is a common cause of post-travel diarrhoea.

Natural history of giardiasis, and complications of the disease

Infection is usually self-limiting, but it has been suggested that giardiasis may trigger functional irritable bowel disease.

Approach to diagnosing giardiasis, and other diagnoses that should be considered

Apart from other bowel infections, causes of malabsorption should be considered, including coeliac disease and pancreatic disease.

'Gold-standard' diagnostic test for giardiasis, and acceptable diagnostic alternatives

Microscopic examination of concentrated faecal samples is the gold standard for all three of these infections. This is labour intensive and requires specific expertise, and intermittent excretion of cysts can hamper diagnosis and require examination of multiple stool samples. The laboratory request should always include travel history or other reasons to request parasitological investigation. Multiplex real-time PCR tests are being introduced by many laboratories to detect all three pathogens simultaneously.

Giardia cysts and trophozoites can usually be seen on faecal microscopy, the sensitivity of which is improved using direct antibody fluorescence. Faecal antigen detection (e.g. by EIAs) is more sensitive, and a variety of molecular assays are increasingly being used. Serology has no role in diagnosis. Trophozoites may be seen in aspirates of contents or biopsies from small bowel.

Treatment for giardiasis, and its effectiveness

Giardiasis is often self-limiting, but treatment of symptomatic patients reduces the severity and duration of the disease. Metronidazole or tinidazole are the treatments of choice, and alternatives include paromomycin, albendazole, or nitazoxanide. Rarely, mepacrine (called quinacrine in the US) is used, for severe cases. Refractory cases may respond to exclusion of dietary lactose for 2 weeks during treatment, and treatment of close contacts to prevent reinfection.

Cryptosporidiosis

Aetiology of cryptosporidiosis

Cryptosporidium parvum and *Cryptosporidium hominis* are the two most common species causing human infections. They are acquired through the faeco-oral route, by ingestion of oocysts containing infective sporozoites. Oocysts are highly resistant to chlorination and can survive for prolonged periods in water and damp soil. Person-to-person spread can also occur. Cryptosporidiosis is a zoonosis which can be contracted from contact with a variety of animals, especially calves in petting zoos and other farm animals, or by ingestion of water contaminated by animal faeces. The sporozoites of cryptosporidia invade the epithelial cells of the small bowel and undergo a complex life cycle that includes auto-reinfection, as well as a sexual life cycle leading to shedding of oocysts in faeces. Severe infections occur in a variety of immunosuppressive states, including severe combined immunodeficiency (SCID), advanced HIV, and inherited immunoglobulin deficiency states, as well as in transplant and chemotherapy patients. In some of these patients, biliary carriage occurs and is difficult to eradicate.

Typical of cryptosporidiosis, and less common symptoms

The typical incubation period of cryptosporidiosis is 3–6 days. The spectrum of disease ranges from asymptomatic infection to watery diarrhoea, which is often associated with abdominal cramps and sometimes with nausea and vomiting. It is more severe than most types of childhood gastroenteritis, and symptoms typically continue for 10–12 days, with prolonged cyst shedding. In immunosuppressed patients, persistent, frequent large-volume watery stool output may be life-threatening. In these patients, especially those with SCID or HIV, biliary involvement can present as pancreatitis or cholangitis leading to biliary stenosis.

Demographics of cryptosporidiosis

Cryptosporidiosis occurs worldwide and is the most common protozoal cause of acute gastroenteritis in the UK, with 3000–6000 laboratory-confirmed cases annually. It can be responsible for large waterborne outbreaks caused by contaminated drinking water (as ordinary water disinfection processes do not kill cryptosporidia), as well as outbreaks associated with swimming pools. It can affect any age group, although it is more common in children under 5 years of age, and more severe in the immunosuppressed. The incidence in people with HIV has decreased since the introduction of highly active antiretroviral therapy.

Natural history of cryptosporidiosis, and complications of the disease

In the immunocompetent host, cryptosporidiosis lasts for about 12 days and then tends to settle. Recurrence of symptoms can occur in up to a third of cases, due to relapse or reinfection. Immunocompromised hosts suffer from intractable diarrhoea that can be very difficult to treat and can lead to substantial weight loss and occasional biliary or pancreatic disease.

Approach to diagnosing cryptosporidiosis, and other diagnoses that should be considered

Cryptosporidiosis should be considered in the differential diagnosis of any community-acquired diarrhoea, especially when prolonged. Coeliac disease should be considered.

'Gold-standard' diagnostic test for cryptosporidiosis, and acceptable diagnostic alternatives

Detection of oocysts in faeces by microscopy requires special stains such as auramine, modified Ziehl–Neelsen, or trichrome stains. Such staining is not part of routine faecal microscopy in many laboratories and may need to be requested specifically. Sensitivity is improved by direct antibody fluorescent techniques and/or examination of multiple samples. Faecal antigen detection by EIA, and direct detection by PCR, are increasingly used in many laboratories. The organisms can be seen in small bowel biopsies, or in brushings from the biliary tree in immunosuppressed patients with biliary complications. Serology has no role in clinical diagnosis.

Treatment for cryptosporidiosis, and its effectiveness

Cryptosporidiosis is self-limiting in immunocompetent hosts, and treatment is not usually required. In immunosuppressed patients, reducing the degree of immunosuppression is the key to management. In patients with immunoglobulin deficiency, replacement immunoglobulin therapy stops the diarrhoea, as does raising the CD4 cell count by 50×10^6 cells/l in patients with HIV, by giving antiretroviral therapy. Protease inhibitors may have additional direct anticryptosporidial activity. Although combinations of paromomycin and azithromycin have been used in the past in severely immunosuppressed patients, there is no direct effect of these or most antimicrobials. Nitazoxanide, a cheap, broad-spectrum, antiparasitic agent available in the tropics, is effective in children and in patients with less severe immunosuppression. It is less easy to obtain and more expensive in Europe and other Western settings.

Amoebiasis

Aetiology of amoebiasis

In amoebiasis, *Entamoeba histolytica* invades the colonic mucosa, producing characteristic ulceration and dysentery (bloody diarrhoea). The first stage is attachment of the trophozoite to the human target cell. Infective cysts are passed in the stool, and transmission is by the direct faeco-oral route. Patients with abnormal lower bowel mucosa (e.g. those with inflammatory bowel disease) are more likely to experience invasive disease, especially if using topical and/or systemic steroids. There is no direct link with other types of immunodeficiency.

Typical symptoms of amoebiasis, and less common symptoms

Most *Entamoeba histolytica* infection is asymptomatic, and only a small proportion of patients go on to develop clinical disease. Intestinal manifestations include amoebic colitis, which causes diarrhoea with blood and mucus, tenesmus, and colicky abdominal pain.

Up to 10% of patients infected with *Entamoeba histolytica* may develop invasive amoebic disease. Amoebic liver abscess (ALA) is the most common form of extra-intestinal disease. This is caused by spread of infection via the portal vein to the liver, and further haematogenous spread. Patients with ALA are usually acutely unwell, presenting with symptoms including upper abdominal pain, right shoulder tip pain, and fever.

Demographics of amoebiasis

There are 48 million clinical cases of amoebiasis per year, with at least 70 000 deaths worldwide. It can be responsible for outbreaks in schools.

Natural history of amoebiasis, and complications of the disease

Amoebic dysentery is usually self-limiting, but fulminant amoebic colitis carries a high mortality. ALA can cause thoracic complications, such as pleural effusion and rupture into the bronchial tree or pericardium. In addition, ALA may rupture into the abdomen or become secondarily infected. Uncommonly, an amoeboma may develop as a granuloma, often localized in the ascending colon.

Approach to diagnosing of amoebiasis, and other diagnoses that should be considered

When diagnosing amoebiasis, exclude other infections that can cause blood in stool, such as shigellosis or campylobacteriosis. Intestinal amoebiasis may mimic inflammatory bowel disease, from which it must be distinguished, because giving corticosteroids to patients with amoebic infection can have disastrous consequences, such as toxic megacolon, or perineal invasion. The main differential diagnoses of ALA are pyogenic liver abscess, and liver neoplasm.

'Gold-standard' diagnostic test for amoebiasis, and acceptable diagnostic alternatives

Invasive colonic disease is confirmed by immediate examination of fresh faeces or scrapings of rectal mucus (i.e. within 30 minutes or less after stool passage (the 'hot stool')). This is essential to visualize mobile trophozoites containing ingested red cells: these rapidly encyst once exposed to the cold. Cysts of *Entamoeba histolytica* are morphologically identical to those of the non-pathogenic amoeba *Entamoeba dispar*, which is much more common, and a frequent reason for over-diagnosis of amoebiasis. The two can be distinguished using commercial antigen detection kits or PCR.

Serology is useful in diagnosis of ALA and severe colonic disease, but may be negative in uncomplicated dysentery. In ALA, peripheral neutrophilia is common, and changes at the right lung base are common on chest X-ray. Ultrasonography of the liver is essential if ALA is suspected. Faecal examinations have no role in diagnosing or excluding ALA.

Treatment for amoebiasis, and its effectiveness

Asymptomatic carriers should be treated with a bowel luminal agent to minimize the spread of disease. The most effective agents are diloxanide furoate or paromomycin, which are poorly absorbed from the intestine and reach optimal amoebicidal concentrations within the intestinal lumen. Symptomatic colonic or liver disease is treated with 'tissue amoebicides' such as metronidazole or tinidazole, which are efficiently absorbed from the small intestine and reach high tissue concentrations. These do not work against remaining intra-luminal amoebae, which must then be eliminated with a bowel luminal agent.

ALA cure can usually be managed with medical therapy alone, but therapeutic aspiration may be needed for large cysts (>10 cm in diameter), especially the minority that involve the left lobe of the liver and have a risk of sudden rupture into the pericardium, causing tamponade.

Further Reading

Checkley W, White AC Jr, Jaganath D, et al. A review of the global burden, novel diagnostics, therapeutics, and vaccine targets for cryptosporidium. *Lancet Infect Dis* 2015; 15: 85–94.

Life cycles and information for patients can be found on the websites of the American Centers for Disease Control and Prevention (https://www.cdc.gov/parasites/) and Public Health England https://www.gov.uk/topic/health-protection/infectious-diseases)

Minetti C, Chalmers RM, Beeching NJ, et al. Giardiasis. *BMJ* 2016; 355: i5369.

Pritt BS and Clark CG. Amebiasis. *Mayo Clin Proc* 2008; 83:1154–60

317 Protozoal infection: Malaria

Nick Beeching, Lynsey Goodwin, and Joanna Peters

Definition of the disease

Malaria is a devastating protozoal infection that affects more than 200 million people worldwide each year, killing up to a million. Five species of *Plasmodium* are recognized causes of human disease: *Plasmodium falciparum, Plasmodium vivax, Plasmodium ovale, Plasmodium malariae, and Plasmodium knowlesi*. In the UK, malaria is the most common imported tropical infection.

Aetiology of the disease

Malaria parasites ('sporozoites') are injected into the human bloodstream by the bite of female *Anopheles* mosquitoes (see Figure 317.1). The sporozoite is rapidly taken up by the liver, where it can multiply silently for weeks to months (extra-erythrocytic schizogony) to form a cyst-like 'pre-erythrocytic schizont' containing thousands of 'merozoites'. Eventually, the schizont ruptures, releasing merozoites into the bloodstream to invade red blood cells, where they mature and multiply in a cyclical pattern, lasting from 24 hours (*Plasmodium knowlesi*) to 72 hours (*Plasmodium malariae*). This culminates in development of intra-erythrocytic schizonts containing 8–32 merozoites,

depending on the species. The erythrocytes and schizonts are then disrupted, releasing merozoites to invade further red cells and start another multiplicative cycle. After several cycles, some intra-erythrocytic parasites differentiate into gametocytes, which fuse and undergo further multiplication within a mosquito to complete the infection cycle.

Symptoms that occur during the erythrocytic cycle are related to red-cell lysis; the release of parasite toxins/antigens; red-cell sequestration; and related tissue anoxia. The degree of parasitaemia (percentage of infected red cells) rarely exceeds 1% for all species except *Plasmodium falciparum*, which can rapidly multiply from a 1% parasitaemia to a >30% parasitaemia and also induces red-cell sequestration in the capillaries of organs such as the brain, the liver, and the kidneys, resulting in organ dysfunction. This combination of massive parasite load and red-cell sequestration makes *Plasmodium falciparum* potentially lethal in non-immune patients (i.e. those seen in the UK).

Malaria may also be transmitted by blood products, needle-stick injury, and IV drug use; in addition, occasionally, it can be transmitted transplacentally. Both perinatal transmission and the deleterious effects of malaria on intrauterine fetal growth are exacerbated by concurrent maternal HIV infection. Heterozygous haemoglobinopathies

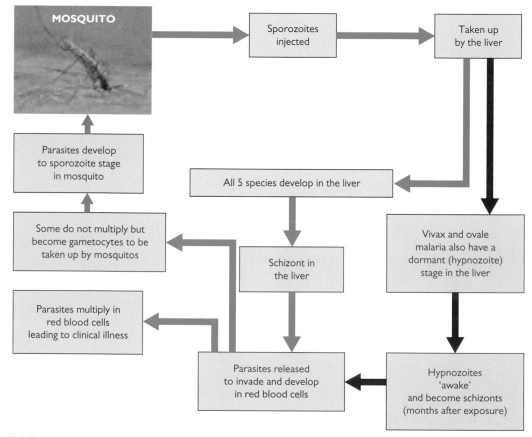

Figure 317.1 Simplified life cycle of malaria.

Adapted with permission from Public Health England: Chiodini P, Hill D, Lalloo D, et al. Guidelines for malaria prevention in travellers from the United Kingdom. London, Health Protection Agency, January 2007. ISBN: 0 901144 83 5.

such as sickle trait (haemoglobin AS) confer partial protection against *Plasmodium falciparum*, but homozygous sickle cell patients may still have lethal infections. In West Africa, most populations lack the Duffy red-cell antigen, which is used by *Plasmodium vivax* merozoites to attach to and enter the erythrocyte, so vivax infections are rare in these countries.

Typical symptoms of the disease, and less common symptoms

In an endemic area, partial immunity develops in survivors of repeated childhood infection, and asymptomatic parasitaemia is not uncommon. The main effects on children in these settings are fever with severe anaemia, respiratory distress, or coma. Rarer sequelae of chronic malaria include hyper-reactive splenomegaly and malarial nephropathy (the latter is caused by *Plasmodium malariae*).

In non-immune people who are returning to Europe from countries where malaria is endemic, the symptoms of uncomplicated malaria are similar those for influenza and may include the abrupt onset of malaise, intermittent rigors, chills, myalgia, and headache. Cough, diarrhoea, and jaundice may also be seen, and patients may not have fever at presentation. The symptoms of malaria are protean. The classical fever patterns (tertian, quartan, etc.) related to the cycle of red-cell lysis and parasite release may not be present in the first 7–10 days of infection. However, severe malaria can rapidly develop in *Plasmodium falciparum* infections, with failure of one or more organs, and may manifest as renal failure, acidosis, haemolytic anaemia, liver failure, respiratory distress syndrome, or brain involvement leading to convulsions and/or coma. Altered consciousness may also occur, due to unrecognized hypoglycaemia (see Box 317.1).

Vivax malaria can occasionally cause severe disease; this is usually respiratory distress syndrome or renal, or brain involvement. Splenic rupture is also reported. The pathophysiology of severe non-falciparum infection is poorly understood but does not relate to erythrocyte sequestration.

Demographics of the disease

Malaria is found throughout the tropics, and is making a comeback in areas where control programmes have failed. Local transmission in Greece in 2012 served as a reminder that malaria used to be endemic around the whole Mediterranean basin, extending as far north as the UK until the 1920s. Seventy-five per cent of cases in the tropics occur in children, especially in Africa. In European settings, the majority of cases occur in people who travel to visit friends or relatives in the tropics. Other tourists, business travellers, and special groups such as military personnel account for about 25% of approximately 2000 cases imported to the UK each year. Overall, about 75% of these are *Plasmodium falciparum* infections, related mostly to travel to sub-Saharan Africa, in contrast to the case in the 1970s and 1980s, when the majority of malaria cases were *Plasmodium vivax* infections imported from South Asia.

Box 317.1 Features of severe falciparum malaria in the European setting

Parasitaemia > 2%
Acidosis (pH < 7.3)
Acute renal failure
Acute Respiratory Distress Syndrome/pulmonary oedema
Coagulopathy/Disseminated Intravascular Coagulation
Haemoglobinuria
Hypoglycaemia (<2.2mol/L)
Reduced consciousness
Severe anaemia (haemoglobin < 80g/L)
Shock secondary to complicating bacteraemia/sepsis syndrome (algid malaria)

Reprinted from *Journal of Infection*, Volume 72, issue 6, David G. Lalloo, Delane Shingadia, David J. Bell, Nicholas J. Beeching, Christopher J.M. Whitty, Peter L. Chiodini, UK malaria treatment guidelines 2016, pp. 635–649, Copyright (2016), with permission from Elsevier

---

Natural history and complications of the disease

The minimum incubation period for malaria is 7–8 days, but is typically up to 2 months for *Plasmodium falciparum* infections, with exceptional cases occurring up to a year after exposure. Incubation periods for other species may be similar but are often longer, especially in vivax and ovale infections, due to the longevity of the dormant 'hypnozoite' liver stages. It is common for the first vivax symptoms to appear 9–10 months after the patient has left the tropics, and this interval may extend for up to 2 years. Untreated non-falciparum infections are usually self-limiting but may recur. In contrast, patients with falciparum malaria can appear deceptively well at presentation but be unconscious 24 hours later, with significant mortality.

Hypoglycaemia is a common complication of falciparum malaria, especially in children, in pregnant women, and in patients treated with quinine. Clinical features compatible with the more severe complications listed in Box 317.1 should be anticipated. Splenomegaly is clinically detectable in less than 50% of imported malaria cases. Malaria does not cause lymphadenopathy. Rashes and clinical bleeding diatheses are rare, although laboratory features of disseminated intravascular coagulation are common in severe malaria.

Approach to managing the disease

Malaria is a medical emergency and should be treated accordingly.

A detailed travel history extending back for at least 2 years is essential in diagnosis. Any ill traveller who has been to the tropics should have blood tests for malaria, with results available in less than half a day (preferably 2 hours). The infecting species should be determined—at least to differentiate falciparum from other species—and the degree of parasitaemia estimated.

All features of severe or complicated malaria (see Box 317.1) should be sought, including observation of respiratory rate to identify underlying respiratory distress syndrome or unrecognized metabolic acidosis, which is a marker for poor prognosis. Patients should be admitted to hospital for initial care, unless a confident diagnosis of uncomplicated non-falciparum malaria is confirmed. Patients with possible or severe falciparum malaria should be managed in a high-dependency or intensive care unit, with advice from an infection specialist if transfer to a regional infection unit is not possible. Common mistakes in such settings are delay in initiating some form of parenteral therapy, over-vigorous infusion of colloids and other IV fluids, and unnecessary transfusions of blood or platelets (see Box 317.2).

Box 317.2 Common errors in recognition and management of malaria

- delayed presentation by patient
- failure of healthcare worker to take a travel history
- failure of healthcare worker to consider malaria in symptomatic patient
- belief that chemoprophylaxis prevents all malaria
- belief that malaria is unlikely to be present, if patient does not remember being bitten by mosquitoes
- belief that absence of splenomegaly excludes malaria
- belief that absence of regular fever pattern excludes malaria
- failure to recognize non-specific clinical presentations of malaria
- failure to obtain good-quality blood film diagnosis immediately (with species diagnosis)
- failure to obtain repeat films or use ancillary diagnostic tests, if first films are negative
- failure to prescribe adequate and appropriate chemotherapy immediately
- failure to anticipate or recognize complications
- failure to treat complications
- failure to follow patient up after treatment

Adapted with permission, from Beeching NJ, Fletcher TE, Wijaya L. Returned travellers. Chapter 15 in Ed. Zuckerman JN. *Principles and Practice of Travel Medicine*, 2nd edition, John Wiley & Sons, Oxford, UK, Copyright © 2013

Other diagnoses that should be considered

In addition to malaria, many other causes of imported fever should be considered, including HIV seroconversion illness, influenza, respiratory infections, and various other tropical infectious possibilities, depending on the area visited. The pre-blood-test probability of a patient having malaria if admitted to hospital is about 60% if returning from sub-Saharan Africa, but only about 10% from South Asia. All patients with imported fever should be risk assessed for the rare possibility of a viral haemorrhagic fever, which can be excluded if the interval between the last possible exposure and the onset of symptoms is more than 21 days.

'Gold-standard' diagnostic test, and alternatives

The gold-standard diagnostic test for malaria is expert microscopy of thick and thin blood films, repeated two to three times over 24 hours if the first film is negative. Few labs have the expertise to examine thick films, which are more sensitive because more blood is examined in the microscopic field. In routine practice, rapid diagnostic tests (RDTs), which are almost as sensitive, are used to detect malarial antigens, such as parasite-specific lactate dehydrogenase, aldose, or histidine-rich protein, in a blood sample. Concurrent thin blood film examination is essential for identification of the parasite and for estimation of the parasitaemia rate. Most RDTs have good sensitivity and specificity for falciparum and vivax infections, but vary for other species, and false-negative results are possible. Molecular techniques are more sensitive and less operator-dependent, but PCR tests for malaria have not yet been standardized enough for use in routine diagnostic practice in the UK. All positive and suspected cases should be confirmed by a reference laboratory.

Other relevant investigations

Routine tests include a full blood count, renal and liver function tests, plasma/blood glucose, blood cultures, and a serum save for possible serology. Blood gas analysis, clotting, and lactate are also important investigations when assessing the severity of falciparum malaria. Thrombocytopenia is common in all forms of malaria, and liver function is often slightly disturbed. There should be a low threshold for performing chest X-ray and other tests, as appropriate.

Patients with vivax or ovale malaria need estimation of glucose-6-phosphate dehydrogenase (G6PD), to exclude deficiency prior to initiation of primaquine therapy.

Prognosis and how to estimate it

The mortality of untreated falciparum infections is high, falling to 1%–2% in the UK when treated. Factors implicated in high mortality include infection in young children, pregnancy, age >60, late presentation, delays in diagnosis and treatment initiation, parasitaemia of 2% or more at presentation, elevated lactate, metabolic acidosis, and presence of other complications (see Box 317.1).

Treatment and its effectiveness

Current national guidelines for treatment of malaria (in the UK, summarized in the British National Formulary) should always be consulted as recommendations change frequently.

Uncomplicated non-falciparum malaria in adults is treated with oral chloroquine or oral artemisinin combination therapy, such as artemether/lumefantrine (Riamet®) or dihydroartemisinin–piperaquine (DHA–PPQ) (Eurartesim®). These options should be accompanied by daily oral primaquine for 2 weeks in patients with vivax or ovale malaria (started as soon as G6PD deficiency has been excluded), to eliminate liver hypnozoites and prevent relapse. Adequate doses of primaquine must be prescribed, typically 30 mg daily for an adult with *Plasmodium vivax* infection. In the US, the same dose is recommended for ovale infections; in the UK, however, a smaller dose of 15 mg daily is considered adequate.

When prescribing chloroquine, check the tablet formulation and base compound content, as many different strength preparations are available. Chloroquine resistance is documented in some cases of vivax malaria, especially cases from Papua New Guinea, Indonesia, and the Solomon Islands, and artemisinin combination therapy may be more appropriate in these cases.

In cases of complicated non-falciparum malaria or dual infection, the current UK guidelines suggest treating as for falciparum malaria, with parenteral therapy.

Chloroquine should never be used to treat imported falciparum malaria, which is usually resistant.

Treatment options for uncomplicated *Plasmodium falciparum* fall into three main categories: artemisinin combination therapy, such as artemether/lumefantrine (Riamet®) or DHA–PPQ (Eurartesim®); atovaquone/proguanil (Malarone®); or quinine plus doxycycline or clindamycin.

Severe or complicated falciparum malaria requires IV therapy. The preferred first-line agent is artesunate, which clears circulating parasites faster than quinine and has fewer side effects. This drug remains off-licence in the EU, but is now available in many British infectious disease units and can be readily supplied to other centres if the patient cannot be transferred.

If artesunate is not available, IV quinine should be started, together with oral doxycycline or clindamycin. A loading dose will be required if the patient has not been taking mefloquine prophylaxis or already received oral quinine in the previous 12 hours. If parenteral therapy is not available, do not delay but give oral quinine (available on any geriatric ward!) immediately, until parenteral preparations can be obtained. ECG monitoring is recommended if there is any history of cardiac problems or arrhythmias. After at least 24 hours of IV therapy and if there are clear signs of improvement, the patient may be switched to a full course of oral artemisinin combination therapy.

Monitor patients with severe malaria closely for hypoglycaemia. Complications are managed conventionally, but avoid overenthusiastic fluid infusion, or respiratory distress will follow in the intensive care unit. Thrombocytopenia resolves after a few days of successful treatment, and platelet transfusion is rarely necessary (or useful, due to immediate consumption). Similarly, anaemia does not need correcting by transfusion, unless very severe or symptomatic. Anticonvulsants are needed for seizures related to cerebral malaria, but steroids or mannitol are not indicated, and prophylactic anticonvulsants have no role in primary seizure prevention. Concurrent bacteraemia should be excluded, especially Gram-negative infections in children, and some experts prescribe broad-spectrum cover anyway in severe malaria (e.g. a third-generation cephalosporin). There is no evidence to support the use of exchange transfusion or red-cell apheresis to reduce circulating parasite load. Daily blood films for parasitaemia counts should be performed to ensure appropriate clearance is occurring, although the parasitaemia may not drop or may even rise during the first 24 hours of successful therapy.

In complex cases, such as malaria during pregnancy and in paediatric populations, specific guidance is available, and urgent specialist infectious disease/tropical medicine advice should be sought on management.

Prevention

Patients who have had acute malaria should be informed they will continue to be at risk in the future when travelling to malarial areas, and appropriate precautions should be taken. This includes maximum measures to reduce the risk of being bitten by mosquitoes, as well as specific and appropriate chemoprophylaxis, the recommendations for which change rapidly. Evidence-based current advice should be sought before travel, from travel clinics or the websites listed in 'Further Reading'.

Public health considerations

All cases of malaria in the UK should be notified promptly to the relevant public health authority.

Further Reading

Beeching NJ, Fletcher TE, and Wijaya L. 'Returned travellers', in Zuckerman JN, ed., *Principles and Practice of Travel Medicine* (2nd edition), 2003. Wiley.

Lalloo DG, Shingadia D, Bell DJ, et al. UK malaria treatment guidelines 2016. *J Infect* 2016; 72: 635–49.

Johnston V, Stockley JM, Dockrell D, et al. Fever in returned travellers presenting in the United Kingdom: Recommendations for investigation and initial management. *J Infect* 2009; 59: 1–18. (This and other guidelines available for free download at http://www.britishinfection.org/guidelines-resources/published-guidelines/)

Public Health England Advisory Committee for Malaria Prevention for UK Travellers. *Guidelines for malaria prevention in travellers from the UK: 2017*. Available at http://www.gov.uk/government/publications/malaria-prevention-guidelines-for-travellers-from-the-uk (accessed 9 Feb 2018).

Public Health England. *Malaria: Guidance, Data and Analysis*; has links to all relevant UK guidelines and resources (http://www.gov.uk/government/collections/malaria-guidance-data-and-analysis)

The Centers for Disease Control and Prevention (US) website has many useful documents, images, etc. (http://www.cdc.gov/MALARIA/)

Travel Health Pro; the website of the National Travel Health Network and Centre provides evidence-based pre-travel medicine advice for professionals and the public (http://travelhealthpro.org.uk/)

318 Worm infection (including hydatid disease)

Sherine Thomas and Nick Beeching

Filarial infections

The main clue to the diagnosis of all helminth infections is peripheral blood eosinophilia, the presence of which should always prompt taking a full travel history. Filarial infections are unusual in the UK, and the main pathogenic groups are summarized in Table 318.1. The most common imported filariasis is *Loa loa* infection from West Africa, characterized by transient 'Calabar swellings', particularly on the face, arms, and upper limbs.

Schistosomiasis

Definition of schistosomiasis

Schistosomiasis, also known as bilharzia, is a parasitic disease caused by the trematode worms of the genus *Schistosoma*. It affects millions worldwide and is considered to be the second most important parasitic infection after malaria. It has a low mortality rate, but causes chronic illness, which can be socio-economically devastating.

Aetiology of schistosomiasis

There are three main species of schistosomes that affect humans (see Table 318.2).

Typical symptoms of schistosomiasis, and less common symptoms

Cercariae penetrating the skin can cause a papular itchy rash, referred to as swimmer's itch. Symptoms with acute infection a few weeks later can include fever, urticaria, splenomegaly, hepatomegaly, cough, and wheeze. This is referred to as Katayama fever.

For other symptoms and complications see Table 318.2.

Approach to diagnosing schistosomiasis

Schistosomiasis should be considered in anyone who has come from or visited endemic areas and had freshwater exposure, including showering in unfiltered lake or river water. Eosinophilia is prominent during the invasive phase, and mild eosinophilia is common in chronic infection. Diagnosis relies on identifying the eggs from adult worms. *Schistosoma haematobium* eggs can be identified from the urine. Bladder activity means that most eggs are voided at around midday; therefore, a 10 am to 2 pm urine collection is likely to yield the best results. Rectal biopsies can also be useful, to directly identify infection. Concentrating stool is more sensitive than direct smear examination in *Schistosoma mansoni* and *Schistosoma japonicum*. Serological tests available from specialist centres are essential, but cannot be used to evaluate treatment effectiveness, as they remain positive for months to years.

Treatment and prognosis of schistosomiasis

Praziquantel is the first-line treatment for schistosomiasis. It is effective, is easily administered, and has very little in the way of side effects, apart from nausea. Clearance of infection needs to be monitored and, in some cases, such as heavy infections, further courses of praziquantel may be required. There are isolated reports of cases of praziquantel resistance and, in the future, artemisinin combined therapy may have a role in treatment.

The fibrotic changes caused by the immunological reactions to trapped eggs can lead to irreversible damage, such as portal hypertension and liver fibrosis, which may need continued monitoring for ongoing complications despite treatment of the underlying infection.

Hydatid disease

Definition of hydatid disease

Hydatid disease or echinococcosis is a zoonotic parasitic infection that affects humans and animals.

Aetiology of hydatid disease

In hydatid disease, humans inadvertently become the secondary host in the life cycle of dog or fox tapeworms. There are two main forms of hydatid disease: cystic disease, which is caused by *Echinococcus multilocularis* (which lives in dogs, wolves, etc., with sheep and other animals being the usual secondary host), and alveolar disease, which is caused by *Echinococcus multilocularis* (which lives in foxes, with rodents as the secondary host). Dogs or foxes infected with adult worms release eggs in their faeces. When these are ingested by an intermediate host, oncospheres liberated in the bowel enter the circulation and get trapped in the capillaries of various organs, where they form cysts. The animals are reinfected when they eat the carcasses of infected dead animals. *Echinococcus granulosus* is present worldwide, and humans are accidental intermediate hosts that become infected by handling soil, dirt, or animal hair that contains eggs. *Echinococcus granulosus* cysts are clearly demarcated with a thick cyst wall lined by a germinal layer that can produce internal daughter cysts. *Echinococcus multilocularis* tissue stages have an external germinal layer and spread through tissue like a cancer.

Typical symptoms of hydatid disease, and its complications

The incubation period for all types of echinococcosis is months to many years. About 70% of *Echinococcus granulosus* cysts in humans form in the liver, and around 20% occur in the lungs. Hepatic cysts are usually asymptomatic; however, if they are symptomatic, the symptoms are usually related to growing mass effects. Alternatively, if the contents of a cyst discharge into the biliary tree, the resulting cholangitis and obstructive jaundice may be mistaken for gallstone disease. Symptoms also occur if secondary bacterial infections occur, mimicking hepatic abscesses. Fluid leaking from cysts can cause a hypersensitivity reaction including urticaria, pruritus, fever, or even anaphylactic reactions.

Cysts in the lungs are usually discovered as an incidental finding, but they may cause dyspnoea, coughing, chest pain, or, occasionally, haemoptysis. Cysts can, rarely, get trapped elsewhere in the body. Cysts in the bone can lead to pathological fractures, and, rarely, cysts in the brain can present with convulsions.

Alveolar hydatid disease presents with a painful, hard liver, weight loss, and fever, resembling liver cancer.

Approach to diagnosing hydatid disease

Imaging is useful for making the diagnosis of hydatid disease. Ultrasound and CT scans of the liver can show typical findings, and MRI scans can be useful for visualization of liquid areas within the tissue. Radiologists with experience of hydatid imaging should be consulted. Serology is useful as an adjunct to imaging and the clinical picture, but lacks sensitivity for extra-hepatic cysts, and specificity is variable. Eosinophilia is not usually a feature of infection but may be present, especially after cyst rupture.

Table 318.1 Main features of filarial infections

Causative species	Vector	Geographical distribution	Natural history and complications of the disease	Diagnosis	Treatment
Lymphatic filariasis					
Wuchereria bancrofti	Mosquitoes: • *Aedes* spp. • *Anopheles* spp. • *Culex* spp. • *Mansonia* spp.	Mainly around the equatorial belt: Africa, South America, Turkey, India, and South East Asia	The adult worms live in the lymphatics of the pelvis Their sheathed microfilariae migrate into the bloodstream where they are present nocturnally They disappear into the pulmonary capillaries by day and, therefore, the vectors that transmit these filariae tend to be night biters; the exception is in some Polynesian islands where the vectors are day biters The mosquitoes then take up the microfilariae when they feed; these are then injected into human hosts when they feed again	Eosinophilia is usually marked in the early stages of infection Microfilariae can be identified in a thick blood film stained with Giemsa (blood taken nocturnally for *Wuchereria bancrofti*) Filarial serology is available at larger tropical centres (Liverpool and London) Ultrasound scans can sometimes identify adult worms in the lymphatics	An experienced tropical medicine or infectious diseases physician should be consulted Treatment options include: • diethylcarbamazine citrate, which has activity against microfilariae and can damage adult worms • albendazole, which has microfilaricidal activity • ivermectin, which has microfilaricidal activity • doxycycline, which kills the endosymbiotic *Wolbachia* bacteria in the worm, increasing the effectiveness of other therapies Chemotherapy typically includes doxycycline for up to 8 weeks followed by a single dose of ivermectin Other combinations may be used, and repeated courses may be required
Brugia malayi	Mosquitoes: • *Aedes* spp. • *Anopheles* spp. • *Mansonia* spp.	South and South East Asia	The incubation period is variable, but usually 8–16 months Symptoms of early disease include recurrent episodes of lymphangitis and transient oedema associated with fever Lymphatic obstruction can occur after many years of recurrent episodes, leading to persistent lymphadenopathy, hydrocoele in males, and elephantiasis		
Brugia timori	Mosquitoes: • *Anopheles* spp.	Lesser Sunda Islands of Indonesia			
Subcutaneous filariasis					
Onchocerca volvulus	Black fly (*Simulium* spp.)	Sub-Saharan Africa and isolated areas of south and central America Black flies breed in rapidly flowing freshwater; therefore, onchocerciasis tends to be concentrated around river areas	Female *Onchocerca volvulus* worms live in subcutaneous tissue, sometimes within nodules, where they produce microfilariae that can migrate through the skin and often to the eyes The microfilariae then only develop further when they are taken up by the black fly and can then be transmitted to another human The adult worms can survive for up to 17 years, but the microfilariae only survive for about 1 year The incubation period is usually 15–18 months Symptoms can be divided into early skin manifestations, including intense itching and papular eruptions, and late skin manifestations, including thickening, oedema, lichenification, and blackening of the skin Regional lymph nodes may be enlarged Subcutaneous nodules containing adult worms are occasionally present Eye disease is the most important feature, with itching, redness, and excess lacrimation occurring early Late disease can lead to varying degrees of visual loss and blindness, hence the name African river blindness		An experienced tropical medicine or infectious diseases physician should be consulted Treatment options include: • ivermectin, which has microfilaricidal activity • doxycycline, which has been shown to kill the endosymbiotic *Wolbachia* bacteria in the filariae; killing these bacteria can maintain freedom from microfilaria for up to 2 years Combination therapy of doxycycline and ivermectin is usually recommended, as above
Loa loa	Deer fly (*Chrysops* spp.)	Rainforest and swamp areas of western Africa (especially Cameroon, on the Ogooue River)	Subcutaneous tissues Can cause transient subcutaneous swellings due to localized angioedema called Calabar swellings Can survive for up to 17 years Adult worms can sometimes be seen crawling across the eye surface, and are referred to as the African eye worm		Treatment options include: • diethylcarbamazine citrate, but patients need to be monitored closely due to the risk of severe and life-threatening side effects • ivermectin, which has microfilaricidal activity

Table 318.2 Features of the three main schistosome species

Schistosoma species	Geographical distribution	Natural history	Symptoms of infection, and complications
Schistosoma haematobium	Middle East and Africa	Parasite eggs are released from infected individuals They hatch on contact with fresh water to release the free swimming miracidia These then infect freshwater snails and transform into sporocysts, which divide and eventually release cercariae from the snail host into the water These penetrate human skin and transform into migrating schistosomula about 8–10 days later The parasites then migrate to the liver and ultimately to the bladder (the perivesical venous plexus), the ureters, and the kidneys Parasites reach maturity in 6–8 weeks, at which time they begin to produce eggs The eggs can migrate to different parts of the body and can become trapped The immunological response to these eggs underlies the pathological features of this infection	Terminal haematuria Dysuria Altered semen Perineal discomfort Vaginal nodules Eggs can be deposited in the bladder and other pelvic organs, where they can lead to a granulomatous reaction, which in turn can lead to an obstructive uropathy, and hydroureter Calcification of the bladder is common, as is a higher risk of bladder cancer Genital tract involvement has also been documented, with occasional cases of secondary infertility due to infection
Schistosoma mansoni	South America, the Caribbean, Africa, and the Middle East	Worm pairs relocate to the mesenteric or rectal veins Adults pairs may produce up to 300 eggs per day during their reproductive lives	Most patients have little in the way of symptoms, but severe manifestations include granuloma of the large bowel, which may ulcerate and bleed Long-standing infections can lead to liver fibrosis and portal hypertension, with associated complications such as variceal bleeds and ascites
Schistosoma japonicum	China and the Philippines	Worm pairs relocate to the mesenteric or rectal veins Adult pairs may produce up to 3000 eggs per day Many of the eggs pass through the walls of the blood vessels, and through the intestinal wall; these eggs are then passed out of the body in faeces	As with *Schistosoma mansoni*, but infection tends to be more severe

Treatment of hydatid disease, and its effectiveness

Albendazole is the mainstay of treatment, either as definitive treatment for a minority of patients with small uncomplicated cysts or in preparation for surgery or controlled aspiration known as PAIR (for **p**ercutaneous **a**spiration, **i**nstillation (of hypertonic saline), and **r**e-aspiration). In the UK all patients should be discussed with an experienced specialist. Medical treatment may need to be prolonged for years in inoperable patients. Success of therapy is mirrored by internal changes in cysts, seen on ultrasound. Surgery or PAIR is best done in a few experienced centres in the UK.

Alveolar hydatid is usually controlled by long-term albendazole therapy, which has transformed the prognosis from inevitable death to control of disease.

Toxocariasis

Definition of toxocariasis

Toxocara canis and *Toxocara cati* are parasitic roundworms that are found in dogs and cats, respectively, and can infect humans.

Aetiology of toxocariasis

Infections in humans occur following ingestion of eggs, usually from sand or soil contaminated by affected faeces; therefore, children appear to be at highest risk of infection. The larvae are released in the intestine and then wander through tissues in the body for 1–2 years.

Typical symptoms of toxocariasis, and its complications

Clinical symptoms are uncommon with this infection, but the symptoms that manifest are due to the migrating larvae. Features of visceral larva migrans (VLM) include fever, abdominal pain, pneumonitis, lymphadenopathy, and behavioural disturbance. Ocular larva migrans (OLM) occurs when the larva invades the eye, producing a granulomatous reaction that can lead to visual disturbances and blindness. Occasionally, the appearance of the retina can be mistaken for a retinoblastoma.

Approach to diagnosing toxocariasis

Eosinophilia may be present, and serological diagnosis can be establishing using an ELISA.

Treatment and prognosis of toxocariasis

The treatment for VLM is albendazole 10 mg/kg per day for 5 days. Topical or systemic steroids are indicated for the treatment of OLM, with little evidence for the benefit of using concurrent anthelmintics.

Further Reading

Agudelo Higuita NI, Brunetti E, and McCloskey C. Cystic echinococcosis. *J Clin Microbiol* 2016; 54: 518–23.

Brunetti E, Kern P, and Vuitton DA. Expert consensus for the diagnosis and treatment of cystic and alveolar echinococcosis in humans. *Acta Trop* 2010; 114: 1–16.

Colley DG, Bustinduy AL, Secor WE, et al. Human schistosomiasis. *Lancet* 2014; 383: 2253–64.

Kearn P. Clinical features and treatment of alveolar echinococcosis. *Curr Opin Infect Dis* 2010; 23: 505–12.

Taylor MJ, Hoerauf A, and Bockarie M. Lymphatic filariasis and onchocerciasis. *Lancet* 2010; 376: 1175–85.

WHO website: includes useful background information and country-specific information about all these conditions (for example, http://www.who.int/topics/schistosomiasis/en/)

319 Prion disease

Richard Knight

Definition of the disease

Prion diseases (also known as transmissible spongiform encephalopathies (TSEs)) affect animals and humans, although only the human diseases will be discussed here (Table 319.1). Despite TSEs having somewhat disparate causes and effects, there are unifying features: TSEs are brain diseases with neurodegenerative pathology, which is typically associated with spongiform change, and, most characteristically, there is tissue deposition of an abnormal structural form of the prion protein. Some of the TSEs are naturally acquired infections and, while others are not, they are potentially transmissible in certain circumstances (Table 319.1).

Aetiology of the disease

Human prion diseases have three broad categories of causes: idiopathic causes, genetic causes, and acquired causes (Table 319.1). The commonest form of prion disease, sporadic Creutzfeldt–Jakob disease (sCJD), is of unknown cause, appearing to be a spontaneous neurodegenerative disease. Genetic prion disease results from pathogenic mutations of *PRNP*, the prion protein gene (located on Chromosome 20). Acquired forms are infections that relate to oral consumption of infected material; surgery; medical treatments; and blood transfusion.

Typical symptoms of the disease, and less common symptoms

Different prion diseases tend to have different clinical manifestations. However, they are all encephalopathic illnesses, typically, dementias with other neurological features (especially cerebellar ataxia and myoclonus). There are no systemic or non-neurological features. **sCJD** usually presents with rapidly progressive dementia, cerebellar ataxia, visual impairment, and myoclonus. Less common presentations include progressive focal abnormalities (especially isolated cerebellar ataxia or cortical blindness) before a more general brain illness ensues. **Genetic prion disease** has a very varied clinical profile, partly dependent on the underlying mutation. Many cases are clinically indistinguishable from sCJD (e.g. the commonest form of genetic Creutzfeldt–Jakob disease; associated with the *PRNP* E200K mutation). Some cases present with a progressive cerebellar ataxia

(e.g. typical Gerstmann–Sträussler–Scheinker disease). Rarely, cases present with severe sleep and autonomic disturbances (e.g. fatal familial insomnia). Patients with **iatrogenic Creutzfeldt–Jakob disease** usually present in the same way as the donor of the infective material does (e.g. with variant Creutzfeldt–Jakob disease (vCJD) in the case of blood transfusion transmissions, and sCJD in the case of dura mater transmissions), the distinction being in the history of relevant exposure. However, human-growth-hormone-related Creutzfeldt–Jakob disease is an exception, consisting of progressive cerebellar ataxia; cognitive or other features are late and may be minor. **vCJD** typically presents with psychiatric or behavioural disturbances. Painful sensory symptoms may also occur. Cerebellar ataxia and clear cognitive impairment occur later (at a mean of around 6 months). Most cases of vCJD have been relatively young (median age at onset: 26 years) compared to sCJD cases (median age at onset: 65 years).

Demographics of the disease

sCJD has a worldwide distribution, with an annual mortality rate of 1–2 per million population per year. Genetic prion disease is also found worldwide but there are foci of relatively high prevalence, for example in Slovakia, Chile, and Israel.

In principle, iatrogenic CJD may occur anywhere. However, most cases related to cadaveric-derived pituitary growth hormone have occurred in the UK, France, and the US, and most cases related to human dura mater grafts in Japan.

vCJD arose as a zoonotic infection, resulting from bovine spongiform encephalopathy (BSE) contamination of food. The majority of cases of vCJD have occurred in the UK (which had the greatest number of cattle affected by BSE) and France but other countries have reported cases (the Netherlands, Italy, the US, Canada, Japan, Spain, Portugal, Eire, Saudi Arabia, and Taiwan).

Natural history and complications of the disease

All prion diseases are invariably progressive and fatal. Increasing neurological impairment leads to total dependence, immobility, and unresponsiveness that will prevent normal fluid and food intake with the expected complications: bronchopneumonia, urinary tract infections, and pulmonary embolism.

Table 319.1 Human prion diseases

Type	Disease	Cause	Comments
Idiopathic	Sporadic Creutzfeldt–Jakob disease	Unknown Currently classed as a spontaneous neurodegenerative disease	Worldwide distribution Mostly affects the middle aged and elderly Annual mortality rate is around 1–2/million
Genetic	Genetic Creutzfeldt–Jakob disease Gerstman–Sträussler–Scheinker disease Fatal familial insomnia	Mutations of the prion protein gene (*PRNP*) Autosomal dominant inheritance	Very varied clinic-pathological phenotypic expression Family history absent in up to 40% of cases
Acquired	Kuru	Cannibalistic funeral rites	Confined to Eastern Highlands of Papua New Guinea
	Iatrogenic Creutzfeldt–Jakob disease	Accidental transmission from person to person, by medical or surgical treatments	Most cases related to cadaveric-derived human growth hormone and dura mater grafts
	Variant Creutzfeldt–Jakob disease	Originally resulting from contamination of human diet by bovine spongiform encephalopathy	Most cases in the UK and France Three cases of secondary transmission via red blood cell transfusion

Table 319.2 Investigations supporting the clinical diagnosis of sporadic and variant Creutzfeldt–Jakob disease

Type of disease	Cerebral MRI*	CSF 14-3-3	CSF RT-QuIC	EEG	Tonsil biopsy
Sporadic	High signal in the putamen and caudate High signal in some cortical areas	Often positive	Nearly always positive	In many cases, generalized, periodic discharges	Not indicated (normal)
Variant	High signal in the posterior thalami (the 'pulvinar sign')	Positive in less than half of cases	Negative	Non-specific changes	Shows deposition of the disease-related abnormal prion protein

*Diffusion-weighted imaging and FLAIR sequences are the most sensitive.

Approach to diagnosing the disease

The general diagnostic approach has three components:

- consider the diagnosis (this requires familiarity with the typical clinical features of the disease)
- exclude other diagnoses (a wide variety of brain disease may present in similar ways)
- undertake tests that will support or confirm the diagnosis (see Table 319.2).

In general, investigation of suspect cases of prion disease will require a wide variety of blood tests, cerebral imaging (e.g. MRI), other imaging (e.g. chest radiology), lumbar puncture with CSF examination, and EEG recording.

Other diagnoses that should be considered

The differential diagnosis for prion disease is potentially very wide, including any cause of a rapidly progressive encephalopathy. The list of potential conditions is long and varied, including infections (e.g. viral encephalitis, progressive multifocal leukoencephalopathy, subacute sclerosing panencephalitis, and HIV), malignancies (e.g. primary brain tumours, cerebral secondaries, and non-metastatic encephalopathies), autoimmune/inflammatory disorders (e.g. Hashimoto's encephalitis and cerebral vasculitis), and atypical, relatively rapidly progressing neurodegenerative brain disease (such as Alzheimer's disease). Many of these are suggested by the history (e.g. symptoms of infection, a known malignancy, a family history), the presence of specific signs (e.g. pyrexia), or the results of initial haematology and biochemistry tests. Cerebral imaging will suggest others (e.g. tumours), and certain CSF results may be helpful (e.g. pleocytosis or identification of infectious agents). The main diagnostic problems tend to start when one is faced with a serious, rapidly progressing brain disease, with no clear clues from the history, no non-neurological signs, and normal or non-specific initially abnormal initial investigations (e.g. a slightly raised CSF total protein).

'Gold-standard' diagnostic test

There is only one absolute diagnostic test for prion disease: neuropathological examination of the brain. This is usually at autopsy; brain biopsy is rarely performed, and its main indication is the confirmation/exclusion of another, potentially treatable diagnosis (e.g. isolated cerebral vasculitis). A brain biopsy that fails to show characteristic prion disease abnormalities does not absolutely exclude the diagnosis. In addition, an appropriate neuropsychiatric illness in someone with a confirmed *PRNP* mutation makes genetic prion disease virtually certain.

Acceptable diagnostic alternatives to the gold standard

There are tests that are supportive of a clinical diagnosis of sCJD and vCJD (Table 319.2). Established clinical diagnostic criteria for prion diseases, based on clinical features and these tests, allow a very confident diagnosis without neuropathology (see http://www.cjd.ed.ac.uk). These criteria define categories of 'probable' prion disease that are very reliable clinical diagnoses. The CSF RT-QuIC test is highly specific for sCJD. Tonsil biopsy may be indicated in suspect vCJD cases, where the clinical picture and the cerebral MRI findings do not meet the criteria for 'probable vCJD'.

Other relevant investigations

The exclusion of other diagnoses may involve a variety of tests, depending on the clinical context.

Prognosis and how to estimate it

All prion diseases are progressive and fatal. The life expectancy in individual cases depends on a number of factors, including the type of prion disease and the intensity of medical supportive management (e.g. the use of gastrostomy feeding and treatment of intercurrent infections). The average duration of sCJD is around only 4 months; occasionally, survival of a year or two is seen. Variant CJD has a slower course, with a median duration of around 14 months. Factors affecting prognosis have been analysed and reported (see Pocchiari et al., 2004).

Treatment and its effectiveness

There is, currently, no proven effective disease-modifying therapy in prion disease.

Further Reading

Knight R and Will R (2004.) Prion diseases. *J Neurol Neurosurg Psychiatry* 2004; 75: i36–i42.

Rinne ML, McGinnis SM, Samuels MA, et al. A startling decline. *N Engl J Med* 2012; 366: 836–42.

Stopschinski BE and Diamond MI. The prion model for progression and diversity of neurodegenerative diseases. *Lancet Neurol* 2017; 16: 323–32

320 Sexually transmitted disease (gonorrhoea)

Martyn Wood and Marilyn Bradley

Definition of the disease

Gonorrhoea is the term used to describe the clinical manifestations of infection with the bacterium *Neisseria gonorrhoeae*.

Aetiology of the disease

Neisseria gonorrhoeae is a Gram-negative diplococcus which usually infects the columnar epithelium of mucous membranes, including the lower male and female genital tracts, the rectum, the pharynx, and the conjunctivae. Transmission is by direct exposure of a mucous membrane to infected secretions, classically via sexual contact. Mother-to-child transmission at birth is also well recognized.

Typical symptoms of the disease, and less common symptoms

The majority of men with urethral *Neisseria gonorrhoeae* infection are symptomatic with either purulent urethral discharge or dysuria, and frequently have both. A small proportion (<10%) are asymptomatic. Fifty per cent of women with endocervical and urethral infection are asymptomatic. Symptomatic women commonly experience altered or increased vaginal discharge, dysuria, lower abdominal pain, and, rarely, intermenstrual or post-coital bleeding. Pharyngeal infection in men and women is usually asymptomatic. The majority of rectal infections in women occur via transmucosal spread and are usually asymptomatic. Rectal infection can occur by direct sexual inoculation in men and women and can cause proctitis or anal discharge.

Less common presentations of gonorrhoea include conjunctivitis from direct inoculation, or disease resulting from haematogenous spread, including arthralgia and localized skin lesions. Disseminated *Neisseria gonorrhoeae* infection is rare and can clinically resemble disseminated *Neisseria meningitidis* infection.

Demographics of the disease

The rate of gonorrhoea infection in the UK peaked in the mid-1970s, with a rapid decline in incidence over the next decade, coinciding with public health campaigns addressing the HIV epidemic. Since the 1990s, the annual incidence of gonorrhoea has increased again. Those who are most at risk of infection include younger age groups (15–29 years), inner-city residents, ethnic minority groups, and men who have sex with men.

Natural history, and complications of the disease

The incubation period for *Neisseria gonorrhoeae* ranges from 2 to 30 days, and infection is usually localized to the lower genital tracts; however, infection can ascend to the upper genital tracts in the form of pelvic inflammatory disease in women, and epididymo-orchitis or prostatitis in men. Both of these conditions can lead to infertility and chronic pelvic pain. Disseminated disease can result in septic arthritis and septicaemia but is uncommon (<1% of infections).

Neisseria gonorrhoeae can be the precipitant of sexually acquired reactive arthritis, which is a condition resulting from infection at a distant (usually genital) site precipitating an autoimmune-mediated sterile inflammation of synovial membranes, tendons, and fascia. In those who carry HLA-B27, susceptibility is increased fiftyfold, with men being most affected.

Approach to diagnosing the disease

Any person presenting with genital symptoms and a history of arthralgia, conjunctivitis, or skin lesions suggestive of *Neisseria* infection should have a full sexual history taken to assess risk and timings for sexual infection exposure. Information from the history should guide which genital and extra-genital areas are sampled for microbiological specimens.

Other diagnoses that should be considered

Chlamydia trachomatis can present in an identical fashion to gonorrhoea infection and should be considered in the differential diagnosis.

'Gold-standard' diagnostic test

The long-established method for detecting gonorrhoea has been the presumptive diagnosis made from observing Gram-negative intracellular diplococci on microscopy of stained discharge or secretions. Subsequent culture on selective media allows identification of *Neisseria gonorrhoeae* and specifically allows determination of antibiotic sensitivities. The detractors to this method are that specimen collection, storage, and preparation require easily accessible microbiology laboratory facilities, and this is not always practicable in a community-screening setting.

Acceptable diagnostic alternatives to the gold standard

There has been a shift from traditional culture methods to nucleic acid amplification test technology (NAATs), which could potentially supplant culture as the gold-standard diagnostic test. These tests are less intolerant of sampling and transportation inconsistencies than culture is. NAATs allow more convenient and flexible testing arrangements, the use of non-invasive testing methods (urine samples and self-taken swabs), and dual testing for *Neisseria gonorrhoeae* and *Chlamydia trachomatis* on the same specimen. Their disadvantage is that antibiotic sensitivities cannot be determined; this is important, as *Neisseria gonorrhoeae* antibiotic resistance remains a significant clinical problem. Rectal and pharyngeal specimens contain higher levels of other *Neisseria* species and potentially may give rise to more false-positive results than standard culture methods.

Other relevant investigations

When suspecting gonorrhoea clinically, a symptomatic patient should always be screened for other sexually acquired pathogens, including *Chlamydia trachomatis*, HIV, and *Treponema pallidum,* as the mode of acquisition is often similar for each of these infections, and gonorrhoea infection facilitates HIV transmission.

Prognosis

Gonorrhoea is a completely curable condition, but late diagnosis and long-standing infections can lead to long-term sequelae such as chronic pain, urethral strictures, and infertility in both men and women.

Treatment and its effectiveness

UK national guidelines recommend that treatment for gonorrhoea be given in any of the following situations:

- presumptive diagnosis made with microscopy
- positive culture for *Neisseria gonorrhoeae*
- positive nucleic acid test (confirmation of the diagnosis by culture is recommended prior to or at the time of treatment)
- on epidemiological grounds, if a recent sexual partner has confirmed gonococcal infection

Antimicrobial resistance has become a significant problem in the last decade, with ciprofloxacin resistance in England and Wales detected in 28% of all cultured samples, and high-level resistance to penicillin and tetracycline also being recognized. As a result, the current recommended first-line treatment for uncomplicated gonorrhoea is dual antibiotic therapy with the third-generation cephalosporin ceftriaxone, given intramuscularly, and the oral macrolide azithromycin. Decreased susceptibility to third-generation cephalosporins and macrolides has been reported, leading to concerns regarding future treatment options.

In all cases, an expert sexual health opinion should be sought when *Neisseria gonorrhoeae* infection is suspected or confirmed, and appropriate sexual contact tracing undertaken.

Further Reading

Bignell C and FitzGerald M. UK national guideline for the management of gonorrhoea in adults, 2011. *Int J STD AIDS* 2011; 22: 541–7.
National Institute for Clinical Excellence. *Gonorrhoea: Summary*. 2017. Available at http://cks.nice.org.uk/gonorrhoea#!topicsummary (accessed 15 Sep 2017).

PART 16

Cancers

321 Cancers related to infection

Daniel Ajzensztejn

Introduction

The development of a cancer is often complex and multifactorial. Environmental factors such as smoking, diet, asbestos exposure, and sun exposure are important causes of cancer, with smoking alone responsible for 25%–30% of cancers. Up to 10% of cancers have a genetic component. Infectious agents are implicated in the development of approximately 15% of cancers. Viruses, bacteria, and parasites can all cause cancers. Cervical, Head & Neck, and hepatocellular carcinoma are the three commonest cancers related to infections.

The role of infectious agents in cancer

Francis Peyton Rous first proposed that an infectious agent could cause cancer in 1911. He was able to demonstrate transmission of sarcoma from chicken to chicken through injection of a cell-free filtrate. Although ridiculed at the time, his work won him a Nobel Prize 57 years later. The infectious agent he discovered is now known as the Rous sarcoma virus. This was the first of several identified cancer-causing viruses, which are also known as oncoviruses.

Viruses that can cause cancer in humans

HPV

For many years, it had been postulated that an infectious agent was involved in the development of cervical cancer. Epidemiological studies linked the disease to early onset of sexual activity and number of sexual partners. Other factors are also important. Smoking, for example, doubles a woman's risk of developing the disease.

HPV is a non-enveloped DNA virus which has now been linked to the development of cervical cancer. More than 140 different HPV types have been recognized to date. HPV-16 and HPV-18 are of particular importance in cervical cancer. Via PCR-based techniques, HPV-16 and HPV-18 have been demonstrated in approximately 70% of cervical cancers. Other high-risk HPV types, including HPV-31, HPV-33, HPV-35, HPV-45, HPV-52, and HPV-58, have also been demonstrated in cervical cancers but to a lesser degree.

Carcinogenesis, the development of cancer, is a multistep process. HPV is important in the initiation of this process, with other factors required for progression to cancer.

HPV viruses replicate in squamous epithelial cells. HPV has also been implicated in several other squamous cell cancers in the anogenital region (penile, vulval, vaginal, and anal carcinomas), the head and neck region, and in some skin cancers (particularly in immunosuppressed individuals, such as renal transplant patients). In the case of oropharyngeal head and neck cancers, tumour HPV status is strongly associated with therapeutic response and survival, with HPV-associated cancers having better outcomes than HPV-negative oropharyngeal cancers.

HPV vaccines

Understanding the viral aetiology of cervical cancer has led to the development of more reliable cervical screening. More importantly, HPV vaccination can prevent some HPV-associated cancers.

To date, there are two commercially available vaccines against HPV. These include virus-like particles which are able to generate a durable immune response to specific HPV types. Both protect against HPV-16 and HPV-18, which cause approximately 70% of cervical cancers. The quadrivalent vaccine also immunizes against HPV-6 and HPV-11, which cause genital warts. Trials are currently also underway with a nonavalent HPV vaccine protecting against HPV-31, HPV-33, HPV-45, HPV-52, and HPV-58 as well as those protected by the quadrivalent vaccine. To be most effective, the vaccine needs to be given prior to infection with HPV. Many countries have introduced vaccination programmes for school-aged girls. In the UK, it is offered to all girls aged 12 and 13. In some countries, the vaccination programme has been extended to include both sexes.

Hepatitis B and hepatitis C viruses

Chronic infection with the hepatitis B virus (HBV) or the hepatitis C virus (HCV) can lead to the development of hepatocellular carcinoma. Although this is a relatively rare disease in the West, it has a high prevalence in sub-Saharan Africa and South East Asia. This means that, on a global scale, it is actually one of the commonest cancers.

HBV

HBV is a hepadnavirus (hepatotropic DNA virus). It has a circular genome composed of partially double-stranded DNA. Viral replication occurs in hepatocytes. The virus then spreads to the blood, where viral antigens and antibodies can be detected in infected individuals.

Acute infection with HBV can cause either an acute liver injury presenting with jaundice, or a subclinical infection. Most acute infections resolve with clearance of the virus from both the liver and blood, with resulting natural immunity to reinfection. In approximately 5% of patients, acute infections are not cleared; such individuals develop persistent viraemia. Globally, there are approximately 400 million individuals with chronic HBV infection. From epidemiological studies, it is known that chronic infection with HBV increases the risk of developing hepatocellular carcinoma a hundredfold.

HCV

HCV is a member of the Flaviviridae family of RNA viruses. In most cases, acute infection with HCV does not cause symptoms. However, in approximately 25% of cases, infected individuals will develop an acute hepatitis presenting with jaundice and malaise. The acute infection is cleared in about 20%–50% of cases. If the infection is not cleared, infected individuals become chronic carriers. Globally, there are approximately 170 million chronic carriers of HCV. Up to 5% of these people will ultimately develop hepatocellular carcinoma. Those at highest risk of developing hepatocellular carcinoma are the approximately two-thirds of chronic carriers who develop a chronic hepatitis, 20% of whom develop liver cirrhosis over a period of 10–20 years. In this subset of patients, there is an annual risk of 1%–4% of going on to develop hepatocellular carcinoma. Infection with particular HCV genotypes, particularly HCV genotype 1b, co-infection with HBV, and alcohol consumption all increase the likelihood of developing hepatocellular carcinoma.

Mechanisms of oncogenesis by HBV and HCV

HBV and HCV both increase the risk of cancer in chronically infected individuals via the host immune response to viral antigens present on the surface of infected hepatocytes. This results in chronic hepatocyte injury similar to that caused by chronic alcohol abuse, alpha-1-antitrypsin deficiency, and Wilson's disease. These conditions all cause chronic liver injury through hepatocyte destruction, regeneration, and fibrosis and are all associated with an increased risk of hepatocellular carcinoma. Although HBV is not directly oncogenic, there is some evidence that HCV is able to independently cause neoplastic transformation of hepatocytes. HCV may also increase the risk of haematological malignancies such as B-cell non-Hodgkin's lymphoma and other lymphoproliferative diseases.

Vaccines and other therapies for HBV and HCV

There is a commercially available HBV vaccine. There is currently no vaccine for HCV. Antiviral therapy can be used in the treatment of chronic carriers. Interferon alfa and antiviral drugs such as lamivudine are used in the treatment of selected chronic HBV carriers. In HCV, treatment with interferon alpha and ribavirin, a synthetic guanosine analogue, can be effective in reducing viral load. It is not yet clear whether this reduces rates of progression to hepatocellular carcinoma. Surgical resection of the tumour and liver transplantation are the only two curative therapies for established hepatocellular carcinoma.

EBV

EBV is a member of the Herpesviridae family of DNA viruses and was the first cancer-causing virus to be identified. The virus was discovered in 1964 and is named after Anthony Epstein and Yvonne Barr, pathologists at the former Middlesex Hospital in London. They identified the virus in cell line cultures taken from pathology specimens collected by a British surgeon, Denis Burkitt, in Uganda. Burkitt had documented the high incidence of B-cell lymphoma in children living in malaria-endemic regions of Africa. This type of lymphoma has since been eponymously named Burkitt's lymphoma. Initial excitement over the identification of a possible cancer-causing virus was soon dampened by the discovery that over 95% of people in the general population had a detectable EBV-specific antibody. Related work led to the link between primary infection with EBV and infectious mononucleosis. Titre levels of EBV-specific antibody were, however, found to be higher in children with Burkitt's lymphoma. This was also seen in some patients with Hodgkin's lymphoma and in Chinese patients with nasopharyngeal cancer, consistent with the original hypothesis of a cancer-causing virus.

Primary infection with EBV is the cause of infectious mononucleosis (also known as glandular fever or 'mono'). The infection is usually spread via saliva and has an incubation period of 4–7 weeks. The virus replicates initially within epithelial cells of the nasopharynx and then infects circulating B-cells. These infected B-cells are recognized and destroyed by T-cells, which account for most of the circulating immune cells during acute infection.

Primary infection is followed by a latent infection characteristic of all herpesvirus infections. During latent infection, the virus is present as episomes in the nuclei of lymphocytes and epithelial cells of the oropharynx, which acts as a reservoir for the virus. B-cells are infected as they circulate through the nasopharynx. Saliva and other secretions contain the virus, thereby enabling viral transmission to uninfected individuals.

EBV latent gene expression codes for several nuclear proteins, certain patterns of which are believed to contribute to cancer development. Their main role is in initiation of oncogenesis. While certain patterns of EBV latent gene expression are associated with cancers, others are associated with healthy carriers of EBV.

In addition to nasopharyngeal carcinoma and Burkitt's lymphoma, several other tumour types, including Hodgkin's lymphoma and gastric cancers, may express EBV at a lower frequency. The sites of these tumours relate to the sites of reservoir of the latent virus.

HHV8

HHV8, also known as Kaposi's sarcoma-associated herpesvirus, is associated with the development of Kaposi's sarcoma (KS). Although the disease was first described in 1872, its causative virus was only identified in 1994. Four epidemiologic patterns of KS have been characterized: (i) AIDS-associated KS is the commonest malignancy in HIV-infected individuals, and development of KS is an AIDS-defining illness; (ii) classic KS, which is predominantly a disease of elderly Mediterranean and East European men; (iii) endemic KS, which is most common in young HIV-seronegative men in sub-Saharan Africa; and (iv) immunosuppression-associated KS, which is related to the suppression of T-cell function. All four types of KS share a degree of underlying immune dysregulation, although, interestingly, individuals with congenital immunosuppression do not appear to be at an increased risk of developing KS.

HIV

Of patients with HIV who develop AIDS, approximately 10% will develop a cancer. This figure includes both AIDS-defining cancers (Kaposi's sarcoma, non-Hodgkin's lymphoma, and cervical cancer) and non-AIDS-defining cancers. The increased risk of cancer development in the context of HIV is believed to be multifactorial, with immunosuppression and co-infection with the other oncogenic viruses described in this chapter playing important roles. A direct oncogenic effect of HIV per se has been hypothesized, particularly with regard to the development of non-EBV-associated lymphomas, but strong evidence for this is lacking.

HTLV-1

Adult T-cell leukaemia (ATL) is an aggressive malignancy of CD4⁺ T-cells. Geographic clustering of the disease, particularly to areas of southern Japan, led to the hypothesis of an infectious aetiology. This was subsequently confirmed when nearly 100% of tested patients were found to be seropositive for HTLV-1. HTLV-1 is a retrovirus which shares several features with HIV, including genetic structure, tropism for CD4⁺ T-cells, and broadly similar routes of transmission. There are, however, marked differences, with over 95% of people infected with HTLV-1 virus going on to become asymptomatic carriers. The mechanism of oncogenesis is complex and multifactorial, as attested to by the fact that only 3%–5% of carriers develop ATL, along with the 30–50-year latency period between infection and development of the disease.

Other viruses that cause cancer in humans

Several other viruses have oncogenic properties. Along with those already discussed, these are summarized in Table 321.1.

Bacteria that cause cancer

Helicobacter pylori

Helicobacter pylori is a Gram-negative microaerophilic bacterium that is found in the upper gastrointestinal tract of approximately 50% of the world's population. *Helicobacter pylori* infection doubles the risk of developing gastric adenocarcinomas of the body and antrum of the stomach. The bacteria can cause an atrophic gastritis, which results in a low-acidity environment that promotes metaplasia and dysplasia. Only 5% of carriers of *Helicobacter pylori* will develop a gastric cancer over a 10-year period; therefore, other factors must also be important. Smoking, infection at a younger age, and male gender all increase the risk, whereas diets rich in fruit and vegetables high in antioxidants, including vitamins C and E, flavonoids, and carotenoids, are protective.

Helicobacter pylori is also associated with the development of gastric mucosa-associated lymphoid tissue (MALT) lymphomas. Gastritis caused by *Helicobacter pylori* results in development of malignant B-cell clones.

Prevention and treatment of cancer associated with Helicobacter pylori

The risk of developing gastric cancer can be reduced through eradication of *Helicobacter pylori*, avoidance of smoking, and maintaining a healthy diet. Established gastric cancers associated with *Helicobacter pylori* are treated in the same manner as other gastric cancers. MALT lymphomas limited to the stomach usually resolve completely with eradication of *Helicobacter pylori*. Surgery and radiotherapy can have a curative role where the disease persists. Chemotherapy can be used where there is evidence of distant spread.

Parasites that cause cancer

Schistosoma haematobium

Schistosoma haematobium, which is endemic in much of Africa and the eastern Mediterranean, is associated with the development of bladder cancer. Unlike non-infective bladder cancers, which are predominantly transitional cell carcinomas, *Schistosoma haematobium*-associated bladder cancer is a squamous cell carcinoma. Infection

Table 321.1 Human viruses with oncogenic properties

Virus family	Type	Human tumour	Cofactors
Flaviviruses	HCV	Hepatocellular carcinoma	–
Hepadnavirus	HBV	Hepatocellular carcinoma	Aflatoxin, alcohol, smoking
Herpesviruses	EBV	Burkitt's lymphoma	Malaria
		Immunoblastic lymphoma	Immunodeficiency
		Nasopharyngeal carcinoma	Nitrosamines, HLA genotype
		Hodgkin's lymphoma	–
		Leiomyosarcomas	–
		Gastric cancers	–
	KSHV (HHV8)	Kaposi's sarcoma	HIV infection
		Pulmonary effusion lymphoma	HIV infection
		Castleman's disease	HIV infection
Papillomaviruses	HPV-16, HPV-18, HPV-33, HPV-39, others	Anogenital cancers and some upper airway cancers	Smoking,? other factors
	HPV-5, HPV-8, HPV-17, others	Skin cancer	Epidermodysplasia verruciformis, sunlight, genetic factors, immune suppression
Polyomavirus	SV40 (monkey virus)	? Brain tumours	–
		? Non-Hodgkin's lymphomas	–
		? Mesotheliomas	–
	JC virus	? Brain tumours	–
	BK virus	? Prostate cancer	–
Retroviruses	HTLV1	Adult T-cell leukaemia/lymphoma	Uncertain

Abbreviations: HCV, hepatitis C virus; HBV, hepatitis B virus; EBV, Epstein–Barr virus; KSHV, Kaposi's sarcoma-associated herpesvirus; HHV8, human herpes virus 8; HIV, human immunodeficiency virus; HPV, human papillomavirus; SV40, simian virus 40; HTLV1, human T-lymphotropic virus type 1.

Adapted with permission from DeVita, Hellman & Rosenberg's Cancer: *Principles & Practice of Oncology*, 8th Edition. Wolters Kluwer Health, copyright © 2008.

occurs through swimming in contaminated water. Larvae burrow into human skin, and migrate via the bloodstream to the liver, where they mature into flukes that travel to the bladder. There, the female fluke lays eggs which traverse the wall of the bladder, causing haematuria. Chronic infection is believed to predispose to cancer through chronic inflammation and fibrosis.

Liver flukes

Parasitic infection by liver flukes of the *Opisthorchis* genus is associated with cholangiocarcinoma. The incidence of cholangiocarcinoma in north-east Thailand, where *Opisthorchis viverrini* is endemic, is 45 times higher than the global average. Many parts of South East Asia where *Clonorchis sinensis* is endemic also have higher than expected rates of the disease. Infection occurs through the consumption of undercooked infected fish. The flukes then establish chronic infection of the bile ducts, where they cause cancer through a combination of inflammation, oxidative stress, and cell proliferation.

Summary

Although accounting for only a relatively small percentage of cancers, infections that can cause cancer are important. Treatment aimed at preventing or eradicating such infections can stop cancer from developing. Vaccinations such as those against HBV and HPV have the potential to dramatically change the epidemiology of diseases. Eradication of *Helicobacter pylori* bacteria can prevent the development of gastric cancer and gastric MALT lymphoma. Eradication of the bacteria is also usually successful as a curative treatment for already established, localized gastric MALT lymphoma. Improved public health measures aimed at reducing contaminated water supplies in parasite endemic regions would bring many health benefits. This would be expected to include a reduction in the incidence of cancers caused by parasites.

Further Reading

Bouvard V, Baan R, Straif K, et al. Special report: Policy. A review of human carcinogens—Part B: Biological agents. *Lancet Oncol* 2009; 10: 321–2.

Buchschacher GL Jr, Wong-Staal F, Howley P, et al. 'Aetiology of Cancer: Viruses', in Lawrence TS, Rosenberg SA, and DeVita VT Jr, eds, *DeVita, Hellman, and Rosenberg's Cancer: Principles and Practice of Oncology* (8th edition), 2008. Lippincott Williams & Wilkins.

322 Principles of oncogenesis

Warren Grant and Martin Scott-Brown

Introduction

It is obvious that the process of developing cancer—oncogenesis—is a multistep process. We know that smoking, obesity, and a family history are strong independent predictors of developing malignancy; yet, in clinics, we often see that some heavy smokers live into their nineties and that some people with close relatives affected by cancer spend many years worrying about a disease that, in the end, they never contract.

For many centuries, scientists have struggled to understand the processes that make cancer cells different from normal cells. There were those in ancient times who believed that tumours were attributable to acts of the gods. Hippocrates suggested that cancer resulted from an imbalance between the black humour that came from the spleen, and the other three humours: blood, phlegm, and bile. It is only in the last 100 years that biologists have been able to characterize some of the pathways that lead to the uncontrolled replication seen in cancer, and subsequently examine exactly how these pathways evolve.

The rampant nature by which cancer invades local and distant tissues, as well its apparent ability to spread between related individuals led some, such as Peyton Rous in 1910, to suggest that cancer was an infectious condition. He was awarded a Nobel Prize in 1966 for the 50 years of work into investigating a link between sarcoma in chickens and a retrovirus that became known as Rous sarcoma virus. He had shown how retroviruses are able to integrate sequences of DNA coding for errors in cellular replication control (oncogenes) by introducing into the human cell viral RNA together with a reverse transcriptase. Viruses are now implicated in many cancers and, in countries where viruses such as HIV and EBV are endemic, the high incidence of malignancies such as Kaposi's sarcoma and Burkitt's lymphoma is likely to be directly related. There are several families of viruses associated with cancer, broadly classed into DNA viruses, which mutate human genes using their own DNA, and retroviruses, like Rous sarcoma virus, which insert viral RNA into the cell, where it is then transcribed into genes.

This link with viruses has not only led to an understanding that cancer originates from genetic mutations, but has also become a key focus in the design of new anticancer therapies. Traditional chemotherapies either alter DNA structure (as with cisplatin) or inhibit production of its component parts (as with 5-fluorouracil.) These broad-spectrum agents have many and varied side effects, largely due to their non-specific activity on replicating DNA throughout the body, not just in tumour cells. New vaccine therapies utilizing gene-coding viruses aim to restore deficient biological pathways, or inhibit mutated ones specific to tumour cells. The hope is that these gene therapies will be effective and easily tolerated by patients, but development is currently progressing with caution. In a trial in France of ten children suffering from X-linked severe combined immunodeficiency and who were injected with a vector that coded for the gene product they lacked, two of the children subsequently died from leukaemia. Further analysis confirmed that the DNA from the viral vector had become integrated into an existing, but normally inactive, proto-oncogene, LM02, triggering its conversion into an active oncogene, and the development of life-threatening malignancy.

To understand how a tiny change in genetic structure could lead to such tragic consequences, we need to understand the molecular biology of the cell and, in particular, to pay attention to the pathways of growth regulation that are necessary in all mammalian cell populations. Errors in six key regulatory pathways are known as the 'hallmarks of cancer' and will be discussed in the rest of this chapter.

Self-sufficiency in growth signals

To maintain tissue integrity, cells must communicate with each other to initiate and inhibit replication as required. This communication is in the form of growth factors—small protein molecules that are secreted and travel through the intercellular space to initiate biological responses by acting as ligands and docking with receptors on the surface of cells. Once stimulated, these transmembrane receptors go on to initiate a cascade of protein phosphorylation that eventually leads to DNA transcription and growth stimulation. Growth factors exist in a sea of other regulatory proteins that control when growth factors are released from cells, in what quantity, and to which tissue they eventually dock. The interactions between these proteins are complex but, in normal cells, growth factors are controlled in a homeostatic fashion to maintain tissue structure and function.

In recent years, a developing interest into how these growth signalling pathways differ in cancer cells has led to some fascinating suggestions. It has become apparent that many cancers manipulate their response to growth factors by upregulating the expression of the growth factor receptors on their cell surfaces or by mutating them and promoting downstream protein phosphorylation independently of any ligand binding. Other cancers produce their own growth factors and excrete them into the extracellular environment, only to see them immediately bind to the cell's own receptors and repeat this self-stimulatory autocrine process.

In around 30% of breast cancers, the HER2/neu transmembrane epidermal growth factor receptor is overexpressed. Overexpression is associated with more rapidly progressive cancers and a 25%–30% shorter overall survival. Recently, the development of Herceptin, which is a humanized monoclonal antibody to the HER2/neu receptor and is given intravenously every 3 weeks, has significantly improved survival in this selected group of patients by blocking HER2/neu activity and preventing initiation of its downstream pro-growth signalling cascade.

Insensitivity to anti-growth signals

Normal cellular replication follows a tightly controlled cycle of events. This cycle is divided up into the synthetic (or S) phase, when DNA is replicated, and the mitotic (or M) phase, when the cell divides into two daughter cells. Between the M phase and the next S phase is a period called G1, and following the S phase is a period called G2 before the cell enters the next M phase. During G1, or the 'first gap' phase of the cycle, between cell birth and the time when DNA synthesis begins, the cell will make critical decisions about whether to begin replicating or to 'rest' in the G0 phase. Should the balance of replication swing in the direction of replication-promoting, or **mitogenic**, proteins, and away from those proteins involved in halting the replication process, the cell will move into the S, or **synthetic**, phase. Once here, the cell cannot return to G1 and is fully committed to undergoing mitosis. It has crossed what is known as the restriction, or R, point, a key cell cycle checkpoint.

Closely regulated cell cycle checkpoints, like the R point, ensure that any cells containing errors in their DNA or that are stimulated to divide at a time when replication is not required, do not complete the cycle. However, the success of cancer cells often involves developing methods to get round these anti-growth checkpoints.

Retinoblastoma protein (pRb) in its hypophosphorylated form acts as a key growth suppressor. It halts the passage of cells through the R point. Through interactions with members of the cyclin family of proteins, it insures that the error-prone products of disordered DNA synthesis are not allowed to pass through the cell cycle and on to other cell generations. Retinoblastomas can develop in the eyes of young children when the gene that encodes pRb, RB1, is mutated. Those with the inherited gene mutation have abnormal RB1 in all their cells, including germ cells, and are likely to develop bilateral retinoblastomas. There is also an association with tumours of the pineal gland and osteosarcomas. In the non-inherited form, abnormal genes still play a key part. However, the abnormal RB1 is only present in the cells of the tumour, which is usually a unilateral retinoblastoma and confers no higher risk of other systemic tumours. Normal pRB can also be inactivated by DNA tumour viruses such as HPV, as these promote the production of oncoproteins that bind to and disable RB1, thus allowing affected cells to replicate uncontrollably.

Evading apoptosis

Apoptosis is programmed cell death. It is a highly preserved function of cells to self-destruct in the presence of unprepared DNA damage or uncontrolled mitotic signals. In normal circumstances, when these situations are detected, a spiralling cascade of proteins from the caspase family set in motion a series of catastrophic structural changes leading eventually to cell breakdown and degradation of cellular material. As previously noted, cancers contain many genetic abnormalities that promote independent and uncontrolled growth. For these errors not to result in immediate cell death, a cancer must have some way of getting round apoptosis. This is why the most common gene mutation in human cancers is in the gene that codes for p53. p53 is a transcription factor that promotes activation of pro-apoptotic genes such as APAF1, CASP1, BAX, and BID. Errors in its ability to detect DNA damage and sustained mitotic signals will lead to a failure to initiate apoptosis and subsequent replication of the damaged DNA and a predisposition to develop cancer. Inherited mutations in the p53 gene are linked to Li–Fraumeni syndrome, a disease characterized by an increased risk of osteosarcomas, breast tumours, lung tumours, and brain tumours, as well as leukaemias.

Sustained angiogenesis

In order for a tumour to receive nutrients and exchange metabolites, as it must do to remain viable, it needs to lie within 100–200 µm of a capillary blood vessel. Lying further from an active blood supply will lead to growth arrest and necrosis. So, for cancers to expand, they need not only to artificially stimulate growth and evade cell death, but also to develop their own vasculature.

Angiogenesis depends on a tight balance of pro- and anti-angiogenic factors. The so-called angiogenic switch represents the on–off interaction between factors which stimulate angiogenesis, such as vascular endothelial growth factor (VEGF) and fibroblast growth factor, and those which inhibit the angiogenic process, such as thrombospondin and angiostatin.

Recently, bevacizumab has entered clinical use in bowel and breast cancer trials. It is an anti-VEGF monoclonal antibody that aims to inhibit the chaotic angiogenesis of tumour cell populations. It is unique in current practice in that it acts upon a circulating ligand. Other monoclonal antibodies attack cell membrane-bound receptors, while more traditional agents act on the internal structure of cancer cells. Current trial protocols involve administering the drug intravenously every 3 weeks for periods up to 1 year or until disease progression. Although it has shown some benefit in stabilizing or shrinking disease in the metastatic setting, there is some suggestion that tumour cell growth may accelerate rapidly once bevacizumab is stopped and the angiogenic switch allowed to flick to the 'on' position.

Tumour invasion and metastases

Cancer is a progressive disease. In cancers such as bowel and breast cancer, we see a clear progression of events over time: growth of the primary lesion, spread to local blood vessels or lymphatics, and subsequent involvement of distant organs such as the liver, the lungs, and the bones. In order to behave in this predictable way, cancer cells must detach from the primary tumour site, extravasate into the local blood supply, evade circulating host defence mechanisms, halt at a suitable site for new growth, permeate through the blood vessel wall, and begin again the cycle of tumour and blood vessel development. The steps that lead to the cancer cell, or 'seed,' finding the tissue, or 'soil' in which it can grow are numerous and involve the manipulation of many factors, including cell adhesion molecules, proteinases that enable endothelial membranes and the extracellular matrix to be broken, cellular growth factors, chemokines, apoptotic signals, and the host immune response.

Clinically, it has proven to be very challenging to prevent the process of cancer spread and metastases. This is likely to be due to our lack of understanding of the complex biology involved. In many cancers, we see that the process of metastasizing is highly inefficient. Blood samples from patients with early breast cancer have been shown to contain large numbers of circulating cancer cells, yet not all of these patients go on to develop metastatic disease. Despite investigating tumour biology and host genetics, we cannot predict accurately who will develop metastases and who will not. In the 1990s there was much excitement in this field as a UK firm, British Biotech, announced the development of a broad-spectrum matrix metalloproteinase inhibitor—marimastat. In animal studies, it had been found to halt tumour cells' ability to break down the extracellular matrix in the process of establishing new growth colonies. Unfortunately, clinical trial data revealed unacceptably high musculoskeletal side effects and this finding, together with public controversy over the way data was presented, led subsequently to the downfall of British Biotech and a sudden halt to the development of these drugs.

Limitless replicative potential

In a normal cell, exposed breaks in the DNA initiate a cascade of regulatory proteins that either repair the damage or initiate apoptosis. This leads to a biological quandary: at the end of every chromosome within the cell is an exposed 'broken' end of DNA. How is this not recognized as damage, and why are cells not in a constant state of apoptosis as a result? The answer lies in a complex of regulatory proteins that surround the end of mammalian chromosomes, at a region known as the **telomere**, and protect it from being recognized as 'damaged' DNA. Each time a cell replicates, the telomere loses DNA from its non-coding free end, shortening the chromosome. Eventually, the cell reaches a critical limit, named, eponymously, the Hayflick limit, where no further replication is possible without damaging functional DNA and initiating cell senescence or apoptosis. In normal tissue, this limits the life of a cell and ensures that more mature cells, that are error-prone, are replaced. Cancer cells manage to prevent this progressive telomere shortening and effectively become immortal by producing telomerase, a key enzyme required to synthesis telomeric DNA. Clinical inhibition of telomerase is currently under early investigation with drug and vaccine programmes.

Further Reading

Mendelsohn J, Howley PM, Israel MA et al. The Molecular Basis of *Cancer* 4e, 2014. Saunders.
Weinberg RA. *The Biology of Cancer*, 2007. Garland Science.

323 Presentations in suspected cancer

David Cutter and Martin Scott-Brown

Introduction

Malignant neoplastic disease includes a vast range of conditions that can originate from and can directly or indirectly affect virtually every organ system of the body. As a consequence of this, the presentation of malignancy can be similarly varied. While a diagnosis of malignancy may be clinically obvious in some cases, in others diagnosis and investigation may be delayed due to non-specific presentations and the attribution of symptoms to non-malignant conditions. Early diagnosis of cancer has an impact on the success of subsequent treatment and overall survival. It is therefore vital to maintain an appropriate level of clinical suspicion when deciding whether and how much to investigate patients with symptoms that could be secondary to an underlying malignancy.

Symptoms directly related to the primary tumour

Many common cancers present with local symptoms that are easily identifiable as possible symptoms of malignancy, for example a breast mass secondary to breast cancer or haemoptysis secondary to lung cancer. In the UK, this has led to the creation of a series of 'red flag' symptoms that should prompt referral for specialist investigation under the '2-week wait' standard introduced for all cancers in 2000. These symptoms are described in more detail in Chapters 326–8. It should be recognized, however, and always born in mind that cancer does not *always* present with 'classic' symptoms. For example, patients with renal cell carcinoma may present with haematuria, loin pain, or a palpable mass, but this 'classic' triad occurs in <10% of cases. Also, some cancers may present with non-specific symptoms that may be present for prolonged periods prior to diagnosis. The common example is ovarian cancer, where little or no symptoms in early disease and vague presentations with abdominal discomfort and bloating, often misdiagnosed as IBS, have led to it being labelled 'the silent killer'.

Symptoms due to metastatic disease

Cancer can first present with a wide range of symptoms secondary to metastatic disease rather than the underlying primary. The chance of presentation with metastatic disease varies widely between different cancer types and histologies. For example, more than 50% of pancreatic cancer patients have distant metastases at diagnosis, compared to less than 10% of differentiated thyroid cancer patients. The pattern of spread also varies, with certain malignancies demonstrating a predilection to metastasize to certain organs for anatomical and biological reasons. For example, colon cancer typically metastasizes to the liver via the portal venous system, whereas ovarian cancer typically spreads transcoelomically over the peritoneal surfaces.

The symptoms and signs precipitated by metastatic disease obviously depend on the site affected. Sign and symptoms associated with various areas are as follows:

- lymph nodes: palpable masses (neck, axillae, groins), lymphoedema, biliary obstruction (porta hepatitis lymphadenopathy)
- liver: anorexia, weight loss, nausea, fever, pain, jaundice
- bone: pain, pathological fracture
- lung: cough, dyspnoea, haemoptysis
- brain: headache, nausea, seizures, focal neurology
- peritoneum: ascites, nausea, vomiting

Constitutional symptoms

Unintentional weight loss

Significant unintentional weight loss (defined as >5% loss of body weight within 6 months) is often regarded as a concerning symptom. Underlying malignancy only accounts for ~25% of cases, however, and the range of other possible causes is diverse. It has been shown that, in the context of normal, simple, baseline examinations (e.g. clinical examination, routine blood tests, chest X-ray, and abdominal ultrasound), the presence of malignancy, and indeed other significant organic illness, is unlikely. Malignancy that does present primarily with weight loss often implies metastatic disease, and the prognosis is generally poor.

Pyrexia of unknown origin

The likely underlying causes of pyrexia of unknown origin (PUO) vary widely depending upon the definition used and the population studied. The proportion of adult cases diagnosed as secondary to an underlying malignancy has decreased over the decades, presumably due to improved diagnosis, and in modern European hospitals is probably now <10%. Where PUO is secondary to a malignancy, it can be of any histology, but risks of haematological malignancy and sarcoma are most increased. PUO is generally associated with more advanced disease and a worse prognosis.

Venous thromboembolic disease

Active malignancy has been estimated to account for almost 20% of incident venous thromboembolic events. The majority of these, however, occur in patients with a preexisting diagnosis of malignancy. In patients with a first episode of deep vein thrombosis and without a known diagnosis of cancer, the risk of new cancer has been estimated at 1%–2% per year, but is thought to be higher in older patients and in those with no other obvious precipitant cause. Therefore, a detailed history should always be taken and any suspicion of underlying cancer investigated as appropriate.

Paraneoplastic syndromes

Malignancies can uncommonly present with the non-metastatic distant signs or symptoms of paraneoplastic syndromes. The cancer that most frequently causes these is small cell lung cancer (SCLC), which is associated with syndrome of inappropriate antidiuretic hormone secretion in up to 40% of cases. Other rarer syndromes seen with SCLC include paraneoplastic cerebellar degeneration and Lambert–Eaton syndrome. Other malignancies that are associated with paraneoplastic syndromes are non-small cell lung cancer (NSCLC), breast cancer, ovarian cancer, and lymphomas.

Paraneoplastic syndromes can be divided into three main groups:

- neurological
- endocrine
- dermatological

Detailed descriptions are beyond the scope of this chapter, and references are supplied for further reading.

Presentation with oncological emergencies

Malignancy can present for the first time as a medical emergency. This could be due to complications of the primary tumour (e.g.

gastrointestinal bleeding) or complications of metastatic disease (e.g. seizures secondary to cerebral metastases or pathological fracture secondary to bone disease). In addition, there are three 'classic' oncological emergencies that are well recognized to be the manner of presentation of a proportion of cancers: spinal cord compression, superior vena cava obstruction, and hypercalcaemia.

Spinal cord compression

Malignant extradural compression of the spinal cord due to involvement of the bony spinal column or adjacent soft tissues occurs in around 5% of patient with a known diagnosis of cancer. In approximately 20% of cases, spinal cord compression is the first presentation of malignancy. The most common malignancies to present with spinal cord compression are lung, prostate, and renal carcinoma, and also malignancies of unknown primary. It presents with a variable onset of sensory and motor signs and symptoms dependant on the severity and level of compression and also whether there is associated pathological fracture or vascular impairment. Urgent investigation with an MRI whole spine, and rapid referral for emergency treatment, are essential, to try and limit neurological sequelae.

Superior vena cava obstruction

Malignant compression of the superior vena cava can also lead to the first presentation of an underlying malignancy. The vast majority (85%–95%) of cases of superior vena cava obstruction are due to cancer, the most common causative types being SCLC, NSCLC, and lymphoma. The syndrome consists of characteristic swelling and oedema, with fixed engorgement of veins, within the distribution of drainage of the superior vena cava (head, neck, arms, and upper thorax). The patient may report symptoms of fullness, breathlessness, and headache, with the symptoms being exacerbated by bending or lying down and being worse in the mornings. While the syndrome requires rapid investigation so that treatment may be given for symptomatic relief, if superior vena cava obstruction is the first presentation of a suspected malignancy, it is vital to obtain histological confirmation of the diagnosis, if at all possible, prior to the commencement of oncological therapy.

Hypercalcaemia

Hypercalcaemia (corrected serum calcium >3.0 mmol/l) occurs in up to 20% of malignancies and can also lead to the presenting symptoms. The most common malignancies to cause hypercalcaemia are breast, lung, prostate, and renal cancers and haematological malignancies (myeloma and lymphomas). The symptoms of hypercalcaemia are often vague and non-specific, including fatigue, drowsiness, confusion, anorexia, nausea and vomiting, polyuria, dehydration, and abdominal pain. Hypercalcaemia should therefore be excluded in many acute clinical presentations and, if confirmed, its presence should be investigated thoroughly to exclude an underlying malignancy.

Screening and incidental presentations

Where screening programmes are in place (e.g. for breast and cervical cancer), patients with new diagnoses present with positive test findings, but usually no clinical symptoms at all. For example, the proportion of new breast cancer diagnoses in UK found as a consequence of mammographic screening is approximately 33%.

The increasing use of more sophisticated medical imaging is leading to an increase in the number of asymptomatic cancers diagnosed incidentally as a consequence of investigation for an unrelated medical problem. While still an uncommon occurrence, this manner of presentation is likely to become more prevalent in the future as the number of investigations performed continues to increase.

Presentation with a family history

While it is only the minority (<5%) of cancer patients that have a truly hereditary malignancy, the inherited cancer predisposition syndromes are increasingly well recognized and described. It is important to recognize the possibility of an inherited genetic defect in a family pedigree so that the patient and their relatives may be referred for genetic counselling, testing, and advice on intervention and prevention, where appropriate. Important examples are the hereditary breast cancer genes BRCA1 and BRCA2, which, when mutated, as well as increasing lifetime breast cancer risk by 10-30-fold, also increase the risks of ovarian, pancreatic, and prostate cancers, thereby affecting both males and females in the family. Multiple cases of early-onset breast cancer (<50 years of age) and bilateral breast cancer are characteristic of families with hereditary breast cancer, and such families should be referred.

Further Reading

Byrne TN, Isakoff SJ, Rincon SP, and Gudewicz TM. Case 27-2012: A 60-year-old woman with painful muscle spasms and hyperreflexia. *N Engl J Med* 2012; 367: 851–61.

Dalmau J, Gilberto Gonzalez R, and Lerwill MF. Case 4-2007: A 56-year-old woman with rapidly progressive vertigo and ataxia. *N Engl J Med* 2007; 356: 612–20.

Darnell RB and Posner JB. Paraneoplastic syndromes involving the nervous system. *N Engl J Med* 2003; 349: 1543–54.

Kerr DJ, Haller DG, Cornelis JH et al (eds). *The Oxford Textbook of Oncology*, 2016. Oxford University Press.

Souhami RL. 'Cancer: Clinical features and management', in Weatherall DJ, ed., *Oxford Textbook of Medicine* (3rd edition), 1996. Oxford University Press.

Introduction

The accurate diagnosis of the precise type and stage of a malignancy is a vital part of cancer management. Treatment options and decisions vary significantly between various stages of the same malignancy (e.g. treatment with radical vs palliative intent) and also between specific histological subtypes of a cancer arising from the same organ (e.g. small-cell lung cancer versus non-small-cell lung cancer (NSCLC)). It is therefore of critical importance that as much accurate information about each individual case is obtained. This is achieved with a variety of diagnostic procedures which allow the multidisciplinary team to reach correct decisions about management. The types of investigations performed typically include radiology and pathology, but clinically important information may also be obtained by other methods, for example surgical staging, clinical examination, endoscopy, and blood tests. As well as directing therapy, accurate staging also allows a more precise estimation of prognosis or the probability of treatment success, knowledge which is of obvious importance to the patient.

Imaging

Imaging plays a vital role in the diagnosis and staging of malignancy. It is often an imaging test that first leads to the suspicion of malignancy, and increasingly sophisticated imaging is being employed more frequently to accurately stage cancer and guide management. Several different modalities are commonly used that have complimentary roles.

Plain radiographs

A plain X-ray is a quick, cheap, and relatively simple investigation and therefore forms an early part of the initial investigation of many malignancies. For example, many lung malignancies are detected by a plain chest X-ray either when investigating relevant symptoms or simply as an incidental finding. Mammography is well established as both a screening tool and part of the diagnostic workup for breast cancer. Plain X-rays are insufficient in themselves to guide modern cancer management, and positive findings are usually confirmed and investigated further by other modalities and tests.

Ultrasound

Ultrasound is another relatively inexpensive, non-invasive investigation that is commonly used in the diagnosis and staging of malignancy. It is often used to guide fine-needle aspiration or core biopsy to obtain a histological diagnosis (e.g. in the diagnosis of breast or neck masses). Specialized ultrasound is also used in some circumstances to aid local staging, for example endoscopic ultrasound to assess oesophageal tumours. Ultrasound is also used to examine the liver for hepatic metastases.

CT scanning

CT scanning has become a 'keystone' for the staging of many malignancies. The speed and availability of modern scanners makes CT an extremely useful tool for imaging the whole body, if required, with one test. While the accuracy of CT assessment is generally good, it can reveal inconclusive findings that require further investigation via other modalities (e.g. small liver abnormalities that require assessment by ultrasound or MRI). CT does have some advantages over MRI, however: for example, it can produce superior images of bony structures and is faster and costs less to run than MRI; in addition, it is quieter and less claustrophobic. Incidental cancers are occasionally noticed on CT scans performed for other reasons (e.g. to investigate suspected renal colic), although the number of non-malignant incidental findings is far greater.

MRI

MRI has much superior soft tissue contrast, compared to CT, and so it allows greater definition of tumours and their relation to fascial planes, bones, vessels, nerves, and adjacent organs. MRI can easily produce images in multiple planes and has the additional advantage of not using ionizing radiation. MRI is commonly used as an adjunct to the local staging of a number of malignancies, including rectal cancer, head and neck cancer, prostate cancer, sarcomas, and CNS malignancies.

FDG-PET scanning

FDG-PET scanning has an evolving role to play in the initial staging of a variety of cancers and also in the assessment of residual/recurrent disease. It has proven to be of particular use in the assessment of NSCLC patients who are otherwise suitable for radical treatment. Prior to the use of FDG-PET in NSCLC staging, up to 50% of operations in apparently early stage disease were proven futile by the presence of disease that was more advanced than had been indicated by other, more conventional staging methods. PET scanning has been demonstrated to reduce the number of futile thoracotomies and this has been proven to be cost effective in CT-node-negative disease. FDG-PET has also been shown to improve diagnostic accuracy and alter patient management in other clinical situations, for example in the staging of colorectal cancer prior to planning metastatectomy, and in the detection of occult primaries in suspected head and neck cancers. There is also some evidence that FDG-PET alters planned radiotherapy treatment volumes in lung, head, and neck cancer, and a trial is underway in early Hodgkin's lymphoma to assess whether a negative FDG-PET after induction chemotherapy can obviate the need for radiotherapy altogether in some cases. The newer technology of FDG-PET/CT is thought to be more accurate than FDG-PET alone by 10%–15% and, as the availability of equipment and expertise improves, it is certain to be put to widespread use.

Pathology

In the majority of cases, a confirmed pathological diagnosis of malignancy is sought before definitive treatment for cancer is undertaken. This is for two main reasons: the first is that benign conditions may mimic malignancy, such that cancer treatment would be entirely inappropriate; the second is that different histological types of malignancy may appear similar clinically and radiologically and yet require very different oncological management, for example lung cancer and lymphoma. As well as confirming the diagnosis, pathological techniques also provide additional prognostic information that can guide management and affect predicted prognosis. The pathologist is, therefore, a vital member of the multidisciplinary team.

Cytology

Cytology is the microscopic examination of stained individual cells and small clusters of cells for diagnosis. The material may be obtained in a number of ways, including via fine-needle aspiration of masses (e.g. of a breast or neck lump), through brushings or scrapes (e.g. bronchial or cervical), and by concentration of fluid samples taken from body cavities (e.g. pleural effusion or ascites) or elsewhere (e.g. sputum or urine). If high-quality cytological samples are available, these are usually sufficient to allow a diagnosis of malignancy and often the major histological type. If the sample is large enough, cells may also be 'spun down' into a pellet that may be embedded in paraffin to allow examination of cells with techniques such as immunohistochemistry. The main advantages of cytology are that it tends to be simpler and less invasive (and therefore suitable for screening) and that it can give a quick result if a cytologist is immediately available. The main disadvantage is that tissue architecture cannot be assessed and so it can be difficult to distinguish between in situ and invasive disease.

Histopathology

Histopathology is the microscopic examination of tissue, rather than individual cells, for diagnosis. The size of tissue examined may vary from small-core needle biopsies through to large, surgically excised specimens. The technique used to obtain the sample and the answers sought from it vary from a simple confirmation of invasive malignancy through to thorough pathological staging of an entire tumour.

Immunohistochemistry

Immunohistochemistry is the process of identifying and localizing proteins on or within cells by using a specific antibody directed at a protein of interest (the antigen) within a sample. In cancer pathology, it has two main uses. The first is the further molecular differentiation of cells, which may look very similar by conventional light microscopy, in order to better confirm the cell type or to give an indication as to the tissue of origin. A good example of this is the relatively common circumstance of a metastatic adenocarcinoma of unknown primary. Using a panel of immunohistochemical markers (including TTF-1, CDX2, CK7, CK20, CEA, ER, etc.) it is possible to estimate the origin of the primary cancer with reasonable positive predictive value. The second use is to assess whether a particular therapeutic intervention is warranted based on the molecular characteristics of the tumour cells. The best example of this is breast cancer, where assessment of the oestrogen and progesterone receptor status and HER2 expression of a tumour is used to determine whether endocrine therapy or trastuzumab is indicated.

Molecular and genetic techniques

Newer molecular and genetic techniques are increasingly being used to aid diagnosis of pathologically complicated tumours and to provide further prognostic and staging information. An example of the diagnostic use of these techniques is in soft tissue sarcomas, which display specific non-random chromosomal changes that now serve as definitive diagnostic criteria (e.g. t(X:18), forming the SYT-SSX transcription factor, diagnostic of synovial sarcoma). An example of how genetic techniques can affect staging is the detection of N-myc amplification in the paediatric cancer neuroblastoma; the detection of this marker influences the prognosis and has therefore been included in the staging criteria. Such techniques are likely to become increasingly commonplace in modern cancer management.

Surgical staging

Often primary surgery for a malignancy acts as both an initial treatment and a staging procedure. The most common examples of this are axillary node sampling for breast cancer and wide lymphadenectomy during colectomy for colon cancer, both of which provide vital staging information regarding the presence or absence of lymph node metastases and so can indicated whether adjuvant chemotherapy is

needed. For suspected ovarian cancer, surgery often represents a diagnostic as well as therapeutic and staging procedure, as histology is often not known preoperatively.

On some occasions, specific surgical procedures are performed to confirm a diagnosis or to stage a malignancy rather than as a therapeutic procedure. Examples of this include neurosurgical biopsy or debulking of a brain tumour to confirm histological diagnosis, and mediastinoscopy to sample lymph nodes prior to definitive treatment for NSCLC.

Clinical and endoscopic staging

For some malignancies, the staging information is derived largely by clinical examination. An example of this is cervical cancer, where clinical examination under anaesthesia (EUA) to assess tumour size and vaginal, parametrial, and uterosacral involvement forms the basis of the FIGO staging system. EUA is often accompanied by proctoscopy and cytoscopy to provide further information.

Other endoscopic examinations are also used to provide diagnosis and staging of malignancies. For example, colonoscopy for colorectal cancer, to provide a histological diagnosis and exclude other synchronous tumours, and bronchoscopy, to confirm a lung cancer, may also provide some information to stage the primary tumour.

Blood tests

While it is not usually the case that a blood test alone can diagnose cancer, serum markers can prove useful is several ways when used in combination with other diagnostic information. They can provide strong evidence as to the origin of metastatic malignancy of unknown primary. For example, sclerotic bone metastases, in combination with a markedly elevated level of prostate-specific antigen, are virtually diagnostic of prostate cancer. Other tumour markers can also provide diagnostic clues and are used in combination with other factors to define the risk of malignancy and so direct further management. For example, for women with adnexal masses, CA125 is used in combination with menopausal status and ultrasound morphology to derive a 'risk of malignancy index' which, while not diagnostic, can triage women between further local investigation and referral to a gynaecological oncologist.

As well as aiding diagnosis, blood tests can also provide prognostic information. For certain malignancies, this is used as part of the staging system. For example, the International Germ Cell Consensus Group Classification uses, amongst other factors, alpha-fetoprotein, human chorionic gonadotrophin, and lactic dehydrogenase to divide metastatic germ cell tumours into good, intermediate, and poor prognostic groups.

Further Reading

https://cancerstaging.org/references-tools/deskreferences/Pages/default.aspx

Peters ML, Pieters RS, Liebmann J, and Graeber G. 'Staging of cancer', in Pieters RS and Liebmann J, eds, *Cancer Concepts: A Guidebook for the Non-Oncologist*, 2013. University of Massachusetts Medical School.

Souhami RL. 'Cancer: Clinical features and management', in Weatherall DJ, ed., *Oxford Textbook of Medicine* (3rd edition), 1996. Oxford University Press.

325 Treatment of cancer

David Cutter and Martin Scott-Brown

Introduction

The variety of conditions that are considered to be 'cancer' is extremely wide, with marked variation in the management approach from disease to disease. A common feature in the management of malignant conditions, however, is the involvement of a wide range of medical professionals at different stages of the patient pathway. This commonly includes physicians, surgeons, radiologists, pathologists, medical oncologists, radiation oncologists, and specialist nurses, as well as a plethora of other allied disciplines. As such, a practice that has been widely adopted is to work as a multidisciplinary team (MDT), with regular meetings to decide the appropriate treatment for each patient with a cancer diagnosis, on an individual and case-by-case basis.

The main treatment modalities for the treatment of cancer are surgery, radiotherapy, and chemotherapy. While these are often combined to form a multimodality therapy, they are all, in isolation, potentially radical (curative) therapies for certain conditions. For example, surgery (in the case of a Stage I colon adenocarcinoma), radiotherapy (in the case of early laryngeal squamous cell carcinoma), and chemotherapy (in the case of acute lymphoblastic leukaemia) are all curative as single-modality treatments. It is commonly the case, however, for a patient to require more than one mode of therapy to achieve the best outcome, for example a combination of surgery, chemotherapy, and radiotherapy for early breast cancer. It can also be the case that two or more different management strategies are thought to give equivalent oncological results, for example surgery or radiotherapy for early prostate cancer. In this situation, the MDT and the patient need to decide on the 'best' management plan for the individual, based on their personal and professional opinions and on the differing toxicity profiles of the alternate treatments.

Surgery

Curative surgery

Surgery is the longest established therapy for cancer and remains the mainstay of radical treatment for most solid tumours. The aim of curative surgery is the complete macroscopic and, as much as possible, microscopic excision of all malignant tissue. The accepted definition of adequate surgical margins varies significantly between cancer types, and also depends on other factors such as tumour size and histological grade/type. The extent of the resection must be balanced against the likely impairment of function and the risks of surgical complications. A detailed knowledge of the natural history of the cancer types and stages and of the possible alternative therapies is therefore essential in formulating a surgical management plan. Often, multimodality therapy may offer the possibility of less extensive or morbid surgery.

Curative surgery is best performed by specialist oncological surgeons who perform a certain number of site-specialized cancer operations each year. The advantage of specific surgical methods and exacting technique has been proven. For example, in rectal cancer the gold-standard operation of 'total mesorectal excision' has been demonstrated to have reduced local recurrence rates when compared with prior surgical techniques. Oncologically adequate primary surgery is a vital part of achieving local cancer control and long-term survival.

Many cancer types metastasize via the lymphatic system. The en bloc resection of regional lymph nodes forms part of the primary treatment for some cancer types. In addition, lymph node dissection provides important staging information and is useful for guiding further therapy. There is, however, considerable controversy over the extent of regional surgery that is appropriate for different cancer sites and types, either where alternative therapy exists (e.g. lymphatic radiotherapy for breast cancer) or where there is uncertainty over the therapeutic benefit (e.g. melanoma).

Cytoreductive surgery

In certain cancers, although all gross disease may not be technically resectable, there is therapeutic value in removing as much disease as possible prior to receiving further therapy. A good example of this is ovarian cancer, where 'maximal cytoreduction', such that there is <2 cm³ of residual disease remaining after surgery, has been demonstrated to improve median survival when performed in combination with chemotherapy.

Surgery for metastatic disease

Solid metastatic cancers are not always incurable and, in certain circumstances, surgery may be used with curative intent for the treatment of limited, and technically resectable, metastatic disease. The most common example of this is the resection of liver metastases from colorectal cancer. For the highly selected minority who are suitable for this treatment, 5-year overall survival rates in contemporary series now exceed 50%. Unfortunately, the majority are not suitable, due to extra-hepatic disease or the extent or location of their liver disease. Surgical resection of isolated or limited lung and brain metastases may also be appropriate on a case-by-case basis. More favourable prognostic factors for these patients include a long disease-free interval, single or few metastases, and smaller bulk of disease.

Palliative surgery

While surgery is less commonly used as a palliative therapy for cancer, there are specific circumstances when it is invaluable for symptom control. Examples include:

- relief of bowel obstruction (or resection for bleeding/perforation)
- palliative loco-regional resection (e.g. to prevent unpleasant local symptoms from a fungating tumour)
- fixation of pathological fractures
- surgical relief of malignant spinal cord compression (demonstrated to be superior to radiotherapy alone in specific circumstances)

The surgeon must know the patient's prognosis and alternative therapeutic options in order to balance the potential benefits, in terms of symptom control and quality of life, against the potential disadvantages and complications of an invasive procedure. It is essential that there is collaboration between surgeons, oncologists, palliative care specialists, and (in some instances) interventional radiologists in these circumstances to decide the best course of management.

Prophylactic surgery

There are some genetic conditions that lead to an extremely high lifetime risk of developing certain types of cancer, for example BRCA mutations leading to breast cancer and familial adenomatous polyposis leading to colon cancer. Prophylactic surgery is a treatment option in these cases, following careful education and counselling about the potential advantages and disadvantages of this approach.

Radiotherapy

Radical and adjuvant radiotherapy

Radiotherapy is the main alternative to surgery as a radical therapy for malignant conditions, either as a single modality or when combined with concurrent chemotherapy. It has replaced, or is an alternative to, surgery for the radical treatment of a variety of cancers, including head and neck cancers, cervical cancer, anal cancer, non-melanomatous skin cancers, bladder cancer, and prostate cancer. Radiotherapy is an effective therapy for lymphoma and germ cell tumours and has been used extensively for these conditions.

Radiotherapy is also used as an adjuvant therapy to eradicate any residual microscopic disease and improve local disease control rates and in some cases, therefore, survival. This is used most commonly for breast cancer, but also for sarcomas, endometrial cancer, and head and neck cancers. Occasionally, radiotherapy is administered neo-adjuvantly (i.e. prior to surgery) to 'down stage' tumours, improve operability, and increase local disease control. The most common example of this is neo-adjuvant chemoradiotherapy for locally advanced rectal cancer.

The commonest form of radiotherapy is external beam radiotherapy, most frequently administered as photons from a linear accelerator. Due to the radiobiology of late toxicity of the normal tissues that are unavoidably irradiated during a radical course of treatment, external beam radiotherapy is usually fractionated (i.e. given in a smaller dose daily over 4–7 weeks) rather than administered as a single treatment. Occasionally, though, external beam radiotherapy is administered as a single large fraction (stereotactic radiosurgery) or in a very few fractions (stereotactic radiotherapy). The radiation dose for a radical treatment is usually in the range of 50–70 Gy, although smaller doses of 40 Gy or less are required for seminomas and lymphomas.

Other commonly used forms of radiotherapy include brachytherapy, which is the placement of radioactive sources at the site for treatment (e.g. intra-prostatic implantation of iodine-125 seeds for localized prostate cancer) and radioisotope therapy (e.g. the use of orally administered iodine-131 for the treatment of differentiated thyroid cancer).

Palliative radiotherapy

Radiotherapy is an effective palliative treatment for symptom control in advanced malignancy. Common uses include:

- relief of pain (especially bone pain, but also from other sites)
- control of bleeding (e.g. haematuria, haemoptysis, PR or PV bleeding)
- treatment for obstruction of hollow organs (e.g. bronchus, oesophagus, or rectum)
- treatment for malignant spinal cord compression
- treatment for superior vena cava obstruction
- treatment for brain and/or leptomeningeal metastases
- treatment of other symptomatic sites (e.g. fungating tumours, skin metastases, nodal disease)

Due to the differing aims of palliative radiotherapy, for convenience, such treatments are often administered as fewer and individually larger fractions, to a lower total dose. For example, a single 8 Gy fraction is commonly used for bone pain, and 20–36 Gy in 5–12 treatments in other circumstances. Occasionally, higher radiotherapy doses are appropriate to attempt to maintain local disease control for as long as possible and hopefully prevent unpleasant symptoms from developing if the prognosis and clinical situation suggest this may be a potential problem. Radioisotopes are also used as a palliative treatment (e.g. strontium for widespread bone pain).

Cytotoxic chemotherapy and endocrine therapy

Radical and adjuvant chemotherapy

In terms of radical therapy, cytotoxic chemotherapy is the third most important modality of treatment and is only curative in isolation for haematological malignancies and germ cell tumours which are exquisitely chemosensitive.

In terms of numbers, cytotoxic chemotherapy plays a much more significant role as an adjuvant therapy for solid tumours to reduce the risk of recurrent disease following primary therapy (usually surgery). The best examples of this are adjuvant chemotherapy for breast cancer and colon cancer.

Endocrine therapy in the form of tamoxifen and, more recently, aromatase inhibitors also plays an important role in the adjuvant therapy of hormone-responsive breast cancers, reducing recurrence rates and improving overall survival.

Palliative chemotherapy

Cytotoxic chemotherapy, as a systemic treatment, has the theoretical advantage of being able to treat all sites of metastatic disease simultaneously and has an established role in the management of advanced malignancy. Chemotherapy has contributed significantly towards improved survival for some disease types; for example, the median survival of patients with metastatic colorectal cancer has improved from 5–6 months, without treatment, to 20–24 months with modern chemotherapy. For other sites, however, the benefits are less marked; for example, palliative chemotherapy for advanced pancreatic cancer improves median survival from 2–3 months to 5–6 months, albeit with some associated benefits in terms of quality of life.

Endocrine therapies are also commonly used as palliative treatments for hormone-responsive advanced breast cancer and prostate cancer, producing significant clinical benefits without the toxicity often associated with cytotoxic chemotherapy.

Newer therapies

Surgical advances and other local therapies

Conventional surgical techniques are constantly evolving with the development of new technology, for example minimally invasive surgery, with the aim of reducing surgical morbidity while maintaining or improving oncological outcomes. A number of other local cancer therapies are also in use and under investigation. These include cryotherapy, most commonly used for locally recurrent prostate cancer, and radiofrequency ablation.

Advances in radiotherapy

While the basic principle behind radiotherapy remains the same today as always, technological advances in the delivery of radiotherapy are allowing improvements in the therapeutic ratio for various malignancies. Intensity-modulated radiotherapy, for example, allows the delivery of more complicated distributions of radiation dose (including concave volumes) to the intended target, while avoiding high doses to adjacent organs and thereby reducing toxicity. This ability has been utilized in prostate cancer to reduce rectal and urinary toxicity and in head and neck cancer to reduce xerostomia from salivary gland irradiation, while maintaining efficacy. A variety of techniques using both conventional linear accelerators and alternative equipment (e.g. tomotherapy and Cyberknife systems) have been developed. Progress in the imaging techniques associated with radiotherapy will also allow improved accuracy of target definition and compensation for organ movement (e.g. with respiration) to maximize the radiotherapy dose to the tumour while minimizing the exposure of normal tissues.

The vast majority of external beam radiotherapy is currently administered with photon beams (X-rays). There is a developing interest in replacing photons with protons and perhaps even heavier charged particles to take advantage of specific physical characteristics of their depth dose curves, allowing the delivery of a high dose of radiation to a tightly defined volume while sparing adjacent structures. In addition to having these dosimetric advantages, certain charged particle beams, such as carbon ions, also possess some biologic advantages in terms of tumour kill potential. The equipment, expertise, and quality control required to perform these therapies is extremely expensive and, at present, particle therapy is mainly utilized for research purposes and some very specific indications, for example paediatric tumours and skull base chordomas and is unlikely to enter mainstream practice, at least in the UK, for the foreseeable future.

Targeting of radioisotopes allows radiotherapy to be administered systemically. The natural avidity of thyroid tissue for iodine has allowed the use of ^{131}I as a 'targeted' therapy for over 50 years. With advances in modern cellular biology, it is now possible to design conjugates that direct radioisotopes to particular cellular targets. An example of such a targeted radiopharmaceutical that has proven effective is ^{90}Y-ibritumomab tiuxetan for non-Hodgkin's lymphoma, and further agents are in preclinical development and early clinical trials.

'Targeted' drug therapies

Over the last decade or so, new generations of non-conventional anticancer drug therapies have emerged from development into clinical practice and are now an increasingly important part of modern cancer treatment. They are often developed with the intent of 'targeting' a specific cellular mechanism or pathway that is known to be important in the mechanisms of cancer. The two main types are the monoclonal antibody therapies and 'small molecule' therapies.

The most widely used monoclonal antibody therapies are trastuzumab and rituximab. Trastuzumab is a humanized monoclonal antibody that interferes with the HER2/neu receptor. This receptor is overexpressed in a proportion of breast cancers, and over-activity of the related cellular pathways (the PI3K/Akt and MAPK pathways) is implicated in many aspects of cancer progression, for example uncontrolled cell division, invasion, and angiogenesis. Adjuvant trastuzumab given for HER2-positive early breast cancer (20%–30% of cases) has been shown to improve both disease-free and overall survival in large randomized trials. Trastuzumab is also used as a palliative treatment for HER2-positive metastatic breast cancer, both as monotherapy and in combination with conventional chemotherapy, where it has been proven to improve response rates, compared to chemotherapy given alone. Rituximab is a chimeric monoclonal antibody that binds to the CD20 protein, which is widely expressed on B-lymphocytes. The exact mode of action is unknown but one mechanism involves the induction of apoptosis in CD20-positive cells, and rituximab is widely used in the treatment of B-cell non-Hodgkin's lymphoma, having been shown to improve results over conventional cytotoxic chemotherapy alone in various forms of the disease. Other examples of monoclonal antibodies used for cancer therapy are cetuximab, which targets the epidermal growth factor receptor; bevacizumab, which targets vascular endothelial growth factor A; and alemtuzumab, which targets CD52.

The majority of the currently used 'targeted small molecule' therapies are directed at a large group of tyrosine kinase (TK) enzymes. The first example used in clinical practice, imatinib, has proven extremely successful in the treatment of chronic myeloid leukaemia (where the target is the TK domain of the pathogenic bcr–abl fusion protein) and gastrointestinal stromal tumours (where the target is the TK c-kit). Other examples of TK inhibitors include the 'multitarget' inhibitors sorafenib and sunitinib, which have shown efficacy in metastatic renal cell carcinoma and hepatocellular carcinoma, diseases where effective therapies were previously lacking.

Research into new systemic therapies is ongoing, with new agents (e.g. mTOR and proteasome inhibitors) under active investigation. As we gain a greater understanding of the underlying cellular basis of cancer, further targets and associated therapies will undoubtedly be developed and added to the therapeutic options available for a variety of cancers.

Further Reading

Chabner BA and Loeffler J. 'Cancer chemotherapy and radiation therapy', in Warrell DA, Cox TM, and Firth JD, eds, *Oxford Textbook of Medicine* (5th edition), 2010. Oxford University Press.

Chang HM, Moudgil R, Scarabelli T et al. Cardiovascular Complications of Cancer Therapy: Best Practices in Diagnosis, Prevention, and Management: Part 1. *J Am Coll Cardiol* 2017; 70: 2536–51.

Chang HM, Okwuosa TM, Scarabelli T et al. Cardiovascular Complications of Cancer Therapy: Best Practices in Diagnosis, Prevention, and Management: Part 2. *J AM Coll Cardiol* 2017; 70: 2552–65.

Gotwals P, Cameron S, Cipolletta D, et al. Prospects for combining targeted and conventional cancer therapy with immunotherapy. *Nat Rev Cancer* 2017; 17: 286–301.

Kerr DJ, Haller DG, Cornelis JH et al (eds). *The Oxford Textbook of Oncology*, 2016. Oxford University Press.

Souhami RL. 'Cancer: Clinical features and management', in Weatherall DJ, ed., *Oxford Textbook of Medicine* (3rd edition), 1996. Oxford University Press.

Definition of the disease

Prostate cancer is the commonest male malignancy, with approximately 35 000 new cases in the UK annually, equating to a lifetime risk of 1 in 10. When diagnosed early, it has a high chance of cure with surgery, external beam radiotherapy, or brachytherapy. Even for metastatic disease, the prognosis is usually several years.

Aetiology of the disease

The mechanism of transformation from normal prostate cells to cancer is poorly understood but appears to have a hormonal basis, with androgen stimulation playing an important role in the pathogenesis. While in most cases there is no clear aetiology, in up to 5% of cases there is a recognizable pattern of inheritance, some of which is attributable to mutations of the BRCA1 tumour suppressor gene.

Approximately 75% of prostate cancers arise in the peripheral zone of the gland, with the remainder arising in the central and transitional zones. Many prostate cancers are multifocal, arising synchronously within different parts of the prostate.

Histologically, over 95% of prostate cancers are adenocarcinomas, derived from prostatic acinar cells.

Typical symptoms of the disease, and less common symptoms

The disease generally presents in one of three ways:

- asymptomatically
- with local symptoms
- with symptoms of metastatic disease

Asymptomatic prostate cancer

Prostate cancer is often diagnosed in asymptomatic individuals on the basis of an elevated level of serum prostate-specific antigen (PSA) or an abnormal-feeling prostate on digital rectal examination (DRE). Alternatively, it may be discovered as the result of an unexpected histological finding following trans-urethral resection of the prostate (TURP) for benign prostatic hypertrophy (BPH).

Prostate cancer with local symptoms

Prostate cancer can cause local symptoms which often initially mimic those of BPH: urinary frequency, poor stream, urgency, hesitancy, incomplete emptying, and nocturia. Rarer but recognized symptoms include incontinence, impotence, haematuria, and haematospermia, all of which are suggestive of more locally advanced disease.

Prostate cancer with symptoms of metastatic disease

Only 5% of patients have metastatic disease at presentation. The disease spreads mainly by the haematogenous route. It has a predilection for bones, particularly the axial skeleton. Bone metastases are usually osteoblastic, although up to 20% are osteoclastic. Sites of bony involvement include, in decreasing order of frequency, the lumbar spine, the proximal femur, the pelvis, the thoracic spine, the ribs, the sternum, and the skull base (which typically presents with cranial nerve palsies). Compared to the case with other malignancies, the spread of prostate cancer to the liver and the lungs is a relatively rare and late event.

Demographics of the disease

Like the prostate gland from which it arises, prostate cancer is exclusively a male disease. The risk of developing the disease increases with age. The disease is rare in those below the age of 40, and only 15% of patients are diagnosed below the age of 65. Post-mortem studies in men dying from other causes show that, by the age of 80, 70% of men will have at least microscopic evidence of prostate cancer.

Natural history, and complications of the disease

Without treatment, the natural history of the disease is variable. Prostate cancer often behaves very indolently. Given that many patients who develop the disease are elderly, it is not difficult to see why more prostate cancer patients die of other causes than from their cancer. In some patients, however, the disease can behave in a more aggressive manner. Staging investigations which can help predict the behaviour of a given cancer are discussed in 'Prognosis and how to estimate it'.

Approach to diagnosing the disease

DRE

The anatomy of the prostate allows the peripheral zone, where the majority of prostate cancers arise, to be palpated on rectal examination. A DRE may reveal a hard, irregular gland, firm nodules, or induration and can detect approximately 55% of prostate cancers.

Serum PSA

PSA, which is expressed by both normal and malignant prostate cells, has become increasingly important in the screening and diagnosing of prostate cancers since the late 1980s. PSA can also be elevated in benign conditions, including BPH, prostatitis, and urinary retention, or following prostate biopsy (see also Table 326.1 and 'Serum PSA testing').

Referral guidelines

The National Institute for Health and Care Excellence (NICE) advise urgent referral for any of the following:

- hard, irregular prostate on DRE
- normal-feeling prostate but rising/raised age-specific PSA, with or without lower urinary tract symptoms
- symptoms and high PSA levels

Other diagnoses that should be considered

BPH is a common cause of urinary symptoms such as urinary frequency, poor stream, urgency, hesitancy, incomplete emptying, and

Table 326.1 Age-specific cut-off PSA measurements	
Age	PSA (ng/ml)
50–59	> 3.0
60–69	> 4.0
70–79	> 5.0

Note: No age-specific reference ranges exist for men over 80.

Reproduced with permission of NHS Cancer Screening Programme © 2009.

nocturia. It is frequently associated with mild PSA elevation, which can instigate investigation to exclude a prostate cancer.

'Gold-standard' diagnostic test

Serum PSA testing

PSA is a highly sensitive test but lacks specificity. Levels above 10 correlate with presence of prostate cancer in up to two-thirds of cases. PSA levels between 4 and 10 prove to be associated with cancer in about one-quarter of cases. While a PSA level less than 4 is reassuring, a percentage of patients with prostate cancer do have PSA results in this range. The specificity of the test can be increased by using an age-specific PSA table (see Table 326.1) or by combining the test with other investigations.

Trans-rectal ultrasound and biopsy

Trans-rectal ultrasound (TRUS) allows visualization of the prostate gland and enables biopsies to be taken. On TRUS, cancers appear hypoechoic. The whole gland should be sampled, with at least 12 biopsies taken. In addition to its diagnostic value, TRUS is also useful for assessing the volume of the prostate and so can assist in treatment choice.

Gleason score

The Gleason score is a histological grade based on the Gleason grade, which allocates tumours a value between 1 and 5, based on the glandular architecture. A Gleason grade of 1 represents a near-normal glandular pattern, while a grade of 5 represents the more aggressive end of the spectrum, with no clear glandular pattern.

The Gleason score is the sum of two Gleason grades: the predominant pattern and the second most common pattern. A typical score would be expressed, for example, as 'Gleason 3 + 3 = 6', 'Gleason 4 + 3 = 7', or 'Gleason 4 + 5 = 9'.

Staging

Prostate cancer can be staged using the TNM system (available online at http://cancerstaging.org/references-tools/quickreferences/Documents/ProstateSmall.pdf). Additionally, prostate cancer can be classified according to the following three categories:

- localized prostate cancer which is completely contained within the prostate (T1 or T2), with no metastatic involvement of regional lymph nodes (N0), or distant sites (M0)
- locally advanced prostate cancer which extends through the prostatic capsule, with extra-capsular extension or invasion of one or both seminal vesicles (T3), invasion of adjacent structures other than seminal vesicles (T4), or involvement of regional lymph nodes (N1), but no distant metastases (M0)
- metastatic prostate cancer which has spread beyond regional lymph nodes, with involvement either of non-regional lymph nodes (M1a), bone (M1b), or other sites with or without associated bone disease (M1c)

Risk stratification

Based on the PSA level, Gleason score, and T stage, patients can be stratified into three categories according to their risk of disease recurrence after definitive local treatment. This risk stratification is also helpful in guiding both imaging investigations and in formulating recommendations for treatment. The three categories are shown in Table 326.2.

Table 326.2 Risk stratification

	PSA level (ng/ml)		Gleason score		T staging
Low risk	<10	and	≤6	and	T1–T2a
Intermediate risk	10–20	or	7	or	T2b
High risk	>20	or	8–10	or	T2c, T3, or T4

Adapted from NICE Guidance 2008.

Multiparametric MRI pelvis

When radical treatment is being considered, it is important to know if the tumour is confined within the prostate (T2 disease) or shows evidence of having breached the prostatic capsule (T3 disease). This is most accurately assessed on multiparametric MRI. It is also helpful in identifying seminal vesicle invasion and enlarged local lymph nodes.

Acceptable diagnostic alternatives to the gold standard

Prostate cancer is not uncommonly an incidental finding found at a review of histology performed after a TURP procedure for presumed BPH. For this reason, histological examination should be performed on all tissue removed at TURP.

When an MRI scan of the prostate is not possible or contraindicated, local disease can be staged on CT or ultrasound, although both are regarded as inferior to MRI.

Other relevant investigations

Nuclear medicine bone scan

A nuclear medicine bone scan is used to determine the presence and location of skeletal metastases. A bone scan should be performed in all patients with intermediate or high-risk disease (see Table 326.2). In the absence of bone pain, a bone scan is not routinely indicated in patients with low-risk disease.

Axial MRI

An axial MRI can be used to exclude skeletal metastasis, as an alternative to a nuclear medicine bone scan or to further investigate indeterminate lesions seen on a bone scan. It is able to detect small axial bone metastases not visible on a bone scan.

Prognosis and how to estimate it

The prognosis of a man diagnosed with prostate cancer varies according to his stage, Gleason grade, and PSA level, as shown in Table 326.2 (also see 'Risk stratification'). Age and comorbidities are, of course, independent factors, which will affect the patient's chance of being alive 5–10 years after being diagnosed.

In a man with low-risk disease, there is a very good chance of the disease being cured with any of the radical treatments discussed in 'Treatment and its effectiveness'. For men with high-risk disease, while long-term cure is still possible, there is a higher likelihood that the cancer will either progress or spread. Partin tables, which take account of the variables in Table 326.2, along with more detailed online nomograms can be used to estimate individual patient outcomes.

Treatment and its effectiveness

Prevention

There is currently no treatment licensed for the prevention of prostate cancer. The recent Phase 3 Prostate Cancer Prevention Trial randomized 18 882 men over 55 with normal DRE and a PSA level under 3 ng/ml to receive either 7 years of finasteride or placebo. Finasteride is an anti-androgen which inhibits the enzyme 5-alpha reductase, thereby blocking the metabolism of testosterone to the more potent androgen, dihydrotestosterone. Despite the not-insignificant toxicity profile that includes impotence, loss of libido, and ejaculatory difficulties, the trial did demonstrate an impressive 24.8% reduction in the prevalence of prostate cancer in the finasteride arm of the study. Of note, however, is that, of those men who did go on to develop cancer, there was a higher proportion of high-grade cancers in the finasteride arm.

Screening

The existence of minimally invasive and cheap initial screening in the form of DRE and PSA testing makes screening for prostate cancer an attractive possibility. Numerous studies have shown that, for patients with a PSA level more than 4 ng/ml, there is a 1:3 chance of detecting prostate cancer at biopsy. Using this cut-off in screening would pick up nearly 70% of prostate cancers. While strong evidence exists that prostate cancer screening is effective in diagnosing more cancers, controversy remains over what impact, if any, detecting more prostate cancers would have on the more important endpoint of improving overall survival. Two large screening trials set up to address this question have recently reported conflicting outcomes. For the present, therefore, there are no plans to introduce a national PSA screening programme in this country, and men should be encouraged to discuss the pros and cons of individual screening with their family doctors.

Treatment of early stage prostate cancer

Early stage prostate cancer, where the disease is confined to the prostate gland, is potentially curable. Radical prostatectomy, radical radiotherapy, and brachytherapy, along with active surveillance, all have a role in the curative treatment of prostate cancer (Table 326.3). There are no randomized trials comparing these treatments head to head; in the absence of these, side effect profiles play an important role in clinician recommendations and patient choice.

Watchful waiting

While so-called watchful waiting should not be regarded as a curative treatment, it is appropriate for some patients. Watchful waiting is the conscious decision not to treat until patients develop symptoms, at which point they are usually treated with hormone therapy. It is particularly suitable for patients with a short life expectancy, such as the elderly or those with significant comorbidities, as these patients are unlikely to die from prostate cancer.

Active surveillance

Active surveillance is a programme of serial DRE, PSA testing, and TRUS-guided biopsies which allow the disease to be reassessed at regular intervals, with a view to deciding if and when treatment becomes necessary. It should be considered in patients who have low-grade tumours and are fit enough to undergo a radical treatment in the event of disease progression. This approach can delay and, in some cases, avoid altogether the risks and side effects of a radical treatment.

Radical prostatectomy

Radical prostatectomy involves the complete resection of the prostate along with the seminal vesicles. Various surgical techniques for this exist, including open retropubic or perineal approaches and laparoscopic or robotically assisted techniques. Surgery is usually reserved for medically fit men who are under 65–70 years old and have T1 or T2 node-negative disease, a low-to-moderate Gleason score, and a PSA level <10, but it can also be used in men with higher-risk disease. In appropriately selected patients, mortality is less than 1%, but major morbidity may be as high as 10%. Approximately 10%–40% of patients will have a degree of urinary incontinence, and up to 60% will have impotence following surgery.

Radical radiotherapy (external beam radiotherapy)

Current NICE guidelines recommend that patients undergoing radical radiotherapy for prostate cancer receive a minimum dose of 74 Gy in no more than 2 Gy per fraction. Patients undergo a 15-minute treatment daily for up to 7.5 weeks. Recent trial evidence suggests shorter regimes with a higher dose per fraction are equally efficacious, and many UK hospitals are now adopting treatment with 60 Gy in 20 fractions over 4 weeks as the current standard of care. There is ongoing research aimed at reducing the number of treatments even further using stereotactic body radiotherapy. Side effects of radiotherapy can be divided into acute side effects (predominantly urinary symptoms, rectal discomfort, bowel symptoms, and fatigue), which generally settle within a few weeks of finishing the treatment, and long-term side effects, which are frequently permanent. Impotence occurs less frequently than following surgery but still affects up to 30%–60% of patients. Other long-term side effects include proctitis (which occurs in approximately 5% or patients), incontinence (which occurs in less than 5% of patients), and long-term changes in bowel habit. Unlike surgery, mortality is not increased by radiotherapy, so there is no age cut-off; however, there is a 2%–3% risk of severe toxicity. In patients with intermittent or high-risk disease, hormonal therapy is usually given in combination with radiotherapy. Pelvic radiotherapy can be considered for patients with a high risk of pelvic lymph node involvement.

Brachytherapy

Brachytherapy is a form of radiotherapy in which the radiation is delivered directly to the prostate using radioactive sources. Two different techniques are used: permanent implantation of radioactive seeds (low-dose-rate brachytherapy) or temporary implantation of radioactive wires (high-dose-rate brachytherapy). Brachytherapy is particularly suitable for men with low-risk disease and relatively small prostate glands and is usually not advised in men with significant obstructive lower urinary tract symptoms or those who have previously undergone TURP. Brachytherapy has a relatively favourable side effect profile, causing lower rates of impotence and incontinence than surgery or external beam radiotherapy but higher rates of obstructive and irritative urinary symptoms. In men with intermediate or high-risk disease, combined treatment with high-dose-rate brachytherapy and external beam radiotherapy can be considered.

Cryotherapy and high-intensity focused ultrasound

Cryotherapy and high-intensity focused ultrasound are new techniques that aim to eradicate prostate cancer by freezing or heating the gland, respectively. They are not currently recommended outside the context of clinical trials, as there is an inadequate amount of long-term outcome data.

Treatment of advanced prostate cancer

Advanced or metastatic disease is, by definition, incurable, and the aim of treatment is therefore to prolong survival and relieve symptoms. Even in this setting, the disease may follow a relatively indolent

Table 326.3 Summary of treatment management options for men with localized prostate cancer		Low risk	Intermediate risk	High risk
Watchful waiting		◆	◆	◆
Radical treatments	Active surveillance	✓	◆	✗
	Prostatectomy	◆	✓	✓*
	External beam Radiotherapy	◆	✓	✓
	Brachytherapy	◆	◆	✗
	High-dose rate brachytherapy with external beam radiotherapy	✗	✓	✓
	Cryotherapy and HIFU	✗†	✗†	✗†

Abbreviations: HIFU, high-intensity focused ultrasound.

Key: ✓, preferred treatment; ◆, treatment option; ✗ not recommended.

*Offer if there is a realistic prospect of long-term disease control.

†Unless as part of a clinical trial comparing use with established interventions.

Adapted from NICE Guidance 2008.

course in some patients. In this section, some of the more commonly used treatments for advanced prostate cancer will be discussed. Each has slightly different indications; therefore, not all drugs will be suitable for every patient. The sequencing of the drugs is individualized based on patient and disease characteristics.

Hormone therapy

Prostate cancer growth is dependent on the presence of testosterone. Therefore, androgen deprivation therapy (ADT) is one approach that can be used for the treatment of men with metastatic prostate cancer.

First-line ADT can be achieved surgically, through bilateral orchidectomy, or medically, by use of subcutaneously administered luteinizing hormone-releasing hormone agonists (LHRHa). These drugs stimulate the production of testosterone in a non-pulsatile (non-physiological) manner, resulting in a disruption of the endogenous hormonal feedback systems and the subsequent downregulation of testosterone production. Anti-androgen tablets should always be started 2 weeks before commencing LHRHa therapy and continued for a further 2 weeks after starting, to prevent transient 'tumour flare', which is caused by an initial increase in testosterone levels during the early days of treatment. Monitoring response to therapy is usually possible by measuring serum PSA, which often falls to undetectable levels. Recently, a luteinizing hormone-releasing hormone antagonist called degaralix has been introduced; it directly blocks the pituitary axis, thus avoiding the initial stimulation of androgen production and negating the need for initial anti-androgens.

If serial PSA testing indicates that the disease appears to be escaping biochemical control, several additional lines of hormonal therapies exist which interfere with various aspects of testosterone metabolism and actions on the tumour:

- anti-androgen tablets can be added to ADT to achieve so-called complete androgen blockade; these drugs block androgen receptors on the cancer cells
- gonadotrophin-releasing hormone antagonists block the release of luteinizing hormone from the pituitary, thereby suppressing testosterone release from the testes
- abiraterone inhibits formation of testosterone by blocking the enzyme CYP17A1; as cortisol production is also inhibited, the drug is therefore given together with prednisolone
- enzalutamide is an inhibitor of androgen receptor signalling

Other hormone therapies that can be used later in the disease course include oestrogens, progestogens, and corticosteroids.

Chemotherapy

Chemotherapy is approved by NICE for the treatment of hormone-refractory metastatic prostate cancer. Docetaxel is generally considered to be the first-line treatment for medically fit patients with metastatic disease. Side effects include tiredness, nausea, vomiting, hair loss, and bone marrow suppression (along with the accompanying risk of neutropenic sepsis).

Palliative radiotherapy

Radiotherapy plays an important role in the management of bone metastases. Pain caused by metastases usually responds very well even to a single fraction of radiotherapy. Spinal cord compression not suitable for spinal surgery can be treated with a short course of radiotherapy (1–5 days of treatment). Radiotherapy is also indicated following surgical fixation of pathological fractures or spinal surgery.

Bisphosphonates and denosumab

Bisphosphonates and denosumab may reduce the incidence of skeletal events, although evidence for this is lacking and their use in this context is not recommended by NICE. They have a role in the treatment of osteoporosis, which is a long-term side effect of androgen deprivation, and in the control of pain associated with metastatic bone disease.

Bone-seeking radioisotopes

Administration of bone-seeking radioisotopes can be helpful in a subset of patients, to control widespread symptomatic osteoblastic bone disease when the disease no longer responds to hormonal manipulation. The use of radium-223 in this context is associated with a small increase in life expectancy.

Immunotherapy

Sipuleucel-T is a personalized cell-based cancer vaccine licensed for the treatment of prostate cancer. It works by programming the immune system to seek out cancer cells expressing prostate acid phosphatase, which is a tissue antigen that is expressed by most prostate cancer cells, irrespective of where they are in the patient. It is prepared specifically for each patient and is thus costly, but it has been shown to improve 3-year survival in patients with metastatic, castration-resistant prostate cancer by 10% compared to placebo (31.7% vs 21.7%) and prolongs mean survival by over 4 months. There is ongoing research using immune checkpoint inhibitors in metastatic prostate cancer.

Further Reading

Horwich A, Parker C, de Reijke T, et al. Prostate cancer: ESMO Clinical Practice Guidelines for diagnosis, treatment and follow-up. *Ann Oncol* 2013; 24: vi106–vi114.

National Institute for Health and Care Excellence. *Prostate Cancer: Diagnosis and Treatment*. 2014. Available at http://www.nice.org.uk/Guidance/CG175 (accessed 16 Sep 2017).

327 Breast cancer

Daniel Ajzensztejn

Definition of the disease

Breast cancer is the commonest female cancer, with a lifetime risk of approximately 1 in 9. There are approximately 40 000 new cases and 11 000 deaths from the disease in England and Wales each year.

Aetiology of the disease

The aetiology of breast cancer is complex, with hormonal, genetic, and modifiable lifestyle factors all involved in developing the disease.

Hormonal risk factors include early menarche, late menopause, usage of hormone replacement therapy, late age at first pregnancy, and nulliparity.

Genetic factors account for up to 10% of breast cancers. Patients with mutations in the BRCA1 tumour suppressor gene have an approximately 50% lifetime risk of developing breast cancer and account for approximately 1% of all breast cancer diagnoses. Carriers also have an increased risk of developing ovarian cancer. BRCA2 tumour suppressor gene mutations account for a further 1% of breast cancers, and carriers have a lifetime risk of approximately 75% of developing breast cancer. Carriers also have an increased risk of prostate cancer, pancreatic cancer, bladder cancer, and non-Hodgkin's lymphoma. Li–Fraumeni syndrome is caused by a germline p53 mutation; carriers of this mutation have a 50% lifetime risk of breast cancer and other malignancies. Several other genetic syndromes have been linked to an increased incidence of breast cancer. There are also families with an increased risk of developing the disease but where the genetic basis of this risk has not yet been fully established.

Modifiable lifestyle factors are also believed to play a role in the development of breast cancer. Obesity results in increased circulating levels of oestrogen, which increases the risk of breast cancer. Healthy diets which are low in alcohol and fats have been suggested to reduce the risk of developing the disease.

Typical symptoms of the disease, and less common symptoms

Breast cancer generally presents in one of three ways:

- asymptomatically
- with locoregional symptoms
- as metastatic disease

Asymptomatic breast cancer

The UK, like many countries, has a national mammographic screening programme, so many breast cancers are picked up prior to onset of symptoms. In addition, screening is able to detect ductal carcinoma in situ (DCIS), a pre-malignant condition which, without treatment, progresses to invasive cancer in up to 50% of cases.

Breast cancer with locoregional symptoms

Locoregional symptoms of breast cancer include:

- lumps
- skin/nipple changes
- lymphadenopathy

Lumps

While most breast lumps are not cancerous, concerning features include lumps which are painless, solitary, unilateral, or hard. Half of all breast cancers arise within the upper outer quadrant of the breast.

Skin/nipple changes

Skin redness, dimpling, change in contour, 'peau d'orange', ulceration, nipple inversion, and nipple discharge may all be the first presentations of breast cancer.

Lymphadenopathy

Although relatively uncommon, axillary lymphadenopathy may be the presenting symptom of breast cancer. Usually, an ipsilateral breast tumour will be found on either examination or imaging. See also see the referral guidelines in 'Approach to diagnosing the disease'.

Metastatic breast cancer

The first presentation of breast cancer may be with metastatic spread. Common sites of spread include the bones, the liver, the lungs, and the brain.

Demographics of the disease

The risk of developing breast cancer increases with age. At age 25, the disease affects approximately 1 in 20 000 women. By the age of 45, the risk has risen to just under 1 in 100. By the time a woman reaches age 85, her lifetime risk of having developed the disease is 1 in 9. The disease can develop in men, but this is relatively rare, accounting for less than 1% of all breast cancer diagnoses.

Natural history, and complications of the disease

Breast cancer is an adenocarcinoma which arises from the glandular tissue of the breast. The disease can be further subdivided histologically. Approximately 75% of breast adenocarcinomas are ductal. Lobular carcinomas account for a further 10%, with medullary, tubular, and several less common subtypes accounting for the remainder.

DCIS is a pre-malignant condition which, without treatment, progresses to invasive ductal carcinoma in up to 50% of cases. Lobular carcinoma in situ (LCIS) is not a true pre-malignant condition. Its presence is, however, indicative of unstable breast tissue, and a finding of LCIS triples a person's lifetime risk of developing breast cancer in either breast (usually, ductal adenocarcinoma)

Invasive breast cancer normally spreads to the axillary lymph nodes in a stepwise progression from the first level through to the third-level axillary nodes. Knowledge of this natural history has revolutionized axillary surgery in recent years through the introduction of sentinel node biopsies (see 'Sentinel node biopsy' in 'Treatment and its effectiveness'). The supraclavicular and internal mammary lymph nodes may also be involved.

Metastatic disease is rare in the absence of node involvement. As mentioned in 'Metastatic breast cancer', common sites of spread are the bones, the liver, the lungs, and the brain.

Approach to diagnosing the disease

NICE guidelines advise urgent referral (within 2 weeks) following an abnormal screening mammogram (see 'Screening') or for any patient who is over the age of 30 and presents with any of the following breast signs or symptoms: a discrete lump; ulceration; a skin nodule; skin distortion; nipple eczema; recent nipple retraction or distortion; and unilateral nipple discharge. Other breast symptoms for which referral is advised (although not necessarily urgently) include a discrete lump in women under the age of 30; asymmetrical nodularity that persists at review after menstruation; an abscess; a persistent refilling or recurrent cyst; intractable pain; and bilateral nipple discharge.

All such patients are seen by a clinician; their history is taken and they then undergo triple assessment, which comprises:

- clinical examination
- imaging (bilateral mammography and ultrasound)
- histology: (assessed on core biopsy)

The assessing clinicians will allocate each a score between 1 and 5, and these scores will be used to recommend further investigation and treatment through multidisciplinary team discussions.

In patients with confirmed breast cancer, blood tests, including a full blood count, liver function tests, and calcium levels, should be performed. Further investigations may include imaging with CT thorax and abdomen along with an isotope bone scan or an MRI of the marrow (the image modality of choice varies according to local protocol). Decisions as to which patients should have such imaging routinely are guided by the risk of finding metastatic disease. In patients with T1 or T2 tumours who have a risk in the order of 2% for having metastatic disease, some clinicians would not routinely perform additional staging investigations. In contrast, patients with T3 or T4 tumours have approximately ten times this risk of metastatic disease, and further staging investigations are routine.

Additional investigations may occasionally be indicated; for example, where full blood count is suggestive of bone marrow involvement, then bone marrow aspiration and trephine should be considered, to exclude metastatic bone marrow infiltration.

The anatomical extent of the cancer is staged using the TNM staging system, which is available online at http://cancerstaging.org/references-tools/quickreferences/Documents/BreastMedium.pdf.

Other diagnoses that should be considered

The majority (90%) of referrals to triple assessment clinics turn out to be related to benign breast disorders and these are therefore the main differentials.

Benign breast disorders that may present similarly to breast cancers include fibrocystic disease, fibroadenomas, intra-ductal papilloma, lipoma, fat necrosis (traumatic), and mastitis.

'Gold-standard' diagnostic test

The triple assessment discussed in 'Approach to diagnosing the disease' is considered the gold standard for the investigation and diagnosis of breast cancer.

Acceptable diagnostic alternatives to the gold standard

Most women enter the national mammographic screening programme at the age of 50 (see 'Screening'). For women at high risk of developing breast cancer, there is NICE guidance for the use of annual breast MRI rather than mammographic screening, with the screening commencing at age 30 (or at age 20 in patients with Li–Fraumeni syndrome).

Other relevant investigations

The oestrogen receptor status of breast cancer cells, as assessed histologically, is used to predict the likely response to hormonal therapies such as tamoxifen and aromatase inhibitors. The progesterone receptor status is also assessed in some centres, although its routine use is not recommended by NICE. HER2 testing by immunohistochemistry and/or fluorescence in situ hybridization should also be performed. Overexpression of the HER2 receptor is associated with a worse prognosis, but also opens additional treatment options such as trastuzumab, a monoclonal antibody that targets the receptor.

In the metastatic setting, tumour markers such as CA 15-3 can be measured at baseline and, if found to be elevated, may be used to assess response to treatment, in addition to radiological methods.

Prognosis and how to estimate it

The prognosis of breast cancer is related to its anatomical extent, as well as other factors. Regional lymph node involvement is the most important prognostic factor in early breast cancer. Other poor prognostic factors include large tumour size, high tumour grade, negative receptor status (oestrogen receptor and/or HER2), and young patient age. Patients with favourable prognostic cancers have a predicted 10-year survival of approximately 95%. Those with poor prognosis cancers have a predicted 10-year survival closer to 20%.

In metastatic breast cancer, even with treatment, the median survival is only 2–3 years. However, there is considerable patient-to-patient variation, with approximately 15% of patients living more than 5 years.

Treatment and its effectiveness

Prevention

Most of the work on prevention of breast cancer has concentrated on women at high risk of developing the disease. In this patient population, there is evidence that selective oestrogen receptor modulators (tamoxifen and raloxifene) reduce the incidence of breast cancer. Their use, however, has not been shown to have an impact on cancer mortality. Risk-reductive surgical techniques such as bilateral oophorectomies and prophylactic mastectomies with or without nipple sparing also have a proven role in high-risk patients.

For the wider female population, while there is some evidence from the MORE osteoporosis prevention trial that raloxifene reduces breast cancer incidence, questions remain as to how long women would need to take the drug and at what age they should start. There are also concerns over the long-term safety of taking such medications. Current advice is therefore to reduce the modifiable risk factors discussed in 'Aetiology of the disease'.

Screening

A breast screening programme was introduced in the UK in 1988. Women between the ages of 50 and 70 are invited for mammograms every 3 years. Beyond this age, women can request mammograms every 3 years but are not invited routinely. The aim of mammographic screening programmes is to detect both preinvasive carcinoma in situ (see 'Natural history, and complications of the disease') and early breast cancers. Such programmes are estimated to reduce breast cancer mortality by approximately 20%. It has been recently recognized that screening also results in the diagnosis and treatment of some cancers that would not have caused problems during a woman's lifetime had the screening not been performed. It is estimated that this over-diagnosis will affect approximately 1% of women screened from age 50–70.

Treatment of early stage breast cancer

Early stage breast cancer is defined as disease confined to the breast and the regional lymph nodes at the time of diagnosis, and accounts for approximately 95% of breast cancer diagnoses. Treatment of early stage breast cancer is aimed at removing macroscopic cancer with surgery, treating local microscopic disease spread with radiotherapy, and treating systemic microscopic disease with systemic therapies such as hormones, chemotherapy, and targeted therapies.

Surgery for early stage breast cancer
Surgical options for early stage breast cancer include:

- mastectomy
- breast-conserving surgery
- axillary node clearance
- sentinel node biopsy

Mastectomy
Historically, the surgery of choice for treatment of breast cancer was modified radical mastectomy. This procedure involves removal of the entire breast, including the nipple and areola complex.

Breast-conserving surgery
Clinical outcomes similar to those obtained with mastectomy can be achieved by combining wide local excision of the tumour with

radiotherapy. For the majority of patients, this approach has become standard care.

Axillary node clearance

Axillary node clearance involves the dissection of first-, second-, and third-level axillary nodes. Despite being associated with complications such as axillary pain, numbness, reduced arm movement, and the development of lymphoedema, this surgery was considered the standard of care for axillary surgery until recently.

Sentinel node biopsy

Sentinel node biopsy involves identifying the first node in the regional lymphatic basin to which the tumour drains. The sentinel node is most reliably identified by using two separate localizing techniques in combination. Peritumoural injection of blue dye and of a radio-isotope can together locate the sentinel node with 95% sensitivity. Axillary node clearance is subsequently performed only where the sentinel node is found to be involved with the tumour.

Radiotherapy for early stage breast cancer

Following breast-conserving surgery, radiotherapy to the conserved breast approximately halves the risk of the disease recurring and reduces the risk of dying from the disease by about a sixth. There are several widely used radiotherapy schedules. The gold standard against which they are compared remains 50 Gy in 25 fractions, with daily treatment Monday–Friday over a 5-week period. This may be followed by a further boost to the tumour bed. The START trial has demonstrated that similar outcomes can be achieved with shorter or less intense regemines (e.g. 40 Gy in 15 fractions over 3 weeks), and these are also widely used.

Adjuvant systemic therapies for early stage breast cancer

Adjuvant systemic therapies for early stage breast cancer include:

- adjuvant hormone therapy
- adjuvant chemotherapy

Adjuvant hormone therapy for early stage breast cancer

Approximately 70% of breast cancers demonstrate oestrogen receptor positivity. Clinical trials in the 1980s revolutionized breast cancer management by showing that the addition of 5 years of tamoxifen to standard treatment in this group of patients was able to reduce rates of local recurrence by approximately 50%, and mortality by about a third. More recent trials have shown 10 years of tamoxifen to be superior to 5 years and this is now the standard treatment in oestrogen-receptor-positive premenopausal women. In postmenopausal women, particularly those with higher-risk node-positive disease, aromatase inhibitors offer some additional benefit compared to tamoxifen.

Adjuvant chemotherapy for early stage breast cancer

There are many chemotherapy regimens used to treat breast cancer. The most common in the United Kingdom is FEC (for **f**luorouracil, **e**pirubicin, and **c**yclophosphamide). In patients with node-positive disease, NICE recommends that docetaxel should also be used as part of their adjuvant therapy. Common side effects of such agents include tiredness, reversible alopecia, nausea, and vomiting. Less common, but serious, side effects include neutropenic sepsis, which requires IV antibiotics for several days until white blood cell counts normalize. Chemotherapy is associated with an approximately 1% mortality, which is largely attributed to neutropenic sepsis. As a result, all patients commencing chemotherapy are given instructions to immediately contact an acute oncology service in the event of elevated temperature, rigours, or other signs of infection.

Adjuvant targeted therapies for early stage breast cancer

Approximately 15% of early breast cancers express high levels of the HER2 receptor. Historically, this phenotype has been associated with a much poorer prognosis. The humanized monoclonal antibody trastuzumab targets this receptor. When the drug is given every 3 weeks for a year to patients with HER2 positive cancers, the risk of relapse is halved, leading to an approximate 30% reduction in mortality. While trastuzumab is generally well tolerated, with few side

effects, there is a small but significant risk of reversible cardiotoxicity, which is usually asymptomatic and responds to cessation of the drug and treatment with an angiotensin-converting enzyme inhibitor. For this reason, all patients are monitored with echocardiograms every 3 months for the duration of their treatment.

Neoadjuvant Therapy

Systemic treatments for breast cancer can also be deliverd prior to surgery. This can include chemotherapy alone or in combination with therapies such as trastuzumab and pertuzumab.

Clinical trials for treatment in early stage breast cancer

The UK National Cancer Research Network (NCRN) was set up in 2001 to provide the NHS with an infrastructure to support high-quality cancer clinical studies to improve the speed, quality, and integration of research resulting in improved patient care. Patients may be offered information about suitable clinical trials as part of their treatment.

Treatment of advanced (metastatic) breast cancer

A multimodality approach is just as important in the treatment of metastatic breast cancer as it is for the treatment of early stage breast cancer.

Palliative systemic therapies for advanced breast cancer

Palliative systemic therapies for advanced breast cancer include:

- hormone therapy
- chemotherapy
- bone directed therapy
- HER2 directed therapy

Hormone therapy for advanced ER positive breast cancer

For the majority of patients with oestrogen-receptor-positive metastatic disease, hormone therapy should be used as first-line palliative therapy. Several different hormone treatments are available, and disease that progresses on one may respond to another. The main advantage of hormone therapies is that most are taken in tablet form and have few side effects, compared to chemotherapy. The main disadvantage is time to onset of action, which may be several months. Thus, hormone therapy may be unsuitable for patients with rapidly progressing disease, particularly liver metastases. Several classes of hormone therapy are available, including selective oestrogen receptor modulators (e.g. tamoxifen), non-steroidal aromatase inhibitors (e.g. anastrozole and letrozole), steroidal aromatase inhibitors (e.g. exemestane), and oestrogen receptor antagonists (e.g. fulvestrant). Selective cyclin-dependent kinase 4 and 6 (CDK4/6) inhibitors are a new class of drug showing promising results in this subset of patients. Older treatments such as sex steroid therapies (e.g. diethylstilbestrol), androgens, and progestogens (e.g. megestrol, medoxyprogesterone) and oestrogen-deprivation therapies (oophorectomy, ovarian irradiation, or the use of analogues of gonadotropin-releasing hormone) still have a role in clinical practice.

Chemotherapy for advanced breast cancer

Chemotherapy is useful in patients with oestrogen-receptor-negative disease or in those for whom hormone therapy is not suitable. NICE guidelines recommend that patients requiring chemotherapy and who have not previously been treated with an anthracycline-containing regimen such as FEC should receive it first line. Second-line chemotherapy should be with single-agent docetaxel. Other chemotherapy regimens such as single-agent capecitabine or vinorelbine can be used as third- or fourth-line treatments.

Bone directed therapy for advanced breast cancer

For patients with bone metastases, denosumab and bisphosphonates have dramatically altered the course of their disease. These drugs have a proven role in preventing or delaying skeletal complications such as pathological fractures and spinal cord compression, as well as the need for radiotherapy and surgery. Bisphosphonates are also useful in managing the hypercalcaemia of malignancy.

HER2 directed therapy for advanced HER2 positive breast cancer

Targeted drugs such as trastuzumab, ado-trastuzumab emtansine, lapatinib, and pertuzumab have all been demonstrated to prolong survival in patients with metastatic HER2-positive disease.

Surgery for advanced breast cancer

Surgery plays an important role in the management of metastatic breast cancer in carefully selected patients with oligometastatic disease. Indications include resection of brain or lung metastases, and spinal surgery for cord compression.

Radiotherapy for advanced breast cancer

Radiotherapy has several important roles in the management of metastatic breast cancer. Bone pain from metastatic deposits often responds very well to even single-fraction radiotherapy treatments. Radiotherapy can also be used to reduce the risk of developing a fracture and for the treatment of cord compression or brain metastases not suitable for surgery (or following recovery from surgery). In addition, radiotherapy can be used to control advanced local disease within the breast and axilla. Specialized radiotherapy techniques such as stereotactic radiosurgery can also have a role in the management of oligometastatic disease.

Clinical trials for treatment in advanced breast cancer

Breast cancer is an area of extensive research, and patients with advanced disease may be offered information about newer targeted treatments and/or chemotherapy drugs as part of the NCRN portfolio of clinical trials.

Further Reading

F. Cardoso, A. Costa, E. Senkus et al. 3rd ESO–ESMO International Consensus Guidelines for Advanced Breast Cancer (ABC 3). *Ann Oncol* 2017; 28: 16–33. doi: 10.1093/annonc/mdw544

National Institute for Health and Care Excellence. *Early and Locally Advanced Breast Cancer: Diagnosis and Treatment.* 2009. Available at http://www.nice.org.uk/Guidance/CG80 (accessed 17 Sep 2017).

National Institute for Health and Care Excellence. *Advanced Breast Cancer: Diagnosis and Treatment.* 2014. Available at http://www.nice.org.uk/Guidance/CG81 (accessed 17 Sep 2017).

Senkus E, Kyriakides S, Ohno S, Penault-Llorca F, Poortmans P, Rutgers E, Zackrisson S, and Cardoso F. Primary breast cancer: ESMO clinical practice guidelines for diagnosis, treatment and follow-up. *Ann Oncol* (2015) 26 (suppl 5): v8–v30. www.esmo.org/Guidelines/Breast-Cancer/Primary-Breast-Cancer.

Yeo B, Turner NC, and Jones AL. An update on the medical management of breast cancer. *BMJ* 2014; 348: g3608.

Ovarian cancer

Definition of ovarian cancer

Ovarian cancer is the fifth most common cancer in females in the UK. In 2008, there were approximately 4000 deaths from ovarian cancer. Ninety per cent of all ovarian cancers are of epithelial origin. Germ cell and sex cord–stromal cell tumours also occur. Primary peritoneal and fallopian tube carcinomas behave clinically like ovarian carcinomas.

Aetiology of ovarian cancer

Risk factors for ovarian cancer include:

- nulliparity
- early menarche
- late menopause
- family history
- α BRCA1 or BRCA2 mutation
- Lynch II syndrome (hereditary non-polyposis colorectal cancer)

Typical symptoms of ovarian cancer, and less common symptoms

Ovarian cancer is frequently asymptomatic. Ultrasound and a CA-125 test can detect ovarian cancer in asymptomatic women. A randomized controlled trial to assess the impact of screening on mortality is in progress. Advanced disease is associated with abdominal bloating, abdominal pain, anorexia, and weight loss. Dyspnoea can occur due to pleural effusion. Sex cord–stromal tumours can cause paraneoplastic syndromes by secreting sex hormones.

Demographics of ovarian cancer

For ovarian cancer, the average age at diagnosis is 59 years. However, the highest incidence is in women between 80 and 84 years.

Natural history of ovarian cancer, and complications of the disease

The majority of patients with ovarian cancer present with advanced disease. Transcoelomic spread to the peritoneum and pleura is common, leading to ascites and pleural effusion, respectively. Omental or serosal deposits can cause bowel obstruction. Lymph node and haematogenous metastases also occur.

Approach to diagnosing ovarian cancer

The presence of an adnexal mass seen on imaging raises the suspicion of ovarian cancer. Diagnosis can only be confirmed pathologically (e.g. cytology of ascitic fluid, or pathological specimen of the ovaries).

Other diagnoses that should be considered aside from ovarian cancer

Other diagnoses that should be considered aside from ovarian cancer include benign ovarian cysts, which are common, particularly in menstruating women. Other differential diagnoses include:

- bowel cancer
- pelvic inflammatory disease
- hydrosalpinx
- uterine cancer
- uterine fibroids

'Gold-standard' diagnostic test for ovarian cancer

Laparotomy is the gold-standard test for the diagnosis and staging of ovarian cancer.

Acceptable diagnostic alternatives to the gold-standard test for ovarian cancer

A patient with a suggestive clinical history and a CA-125 level >2000 should be regarded as having ovarian cancer until proven otherwise. If a patient is not fit for surgery, ascitic fluid cytology can be diagnostic. Pelvic ultrasound or MRI may be helpful.

Other relevant investigations for ovarian cancer

CA-125 is raised in 90% of women with ovarian cancer. However, it can also be raised due to endometriosis, uterine fibroids, benign ovarian tumours, or other cancers. It is most useful as a surrogate for response to treatment. Measure beta-human chorionic gonadotropin, alpha-fetoprotein, and lactate dehydrogenase if you suspect a germ cell tumour.

Prognosis of ovarian cancer, and how to estimate it

For ovarian cancer, the overall 5-year survival is approximately 40%. Poor prognostic factors include:

- Stage III/IV disease
- clear cell type
- a high-grade tumour
- a residual tumour >3 cm in diameter after surgery

Treatment of ovarian cancer, and its effectiveness

For ovarian cancer, total abdominal hysterectomy, bilateral salpingo-oophorectomy, and omentectomy are the mainstays of treatment. Adjuvant chemotherapy is usually indicated. In advanced disease, primary chemotherapy can be given prior to interval debulking surgery. Chemotherapy or hormone therapy is used to treat metastatic or recurrent disease.

Testicular cancer

Definition of testicular cancer

Testicular cancer is a rare disease: there were 2138 new cases of testicular cancer diagnosed in 2008 in the UK, and only 70 deaths. Ninety-five per cent of testicular cancers are germ cell tumours. Stromal cell tumours and lymphomas make up the remaining 5%. Germ cell tumours can be either seminomas or non-seminomas. Non-seminomas are subtyped according to the WHO classification system.

Aetiology of testicular cancer

In testicular cancer, germ cell tumours arise from a carcinoma in situ. Having an undescended testis increases the risk of testicular cancer by tenfold. The risk is also increased in the contralateral testis. If orchidopexy is performed before 2 years of age, the risk is partially normalized. The incidence of testicular cancer is higher in first-degree relatives of men with testicular cancer. Other risk factors include infertility, Down's syndrome, and Klinefelter syndrome.

Typical symptoms of testicular cancer, and less common symptoms

Patients with testicular cancer typically present with a painless testicular mass. Rarely, an extremely high level of beta-human chorionic gonadotropin causes gynaecomastia and/or hyperthyroidism (because beta-human chorionic gonadotropin has a subunit in common with thyroid-stimulating hormone). Metastatic pulmonary disease may cause dyspnoea and haemoptysis.

Demographics of testicular cancer

Testicular cancer is more common in Caucasian men than in African or Asian men. The peak incidence is at 25–34 years of age. Seminomatous tumours present on average 10 years later than non-seminomatous tumours.

Natural history of testicular cancer, and complications of the disease

Testicular cancer is highly curable, even in the presence of metastases. Local spread commonly involves the rete testis. The pattern of lymphatic spread is predictable, particularly for seminomatous tumours. The lung is the most common site for distant metastases. Late complications of treatment occur, including secondary malignancies.

Approach to diagnosing testicular cancer

A testicular mass needs prompt investigation. Biopsy should be avoided due to the risk of bleeding and tumour seeding. Patients should proceed to surgery if a mass is clinically suspicious.

Other diagnoses that should be considered aside from testicular cancer

Other diagnoses that should be considered aside from testicular cancer include:

- epididymitis
- epididymal cyst
- hydrocele
- varicocele
- spermatocele
- metastasis of other cancers
- orchitis

'Gold-standard' diagnostic test for testicular cancer

For testicular cancer, testicular ultrasound is the gold-standard investigation, followed by orchidectomy.

Acceptable diagnostic alternatives to the gold-standard test for testicular cancer

When diagnosing testicular cancer, it is rarely relevant to have any test other than testicular ultrasound followed by orchidectomy.

Other relevant investigations for testicular cancer

In testicular cancer, tumour markers are prognostic and are surrogate markers for response to treatment. Beta-human chorionic gonadotropin is secreted by both seminomas and non-seminomas. Alpha-fetoprotein is secreted by embryonal or yolk sac elements in non-seminomas. Lactate dehydrogenase is a non-specific, prognostic marker in testicular cancer. Staging investigations include CT chest, abdomen, and pelvis.

Prognosis of testicular cancer, and how to estimate it

For testicular cancer, the prognosis is good, with a 5-year survival rate of 98%. Non-pulmonary visceral metastases and very high tumour markers at diagnosis are associated with a worse prognosis.

Treatment of testicular cancer, and its effectiveness

For testicular cancer, radical orchidectomy is the primary treatment. Adjuvant chemotherapy or radiotherapy reduces the risk of recurrence. Metastatic and recurrent disease is treated with chemotherapy. Testicular cancers, particularly seminomas, are highly chemosensitive.

Further Reading

Krege S, Beyer J, Souchon R, et al. European consensus conference on diagnosis and treatment of germ cell cancer. A report of the second meeting of the European Germ Cell Cancer Consensus group (EGCCCG): Part I. Eur Urol 2008; 53: 478–96.

Schwartz PE (ed.). Advances in Ovarian Cancer Management, 2012. Future Medicine Ltd.

Introduction

Treatment in cancer is aimed at improving survival (curing where possible) and/or improving symptoms. Symptoms may be caused by the cancer itself (primary tumour, metastases, or paraneoplastic phenomenon) or by the treatments patients undergo to treat the cancer (surgery, radiotherapy, chemotherapy, hormone therapy, and biological therapy). Therefore, symptom control is one of the key roles of oncologists as they treat cancer patients.

The most important part of symptom control in cancer patients is to elucidate the underlying cause of the symptom. Symptom control is most effective when the underlying cause is targeted; for example, shoulder pain may be treated most effectively by local radiotherapy if it is due to a bone metastasis in the humeral head, by dexamethasone if it is referred pain due to diaphragmatic irritation from hepatomegaly, and by amitriptyline or gabapentin if it is neuropathic pain due to cervical nerve root irritation.

Covering all symptom control in cancer patients is beyond the remit of this chapter; however, we will cover the control of pain and nausea and vomiting, as these are very common symptoms in cancer patients.

Pain in the cancer patient

Three-quarters of cancer patients experience pain at some point in their illness. Acute, severe pain can produce fear and anxiety for the patient and their carers. Chronic pain is extremely debilitating, is associated with depression, and impairs a patient's ability to cope with ongoing treatment. Multiple, concurrent pains are common, particularly in advanced cancer, and it is important to consider the cause and appropriate management of each pain separately.

History taking for pain in the cancer patient

The history should include the number and location of pain sites, the character of the pain (e.g. nociceptive or neuropathic, constant or episodic, with triggering or relieving factors), and its response to analgesics. Also, ascertain the impact of the pain on the patient.

Examination for pain in the cancer patient

During the examination, examine painful areas gently and carefully, to avoid exacerbating pain. Ascertain whether the pain is due to masses or organomegaly, whether the pain arises from soft tissue or bone, and whether there are associated sensory changes which may suggest a neuropathic element.

Causes of pain in the cancer patient

Pain is often caused by the tumour/metastases compressing normal structures. Bone metastases can be painful but will also result in neuropathic pain if they are compressing nerves. Intracranial disease can cause raised intracranial pressure resulting in headache. Liver metastases become painful once they cause stretching of the liver capsule. Primary bowel tumours or peritoneal disease can cause pain secondary to bowel obstruction. Cancer also predisposes patients to pulmonary embolism, which can present with pleuritic chest pain, so we must not overlook non-malignant causes of pain that may be present in the cancer patient.

General principles of pain management in the cancer patient

It is vital to ensure that reversible causes of pain are excluded and treated (e.g. constipation or infection). If the underlying cause has been identified, consider whether this can be helped by disease-modifying treatment (e.g. radiotherapy, chemotherapy, hormone therapy, or surgery).

Ensure the patient has adequate analgesia and understands how best to use it. Give regular analgesics to maintain an analgesic effect. Always have additional analgesia written up for pain that breaks through the regular analgesic regimen ('breakthrough pain'). Add additional analgesics one at a time, so that you are able to assess the efficacy of each drug. Ineffective drugs or those that are no longer making a significant contribution to analgesia should be stopped. Titrate opioids to effect or tolerance before adding in additional drugs, to avoid unnecessarily complicated regimes. In difficult cancer pain, combinations are often necessary to achieve adequate analgesia with minimum side effects. Consider referral to the palliative care or pain team.

The WHO analgesic ladder (see Table 329.1) provides a systematic approach to pain management in cancer.

An adjuvant is a drug (e.g. corticosteroids, tricyclic antidepressants, anticonvulsants) which is not analgesic in its prime function but has analgesic actions in particular kinds of pain. It may be appropriate at any stage of the ladder. In practice, however, this recommendation is a guideline, and the choice of analgesic should be determined by the cause and nature of the pain and the significance of potential adverse effects for a particular patient.

Management of specific pains in the cancer patient

Neuropathic pain is associated with nerve compression or injury. It usually responds to standard analgesics; however, there may be a ceiling of unacceptable side effects with opioids before complete analgesia is achieved, so adjuvants may be necessary (e.g. dexamethasone, amitriptyline, gabapentin); in difficult neuropathic pain, consider referral to the pain team.

Bone pain may be usefully treated with radiotherapy, bisphosphonates, hormonal therapy, or radioisotopes. Vertebroplasty or surgical fixation may also be beneficial.

Liver metastases stretching the liver capsule may cause intense right upper quadrant pain that may be exacerbated by inspiration; there may also be a palpable, tender liver. This pain may respond to NSAIDs and opioids, but a corticosteroid may be highly effective as an adjuvant and reduce the need for opioids.

Nausea and vomiting in the cancer patient

Nausea and vomiting is very common in cancer patients (up to 50%), especially in those receiving chemotherapy (70%–80%). Nausea and vomiting contributes significantly to the morbidity of cancer and its treatment. It is important to determine the underlying causes of the vomiting, as this guides treatment. In many cases, the causes for vomiting are multifactorial, so this requires an understanding of the sites

Table 329.1 The WHO analgesic ladder

Step 1	Non-opioid (e.g. paracetamol, ibuprofen) ± adjuvants
Step 2	Opioid for mild to moderate pain (e.g. codeine, tramadol) + non-opioid ± adjuvants
Step 3	Opioid for moderate to severe pain (e.g. morphine) + non-opioid ± adjuvants

Reprinted from WHO, WHO Pain Relief Ladder, Copyright (2009). http://www.who.int/cancer/palliative/painladder/en/.

Table 329.2 Common anti-emetics

Anti-emetic	Receptor profile and site of action	Clinical indication
Metoclopramide 10 mg tds PO/SC (pre-meal) 30–100 mg/24 hour SC infusion	Pro-kinetic UGI tract D_2 antagonist 5-HT_4 agonist 5-HT_3>100 mg/24 hour CTZ D_2 antagonist 5-HT_3>100 mg/24 hour	Gastric stasis Functional GI obstruction Chemical/metabolic Cytotoxic chemotherapy Hypercalcaemia Uraemia Opioids
Domperidone 10 mg tds PO (pre-meal) 60 mg bd PR	Pro-kinetic UGI tract D_2 antagonist No action inside blood-brain barrier so no extrapyramidal side effects.	Gastric stasis
Haloperidol 1.5–10 mg nocte PO/SC	CTZ D_2 antagonist	Chemical/metabolic Cytotoxic chemotherapy Hypercalcaemia Uraemia Opioids
Cyclizine 50 mg tds PO/SC 100–150 mg/24 hour	Vomiting centre ACh H_1	Mechanical GI obstruction ↑ ICP
SC infusion	Vestibular nuclei ACh H_1	Movement related
Granisetron 1–2 mg od PO/SC	CTZ 5-HT_3	Cytotoxic chemotherapy Radiotherapy
Ondansetron 8 mg bd PO/SC	GI tract 5-HT_3	GI obstruction (2nd line)
Levomepromazine 6.25–75 mg nocte PO/SC	Vomiting centre D_2 5-HT_2 $α_1$ ACh	Broad spectrum 2nd line
Dexamethasone 4–8 mg od/bd PO/SC	Cerebral cortex Mechanism unknown Anti-inflammatory Adjunct in difficult emesis	Cytotoxic chemotherapy Radiotherapy ↑ ICP Functional GI obstruction

Abbreviations: $α_1$, alpha-1 adrenergic receptor; 5-HT_2, serotonin 5-HT_2 receptor; 5-HT_3, serotonin 5-HT_3 receptor; 5-HT_4, serotonin 5-HT_4 receptor; ACh, acetylcholine; bd, bid die (twice daily); CTZ, chemoreceptor trigger zone; D_2, dopamine receptor 2; GI, gastrointestinal; H_1, histamine H_1 receptor; ICP, intracranial pressure; nocte, at night; od, omni die (every day); PO, per oram (by mouth); PR, per rectum (rectally); SC, subcutis (subcutaneous); tds, ter die sumendum; UGI, upper gastrointestinal tract.

Reproduced with permission from Scott-Brown, Spence, Johnstone, *Emergencies in Oncology*, Oxford University Press, Oxford, UK, Copyright © 2007

of action of the anti-emetics and a logical approach to their use to achieve control of this distressing symptom (see Table 329.2).

Chemical/metabolic nausea is often continuous and is not relieved by vomiting. Causes include chemotherapy and abdominal or cranial radiotherapy, uraemia, hypercalcaemia, and drugs (e.g. opioids or antibiotics).

Gastric stasis/bowel obstruction is usually associated with abdominal distension (particularly after eating), and intermittent nausea which is relieved by vomiting. It can be caused by drugs (e.g. opioids or anticholinergic drugs), gastrointestinal tumours, peritoneal carcinomatosis, or adhesions secondary to previous abdominal surgery.

The nausea associated with raised intracranial pressure is commonly worse in the morning, with headache and, occasionally, neurological signs.

Vestibular disease or base of skull pathology usually results in nausea exacerbated by movement.

History taking for nausea and vomiting in the cancer patient

A detailed history will often elucidate the cause of nausea. Important points include:

- Is nausea or vomiting the major symptom?
- Is the nausea relieved by vomiting?
- Has the patient recently received chemotherapy or radiotherapy or recently commenced on a new drug?
- Are there other associated symptoms (e.g. colicky abdominal pain, headache, vertigo)?

Examination for nausea and vomiting in the cancer patient

The examination should assess both the impact of vomiting (e.g. hypovolaemia) as well as the cause of the nausea/vomiting (e.g. look for organomegaly, abdominal distension, bowel sounds; perform both a neurological examination and fundoscopy).

Investigation for nausea and vomiting in the cancer patient

A systematic approach to investigations is useful, as these can often help to elucidate the cause, including blood tests (e.g. urea and electrolytes, calcium level, bilirubin level) and imaging (e.g. abdominal X-ray, CT brain, CT abdomen, contrast swallow/meal).

Management of nausea and vomiting in the cancer patient

Most patients with nausea and vomiting can be managed as outpatients, as long as the patient has an adequate oral intake to maintain hydration status, is not hypotensive, and does not have an electrolyte imbalance.

If the patient is severely dehydrated (e.g. hypotensive or tachycardic), drowsy, or confused, start IV rehydration and perform blood tests immediately. If the patient is oliguric, give IV fluids and insert a urinary catheter to monitor urinary output (aim for an output >0.5 ml/kg per hour).

If the patient is distressed by severe nausea and/or vomiting, consider giving a broad-spectrum anti-emetic such as cyclizine 50 mg subcutaneously or intravenously, prior to further assessment. In persistent vomiting, absorption by oral route may be poor, so give essential medication by subcutaneous or IV routes.

Review current medications and consider stopping drugs which may be causative, but do not stop opioids if the patient has been in pain but add an anti-emetic. Treat correctable causes (e.g. hypercalcaemia, raised intracranial pressure, uraemia, gastritis, constipation).

Anti-emetics should be given on a regular basis, with the dose adjusted as needed. If oral absorption is poor because of continuous vomiting, give the anti-emetic subcutaneously, intravenously, or per rectum. If there is little response to the first anti-emetic after 24 hours, then optimize the dose, taking account of the doses required. If there is still no response, change to an alternative anti-emetic with a different receptor profile. Finally, add in a second anti-emetic with a different receptor profile.

Antimuscarinic drugs (e.g. cyclizine) block the cholinergic pathway through which prokinetic drugs (e.g. metoclopramide, domperidone) act. Although the central effects of metoclopramide are not inhibited by cyclizine, a combination of cyclizine and metoclopramide is best avoided.

If nausea/vomiting remains difficult to control, seek advice from the palliative care team.

Further Reading

Faull C, de Caestecker S, and Nicholson A et al. *Handbook of Palliative Care* (3rd edition). 2012. Wiley-Blackwell

Twycross RG, Wilcock A, and Toller CS. *Symptom Management in Advanced Cancer* (4th edition), 2007. Palliativedrugs.com Ltd.

Watson M, Lucas C, and Hoy A et al. *Oxford Handbook of Palliative Care* (2nd edition), 2012. Oxford University Press.

330 Dying from cancer

Martin Scott-Brown

Introduction

For many patients, dying from cancer has been an ever-present reality from the time they were diagnosed with incurable recurrent or metastatic cancer. Treatment may have delayed the inevitable, but there does come a point where aggressive management no longer improves the prognosis or can only prolong life that is of such a poor quality that it is not valued by the patient. It sometimes is easier to continue with treatment than to take the time with the patient to discuss the reasons why further treatment is not appropriate. For patients with advanced cancer and whose condition is deteriorating, the following questions should be considered before initiating treatment aimed at prolonging life:

- Is this the final stage of a progressive deterioration or an acute event? Are the causes of this deterioration reversible? The ICU is usually not appropriate for patients with advanced cancer.
- Are there any further oncological treatments that may improve the prognosis?
- What is the patient's perception of their quality of life? Is there a realistic chance of return to a quality of life that will be of value to the patient?
- Is the patient dying?

Treatment of correctable causes (e.g. obstructive uropathy, chest infection) may still not be in the patient's best interest if they recover only to face a period of further deterioration and distressing symptoms before they die. However, patients and their families must be included in discussions as to the level of further intervention and the reasons for stopping active treatment.

The diagnosis of dying

It is not always easy to 'diagnose' those patients who are dying, and the diagnosis of dying is a skill often obtained only through experience. It is important to make the diagnosis, as it then avoids inappropriate treatment and unnecessary investigations. The following can be helpful indicators in the context of advanced cancer:

- the patient is profoundly weak and bed bound
- the patient is semi-comatose
- the patient is unable to take oral medication
- the patient is unable to take more than sips of water

Management of the dying patient

The priorities at this stage are:

- good symptom control
- clear, sensitive communication with the patient and their family

As oncologists, we know that many of our patients will die from their cancers. Our treatments may not prevent their death; however, our expertise must be used to enable them to die with their symptoms controlled.

General management

Initiate the hospital's care pathway for dying patients. Previously, the Liverpool care pathway was widely used; following certain criticisms (mainly around patient and relative communication), updated pathways largely based on the Liverpool care pathway but not using the name are used by many hospitals

Document the 'do not attempt cardiopulmonary resuscitation' decision. Involve the hospital palliative care team if there are:

- difficult symptom control issues
- difficult communication issues with the patient or family

Avoid investigations that are not going to alter management (e.g. blood tests). Stop inappropriate nursing interventions (e.g. monitoring vital signs). Stop medication that will have no impact on the patient's symptoms. If possible, convert essential medication to the subcutaneous (SC) route (using a syringe driver if necessary). Consider a urinary catheter.

Communication

Wherever possible, enable the patient to discuss their prognosis and ongoing plan of care. Involve the family in all discussions (with the patient's permission). Offer the input of the hospital chaplaincy team or representative of his or her own faith. Patients and families will often ask, 'How long?' This is very difficult to answer; however, the following is a good rule of thumb:

- if the patient is deteriorating every week, the prognosis is probably 'weeks'
- if the patient is deteriorating every day, the prognosis is probably 'days'
- if the patient is deteriorating every hour, the prognosis is probably 'hours'

Patients who are in their last 'hours' usually develop a deepening coma, variable respiratory pattern, and poor peripheral circulation.

Symptom control

Pain

As long as the patient is responsive, pain can be assessed in the usual way. Once they become unresponsive, you have to rely on non-verbal cues (e.g. grimacing, groaning, and muscle tension in areas of pain). Family members will often report perceptions that the patient is in pain. If there is any doubt, give a breakthrough dose of SC morphine and monitor the apparent level of distress. If the patient is unable to take oral medication, convert regular per oram opioids to an SC infusion of diamorphine. The opioid level may need to be reduced if the patient is dying of renal failure. Patients may develop a generalized musculoskeletal pain when they are bed bound and dying. This usually responds well to low-dose diamorphine SC 10–20 mg per 24 hours. If a patient has been on oral NSAIDs, these can be converted to tenoxicam SC 20 mg once daily or diclofenac per rectum 50 mg twice daily; alternatively, the dose of opioid can be increased to compensate. If the patient is using co-analgesics such as tricyclic antidepressants or anticonvulsants, the opioid levels may need to be increased once the levels of these drugs have been significantly reduced.

Breathlessness

Many patients fear dying with severe breathlessness. Reassure patients that breathlessness can be relieved, although, occasionally, patients may have to be sedated to achieve adequate relief. Slowly progressive breathlessness can be managed with a SC infusion of morphine (10–20 mg per 24 hours) plus midazolam (10–20 mg per 24 hours). This can be titrated up to achieve the desired effect. Patients who are dying consequent to rapidly deteriorating respiratory function are in severe distress and need urgent attention. Sedation is usually the only way to provide relief, and midazolam needs to be titrated rapidly (up to 60 mg per 24 hours)

Vomiting

The control of nausea and vomiting is no different in the terminal phase; however, medication should be given via the SC route.

Restlessness and agitation

In the terminal phase of cancer, there are many potential causes of restlessness, agitation, and cognitive failure (including renal failure, opioid toxicity, and cerebral metastases). It is not usually possible to identify a single cause, but it is worth excluding urinary retention and considering a reduction in opioids if the patient is not in pain and there are signs of opioid toxicity. Attention to the patient's surroundings is important, with familiar faces and a peaceful, quiet environment. Appropriate drugs can also be helpful to gain control of the symptoms (e.g. midazolam, haloperidol, and levomepromazine). Seek specialist palliative care advice when agitation does not settle.

Upper respiratory tract secretions ('death rattle')

Upper respiratory tract secretions (the 'death rattle') can be reduced using anti-cholinergic drugs (e.g. hyoscine butylbromide 20 mg SC, followed by 40–80 mg per 24 hours by SC infusion), but they are usually difficult to control completely. Reassure the family that, if the patient is unconscious, they will not be distressed by the secretions. Early treatment often achieves better control. Repositioning the patient on their side may be helpful. Avoid suction except in severe cases.

Nutrition and hydration

If nutrition and hydration need to be given by a non-oral route, then, under UK law, they constitute medical treatments rather than basic human rights. For patients and families, however, they remain deeply symbolic of survival, and this area often needs very sensitive communication. If the patient is still responsive and competent, then their wishes are paramount. At this stage, comfort is the primary goal and this can usually be achieved without recourse to artificial nutrition or hydration, as it is normal for patients who are dying to lose interest in food and fluid. Symptoms of thirst can usually be alleviated by sips of water from a cup or sponge and good mouth care. If patients remain symptomatically thirsty in spite of these measures, then IV or SC fluids can be considered (1–2 l per 24 hours). If the family cannot accept that parenteral fluids are not necessary, then it may be appropriate to continue them rather than provoke conflict and risk a complicated bereavement.

Further Reading

The Marie Curie Palliative Care Institute 'Terminal Care Pathway' (http://www.mcpcil.org.uk/)

National Institute for Health and Care Excellence. *End of Life Care for Adults*. 2011. Available at https://www.nice.org.uk/guidance/qs13/chapter/introduction-and-overview.

National Institute for Health and Care Excellence. *Care of Dying Adults* in the Last Days of Life. 2015. Available at https://www.nice.org.uk/guidance/ng31/resources/care-of-dying-adults-in-the-last-days-of-life-pdf-1837387324357

PART 17

Dietary, lifestyle, and environmental factors affecting health

331 Normal nutritional function

Michelle Ellinson and Tommy Rampling

Introduction

Normal nutritional function requires a healthy diet. Healthy eating incorporates a variety of nutrients that are essential for energy expenditure, prevention of disease, and maintenance of normal physiological function. An unhealthy diet can result in malnutrition, and this contributes to illness and death throughout the world. The core principle of healthy eating is obtaining an adequate balance, and the diseases resulting from overnourishment differ greatly from those resulting from undernourishment.

In resource-limited settings diets tend to rely heavily on staple crops, and can be very seasonal. Energy sources are predominantly cereals, whereas meat and fish are limited. Malnutrition tends to occur from a lack of essential nutrients, leading to conditions such as vitamin deficiencies, kwashiorkor, and iodine deficiency syndromes. In high-resource settings, people have more freedom to choose what they eat. Thus, diets tend to be high in fat and dense in energy. Obesity, diabetes, coronary heart disease, cancer, and hypertension are major contributors to morbidity and mortality.

A healthy diet should contain adequate proportions of carbohydrates, fats, proteins, vitamins, and trace elements. The intake of these constituents is sporadic, with meals constituting major boluses of potential energy. Energy expenditure, conversely, is continuous. The human body has, therefore, developed complex mechanisms directing nutrients into storage when in excess, and mobilizing these stores as they are needed, and it is essential that sufficient energy is always available to maintain the basal metabolic rate, which is the amount of energy expended while at rest in a neutrally temperate environment. This energy is sufficient only for the functioning of the vital organs, such as the heart, the lungs, the liver, the kidneys, and the CNS.

Carbohydrates

Carbohydrates are monomers, dimers, and polymers of saccharide molecules, and can be classified as such. Monosaccharides, such as glucose and fructose, and disaccharides, such as sucrose, lactose, and maltose, are termed 'simple sugars'. Oligosaccharides contain between three and ten monosaccharide units, and polysaccharides contain more than ten units. Starch is a polysaccharide complex carbohydrate that is found mainly in plants and should be part of the staple diet. There are various types of starch, depending on the linkage and hydrolysis of the units, and the resistance of the starch to digestion within the intestine. Foods such as white bread and potatoes contain starch that is rapidly digested in the small intestine, whereas foods such as beans, peas, lentils, and pasta take longer to be digested in the small intestine, thus producing a lower glycaemic response in the blood. Resistant starches are foods that are not digested in the small intestine, and instead become fermented in the large intestine by the bacteria. Dietary fibre, which contains non-starch polysaccharides, is an example of a resistant starch and is essential for maintenance of a healthy large bowel, lowering of cholesterol, increasing bowel motility, and reduction in constipation. Foods that are a good source of fibre include fruits, vegetables, and cereals.

After a meal, the body goes into the absorptive state, and the liver, the adipose tissue, the skeletal muscles, and the brain utilize the glucose. The liver retains up to 60% of the glucose via the hepatic portal system and converts it to glycogen. In addition, pyruvate carboxylase is downregulated, so there is decreased gluconeogenesis. Insulin levels increase as there is increased production by the beta cells in the islets of Langerhans in the pancreas. Once insulin is in circulation, there are insulin receptors on the cell membrane which cause migration of glucose transporters (e.g. GLU4) towards the cell membrane to allow uptake of glucose by the cell. Glucose stimulates the release of insulin and therefore decreases the release of glucagon. An increase in insulin also results from an increase in the amino acid arginine, and the hormone secretin, which is released within the gastrointestinal tract. The adipose tissue undergoes an influx of glucose into the adipocytes, where glucose is phosphorylated to create glucose-6-phosphate. Skeletal muscle also absorbs the glucose, which is stored as glycogen. In the well-fed state, the brain uses glucose as the primary fuel. The brain is unable to store glycogen and therefore relies on glucose crossing the blood–brain barrier to enter the endothelial cells lining the blood vessels.

It is recommended to have between four and six servings of carbohydrates per day. The energy content of 1 g of carbohydrate is 4 calories, which is relatively low compared to 9 calories per 1 g of fat. Therefore, adding fat to carbohydrates will increase the calorie content of the carbohydrate-containing food.

Proteins

Proteins are macromolecules consisting of chains of amino acids. Proteins have numerous functions in the body: they serve as constituents of cellular membranes, transport molecules, coenzymes, hormones, and immune mediators, as well as maintain pH balance. There are 20 different amino acids from which proteins can be constructed. Of these, nine are essential dietary requirements, as the body is unable to efficiently manufacture them at the rate in which they are utilized. Nitrogen is one of the constituents of the protein molecule, and a positive nitrogen balance occurs when the amount of nitrogen consumed is greater than the amount excreted in urine, faeces, or sweat. Examples of this occurring would be during growth and tissue repair. Negative nitrogen balance occurs when the amount excreted is greater than the amount consumed, as happens, for example, during surgery, illness, or a decrease in protein intake. In 1991, the Department of Health recommended that the intake for protein in healthy adults be 0.75 g/kg of ideal weight per day.

Foods containing high concentrations of protein include meats, fish, dairy products, eggs, beans, nuts, and pulses. A balanced diet should aim for two servings of protein per day, choosing lean meats and low-fat dairy products if aiming to maintain weight within the healthy weight for height range.

Dietary protein is digested in the small intestine and absorbed as peptides and amino acids. On entering the enterocytes of the small intestine, some of the amino acids are preferentially selected and removed for use as oxidative fuel. The amino acids that remain travel via the portal vein to the liver, where further selective oxidation occurs. This accounts for consumption of up to 60% of the incoming amino acids. The liver is also responsible for large volumes of protein synthesis. The amino acid molecules are reformed into useable human protein structures, such as albumin, and most proteins involved in the coagulation pathways.

The liver is also the only significant site of urea synthesis. The individual atoms that make up urea molecules come from carbon dioxide, aspartate, ammonia, and water. It is formed in an anabolic process known as the urea cycle. The function of urea is to serve as a safe vehicle for excreting nitrogen waste, most notably amino acids and ammonia. When amino acids are released from proteolysis in peripheral tissues, they must transport, or transfer their amino nitrogen to the liver. The predominant amino acid carriers of nitrogen, released from proteolysis in muscle and adipose tissue are alanine and glutamine, and hepatic removal of these two far exceeds that of other amino acids.

Transamination of pyruvate and 2-oxoglutarate allows the transfer of amino acids into tissues via gluconeogenesis, producing glucose that can be recycled to the peripheral tissues. Once formed, alanine can be transaminated further to form aspartate for use in the urea cycle.

The other route of entry of nitrogen into the urea cycle is ammonia. Ammonia is a basic metabolic waste product that can raise intracellular pH to toxic levels. Ammonia may be formed in the peripheral tissues by oxidative deamination of glutamate. Defects of the urea cycle, for example in liver dysfunction, can have serious manifestations, such as hepatic encephalopathy. Therefore, although urea is a waste product and its synthesis requires energy, its synthesis is still an essential function of the liver.

Fats

Fats provide the most calories per gram (i.e. 9 calories/g). The majority of the fat molecule is made up of triglycerides. Fat in the diet may be visible, such as butter, or fat on meat/chicken, or invisible, such as hidden sources of fat in cakes and biscuits. The melting point of fat depends on the length and saturation of the fatty acid chain. Monounsaturated fats such as olive oil have one double bond between two carbon atoms; polyunsaturated fats such as fish oils have two or more double bonds within the chain. Fats provide essential fatty acids which the body cannot synthesize, and are derived from two different parent fatty acids known as omega-3 (i.e. alpha-linolenic acid) and omega-6 (i.e. linoleic acid).

Fats in the body have structural and storage capacity. Cellular membranes are made up of a phospholipid outer layer, with the fatty acid chain pointing inwards. Protein molecules that serve as receptors or enzymes are inserted between the layers. Vitamins and cholesterol molecules are also situated on cellular membranes.

Storage fats, also known as lipids, are stored within adipose tissue as an energy reserve. Fatty acids stored in adipose tissue tend to be by-products of the diet rather than fatty acids that have been generated within the body.

Cholesterol is metabolized to form steroids in the adrenal glands, and bile acids in the liver.

The need for specifying the upper limits of dietary intake of total fat can be seen with the correlation of a diet high in saturated fatty acids with high blood cholesterol and therefore heart disease. Decreasing the total fat in the diet can reduce the concentration of plasma cholesterol and the risk of developing atherosclerosis. There is also a genetic component to high plasma cholesterol concentrations such as familial hypercholesterolaemia. High-fat diets lead to raised plasma cholesterol and obesity. If saturated fatty acids are replaced by unsaturated fatty acids, the total LDL would decrease. In order to decrease cholesterol intake, diets need to be modified so that the diet will contain total fat that contributes to a maximum of 35% of total energy and that saturated fatty acids contribute to a maximum of 10% of total energy. Patients who have suffered a myocardial infarction should be given dietary advice on the 'Mediterranean diet', which is a diet that focuses on a decrease in saturated fat intake and an increase in the consumption of fruit and vegetables and monounsaturated/polyunsaturated fatty acids.

Dietary fats are generally broken down in the small intestine by bile salts, which emulsify the fats. The hormone cholecystokinin, which is released by the duodenum, causes the gall bladder to release bile salts. Pancreatic lipase breaks down the fatty acids as well as cholesteryl esters, resulting in the production of free cholesterol and fatty acids. The free fatty acids and cholesterol then combine with the bile salts to form micelles which are absorbed in the intestine. Steatorrhoea occurs when there is lipid malabsorption, which could result in deficiencies in the fat-soluble vitamins (vitamins A, D, E, and K) as well as the essential fatty acids.

Further Reading

Dehghan M, Mente A, Zhang X et al. Associations of fats and carbohydrate intake with cardiovascular disease and mortality in 18 countries from five continents (PURE): a prospective cohort study. *Lancet* 2017; 390: 2050–62.

Mueller C, Compher C, and Ellen DM. ASPEN clinical guidelines: Nutrition screening, assessment, and intervention in adults. *J Parenter Enteral Nutr* 2011; 35: 16–24.

National Institute for Health and Care Excellence. *Behaviour Change: Individual Approaches.* 2014. Available at http://www.nice.org.uk/Guidance/PH49 (accessed 17 Sep 2017).

332 Starvation and malnutrition

Satish Keshav and Alexandra Kent

Definition of the disease

Starvation is a state of severe malnutrition due to a reduction in macro- and micronutrient intake. The basis underlying starvation is an imbalance between energy intake and energy expenditure.

Aetiology of the disease

The commonest cause of starvation is lack of available food, usually due to environmental, social, and economic reasons; other causes include:

- anorexia nervosa
- depression and other psychiatric disorders
- coma and disturbance of consciousness
- intestinal failure
- mechanical failure of digestion, including poor dentition and intestinal obstruction

Protein energy malnutrition is usually seen in developing countries; the two forms seen are:

- marasmus: this is caused by inadequate calories, and leads to emaciation
- kwashiorkor: this was originally thought to be caused by protein malabsorption, although it is now thought that it is likely to be caused by deficiency of micronutrients, particularly those with antioxidant function, such as glutathione, vitamin E, and polyunsaturated fatty acids

Typical symptoms of the disease, and less common symptoms

Individuals experiencing starvation undergo catabolysis, whereby the body breaks down fat and muscle tissue to provide energy sources for vital organs, such as the heart and brain. Muscle atrophy leads to weakness, and gastrointestinal atrophy reduces hunger. As the patient becomes more starved, they often lose the ability to sense thirst, and so become dehydrated. Movement becomes painful, and patients become fatigued and apathetic. Depression and irritability may occur. Infections are more common, and cause catabolism, hastening death, which eventually ensues.

Marasmus leads to extensive tissue and muscle wasting, often with loose skin folds and drastic loss of adipose tissue. A patient with kwashiorkor is defined by the presence of pedal oedema, and often presents with hepatomegaly, a distended abdomen, dermatoses, anorexia, thin hair, and irritability.

Symptoms related to specific nutrient deficiencies are shown in Table 332.1.

Demographics of the disease

The WHO states that malnutrition is the biggest contributor to child mortality, associated with ~54% of cases of deaths in children in developing countries in 2001. Currently, it is estimated that there are 963 million undernourished people in the world, which reduces to approximately 1 in 7 people, and is equal to the joint populations of the US, Canada, and the European Union. One person dies every second as a result of hunger; this is equal to 4000 every hour, 100 000 each day, and 36 million each year. It is estimated that 684 000 child deaths per year could be prevented worldwide, by increasing access to vitamin A and zinc. In the developed world, studies have suggested that 40% of hospital inpatients are malnourished, of which 70% of cases are unrecognized.

Natural history, and complications of the disease

Fluid and electrolyte disturbance

As patients become starved or malnourished, they often lose their thirst reflex and so become dehydrated. This puts them at risk of electrolyte disturbance and renal impairment, especially hypokalaemia, hypochloraemia, metabolic alkalosis, and ketonuria.

Impaired immune system

The weakened body of a starved/malnourished patient is more prone to infection, due to a dysfunctional immune system. This results in a reduced production of IgA, T-cells, cytokines, and complement, as well as a decrease in phagocytosis, amongst other effects.

Infections

In starvation/malnutrition, resultant infections, particularly diarrhoea, worsen nutrient absorption, increase metabolic needs, and can cause anorexia.

Cardiovascular complications

Cardiovascular complications of starvation/malnutrition include orthostatic hypotension, bradycardia, arrhythmias, and heart failure.

Gastrointestinal complications

Starvation/malnutrition can cause constipation, parotid gland hypertrophy, fatty liver, gallstones, and pancreatitis.

Growth retardation

Malnutrition and illnesses associated with starvation can lead to physical and mental growth retardation, and have been shown to have a significant effect on a child's long-term future, including potential future earnings.

Endocrine effects

The endocrine effects of starvation/malnutrition include delayed puberty, amenorrhoea, hypercortisolaemia, low T3 levels, and diabetes insipidus.

Dermatological complications

Patients who are starved/malnourished will have thin, brittle hair, alopecia, and brittle nails. Lanugo hair will grow in an attempt to insulate the body.

Approach to diagnosing the disease

Many patients seen in a hospital setting are at risk of malnutrition. Any patient with signs of starvation should have a full history taken and complete examination assessing for any signs or symptoms of nutritional deficiency. The Malnutrition Universal Screening Tool can help to assess nutritional status. This combines information about the patient's current BMI, unplanned weight loss in the preceding 3–6 months, and the effect of any acute disease state. The overall score reflects the patient's overall risk of malnutrition and can guide therapy.

Table 332.1 Vitamin deficiencies

Vitamin	Condition	Symptoms/signs
Vitamin A		Night blindness
		Poor growth
Vitamin B₁ (thiamine)	Beriberi	Weakness
		Muscle pain
		Heart failure
		Peripheral neuropathy
		Wernicke's encephalopathy
Vitamin B₃ (niacin)	Pellagra	Dermatitis
		Aggression
		Insomnia
		Weakness
		Confusion
		Diarrhoea
		Ataxia
		Glossitis
		Dementia
		Dilated cardiomyopathy
Vitamin B₁₂		Macrocytic anaemia
		Peripheral demyelination
		Sleep disturbances
		Subacute combined degeneration of the spinal cord
Vitamin C	Scurvy	Malaise
		Lethargy
		Myalgia
		Bruising
		Gum disease
		Neuropathy
Vitamin D	Osteomalacia (adults)	Bone pain
	Rickets (children)	Increased fractures
		Dental problems
		Skeletal deformities (bow legs)
		Craniotabes
		Hypocalcaemia
		Growth disturbance
		Metaphyseal cartilage hyperplasia
Calcium		Osteoporosis
		Rickets
		Tetany
Folate		Macrocytic anaemia
		Weakness
		Headaches
		Irritability
Iodine	Goitre*	Low thyroid hormones
		Raised thyroid-stimulating hormone
	Cretinism	Mental retardation
		Stunted growth
		Deaf–mutism
Iron		Microcytic anaemia
Selenium	Keshan disease	Myocardial necrosis
	Kashin–Beck disease	Atrophy
		Degeneration and necrosis of cartilage
		Selenium aids conversion of thyroxine into triiodothyronine, so deficiency can cause signs of hypothyroidism
Zinc		Anorexia
		Lethargy
		Diarrhoea
		Growth and mental retardation
		Alopecia
		Dermatitis
		Neuropathy
		Anaemia
		Hepatosplenomegaly
		Macular degeneration

*May occur with or without cretinism.

Other diagnoses that should be considered

Starvation is due to poor oral intake, and the underlying cause(s) should be ascertained: these include disinterest, poor dentition, an inability to shop or prepare food, or psychiatric causes (e.g. depression, anorexia nervosa).

'Gold-standard' diagnostic test

There is no specific test that can diagnose starvation. The diagnosis is made on a combination of history, examination, and nutritional assessments.

Investigations

Laboratory studies for starvation/malnutrition should include a full blood count, renal function tests, electrolyte levels, liver function tests, albumin levels, a bone profile, haematinics, and levels of vitamin and trace elements (e.g. zinc, selenium). Starved patients will have ketones in their urine. Patients should undergo investigations to detect potential associated infections, such as a chest X-ray, stool culture, blood culture, and so on. An ECG should be performed to assess for small QRS complexes, the QT interval, arrhythmias, and bradycardia. If there is no clear reason for the starvation, such as poor access to food, it is important to perform a psychiatric assessment.

Prognosis and how to estimate it

The prognosis for starvation is variable and difficult to estimate. Approximately 50% of patients with anorexia nervosa will recover fully, ~30% will improve, and ~20% have a relapsing condition. Unfortunately, many elderly patients will have undiagnosed malnutrition and die from concurrent sepsis, with the malnutrition often under-treated.

Ultimately, patients can deteriorate to the point where their physiological mechanism for protein synthesis and handling is redundant. At this point, food and protein replacement is futile, and the patient is facing an inevitable death.

Treatment and its effectiveness

The mainstay of treatment comprises replacing fluid, correcting electrolyte derangements, and providing protein, carbohydrates, and calories. Protein, energy, and nutrient requirement vary according to age, sex, and activity levels, and should be adapted for each patient. This should all be done under the close supervision of nutritional specialists and dieticians. Physicians should identify complications of malnutrition and starvation early and initiate rapid treatment, as delayed treatment can be fatal (see 'Natural history, and complications of the disease'), with infections, dehydration, and circulatory failure being associated with higher mortality.

Doctors should involve the dietetics department in the management of sick patients early in their admission to prevent complications associated with malnutrition and starvation.

Further Reading

Fukatsu K and Kudsk KA. Nutrition and gut immunity. *Surg Clin North Am* 2011; 91: 755–70, vii.

Holick MF. Vitamin D deficiency. *N Engl J Med* 2007; 357: 266–81.

Mann J and Truswell S. (3rd edition) *Essentials of Human Nutrition*. 2007. Oxford University Press.

Maqbool A, Olsen IE and Stallings VA. 'Clinical assessment of nutritional status', in Duggan C, Watkins JB, and Walker WA, eds, *Nutrition in Pediatrics: Basic Science, Clinical Applications* (4th edition), 2008. BC Decker Inc.

Ormerod C, Farrer K, Harper L, et al. Refeeding syndrome: A clinical review. *Br J Hosp Med (Lond)* 2010; 71: 686–90.

White JV, Guenter P, Jensen G, et al. Consensus statement: Academy of Nutrition and Dietetics and American Society for Parenteral and Enteral Nutrition: Characteristics recommended for the identification and documentation of adult malnutrition (undernutrition). *J Parenter Enteral Nutr* 2012; 36: 275–83.

333 Vitamin deficiencies

Aminda De Silva, J. A. Saunders, and M. A. Stroud

Definition of the disease

Vitamins are organic compounds required by the body in small amounts to perform specific cellular functions. Nine vitamins (thiamine (vitamin B_1), riboflavin (vitamin B_2), pyridoxine (vitamin B_6), cyanocobalamin (vitamin B_{12}), niacin (nicotinic acid; vitamin B_3), pantothenic acid (vitamin B_5), biotin (vitamin B_7; vitamin H), folic acid (folate; vitamin B_9), and ascorbic acid (vitamin C)) are water soluble, while four (vitamins A, D, E, and K) are fat soluble.

The importance of vitamins was first appreciated through recognition of their clinical deficiency state (e.g. the existence of scurvy was linked to diets low in fresh fruit and vegetables, and this then led to the identification of vitamin C). However, this approach has led to the concept that the primary purpose of a vitamin is to prevent the associated clinical deficiency state and, consequently, unless patients exhibit signs of a specific clinical deficiency state, they are thought to be replete in the corresponding vitamin. This is a misunderstanding. In reality, most vitamins have many different functions which are incompletely understood, and impaired biochemical function and even functional problems affecting metabolic, immunological, or cognitive status can occur with marginal vitamin depletion long before overt clinical deficiency becomes evident. A high index of suspicion is thus essential in all patients who have malnutrition or malabsorption, to ensure that levels that might compromise health, resistance to disease, and recovery from injury or illness are not left untreated.

Aetiology and demographics of the disease

Vitamins cannot be synthesized by humans but are obtained from the diet. Deficiencies of water-soluble vitamins (except vitamin B_{12}) may develop after weeks to months of undernutrition, whereas deficiencies of fat-soluble vitamins and vitamin B_{12} may take more than a year to develop because of relatively large body stores.

In developed countries, traditional medical thinking suggests that vitamin deficiencies result mainly from poverty, food faddism, poor diets, malabsorption, drugs, alcoholism, or prolonged and inadequately supplemented parenteral feeding, with groups at particular risk including pregnant women, children, the institutionalized, and the frail elderly. However, mild functional vitamin deficiency is probably very common, since, although it would be expected that our nutritional needs would easily be met from food alone, our biology did not evolve in the context of the modern western diet, which may have a low micronutrient content. Furthermore, the relatively high activity levels of our ancestors meant that, in general, they would have consumed quite a lot of food daily. This therefore raises the question as to whether some sedentary individuals, eating relatively little, may not be meeting their full 'functional' vitamin requirements even if they are not thin and, certainly, there is good biochemical evidence that many apparently healthy, older individuals are not functionally replete in one or more of the vitamins needed for adequate hepatic transamination (i.e. vitamin B_{12}, vitamin B_6, and/or folate). In addition, the fact that folic acid supplements in early pregnancy dramatically reduce the incidence of neural-tube defects suggests that vitamin intake in this group is also suboptimal.

In developing countries, deficiencies often result from all these factors, which are often coupled with simple lack of access to adequate nutrition.

Typical symptoms of the disease, and less common symptoms

Typical problems related to vitamin deficiency are summarized in Table 333.1.

Natural history and complications of the disease

Deficiencies in water-soluble vitamins

Vitamin B_1 (thiamine) deficiency

Individuals with high alcohol intakes are at particular risk of vitamin B_1 (thiamine) deficiency. The provision of carbohydrate to malnourished individuals can precipitate thiamine deficiency, leading to the reversible Wernicke's encephalopathy (ataxia, ophthalmoplegia, and confusion), which, if not rapidly corrected, can then lead to the irreversible Korsakoff's dementia and impairment of short-term memory.

Beriberi (cardiac failure and peripheral neuropathy) can also occur, although it happens less often than the Wernicke–Korsakoff syndrome, but can go unrecognized, as poor cardiac function is often put down to other problems. Thiamine overdosage (more than 3 g/day) can lead to toxicity, with headaches, irritability, and insomnia, as well as weakness.

Vitamin B_2 (riboflavin) deficiency

Vitamin B_2 (riboflavin) deficiency is probably more common than generally appreciated, due to the non-specific nature of symptoms. Vegans are at particular risk.

Vitamin B_3 (niacin; nicotinic acid) deficiency

Vitamin B_3 (niacin; nicotinic acid) deficiency is most commonly seen in alcoholics and in patients with long-term malabsorption. Rarely, this deficiency can be seen in three specific settings: carcinoid syndrome, prolonged use of isoniazid, and Hartnup disease. High doses can be toxic to the liver and the kidneys.

Vitamin B_5 (pantothenic acid) deficiency

Deficiency of vitamin B_5 (pantothenic acid) in humans is extremely rare. No reports of toxicity with overdosage have been identified.

Vitamin B_6 (pyridoxine) deficiency

Vitamin B_6 (pyridoxine) is required for amino acid metabolism. Some genetic syndromes (e.g. homocystinuria) may mimic pyridoxine deficiency. Some drugs (e.g. isoniazid) interact with pyridoxal phosphate, producing a deficiency.

Vitamin B_7 (biotin/vitamin H) deficiency

Vitamin B_7 (biotin/vitamin H) deficiency can be seen in patients on haemodialysis, and with long-term therapy with some anticonvulsants. Toxicity has not been reported.

Vitamin B_{12} and folate deficiency

Vitamin B_{12} and folate deficiencies are common and can be particularly seen in patients with poor diet and alcoholism, pernicious anaemia, or terminal ileal Crohn's disease, as well as in those who are post gastrectomy. Bacterial overgrowth also utilizes vitamin B_{12} within the small bowel. Overdosage does not seem to be a problem.

Table 333.1 Vitamin deficiency and associated syndromes

Vitamin	Symptoms of deficiency	Rare manifestations
Water-soluble vitamins		
Thiamine (vitamin B$_1$)	Subclinical deficiency: • headache • tiredness • anorexia • muscle wasting Severe deficiency: • dry beriberi: symmetrical peripheral polyneuropathy (sensory and motor) • wet beriberi: neuropathy and congestive cardiac failure • Wernicke's encephalopathy • Korsakoff syndrome	Leigh's syndrome: necrotizing encephalomyopathy
Riboflavin (vitamin B$_2$)	Sore throat Oedema of mucous membranes Cheilosis Stomatitis Glossitis Normocytic–normochromic anaemia Seborrhoeic dermatitis	
Niacin (vitamin B$_3$)	Glossitis Diarrhoea Vomiting Insomnia Fatigue Visual loss Anxiety Delusions Dementia Encephalopathy	Pellagra: photosensitive pigmented dermatitis, diarrhoea, and dementia; can be fatal.
Pantothenic acid (vitamin B$_5$)	Paraesthesiae Dysesthesiae Gastrointestinal disturbances Irritability Malaise	Implicated in 'burning feet' syndrome of prisoners of war
Pyridoxine (vitamin B$_6$)	Marginal deficiencies: • stomatitis • glossitis • cheilosis • irritability • mood disturbance Severe deficiency: • hypochromic anaemia • convulsions	
Biotin (vitamin B$_7$; vitamin H)	Myalgia Dysesthesias Nausea Glossitis Anorexia Hair loss Desquamating dermatitis	
Folic acid (folate; vitamin B$_9$)	Anaemia Lemon-yellow tinge Glossitis	Megaloblastic anaemia Neural-tube defects at time of conception Hyperhomocysteinaemia
Cyanocobalamin (vitamin B$_{12}$)	Anaemia Lemon-yellow discolouration Glossitis Stomatitis Progressive peripheral polyneuropathy Cognitive slowing	Subacute combined degeneration of the dorsal and lateral spinal columns Dementia Optic atrophy Megaloblastic anaemia Increased risk of osteoporosis Hyperhomocysteinaemia
Ascorbic acid (vitamin C)	Early symptoms: • fatigue • weakness • aching joints • muscles	Late stages: • anaemia • petechial and sheet haemorrhages • delayed wound healing • bleeding gums

Table 333.1 (Continued)

Vitamin	Symptoms of deficiency	Rare manifestations
Fat-soluble vitamins		
Vitamin A	Xerophthalmia Poor bone growth Skin problems Impairment of humoral and cell-mediated immunity Impaired hearing Taste and smell Reduced male fertility	In pregnancy, deficiency can result in malformations in offspring
Vitamin D	Subclinical deficiency may contribute to: • osteoporosis • bone pain • reduced immune function • hypophosphataemia • hypocalcaemia	Persistent hypocalcaemia causes secondary hyperparathyroidism leading to osteomalacia Implicated in aetiology of several cancers
Vitamin E	Ataxia Hyporeflexia Dorsal column signs Skeletal myopathy Haemolysis	
Vitamin K	Prolongation of clotting time	Skeletal deformities or calcium deposition in the vasculature

Vitamin C deficiency

Marginal vitamin C deficiency compromises wound healing and limits antioxidant defences, while overt deficiency leads to scurvy, which in UK practice can be seen not uncommonly in alcoholics, patients with anorexia nervosa, and in those with long-term gastrointestinal disease with malabsorption. Scurvy manifests as gum hypertrophy, inflammation, loss of teeth, and skin rashes. Vitamin C toxicity does not seem to cause problems.

Deficiencies in fat-soluble vitamins

Vitamin A deficiency

Most people associate vitamin A deficiency with night blindness. This is rare in the UK, except in patients with severe fat malabsorption and, even worldwide, depletion to levels severe enough to cause retinal problems is rare. However, less severe depletion leading to increased vulnerability to gastrointestinal and respiratory infections and measles is common, with good evidence that oral vitamin A supplementation can reduce mortality by around 50%. Excess vitamin A can cause hepatotoxicity.

Vitamin D deficiency

Severe vitamin D deficiency leads to osteomalacia in adults, who may present with fractures but more commonly suffer from pelvic bone pain, muscle aches, and general weakness.

Many cells within the body exhibit vitamin D receptors and hence there must be many functions of this vitamin that are still poorly understood. At least 16 types of cancer, including breast, colon, ovary, and prostate cancer, have been linked to vitamin D deficiency due to poor sunlight exposure.

Deficiency occurs as a result of overt fat malabsorption and malnutrition, chronic kidney disease, or poor sunlight exposure. Modern life at high latitudes may not provide enough skin exposure to sunlight to permit full functional levels.

Overdosage can lead to metastatic calcification, hypercalcaemia, or pseudogout.

Vitamin E deficiency

Vitamin E has a role as an antioxidant and in immunity. Deficiency due to malabsorption can lead to neuropathy, myopathy, and compromised immunity.

Vitamin K deficiency

Deficiency in vitamin K is unusual, as this vitamin is produced by gut flora. However, long-term antibiotic use can diminish the numbers of the colonic bacteria that synthesize absorbable vitamin K, and therefore can contribute to vitamin deficiency. Overdosage can lead to difficulty in achieving therapeutic effectiveness with warfarin.

Approach to diagnosing the disease

The most difficult step in diagnosing vitamin deficiency is frequently simply considering the diagnosis in the first place, especially since, as noted, deficiency is often subclinical without the signs and symptoms of the specific deficiency syndromes. A high index of suspicion for vitamin deficiency or risk of deficiency is therefore needed, with suspicions aroused for malnourished patients or those at risk on nutritional screening (i.e. all individuals with a body mass index of less than 20 kg/m², unintentional weight loss of over 5% in the previous 3 months, or those who have been eating or will be eating very little). Findings of brittle nails, angular stomatitis, glossitis, hair thinning, or oedema of unknown cause should prompt particular concerns and either specific investigation or pragmatic treatment.

After taking the initial step of considering vitamin deficiency, it would be good, if possible, to confirm any deficiency with simple blood tests. However, although most hospital pathology services can provide measurements of vitamin B_{12}, folic acid, and vitamin D, blood samples to confirm deficiencies of other vitamins or trace elements usually need to be sent to specialist centres; in addition, interpretation of results is problematic since:

- plasma or even red-cell vitamin levels may not reflect true functional tissue availability in vivo
- acute phase responses alter levels of binding proteins, and the degree of binding may increase or decrease levels found in plasma
- inflammation within the liver may lead to leakage of vitamins into the circulation, leading to artificially high levels (e.g. of vitamin B_{12})

In view of these difficulties, a pragmatic approach will often need to be taken in making a diagnosis of vitamin deficiency in clinical practice.

Other diagnoses that should be considered

The differential diagnoses of the many vitamin deficiency syndromes are extremely broad and overlap with each other, as the associated symptoms and signs are generally fairly non-specific.

'Gold-standard' diagnostic tests

The gold-standard diagnostic tests for vitamin deficiency are shown in in Table 333.2.

Acceptable diagnostic alternatives to the gold standard

Acceptable diagnostic alternatives to the gold-standard tests for vitamin deficiency are shown in Table 333.2.

Other relevant investigations

Other relevant investigations for vitamin deficiency are shown in Table 333.2.

Treatment and its effectiveness

Vitamin deficiencies should be treated in the wider context of dealing with malnutrition. General principles include ensuring generous micronutrient and vitamin supplementation during early feeding while avoiding excess provision of micronutrients that might encourage microbial growth or increase free radical damage. Additional specific vitamin supplements should be given to patients with overt deficiency states.

Giving single vitamin supplements to malnourished individuals can pose potential problems, both from direct toxicity of the vitamin itself (e.g. hepatotoxicity from vitamin A overdosage) but also by the possible unmasking of other deficiencies by driving certain metabolic pathways and, in the process, depleting substrates for these pathways, while possibly generating toxic excess products. A prime example of

Table 333.2 Vitamins: Deficiency and diagnosis

Vitamin	Gold standard	Acceptable diagnostic alternatives	Other relevant investigations
Water-soluble vitamins			
Thiamine (vitamin B_1)	Thiamine status may be assessed by measurement of thiamine levels in blood or urine, before and after loading	Erythrocyte transketolase activity or its activation coefficient in haemolysed red blood cells is a functional measure of thiamine status	
Pyridoxine (vitamin B_6)	High-pressure liquid chromatography	Pyridoxal phosphate has been determined enzymatically using tyrosine apodecarboxylase or by fluorimetric methods	Vitamin B_6 status has also been assessed using erythrocyte aminotransferases and the tryptophan loading test
Folic acid (folate; vitamin B_9)	Red-cell folate levels are more stable and reflect long-term intake	Serum folate is a short-term indicator of folate status	
Cyanocobalamin (vitamin B_{12})	As plasma levels may not be reliable, other markers have been identified (including methylmalonic acid, homocysteine, holotranscobalamin, anti-intrinsic factor antibodies) to establish functional activity	Measurement of vitamin B_{12} in plasma is routinely used to determine deficiency, but may not be a reliable indication in all cases; in pregnancy, for example, tissue levels are normal but serum levels are low Carrier levels are also influenced by the oral contraceptive pill, which may lead to apparently low blood levels when there is no real functional deficiency	Several methods have been devised (Schilling test, cobalamin absorbance test, serum gastrin deoxyuridine suppression test) to distinguish different causes of deficiency
Ascorbic acid (vitamin C)	Leucocytes contain higher concentrations of vitamin C than plasma, whole blood, or serum but measurement of leucocyte vitamin C is technically more difficult than estimation of plasma or urinary levels	Plasma and urinary vitamin C levels may be measured but reflect recent dietary intake rather than the level of vitamin C in body stores	
Fat-soluble vitamins			
Vitamin A	Hepatic concentration of retinyl esters is the most objective measure of vitamin A status, but cannot be readily determined in living individuals	The plasma retinol concentration is under homeostatic control by the synthesis of retinol-binding protein, and therefore is an insensitive indicator of status, except in cases of extreme depletion, when other signs of deficiency are already evident	Retinal function tests and assessment of retinol-binding proteins can also be used to assess vitamin A status
Vitamin D	The conventional marker of vitamin D status is plasma 25-hydroxyvitamin D; this marker is employed because it reflects the main storage form of precursor substrate for vitamin D, 1,25-dihydroxyvitamin D, the formation of which is under homeostatic control		DEXA
Vitamin E	Measurement of serum plasma concentration of alpha-tocopherol provides the simplest and most direct evidence of vitamin E status		
Vitamin K	A radioimmunoassay which measures the ratio of prothrombin to partially carboxylated prothrombin in plasma (the latter is formed during vitamin K deficiency) is now available	Functional tests of blood clotting can be used to assess vitamin K status	

this problem is that, due to the interaction between B_{12} and folate, the administration of one can lead to severe depletion of the other.

We would therefore recommend that, since there are only limited means of determining which vitamin levels are compromised, a balanced preparation of all vitamins and micronutrients should be administered in suspected cases of deficiency. Care should be taken when prescribing, however, as some oral multivitamin preparations lack some vitamins and trace elements and, currently, there are no complete liquid vitamin preparations.

Some specific examples of patients for whom supplementation is essential are patients at risk of refeeding syndrome, patients suffering with alcoholic liver disease, patients who are elderly, and patients with non-healing wounds; in these cases, vitamin B_1 (thiamine) and multivitamin supplements should be provided.

If the result of a vitamin assay shows probable depletion, given the limitations in interpretation as outlined in 'Approach to diagnosing the disease', it is usually appropriate to provide additional specific supplementation for around 2 weeks before rechecking levels. In general, total provision should be both balanced and supra normal in order to meet normal maintenance needs, possible raised demands of illness, and correction of depletion.

Successful treatment of vitamin deficiency depends on the underlying cause; simple inadequate nutritional intake due to poor diet is easy to correct, while complex malabsorptive disorders may require long-term IV nutrition.

Further Reading

Food Standards Agency. *Safe Upper Levels for Vitamins and Minerals: Report of the Expert Group on Vitamins and Minerals*, 2003. Food Standards Agency.

Powell-Tuck J and Eastwood M. 'Vitamins and trace elements', in Warrell DA, Cox TM, and Firth JD, eds, *Oxford Textbook of Medicine* (5th edition), 2010. Oxford University Press.

Matt Wise and Paul Frost

Rationale for nutritional support in the critically ill

Major injury evokes a constellation of reproducible hormonal, metabolic, and haemodynamic responses which are collectively termed 'the adaptive stress response', the purpose of which is to facilitate tissue repair and restore normal homeostasis.

The stress response is characterized by activation of the sympathetic nervous system, with concomitant increases in circulating catecholamines and increased secretion of pituitary hormones. Adrenocorticotropic hormone stimulates the release of cortisol, promoting protein catabolism as well as lipolysis and gluconeogenesis.

Additionally, injury and sepsis are associated with the release of cytokines such as tumour necrosis factor alpha, interleukin 1, and interleukin-6. These cytokines contribute to glucose intolerance and protein catabolism. The net effect of critical illness is an increased energy requirement coupled with a loss of total body protein.

If critical illness is prolonged, the adaptive stress response may become maladaptive, in essence exerting a parasitic effect leaching away structural proteins, (typically around 17% of muscle mass is lost after about 3 weeks) and impairing host immunity. This may be manifested by diaphragmatic weakness and prolonged ventilator weaning; impaired wound healing; and an increased propensity to infection.

Primarily, therapy should be directed towards the underlying illness, as nutritional support per se will not reverse the stress response and its sequelae. Nonetheless, adequate nutritional support in the early stages of critical illness may attenuate protein catabolism and its adverse effects.

Nutritional assessment of the critically ill

The main aims of nutritional assessment in the critically ill are to detect prior malnutrition, estimate energy and protein requirements, and monitor the effectiveness of nutritional replacement.

Detecting malnutrition in the critically ill

Malnutrition can be defined as a pathological state resulting from a relative or absolute deficiency in one or more essential nutrients. Malnutrition is associated with increased mortality and morbidity, and it is essential to screen all acutely ill patients for this condition. Although a variety of anthropometric (e.g. mid-arm circumference, triceps skinfold thickness), biochemical (e.g. levels of retinol-binding globulin, transferrin, pre-albumin); immunological (e.g. delayed hypersensitivity), and functional (e.g. skeletal muscle function) parameters have been utilized in the assessment of nutritional status, none is ideal, as they all lack sensitivity and specificity.

Nutritional assessment is best done using a combination of simple clinical parameters such as those incorporated in the Malnutrition Universal Screening Tool (MUST). MUST is a five-step screening tool which can be used to determine whether an adult is malnourished, at risk of malnutrition, or obese; it also provides guidelines for developing an appropriate management plan. Step 1 is to measure the BMI, Step 2 is to assess unintentional weight loss over the last 3–6 months, and Step 3 is to assess the acute disease and its effect on nutritional intake. At each of these steps, the result is given a score between 0 and 2. In Step 4, the scores obtained for the three steps are added together to provide a final score indicating the overall risk of malnutrition. This score then dictates the nutritional management plan, which is determined in Step 5. The majority of critically ill patients screened in this way have been shown to be at high risk of malnutrition and require nutritional support.

Energy and protein requirements in the critically ill

The energy required during critical illness depends on the type, severity, and phase of the illness, as well as the patient's activity levels. Burns, polytrauma, and septic shock are characterized by an enhanced hypermetabolic response and an increased energy expenditure, compared to other types of critical illness. As recovery occurs, the metabolic response to the illness converts from a catabolic to an anabolic phase, which is associated with an increase of fat and protein stores, and weight gain. Moreover, as activities such as spontaneous breathing and mobilization increase, energy expenditure increases further and should be accounted for when calculating nutritional requirements.

While underfeeding is obviously undesirable, gross overfeeding can cause hyperglycaemia, hepatic steatosis, and immune dysfunction, as well as increase carbon dioxide production and contribute to respiratory failure.

Indirect calorimetry devices allow non-invasive measurement of respiratory gas exchange, from which the energy expenditure can be calculated. While there are a number of formulae available for this purpose, the following equation, called the modified Weir equation, is most often utilized:

$$EE = (3.94 \times VO_2) + (1.1 \times VCO_2)$$

where EE is energy expenditure (in kilocalories per day), VO_2 is oxygen consumption (in millilitres per minute), and VCO_2 is carbon dioxide production (in millilitres per minute).

Although indirect calorimetry can reduce incidences of over- and underfeeding by providing accurate measurements of energy expenditure, there are a number of potential sources of error when using this technique. In critically ill patients, steady state conditions are easily disturbed by intercurrent illness such as seizures or sepsis; pain; anxiety; catecholamine use; altered ventilation; airway leaks; and increased inspired oxygen concentrations. Over the course of the day, measurements of energy expenditure may vary by as much as 23%.

Predictive equations can also be utilized to estimate energy expenditure in the critically ill. Examples include the Harris–Benedict equation and the Schofield equation. The Schofield equation estimates a basal metabolic rate based on age, sex, and weight, and per cent adjustments are made according to 'stress factors' for particular illnesses, the level of the patient's activity, and diet-induced thermogenesis. Such equations are frequently inaccurate in critically ill patients, often overestimating caloric requirements.

Amino acids released during protein catabolism are largely recycled, so the minimal daily protein requirement for adults is only about 20 g/day. During critical illness, this value varies, depending on the stage and severity of the illness, but is unlikely to be in excess of 80 g/day. Protein given in excess of this is used or is stored as energy.

A 24-hour urinary urea nitrogen test (UUN) can be used to calculate the nitrogen balance and hence determined the patient's protein requirements (1 g of nitrogen is equal to 6.25 g of protein). Nitrogen intake should be around 25% greater than the measured UUN to take account of other protein losses, for example from the digestive tract and skin. Nitrogen balance studies are of limited usefulness if extra-renal nitrogen losses are increased, for example from burns, wounds, drains, or stomas, or if the UUN cannot be measured because of renal failure.

An expert group from the European Society of Enteral and Parenteral Nutrition (ESPEN) have recognized the limitations of estimating energy and protein requirements in critically ill patients and have made pragmatic recommendations. Thus, during the initial acute phase of critical illness, an exogenous energy supply in excess of 20–25 kcal per kilogram of body weight per day may be harmful but, during recovery (the anabolic flow phase), the aim should be to provide a total of 25–30 total kcal per kilogram of body weight per day. (This is inclusive of protein, which is usually administered at between 1.2 g/kg per day and 1.5 g/kg per day).

Monitoring the effectiveness of nutritional replacement in the critically ill

ICU patients receiving nutritional support need to be screened daily to ensure that nutritional goals are being met and that there are no complications associated with feeding.

Nutritional delivery in the critically ill

Nutrition can be administered directly into the gastrointestinal tract, as enteral nutrition, or given intravenously, as parenteral nutrition. In critically ill patients, there is a paucity of evidence that clearly demonstrates the superiority of enteral nutrition over parenteral nutrition. Indeed, because of gastrointestinal intolerance, it is frequently difficult to administer the prescribed amount of feed by the enteral route. Moreover, the increased rates of infection that have been historically described as being associated with parenteral nutrition may actually have been related to the under-treatment of hyperglycaemia, or excess lipid administration. Nonetheless, safety, cost, and feasibility generally favour enteral nutrition over parenteral nutrition as the preferred route of nutritional support in the ICU.

Enteral nutrition

Enteral nutrition is indicated in all critically ill patients who are not expected to be on a full oral diet within 3 days. It is usually administered via a gastrointestinal feeding tube and should be initiated within 24 hours of ICU admission, providing the patient has a functioning gastrointestinal tract and is haemodynamically stable.

Feed formulae for enteral nutrition

Polymeric feeds for enteral nutrition contain a mixture of nutrients similar to those encountered in a normal diet, and the majority of critically ill patients can be fed with such formulations. There are many commercially available polymeric feeds; typically, they are iso-osmotic (approximately 300 mOsmol/kg) and contain 1 kcal/ml as a mixed fuel system (45%–60% carbohydrates, 20%–35% lipids, and 15%–20% proteins). Micronutrients (i.e. trace elements and vitamins) are added so that full feeding matches recommended daily allowances for these micronutrients. These solutions are gluten-free, lactose-free, and sucrose-free.

Semi-elemental and elemental feeds are designed for patients with impaired digestion or absorption. These feeds contain predigested nutrients in the form of oligopeptides or amino acids, medium-chain triglycerides, and glucose. Such formulations have a high osmolality (approximately 630 mOsmol/kg) and often induce diarrhoea. These feeds should only be prescribed in the ICU for a specific indication (e.g. short bowel syndrome, pancreatitis, inflammatory bowel syndrome).

Soluble fibre, such as guar gum and pectins, is an important source of energy for the colonic enterocyte, while insoluble fibre, such as soy polysaccharides) increases stool bulk and shortens intestinal transit times. Despite these important properties, the efficacy of fibre in critically ill patients has not been proven, and not all polymeric feeds contain fibre.

Special-formulae feeds have been designed for patients with specific organ failures; for example, patients with chronic respiratory failure may benefit from feeds containing more fat than carbohydrate. The reason for this is that the respiratory quotient of fat is less than that for carbohydrate so that less carbon dioxide is produced from the oxidation of this feed. Other feeds have lower sodium and potassium contents and so may be helpful in the setting of renal or hepatic failure.

Immunonutrition

In recent years, it has been suggested that certain nutrients may have a beneficial effect on immune function in critically ill patients. These substances have been termed 'nutraceuticals'.

Glutamine

Glutamine is the most abundant non-essential amino acid in the body; it becomes conditionally dependent (i.e. requiring exogenous supplementation) during critical illness, as it is the preferred oxidative substrate for rapidly proliferating cells such as lymphocytes and enterocytes. Moreover, as a nucleotide precursor, it is intimately connected to protein synthesis. Consequently, glutamine is essential for preserving normal intestinal mucosal structure and function and may prevent translocation of harmful bacteria and bacterial products. Additionally, as an essential precursor of glutathione, glutamine has an important role as an antioxidant and as a regulator of ammonia balance and acid–base balance.

There is moderate evidence that glutamine reduces infection rates and days of mechanical ventilation in critically ill patients but it seems to have minimal or no effect on length of intensive care stay or risk of death.

Arginine, nucleotides, and omega-3 fatty acids

The amino acid arginine can modulate immune cells in several ways; for example, it can increase the number and activity of T-cells and enhance neutrophil phagocytosis. In addition, arginine metabolism is responsible for nitric oxide synthesis, which is of central importance in the inflammatory response. Although arginine levels are decreased in septic patients, supplementation does not appear to be beneficial.

Nucleotides are used in the synthesis of essential substances such as nucleic acids and adenosine triphosphate and have been shown to have immunostimulating effects on T-cells in vitro.

Omega-3 fatty acids are found in fish oil and have anti-inflammatory effects. Dietary substitution of omega-6 fatty acids, which are found in vegetable oils, by omega-3 fatty acids favours the synthesis of less active eicosanoids such as prostaglandin E3 and leukotriene B5, which may attenuate the inflammatory response.

A commercially produced feed enriched with arginine, omega-3 fatty acids, and nucleotides improved mortality in patients undergoing upper gastrointestinal surgery, as compared to a standard feed. Similarly, in patients with acute respiratory distress syndrome, a nutritional formula containing omega-3 fatty acids and antioxidants reduced the number of ventilator days, the length of the ICU stay, and the number of organ failures.

Administration of enteral nutrition

The majority of patients in the ICU are fed with a fine-bore (internal diameter 1.5 mm) nasogastric tube. These tubes are inserted with the aid of a wire stylet, and their position in the stomach is confirmed radiologically.

Post-pyloric feeding is indicated following upper gastrointestinal surgery (e.g. oesophagectomy) or if the small bowel is normal but there is refractory gastroparesis. Jejunal tubes can be placed intraoperatively (feeding jejunostomy) or endoscopically (nasojejunal tube).

The rate of accidental removal of nasoenteric tubes, either by agitated, uncooperative patients or during routine care, can be decreased by using a nasoenteric 'bridle.' This is fashioned from soft tape, which is passed through the nostrils and looped around the nasal septum and provides an anchor to which the nasoenteric tube can be secured.

Commercial feeds are usually presented in 500 ml containers, which are convenient for storage as well as being easy to handle at the bedside. Tubing is used to connect the container to the nasoenteric tube, and the feed is administered continuously using a pump. Enteral nutrition is usually managed according to locally agreed feeding protocols. The patient should be fed in a semi-recumbent position, as this is associated with a decreased incidence of ventilator-associated pneumonia. Typically, gastric residual volumes are checked every 4 hours. If the volumes are excessive (i.e. >300 ml), then consideration should be given to the causes of gastroparesis (e.g. sepsis, morphine derivatives) and to the instigation of prokinetic agents. Metoclopramide and erythromycin given intravenously improve gastrointestinal motility and tolerance to enteral nutrition. However, although gastroparesis is common in the ICU (e.g. affecting 40% of patients with head injuries), these drugs should not be used routinely; rather, they should be reserved for patients with high gastric residual volumes.

Complications of enteral feeding

Malposition of the feeding tube can have devastating consequences; for example, endobronchial placement can lead to pneumothorax or to the infusion of feed into the lungs. Tube insertion can cause significant bleeding and injury to the nasal pharynx, the oral pharynx, the oesophagus, or the stomach; in addition, it can cause sinusitis. Moreover, the aspiration of feed may lead to pneumonia. Finally, the feed may cause gastrointestinal intolerance, which can manifest as abdominal distension, nausea, vomiting, and diarrhoea.

Parenteral nutrition

Patients should receive parenteral nutrition when enteral nutrition is likely to fail or is contraindicated. Conditions where these circumstances can arise include prolonged ileus following major intra-abdominal surgery; high-output fistulae; short bowel syndrome; pancreatitis; enteritis; and thoracic duct injury with chylothorax.

Parenteral nutrition should be progressively introduced, starting at no more than 50% of estimated requirement and then increased to full feed over 3 days. Ideally, daily energy requirements should be measured but, when this is not possible, a target of 25 kcal per kilogram of body weight per day should be selected. Parenteral nutrition is given as a complete formulation in a single bag and infused continuously via a dedicated central or peripheral venous catheter.

In parenteral nutrition, carbohydrates and lipids are the principal energy sources, while amino acids are given to attenuate protein catabolism and reduce the loss of lean muscle mass.

Parenteral lipid solutions are composed of triglycerides, with phospholipids as emulsifiers. As an alternative energy substrate, lipids have a glucose-sparing effect and so help prevent hyperglycaemia. Moreover, lipid solutions provide linoleic and linolenic acid; deficiencies of these essential fatty acids can result in dermatitis, increased susceptibility to infection, and delayed wound healing. A number of lipid formulations are commercially available but, in the ICU, soybean oil-based emulsions, often referred to as long-chain triglycerides, tend to predominate.

Parenteral nutrition protein is provided as a balanced amino acid solution (i.e. one that is composed to maintain normal fasting plasma levels of essential amino acids).

According to ESPEN guidelines, parenteral nutrition for ICU patients should contain glucose, at a minimum of 2 g per kilogram of body weight per day (no more than 5–6 g per kilogram of body weight per day), and lipids, at 0.7–1.5 g per kilogram of body weight per day. A balanced amino acid mixture should be infused at 1.3–1.5 g per kilogram of ideal body weight per day (this solution should contain glutamine at 0.2–0.4 g per kilogram of body weight per day). Finally, parenteral nutrition should contain one daily dose of multivitamins and trace elements.

Parenteral nutrition monitoring

In the ICU, parenteral nutrition monitoring includes 4-hourly vital signs (temperature, pulse, blood pressure, and respiratory rate), 1–6-hourly glucose levels, a daily full blood count, a daily INR, and daily liver function tests, as well as daily measurements of plasma electrolytes and magnesium, phosphate, and calcium levels. Baseline levels of trace elements, folate, ferritin, and vitamin B_{12} should also be monitored.

Complications of parenteral nutrition

Complications of parenteral nutrition include catheter complications such as trauma, malposition, arrhythmias, air embolus, infection, and occlusion. In addition, solution-related complications, such as hyperglycaemia, electrolyte disturbances, metabolic acidosis, vitamin and trace element deficiencies, pulmonary oedema, and hepatic dysfunction, can occur.

Refeeding syndrome

Refeeding syndrome can occur when previously severely malnourished patients receive high carbohydrate loads. It is characterized by hypophosphataemia, hypokalaemia, hypomagnesaemia, and fluid abnormalities. These disturbances can lead to cardiorespiratory failure, cardiac arrhythmias, coma, and even death. Management includes electrolyte repletion and a reduction in feeding rate.

Further Reading

Casaer MP and Van den Berghe G. Nutrition in the acute phase of critical illness. *N Engl J Med* 2014; 370: 1227–36.

Preiser J-C, van Zanten ARH, Berger MM, et al. Metabolic and nutritional support of critically ill patients: Consensus and controversies. *Crit Care* 2015; 19: 35.

335 Poor diets

Rob Andrews and Clare England

Introduction

Apart from breast milk, no single food contains all the essential nutrients the body needs to be healthy and function efficiently. The nutritional value of a person's diet depends on the overall balance of foods eaten over a period of time, as well as on the needs of the individual.

Over the last 60 years, there has been increasing agreement about the balance of nutrients and foods that make up a 'good' diet. This consists primarily of wholegrains (i.e. cereal grains, or foods made from them, containing bran, germ, and endosperm, e.g. wholemeal breads, oatmeal, and dark rye); vegetables and fruit, including nuts and pulses; moderate amounts of fish and low-fat dairy foods; and limited amounts of meat. The consumption of saturated fat should be low, with saturated fat being replaced by mono- and polyunsaturated vegetable fats and fish oils. Trans-fatty acids should be minimized, and added sugar should provide no more than 10% of energy intake. However, as omnivores, humans can survive on a wide range of different foods, and many people worldwide eat diets that fall far short of this ideal.

The effect of poor diets

Poor diets are patterns of food intake that do not provide the right balance of nutrients for health. A poor diet can lead to an individual becoming deficient in or taking an excess of one or more nutrients. Excessive energy intake is associated with diabetes, cardiovascular disease, and cancer, whereas diets rich in fibre, fruit, and vegetables are associated with reduced risk. In 2001, some 33.9 million reported deaths worldwide were due to chronic diseases in which diet is known to have an impact, and about 3.9 million deaths in children under 5 each year are associated with undernutrition. Worldwide, there is a move away from 'traditional' diets rich in a variety of vegetables and wholegrains towards a pattern that has been described as a 'Western' dietary pattern: high in red and processed meats, high-fat dairy foods, refined grains, processed foods, and sugary foods and drinks, and low in fibre, fruit, and vegetables, contributing to the levels of chronic disease worldwide.

Nutrient excesses and deficiencies

Energy excess

Energy needs are affected by one's genome, activity levels, health, and environment. As a benchmark, 1900 –2550 kcal/day will provide most adults with sufficient energy.

Energy intake in excess of requirements leads to obesity. The prevalence of obesity has increased worldwide and no longer occurs only in developed countries. Developing countries are experiencing a rapid shift to industrialized, more urbanized economies, alongside the globalization of mass media and increased advertising. This leads to changes to traditional dietary patterns, referred to as the 'nutrition transition'. The results of this are an increased consumption of animal fats, and foods high in fat and sugar and low in fibre. Simultaneously, there is a reduction in physical activity. These two changes result in increased obesity levels. This has produced a worldwide rise in diseases linked with obesity: diabetes, coronary heart disease, stroke, and certain cancers (e.g. oesophageal cancer, pancreatic cancer, colorectal cancer, breast cancer, endometrial cancer, and renal cancer).

To prevent obesity, the WHO recommends a shift away from diets containing a high proportion of high-fat, high-sugar, energy-dense foods and high-sugar drinks towards greater consumption of foods that are lower energy and micronutrient (vitamins and minerals) rich—vegetables, legumes, fruit, and wholegrains—alongside an increase in physical activity.

Energy/protein deficiency

Despite the global rise in obesity, energy deficiency remains widespread. In 2007 some 923 million people worldwide had energy intakes below that required for an active, healthy life; this represents an increase of 75 million over 2 years. Most of these people live in developing countries. In the UK, energy deficiency is most commonly seen in the elderly, 70% of whom are not diagnosed.

Energy deficiency results in weight loss due to loss of body fat and muscle mass. Essential tissue is preserved for as long as possible. Involuntary energy deficiency is accompanied by deficiencies in protein and micronutrients. Protein-energy malnutrition (PEM) results in general muscle wasting which causes the muscle fibres to shrink. The spaces between the cells fill with extracellular fluid, leading to oedema and thus masking tissue loss. Protein is lost from the skin and internal organs, increasing the risk of infections, although brain tissue is preserved. In severe PEM, the gut ceases to function normally, and diarrhoea can occur in the absence of infection, causing life-threatening dehydration.

Fetal, chronic infant, and childhood undernutrition causes retarded growth and stunting and increases the risk of coronary heart disease, stroke, diabetes, and hypertension in later life. Chronically undernourished people reduce non-essential activity, are more likely to take naps, and tend to be less socially active than their better-nourished peers.

Undernutrition coexisting with overnutrition

Undernutrition remains prevalent in developing countries but there is also a rise in the number of people affected by obesity. In China, overweight has increased fastest amongst low-income and rural adults, due to a shift towards diets consisting primarily of cheap refined starches, vegetable oils, and cheap and processed meats. These energy-dense diets are low in fibre, vegetables, and fruit and can be deficient in essential micronutrients. Individuals living on these diets can simultaneously be overweight and at risk of poor health due to deficiency. The burden of ill health is further worsened if an individual experienced chronic undernutrition early in life: excessive weight gain in people affected by stunting further increases the risk of diabetes, cardiovascular disease, and certain cancers. An estimated 2 billion people suffer from 'hidden' hunger, meeting or exceeding calorie and protein needs but being deficient in one or several micronutrients.

Effective interventions include government regulation to ensure a healthier composition of staple foods, and programmes involving diet and physical activity advice in the workplace, community, schools, and primary healthcare settings. Pricing strategies to encourage healthier choices have been found to be moderately effective.

Protein excess

The reference dietary value for protein in the UK is 0.75 g of protein per kilogram of body weight. Most non-vegetarians, and many lacto-vegetarians, in the developed world eat intakes in excess of this and may easily exceed twice this if physically active.

In the UK, guidance exists to avoid daily protein intakes in excess of 1.5 g of protein per kilogram of body weight, due to concerns of the effect on renal function, bone health, blood pressure, kidney stones, and certain cancers. An FAO/WHO panel discounted these concerns in individuals at low risk of kidney failure in 2007, concluding there is no need for protein restriction. High intakes of red and processed meats have been linked with colorectal cancer, although this does not appear to be due to high intakes of protein per se.

Athletes, keen to increase muscle mass, may consume 3 g of protein per kilogram of body weight from food and a further 1 g of protein per kilogram of body weight from supplements. These levels are not harmful in the short term, but it is unknown what impact, if any, they have on chronic diseases later in life. Protein intakes at this level result in increased oxidation of amino acids rather than increased synthesis of muscle, making them ineffective for the purpose used. An upper level of around 2.0–2.5 g of protein per kilogram of body weight is more appropriate.

Very high intakes of protein (>45% energy intake; >5 g of protein per kilogram of body weight) can cause 'rabbit starvation', symptoms of which are nausea, diarrhoea, hyperaminoacidaemia, hyperinsulinaemia, and hyperammonaemia and which can lead to death.

Vitamin and mineral deficiencies

Micronutrients (vitamins and minerals) are nutrients that are needed in small quantities throughout life. They are necessary for a wide range of processes, including immunity; brain and nervous system development; cognitive processes; skeletal and muscular growth and function; gastrointestinal function; and vision. Deficiencies lead to specific illnesses as well as an increased susceptibility to infection, delayed recovery, and reduced response to vaccination. This can contribute to further deficiency. There are various approaches to tackling micronutrient deficiency worldwide. The main approaches are food fortification of commonly eaten staples (e.g. cereal foods fortified with folic acid; salt fortified with iodine); the mass provision of supplements, such as vitamin A, via community-based volunteers or during immunization programmes; improving access to food by encouraging home gardening and local cooperatives; and providing nutritional education to change habits and promote dietary diversity. Also important is the treatment of illnesses that result in nutrient deficiencies, such as diarrhoea, malaria, and worms.

It is unclear how many people are affected by micronutrient deficiencies. However, some 500 000 children become blind annually due to xerophthalmia (vitamin A deficiency), and half of pregnant women worldwide are anaemic (half due to iron deficiency), with anaemia being associated with 20% of maternal deaths. In addition, 1.9 billion people do not get enough iodine, and iodine deficiency disorders (e.g. cretinism, deaf mutism, mental retardation, and increased risk of miscarriage) affect 13% of the world's population. Folate deficiency, which is responsible for neural tube defects, appears to be widespread, ranging from 26%–80%, and is probably the most common micronutrient deficiency in developed countries; it is caused by low intakes of green leafy vegetables and wholegrains.

Low vegetable and fruit consumption

Low fruit and vegetable consumption is estimated to contribute to 2.6 million deaths, 11% of strokes, and 31% of ischaemic heart disease. About 1.8% of the global burden of disease is attributable to low consumption of fruit and vegetables, with the greatest burden seen in middle-income European countries, and South East Asia

The WHO recommends consuming 400 g of fruit and vegetables per day, not including starchy vegetables like potatoes, yams, taro, and cassava. This represents a minimum amount and is of particular importance for reducing the risks of developing cardiovascular disease, diabetes, and obesity, as well as avoiding micronutrient deficiencies. Attempts have been made to quantify the protective effects of increased fruit and vegetable intake on health: an increment of one serving per day is associated with a 6% reduction in ischaemic stroke and a 4% lower risk of fatal ischaemic heart disease. Small inverse associations have been found for overall cancer risk.

Fruits and vegetables are high in fibre, vitamins, phytonutrients, and potassium and low in energy. The health benefits from increased consumption of fruits and vegetables seem to be due to the foods as a whole rather than to individual nutrients.

To increase consumption, many countries run public health campaigns, such as the 'five a day' message. In the UK, consumption is, on average, 2.8 servings/day. People cite barriers such as disliking vegetables and fruit, not being confident in preparing vegetables, lack of time, and lack of availability. Worldwide, though, the greatest barrier is cost.

Poor diets, and types of fat

An unsaturated fat is a fat or fatty acid in which there are one or more double bonds in the fatty acid chain. A fat molecule is mono-unsaturated if it contains one double bond, and polyunsaturated if it contains more than one double bond. Unsaturated fatty acids show geometric isomerism: the doubly bonded carbon atoms either have their attached hydrogens on the same side (cis) or have them on opposite sides (trans). Cis fatty acids are bent and cannot stack easily, so they have a lower melting point. Where double bonds are formed, hydrogen atoms are eliminated. Thus, a saturated fat is 'saturated' with hydrogen atoms.

Diets high in saturated fats are strongly associated with coronary heart disease, perhaps because these fatty acids raise total and LDL cholesterol. The main sources are meat and dairy products; this fact perhaps explains why the traditional Northern European, American, and Australian diets are associated with a higher risk of coronary heart disease.

Trans-fatty acids, produced by the partial hydrogenation of vegetable oils, raise LDL cholesterol, lower HDL cholesterol, and raise triglycerides, making them particularly atherogenic. They may promote inflammation, having been associated with increased levels of interleukin 6 and C-reactive protein. Diets high in deep-fried fast foods, manufactured baked goods, sweets, and savoury snack foods may be high in trans fats. In northern India, the consumption of vanaspati, made from vegetable oil and containing over 40% trans fats, can be as high as 20 g per person per day; its use is widespread in food manufacturing and street foods. In recent years, legislation, voluntary changes by food manufacturers, and better food labelling has reduced the amount of trans fats used in many countries.

Ideally, saturated fats should make up less than 10% of total energy intake and should be replaced with monounsaturated fats such as rapeseed or olive oil. High-fat dairy produce should be replaced with low-fat dairy; consumption of fatty meats should be kept low; and it is recommended that people aim to eat between one and two portions of fish each week, with one of these being a portion of oily fish (e.g. mackerel, sardines, herring, salmon, or trout). Trans fats should account for less than 2% of total energy intake.

Poor diets associated with food preparation

High consumption of meats preserved by smoking, salting, or the addition of nitrates or nitrites (i.e. bacon, ham, and salami) was strongly linked to an increased risk of colorectal cancer and less strongly linked with cancers of the oesophagus, stomach, lung, and prostate by the World Cancer Research Fund. It has been proposed that this is due to the formation of mutagenic N-nitroso compounds during the preservation of the meat, and to haem-induced carcinogenesis. However, high consumption of preserved meat products has also been linked to a generally poorer diet containing low levels of fruit and vegetables, and high levels of refined carbohydrates and alcohol.

High consumption of red meat has been strongly associated with colorectal cancer and less strongly associated with stomach cancer. This may be due to cooking methods, as the high temperature cooking of meat, to 150°C or higher, also produces mutagenic heterocyclic amines and polycyclic aromatic hydrocarbons.

Heavy metals from cookware may contaminate food, although it is not known how this impacts upon the burden of disease worldwide. Lead can leach from glazed earthenware into leben, a traditional Tunisian acidified milk drink, and can contaminate food when unheated spices are ground in earthenware pots in Mexico.

'Junk food'

The term 'junk food' is a shorthand term for foods that either have little nutritional value or are high in nutrients considered undesirable. This is an inexact definition, and classification depends on what cultural role foods play in the diet: chips are considered to be 'junk food', but roast potatoes are not; takeaway fried chicken is considered to be 'junk food', but Wiener schnitzel is not. The term is also used to refer to cheap, highly processed, ready-to-eat or takeaway foods that are energy dense, high in fat and salt/sugar, and low in fibre and contain few micronutrients.

Inexact or not, the term is widely used. A dietary pattern of high levels of processed, low-nutrient, energy-dense foods is identified as a 'junk food pattern' and is associated with hyperactivity, smoking, and sedentary behaviour in children and adolescents.

Further Reading

Hooper L, Summerbell CD, Thompson, R, et al. Reduced or modified dietary fat for preventing cardiovascular disease. *Cochrane Database Syst Rev* 2012; 5: CD002137.

Miller V, Mente, A, Dehghan M et al. Fruit, vegetable, and legume intake, and cardiovascular disease and deaths in 18 countries (PURE): a prospective cohort study. *Lancet* 2017; 390: 2037–49.

Popkin B M, Adair LS, and Ng SW. Global nutrition transition and the pandemic of obesity in developing countries. *Nutri Rev* 2012; 70: 3–21.

Zitvogel L, Pietrocola F, and Kroemer G. Nutrition, inflammation and cancer. *Nat Immunol* 2017; 18: 843–50.

Introduction

Obesity has been around for more than 20 000 years, as evidenced by statuettes produced in the Stone Age. Body mass index (BMI), calculated as weight divided by the square of the height, is one of the simplest and most common ways of defining obesity. A BMI between 18.5 and 24.9 is classed as normal. BMI values of 25.0–29.9 suggest overweight, and any values over 30 are deemed obese (see Table 336.1). Across populations, BMI is closely associated with whole body adiposity, and the cut-off levels for overweight and obesity reflex the increasing risk of metabolic, cardiovascular, and other complications of obesity as BMI increases above the normal range.

Obesity is widely agreed to be caused by a prolonged period of energy imbalance. In 95% of cases, it is due to the impact of an obesogenic lifestyle (overconsumption of energy and/or insufficient energy expenditure) on a variable background of genetic susceptibility. The remaining cases are caused by certain drugs, specific endocrine diseases, and monogenic syndromes (see Box 336.1).

Epidemiology of obesity

Worldwide, obesity is common and rapidly increasing. Currently, more than 1 billion adults are overweight (BMI 25.0–29.9) and at least 300 million of them are clinically obese (BMI >30). Obesity is most prevalent in Westernized countries, with up to one-third of adults being affected, but it is rapidly increasing in the developing world. The global distribution of overweight, including obesity, is shown in Figure 336.1.

Most countries are showing a steady rise in the prevalence of overweight and obesity. In the UK and USA it is predicted that by 2020 37% of men and 40% of women will be obese.

Cost of obesity to society

The cost to society of obesity is huge, with it accounting for 6% of direct health expenditure in Europe. In the UK, the current cost to the National Health Service is estimated to be £4.2 billion and is forecasted to more than double by 2050.

Box 336.1 Causes of human obesity

Common or lifestyle-related obesity >95% of cases
- genetic susceptibility (polygenic)
- obesogenic lifestyle (overconsumption of energy and/or insufficient energy expenditure)

Secondary obesity (<5%)

Obesogenic drugs
- corticosteroid
- diabetes medication
- antipsychotic drugs

Endocrine disorders
- hypothyroidism
- Cushing's disease
- hypopituitism

Inherited syndromes
- Prader–Willi syndrome
- fragile X syndrome
- Alström syndrome

Monogenic disorders
- leptin
- melanocortin-4 receptor

Cost of obesity to the individual

Obesity subjects a person to unwanted social, psychological, and physical disadvantages. The combination of these factors inevitably creates negative impacts on the individual's quality of life. Socially, obesity is still associated with undesirable stigma, and this affects all aspects of life. Over the last 50 years, many surveys and reports have found that obese children perform less well and are more likely to be placed into remedial classes at school; obese adolescents, especially young overweight women, have lower acceptance rates for universities and receive less financial support from home; and obese adults are subjected to a higher percentages of prejudice in their employment and are often perceived as lacking in self-control and drive. Obesity has also been shown to impinge on personal relationships as well as marriage prospects.

Health hazards of obesity

Obesity has been linked with various diseases. Associations are recognized with type 2 diabetes mellitus (T2DM), hypertension, dyslipidaemia, and coronary heart disease, as well as osteoarthritis, polycystic ovarian syndrome, obstructive sleep apnoea, and obesity-hypoventilation syndrome. Obesity has also been implicated in several malignancies and in chronic renal failure. Population surveys have estimated that obesity accounts for 60% of the risk of developing T2DM, 30%–40% of the risk of developing hypertension or endometrial cancer, 20%–25% of the risk for coronary heart disease and stroke, and approximately 10% of the risk of developing carcinoma of the breast or of the colon (see Figure 336.2).

Psychiatric diseases associated with obesity include anxiety, depression, bipolar disease, and two distinct eating disorders: binge eating disorder and night-eating syndrome. In women, obesity is associated with a higher risk of major depression; in contrast, the risk

Table 336.1 The WHO international classification of adult underweight, overweight, and obesity according to BMI

Classification by BMI (kg/m²)	
Underweight <18.5	
Severe thinness	<16.0
Moderate thinness	16.0–16.9
Mild thinness	17.0–18.49
Normal weight 18.5–24.9	
Overweight ≥25.0	
Pre-obese	25.0–29.9
Obese ≥30.0	
Obese class I	30.0–34.9
Obese class II	35.0–39.9
Obese class III	≥40.0

Reprinted from the WHO Global Database on Body Mass Index, 9780199568741. With permission from the World Health Organization.

(A)

Prevalence of overweight*, ages 18+, 2016 (age standardized estimate) Male

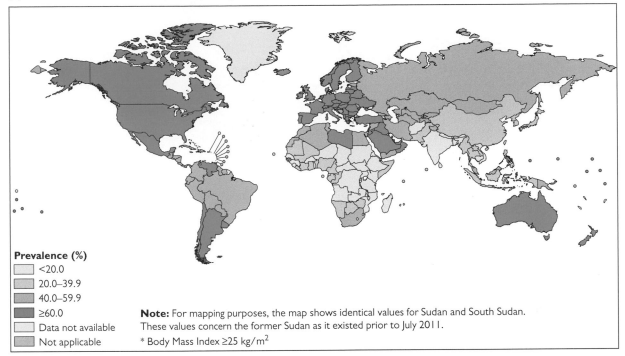

Prevalence (%)
- <20.0
- 20.0–39.9
- 40.0–59.9
- ≥60.0
- Data not available
- Not applicable

Note: For mapping purposes, the map shows identical values for Sudan and South Sudan. These values concern the former Sudan as it existed prior to July 2011.

* Body Mass Index ≥25 kg/m²

The boundaries and names shown and the designations used on this map do not imply the expression of any opinion whatsoever on the part of the World Health Organization concerning the legal status of any country, territory, city or area or of its authorities, or concerning the delimination of its frontiers or boundaries. Dotted and dashed lines on maps represent approximate border lines for which there may not yet be full agreement.

(B)

Prevalence of overweight*, ages 18+, 2016 (age standardized estimate) Female

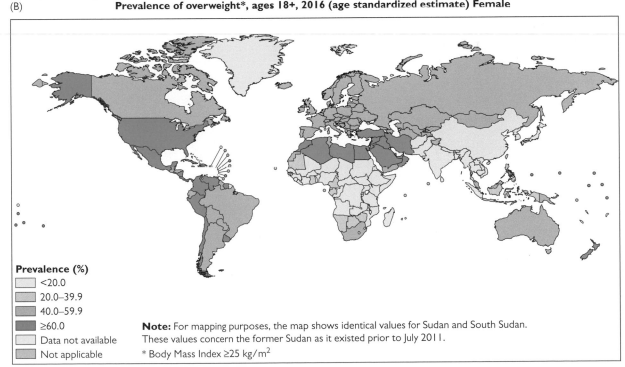

Prevalence (%)
- <20.0
- 20.0–39.9
- 40.0–59.9
- ≥60.0
- Data not available
- Not applicable

Note: For mapping purposes, the map shows identical values for Sudan and South Sudan. These values concern the former Sudan as it existed prior to July 2011.

* Body Mass Index ≥25 kg/m²

The boundaries and names shown and the designations used on this map do not imply the expression of any opinion whatsoever on the part of the World Health Organization concerning the legal status of any country, territory, city or area or of its authorities, or concerning the delimination of its frontiers or boundaries. Dotted and dashed lines on maps represent approximate border lines for which there may not yet be full agreement.

Figure 336.1 Mean body mass index (kg/m²) for ages 18+ in 2014 (age-standardized estimate), for (A) women and (B) men. Data from the WHO; the boundaries and names shown and the designations used on this map do not imply the expression of any opinion whatsoever on the part of the WHO concerning the legal status of any country, territory, city or area or of its authorities, or concerning the delimination of its frontiers or boundaries. Dotted and dashed lines on maps represent approximate border lines for which there may not yet be full agreement.

Reprinted from The Global Health Observatory Map Gallery, Copyright World Health Organization 2017 http://gamapserver.who.int/mapLibrary.

(C)

Prevalence of obesity*, ages 18+, 2016 (age standardized estimate) Female

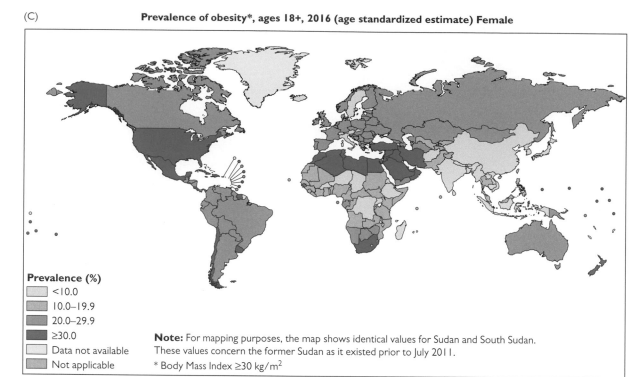

Prevalence (%)
- <10.0
- 10.0–19.9
- 20.0–29.9
- ≥30.0
- Data not available
- Not applicable

Note: For mapping purposes, the map shows identical values for Sudan and South Sudan. These values concern the former Sudan as it existed prior to July 2011.

* Body Mass Index ≥30 kg/m²

The boundaries and names shown and the designations used on this map do not imply the expression of any opinion whatsoever on the part of the World Health Organization concerning the legal status of any country, territory, city or area or of its authorities, or concerning the delimitation of its frontiers or boundaries. Dotted and dashed lines on maps represent approximate border lines for which there may not yet be full agreement.

(D)

Prevalence of obesity*, ages 18+, 2016 (age standardized estimate) Male

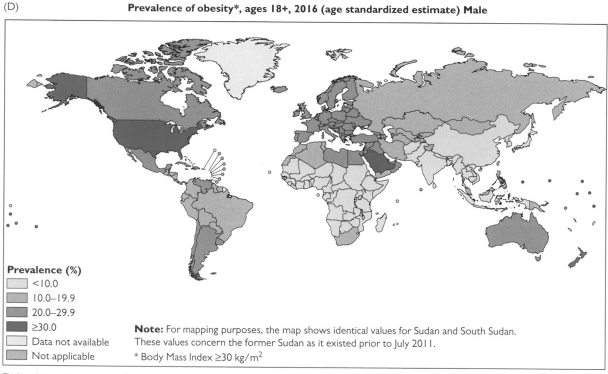

Prevalence (%)
- <10.0
- 10.0–19.9
- 20.0–29.9
- ≥30.0
- Data not available
- Not applicable

Note: For mapping purposes, the map shows identical values for Sudan and South Sudan. These values concern the former Sudan as it existed prior to July 2011.

* Body Mass Index ≥30 kg/m²

The boundaries and names shown and the designations used on this map do not imply the expression of any opinion whatsoever on the part of the World Health Organization concerning the legal status of any country, territory, city or area or of its authorities, or concerning the delimination of its frontiers or boundaries. Dotted and dashed lines on maps represent approximate border lines for which there may not yet be full agreement.

Figure 336.1 Continued

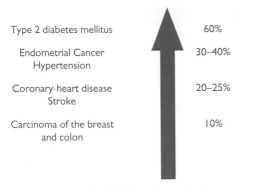

Type 2 diabetes mellitus	60%
Endometrial Cancer Hypertension	30–40%
Coronary-heart disease Stroke	20–25%
Carcinoma of the breast and colon	10%

Figure 336.2 Percentage of risk of disease due to obesity.

in men is decreased. As well as affecting the patients' quality of life, these disorders can reduce their adherence to obesity management and thus affect the clinical outcomes.

Obesity also significantly shortens life expectancy, especially in men. The risk from premature death increases with each increment in BMI, such that individuals with a BMI >30 are at a two- to fourfold increased risk of dying prematurely. In England, obesity has been estimated to shorten life on average by 9 years. Physical inactivity further increases this risk of dying early, with the combination of physical inactivity and obesity thought to account for 30% of all premature deaths worldwide.

Prevention of obesity

Given the long list of diseases that it causes and the poor record of treating it, obesity is a disease that needs to be prevented. Prevention should be distinguished from treatment, with it aiming to reduce or stabilize weight or, in the case of children, limiting weight gain so that overweight children grow into normal-weight adults. Prevention of obesity comprises three stages: primary (to prevent normal-weight subjects from becoming overweight), secondary (to prevent overweight patients from becoming obese), and tertiary (to prevent obese subjects from developing the comorbidities of obesity).

Primary and secondary prevention

Many primary and secondary prevention strategies have been tried. The majority of these have failed to improve obesogenic behaviours and/or reduce the prevalence of overweight or obesity. Those that have succeeded involve multidisciplinary teams, are population wide, sustainable, and address social, ethnic, and cultural diversity.

Breastfeeding reduces the risk of overweight and obesity by as much as 20% for 4 years and should be encouraged. Strategies to encourage the whole family to exercise are also helpful for limiting weight gain in preschool children. School-led programmes, with parental support, that promote healthy eating and increased exercise to replace sedentary play have been successful, although the benefits are often short-lived. A few workplace and community-based programmes that target adults have been successful but few have had lasting effects.

Tertiary prevention

In people with established obesity, it is imperative to prevent subsequent development of comorbidities. Lifestyle modifications are still the central theme in this population and have met with some success. The majority of programmes have targeted the prevention of diabetes. One such example is the Diabetes Prevention Program study, which showed that, with lifestyle modification, including a low-fat, low-calorie diet and moderate exercise of 150 minutes per week, that they could reduce the incidence of diabetes by 58% in a group of overweight participants with impaired glucose tolerance. These results indicate that changes in diet and physical activity can be introduced and sustained in a clinical trial. The challenge is to find methods for achieving similar changes in the community.

Special circumstances

Certain population are at increased risk of gaining weight and, where possible, help should be provided.

Smoking cessation

Many smokers are reluctant to stop smoking for fear of weight gain. Although most people will gain less than 4.5 kg, 13% of the people may gain as much as 11 kg. Weight gain mostly occurs within the first 2 months of smoke cessation and is due to increased energy intake, reduced metabolic rate, and reduced physical activity. Prevention strategies should be considered to lessen the possibility of weight gain after smoking cessation.

Exercise should be recommended, as it reducing craving and withdrawal symptoms and halves weight gain. Greater benefits are seen when it is used as part of a cognitive behavioural smoking cessation programme.

Bupropion, an atypical antidepressant, may be considered as a supplement to help patient minimize weight gain after smoking cessation, although the evidence of its effectiveness is not robust. Nicotine replacement therapy is commonly given as part of the cessation programme and can be very effective in limiting weight gain. However, on withdrawal of nicotine replacement, the patients can gain as much weight as those who were not on the replacement.

Pregnancy

There is substantial evidence that obesity in pregnancy contribute to increased morbidity and mortality for both mothers and babies. The CEMACH maternal death enquiry has found that 35% of women who died were obese, and 30% of mothers who had stillbirths were also obese.

Prior to pregnancy, obese women should be provided with information about the possible complications of obesity, and encouraged to lose weight before conception. Diet, exercise, and behavioural therapy again should comprise the first-line therapy. If pharmacological therapy is required, then metformin and orlistat can be safely used.

Weight loss is not advocated during pregnancy; the aim instead is to limit weight gain to 7–11 kg for overweight women, and to 7 kg for obese women. Screening for glucose intolerance should be carried out at presentation and repeated later in pregnancy if the initial screening test is negative; in addition, blood pressure should be monitored closely, as obese women are at increased risk of pre-eclampsia.

Family histories of T2DM and obesity

In those with a family history of T2DM and obesity, the risk of developing obesity and its associated comorbidities is higher than in the general population. These patients should be provided with information on the importance of weight management and possible complications related to obesity. Lifestyle modification is likely to be the most cost-effective way of obesity prevention.

Iatrogenic obesity

Weight gain can be a side effect of many treatments such as corticosteroids, anti-diabetic medications, and some antipsychotic drugs. Where possible, a non-obesogenic drug should be used (Table 336.2); if this is not possible, then the lowest dose for the least time possible should be used.

Endocrine diseases such as hypothyroidism, Cushing's disease, and hypopituitism can cause weight gain and, where appropriate, looked for. Weight generally falls on treatment of these conditions.

Treating obesity or limiting the impact of obesity

Established obesity is very difficult to treat with the currently available medical treatment, and often the effects are not long-lasting.

Lifestyle modification

Lifestyle modification is essentially the first-line treatment in all cases of obesity. A low-fat, low-calorie diet of 1000–1500 kcal per day in combination with moderate exercise of 150 minutes a week, with additional support from health professionals often produces good

Table 336.2 Weight gain and medications

Drug class	May cause weight gain	Less weight gain, weight neutral or weight loss
Antipsychotics	Clozapine	Ziprasidone
	Risperidone	Aripiprazole
	Olanzapine	
Antidepressants and mood stabilizers	Citalopram	Bupropion
	Lithium	Sertaline
	MAOIs	Fluoxetine
	TCAs	
	Venlafaxine	
	Mirtazapine	
	Paroxetine	
Anticonvulsants	Carbamazepine	Lamotrigine
	Gabapentin	Topiramate
	Valproate	
Diabetes drugs	Insulin	Metformin
	Sulfonylureas	Acarbose
	Thiazolidinediones	Exenatide and liraglutide
		Sitagliptin, vildagliptin & saxagliptin
Antihypertensives	Alpha blockers	ACE inhibitors
	Beta blockers	Calcium channel blockers
Oral contraceptives	Progesterone-only pill	Barrier method
	Combination pill with progesterone	IUDs

Abbreviations: ACE, angiotensin-converting enzyme; IUD, intrauterine device; MOAI, monoamine oxidase inhibitor; TCA, tricyclic antidepressant.

Reproduced with permission from Prescriber: Guide to current recommended management of Obesity, September 2012, John Wiley and Sons Ltd.

Table 336.3 Drugs used to treat obesity in the NHS

Name	Average weight loss (kg)	Patients selection	Side effect
Orlistat	2.9	In patients with or without diabetes mellitus	Gastrointestinal symptoms & Steatorrhoea
Metformin	0.5–4		Gastrointestinal symptoms
Topiramate	6–9		Mood changes and cognitive dysfunction
Exenatide/ Liraglutide	2–3	In patients with diabetes mellitus only	Gastrointestinal symptoms
Pramlintide	4–6		Gastrointestinal symptoms and hypoglycaemia

Reproduced with permission from Prescriber: Guide to current recommended management of Obesity, September 2012, John Wiley and Sons Ltd.

results for people in a weight management program. However, lifestyle change can be difficult to adhere to in the long run for some, and they may require medical intervention to achieve weight loss.

Eating disorders have higher prevalence in the obese population. They can impinge on the obesity treatments and reduce their long-term effectiveness. Studies have shown that behavioural interventions, cognitive behavioural therapy, and interpersonal psychotherapy are useful treatment tools for patients with eating disorders, as these methods are effective for both treating eating disorders and achieving weight reductions, especially when used as part of a weight management program.

Complementary and alternative medicine

Complementary and alternative medicine therapies have become popular for weight reduction as they are viewed as natural and easily accessible and are perceived to be effective. The methods of choice for weight control are yoga, meditation, massage, acupuncture, and eastern martial arts such as tai chi and qi gong, as well as hypnotherapy, homeopathy, and herbal remedies.

Many reviews of non-prescription supplements have shown that the weight reduction achieved is statistically significant, but the effect is modest. With inappropriate use, some supplements can have unwanted adverse effects, such as increased risks of psychiatric symptoms, gastrointestinal symptoms, and palpitations. Hypnotherapy has shown to produce reasonable weight reduction (5–6 kg) when used as an adjunct to dietary advice or in combination with cognitive behavioural therapy as part of a weight management plan. However, the results are, again, clinically debatable and, due to the general lack of substantial randomized controlled trials or larger clinical trials, complementary and alternative medicine is not recognized as a definitive treatment for obesity. However, it may be used to supplement pharmaceutical agents and surgical interventions to obesity.

Weight loss drugs

When weight reduction is not achieved through lifestyle modification alone, anti-obesity medications (Table 336.3) are often considered. These are available for obese individuals who have been on lifestyle modification for at least 6 months duration with minimum weight reduction. The current National Institute for Health and Care

Excellence (2006) guideline on obesity prevention suggests that orlistat, the only remaining simple anti-obesity agent, following the recent withdraw of sibutramine due to increased cardiovascular risks, should be considered for both first- and second-line treatment after lifestyle modification. Orlistat should only be continued if patients have achieved the required weight loss, which is 3% weight loss at 3 months or 5% weight loss at 6 months, while on treatment. More specialized anti-obesity agents, such as metformin, selective serotonin reuptake inhibitors, and topiramate, are often tried in specialist obesity clinics if patients fail to achieve weight loss with this treatment plan. Saxenda® (liraglutide 3mg), a GLP-1 analogue, was marketed in January 2017 in the UK as a weight loss medication for obese patients with a BMI >30 or BMI greater than or equal (please us sign) 27 in the presence of at least one weight related comorbid condition. In clinical studies it produced on average a 5-7 Kg weight loss. Mysimba® (naltrexone-bupropion), recently launched in the UK can be used in a similar population and on average causes a 3-5 kg weight loss. Both of these drugs are only currently available on private prescription in the UK.

Bariatric surgery

Bariatric surgery has now, in selected groups, been shown to improve the cardiovascular risk factor profile, reduce cancer incidence, and reduce mortality. In recent years, bariatric surgery has been made available on the NHS for those who have a BMI >40 and those who have a BMI >35 and have comorbidities (e.g. T2DM, hypertension, cardiovascular disease, and obstructive sleep apnoea), or BMI> 30 with T2DM diagnosed in the last 10 years after they have received medical intervention and are deemed suitable for surgery. There are three types of bariatric surgery that are performed in the UK: gastric banding and vertical sleeve gastrectomy, both of which are restrictive procedures, and the Roux-en-Y gastric bypass, which is a malabsorptive procedure.

Surgery is currently the only treatment that has shown to produce long-lasting weight reduction and lasting improvement on comorbidities.

However, even in the hands of an experienced surgeon, bariatric surgery is still associated with a mortality rate of up to 0.3%. Postoperatively, patients require long-term follow-up and monitoring for potential surgery-related complications. Therefore, this approach should only be considered as a last resort and offered to people who are unable to maintain long-term weight loss.

Further Reading

Akabas SR, Lederman SA, and Moore BJ (eds). *Textbook of Obesity: Biological, Psychological, and Cultural Influences*, 2012. Wiley–Blackwell.

Bray GA and Bouchard C (eds). *Handbook of Obesity: Clinical Applications* (3rd edition), 2008. Taylor & Francis.

National Institute for Health and Care Excellence. *Obesity Prevention*. 2006. Available at http://www.nice.org.uk/Guidance/CG43 (accessed 20 Aug 2017).

Wang YC, McPherson K, Marsh T, et al. Gortmaker SL, Brown M. Health and economic burden of the projected obesity trends in the USA and the UK. *Lancet* 2011; 378(9793):815–25.

Williams G and Fruhbeck G (eds). *Obesity: Science to Practice*, 2009. Wiley.

337 Physical activity and its role in disease prevention

Melvyn Hillsdon and Tim Anstiss

All parts of the body which have a function if used in moderation and exercised in labours in which each is accustomed, become thereby healthy, well-developed and age more slowly, but if unused they become liable to disease, defective in growth and age quickly.

Hippocrates

Introduction

Regular physical activity is one of the most powerful protective and therapeutic factors known to medicine, and this has been recognized for millennia. It protects people from a wide range of health problems and benefits over 20 conditions and diseases, including coronary heart disease, stroke, diabetes, chronic pain, depression, frailty, and cancer. It is also associated with positive mental well-being and a healthy body weight. Among older people, physical activity is associated with better health and cognitive function and can reduce the risk of falls in those with mobility problems.

Taking insufficient physical activity has been estimated to be the fourth leading risk factor for deaths and burden of disease globally, ahead of overweight or obesity. Lack of physical activity may contribute to almost one in ten premature deaths from coronary heart disease (CHD) and one in six deaths from all causes. Population levels of physical inactivity are also hugely costly, with direct costs to the National Health Service estimated at over £900 million in 2009/10. Inactivity is detectable and reducible in individuals and groups.

Definition and measurement

Physical activity can be defined as any bodily movement produced by contraction of skeletal muscles and resulting in caloric expenditure. It includes, but is not limited to, exercise, which can be defined as a subcategory of physical activity that is planned, structured, and repetitive. Physical activity includes occupational physical activity, recreational physical activity, transport physical activity, domestic physical activity (housework, gardening, etc.), and sport. The amount of physical activity a person takes can be measured in terms of frequency, intensity, duration, and type (e.g. aerobic, strength, flexibility, and speed).

Mechanism of benefit from exercise

Recommended amounts

A distinction should be made between physical activity (which is a behaviour) and fitness (which is a measure of a person's capacity to do physical activity, e.g. the maximum amount of oxygen that their muscles can take up per kilogram of body weight per minute, or their maximum strength). Physical activities, such as walking, running, playing sport, or lifting weights, will typically result in improved fitness, but a significant percentage of the variation in fitness levels is genetically determined. Becoming more active and becoming more fit are both likely to yield health and well-being benefits, and a skilled practitioner can tailor a physical activity programme to deliver the specific health, well-being, and functional benefits desired by the patient.

Some of the benefits of a session of physical activity only last a few hours—for instance, the blood-thinning effects, the blood-pressure-lowering effect, the reduction in sugar and fats in the blood, the muscular relaxation effects, and the psychological well-being effects (e.g. the feelings of pleasant fatigue). They cannot be stored up but, like medication, need to be taken regularly to have a health benefit. This has been called the 'last dose' effect.

UK and global physical activity guidelines recommend that all adults should aim to be physically active each day and, over the course of a week, should undertake at least 150 minutes (2.5 hours) of moderate intensity (equivalent to brisk-to-fast walking) physical activity in bouts of 10 minutes or more. Comparable benefits can be achieved through 75 minutes of vigorous intensity activity spread across the week, or combinations of moderate and vigorous intensity activity. In addition to taking moderate or vigorous aerobic activity, current UK guidelines recommend that adults aged 19 and over should also undertake muscle strengthening resistance-type activity on at least two days a week to increase bone strength and muscular fitness. Current UK guidelines also recommend that adults aged 65 and over at risk of falls should perform activities to improve balance and co-ordination at least twice each week.

Size of the risk, and strength of the evidence

There is strong evidence that physical inactivity reduces life expectancy and is a major cause of non-communicable diseases, including coronary heart disease (CHD), type 2 diabetes, breast cancer, and colon cancer. Globally, inactivity increases the risk of premature mortality by 28%, the risk of CHD by 16%, type 2 diabetes by 20%,

Table 337.1 The strength of the evidence for the health benefits of regular physical activity

Health benefit	Strength of evidence
Lower risk of:	
• premature death	Strong
• coronary heart disease	Strong
• stroke	Strong
• high blood pressure	Strong
• adverse blood lipid profile	Strong
• type 2 diabetes	Strong
• metabolic syndrome	Strong
• colon cancer	Strong
• breast cancer	Strong
• depression	Strong
Prevention of weight gain	Strong
Weight loss in conjunction with a reduced calorie intake	Strong
Prevention of falls	Strong
Better cognitive function in older adults	Strong
Better physical function for older adults	Moderate to strong
Lower risk of:	
• hip fracture	Moderate
• lung cancer	Moderate
• endometrial cancer	Moderate
Increased bone density	Moderate
Improved sleep quality	Moderate
Weight maintenance following weight loss	Moderate

Data from Physical Activity Guidelines Advisory Committee. Physical Activity Guidelines Advisory Committee Report, 2008. Washington, DC: U.S. Department of Health and Human Services, 2008.

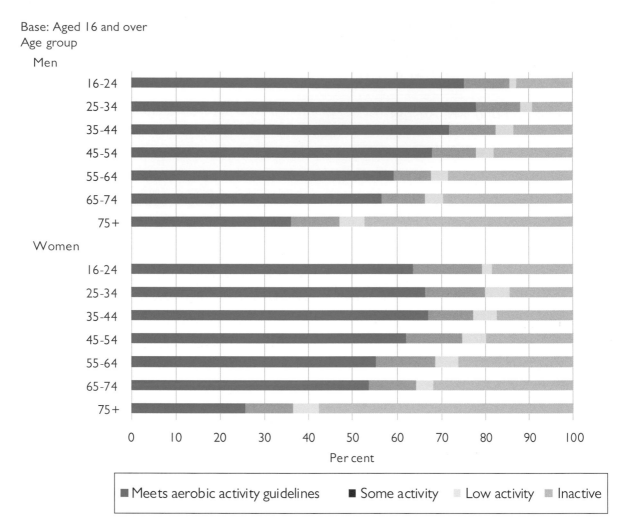

Figure 337.1 Summary activity levels in English adults, by age and sex.

Reproduced from 'Health Survey for England 2016: Physical activity in Adults', 13 December 2017. Source: NHS Digital. Copyright © 2017 Health and Social Care Information Centre. The Health and Social Care Information Centre is a non-departmental body created by statute, also known as NHS Digital. Contains public sector information licensed under the Open Government Licence v3.0. HYPERLINK "http://www.nationalarchives.gov.uk/doc/open-government-licence" www.nationalarchives.gov.uk/doc/open-government-licence.

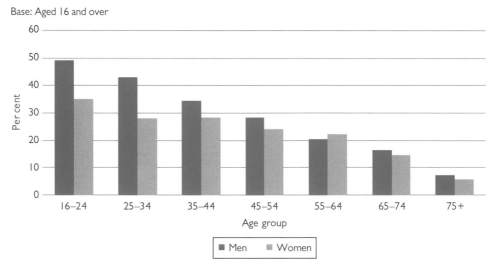

Figure 337.2 Proportion of English adults meeting both the aerobic and muscle-strengthening guidelines, by age and sex.

Reproduced from 'Health Survey for England 2016: Physical activity in Adults', 13 December 2017. Source: NHS Digital. Copyright © 2017 Health and Social Care Information Centre. The Health and Social Care Information Centre is a non-departmental body created by statute, also known as NHS Digital. Contains public sector information licensed under the Open Government Licence v3.0. HYPERLINK "http://www.nationalarchives.gov.uk/doc/open-government-licence" www.nationalarchives.gov.uk/doc/open-government-licence.

breast cancer by 33%, and colon cancer by 32%. The strength of the evidence linking regular physical activity to a range of health benefits is summarized in Table 337.1.

Disease burden

It is estimated that 9% of deaths worldwide are due to physical inactivity, equivalent to 5.3 million deaths per year globally and similar to the global burden of mortality associated with smoking. It is also estimated that physical inactivity is the cause of 6%–10% of cases of CHD, type 2 diabetes, breast cancer, and colon cancer.

It is estimated that physical inactivity contributed over £1 billion to the direct health cost burden to the NHS. In England alone, over 35 000 deaths (from just five conditions: postmenopausal breast cancer, lower gastrointestinal cancer, cerebrovascular disease, cardiovascular disease, and diabetes) might be avoided if the population were physically active at recommended levels.

Prevalence of inactivity as a risk factor

Data from 20 countries report prevalence rates of inactivity range between 37% and 79%. The most recent Health Survey for England (2016) found that 66% of men and 58% of women aged 16 and over met the aerobic guidelines of at least 150 minutes of moderate activity or 75 minutes of vigorous activity per week or an equivalent combination of both, in bouts of 10 minutes or more (see Figure 337.1). The proportion of adults meeting the aerobic activity guidelines varied by quintile of the Index of Multiple Deprivation (IMD), ranging from 50% in the most deprived quintile to 68% in the least deprived quintile. Fewer adults - 31% of men and 23% of women aged 16 and over - met both the aerobic and muscle-strengthening guidelines (see Figure 337.2). As mentioned above, current UK guidelines recommend that adults aged 65 and over at risk of falls should perform activities to improve balance and co-ordination at least twice each week. Of those adults aged 65 and over taking low levels of aerobic activity, only 11% of met the balance and co-ordination guidelines, and of those adults aged 65 and over classed as inactive, only 2% met the balance and co-ordination guidelines.

Screening for inactivity

Tests are available to help clinicians determine the presence of physical inactivity as a risk factor and can be used as part of a comprehensive screening battery (e.g. for cardiovascular disease). Results of the test can be used to inform evidence-based interventions to improve patient health and well-being. A simple, pragmatic self-report measure has been developed that classifies people into four levels of physical activity and has predictive validity for all-cause mortality and incident cardiovascular disease. Individuals are classified as 'active', 'moderately active', 'moderately inactive', or 'inactive'. Compared to the inactive group, the active group had an approximately 30% lower risk of all-cause mortality and cardiovascular disease, even after adjustment for age and other risk factors.

The questionnaire has been adapted for screening patients for physical inactivity in primary care (see http://webarchive.nationalarchives.gov.uk/20130107105354/http://www.dh.gov.uk/en/ Publicationsandstatistics/Publications/PublicationsPolicyAndGuidance/ DH_063812) and is the basis of a physical activity care pathway developed by the Department of Health in England (see http://webarchive. nationalarchives.gov.uk/ + /www.dh.gov.uk/en/ Publichealth/ Healthimprovement/PhysicalActivity/DH_099438).

The effectiveness of interventions to reduce inactivity

An individual's level of physical activity is determined by factors operating at individual, social, and environmental levels. Interventions to increase physical activity have primarily been at the individual level. A review of interventions found that informational interventions (e.g. prompts to encourage stair use), community-wide campaigns, and behavioural and social interventions can be effective at increasing physical activity levels. Based on available evidence, the National Institute for Health and Clinical Excellence recommends that primary care practitioners should take the opportunity, whenever possible, to identify inactive adults and advise them to aim for 30 minutes of moderate activity on 5 days of the week (or more)—taking into account an individual's needs, preferences, and circumstances, and providing patients with written information about the benefits of physical activity, and local opportunities to become and stay more active.

Behaviour-change interventions are modestly effective at increasing physical activity in the short- and long- term. Person-centred, autonomy-supporting communication styles, such as motivational interviewing, together with techniques of behavioural self-regulation such as self-monitoring and goal-setting, are more likely to bring about sustained increases in physical activity.

Summary

Physical inactivity is a prevalent and powerful risk factor for a wide range of disease. Its presence can be detected, and effective, brief interventions exist to help clinicians reduce this risk factor and improve their patients' health and well-being, while reducing disease progression and the risk of complications in some patients.

Further Reading

Lee IM, Shiroma EJ, Lobelo F, et al. Effects of physical inactivity on major non-communicable diseases worldwide: An analysis of burden of disease and life expectancy. *Lancet* 2012; 380: 219–29.

National Institute for Health and Care Excellence. *Physical Activity: Brief Advice for Adults in Primary Care.* 2013. Available at https://www. nice.org.uk/Guidance/PH44 (accessed 18 Sep 2017).

NHS Digital. Health Survey for England 2016: Physical activity in adults. Available at https://digital.nhs.uk/media/34516/Health-Survey...activity/.../HSE16-Adult-phy-act.

Samdal GB, Eide GE, Barth T, et al. Effective behaviour change techniques for physical activity and healthy eating in overweight and obese adults; systematic review and meta-regression analyses. *Int J Behav Nutr Phys Act* 2017;14: 42.

WHO. *Global Recommendations on Physical Activity for Health*, 2010. WHO.

Why is smoking dangerous?

The UK government, in its White Paper in 1998, declared that 'smoking is the greatest single cause of preventable illness and premature death in the UK'. Cigarette smoke is inhaled because it contains nicotine, which is highly addictive. Nicotine itself has some adverse physiological effects but it is mainly the 4000+ chemicals (including acetone, arsenic, paint stripper, pesticides, and over 60 known carcinogens), added to make the cigarette such an extremely potent nicotine delivery device, that cause so much damage.

A smoker dies on average 8–10 years before a non-smoker. The commonest causes of premature death in smokers are cardiovascular disease, lung cancer, and COPD. However, smoking also leads to much morbidity, causing or worsening many illnesses in every system of the body, such as:

- in the cardiovascular system, myocardial infarctions, ischaemic heart disease, hypertension, arrhythmias, cardiomyopathies, peripheral vascular disease, aneurysms, and venous stasis/thromboses
- in the respiratory system, chest infections, rhinitis, COPD, asthma, and several interstitial lung diseases
- in the gastrointestinal system, peptic ulcer disease, reflux, pancreatitis, and Crohn's disease
- in the musculoskeletal system, osteoporosis, delayed fracture healing, and Perthe's disease
- in the neurological system, strokes, probable dementia, and multiple sclerosis
- in the reproductive system, erectile dysfunction, reduced fertility (male and female), poor pregnancy outcomes, and increased infant mortality
- in the skin and soft tissues, poor wound healing, premature ageing, psoriasis, hidradenitis suppurativa, peridontitis, and hair loss
- in the endocrine system, Graves' disease, insulin resistance, and testicular and ovarian dysfunction
- in the eyes, cataracts, optic nerve toxicity (tobacco-related amblyopia), and macular degeneration
- in the ears, otitis media

In addition, smoking is associated with a number of cancers, including lung cancer, nasopharyngeal cancer, laryngeal cancer, oesophageal cancer, stomach cancer, pancreatic cancer, colonic cancer, kidney cancer, bladder cancer, cervical cancer, and acute myeloid leukaemia.

Stopping smoking at any age has been shown to improve health and increase life expectancy. Even with advanced smoking-related diseases, observational studies show clinically meaningful benefits in stopping smoking. Some generic health benefits in stopping smoking are given in Table 338.1.

Magnitude and demographics of smoking

Taxation, advertising bans, public health messages, legislation for minimal age, and banning smoking in work and enclosed public places has helped to reduce tobacco use in many high-income countries. In Britain in 2008, just 22% of men smoked compared with 65% in 1948. Furthermore, the rates of some major tobacco-related diseases, such as lung cancer, are now falling (at least in men). Around 24% of adult women smoke.

The rate of decline in smoking has slowed; for example, in US adults, smoking declined on average by only 0.39% per year after 1990, with no significant drop in prevalence from 2004 to 2006, and the cost to the NHS per quitter in the UK has risen over the last 5 years.

Moreover, the world is still in the midst of an epidemic of tobacco-related illness. The substantial decline in smoking in the West has not

Table 338.1 Some generic health benefits in stopping smoking	
Time since quitting	**Beneficial health changes that take place**
24 hours	Lungs start to clear out mucus and other smoking debris
48 hours	Carbon monoxide will be eliminated from the body Ability to taste and smell is greatly improved
72 hours	Breathing becomes easier Bronchial tubes begin to relax and energy levels increase
2–12 weeks	Blood circulation improves
3–9 months	Coughs, wheezing, and breathing problems improve as lung function is increased by up to 10%
1 year	Risk of heart attack falls to about half that of a smoker
10 years	Risk of lung cancer falls to half that of a smoker
15 years	Risk of heart attack falls to the same as someone who has never smoked

happened elsewhere: 1.2 billion people (about 40% of all men and 10% of women) worldwide are smoking 5 trillion cigarettes annually, particularly in low- and middle-income countries. Cigarette production and consumption in developing countries are rising by just under 1% a year. About 6 million people now die each year because of tobacco and, without a rapid change in the epidemic's course, this figure is estimated to rise to 8.3 million, and tobacco will be the biggest worldwide killer by 2030.

How do you reduce smoking uptake and help patients quit?

Helping populations reduce smoking

National and international control strategies are best summarized by the WHO Framework Convention on Tobacco Control (available at http://www.who.int/fctc/text_download/en/); 168 nations have now ratified it, committing themselves to a broad set of initiatives addressing issues such as advertising and promotion; minimum price and taxes; labelling; protection against second-hand smoke; education and cessation; gender issues; illicit trade; and sales to minors. Despite continuing opposition by the tobacco industry, the framework sets deadlines for implementing measures and, in 2008, the process was reinforced by a package of six measures known as MPOWER, drawn up by the WHO to help countries cut demand for cigarettes.

The bans on smoking in enclosed public spaces consistently show high (and progressively higher) levels of public support (even in smokers), very good compliance, improvements in the health of hospitality workers, improvements in public health (e.g. reduction in hospital admissions for myocardial infarctions in Scotland), and no clear evidence of adverse economic impact or a switch to increased smoking at home.

Efforts to reduce smoking at more local community levels using mass media campaigns, the internet, mobile texts, or telephone quit lines have a very weak but positive effect on quit rates. They are probably still cost-effective because they can reach large numbers of smokers. The best content of these packages is still not known.

Preventing uptake of smoking in children is difficult; mass media campaigns or educational programmes seem to have little effect. Some promising interventions include using a respected classroom peer to advocate non-smoking.

Helping individuals stop smoking

Around 70% of smokers say they want to stop. The least effective way for an individual smoker to try to quit is to go 'cold turkey' and try without behavioural support. However, it remains the most popular method and, because of the large numbers involved, more smokers quit by this method than any other.

Any health professional can have a positive impact on someone's chances of quitting. Meta-analyses of 20 randomized controlled trials suggests nursing-delivered interventions significantly increase the odds of quitting (odds ratio 1.47, 95% confidence interval 1.29–1.68), particularly for hospitalized patients but also in non-hospitalized patients.

Pooled data from randomized and observational trials since 1972 confirm that even brief doctor advice is better than no advice in improving validated quit rates over at least 6 months (odds ratio 1.74, 95% confidence interval 1.48–2.05). There is also a clear dose response with better quit rates following more intensive advice and when offering follow-up visits.

Community pharmacists have a role in smoking cessation and can reach large numbers of smokers but more research is needed to establish what training and type of intervention is most effective.

Pharmacotherapy to aid smoking cessation

Nicotine replacement therapy (NRT) has been licensed since 1982, with inhalators, microtabs, lozenges (short-acting), and transdermal patches (long-acting) all being used today. Repeat Cochrane reviews of well-designed randomized controlled trials suggests all types of NRT roughly double a smoker's chance of quitting over at least 1 year. Trials sponsored by manufacturers of NRT are more likely to show positive results but compulsory registration of all trials should reduce publication bias in future.

Varenicline is an oral partial agonist of the alpha-4 beta-2 subtype nicotinic acetylcholine receptor. It has both agonistic and antagonistic properties, so it can both reduce craving and withdrawal and block the rewarding effects of smoking. It appears to be at least as or probably more effective than effective NRT and probably superior to bupropion. Overall, it is well tolerated, its main side effects being nausea and sleep disturbance. Recent major studies show it causes no more increased neuro-psychiatric effects above NRT or placebo, even in those with neuro-psychiatric illness. More studies in patient subgroups, using prolonged dosing (for more than 12 weeks) and even in combination with NRT, are eagerly awaited.

The atypical antidepressant bupropion also roughly doubles the odds of quitting. Its main side effect is a seizure rate of around 1 in 1000. It is much more widely used in the US and Europe than in the UK. Nortriptyline has been recommended as a second-line treatment for smoking cessation but no other antidepressant or anxiolytic has been shown to help cessation.

Two large trials suggest that the generic plant-based alkaloid cytisine is well tolerated and can aid smoking cessation, being at least as effective as varenicline and NRT. Further work on dosing, side effects, and longer-term quit rates is ongoing.

E-cigarettes, which are much safer than cigarettes as they superheat nicotine containing liquids, have been reported by smokers to help them quit: two open-label trials suggest they may be as effective as NRT in the short to medium term. However, they are not subject to medicines manufacturing standards, their long-term safety especially the condensate, is not proven, they are increasingly owned by the tobacco industry, and their role in 'renormalizing' smoking (e.g. in public) is controversial although there is no evidence they lead to smoking uptake.

New pharmacological treatments, including novel ways to deliver nicotine, selective inhibitors of the nicotine metabolizing enzyme CYP2A6, and nicotine vaccines, are being evaluated.

The success claimed by practitioners of aversive smoking, and alternative therapies such as acupuncture and hypnotherapy, has not yet been shown to be superior to placebo or sham treatments in pooled analyses of well-designed randomized trials, and these methods are not recommended.

Who should be offered smoking cessation treatment?

In the UK, the National Institute for Health and Care Excellence (NICE) guidelines recommend that 'everyone who smokes should

Table 338.2 Typical validated sustained quit rates by level of intervention

Intervention	Quit rates at 1 year (%)
None (spontaneous quit rate)	2–3
Generic health professional: • minimal counselling (<3 min) • brief counselling (3–10 min) • counselling (>10 min)	4 5 8–10
Interactive internet programmes	6
Interactive telephone programmes	10
Group classes or individual sessions with specialist without medication	15
Group classes or individual sessions with specialist combined with medication	25

be advised to quit, unless there are exceptional circumstances' and 'smoking cessation advice and support should be available in the community, primary and secondary care settings for everyone who smokes'.

Few health professionals have received specific training on smoking cessation, such as how to recognize symptoms of nicotine withdrawal, what pharmacotherapy is most appropriate (or is contraindicated), what key facts are specific to each illness, and so on. Not all hospitals have access to in-house specialists and there is evidence that those who do have them may not be using them appropriately. A healthcare provider sees 70% of all smokers at least once every year, yet only 39% of tobacco users reported being offered any advice or assistance to quit, and the majority of quit attempts and even pharmacotherapy prescriptions remain patient instigated. Within hospitals, in developed countries, another meta-analysis concluded that 'levels of smoking cessation care are less than optimal, and the levels of some important care practices are particularly low.'

Following brief advice, if the smoker expresses a desire to quit, they should ideally be referred to a specialist service that can tailor advice. Services combining intensive early support (at least weekly sessions for the first month) with pharmacotherapy and then with less intensive follow-up (e.g. at 6 months and at 1 year (to allow for annual celebrations, anniversaries)) are extremely effective (see Table 338.2), with numbers needed to treat of only around 6–7. They are also cost-effective and well below the benchmark used by NICE, for cost per quality-adjusted life-year gained, to justify treatment on the NHS.

Amelioration of the impact of smoking-reduction strategies

Traditionally, smoking cessation was deemed only effective if a patient completely stopped. Some work (e.g. on patients with COPD) has shown similar long-term validated and sustained quit rates in those smokers advised to cut down their smoking, compared to those advised to stop completely.

The relative health benefits from reducing smoking and strategies to prevent relapse are being examined. Other studies identifying those at highest risk of relapse, the neurogenetics of nicotine addiction, the interaction between certain genes and smoking in causing certain cancers, and so on, are being reported each year.

Further Reading

Carter BD, Abnet CC, Feskanich D, et al. Smoking and mortality: Beyond established causes. *N Engl J Med* 2015; 372: 631–40.

National Institute for Health and Care Excellence. *Smoking Cessation: Supporting People to Stop Smoking.* 2013. Available at http://www.nice.org.uk/Guidance/QS43 (accessed 20 Aug 2017).

Pirie K, Peto R, Reeves GK, Green J, Beral V. The 21st century hazards of smoking and benefits of stopping: A prospective study of one million women in the UK. *Lancet* 2013; 381: 133–41.

339 Alcohol

Sir Ian Gilmore and William Gilmore

Demographics of alcohol consumption in the UK and beyond

Alcohol has been used for thousands of years and, indeed, in very different ways. Two thousand years ago, the occupying Romans sipped wine regularly but reasonably moderately, and marvelled at the local English serfs who celebrated bringing in their crops with brief episodes of unrivalled drunkenness. Its use was not only tolerated but sometimes encouraged by the ruling classes as a way of subjugating the population and dulling their awareness of the conditions in which they had to live and work. The adverse impact of gin consumption was famously recorded by Hogarth's painting of 'Gin Lane' but, at the same time, beer was reckoned a safer alternative to water for fluid intake and was linked to happiness and prosperity in the sister painting of 'Beer Street'. It was against the 'pernicious use of strong liquors' and not beer that the president of the Royal College of Physicians, John Friend, petitioned Parliament in 1726. Some desultory attempts were made by Parliament in the eighteenth century to introduce legislation in order to tax and control alcohol production but they were eventually repealed. It was really the onset of the Industrial Revolution in nineteenth-century England that brought into sharp relief the wasted productivity and lost opportunity from excess consumption. England moved from a rural, relatively disorganized workforce to an urban, more closely scrutinized and supervised one—for instance, in factories, where men needed their wits about them to work heavy machinery, workers who were absent (in body or mind) were noticed. And, in Victorian Britain, there arose a greater social conscience—an awareness, for example, of the harm, through neglect, inflicted on the children of those who spent their wages and their days in an alcoholic stupor. Nonetheless, per capita consumption of alcohol in the UK at the end of the nineteenth century was greater than it is today (see Figure 339.1). It fell progressively through the first half of the twentieth century, with two marked dips. The first

coincided with the introduction of licensing hours' restrictions during the First World War, and the second with the economic depression of the 1930s.

Following the Second World War, there was a doubling of consumption between 1950 and the present day, to about 10 l of pure alcohol per capita. There has been a small fall of 9% in the last 5 years; this may be, in part, related to the changing ethnic mix and increasing number of non-drinkers. There has always been a mismatch between self-reported consumption in lifestyle questionnaires, and the data from customs and excise, with the latter being 40% greater. From the latter, it can be estimated that the average consumption of non-teetotal adults in England is 25 units (0.25 l of pure alcohol) per week, which is well above recommended limits of 14 units for women, and 21 units for men. Of course, average figures hide population differences, and it is estimated that the heaviest-consuming 10% of the population account for 40% of that drunk. While men continue to drink, on average, about twice the amount that women do, the rate of rise of consumption in women has been steeper. Average consumption is comparable across socio-economic groups but there is evidence of both more teetotallers and more drinking in a harmful way in the poorest group. In 2007, 13% of those aged 11–15 admitted to having drunk alcohol during the previous week. This figure is falling, but those who do drink are drinking more. The average weekly consumption of pupils who drink is 13 units/week.

Binge drinking estimates are unreliable, as they depend on self-reporting in questionnaires; in the UK, they are taken as drinking twice the daily recommended limits of 4 units for men, and 3 units for women, on the heaviest drinking day in the previous week. In 2010, 19% of men, and 12% of women, admitted to binge drinking, with the figures being 24% and 17%, respectively, for those aged 16–24. The preferred venue for drinking in the UK has changed markedly, mainly in response to the availability of cheap supermarket drink. Thirty years ago, the vast majority of alcohol was consumed in pubs

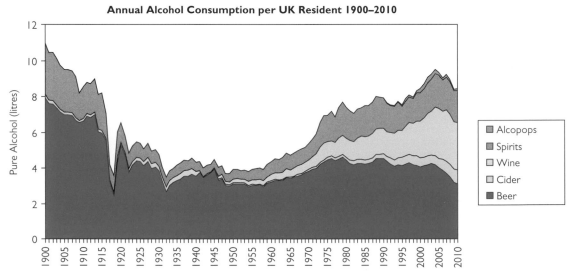

Annual Alcohol Consumption per UK Resident 1900–2010

Figure 339.1 Annual alcohol consumption per UK resident from 1900 to 2010 (litres of pure alcohol consumed, by beverage type).
With permission from Alcohol Misuse, Department of Health.

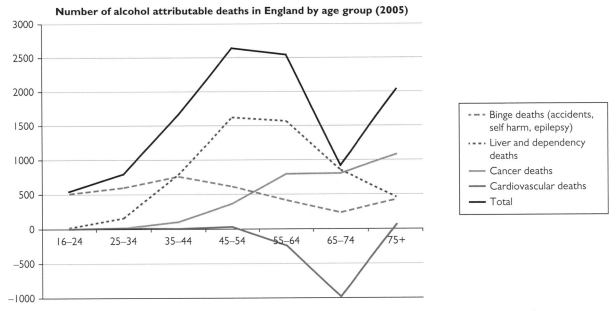

Figure 339.2 Number of alcohol-attributable deaths in England in 2005 by age group and cause. With permission from Alcohol Misuse, Department of Health.

and restaurants, whereas, in 2009, the market share of off-licence outlets was 65%. However, drinkers under 24 years of age still drink predominantly away from home.

The UK per capita consumption of alcohol is close to the European average, but consumption has been falling in Mediterranean countries and rising in northern and eastern Europe. Europe has the highest consumption of all continents, but there is undoubtedly massive under-reporting in many countries, particularly because of local unregulated production and consumption. It is estimated that less than 10% of consumption is captured in statistics in parts of Africa.

The health impact of alcohol consumption

The UK's accelerating consumption in the last half century has been accompanied by an increasing toll on morbidity and mortality. The economic costs of alcohol misuse in England alone is about £3.5 billion, although this figure is dwarfed by crime costs of £11 billion, and lost productivity of £7 billion. Of course, these figures could be offset against the economic benefits of alcohol in terms of jobs and trade, but the net figure would still be grossly in the red. The annual number of alcohol-related deaths in 2010, reported by the Office for National Statistics, was 6669, although some estimate that the figure could be as high as 40 000 if the attributable fraction of all alcohol-related diseases, such as cancer and heart disease, were taken into account. In the UK, the number of deaths from liver disease, which is a surrogate marker for alcohol-related harm as it is responsible for about 80% of liver deaths, has risen fourfold in the last 40 years and has now exceeded that for European Union. Even more striking is the age distribution of alcohol-related deaths, with the majority of such deaths occurring in younger age groups (see Figure 339.2). Cigarette smoking continues to be an even bigger factor overall than alcohol in premature deaths, but alcohol is more significant in those under 60 years of age, highlighting the fact that alcohol is often responsible for morbidity and mortality when people would otherwise be at their most productive. On average, the number of years lost in England for each alcohol-attributable death is 20 in men, and 15 in women.

Hospital admissions mirror this rise in mortality in recent years, and these now are estimated by the North West Public Health Observatory to exceed one million per annum in England. These are not, as might be imagined, mainly from the acute effects of drunkenness but from chronic sequelae and dependence, as figures from Liverpool show (Figure 339.3).

These figures emphasize the burden of alcohol dependence, which is rising alongside physical diseases and for which the incidence has risen from 1.0 million to 1.6 million people in England in the last decade. The wide range of conditions linked to alcohol is shown in Box 339.1. The risks can be divided into those acute harms that accompany bingeing, such as violence, accidents, and sudden death, and the chronic ill effects, such as cirrhosis and cancer. There is increasing awareness of alcohol as a risk factor in various cancers; in a recent European study, it was estimated that 1 cancer in 10 in men, and 1 in 30 in women, are caused by alcohol. Furthermore, there can be significant risks of consumption within limits thought of as safe; for example, a women consuming a bottle of wine each week (10 units; 80 g of alcohol) increases her risk of breast cancer by about 10%.

The apparent reduction in all-risk mortality from moderate alcohol consumption before a steep rise in mortality linked to heavy drinking (the so-called J-shaped curve) remains contested by some, on the grounds that studies fail to take sufficient account of confounding factors of diet and exercise in light drinkers. However, on the basis of several meta-analyses, it is likely that moderate drinking reduces deaths from coronary heart disease and ischaemic stroke. This effect is likely to be mediated through changes in HDL cholesterol. However, this benefit is seen only in those aged 55 or more, and the benefit is likely to be derived from very low levels of consumption (less than one unit daily).

A very significant burden of harm that is difficult to quantify is the harm to others, sometimes referred to (unsatisfactorily) as passive drinking. This harm is felt across the age spectrum. The full fetal alcohol syndrome, where there is profound neurocognitive damage and a characteristic facial appearance including wide-set eyes and a flat-bridged nose and which results from heavy in utero exposure, is relatively uncommon in the UK (about 100 cases reported each year). However, it is thought likely that many more subtle alcohol-related abnormalities may be present in up to 1 in 100 births; these make up what is now called fetal alcohol spectrum disorder, where hyperactivity and inattention may be prominent features. The impact of alcohol dependence on other family members, including children, is thought to be underestimated, and alcohol is a significant factor in at least half of cases of domestic violence. These and other alcohol-related causes of damage to others are listed in Box 339.2.

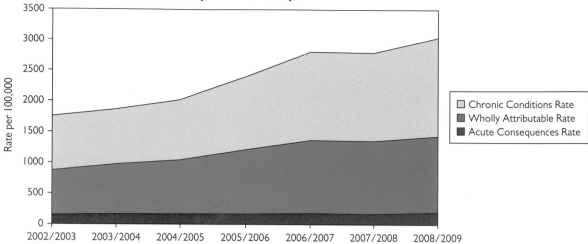

Alcohol Related Admissions for Liverpool PCT (residents) 2002/03 to 2008/09 by Condition Group.

Legend:
- Chronic Conditions Rate
- Wholly Attributable Rate
- Acute Consequences Rate

Figure 339.3 Alcohol-related hospital admissions for Liverpool residents (2002/03 to 2008/09) by condition group. With permission from Liverpool Primary Care Trust.

Box 339.1 Examples of alcohol damage to the drinker

- cardiovascular diseases
- cancers
- liver diseases
- gastritis
- degeneration of the nervous system
- diabetes
- nutrition-related conditions
- epileptic seizure
- unipolar depressive disorder
- tolerance
- dependence
- alcohol-related brain damage
- poisoning
- inhalation of gastric contents
- self-harm
- accidents and injuries

Box 339.2 Examples of alcohol damage to others

- fetal alcohol spectrum disorder
- violence
- accidents
- crime
- antisocial behaviour
- low birth weight
- spontaneous miscarriage
- family problems
- road traffic accidents
- work problems

Evidence-based public health policy for prevention of harm from alcohol

Public health policies to reduce the harm from alcohol must draw on best evidence and, in principle, use the minimum amount of intervention needed to produce the desired result. This has been adopted in the Nuffield Council on Bioethics Intervention Ladder (Box 339.3) and in 'nudge theory'. However, when dealing with a substance so pervasive in our culture as alcohol, which is so cheap, so readily available, and of such addictive potential, it is unlikely that lower rungs of the ladder will be effective.

There is overwhelming evidence that price is a key driver of both consumption and harm and, in the face of market competition, this requires regulation. The commonest way to regulate price in most countries has been through general taxation or a specific alcohol duty. This approach is effective but adds to the cost of all beverages, whether cheap or expensive, and whether consumed in pubs or at home. This has led to interest in setting a minimum floor below which a set amount of alcohol in a beverage cannot be sold: a minimum unit price (MUP). This has been used to regulate beer prices in some provinces in Canada, and, at the University of Sheffield, the results of modelling the impact of an MUP in the UK

suggest that the health gain could be large if a unit of alcohol (8 g) could not be sold for less than, say, £0.50 (€0.60, $0.80). The heaviest drinkers and those who are underage favour the cheapest alcohol, so an MUP effectively targets those most vulnerable to harm. There are plans to instigate this in the four nations within the UK and in the Republic of Ireland, but it is likely to face challenge in the European Court because it runs counter to the principle of free competition in markets.

The next area where evidence is strong for the effectiveness of public health intervention is on physical availability. This can be targeted through regulation of hours of opening, location, and density of retail outlets, and also by strengthening existing measures to prevent sales to underage drinkers and those already drunk. There is also an opportunity for change further down the ladder of intervention, such as putting alcoholic products in shops within a defined area with separate checkout facilities.

Drink-driving countermeasures are known to be effective. The introduction of random breath tests of drivers has been shown to reduce alcohol-related road traffic accidents. This can be complemented with the reduction of blood alcohol concentration limits, and requiring drivers under the legal age of purchase to have a blood alcohol concentration limit of zero.

The promotion of alcoholic beverages is a multimillion-pound business, and one where there is evidence, particularly in children, that harm ensues. The evidence suggests that children are likely to drink younger, and to drink more when they start, if exposed to alcohol marketing. In many countries, advertising standards are monitored by forms of industry self-regulation, but these clearly fail. Regulation is getting progressively more difficult as the methods of marketing

Box 339.3 Nuffield Council on Bioethics Intervention Ladder: A range of intervention options available to policymakers

Eliminate choice. Regulate in such a way as to entirely eliminate choice, for example through compulsory isolation of patients with infectious diseases.

Restrict choice. Regulate in such a way as to restrict the options available to people with the aim of protecting them, for example removing unhealthy ingredients from foods, or unhealthy foods from shops or restaurants.

Guide choice through disincentives. Fiscal and other disincentives can be put in place to influence people not to pursue certain activities, for example through taxes on cigarettes, or by discouraging the use of cars in inner cities through charging schemes or limitations of parking spaces.

Guide choices through incentives. Regulations can be offered that guide choices by fiscal and other incentives, for example offering tax-breaks for the purchase of bicycles that are used as a means of travelling to work.

Guide choices through changing the default policy. For example, in a restaurant, instead of providing chips as a standard side dish (with healthier options available), menus could be changed to provide a more healthy option as standard (with chips as an option available).

Enable choice. Enable individuals to change their behaviours, for example by offering participation in an NHS 'stop smoking' programme, building cycle lanes, or providing free fruit in schools.

Provide information. Inform and educate the public, for example as part of campaigns to encourage people to walk more or eat five portions of fruit and vegetables per day.

Do nothing or simply monitor the current situation.

The Nuffield Council on Bioethics report on Public health: ethical issues, Box 3.2

become more varied and pervasive, particularly through the internet. However, there are simple steps that could be taken, for example banning the drinks industry from engaging in sports sponsorship, as in France, or restricting cinema alcohol advertisements to films suitable only for those over 18 years of age.

There continues to be little evidence that public education and information are useful tools for reducing alcohol-related harm. This may be because they are given in the wrong format or in insufficient quantity. There is evidence that knowledge may be improved but, when used alone, information does not seem to bring about sustained behaviour change. It may be, however, that it has a role in informing the public of the scale of the problem so that firmer measures, such as regulation, are more acceptable when implemented.

Box 339.4 Identification and brief advice in a hospital setting

The Alcohol Health Work project at St Mary's Hospital, London, has been running since 1988. They have developed an evolving, brief, and effective screening tool for use in accident and emergency (A & E)—the Paddington Alcohol Test (PAT). On presentation to A & E, medical and nursing staff use the PAT to screen the alcohol consumption of patients attending for reasons commonly associated with alcohol misuse and offer brief advice. Those that screen positive are referred (with patient's agreement) to an alcohol nurse specialist (ANS). Referrals to the ANS may also be made from other wards in the hospital. The ANS provides a patient-centred assessment offering either advice and information or, in some cases, referral to community alcohol services. In 2007–8, 848 patients accepted referral to the ANS, with 63% attending. Public Health England, Alcohol Learning Resources.

Diagnosis and treatment of alcohol misuse

The scale of the problem from alcohol misuse is so great in some developed countries, such as the UK and Ireland, that we cannot afford to wait to see if public health measures are effective in reducing misuse and harm—there is an urgent need for the early detection and treatment of drinkers who are already at risk of or suffering physical, mental, or social damage. Interventions are effective and good value for money, but the problem lies in getting access to these treatments. There is, overall, a lack of treatment services; in addition, healthcare workers are often slow to refer patients to such treatment services, in the mistaken belief that nothing can be done.

When patients are detected before the signs of severe alcohol dependence appear, real and lasting benefits can accrue from administering structured brief advice. This can be given by a trained health worker in about 15 minutes and may be repeated. It has been shown to be effective even 12 months after it was given, and only eight patients need to be treated for there to be benefit in one. This is more effective, for example, than smoking cessation programmes and is highly cost-effective. This programme of identification and brief advice (IBA) has been shown to work in different settings, including primary care, A & E departments, and criminal justice settings (an example of good practice is included in Box 339.4). The key is to increase the frequency with which the initial identification of alcohol misuse takes place, and this will not happen until opportunistic screening for hazardous or harmful drinking begins to be carried out on a routine basis when individuals come into contact with health services for apparently unrelated reasons.

As approximately 80% of the UK population visits their GP at least once a year, the GP's office is an opportune setting for IBAs. However, at present, there are no financial incentives for GPs in primary care to undertake this, on top of time constraints and a lack of training in this area. At a local level, some primary care trusts have introduced locally enhanced services that cover alcohol screening and brief intervention but there is a possibility of this being lost in the changing landscape of primary care funding.

It is less certain whether IBAs are effective in cases of more severe dependence, as detected by tools such as the Alcohol Use Disorder Identification Tool; however, specialist alcohol treatment services have been shown to be of proven benefit in these patients and should be available to take referrals. It is only by matching problem drinkers with the correct avenue of treatment that it will prove possible to break the 'revolving door' cycle of recurrent admissions into acute hospitals, a cycle that so many of these patients currently experience.

Conclusions

Alcohol use poses a really important public health challenge to many developing and developed countries, and this is particularly true in the UK at present. Any potential cardiovascular benefit of light consumption is swamped by the consequences of heavy drinking, and there is little sign that attempts at public health messages or setting recommended limits is having an impact. The consequences of societal harm to health, crime, and productivity are so great as to justify legislative measures around price, marketing, and availability, even though such measures are at odds with politicians' natural instincts to respect free will and personal choice. This move to increase regulation is being seen first in Scotland, where the amount of alcohol-related harm is currently greatest, but other parts of the UK are following. There is also a need to improve services to detect those with early signs of physical or mental harm, as early intervention can be both effective for the individual and economically sound for the country.

Further Reading

Babor T, Caetano R, Casswell S, et al. *Alcohol: No Ordinary Commodity. Research and Public Policy* (2nd edition), 2010. Oxford University Press.

National Institute for Health and Care Excellence. *Alcohol-Use Disorders: Diagnosis, Assessment and Management of Harmful Drinking and Alcohol Dependence.* Available at http://www.nice.org.uk/guidance/CG115 (accessed 18 Sep 2017).

340 Environmental radiation

Mark P. Little

Introduction

Risks associated with ionizing radiation have been known for almost as long as ionizing radiation itself. Within a year of the discovery of X-rays by Röntgen in 1895, skin burns had been reported and, within 7 years, a case of skin cancer was observed, all associated with high-dose X-ray exposure. In general, the risks associated with ionizing radiation can be divided into what have been termed (by the International Commission on Radiological Protection) stochastic effects (e.g. genetic risks in offspring, and somatic effects (cancer) in the directly exposed population), and deterministic, or tissue-reaction, effects. Deterministic effects are typically associated with high-dose exposures, and will not be considered further here.

Types of ionizing radiation, sources of exposure, and units

Ionizing radiation is any electromagnetic wave or particle that can remove an electron from an atom or molecule. The process of ionization in living material necessarily changes atoms and molecules, at least transiently, and may thus damage cells. If cellular damage occurs and is not adequately repaired, the cell may die or senesce, or the damage may result in a viable but modified cell which can go on to become cancerous, if it is a somatic cell, or lead to inherited disease, if it is a germ cell.

The basic quantity used to measure absorbed dose from radiation is the gray (Gy), defined as one joule (J) of initial energy (of charged particles released by the ionization events) per kilogram of tissue. The biological effects per unit of absorbed dose differ with the type of radiation, so that a weighted quantity called the equivalent dose is used, which is measured in sieverts (Sv). Low-level linear-energy transfer (LET) radiation (e.g. photons, electrons, muons) is assigned a radiation weighting factor of 1, whereas high-LET radiation (e.g. neutrons, protons, alpha particles) is assigned radiation weighting factors of between 5 and 20, depending on the energy of the particles.

All living organisms are continually exposed to ionizing radiation, for example from cosmic and terrestrial gamma rays, ingestion of potassium-40, and radon exposure. Worldwide, the average human exposure to radiation from natural sources is 2.4 mSv per year, about half of which is due to the effects of radon daughters (Table 340.1).

Major studies examining environmental exposure in relation to cancer

Natural radiation exposure

Indoor radon exposure

Although it has long been recognized that radon causes lung cancer in underground miners, the possible hazard of exposure to radon at the generally low levels found in homes was not appreciated until more recently. There have been a number of studies of lung cancer in relation to indoor radon exposure, culminating in two sets of independent pooled analyses, one in North America and the other European, both of which clearly demonstrate a significant association between radon daughter exposure and lung cancer. There have also been studies of radon daughter exposure in relation to other malignancies, in particular leukaemia, but these have, for the most part, been inconclusive.

Gamma radiation exposure: High-background studies

Natural background radiation varies tremendously between and within countries. An area with high natural background radiation is defined as an area or a complex of dwellings where the sum of cosmic radiation and natural radioactivity in the soil, air, water, food, and so on, leads to chronic exposures that result in an annual effective dose that is above a defined level. Studies of the health effects of high-background radiation exposure have thus far been inconclusive.

Man-made radiation exposure

Studies of populations exposed to fallout from nuclear weapons testing have suggested that such populations have an increased risk of thyroid and other cancers. A substantial increase in the incidence of thyroid cancer has also been observed amongst those exposed to radioactive iodines in childhood and adolescence in the most highly contaminated territories of Ukraine, Belarus, and Russia following the Chernobyl accident. Iodine deficiency may have increased the risk of developing thyroid cancer following exposure to radioactive iodines, while prolonged stable iodine supplementation in the years after exposure may reduce this risk. There is evidence of risk associated with obstetric *in utero* exposure to diagnostic X-rays, and with paediatric exposure to computerized tomography, although this is still controversial.

Prevention of disease

Heritable genetic and cancer-related effects are the main late health consequences of environmental exposure to ionizing radiation; somatic risks dominate the overall estimate of health detriment. For both somatic and genetic effects, the probability of their occurrence, but not their severity, is taken to depend on the radiation dose. The dose response may be non-linear (e.g. for leukaemia). For most

Table 340.1 Current sources of exposure, annual effective doses (in millisieverts per year), and typical ranges

Source	Source sub-type	Worldwide average (mSv/year)	Typical range (mSv/year), other notes
Natural	External exposure		
	Cosmic rays	0.4	0.3–1.0
	Terrestrial gamma rays	0.5	0.3–0.6
	Internal exposure		
	Inhalation (mostly via radon)	1.2	0.2–10
	Ingestion	0.3	0.2–0.8
	Total natural	2.4	1–10
Man-made	Diagnostic medical	0.4	0.04–1.0
	Atmospheric nuclear testing	0.005	Decrease from maximum of 0.15 in 1963
	Chernobyl accident	0.002	Decrease from maximum of 0.04 in 1986
	Nuclear power production	0.0002	Has increased with expansion of programme, but decreased with improved practice

From Sources and effects of ionizing radiation. UNSCEAR 2000 report to the General Assembly, with scientific annexes. by United Nations Scientific Committee on the Effects of Atomic Radiation (UNSCEAR), Volume I: Sources. Vol. E.00.IX.3. pp. 1–654, © 2000 United Nations. Reprinted with the permission of the United Nations.

Table 340.2 Cancer and heritable genetic risk estimates associated with low-dose irradiation for a UK population

		Risk/100 Gy
Somatic (cancer) mortality risks*		
Relative risk transport	Leukaemia	0.50 (0.11, 0.97)[†]
	Solid cancer	5.45 (3.06, 7.99)[†]
Absolute risk transport	Leukaemia	0.52 (0.15, 0.90)[†]
	Solid cancer	4.48 (2.28, 6.83)[†]
Heritable genetic risk‡		
Autosomal dominant, X linked	Risk to first generation	0.075–0.15
	Risk to second generation	0.05–0.10
Autosomal recessive	Risk to first generation	~0
	Risk to second generation	~0
Chronic multifactorial disease	Risk to first generation	0.025–0.12
	Risk to second generation	0.025–0.12
Developmental abnormalities	Risk to first generation	0.20
	Risk to second generation	0.04–0.10
Total	Risk to first generation	0.30–0.47
	Risk to second generation	0.12–0.32

*Risk calculated for a UK population, assuming a test dose of 0.1 Gy administered, and using a generalized excess absolute or relative risk model which is linear–quadratic in dose.

[†]Ninety per cent Bayesian credibility interval.

‡Risk calculated for radiation exposure only in one generation, with a dose and dose-rate effectiveness factor of 3 applied.

Data from

United Nations Scientific Committee on the Effects of Atomic Radiation (UNSCEAR) (2001). Hereditary effects of radiation. UNSCEAR 2001 report to the General Assembly, with scientific annex. Volume E.01.IX.2. pp. 1–160.

United Nations Scientific Committee on the Effects of Atomic Radiation (UNSCEAR) (2008). UNSCEAR 2006 Report. Annex A. Epidemiological Studies of Radiation and Cancer. pp. 13–322. ISBN 978-92-1-142263-4.

stochastic effects, it is generally accepted that, at sufficiently low doses, there is a non-zero linear component to the dose response (i.e. there is no threshold), but contrary opinions have also been expressed.

Heritable genetic effects

The heritable genetic risks associated with radiation exposure are estimated directly from animal studies in combination with data on baseline incidence of disease in human populations. There is little or no evidence of human radiation-induced genetic disease, and the results of the most comprehensive of human epidemiological studies, namely that carried out on the children of the Japanese atomic bomb survivors, are negative. Table 340.2 summarizes estimates of risk, based on a mutational doubling dose of 1 Gy. This is derived from human data on spontaneous mutation rates, and mouse data on induced mutation rates.

Somatic effects (cancer)

Most of the information on radiation-induced cancer risk comes from (a) the Japanese atomic bomb survivors, (b) medically exposed populations, and (c) occupationally exposed groups. The Life Span Study cohort of Japanese atomic bomb survivors is unusual amongst exposed populations in that both genders and a wide range of ages were exposed, comparable with those of a general population. Most medically treated groups are more restricted in the age and gender mix. Table 340.2 summarizes estimates of cancer mortality risk for a UK population.

Non-cancer late health effects

For some time, there has been evidence of excess cardiovascular morbidity associated with high-dose radiotherapeutic procedures. The mechanisms for such effects at high radiation doses are reasonably well understood, being probably inflammatory in nature, resulting from inactivation of large numbers of cells and associated functional impairment of the affected tissue. There is emerging evidence of excess risks of non-cancer late health effects, specifically circulatory disease and cataract, in the Japanese atomic bomb survivors and in some of those who are occupationally exposed. The most current biological data imply that the mechanisms for circulatory disease are unlikely to involve somatic cell mutation, but this mechanism cannot be excluded for cataract.

Screening for disease

As described in 'Prevention of disease' and shown in Table 340.2, the main diseases that should be screened for are cancers in the directly exposed population. Genetic effects will occur at relatively low prevalence and may not be easily detectable, especially given the multifactorial nature of many diseases. The cancers to be screened for will be determined by the organ-specific doses. When the exposure is uniform whole body, as is often the case following environmental radiation exposure, the main radiogenic cancer sites should be examined (e.g. breast, thyroid, bone marrow, lung, and skin). However, the use of X-rays or mammograms for screening purposes should only be conducted after careful analysis of the risks and benefits—for example, the use of annual mammographic screens of the general female population for breast cancer is justified above the age of 40 (the breast cancer deaths averted by screening exceed the breast cancers induced by the mammographic X-rays), but not below that age. Cataract should also be assessed.

Further Reading

Little MP, Azizova TV, Bazyka D, et al. Systematic review and meta-analysis of circulatory disease from exposure to low-level ionizing radiation and estimates of potential population mortality risks. *Environ Health Perspect* 2012; 120: 1503–11.

Little MP. Radiation and circulatory disease. *Mut Res Reviews* 2016; 770: 299–318.

Little MP, Wakeford R, Tawn EJ, et al. Risks associated with low doses and low dose rates of ionizing radiation: Why linearity may be (almost) the best we can do. *Radiology* 2009; 251: 6–12.

341 Air pollution

Anthony Frew

Why is air pollution dangerous?

Any public debate about air pollution starts with the premise that air pollution cannot be good for you, so we should have less of it. However, it is much more difficult to determine how much is dangerous, and even more difficult to decide how much we are willing to pay for improvements in measured air pollution. Recent UK estimates suggest that fine particulate pollution causes about 6500 deaths per year, although it is not clear how many years of life are lost as a result. Some deaths may just be brought forward by a few days or weeks, while others may be truly premature. Globally, household pollution from cooking fuels may cause up to two million premature deaths per year in the developing world.

The hazards of black smoke air pollution have been known since antiquity. The first descriptions of deaths caused by air pollution are those recorded after the eruption of Vesuvius in AD 79. In modern times, the infamous smogs of the early twentieth century in Belgium and London were clearly shown to trigger deaths in people with chronic bronchitis and heart disease. In mechanistic terms, black smoke and sulphur dioxide generated from industrial processes and domestic coal burning cause airway inflammation, exacerbation of chronic bronchitis, and consequent heart failure. Epidemiological analysis has confirmed that the deaths included both those who were likely to have died soon anyway and those who might well have survived for months or years if the pollution event had not occurred.

Clean air legislation has dramatically reduced the levels of these traditional pollutants in the West, although these pollutants are still important in China, and smoke from solid cooking fuel continues to take a heavy toll amongst women in less developed parts of the world.

New forms of air pollution have emerged, principally due to the increase in motor vehicle traffic since the 1950s. The combination of fine particulates and ground-level ozone causes 'summer smogs' which intensify over cities during summer periods of high barometric pressure. In Los Angeles and Mexico City, ozone concentrations commonly reach levels which are associated with adverse respiratory effects in normal and asthmatic subjects.

Ozone directly affects the airways, causing reduced inspiratory capacity. This effect is more marked in patients with asthma and is clinically important, since epidemiological studies have found linear associations between ozone concentrations and admission rates for asthma and related respiratory diseases. Ozone induces an acute neutrophilic inflammatory response in human and animal airways together with release of chemokines (e.g. interleukin 8 and growth-related oncogene-alpha). Nitrogen oxides have less direct effect on human airways, but they increase the response to allergen challenge in patients with atopic asthma. Nitrogen oxide exposure also increases the risk of becoming ill after exposure to influenza. Alveolar macrophages are less able to inactivate influenza viruses, and this leads to an increased probability of infection after experimental exposure to influenza.

In the last two decades, major concerns have been raised about the effects of fine particulates. An association between fine particulate levels and cardiovascular and respiratory mortality and morbidity was first reported in 1993 and has since been confirmed in several other countries. Globally, about 90% of airborne particles are formed naturally, from sea spray, dust storms, volcanoes, and burning grass and forests. Human activity accounts for about 10% of aerosols (in terms of mass). This comes from transport, power stations, and various industrial processes. Diesel exhaust is the principal source of fine particulate pollution in Europe, while sea spray is the principal source in California, and agricultural activity is a major contributor in inland areas of the US. Dust storms are important sources in the Sahara, the Middle East, and parts of China. The mechanism of adverse health effects remains unclear but, unlike the case for ozone and nitrogen oxides, there is no safe threshold for the health effects of particulates. Since the 1990s, tax measures aimed at reducing greenhouse gas emissions have led to a rapid rise in the proportion of new cars with diesel engines. In the UK, this rose from 4% in 1990 to one-third of new cars in 2004 while, in France, over half of new vehicles have diesel engines. Diesel exhaust particles may increase the risk of sensitization to airborne allergens and cause airways inflammation both in vitro and in vivo.

Extensive epidemiological work has confirmed that there is an association between increased exposure to environmental fine particulates and death from cardiovascular causes. Various mechanisms have been proposed: cardiac rhythm disturbance seems the most likely at present. It has also been proposed that high numbers of ultrafine particles may cause alveolar inflammation which then exacerbates preexisting cardiac and pulmonary disease. In support of this hypothesis, the metal content of ultrafine particles induces oxidative stress when alveolar macrophages are exposed to particles in vitro. While this is a plausible mechanism, in epidemiological studies, it is difficult to separate the effects of ultrafine particles from those of other traffic-related pollutants.

Air pollution: The magnitude of the problem

There are several different components of air pollution, with distinct exposure profiles. Black smoke and sulphur dioxide are principally generated by the burning of coal for industrial and domestic purposes. In the developing world, many women and children are exposed to fumes from solid cooking fuels, with those of biological origin being particularly toxic. Poor ventilation of huts and other enclosed cooking spaces is an additional factor in increasing exposure.

Nitrogen oxides are primary pollutants generated by the burning of fossil fuels. Maximum levels are found in cities and along major roads, with lower levels in the countryside. Indoor exposure levels reflect external levels but can vary considerably if there are local internal sources (e.g. gas cookers, unflued heaters, motor vehicles in garages).

Ozone is a secondary pollutant which is generated from atmospheric oxygen exposed to nitrogen oxides in the presence of sunlight. Consequently, levels are highest on sunny days, and there is considerable variation at different times of day, with peaks in the afternoon and troughs at night. Ozone is more widely distributed than nitrogen oxides, and levels tend to be higher in the countryside than in towns, because ozone is absorbed by other pollutants generated in cities. In the UK, levels associated with adverse health effects are only rarely encountered. This contrasts with the case in cities like Los Angeles and Mexico City, where ozone levels commonly reach the point where even normal healthy individuals may be affected.

Fine and ultrafine particulates are mostly generated by incomplete combustion of fossil fuels, resulting in carbon particles which vary in size and shape. Diesel engines produce much more particulate than gasoline engines do; due to the high temperatures in the engine, small amounts of transitional metals and volatile organic compounds adhere to the surface of the carbon particles. This makes characterization of particulates very difficult. For most practical and regulatory purposes, exposure is measured by mass per unit volume of air, while biological activity depends primarily on the exposed surface area, which depends on the square of the particle radius (weight being a function of the cube of the radius).

Radon is a naturally occurring radioactive gas which forms during the decay of uranium and thorium. It is the second most important cause of lung cancer (after cigarette smoking), causing about 21 000 deaths per year in the US. Radon exposure is highest in uranium miners, and in locations where granite is at the surface or used in buildings. It also accumulates in domestic houses, especially in areas with restricted ventilation (e.g. basements and attics).

Controlling pollution exposure

The principal means of controlling pollution exposure is through understanding and regulating the sources of pollution. In doing so, it is vital to recognize that pollution does not respect national boundaries. Indeed, much of the pollution that affects the UK is generated in the Ruhr and other industrial areas of Northern Europe, while the prevailing weather systems export much of the UK's pollution towards Scandinavia. Sources such as coal-fired power stations can be replaced by 'cleaner' power stations burning gas; this will reduce the particulate levels but still contribute to levels of nitrogen oxides and ozone. Nuclear power has its own issues, but does not contribute to air pollution, while wind and tidal power is essentially pollution-free, except for any products released during manufacture of the turbines.

Diesel engines contribute a substantial proportion of fine particulate matter (PM10: respirable particles with a diameter of <10 μm) in urban settings. Particle traps will dramatically reduce the amount of PM10 released. Engineering solutions, such as increasing the engine compression ratio, will alter the type of particle generated (i.e. they produce more small particles <2.5 μm in diameter (ultrafine particles)), although the health impact of such changes has not been fully worked out.

Where source control is not practical (e.g. for ozone), understanding the diurnal cycle and time trends may allow those affected to adjust their activities to the most appropriate times. For example, there are higher ozone levels in the afternoon, so less exposure will occur if exercise is taken in the morning or late evening.

A number of steps have been taken to reduce release of volatile organic compounds (VOCs) and products of incomplete combustion which, together with sunlight, trigger the generation of ground-level ozone. Engineering solutions to reduce VOC emissions, such as improving fuel efficiency and using catalytic converters, seem to be the best way forward at present. In the long term, there needs to be a consensus about how the seemingly inexorable increase in the use of personal motorized transport can be mitigated or reduced. This is clearly part of a much wider debate about the way future generations wish to live, work, and play.

Amelioration of the impact of air pollution

Given that the impact of the various pollutants is different, a number of separate strategies have been considered to alleviate their potential impact.

In sub-Saharan Africa, steps are being taken to encourage switching away from traditional solid fuels that are associated with respiratory morbidity. While ozone and nitrogen oxides induce oxidant stress, and deplete antioxidants in bronchoalveolar lavage fluid, clinical trials of increased dietary intake of antioxidant vitamins have not shown any evidence that this will protect against ozone-induced inflammation. As regards the ability of pollution to trigger asthma, management consists of reducing exposure and using standard antiasthma medication to prevent and control exacerbations. The principal risk with fine particulates is cardiac mortality and morbidity. However, there is no obvious way to mitigate this cardiac risk apart from limiting exertion (and hence exposure) during pollution episodes. The main problem is that we do not understand the mechanism involved, mainly because the individual events seem to be rare (albeit catastrophic for those affected).

Further Reading

Bentayeb M, Simoni M, Baiz N, et al. Adverse respiratory effects of outdoor air pollution in the elderly. *Int J Tuberc Lung Dis* 2012; 16: 1149–61.

Chen H, Goldberg MS, and Villeneuve PJ. A systematic review of the relation between long-term exposure to ambient air pollution and chronic diseases. *Rev Environ Health* 2008; 23: 243–97.

Landrigan PJ, Fuller R, Acosta NJR, et al. The Lancet Commission on pollution and health. *Lancet* 2018; 391: 462–512.

Langrish JP, Bosson J, Unosson J, et al. Cardiovascular effects of particulate air pollution exposure: time course and underlying mechanisms. *J Intern Med* 2012; 272: 224–39.

Laumbach RJ. Outdoor air pollutants and patient health. *Am Fam Physician* 2010; 81: 175–80.

Kelly FJ and Fussell JC. Air pollution and public health: emerging hazards and improved understanding of risk. *Environ Geochem Health* 2015; 37:631–49.

Mortimer K, Gordon SB, Jindal SK, et al. Household air pollution is a major avoidable risk factor for cardiorespiratory disease. *Chest* 2012; 142: 1308–15.

World Health Organization. *Preventing disease through healthy environments*. 2016. Available at: http://apps.who.int/iris/bitstream/10665/204585/1/9789241565196_eng.pdf

Why are non-prescription drugs dangerous?

The use of non-prescription drugs is widespread and has a major impact on the health of the individual user and society. In 2006, the British Crime Survey reported that 10% of adults had used one or more illicit drugs in the preceding year, with 3% reporting using a Class A drug. Over 11 million people in the UK are estimated to have used an illicit drug at least once in their lifetime (35%). Drugs abused vary in their intrinsic potential to cause addiction and, with it, more regular and harmful use. Drug users are influenced by trends and fashions, adopting new compounds such as crack cocaine and experimenting with routes of ingestion. Some drugs may become less popular over time, such as LSD, and others, such as cannabis, experience a revival as more potent strains (e.g. Skunk) are developed. A problem drug user is best defined as a person whose drug taking is no longer controlled or undertaken for recreational purposes and where drugs have become a more essential element of the individual's life.

The true economic and social cost of drug use is likely to be substantially greater than the published figures, which are derived from a variety of health and crime surveys which may overlook vulnerable groups such as the homeless. The majority of non-prescription drugs used in the UK are illegal and covered by the Misuse of Drugs Act 1971. The drugs most commonly abused gave rise in 2003–4 to an estimated financial cost in England and Wales of 15.4 billion pounds to the economy, with Class A drugs such as heroin and cocaine accounting for the majority of this. Some 90% of the cost is due to drug-related crime, with only 3% (£488 million) due to health service expenditure, which is mainly on inpatient care episodes. This still represents a major health pressure, which in 2006–7 amounted to 38 000 admissions, in England, for primary and secondary drug-related mental or behavioural problems, and over 10 000 admissions recorded for drug poisoning.

Clinicians in all specialities can expect to encounter harmful drug use, especially those working in primary care, A & E, and psychiatric services. Presenting problems are protean, ranging from mood disorders, delirium, and psychosis to sepsis, malnutrition, and hepatitis. Blood-borne infections such as hepatitis C and HIV are widespread, as contaminated needles and syringes are shared by up to a quarter of problem drug users. Even smoking drugs such as crack cocaine can lead to increased transmission of hepatitis C through oral ulceration and contact with hot contaminated smoking pipes. Amongst the UK population, over half of IV drug users have hepatitis C, a quarter have antibodies to hepatitis B, and, by 2006, 4662 had been diagnosed with HIV.

Non-prescription drug abuse is a leading cause of death and morbidity amongst the young adult population (those aged 16–35). In 2006 there were 1573 deaths where the underlying cause was poisoning, drug abuse, or dependence on substances controlled under the Misuse of Drugs Act. The vast majority (79%) were male. Young men, in particular, are at greater risk of violent death through associated criminal activity such as drug supplying and from deliberate and accidental overdose. The male-to-female ratio for deaths associated with mental and behavioural disorder is 6:1.

Magnitude/demographics of non-prescription drug use

In order to understand the risks of non-prescription drug taking, it is necessary to have knowledge of the legal classification system used to correlate data on health and social harm. The law defines three major classes of illicit drugs (A, B, and C), according to their perceived dangerousness. Some drugs can appear in both higher and lower classes, depending on how the drug is prepared for use. Drugs are reviewed by the home secretary, and their classification may change when evidence suggests the risk warrants it. The most harmful drugs are Class A drugs and include the opiates heroin and methadone, stimulants such as cocaine, crack cocaine, and ecstasy (MDMA), the hallucinogens, LSD, and, recently added, all forms (fresh and prepared) of magic mushrooms. Amphetamines prepared for injection are also considered to be Class A drugs.

Although, broadly, all Class A drugs are harmful, the impact and scale of opiate and cocaine use are vastly greater than those caused by magic mushrooms. There were an estimated 327 000 problem users of Class A substances in England in 2003–4, with the majority (60%) using heroin and/or cocaine. Equally, the lower classification of cannabis as a Class B drug conceals a growing problem of chronic, drug-induced psychosis. The newer forms of potent cannabis plants now commonly contain five times the amount of active substance, THC, than was found in strains in the 1970s. Current users will invariably be smoking the more potent form 'Skunk ', and many have little knowledge of the increased risk, especially the risk in children of developing schizophrenia-like disorders. Ten per cent of children asked thought it was ok to try cannabis, and 75 % of those in formal treatment under the age of 18 are receiving therapy for cannabis abuse.

Some drugs, such as anabolic steroids (designated as Class C drugs) are hardly thought of as harmful by users, despite evidence of serious health risks, and remain, in their various forms, a common problem in the world of performance sports. Solvents and glues are highly toxic yet remain unclassified, although it is an offence to supply them if it is likely that they will be abused.

Criminal prosecution is possible for any class of drug possession but the tariffs are greatest for Class A drugs, and imprisonment for supplying or allowing drug use on your premises is to be expected. Possession with intent to supply carries a term of 2.5 years at present in UK.

The demographics available support the clinical impression that problem drug use is positively correlated with socially vulnerable groups. Contributing factors include financial deprivation, male gender, alcohol abuse, unemployment, school exclusion, and criminality. Those at greater risk of Class A drug use also include young adults and children who have ever been homeless, truanted, looked after in care homes, or fostered. Parental attitudes also condition children to accept drug use. Families with substance-abusing parents show higher rates of drug use amongst children. Overall, vulnerable groups represent only 28% of those surveyed but account for 61% of users of Class A drugs.

Prevention of drug abuse

Prevention of drug abuse by means of health promotion initiatives and education in schools, as with smoking and alcohol education, has certainly increased awareness amongst children and young adults of the risks associated with drug misuse. Surveys show that very few (2%) children aged 11 are uninformed about drug abuse. Despite this, large numbers of 14-year-olds admit to having taking illicit substances. The drug that those aged 14–15 most commonly report to have taken is cannabis (22%), although younger children are more likely to abuse solvents. Children surveyed give a variety of reasons for using drugs. Many admit experimenting with friends. Boys are more likely to try harder drugs and report doing so to get high or feel good.

Health education programmes have been successful in many areas of public health. Providing information does change attitudes. Clinicians play an important role in promoting healthy lifestyles and motivating patients to change habits and make use of available treatment services. NHS initiatives have, for example, reduced the prevalence of cigarette smoking from 28% to 21%; most smokers who wish to give up support initiatives that help them quit. A similar attitude is found amongst problem drug users, with up to three-quarters saying they want to stop.

The UK government has made the identification of and accessing treatment by drug abusers a major target, and doing so is now one of the eight key performance indicators for the NHS. The investment of resources into this was enhanced by the establishment of a special health authority for England: the National Treatment Authority (NTA). Funding from the Department of Health and the Home Office has been pooled into a treatment budget which was allocated annually to 150 local drug action teams (DATs). These are partnerships of social services, housing, education, health, and prison and probation services, as well as private and voluntary sector providers. The DATs determined how resources were spent locally and, as well as commissioning treatment services, were responsible for monitoring and reporting on performance. The result of this major investment in what had, for decades, been a poorly resourced area of healthcare is published in the NTA annual reports. The NTA and its functions were absorbed into the Department of Public Health in 2012.

The treatment system appears from recent data to be very effective in identifying young problem drug users (using heroin and crack cocaine). The time taken from first use of drugs and receiving treatment has fallen by a year to 2.9 years for those aged 18–24. GP and criminal justice referrals appear to be effective in targeting treatment-naive problem drug users. This is reflected in the reduced number of young adults in services being treated for problem drug use between 2006 and 2008 (from 68% to 53%).

There has been a significant reduction in some forms of drug misuse reported by children aged 11–15 between 2001 and 2007. The percentage reporting being offered drugs has fallen from 42% to 36%, and the percentage of those admitting to any form of drug misuse within the previous month has decreased from 12% to 10%. The sharpest fall has been in the percentage of those using cannabis (from 13% to 9%), although the use of Class A drugs remains static at 4%. It seems likely that the reduction is as a result of targeted health education within schools, with parents and teachers showing a greater awareness of the risk of problem drug use amongst children, as well as the increased availability of treatment.

While the overall impact of new treatment services is presently being assessed, the initial results appear impressive. Over half of the estimated 330 000 heroin and crack addicts in England are now receiving effective treatment. The population of problem drug users is getting older, as fewer younger people progress into or remain involved with heroin and crack cocaine. Twenty per cent of those entering treatment in 2008 are now over 40 years old.

The majority of treatments are carried out by community teams. Only 3% of drug users receive inpatient care or rehabilitation. Individuals are assessed and offered a variety of therapeutic interventions, according to their needs. In 2008, some 43% were prescribed medication, with the commonest medication being methadone, which reflects the large number (49%) presenting to services with recent or current IV drug abuse.

The majority of those entering services will also be offered a range of psychosocial interventions based on motivational techniques which are based on increasing the user's sense of discomfort with their habit (dissonance) and guiding them through selective feedback to a point where they can commit to stopping. These cognitive therapy methods are well established for the treatment of other disorders such as alcohol abuse and depressive disorders.

Amelioration of the impact of drug abuse

Not all those entering treatment can be expected to achieve recovery; on average, 12% will successfully complete treatment and be free from dependency, a figure which has doubled since 2005. A troubling 10% will prematurely leave treatment, although some may return later. A major goal of all clinicians is to use the opportunities presented by any contact with a health service to promote safer drug use. There is a range of harm reduction initiatives on offer, including the website http://www.harmreduction-works.org.uk.

Dispelling myths and encouraging patients to believe that simple changes in their habits, such as washing out syringes with thin bleach or getting vaccinated against hepatitis B, are tasks every clinician should embrace. A drug user may have no idea about the risk of sharing syringes or have received poor advice from other users about how to clean equipment. Many wrongly believe that boiling water will kill HIV when, in fact, it tends to preserve the virus under a protective film of denatured blood proteins. Drug users need to know how long the viruses survive inside dirty syringes. Viable HIV can be recovered for up to 6 weeks from the void spaces in most syringes. Although hepatitis C virus (HCV) is much less resilient, it is far more likely to transmit, as the typical viral load is vastly greater. Most crack cocaine addicts are surprised to find they are at risk of HCV transmission by sharing smoking pipes or that injecting crack causes much more damage to veins due to higher acidity and local anaesthetic effects.

Harm reduction strategies have been offered to IV drug users for many years. The best known are the needle exchange schemes. Uptake by addicts varies across the UK but rarely exceeds 25%. There remain a large number (48%) who report dangerous habits such as sharing injecting equipment (works).

Heroin users can reduce their risk of accidental overdose by being made aware of signs that they or other users may be becoming more vulnerable. Typical warning signs are longer history of use, not being in treatment, simultaneous use of benzodiazepines or alcohol, recent release from prison or a completed detoxification, and near miss events where consciousness was impaired, as revealed by pressure injuries and lost days.

The reluctant user needs to survive until they can be encouraged into treatment.

Further Reading

Boyer EW. Management of opioid analgesic overdose. *N Engl J Med* 2012; 367: 146–55.

Fingleton NA, Watson MC, Duncan EM, et al. Non-prescription medicine misuse, abuse and dependence: a cross-sectional survey of the UK general population. *J Pub Health* 2016; 38: 722–30. https://www.slideshare.net/croaker260/2014-street-drugreview

Markel H. The accidental addict. *N Engl J Med* 2005; 352: 966–8.

Public Health England: *Drug Treatment in England 2013–14* (http://www.nta.nhs.uk/uploads/drug-treatment-in-england-2013-14-commentary.pdf)

Public Health England: *Alcohol Treatment in England 2013–14* (http://www.nta.nhs.uk/uploads/adult-alcohol-statistics-2013-14-commentary.pdf)

Schuckit MA. Treatment of opiod-use disorders. *N Engl J Med* 2016; 375: 357–68.

PART 18

Prevention of disease

343 Prevention of cardiovascular disease

Amitava Banerjee and Kaleab Asrress

Introduction

The global scale of the cardiovascular disease epidemic is unquestionable, causing a greater burden of mortality and morbidity than any other disease, regardless of country or population. With demographic change and ageing populations, the prevalence of cardiovascular disease and its risk factors is set to increase. The commonest cardiovascular diseases are atherosclerotic, affecting all arterial territories. Figure 343.1 illustrates the major contributors to cardiovascular disease, showing the predominance of coronary artery disease and cerebrovascular disease (stroke and transient ischaemic attack (TIA)).

The 'burden of disease' approach has highlighted the fact that cardiovascular disease and non-communicable diseases are not simply diseases of affluence but affect people of all countries, with enormous costs in terms of public health, healthcare, and overall economies. Coronary artery disease is the leading cause of mortality in all regions of the world apart from sub-Saharan Africa, followed by cerebrovascular disease. It should be noted, however, that there has been a major decline in age-standardised cardiovascular disease mortality in Western Europe, the US, and Japan over the past 40 years. There are multiple factors underlying these favourable trends but understanding the epidemiology and characterizing individual risk factors for cardiovascular disease has been central in formulating preventive and treatment strategies. The INTERHEART study showed that 90% of cardiovascular risk can be explained by nine easily identifiable risk factors; an awareness of these, and the discovery of novel factors, will continue to serve in the fight to reduce the burden of cardiovascular disease. These risk factors for cardiovascular disease, traditional and novel, are discussed in Chapter 86. Geoffrey Rose first championed population-wide approaches versus strategies which target only high-risk individuals. Prevention aims to 'catch the disease' upstream, therefore delaying, reducing, or eliminating the risk of coronary artery disease. Surrogate markers for coronary artery disease have emerged in efforts to detect disease at earlier stages, and in order to better understand the pathophysiology. For example, coronary artery calcium scoring is emerging as a marker of future risk of coronary artery disease. Risk stratification scores are increasingly used as tools to individualize a person's future risk of coronary artery disease in order to better target treatment and prevention strategies.

Causes of coronary artery disease

Large-scale epidemiologic studies over the last 50 years have firmly established the commonest risk factors for coronary artery disease, notably cigarette smoking, hypertension, diabetes mellitus, hypercholesterolaemia, and a family history of coronary artery disease. The 'risk factors approach' to coronary artery disease has looked at these factors, individually and in combination, in the causation of disease (Figure 343.2). The complex causation pathways involve interplay of individual factors, whether genetic or environmental. More recently, there has been increasing interest in 'epigenetics' or the way in which the environment interacts with genes in the process underlying coronary artery disease and other cardiovascular diseases.

Prevention of coronary artery disease

There is increasing recognition that the processes underlying coronary artery disease begin early in life, and possibly in utero.

Primary prevention of coronary artery disease

Primary prevention involves the prevention of disease before its biological onset. Primary prevention strategies include reducing environmental exposures, improving human resistance to disease, and providing education and tend to act at a broader, population-wide level. In the case of coronary artery disease, examples of primary prevention are the use of the aspirin and statins in individuals with no coronary artery disease but early stage risk factors. The polypill is a 'combination approach' to primary prevention, originally suggested by Wald and Law in 2002, which treats multiple risk factors with one pill that has a larger, cumulative effect on prevention than its individual components do. Several different formulations are in development, and clinical trials are underway to test the utility and safety of the polypill approach.

However, there is controversy regarding the evidence base for primary prevention in coronary artery disease. For example, although earlier meta-analyses of the use of statins in primary prevention of coronary artery disease have shown a beneficial effect, several of the statin trials recruited individuals with preexisting disease (and are therefore not true primary prevention trials). Current guidance only advocates the use of statins for primary prevention in adults with a 20% or greater 10-year risk of developing cardiovascular disease. The most effective and cost-effective intervention for primary prevention in lower-risk adults is currently unclear. However, many of these calculations are based on the cost of interventions, and as potent drugs such as statins come off patent, many primary prevention strategies previously felt not to be cost effective become viable.

Secondary prevention of coronary artery disease

Secondary prevention aims to identify and treat existing disease in order to reduce morbidity and mortality. The reason for highlighting the secondary prevention group is that these patients have very high rates of further events, much higher than those who have not

Global deaths from CVD (millions)

- Coronary artery disease
- Hypertensive heart disease
- Rheumatic heart disease
- Cerebrovascular disease
- Inflammatory heart disease
- Other forms of heart disease

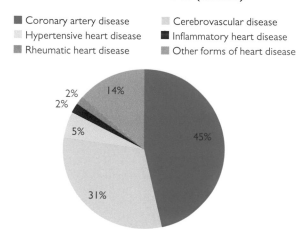

Figure 343.1 Annual global deaths from cardiovascular disease; CVD, cardiovascular disease.

Reprinted from *Global Atlas on Cardiovascular Disease Prevention and Control*, Puska P, Norrving B, p. 4, Copyright (2011) World Health Organization.

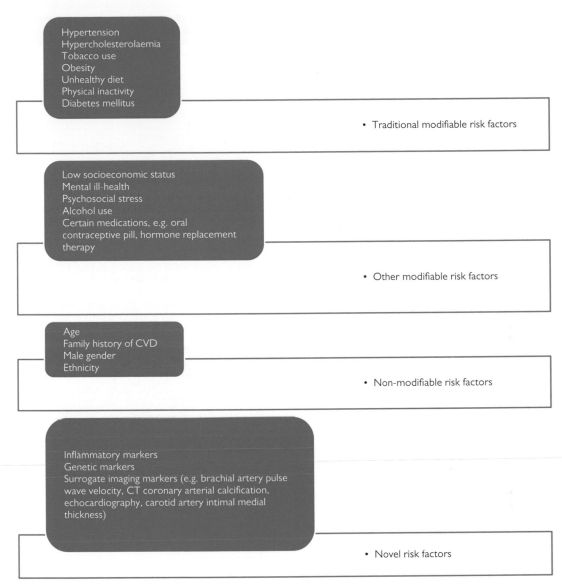

- Traditional modifiable risk factors

  Hypertension
  Hypercholesterolaemia
  Tobacco use
  Obesity
  Unhealthy diet
  Physical inactivity
  Diabetes mellitus

- Other modifiable risk factors

  Low socioeconomic status
  Mental ill-health
  Psychosocial stress
  Alcohol use
  Certain medications, e.g. oral
  contraceptive pill, hormone replacement
  therapy

- Non-modifiable risk factors

  Age
  Family history of CVD
  Male gender
  Ethnicity

- Novel risk factors

  Inflammatory markers
  Genetic markers
  Surrogate imaging markers (e.g. brachial artery pulse
  wave velocity, CT coronary arterial calcification,
  echocardiography, carotid artery intimal medial
  thickness)

Figure 343.2 Risk factors for coronary artery disease; CVD, cardiovascular disease.

had symptoms from cardiovascular disease. Secondary prevention may involve the treatment of individuals with single potent or multiple risk factors (together creating such a risk that the individual falls into the same risk category as those with established cardiovascular disease) and/or disease. The treatment of hypertension and hypercholesterolaemia in asymptomatic individuals with multiple risk factors (especially if they include diabetes) risk factors, or in individuals with symptoms such as angina or intermittent claudication, is classified as secondary prevention. The evidence base for secondary prevention strategies, such as the use of aspirin, statins, and/or antihypertensive therapy, is stronger than for primary prevention.

Tertiary prevention of coronary artery disease

Tertiary prevention aims to soften the impact of an ongoing illness or injury that has lasting effects. Tertiary prevention targets individuals with established, symptomatic coronary artery disease, to prevent further disease progression, morbidity, and mortality. After a myocardial infarction, interventions that improve prognosis include smoking cessation, increased physical exercise, and participation in a comprehensive cardiovascular rehabilitation programme.

Primordial prevention of coronary artery disease

Primordial prevention lies upstream in the continuum and can be defined as 'prevention of risk factors themselves'. This process may begin with change in social and environmental conditions in which these factors are observed to develop, and continues for high-risk children, adolescents, and young adults. Primordial prevention aims to change the socio-economic status of society. Improved socio-economic status has an inverse correlation with lifestyle risk factors such as smoking, poor nutritional status, and lack of exercise.

The Barker hypothesis, also known as the 'developmental origins of adult disease' hypothesis, was first described in detail in the early 1990s to explain how the intrauterine environment may have far-reaching effects on later adult life. The risk of coronary artery disease is higher in people who have low birthweight, and this risk decreases progressively across the range of birthweights; these findings have been replicated in several populations throughout the world. Placental growth, maternal nutrition, and early postnatal growth have all been associated with increased risk of coronary artery disease, and there is also evidence of association for stroke, hypertension, and insulin resistance. A pragmatic recommendation for primordial coronary artery disease prevention on the basis of the Barker hypothesis is the need for to educate women of childbearing age about the importance of health and nutrition during and after pregnancy.

High-risk versus population approaches to the prevention of coronary artery disease

The level of patient care changes with the level of prevention. Primordial and primary prevention are activities at the population level, whereas secondary and tertiary prevention involves the treatment of individual patients. The latter two activities tend to occur in the inpatient setting, whereas the former two occur at the societal level.

Geoffrey Rose championed the concept that small changes in risk factor levels in low-risk individuals (the 'population approach') across a population may have a greater impact on disease prevention than large changes in the same risk factors in high-risk individuals (the 'high-risk approach'). The reality is that both approaches are required for the adequate treatment and prevention of cardiovascular disease. For example, education about lifestyle, smoking cessation, and exercise are necessary alongside improved access to secondary and tertiary prevention strategies such as drugs, primary angioplasty, and coronary artery bypass graft surgery.

A unified approach to the prevention of coronary artery disease

There are shared risk factors across several cardiovascular diseases. For example, atherosclerotic diseases (namely coronary disease, cerebrovascular disease, peripheral artery disease, and aortic disease) all share the same traditional risk factors of hypertension, history of smoking, diabetes mellitus, hypercholesterolaemia, and a family history of cardiovascular disease. Therefore, health professionals and the health systems they work in must recognize the synergism which can result from prevention in 'vascular medicine'. Adequate secondary prevention with aspirin, angiotensin-converting-enzyme inhibitors, and statins after a stroke will not only reduce the risk of future stroke and TIA but also reduce the risk of coronary and peripheral vascular disease in such patients.

However, different approaches are required for individual risk factors, depending on the type of vascular disease. Hypertension is relatively more important in the development of cerebrovascular disease, so strict blood pressure monitoring and control may be more important after stroke than for acute coronary syndrome. Nonetheless, at the level of primary prevention, greater benefit can be achieved by using the same approach for all risk factors across all types of vascular disease.

Risk prediction in the prevention of cardiovascular disease

The decision to initiate preventive therapy (whether life-long statin treatment or coronary stent insertion) is based on the assessment of the risks and benefits of the particular treatment, alongside the patient's personal preferences. An assessment of a patient's baseline risk of disease without therapy can help when the risk associated with a treatment is above a certain threshold. Research and clinical practice in vascular disease has been at the forefront of development of risk prediction tools to quantify and personalize an individual's future risk of cardiovascular events.

The Framingham Heart Study led to the first 'risk calculator' for quantifying an individual's future risk of coronary artery disease on the basis of their risk factor profile. There has been increasing recognition that overall risks and the contributions of individual risk factors vary between populations and over time, leading to prospective studies in different populations with the development of population-specific risk prediction tools. In the UK, the Q-RISK and ASSIGN risk calculators are recent examples of cardiovascular calculators developed for the UK populations, with the novel addition of risk factors such as social deprivation, ethnicity, and family history. Tools have also been derived and validated for use in lower-income settings without laboratory testing facilities for cardiovascular risk factors.

Disease- and situation-specific risk prediction tools have also emerged for the range of cardiovascular diseases. The potentially

Table 343.1 The ABCD[2] algorithm for stroke risk prediction following a transient ischaemic attack

Symbol	Clinical feature	Criterion	Point
A	Age	≥60	1
B	Blood pressure	≥140/90 mmHg	1
C	Clinical features of the TIA	unilateral weakness	2
		speech disturbance without weakness	1
D1	Duration of symptoms	≥60 min	2
		10–59 min	1
		<10 min	0
D2	Diabetes Mellitus	diagnosed with diabetes?	1

Abbreviations: TIA, transient ischaemic attack.

Reprinted from *The Lancet*, Volume 369, issue 9558, S Claiborne Johnston et al Validation and refinement of scores to predict very early stroke risk after transient ischaemic attack, pp. 283-292, Copyright (2007), with permission from Elsevier.

high risk of stroke within the first 2 days after a TIA led to the prospective study of outcomes after TIA in the Oxford Vascular Study, and the subsequent development of the ABCD and ABCD[2] scores for risk stratification after TIA. These scores have enabled clinicians to decide whether to admit and treat post-TIA patients. Using the

Table 343.2 The CHADS$_2$, CHA$_2$DS$_2$-VASc, and HAS-BLED scores for assessing stroke and bleeding risk

CHADS$_2$[1]	Score
Congestive cardiac failure*	1
Hypertension (blood pressure consistently >140/90 mmHg or treated hypertension on medication)	1
Age ≥75 years	1
Diabetes mellitus	1
Stroke/transient ischemic attack/thromboembolism	2
Maximum score	6
CHA$_2$DS$_2$-VASc[2]	
Congestive cardiac failure*	1
Hypertension (blood pressure consistently >140/90 mmHg or treated hypertension on medication)	1
Age ≥75 years	2
Diabetes mellitus	1
Stroke/transient ischemic attack/thromboembolism	2
Vascular disease (previous MI, peripheral arterial disease or aortic plaque)	1
Age 65–74 years	1
Sex category (i.e. female)	1
Maximum score	9
HAS-BLED[3]	
Hypertension (systolic>160 mmHg)	1
Abnormal renal and liver function (1 point each)	1 or 2
Stroke	1
Bleeding tendency or predisposition	1
Labile INR (if on warfarin)	1
Elderly (age>65)	1
Drug or alcohol (1 point each)	1 or 2
Maximum score	9

Abbreviations: INR, international normalized rate; MI, myocardial infarction.

[1]CHADS$_2$ score and risk of stroke and thromboembolism: 0 = low risk; 1 = moderate risk; ≥2 = high risk. [2]CHA$_2$DS$_2$-VASc score and risk of stroke and thromboembolism: 0 = low risk; 1 = moderate risk; ≥2 = high risk; [3]HAS-BLED score and risk of major bleeding: 0–2 = low risk; ≥3 = high risk.

*Congestive cardiac failure is moderate to severe systolic left ventricular dysfunction, defined arbitrarily as a left ventricular ejection fraction (LVEF) ≤40%.

Reproduced with permission from A. John Camm et al., 2012 focused update of the ESC Guidelines for the management of atrial fibrillation, *European Heart Journal*, Volume 33, Issue 21, pp. 2719–2747, Copyright © 2012 Oxford University Press.

Table 343.3 Approach to thromboprophylaxis in patients with atrial fibrillation

Risk category	CHA₂DS₂-VASc score	Recommended
One 'major' or ≥2 'clinically relevant non-major' risk factors	≥2	OAC, given as well-controlled VKA (INR 2.0–3.0) or direct-acting oral anticoagulant (DOAC)*
One 'clinically relevant non-major' risk factor	1	OAC or aspirin 75–325 mg daily. Preferred: OAC
No risk factors	0	Either aspirin 75–325 mg daily or no antithrombotic therapy. Preferred: no antithrombotic therapy

Note: CHA₂DS₂-VASc = cardiac failure, hypertension, age ≥75 (doubled), diabetes, stroke (doubled)-vascular disease, age 65–74, and sex category (female); INR = international normalized ratio; OAC = oral anticoagulation, such as a vitamin K antagonist (VKA) adjusted to an intensity range of INR 2.0–3.0 (target 2.5).

*OAC, such as a VKA, adjusted to an intensity range of INR 2.0–3.0 (target 2.5), or a direct-acting oral anticoagulant.

Reproduced with permission from A. John Camm et al., 2012 focused update of the ESC Guidelines for the management of atrial fibrillation, *European Heart Journal*, Volume 33, Issue 21, pp. 2719-2747, Copyright © 2012 Oxford University Press.

ABCD2 algorithm, 2-day risks for a subsequent stroke are 1% for a score of 0–3, 4% for a score of 4–5, and 8% for a score of 6–7 (Table 343.1).

The CHADS₂ and CHADS-Vasc tools are used to predict risk of stroke and thromboembolism in patients with atrial fibrillation (AF) and influence the decision to start oral anticoagulation (OAC) with warfarin or novel anticoagulants such as dabigatran. Table 343.2 summarizes these two risk stratification scores as well as the novel HAS-BLED score, which can be used to assess bleeding risk in patients with AF prior to initiation of OAC. Table 343.3 shows how the CHADS₂ and CHADS-Vasc tools are used in clinical practice. The risk of the outcome without therapy and the risk of an adverse outcome with the therapy (measured using the HAS-BLED score) are balanced to make the treatment decision regarding OAC.

Risk scores should only be used in patients who have characteristics similar to those of the patient cohort in which the risk score was originally validated. For example, risk scores for predicting coronary artery disease should not be used to predict stroke, as they have not been validated for that purpose.

In patients with one 'clinically relevant non-major' stroke risk factor (i.e. CHA₂DS₂-VASc score = 1), dabigatran 110 mg twice daily may be considered, as its efficacy is similar to that of vitamin K antagonists with respect to the prevention of stroke and systemic embolism but it has lower rates of intracranial haemorrhage and major bleeding when compared with vitamin K antagonists and (probably) aspirin.

Further Reading

Jellinger PS, Handelsman Y, Rosenblit PD, et al. American association of clinical endocrinologists and American college of endocrinology guidelines for management of dyslipidemia and prevention of cardiovascular disease. *Enocr Pract* 2017; 23(Suppl 2): 1–87.

Joint British Societies' consensus recommendations for the prevention of cardiovascular disease (JBS3). *Heart* 2014; 100: ii1–ii67.

Piepoli MF, Hoes AW, Agewall S, et al. 2016 European Guidelines on cardiovascular disease prevention in clinical practice: The Sixth Joint Task Force of the European Society of Cardiology and Other Societies on Cardiovascular Disease Prevention in Clinical Practice (constituted by representatives of 10 societies and by invited experts)Developed with the special contribution of the European Association for Cardiovascular Prevention & Rehabilitation (EACPR). *Eur Heart J* 2016; 37:2315–81.

National Institute for Health and Care Excellence. *Hypertension in Adults: Diagnosis and Management*. 2011. Available at http://www.nice.org.uk/Guidance/CG127 (accessed 19 Sep 2017).

National Institute for Health and Care Excellence. *Cardiovascular disease: risk assessment and reduction, including lipid modification Clinical guideline [CG181]* 2014. Last updated: September 2016. Available at https://www.nice.org.uk/guidance/cg181.

The Task Force for the management of arterial hypertension of the European Society of Hypertension (ESH) and of the European Society of Cardiology (ESC). 2013 ESH/ESC Guidelines for the management of arterial hypertension. *Eur Heart J* 2013; 34: 2159–219.

Whelton PK, Carey RM, Aronow WS, et al. 2017 ACC/AHA/AAPA/ABC/ACPM/AGS/APhA/ASH/ASPC/NMA/PCNA guideline for the prevention, detection, evaluation, and management of high blood pressure in adults: executive summary: a report of the American College of Cardiology/American Heart Association Task Force on Clinical Practice Guidelines. Available at http://hyper.ahajournals.org/content/hypertensionaha/early/2017/11/10/HYP.0000000000000066.full.pdf.

344 Prevention of respiratory disease

Mona Bafadhel

Introduction

The prevention of disease at a population health level rather than an individual health level is aimed at reducing causes of 'preventable' death and, under the auspices of public health and epidemiology, is an integral part of primary, secondary, and tertiary care.

Classification of death is usually according to the type of primary disease or injury. However, there are a number of recognized risk factors for death, and modifications in behaviour or risk factors can substantially reduce preventable causes of death and the associated healthcare and economic burden of chronic disease management.

According to the WHO, hundreds of millions of people from infancy to old age suffer from preventable chronic respiratory diseases. There are over four million deaths annually from preventable respiratory diseases, and common respiratory disorders (e.g. lower respiratory tract infections, chronic obstructive pulmonary disease, lung cancer, and tuberculosis) account for approximately 20% of all deaths worldwide.

In this chapter, we discuss the prevention of respiratory disease, covering diseases associated with smoking (one of the biggest risk factors associated with preventable deaths), air pollution, and other lifestyle factors associated with respiratory disease; changes in legislation concerning smoking and work-related respiratory disease; and, finally, the prevention of respiratory diseases through the use of immunization and screening tools.

The history and burden of smoking

History of smoking

The spread of tobacco agriculture within Europe, Africa, and South East Asia occurred after the return of Christopher Columbus, following his journey to the Americas. However, the widespread introduction of tobacco and the act of smoking was not met without opposition; smoking was banned by the Pope in 1590 and the cultivation of tobacco was suppressed by King James I in 1604. However, with its increasing popularity, economic revenue, and mass production, the era of the modern-day cigarette was firmly in place in the early twentieth century.

Smoking habits

Men are more likely to smoke than women, although in the UK the gender gap has narrowed over time. There is currently a downward trend in the number of people starting to smoke and, more recently, an increase in the number of people giving up smoking (Figure 344.1).

Smoking cessation

Smoking cessation is imperative in the practice of healthcare and disease prevention. Interventions to aid smoking cessation include unassisted methods such as healthcare provider advice, group cessation clinics, and one-to-one smoking cessation counselling. Nicotine replacement therapy (NRT), nicotinic receptor partial agonists (e.g. varenicline), and antidepressant medication (e.g. bupropion) are approved as smoking cessation aids. Success rates for each of these methods is varied and ranges from 10% with healthcare provider advice alone to 33% in persons who use NRT medication (the success rate being defined as the percentage of persons who remained 'quitters' after a 6-month period). Support and advice, including discussions of the short- and long-term effects of smoking cessation, need to be provided in order to maintain smoking cessation.

Legislation

Smoking legislation exists to protect individuals from the effect of second-hand smoke; the WHO Framework Convention Tobacco Control Treaty was developed in response to the tobacco epidemic, and serves to affirm the highest standard of health to all individuals, providing both measures to reduce tobacco demand (cost and taxes) and protection

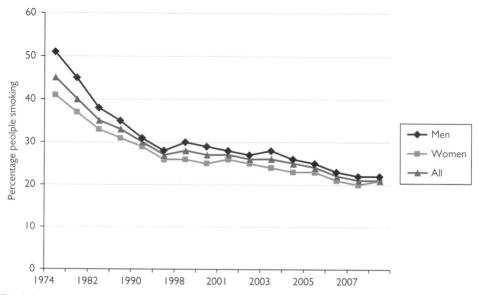

Figure 344.1 The decline in smoking in recent years.
Data from an Office of National Statistics survey (http://www.ons.gov.uk/ons/dcp171776_302558.pdf).

from the effects of tobacco exposure. In the UK, the ban on smoking in public places was first introduced in Scotland (March 2006), then Wales and Northern Ireland (April 2007), and, finally, in England (July 2007). This ban involves the prohibition of smoking in all enclosed public spaces (e.g. workplaces, restaurants, bars, and pubs). Since its introduction, there has been a decline in cigarette sales, and reduced trends of all-cause smoking-related hospitalization.

The evidence for the role of smoking in respiratory disease

Lung cancer

In the UK, lung cancer is the most common cause of death from cancer and is responsible for over one-fifth of all cancer deaths. Variations in lung cancer mortality rates within the UK reflect the variations in smoking trends within geographical areas, with smoking and lung cancer rates higher in Scotland than in England and Wales. In 1956, Doll and Hill published their epidemiological findings which linked lung cancer with smoking. Heavy smokers (defined as those smoking more than 25 grams of tobacco or 25 cigarettes per day) were approximately 20 times more likely to die from lung cancer than never smokers in a 5-year follow-up period. Worldwide, almost 90% of lung cancer is attributed to smoking; after a lag time of 20 years, there is now a steady increase in the number of women being diagnosed with lung cancer. Prevention of lung cancer is the most cost-effective way of combating this disease; primary prevention with smoking cessation is unequivocally an important tool in this process, as general population screening methods have not demonstrated clear benefits.

Chronic obstructive pulmonary disease

Chronic obstructive pulmonary disease (COPD) is currently the fifth leading cause of death worldwide, and is predicted to be the third leading cause of death worldwide by 2020. It is the only common disease worldwide that continues to increase in incidence and prevalence, and rates in women are increasing three times faster than men. In the UK, approximately 1 million people are diagnosed with COPD, but there are believed to be a further 2 million persons that have not been formally diagnosed. This leads to an estimate that, in the UK alone, 1 in 10 people over the age of 40 are likely to have COPD, making it one of the most prevalent respiratory diseases. COPD is diagnosed by clinical history and spirometry and largely encompasses the terms emphysema, chronic bronchitis, and chronic asthma. The severity of COPD can also be diagnosed by spirometry, symptoms and history of exacerbations. It is an irreversible airways disease associated with a progressive decline in lung function and is accelerated in people who continue to smoke. Smoking is the main cause of COPD, although there is increasing recognition of biomass fuels and air/dust pollution as causal agents. In 1977, Fletcher and Peto published a landmark study evaluating the effects of smoking on the development of COPD; in it, they showed that regular smokers exhibited an accelerated decline in forced expiratory volume in 1 second but that this slowed to the rate of natural decline after smoking cessation.

Preventing common respiratory infections

Vaccinations

Acute respiratory infections are estimated to be responsible for 4 million deaths worldwide and are the leading causes of death in children under the age of 5. Vaccines are currently available for the prevention of disease from the following pathogens, with which there are associated respiratory disease burdens:

- *Haemophilus influenzae* B
- *Streptococcus pneumoniae*
- influenza virus

Haemophilus influenzae B

The *Haemophilus influenzae* type b bacterium is commonly present in the nose and throat, and is transmitted through droplet spread. Infection with *Haemophilus influenzae* type b may be mild and asymptomatic; in the developed world, it can cause fatal pneumonia, while, in developing countries, it can be responsible for non-epidemic meningitis. *Haemophilus influenzae* type b infection can be prevented by vaccination.

Streptococcus pneumoniae

Streptococcus pneumoniae is a leading cause of morbidity and mortality worldwide, with pneumococcal bacteraemia episodes being common at the extremes of age. So far, there are 40 serogroups and 90 serotypes, with differences worldwide with respect to which serotypes cause disease and thus which vaccine programmes are likely to be effective. *Streptococcus pneumoniae* is carried in the human nasopharynx and spreads via droplets. Within the first year of life, almost everyone is colonized with at least one strain. In adulthood, at least 30% of cases of community-acquired pneumonia are related to *Streptococcus pneumoniae*. Vaccination is 60% effective in immunocompetent individuals, with an efficacy in the region of 20% in immunocompromised individuals.

Influenza

Influenza is highly contagious and readily transmitted via droplets. There are up to 600 million cases of influenza each year, with approximately 0.5 million deaths per year. Seasonal influenza epidemics reflect that there is continuous antigenic virus change, with the emergence of strains that cause epidemics and pandemics. Circulating influenza A human strains can acquire new genes from avian or other animal reservoirs, such as pigs, and these can cause worldwide pandemics, as was the case in 1918, 1957, 1968, and 2009. Facing this requires continually updated strain changes of influenza vaccines or the production of a universal vaccine, with vigilance and hygiene practices as routine practices. Mortality from influenza can be unpredictable, but vaccination programmes for the population at risk, including the elderly and the immunocompromised, allow for success in mortality rate reduction.

Respiratory syncytial virus

Respiratory syncytial virus (RSV) is the most important cause of viral lower respiratory tract infection in infants and children, commonly causing hospitalizations due to bronchiolitis and childhood pneumonia. Humans are the only reservoir for RSV, but the virus can persist for several hours on inanimate objects. It is common for children to have more than one RSV infection, which increases the risk of childhood wheezing episodes and the development of asthma.

TB

One-third of the world's population (2 billion people) is infected by *Mycobacterium tuberculosis* and thus exposed to the risk of developing TB. It is estimated that there are 9 million new cases of TB each year, and almost 2 million deaths from TB annually worldwide. BCG, a vaccine using Bacillus Calmette–Guérin, a derivative of *Mycobacterium bovis*, protects children from severe pulmonary forms of TB but has no lasting effects of protection into adulthood. The emergence of multidrug-resistant TB, extremely resistant TB, and coexistent infection with HIV underscores the importance of developing better and improved TB vaccines. TB is highly contagious; each infectious carrier of pulmonary TB will infect 15 people on average each year, as the infection spreads via droplets and the number of bacilli required to initiate an infection is low. To prevent this common and treatable yet potentially fatal infection, an effective vaccine, together with surveillance and screening programmes, is required in both the developing and the developed world.

Lifestyle factors involved in preventable respiratory disease

Obesity

Obesity is the most common risk factor for obstructive sleep apnoea (OSA), the commonest cause for sleep-related respiratory disorders. It is caused by obstruction of the upper airway, where obstruction is caused by an increased muscle relaxation that occurs during sleep.

It is characterized by repeated pauses in breathing; such pauses are termed 'apnoeas'. OSA is associated with an increased risk of systemic and pulmonary hypertension, cardiovascular disease, and metabolic syndrome. Risk factors for OSA include reduced muscular tone and increased soft tissue mass surrounding the upper airway. With the worldwide increase in obesity, OSA is becoming more prevalent. Weight reduction can reverse OSA, and at-risk individuals should be recognized early to prevent associated cardiovascular and metabolic risks.

Air pollution

Air pollution (outdoor or indoor) is defined as the introduction of chemicals, particulate matter, and/or biological materials that can cause harm or discomfort to humans and other living organisms. For outdoor air, pollution air quality standards govern atmospheric concentrations for specific known pollutants; various thresholds can also be set, to communicate to the public the relative risks of outdoor activity. Indoor air pollution, with exposure to biomass smoke, is considered a risk factor for the development of COPD, lung cancer, and acute lower respiratory infections. The levels of small soot or dust particles generated by burning solid fuels can exceed acceptable levels for outdoor pollution by 100 times. The reliance on burning wood, dung, crop waste, and coal to meet energy needs, in environments that have poor ventilation, continues to rise in developing countries. Indoor air pollution doubles the risk of pneumonia, triples the risk of COPD, and almost doubles the risk of lung cancer in non-smoking women. Provisions of measures that reduce indoor air pollution include using improved stoves and hoods that vent to the outdoors, and switching to more sustainable and cleaner alternatives.

Occupational exposure

Through regulation, it is possible to reduce occupational exposure to known carcinogens and the associated risk of respiratory disease. The most widely known occupational respiratory disease, with clear legislative recommendations for prevention, management, and counselling for compensation, is that related to asbestos. Exposure to asbestos fibres causes asbestosis (a progressive pulmonary fibrosis) and mesothelioma (pleural cancer) and increases the risk of both lung cancer and benign disease such as pleural plaques. Occupational exposure to dusts, fumes, natural, and non-natural elements also increases the risk of diseases such as asthma; hence, legal requirements for providing education and respiratory protection to at-risk individuals within the workplace can prevent respiratory illness.

Conclusion

Respiratory illness is common, and is a great burden on healthcare worldwide. Population-based methods to reduce this burden must begin with prevention, as simple measures such as education, vaccinations, screening, and hygiene can reduce the prevalence and incidence of many preventable respiratory diseases in a cost-effective manner.

Further Reading

Broaddus VC, Robert J. Mason RJ, Ernst JD, et al. *Murray and Nadel's Textbook of Respiratory Medicine* (6th edition), 2015. Saunders.
Maskell N and Ann Millar A (eds). *Oxford Desk Reference: Respiratory Medicine*, 2009. Oxford University Press.

Introduction

A number of factors are known to predispose to renal disease, such as diabetes mellitus, hypertension, and exposure to certain drugs (see Box 345.1) or substances (e.g. mercury and other heavy metals). In people who are at risk for these reasons, renal function should be regularly monitored as part of routine care.

Prevention of kidney disease

Kidney diseases are identified by elevations in the serum creatinine; the presence in the urine of blood, protein, or elevated levels of certain electrolytes; or evidence of anatomical abnormalities. Due to the large functional reserve of the kidneys, symptoms of impaired renal function usually occur late in the course of disease, highlighting the importance of early detection and, where available, the use of ameliorating therapies. Therapies exist for some forms of acute and chronic kidney diseases and range from inexpensive (e.g. normal saline to ensure adequate hydration prior to IV contrast administration) to very expensive (e.g. enzyme replacement in Fabry's disease). Once chronic damage is established, it may be possible to slow the rate of progression to end-stage renal disease or prevent its occurrence entirely. Even when end-stage renal disease has developed, it may be possible to prevent the development of the metabolic consequences of deranged kidney function, such as acidosis, anaemia, and defective bone mineralization, all of which increase morbidity and mortality (these are discussed in Chapter 163).

Prevention of acute kidney injury

The majority of cases of acute kidney injury are predictable and are caused by impaired renal perfusion leading to tubular damage, or by the effects of substances that are toxic to the tubules. The important reabsorptive and secretory functions of tubular cells may also expose them to high concentrations of toxins, including various medications that can lead to direct damage.

Acute kidney injury is commonly seen in hospitalized patients, and particular groups of patients are at risk, as discussed in 'Introduction' (also see Box 345.2). In many cases, the kidney injury is secondary to the underlying disease process or processes responsible for the admission, but careful attention to optimizing renal perfusion and the avoidance of further insults can reduce renal damage and decrease the likelihood of needing renal replacement therapy.

In clinical practice, a combination of these risk factors often coexist, and some common scenarios include renal impairment arising as a result of hypotension, sepsis, or the use of IV contrast or nephrotoxic drugs.

In many situations, acute kidney injury may be prevented if the risk of the injury is appreciated, patients are identified early, and measures are taken to ensure adequate renal perfusion and to avoid further renal insults. Approaches include:

- prompt fluid resuscitation in volume-depleted patients; postural hypotension is a good marker for ongoing intravascular depletion,

---

Box 345.1 Risk factors for kidney disease

Vascular
- hypertension
- heart failure/coronary artery disease
- cerebrovascular disease
- peripheral vascular disease

Multisystem diseases
- diabetes mellitus
- SLE
- vasculitis
- myeloma
- rheumatoid arthritis
- scleroderma

Infectious agents
- HIV
- hepatitis B
- hepatitis C

Urological conditions
- bladder outflow obstruction
- neurogenic bladder
- urinary diversion surgery
- urinary anatomical abnormalities
- recurrent urinary tract stone formation

Drugs
- angiotensin-converting enzyme inhibitors and angiotensin receptor blockers
- NSAIDs
- lithium
- mesalazine
- calcineurin inhibitors (ciclosporin, tacrolimus)
- antibiotics (e.g. gentamicin and amphotericin)
- chemotherapy agents (e.g. cisplatin)
- radio-opaque contrast

Box 345.2 Risk factors for acute kidney injury

Reduced nephron mass
- preexisting chronic kidney disease
- elderly patients

Systemic diseases
- diabetes mellitus
- myeloma

Impaired renal perfusion
- volume depletion
  - vomiting or diarrhoea
  - burns
  - haemorrhage
- volume redistribution
  - sepsis
  - cardiac failure
- renal artery stenosis
- hypotension

Nephrotoxic medications
- antibiotics
- chemotherapy agents
- antihypertensives
- NSAIDs

Impaired drainage
- prostatic obstruction
- spinal cord injury

and repeated clinical assessment is essential in order to deliver appropriate fluid replacement

- careful prescription of maintenance IV fluid in patients with inadequate oral intake
- daily weighing, where possible; this is very helpful for monitoring fluid balance, and can be used in addition to taking input and output measures
- maintenance of an adequate mean arterial blood pressure, using invasive monitoring and inotropes if needed
- stopping angiotensin-converting-enzyme inhibitors (ACE-Is) and angiotensin receptor blockers (ARBs) in acutely unwell or dehydrated patients
- avoiding NSAIDs for post-operative analgesia in at-risk patients
- performing regular checks of renal function
- monitoring levels of nephrotoxic agents (e.g. gentamicin, ciclosporin, tacrolimus) if clinical need necessitates their use
- excluding bladder outflow obstruction

Patients with a reduced glomerular filtration rate (GFR) are at greater risk of contrast-induced nephropathy, particularly if there is concomitant dehydration or diabetes mellitus. Alternative imaging modalities should be used where possible; if contrast is necessary, the minimum possible volume should be used. Hyperosmolar and ionic contrast media should be avoided. Adequate pre-hydration is essential and should be continued for at least 24 hours after the procedure.

Prevention of chronic kidney diseases

Genetic kidney diseases

A large number of genetic diseases involve the kidneys; some are specific to the kidneys, whereas in others, renal damage occurs in the context of more generalized disease. With improvements in DNA sequencing technologies, it is becoming easier to screen for mutations prenatally and to provide counselling. For some diseases, evidence is accumulating that early interventions may slow the rate of decline in renal function associated with the disease. As a result, these patients may never reach end-stage kidney disease or even develop significant renal dysfunction during their lifespan. An example may be polycystic kidney disease (see Chapter 169), where renal impairment develops over time due to progressive cyst expansion, which compresses and compromises normal renal tissue. Early inhibition of cyst growth with vaptans, ACE-I, somatostatin analogues, or other therapies currently under investigation may prevent disease. Table 345.1 lists some genetic diseases and currently available or experimental therapies.

Acquired kidney diseases

In the developed world, diabetes and lifestyle diseases are responsible for the majority of patients who reach end-stage kidney disease. Most of these conditions are associated with either elevations of the serum creatinine (a reduction in GFR) or the presence of albuminuria or proteinuria. Several large studies demonstrate that population-based screening strategies can identify asymptomatic people with albuminuria or reduced estimated GFR and it may be that early

Table 345.1 Genetic disease causing renal impairment

Disease	Mutation	Potential therapies
Adult polycystic kidney disease	Polycystin	Angiotensin-converting enzyme inhibitors Vaptans Triptolide
Cystinosis	Cystinosin	Cysteamine
Fabry's disease	Alpha-galactosidase	Alpha-galactosidase
Familial juvenile hyperuricaemic nephropathy	Uromodulin	Allopurinol

treatment will prevent progression to significant chronic renal impairment in these patients.

For patients with diabetes, there is good evidence that optimizing glycaemic control and the early use of ACE-Is or ARBs can reduce the rate of renal progression. Good blood pressure control can slow the rate of renal deterioration in patients with renal impairment, and current evidence would suggest using ACE-Is or ARBs if there is evidence of proteinuria.

Screening for kidney disease

In the UK, there has been widespread adoption of routine estimated GFR reporting to assist in the identification of chronic kidney disease; however, the current classification scheme is contentious, as many patients, particularly those with chronic kidney disease, may have renal function in the normal range for their age and sex, as determined by population-based studies. These people do not have any significant chronic kidney disease and there is no evidence that they will progress to end-stage disease.

In addition to questions regarding the validity of the current classification system, in many cases there is little or no evidence that any treatments will alter the progression of disease. Key exceptions where treatments can prevent progression of renal disease are diabetic nephropathy, hypertensive nephropathy, and some of the proteinuric glomerulonephritides. It is also worth mentioning that treatment of these conditions generally reduces the risk of a cardiovascular event to a greater degree than the risk of progression to end-stage renal disease.

Further Reading

Acute kidney injury: prevention, detection and management Clinical guideline Published: 28 August 2013 nice.org.uk/guidance/cg169
Brown WW, Peters RM, Ohmit SE, et al. Early detection of kidney disease in community settings: The Kidney Early Evaluation Program (KEEP). *Am J Kidney Dis* 2003; 42: 22–35.
Steddon S, Chesser A, Cunningham J, et al. *Oxford Handbook of Nephrology and Hypertension* (2nd edition), 2014. Oxford University Press.

346 Prevention of gastrointestinal disease

Satish Keshav and Alexandra Kent

Introduction

Disease prevention is usually directed where there is considerable morbidity or mortality, and etiological factors that can be controlled, treated, or reduced. The greatest morbidity and mortality from gastrointestinal disease is related to infectious diarrhoea and gastrointestinal cancer, both of which can be prevented. In addition, alcohol consumption and viral hepatitis are preventable causes of liver disease, liver failure, and hepatic cancer.

Alcohol

It is well recognized that excess alcohol consumption is associated with a wide range of different disease processes. In addition to liver disease, alcohol consumption is also an etiological factor in many cancers, and is estimated to be the cause of 6% of cancer deaths. Excess alcohol consumption probably doubles the risk of oesophageal cancer, although some studies estimate the risk to be 5–10 times that of an abstinent person. It also increases the risk of bowel and liver cancer. The concept that red wine can reduce cancer risk has been disputed by large studies, and should not be supported in clinical practice. Gastrointestinal physicians will see many patients with deranged liver function related to alcohol consumption, and it is important that the patient is educated appropriately: reducing alcohol consumption not only reduces the risk of liver disease and cirrhosis, but also reduces the risk of cancer. Prevention is difficult and dependent on patient commitment, so support services should be made available. Alcohol is discussed in more detail in Chapters 211 and 339.

Smoking

Smoking is an etiological factor in many diseases: 50% of smokers die from cancer or smoking-related diseases, and 25% of these deaths will be in patients under the age of 70 years. Smoking has been closely associated with oesophageal, gastric, and liver cancer and, consequently, smoking prevention should reduce the incidence of these and other smoking-related conditions. Smoking also has a significant effect in inflammatory bowel disease. Epidemiological studies have shown smoking to be associated with a worse outlook in Crohn's disease, with disease flares and an increased risk of surgery. Conversely, ulcerative colitis is more frequent with non-smokers, and often presents for the first time when former smokers stop. An interesting corollary of this is that life-expectancy in ulcerative colitis is equal to or greater than in the general population.

Peptic ulcer disease

The two main treatment options for patients with peptic ulcer disease are proton-pump inhibitors and eradication of *Helicobacter pylori,* as both treatments improve ulcer healing. However, there is no evidence that either treatment can be used a primary preventive measure. A recent Cochrane review established that, in the setting of NSAID-induced ulceration, proton-pump inhibitors, misoprostol, and double-dose H2 antagonists can reduce the incidence of gastric and duodenal ulceration. The cost-effectiveness of such preventive measures is unknown. Usually, prophylactic treatment is reserved for patients who would have a poor prognosis should they develop peptic ulcers, for example, elderly patients receiving anticoagulation medication. Selective COX-2 inhibitors were initially thought to be anti-inflammatory drugs that would not cause the gastrointestinal ulceration associated with NSAIDs. Unfortunately, they are still associated with gastrointestinal ulceration and perforation, although the risk is lower than with NSAIDs. There is a well-established association between *Helicobacter pylori* and gastric cancer, and several observational studies from Japan and China have shown that eradication of *Helicobacter pylori* reduces the incidence of stomach cancer. However, this result cannot be transferred to general medical practice without larger studies, as these findings may relate to the higher incidence of stomach cancer in these countries.

Colorectal cancer

The most effective preventive measure for colorectal cancer is the establishment of screening programmes. Currently, in the UK, those aged 60–69 are offered faecal occult blood tests, with a colonoscopy offered to people with positive results, as part of the National Bowel Cancer Screening Programme. The aim is to identify people with early and therefore treatable cancers, and also people with colorectal adenomatous polyps. Adenomatous polyps are then monitored through adenoma screening programmes. Other conditions requiring colorectal cancer surveillance include inflammatory bowel disease, acromegaly, familial adenomatous polyposis, hereditary non-polyposis colorectal cancer, juvenile polyposis, Peutz–Jeghers syndrome, a strong family history of colorectal cancer, and ureterosigmoidostomy (for further details regarding screening in gastrointestinal disease, see Chapter 354). Other etiological factors known to increase the risk of bowel cancer include diets high in fat and cholesterol, and red meat, especially processed meat. Smoking, obesity, and alcohol increase the risk of colorectal cancer. Many patients who attend hospital harbour concerns of developing cancer, and all of these factors can be discussed with them as potential preventive measures. Diabetes mellitus has also been shown to increase the risk of adenomatous polyps. Conversely, studies have shown that regular aspirin ingestion can reduce the incidence of colorectal adenomatous polyps and colon cancer.

Oesophageal adenocarcinoma

There is clear evidence that recurrent acid reflux can lead to inflammation in the oesophagus, which can lead to the development of Barrett's oesophagus. Approximately 10% of patients undergoing endoscopy for reflux symptoms have Barrett's oesophagus, and approximately of these 5% have associated dysplasia. Adenocarcinoma arises from Barrett's dysplasia; therefore, patients with Barrett's oesophagus may enter a screening programme (see Chapter 354 for further details). There is no definitive evidence that this will reduce the incidence of oesophageal adenocarcinoma as yet, but the combination of earlier diagnosis and treatment of high-grade dysplasia is expected to have this effect. Patients with Barrett's oesophagus are maintained on long-term proton-pump inhibitors, to reduce acid exposure, with the aim of reducing progression or the development of dysplasia.

Hepatitis B

There is a growing incidence of hepatitis B infection in the UK, due to immigration. The major routes of transmission are vertical, from mother to child, mainly in the Far East, and horizontal, from shared needles, unprotected sexual intercourse, and non-sterile shared equipment, for instance in tattooing. The development of a vaccine for hepatitis B offers the chance to eliminate the risk of transmission. Currently, it is offered to at-risk populations. These include medical workers, IV drug users, family members or partners of hepatitis patients, and immunosuppressed patients.

Hepatitis C

Hepatitis C is a growing concern, with patients presenting with liver complications many years after contracting the virus. Research hopes to develop a vaccine but, even if such research is successful, reaching patients at risk of contracting the virus will be difficult. Prevention includes promoting sterile-needle programmes amongst users of IV drugs. There is limited evidence of sexual transmission, and blood products are now routinely screened.

Non-alcoholic fatty liver disease

There is a growing incidence of non-alcoholic fatty liver disease (NAFLD) worldwide, with estimates of 20% of the population being affected in the UK. Risk factors for the development of NAFLD include obesity, diabetes, impaired glucose tolerance, hyperlipidaemia, and hypertension. These are obviously also etiological factors for ischaemic heart disease; thus, patients receive additional benefit from controlling each factor. Weight loss, together with control of blood pressure, cholesterol levels, and diabetes, is expected to slow the progression of liver disease, preventing the development of steatohepatitis and subsequent cirrhosis.

Gastrointestinal infection

The most important preventive measure to reduce the incidence of gastrointestinal infections is to maintain good sanitation, with hand-washing and hygienic food preparation. The main barrier to this worldwide is the lack of safe, uncontaminated drinking water, poor sanitary facilities, and poverty.

Further Reading

Botteri E, Iodice S, Bagnardi V, et al. Smoking and colorectal cancer: A meta-analysis. *JAMA* 2008; 300: 2765–78.

Haas SL, Ye W, and Löhr JM. Alcohol consumption and digestive tract cancer. *Curr Opin Clin Nutr Metab Care* 2012; 15: 457–67.

Hou N, Huo D, and Dignam JJ. Prevention of colorectal cancer and dietary management. *Chin Clin Oncol* 2013; 2: 13.

Lordick F, Mariette C, Haustermans K et al. ESMO Clinical Practice Guidelines for diagnosis, treatment and follow-up. *Ann Oncol* 2016; 27: v50-v57.

Talley NJ, Locke GR, Moayyedi P, et al. (eds). *GI Epidemiology: Diseases and Clinical Methodology* (2nd edition), 2014. Wiley-Blackwell.

347 Prevention of neurological disease

Karen Morrison

Introduction

Neurological disease is very common. It is estimated that one-third of consultations with general practitioners involve neurological complaints, and neurological disorders are present in one-third of patients admitted to hospital. Table 347.1 shows the prevalence of some of the most common neurological diseases.

In considering how to reduce the incidence of neurological disease, one must take into account the feasibility of prevention, and the overall morbidity caused by the disease. In stroke, which is very common, interventions which reduce incidence by a small percentage have the potential to have a large impact on a population basis. A disorder such as migraine, while not life-limiting, accounts for significant morbidity and time off work (one study suggests that there are the equivalent of 112 million bedridden days per year due to migraine alone), so, again, interventions that reduce the frequency of episodes even by a small percentage can have great overall impact. In this chapter, we consider the major categories of neurological disease based on pathogenesis, and current and future approaches to prevention.

Prevention in vascular neurological disease

Prevention of stroke

Stroke is the main cause of neurological morbidity in adults and the third most common cause of death worldwide after ischaemic heart disease and cancer (all forms combined). Preventive strategies for stroke, due to either ischaemia or haemorrhage, are discussed in Chapter 348.

Prevention of epileptic seizures

Epilepsy is another of the common, serious brain disorders, with a prevalence of just under 1% of the population. Most cases of epilepsy are termed 'cryptogenic' or 'idiopathic', with no underlying structural brain abnormality identified. While surgically resected specimens from some patients with seizures can show anatomical changes such as mesial temporal sclerosis, with neuronal dropout and reactive gliosis, these morphological changes don't explain how seizures develop and propagate. There has been extensive debate over the years as to whether 'seizures begat seizures', that is, does having one epileptic seizure in some way prime or 'kindle' the brain so that further seizures are more likely to occur? If such priming does occur, it is even more important to try to prevent seizures in those who have already suffered an event.

Overall, around 60% of people with epilepsy are well controlled (rendered seizure-free) by using a single drug at appropriate therapeutic dose; 70% are well controlled on two drugs; and around 75% on three drugs. The various classes of antiepileptic drugs have been detailed in Chapter 226. Other measures that can be effective at reducing seizure frequency include ensuring sufficient sleep, maintaining a regular routine with regular meals, and avoiding triggers as appropriate, such as flickering lights where photosensitivity has been demonstrated. Some seizures are the result of underlying structural or metabolic disease (see Table 347.2); in such instances, prevention of further attacks relies on treatment of the underlying cause, in addition to providing anticonvulsant therapy. Neurosurgery to remove an identified epileptogenic focus (such as may occur with congenital brain malformations) can be extremely effective at reducing the frequency, or even eliminating, seizures in appropriately selected patients.

One of the causes of refractory epilepsy is non-compliance with medication. Current first-line anticonvulsant drugs have many fewer long-term side effects than previously used drugs such as phenytoin and phenobarbital, although side effects such as somnolence and mental dulling or weight gain are still reported and undoubtedly influence compliance. An important specific area is that of epilepsy and pregnancy. Overall, there is no increased risk of seizures in pregnancy, but some women, concerned about the possible teratogenic effects of anticonvulsants, will reduce or stop their medications in pregnancy and thus be at increased risk of seizures. Women need clear advice on the safest and most appropriate anticonvulsants to take during pregnancy and breastfeeding, and should be referred for appropriate specialist advice, ideally prior to conceiving.

Another area of epilepsy prevention to consider is that of prophylactic use of anticonvulsants following head trauma or in relation to brain surgery. Factors that increase the risk of a seizure following head injury include the severity of the injury, whether there is depression of a skull fracture, the presence of focal neurological signs and/or intracranial haematoma, and the duration

Table 347.1 Prevalence of some common neurological disorders

Disorder	Prevalence per 100 000 population
Migraine	2000
Other severe headache	1500
Epilepsy	650
Acute cerebrovascular disease	600
Lumbosacral pain	500
Dementia	250
Parkinson's disease	200
Single seizure	60
Multiple sclerosis	60

Table 347.2 Some causes of epilepsy

Causes	Notes
Idiopathic	No underlying metabolic or structural brain disease
Structural brain disease	e.g. congenital neuronal migration disorder
Epilepsy post head trauma	
Intracranial space-occupying lesion	e.g. brain tumour, brain abscess
Epilepsy due to monogenic gene mutations	e.g. mutations in GABA$_A$ receptor, K$^+$ channel mutations
Metabolic causes: • hyperglycaemia • hypoxia • uraemia • hypernatraemia • hypokalaemia • hypocalcaemia • liver disease	
Drugs	e.g. phenothiazines, tricyclic antidepressants
Drug withdrawal	e.g. benzodiazepines, alcohol withdrawal

of post-traumatic amnesia. Age is a further important factor, with young children having the highest risk of seizures post head trauma, and the risk progressively decreasing throughout life. There is reasonable evidence to support the use of prophylactic anticonvulsant medications for 6 months following severe head injury or brain surgery, but the evidence for prophylaxis decreasing the risk of later post-traumatic seizures is less secure.

Prevention of degenerative brain disease

Degenerative brain disease is an increasing burden to individuals and society in our ageing population. The most common diseases in this category are dementia and Parkinson's disease. Other degenerative disorders include motor neuron disease (also known as amyotrophic lateral sclerosis), inherited disorders such as Huntington's disease, and the Parkinson's related disorders of multiple system atrophy and progressive supranuclear palsy. While these latter diseases are, fortunately, quite rare, they cause huge suffering to individuals, carers, and families; thus, any interventions that might reduce their incidence would be highly valuable. Some of the theories proposed to account for the increasing incidence of these disorders with age include decreased mitochondrial efficiency and function, increased cellular oxidative stress with decreased repair mechanisms, and the impairment of pathways of autophagy and protein turnover.

Prevention of Alzheimer's disease

Alzheimer's disease, named after Alois Alzheimer, the German psychiatrist who first published on the disease in 1907, is the commonest form of dementia. The prevalence increases exponentially with age from 65 onwards, such that between 5% and 10% of people aged between 65 and 74 years are affected, rising to between 30% and 40% of the population aged over 85 years. The key features of memory loss, personality decline, and cognitive decline progress over years such that, by the advanced stages of the disease, individuals can no longer recognize close family and friends, are mute, incontinent, and cachectic, and may suffer seizures. Neuropathologically, Alzheimer's disease is characterized by intra-neuronal protein aggregates of hyperphosphorylated tau protein (neurofibrillary tangles), aggregation of plaques of amyloid beta protein in the brain parenchyma and in blood vessel walls, and neuronal degeneration and loss.

There has been, and continues to be, extensive research aimed at identifying risk factors for Alzheimer's disease so that preventive strategies can be undertaken. Some of these factors, confirmed in large, prospective studies, are listed in Box 347.1.

Some of the possible preventive interventions are listed in Box 347.2. While there is good evidence that treating or preventing vascular disease will reduce the subsequent risk of developing Alzheimer's disease, the evidence is less clear for strategies such as use of NSAIDs, statin therapy, or hormone replacement therapy, with most of the evidence coming from retrospective population or clinic studies rather than prospective studies.

Box 347.2 Suggested strategies to prevent Alzheimer's disease

- vascular disease: treat hypertension, avoid smoking
- retain intellectual abilities: crosswords, Sudoku, 'if you don't use it you lose it'
- maintain social interactions
- maintain an active lifestyle
- hormone replacement therapy in postmenopausal women
- statin therapy
- anti-inflammatory drug use

Prevention of Parkinson's disease

Parkinson's disease, another common neurodegenerative disorder, is characterized clinically by tremor, rigidity, and bradykinesia, with the underlying pathological feature of degeneration of dopaminergic cells and accumulation of intra-neuronal inclusions in the neurons of the substantia nigra of the midbrain. Parkinson's disease mostly occurs in people over 60 years of age, but early onset disease (onset less than the age of 40 years) is well recognized, particularly in some rare inherited forms of the disease, for example disease due to mutations in PARK2. Epidemiological studies have identified environmental risk factors for the disease (see Box 347.3), while, in the last decade, an increasing number of genetic variants have been identified (e.g. variants in SCNA, LRRK2, and GBA) that also increase susceptibility to sporadic Parkinson's disease.

The observation of decreased incidence of Parkinson's disease in cigarette smokers has been noted for at least 20 years. At one time, this was thought due to the fact that cigarette smokers die prematurely from vascular disease and cancer, such that they do not reach an age at which they are likely to develop Parkinson's disease. It is now clear that this is not the explanation and that cigarette smoking does indeed protect against developing Parkinson's disease, with greater protection accruing to those who have smoked for the longest time. The mechanism for the protective effect is not known. One theory relates to the fact that nicotine can stimulate postsynaptic dopamine receptors and so protect against their downregulation. Caffeine also protects against developing Parkinson's disease; as its chemical structure is similar to that of nicotine, it may act via a similar mechanism. The discovery that MPTP can cause a severe form of parkinsonism came in the 1980s, when a group of IV drug addicts developed the disease on injecting a contaminated synthetic heroin preparation. Although MPTP has been very useful in developing animal models to investigate underlying pathways and mechanisms in the disease, its identification as a selective toxin for dopaminergic neurons has not as yet led to any specific preventive strategies.

Prevention of multiple sclerosis

Multiple sclerosis (MS) is being included here, as it is the most common disorder which results in severe physical disability in young adults in the UK (see Chapter 231). The underlying pathology in the

---

Box 347.1 Risk factors for Alzheimer's disease

- age: the most consistent risk factor
- poor educational attainment
- vascular disease: hypertension, hypercholesterolaemia, diabetes mellitus
- family history of Alzheimer's disease
- genetic factors: polymorphisms of apolipoprotein E (the risk of developing Alzheimer's disease is 2–3× greater for APOE4 heterozygotes and 6–8× greater for APOE4 homozygotes, compared to that for those not carrying this allele)
- menopause in women
- rare genetic mutations (for familial forms of Alzheimer's disease): mutations in amyloid precursor protein, presenilin 1, or presenilin 2
- previous significant head trauma

Box 347.3 Environmental causes of Parkinson's disease

Increased risk
- pesticide use, particularly rotenone
- rural residence, farming
- drinking well water
- MPTP (a mitochondrial protoxin)
- heavy metal exposure (e.g. manganese, lead)
- repeated head injury (e.g. boxing)
- encephalitis lethargica

Decreased risk
- cigarette smoking
- coffee drinking

most common form of the disease is the formation of inflammatory plaques resulting in demyelination of axons within the CNS. In time (usually between 4 and 6 weeks) these inflammatory plaques resolve, the myelin sheath is repaired, and normal neuronal function returns. However, with repeated 'attacks' of demyelination, remyelination is incomplete, and axonal loss occurs, resulting in the patient accumulating long-term disability.

The cause of MS is still uncertain, although there is evidence that immune mediated mechanisms are involved, with both B-cells and T-cells implicated. There are both genetic and environmental risk factors for the disease. The disease is more common in identical twins than in non-identical twins, and the risk of developing MS if a sibling has the disease is between 3% and 5%, which is about 30–50 times higher than the background risk in the population. Considering environmental factors, the disease has a higher incidence in regions with a temperate climate. One explanation for this is that certain viruses found in these regions may trigger the disease. However, studies of EBV, measles, and various herpes viruses have yielded varying results, and there is still no firm evidence to implicate any specific infectious agent. Another explanation for the geographical distribution of the disease is that a lack of vitamin D is implicated in its pathogenesis. There is some recent evidence that adequate vitamin D levels can be protective against developing MS, but the mechanism for this effect is not clear, and it remains uncertain as to whether vitamin D supplementation can influence MS progression.

While there are no clearly identified interventions that can prevent a first episode of demyelination, there is now huge research effort directed towards immunomodulatory therapies that can reduce the chances of subsequent attacks. Currently, there are several immunosuppressive treatments, both IV and oral, that reduce the risk of relapses in the disease, and many studies in progress of immune modulators that show great promise in reducing the axonal loss and thus slow or prevent the axonal damage in the secondary progressive phase of the disease.

Prevention of infectious diseases of the brain

Prevention of bacterial meningitis

Other important causes globally of serious neurological disease are meningitis and encephalitis. Bacterial meningitis is, thankfully, not common in the developed world (i.e. its incidence is 3 per 100 000) but, worldwide, it is, particularly in sub-Saharan Africa, in the so-called 'meningitis belt', where epidemics affecting up to 800 per 100 000 have been reported. The main causes of bacterial meningitis in the UK are listed in Table 347.3. Untreated, bacterial meningitis is fatal. Overall, mortality from the disease in the UK is still about 10%.

The key to successful treatment in bacterial meningitis is to recognize the symptoms (i.e. rapid onset of generalized headache, fever, photophobia, and neck stiffness, with possibly a purpuric skin rash in meningococcal disease) and to treat promptly with high-dose, appropriate IV antibiotics. Often, the antibiotics used to treat are chosen empirically to cover a broad spectrum of organisms, and are

then later refined once the causative organism is identified from CSF analysis. The role of corticosteroid therapy in the treatment of meningitis has been the subject of intense debate. The consensus now is that adjuvant treatment with dexamethasone should be given just before the first dose of antibiotics and continued for 4 days. The benefit of such additional steroid therapy is probably greatest in those with pneumococcal disease. Some forms of bacterial meningitis, such as that due to the pneumococcus, are notifiable diseases, requiring reporting of the case to the relevant public health body. Close contacts of identified or suspected cases should be treated with prophylactic antibiotics, for example 2 days of oral rifampicin for close contacts of people with meningococcal meningitis, or 4 days of rifampicin and trimethoprim for contacts of haemophilus meningitis cases. However, although such prophylaxis reduces the risks of immediate infection with the disease, clearly this does not protect these individuals from future infections.

Key advances have been, and continue to be, made in vaccine development to prevent cases of bacterial meningitis. The Haemophilus influenzae type b (or Hib) vaccine is now used as part of routine childhood vaccination programmes in developed countries, as is the pneumococcal conjugate vaccine, which is active against seven of the common serotypes of the pathogen. Pneumococcal vaccination is often now also offered to those adults who have not had the vaccine in childhood but are living in close proximity to others (e.g. military recruits, students). There is also now a polyvalent vaccine, which is active against 23 serotypes of pneumococci, but its use tends to be reserved for specific high-risk groups, for example patients post splenectomy. Of great global importance has been the recent successful development of the MenAfriVac vaccine, a vaccine that is active against Group A meningococcus, a key organism responsible for bacterial meningitis in the 'meningitis belt'. This vaccine, which does not have to be refrigerated and thus can be efficiently delivered to those most at need, allows large numbers of people at risk to have effective vaccination for a year, at a cost of less than $1 a dose.

Prevention of cerebral malaria

Malaria is the world's most important parasitic disease, with 40% of the world's population living in endemic areas. Cerebral malaria, caused by the plasmodium falciparum parasite, is one of the most serious forms of malaria, with about a fifth of cases being fatal, and young children being particularly susceptible to severe infection. Of those who survive the acute illness, around 10% will have severe sequelae, such as hemiplegia, ataxia, seizures, or cognitive impairment. Preventive strategies against infection include the use of insecticide-treated mosquito nets, and indoor spraying of insecticide in endemic areas. Some drugs used to treat malaria can prevent contraction of the disease, and tend to be taken by visitors to endemic areas. These drugs, such as chloroquine, mefloquine, doxycycline, or a combination of atovaquone and proguanil, are not often taken by long-term residents in endemic areas. The drugs are expensive, they have side effects, particularly with long-term use, and there is also the issue that they may increase the scourge of drug resistance in the parasite.

Efforts have been underway for years to develop an effective and cheap malaria vaccine but, as yet, this remains elusive. Many commercial, charitable, and government-backed organizations are working towards this goal. The Malaria Vaccine Advisory Committee of the WHO has a landmark objective to 'develop and licence a first generation malaria vaccine that has protective efficacy against severe disease and death' by 2015.

Prevention and genetic neurological disease

In this chapter, we will also briefly mention genetic neurological disease, as the contribution of genetically mediated disease to overall neurological disease burden is high. There are a great many inherited single-gene disorders which have prominent neurological symptoms, while many other 'sporadic' neurological disorders have significant genetic susceptibility factors acting along with environmental influences.

With the possibility of a molecular diagnosis of a genetic neurological disorder such as Huntington's disease comes the opportunity for testing of relatives to determine carrier status. Huntington's disease,

Table 347.3	Causes of bacterial meningitis in the UK
Age of patient	**Organism**
Newborn	Group B streptococcus
	Escherichia coli
	Listeria
	Proteus mirabilis
3 months old to 17 years old	*Neisseria meningitidis*
	Pneumococcus
	Haemophilus influenzae
17–50 years old	Pneumococcus
	Neisseria meningitidis
Over 50 years old	Pneumococcus
	Listeria
	Gram-negative bacilli

an autosomal dominant disorder, usually presents in adult life with progressive cognitive changes and choreiform movements and there is currently no curative therapy. The age at onset is dependent on the specific number of expanded (CAG) trinucleotide repeats encoding glutamine residues within the huntingtin protein, which is encoded by HTT (chromosomal location 4p16.3). In considering prevention in Huntington's disease, it is possible to perform genetic testing of those at risk of this autosomal dominant disease. This is usually performed after extensive counselling through clinical genetics services and according to nationally agreed standardized protocols. If such carrier testing is performed before those carriers themselves have had children, they can then be offered options for prenatal diagnosis for subsequent pregnancies, with fetal tissue obtained through chorionic villous sampling. Previously, such prenatal diagnosis was performed based on analysis of linked genetic markers, with those genetic markers being typed in DNA samples from both parents and from the chorionic villous or amniotic fluid samples. Now, with direct mutation analysis possible, the fetal tissue can be directly screened for the expanded trinucleotide repeat, and families given direct information on the carrier status of the fetus.

A recent new development is that of pre-implantation genetic diagnosis, in which eggs and sperm are harvested from the parents, in vitro fertilization takes place, embryos are grown to the 8- or 16-cell stage, and then genetic analysis performed on 1 or 2 cells taken from these embryos. Subsequently, only those embryos that are free from the mutation are transplanted back into the mother's uterus, allowing the birth of a child free of the disease. Protocols have also been developed to allow individuals to have such pre-implantation genetic diagnosis without the parental genotypes being revealed to the parents. This 'non-disclosure' or 'exclusion testing' means that a couple can be guaranteed to have a child free from Huntington's but not have to learn if one of them is indeed a carrier themselves.

It should be emphasized that procedures for prenatal diagnosis are carefully regulated by law, and that couples who are proceeding with these procedures require extensive and appropriate counselling via clinical genetic services. The example of Huntington's disease has been used in this section as it was one of the first Mendelian neurological disorders for which carrier screening and prenatal diagnosis was widely adopted. The reader is referred to the website http://www.hfea.gov.uk/preimplantation-genetic-diagnosis.html for information on the very many other genetic diseases, many of them neurological, for which such pre-implantation genetic diagnosis has been given regulatory approval in the UK.

Lifestyle modifications for the prevention of neurological disease: alcohol and other substances of abuse

No chapter on the prevention of neurological disease would be complete without a consideration of some of the neurological effects of excessive alcohol and of other drugs of abuse. Current recommended levels of alcohol consumption in the UK are, for men, no more than 21 units per week, with no more than 4 units per day, and, for women, no more than 14 units per week, with no more than 3 units per day. Clearly, if excess alcohol consumption leads

Table 347.4 Some neurological manifestations of chronic excessive alcohol intake

Manifestation	Notes
Cognitive decline	May lead to frank dementia
Cerebellar dysfunction	
Peripheral neuropathy	Often painful
Wernicke's encephalopathy	Confusional state
Korsakoff's psychosis	Amnesia, executive dysfunction
Depression	
Seizures	
Alcoholic myopathy	Painful

to intoxication, there can be neurological sequelae consequent on trauma. Several studies have shown that head injuries in those who are intoxicated are more serious, with more damage evident on CT brain scanning, and greater memory and other neuropsychological impairments in the long term than in sober patients.

Table 347.4 lists some of the neurological disorders consequent on prolonged excessive alcohol consumption. While some of these disorders are partially reversible if an individual stops drinking alcohol, others are not, and treatments are only partially effective. The best approach in this case is, undoubtedly, prevention. While various government initiatives have been tried to encourage more responsible alcohol consumption, these have tended to focus on the acute consequences of intoxication (e.g. drink-driving campaigns) or the long-term consequences of liver disease. As listed in Table 347.4, alcohol excess can have many, varied consequences on the brain and peripheral nerves. One strategy that has clearly been shown to reduce excessive, prolonged drinking is for governments to tax alcohol heavily, but this is not a universally popular solution to the problem and so is often not implemented in democratic societies.

Other illegal substances of abuse can also have devastating long-term consequences on brain function. Cocaine and amphetamine use has been linked to increasing the risk of stroke. Much recent attention has focused on the possible link between marijuana use and subsequent cognitive decline. Particularly concerning is data that shows that those who were heavy users of marijuana before the age of 18 show mental decline even after stopping the drug, suggesting that use of the drug during adolescence can have long-term consequences on subsequent brain development.

Further Reading

GBD 2015 Neurological Disorders Collaborator Group. Global, regional, and national burden of neurological disorders during 1990–2015: a systematic analysis for the Global Burden of Disease Study 2015. *Lancet Neurol* 2017; 16: 877–97.

Gorelick PB, Testai F, Hankey G, et al. (eds). *Hankey's Clinical Neurology* (2nd edition), 2014. CRC Press.

Lindsay KW, Bone I, and Fuller G. *Neurology and Neurosurgery Illustrated* (5th edition), 2010. Churchill Livingstone.

Karen Morrison

Prevention of thromboembolic stroke

Stroke is the main cause of neurological morbidity in adults and the third most common cause of death worldwide after ischaemic heart disease and cancer (all forms combined). It is more common in older people, with three-quarters of strokes occurring in people over 65 years of age, and estimates are that overall stroke morbidity will double by the early 2020s. The worldwide figure of increasing incidence of stroke detection masks the fact that mortality from stroke has actually been falling in developed countries since the latter half of the twentieth century while the mortality has continued to rise in China, Asia, and eastern Europe. Although the incidence of stroke is greater in men that women in each decade, the absolute number of fatal strokes is greater in elderly women than men, reflecting the larger number of women in this population group.

As discussed in Chapter 227, the term 'stroke' denotes a neurological disease disorder, usually of abrupt onset, which lasts more than 24 hours, as a result of perturbation of the brain's blood supply. This disruption of blood supply is due to cerebral infarction in most (80%–85%) cases, with underlying causes that include atheroma, diabetes, smoking, obesity, and cardiac embolism, and due to cerebral haemorrhage (often as a result of underlying hypertension) in the remaining 15%–20% of cases. Other rare causes of stroke include specific types of stroke that occur during pregnancy, such as amniotic fluid embolism, stroke due to venous sinus thrombosis (the risk factors for which also include pregnancy and the puerperium, corticosteroid use, and various hypercoagulable states, including those associated with inflammatory bowel disease) and strokes due to substance misuse (particularly recognized with cocaine and amphetamine abuse). Box 348.1 lists some of the ischaemic stroke risk factors for which there is good or reasonably good evidence. For other factors, such as diet (high salt, or diets low in nutrients such as potassium, calcium, fresh fruit, or antioxidants such as vitamin C or E), type A behaviour, snoring, sleep apnoea, or dental disease, the evidence is less certain.

Despite the many risk factors for which there is reasonable evidence for a causative role in stroke, there is considerably less evidence for modification of these factors having a significant effect on incidence. The key preventive strategies, for which there is good data for reducing stroke risk, are listed in Box 348.2.

Clearly, the higher an individual's risk of having a stroke, the more they have to gain from prevention, so one strategy would be to concentrate efforts on reducing stroke risk in those at very high risk, as this could be perceived as being most 'cost-effective'. However, most strokes arise in people at moderate risk of stroke; so, at a population level, preventive measures should be introduced to all those at moderate risk too, as this will have a much greater effect on overall incidence. Specifically for hypertension, it has been estimated that treatment reduces an individual's risk of having a stroke by about 40% within 1 or 2 years of starting treatment. Individuals who have had a recent stroke or transient ischaemic attack (TIA) are at much higher absolute risk of stroke than the general population, so it is even more important that hypertension in these individuals is appropriately treated. Also, as the absolute risk of stroke increases with age, elderly patients with hypertension ought to be treated, as they stand to gain even more benefit, although they are also at higher risk of drug side effects. There is no good evidence to inform the decision as to when to start antihypertensive treatment following an acute stroke. Most physicians tend to wait for 1 or 2 weeks post stroke to start treatment, as there is some evidence that blood pressure can be elevated acutely secondary to stroke. Recent data suggests that variability in blood pressure is a key risk factor for stroke; thus, antihypertensive therapies that reduce this variability, such as angiotensin-converting-enzyme

inhibitors, may have a greater effect in preventing stroke than the traditional therapies of diuretics and beta blockers. All ischaemic stroke and TIA patients should be advised to reduce their dietary intake of saturated fat and, on the basis of recent evidence from large trials, to take statin therapy. In addition to lowering blood lipids, statins also reduce variability in blood pressure, and this may account for some of their benefit in stroke prevention.

Several large trials have clearly shown the benefit of antiplatelet therapy in secondary prevention of stroke following a stroke or TIA. Aspirin, 75 mg daily for life, is the antiplatelet therapy of first choice,

---

Box 348.1 Risk factors for ischaemic strokes

Potentially modifiable or treatable

- hypertension: stroke risk is increased with both raised diastolic and systolic blood pressure, with isolated systolic hypertension, and with visit-to-visit variability in systolic blood pressure
- The WHO estimates that 62% of all strokes are attributable to hypertension
- diabetes: in addition to increasing the risk of stroke, people with diabetes are more likely to die if they suffer a stroke, compared to non-diabetics
- previous stroke or transient ischaemic attack
- smoking
- excess alcohol consumption
- obesity
- oral contraceptive use (particularly if the patient also suffers migraine with aura)
- blood lipoprotein disorders, although the relationship of stroke with raised plasma total cholesterol, increased LDL cholesterol, and decreased HDL cholesterol is less clear than with coronary artery disease
- cardiac disease (e.g. atrial fibrillation)
- lack of physical exercise
- plasma fibrinogen levels: strongly associated with stroke incidence but may be due to confounding with several of the factors listed in this section

Non-modifiable

- age: increased incidence with age
- gender: increased incidence in males, although much less excess compared with coronary events and peripheral vascular disease; equal sex incidence in the very young and the very old
- family history of vascular disease
- race: higher incidence in black populations than in white populations, and greater incidence in people of Pacific origin than in those of European origin (certainly, in people **living** in Western countries; there is a dearth of incidence data from South Asia, South East Asia, Africa, and South America)

Box 348.2 Key preventive strategies in ischaemic stroke

- treat hypertension
- maintain good diabetic control
- treat atrial fibrillation with warfarin or novel anticoagulants
- give aspirin following acute stroke
- stop smoking
- lower plasma cholesterol

as it is effective, safe, and inexpensive. In one large study, immediate antiplatelet therapy following acute ischaemic stroke reduced the chances of a vascular event (myocardial infarction, angina, stroke, TIA) by 11%, corresponding to the avoidance of 12 events for every 1000 patients treated for 1 month. In those with a past history of stroke or TIA, antiplatelet drugs reduced the risk of subsequent vascular events from 22% to 18%, equivalent to avoiding 37 serious vascular events per 1000 patients treated over 3 years. Clopidogrel is equally effective for secondary stroke prevention, and is recommended for patients intolerant of aspirin. The combination of aspirin and dipyridamole is slightly more effective than aspirin alone, but there is little data to support its cost-effectiveness; thus, aspirin alone is the antiplatelet therapy of choice. Anticoagulation with warfarin is indicated for most patients with TIA or ischaemic stroke who are in atrial fibrillation, provided that there are no contraindications, such as recent gastrointestinal bleeding, a history of uncontrolled hypertension, or alcoholic liver disease, or where there is difficulty with access to a reliable anticoagulation clinic.

Considering primary stroke prevention, recent meta-analyses show no evidence for a reduction in total stroke in people who are at low risk (asymptomatic, no vascular risk factors, no history of previous symptomatic vascular disease) with aspirin therapy, so this is not recommended.

Prevention of cerebral haemorrhage

Cerebral haemorrhage accounts for about one-fifth of all strokes, and over 90% of cases of cerebral haemorrhage are due to rupture of intracranial aneurysms. Aneurysmal subarachnoid haemorrhage has a poor prognosis. Over 40% of people die within a month of admission to hospital and, of those who survive, half are left severely disabled. Risk factors for the presence of aneurysms include smoking, alcohol consumption, hypertension, and a family history of the disorder. Preventive strategies to reduce the incidence

include tackling risk factors if possible, and screening to identify and treat aneurysms prior to rupture. Estimates for the annual risk of bleeding from unruptured aneurysms vary greatly, depending on assumptions and biases in different studies, and range from 1 in 20 to 1 in 200. The risk is greater for aneurysms greater than 10 mm in diameter, for symptomatic aneurysms, and for those detected in the posterior circulation, so these are probably the aneurysms to target for intervention, either by intra-arterial coiling of the aneurysm (the preferred procedure) or by neurosurgical clipping of the aneurysmal neck.

Specific issues arise in advice regarding screening relatives of those with a family history of ruptured intracranial aneurysms. The general view is to offer screening, either by MRI or CT scanning, to detect unruptured intracranial aneurysms in families with two or more first-degree relatives affected by subarachnoid haemorrhage. There is no clear data to inform the answer to the question of how frequently scanning should be repeated in those at risk.

Further Reading

Freedman B, Potpara TS, and Lip GYH. Atrial fi brillation 1 stroke prevention in atrial fi brillation. *Lancet* 2016; 388: 806–17

Grotta JC. Carotid stenosis. *N Engl J Med* 2013; 369: 1143–50.

Intercollegiate Stroke Working Party. *National Clinical Guideline for Stroke* (4th edition), 2012. Royal College of Physicians.

Kernan WN, Ovbiagele B, Black HR, et al. Guidelines for the prevention of stroke in patients with stroke and transient ischemic attack: A guideline for healthcare professionals from the American Heart Association/American Stroke Association. *Stroke* 2014; 45: 2160–236.

Meschia JF, Bushnell C, Boden-Albala B, et al. Guidelines for the primary prevention of stroke: A statement for healthcare professionals from the American Heart Association/American Stroke Association. *Stroke* 2014; 45: 3754–832.

349 Prevention of infection

Tony Bentley

Introduction

Medicine is the science of diagnosing, treating, and preventing disease; its focus is the needs of an individual patient. Public health is the science and practice of protecting and improving the health of a community—medicine on a larger scale. The aim of government should be to create the health and happiness of its people. Politics is, therefore, public health medicine on a grand scale. Likewise, prevention of infection can be seen as an individual issue, a population issue, or a global issue. The principles of prevention of infection, whether at the level of the individual patient or at the level of a population, are the avoidance of infectious agents, the maintenance of innate immunity, and the stimulation of acquired immunity.

Cholera: Prevention of infection by the application of engineering in support of public health

The cholera bacterium is a member of the genus *Vibrio*. Vibrios are Gram-negative bacteria that live in surface water and occur in both marine and freshwater habitats. The two most important pathogens in this genus are *Vibrio cholerae* and *Vibrio parahaemolyticus*.

Asiatic cholera, or epidemic cholera, occurs when *Vibrio cholerae* is transmitted to humans from contaminated water or food. Currently, the most widely distributed strain is *Vibrio cholerae* O139 'Bengal'. The toxin produced by *Vibrio cholerae* binds to the epithelial cells of the mucosal lining of the small intestine. Part of the toxin then becomes detached and is taken into the cell by endocytosis; there, it acts by switching on production of cyclic AMP. The massive secretion of water and electrolytes that then occurs can result in severe and rapid dehydration.

The prevention of cholera and many other waterborne infections is by proper sanitation. Sanitation can be considered to be a way of promoting the health of a population through hygiene, thereby preventing contact with the hazards associated with waste. Human health can be affected by waste arising from human and animal faeces, domestic wastewater, and industrial and agricultural waste. In addition to bacteria and viruses, there are other hazards in waste, including other biological or chemical causes of disease. The hygienic measures used to prevent infection include engineering solutions such as latrines and septic tanks, closed drainage systems, and sewerage and wastewater treatment.

In the management of a cholera outbreak, hygiene begins with the proper management of affected patients, as large numbers of *Vibrio cholerae* bacilli are excreted in their faeces. Proper disposal of faecal material and contaminated clothing and bedclothes is essential. Environmental cleaning and handwashing with soap and water must accompany this.

Polio: Prevention of infection by science and political will

Polioviruses are members of the enterovirus group, infecting, and being shed from, the gastrointestinal tract of humans. Paralytic poliomyelitis occurs in approximately 1% of individuals infected by the poliovirus, as a consequence of chance viral spread to the CNS, and consequent neuronal damage. Major epidemics of polio began in Europe and the US in the last decades of the nineteenth century. As polio became one of the most feared diseases of childhood during the twentieth century, a race to develop an effective vaccine began.

For a vaccine to be successful, sufficient immunity needs to be produced to efficiently prevent disease and to block person-to-person spread. Two vaccines are now being used throughout the world in a concerted attempt to eradicate polio under the WHO Global Polio Eradication Initiative launched in 1988. The inactivated virus vaccine (the Salk vaccine) produces protective levels of antibody to all three serotypes of poliovirus after two injections, in more than 90% of individuals. The attenuated oral vaccine (the Sabin vaccine) multiplies in the gut lymphoid tissue and produces immunity to all three virus serotypes in approximately 95% of individuals after three doses. Oral polio vaccine is inexpensive and easy to administer but may, in 1 in 750 000 recipients, revert to a neurovirulent form.

By the end of 2006, only four countries remained (Nigeria, India, Pakistan, and Afghanistan) which had never interrupted endemic transmission of wild poliovirus. In February 2006, epidemics occurred in Yemen and Indonesia, which were successfully stopped. Globally in 2006, fewer than 2000 cases were reported.

Blood-borne viruses: Lifestyle, and the development of modern pandemics

Hepatitis B virus (HBV), hepatitis C virus (HCV), and HIV have much in common in the way they are transmitted from person to person (i.e. via sexual transmission, vertical transmission (from mother to baby), transmission by injecting drug use, and transmission by certain healthcare practices). The contribution of each of these modes of spread varies between the three.

HBV is thought to have infected 2 billion people worldwide, causing up to 1 million deaths each year by cirrhosis and hepatocellular carcinoma. In developing countries, particularly in Asia and Africa, HBV infection is usually acquired perinatally or in childhood. When acquired at a young age, HBV infection is more likely to become chronic, thus putting further generations at risk from mother-to-infant transmission. In the West, HBV infection is more commonly caught in adulthood as a consequence of sexual transmission or injecting drug use. These modes of transmission, of course, also exist in developing countries, as do those within healthcare settings, such as contaminated surgical instruments, unscreened blood transfusions, and, in particular, unsafe injection practice using contaminated needles.

Hepatitis B vaccination has been available for over 25 years. It was the first vaccine introduced with the specific aim of preventing a cancer and has been highly successful in reducing mother-to-infant transmission (e.g. in Taiwan, where the first national vaccination programme was initiated in 1984). In Italy, HBV vaccine was first recommended and then made compulsory for both infants and adolescents, resulting in a significant decline in the incidence of acute HBV infection in young adults.

HCV was discovered in 1989. It is a cause of both acute and chronic hepatitis and is now recognized as the leading cause of liver transplantation in the developed world. HCV has a worldwide distribution but, like HBV, has higher seroprevalence rates in Asia and Africa. Seroprevalence rates vary from country to country (e.g. 0.9% in India, 3.2% in China, and 22% in Egypt). Seroprevalence surveys in the US have revealed how the incidence has decreased in recent decades to an overall rate of approximately 0.2%. In Western countries, the majority of infections occur as a result of injecting drug use, particularly in those sharing preparation equipment. HCV infection usually occurs rapidly after the start of injecting use behaviour. Thus, in long-term injecting drug users, rates can be as high as 60%–90%. A combination of donor selection, avoidance of non-voluntary (i.e. paid) donors, and the screening of blood donations for HCV ensure the safety of blood supplies in those countries that can afford these measures.

HIV arose, probably early in the twentieth century, as a consequence of genetic reassortment in wild chimps in Africa co-infected with two distinct simian immunodeficiency viruses. The new virus had the capacity to infect humans and probably did so as a consequence of the killing and consumption of chimps as bushmeat. Human-to-human transmission of HIV is predominantly by sexual transmission. In Africa, the virus was spread along main truck routes by the interactions of drivers and prostitutes. Transfer around the world most likely occurred by workers and other travellers returning from Central Africa to places such as Haiti and the US. Once introduced into relatively closed but promiscuous communities, such as the gay community in San Francisco in the early 1980s, significant spread occurred. As a consequence, the associated illnesses caused by the immunodeficiency induced by HIV were recognized, the acquired immunodeficiency syndrome (AIDS) defined, and the virus isolated and identified. Other means of transmission of HIV that contributed to its global spread include the manufacture of factor VIII, which is used for the treatment of haemophiliacs, from pooled donor blood and, as for HBV and HCV, injecting drug abuse, and the use of contaminated needles in healthcare settings.

Healthcare-associated infection: The failure of modern medicine to prevent infection

Over the past 5 years, healthcare-associated infection has come to the top of the agendas of both politicians and those responsible for hospital accreditation in the UK and many other countries. The term 'healthcare-associated infection' now refers to infections associated with healthcare wherever it is delivered, and the term 'hospital-acquired infection' is no longer considered appropriate. Most of the focus of recent political initiatives, however, remains on *Clostridium difficile*-associated diarrhoea and bloodstream infections due to MRSA.

Significant success has been achieved in reducing the incidence of both *Clostridium difficile*-associated diarrhoea and MRSA bacteraemias as a consequence of this political pressure. Two questions need to be asked. Why was it that, almost 150 years after the era of Ignaz Semmelweis, Joseph Lister, and Florence Nightingale, did it require political interference in healthcare to deliver these improvements, and have those efforts been too narrowly focused and allowed other healthcare-associated infections to remain unchecked?

MRSA

MRSA was first reported in 1961 very soon after the introduction of methicillin into clinical practice. It was not until the early 1980s that outbreaks of MRSA with epidemic potential were first recognized. These were subject, in the early days, to attempted containment based on an aggressive search-and-destroy strategy. Control of the spread of generally virulent, potentially epidemic, MRSA is important, as these isolates are not susceptible to the cheap and effective antibiotics that are commonly used for both prophylaxis and treatment of a wide range of common infections.

In attempting to control MRSA, it should be remembered that, first and foremost, MRSA is a strain of *Staphylococcus aureus*. As a bacterium, *Staphylococcus aureus* is well adapted to the human body, colonizing the anterior nares, the groin, and the perineum in up to 30% of the population. It has the capacity to spread from person to person. The possession of virulence factors means that it remains potentially pathogenic, capable of causing a range of infections, from superficial cutaneous infection to septicaemia. Many strains of MRSA have characteristics (e.g. adhesion, dispersal, and survival within the environment) that make for potential epidemic spread. This has led to rapid local, regional, and global spread of certain clones. Sixteen such clones have been characterized in the UK, including EMRSA-3, EMRSA-15, and EMRSA-16.

The first stage of controlling an MRSA outbreak is to ensure it is known which patients are colonized or infected with MRSA. This is achieved by opportunistically screening appropriate patients (e.g. on admission to hospital). Any screening programme needs to be supported by the maintenance of a database linked to the hospital's patient administration system, for future episodes of care. Patients who are at high-risk of MRSA colonization and could be cost-effectively screened include those with a prior history of MRSA carriage; the elderly; those with multiple previous hospital admissions; those with skin damage (ulceration or surgical wounds); those being admitted from nursing or residential homes; and those being admitted to high-risk clinical environments, such as elective orthopaedics, vascular surgery, and augmented care. The carriage rate of MRSA within these groups in the UK is approximately 7%. The cost-effectiveness of a wider screening programme which was recently adopted in England and includes all admissions to hospital, including those attending for day case surgery, is less likely to be cost-effective. The carriage rate in this wider population is approximately 0.7%–1.0%.

Once the patients have been identified, the risk of spread needs to be reduced by prompt patient isolation, application of a decolonization protocol (e.g. nasal mupirocin and anti-staphylococcal body wash), reduction of patient movement, and effective hand hygiene. Other patients within a clinical environment should have their risk of acquiring MRSA reduced by reducing the incidence of unnecessary IV devices, urinary catheters, and wound manipulation, as well as unnecessary antibiotic exposure. MRSA bacteraemias that do occur should be subject to a root cause analysis to understand why the event happened and to ensure lessons can be learnt.

It is often quoted that about 40% of *Staphylococcus aureus* bacteraemias (SABs) in the UK are caused by MRSA. This figure was based on data, reported voluntarily to the UK's Health Protection Agency, for 1999–2003. The data also shows that the number of methicillin-sensitive SABs continued to increase between 2003 and 2007, while the absolute number and overall percentage of MRSA bacteraemias has fallen as a consequence of the MRSA-focused efforts. It is important to note both that the majority of SABs are acquired in the community and that the majority of SABs are healthcare associated. The most common healthcare-associated sources of SAB are vascular catheters and wounds, skin and soft tissue infections, and catheter-related urosepsis.

SAB is associated with a significant mortality, which is higher in both community-acquired bacteraemia and MRSA bacteraemia. In order to effectively reduce healthcare-associated SABs, a joint acute/community strategy focusing on all strains of *Staphylococcus aureus*, rather than MRSA in isolation, will be required.

Clostridium difficile-associated diarrhoea

Diphtheritic colitis, or pseudomembranous colitis, has been recognized for over 100 years. However, in the first half of the twentieth century, cases were uncommon, and the cause was not understood. Following the introduction of broad-spectrum antibiotics (particularly tetracyclines and chloramphenicol) into medical practice in the early 1950s, the number of case reports increased. A further increase in incidence was seen in the late 1960s but was attributed to the use of lincomycin and clindamycin. In the 1970s, the causal link with toxins produced by *Clostridium difficile* was made. Despite an understanding of the pathogenesis of *Clostridium difficile*-associated diarrhoea, there was a continued rise in cases in the years between 1990 and 2004, punctuated by several very significant local and regional epidemics.

Although colonization of the gastrointestinal tract by *Clostridium difficile* is via an environmental source, *Clostridium difficile*-associated diarrhoea occurs when the normal bacterial flora is disturbed by antibiotics, and overgrowth of *Clostridium difficile* occurs. The release of *Clostridium difficile* toxin A (an enterotoxin) and *Clostridium difficile* toxin B (a cytotoxin) causes disease of varying severity, ranging from mild diarrhoea to fulminant pseudomembranous colitis and perforation. Currently implicated antibiotics include third-generation cephalosporins (e.g. cefuroxime) and quinolones (e.g. ciprofloxacin).

To ensure patient safety, the control of *Clostridium difficile* requires the implementation of a range of actions. The complete care bundle includes:

- active case surveillance by nursing and medical staff
- the provision of a rapid diagnostic testing service
- prompt isolation of patients, in single rooms, cohort bays, or isolation wards, as justified by the number of cases
- enhanced environmental cleaning using a combination of a detergent and chlorine-based disinfectant

- appropriate use of personal protective equipment, and increased hand hygiene using soap and water
- active case management to reduce duration of symptoms and excretion of spores, by using appropriate therapeutic antibiotics (e.g. oral metronidazole or vancomycin) and nutritional support
- aggressive antibiotic stewardship:
  - right drug–right indication
  - avoidance of broad-spectrum agents
  - minimum duration
  - single-dose prophylaxis
  - monitoring overall consumption
- adequate discharge information to future carers, to reduce the risk of recurrence, which can occur in up to 20% of cases

Further Reading

Harris JB, LaRocque RC, Qadri F, et al. Cholera. *Lancet* 2012; 379: 2466–76.

Leffler DA and Lamont JT. *Clostridium difficile* infection. *N Engl J Med* 2015; 372: 1539–48.

National Institute for Health and Care Excellence. *Infection Prevention and Control*. 2014. Available at http://www.nice.org.uk/guidance/qs61/resources/guidance-infection-prevention-and-control-pdf (accessed 20 Sep 2017).

Trepo C, Chan HLY, and Lok A. Hepatitis B virus infection. *Lancet* 2014; 384: 2053–63.

350 Prevention of cancer

Warren Grant and Martin Scott-Brown

Introduction

In the UK, the four commonest cancers—lung cancer, breast cancer, colon cancer, and prostate cancer—result in around 62 000 deaths every year. Although deaths from cancer have fallen in the UK over the last 20 years, the UK still suffers from higher cancer death rates than many other countries in Western Europe. In 1999, the UK government produced a White Paper called *Saving Lives: Our Healthier Nation* that outlined a national target to reduce the death rate from cancer by at least 20% in people under 75 by 2010. The subsequent NHS Cancer Plan of 2000 designed a framework by which to achieve this target through effective prevention, screening, and treatment programmes as well as restructuring and developing new diagnostic and treatment facilities. But do we know enough about the biology of the development of cancer for government health policies alone to force dramatic changes in survival? The science behind the causes of cancer tells us that its origin lies in acquired or inherited genetic abnormalities. Inherited gene mutation syndromes and exposure to environmental mutagens cause cancer, largely through abnormalities in DNA repair mechanisms, leading to uncontrolled cell proliferation. Although screening those thought to be at highest risk, and regulating exposure to environmental carcinogens such as tobacco or ionizing radiation have, and will continue to reduce cancer deaths, there are many other environmental factors that have been shown to increase the population risk of cancer. These will be outlined in this chapter. However, the available evidence is largely from retrospective and cross-sectional population-based studies and therefore limits our ability to apply this knowledge to the risk of the individual patient we may see in clinic. Although we may be able to put him or her into a high-, intermediate-, or low-risk category, the question 'will I get cancer, doc?' is one that we cannot answer with certainty.

The NHS Cancer Plan of 2000, designed to reduce cancer deaths in this country and to bring UK treatment results in line with those other countries in Europe, focuses on preventing malignancy as part of its comprehensive cancer management strategy. It highlights that the rich are less likely to develop cancer, and will survive longer if they are diagnosed than those who live in poverty. This may reflect available treatment options, but is more likely to be related to the lifestyle of those with regular work, as these may be more health aware. The Cancer Plan, however, suggests that relieving poverty may be more labour intensive and less rewarding than encouraging positive risk-reducing behaviour in all members of the population.

Eating well can reduce the risk of developing many cancers, particularly of the stomach and bowel. The Cancer Plan outlines the 'Five-a-Day' programme which was rolled out in 2002, and encouraged people to eat at least five portions of fruit and vegetables per day. Obese people are also at higher risk of cancers, in particular endometrial cancer. A good diet and regular exercise not only reduce obesity but are also independent risk-reducing factors. Alcohol misuse is thought to be a major risk factor in around 3% of all cancers, with the highest risk for cancers of the mouth and throat. As part of the Cancer Plan, the Department of Health promotes physical activity and general health programmes, as well as alcohol and smoking programmes particularly in deprived areas.

Focusing on these healthy lifestyle points highlighted can potentially reduce an individual lifetime risk of all cancers. However, our knowledge of the biology of four cancers in particular has led to the development of specific life-saving interventions. Outlined in this chapter are details regarding ongoing prevention strategies for carcinomas of the lung, the breast, the bowel, and the cervix.

Lung cancer

Cancer of the bronchus is the leading cause of cancer death in both men and women in the UK. Its incidence currently stands at 82 per 100 000 males, and 50 per 100 000 females. Several etiological factors have been identified, including ionizing radiation, asbestos, and other industrial pollutants but, by far, the leading causative factor is tobacco smoking. Tobacco products gained favour in the returning soldiers of the First World War. Since then, a significant age-related trend in deaths from lung cancer in men has developed. In the last 50 years, more women have taken up the habit, and thus their death rates have increased over time. Despite other cancers, such as breast cancer, being more commonly diagnosed in women, lung cancer remains the commonest cause of cancer death in women in the UK. In 2000 there were 38 400 new cases of lung cancer in men and women in the UK, and 33 600 deaths from the disease.

How can we prevent lung cancer?

In 1954, Doll and Hill established that, in British doctors, the fall in death rates from lung cancer was linked to smoking cessation: after 12 years of non-smoking, the risk of lung cancer was almost as low as that for those who had never smoked, except for those who had smoked >20 cigarettes a day, as the risk never fell to this low level in that group. Doll and Hill's work has led to several government initiatives to reduce population exposure to tobacco smoke. The carcinogens in tobacco smoke cause mutations in many genes, but current research suggests a significant effect on TP53, a key tumour suppressor gene that recognizes DNA damage and initiates apoptosis.

In the UK, it is currently illegal to smoke in public places. There is also a ban on tobacco advertising and a tight control on taxation and sale of tobacco products. In local communities, smoking cessation clinics have been developed in general practice, and workplace cessation programmes have also been rolled out.

Fifty years after his first publication, and as the knowledge of the link between tobacco and carcinogenesis had grown, Doll wrote a seminal paper showing that younger populations, who had lower numbers of heavy smokers, had significantly reduced their risk of developing lung cancer. With tobacco smoking now much less of a social activity, and much more expensive than it ever was, it is hoped that this effect will spread to the entire population and that the incidence of lung cancer will continue to fall in the years to come.

Breast cancer

In the UK, breast cancer affects approximately 11% of women. It is the commonest cancer in women, accounting for 30% of all cancer diagnoses. Up to 10% of patients may inherit breast cancer because of dominant genetic mutations. Two of the commonest genetic errors, which account for 80% of the inherited cases, are those that affect the BRCA1 and BRCA2 genes. There are likely to be other risky genetic abnormalities, and tests for some of them have been combined into disease screening programmes in the US. However, 90% of breast cancer cases appear sporadically, with no detectable inherited cause. These sporadic cases are more common in women of older age. Risk factors include early onset of menstruation, late menopause, and later first pregnancy. Chronic systemic exposure to exogenous oestrogens (e.g. oral contraceptives or hormone replacement therapy) does increase the risk of breast cancer but only by adding a further 6 cases per 1000 women. Those who stop taking the oral contraceptives or hormone replacement therapy return to the baseline risk after a period of 10 years.

How can we prevent breast cancer?

Women thought to be at high risk of developing breast cancer, most commonly due to known genetic mutations, should be counselled for bilateral mastectomy. This would aim to reduce their risk of breast cancer by around 90%. Modern surgical techniques can yield tissue reconstructions of identical size and shape. The use of chemoprevention in these high-risk cases is less clear. Trials using tamoxifen have not produced consistent results. A recent placebo-controlled trial in the UK that recruited around 2 500 women with a family history of breast cancer showed no difference in the incidence of breast cancer between the tamoxifen and placebo arms at 6 years from randomization. Although a much larger American trial of 13 000 women was stopped early because of a significant benefit in the tamoxifen arm, there was also a significant increase in the incidence of thromboembolic side effects. The use of raloxifene has also been investigated in postmenopausal women, with a suggestion of some protective effect. Again, an increased risk in thromboembolic events was seen.

Despite our knowledge of genetic and environmental causes of breast cancer, the single most powerful tool in preventing breast cancer deaths is its early detection and treatment, rather than its prevention. The UK breast cancer screening programme, first set up in 1988, will save 1250 lives per year by 2010, and involves an invitation to undergo bilateral two-view mammography for all women between the ages of 50–70. The programme will soon be extended to those aged 47–73. Since screening was introduced, the incidence of breast cancer has risen from around 80 in 100 000 per year to nearly 100 in 100 000 per year but the death rate from it has fallen from 40 in 100 000 per year to around 30 in 100 000 per year.

Colorectal cancer

Colorectal cancer is the second most common cancer (after lung) in terms of incidence and mortality in England and Wales and is commoner in men than in women. Each year, around 30 000 people in England will be diagnosed with cancers of the colon or rectum, and 13 000 will die of these diseases. Those with a family history have a significantly increased risk of developing colorectal cancer themselves, and around 5% of cases have identifiable genetic abnormalities conferring a very high risk of contracting the disease. Patients with familial adenomatous poliposis have hundreds of colonic polyps and will inevitably develop cancer before the age of 40 unless the colon is removed. Those with hereditary non-polyposis colorectal cancer are likely to develop cancer at a young age, presenting with abdominal pain or rectal bleeding, but are less likely to develop polyps.

Other risk factors for colorectal carcinoma are likely to relate to chronic inflammation and the disordered structure of the mucosal crypts on the surface of the bowel. Patients with inflammatory bowel disease have an increased risk of developing colorectal cancer, and this risk is proportional in magnitude to the duration of the diagnosis. Lifestyle and diet are environmental factors that are thought to explain some of the geographic differences in the incidence of bowel cancer. Fewer than 2 cases per 100 000 people are seen in India, rising to 55 per 100 000 men in New Zealand. Higher socio-economic class, smoking, and diets rich in processed meats and low in fibre are thought to be key risk factors.

How can we prevent colorectal cancer?

Modifying environmental factors may prevent cancer diagnoses in some patients. Non-smoking, healthy-eating, active-living individuals are less likely to die from colon cancer by a factor of between 2 and 8. There is also some limited evidence to suggest that those who add folic acid or selenium to their diets may have lower rates of colon cancer. Recent evidence has also suggested that regular aspirin may act as a chemoprotective agent, by inhibiting the COX-1 and COX-2 enzymes and suppressing polyp formation. The targeted COX-2 inhibitors such as celecoxib may also have a role in chemoprevention but worries about cardiac toxicity have slowed research in this area.

Colon cancer is curable in over 80% of patients if caught early, compared with less than 40% if lymph nodes contain metastatic deposits at the time of diagnosis. With this in mind, the National Bowel Cancer Programme was set up as a government initiative to reduce deaths from colon cancer in 2003. Its three constituent parts were the development of a national screening programme, the streamlining of care for symptomatic patients, and the improvement of access to treatment. After many years of evaluating the appropriate screening test to use and which people are most likely to benefit, the UK's bowel screening programme currently asks all men and women between ages 60 and 69 to provide a stool sample for occult blood testing every 2 years. Those with a positive test result will go on to have further examination by colonoscopy. It is hoped that this scheme alone will reduce cancer deaths by 16%.

Cervical cancer

Squamous carcinoma of the cervix is a relatively rare cancer in the UK. Its incidence is around 12 per 100 000 women, with 4 per 100 000 dying of the disease each year. However, it is probably one of the most preventable of all the carcinomas. In 2008 Dr Harald zur Hausen of the German Cancer Research Centre in Heidelberg received the Nobel Prize in Medicine for discovering the link between HPV, a double-stranded DNA virus, and cervical cancer. HPV positivity is seen in virtually all of the 500 000 worldwide cases reported annually, particularly serotypes 16, 18, 31, and 45. Once a cell is infected, if the viral DNA is not cleared by a functioning DNA repair mechanism, sections of it are incorporated into human DNA and interfere with the function of the tumour suppressor genes TP53 and RB.

How can we prevent cervical cancer?

HPV is a sexually transmitted infection. Sexual abstinence offers almost 100% protection against developing cervical carcinoma. Cervical screening has been offered on the NHS in the form of smear test to all women between the ages of 25 and 64 since 1988. This facilitated diagnosis and treatment of early precancerous lesions: cervical intra-epithelial neoplasia I–III. It is estimated that the screening programme alone saves 5000 lives a year. In 2008 the UK introduced a national HPV vaccine campaign aiming to prevent infection in young girls before they become sexually active. The vaccine, Cervarix ®, is a bivalent agent targeted against HPV-16 and HPV-18 virus-like particles and is routinely offered to girls in Year 8 (aged 12–13). Together with a one-off 'catch-up' vaccination campaign that will target 17- and 18-year-old girls from autumn 2009, and continuation of the cervical screening programme, cervical carcinoma may be eliminated from the UK over the course of the next 50 years. Cervical adenocarcinoma currently accounts for 10%–15% of cervical cancer cases. It does not have the same link to HPV and is likely to persist. In sub-Saharan Africa, where cervical cancer is common and there is largely no framework for national screening programmes, the role of HPV vaccination or one-off HPV testing is currently being investigated as a preventive strategy.

Further Reading

American Cancer Society: *Breast Cancer Prevention and Early Detection* (http://www.cancer.org/acs/groups/cid/documents/webcontent/003165-pdf.pdf)

American Cancer Society: *Cervical Cancer Prevention and Early Detection* (http://www.cancer.org/acs/groups/cid/documents/webcontent/003167-pdf.pdf)

American Cancer Society: *Colorectal Cancer Prevention and Early Detection* (http://www.cancer.org/acs/groups/cid/documents/webcontent/003170-pdf.pdf)

American Cancer Society: *Lung Cancer Prevention and Early Detection* (http://www.cancer.org/acs/groups/cid/documents/webcontent/acspc-039558-pdf.pdf)

American Cancer Society: *Prostate Cancer Prevention and Early Detection* (http://www.cancer.org/acs/groups/cid/documents/webcontent/003182-pdf.pdf)

Department of Health. *The NHS Cancer Plan: A Plan for Investment, A Plan for Reform*, 2000. Department of Health.

Kushi LH, Doyle C, McCullough M, et al. American Cancer Society guidelines on nutrition and physical activity for cancer prevention. *CA: Cancer J Clin* 2012; 62: 30–67.

PART 19

Screening for disease

Amitava Banerjee and Kaleab Asrress

Introduction

Screening involves testing asymptomatic individuals who have risk factors, or individuals who are in the early stages of a disease, in order to decide whether further investigation, clinical intervention, or treatment is warranted. Therefore, screening is classically a primary prevention strategy which aims to capture disease early in its course, but it can also involve secondary prevention in individuals with established disease. In the words of Geoffrey Rose, screening is a 'population' strategy. Examples of screening programmes are blood pressure monitoring in primary care to screen for hypertension, and ultrasound examination to screen for abdominal aortic aneurysm.

The effectiveness and feasibility of screening are influenced by several factors. First, the diagnostic accuracy of the screening test in question is crucial. For example, exercise ECG testing, although widely used, is not recommended in the current National Institute for Health and Care Excellence (NICE) guidelines for the investigation of chest pain, due to having low sensitivity and specificity in the detection of coronary heart disease (National Institute for Health and Care Excellence, 2010). Moreover, exercise ECG testing has even lower diagnostic accuracy in asymptomatic patients with coronary heart disease. Figure 351.1 shows an analysis from a recent systematic review of prospective diagnostic accuracy studies of exercise stress testing for coronary artery disease. A positive likelihood ratio quantifies the likelihood of presence of disease if a test is positive; by convention, a positive likelihood ratio ≥5 constitutes a clinically useful diagnostic test. Conversely, a negative likelihood ratio quantifies the likelihood of absence of disease if a test is negative; a negative likelihood ratio ≤0.2 is acceptable.

Second, physical and financial resources influence the decision to screen. For example, the cost and the effectiveness of CT coronary angiography and other new imaging modalities to assess coronary vasculature must be weighed against the cost of existing investigations (e.g. coronary angiography) and the need for new equipment and staff training and recruitment. Finally, the safety of the investigation is an important factor, and patient preferences and physician preferences should be taken into consideration. However, while non-invasive screening examinations are preferable from the point of view of patients and clinicians, sometimes invasive screening tests

may be required at a later stage in order to give a definitive diagnosis (e.g. pressure wire studies to measure fractional flow reserve in a coronary artery).

The WHO's principles of screening, first formulated in 1968, are still very relevant today (Box 351.1). Decision analysis has led to 'pathways' which guide investigation and treatment within screening programmes. There is increasing recognition that there are shared risk factors and shared preventive and treatment strategies for vascular disease, regardless of arterial territory. The concept of 'vascular medicine' has gained credence, leading to opportunistic screening in other vascular territories if an individual presents with disease in one territory. For example, post-myocardial infarction patients have higher incidence of cerebrovascular and peripheral arterial disease, so carotid duplex scanning and measurement of the ankle–brachial pressure index may be valid screening approaches for arterial disease in other territories.

Screening for risk factors for cardiovascular disease

Risk factors for cardiovascular disease have been discussed in Chapter 86, and are summarized in Box 351.2. In Table 351.1, the effects and costs of various interventions for primary prevention interventions in cardiovascular disease are outlined. For example, aspirin therapy, lipid-lowering therapy, and blood-pressure-lowering therapy reduce the 1-year risk of coronary heart disease by 18%, 30%, and 15%, respectively, at costs of £26, £437, and £109, respectively. Primary prevention involves (i) population approaches to address behavioural risk factors (e.g. smoking, diet), emphasizing surveillance, education, and health policy interventions, and (ii) the individualized treatment of risk factors (e.g. hypertension). Opportunistic screening for risk factors can form part of both approaches to primary prevention.

Different guidelines use different risk stratification tools to predict future cardiovascular risk upon which further management will be based. Guidelines for primary prevention and screening have tended to be pragmatic and based on the availability of infrastructure and resources rather than being evidence based. For example, in the NHS setting, cardiovascular disease prevention and risk factor assessment are generally part of existing 'NHS Health Checks', where, every

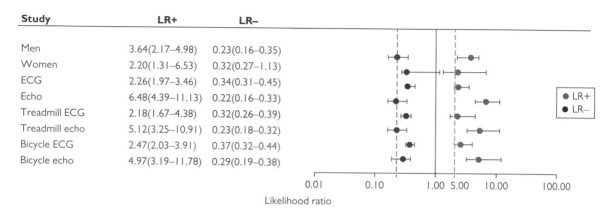

Study	LR+	LR−
Men	3.64(2.17–4.98)	0.23(0.16–0.35)
Women	2.20(1.31–6.53)	0.32(0.27–1.13)
ECG	2.26(1.97–3.46)	0.34(0.31–0.45)
Echo	6.48(4.39–11.13)	0.22(0.16–0.33)
Treadmill ECG	2.18(1.67–4.38)	0.32(0.26–0.39)
Treadmill echo	5.12(3.25–10.91)	0.23(0.18–0.32)
Bicycle ECG	2.47(2.03–3.91)	0.37(0.32–0.44)
Bicycle echo	4.97(3.19–11.78)	0.29(0.19–0.38)

Figure 351.1 Sensitivity analysis of subgroup analysis of positive and negative likelihood ratios for exercise testing; LR, likelihood ratio.

Reproduced with permission from Banerjee et al., Diagnostic accuracy of exercise stress testing for coronary artery disease: a systematic review and meta-analysis of prospective studies, International Journal of Clinical Practice, volume 66, issue 5, pp. 477–92, copyright © 2012 John Wiley and Sons.

Box 351.1 Principles of screening

1. The condition should be an important health problem.
2. There should be a treatment for the condition.
3. Facilities for diagnosis and treatment should be available.
4. There should be a latent stage of the disease.
5. There should be a test or examination for the condition.
6. The test should be acceptable to the population.
7. The natural history of the disease should be adequately understood.
8. There should be an agreed policy on whom to treat.
9. The total cost of finding a case should be economically balanced in relation to medical expenditure as a whole.
10. Case-finding should be a continuous process, not just a 'once and for all' project.

Reprinted from *Principles and practice of screening for disease*, Wilson JMG, Jungner G., Copyright (1968) World Health Organization

5 years, everyone between the ages of 40 and 74 is eligible for an NHS Health Check, which includes a number of simple tests to check for risk factors for heart and kidney disease, stroke, and diabetes.

Cardiovascular risk scores such as the Framingham risk score can be used to predict the future risk of cardiovascular events; in line with consensus guidelines, if a person's risk is above the recommended risk threshold, treatment and/or further investigation should be initiated. The 2014 NICE guidelines for cardiovascular disease state that 'people should be prioritized for a full formal risk assessment if their estimated 10-year risk of [cardiovascular disease] is 20% or more' and do not recommend opportunistic screening in unselected populations as the main strategy (National Institute for Health and Care Excellence, 2014). Ideally, risk scores should be locally or nationally validated. For example, Q-RISK and ASSIGN scores are now widely used in the UK, rather than the Framingham scores, since they were developed and validated in UK populations and therefore have greater predictive accuracy there.

Cardiovascular diseases share risk factors across arterial territories and disease processes, and, occasionally, appropriate and timely recognition and treatment of cardiovascular risk factors can have positive effects on health beyond the cardiovascular system. For example, hypertension is a risk factor for coronary heart disease and stroke as well as atrial fibrillation. Similarly, treatment with aspirin on the basis of increased risk of coronary heart disease may yield benefits in terms of cancer prevention. Therefore, opportunistic risk screening can have synergistic benefits.

Screening for risk factors does have costs in terms of human and physical resources, as well as psychological and lifestyle effects on individuals, and is only worthwhile if interventions are possible on the basis of the results of screening tests. In the words of epidemiologist and public health pioneer Geoffrey Rose, prevention occurs at the level of 'populations' as well as at the level of 'high-risk individuals', and it has been suggested by some that interventions could be made in large parts of the population in order to alter risk factors without screening for those factors. For example, government-mandated reductions in salt and saturated fats are examples of national health policies which have been successfully implemented without

Box 351.2 Major determinants of cardiovascular risk

- hypertension
- age
- gender
- lipid profile
- smoking
- diabetes mellitus
- family history
- ethnicity
- alcohol intake
- diet
- waist circumference
- psychosocial factors

associated screening of individuals. As risk factor levels for cardiovascular disease have increased globally in recent years, such considerations will grow in importance. The Global Burden of Disease Study showed that in 2010, the three leading risk factors for global disease burden of mortality and morbidity were high blood pressure (7.0%), tobacco smoking (including second-hand smoke; 6.3%), and alcohol use (5.5%), whereas, in 1990, the same study showed that the leading risk factors were childhood underweight (7.9%), household air pollution from solid fuels (7.0%), and tobacco smoking (including second-hand smoke; 6.1%).

The polypill in primary and secondary prevention of cardiovascular disease

The 'polypill' has been suggested to cumulatively reduce cardiovascular disease risk by combining aspirin, a beta blocker, a statin, and an angiotensin-converting enzyme (ACE) inhibitor in varying doses. The polypill could be used in both primary and secondary prevention. It has been hypothesized that a polypill could reduce cardiovascular disease events by 75% in those with vascular disease, which would constitute secondary prevention. If it were used in all those older than 55 years without cardiovascular disease, it is estimated that a polypill would safely reduce ischaemic heart disease events by 88%, and strokes by 80%, which is a primary prevention strategy. Several versions of the polypill are now being trialled by different research groups in different settings involving both primary and secondary prevention.

The polypill, when used in primary prevention, can 'tailor' the intervention to the individual with the aim of maximizing benefits and minimizing risks. However, these factors must be balanced with the disadvantages of high screening costs and imprecise long-term risk prediction in primary prevention. Risk factor thresholds ignore the fact that the relationship between most risk factors (e.g. blood pressure, cholesterol, smoking) and cardiovascular disease is continuous and linear. Therefore, intervening in only those individuals with high risk factor levels excludes the large proportion of cardiovascular events that occur amongst people with 'average' risk factor levels and probably represents the majority of the population (the so-called prevention paradox). Moreover, average risk factor levels seen in Westernized societies and in many urban settings in low-income countries may be biologically abnormal, as highlighted by the Global Burden of Disease Study. Therefore, the individual 'high-risk strategy' may have less overall benefit than a 'population-based strategy' that involves lowering risk factor levels in entire populations.

Importantly, it is unlikely that the long-term use of multiple drugs given separately in 'healthy' asymptomatic individuals to lower multiple risk factor levels will be feasible in whole populations, even in motivated individuals. Advocates of the polypill have suggested that, if the polypill were administered once daily, it could intervene simultaneously across several common risk factors and theoretically reduce cardiovascular disease to a large extent. Amongst people without existing cardiovascular disease, the most discriminatory screening factor is age, because >90% of cardiovascular disease deaths occur in people aged ≥55 years, as illustrated by multiple national and international epidemiologic studies of cardiovascular disease, including the Global Burden of Disease Study. The use of the polypill in people aged ≥55 years, especially in those with at least one additional risk factor (i.e. those at moderate risk), could therefore prevent the majority of cardiovascular disease events in both high- and low-income countries. However, opponents to widespread use of the polypill in primary prevention cite 'over-medicalization' and 'over-treatment' as major concerns.

The data for the components of the polypill in secondary prevention of cardiovascular disease is much stronger, in the form of high-quality randomized evidence supporting the use of aspirin, statins, beta blockers, and blockers of the renin–angiotensin system (e.g. ACE inhibitors and angiotensin receptor blockers). It has been estimated that 50% of the decline in cardiovascular mortality observed in developed countries during the last 20 years is attributable to medical therapy. However, despite clear evidence of effectiveness, rates of use of secondary prevention therapies and adherence to these therapies are disappointing, even in high-income countries, due to multiple barriers to implementation of secondary prevention, including (i) inadequate prescription of proven therapies in individuals who may benefit; (ii) poor long-term adherence to prescribed medications (often <50%),

Table 351.1 Intervention costs and effects

Intervention	Annual cost per person (£)	Measure of effect	Relative risk
Thiazide diuretic	45	RR CAD; RR stroke	0.86; 0.62
Beta blocker	68	RR CAD; RR stroke	0.89; 0.83
Calcium-channel blocker	140	RR CAD; RR stroke	0.85; 0.66
ACE inhibitor	136	RR CAD; RR stroke	0.83; 0.78
Aspirin	26	RR CAD; RR stroke (ischaemic); RR stroke (haemorrhagic); RR GI bleed	0.82; 0.86; 1.32; 1.54
Statin	440	RR CAD; RR stroke	0.70; 0.81
Phyosterol margarine	165	Total cholesterol	0.925
Dietary advice	Year 1:84 Year 2+:110	Systolic BP; Total cholesterol	0.984; 0.969
Lifestyle programme	Year 1: 164 Year 2+:110	Systolic BP; Total cholesterol	0.974; 0.967
Community heart health programme	Year 1: 1.51 Year 2+:1.02	Systolic BP; Total cholesterol	0.975; 0.995
Mandatory salt reduction	0.52	mg Na/day men; mg Na/day women	0.894; 0.967
Voluntary salt reduction (current practice)	0.31	mg Na/day men; mg Na/day women	0.50; 0.34
Lipid-lowering (current practice)	437	RR CAD; RR stroke	0.70; 0.81
BP-lowering (current practice)	109	RR CAD; RR stroke	0.85; 0.70

Note: All costs are in 2008 GB pounds sterling.

Abbreviations: ACE, angiotensin-converting enzyme; BP, blood pressure; CAD, coronary artery disease; RR, relative risk.

Adapted with permission from Cobiac LJ, Magnus A, Lim S, Barendregt JJ, Carter R, Vos T. Which interventions offer best value for money in primary prevention of cardiovascular disease? *PLoS One,* 7:e41842 2012.

which is caused by sociocultural, psychological, economic, and clinical factors related to patients, healthcare providers, healthcare systems, and their interactions; and (iii) cost and affordability.

Screening for surrogate markers of cardiovascular disease

Risk factors are markers that are statistically related to the risk of developing cardiovascular disease; they do not necessarily identify the disease itself. From the research and trial perspective, surrogate markers do not always correlate with 'hard' disease outcomes (such as cardiovascular disease events) and are therefore not as reliable in 'real-world' clinical practice.

However, surrogate markers of disease make it possible to identify and track disease progression. Reliable markers for the disease might ultimately allow disease progression to replace endpoint events as a guide to the risk of disease and response to therapy, as well as identifying earlier phases of the disease for intervention. Ultimately, the predictive and prognostic accuracy of surrogate markers in screening are weighed against their cost before their use in a given population. However, even relatively new technologies can be introduced into health systems relatively quickly if they are incorporated into consensus clinical guidelines, as illustrated by coronary artery calcium scoring (see 'Coronary artery calcium score').

Carotid intima–media thickness

Carotid intima–media thickness, which is determined via B-mode ultrasound, has been shown to be a safe, non-invasive, and relatively inexpensive means of assessing subclinical atherosclerosis. It correlates with the presence of coronary atherosclerosis and represents an independent risk factor for coronary events as well as stroke and transient ischaemic attacks.

Left ventricular hypertrophy

Left ventricular hypertrophy, which can be detected on echocardiography or ECG, is associated with several disease processes but most commonly hypertension. It is an independent predictor of cardiovascular events: when reductions in left ventricular mass result from antihypertensive therapy, they are associated with reductions in cardiovascular events, independently of blood pressure reduction. There is evidence that echocardiography is more sensitive and more

specific than ECG in the diagnosis of left ventricular hypertrophy; however, the benefits of this increased diagnostic accuracy must be weighed against the increased cost of providing increased access to echocardiography services.

Structural and functional changes in the arterial wall precede and accompany atherosclerotic processes. Therefore, measuring arterial stiffness is another way to assess cardiovascular risk. Large-artery stiffness, as assessed by **pulse pressure** and **pulse wave velocity**, is age dependent and reflects structural alterations that are accelerated by hypertension and atherosclerosis. **Pulse contour analysis** provides information about small-artery stiffness. These techniques provide a way to identify premature disease and to track the progression of disease and the impact of therapy.

Coronary artery calcium score

The coronary artery calcium score is a measure of coronary arterial calcification and is determined by performing CT of the heart. This score is a strong predictor of coronary heart disease events and overall mortality, providing predictive information beyond that of standard risk factors across different racial and age groups. According to the NICE clinical guidelines for chest pain of recent onset (National Institute for Health and Care Excellence, 2010), this score can be used to rule out cardiovascular disease in patients who present with chest pain but, on the basis of traditional risk factors, have a low estimated likelihood of coronary artery disease (10%–29%; see Figure 351.2).

Age- and sex-specific factors

Table 351.2 describes the algorithm recommended by the NICE guidelines for estimating the baseline likelihood of coronary heart disease in an age- and sex-specific manner. In individuals in whom the estimated likelihood of coronary heart disease is ≥30%, diagnostic testing in the form of non-invasive functional imaging or invasive coronary angiography should be carried out if the estimated likelihood is 30%–60% or 61%–90%, respectively.

Screening for established cardiovascular disease

Screening for symptomatic individuals with coronary heart disease, as discussed in 'Screening for surrogate markers of cardiovascular disease', involves using the coronary artery calcium score, functional

Stable chest pain pathway

2. Diagnostic testing for people in whom stable angina cannot be diagnosed or excluded by clinical assessment alone

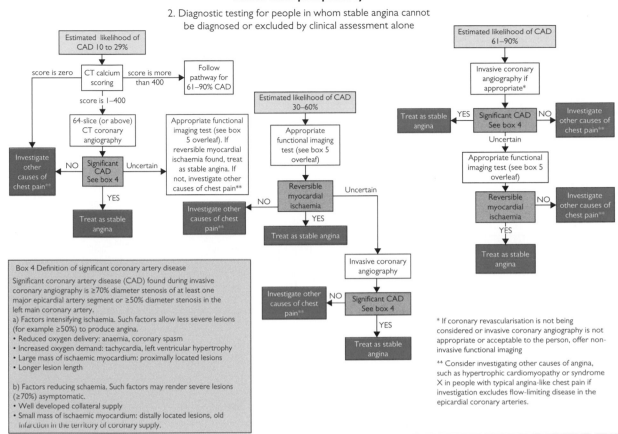

Figure 351.2 NICE stable chest pain pathway.

Pathway from appendix 1 of https://www.nice.org.uk/guidance/gid-mt252/documents/heartflow-ffrct-for-the-computation-of-fractional-flow-reserve-from-coronary-ct-angiography-final-scope2.

imaging, or angiography, based on risk stratification and the use of guidelines (such as the algorithm shown in Table 351.2).

Atrial fibrillation

Atrial fibrillation (AF) increases the risk of stroke, thromboembolism, morbidity, and mortality, with huge implications for healthcare expenditure. Demographic transitions and ageing populations are projected to greatly increase the global burden of AF and its sequelae. For stroke and thromboembolism, prevention can be primary (to reduce risk of first stroke) or secondary (preventing recurrent strokes). Prevention can occur at the level of AF itself, with primary prevention restricting the development of AF by reducing the cardiovascular risk factor burden and by the use of upstream therapies, while secondary prevention involves reducing risk factors and the risk of stroke in individuals with established AF. For example, in stroke prevention, a recent analysis has shown that direct-acting anticoagulants (apixaban, rivaroxaban, and dabigatran) have broadly similar efficacies in the secondary prevention of ischaemic stroke, haemorrhagic stroke, vascular death, major bleeding, and intracranial bleeding in AF patients. On the other hand, in the primary prevention of stroke, the three drugs showed some differences in relation to efficacy and bleeding. Thus, it is critical to clarify the level of prevention when considering the impact of different screening and prevention strategies.

Table 351.2 Percentage of people estimated to have coronary artery disease according to typicality of symptoms, age, sex, and risk factors

Age, years	Non-anginal chest pain				Atypical angina				Typical angina			
	Men		Women		Men		Women		Men		Women	
	Low	High	Low	High	Low	High	Low	High	Low	High	Low	High
35	**3**	**35**	**1**	**19**	8	59	2	39	30	88	10	78
45	**9**	**47**	**2**	**22**	21	70	5	43	51	92	20	79
55	**23**	**59**	**4**	**25**	45	79	10	47	80	95	38	82
65	**49**	**69**	**9**	**29**	71	86	20	51	93	97	56	84

For men older than 70 year with atypical or typical symptoms, assume an estimate >90%. For women older than 70, assume an estimate of 61–90% except women at high risk and with typical symptoms, where a risk of >90% should be assumed. Values are per cent of people at each mid-decade age with significant coronary artery disease (CAD). High = high risk = diabetes, smoking, and hyperlipidaemia (total cholesterol >6.47 mmol/litre). Low = Low risk = none of these three. The area in bold represents people with symptoms of non-anginal chest pain, who would not be investigated for stable angina routinely. Note: these results are likely to overestimate CAD in primary care populations. If there are resting ECG ST-T changes or Q waves, the likelihood of CAD is higher in each cell of the table.

From page 8 of https://www.nice.org.uk/guidance/cg95/resources/guidance-chest-pain-of-recent-onset-pdf.

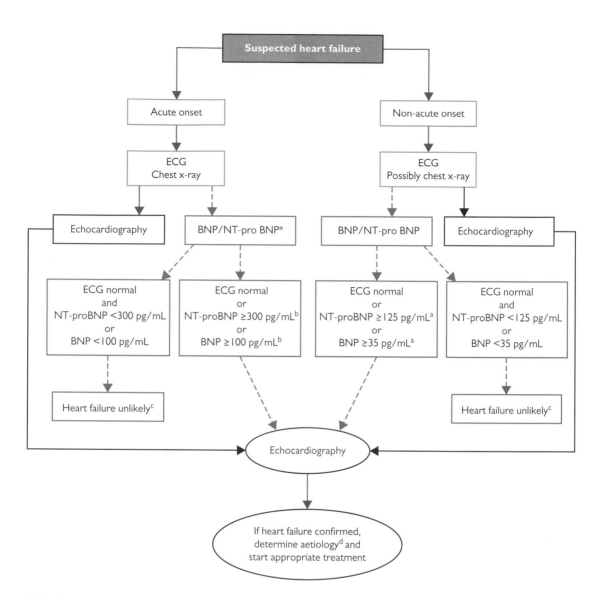

Figure 351.3 European Society of Cardiology guidelines for diagnosis in patients with suspected heart failure, showing alternative 'echocardiography first' (black) or 'natriuretic peptide first' (blue) approaches; BNP, B-type natriuretic peptide; NT-pro BNP, N-terminal pro B-type natriuretic peptide.

Reproduced with permission from John J. V. McMurray et al., ESC Guidelines for the diagnosis and treatment of acute and chronic heart failure 2012, *European Heart Journal*, Volume 33, Issue 14, pp. 1787–1847, Copyright © 2012 Oxford University Press.

A recent consensus statement from the Royal College of Physicians of Edinburgh concluded that 'the most cost-effective method for the detection of AF in primary care is by opportunistic screening of people aged 65 years or older by radial pulse checking followed as soon as practicable by a 12-lead ECG for those with an irregular pulse. ... Diagnostic ECGs should be analysed by a competent individual supported by audit and feedback.' (Stott, Dewar, Garratt, et al., 2012, p. 34). The statement also says, 'Where clinical suspicion of paroxysmal AF exists, including after ischaemic stroke or transient ischaemic attack ... , longer ECG monitoring periods (at least 24 hours) or event recorders should be used' (Stott, Dewar, Garratt, et al., 2012, p. 34). Early recognition of AF is made much more difficult by its often silent nature, with about one-third of patients being unaware of their asymptomatic arrhythmia. The fact that symptoms are unreliable for estimating AF burden and identifying patients with AF has

led to recommendations for the use of longer-term continuous ECG monitoring and even implantable loop recorders, particularly in the setting of cryptogenic stroke, where the role of AF is likely to have been greatly underestimated.

Asymptomatic left ventricular dysfunction

Asymptomatic left ventricular dysfunction progresses to symptomatic heart failure at rates of up to 10% per year, if untreated. Therefore, early detection, if achievable, is important because randomized trials have shown that appropriate drug therapy can significantly improve survival and cardiovascular outcomes. Possible screening strategies may involve ECG, imaging modalities (e.g. echocardiography), biomarkers (e.g. BNP), or a combination of these approaches. Because the signs and symptoms of heart failure are so non-specific, many patients who have suspected heart failure and are referred for echocardiography are not found to have an important cardiac abnormality.

Where the availability of echocardiography is limited, the European Society of Cardiology guidelines recommend measuring the blood concentration of natriuretic peptides, a family of hormones which are secreted at increased levels when the heart is diseased or the load on any chamber is increased (Figure 351.3). A normal natriuretic peptide level has a high specificity; that is, in an untreated patient, it virtually excludes significant cardiac disease, removing the need for echocardiography. Guidelines have tended to focus on patients with 'suspected heart failure' and not those who are 'asymptomatic'.

Community-based studies have highlighted the high prevalence of heart failure (both systolic and diastolic) in patients with risk factors for cardiovascular disease. For example, the ECHOES study showed that definite systolic dysfunction (defined as an ejection fraction <40%) was found in 22.1% of patients with coronary artery disease, and 5.8% with diabetes, although approximately half of the patients in whom the dysfunction was found were asymptomatic. However, at present, further trials of targeted echocardiography are required before widespread echocardiographic screening is advocated. Testing for BNP levels is likely to provide the most cost-effective method of screening for heart failure in populations, although further prospective trial and cost-effectiveness data are required.

Abdominal aortic aneurysm

Abdominal aortic aneurysm (AAA) rupture is a cause of sudden death. Detection and surveillance are thought to be cost-effective methods for preventing AAA rupture, by ensuring timely AAA surgical repair. AAA screening is gradually being rolled out across the NHS in the UK. Men aged 65 and over are eligible for AAA screening by abdominal ultrasound scanning. The NHS AAA Screening Programme aims to reduce deaths from ruptured AAA amongst men aged 65 and over by up to 50%.

Summary

In this chapter, we have focused on screening for cardiovascular disease via risk factors, surrogate markers, and detecting established disease. The high burden of cardiovascular risk factors and diseases in all populations in both high- and low-income settings make these considerations of optimal screening strategies universally important. Currently, screening strategies have tended to focus on risk factors rather than established disease, due to many factors, including resource constraints, lack of prospective evidence, and sociocultural factors. In addition, the body of randomized evidence in diagnostic and prognostic studies has lagged behind the exponential growth of trials in the therapeutic arena. Given the importance of screening in both high-risk and population approaches to the prevention of cardiovascular disease, more research is urgently needed.

Further Reading

Greenland P, Alpert JS, Beller GA, et al. 2010 ACCF/AHA guideline for assessment of cardiovascular risk in asymptomatic adults: A report of the American College of Cardiology Foundation/American Heart Association Task Force on Practice Guidelines. Developed in collaboration with American Society of Echocardiography, American Society of Nuclear Cardiology, Society of Atherosclerosis Imaging and Prevention, Society for Cardiovascular Angiography and Interventions, Society of Cardiovascular Computed Tomography, and Society for Cardiovascular Magnetic Resonance. *J Am Coll Cardiol* 2010; 56: 14–21.

Kavey REW, Daniels SR, Lauer RM, et al. American Heart Association Guidelines for primary prevention of atherosclerotic cardiovascular disease beginning in childhood. *Circulation* 2003; 107: 1562–6.

National Institute for Health and Care Excellence. *Chest Pain of Recent Onset: Assessment and Diagnosis*. 2010. Available at http://www.nice.org.uk/guidance/cg95/resources/chest-pain-of-recent-onset-assessment-and-diagnosis-pdf-975751036117 (accessed 21 Sep 2017).

National Institute for Health and Care Excellence. *Cardiovascular Disease: Risk Assessment and Reduction, Including Lipid Modification*. 2014. Available at http://www.nice.org.uk/guidance/cg181/resources/cardiovascular-disease-risk-assessment-and-reduction-including-lipid-modification-35109807660997 (accessed 21 Sep 2017).

Stott DJ, Dewar RI, Garratt CJ, et al. RCPE UK Consensus Conference on 'Approaching the comprehensive management of atrial fibrillation: evolution or revolution?'. *J R Coll Physicians Edinb* 2012; 42: 34–5.

Abdul Nasimudeen

Introduction

Routine screening for respiratory diseases is currently not available to the general healthy population, with the exception of screening for cystic fibrosis. In this chapter, we discuss the screening strategies in place for cystic fibrosis, TB, and other conditions, such as COPD, lung cancer, alpha-1 antitrypsin deficiency, pulmonary hypertension, pulmonary arteriovenous malformation, and obstructive sleep apnoea, for which screening can be applied. While screening has the potential to improve quality of life through early diagnosis and management, it is not an easy process and cannot offer a guarantee of protection.

Cystic fibrosis

Neonatal screening has helped early diagnosis of cystic fibrosis before any symptoms may have developed and there is evidence to suggest screening provides better pulmonary outcomes. The UK National Screening Committee currently recommends screening for this condition by testing the blood for immunoreactive trypsinogen (IRT) as part of the Guthrie test on all newborn infants. This is not diagnostic, and further tests are required to confirm the diagnosis. Screening helps affected parents to have genetic counselling to avoid the birth of a second child with cystic fibrosis in a family where the first child may have been undiagnosed.

False-positive levels of IRT are possible in those who are heterozygous for the cystic fibrosis mutation and in those from non-Caucasian origin. These can lead to long-term psychosocial consequences for the families involved in the screening until further diagnostic testing is done. False-negative results are also possible, as ITR levels start to fall variably after the first 4 weeks of birth. A negative IRT test after 8 weeks is no longer informative.

Carrier screening looking for mutation analysis is available for those who have a relative known to have cystic fibrosis and a relative or a partner known to be a carrier of cystic fibrosis. Prenatal screening trials have been done in the past using different approaches in hospital and primary care settings. Stepwise screening and couple screening methods have been used, with the former first testing the pregnant woman and then only testing her partner if she is found to be a carrier. There is now evidence to suggest that prenatal screening of at-risk couples identified by the newborn screening programme has resulted in a reduction in the live-birth prevalence of cystic fibrosis.

TB

Studies have shown that mass screening of general population with chest X-rays (CXRs) makes no difference to the number of new cases of TB in that group. The best way of control is preventing the spread from smear-positive cases, and screening contacts. The National Institute of Health Excellence recommends screening the contacts of all cases of active TB, new entrants, healthcare workers, homeless workers, and prisoners.

The Mantoux test is recommended for all close contacts with no evidence of previous BCG, and those under 35 years of age and with previous BCG vaccination. Contacts over 35 years of age and with previous BCG vaccination are screened with a CXR. Further clinical assessments may then be necessary with interferon gamma assays (IGRA) and additional CXRs to determine whether latent disease or active infection is present.

New entrants screening is currently applied only to persons coming from countries with a high incidence of TB (e.g. sub-Saharan Africa or a country with an incidence of >500 in 100 000 population). Patients should be identified from port of arrival reports, registration with primary care, entry to education, and links with voluntary groups. All new immigrants are recommended to have a CXR unless they are <11 years of age or pregnant, in which case they should have a Mantoux test, followed by a clinical assessment for active and latent TB, and risk assessment for HIV.

NHS employee screening is via a pre-employment questionnaire. Asymptomatic individuals with evidence of BCG vaccination are given general advice, whereas vaccination is offered to those with no evidence of active or latent infection. Active case finding in homeless people is recommended using CXRs, based on symptoms, and prisoners should be screened using a health questionnaire on entry followed by a CXR and three sputum samples for TB microscopy.

Screening of contacts in countries such as the UK is not just to identify active cases and initiate treatment but also to identify patients with latent TB who may be able to receive treatment which reduces the risk of acquiring an active infection in the first 2 years after exposure, the time when the risk is considered to be high. In the future, IGRA may replace Mantoux as the first-line screening tool, and trials may show that new entrant screening should ideally include migrants from countries such as India and Pakistan (this population is currently left out, due to having a lower incidence of TB).

Lung cancer

Currently, there is insufficient evidence to recommend for or against screening for lung cancer, even in asymptomatic high-risk individuals, with a low-dose CT (LDCT) scan, a CXR, sputum cytology, or a combination of these tests. The sensitivity and specificity of CXR for diagnosing lung cancer are 26% and 93%, respectively. An LDCT scan is up to four times more sensitive than a CXR but the false-positive rates range from 5% to 41%.

Screening high-risk patients (>50 years of age, >20 pack-year smoking history) using CXRs, with or without sputum cytology, have shown no mortality benefit. The main drawbacks of lung cancer screening trials are lack of control for occupational exposures and family history, possible bias from the screening of healthy individuals, and the lack of completely unscreened control groups. Several cohort studies of LDCT have shown that an LDCT is significantly more sensitive than a CXR for identifying lung cancer and also identifies a significantly higher proportion of small (early stage, resectable) lung cancers than a CXR does. However, the effectiveness of an LDCT in decreasing lung cancer mortality cannot be evaluated from these studies because of the absence of randomization and the lack of an unscreened control group for which mortality was an outcome. International Early Lung Cancer Action Program investigators looking at the survival of patients with Stage 1 lung cancer detected on CT screening concluded that annual spiral CT screening can detect curable lung cancer but the main drawbacks were that the study had no control group; it lacked an unbiased outcome measure and did not mention the harms of screening.

Screening smokers via CT can show other incidental non-malignant conditions needing further investigation and high-risk procedures such as lung biopsies. This can sometimes lead to over-diagnosis and to patients having to deal with the psychological issues arising from stress and anxiety. The National Lung Cancer Screening Trial launched in 2002 is currently comparing the utility of CT scans and

CXRs for screening. More than 50 000 patients have been enrolled and the results will not be available until later this year. This study has also tried to address some important issues, such as all causes of death in groups screened for lung cancer, the cost-effectiveness of screening, the quality of life for those who test positive, and the influence of screening on smoking behaviour and beliefs.

The identification of biomarkers has led to a greater understanding of the molecular pathways of lung cancer. Mutations in K-ras and p53, and proteins such as carcinoembryonic antigen, CYFRA21-1, plasma kallikrein B1, neuron-specific enolase, and so on, have been proposed as potential biomarkers for lung cancer. However, despite extensive studies thus far, few have turned out to be useful and, even those used do not show enough sensitivity, specificity, and reproducibility for general use.

COPD

Most individuals with airflow limitation do not recognize or report symptoms, and spirometry forms the mainstay in screening for COPD, although, currently, there are no recommendations to screen asymptomatic high-risk healthy adults. In individuals who present with respiratory symptoms, spirometry would be indicated as part of a diagnostic test for COPD, asthma, or other pulmonary diseases. Screening and early detection for those with mild or moderate airflow obstruction could benefit from smoking cessation advice and annual influenza vaccination.

Pharmacological therapy to these individuals may help prevent exacerbations but may not change hospitalization rates in those with severe disease. It is not known whether pharmacological therapy in patients who are asymptomatic but meet spirometric criteria for moderate-to-severe disease would have the same benefit as in those who are symptomatic with severe airflow obstruction. The costs associated with screening for COPD are large, even in those considered as high risk. There is a risk of false-positive diagnosis in those over 70 years of age, due to the natural decline of lung function.

Although influenza vaccination may reduce exacerbations, there is not much evidence to indicate that spirometry screening improves influenza vaccination rates or promotes smoking cessation. In the future, screening programmes should aim to prevent disease progression, exacerbations, and COPD-related complications. It should also aim to improve exercise tolerance and health status and provide a reduction in mortality.

Alpha-1 antitrypsin deficiency

Despite its prevalence, alpha-1 antitrypsin deficiency remains grossly under-diagnosed, the reason being its highly variable symptom development, as it can present with symptoms similar to COPD or asthma, or have no symptoms at all. Initially, a blood test is done to measure alpha-1 antitrypsin concentrations; patients found to have suboptimal or low levels of alpha-1 antitrypsin should then undergo DNA testing to identify which of the various alpha-1 antitrypsin deficiency genotypes they have.

Current European Respiratory Society and American Thoracic Society guidelines recommend a high level of suspicion for:

- symptomatic individuals with early onset (<45 years of age) emphysema, regardless of smoking history
- individuals with emphysema in the absence of a recognized risk factor
- individuals with predominantly basal emphysema on a CT scan
- individuals who have asthma with incomplete reversibility of airflow obstruction after aggressive treatment with bronchodilators
- asymptomatic individuals with airflow obstruction on lung function testing and with identifiable risk factors such as smoking or occupational exposure
- individuals with unexplained liver disease
- adults with necrotizing panniculitis
- individuals with bronchiectasis with no obvious cause
- siblings of individuals with alpha-1 antitrypsin deficiency

They also recommend that such individuals undergo diagnostic testing for alpha-1 antitrypsin deficiency.

Recognition of alpha-1 antitrypsin deficiency can prompt specific interventions such as genetic counselling, screening of family members, smoking cessation advice, and consideration of augmentation therapy. Evidence from previous studies suggests that targeted detection has generally produced a higher rate of detecting disease than large-scale population-based screening has. In the future, improved awareness campaigns and easy and cheaper sampling techniques may improve the detection rates, resulting in better treatment options such as augmentation therapy, which may well help preserve lung function in asymptomatic individuals.

Pulmonary hypertension

Heritable pulmonary arterial hypertension (PAH) is an autosomal dominant condition with incomplete penetrance. Mutations in BMPR2, which resides in the chromosomal region 2q32, have been identified in up to 70% of patients when PAH occurs within families. The same mutations have been identified in patients with idiopathic (sporadic) forms of PAH as well. Mutations in ALK1 and ENG have been identified in patients with a family history of hereditary haemorrhagic telangiectasia (HHT). Individuals can still end up transmitting the mutations to their children but may never acquire the disease due to variable penetrance. One way of screening would be to do genetic testing and counselling of these individuals, with detailed explanation of the limitations and risks involved. Linkage analysis of at-risk relatives, in the absence of any identified mutations or gene sequencing, is another way of identifying patients at risk of developing heritable PAH.

Echocardiography should always be performed in cases of suspected pulmonary hypertension. Pulmonary hypertension is defined as a mean pulmonary arterial pressure ≥25 mm Hg on Doppler measurements but these values can be inaccurate in some individuals. Underestimation of pulmonary hypertension can happen in patients with severe tricuspid regurgitation, and overestimation by >10 mm Hg is also common; hence, Doppler echo is not ideal for screening asymptomatic or patients with mild pulmonary hypertension. One study by Grünig et al. (2000) looking at asymptomatic carriers of a mutated primary pulmonary hypertension (PPH) gene did suggest that stress echocardiographic measurements of pulmonary artery systolic pressure may be useful for identify persons at risk of PPH even before the pulmonary arterial pressure at rest is elevated.

ECG may provide supportive evidence for pulmonary hypertension. In patients with idiopathic PAH, right ventricular hypertrophy and right axis deviation is present in 87% and 79% of patients, respectively, but the sensitivity and specificity rates of 55% and 70% makes ECG a poor screening tool. The CXR may be abnormal in up to 90% of patients with idiopathic PAH, but the degree of pulmonary hypertension does not correlate with the extent of radiographic abnormalities.

Patients suspected of or diagnosed with pulmonary hypertension may well need further tests such as a CT scan, a lung function test, a V/Q scan, and so on, but none of these tests provide a useful screening tool at present. Prenatal testing for heritable PAH is a possibility in future, given the genetic background, but this is controversial, as the intellect of PAH patients is normal, and effective treatments are available.

Pulmonary arteriovenous malformation

Due to the high incidence of unsuspected pulmonary and cerebral arteriovenous malformation in family members of patients with HHT, it is recommended that family members carrying the mutation for this disease should be screened for pulmonary arteriovenous malformation via chest radiography and/or measurement of shunt fraction. Contrast echocardiography or V/Q scanning could also be used as first-line screening in patients with a high index of suspicion.

Although screening with CT is very sensitive, it does carry a risk of radiation exposure and cost issues. Contrast echocardiography carries a risk of diagnosing microvascular shunts which may not need intervention. Routine genetic screening of HHT family members may play an increasingly important role in future but is currently limited by the lack of a predominant mutation.

Obstructive sleep apnoea

Obstructive sleep apnoea (OSA), if undiagnosed, does carry a significant cardiovascular mortality and morbidity, with a high risk of automobile and workplace accidents. Although polysomnography remains the gold standard for diagnosis, currently in UK hospital settings, the Epworth Sleep Score and nocturnal oximetry are widely used as a screening tool for the diagnosis of OSA.

A recent study concluded that simple variables such as sex, blood pressure, BMI, and self-reported snoring could all provide valid tools for the assessment of sleep disordered breathing.

In the future, due to increasing number of patients with obesity, conditions such as OSA are likely to increase and screening programmes using the tools described in this section should be used in primary care settings to improve the diagnosis and outcome measures.

Further Reading

Grünig E, Janssen B, and Mereles D. Abnormal pulmonary artery pressure response in asymptomatic carriers of primary pulmonary hypertension gene. *Circulation* 2000; 102: 1145–50.

McGoon M, Gutterman D, Steen V, et al. Screening, early detection, and diagnosis of pulmonary arterial hypertension: ACCP evidence-based clinical practice guidelines. *Chest* 2004; 126: 14S–34S.

National Institute for Health and Care Excellence. *Tuberculosis: Clinical Diagnosis and Management of Tuberculosis, and Measures for its Prevention and Control*. 2011. Available at https://www.nice.org.uk/guidance/CG117 (accessed 20 Aug 2017).

Stoller JK, Snider GL, Brantly ML, et al. American Thoracic Society/European Respiratory Society Statement: Standards for the diagnosis and management of individuals with alpha-1 antitrypsin deficiency. *Am J Respir Crit Care Med* 2003; 168: 818–900.

UK National Screening Committee policy on cystic fibrosis in newborns (http://www.screening.nhs.uk/cysticfibrosis-newborn)

US Preventive Services Task Force (http://www.uspreventiveservicestaskforce.org)

353 Screening for kidney disease

Aron Chakera, William G. Herrington, and Christopher A. O'Callaghan

What kidney diseases can we screen for?

Renal disease is common and, with routine reporting of estimated glomerular filtration rates, impairment of renal function is increasingly being recognized.

As renal impairment is usually asymptomatic until very advanced, chronic kidney disease (CKD) guidelines have been developed to improve the identification and screening of at-risk populations.

Target groups include patients with vascular risk factors (e.g. diabetes mellitus and hypertension); patients with certain multisystem diseases which can cause renal impairment; patients with urological conditions; patients on nephrotoxic medication; and immediate relatives of patients with established renal disease (see Table 353.1).

Kidney function should also be checked during intercurrent illness and perioperatively in all patients with CKD or suspected CKD. The frequency of screening is dictated by the CKD stage (see Table 353.2).

How do we screen for kidney disease?

Screening for kidney disease should include a serum creatinine measurement and, in most circumstances, a urine dipstick. Diabetic patients should also have an albumin-to-creatinine ratio or an Albustix® measurement to identify microalbuminuria, which will not be detected on standard urine dipsticks.

What is the impact of kidney disease screening in the real world?

The costs of a serum creatinine test and a urine dipstick are low. The tests are simple to perform, minimally invasive, and readily available.

Table 353.2 Current Renal Association guidelines for screening frequency

eGFR	Screening frequency
>90	annual
60–89	annual
30–59 *(known to be stable*)*	annual
30–59 *(newly diagnosed or progressive†)*	6-monthly
15–29 *(known to be stable*)*	6-monthly
15-29 *(newly diagnosed or progressive†)*	3-monthly
<15	3 monthly

Abbreviations: eGFR, estimated glomerular filtration rate; GFR, glomerular filtration rate.
*Stable kidney function defined as change of GFR of <2 ml/min/1.73 m² over 6 months or more.
†Progressive kidney damage defined as change of GFR of >2 ml/min/1.73 m² over 6 months or more.
Reproduced with permission of the Renal Association.

The introduction of national guidelines is raising the awareness and detection of CKD in the community. Earlier detection of kidney disease may allow treatment to prevent the progression of renal impairment. For example, there is increasing evidence that starting angiotensin-converting-enzyme inhibitors or angiotensin receptor blockers in diabetics with microalbuminuria slows progression to overt nephropathy.

Screening programmes can also identify patients at risk of end-stage disease, in time to allow the patient and physician to prepare for renal replacement therapy or to ensure that appropriate advanced directives are in place.

Issues and the future of kidney disease screening programmes

The impact of the new CKD screening guidelines on patient outcomes still needs to be validated. There is ongoing debate about which patients need referral for specialist opinions and which can be managed safely in primary care. This will potentially have significant impact on resource allocation and workload.

As the serum creatinine test is acknowledged to be an imperfect measure of renal function, particularly when the estimated glomerular filtration rate is above 60 ml/min 1.73 m⁻², there is a need for new markers to be developed. One promising measure is the serum cystatin C level.

Further Reading

National Institute for Health and Care Excellence. *Chronic Kidney Disease in Adults: Assessment and Management.* 2014. Available at http://www.nice.org.uk/guidance/cg182 (accessed 21 Sep 2017).
National Kidney Foundation. K/DOQI Clinical practice guidelines for chronic kidney disease: Evaluation, classification and stratification. *Am J Kidney Dis* 2002; 39: S1–S266.

Table 353.1 Target groups for renal screening

Vascular	Multisystem diseases	Urological conditions	Nephrotoxic drugs
Hypertension	Diabetes mellitus	Bladder outflow obstruction	Angiotensin-converting enzyme inhibitors and angiotensin receptor blockers
Heart failure	SLE	Neurogenic bladder	
Coronary artery disease	Vasculitis	Urinary diversion surgery	
Cerebrovascular disease	Myeloma	Urinary anatomical abnormalities	NSAIDs
Peripheral vascular disease	Rheumatoid arthritis	Recurrent stone formers	Lithium
	Scleroderma	Stone disease due to primary hyperoxaluria, cystinuria, Dent's disease, or infections	Mesalazine
			Calcineurin inhibitors (ciclosporin, tacrolimus)
			Proton-pump inhibitors

Barrett's oesophagus

Barrett's oesophagus (BO) is where the normal squamous epithelium in the oesophagus has been replaced by metaplastic columnar epithelium. This is generally diagnosed endoscopically and requires histological confirmation. Chronic heartburn affects a large number of the population, and BO is found in approximately 10% of those undergoing endoscopy for reflux symptoms. However, the risk of adenocarcinoma in patients with gastro-oesophageal reflux is <1 in 1000 per year; therefore, performing BO screening in patients presenting with heartburn is not appropriate. In patients with BO, approximately 5% will develop dysplasia, and 10%–50% of the low-grade dysplasias will progress to high-grade dysplasia or adenocarcinoma within 2–5 years. In addition, a high-grade dysplasia contains a focus of adenocarcinoma in 30%–40% of cases. Screening has been developed to reduce the development of adenocarcinoma via the early detection of high-grade dysplasias or cancer in situ.

How do we screen for BO?

Current guidelines from the British Society of Gastroenterology (BSG) advocate the following screening programme:

- symptomatic therapy with a proton-pump inhibitor should be offered to those with BO, and the dose escalated to control symptoms; however, it must be recognized that studies have shown that symptom control does not necessarily correlate with prevention of acid reflux
- quadrantic biopsies should be taken every 2 cm from the segment of BO, and from any visible lesion
- BO with no dysplasia should undergo a surveillance endoscopy after 2 years
- biopsies which are 'indefinite for dysplasia' should lead to a repeat endoscopy with further multiple biopsies; if the second set of biopsies plus a third set at 6 months continue to show no definite dysplasia, the patient can return to 2-yearly surveillance
- low-grade dysplasia should be treated with high-dose acid suppression for 8–12 weeks and then be re-biopsied; persistent low-grade dysplasia requires 6-monthly surveillance
- if high-grade dysplasia persists after acid suppression and re-biopsy, the patient should be offered treatment; treatment options include mucosal resection, photodynamic therapy, radiofrequency ablation, and oesophagectomy

This advice should be purely used as a guideline, with each patient being assessed individually as to their suitability for undergoing routine endoscopies. Factors associated with a higher risk of developing cancer include age >45 years, male gender, extended segment BO (>8 cm), mucosal damage (oesophagitis, ulceration), family history of cancer, long duration of reflux, and early age of reflux symptoms.

What is the impact of screening for BO?

Currently, survival rates for patients with BO are identical to those for age- and sex-matched populations, with most patients dying from causes unrelated to their BO. However, adenocarcinoma of the oesophagus and gastro-oesophageal junction is the fastest growing cancer of the Western world; thus, screening has been implemented in an attempt to curb this growth. Currently, there is little evidence to confirm or refute the evidence for screening of BO.

The future of BO screening programmes

The real impact of BO screening programmes will become more evident as the screening program continues. The Barrett's Oesophagus Surveillance Study and other such studies will eventually give evidence as to the actual benefit to patients (in increased life-years) and the NHS (in cost-effectiveness).

Colorectal cancer

Colorectal cancer is the third most common cancer in the UK, and the second commonest cause of cancer-related death. Approximately 1 in 20 people will develop colorectal cancer in their lifetime. The main aim of colorectal cancer screening is the early detection of polyps and cancers, at a time when treatment is likely to be more effective.

How do we screen for colorectal cancer?

The NHS National Bowel Cancer Screening Programme was introduced in 2006 and offers faecal occult blood (FOB) testing every 2 years to all men and women aged 60–69. Patients who are ≥70 and want FOB testing can obtain screening kits via a telephone helpline. Patients with positive FOB tests are subsequently offered a colonoscopy.

What is the impact of screening for colorectal cancer?

The screening programme has estimated the costs in 2008–9 to be £55 000 000. It has been estimated that, if 1000 people undergo FOB testing, approximately 20 will have positive results. Of those with positive results, ~10% will have an underlying colorectal cancer. This equates to 2 of the original 1000 patients (i.e. 0.2% of those screened). Furthermore ~6 (0.6%) will have colonic polyps, which can be removed at colonoscopy and dictate the need for further surveillance (see 'Screening in patients with adenomatous colorectal polyps'). Studies have shown that screening reduces the risk of death from colorectal cancer by ~16%.

The future of colorectal screening programmes

The colorectal cancer screening programme is still in its early days; the full extent of cancer prevention it provides will be recognized over the next few years. Despite the fact that changing lifestyle measures have reduced the rate of colorectal cancer, it is expected that population growth, alongside screening programmes and increased public awareness, will lead to a higher number of cases over the next 20 years.

Screening for gastrointestinal cancer in specific groups

Various groups have been shown to have an increased risk of gastrointestinal (GI) cancer, including those with inflammatory bowel disease, acromegaly, or a family history of colorectal cancer, amongst others. Guidelines have been put in place to ensure these patients are monitored regularly, aiming to reduce their risk of GI cancer to that of the general population.

Screening for GI cancer in patients who have had a colorectal cancer resection

There is no evidence that screening for GI cancer after colorectal cancer resection improves survival. However, the BSG advise that a colonoscopy should be performed 5 years after a colorectal cancer resection, and 5-yearly thereafter, up to the age of 70 years. In addition, it is reasonable to offer liver imaging within 2 years of the surgery to those ≤70 years, to identify operable liver metastases early.

Studies are ongoing in order to detect the benefit of more aggressive surveillance in this patient group.

Screening for GI cancer in patients with adenomatous colorectal polyps

It is widely accepted that most colorectal cancers develop from asymptomatic adenomatous polyps. The National Polyp Study in the US showed a reduction in incidence of colorectal cancer by 70%–90% in patients undergoing polyp surveillance. If polyps are seen at the time of colonoscopy, they should be removed. BSG guidelines advocate follow-up of these patients, as follows:

- 1–2 small (<1 cm) polyps: no follow-up or colonoscopy for 5 years
- 3–4 polyps, or one polyp which is ≥1 cm in diameter: 3-yearly colonoscopy, until two consecutive negative colonoscopies
- ≥5 or ≥3 polyps, with one of them being ≥1 cm: 12-monthly colonoscopy
- large lesions: these should be re-examined at 3 months

The degree of dysplasia also affects time between colonoscopies, with high-grade dysplasia requiring rapid re-examination of the polyp site. Surveillance is usually ceased at 75 years, when the life expectancy is seen to be shorter than the average time taken for adenomas to become malignant.

Screening for GI cancer in patients with inflammatory bowel disease

Patients with inflammatory bowel disease affecting their colon are at an increased risk of colorectal cancer, and colonoscopy has been advocated to increase detection of dysplasia. The following guidelines have been provided:

- surveillance colonoscopies should be performed when the disease is in remission, as differentiating between inflamed and dysplastic tissue is difficult
- colonoscopy should be performed 8–10 years after diagnosis, to assess the extent of the disease
- surveillance colonoscopy should be commenced 8–10 years after symptom onset in patients with extensive colitis
- surveillance colonoscopy should be commenced 15–20 years after symptom onset in patients with left-sided disease
- patients with associated primary sclerosing cholangitis have an even greater risk of colorectal cancer, and should undergo an annual colonoscopy

The BSG recommends that, during the colonoscopy, two to four biopsies should be taken every 10 cm and from suspicious areas. More recent advances in endoscopic procedures (chromoendoscopy, narrow-band imaging) are more effective at identifying abnormal mucosa. Subsequent studies suggest surveillance is more effective if these modalities are used, with biopsies targeting abnormal tissue.

Screening for GI cancer in patients with acromegaly

Screening of acromegalic patient for colorectal cancer commences at the age of 40 years, and is influenced by the activity of underlying acromegaly. Patients found to have adenomatous polyps at the index endoscopy, or those with IGF-1 levels above the maximum normal range, should undergo 3-yearly surveillance. Those with a negative initial endoscopy or normal IGF-1 levels require 5-yearly surveillance.

Screening for GI cancer in patients who have undergone a ureterosigmoidostomy

Patients who have undergone a ureterosigmoidostomy are at risk of developing adenomas and subsequent adenocarcinomas at the anastomosis. The earliest recorded case of a ureterosigmoidostomy-related adenoma occurred 10 years post-operatively. Therefore, screening in these patients, via flexible sigmoidoscopy, should commence 10 years post-operatively. This screening should only be stopped if the patient undergoes a further procedure with an alternative diversion and removal of the ureteric anastomosis.

Screening for GI cancer in patients with a family history of colorectal cancer

Patients are considered to have a significant family history of colorectal cancer and thus require colonoscopic surveillance if they have either one first-degree relative who has colorectal cancer and is <45 years old, or two first-degree relatives affected by colorectal cancer. The lifetime risk of dying from colorectal cancer is as follows: 1:50 for those in the general population, 1:17 for those with any family history, 1:10 for those with one affected relative <45 years old, and 1:6 for those with two affected relatives. Patients with a significant family history of colorectal cancer should be offered a colonoscopy at 35–40 years, with a repeat at 50 years of age.

Screening for GI cancer in patients with hereditary non-polyposis colorectal cancer

Patients with hereditary non-polyposis colorectal cancer (HNPCC) should be referred to a regional genetics centre in order to undergo formal assessment, with genetic mutation analysis. Thereafter, the specialist centre can organize family screening as required. In patients with HNPCC, there is a lifetime risk of colorectal cancer of ~80%, and 13%–20% for gastric cancer. Colonoscopic cancer surveillance in these patients should start at age 25, and gastroscopic surveillance at age 50 (in families affected by gastric cancer), or 5 years earlier than the first case within the family. Surveillance should continue with colonoscopies every 2 years until the age of 75. Surveillance is not required in family members who do not carry the genetic mutation shown to be the cause of colorectal cancer in other members of their family.

Screening for GI cancer in patients with familial adenomatous polyposis

Patients with familial adenomatous polyposis should be referred to a regional genetics centre in order to undergo formal assessment, with genetic mutation analysis. Thereafter, the specialist centre can organize family screening as required. Patients with familial adenomatous polyposis will almost universally develop colorectal cancer, with gastroduodenal cancers occurring in ~7%. Surgery in these patients is strongly recommended before age 25, preferably with a proctocolectomy and ileo-anal pouch. Patients deferring surgery should be offered annual colonoscopies and 6-monthly sigmoidoscopies. If the anorectum is retained the patient should have annual surveillance, due to the risk of cancer in the remaining bowel.

Upper GI endoscopy should be performed 3-yearly from the age of 30, although patients with large numbers of polyps should have more frequent endoscopies.

Screening for GI cancer in patients with juvenile polyposis

Patients with juvenile polyposis should be referred to a regional genetics centre in order to undergo formal assessment, with genetic mutation analysis. Thereafter, the specialist centre can organize family screening as required. Of those with this disease, 10%–38% develop colorectal cancer, and ~21% develop gastric cancer. Patients with juvenile polyposis should be offered colonoscopic screening from ages 15–18, and upper GI endoscopy from age 25, on an annual or biannual basis.

Screening for GI cancer in patients with Peutz–Jeghers syndrome

Patients with Peutz–Jeghers syndrome should be referred to a regional genetics centre in order to undergo formal assessment, with genetic mutation analysis. Thereafter, the specialist centre can organize family screening as required. Of those with this disease, 10%–20% will develop colorectal cancer; therefore, patients with Peutz–Jeghers syndrome should undergo colonoscopic surveillance from age 18, with upper GI endoscopy 3-yearly from age 25.

Hepatocellular cancer

Cirrhosis is a risk factor for the development of hepatocellular cancer (HCC), with an annual risk of 1%–6%.

How do we screen for HCC?

Currently, the strategies involved in HCC screening are 6-monthly liver ultrasounds, and alpha-fetoprotein levels. This should, in theory, be offered to all patients with evidence of cirrhosis. However, in general, screening is reserved for patients who are suitable for active treatment should a small HCC be found (e.g. those with Child–Pugh Class A or B liver disease). Many patients with cirrhosis have decompensated disease with poor synthetic function, resulting in a poor prognosis. As with all screening programmes, thought should be given to whether the patient will benefit from early detection of an underlying cancer.

What is the impact of HCC screening?

The evidence for screening for HCC in cirrhotic patients is limited, with few controlled studies. Small studies have shown improved early detection and overall survival in patients with hepatitis B cirrhosis. Early detection of HCC is advantageous, as the prognosis in advanced disease is very poor. Unfortunately, a large percentage of HCCs are found in patients with undiagnosed cirrhosis, meaning that screening will fail to pick up these patients. Each centre should develop its own surveillance programme, based on the available expertise; but, in general, 6-monthly alpha-fetoprotein tests and ultrasound scans are advocated.

Further Reading

Bénard F, Barkun AN, Martel M et al. Systematic review of colorectal cancer screening guidelines for average-risk adults: Summarizing the current global recommendations. *World J Gastroenterol* 2018; 24: 124–38.

Cairns SR, Scholefield JH, Robert J Steele RJ, et al. Guidelines for colorectal cancer screening and surveillance in moderate and high risk groups (update from 2002). *Gut* 2010; 59: 666–90.

Spechler SJ. Barrett's esophagus. *N Engl J Med* 2002; 346: 836–42.

355 Screening for neurological disease

Sarah Cader

What neurological diseases can we screen for?

Given the nature of some neurological diseases to become progressively disabling, early detection and treatment would be very welcome. However, screening for neurological illnesses in the general population has a number of problems. There are only a few neurological conditions that exist in a detectable asymptomatic state prior to development of clinical disease, and a small number of other conditions have early symptomatic stages before the full impact of the disease manifests. In addition, in many neurological conditions, there are no definitive treatments available. There are, of course, many genetic conditions that have neurological manifestations and could be screened for, and early access to neurological assessment for some progressive conditions may enable early intervention.

Potential target groups include patients with neurogenetic disorders, patients with neurodegenerative disorders, patients with inflammatory disorders, and patients with metabolic disorders (see Table 355.1).

Table 355.1 lists the more common neurological conditions for which there may be a potential role for screening and intervention. Acute neurological conditions, such as infections and acute inflammatory disorders, would not merit screening as they are rapid in onset, and many have good treatments. There are also a number of relatively benign chronic conditions, such as migraine and epilepsy, that are readily treatable and do not typically progress.

How can we screen for neurological diseases?

A full neurological examination should be undertaken for all patients presenting to hospital. This may allow early detection of subtle neurological defects that the patient has not yet become aware or had ignored. It can provide clues to systemic conditions or be an indicator of an emerging neurological diagnosis.

For the most part, it is not appropriate to screen the general asymptomatic population for these conditions, as they are not common conditions. However, it would be worthwhile being aware of the conditions in Table 355.1 so that they are considered in all patients.

Screening for neurogenetic disorders

Screening for patients with genetic disorders is potentially exciting as it is likely that there will be a specific and sensitive test for the condition that can be used before the emergence of any clinical symptoms.

Many of these patients will have a family history that will indicate the risk. Certainly, in the case of Huntington's disease, genetic screening is done for predictive testing in relatives of affected individuals. In Huntington's disease, there is an unstable CAG trinucleotide repeat in Chromosome 4. If there are >40 repeats, then the individuals will develop the disease, although the onset is earlier in those with longer segments. Charcot–Marie–Tooth disease, or hereditary motor and sensory neuropathy, is caused by a number of different mutations. Testing is usually for the commoner mutations in PMP22 and MPZ, and is confined usually to patients presenting with a neuropathy following supportive nerve conduction studies or with affected family members. There have been many mutations that have been shown to cause mitochondrial disorders, and these can occur in both mitochondrial DNA and the nuclear DNA encoding for mitochondria. Initial screening is, therefore, usually for evidence of an underlying mitochondrial defect, and this will be evident on electromyography, from a muscle biopsy, or in blood lactate levels. If the clinical signs and bedside testing indicate that a mitochondrial diagnosis is possible, then the patient's tissue and blood can be sent for screening of the genome or more targeted mutation analysis. Muscular dystrophies comprise a large group of muscle disorders that are caused by an underlying defect in the genes encoding muscle development. Genetic testing usually provides a definite diagnosis, but it needs to be targeted according to the clinical picture and whether any family members are affected. There may be additional clues from testing for creatine kinase, a muscle enzyme.

Screening for neurodegenerative disorders

The incentive to screen for neurodegenerative conditions is large, given the potential to interrupt the disease early in its course before progression has been established. Unfortunately, screening for these conditions is not easy, and they are rather insidious in onset. There are familial variants that could be screened with genetic testing, but they tend to be rare in comparison. Early onset Alzheimer's disease can be caused by mutations in PSEN1, PSEN2, and APP. Sporadic and late-onset Alzheimer's does not have any specific genetic test. Early stage of dementia can be difficult to diagnose accurately, so diagnosis is often not made until cognitive impairment is established. Brain biopsy might detect early pathological changes but taking a brain biopsy is not practical in most patients. In Parkinson's disease, diagnosis is based on a triad of bradykinesia, rigidity, and tremor. However, radioisotope imaging for the dopamine transporter can demonstrate evidence of dopamine depletion even relatively early in the condition, when the only symptom may be a tremor. The test will not reliably distinguish Parkinson's disease from other causes of parkinsonism, such as multisystem atrophy or progressive supranuclear palsy. Genetic mutations have been identified for some familial, early onset cases in a number of genes, such as PARK2. Genetic mutations have only been identified in a small proportion of patients with motor neuron disease, most commonly in SOD1; diagnosis is usually made late, progression is rapid, and there is currently no method to screen patients for the risk of developing this disease. Spongiform encephalopathies, on the other hand, have a typically long latency. Familial Creutzfeldt–Jakob disease, Gerstmann–Sträussler–Schienker disease, and familial fatal insomnia are hereditary spongiform encephalopathies that are due to mutations in PRNP, the gene that codes for the human prion protein. Genetic screening can be done in those with affected family members. Sporadic forms of these diseases may be due to post-translational structural protein changes or spontaneous somatic gene mutations. These changes may be present for some time before any symptoms emerge. Homozygosity for methionine at codon 129 of PRNP gene appears to confer susceptibility to Creutzfeldt–Jakob disease.

Neurogenetic disorders	Neurodegenerative disorders	Inflammatory and autoimmune disorders	Metabolic disorders
Huntington's disease	Alzheimer's disease	Multiple sclerosis	Vitamin B$_{12}$ deficiency
Charcot–Marie–Tooth disease	Parkinson's disease	SLE	Wilson's disease
Mitochondrial disease	Motor neuron disease	Sarcoidosis	Copper deficiency
Muscular dystrophy	Spongiform encephalopathies	Vasculitis	Lead neuropathy
		Temporal arteritis	Iron overload
			Thyroid disease
			Drug-induced myopathy
			Diabetes

Table 355.1 Neurological conditions for which there may be a potential role for screening and intervention

Screening for inflammatory and autoimmune disorders

Inflammatory disorders are often multisystem and may be detectable before any significant symptoms appear. Temporal arteritis can lead to blindness, but testing the erythrocyte sedimentation rate (ESR) in older patients presenting with headache is a useful screening tool that may prevent any problems. Similarly, patients with other vasculitides, as well as with SLE and many other autoimmune conditions, may have a raised ESR, or be positive for autoimmune antibodies (e.g. antineutrophil cytoplasmic antibodies). If this is the case, then immunosuppressive treatment can be instigated early to prevent more serious clinical problems. Sarcoidosis can be more troublesome to screen, as angiotensin-converting enzyme is neither particularly sensitive nor specific. A chest radiograph may show hilar lymphadenopathy, and there may be abnormalities in liver enzymes. However, these will only be present during a flare, and have no predictive value as to the onset of neurosarcoid. Evidence of multiple sclerosis may be found on MRI in patients that have minimal symptoms. It may be possible to treat these patients before a definite diagnosis of the disease is made or any progression occurs.

Screening for metabolic disorders

Some neurological disorders are due to deficiencies or toxic levels of certain substances. Most of the tests in these cases are simple to perform and involve a simple blood test. Testing for vitamin B_{12} and thyroid hormone levels is widespread, since there is considerable awareness of the problems their deficiencies can cause. Testing for trace metals and less common conditions tends to be reserved for patients that present to the neurologist with consistent symptoms, and so are not screened as such. Paediatric specialists will, however, often do an extended spectrum of screening tests for the common inborn errors of metabolism.

What is the impact of screening for neurological diseases in the real world?

Neither the genetic or neurodegenerative conditions have many effective treatments. Management is largely supportive, and widespread screening for relatively rare conditions is not cost-effective.

In multiple sclerosis, there is some evidence that early intervention may prevent the onset of clinically definite disease, but this is limited. In other inflammatory disorders, early immunosuppression will prevent progression and accumulation of disability. In practice, patients do not get such treatment until they have symptoms that would necessitate the use of potentially strong drugs.

Most metabolic disorders are rare and so do not justify routine screening. Screening for vitamin deficiencies, diabetes, and thyroid disease is routinely done, and early detection has no doubt prevented the onset of a considerable degree of neurological morbidity. These are common conditions that are easily tested.

Issues and the future of neurological screening programmes

There are no screening programmes in neurology. As studies emerge, it may become apparent that early intervention in some conditions does indeed prevent development of the disease. This is may be first available for multiple sclerosis, which is one of the commonest neurological conditions, and MRI is safe and sensitive, albeit relatively expensive.

The main issues remain across neurology. There are often inadequate treatments for many diseases and there is difficulty in early diagnosis when symptoms may only show subtle differences at early stages. In neurology, there is a wide range of relatively rare conditions, and screening in these circumstances is very difficult.

Further Reading

Fuller G and Manford MR. *Neurology: An Illustrated Colour Text*, (3rd edition), 2010. Churchill Livingstone.

Manji H, Connolly S, Kitchen N, et al. *Oxford Handbook of Neurology* (2nd edition), 2014. Oxford University Press.

Screening for cancer

Warren Grant and Martin Scott-Brown

Aims of screening for cancer

Many of us spend a lot of time wanting not to contract diseases! We are likely to alter our lifestyles as a result. Physicians, particularly in primary care, are challenged on a daily basis by worried people who feel they may not be able to avoid conditions such as cancer. These individuals often believe they should at least have it 'caught early' before it causes them any harm. The physician then enters the world of preventive care. It incorporates medical traditions such as 'the annual medical' and is the motivation behind the GP that takes your blood pressure when you attend with an infected toenail.

Preventive care encompasses immunization, screening, lifestyle change, and chemoprevention (i.e. using medicine to prevent disease). Each of these aspects involves active participation by the patient. In cancer, screening is a key method of preventing symptomatic disease, but is subtly different from the patient-led preventive care consultation. The aim in cancer screening is not just to prevent the incidence of disease or diagnose it in an early stage but, most importantly, to reduce mortality. Designing screening programmes leads to challenging questions such as:

- is it worth diagnosing the cancer before symptoms develop?
- will screening reduce mortality or just create more people living with the disease?
- who should be screened?
- what form should the screening test take?
- is screening cheaper than treating symptomatic disease?
- how will screening affect individuals without the diagnosis?

Effective cancer screening programmes require a centralized organization to coordinate implementation, robust statistical evidence of benefit, and extensive cost and resource planning for the inevitable increase in use of diagnostic and treatment services. This chapter will outline the three UK population cancer screening programmes and highlight the key issues considered in their design.

The history of screening for cancer

Cancer screening began with the Pap smear. George Papanicolaou published his seminal paper 'The diagnostic value of vaginal smears in carcinoma of the uterus' in *American Journal of Obstetrics and Gynaecology* in 1941. He had first announced his ideas based on exfoliative cytology back in 1928 but, at this time, his colleagues held such strong doubts about the validity of such a test that he laid his ideas to rest for the forthcoming decade.

Since then, the only evidence-based programmes to have been developed are in breast, cervical, and bowel cancers. This reflects not only the challenging and lengthy process of assessing potential screening tests, but also how certain cancers are more suitable for screening than others.

Which cancers are suitable for screening?

In 1968 Wilson and Junger of the WHO outlined a series of principles that should lie behind the development of a screening programme:

- the condition to be screened should be an important public health problem in terms of frequency and severity
- its natural history should be well understood
- it should be recognizable at an early stage
- treatment outcomes should be better at an early stage of the disease

- a suitable test exists (i.e. one that can reliably detect the disease)
- an acceptable test exists (i.e. one that is cost-effective and safe for patients)
- adequate facilities should exist to cope with the abnormalities detected
- screening should be done at repeated intervals when the onset of the disease is insidious
- the chance of harm should be less than the chance of benefit
- the financial cost should be balanced against the benefit

These ten principles clarify the aims and objectives of disease screening. They also highlight key problems in the development of such a programme for cancer. For example, the incidence of prostate cancer has increased over recent years, and many countries are looking for ways of preventing an increase in prostate cancer deaths. However, the design of a suitable screening programme falls at the second principle. Prostate cancer's indolent natural history makes decisions about when to screen very complicated. Should all men over 18 be screened because we know early diagnosis of organ-confined disease offers more treatment options and that disease in younger men is more likely to be fatal? Or should we just screen men aged over 50 once a year to save cost? What about screening the symptomatic? Maybe this is enough to reduce mortality. But what about the onset of symptoms in young men? These individuals are more likely to have aggressive disease, and symptomatic treatment may be too late to prevent mortality. The issues with prostate cancer screening highlight themes common to screening in many other less prevalent cancers (e.g. ovarian or gastric cancers).

Screening for breast cancer

In the UK, breast cancer screening was set up by the Department of Health in 1988, in response to the report of a working group lead by Professor Sir Patrick Forrest. The Forrest Report, as it became known, was published in 1986 and set out ideas about population screening in the UK for breast cancer. It concluded that screening by mammography could lead to prolongation of life for women aged 50 and over.

Women were first invited for screening in 1988 and by 1990 national coverage had been achieved. The programme is currently costed at around £75 million per year, which works out at around £37.50 per woman invited, or £45.50 per woman screened.

Recent developments in the programme mean that women between the ages of 47 and 73 will be invited to attend for two-view mammographic assessment every 3 years. After the age of 73, women can attend for screening by open invitation, but are no longer routinely invited. Some screening does occur in the high-risk population under 47. This is often instigated by the local genetic counselling team, oncologists, or GPs. The idea of the screening programme is to detect radiological changes of cancer at a very early stage. Those who are found to have abnormal tests go on to have further diagnostic investigations, including a core biopsy. This has been shown to reduce mortality and, by 2010, saved 1250 lives each year. But breast screening will also cause some women to undergo invasive biopsy tests for benign breast lesions.

Screening for cervical cancer

In some cancers, there is a biological window of opportunity where precancerous abnormalities can be reliably detected. In these cases, screening can lead to treatment to prevent the onset of invasive cancer. This is the basis for cervical cancer screening.

In the UK, a liquid-based cytology (LBC) test is used to screen all women between the ages of 25 and 64 at 3–5 year intervals. It involves obtaining a specimen via a speculum examination and taking a 'smear' of the cells on the cervical surface. This specimen is then added to a fluid solution for preservation before it is sent to a laboratory for analysis.

In recent years, both the interval between screening invitations and the nature of the assessment test used have undergone extensive review and development to improve the quality of the programme. Initially, all women were screened every 3 years. Since 2003, those aged 50 or over have been offered 5-yearly invitations. This has obvious cost benefits by reducing the number of tests carried out, and may increase the specificity of the testing programme. But it will also increase the chance of length time bias and more aggressive cancers may be missed.

Smear testing began in the 1960s but initially was only used by those who presented to a doctor. As a result, those women thought to be at highest risk were likely not to have the test, and those who did have it and had a positive result had no formal framework to ensure that their condition was managed in a standard way. The computerized national screening programme was rolled out in 1988.

In September 2008 the HPV vaccine was introduced in the UK for girls aged 12–13. This virus is a key etiological factor in cervical cancer and, inevitably, the vaccine will reduce its incidence, but it will take many years to do so. As a result, the LBC screening programme is likely to continue for the foreseeable future.

Screening for bowel cancer

A bowel cancer screening programme was initiated across the UK, with national coverage achieved by the end of 2009. It is aimed at diagnosing cancer at an early stage by using faecal occult blood (FOB) testing. This technique was tested in a successful pilot based in Coventry and North Warwickshire in 2007. A kit is sent to the homes of all men and women aged 60–69 with instructions about how to use it. The sample is then sent to a hub laboratory, and the results are communicated to the patient within 2 weeks. Those with a positive test will see a specialist nurse and are likely to undergo colonoscopy, the gold-standard diagnostic test for bowel cancer. The total cost of the programme will be around £55 million per year. One of the major issues in designing the programme was establishing a reliable screening test. Although, due to its high sensitivity and specificity, colonoscopy is the gold-standard diagnostic test for bowel cancer, it is relatively expensive. Other radiological investigations have similar problems. FOB tests are cheap, easy to mass-produce, and have been shown to have a high sensitivity for bowel cancer. But what about reliability? If a major feasibility study for bowel cancer screening involved the Haemoccult tester (Beckman Coulter Inc., Fullerton, California) and you wish to use a tester of a different brand, should you run another major randomized control trial? In practice, this has not been done.

Ensuring a useful cancer screening test

The accuracy of a screening test, that is, its ability to differentiate diseased from non-diseased individuals, is measured by its **sensitivity** and **specificity** (see Table 356.1).

Sensitivity is the proportion of individuals **with** the disease who are correctly identified by the test. Specificity is proportion of individuals **without** the disease who are correctly identified by the test. Ideally, a screening test would score 100% sensitivity and specificity, but no test currently does this. This results in some individuals being diagnosed as having the screened condition when they do not, and some individuals with the screened condition not being diagnosed. In a quest to reduce the numbers of these unfortunate individuals, every effort is made to increase sensitivity and specificity; however, in practice, they are inversely related. If, for example, the value of a positive result for a blood test such as the PSA test in prostate cancer is reduced (e.g. from 4 ng/ml to 3 ng/ml), more cases of prostate cancer are likely to be diagnosed and thus the sensitivity would rise. At the same time, some individuals who do not have prostate cancer are likely to be diagnosed as having the condition because they have benignly elevated PSA levels (e.g. because of prostatitis). Balancing these two factors is key to a successful cancer screening programme.

When evaluating a screening programme, it is also important to understand the **positive predictive value** of the test involved. The positive predictive value is the proportion of individuals who actually have the disease, having had a positive test result. It is based on the sensitivity and specificity of the screening test and also, importantly, on the prevalence of the disease. To put it another way, if the positive predictive value of a test is only 10%, this could be because the test is not accurate in detecting the disease (low sensitivity), inaccurate in defining people who do not have the disease (low specificity), or it could be that the population screened are of low risk for the disease. Therefore, factors that increase the positive predictive value include increasing the sensitivity and the specificity of the test, as well as focusing on high-risk individuals. A high positive predictive value may not always correlate with a good screening test. It may be that only large, advanced tumours are detected, and screening them is likely to be of no benefit to patient survival. A test with a low positive predictive value may reflect screening in a low-prevalence population but with a greater cancer detection rate (increased sensitivity) diagnosing a broader selection of tumours. These patients will benefit from screening.

Bias in screening for cancer

As mentioned earlier, screening for cancer is designed to increase survival in those who have the disease and who have been screened, compared to those who have not been screened. Assessing survival in this context raises some statistical challenges and is subject to two types of bias—**length time and lead time** (see 'Bias in screening for cancer'). Generally, randomized control trials (RCTs) are thought of as the gold standard when it comes to evaluating a screening programme. Case-control studies are a cheaper, smaller alternative to RCTs but are prone to selection bias. In the ideal trial, large numbers of individuals would be allocated randomly to either have the screening test or not. This selected population would then be followed up until enough data on the key outcome have been collated. In cancer screening, this outcome is survival. This type of trial is expensive, can take many years to complete (depending on the biology of the cancer), and requires many thousands of participants to give statistically significant results. As an example, four RCTs evaluating screening for bowel cancer have involved over 300 000 people and taken around 15 years to complete. When analysing such trials, it is important to note that the relevant outcome is a change in **disease-specific** survival. Trials that present data on overall survival can often be misinterpreted.

Results of trials that suggest there is a survival advantage in those who have had the screening test may be reflecting **lead time bias**. Lead time is, in essence, what a screening programme is trying to promote, that is, an extension in the period of time before an individual would have normally presented with symptoms from the disease being screened. However, an apparent increase in length of survival, without taking account of mortality rate, can merely reflect an earlier diagnosis of a condition that individuals then live with for longer, before dying at the same rate and at the same age as the population without screening. As mentioned, prospective RCTs that take account of disease-specific mortality rates help to get round problems of lead time bias.

Table 356.1 Determining the sensitivity, specificity, and negative/positive predictive value of a test

Test result	Disease	No disease	Total
Positive	A	B	A + B
Negative	C	D	C + D
Total	A + C	B + D	A + B + C + D

Note: sensitivity = $A/(A + C)$; specificity = $D/(B + D)$; positive predictive value = $A/(A + B)$; negative predictive value = $D/(C + D)$.

Length time bias suggests that aggressive, fast-growing cancers are less common after a screening programme is introduced, and results in the phenomenon of slower-growing, less aggressive cancers being more common in the screened population. It occurs because of the interval between screening invitations. During this time, some individuals will develop aggressive, fast-growing tumours and may go on to develop symptoms or even die from them before their next screening invitation. Those individuals who develop slower-growing tumours are more likely to be picked up at screening. The ideal screening interval, therefore, will be short enough to detect the onset of new disease, at a time when it can successfully be treated, without putting too large a resource burden on the organizing agency or inconveniencing the population to be screened and encouraging them not to attend (e.g. breast cancer screening every 3 years).

Further Reading

Cancer Screening Overview (PDQ®)–Health Professional Version. Found at: https://www.cancer.gov/about-cancer/screening/hp-screening-overview-pdq

Duffy S, Hill C, and Esteve J. *Quantitative Methods for the Evaluation of Cancer Screening*, 2001. Arnold.

Index

Note: Tables, figures, and boxes are indicated by an italic *t*, *f*, and *b* following the page number.